Measurement of Joint Motion
A Guide to Goniometry
fourth edition

Cynthia C. Norkin, EdD, PT
Former Associate Professor and Director
School of Physical Therapy
College of Health and Human Services
Ohio University
Athens, Ohio

D. Joyce White, DSc, PT
Associate Professor of Physical Therapy
School of Health and Environment
University of Massachusetts Lowell
Lowell, Massachusetts

Photographs by Jocelyn Greene Molleur and Lucia Grochowska Littlefield
Technical Advisor George Kalem, III
Illustrations by Timothy Wayne Malone

F.A. Davis Company • Philadelphia

F. A. Davis Company
1915 Arch Street
Philadelphia, PA 19103
www.fadavis.com

Copyright © 2009 by F. A. Davis Company

Printed in the United States of America

Last digit indicates print number: 10 9 8 7 6

Acquisitions Editor: Melissa Duffield
Publisher: Margaret Biblis
Manager of Content Development: George W. Lang
Developmental Editor: Karen Carter
Art and Design Manager: Carolyn O'Brien

As new scientific information becomes available through basic and clinical research, recommended treatments and drug therapies undergo changes. The author(s) and publisher have done everything possible to make this book accurate, up to date, and in accord with accepted standards at the time of publication. The author(s), editors, and publisher are not responsible for errors or omissions or for consequences from application of the book, and make no warranty, expressed or implied, in regard to the contents of the book. Any practice described in this book should be applied by the reader in accordance with professional standards of care used in regard to the unique circumstances that may apply in each situation. The reader is advised always to check product information (package inserts) for changes and new information regarding dose and contraindications before administering any drug. Caution is especially urged when using new or infrequently ordered drugs.

Library of Congress Cataloging-in-Publication Data

Norkin, Cynthia C.
Measurement of joint motion : a guide to goniometry / Cynthia C. Norkin, D. Joyce White ; photographs by Jocelyn Greene Molleur and Lucia Grochowska Littlefield ; illustrations by Timothy Wayne Malone. -- 4th ed.
    p. ; cm.
  Includes bibliographical references and index.
  ISBN-13: 978-0-8036-2066-7
  ISBN-10: 0-8036-2066-7
  1. Joints--Range of motion--Measurement. I. White, D. Joyce. II. Title.
  [DNLM: 1. Arthrometry, Articular--methods. 2. Joint Diseases--diagnosis. 3. Joints--physiology.
WE 300 N841m 2009]
  RD734.N67 2009
  612.7'5--dc22

                                                                    2008036707

To our families and students, who give meaning and enjoyment to our lives.
—*CCN and DJW*

Preface

The measurement of joint motion is an important component of a thorough physical examination of the extremities and spine, one which helps health professionals identify impairments and assess rehabilitative status. The need for a comprehensive text with sufficient written detail and photographs to allow for the standardization of goniometric measurement methods—both for the purposes of teaching and clinical practice led to the development of the first edition of the *Measurement of Joint Motion: A Guide to Goniometry* in 1985. Our approach included a discussion and illustration of testing position, stabilization, end-feel, and goniometer alignment for each measurable joint in the body. The resulting text was extremely well received by a variety of health professional educational programs and was used as a reference in many clinical settings.

In the years following initial publication, a considerable amount of research on the measurement of joint motion appeared in the literature. Consequently, a second edition, published in 1995, included a chapter on the reliability and validity of joint measurement as well as joint-specific research sections in each existing chapter. We also expanded the text by adding structure, osteokinematics, arthrokinematics, capsular and noncapsular patterns of limitation, and functional ranges of motion for each joint.

The third edition included extensive new research findings related to joint motion. New to the third edition was the inclusion of muscle length testing at joints where muscle length is often a factor affecting range of motion. This addition integrated the measurement procedures used in this book with the American Physical Therapy Association's *Guide to Physical Therapy Practice*. Inclinometer techniques for measuring range of motion of the spine were added to coincide with current practice in some clinical settings. Illustrations were included to accompany anatomical descriptions so that the reader had a visual reminder of the joint structures involved in range of motion. New illustrations of bony anatomical landmarks and photographs of surface anatomy were added to help the reader align the goniometer accurately.

In the fourth edition we reorganized the content in Chapters 4 to 13 to create a more logical progression from anatomical descriptions of joint structures and landmarks used in goniometer alignment directly to the measurement procedures. Information summarizing research findings now follows, rather than precedes, the measurement procedures. This restructuring makes it easier for readers that are focused on learning measurement technique, as well as readers that are focused on reviewing the research literature for evidence-based practice, to find what they are seeking. Similar to earlier editions we have incorporated new information on normative range of motion values for various age and gender groups, as well as the range of motion needed to perform common functional tasks. We added current information on the effects of subject characteristics, such as body mass, occupational and recreational activities, and the effects of the testing process, such as the testing position and type of measuring instrument, on range of motion. In the fourth edition we added and restructured more measurement techniques to the spine chapters and added several commonly used methods to assess finger and thumb range of motion. The TMJ chapter was enhanced with clear photographs and illustrations of measurement techniques. In addition, over 90 new photographs and illustrations replaced many of the older, dated art work.

This book continues to present goniometry logically and clearly. Chapter 1 discusses basic concepts regarding the use of goniometry to assess range of motion and muscle length in patient evaluation. Arthrokinematic and osteokinematic movements, elements of active and passive range of motion, hypomobility, hypermobility, and factors affecting joint motion are included. The inclusion of end-feels and capsular and noncapsular patterns of joint limitation introduces readers to current concepts in orthopedic manual therapy and encourages them to consider joint structure while measuring joint motion.

Chapter 2 takes the reader through a step-by-step process to master the techniques of goniometric evaluation, including: positioning, stabilization, instruments used for measurement, goniometer alignment, and the recording of results. Exercises that help develop necessary psychomotor skills and demonstrate direct application of theoretical concepts facilitate learning.

Chapter 3 discusses the validity and reliability of measurement. The results of validity and reliability studies on the measurement of joint motion are summarized to help the reader focus on ways of improving and interpreting goniometric measurements. Mathematical methods of evaluating reliability are shown along with examples and exercises so that the readers can assess their reliability in taking measurements.

Chapters 4 to 13 present detailed information on goniometric testing procedures for the upper and lower extremities, spine, and temporomandibular joint. When appropriate, muscle length testing procedures are also included. The text presents the anatomical landmarks, testing position, stabilization, testing motion, normal end-feel, and goniometer alignment for each joint and motion, in a format that reinforces a consistent approach to evaluation. The extensive use of photographs and captions eliminates the need for repeated demonstrations by an instructor and provides the reader with a permanent reference for visualizing the procedures. Also included is information on joint structure, osteokinematic and arthrokinematic motion, and capsular patterns of restrictions. A review of current literature regarding normal range of motion values; the effects of age, gender, and other factors on range of motion; functional range of motion; and reliability and validity of measurement procedures are also presented for each body region to assist the reader to comply with evidence-based practice.

We hope this book makes the teaching and learning of goniometry easier and improves the standardization and thus the reliability and validity of this examination tool. We believe that the fourth edition provides a comprehensive coverage of the clinical measurement of joint motion and muscle length. We hope that the additions will motivate health professionals to conduct research and to use research results in evaluation. We encourage our readers to provide us with feedback on our current efforts to bring you a high-quality, user-friendly text.

CCN
DJW

Acknowledgments

We are very grateful for the contributions of the many people who were involved in the development and production of this text. Photographer Jocelyn Molleur applied her skill and patience during many sessions at the physical therapy laboratory at the University of Massachusetts Lowell to produce the high-quality photographs that appear in both the third and fourth editions. Her efforts combined with those of Lucia Grochowska Littlefield, who took the photographs for the first edition, are responsible for an important feature of the book. Timothy Malone, an artist from Ohio, used his talents, knowledge of anatomy, and good humor to create the excellent illustrations that appear in this edition. We also offer our thanks to Colleen DeCotret, Alexander White, Claudia Van Bibber, and University of Massachusetts Lowell physical therapy students: Rachel Blakeslee, Rebecca D'Amour, and Chris Fournier who graciously agreed to be subjects for the new photographs and provided painstaking research support for the fourth edition.

We wish to express our appreciation to these dedicated professionals at F. A. Davis: Margaret Biblis, Publisher, and Melissa Duffield, Acquisitions Editor, for their encouragement and commitment to excellence. Our thanks are also extended to George Lang, Manager of Content Development; David Orzechowski, Managing Editor; Robert Butler, Production Manager; Karen Carter, Developmental Editor; Carolyn O'Brien, Manager of Art and Design; Katharine L. Margeson, Illustration Coordinator; Elizabeth Stepchin, Developmental Associate; Stephanie Casey, Administrative Assistant; and Jean-Francois Vilain, Former Publisher for the first and second editions. We are very grateful to the numerous students, faculty, and clinicians who over the years have used the book or formally reviewed portions of the manuscript and offered insightful comments and helpful suggestions that have improved this text.

Finally, we wish to thank our families: Cynthia's daughter, Alexandra, and her daughters, Taylor and Kimberly; and Joyce's husband, Jonathan, sons, Alexander and Ethan, and parents, Dorothy and Emerson, for their continuing encouragement and support. We will always be appreciative.

Reviewers

Joni Goldwasser Barry, PT, DPT, NCS
Assistant Professor
School of Health Professions
Maryville University
St. Louis, Missouri

Rebekah R. Bower, MS, ATC, LAT
Education Coordinator
Athletic Training Education Program
Health, Phys. Ed. & Recreation Department
Wright State University
Dayton, Ohio

Marc Campo, PT, MS, OSC, Cert. MDT
Assistant Professor
Physical Therapy Department
Mercy College
Dobbs Ferry, New York

Gary Steven Chleboun, PhD, PT
Professor
School of Physical Therapy
Ohio University
Athens, Ohio

Liz L. Harrison, DPT, BPT, MSc, PhD
Professor and Associate Dean
School of Physical Therapy
University of Saskatchewan
Saskatoon, Saskatchewan, Canada

Suchita Kulkarni-Lambore, PT, PhD
Associate Professor
Physical Therapy Department
Chatham College
Pittsburgh, Pennsylvania

Teresa Seefeld, PT, ATC
Assistant Professor
Athletic Training Department
University of Mary
Bismarck, North Dakota

Contents

PART 1

INTRODUCTION TO GONIOMETRY

OBJECTIVES

On completion of Part I, the reader will be able to:

1. **Define:**
   - Goniometry
   - Planes and axes
   - Range of motion
   - End-feel
   - Muscle length testing
   - Reliability
   - Validity

2. **Identify the appropriate planes and axes for each of the following motions:**

   Flexion–extension, abduction–adduction, and rotation

3. **Compare:**
   - Active and passive ranges of motion
   - Arthrokinematic and osteokinematic motions
   - Soft, firm, and hard end-feels
   - Hypomobility and hypermobility
   - Capsular and noncapsular patterns of restricted motion
   - One-joint, two-joint, and multijoint muscles
   - Reliability and validity
   - Intratester and intertester reliability

4. **Explain the importance of:**
   - Testing positions
   - Stabilization

   - Clinical estimates of range of motion
   - Palpating bony landmarks
   - Recording starting and ending positions

5. **Describe the parts of universal, fluid, and pendulum goniometers**

6. **List:**
   - Six-step explanation sequence
   - 12-step testing sequence
   - 10 items included in recording

7. **Perform a goniometric evaluation of the elbow joint including:**
   - Clear explanation of the procedure
   - Positioning of a subject in the testing position
   - Adequate stabilization of the proximal joint component
   - Correct determination of the end of the range of motion
   - Correct identification of the end-feel
   - Palpation of the correct bony landmarks
   - Accurate alignment of the goniometer
   - Correct reading of the goniometer and recording of the measurement

8. **Perform and interpret intratester and intertester reliability tests including standard deviation, coefficient of variation, correlation coefficients, and standard error of measurement.**

Chapter 1

Basic Concepts

This book is designed to serve as a guide to learning the technique of human joint measurement called goniometry. Background information on principles and procedures necessary for an understanding of goniometry is found in Part 1. Practice exercises are included at appropriate intervals to help the examiner apply this information and develop the psychomotor skills necessary for competency in goniometry. The validity and reliability of goniometric measurements are explored to encourage thoughtful and appropriate use of these techniques in clinical practice. Procedures for the goniometric examination of joint range of motion and muscle length testing of the upper extremity, lower extremity, and spine and temporomandibular joint are presented in Parts II, III, and IV, respectively.

Goniometry

The term goniometry is derived from two Greek words, *gonia*, meaning angle, and *metron*, meaning measure. Therefore, goniometry refers to the measurement of angles, in particular the measurement of angles created at human joints by the bones of the body. The examiner obtains these measurements by placing the parts of the measuring instrument, called a goniometer, along the bones immediately proximal and distal to the joint being evaluated. Goniometry may be used to determine both a particular joint position and the total amount of motion available at a joint.

Example: The elbow joint is evaluated by placing the parts of the measuring instrument on the humerus (proximal segment) and the forearm (distal segment) and measuring either a specific joint position or the total arc of motion (Fig. 1.1).

Goniometry is an important part of a comprehensive examination of joints and surrounding soft tissue. A comprehensive examination typically begins by interviewing the subject and reviewing records to obtain an accurate description of current symptoms; functional abilities; occupational, social, and recreational activities; and medical history. Observation of the body to assess bone and soft tissue contour, as well as skin and nail condition, usually follows the interview. Gentle

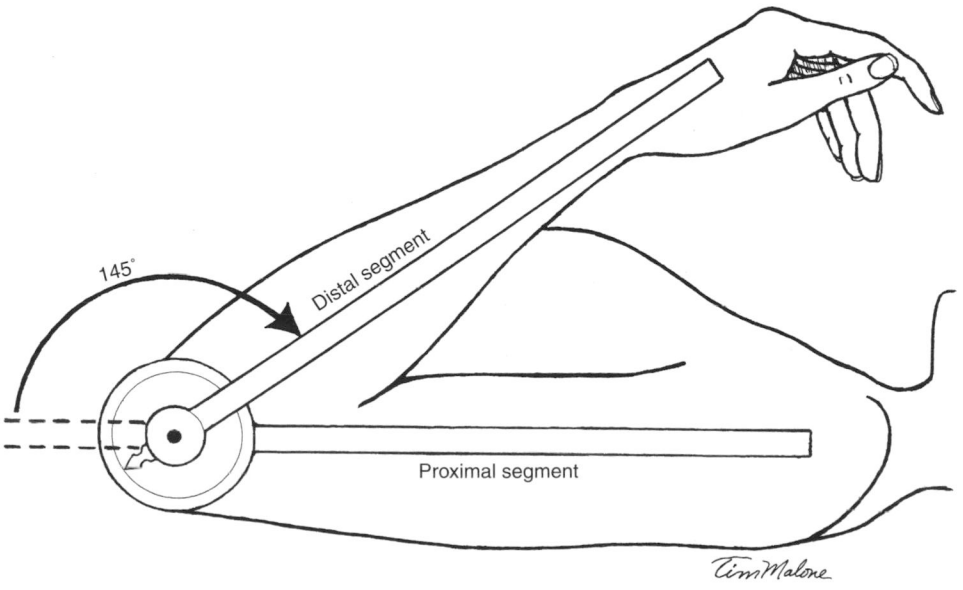

145°

Distal segment

Proximal segment

Tim Malone

FIGURE 1.1 The left upper extremity of a subject in the supine position is shown. The parts of the measuring instrument have been placed along the proximal (humerus) and distal (radius) segments and centered over the axis of the elbow joint. When the distal segment has been moved toward the proximal segment (elbow flexion), a measurement of the arc of motion can be obtained.

palpation is used to determine skin temperature and the quality of soft tissue deformities and to locate pain symptoms in relation to anatomical structures. Anthropometric measurements such as leg length, circumference, and body volume may be indicated.

The performance of active joint motions by the subject during the examination allows the examiner to screen for abnormal movements and gain information about the subject's willingness to move. If abnormal active motions are found, the examiner performs passive joint motions in an attempt to determine reasons for joint limitation. Performing passive joint motions enables the examiner to assess the tissue that is limiting the motion, detect pain, and make an estimate of the amount of motion. Goniometry is used to measure and document the amount of active and passive joint motion as well as abnormal fixed joint positions. Resisted isometric muscle contractions, joint integrity and mobility tests, and special tests for specific body regions are used in conjunction with goniometry to help identify the injured anatomical structures. Tests to assess muscle performance and neurological function are often included. Diagnostic imaging procedures and laboratory tests may be required.

Goniometric data used in conjunction with other information can provide a basis for the following:

- Determining the presence or absence of impairment
- Establishing a diagnosis
- Developing a prognosis, treatment goals, and plan of care
- Evaluating progress or lack of progress toward rehabilitative goals
- Modifying treatment
- Motivating the subject
- Researching the effectiveness of therapeutic techniques or regimens (for example, measuring outcomes following exercises, medications, and surgical procedures)
- Fabricating orthoses and adaptive equipment

◯ Joint Motion

Arthrokinematics

Motion at a joint occurs as the result of movement of one joint surface in relation to another. **Arthrokinematics** is the term used to refer to the movement of joint surfaces. The movements of joint surfaces are described as slides (or glides), spins, and rolls.[1,2] A **slide (glide)**, which is a translatory motion, is the sliding of one joint surface over another, as when a braked wheel skids (Fig. 1.2). A **spin** is a rotary motion, similar to the spinning of a toy top. All points on the moving joint surface rotate around a fixed axis of motion (Fig. 1.3). A **roll** is a rotary motion similar to the rolling of the bottom of a rocking chair on the floor or the rolling of a tire on the road (Fig. 1.4).

In the human body, slides, spins, and rolls usually occur in combination with each other and result in angular movement of the shafts of the bones. The combination of the sliding and rolling is referred to as roll-sliding or roll-gliding[3] and

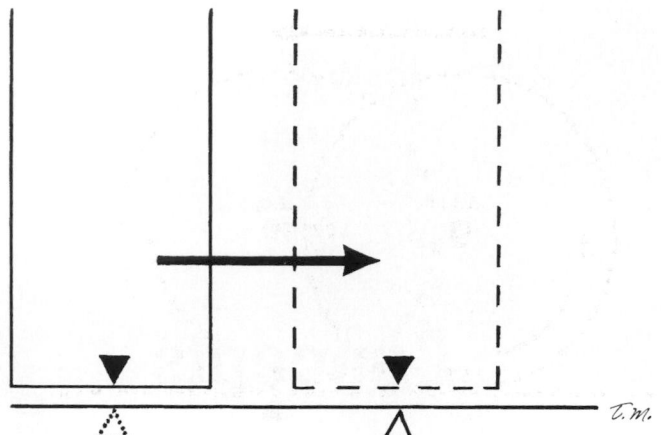

FIGURE 1.2 A slide is a translatory motion in which the same point on the moving joint surface comes in contact with new points on the opposing surface, and all the points on the moving surface travel the same amount of distance.

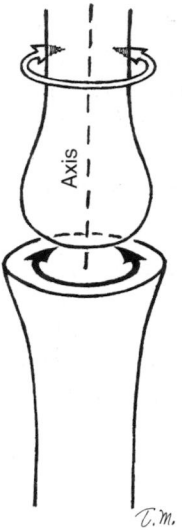

FIGURE 1.3 A spin is a rotary motion in which all the points on the moving surface rotate around a fixed central axis. The points on the moving joint surface that are closer to the axis of motion will travel a smaller distance than the points further from the axis.

allows for increased motion at a joint by postponing the joint compression and separation that would occur at either side of the joint during a pure roll. The direction of the rolling and sliding components of a roll-slide will vary depending on the shape of the moving joint surface.[2,3] If a convex joint surface is moving, the convex surface will roll in the same direction as the angular motion of the shaft of the bone but will slide in the opposite direction (Fig. 1.5A). If a concave joint surface is moving, the concave surface will roll and slide in the same direction as the angular motion of the shaft of the bone (Fig. 1.5B).

Arthrokinematic motions are examined for amount of motion, tissue resistance at the end of the motion (end-feel),

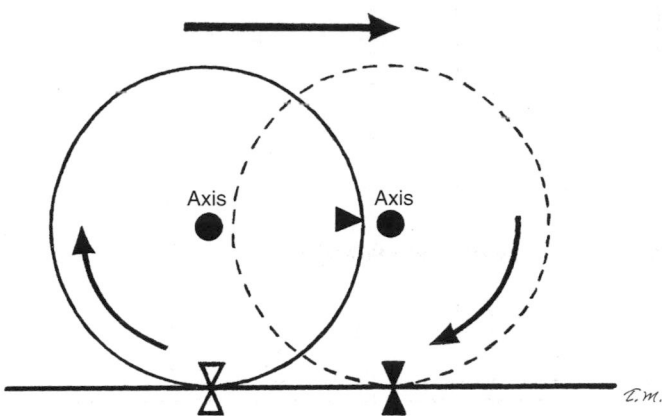

FIGURE 1.4 A roll is a rotary motion in which new points on the moving joint surface come in contact with new points on the opposing surface. The axis of rotation has also moved, in this case to the right.

and effect on the patient's symptoms.[4] The ranges of arthrokinematic motions are very small and cannot be measured with a goniometer or standard ruler. Instead, arthrokinematic motions are subjectively compared to the same motion on the contralateral side of the body, or compared to an examiner's past experience testing people of similar age and gender as the patient. These motions are also called accessory or joint play motions.

Osteokinematics

Osteokinematics refers to the gross movement of the shafts of bones rather than the movement of joint surfaces. The movements of the shafts of bones are usually described in

terms of the rotary or angular motion produced, as if the movement occurs around a fixed axis of motion. Goniometry measures the angles created by the rotary motion of the shafts of the bones. Some translatory shifting of the axis of motion usually occurs during movement; however, most clinicians find the description of osteokinematic movement in terms of just rotary motion to be sufficiently accurate and use goniometry to measure osteokinematic movements.

Planes and Axes

Osteokinematic motions are classically described as taking place in one of the three **cardinal planes** of the body (sagittal, frontal, transverse) around three corresponding **axes** (medial–lateral, anterior–posterior, vertical). The three planes lie at right angles to one another, whereas the three axes lie at right angles both to one another and to their corresponding planes.

The **sagittal plane** proceeds from the anterior to the posterior aspect of the body. The median sagittal plane divides the body into right and left halves. The motions of flexion and extension occur in the sagittal plane (Fig. 1.6). The axis around which the motions of flexion and extension occur may be envisioned as a line that is perpendicular to the sagittal plane and proceeds from one side of the body to the other. This axis is called a **medial–lateral axis**. All motions in the sagittal plane take place around a medial–lateral axis.

The **frontal plane** proceeds from one side of the body to the other and divides the body into front and back halves. The motions that occur in the frontal plane are abduction and adduction (Fig. 1.7). The axis around which the motions of abduction and adduction take place is an **anterior–posterior axis**. This axis lies at right angles to the frontal plane and proceeds from

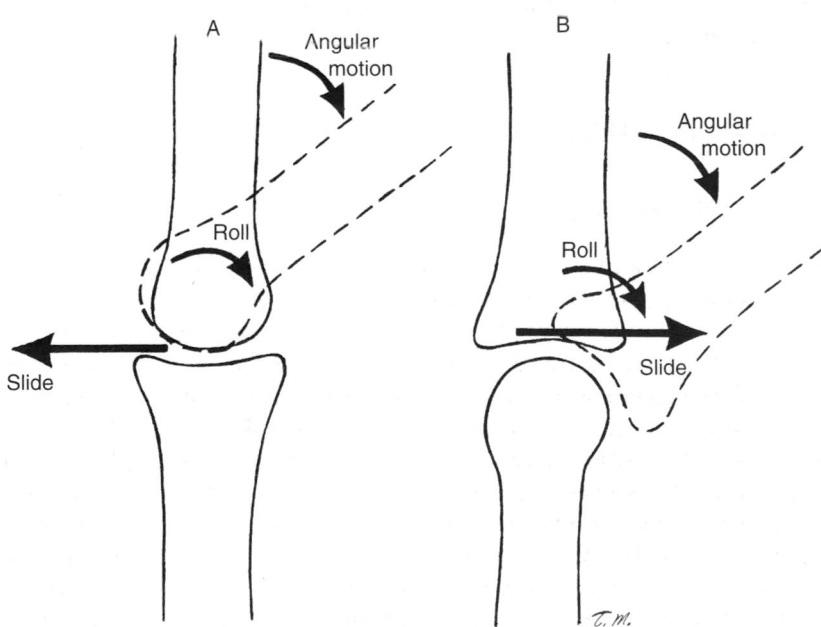

FIGURE 1.5 (A) If the joint surface of the moving bone is convex, sliding is in the opposite direction to the rolling and angular movement of the bone. (B) If the joint surface of the moving bone is concave, sliding is in the same direction as the rolling and angular movement of the bone.

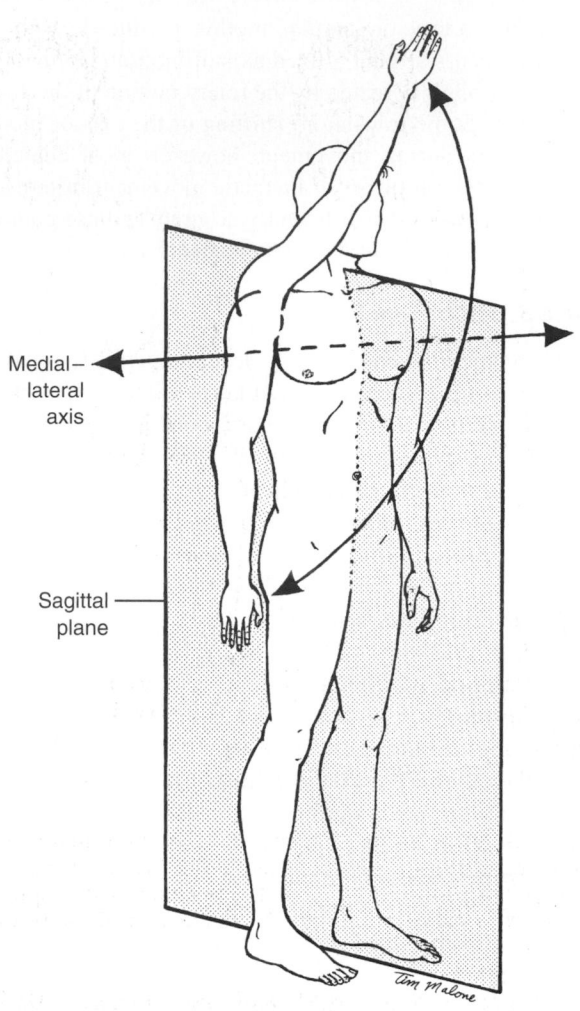

FIGURE 1.6 The shaded areas indicate the sagittal plane. This plane proceeds from the anterior aspect of the body to the posterior aspect. Motions in this plane, such as flexion and extension of the upper and lower extremities, take place around a medial–lateral axis.

the anterior to the posterior aspect of the body. Therefore, the anterior–posterior axis lies in the sagittal plane.

The **transverse plane** is horizontal and divides the body into upper and lower portions. The motion of rotation occurs in the transverse plane around a vertical axis (Fig. 1.8A and B). The **vertical axis** lies at right angles to the transverse plane and proceeds in a cranial to caudal direction.

The motions described previously are considered to occur in a single plane around a single axis. Combination motions such as circumduction (flexion–abduction–extension–adduction) are possible at many joints, but because of the limitations imposed by the uniaxial design of the measuring instrument, only motion occurring in a single plane can be measured in goniometry.

The type of motion that is available at a joint varies according to the structure of the joint. Some joints, such as the interphalangeal joints of the digits, permit a large amount of motion in only one plane around a single axis: flexion and extension in the sagittal plane around a medial–lateral axis. A

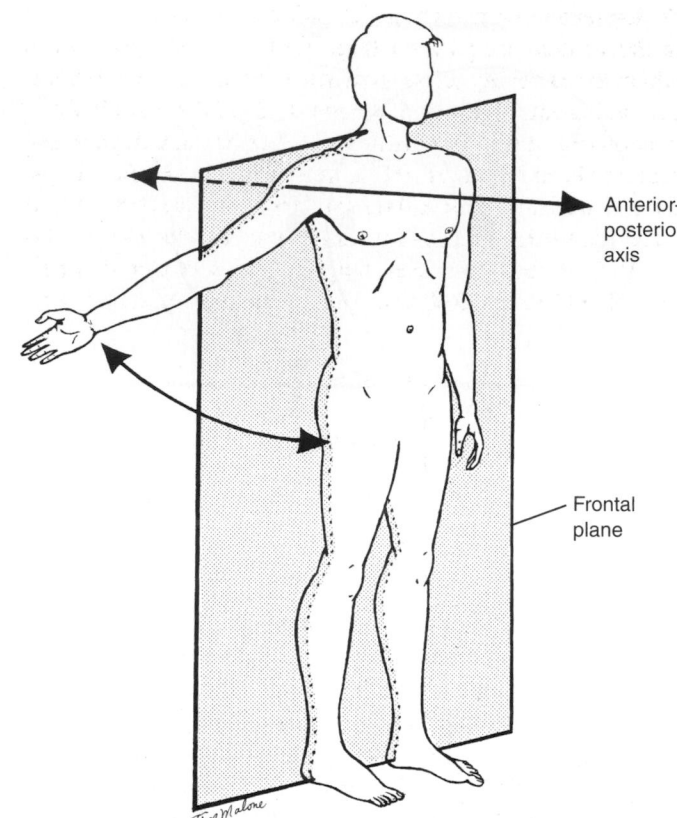

FIGURE 1.7 The frontal plane, indicated by the shaded area, proceeds from one side of the body to the other. Motions in this plane, such as abduction and adduction of the upper and lower extremities, take place around an anterior–posterior axis.

joint that allows motion in only one plane is described as having 1 **degree of freedom of motion.** The interphalangeal joints of the digits have 1 degree of freedom of motion. Other joints, such as the glenohumeral joint, permit motion in three planes around three axes: flexion and extension in the sagittal plane around a medial–lateral axis, abduction and adduction in the frontal plane around an anterior–posterior axis, and medial and lateral rotation in the transverse plane around a vertical axis. The glenohumeral joint has three degrees of freedom of motion.

The planes and axes for each joint and joint motion to be measured are presented in Chapters 4 through 13.

⟲ Range of Motion

Range of motion (ROM) is the arc of motion that occurs at a joint or a series of joints.[5] The starting position for measuring all ROM, except rotations in the transverse plane, is anatomical position. Three notation systems have been used to define ROM: the 0 to 180 degree system, the 180 to 0 degree system, and the 360 degree system.

In the **0 to 180 degree notation system**, the upper-extremity and lower-extremity joints are at 0 degrees for flexion–extension and abduction–adduction when the body is in the anatomical position (Fig. 1.9A). A body position in which the extremity joints are halfway between medial (internal) and lateral (external) rotation is 0 degrees for the ROM in rotation (Fig. 1.9B). Normally, a ROM begins at 0 degrees and proceeds in an arc toward 180 degrees. This 0 to 180 degree system of notation, also called the **neutral zero method,** is widely used throughout the world. First described by Silver[6] in 1923, its use has been supported by many authorities, including Cave and Roberts,[7] Moore,[8] the American Academy

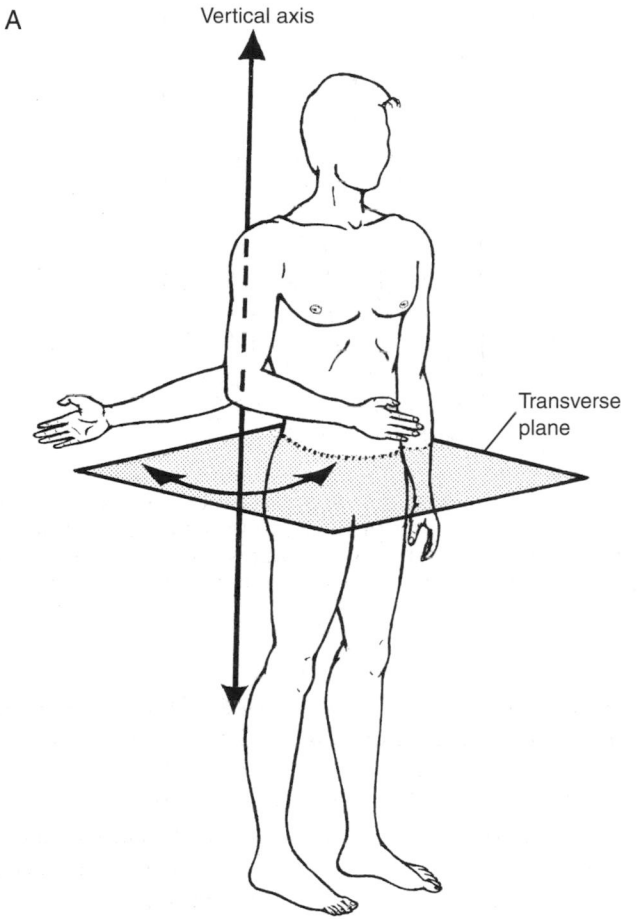

A

Vertical axis

Transverse plane

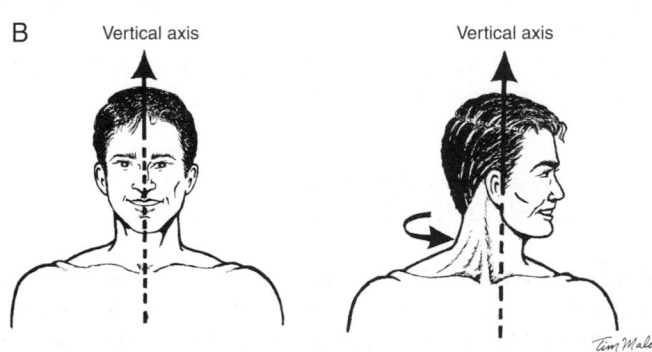

B

Vertical axis   Vertical axis

FIGURE 1.8 The transverse plane is indicated by the shaded area. Movements in this plane take place around a vertical axis. These motions include rotation of the shoulder (A), head (B), and hip, as well as pronation and supination of the forearm.

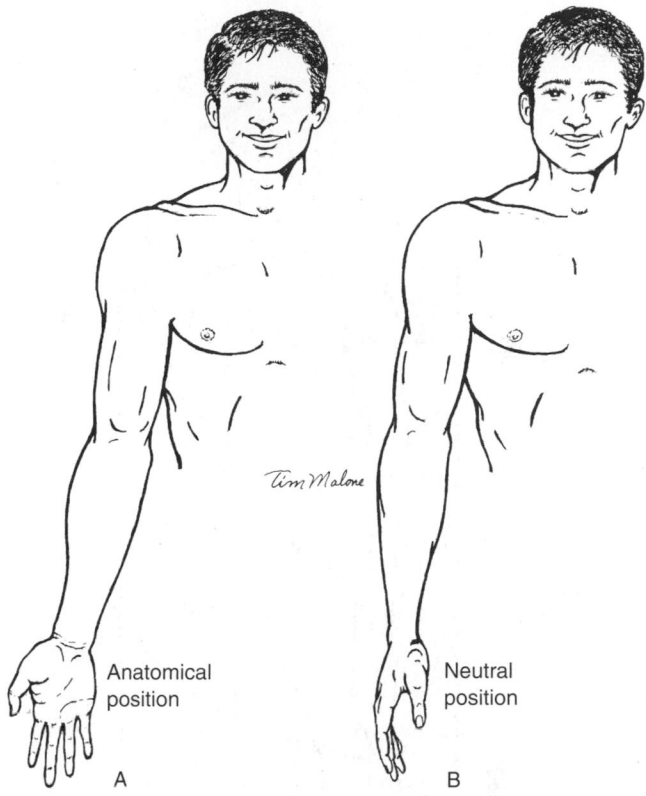

Anatomical position

Neutral position

A

B

FIGURE 1.9 (A) In the anatomical position, the forearm is supinated so that the palms of the hands face anteriorly. (B) When the forearm is in a neutral position (with respect to rotation), the palm of the hand faces the side of the body.

of Orthopaedic Surgeons,[9,10] and the American Medical Association.[11]

Example: The ROM for shoulder flexion, which begins with the shoulder in the anatomical position (0 degrees) and ends with the arm overhead in full flexion (180 degrees), is expressed as 0 to 180 degrees.

In the preceding example, the portion of the extension ROM from full shoulder flexion back to the zero starting position does not need to be measured because this ROM represents the same arc of motion that was measured in flexion. However, the portion of the extension ROM that is available beyond the zero starting position must be measured (Fig. 1.10). Documentation of extension ROM usually incorporates only the extension that occurs beyond the zero starting position. The term **extension,** as it is used in this manual, refers to both the motion that is a return from full flexion to the zero starting position and the motion that normally occurs beyond the zero starting position. The term **hyperextension** is used to describe a greater than normal extension ROM.

Two other systems of notation have been described. The **180 to 0 degree notation system** defines anatomical position as 180 degrees.[12] ROM begins at 180 degrees and proceeds in an arc toward 0 degrees. The **360 degree notation system** also defines anatomical position as 180 degrees.[13,14] The motions of flexion and abduction begin at 180 degrees and proceed in an arc

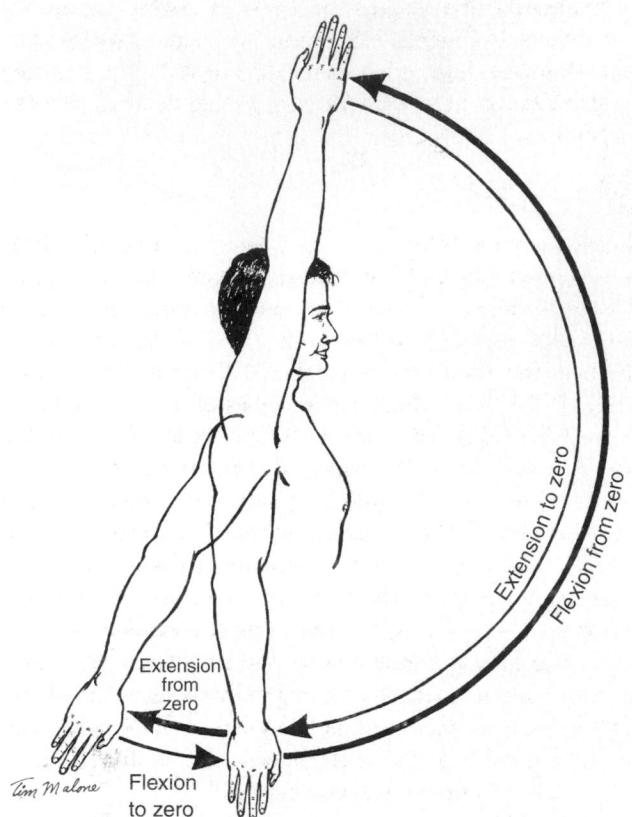

FIGURE 1.10 Flexion and extension of the shoulder begin with the shoulder in the anatomical position. The ROM in flexion proceeds anteriorly from the zero position through an arc toward 180 degrees. The long, bold arrow shows the ROM in flexion, which is measured in goniometry. The ROM in extension proceeds posteriorly from the zero position through an arc toward 180 degrees. The short, bold arrow shows the ROM in extension, which is measured in goniometry.

toward 0 degrees. The motions of extension and adduction begin at 180 degrees and proceed in an arc toward 360 degrees. These two notation systems are more difficult to interpret than the 0 to 180 degree notation system and are infrequently used. Therefore, we have not included them in this text.

Active Range of Motion

Active range of motion (AROM) is the arc of motion attained by a subject during unassisted voluntary joint motion. Having a subject perform active ROM provides the examiner with information about the subject's willingness to move, coordination, muscle strength, and joint ROM. If pain occurs during active ROM, it may be due to contracting or stretching of "contractile" tissues, such as muscles, tendons, and their attachments to bone. Pain may also be due to stretching or pinching of noncontractile (inert) tissues, such as ligaments, joint capsules, bursa, fascia, and skin. Testing active ROM is a good screening technique to help focus a physical examination. If a subject can complete active ROM easily and painlessly, further testing of that motion is probably not needed.

If, however, active ROM is limited, painful, or awkward, the physical examination should include additional testing to clarify the problem.

Passive Range of Motion

Passive range of motion (PROM) is the arc of motion attained by an examiner without assistance from the subject. The subject remains relaxed and plays no active role in producing the motion. Normally passive ROM is slightly greater than active ROM[15–17] because each joint has a small amount of available motion that is not under voluntary control. The additional passive ROM that is available at the end of the normal active ROM is due to the stretch of tissues surrounding the joint and the reduced bulk of relaxed compared to contracting muscles. This additional passive ROM helps to protect joint structures because it allows the joint to absorb extrinsic forces.

Testing passive ROM provides the examiner with information about the integrity of the joint surfaces and the extensibility of the joint capsule and associated ligaments, muscles, fascia, and skin. To focus on these issues, passive ROM rather than active ROM should be tested in goniometry. Unlike active ROM, passive ROM does not depend on the subject's muscle strength and coordination. Comparisons between passive ROMs and active ROMs provide information about the amount of motion permitted by the associated joint structures (passive ROM) relative to the subject's ability to produce motion at a joint (active ROM). In cases of impairment such as muscle weakness, passive ROMs and active ROMs may vary considerably.

Example: An examiner may find that a subject with a muscle paralysis has a full passive ROM but no active ROM at the same joint. In this instance, the joint surfaces and the extensibility of the joint capsule, ligaments, muscles, tendons, fascia, and skin are sufficient to allow full passive ROM. The lack of muscle strength prevents active motion at the joint.

The examiner should test passive ROM prior to performing a manual muscle test of muscle strength because the grading of manual muscle tests is based on completion of the joint ROM. An examiner must know the extent of the passive ROM before initiating a manual muscle test.

If pain occurs during passive ROM, it is often due to moving, stretching, or pinching of noncontractile (inert) structures. Pain occurring at the end of passive ROM may be due to stretching of contractile structures as well as noncontractile structures. Pain during passive ROM is not due to active shortening (contracting) of contractile tissues. By comparing which motions (active versus passive) cause pain and noting the location of the pain, the examiner can begin to determine which injured tissues are involved. Having the subject perform resisted isometric muscle contractions midway through the ROM, so that no tissues are being stretched, can help to isolate contractile structures. Having the examiner perform joint play mobility and joint integrity tests on the subject can help determine which noncontractile structures are involved. Careful consideration of the end-feel and location of tissue tension and pain during passive ROM also adds information about structures that are limiting ROM.

End-Feel

The amount of passive ROM is determined by the unique structure of the joint being tested. Some joints are structured so that the joint capsules limit the end of the ROM in a particular direction, whereas other joints are so structured that ligaments limit the end of a particular ROM. Other normal limitations to motion include passive tension in soft tissue such as muscles, fascia, and skin; soft tissue approximation; and contact of joint surfaces.

The type of structure that limits a ROM has a characteristic feel that may be detected by the examiner who is performing the passive ROM. This feeling, which is experienced by an examiner as a barrier to further motion at the end of a passive ROM, is called the **end-feel.** Developing the ability to determine the character of the end-feel requires practice and sensitivity. Determination of the end-feel must be carried out slowly and carefully to detect the end of the ROM and to distinguish among the various normal and abnormal end-feels. The ability to detect the end of the ROM is critical to the safe and accurate performance of goniometry. The ability to distinguish among the various end-feels helps the examiner identify the type of limiting structure. Cyriax,[18] Kaltenborn,[3] and Paris[19] have described a variety of normal (physiological) and abnormal (pathological) end-feels. Table 1.1, which describes normal end-feels, and Table 1.2, which describes abnormal end-feels, have been adapted from the works of these authors.

In Chapters 4 through 13 we describe what we believe are the normal end-feels and the structures that limit the ROM for each joint and motion. Because of the paucity of specific literature in this area, these descriptions are based on our experience in evaluating joint motion and on information obtained from established anatomy[20,21] and biomechanics texts.[22–28] Considerable controversy exists among experts concerning the structures that limit the ROM in some parts of the body. Also, normal individual variations in body structure may cause instances in which the end-feel differs from our description.

Examiners should practice trying to distinguish among the end-feels. In Chapter 2, Exercise 1 is included for this purpose. However, some additional topics regarding positioning and stabilization must be addressed before this exercise can be completed.

Hypomobility

The term **hypomobility** refers to a decrease in passive ROM that is substantially less than normal values for that joint, given the subject's age and gender. The end-feel occurs early in the ROM and may be different in quality from what is expected. The limitation in passive ROM may be due to a variety of causes including abnormalities of the joint surfaces; passive shortening of joint capsules, ligaments, muscles, fascia, and skin; and inflammation of these structures. Hypomobility has been associated with many orthopedic conditions such as osteoarthritis,[29,30] rheumatoid arthritis,[31] adhesive capsulitis,[32,33] and spinal disorders.[34, 35] Decreased ROM is a common consequence of immobilization after fractures[36,37] and scar development after burns.[38,39] Neurological conditions such as stroke, head trauma, cerebral palsy, and complex regional pain syndrome[40] can also result in hypomobility owing to loss of voluntary movement, increased muscle tone, immobilization, and pain. In addition, metabolic conditions such as diabetes have been associated with limited joint motion.[41–43]

Capsular Patterns of Restricted Motion

Cyriax[18] has proposed that pathological conditions involving the entire joint capsule cause a particular pattern of restriction involving all or most of the passive motions of the joint. This pattern of restriction is called a **capsular pattern**. The restrictions do not involve a fixed number of degrees for each motion, but rather a fixed proportion of one motion relative to another motion.

Example: The capsular pattern for the elbow joint is a greater limitation of flexion than of extension. The elbow joint normally has a passive flexion ROM of

TABLE 1.1 Normal End-Feels

End-Feel	Description	Example
Soft	Soft tissue approximation	Knee flexion (contact between soft tissue of posterior leg and posterior thigh)
Firm	Muscular stretch	Hip flexion with the knee straight (passive elastic tension of hamstring muscles)
	Capsular stretch	Extension of metacarpophalangeal joints of fingers (tension in the anterior capsule)
	Ligamentous stretch	Forearm supination (tension in the palmar radioulnar ligament of the inferior radioulnar joint, interosseous membrane, oblique cord)
Hard	Bone contacting bone	Elbow extension (contact between the olecranon process of the ulna and the olecranon fossa of the humerus)

TABLE 1.2	Abnormal End-Feels	
End-Feel	**Description**	**Example**
Soft	Occurs sooner or later in the ROM than is usual or in a joint that normally has a firm or hard end-feel. Feels boggy.	Soft tissue edema Synovitis
Firm	Occurs sooner or later in the ROM than is usual or in a joint that normally has a soft or hard end-feel.	Increased muscular tonus Capsular, muscular, ligamentous, and fascial shortening
Hard	Occurs sooner or later in the ROM than is usual or in a joint that normally has a soft or firm end-feel. A bony grating or bony block is felt.	Chondromalacia Osteoarthritis Loose bodies in joint Myositis ossificans Fracture
Empty	No real end-feel because pain prevents reaching end of ROM. No resistance is felt except for patient's protective muscle splinting or muscle spasm.	Acute joint inflammation Bursitis Abscess Fracture Psychogenic disorder

0 to 150 degrees. If the capsular involvement is mild, the subject might lose the last 15 degrees of flexion and the last 5 degrees of extension so that the passive flexion ROM is 5 to 135 degrees. If the capsular involvement is more severe, the subject might lose the last 30 degrees of flexion and the first 10 degrees of extension so that the passive flexion ROM is 10 to 120 degrees.

Capsular patterns vary from joint to joint (Table 1.3). The capsular patterns for each joint, as presented by Cyriax[18] and Kaltenborn,[3] are listed in the beginning of Chapters 4 through 13. Studies are needed to test the hypotheses regarding the cause of capsular patterns and to determine the capsular pattern for each joint. Several studies[44–46] have examined the construct validity of Cyriax's capsular pattern in patients with arthritis or arthrosis of the knee. Although differing opinions exist, the findings seem to support the concept of a capsular pattern of restriction for the knee but with more liberal interpretation of the proportions of limitation than suggested by Cyriax.[18] Two studies[46,47] examining capsular patterns for the hip found decreases in all hip motions in osteoarthritic hips as compared to nonosteoarthritic hips, but raised questions concerning specific patterns of limitation proposed by Kaltenborn[3] and Cyriax.[18]

Hertling and Kessler[48] have thoughtfully extended Cyriax's concepts on causes of capsular patterns. They suggest that conditions resulting in a capsular pattern of restriction can be classified into two general categories: (1) conditions in which there is considerable joint effusion or synovial inflammation, and (2) conditions in which there is relative capsular fibrosis.

Joint effusion and synovial inflammation accompany conditions such as traumatic arthritis, infectious arthritis, acute rheumatoid arthritis, and gout. In these conditions the joint capsule is distended by excessive intra-articular synovial fluid, causing the joint to maintain a position that allows the greatest intra-articular joint volume. Pain triggered by stretching the capsule and muscle spasms that protect the capsule from further insult inhibit movement and cause a capsular pattern of restriction.

Relative capsular fibrosis often occurs during chronic low-grade capsular inflammation, immobilization of a joint, and the resolution of acute capsular inflammation. These conditions increase the relative proportion of collagen compared with that of mucopolysaccharide in the joint capsule, or they change the structure of the collagen. The resulting decrease in extensibility of the entire capsule causes a capsular pattern of restriction.

Noncapsular Patterns of Restricted Motion

A limitation of passive motion that is not proportioned similarly to a capsular pattern is called a **noncapsular pattern** of restricted motion.[18,48] A noncapsular pattern is usually caused by a condition involving structures other than the entire joint capsule. Internal joint derangement, adhesion of a part of a joint capsule, ligament shortening, muscle strains, and muscle contractures are examples of conditions that typically result in noncapsular patterns of restriction. Noncapsular patterns usually

TABLE 1.3 Capsular Pattern of Extremity Joints

Joint	Restricted Motions
Glenohumeral joint	Greatest loss of lateral rotation, moderate loss of abduction, minimal loss of medial rotation.
Elbow complex (humeroulnar, humeroradial, proximal radioulnar joints)	Loss of flexion greater than loss of extension. Rotations full and painless except in advanced cases.
Forearm (proximal and distal radioulnar joints)	Equal loss of supination and pronation, only occurring if elbow has marked restrictions of flexion and extension.
Wrist (radiocarpal and midcarpal joints)	Equal loss of flexion and extension, slight loss of ulnar and radial deviation (Cyriax).
	Equal loss of all motions (Kaltenborn).
Hand	
Carpometacarpal joint—digit 1	Loss of abduction (Cyriax). Loss of abduction greater than extension (Kaltenborn).
Carpometacarpal joint—digits 2–5	Equal loss of all motions.
Metacarpophalangeal and interphalangeal joints	Equal loss of flexion and extension (Cyriax).
	Restricted in all motions, but loss of flexion greater than loss of other motions (Kaltenborn).
Hip	Greatest loss of medial rotation and flexion, some loss of abduction, slight loss of extension. Little or no loss of adduction and lateral rotation (Cyriax).
	Greatest loss of medial rotation, followed by less restriction of extension, abduction, flexion, and lateral rotation (Kaltenborn).
Knee (tibiofemoral joint)	Loss of flexion greater than extension.
Ankle (talocrural joint)	Loss of plantarflexion greater than dorsiflexion.
Subtalar joint	Loss of inversion (varus).
Midtarsal joint	Loss of inversion (adduction and medial rotation); other motions full.
Foot	
Metatarsophalangeal joint—digit 1	Loss of extension greater than flexion.
Metatarsophalangeal joint—digits 2–5	Loss of flexion greater than extension.
Interphalangeal joints	Loss of extension greater than flexion.

Reproduced with permission from Dyrek, DA: Assessment and treatment planning strategies for musculoskeletal deficits. In O'Sullivan, SB, and Schmitz, TJ (eds): Physical Rehabilitation: Assessment and Treatment, ed 3. FA Davis, Philadelphia, 1994.
Capsular patterns are from Cyriax[18] and Kaltenborn.[3]

involve only one or two motions of a joint, in contrast to capsular patterns, which involve all or most motions of a joint.[3,18]

Example: A strain of the biceps muscle may result in pain and restriction at the end of the range of passive elbow extension. The passive motion of elbow flexion would not be affected.

Hypermobility

The term **hypermobility** refers to an increase in passive ROM that exceeds normal values for that joint, given the subject's age and gender. For example, in adults the normal ROM for extension at the elbow joint is about 0 degrees.[10] A ROM measurement of 30 degrees or more of extension at the elbow is well beyond normal ROM and is indicative of a hypermobile joint in an adult. Children have some normally occurring specific instances of increased ROM as compared with adults. For example, neonates 6 to 72 hours old have been found to have a mean ankle dorsiflexion passive ROM of 59 degrees,[50] which contrasts with mean adult ROM values of between 12 and 20 degrees.[9,51] The increased motion that is present in these children is normal for their age. If the increased motion persists beyond the expected age range, it would be considered abnormal and hypermobility would be present.

Hypermobility is due to the laxity of soft tissue structures such as ligaments, capsules, and muscles that normally prevent excessive motion at a joint. In some instances the hypermobility may be due to abnormalities of the joint surfaces. A frequent cause of hypermobility is trauma to a joint. Hypermobility also occurs in serious hereditary disorders of connective tissue such as Ehlers-Danlos syndrome, Marfan syndrome, rheumatic diseases, and osteogenesis imperfecta. One of the typical physical abnormalities of Down syndrome is hypermobility. In this instance generalized hypotonia is thought to be an important contributing factor to the hypermobility.

Hypermobility syndrome (HMS) or benign joint hypermobility syndrome (BJHS) is used to describe otherwise-healthy individuals who have generalized hypermobility accompanied by musculoskeletal symptoms.[52,53] An inherited abnormality in collagen and regular physical exercise are thought to be responsible for the joint laxity in these individuals.[54,55] Traditionally, the diagnosis of HMS involves the exclusion of other conditions, a score of at least "4" on the Beighton scale (Table 1-4), and arthralgia for longer than 3 months in four or more joints.[56–58] Some researchers have noted that these criteria are inadequate for children because scores greater than "4" on the Beighton scale have been found in 65 percent of a sample of 1120 children ages 4 to 7 years in Brazil.[55] Other criteria have also been proposed, including additional joint motions and extra-articular signs.[53,54,58]

TABLE 1.4 Beighton Hypermobility Score

The Ability to	Points
Passively appose thumb to forearm	
Right	1
Left	1
Passively extend fifth MCP joint more than 90 degrees	
Right	1
Left	1
Hyperextend elbow more than 10 degrees	
Right	1
Left	1
Hyperextend knee more than 10 degrees	
Right	1
Left	1
Place palms on floor by flexing trunk with knees straight	1
Total Beighton Score = sum of points.	0–9

Adapted from Beighton, P, Solomon, L, and Soskolne, CL: Articular mobility in an African population. Ann Rheum Dis 32:23, 1973.

According to Grahame,[53] the following joint motions should also be considered: shoulder lateral rotation greater than 90 degrees, cervical spine lateral flexion greater than 60 degrees, distal interphalangeal joint hyperextension greater than 60 degrees, and first metatarsophalangeal joint extension greater than 90 degrees.

Factors Affecting Range of Motion

ROM varies among individuals and is influenced by factors such as age, gender, and whether the motion is performed actively or passively. A fairly extensive amount of research on the effects of age and gender on ROM has been conducted for the upper and lower extremities as well as the spine. Other factors relating to subject characteristics such as body mass index (BMI), occupational activities, and recreational activities may affect ROM, but have not been as extensively researched as age and gender. In addition, factors relating to the testing process, such as the testing position, type of instrument employed, experience of the examiner, and even time of day have been identified as affecting ROM measurements. A brief summary of research findings that examine age and gender effects on ROM is presented later in this chapter. To assist the examiner, more detailed information about the effects of age and gender on the featured joints is presented at the end of Chapters 4 through 13. Information on the effects of subject characteristics and the testing process is included if available.

Ideally, to determine whether a ROM is impaired, the value of the ROM of the joint under consideration should be compared with ROM values from people of the same age and gender and from studies that used the same method of measurement. Often such comparisons are not possible because age-related and gender-related norms have not been established for all groups. In such situations the ROM of the joint should be compared with the same joint of the individual's contralateral extremity, providing that the contralateral extremity is not impaired or used selectively in athletic or occupational activities. Most studies have found little difference between the ROM of the right and left extremities.[29,51,59–65] A few studies[16,66–68] have found slightly less ROM in some joints of the upper extremity on the dominant or right side as compared with the contralateral side, which Allender and coworkers[66] attribute to increased exposure to stress. If the contralateral extremity is inappropriate for comparison, the individual's ROM may be compared with average ROM values in handbooks of the American Academy of Orthopaedic Surgeons[9,10] and other standard texts.[11,69–73] However, in many of these texts, the populations from which the values were derived, as well as the testing positions and type of measuring instruments used, are not identified.

Mean ROM values published in several standard texts and studies are summarized at the beginning of the Range of Motion Testing Procedures for each motion and in tables at the end of Chapters 4 through 13. The ROM values presented should serve as only a general guide to identifying normal versus impaired ROM. Considerable differences in mean

ROM values are sometimes noted between the various references.

Age

Numerous studies have been conducted to determine the effects of age on ROM of the extremities and spine. General agreement exists among investigators regarding the age-related effects on the ROM of the extremity joints of new-borns, infants, and young children up to about 2 years of age.[50,74–78] These age effects are joint and motion specific but do not seem to be affected by gender; both males and females are affected similarly. The youngest age groups have more hip flexion, hip abduction, hip lateral rotation, ankle dorsiflexion, and elbow motion as compared to adults. Limitations in hip extension, knee extension, and plantar flexion are considered to be normal for these youngest age groups. Mean values for these age groups differ by more than 2 standard deviations from mean values for adults published by the American Academy of Orthopaedic Surgeons,[9] the American Medical Association,[11] and Boone and Azen.[51] Therefore, age-appropriate norms should be used whenever possible for newborns, infants, and young children up to 2 years of age.

Most investigators who have studied a wide range of age groups have found that older adult groups have somewhat less ROM of the extremities than younger adult groups. These age-related changes in the ROM of older adults also are joint and motion specific and may affect males and females differently. Allander and associates[66] found that wrist flexion–extension, hip rotation, and shoulder rotation ROM decreased with increasing age, whereas flexion ROM in the metacarpophalangeal (MCP) joint of the thumb showed no consistent loss of motion. Roach and Miles[79] generally found a small decrease (3 to 5 degrees) in mean active hip and knee motions between the youngest age group (25 to 39 years) and the oldest age group (60 to 74 years). Except for hip extension ROM, these decreases represented less than 15 percent of the arc of motion. Stubbs, Fernandez, and Glenn[67] found a decrease of between 4 percent and 30 percent in 11 of 23 joints studied in men between the ages of 25 and 54 years. James and Parker[15] found systematic decreases in 10 active and passive lower-extremity motions in subjects who were between 70 and 92 years of age.

As with the extremities, age-related effects on spinal ROM appear to be motion specific. Investigators have reached varying conclusions regarding how large a decrease in ROM occurs with increasing age. Moll and Wright[80] found an initial increase in thoracolumbar spinal mobility (flexion, extension, lateral flexion) in subjects from 15 to 34 years of age, followed by a progressive decrease with increasing age. These authors concluded that age alone may decrease spinal mobility from 25 percent to 52 percent by the seventh decade, depending on the motion. Loebl[81] found that thoracolumbar spinal mobility (flexion–extension) decreases with age an average of 8 degrees per decade. Fitzgerald and colleagues[82] found a systematic decrease in lateral flexion and extension of the lumbar spine at 20-year intervals but no differences in rotation and forward flexion. Youdas and associates[83] found that with each decade both females and males lose approximately 5 degrees of active motion in neck extension and 3 degrees in lateral flexion and rotation. Chen and colleagues,[84] in a review of the literature regarding the effects of aging on cervical spine ROM, concluded that active cervical ROM decreased by 4 degrees per decade, which is similar to the findings of Youdas and associates.

Gender

The effects of gender on the ROM of the extremities and spine also appear to be joint and motion specific. If gender differences in the amount of ROM are found, females are more often reported to have slightly greater ROM than males. In general, gender differences appear to be more prevalent in adults than in young children.

Bell and Hoshizaki[85] found that females across an age range of 18 to 88 years had more flexibility than males in 14 of 17 joint motions tested. Beighton, Solomon, and Soskolne,[56] in a study of an African population, found that females between 0 and 80 years of age were more mobile than their male counterparts. Walker and coworkers,[86] in a study of 28 joint motions in 60 to 84 year olds, reported that 8 motions were greater in females and 4 motions were greater in males, whereas the other motions showed little gender difference. Kalscheur and associates[87] measured 24 upper-extremity and cervical motions in men and women between the ages of 63 and 86 years. Gender differences were noted for 14 of the motions, and in all cases the older women had greater active ROM than the older men. Looking at the thoracolumbar spine, Moll and Wright[80] found that female left lateral flexion exceeded male left lateral flexion by 11 percent. However, male mobility exceeded female mobility in thoracolumbar flexion and extension.

◯ Muscle Length Testing

Maximal **muscle length** is the greatest extensibility of a muscle-tendon unit.[5] It is the maximal distance between the proximal and the distal attachments of a muscle to bone. Clinically, muscle length is not measured directly; instead, it is measured indirectly by determining the maximal passive ROM of the joint(s) crossed by the muscle.[88–90] Muscle length, in addition to the integrity of the joint surfaces and the extensibility of the capsule, ligaments, fascia, and skin, affects the amount of passive ROM of a joint. The purpose of testing muscle length is to ascertain whether hypomobility or hypermobility is caused by the length of the inactive antagonist muscle or other structures. By ascertaining which structures are involved, the health professional can choose more specific and more effective treatment procedures.

Muscles can be categorized by the number of joints they cross from their proximal to their distal attachments. **One-joint muscles** cross and therefore influence the motion of only one joint. **Two-joint muscles** cross and influence the motion of two joints, whereas multi-joint muscles cross and influence multiple joints.

No difference exists between the indirect measurement of the length of a one-joint muscle and the measurement of passive joint ROM in the direction opposite to the muscle's active motion. Usually, one-joint muscles have sufficient length to allow full passive ROM at the joint they cross. If a one-joint muscle is shorter than normal, passive ROM in the direction opposite to the muscle's action is decreased and the end-feel is firm owing to a muscular stretch. At the end of the ROM the examiner may be able to palpate tension within the muscle-tendon unit if the structures are superficial. In addition, the subject may complain of pain in the region of the tight muscle and tendon. These signs and symptoms help to confirm muscle shortness as the cause of the joint limitation.

If a one-joint muscle is abnormally lax, passive tension in the capsule and ligaments may initially maintain a normal ROM. However, with time, these joint structures often lengthen as well and passive ROM at the joint increases. Because the indirect measurement of the length of one-joint muscles is the same as the measurement of passive joint ROM, we have not presented specific muscle length tests for one-joint muscles.

Example: The length of one-joint hip adductors such as the adductor longus, adductor magnus, and adductor brevis is assessed by measuring passive hip abduction ROM. The indirect measurement of the length of these hip adductor muscles is identical to the measurement of passive hip abduction ROM (Fig. 1.11).

In contrast to one-joint muscles, the length of two-joint and multi-joint muscles is usually not sufficient to allow full passive ROM to occur simultaneously at all joints crossed by these muscles.[91] This inability of a muscle to lengthen and allow full ROM at all of the joints the muscle crosses is termed **passive insufficiency.** If a two-joint or multi-joint muscle crosses a joint the examiner is assessing for ROM, the subject must be positioned so that passive tension in the muscle does not limit the joint's ROM. To allow full ROM at the joint under consideration and to ensure sufficient length in the muscle, the muscle must be put on slack at all of the joints the muscle crosses that are not being assessed. A muscle is put on slack by passively approximating the origin and insertion of the muscle.

Example: The triceps is a two-joint muscle that extends the elbow and shoulder. The triceps is passively insufficient during full shoulder flexion and full elbow flexion. When an examiner assesses elbow flexion ROM, the shoulder must be in a neutral position so there is sufficient length in the triceps to allow full flexion at the elbow (Fig. 1.12).

To assess the length of a two-joint muscle, the subject is positioned so that the muscle is lengthened over the proximal or distal joint that the muscle crosses. One joint is held in position while the examiner attempts to further lengthen the muscle by moving the second joint through full ROM. The end-feel in this situation is firm owing to the development of passive tension in the stretched muscle. The length of the two-joint muscle is indirectly assessed by measuring the passive ROM in the direction opposite to the muscle's action at the second joint.

Example: To assess the length of a two-joint muscle such as the triceps, the shoulder is positioned and held in full flexion. The elbow is flexed until tension is felt in the triceps, creating a firm end-feel. The length of the triceps is determined by measuring passive ROM of elbow flexion with the shoulder in flexion (Fig. 1.13).

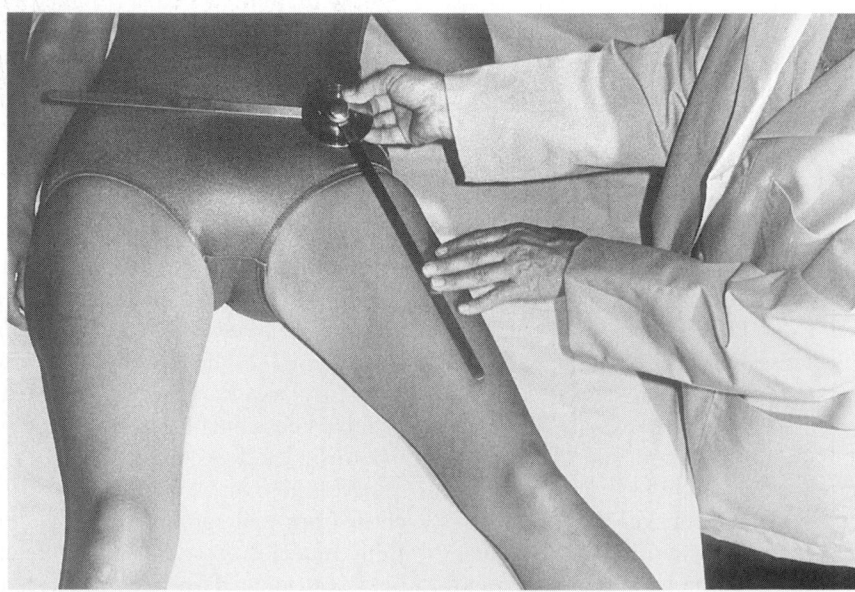

FIGURE 1.11 The indirect measurement of the muscle length of one-joint hip adductors is the same as measurement of passive hip abduction ROM.

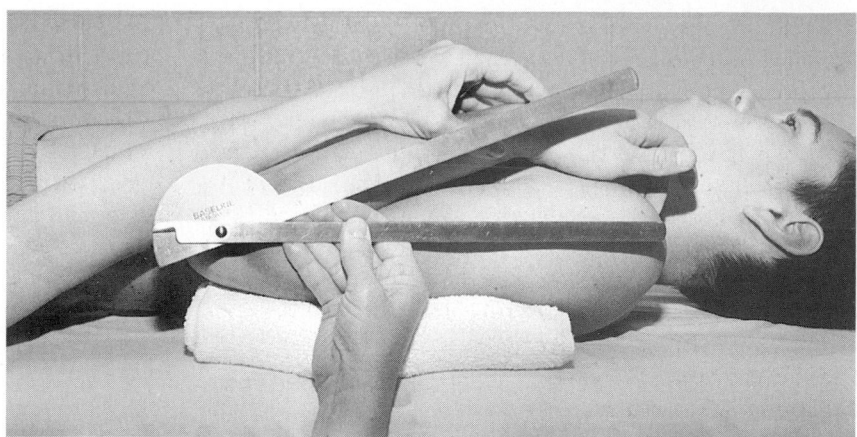

FIGURE 1.12 During the measurement of elbow flexion ROM, the shoulder must be in neutral to avoid passive insufficiency of the triceps, which would limit the ROM.

The length of multi-joint muscles is assessed in a manner similar to that used in assessing the length of two-joint muscles. However, the subject is positioned and held so that the muscle is lengthened over all of the joints that the muscle crosses except for one last joint. The examiner attempts to further lengthen the muscle by moving the last joint through full ROM. Again, the end-feel is firm owing to tension in the stretched muscle. The length of the multi-joint muscle is indirectly determined by measuring passive ROM in the direction opposite to the muscle's action at the last joint to be moved. Commonly used muscle length tests that indirectly assess two-joint and multi-joint muscles have been included in Chapters 4 through 12 as appropriate.

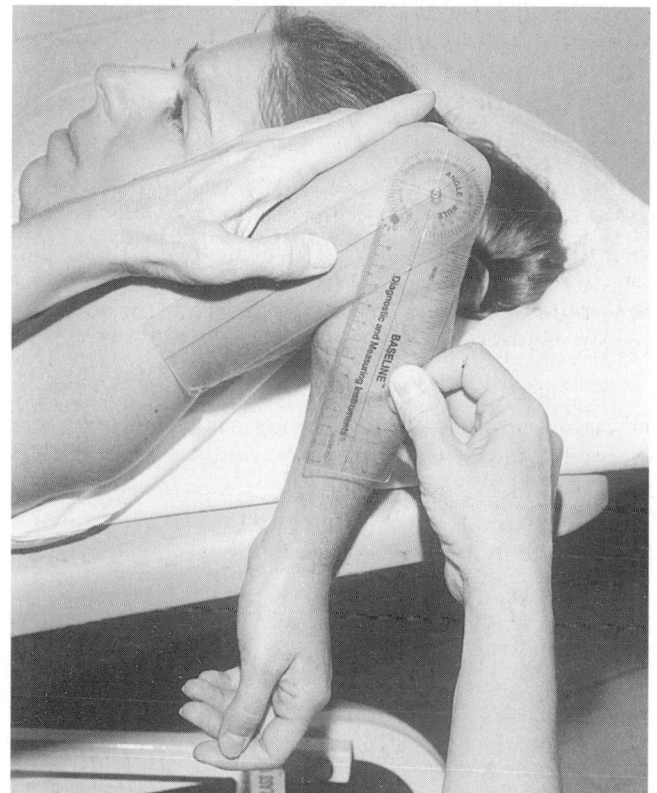

FIGURE 1.13 To assess the length of the two-joint triceps muscle, elbow flexion is measured while the shoulder is positioned in flexion.

REFERENCES

1. MacConaill, MA, and Basmajian, JV: Muscles and Movement: A Basis for Human Kinesiology, ed 2. Robert E. Krieger, New York, 1977.
2. Kisner, C, and Colby, LA: Therapeutic Exercise, ed 5. FA Davis, Philadelphia, 2007.
3. Kaltenborn, FM: Manual Mobilization of the Extremity Joints, ed 5. Olaf Norlis Bokhandel, Oslo, 1999.
4. White, DJ: Musculoskeletal Examination. In O'Sullivan, SB, and Schmitz, TJ (eds): Physical Rehabilitation, ed 5. FA Davis, Philadelphia, 2007.
5. American Physical Therapy Association: Guide to Physical Therapist Practice, ed 2. Phys Ther 81:9, 2001.
6. Silver, D: Measurement of the range of motion in joints. J Bone Joint Surg 21:569, 1923.
7. Cave, EF, and Roberts, SM: A method for measuring and recording joint function. J Bone Joint Surg 18:455, 1936.
8. Moore, ML: The measurement of joint motion. Part II: The technic of goniometry. Phys Ther Rev 29:256, 1949.
9. American Academy of Orthopaedic Surgeons: Joint Motion: Methods of Measuring and Recording. AAOS, Chicago, 1965.
10. Greene, WB, and Heckman, JD (eds): The Clinical Measurement of Joint Motion. American Academy of Orthopaedic Surgeons, Rosemont, IL, 1994.
11. American Medical Association: Guides to the Evaluation of Permanent Impairment, ed 5. Cocchiarella, L, and Andersson, GBJ (editors). AMA, Chicago, 2001.
12. Clark, WA: A system of joint measurement. J Orthop Surg 2:687, 1920.
13. West, CC: Measurement of joint motion. Arch Phys Med Rehabil 26:414, 1945.
14. Cole, TM, and Tobis, JS: Measurement of Musculoskeletal Function. In Kottke, FJ, and Lehmann, JF (eds): Krusenn's Handbook of Physical Medicine and Rehabilitation, ed 4. WB Saunders, Philadelphia, 1990.
15. James, B, and Parker, AW: Active and passive mobility of lower limb joints in elderly men and women. Am J Phys Med Rehabil 68:162, 1989.
16. Gunal, I, et al: Normal range of motion of the joints of the upper extremity in male subjects, with special reference to side. J Bone Joint Surg (Am) 78(A):1401, 1996.
17. Smahel, Z, and Klimova, A: The influence of age and exercise on the mobility of hand joints: 1: Metacarpophalangeal joints of the three-phalangeal fingers. Acta Chirurgiae Plasticae 46:81, 2004.
18. Cyriax, J: Textbook of Orthopaedic Medicine: Diagnosis of Soft Tissue Lesions, ed 8. Bailliere Tindall, London, 1982.
19. Paris, SV: Extremity Dysfunction and Mobilization. Institute Press, Atlanta, 1980.
20. Standring, S (ed): Grey's Anatomy, ed 39. Elsevier, New York, 2005.
21. Moore, KL, and Dalley, AF: Clinically Oriented Anatomy, ed 5. Lippincott, Williams & Wilkins, Baltimore, 2005.
22. Kapandji, IA: Physiology of the Joints, Vol 1, ed 2. Churchill Livingstone, London, 1970.
23. Kapandji, IA: Physiology of the Joints, Vol 2, ed 2. Williams & Wilkins, Baltimore, 1970.
24. Kapandji, IA: Physiology of the Joints, Vol 3, ed 2. Churchill Livingstone, London, 1970.
25. Steindler, A: Kinesiology of the Human Body. Charles C. Thomas, Springfield, IL, 1955.
26. Gowitzke, BA, and Milner, M: Understanding the Scientific Basis for Human Movement, ed 3. Williams & Wilkins, Baltimore, 1988.
27. Levangie, PL, and Norkin, CC: Joint Structure and Function: A Comprehensive Analysis, ed 4. FA Davis, Philadelphia, 2005.
28. Newmann, DA: Kinesiology of the Musculoskeletal System. Mosby, St. Louis, Mo, 2002.
29. Steultjens, MPM, et al: Range of joint motion and disability in patients with osteoarthritis of the knee or hip. Rheumatology 39:955, 2000.
30. Messier, SP, et al: Osteoarthritis of the knee: Effects on gait, strength, and flexibility. Arch Phys Med Rehabil 73:29, 1992.
31. Goodson, A, et al: Direct, quantitative clinical assessment of hand function: Usefulness and reproducibility. Manual Ther 12:144, 2007.
32. Stam, HW: Frozen shoulder: A review of current concepts. Physiotherapy 80:588, 1994.
33. Roubal, PJ, Dobritt, D, and Placzek, JD: Glenohumeral gliding manipulation following interscalene brachial plexus block in patients with adhesive capsulitis. J Orthop Sports Phys Ther 24:66, 1996.
34. Hagen, KB, et al: Relationship between subjective neck disorders and cervical spine mobility and motion-related pain in male machine operators. Spine 22:1501, 1997.
35. Hermann, KM, and Reese, CS: Relationship among selected measures of impairment, functional limitation, and disability in patients with cervical spine disorders. Phys Ther 81:903, 2001.
36. MacKenzie, EJ, et al: Physical impairment and functional outcomes six months after severe lower extremity fractures. J Trauma 34:528, 1993.
37. Chesworth, BM, and Vandervoort, AA: Comparison of passive stiffness variables and range of motion in uninvolved and involved ankle joints of patients following ankle fractures. Phys Ther 75:254, 1995.
38. Richard, RL, and Ward, RS: Burns. In O'Sullivan, SB and Schmitz, TJ (eds): Physical Rehabilitation: Assessment and Treatment, ed 5. FA Davis, Philadelphia, 2005.
39. Johnson, J, and Silverberg, R: Serial casting of the lower extremity to correct contractures during the acute phase of burn care. Phys Ther 75:262, 1995.
40. Field, J: Measurement of finger stiffness in algodystrophy. Hand Clin 19:511, 2003.
41. Schulte, L, et al: A quantitative assessment of limited joint mobility in patients with diabetes. Arthritis Rheum 10:1429, 1993.
42. Rao, SR, et al: Increased passive ankle stiffness and reduced dorsiflexion range of motion in individuals with diabetes mellitus. Foot & Ankle International 27:617, 2006.
43. Sauseng, S, Kastenbauer, T, and Irsigler, K: Limited joint mobility in selected hand and foot joints in patients with type 1 diabetes mellitus: A methodology comparison. Diab Nutr Metab 15:1, 2002.
44. Fritz, JM, et al: An examination of the selective tissue tension scheme, with evidence for the concept of a capsular pattern of the knee. Phys Ther 78:1046, 1998.
45. Hayes, KW, Petersen, C, and Falconer, J: An examination of Cyriax's passive motion tests with patients having osteoarthritis of the knee. Phys Ther 74:697, 1994.
46. Biji, D, et al: Validity of Cyriax's concept capsular pattern for the diagnosis of osteoarthiritis of hip and/or knee. Scand J Rheumatol 27:347, 1998.
47. Klassbo, M, and Harms-Ringdahl, K: Examination of passive ROM and capsular pattern in the hip. Physiotherapy Research International 8:1, 2003.
48. Dyrek, DA: Assessment and treatment planning strategies for musculoskeletal deficits. In O'Sullivan, SB, and Schmitz, TJ (eds): Physical Rehabilitation: Assessment and Treatment, ed 3. FA Davis, Philadelphia, 1994.
49. Hertling, DH, and Kessler, RM: Management of Common Musculoskeletal Disorders, ed 4. Lippincott, Williams & Wilkins, Philadelphia, 2005.
50. Waugh, KG, et al: Measurement of selected hip, knee and ankle joint motions in newborns. Phys Ther 63:1616, 1983.
51. Boone, DC, and Azen, SP: Normal range of motion of joints in male subjects. J Bone Joint Surg Am 61:756, 1979.
52. Everman, DB, and Robin, NH: Hypermobility syndrome. Pediatr Rev 19:111, 1998.
53. Grahame, R: Hypermobility not a circus act. Int J Clin Pract 54:314, 2000.
54. Russek, LN: Hypermobility syndrome. Phys Ther 79:59, 1999.
55. Lamari, NM, Chueire, AG, and Cordeiro, JA: Analysis of joint mobility patterns among preschool children. Sao Paulo Med:123:119, 2005.
56. Beighton, P, Solomon, L, and Soskolne, CL: Articular mobility in an African population. Ann Rheum Dis 32:23, 1973.
57. Remvig, L, Jensen, DV, and Ward, RC: Are diagnostic criteria for general joint hypermobility and benign joint hypermobility syndrome based on reproducible and valid tests? A review of the literature. J Rheumatol 34:798, 2007.
58. Bird, HA: Joint hypermobility: Report from Special Interest Groups of the annual meeting of the British Society of Rheumatology. Br J Rheumatol 31:205, 1992.
59. Roaas, A, and Andersson, GB: Normal range of motion of the hip, knee and ankle joints in male subjects, 30–40 years of age. Acta Othop Scand 53:205, 1982.
60. Chang, DE, Buschbacher, LP, and Edlich, RF: Limited joint mobility in power lifters. Am J Sports Med 16:280, 1988.
61. Ahlberg, A, Moussa, M, and Al-Nahdi, M: On geographical variations in the normal range of joint motion. Clin Orthop Rel Res 234:229, 1988.
62. Schwarze, DJ, and Denton, JR: Normal values of neonatal limbs: An evaluation of 1000 neonates. J Res Pediatr Orthop 13:758, 1993.
63. Stefanyshyn, DJ, and Ensberg, JR: Right to left differences in the ankle joint complex range of motion. Med Sci Sports Exerc 26:551, 1993.
64. Mosley, AM, Crosbie, J, and Adams, R: Normative data for passive ankle plantar flexion-dorsiflexion flexibility. Clin Biomech 16:514, 2001.

65. Escalanate, A, et al: Determinants of hip and knee flexion range: Results from the San Antonio Longitudinal Study of Aging. Arthritis Care Res 12:8, 1999.

66. Allender, E, et al: Normal range of joint movements in shoulder, hip, wrist and thumb with special reference to side: A comparison between two populations. Int J Epidemiol 3:253, 1974.

67. Stubbs, NB, Fernandez, JE, and Glenn, WM: Normative data on joint ranges of motion for 25- to 54-year old males. Int J Ind Ergonomics 12:265, 1993.

68. Escalante, A, Lichtenstein, MJ, and Hazuda, HP: Determinants of shoulder and elbow flexion range: Results from the San Antonio longitudinal study of aging. Arthritis Care Res 12:277, 1999.

69. Hoppenfeld, S: Physical Examination of the Spine and Extremities. Appleton-Century-Crofts, New York, 1976.

70. Kendall, FP, et al: Muscles: Testing and Function with Posture and Pain, ed 5. Lippincott, Williams & Wilkins, Philadelphia, 2005.

71. Esch, D, and Lepley, M: Evaluation of Joint Motion: Methods of Measurement and Recording. University of Minnesota Press, Minneapolis, 1974.

72. Palmer, ML, and Epler, M: Fundamentals of Musculoskeletal Assessment Techniques. Lippincott, Williams & Wilkins, Philadelphia, 1998.

73. Reese, NB, and Bandy, WD: Joint Range of Motion and Muscle Length Testing. WB Saunders, Philadelphia, 2002.

74. Drews, JE, Vraciu, JK, and Pellino, G: Range of motion of the joints of the lower extremities of newborns. Phys Occup Ther Pediatr 4:49, 1984.

75. Phelps, E, Smith, LJ, and Hallum, A: Normal range of hip motion of infants between nine and 24 months of age. Dev Med Child Neurol 27:785, 1985.

76. Wanatabe, H, et al: The range of joint motions of the extremities in healthy Japanese people: The differences according to age. Nippon Seikeigeka Gakkai Zasshi 53:275, 1979. Cited in Walker, JM: Musculoskeletal development: A review. Phys Ther 71:878, 1991.

77. Schwarze, DJ, and Denton, JR: Normal values of neonatal limbs: An evaluation of 1000 neonates. J Pediatr Orthop 13:758, 1993.

78. Broughton, NS, Wright, J, and Menelaus, MB: Range of knee motion in normal neonates. J Pediatr Orthop 13:263, 1993.

79. Roach, KE, and Miles, TP: Normal hip and knee active range of motion: The relationship to age. Phys Ther 71:656, 1991.

80. Moll, JMH, and Wright, V: Normal range of spinal mobility. Ann Rheum Dis 30:381, 1971.

81. Loebl, WY: Measurement of spinal posture and range of spinal movement. Ann Phys Med 9:103, 1967.

82. Fitzgerald, GK, et al: Objective assessment with establishment of normal values for lumbar spinal range of motion. Phys Ther 63:1776, 1983.

83. Youdas, JW, et al: Normal range of motion of the cervical spine: An initial goniometric study. Phys Ther 72:770, 1992.

84. Chen, J, et al: Meta-analysis of normative cervical motion. Spine 24:1571, 1999.

85. Bell, RD, and Hoshizaki, TB: Relationship of age and sex with range of motion: Seventeen joint actions in humans. Can J Appl Sci 6:202, 1981.

86. Walker, JM, et al: Active mobility of the extremities in older subjects. Phys Ther 64:919, 1984.

87. Kalscheur, JA, Costello, PS, and Emery, LJ: Gender differences in range of motion in older adults. Physical & Occupational Therapy in Geriatrics 22:77, 2003.

88. Gajdosik, RL, et al: Comparison of four clinical tests for assessing hamstring muscle length. J Orthop Sports Phys Ther 18:614, 1993.

89. Tardieu, G, Lespargot, A, and Tardieu, C: To what extent is the tibia-calcaneum angle a reliable measurement of the triceps surae length: Radiological correction of the torque-angle curve. Eur J Appl Physiol 37:163, 1977.

90. Gajdosik, RL: Passive extensibility of skeletal muscle: Review of the literature with clinical implications. Clin Biomech 16:87, 2001.

91. Gajdosik, RL, Hallett, JP, and Slaughter, LL: Passive insufficiency of two-joint shoulder muscles. Clin Biomech 9:377, 1994.

Chapter 2

Procedures

Competency in goniometry requires that the examiner acquire the following knowledge and develop the following skills.

The examiner must have knowledge of the following for each joint and motion:

1. Joint structure and function
2. Normal end-feels
3. Testing positions
4. Stabilization required
5. Anatomical bony landmarks
6. Instrument alignment

The examiner must have the skill to perform the following for each joint and motion:

1. Position and stabilize correctly
2. Move a body part through the appropriate range of motion (ROM)
3. Determine the end of the ROM and end-feel
4. Palpate the appropriate bony landmarks
5. Align the measuring instrument with landmarks
6. Read the measuring instrument
7. Record measurements correctly

⟳ Positioning

Positioning is an important part of goniometry because it is used to place the joints in a zero starting position and helps to stabilize the proximal joint segment. Positioning affects the amount of tension in soft tissue structures (capsule, ligaments, muscles) surrounding a joint. A testing position in which one or more of these soft tissue structures become taut results in a more limited ROM than a position in which the same structures become lax. As can be seen in the following example, the use of different testing positions alters the ROM obtained for hip flexion.

Example: A testing position in which the knee is flexed yields a greater hip flexion ROM than a testing position in which the knee is extended. When the knee is extended, hip flexion is prematurely limited by tension in the hamstring muscles.

It is important that examiners use the same testing position during successive measurements of a joint ROM so that the relative amounts of tension in the soft tissue structures are the same as in previous measurements. In this manner, a comparison of ROM measurements taken in the same position should yield similar results. When different testing positions are used for successive measurements of a joint ROM, more variability is added to the measurement[1–10] and no basis for comparison exists. If testing positions vary, it is difficult to determine if differences in successive measurements are the result of changes in the testing position or a true change in joint ROM.

Testing positions refer to the positions of the body that we recommend for obtaining goniometric measurements. The series of testing positions that are presented in this text are designed to do the following:

1. Place the joint in a starting position of 0 degrees
2. Permit a complete ROM
3. Provide stabilization for the proximal joint segment

If a testing position cannot be attained because of restrictions imposed by the environment or limitations of the subject, the examiner must use creativity to decide how to obtain a particular joint measurement. The alternative testing position that is created must serve the same three functions as the recommended testing position. The examiner must describe the position precisely in the subject's records so that the same position can be used for all subsequent measurements.

Testing positions involve a variety of body positions such as supine, prone, sitting, and standing. When an examiner intends to test several joints and motions during one testing session, the goniometric examination should be planned to avoid moving the subject unnecessarily. For example, if the subject is prone, all possible measurements in this position should be taken before the subject is moved into another position. Table 2.1, which lists joint measurements by body

TABLE 2.1	Joint Measurements by Body Position			
	Prone	**Supine**	**Sitting**	**Standing**
Shoulder	Extension	Flexion		
		Abduction		
		Medial rotation		
		Lateral rotation		
Elbow		Flexion		
Forearm			Pronation	
			Supination	
Wrist			All motions	
Hand			All motions	
Hip	Extension	Flexion	Medial rotation	
		Abduction	Lateral rotation	
		Adduction		
Knee		Flexion		
Ankle and foot	Subtalar inversion	Dorsiflexion	Dorsiflexion	
	Subtalar eversion	Plantar flexion	Plantar flexion	
		Inversion	Inversion	
		Eversion	Eversion	
		Midtarsal inversion	Midtarsal inversion	
		Midtarsal eversion	Midtarsal eversion	
Toes		All motions	All motions	
Cervical spine			Flexion	
			Extension	
			Lateral flexion	
		Rotation (I)	Rotation	
Thoracolumbar spine			Rotation	Flexion
				Extension
				Lateral flexion
				Rotation (I)
Temporomandibular joint			Depression	
			Protrusion	
			Lateral excursion	

I = measured with inclinometer(s)

position, has been designed to help the examiner plan a goniometric examination.

⭕ Stabilization

The testing position helps to stabilize the subject's body and proximal joint segment so that a motion can be isolated to the joint being examined. Isolating the motion to one joint helps to ensure that a true measurement of the motion is obtained, rather than a measurement of combined motions that occur at

a series of joints. Positional stabilization may be supplemented by manual stabilization provided by the examiner.

Example: Measurement of medial rotation of the hip joint is performed with the subject in a sitting position (Fig. 2.1A). The pelvis (proximal segment) is partially stabilized by the body weight, but the subject is moving her trunk and pelvis during hip rotation. Additional stabilization should be provided by the examiner and the subject (Fig. 2.1B). The examiner provides manual stabilization for the pelvis by exerting a downward pressure on the iliac crest of the side

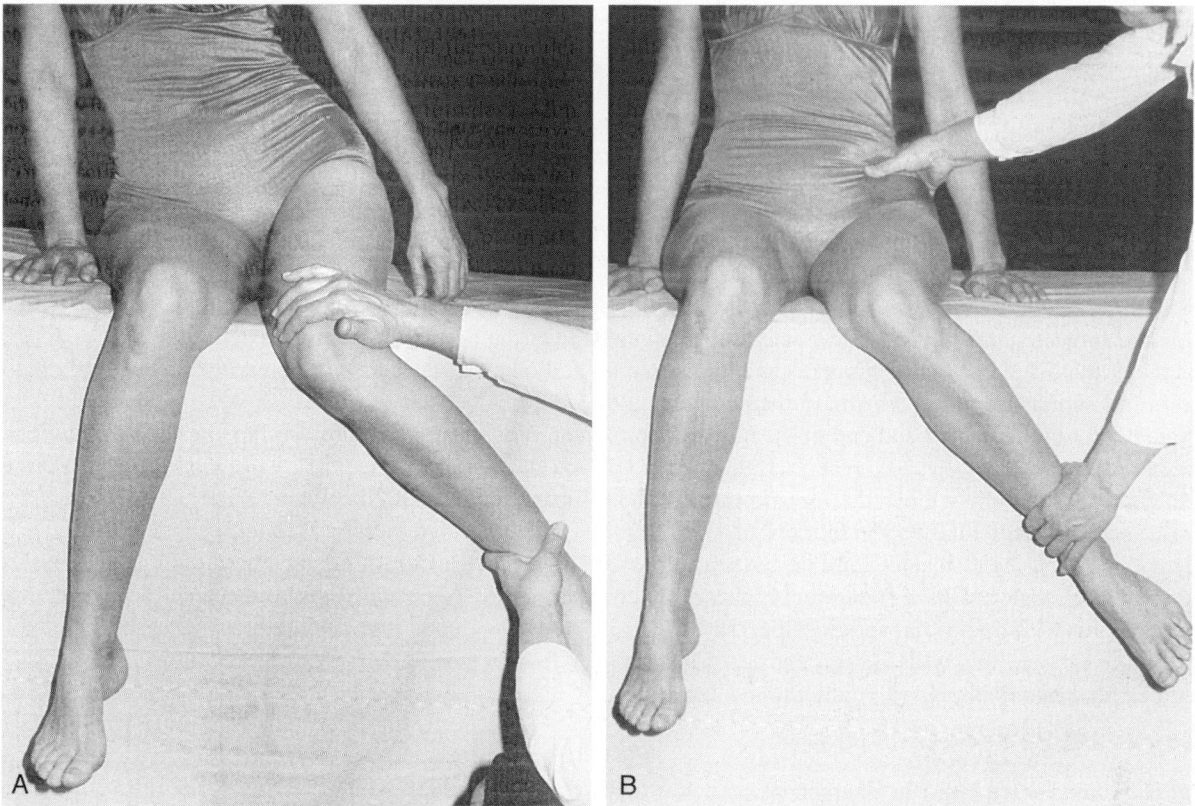

FIGURE 2.1 (A) The consequences of inadequate stabilization. The examiner has failed to stabilize the subject's pelvis and trunk; therefore, a lateral tilt of the pelvis and lateral flexion of the trunk accompany the motion of hip medial rotation. The range of medial rotation appears greater than it actually is because of the added motion from the pelvis and trunk. (B) The use of proper stabilization. The examiner uses her right hand to stabilize the pelvis (keeping the pelvis from raising off the table) during the passive range of motion (ROM). The subject assists in stabilizing the pelvis by placing her body weight on the left side. The subject keeps her trunk straight by placing both hands on the table.

being tested. The subject is instructed to shift her body weight over the hip being tested to help keep the pelvis stabilized.

For most measurements, the amount of manual stabilization applied by an examiner must be sufficient to keep the proximal joint segment fixed during movement of the distal joint segment. If both the distal and the proximal joint segments are allowed to move during joint testing, the end of the ROM is difficult to determine. Learning how to stabilize requires practice because the examiner must stabilize with one hand while simultaneously moving the distal joint segment with the other hand. Sometimes in the case of the hip a second person may be necessary to help either with stabilizing the proximal joint segment or with holding the distal joint segment after the end of the ROM has been determined, so that the goniometer can be accurately aligned. The techniques of stabilizing the proximal joint segment and of determining the end of a ROM (end-feel) are basic to goniometry and must be mastered prior to learning how to use the goniometer. **Exercise 1 on page 22** is designed to help the examiner learn how to stabilize and determine the end of the ROM and end-feel.

⊘ Measurement Instruments

A variety of instruments are used to measure joint motion. These instruments range from simple paper tracings and tape measures to electrogoniometers and motion analysis systems. An examiner may choose to use a particular instrument based upon the purpose of the measurement (clinical versus research); the motion being measured; and the instrument's accuracy, availability, cost, ease of use, and size.

Universal Goniometer

The **universal goniometer** is the instrument most commonly used to measure joint position and motion in the clinical setting. Moore[11,12] designated this type of goniometer as "universal" because of its versatility. It can be used to measure joint position and ROM at almost all joints of the body. The majority of measurement techniques presented in this book demonstrate the use of the universal goniometer.

Universal goniometers may be constructed of plastic (Fig. 2.2) or metal (Fig. 2.3) and are produced in many sizes

Exercise 1

Determining the End of the Range of Motion and End-Feel

This exercise is designed to help the examiner determine the end of the ROM and to differentiate among the three normal end-feels: soft, firm, and hard.

ELBOW FLEXION: Soft End-Feel

ACTIVITIES: See Figure 5.13 in Chapter 5.

1. Select a subject.
2. Position the subject supine with the arm placed close to the side of the body. A towel roll is placed under the distal end of the humerus to allow space for full elbow extension. The forearm is placed in full supination with the palm of the hand facing the ceiling.
3. With one hand, stabilize the distal end of the humerus (proximal joint segment) to prevent flexion of the shoulder.
4. With the other hand, slowly move the forearm through the full passive range of elbow flexion until you feel resistance limiting the motion.
5. Gently push against the resistance until no further flexion can be achieved. Carefully note the quality of the resistance. This soft end-feel is caused by compression of the muscle bulk of the anterior forearm with that of the anterior upper arm.
6. Compare this soft end-feel with the soft end-feel found in knee flexion (see ROM Testing Procedures for Knee Flexion and Figure 9.6 in Chapter 9).

ANKLE DORSIFLEXION: Firm End-Feel

ACTIVITIES: See Figure 10.11 in Chapter 10.

1. Select a subject.
2. Place the subject sitting so that the lower leg is over the edge of the supporting surface and the knee is flexed at least 30 degrees.
3. With one hand, stabilize the distal end of the tibia and fibula to prevent knee extension and hip motions.
4. With the other hand on the plantar surface of the metatarsals, slowly move the foot through the full passive range of ankle dorsiflexion until you feel resistance limiting the motion.
5. Push against the resistance until no further dorsiflexion can be achieved. Carefully note the quality of the resistance. This firm end-feel is caused by tension in the Achilles tendon, the posterior portion of the deltoid ligament, the posterior talofibular ligament, the calcaneo-fibular ligament, the posterior joint capsule, and the wedging of the talus into the mortise formed by the tibia and fibula.
6. Compare this firm end-feel with the firm end-feel found in metacarpophalangeal (MCP) extension of the fingers (see ROM Testing Procedures for Fingers MCP Extension and Figure 7.12 in Chapter 7).

ELBOW EXTENSION: Hard End-Feel

ACTIVITIES:

1. Select a subject.
2. Position the subject supine with the arm placed close to the side of the body. A small towel roll is placed under the distal end of the humerus to allow full elbow extension. The forearm is placed in full supination with the palm of the hand facing the ceiling.
3. With one hand resting on the towel roll and holding the posterior, distal end of the humerus, stabilize the humerus (proximal joint segment) to prevent extension of the shoulder.
4. With the other hand, slowly move the forearm through the full passive range of elbow extension until you feel resistance limiting the motion.
5. Gently push against the resistance until no further extension can be attained. Carefully note the quality of the resistance. When the end-feel is hard, it has no give to it. This hard end-feel is caused by contact between the olecranon process of the ulna and the olecranon fossa of the humerus.
6. Compare this hard end-feel with the hard end-feel usually found in radial deviation of the wrist (see ROM Testing Procedures for Radial Deviation and Figure 6.12 in Chapter 6).

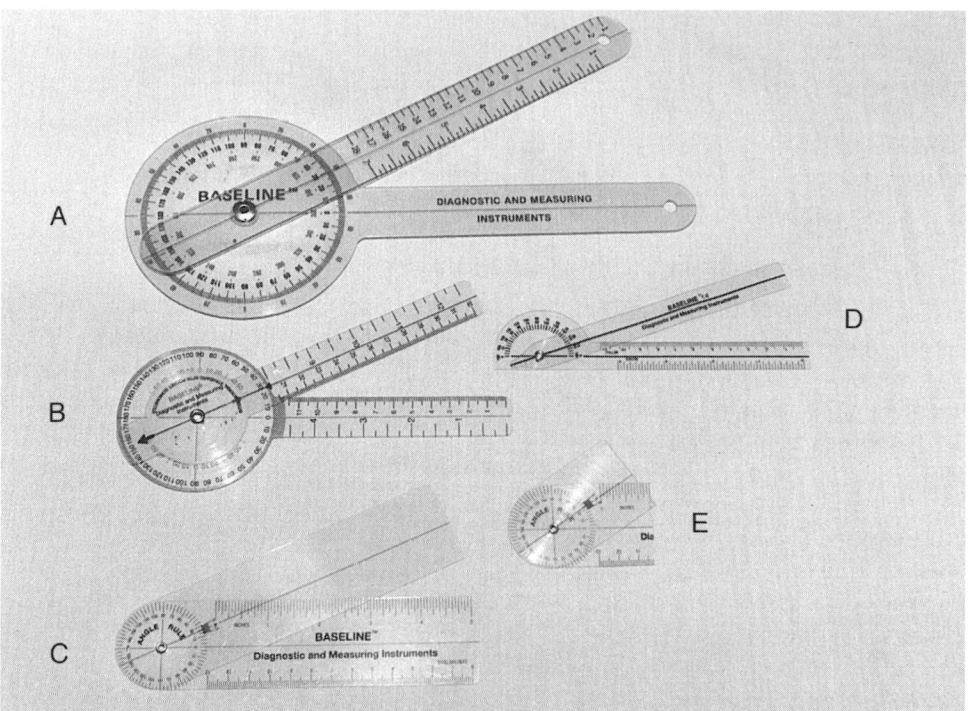

FIGURE 2.2 Plastic universal goniometers are available in different shapes and sizes. Some goniometers have full-circle bodies (A,B,C,E), whereas others have half-circle bodies (D). The 14-inch goniometer (A) is used to measure large joints such as the hip, knee, and shoulder. Six- to 8-inch goniometers (B,C,D) are used to assess midsized joints such as the wrist and ankle. The small goniometer (E) has been cut in length from a 6-inch goniometer (C) to make it easier to measure the fingers and toes.

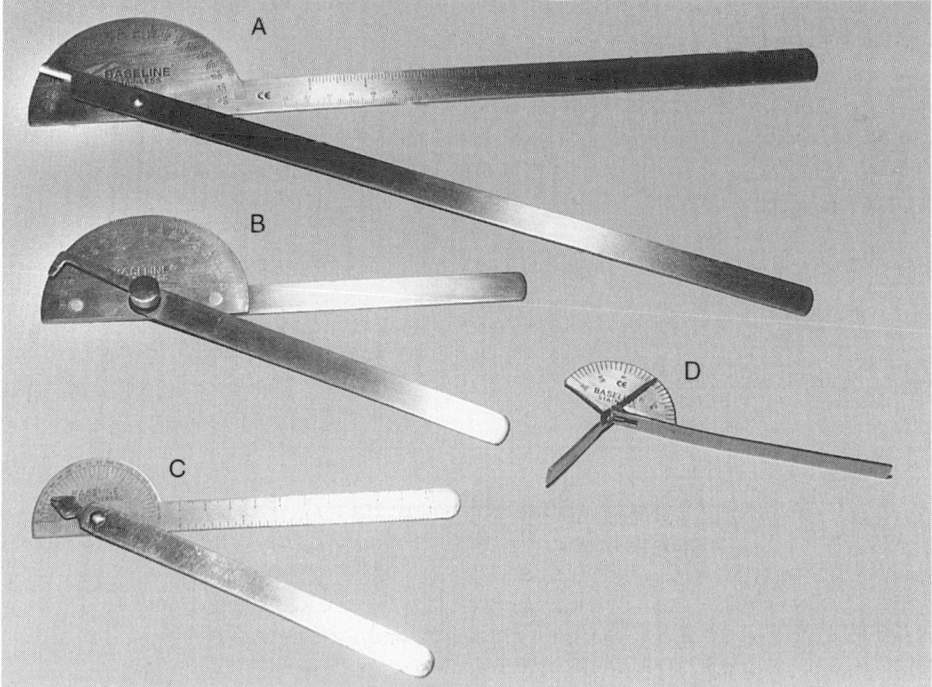

FIGURE 2.3 These metal goniometers are of different sizes but all have half-circle bodies. Metal goniometers with full-circle bodies are also available. The smallest goniometer (D) is specifically designed to lie on the dorsal or ventral surface of the fingers and toes while measuring joint motion. Goniometers A and B have a cut-out portion on the moving arm, whereas goniometers C and D have pointers on the moving arm to enable the reading of the scale on the bodies.

and shapes but adhere to the same basic design. Typically the design includes a body and two thin extensions called arms—a stationary arm and a moving arm (Fig. 2.4).

The **body** of a universal goniometer resembles a protractor and may form a half circle or a full circle (Fig. 2.5). The scales on a half-circle goniometer read from 0 to 180 degrees and from 180 to 0 degrees. The scales on a full-circle instrument may read either from 0 to 180 degrees and from 180 to 0 degrees, or from 0 to 360 degrees and from 360 to 0 degrees. Sometimes full-circle instruments have both 180-degree and 360-degree scales.

Increments on the scales may vary from 1 to 10 degrees, but 1- and 5-degree increments are the most common.

Traditionally, the **arms** of a universal goniometer are designated as moving or stationary according to how they are attached to the body of the goniometer (Fig. 2.4). The **stationary arm** is a structural part of the body of the goniometer and cannot be moved independently from the body. The **moving arm** is attached to the center of the body of most plastic goniometers by a rivet that permits the arm to move freely on the body. The moving arm may have one or more of the following features: a pointed end, a black or white line extending the length of the arm, or a cut-out portion (window). Goniometers that are used to measure ROM on radiographs have an opaque white line extending the length of the arms and opaque markings on the body. These features help the examiner to read the scales.

The length of the arms varies among instruments from approximately 1 to 14 inches. These variations in length represent an attempt on the part of the manufacturers to adapt the size of the instrument to the size of the joints.

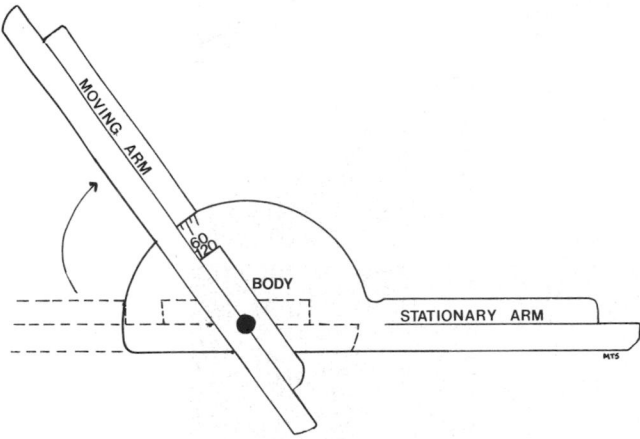

FIGURE 2.4 The body of this universal goniometer forms a half circle. The stationary arm is an integral part of the body of the goniometer. The moving arm is attached to the body by a rivet so that it can be moved independently from the body. In this example, a cut-out portion, sometimes referred to as a "window," is found in the center and at the end of the moving arm. The windows permit the examiner to read the scale on the body of the goniometer.

Example: A universal goniometer with 14-inch arms is appropriate for measuring motion at the knee joint because the arms are long enough to permit alignment with the greater trochanter of the femur and the lateral malleolus of the tibia (Fig. 2.6A). A universal goniometer with short arms would be difficult to use because the arms do not extend a sufficient distance along the femur and tibia to permit alignment with the bony landmarks (Fig. 2.6B). A goniometer with long arms would be awkward for measuring the MCP joints of the hand.

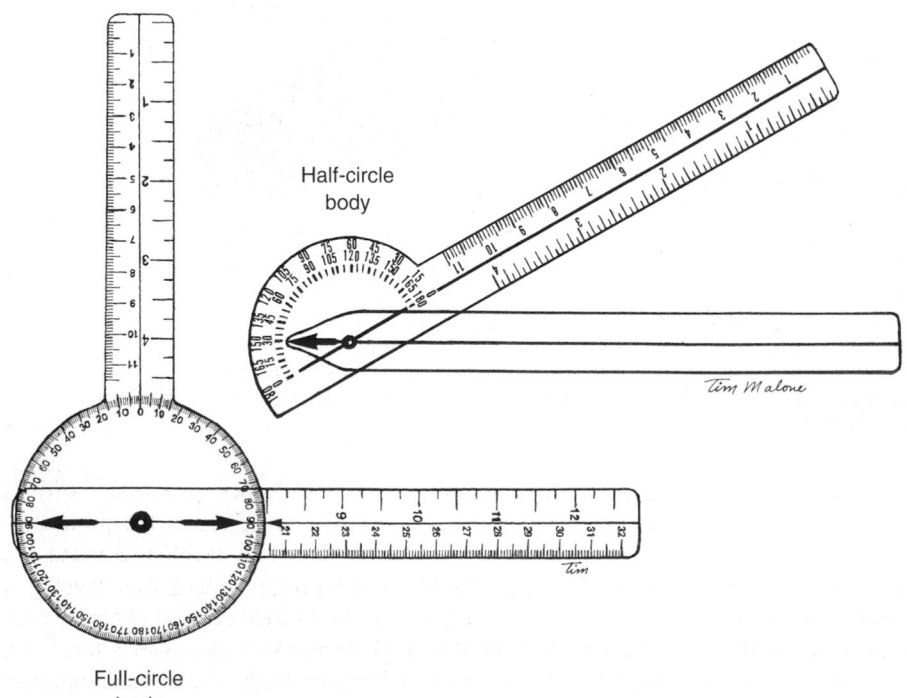

Half-circle body

Full-circle body

FIGURE 2.5 The body of the goniometer may be either a half circle (top) or a full circle (bottom).

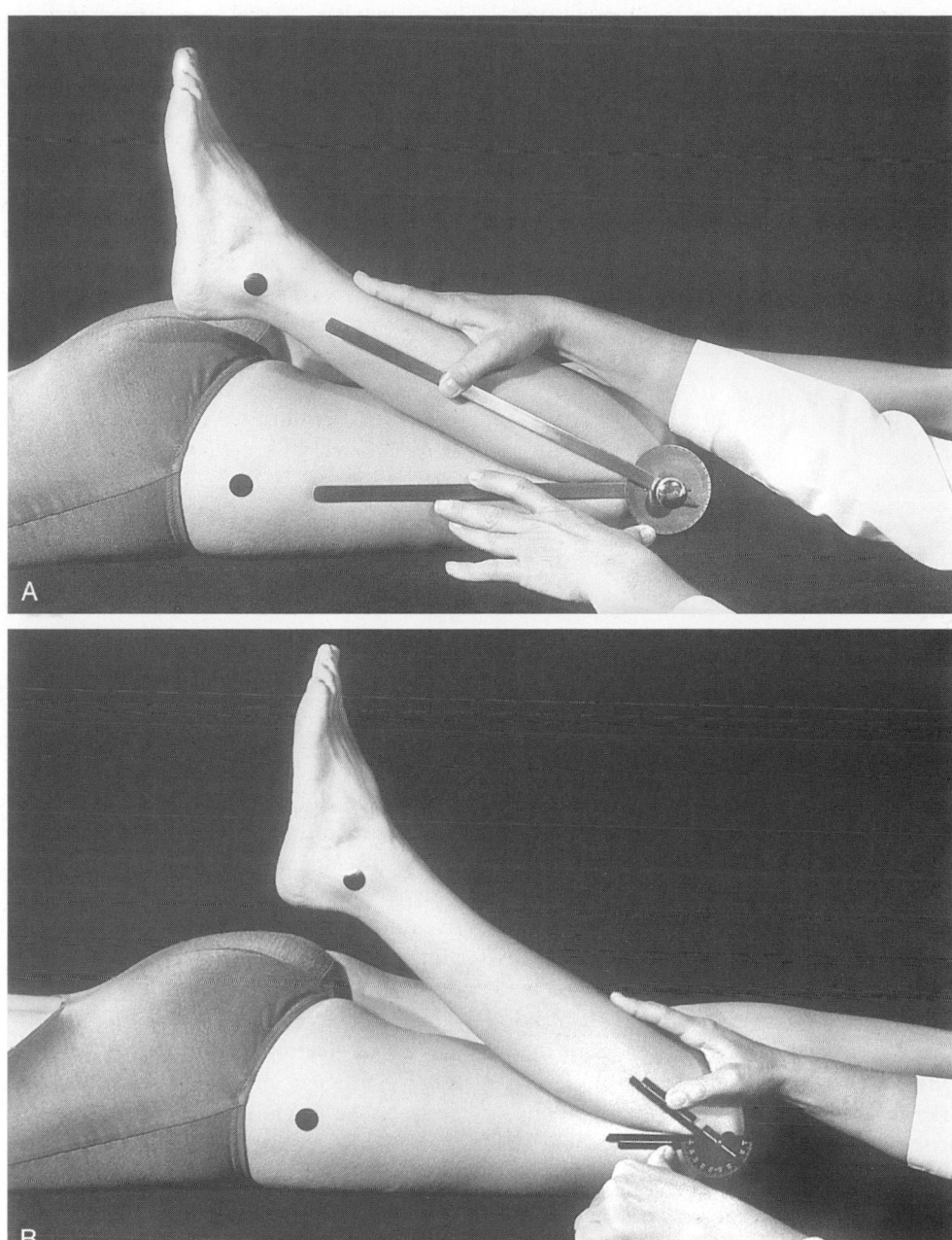

FIGURE 2.6 Selecting the right-sized goniometer makes it easier to measure joint motion. (A) The examiner is using a full-circle instrument with long arms to measure knee flexion ROM. The arms of the goniometer extend along the distal and proximal segments of the joint to within a few inches of the bony landmarks (black dots) that are used to align the arms. The proximity of the ends of the arms to the landmarks makes alignment easy and helps ensure that the arms are aligned accurately. (B) The small half-circle metal goniometer is a poor choice for measuring knee flexion ROM because the landmarks are so far from the ends of the goniometer's arms that accurate alignment is difficult.

Gravity-Dependent Goniometers (Inclinometers)

Although not as common as the universal goniometer, several other types of manual goniometers may be found in the clinical setting. **Gravity-dependent goniometers** or **inclinometers** use gravity's effect on pointers and fluid levels to measure joint position and motion (Fig. 2.7). The **pendulum goniometer** consists of a 360-degree protractor with a weighted pointer hanging from the center of the protractor. This device was first described by Fox and Van Breeme[13] in 1934. The **fluid (bubble) goniometer**, which was developed by Schenkar[14] in 1956, has a fluid-filled circular chamber containing an air bubble. It is similar to a carpenter's level but, being circular, has a 360-degree scale. Other inclinometers such as the Myrin OB Goniometer and the cervical range of

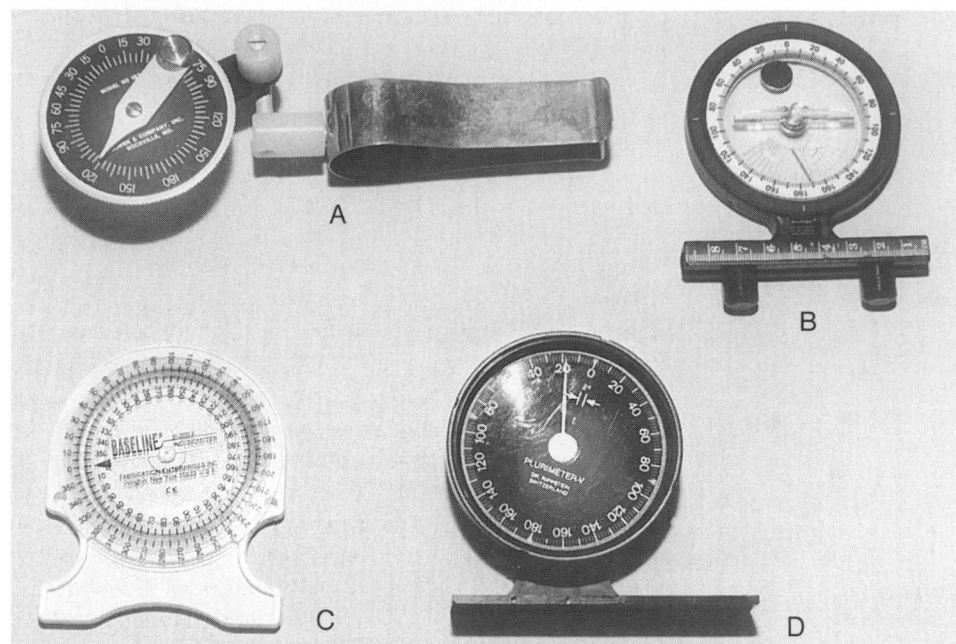

FIGURE 2.7 Each of these gravity-dependent goniometers uses a weighted pointer (A,B,D) or bubble (C) to indicate the position of the goniometer relative to the vertical pull of gravity. All of these inclinometers have a rotating dial so that the scale can be zeroed with the pointer or bubble in the starting position.

motion device (CROM) use a pendulum needle that reacts to gravity to measure motions in the frontal and sagittal planes and use a compass needle that reacts to the earth's magnetic field to measure motions in the horizontal plane. A fairly large selection of manual inclinometers and a few digital inclinometers are commercially available. Generally these instruments are more expensive than universal goniometers.

Inclinometers are either attached to or held on the distal segment of the joint being measured. The angle between the long axis of the distal segment and the line of gravity is noted. Inclinometers may be easier to use in certain situations than universal goniometers because they do not have to be aligned with bony landmarks or centered over the axis of motion. However, it is critical that the proximal segment of the joint being measured be positioned vertically or horizontally to obtain accurate measurements; otherwise, adjustments must be made in determining the measurement.[12,15] Inclinometers are also difficult to use on small joints[16] and where there is soft tissue deformity or edema.[12,15]

Although universal and gravity-dependent goniometers may be available within a clinical setting, they should not be used interchangeably.[17–20] For example, an examiner should not use a universal goniometer on Tuesday and an inclinometer on Wednesday to measure a subject's knee ROM. The two instruments may provide slightly different results, making comparisons for judging changes in ROM inappropriate.

Electrogoniometers

Electrogoniometers, introduced by Karpovich and Karpovich[21] in 1959, are used primarily in research to obtain dynamic joint measurements. Most devices have two arms, similar to those of the universal goniometer, which are attached to the proximal and distal segments of the joint being measured.[22–25]

A potentiometer is connected to the two arms. Changes in joint position cause the resistance in the potentiometer to vary. The resulting change in voltage can be used to indicate the amount of joint motion. Potentiometers measuring angular displacement have also been integrated with strain gauges[26,27] and isokinetic dynamometers[28] for measuring resistive torque. Flexible electrogoniometers with two plastic endblocks connected by a flexible strain gauge have been designed to measure angular displacement between the endblocks in one or two planes of motion.[19,29]

Some electrogoniometers resemble pendulum goniometers.[30,31] Changes in joint position cause a change in contact between the pendulum and the small resistors. Contact with the resistors produces a change in electric current, which is used to indicate the amount of joint motion.

Electrogoniometers are expensive and take time to calibrate accurately and attach to the subject. Given these drawbacks, electrogoniometers are used more often in research than in clinical settings. Radiographs, photographs, film, videotapes, and computer-assisted video motion analysis systems are other joint measurement methods used more commonly in research settings.

Visual Estimation

Although some examiners make visual estimates of joint position and motion rather than use a measuring instrument, we do not recommend this practice. Several authors suggest the use of visual estimates in situations in which the subject has excessive soft tissue covering physical landmarks.[32,33] Most authorities report more accurate and reliable measurements with a goniometer than with visual estimates.[34–40] Even when produced by a skilled examiner, visual estimates yield only subjective information in contrast to goniometric measurements, which yield objective information. However, estimates are useful in the learning process. Visual estimates made prior to goniometric measurements help to reduce errors attributable to incorrect reading of the goniometer. If the goniometric measurement is not in the same quadrant as the estimate, the examiner is alerted to the possibility that the wrong scale is being read.

After the examiner has read and studied this section on measurement instruments, **Exercise 2** should be completed. Given the adaptability and widespread use of the universal goniometer in the clinical setting, this book focuses on teaching the measurement of joint motion using a universal goniometer.

Alignment

Goniometer alignment refers to the alignment of the arms of the goniometer with the proximal and distal segments of the joint being evaluated. Instead of depending on soft tissue contour, the examiner should use bony **anatomical landmarks** to more accurately visualize the joint segments. These landmarks, which have been identified for all joint measurements, should be exposed so that they may be identified easily and also palpated (Fig. 2.8). The landmarks should be learned and adhered to when taking all measurements. The careful visualization, palpation, and alignment of the arms of the goniometer with the landmarks improve the accuracy and consistency of the measurements.

The stationary arm is often aligned parallel to the longitudinal axis of the proximal segment of the joint, and the moving arm is aligned parallel to the longitudinal axis of the distal segment of the joint (Fig. 2.9). In some situations, because of limitations imposed by either the goniometer or the subject (Fig. 2.10A), it may be necessary to reverse the alignment of the two arms so that the moving arm is aligned with the proximal part and the stationary arm is aligned with the distal part (Fig. 2.10B). Therefore, we have decided to use the term **proximal arm** to refer to the arm of the goniometer that is aligned with the proximal segment of the joint. The term **distal arm** refers to the arm aligned with the distal

Exercise 2

The Universal Goniometer

The following activities are designed to help the examiner become familiar with the universal goniometer.

EQUIPMENT: Full-circle and half-circle universal goniometers made of plastic and metal.

ACTIVITIES:

1. Select a goniometer.
2. Identify the type of goniometer selected (full-circle or half-circle) by noting the shape of the body.
3. Differentiate between the moving and the stationary arms of the goniometer. (Remember that the stationary arm is an integral part of the body of the goniometer.)
4. Observe the moving arm to see if it has a cut-out portion.
5. Find the line in the middle of the moving arm and follow it to a number on the scale.
6. Study the body of the goniometer and answer the following questions:
   a. Is the scale located on one or both sides?
   b. Is it possible to read the scale through the body of the goniometer?
   c. What intervals are used?
   d. Does the body contain one, two, or more scales?
7. Hold the goniometer in both hands. Position the arms so that they form a continuous straight line. When the arms are in this position, find the scale that reads 0 degrees.
8. Keep the stationary arm fixed in place and shift the moving arm while watching the numbers on the scale, either at the tip of the moving arm or in the cut-out portion. Shift the moving arm from 0 to 45, 90, 150, and 180 degrees.
9. Keep the stationary arm fixed and shift the moving arm from 0 degrees through an estimated 45-degree arc of motion. Compare the visual estimate with the actual arc of motion by reading the scale on the goniometer. Try to estimate other arcs of motion and compare the estimates with the actual arc of motion.
10. Keep the moving arm fixed in place and move the stationary arm through different arcs of motion.
11. Repeat steps 2 to 10 using different goniometers.

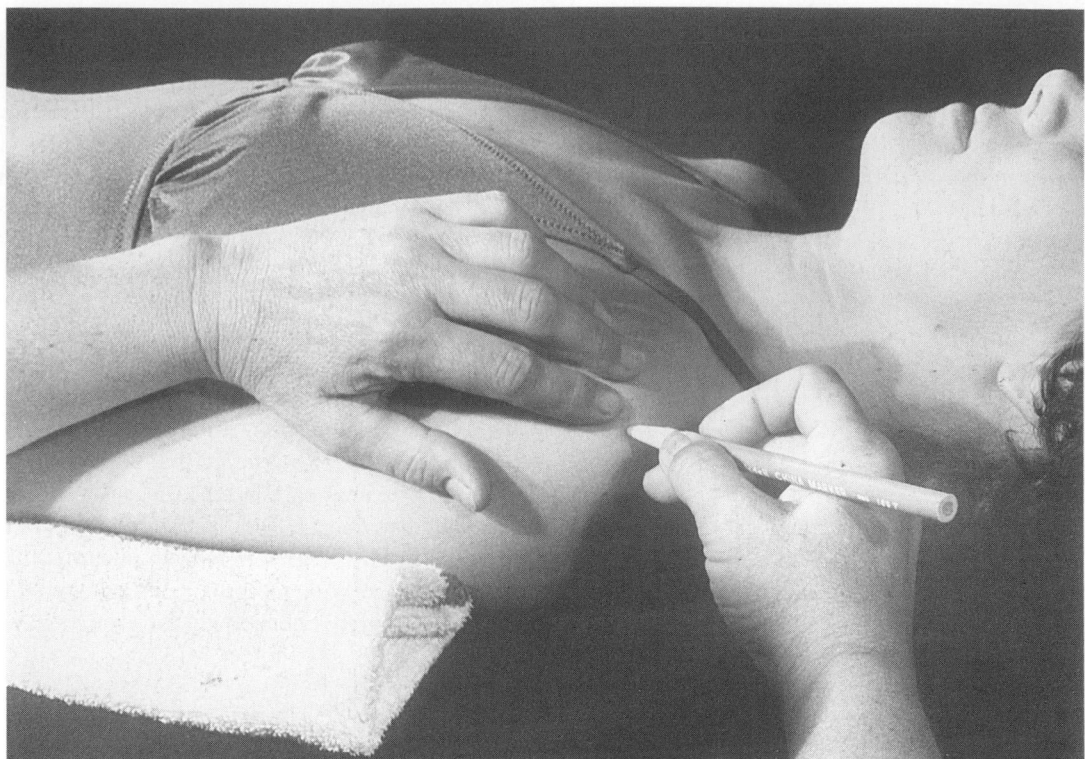

FIGURE 2.8 The examiner is using a grease pencil to mark the location of the subject's left acromion process. Note that the patient's clothing has been removed so that the bony landmark can be easily visualized. The examiner is using the index and middle fingers of her left hand to palpate the bony landmark.

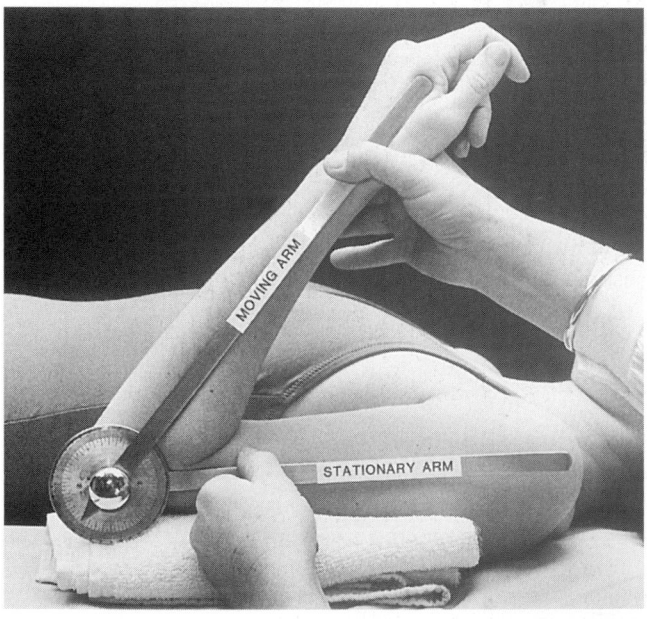

FIGURE 2.9 When using a full-circle goniometer to measure ROM of elbow flexion, the stationary arm is usually aligned parallel to the longitudinal axis of the proximal part (subject's humerus) and the moving arm is aligned parallel to the longitudinal axis of the distal part (subject's forearm). However, if the arms of the goniometer are reversed, the same angle will be measured.

segment of the joint (Fig. 2.11). The anatomical landmarks provide reference points that help to ensure that the alignment of the arms is correct.

The **fulcrum** of the goniometer may be placed over the approximate location of the axis of motion of the joint being measured. However, because the axis of motion changes during movement, the location of the fulcrum must be adjusted accordingly. Moore[12] suggests that careful alignment of the proximal and distal arms ensures that the fulcrum of the goniometer is located at the approximate axis of motion. Therefore, alignment of the arms of the goniometer with the proximal and distal joint segments should be emphasized more than placement of the fulcrum over the approximate axis of motion.

Errors in measuring joint position and motion with a goniometer can occur if the examiner is not careful. When aligning the arms and reading the scale of the goniometer, the examiner must be at eye level with the goniometer to avoid parallax. If the examiner is higher or lower than the goniometer, the alignment and scales may be distorted. Often a goniometer will have several scales, one going from 0 to 180 degrees and another going from 180 to 0 degrees. Examiners must carefully determine which scale is correct for the measurement. If a visual estimate is made before the measurement is taken, gross errors caused by reading the wrong scale

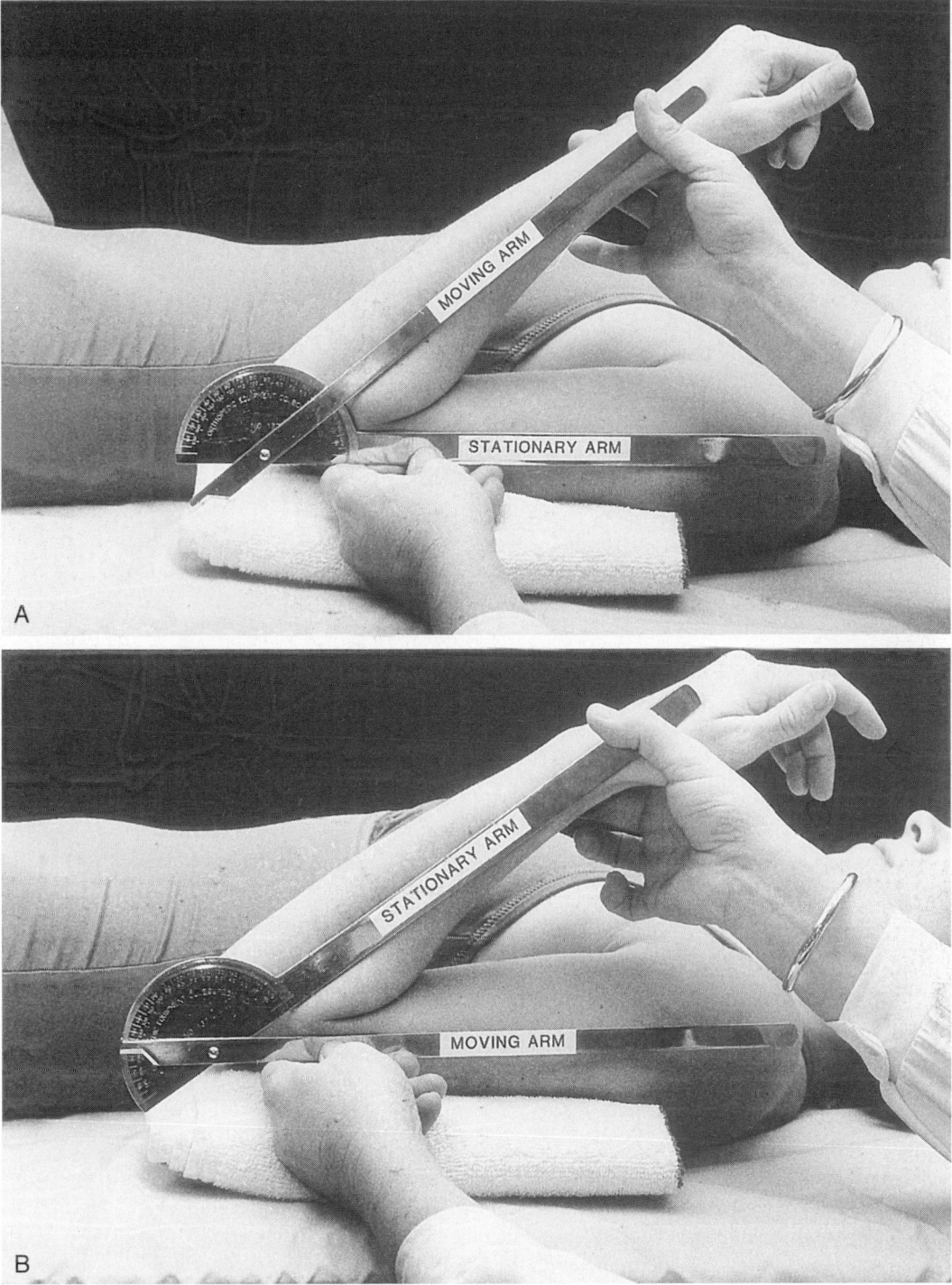

FIGURE 2.10 (A) When the examiner uses a half-circle goniometer to measure left elbow flexion, aligning the moving arm with the subject's forearm causes the pointer to move beyond the goniometer body, which makes it impossible to read the scale. (B) Reversing the arms of the instrument so that the stationary arm is aligned parallel to the distal part and the moving arm is aligned parallel to the proximal part causes the pointer to remain on the body of the goniometer, enabling the examiner to read the scale along the pointer.

will be obvious. Another source of error is misinterpretation of the intervals on the scale. For example, the smallest interval of a particular goniometer may be 5 degrees, but an examiner may believe the interval represents 1 degree. In this case the examiner would incorrectly read 91 degrees instead of 95 degrees.

After the examiner has read this section on alignment, Exercise 3 should be completed.

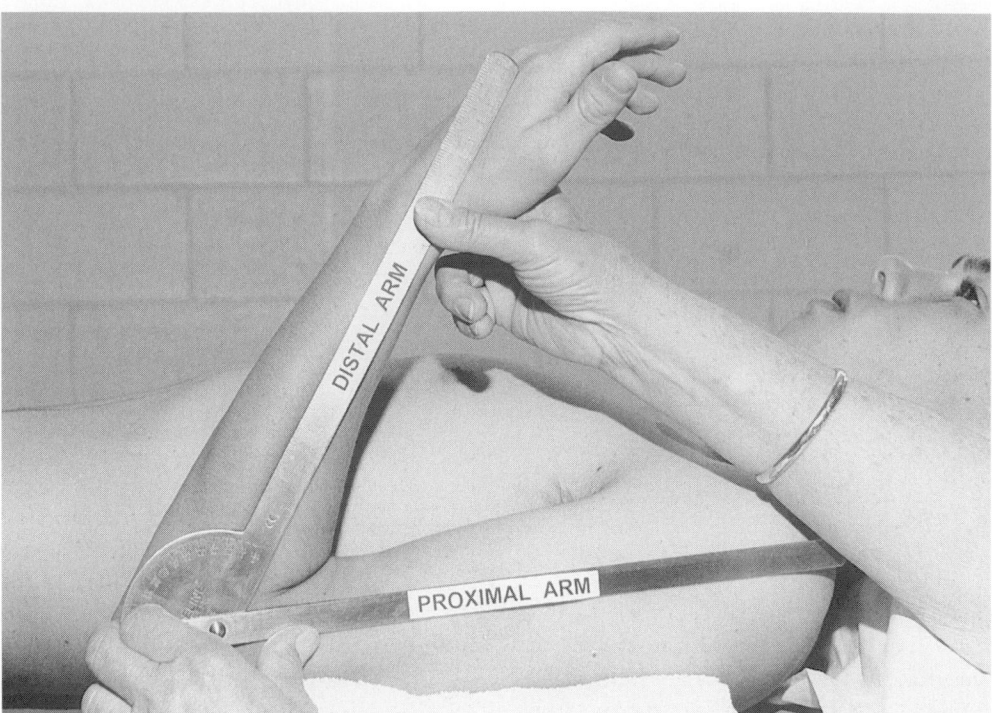

FIGURE 2.11 Throughout the book we use the term "proximal arm" to indicate the arm of the goniometer that is aligned with the proximal segment of the joint being examined. The term "distal arm" is used to indicate the arm of the goniometer that is aligned with the distal segment of the joint. During the measurement of elbow flexion, the proximal arm is aligned with the humerus, and the distal arm is aligned with the forearm.

Exercise 3

Goniometer Alignment for Elbow Flexion

The following activities are designed to help the examiner learn how to align and read the goniometer.

EQUIPMENT: Full-circle and half-circle universal goniometers of plastic and metal in various sizes and a skin-marking pencil.

ACTIVITIES: See Figures 5.9 to 5.15 in Chapter 5.

1. Select a goniometer and a subject.
2. Position the subject so that he or she is supine. The subject's right arm should be positioned so that it is close to the side of the body with the forearm in supination (palm of hand faces the ceiling). A towel roll placed under the distal humerus helps to ensure that the elbow is fully extended.
3. Locate and mark each of the following landmarks with the pencil: acromion process, lateral epicondyle of the humerus, radial head, and radial styloid process.
4. Align the proximal arm of the goniometer along the longitudinal axis of the humerus, using the acromion process and the lateral epicondyle as reference landmarks. Make sure that you are positioned so that the goniometer is at eye level during the alignment process.
5. Align the distal arm of the goniometer along the longitudinal axis of the radius, using the radial head and the radial styloid process as reference landmarks.
6. The fulcrum should be close to the lateral epicondyle. Check to make sure that the body of the goniometer is not being deflected by the supporting surface.
7. Recheck the alignment of the arms and readjust the alignment as necessary.
8. Read the scale on the goniometer.
9. Remove the goniometer from the subject's arm and place it nearby so it is handy for measuring the next joint position.

10. Move the subject's forearm into various positions in the flexion ROM, including the end of the flexion ROM. At each joint position, align and read the goniometer. Remember that you must support the subject's forearm while aligning the goniometer.
11. Repeat steps 3 to 10 on the subject's left upper extremity.
12. Repeat steps 4 to 10 using goniometers of different sizes and shapes.
13. Answer the following questions:
    a. Did the length of the goniometer arms affect the accuracy of the alignment? Explain.
    b. What length goniometer arms would you recommend as being the most appropriate for this measurement? Why?
    c. Did the type of goniometer used (full-circle or half-circle) affect either joint alignment or the reading of the scale? Explain.
    d. Did the side of the body that you were testing make a difference in your ability to align the goniometer? Why?

⊘ Recording

Goniometric measurements are recorded in numerical tables, in pictorial charts, or within the written text of an evaluation. Regardless of which method is used, recordings should provide enough information to permit an accurate interpretation of the measurement. The following items are recommended to be included in the recording:

1. Subject's name, age, and gender
2. Examiner's name
3. Date and time of measurement
4. Make and type of goniometer used
5. Side of the body, joint, and motion being measured (for example, left knee flexion)
6. ROM, including the number of degrees at the beginning and end of the motion
7. Type of motion being measured (that is, passive or active motion)
8. Any subjective information, such as discomfort or pain, that is reported by the subject during the testing
9. Any objective information obtained by the examiner during testing, such as a protective muscle spasm, crepitus, or capsular or noncapsular pattern of restriction
10. A complete description of any deviation from the recommended testing positions

If a subject has normal pain-free ROM during active or passive motion, the ROM may be recorded as normal (N) or within normal limits (WNL). To determine whether the ROM is normal, the examiner should compare the ROM of the joint being tested with ROM values from people of the same age and gender, and from studies that used the same method of measurement. A selection of normal ROM values for adults is presented at the beginning of testing procedures for each motion. Text and ROM tables that report normal values by age with information on gender and methods of measurement are presented in Research Findings in Chapters 4 through 13. The ROM of the joint being tested may also be compared with the same joint of the subject's contralateral extremity, provided that the contralateral extremity is neither impaired nor used selectively in athletic or occupational activities.

If passive ROM appears to be decreased or increased when compared with normal values, the ROM should be measured and recorded. Recordings should include both the starting and the ending joint positions to define the ROM. A recording that includes only the total ROM, such as 50 degrees of flexion, gives no information as to where a motion begins and ends. Likewise, a recording that lists –20 degrees (minus 20 degrees) of flexion is open to misinterpretation because the lack of flexion could occur at either the end or the beginning of the ROM.

A motion such as flexion that begins at 0 degrees and ends at 50 degrees of flexion is recorded as 0–50 degrees of flexion (Fig. 2.12A). A motion that begins with the joint flexed at 20 degrees and ends at 70 degrees of flexion is recorded as 20–70 degrees of flexion (Fig. 2.12B). The total ROM is the same (50 degrees) in both instances, but the arcs of motion are different.

Because both the starting and the ending joint positions have been recorded, the measurement can be interpreted correctly. If we assume that the normal ROM for this movement is 0 to 140 degrees, the subject who has a flexion ROM of 0–50 degrees lacks motion at the end of the flexion ROM. The subject with a flexion ROM of 20–70 degrees lacks motion both at the beginning and at the end of the flexion ROM. The term **hypomobile** may be applied to both of these joints because both joints have a less-than-normal ROM.

Sometimes the opposite situation exists, in which a joint has a greater-than-normal range of motion and is **hypermobile.** If an elbow joint is hypermobile, the starting position for measuring elbow flexion may be in hyperextension rather than at 0 degrees. If the elbow was hyperextended 20 degrees in the starting position, the beginning of the flexion ROM would be recorded as 20 degrees of hyperextension (Fig. 2.13). To clarify that the 20 degrees represents hyperextension rather than limited flexion, a "0" representing the zero starting position, which is now within the ROM, is included. A ROM that begins at 20 degrees of hyperextension and ends at 140 degrees of flexion is recorded as 20–0–140 degrees of flexion.

Some authorities have suggested the use of plus (+) and minus (−) signs to indicate hypomobility and hypermobility. However, the use of these signs varies depending

A

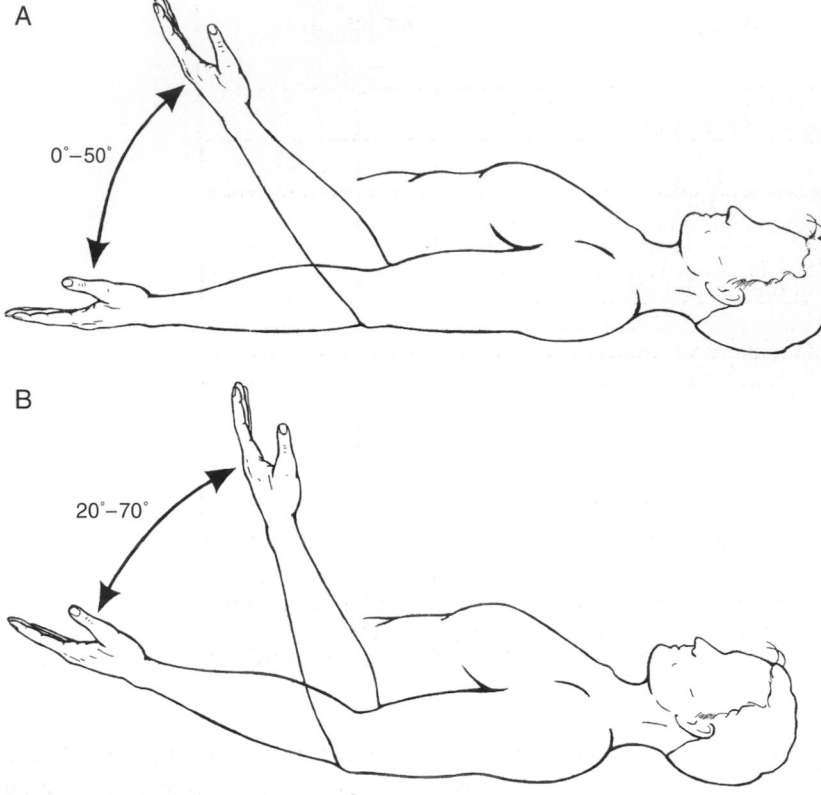

0°–50°

B

20°–70°

FIGURE 2.12 A recording of ROM should include the beginning of the range as well as the end. (A) In this illustration, the motion begins at 0 degrees and ends at 50 degrees so that the total ROM is 50 degrees. (B) In this illustration, the motion begins at 20 degrees of flexion and ends at 70 degrees, so that the total ROM is 50 degrees. For both subjects, the total ROM is the same, 50 degrees, even though the arcs of motion are different.

on the authority consulted. To avoid confusion, we have omitted the use of plus and minus signs. A ROM that does not start with 0 degrees or ends prematurely indicates hypomobility. The addition of zero, representing the usual starting position within the ROM, indicates hypermobility.

Numerical Tables

Numerical tables typically list joint motions in a column down the center of the form (Fig. 2.14). Space to the left of the central column is reserved for measurements taken on the left side of the subject's body; space to the right is reserved for measurements taken on the right side of the body. The examiner's initials and the date of testing are

noted at the top of the measurement columns. Subsequent measurements are recorded on the same form and identified by the examiner's initials and the date at the top of the appropriate measurement column. This format makes it easy to compare a series of measurements to identify problem motions and then to track rehabilitative response over time.

Pictorial Charts

Pictorial charts may be used in isolation or combined with numerical tables to record ROM measurements. Pictorial charts usually include a diagram of the normal starting and ending positions of the motion (Fig. 2.15).

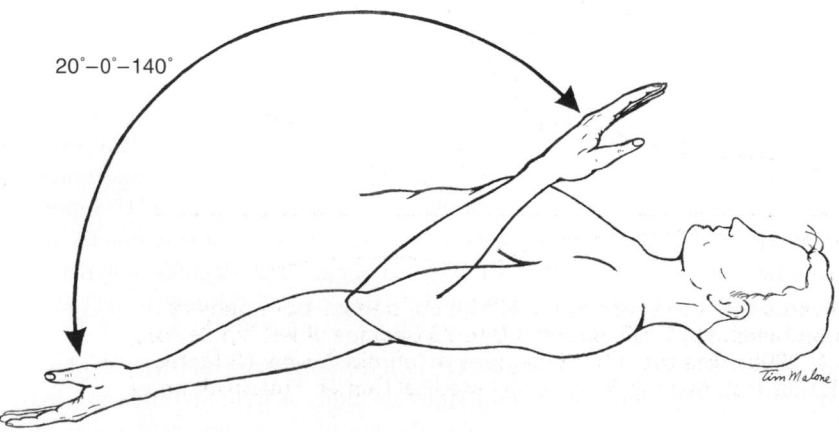

20°–0°–140°

FIGURE 2.13 This subject has 20 degrees of hyperextension at his elbow. In this case, motion begins at 20 degrees of hyperextension and proceeds through the 0-degree position to 140 degrees of flexion.

		JW	JW	Examiner	JW			
		4/1/08	3/18/08	Date	3/18/08			
				Hip				
		0-98	0-73	Flexion	0-118			
		0-5	0-5	Extension	0-12			
		0-28	0-18	Abduction	0-32			
		0-12	0-6	Adduction	0-15			
		0-35	0-24	Medial Rotation	0-42			
		0-40	0-35	Lateral Rotation	0-44			
				Comments:				

Name Paul Jones   Age 57   Gender M

Left   Right

FIGURE 2.14 This numerical table records the results of ROM measurements of a subject's left and right hips. The examiner has recorded her initials and the date of testing at the top of each column of ROM measurements. Note that the right hip was tested once, on March 18, 2008, and the left hip was tested twice, once on March 18, 2008, and again on April 1, 2008.

Sagittal–Frontal–Transverse–Rotation Method

Another method of recording, which may be included in a written text or formatted into a table, is the **sagittal–frontal–transverse–rotation (SFTR) recording method**, developed by Gerhardt and Russe.[41,42] Although it is not commonly used in the United States, it is used in a few countries in Europe and has been described by the American Medical Association.[43] In the SFTR method, three numbers are used to describe all motions in a given plane. The first and last numbers indicate the ends of the ROM in that plane. The middle

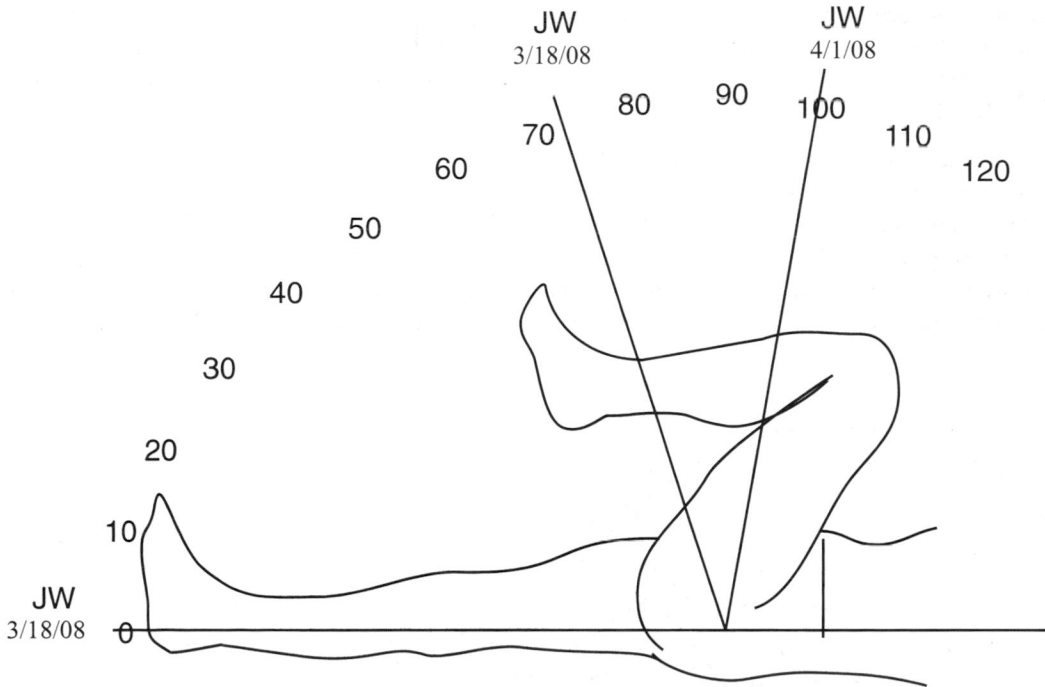

FIGURE 2.15 This pictorial chart records the results of flexion ROM measurements of a subject's left hip. For measurements taken on March 18, 2008, note the 0 to 73 degrees of left hip flexion; for measurements taken on April 1, 2008, note the 0 to 98 degrees of left hip flexion. (Adapted with permission from Range of Motion Test, New York University Medical Center, Rusk Institute of Rehabilitation Medicine.)

number indicates the starting position, which would be 0 in normal motion.

In the **sagittal plane,** represented by S, the first number indicates the end of the extension ROM, the middle number indicates the starting position, and the last number indicates the end of the flexion ROM.

Example: If a subject has 50 degrees of shoulder extension and 170 degrees of shoulder flexion, these motions would be recorded: Shoulder S: 50–0–170 degrees.

In the **frontal plane,** represented by F, the first number indicates the end of the abduction ROM, the middle number indicates the starting position, and the last number indicates the end of the adduction ROM. The ends of spinal ROM in the frontal plane (lateral flexion) are listed to the left first and to the right last.

Example: If a subject has 45 degrees of hip abduction and 15 degrees of hip adduction, these motions would be recorded: Hip F: 45–0–15 degrees.

In the **transverse plane,** represented by T, the first number indicates the end of the horizontal abduction ROM, the middle number indicates the starting position, and the last number indicates the end of the horizontal adduction ROM.

Example: If a subject has 30 degrees of shoulder horizontal abduction and 135 degrees of shoulder horizontal adduction, these motions would be recorded: Shoulder T: 30–0–135 degrees.

Rotation is represented by R. Lateral rotation ROM, including supination and eversion, is listed first; medial rotation ROM, including pronation and inversion, is listed last. Rotation ROM of the spine to the left is listed first; rotation ROM to the right is listed last. Limb position during measurement is noted if it varies from anatomical position. "F90" would indicate that a measurement was taken with the limb positioned in 90 degrees of flexion.

Example: If a subject has 35 degrees of lateral rotation ROM of the hip and 45 degrees of medial rotation ROM of the hip, and these motions were measured with the hip in 90 degrees of flexion, these motions would be recorded: Hip R: (F90) 35–0–45 degrees.

Hypomobility is noted by the lack of 0 as the middle number or by less-than-normal values for the first and last numbers, which indicate the ends of the ROM.

Example: If elbow flexion ROM was limited and a subject could move only between 20 and 90 degrees of flexion, it would be recorded: Elbow S: 0–20–90 degrees. The starting position is 20 degrees of flexion, and the end of the ROM is 90 degrees of flexion.

A fixed-joint limitation, ankylosis is indicated by the use of only two numbers. The zero starting position is included to clarify in which motion the fixed position occurs.

Example: An elbow fixed in 40 degrees of flexion would be recorded: Elbow S: 0–40 degrees.

American Medical Association Guides to Evaluation Method

Another system of recording restricted motion has been described by the American Medical Association in the Guides to the Evaluation of Permanent Impairment.[43] This book provides ratings of permanent impairment for all major body systems, including the respiratory, cardiovascular, digestive, and visual systems. The longest chapter focuses on impairment evaluation of the extremities, spine, and pelvis. Restricted active motion, ankylosis, amputation, sensory loss, vascular changes, loss of strength, pain, joint crepitation, joint swelling, joint instability, and deformity are measured and converted to percentage of impairment for the body part. The total percentage of impairment for the body part is converted to the percentage of impairment for the extremity and, finally, to a percentage of impairment for the entire body. Often these permanent impairment ratings are used, along with other information, to determine the patient's level of disability and the amount of monetary compensation to be expected from the employer or the insurer. Physicians and therapists working with patients with permanent impairments who are seeking compensation for their disabilities should refer to this book for more detail.

The system of recording restricted motion found in the Guides to the Evaluation of Permanent Impairment also uses the 0 to 180 degree notation method. The neutral starting position is recorded as 0 degrees with motions progressing toward 180 degrees. However, the recording system proposed in the Guides to the Evaluation of Permanent Impairment does differ from other recording systems described in our text. In this system, when extension exceeds the neutral starting position, it is referred to as hyperextension and is expressed with the plus (+) symbol. For example, motion at the metacarpophalangeal (MCP) joint of a finger from 15 degrees of hyperextension to 45 degrees of flexion would be recorded as +15 to 45 degrees. The plus (+) symbol is used to emphasize the fact that the joint has hyperextension.

In this system, the minus (−) symbol is used to emphasize the fact that a joint has an extension limitation. When the neutral (zero) starting position cannot be attained, an extension limitation exists and is expressed with the minus symbol. For example, motion at the MCP joint of a finger from 15 degrees of flexion to 45 degrees of flexion would be recorded as −15 to 45 degrees. It should be noted that the American Academy of Orthopaedic Surgeons[40] does not use the minus (−) symbol to indicate an extension limitation or hypomobility.

○ Procedures

Prior to beginning a goniometric evaluation, the examiner must do the following:

- Determine which joints and motions need to be tested
- Organize the testing sequence by body position
- Gather the necessary equipment, such as goniometers, towel rolls, and recording forms
- Prepare an explanation of the procedure for the subject

Explanation Procedure

The listed steps and the example that follow provide the examiner with a suggested format for explaining the goniometric testing procedure to a subject.

Steps

1. Introduce self and explain purpose
2. Explain and demonstrate goniometer
3. Explain and demonstrate anatomical landmarks
4. Explain and demonstrate testing position
5. Explain and demonstrate examiner's and subject's roles
6. Confirm subject's understanding

Lay rather than technical terms are used in the example so that the subject can understand the procedure. During the explanation, the examiner should try to establish a good rapport with the subject and enlist the subject's participation in the evaluation process. After reading the example, the examiner should practice **Exercise 4 on page 36.**

Example: Explanation of Goniometric Testing Procedure for Measuring Elbow Flexion

1. Introduce Self and Explain Purpose

Introduction: My name is _____. I am a (occupational title).

Explanation: I understand that you have been having some difficulty moving your elbow. I am going to measure the amount of motion that you have at your elbow joint to see if it is equal to, less than, or greater than normal. I will use this information to plan a treatment program and assess its effectiveness.

Demonstration: The examiner flexes and extends his or her own elbow so that the subject is able to observe a joint motion.

2. Explain and Demonstrate Goniometer

Explanation: The instrument that I will be using to obtain the measurements is called a goniometer. It is similar to a protractor, but it has two extensions called arms. It is placed on the outside of your body, next to your elbow.

Demonstration: The examiner shows the goniometer to the subject and encourages the subject to ask questions. The examiner shows the subject how the goniometer is used by holding it next to his or her own elbow.

3. Explain and Demonstrate Anatomical Landmarks

Explanation: To obtain accurate measurements, I will need to identify some anatomical landmarks. These landmarks help me to align the arms of the goniometer. Because these landmarks are important, I may

have to ask you to remove certain articles of clothing, such as your shirt. Also, to locate some of the landmarks, I may have to press my fingers against your skin.

Demonstration: The examiner shows the subject an easily identified anatomical landmark such as the radial styloid process.

4. Explain and Demonstrate Recommended Testing Positions

Explanation: Certain testing positions have been established to help make joint measurements easier and more accurate. Whenever possible, I would like you to assume these positions. If you need some help in getting into a particular position, I will be happy to assist you. Please let me know if you need assistance.

Demonstration: The sitting or supine positions.

5. Explain and Demonstrate Examiner's and Subject's Roles During Active Motion

Explanation: I will ask you to move your arm in exactly the same way that I move your arm.

Demonstration: The examiner takes the subject's arm through a passive ROM and then asks the subject to perform the same motion.

6. Explain and Demonstrate Examiner's and Subject's Roles During Passive Motion

Explanation: I will move your arm and take a measurement. You should relax and let me do all of the work. These measurements should not cause discomfort. Please let me know if you have any discomfort and I will stop moving your arm.

Demonstration: The examiner moves the subject's arm gently and slowly through the range of elbow flexion.

7. Confirm Subject's Understanding

Explanation: Do you have any questions? Are you ready to begin?

Testing Procedure

The testing procedure is initiated after the explanation has been given and the examiner is assured that the subject understands the nature of the testing process. The testing procedure consists of the following 12-step sequence of activities.

Steps

1. Place the subject in the testing position.
2. Stabilize the proximal joint segment.
3. Move the distal joint segment to the zero starting position. If the joint cannot be moved to the zero starting position, it should be moved as close as possible to the zero starting position. Slowly move the distal joint segment to the end of the passive ROM and determine the end-feel. Ask the subject if there was any discomfort during the motion.
4. Make a visual estimate of the ROM.
5. Return the distal joint segment to the starting position.
6. Palpate the bony anatomical landmarks.
7. Align the goniometer.
8. Read and record the starting position. Remove the goniometer.

9. Stabilize the proximal joint segment.
10. Move the distal segment through the full ROM.
11. Replace and realign the goniometer. Palpate the anatomical landmarks again if necessary.
12. Read and record the ROM.

Exercise 5, which is based on the 12-step sequence, affords the examiner an opportunity to use the testing procedure for an evaluation of the elbow joint. This exercise should be practiced until the examiner is able to perform the activities sequentially without reference to the exercise.

Exercise 4

Explanation of Goniometric Testing Procedure

EQUIPMENT: A universal goniometer.

ACTIVITIES: Practice the following six steps with a subject.

1. Introduce yourself and explain the purpose of goniometric testing. Demonstrate a joint ROM on yourself.
2. Show the goniometer to your subject and demonstrate how it is used to measure a joint ROM.
3. Explain why bony landmarks must be located and palpated. Demonstrate how you would locate a bony landmark on yourself, and explain why clothing may have to be removed.
4. Explain and demonstrate why changes in position may be required.
5. Explain the subject's role in the procedure. Explain and demonstrate your role in the procedure.
6. Obtain confirmation of the subject's understanding of your explanation.

Exercise 5

Testing Procedure for Goniometric Measurement of Elbow Flexion ROM

EQUIPMENT: A universal goniometer, skin-marking pencil, recording form, and pencil.

ACTIVITIES: See Figures 5.9 to 5.15 in Chapter 5.

1. Place the subject in a supine position, with the arm to be tested positioned close to the side of the body. Place a towel roll under the distal end of the humerus to allow full elbow extension. Position the forearm in full supination, with the palm of the hand facing the ceiling.
2. Stabilize the distal end of the humerus to prevent flexion of the shoulder.
3. Move the forearm to the zero starting position and determine whether there is any motion (extension) beyond zero. Move to the end of the passive range of flexion. Evaluate the end-feel. Usually the end-feel is soft because of compression of the muscle bulk on the anterior forearm in conjunction with that on the anterior humerus. Ask the subject if there was any discomfort during the motion. Refer to Figure 5.13.
4. Make a visual estimate of the beginning and end of the ROM.
5. Return the forearm to the starting position.
6. Palpate the bony anatomical landmarks (acromion process, lateral epicondyle of the humerus, radial head, and radial styloid process) and mark with a skin pencil. Refer to Figures 5.9 to 5.12.
7. Align the arms and the fulcrum of the goniometer. Align the proximal arm with the lateral midline of the humerus, using the acromion process and lateral epicondyle for reference. Align the distal arm along the lateral midline of the radius, using the radial head and the radial styloid process for reference. The fulcrum should be close to the lateral epicondyle of the humerus.
8. Read the goniometer and record the starting position. Refer to Figure 5.14. Remove the goniometer.
9. Stabilize the proximal joint segment (humerus).
10. Perform the passive ROM, making sure that you complete the available range.
11. When the end of the ROM has been attained, replace and realign the goniometer. Palpate the anatomical landmarks again if necessary. Refer to Figure 5.15.
12. Read the goniometer and record your reading. Compare your reading with your visual estimate to make sure that you are reading the correct scale on the goniometer.

REFERENCES

1. Rothstein, JM, Miller, PJ, and Roettger, F: Goniometric reliability in a clinical setting. Phys Ther 63:1611, 1983.
2. Ekstrand, J, et al: Lower extremity goniometric measurements: A study to determine their reliability. Arch Phys Med Rehabil 63:171, 1982.
3. Sabar, JS, et al: Goniometric assessment of shoulder range of motion: Comparison of testing in supine and sitting positions. Arch Phys Med Rehabil 79:64,1998.
4. Marshall, MM, Morzall, JR, and Shealy, JE: The effects of complex wrist and forearm posture on wrist range of motion. Human Factors 41:205, 1999.
5. Werner, SL, and Plancher, KD: Biomechanics of wrist injuries in sports. Clin Sports Med 17:407, 1998.
6. Simoneau, GG, et al: Influence of hip position and gender on active hip internal and external rotation. J Orthop Sports Phys Ther 28:158, 1998.
7. Bierma-Zeinstra, SMA, et al: Comparison between two devices for measuring hip joint motions. Clin Rehabil 12:497, 1998.
8. Van Dillen, LR, et al: Effect of knee and hip position on hip extension range of motion in individuals with and without low back pain. J Orthop Sports Phys Ther 30:307, 2000.
9. Mecagni, C, et al: Balance and ankle range of motion in community-dwelling women aged 64–87 years: A correlation study. Phys Ther 80:1004, 2000.
10. Bennell, K, et al: Hip and ankle range of motion and hip muscle strength in young female ballet dancers and controls. Br J Sports Med 33:340, 1999.
11. Moore, ML: The measurement of joint motion. Part II: The technic of goniometry. Phys Ther Rev 29:256, 1949.
12. Moore, ML: Clinical assessment of joint motion. In Basmajian, JV (ed): Therapeutic Exercise, ed 3. Williams & Wilkins, Baltimore, 1978.
13. Fox, RF, and Van Breemen, J: Chronic Rheumatism, Causation and Treatment. Churchill, London, 1934, p 327.
14. Schenkar, WW: Improved method of joint motion measurement. N Y J Med 56:539, 1956.
15. Miller, PJ: Assessment of joint motion. In Rothstein, JM (ed): Measurement in Physical Therapy. Churchill Livingstone, New York, 1985.
16. Clarkson, HM: Musculoskeletal Assessment: Joint Range of Motion and Manual Muscle Strength, ed 2. Lippincott Williams & Wilkins, Philadelphia, 2000.
17. Petherick, M, et al: Concurrent validity and intertester reliability of universal and fluid-based goniometers for active elbow range of motion. Phys Ther 68:966, 1988.
18. Rheault, W, et al: Intertester reliability and concurrent validity of fluid-based and universal goniometers for active knee flexion. Phys Ther 68:1676, 1988.
19. Goodwin, J, et al: Clinical methods of goniometry: A comparative study. Disabil Rehabil 14:10, 1992.
20. Rome, K, and Cowieson, F: A reliability study of the universal goniometer, fluid goniometer, and electrogoniometer for the measurement of ankle dorsiflexion. Foot Ankle 17:28, 1996.
21. Karpovich, PV, and Karpovich, GP: Electrogoniometer: A new device for study of joints in action. Fed Proc 18:79, 1959.
22. Kettelkamp, DB, et al: An electrogoniometric study of knee motion in normal gait. J Bone Joint Surg Am 52:775, 1970.
23. Knutzen, KM, Bates, BT, and Hamill, J: Electrogoniometry of postsurgical knee bracing in running. Am J Phys Med Rehabil 62:172, 1983.
24. Carey, JR, Patterson, JR, and Hollenstein, PJ: Sensitivity and reliability of force tracking and joint-movement tracking scores in healthy subjects. Phys Ther 68:1087, 1988.
25. Torburn, L, Perry, J, and Gronley, JK: Assessment of rearfoot motion: Passive positioning, one-legged standing, gait. Foot Ankle 19:688:1998.
26. Vandervoort, AA, et al: Age and sex effects on mobility of the human ankle. J Gerontol 47:M17, 1992.
27. Chesworth, BM, and Vandervoort, AA: Comparison of passive stiffness variables and range of motion in uninvolved and involved ankle joints of patients following ankle fractures. Phys Ther 75:253, 1995.
28. Gajdosik, RL, Vander Linden, DW, and Williams, AK: Influence of age on length and passive elastic stiffness characteristics of the calf muscles-tendon unit of women. Phys Ther 79:827, 1999.
29. Ball, P, and Johnson, GR: Reliability of hindfoot goniometry when using a flexible electrogoniometer. Clin Biomech 8:13, 1993.
30. Clapper, MP, and Wolf, SL: Comparison of the reliability of the Ortho-ranger and the standard goniometer for assessing active lower extremity range of motion. Phys Ther 68:214, 1988.
31. Greene, BL, and Wolf, SL: Upper extremity joint movement: Comparison of two measurement devices. Arch Phys Med Rehabil 70:288, 1989.
32. American Academy of Orthopaedic Surgeons: Joint Motion: A Method of Measuring and Recording. AAOS, Chicago, 1965.
33. Rowe, CR: Joint measurement in disability evaluation. Clin Orthop 32:43, 1964.
34. Watkins, MA, et al: Reliability of goniometric measurements and visual estimates of knee range of motion obtained in a clinical setting. Phys Ther 71:90, 1991.
35. Youdas, JW, Carey, JR, and Garrett, TR: Reliability of measurements of cervical spine range of motion: Comparison of three methods. Phys Ther 71:98, 1991.
36. Low, JL: The reliability of joint measurement. Physiotherapy 62:227, 1976.
37. Moore, ML: The measurement of joint motion. Part I: Introductory review of the literature. Phys Ther Rev 29:195, 1949.
38. Salter, N: Methods of measurement of muscle and joint function. J Bone Joint Surg Br 34:474, 1955.
39. Minor, MA, and Minor, SD: Patient Evaluation Methods for the Health Professional. Reston Publishing, Reston, VA, 1985.
40. Greene, WB, and Heckman JD (eds): The Clinical Measurement of Joint Motion. American Academy of Orthopaedic Surgeons, Rosemont, IL, 1994.
41. Gerhardt, JJ, and Russe, OA: International SFTR Method of Measuring and Recording Joint Motion. Hans Huber, Bern, 1975.
42. Gerhardt, JJ: Clinical measurement of joint motion and position in the neutral-zero method and SFTR: Basic principles. Int Rehabil Med 5:161, 1983.
43. Cocchisrella, L and Andersson, GBJ (eds): Guides to the Evaluation of Permanent Impairment, ed 5. American Medical Association, Milwaukee, 2001.

VALIDITY AND RELIABILITY

Validity

For goniometry to provide meaningful information, measurements must be valid and reliable. Currier[1] states that **validity** is "the degree to which an instrument measures what it is purported to measure; the extent to which it fulfills its purpose." Stated in another way, the validity of a measurement refers to how well the measurement represents the true value of the variable of interest. The purpose of goniometry is to measure the angle created at a joint by the adjacent bones of the body. Therefore, a valid goniometric measurement is one that truly represents the actual joint angle. The joint angle is used to describe a specific joint position or, if a beginning and ending joint position are compared, a range of motion (ROM).

Face Validity

There are four main types of validity: face validity, content validity, criterion-related validity, and construct validity.[2–5] Most support for the validity of goniometry is in the form of face, content, and criterion-related validity. **Face validity** indicates that the instrument generally appears to measure what it proposes to measure—that it is plausible.[2–5] Much of the literature on goniometric measurement does not specifically address the issue of validity; rather, it assumes that the angle created by aligning the arms of a universal goniometer with bony landmarks truly represents the angle created by the proximal and distal bones composing the joint. One infers that changes in goniometer alignment reflect changes in joint angle and represent a range of joint motion. Portney and Watkins[3] report that face validity is easily established for some tests, such as the measurement of ROM, because the instrument measures the variable of interest through direct observation.

Content Validity

Content validity is determined by judging whether or not an instrument adequately measures and represents the domain of content—the substance—of the variable of interest.[2–5] Both content and face validity are based on subjective

opinion. However, face validity is the most basic and elementary form of validity, whereas content validity involves more rigorous and careful consideration. Gajdosik and Bohannon[6] state, "Physical therapists judge the validity of most ROM measurements based on their anatomical knowledge and their applied skills of visual inspection, palpation of bony landmarks, and accurate alignment of the goniometer. Generally, the accurate application of knowledge and skills, combined with interpreting the results as measurement of ROM only, provide sufficient evidence to ensure content validity."

Criterion-Related Validity

Criterion-related validity justifies the validity of the measuring instrument by comparing measurements made with the instrument to a well-established gold standard of measurement—the criterion.[2–5] If the measurements made with the instrument and criterion are taken at approximately the same time, **concurrent validity** is tested. Concurrent validity is a type of criterion-related validity.[3,7] Criterion-related validity can be assessed objectively with statistical methods. In terms of goniometry, an examiner may question the construction of a particular goniometer on a very basic level and consider whether the degree units of the goniometer accurately represent the degree units of a circle. The angles of the goniometer can be compared with known angles of a protractor—the criterion. Usually the construction of goniometers is adequate, and the issue of validity focuses on whether the goniometer accurately measures the angle of joint position and ROM in a subject.

Criterion-Related Validity Studies of Extremity Joints

The best gold standard used to establish criterion-related validity of goniometric measurements of joint position and ROM is radiography. Several studies that examined extremity joints for the concurrent validity of goniometric and radiographic measurements are discussed below. When available, summaries of additional studies comparing goniometry to radiographs and/or photographs are included in the Research Findings sections of Chapters 4 to 13. Gogia and associates[8] measured the knee position of 30 subjects with radiography and with a universal goniometer. Knee positions ranged from

0 to 120 degrees. High correlation (correlation coefficient [r] = 0.97) and agreement (intraclass correlation coefficient [ICC] = 0.98) were found between the two types of measurements. Therefore goniometric measurement of knee joint position was considered to be valid. Enwemeka[9] studied the validity of measuring knee ROM with a universal goniometer by comparing the goniometric measurements taken on 10 subjects with radiographs. No significant differences were found between the two types of measurements when ROM was within 30 to 90 degrees of flexion (mean difference between the two measurements ranged from 0.5 to 3.8 degrees). However, a significant difference was found when ROM was within 0 to 15 degrees of flexion (mean difference 4.6 degrees). Ahlback and Lindahl[10] found that a joint-specific goniometer used to measure hip flexion and extension in 14 subjects closely agreed with radiographic measurements. Kato and coworkers[11] compared the accuracy of three types of goniometers aligned on the lateral and dorsal surfaces of the proximal interphalangeal joints of the 16 fixated fingers to radiographs. Mean differences between the goniometers and radiographs ranged from 0.5 to 3.3 degrees.

Criterion-Related Validity Studies of the Spine

Various instruments used to measure ROM of the spine have also been compared with a radiographic criterion, although some researchers question the use of radiographs as the gold standard given the variability of ROM measurement taken from spinal radiographs.[12] Three studies that contrasted cervical range of motion measurements taken with gravity-dependent goniometers with those recorded on radiographs found concurrent validity to be high. Herrmann,[13] in a study of 11 subjects, noted a high correlation (r = 0.97) and agreement (ICC = 0.98) between radiographic measures and pendulum goniometer measures of head and neck flexion–extension. Ordway and colleagues[14] simultaneously measured cervical flexion and extension in 20 healthy subjects with a cervical range of motion device (CROM), a computerized tracking system, and radiographs. There were no significant differences between measurements taken with the CROM and radiographic angles determined by an occipital line and a vertical line, although there were differences between the CROM and the radiographic angles between the occiput and C-7. Tousignant and coworkers[15] measured cervical flexion and extension in 31 subjects with a CROM goniometer and radiographs that included cervical and upper thoracic motion. They found a high correlation between the two measurements (r = 0.97).

Studies that compared clinical ROM measurement methods for the lumbar spine with radiographic results report high to low validity. Macrae and Wright[16] measured lumbar flexion in 342 subjects by using a tape measure, according to the Schober and modified Schober method, and compared these results with those shown in radiographs. Their findings support the validity of these measures: correlation coefficient values between the Schober method and the radiographic evidence were 0.90 (standard error = 6.2 degrees) and between the modified Schober and the radiographs were 0.97 (standard error = 3.3 degrees). Portek and associates,[17] in a study of 11 males, found no significant difference between lumbar flexion and extension ROM measurement taken with a skin distraction method and single inclinometer compared with radiographic evidence, but correlation coefficients were low (0.42 to 0.57). Comparisons may have been inappropriate because measurements were made sequentially rather than concurrently, with subjects in varying testing positions. Radiographs and skin distraction methods were performed on standing subjects, whereas inclinometer measurements were performed in subjects sitting for flexion and prone for extension.

Burdett, Brown, and Fall,[18] in a study of 27 subjects, found a fair correlation between measurements taken with a single inclinometer and radiographs for lumbar flexion (r = 0.73) and a very poor correlation for lumbar extension (r = 0.15). Mayer and coworkers[19] measured lumbar flexion and extension in 12 patients with a single inclinometer, double inclinometer, and radiographs. No significant difference was noted between measurements. Saur and colleagues,[20] in a study of 54 patients, found lumbar flexion ROM measurement taken with two inclinometers correlated highly with radiographs (r = 0.98). Extension ROM measurement correlated with radiographs to a fair degree (r = 0.75). Samo and associates[21] used double inclinometers and radiographs to measure 30 subjects held in a position of flexion and extension. Radiographs resulted in flexion values that were 11 to 15 degrees greater than those found with inclinometers and extension values that were 4 to 5 degrees less than those found with inclinometers.

Construct Validity

Construct validity is the ability of an instrument to measure an abstract concept (construct)[3] or to be used to make an inferred interpretation.[7] There is a movement within rehabilitative medicine to develop and validate measurement tools to identify functional limitations and predict disability.[22] Joint ROM may be one such measurement tool. In Chapters 4 through 13 on measurement procedures, we have included the results of research studies that report joint ROM observed during functional tasks. These findings begin to quantify the joint motion needed to avoid functional limitations. Several researchers have artificially restricted joint motion with splints or braces and examined the effect on function.[23–25] It appears that many functional tasks can be completed with severely restricted elbow or wrist ROM, providing other adjacent joints are able to compensate.

Some studies have measured the correlation between ROM values and the ability to perform functional tasks in patient populations. A study by Hermann and Reese[26] examined the relationship among impairments, functional limitations, and disability in 80 patients with cervical spine disorders. The highest correlation (r = 0.82) occurred between impairment measures and functional limitation measures, with ROM contributing more to the relationship than the other two impairment measures of cervical muscle force and pain. Triffitt[27] found significant correlations between the amount of shoulder ROM and the ability to perform nine functional activities in 125 patients with shoulder symptoms. Wagner and colleagues[28] measured passive ROM of wrist flexion, extension, radial and ulnar deviation, and the strength of the wrist extensor and flexor muscles in 18 boys with Duchenne muscular dystrophy. A highly significant negative correlation was found between difficulty performing functional hand tasks and radial deviation ROM ($r = -0.76$ to -0.86) and between difficulty performing functional hand tasks and wrist extensor strength ($r = -0.61$ to -0.83).

⬭ Reliability

The **reliability** of a measurement refers to the amount of consistency between successive measurements of the same variable on the same subject under the same conditions. A goniometric measurement is highly reliable if successive measurements of a joint angle or ROM, on the same subject and under the same conditions, yield the same results. A highly reliable measurement contains little measurement error. Assuming that a measurement is valid and highly reliable, an examiner can confidently use its results to determine a true absence, presence, or change in dysfunction. For example, a highly reliable goniometric measurement could be used to determine the presence of joint ROM limitation, to evaluate patient progress toward rehabilitative goals, and to assess the effectiveness of therapeutic interventions.

A measurement with poor reliability contains a large amount of measurement error. An unreliable measurement is inconsistent and does not produce the same results when the same variable is measured on the same subject under the same conditions. A measurement that has poor reliability is not dependable and should not be used in the clinical decision-making process.

Summary of Goniometric Reliability Studies

The reliability of goniometric measurement has been the focus of many research studies. Given the variety of study designs and measurement techniques, it is difficult to compare the results of many of these studies. However, some findings noted in several studies can be summarized. An overview of such findings is presented here. More information on reliability studies that pertain to the featured joint is reviewed in Chapters 4 through 13. Readers may also wish to refer to several review articles and book chapters on this topic.[6,29–31]

The measurement of joint position and ROM of the extremities with a universal goniometer has generally been found to have good-to-excellent reliability. Numerous reliability studies have been conducted on joints of the upper and lower extremities. Some studies have examined the reliability of measuring joints held in a fixed position, whereas others have examined the reliability of measuring passive or active

ROM. Studies that measured a fixed joint position usually have reported higher reliability values than studies that measured ROM.[8,13,32,33] This finding is expected because more sources of variation and error are present in measuring ROM than in measuring a fixed joint position. Additional sources of error in measuring ROM include movement of the joint axis, variations in manual force applied by the examiner during passive ROM, and variations in a subject's effort during active ROM.

The reliability of goniometric ROM measurements varies somewhat depending on the joint and motion. ROM measurements of upper-extremity joints have been found by several researchers to be more reliable than ROM measurements of lower-extremity joints,[34,35] although opposing results have also been reported.[36] Even within the upper or lower extremities there are differences in reliability between joints and motions. For example, Hellebrandt, Duvall, and Moore,[37] in a study of upper-extremity joints, noted that measurements of wrist flexion, medial rotation of the shoulder, and abduction of the shoulder were less reliable than measurements of other motions of the upper extremity. Low[38] found ROM measurements of wrist extension to be less reliable than measurements of elbow flexion. Greene and Wolf[39] reported ROM measurements of shoulder rotation and wrist motions to be more variable than elbow motion and other shoulder motions. Reliability studies on ROM measurement of the cervical and thoracic spine in which a universal goniometer was used have generally reported lower reliability values than studies of the extremity joints.[18,40–43] Many devices and techniques have been developed to try to improve the reliability of measuring spinal motions. Gajdosik and Bohannon[6] suggested that the reliability of measuring certain joints and motions might be adversely affected by the complexity of the joint. Measurement of motions that are influenced by movement of adjacent joints or multijoint muscles may be less reliable than measurement of motions of simple hinge joints. Difficulty palpating bony landmarks and passively moving heavy body parts may also play a role in reducing the reliability of measuring ROM of the lower extremity and spine.[6,34]

Many studies of joint measurement methods have found intratester reliability to be higher than intertester reliability.[18,32–38,40,41,43–63] Reliability was higher when successive measurements were taken by the same examiner than when successive measurements were taken by different examiners. This is true for studies that measured joint position and ROM of the extremities and spine with universal goniometers and other devices such as joint-specific goniometers, pendulum goniometers, tape measures, and flexible rulers. Only a few studies found intertester reliability to be higher than intratester reliability.[64–67] In most of these studies, the time interval between repeated measurements by the same examiner was considerably greater than the time interval between measurements by different examiners.

The reliability of goniometric measurements is affected by the measurement procedure. Several studies found that intertester reliability improved when all the examiners used consistent, well-defined testing positions and measurement methods.[45,47,48,68] Intertester reliability was lower if examiners used a variety of positions and measurement methods.

Several investigators have examined the reliability of using the mean (average) of several goniometric measurements compared with using one measurement. Low[38] recommends using the mean of several measurements made with the goniometer to increase reliability over one measurement. Early studies by Cobe[69] and Hewitt[70] also used the mean of several measurements. However, Boone and associates[34] found no significant difference between repeated measurements made by the same examiner during one session and suggested that one measurement taken by an examiner is as reliable as the mean of repeated measurements. Rothstein, Miller, and Roettger,[48] in a study on knee and elbow ROM, found that intertester reliability determined from the means of two measurements improved only slightly from the intertester reliability determined from single measurements.

The authors of some texts on goniometric methods suggest the use of universal goniometers with longer arms to measure joints with large body segments such as the hip and shoulder.[29,71,72] Goniometers with shorter arms are recommended to measure joints with small body segments such as the wrist and fingers. Robson,[73] using a mathematical model, determined that goniometers with longer arms are more accurate in measuring an angle than goniometers with shorter arms. Goniometers with longer arms reduce the effects of errors in the placement of the goniometer axis. However, Rothstein, Miller, and Roettger[48] found no difference in reliability among large plastic, large metal, and small plastic universal goniometers used to measure knee and elbow ROM. Riddle, Rothstein, and Lamb[46] also reported no difference in reliability between large and small plastic universal goniometers used to measure shoulder ROM.

Numerous studies have compared the measurement values and reliability of different types of devices used to measure joint ROM. Universal, pendulum, and fluid goniometers; joint-specific devices; tape measures; and wire tracing are some of the devices that have been compared. Studies comparing clinical measurement devices have been conducted on the shoulder,[37,39] elbow,[32,37,39,57,74,75] wrist,[32,39] hand,[33,60,76,77] hip,[78,79] knee,[48,78,80,81] ankle,[78,82] cervical spine,[40,41,65,83] and thoracolumbar spine.[17,21,42,63,84–91] Many studies have found differences in values and reliability between measurement devices, whereas some studies have reported no differences.

In conclusion, on the basis of reliability studies and our clinical experience, we recommend the following procedures to improve the reliability of goniometric measurements (Table 3.1). Examiners should use consistent, well-defined testing positions and carefully palpated anatomical landmarks to align the arms of the goniometer. During successive measurements of passive ROM, examiners should strive to apply the same amount of manual force to move the subject's body. During successive measurements of active ROM, the subject should be urged to exert the same effort to perform a motion. To reduce measurement variability, it is prudent to take repeated measurements on a subject with the same type of measurement device. For example, an examiner should take all repeated measurements of a ROM with a universal goniometer, rather than taking the first measurement with a universal goniometer and the second measurement with an inclinometer. We believe most examiners find it easier and more accurate to use a large universal goniometer when measuring joints with large body segments and a small goniometer when measuring joints with small body segments. Inexperienced examiners may wish to take several measurements and record the mean (average) of those measurements to improve reliability, but one measurement is usually sufficient for more experienced examiners using good technique. Finally, it is important to remember that successive measurements are more reliable if taken by the same examiner rather than by different examiners.

The mean standard deviation of repeated ROM measurement of extremity joints taken by one examiner using a universal goniometer has been found to range from 4 to 5 degrees.[34,36] Therefore, to show improvement or worsening of a joint motion measured by the same examiner, a difference of about 5 degrees (1 standard deviation) to 10 degrees (2 standard deviations) is necessary. The mean standard deviation increased to 5 to 6 degrees for repeated measurements taken by different examiners,[34,36] so that a difference of about 6 (1 standard deviation) to 12 degrees (2 standard deviations) is necessary to show true change in this situation. These values serve as a general guideline only and will vary depending on the joint and motion being tested, the examiners and procedures used, and the individual being tested. Refer to the Research Findings section of Chapters 4 to 13 for more joint-specific information on reliability.

TABLE 3.1 Recommendations for Improving the Reliability of Goniometric Measurements

- Use consistent, well-defined positions.
- Use consistent, well-defined, and carefully palpated anatomical landmarks to align the goniometer.
- Use the same amount of manual force to move subject's body part during successive measurements of passive ROM.
- Urge subject to exert the same effort to move the body part during successive measurements of active ROM.
- Use the same device to take successive measurements.
- Use a goniometer that is suitable in size to the joint being measured.
- If examiner is less experienced, record the mean of several measurements rather than a single measurement.
- Have the *same* examiner, rather than a *different* examiner, take successive measurements.

Statistical Methods of Evaluating Measurement Reliability

Clinical measurements are prone to three main sources of variation: (1) true biological variation, (2) temporal variation, and (3) measurement error.[92] **True biological variation** refers to variation in measurements from one individual to another, caused by factors such as age, sex, race, genetics, medical history, and condition. **Temporal variation** refers to variation in measurements made on the same individual at different times, caused by changes in factors such as a subject's medical (physical) condition, activity level, emotional state, and circadian rhythms. **Measurement error** refers to variation in measurements made on the same individual under the same conditions at different times, caused by factors such as the examiners (testers), measuring instruments, and procedural methods. For example, the skill level and experience of the examiners, the accuracy of the measurement instruments, and the standardization of the measurement methods affect the amount of measurement error. Reliability reflects the degree to which a measurement is free of measurement error; therefore, highly reliable measurements have little measurement error.

Statistics can be used to assess variation in numerical data and hence to assess measurement reliability.[92,93] A digression into statistical methods of testing and expressing reliability is included to assist the examiner in correctly interpreting goniometric measurements and in understanding the literature on joint measurement. Several statistics—the standard deviation, coefficient of variation, Pearson product moment correlation coefficient, intraclass correlation coefficient, and standard error of measurement—are discussed. Examples that show the calculation of these statistical tests are presented. For additional information, including the assumptions underlying the use of these statistical tests, the reader is referred to the cited references.

At the end of this chapter, two exercises are included for examiners to assess their reliability in obtaining goniometric measurements. Many authors recommend that clinicians conduct their own studies to determine reliability among their staff and patient population. Miller[30] has presented a step-by-step procedure for conducting such studies.

Standard Deviation

In the medical literature, the statistic most frequently used to indicate variation is the standard deviation.[92,93] The **standard deviation** is the square root of the mean of the squares of the deviations from the data mean. The standard deviation is symbolized as **SD**, **s**, or **sd**. If we denote each data observation as x and the number of observations as n, and the summation notation Σ is used, then the mean that is denoted by $\bar{x}$, is as follows:

$$\text{mean} = \bar{x} = \frac{\Sigma x}{n}$$

Two formulas for the standard deviation are given below. The first is the definitional formula; the second is the computational formula. Both formulas give the same result. The definitional formula is easier to understand, but the computational formula is easier to calculate.

$$\text{Standard deviation} = SD = \sqrt{\frac{\Sigma (x - \bar{x})^2}{n - 1}}$$

$$SD = \sqrt{\frac{\Sigma(x)^2 - \frac{(\Sigma x)^2}{n}}{n - 1}}$$

The standard deviation has the same units as the original data observations. If the data observations have a normal (bell-shaped) frequency distribution, 1 standard deviation above and below the mean includes about 68 percent of all the observations, and 2 standard deviations above and below the mean include about 95 percent of the observations.

It is important to note that several standard deviations may be determined from a single study and represent different sources of variation.[92] Two of these standard deviations are discussed here. One standard deviation that can be determined represents mainly *inter*subject variation around the mean of measurements taken of a group of subjects, indicating biological variation. This standard deviation may be of interest in deciding whether a subject has an abnormal ROM in comparison with other people of the same age and gender. Another standard deviation that can be determined represents *intra*subject variation around the mean of measurements taken of an individual, indicating measurement error. This is the standard deviation of interest to indicate measurement reliability.

An example of how to determine these two standard deviations is provided. Table 3.2 presents ROM measurements taken on five subjects. Three repeated measurements (observations) were taken on each subject by the same examiner.

The **standard deviation indicating biological variation** (intersubject variation) is determined by first calculating the mean ROM measurement for each subject. The mean ROM measurement for each of the five subjects is found in the last column of Table 3.2. The grand mean of the mean ROM measurement for each of the five subjects equals 56 degrees. The grand mean is symbolized by $\bar{X}$. The standard deviation is determined by finding the differences between each of the five subjects' means and the grand mean. The differences are squared and added together. The sum is used in the definitional formula for the standard deviation. Calculation of the standard deviation indicating biological variation is found in Table 3.3.

In the example, the standard deviation indicating biological variation equals 13.6 degrees. This standard deviation denotes primarily intersubject variation. Knowledge of intersubject variation may be helpful in deciding whether a subject has an abnormal ROM in comparison with other people of the same age and gender. If a normal distribution of the measurements is assumed, one way of interpreting this standard deviation is to predict that about 68 percent of all the subjects' mean ROM measurements

TABLE 3.2	Three Repeated ROM Measurements (in Degrees) Taken on Five Subjects				
Subject	First Measurement	Second Measurement	Third Measurement	Total	Mean of Three Measurements ($\bar{x}$)
1	57	55	65	177	59
2	66	65	70	201	67
3	66	70	74	210	70
4	35	40	42	117	39
5	45	48	42	135	45

Grand mean $(\bar{X}) = \dfrac{(59 + 67 + 70 + 39 + 45)}{5} = 56$ degrees.

TABLE 3.3	Calculation of the Standard Deviation Indicating Biological Variation in Degrees			
Subject	Mean of Three Measurements ($\bar{x}$)	Grand Mean ($\bar{X}$)	($\bar{x} - \bar{X}$)	($\bar{x} - \bar{X}$)^2
1	59	56	3	9
2	67	56	11	121
3	70	56	14	196
4	39	56	−17	289
5	45	56	−11	121

$\Sigma(\bar{x} - \bar{X})^2 = 9 + 121 + 196 + 289 + 121 = 736$ degrees; $SD = \sqrt{\dfrac{\Sigma(\bar{x} - \bar{X})^2}{(n-1)}} = \sqrt{\dfrac{736}{(5-1)}} = 13.6$ degrees.

would fall between 42.4 degrees and 69.6 degrees (plus or minus 1 standard deviation around the grand mean of 56 degrees). We would expect that about 95 percent of all the subjects' mean ROM measurements would fall between 28.8 degrees and 83.2 degrees (plus or minus 2 standard deviations around the grand mean of 56 degrees).

The standard deviation indicating measurement error (intrasubject variation) also is determined by first calculating the mean ROM measurement for each subject. However, this standard deviation is determined by finding the differences between each of the three repeated measurements taken on a subject and the mean of that subject's measurements. The differences are squared and added together. The sum is used in the definitional formula for the standard deviation. Using the information on subject 1 in the example, the calculation of the standard deviation indicating measurement error is shown in Table 3.4.

Referring to Table 3.2 for information on the each of the other subjects and using the same procedure as shown in Table 3.4, the standard deviation for subject 1 = 5.3 degrees, the standard deviation for subject 2 = 2.6 degrees, the

standard deviation for subject 3 = 4.0 degrees, the standard deviation for subject 4 = 3.6 degrees, and the standard deviation for subject 5 = 3.0 degrees. The mean standard deviation for all of the subjects combined is determined by

TABLE 3.4	Calculation of the Standard Deviation Indicating Measurement Error in Degrees for Subject 1		
Measurements (x)	Mean ($\bar{x}$)	($x - \bar{x}$)	($x - \bar{x}$)^2
57	59	−2	4
55	59	−4	16
65	59	6	36

$SD = \sqrt{\dfrac{\Sigma(x - \bar{x})^2}{(n-1)}} = \sqrt{\dfrac{56}{2}} = 5.3$ degrees

summing the five subjects' standard deviations and dividing by the number of subjects, which is 5:

$$SD = \frac{5.3 + 2.6 + 4.0 + 3.6 + 3.0}{5} = \frac{18.5}{5} = 3.7 \text{ degrees}$$

In the example, the standard deviation indicating intra-subject variation equals 3.7 degrees. This standard deviation is appropriate for indicating measurement error, especially if the repeated measurements on each subject were taken within a short period of time. Note that in this example the standard deviation indicating measurement error (3.7 degrees) is much smaller than the standard deviation indicating biological variation (13.6 degrees). One way of interpreting the standard deviation for measurement error is to predict that about 68 percent of the repeated measurements on a subject would fall within 3.7 degrees (1 standard deviation) above and below the mean of the repeated measurements of a subject because of measurement error. We would expect that about 95 percent of the repeated measurements on a subject would fall within 7.4 degrees (2 standard deviations) above and below the mean of the repeated measurements of a subject, again because of measurement error. The smaller the standard deviation, the less the measurement error and the better the reliability.

Coefficient of Variation

Sometimes it is helpful to consider the percentage of variation rather than the standard deviation, which is expressed in the units of the data observation (measurement). The **coefficient of variation** is a measure of variation that is relative to the mean and standardized so that the variations of different variables can be compared. The coefficient of variation is the standard deviation divided by the mean and multiplied by 100 percent. It is a percentage and is not expressed in the units of the original observation. The coefficient of variation is symbolized by **CV** and the formula is as follows:

$$\text{coefficient of variation} = CV = \frac{SD}{\bar{x}} (100)\%$$

For the example presented in Table 3.2, the coefficient of variation indicating biological variation uses the standard deviation for biological variation (standard deviation = 13.6 degrees).

$$CV = \frac{SD}{\bar{x}} (100)\% = \frac{13.6}{56}(100)\% = 24.3\%$$

The coefficient of variation indicating measurement error uses the standard deviation for measurement error (standard deviation = 3.7 degrees).

$$CV = \frac{SD}{\bar{x}} (100)\% = \frac{3.7}{56} (100)\% = 6.6\%$$

In this example the coefficient of variation for measurement error (6.6 percent) is less than the coefficient of variation for biological variation (24.3 percent).

Another name for the coefficient of variation indicating measurement error is the **coefficient of variation of replication.**[94] The lower the coefficient of variation of replication, the lower the measurement error and the better the reliability.

This statistic is especially useful in comparing the reliability of two or more variables that have different units of measurement (for example, comparing ROM measurement methods recorded in inches versus degrees).

Correlation Coefficients

Correlation coefficients are traditionally used to measure the relationship between two variables. They result in a number from -1 to $+1$, which indicates how well an equation can predict one variable from another variable.[2-4,92] A $+1$ describes a perfect positive linear (straight-line) relationship, whereas a -1 describes a perfect negative linear relationship. A correlation coefficient of 0 indicates that there is no linear relationship between the two variables. Correlation coefficients are used to indicate measurement reliability because it is assumed that two repeated measurements should be highly correlated and approach $+1$. One interpretation of correlation coefficients used to indicate reliability is that 0.90 to 0.99 equals high reliability, 0.80 to 0.89 equals good reliability, 0.70 to 0.79 equals fair reliability, and 0.69 and below equals poor reliability.[95] Another interpretation offered by Portney and Watkins[3] states that correlation coefficients higher than 0.75 indicate good reliability, whereas those less than 0.75 indicate poor to moderate reliability.

Pearson Product Moment Correlation Coefficient

Because goniometric measurements produce ratio level data, the **Pearson product moment correlation coefficient** has been the correlation coefficient usually calculated to indicate the reliability of pairs of goniometric measurements. The Pearson product moment correlation coefficient is symbolized by **r**, and its formula is presented following this paragraph. If this statistic is used to indicate reliability, x symbolizes the first measurement and y symbolizes the second measurement.

$$r = \frac{\Sigma(x - \bar{x})(y - \bar{y})}{\sqrt{\Sigma(x - \bar{x})^2} \sqrt{\Sigma(y - \bar{y})^2}}$$

Referring to the example in Table 3.2, the Pearson correlation coefficient can be used to determine the relationship between the first and the second ROM measurements on the five subjects. Calculation of the Pearson product moment correlation coefficient for this example is found in Table 3.5. The resulting value of $r = 0.98$ indicates a highly positive linear relationship between the first and the second measurements. In other words, the two measurements are highly correlated.

$$r = \frac{\Sigma(x - \bar{x})(y - \bar{y})}{\sqrt{\Sigma(x - \bar{x})^2} \sqrt{\Sigma(y - \bar{y})^2}}$$

$$= \frac{650.6}{\sqrt{738.8} \sqrt{597.2}} = \frac{650.6}{(27.2)(24.4)} = 0.98$$

The Pearson product moment correlation coefficient indicates association between the pairs of measurements rather than agreement. Therefore, to decide whether the two

| TABLE 3.5 | Calculation of the Pearson Product Moment Correlation Coefficient for the First (x) and Second (y) ROM Measurements in Degrees | | | | | |

Subject	x	y	$(x - \bar{x})$	$(y - \bar{y})$	$(x - \bar{x})(y - \bar{y})$	$(x - \bar{x})^2$	$(y - \bar{y})^2$
1	57	55	3.2	−0.6	−1.92	10.24	0.36
2	66	65	12.2	9.4	114.68	148.84	88.36
3	66	70	12.2	14.4	175.68	148.84	207.36
4	35	40	−18.8	−15.6	293.28	353.44	243.36
5	45	48	−8.8	−7.6	68.88	77.44	57.76
					$\Sigma = 650.60$	$\Sigma = 738.80$	$\Sigma = 597.20$

$$\bar{x} = \frac{57 + 66 + 66 + 35 + 45}{5} = 53.8 \text{ degrees}; \quad \bar{y} = \frac{55 + 65 + 70 + 40 + 48}{5} = 55.6 \text{ degrees}.$$

measurements are identical, the equation of the straight line best representing the relationship should be determined. If the equation of the straight line representing the relationship includes a slope b equal to 1 and an intercept a equal to 0, then an r value that approaches $+1$ also indicates that the two measurements are identical. The equation of a straight line is $y = a + bx$, with x symbolizing the first measurement, y the second measurement, a the intercept, and b the slope. The equation for a slope is

$$\text{slope} = b = \frac{\Sigma (x - \bar{x})(y - \bar{y})}{\Sigma (x - \bar{x})^2}$$

The equation for an intercept is *intercept* $= a = \bar{y} - b\bar{x}$

For our example, the slope and intercept are calculated as follows:

$$b = \frac{\Sigma (x - \bar{x})(y - \bar{y})}{\Sigma (x - \bar{x})^2} = \frac{650.6}{738.8} = 0.88$$

$$intercept = a = \bar{y} - b\bar{x} = 55.6 - 0.88(53.8) = 8.26$$

The equation of the straight line best representing the relationship between the first and the second measurements in the example is $y = 8.26 + 0.88x$. Although the r value indicates high correlation, the two measurements are not identical given the linear equation.

One concern in interpreting correlation coefficients is that the value of the correlation coefficient is markedly influenced by the range of the measurements.[3,93,96] The greater the biological variation between individuals for the measurement, the more extreme the r value, so that r is closer to -1 or $+1$. Another limitation is the fact that the Pearson product moment correlation coefficient can evaluate the relationship between only two variables or measurements at a time.

Intraclass Correlation Coefficient

To avoid the need for calculating and interpreting both the correlation coefficient and a linear equation, some investigators use the **intraclass correlation coefficient (ICC)** to evaluate reliability. The ICC also allows the comparison of two or more measurements at a time; one can think of it as an average correlation among all possible pairs of measurements.[96]

This statistic is determined from an analysis of variance model, which compares different sources of variation. The ICC is conceptually expressed as the ratio of the variance associated with the subjects, divided by the sum of the variance associated with the subjects plus error variance.[97] The theoretical limits of the ICC are between 0 and $+1$; $+1$ indicates perfect agreement (no error variance), whereas 0 indicates no agreement (large amount of error variance).

There are six different formulas for determining ICC values based on the design of the study, the purpose of the study, and the type of measurement.[3,97,98] Three models have been described, each with two different forms. In Model 1, each subject is tested by a different set of testers, and the testers are considered representative of a larger population of testers—to allow the results to be generalized to other testers. In Model 2, each subject is tested by the same set of testers, and again the testers are considered representative of a larger population of testers. In Model 3, each subject is tested by the same set of testers, but the testers are the only testers of interest—the results are not intended to be generalized to other testers. The first form of all three models is used when single measurements (1) are compared, whereas the second form is used when the means of multiple measurements (k) are compared. The different formulas for the ICC are identified by two numbers enclosed by parentheses. The first number indicates the model, and the second number indicates the form. For further discussion, examples, and formulas, the reader is urged to refer to the referenced texts[3] and articles.[97–99]

In our example, a repeated measures analysis of variance was conducted and the ICC (3,1) was calculated as 0.94. This ICC model was used because each measurement was taken by the same tester, there was only an interest in applying the results to this tester, and single measurements were compared rather than the means of several measurements. This ICC value indicates a high reliability between the three repeated measurements. However, this value is slightly lower than the Pearson product moment correlation coefficient, perhaps due to the variability added by the third measurement on each subject.

Like the Pearson product moment correlation coefficient, the ICC is also influenced by the range of measurements between the subjects. As the group of subjects becomes more homogeneous, the ability of the ICC to detect agreement is reduced and the ICC can erroneously indicate poor reliability.[3,97,100] Because correlation coefficients are sensitive to the range of the measurements and do not provide an index of reliability in the units of the measurement, some experts prefer the use of the standard deviation of the repeated measurements (intrasubject standard deviation) or the standard error of measurement to assess reliability.[4,100,101]

Standard Error of Measurement

The standard error of measurement is the final statistic that we review here to evaluate reliability. It has received support because of its practical interpretation in estimating measurement error in the same units as the measurement. According to DuBois,[102] "The **standard error of measurement** is the likely standard deviation of the error made in predicting true scores when we have knowledge only of the obtained scores." The true scores (measurements) are forever unknown, but several formulas have been developed to estimate this statistic. The standard error of measurement is symbolized as **SEM**, **SE$_{meas}$**, or **S$_{meas}$**. If the standard deviation indicating biological variation is denoted SD$_x$, a correlation coefficient such as the intraclass correlation coefficient is denoted ICC, and the Pearson product moment correlation coefficient is denoted r, the formulas for the SEM are as follows:

$$SEM = SD_x \sqrt{1 - ICC}$$

or

$$SEM = SD_x \sqrt{1 - r}$$

The SEM can also be determined from a repeated measures analysis of variance model. The SEM is equivalent to the square root of the mean square of the error.[103,104] Because the SEM is a special case of the standard deviation, 1 standard error of measurement above and below the observed measurement includes the true measurement 68 percent of the time. Two standard errors of measurement above and below the observed measurement include the true measurement 95 percent of the time.

It is important to note that another statistic, the standard error of the mean, is often confused with the standard error of measurement. The standard error of the mean is symbolized as SEM, SE$_M$, SE$_{\bar{x}}$, or S$_{\bar{x}}$.[2,4,92,93] The use of the same or similar symbols to represent different statistics has added much confusion to the reliability literature. These two statistics are not equivalent, nor do they have the same interpretation. The standard error of the mean is the standard deviation of a distribution of means taken from samples of a population.[1,2,93] It describes how much variation can be expected in the means from future samples of the same size. Because we are interested in the variation of individual measurements when evaluating reliability rather than the variation of means, the standard deviation of the repeated measurements or the standard error of measurement are the appropriate statistical tests to use.[105]

Let us return to the example and calculate the standard error of the measurement. The value for the ICC is 0.94. The value for SD$_x$, the standard deviation indicating biological variation among the 5 subjects, is 13.6.

$$SEM = SD_x \sqrt{1 - ICC}$$

$$13.6 \sqrt{1 - 0.94} = 13.6 \sqrt{0.06} = 3.3 \text{ degrees}$$

Likewise, if we use the results of the repeated measures analysis of variance to calculate the SEM, the SEM equals the square root of the mean square of the error = $\sqrt{10.9}$ = 3.3 degrees. In this example, about two-thirds of the time the true measurement would be within 3.3 degrees of the observed measurement.

Exercises to Evaluate Reliability

Exercises 6 and 7 have been included to help examiners assess their reliability in obtaining goniometric measurements. Calculations of the standard deviation and coefficient of variation are included in the belief that understanding is reinforced by practical application. **Exercise 6** examines **intratester reliability**. Intratester reliability refers to the amount of agreement between repeated measurements of the same joint position or ROM by the same examiner (tester). An intratester reliability study answers the question: How accurately can an examiner reproduce his or her own measurements? **Exercise 7** examines **intertester reliability**. Intertester reliability refers to the amount of agreement between repeated measurements of the same joint position or ROM by different examiners (testers). An intertester reliability study answers the question: How accurately can one examiner reproduce measurements taken by other examiners?

Exercise 6

Intratester Reliability

1. Select a subject and a universal goniometer.
2. Measure elbow flexion ROM on your subject three times, following the steps outlined in Chapter 2, Exercise 5.
3. Record each measurement on the recording form (see opposite page) in the column labeled x. A measurement is denoted by x.
4. Compare the measurements. If a discrepancy of more than 5 degrees exists between measurements, recheck each step in the procedure to make sure that you are performing the steps correctly, and then repeat this exercise.
5. Continue practicing until you have obtained three successive measurements that are within 5 degrees of each other.
6. To gain an understanding of several of the statistics used to evaluate intratester reliability, calculate the standard deviation and coefficient of variation by completing the following steps.
   a. Add the three measurements together to determine the sum of the measurements. Σ is the symbol for summation. Record the sum at the bottom of the column labeled x.
   b. To determine the **mean**, divide this sum by 3, which is the number of measurements. The number of measurements is denoted by n. The mean is denoted by $\bar{x}$. Space to calculate the mean is provided on the recording form.
   c. To continue the process of calculating the **standard deviation**, subtract the mean from each of the three measurements and record the results in the column labeled $x - \bar{x}$. Space to calculate the standard deviation is provided on the recording form.
   d. Square each of the numbers in the column labeled $x - \bar{x}$, and record the results in the column labeled $(x - \bar{x})^2$.
   e. Add the three numbers in column $(x - \bar{x})^2$ to determine the sum of the squares. Record the results at the bottom of the column labeled $(x - \bar{x})^2$.
   f. Divide this sum by 2, which is the number of measurements minus 1 $(n - 1)$. Then find the square root of this number.
   g. To determine the **coefficient of variation,** divide the standard deviation by the mean. Multiply this number by 100 percent. Space to calculate the coefficient of variation is provided on the recording form.
7. Repeat this procedure with other joints and motions after you have learned the testing procedures.

RECORDING FORM FOR EXERCISE 6. INTRATESTER RELIABILITY

Follow the steps outlined in Exercise 6. Use this form to record your measurements and the result of your calculations.

Subject's Name _____ Date _____

Examiner's Name _____

Joint and Motion _____ Right or Left Side _____

Passive or Active Motion _____ Type of Goniometer _____

Measurement	x	$x - \bar{x}$	$(x - \bar{x})^2$	x^2
1				
2				
3				
$n = 3$	$\Sigma x =$		$\Sigma(x - \bar{x})^2 =$	$\Sigma x^2 =$

$$\text{Mean of the three measurements} = \bar{x} = \frac{\Sigma x}{n} =$$

$$\text{Standard deviation} = \sqrt{\frac{\Sigma (x - \bar{x})^2}{n - 1}} =$$

$$\text{or use SD} = \sqrt{\frac{\Sigma x^2 - \frac{(\Sigma x)^2}{n}}{n - 1}}$$

$$\text{Coefficient of variation} = \frac{\text{SD}}{\bar{x}} (100)\% =$$

Exercise 7

Intertester Reliability

1. Select a subject and a universal goniometer.
2. Measure elbow flexion ROM on your subject once, following the steps outlined in Chapter 2, Exercise 5.
3. Ask two other examiners to measure the same elbow flexion ROM on your subject, using your goniometer and following the steps outlined in Chapter 2, Exercise 5.
4. Record each measurement on the recording form (see opposite page) in the column labeled x. A measurement is denoted by x.
5. Compare the measurements. If a discrepancy of more than 5 degrees exists between measurements, repeat this exercise. The examiners should observe one another's measurements to discover differences in technique that might account for variability, such as faulty alignment, lack of stabilization, or reading the wrong scale.
6. To gain an understanding of several of the statistics used to evaluate intertester reliability, calculate the mean deviation, standard deviation, and coefficient of variation by completing the following steps.
    a. Add the three measurements together to determine the sum of the measurements. Σ is the symbol for summation. Record the sum at the bottom of the column labeled x.
    b. To determine the **mean,** divide this sum by 3, which is the number of measurements. The number of measurements is denoted by n. The mean is denoted by $\bar{x}$. Space to calculate the mean is provided on the recording form.
    c. To continue the process of calculating the **standard deviation**, subtract the mean from each of the three measurements, and record the results in the column labeled $x - \bar{x}$. Space to calculate the standard deviation is provided on the recording form.
    d. Square each of the numbers in the column labeled $x - \bar{x}$, and record the results in the column labeled $(x - \bar{x})^2$.
    e. Add the three numbers in column $(x - x)^2$ to determine the sum of the squares. Record the results at the bottom of column $(x - \bar{x})^2$.
    f. Divide this sum by 2, which is the number of measurements minus 1 $(n - 1)$. Then find the square root of this number.
    g. To determine the **coefficient of variation,** divide the standard deviation by the mean. Multiply this number by 100 percent. Space to calculate the coefficient of variation is provided on the recording form.
7. Repeat this exercise with other joints and motions after you have learned the testing procedures.

RECORDING FORM FOR EXERCISE 7. INTERTESTER RELIABILITY

Follow the steps outlined in Exercise 7. Use this form to record your measurements and the results of your calculations.

Subject's Name _____ Date _____

Examiner 1. Name _____

Examiner 2. Name_____ Joint and Motion _____

Examiner 3. Name _____ Right or Left Side _____

Passive or Active Motion _____ Type of Goniometer _____

Measurement	x	$x - \bar{x}$	$(x - \bar{x})^2$	x^2
1				
2				
3				
$n = 3$	$\Sigma x =$		$\Sigma(x - \bar{x})^2 =$	$\Sigma x^2 =$

$$\text{Mean of the three measurements} = \bar{x} = \frac{\Sigma x}{n} =$$

$$\text{Standard deviation} = \sqrt{\frac{\Sigma\,(x - \bar{x})^2}{n - 1}}$$

$$\text{or use SD} = \sqrt{\frac{\Sigma x^2 - \dfrac{(\Sigma x)^2}{n}}{n - 1}}$$

$$\text{Coefficient of variation} = \frac{\text{SD}}{\bar{x}}(100)\% =$$

REFERENCES

1. Currier, DP: Elements of Research in Physical Therapy, ed 3. Williams & Wilkins, Baltimore, 1990, p 171.
2. Kerlinger, FN: Foundations of Behavioral Research, ed 2. Holt, Rinehart, & Winston, New York, 1973.
3. Portney, LG, and Watkins, MP: Foundations of Clinical Research: Applications to Practice, ed 2. Prentice-Hall, Upper Saddle River, NJ, 2000.
4. Rothstein, JM: Measurement and Clinical Practice: Theory and Application. In Rothstein, JM (ed): Measurement in Physical Therapy. Churchill Livingstone, New York, 1985.
5. Sims, J, and Arnell, P: Measurement validity in physical therapy research. Phys Ther 73:102, 1993.
6. Gajdosik, RL, and Bohannon, RW: Clinical measurement of range of motion: Review of goniometry emphasizing reliability and validity. Phys Ther 67:1867, 1987.
7. American Physical Therapy Association: Standards for tests and measurements in physical therapy practice. Phys Ther 71:589, 1991.
8. Gogia, PP, et al: Reliability and validity of goniometric measurements at the knee. Phys Ther 67:192, 1987.
9. Enwemeka, CS: Radiographic verification of knee goniometry. Scand J Rehabil Med 18:47, 1986.
10. Ahlback, SO, and Lindahl, O: Sagittal mobility of the hip-joint. Acta Orthop Scand 34:310, 1964.
11. Kato, M, et al: The accuracy of goniometric measurements of proximal interphalangeal joints in fresh cadavers: Comparison between methods of measurement, types of goniometers, and fingers. J Hand Ther 20:12, 2007.
12. Chen, J, et al: Meta-analysis of normative cervical motion. Spine 24:1571, 1999.
13. Herrmann, DB: Validity study of head and neck flexion-extension motion comparing measurements of a pendulum goniometer and roentgenograms. J Orthop Sports Phys Ther 11:414, 1990.
14. Ordway, NR, et al: Cervical sagittal range-of-motion analysis using three methods: Cervical range-of-motion device, space, and radiography. Spine 22:501, 1997.
15. Tousignant, M, et al: Criterion validity of the cervical range of motion (CROM) goniometer for cervical flexion and extension. Spine 25:324, 2000.
16. Macrae, JF, and Wright, V: Measurement of back movement. Ann Rheum Dis 28:584, 1969.
17. Portek, I, et al: Correlation between radiographic and clinical measurement of lumbar spine movement. Br J Rheumatol 22:197, 1983.
18. Burdett, RG, Brown, KE, and Fall, MP: Reliability and validity of four instruments for measuring lumbar spine and pelvic positions. Phys Ther 66:677, 1986.
19. Mayer, TG, et al: Use of noninvasive techniques for quantification of spinal range-of-motion in normal subjects and chronic low-back dysfunction patients. Spine 9:588, 1984.
20. Saur, PM, et al: Lumbar range of motion: Reliability and validity of the inclinometer technique in the clinical measurement of trunk flexibility. Spine 21:1332, 1996.
21. Samo, DG, et al: Validity of three lumbar sagittal motion measurement methods: Surface inclinometers compared with radiographs. J Occup Environ Med 39:209, 1997.
22. Campbell, SK: Commentary: Measurement validity in physical therapy research. Phys Ther 73:110, 1993.
23. Vasen, AP, et al: Functional range of motion of the elbow. J Hand Surg 20A:288, 1995.
24. Cooper, JE, et al: Elbow joint restriction: Effect on functional upper limb motion during performance of three feeding activities. Arch Phys Med Rehabil 74:805, 1993.
25. Nelson, DL: Functional wrist motion. Hand Clin 13:83, 1997.
26. Hermann, KM, and Reese, CS: Relationships among selected measures of impairment, functional limitation, and disability in patients with cervical spine disorder. Phys Ther 81:903, 2001.
27. Triffitt, PD: The relationship between motion of the shoulder and the stated ability to perform activities of daily living. J Bone Joint Surg 80:41, 1998.
28. Wagner, MB, et al: Assessment of hand function in Duchenne muscular dystrophy. Arch Phys Med Rehabil 74:801, 1993.
29. Moore, ML: Clinical assessment of joint motion. In Basmajian, JV (ed): Therapeutic Exercise, ed 3. Williams & Wilkins, Baltimore, 1978.
30. Miller, PJ: Assessment of joint motion. In Rothstein, JM (ed): Measurement in Physical Therapy. Churchill Livingstone, New York, 1985.

31. Lea, RD, and Gerhardt, JJ: Current concepts review: Range-of-motion measurements. J Bone Joint Surg Am 77:784, 1995.
32. Grohmann, JEL: Comparison of two methods of goniometry. Phys Ther 63:922, 1983.
33. Hamilton, GF, and Lachenbruch, PA: Reliability of goniometers in assessing finger joint angle. Phys Ther 49:465, 1969.
34. Boone, DC, et al: Reliability of goniometric measurements. Phys Ther 58:1355, 1978.
35. Pandya, S, et al: Reliability of goniometric measurements in patients with Duchenne muscular dystrophy. Phys Ther 65:1339, 1985.
36. Bovens, AMP, et al: Variability and reliability of joint measurements. Am J Sport Med 18:58, 1990.
37. Hellebrandt, FA, Duvall, EN, and Moore, ML: The measurement of joint motion. Part III: Reliability of goniometry. Phys Ther Rev 29:302, 1949.
38. Low, JL: The reliability of joint measurement. Physiotherapy 62:227, 1976.
39. Greene, BL, and Wolf, SL: Upper extremity joint movement: Comparison of two measurement devices. Arch Phys Med Rehabil 70:299, 1989.
40. Tucci, SM, et al: Cervical motion assessment: A new, simple and accurate method. Arch Phys Med Rehabil 67:225, 1986.
41. Youdas, JW, Carey, JR, and Garrett, TR: Reliability of measurements of cervical spine range of motion: Comparison of three methods. Phys Ther 71:2, 1991.
42. Fitzgerald, GK, et al: Objective assessment with establishment of normal values for lumbar spine range of motion. Phys Ther 63:1776, 1983.
43. Nitschke, JE, et al: Reliability of the American Medical Association Guides' model for measuring spinal range of motion. Spine 24:262, 1999.
44. Mayerson, NH, and Milano, RA: Goniometric measurement reliability in physical medicine. Arch Phys Med Rehabil 65:92, 1984.
45. Watkins, MA, et al: Reliability of goniometric measurements and visual estimates of knee range of motion obtained in a clinical setting. Phys Ther 71:90, 1991.
46. Riddle, DL, Rothstein, JM, and Lamb, RL: Goniometric reliability in a clinical setting: Shoulder measurements. Phys Ther 67:668, 1987.
47. Ekstrand, J, et al: Lower extremity goniometric measurements: A study to determine their reliability. Arch Phys Med Rehabil 63:171, 1982.
48. Rothstein, JM, Miller, PJ, and Roettger, RF: Goniometric reliability in a clinical setting: Elbow and knee measurements. Phys Ther 63:1611, 1983.
49. Solgaard, S, et al: Reproducibility of goniometry of the wrist. Scand J Rehabil Med 18:5, 1986.
50. Patel, RS: Intratester and intertester reliability of the inclinometer in measuring lumbar flexion [abstract]. Phys Ther 72:S44, 1992.
51. Lovell, FW, Rothstein, JM, and Personius, WJ: Reliability of clinical measurements of lumbar lordosis taken with a flexible rule. Phys Ther 69:96, 1989.
52. Bartlett, JD, et al: Hip flexion contractures: A comparison of measurement methods. Arch Phys Med Rehabil 66:620, 1985.
53. Jonson, SR, and Gross, MT: Intraexaminer reliability, interexaminer reliability, and mean values for nine lower extremity skeletal measures in healthy naval midshipmen. J Orthop Sports Phys Ther 25:253, 1997
54. Elveru, RA, Rothstein, JM, and Lamb, RL: Goniometric reliability in a clinical setting. Phys Ther 68:672, 1988.
55. Diamond, JE, et al: Reliability of a diabetic foot evaluation. Phys Ther 69:797, 1989.
56. MacDermid, JC, et al: Intratester and intertester reliability of goniometric measurement of passive lateral shoulder rotation. J Hand Ther 12:187, 1999.
57. Armstrong, AD, et al: Reliability of range-of-motion measurement in the elbow and forearm. J Shoulder Elbow Surg 7:573, 1998.
58. Boon, AJ, and Smith, J: Manual scapular stabilization: Its effect on shoulder rotational range of motion Arch Phys Med Rehabil 81:978, 2000.
59. Horger, MM: The reliability of goniometric measurements of active and passive wrist motions. Am J Occup Ther 44:342, 1990.
60. Ellis, B, Bruton, A, and Goddard, JR: Joint angle measurement: A comparative study of the reliability of goniometry and wire tracing for the hand. Clin Rehabil 11:314, 1997.
61. Pellecchia, GL, and Bohannon, RW: Active lateral neck flexion range of motion measurements obtained with a modified goniometer. Reliability and estimates of normal. J Manipulative Physiol Ther 21:443, 1998.
62. Nilsson, N: Measuring passive cervical motion: A study of reliability. J Manipulative Physiol Ther 18:293, 1995.
63. Williams, R, et al: Reliability of the modified-modified Schober and double inclinometer methods for measuring lumbar flexion and extension. Phys Ther 73:26, 1993.

64. Defibaugh, JJ: Measurement of head motion. Part II: An experimental study of head motion in adult males. Phys Ther 44:163, 1964.

65. Balogun, JA, et al: Inter- and intratester reliability of measuring neck motions with tape measure and Myrin Gravity-Reference Goniometer. J Orthop Sports Phys Ther 10:248, 1989.

66. Capuano-Pucci, D, et al: Intratester and intertester reliability of the cervical range of motion. Arch Phys Med Rehabil 72:338, 1991.

67. LaStayo, PC, and Wheeler, DL: Reliability of passive wrist flexion and extension goniometric measurements: A multicenter study. Phys Ther 74:162, 1994.

68. Mayer, TG, et al: Spinal range of motion. Spine 22:1976, 1997.

69. Cobe, HM: The range of active motion at the wrist of white adults. J Bone Joint Surg Br 10:763, 1928.

70. Hewitt, D: The range of active motion at the wrist of women. J Bone Joint Surg Br 10:775, 1928.

71. Palmer, ML, and Epler, M: Clinical Assessment Procedures in Physical Therapy, ed 2. JB Lippincott, Philadelphia, 1998.

72. Clarkson, HM: Musculoskeletal Assessment: Joint Range of Motion and Manual Muscle Strength, ed 2. Williams & Wilkins, Baltimore, 2000.

73. Robson, P: A method to reduce the variable error in joint range measurement. Ann Phys Med 8:262, 1966.

74. Goodwin, J, et al: Clinical methods of goniometry: A comparative study. Disabil Rehabil 14:10, 1992.

75. Petherick, M, et al: Concurrent validity and intertester reliability of universal and fluid-based goniometers for active elbow range of motion. Phys Ther 68:966, 1988.

76. Brown, A, et al: Validity and reliability of the Dexter hand evaluation and therapy system in hand-injured patients. J Hand Ther 13:37, 2000.

77. Weiss, PL, et al: Using the Exos Handmaster to measure digital range of motion: Reliability and validity. Med Eng Phys 16:323, 1994.

78. Clapper, MP, and Wolf, SL: Comparison of the reliability of the Orthoranger and the standard goniometer for assessing active lower extremity range of motion. Phys Ther 68:214, 1988.

79. Ellison, JB, Rose, SJ, and Sahrman, SA: Patterns of hip rotation: A comparison between healthy subjects and patients with low back pain. Phys Ther 70:537, 1990.

80. Rheault, W, et al: Intertester reliability and concurrent validity of fluid-based and universal goniometers for active knee flexion. Phys Ther 68:1676, 1988.

81. Bartholomy, JK, Chandler, RF, and Kaplan, SE: Validity analysis of fluid goniometer measurements of knee flexion [abstract]. Phys Ther 80:S46, 2000.

82. Rome, K, and Cowieson, F: A reliability study of the universal goniometer, fluid goniometer, and electrogoniometer for the measurement of ankle dorsiflexion. Foot Ankle Int 17:28, 1996.

83. White, DJ, et al: Reliability of three methods of measuring cervical motion [abstract]. Phys Ther 66:771, 1986.

84. Reynolds, PMG: Measurement of spinal mobility: A comparison of three methods. Rheumatol Rehabil 14:180, 1975.

85. Miller, MH, et al: Measurement of spinal mobility in the sagittal plane: New skin distraction technique compared with established methods. J Rheumatol 11:4, 1984.

86. Gill, K, et al: Repeatability of four clinical methods for assessment of lumbar spinal motion. Spine 13:50, 1988.

87. Lindahl, O: Determination of the sagittal mobility of the lumbar spine. Acta Orthop Scand 37:241, 1966.

88. White, DJ, et al: Reliability of three clinical methods of measuring lateral flexion in the thoracolumbar pine [abstract]. Phys Ther 67:759, 1987.

89. Mayer, RS, et al: Variance in the measurement of sagittal lumbar range of motion among examiners, subjects, and instruments. Spine 20:1489, 1995.

90. Chen, SP, et al: Reliability of the lumbar sagittal motion measurement methods: Surface inclinometers. J Occup Environ Med 39:217, 1997.

91. Breum, J, Wilberg, J, and Bolton, JE: Reliability and concurrent validity of the BROM II for measuring lumbar mobility. J Manipulative Physiol Ther 18:497, 1995.

92. Colton, T: Statistics in Medicine. Little, Brown, Boston, 1974.

93. Dawson-Saunders, B, and Trapp, RG: Basic and Clinical Biostatistics. Appleton & Lange, Norwalk, CT, 1990.

94. Francis, K: Computer communication: Reliability. Phys Ther 66:1140, 1986.

95. Blesh, TE: Measurement in Physical Education, ed 2. Ronald Press, New York, 1974. Cited by Currier, DP: Elements of Research in Physical Therapy, ed 3. Williams & Wilkins, Baltimore, 1990.

96. Bland, JM, and Altman, DG: Measurement error and correlation coefficients [statistics notes]. BMJ 313:41, 1996.

97. Lahey, MA, Downey, RG, and Saal, FE: Intraclass correlations: There's more there than meets the eye. Psychol Bull 93:586, 1983.

98. Shout, PE, and Fleiss, JL: Intraclass correlations: Uses in assessing rater reliability. Psychol Bull 86:420, 1979.

99. Krebs, DE: Computer communication: Intraclass correlation coefficients. Phys Ther 64:1581, 1984.

100. Stratford, P: Reliability: Consistency or differentiating among subjects? [letters to the editor]. Phys Ther 69:299, 1989.

101. Bland, JM, and Altman, DG: Measurement error [statistics notes]. BMJ 312:1654, 1996.

102. DuBois, PH: An Introduction to Psychological Statistics. Harper & Row, New York, 1965, p 401.

103. Stratford, P: Use of the standard error as a reliability index of interest: An applied example using elbow flexor strength data. Phys Ther 77:745, 1997.

104. Eliasziw, M, et al: Statistical methodology for the concurrent assessment of interrater and intrarater reliability: Using goniometric measurement as an example. Phys Ther 74:777, 1994.

105. Bartko, JJ: Rationale for reporting standard deviations rather than standard errors of the mean. Am J Psychiatry 142:1060, 1985.

UPPER-EXTREMITY TESTING

OBJECTIVES

OBJECTIVES

ON COMPLETION OF PART II, THE READER WILL BE ABLE TO:

1. **Identify:**
   - Appropriate planes and axes for each upper-extremity joint motion
   - Structures that limit the end of the range of motion
   - Expected normal end-feels

2. **Describe:**
   - Testing positions used for each upper-extremity joint motion and muscle length test
   - Goniometer alignment
   - Capsular pattern of restricted motion
   - Range of motion necessary for selected functional activities

3. **Explain:**
   - How age, gender, and other factors can affect the range of motion
   - How sources of error in measurement can affect testing results

4. **Perform a goniometric measurement of any upper-extremity joint including:**
   - A clear explanation of the testing procedure
   - Proper positioning of the subject

- Adequate stabilization of the proximal joint component
- Correct determination of the end of the range of motion
- Correct identification of the end-feel
- Palpation of the appropriate bony landmarks
- Accurate alignment of the goniometer and correct reading and recording

5. **Plan goniometric measurements of the shoulder, elbow, wrist, and hand that are organized by body position.**

6. **Assess intratester and intertester reliability of goniometric measurements of the upper-extremity joints using methods described in Chapter 3.**

7. **Perform tests of muscle length at the shoulder, elbow, wrist, and hand including:**
   - A clear explanation of the testing procedure
   - Proper positioning of the subject in the starting position
   - Adequate stabilization
   - Use of appropriate testing motion
   - Correct identification of the end-feel
   - Accurate alignment of the goniometer and correct reading and recording

The testing positions, stabilization techniques, end-feels, and goniometer alignment for the joints of the upper extremities are presented in Chapters 4 through 7. The goniometric evaluation should follow the 12-step sequence presented in Exercise 5 in Chapter 2.

Chapter 4

The Shoulder

○ Structure and Function

Glenohumeral Joint

Anatomy

The glenohumeral joint is a synovial ball-and-socket joint. The ball is the convex head of the humerus, which faces medially, superiorly, and posteriorly with respect to the shaft of the humerus (Fig. 4.1).[1,2] The socket is formed by the concave glenoid fossa of the scapula and faces laterally, superiorly, and anteriorly. The socket is shallow and smaller than the humeral head but is deepened and enlarged by the fibrocartilaginous glenoid labrum. The joint capsule is thin and lax, blends with the glenoid labrum, and is reinforced by the tendons of the rotator cuff muscles and by the glenohumeral (superior, middle, inferior) and coracohumeral ligaments (Fig. 4.2).

Osteokinematics

The glenohumeral joint has 3 degrees of freedom. The motions permitted at the joint are flexion–extension, abduction–adduction, and medial–lateral rotation.[1,2] In addition, horizontal abduction and horizontal adduction are functional motions performed at the level of the shoulder and are created by combining abduction and extension, and adduction and flexion, respectively. Full range of motion (ROM) of the shoulder requires humeral, scapular, and clavicular motion at the glenohumeral, sternoclavicular, acromioclavicular, and scapulothoracic joints.

Arthrokinematics

Motion at the glenohumeral joint occurs as a rolling and sliding of the head of the humerus on the glenoid fossa. The convex joint surface of the head of the humerus slides in the opposite direction and rolls in the same direction as the osteokinematic movements of the shaft of the humerus.[2,3] The sliding motions help to maintain contact between the head of the humerus and the glenoid fossa of the scapular during the rolling motions and reduce translational movement of the axis of rotation in the humerus. During abduction the surface of the humeral head slides inferiorly while rolling superiorly.[2–5] The opposite motions occur during adduction. In medial rotation and flexion, the surface of the humeral head slides posteriorly and rolls anteriorly.[4,5] In lateral rotation and extension, the surface of the humeral head slides anteriorly and rolls posteriorly on the glenoid fossa.[4,5] Arthrokinematic motions during flexion and extension have also been described as a spin.[3]

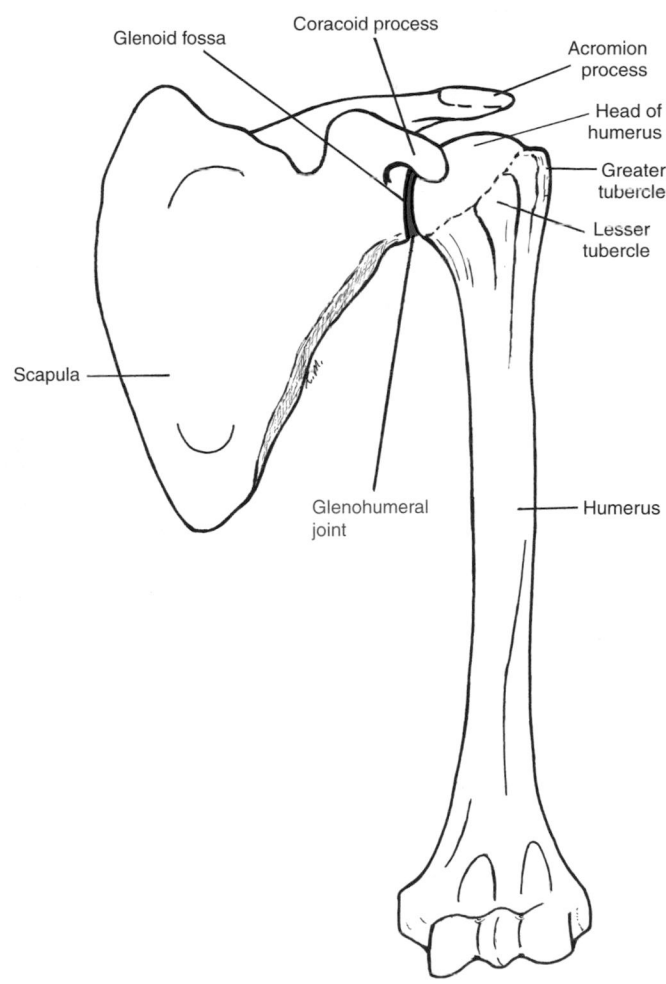

FIGURE 4.1 An anterior view of the left glenohumeral joint.

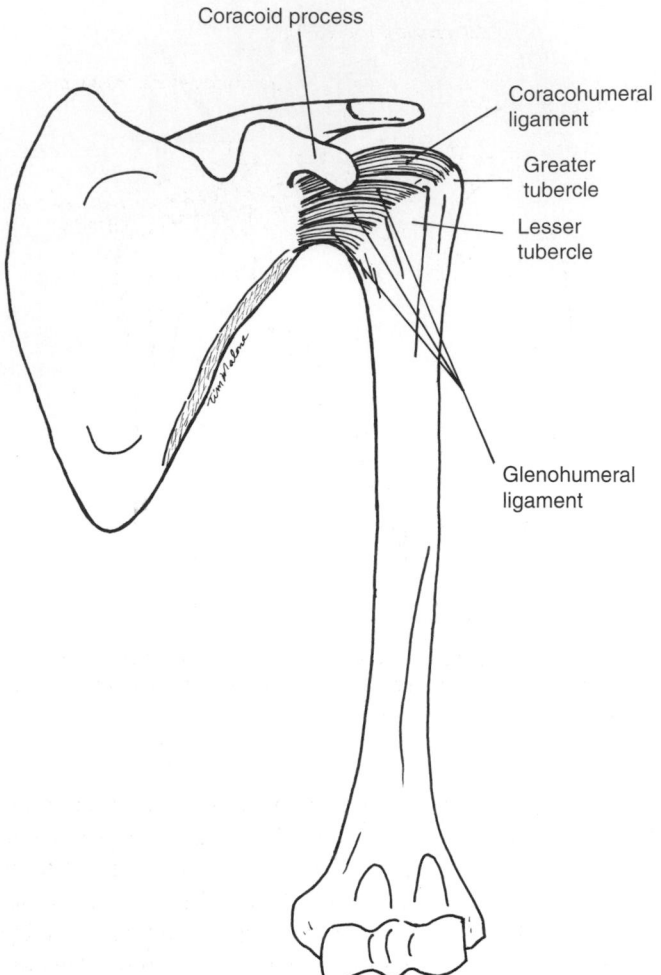

FIGURE 4.2 An anterior view of the left glenohumeral joint showing the coracohumeral and glenohumeral ligaments.

Capsular Pattern

The greatest restriction of passive motion is in lateral rotation, followed by some restriction in abduction and less restriction in medial rotation.[5,6]

Sternoclavicular Joint

Anatomy

The sternoclavicular (SC) joint is a synovial joint linking the medial end of the clavicle with the sternum and the cartilage of the first rib (Fig. 4.3A). The joint surfaces are saddle-shaped.[1,2] The clavicular joint surface is convex cephalocaudally and concave anteroposteriorly. The opposing joint surface, located at the notch formed by the manubrium of the sternum and the first costal cartilage, is concave cephalocaudally and convex anteroposteriorly. An articular disc divides the joint into two separate compartments.

The associated joint capsule is strong and reinforced by anterior and posterior sternoclavicular ligaments (Fig. 4.3B). These ligaments limit anterior–posterior movement of the medial end of the clavicle. The costoclavicular ligament, which extends from the inferior surface of the medial end of the clavicle to the first rib, limits clavicular elevation and

protraction. The interclavicular ligament extends from one clavicle to another and limits excessive inferior movement of the clavicle.[7]

Osteokinematics

The SC joint has 3 degrees of freedom, and motion consists of movement of the clavicle on the sternum. These motions are described by the movement at the lateral end of the clavicle. Clavicular motions include elevation–depression, protraction–retraction, and anterior–posterior rotation.[2,7]

Arthrokinematics

During clavicular elevation and depression, the convex portion of the joint surface of the clavicle slides on the concave manubrium in the opposite direction and rolls in the same direction as movement of the lateral end of the clavicle.[2–5] In protraction and retraction, the concave portion of the clavicular joint surface slides and rolls on the convex surface of the manubrium in the same direction as the lateral end of the clavicle.[2–5] In rotation, the clavicular joint surface spins on the opposing joint surface. In summary, the clavicle slides inferiorly in elevation, superiorly in depression, anteriorly in protraction, and posteriorly in retraction.

Acromioclavicular Joint

Anatomy

The acromioclavicular (AC) joint is a synovial joint linking the scapula and the clavicle. The scapular joint surface is a

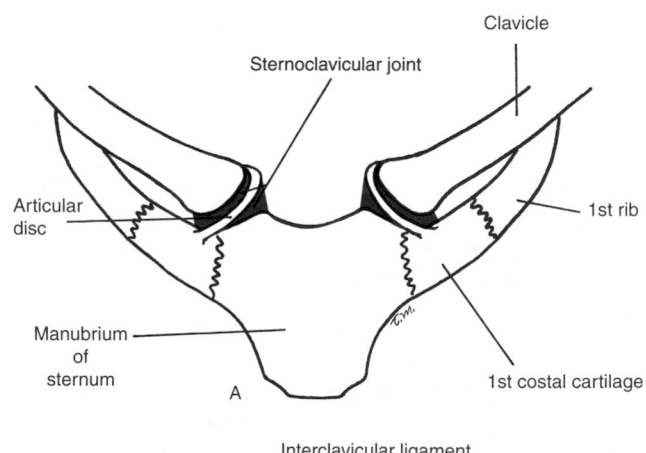

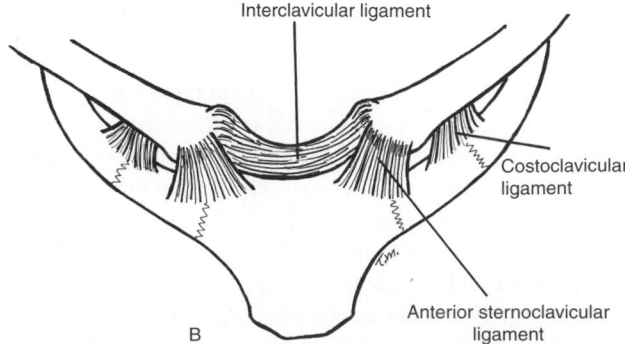

FIGURE 4.3 **(A)** An anterior view of the sternoclavicular joint showing the bone structures and articular disc. **(B)** An anterior view of the SC joint showing the interclavicular, sternoclavicular, and costoclavicular ligaments.

shallow concave facet located on the medial aspect of the acromion of the scapula (Fig. 4.4).[4,5] The clavicular joint surface is a slightly convex facet located on the lateral end of the clavicle. However, in some individuals the joint surfaces may be flat or the reverse pattern of convex–concave shapes.[1] The joint contains a fibrocartilaginous disc and is surrounded by a weak joint capsule. The superior and inferior acromioclavicular ligaments reinforce the capsule (Fig. 4.5). The coracoclavicular ligament, which extends between the clavicle and the scapular coracoid process, provides additional stability.

Osteokinematics

The AC joint has 3 degrees of freedom and permits movement of the scapula on the clavicle in three planes.[2] Numerous terms have been used to describe these motions. **Tilting** (tipping) is movement of the scapula in the sagittal plane around a coronal axis. During anterior tilting the superior border of the scapula and glenoid fossa move anteriorly, whereas the inferior angle moves posteriorly. During posterior tilting (tipping) the superior border of the scapula and glenoid fossa move posteriorly, whereas the inferior angle moves anteriorly.

Upward and **downward rotations** of the scapula occur in the frontal plane around an anterior–posterior axis. During upward rotation the glenoid fossa moves cranially, whereas during downward rotation the glenoid fossa moves caudally.

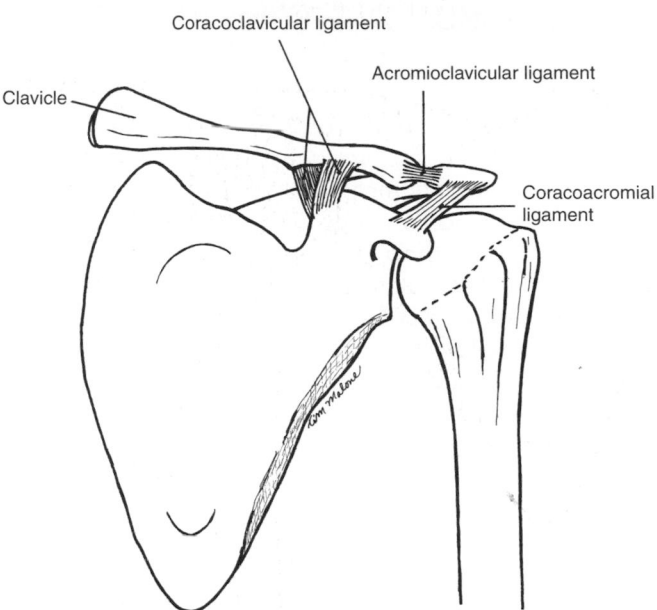

FIGURE 4.5 An anterior view of the left acromioclavicular joint showing the coracoclavicular, acromioclavicular, and coracoacromial ligaments.

Protraction and **retraction** of the scapula occur in the transverse plane around a vertical axis. During protraction (also termed medial rotation, or winging) the glenoid fossa moves medially and anteriorly, whereas the vertebral border of the scapula moves away from the spine. During retraction (also termed lateral rotation) the glenoid fossa moves laterally and posteriorly, whereas the vertebral border of the scapula moves toward the spine. The terms abduction–adduction have been used by various authors to indicate the motions of upward rotation–downward rotation as well as protraction–retraction.[5,7]

Arthrokinematics

If the acromial facet is concave in shape, the acromial facet will slide and roll on the lateral end of the clavicle in the same direction as osteokinematic movement of the scapula.[5]

Scapulothoracic Joint

Anatomy

The scapulothoracic joint is considered to be a functional rather than an anatomical joint. The joint surfaces are the anterior surface of the scapula and the posterior surface of the thorax.

Osteokinematics

The motions that occur at the scapulothoracic joint are caused by the independent or combined motions of the sternoclavicular and acromioclavicular joints. These motions include scapular elevation–depression, upward–downward rotation, anterior–posterior tilting, protraction–retraction, and medial–lateral rotation.[1,2]

Arthrokinematics

Motion consists of a sliding of the scapula on the thorax.

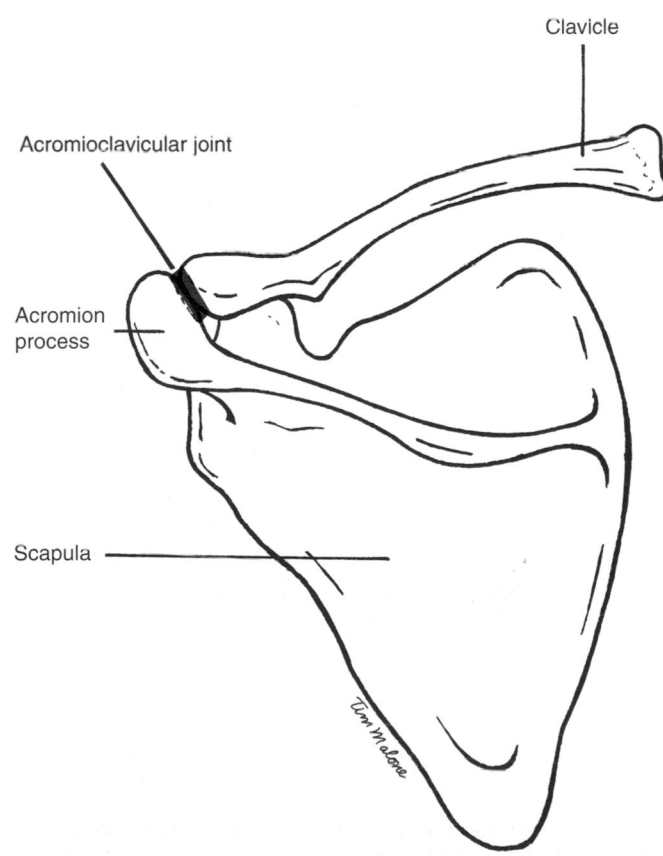

FIGURE 4.4 A posterior–superior view of the left acromioclavicular joint.

60 PART II ● Upper-Extremity Testing

RANGE OF MOTION TESTING PROCEDURES: Shoulder

Full ROM of the shoulder requires movement at the glenohumeral, SC, AC, and scapulothoracic joints. To make measurements more informative, we suggest using two methods of measuring the ROM of the shoulder. One method measures passive motion primarily at the glenohumeral joint. The other method measures passive ROM at all the joints included in the shoulder complex.

We have found the method that measures primarily glenohumeral motion is helpful in identifying glenohumeral joint problems within the shoulder complex. The ability to differentiate and quantify ROM at the glenohumeral joint from other joints in the shoulder complex is important in diagnosing and treating many shoulder conditions. This method of measuring glenohumeral motion requires the use of passive motion and careful stabilization of the scapula. Active motion is avoided because it results in synchronous motion throughout the shoulder complex, making isolation of glenohumeral motion difficult. Certain studies have begun establishing some normative values (Table 4.2 in Research Findings) and assessing the reliability of this glenohumeral measurement method.

The second method measures full motion of the shoulder complex and is useful in evaluating the functional ROM of the shoulder. This more traditional method of assessing shoulder motion incorporates the stabilization of the thoracic spine and rib cage. Tissue resistance to further motion is typically due to the stretch of structures connecting the clavicle to the sternum, and the scapula to the ribs and spine. ROM values for shoulder complex motion are presented in Tables 4.1, 4.3, and 4.4 in Research Findings. Both methods of measuring the ROM of the shoulder are presented in the following discussions of stabilization techniques and end-feels. However, the alignment of the goniometer is the same for measuring glenohumeral and shoulder complex motions.

Landmarks for Testing Procedure

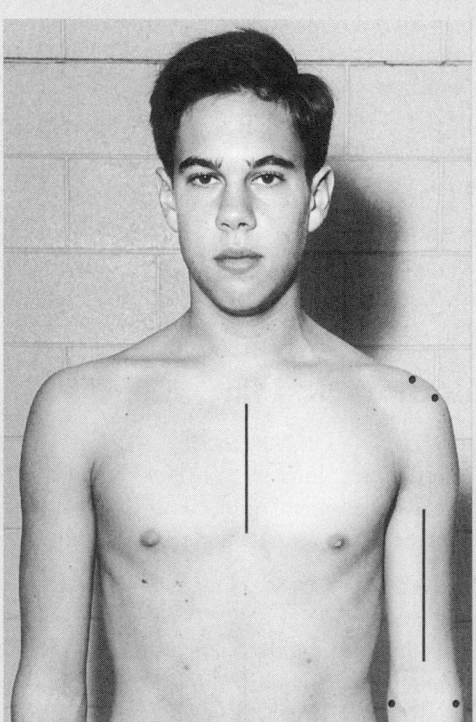

FIGURE 4.6 An anterior view of the humerus, clavicle, sternum, and scapula showing surface anatomy landmarks for aligning the goniometer.

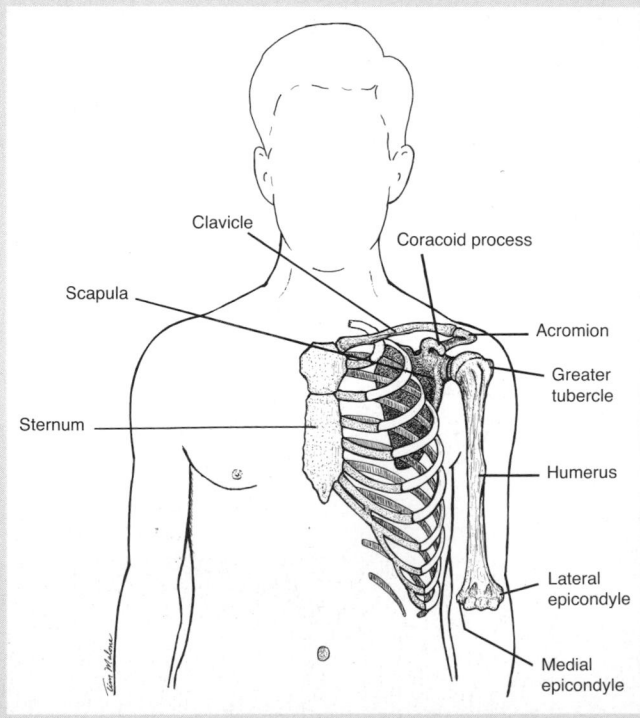

FIGURE 4.7 An anterior view of the humerus, clavicle, sternum, and scapula showing bony anatomical landmarks for aligning the goniometer.

Landmarks for Testing Procedure (continued)

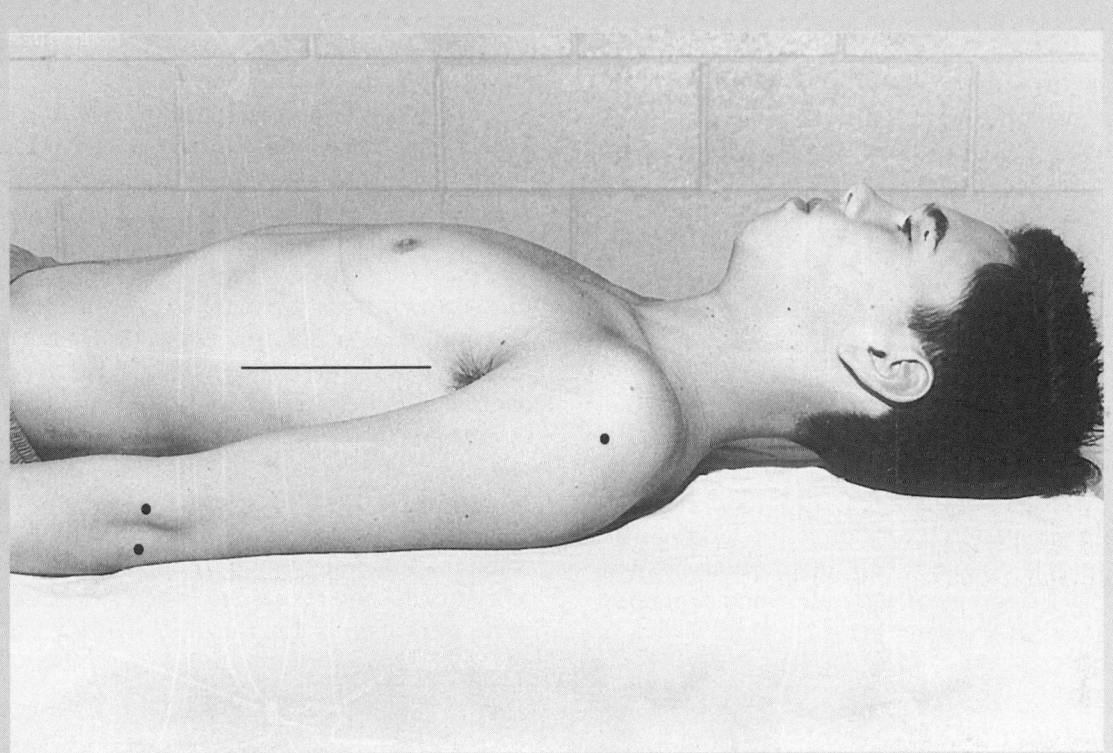

FIGURE 4.8 A lateral view of the upper arm showing surface anatomy landmarks for aligning the goniometer.

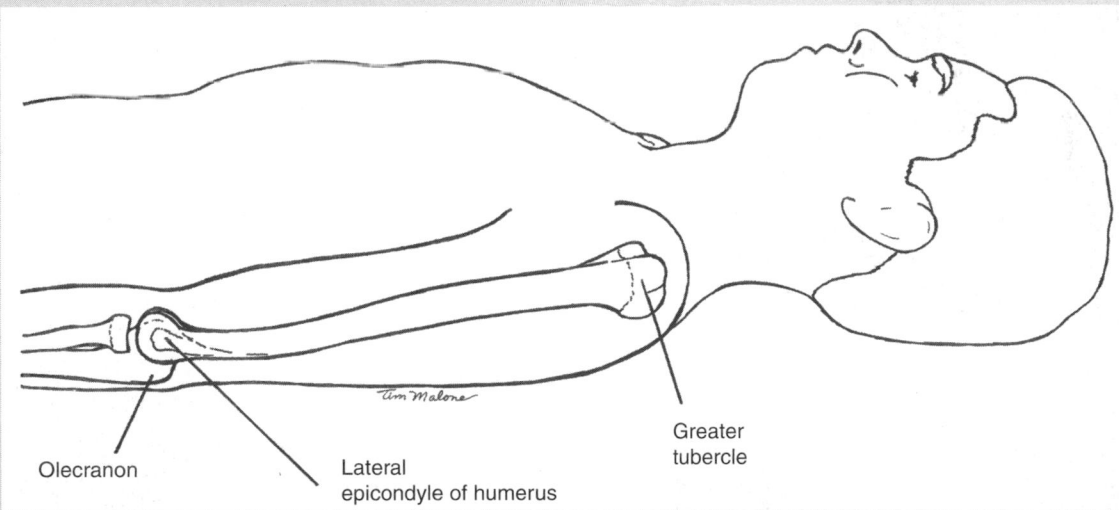

Olecranon

Lateral
epicondyle of humerus

Greater
tubercle

FIGURE 4.9 A lateral view of the upper arm showing bony anatomical landmarks for aligning the goniometer.

● FLEXION

Motion occurs in the sagittal plane around a medial–lateral axis. Normal shoulder complex flexion ROM for adults is 180 degrees according to the American Academy of Orthopaedic Surgeons (AAOS),[8,9] 180 degrees according to the American Medical Association (AMA),[10] and 165 degrees according to Boone and Azen.[11] Normal glenohumeral flexion ROM for adults is 106 degrees according to Lannan, Lehman, and Toland[12] and 97 degrees according to Rundquist and coworkers[13] for a small sample of older subjects. See Tables 4.1 to 4.4 in Research Findings for additional normal ROM values by age and gender.

Testing Position

Place the subject supine, with the knees flexed to flatten the lumbar spine. Position the shoulder in 0 degrees of abduction, adduction, and rotation. Place the elbow in extension so that tension in the long head of the triceps muscle does not limit the motion. Position the forearm in 0 degrees of supination and pronation so that the palm of the hand faces the body.

Stabilization
Glenohumeral Flexion
Stabilize the scapula to prevent posterior tilting, upward rotation, and elevation of the scapula.

Shoulder Complex Flexion
Stabilize the thorax to prevent extension of the spine and movement of the ribs. The weight of the trunk may assist stabilization.

Testing Motion
Flex the shoulder by lifting the humerus off the examining table, bringing the hand up over the subject's head. Maintain the extremity in neutral abduction and adduction during the motion. Slight rotation is allowed to occur as needed to attain maximal flexion.

Glenohumeral Flexion
The end of glenohumeral flexion ROM occurs when resistance to further motion is felt and attempts to overcome the resistance cause upward rotation, posterior tilting, or elevation of the scapula (Fig. 4.10).

Shoulder Complex Flexion
The end of shoulder complex flexion ROM occurs when resistance to further motion is felt and attempts to overcome the resistance cause extension of the spine or motion of the ribs (Fig. 4.11).

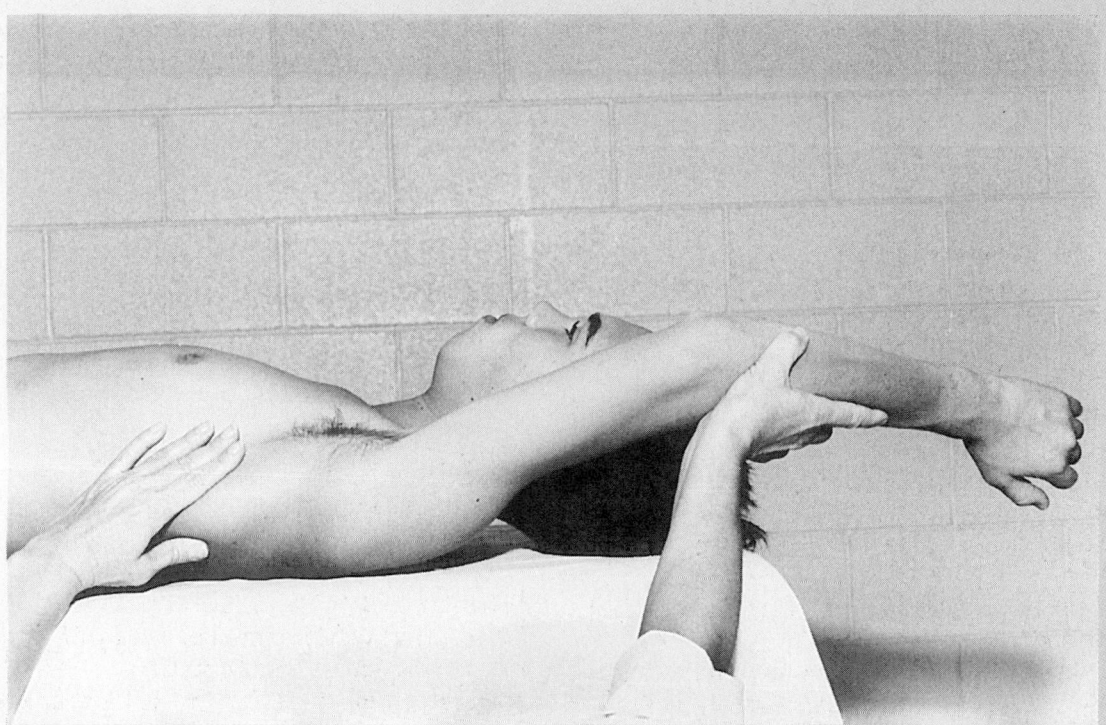

FIGURE 4.10 The end of glenohumeral flexion ROM. The examiner stabilizes the lateral border of the scapula with her hand. The examiner is able to determine that the end of the ROM has been reached because any attempt to move the extremity into additional flexion causes the lateral border of the scapula to move anteriorly and laterally.

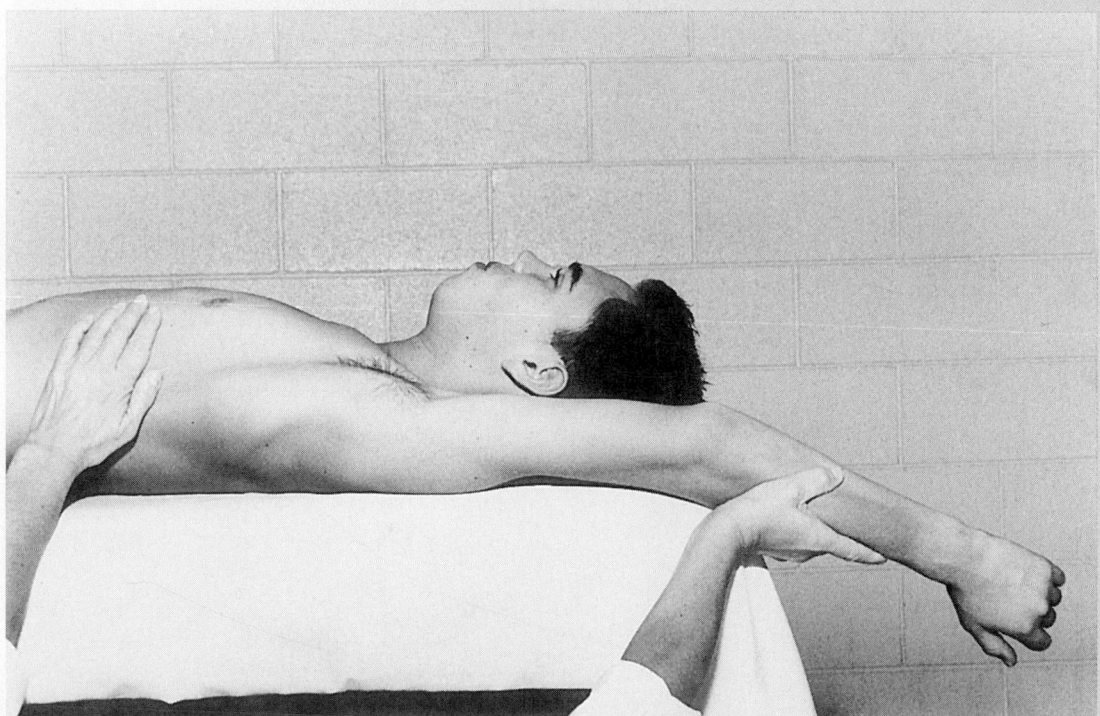

FIGURE 4.11 The end of shoulder complex flexion ROM. The examiner stabilizes the subject's trunk and ribs with her hand. The examiner is able to determine that the end of the ROM has been reached because any attempt to move the extremity into additional flexion causes extension of the spine and movement of the ribs.

Normal End-Feel
Glenohumeral Flexion
The end-feel is firm because of tension in the posterior band of the coracohumeral ligament; the posterior joint capsule; and the posterior deltoid, teres minor, teres major, and infraspinatus muscles.

Shoulder Complex Flexion
The end-feel is firm because of tension in the costoclavicular ligament and SC capsule and ligaments, and the latissimus dorsi, sternocostal fibers of the pectoralis major and pectoralis minor, and rhomboid major and minor muscles.

Goniometer Alignment
This goniometer alignment is used for measuring glenohumeral and shoulder complex flexion (Figs. 4.12 through 4.14).

1. Center **fulcrum** of the goniometer over the lateral aspect of the greater tubercle.
2. Align **proximal arm** parallel to the midaxillary line of the thorax.
3. Align **distal arm** with the lateral midline of the humerus. Depending on how much flexion and rotation occur, the lateral epicondyle of the humerus or the olecranon process of the ulnar may be helpful references.

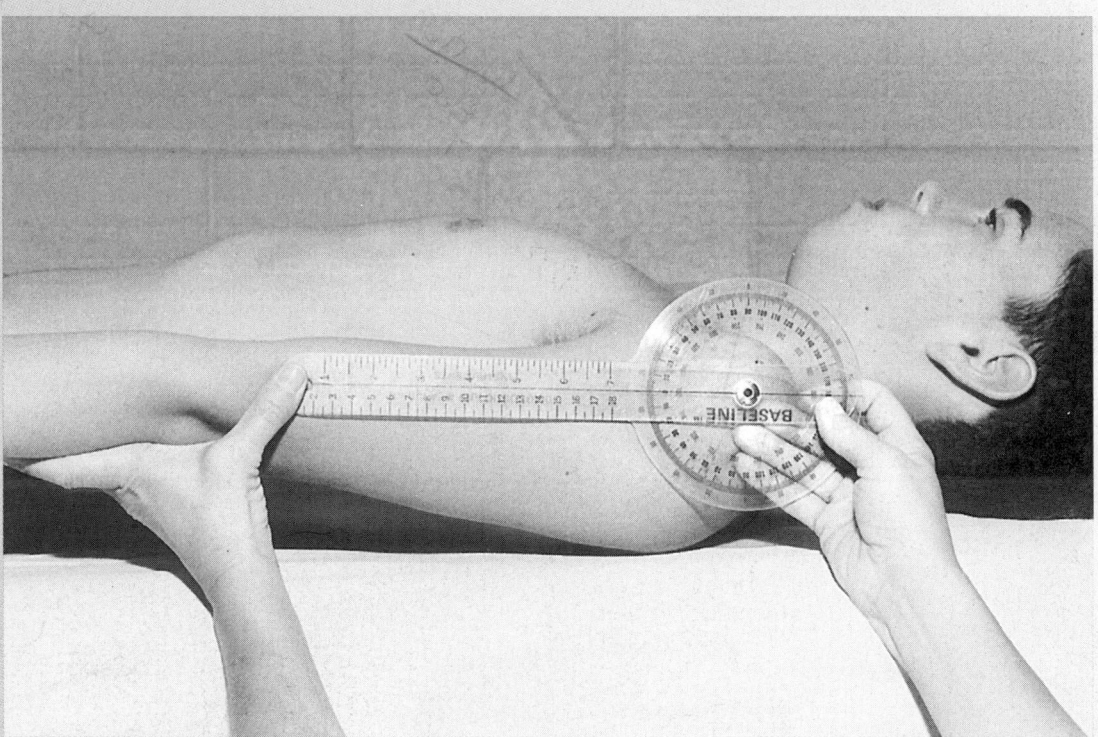

FIGURE 4.12 The alignment of the goniometer at the beginning of glenohumeral and shoulder complex flexion ROM.

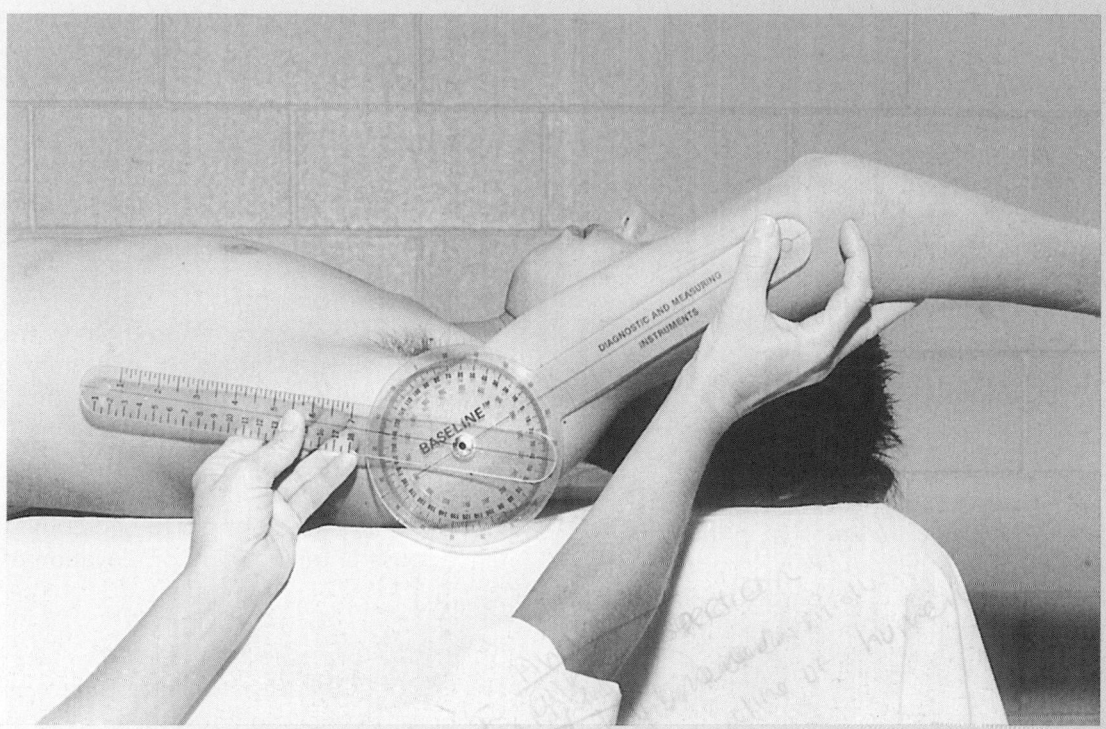

FIGURE 4.13 The alignment of the goniometer at the end of glenohumeral flexion ROM. The examiner's hand supports the subject's extremity and maintains the goniometer's distal arm in correct alignment over the lateral epicondyle. The examiner's other hand releases its stabilization and aligns the goniometer's proximal arm with the lateral midline of the thorax.

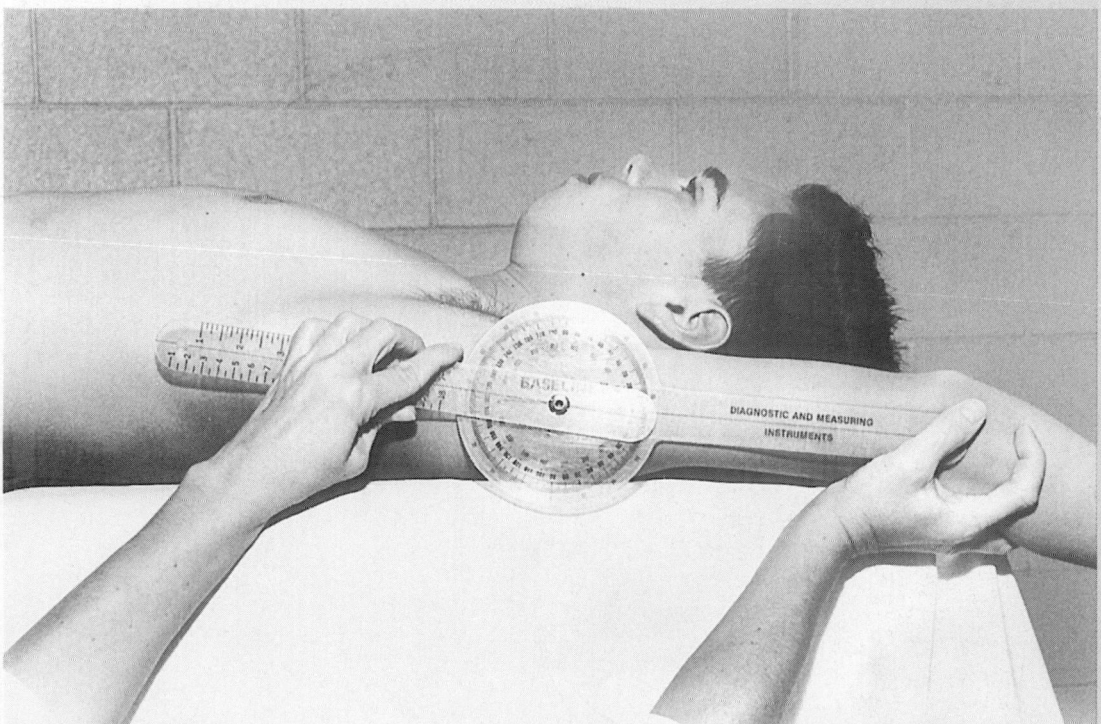

FIGURE 4.14 The alignment of the goniometer at the end of shoulder complex flexion ROM. More motion is noted during shoulder complex flexion than in glenohumeral flexion.

● EXTENSION

Motion occurs in the sagittal plane around a medial–lateral axis. Normal shoulder complex extension ROM for adults is 50 degrees according to the AMA,[10] 57 degrees according to Boone and Azen,[11] and 60 degrees according to the AAOS.[8] Normal glenohumeral extension ROM for adults is 20 degrees as cited by Lannan, Lehman, and Toland.[12] See Tables 4.1 to 4.4 in Research Findings for additional normal ROM values by age and gender.

Testing Position

Position the subject prone, with the face turned away from the shoulder being tested. A pillow is not used under the head. Place the shoulder in 0 degrees of abduction, adduction, and rotation. Position the elbow in slight flexion so that tension in the long head of the biceps brachii muscle will not restrict the motion. Place the forearm in 0 degrees of supination and pronation so that the palm of the hand faces the body.

Stabilization
Glenohumeral Extension

Stabilize the scapula at the inferior angle or at the acromion and coracoid processes to prevent elevation and anterior tilting (inferior angle moves posteriorly) of the scapula.

Shoulder Complex Extension

The examining table and the weight of the trunk stabilize the thorax to prevent forward flexion of the spine. The examiner can also stabilize the trunk to prevent rotation of the spine.

Testing Motion

Extend the shoulder by lifting the humerus off the examining table. Maintain the extremity in neutral abduction and adduction during the motion.

Glenohumeral Extension

The end of ROM occurs when resistance to further motion is felt and attempts to overcome the resistance cause anterior tilting or elevation of the scapula (Fig. 4.15).

Shoulder Complex Extension

The end of ROM occurs when resistance to further motion is felt and attempts to overcome the resistance cause forward flexion or rotation of the spine (Fig. 4.16).

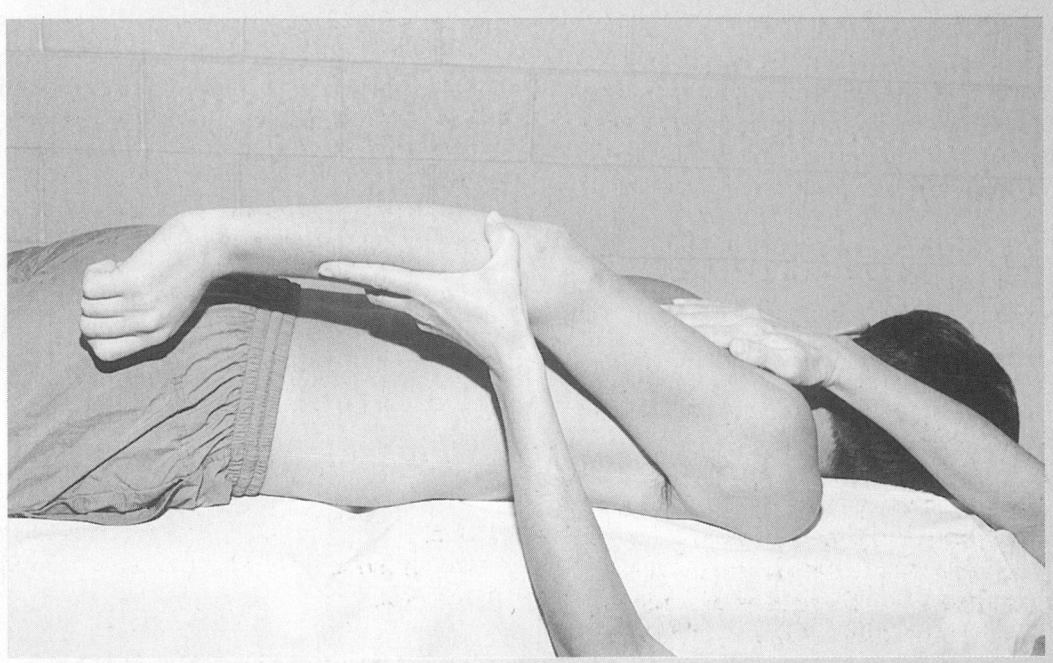

FIGURE 4.15 The end of glenohumeral extension ROM. The examiner is stabilizing the inferior angle of the scapula with her hand. The examiner is able to determine that the end of the ROM in extension has been reached because any attempt to move the humerus into additional extension causes the scapula to tilt anteriorly and to elevate, causing the inferior angle of the scapula to move posteriorly. Alternatively, the examiner may stabilize the acromion and coracoid processes of the scapula.

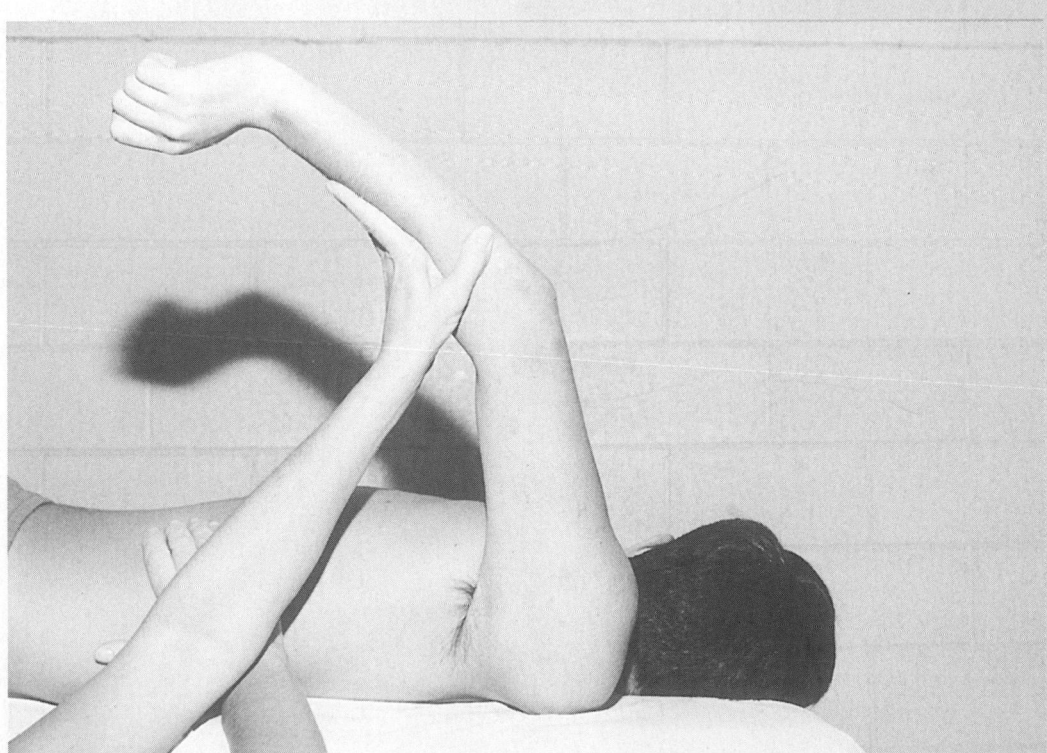

FIGURE 4.16 The end shoulder complex extension ROM. The examiner stabilizes the subject's trunk and ribs with her hand. The examiner is able to determine that the end of the ROM has been reached because any attempt to move the extremity into additional extension causes flexion and rotation of the spine.

Normal End-Feel
Glenohumeral Extension
The end-feel is firm because of tension in the anterior band of the coracohumeral ligament; anterior joint capsule; and clavicular fibers of the pectoralis major, coracobrachialis, and anterior deltoid muscles.

Shoulder Complex Extension
The end-feel is firm because of tension in the SC capsule and ligaments and in the serratus anterior muscle.

Goniometer Alignment
This goniometer alignment is used for measuring glenohumeral and shoulder complex extension (Figs. 4.17 to 4.19).

1. Center **fulcrum** of the goniometer over the lateral aspect of the greater tubercle.
2. Align **proximal arm** parallel to the midaxillary line of the thorax.
3. Align **distal arm** with the lateral midline of the humerus, using the lateral epicondyle of the humerus for reference.

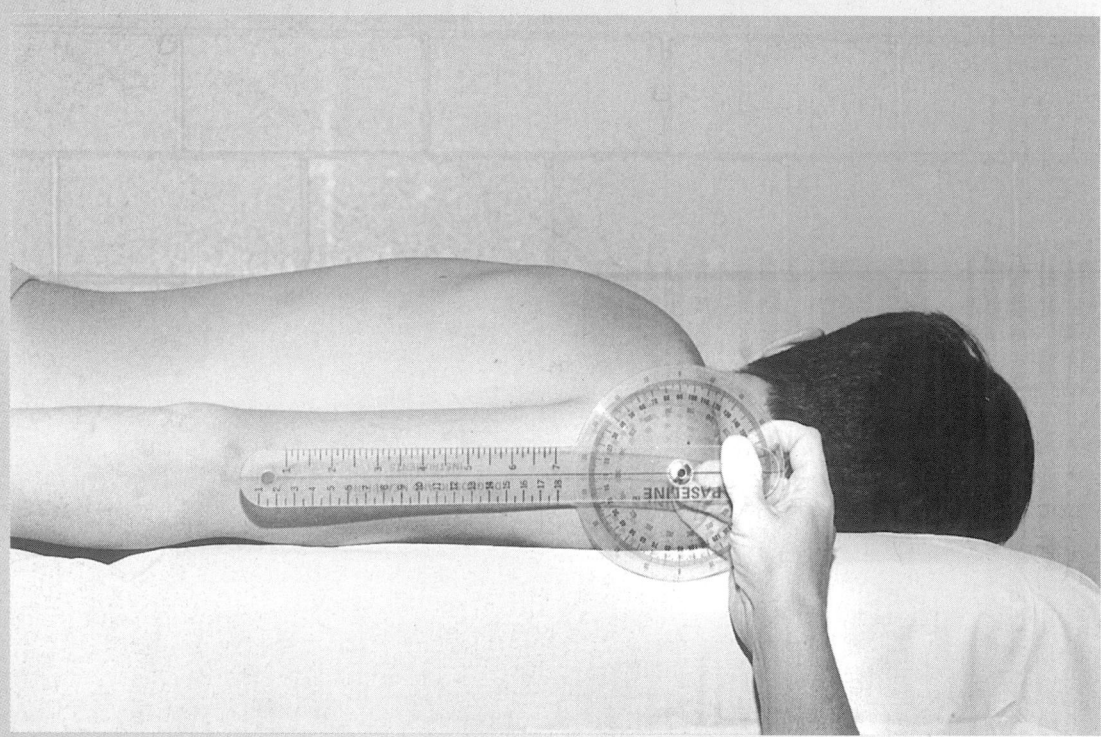

FIGURE 4.17 The alignment of the goniometer at the beginning of glenohumeral and shoulder complex extension ROM.

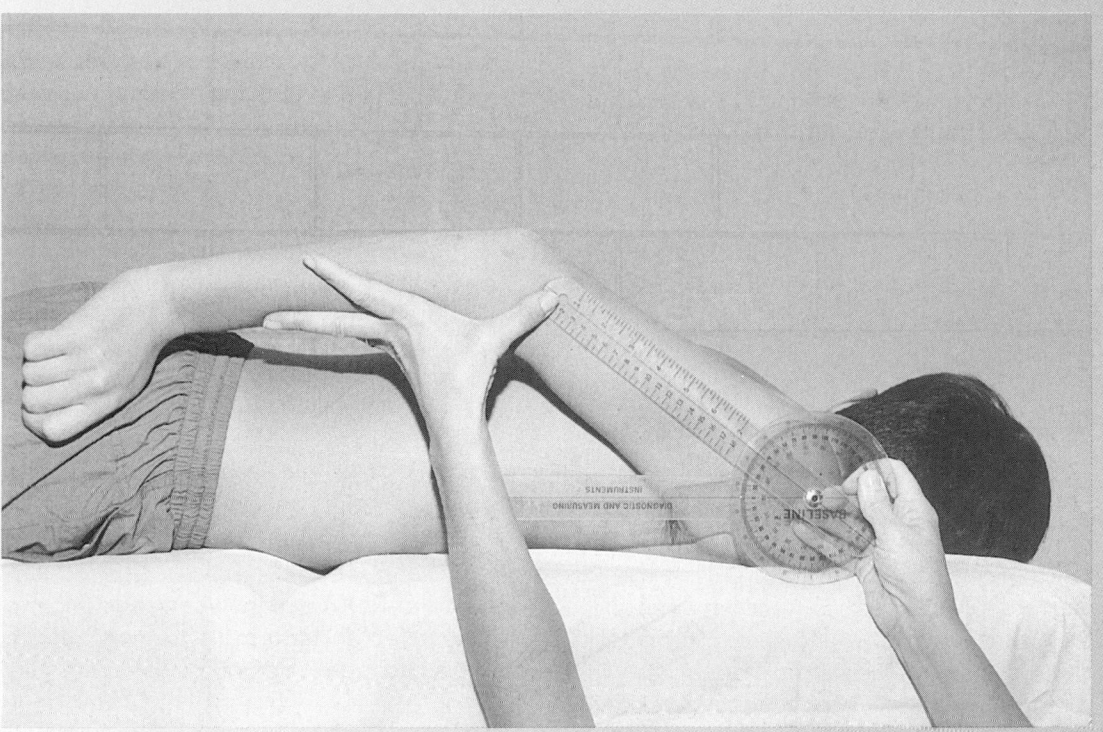

FIGURE 4.18 The alignment of the goniometer at the end of glenohumeral extension ROM. The examiner's left hand supports the subject's extremity and holds the distal arm of the goniometer in correct alignment over the lateral epicondyle of the humerus.

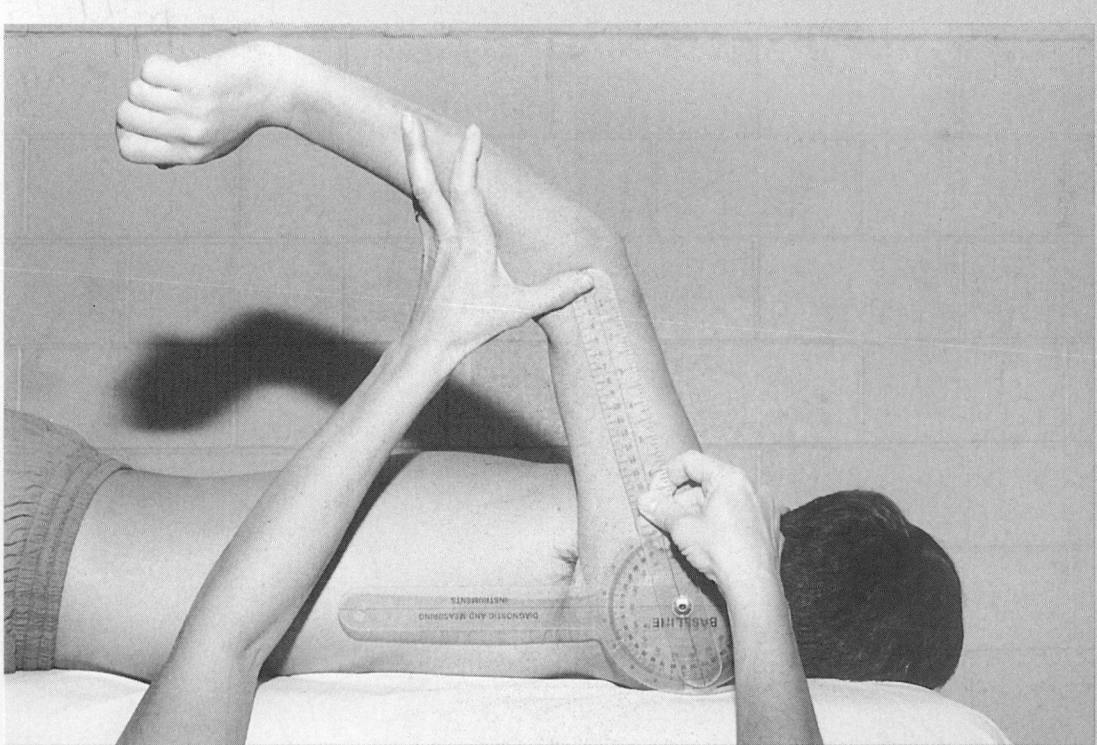

FIGURE 4.19 The alignment of the goniometer at the end of shoulder complex extension ROM. The examiner's hand that formerly stabilized the subject's trunk now positions the goniometer.

● ABDUCTION

Motion occurs in the frontal plane around an anterior–posterior axis. Normal shoulder complex abduction ROM for adults is 180 degrees according to the AAOS[8] and AMA[10] and 183 degrees according to Boone and Azen.[11] Normal glenohumeral abduction ROM for adults is 129 degrees as noted by Lannan, Lehman, and Toland,[12] 100 degrees according to Rundquist and coworkers[13] for a small sample of older subjects, and ranging from 90 to 120 degrees in Levangie and Norkin.[2] See Tables 4.1 to 4.4 in Research Findings for additional normal ROM values by age and gender.

Testing Position

Position the subject supine, with the shoulder in lateral rotation and 0 degrees of flexion and extension so that the palm of the hand faces anteriorly. If the humerus is not laterally rotated, contact between the greater tubercle of the humerus and the upper portion of the glenoid fossa or the acromion process will restrict the motion. The elbow should be extended so that tension in the long head of the triceps does not restrict the motion.

Stabilization
Glenohumeral Abduction

Stabilize the scapula to prevent upward rotation and elevation of the scapula.

Shoulder Complex Abduction

Stabilize the thorax to prevent lateral flexion of the spine. The weight of the trunk may assist stabilization.

Testing Motion

Abduct the shoulder by moving the humerus laterally away from the subject's trunk. Maintain the upper extremity in lateral rotation and neutral flexion and extension during the motion.

Glenohumeral Abduction

The end of ROM occurs when resistance to further motion is felt and attempts to overcome the resistance cause upward rotation or elevation of the scapula (Fig. 4.20).

Shoulder Complex Abduction

The end of ROM occurs when resistance to further motion is felt and attempts to overcome the resistance cause lateral flexion of the spine (Fig. 4.21).

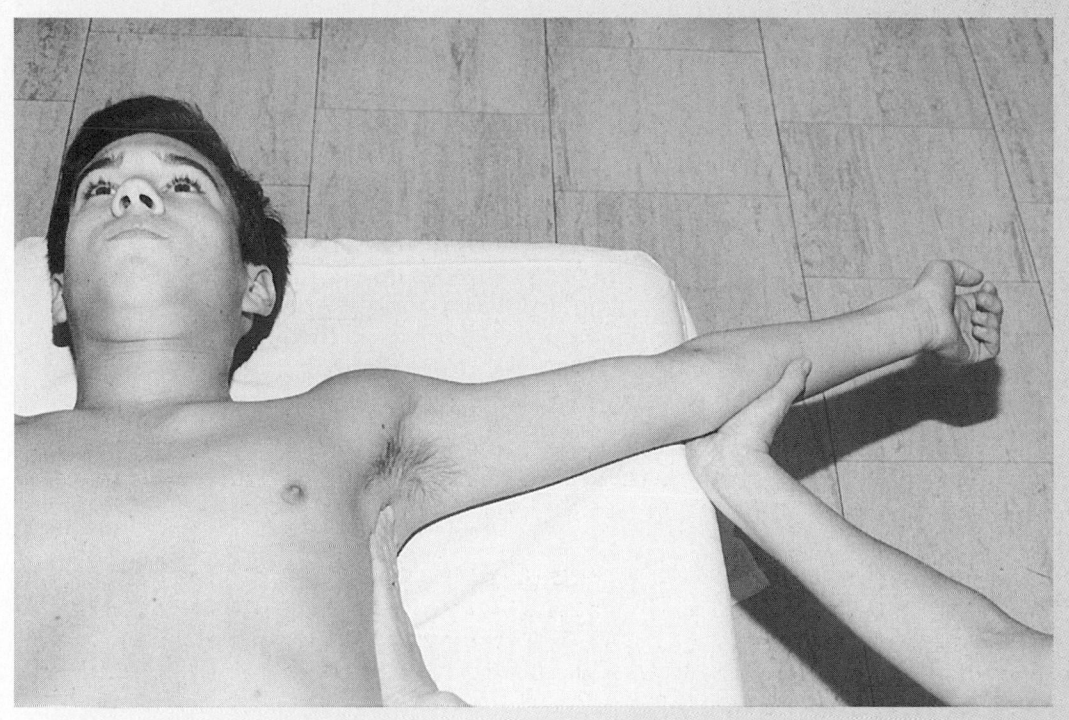

FIGURE 4.20 The end of the ROM of glenohumeral abduction. The examiner stabilizes the lateral border of the scapula with her hand to detect upward rotation of the scapula. Alternatively, the examiner may stabilize the acromion and coracoid processes of the scapula to detect elevation of the scapula.

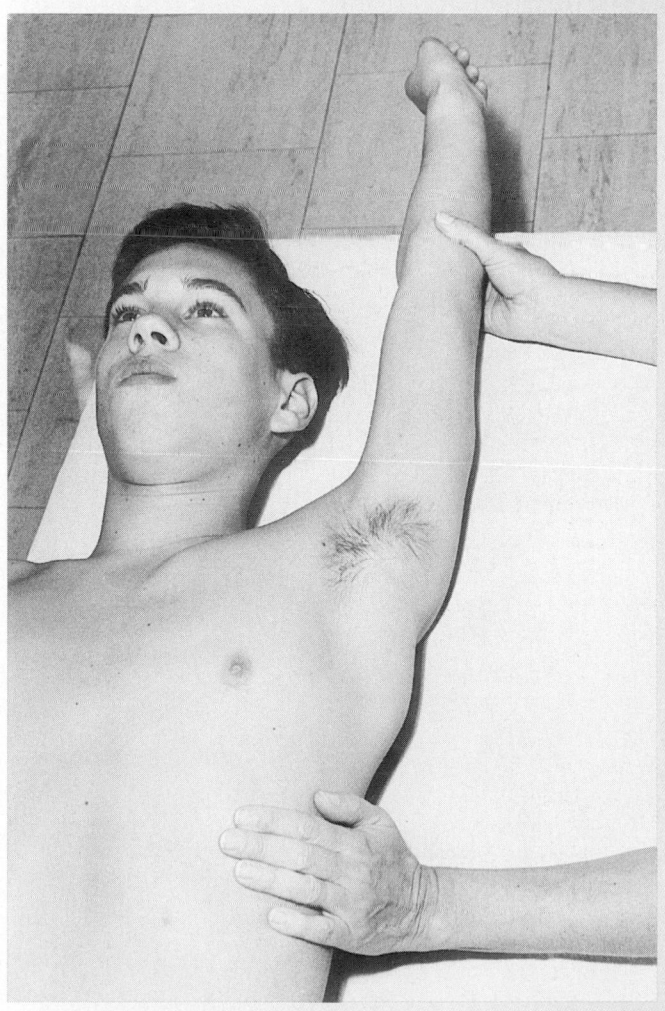

FIGURE 4.21 The end of the ROM of shoulder complex abduction. The examiner stabilizes the subject's trunk and ribs with her hand to detect lateral flexion of the spine and movement of the ribs.

Normal End-Feel

Glenohumeral Abduction

The end-feel is usually firm because of tension in the middle and inferior bands of the gleno- humeral ligament, inferior joint capsule, and the teres major and clavicular fibers of the pectoralis major muscles.

Shoulder Complex Abduction

The end-feel is firm because of tension in the costocla- vicular ligament; sternoclavicular capsule and ligaments; and latissimus dorsi, sternocostal fibers of the pectoralis major, and major and minor rhomboid muscles.

Goniometer Alignment

This goniometer alignment is used for measuring glenohumeral and shoulder complex abduction (Figs. 4.22 to 4.24).

1. Center **fulcrum** of the goniometer close to the anterior aspect of the acromial process.
2. Align **proximal arm** so that it is parallel to the mid- line of the anterior aspect of the sternum.
3. Align **distal arm** with the anterior midline of the humerus. Depending on the amount of abduction and lateral rotation that has occurred, the medial epicondyle may be a helpful reference.

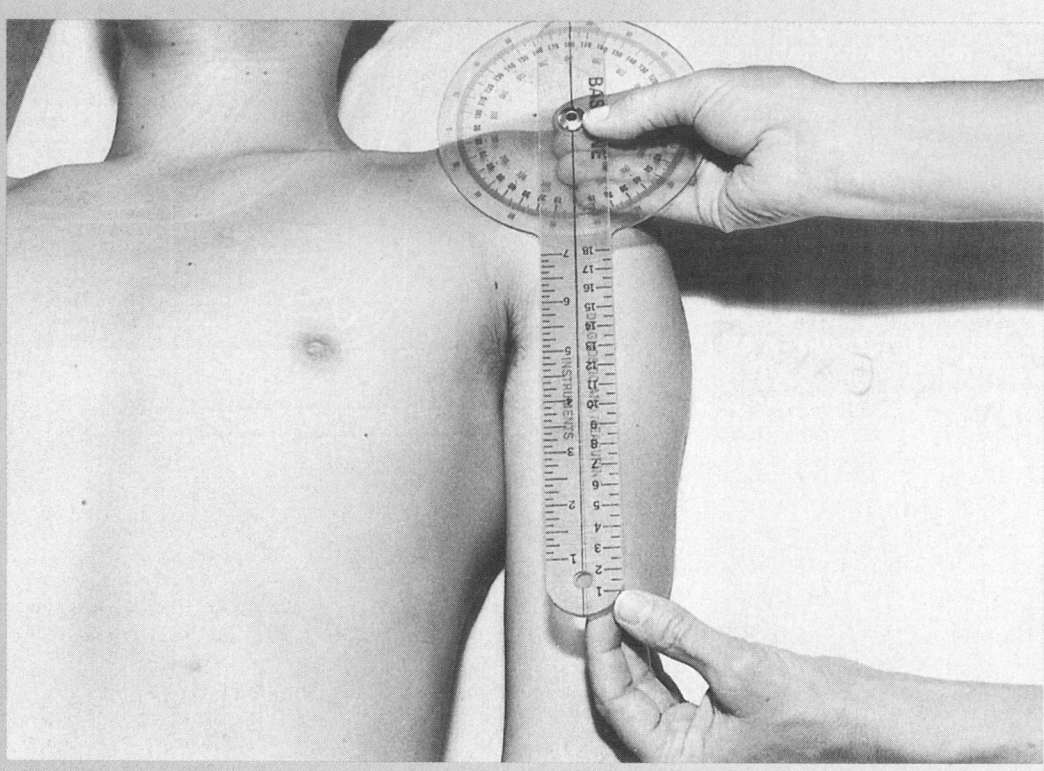

FIGURE 4.22 The align- ment of the goniometer at the beginning of gleno- humeral and shoulder complex abduction ROM.

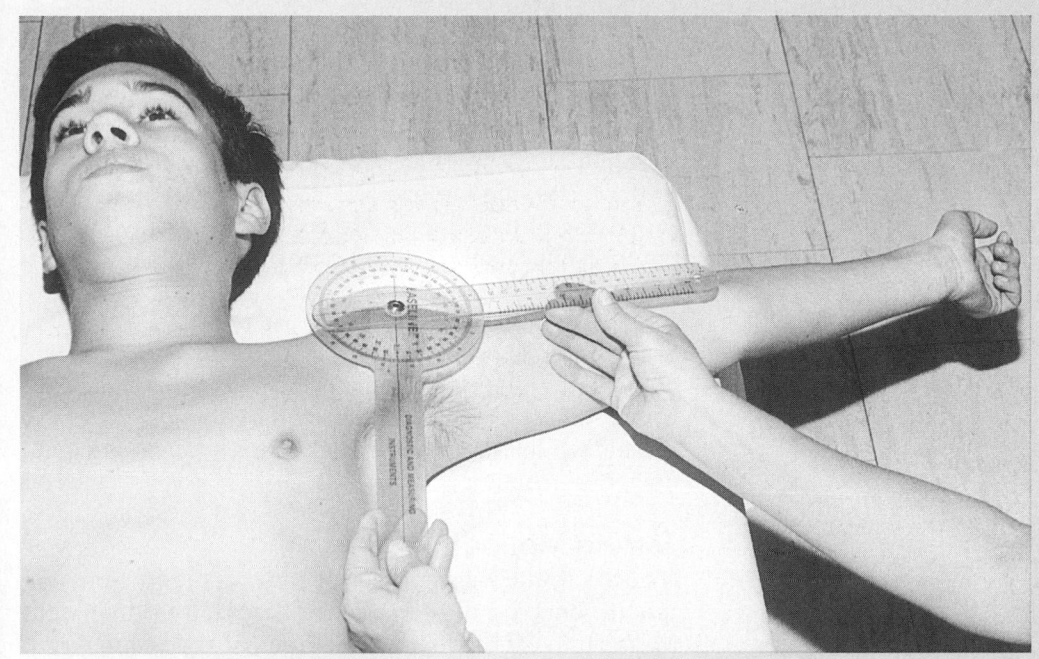

FIGURE 4.23 The alignment of the goniometer at the end of glenohumeral abduction ROM. The examining table or the examiner's hand can support the subject's extremity and align the goniometer's distal arm with the anterior midline of the humerus. The examiner's other hand has released its stabilization of the scapula and is holding the proximal arm of the goniometer parallel to the sternum.

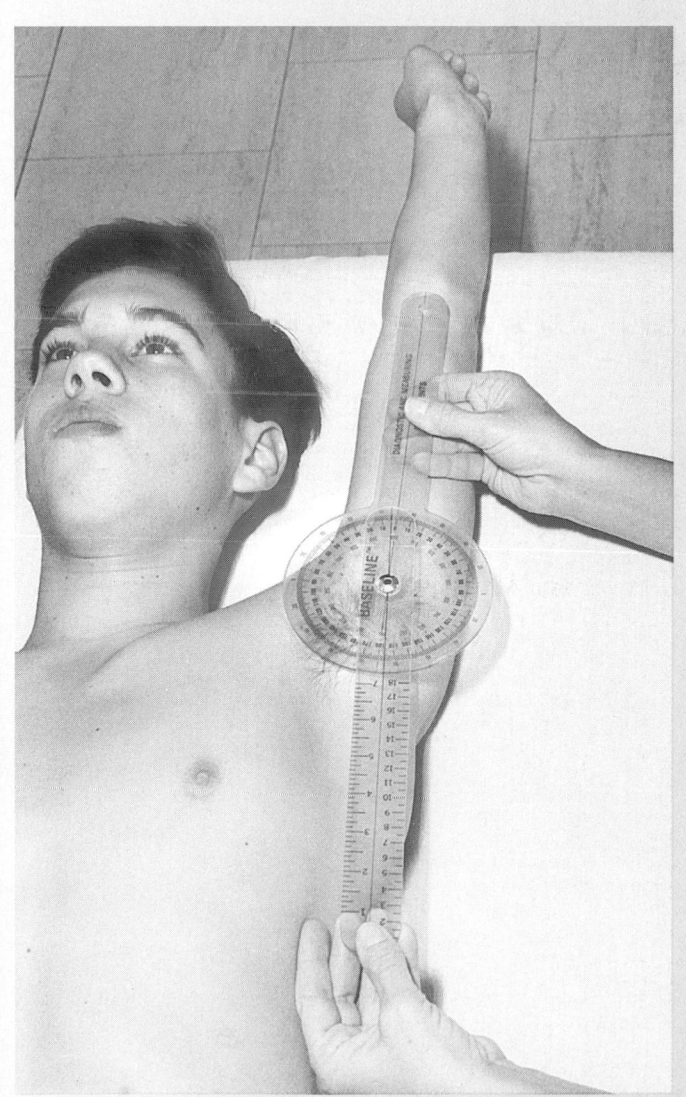

FIGURE 4.24 The alignment of the goniometer at the end of shoulder complex abduction ROM. The humerus has laterally rotated, and the medial epicondyle is now a helpful anatomical landmark for aligning the distal arm of the goniometer. Note that the placement of the stationary and moving arms of the goniometer with the proximal and distal joint segments have switched from that in Fig. 4.23, but both placements will give an accurate measurement of the angle at the end of motion.

● ADDUCTION

Motion occurs in the frontal plane around an anterior-posterior axis. Adduction is not usually measured and recorded because it is the return to the zero starting position from full abduction.

● MEDIAL (INTERNAL) ROTATION

When the subject is in anatomical position, the motion occurs in the transverse plane around a vertical axis. When the subject is in the testing position, the motion occurs in the sagittal plane around a medial-lateral (coronal) axis. Normal shoulder complex medial rotation for adults is 67 degrees according to Boone and Azen,[11] 70 degrees according to the AAOS,[8] and 90 degrees according to the AMA.[10] Normal glenohumeral medial rotation for adults is 49 degrees according to Lannan, Lehman, and Toland,[12] and for older children it is 54 degrees according to Ellenbecker[14] and 63 degrees according to Boon and Smith.[15] See Tables 4.1 to 4.4 in Research Findings for additional normal ROM values by age and gender.

Testing Position

Position the subject supine, with the arm being tested in 90 degrees of shoulder abduction. Place the forearm perpendicular to the supporting surface and in 0 degrees of supination and pronation so that the palm of the hand faces the feet. Rest the full length of the humerus on the examining table. The elbow is not supported by the examining table. Place a pad under the humerus so that the humerus is level with the acromion process.

Stabilization

Glenohumeral Medial Rotation

In the beginning of the ROM, stabilization is often needed at the distal end of the humerus to keep the shoulder in 90 degrees of abduction. Toward the end of the ROM, the clavicle and corocoid and acromion processes of the scapula are stabilized to prevent anterior tilting and protraction of the scapula.

Shoulder Complex Medial Rotation

Stabilization is often needed at the distal end of the humerus to keep the shoulder in 90 degrees of abduction. The thorax may be stabilized by the weight of the subject's trunk or with the examiner's hand to prevent flexion or rotation of the spine.

Testing Motion

Medially rotate the shoulder by moving the forearm anteriorly, bringing the palm of the hand toward the floor. Maintain the shoulder in 90 degrees of abduction and the elbow in 90 degrees of flexion during the motion.

Glenohumeral Medial Rotation

The end of ROM occurs when resistance to further motion is felt and attempts to overcome the resistance cause an anterior tilt or protraction of the scapula (Fig. 4.25).

Shoulder Complex Medial Rotation

The end of ROM occurs when resistance to further motion is felt and attempts to overcome the resistance cause flexion or rotation of the spine (Fig. 4.26).

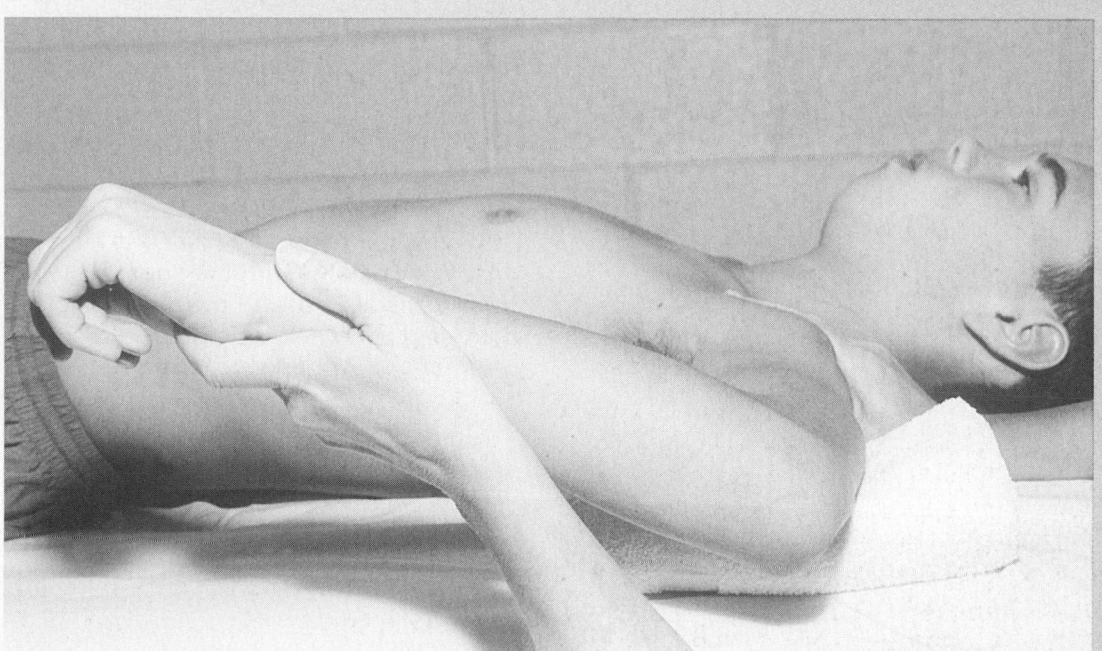

FIGURE 4.25 The end of glenohumeral medial (internal) rotation ROM. The examiner stabilizes the acromion and coracoid processes of the scapula. The examiner is able to determine that the end of the ROM has been reached because any attempt to move the extremity into additional medial rotation causes the scapula to tilt anteriorly or protract. The examiner should also maintain the shoulder in 90 degrees of abduction and the elbow in 90 degrees of flexion during the motion.

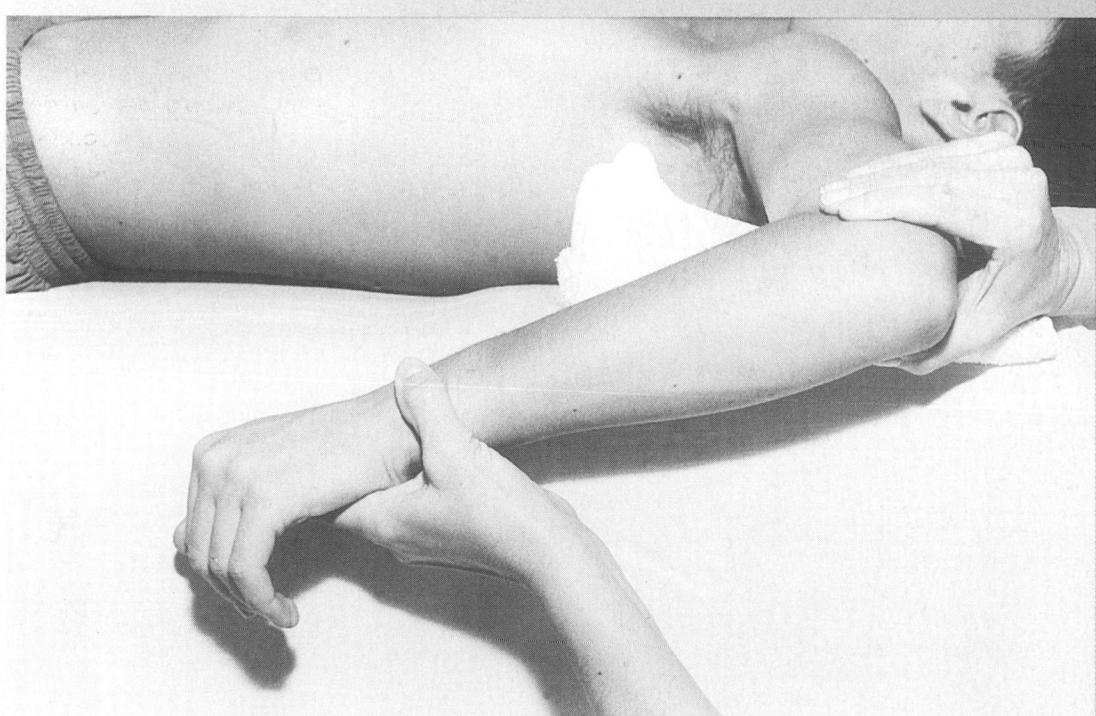

FIGURE 4.26 The end of shoulder complex medial (internal) rotation ROM. The examiner stabilizes the distal end of the humerus to maintain the shoulder in 90 degrees of abduction and the elbow in 90 degrees of flexion during the motion. Resistance is noted at the end of medial rotation of the shoulder complex because attempts to move the extremity into further motion cause the spine to flex or rotate. The clavicle and scapula are allowed to move as they participate in shoulder complex motions.

Normal End-Feel

Glenohumeral Medial Rotation

The end-feel is firm because of tension in the posterior joint capsule and the infraspinatus and teres minor muscles.

Shoulder Complex Medial Rotation

The end-feel is firm because of tension in the sternoclavicular capsule and ligaments, the costoclavicular ligament, and the major and minor rhomboid and trapezius muscles.

Goniometer Alignment

This goniometer alignment is used for measuring glenohumeral and shoulder complex medial rotation (Figs. 4.27 to 4.29).

1. Center **fulcrum** of the goniometer over the olecranon process.
2. Align **proximal arm** so that it is either perpendicular to or parallel with the floor.
3. Align **distal arm** with the ulna, using the olecranon process and ulnar styloid for reference.

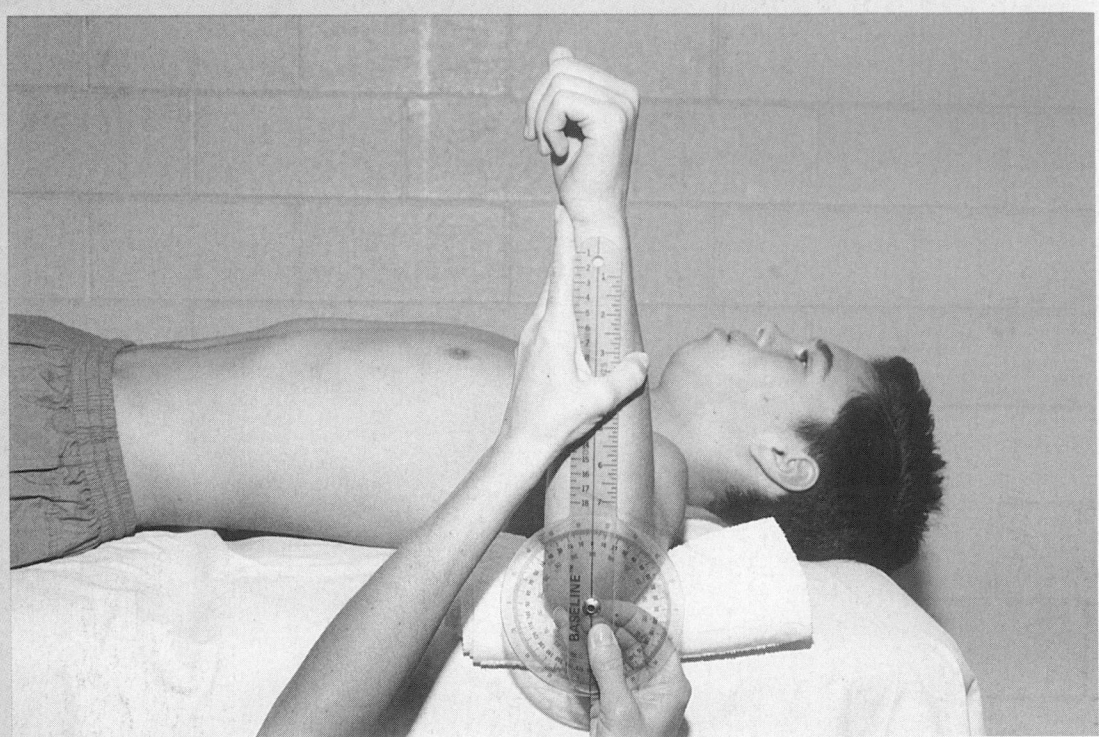

FIGURE 4.27 The alignment of the goniometer at the beginning of medial rotation ROM of the glenohumeral and shoulder complex.

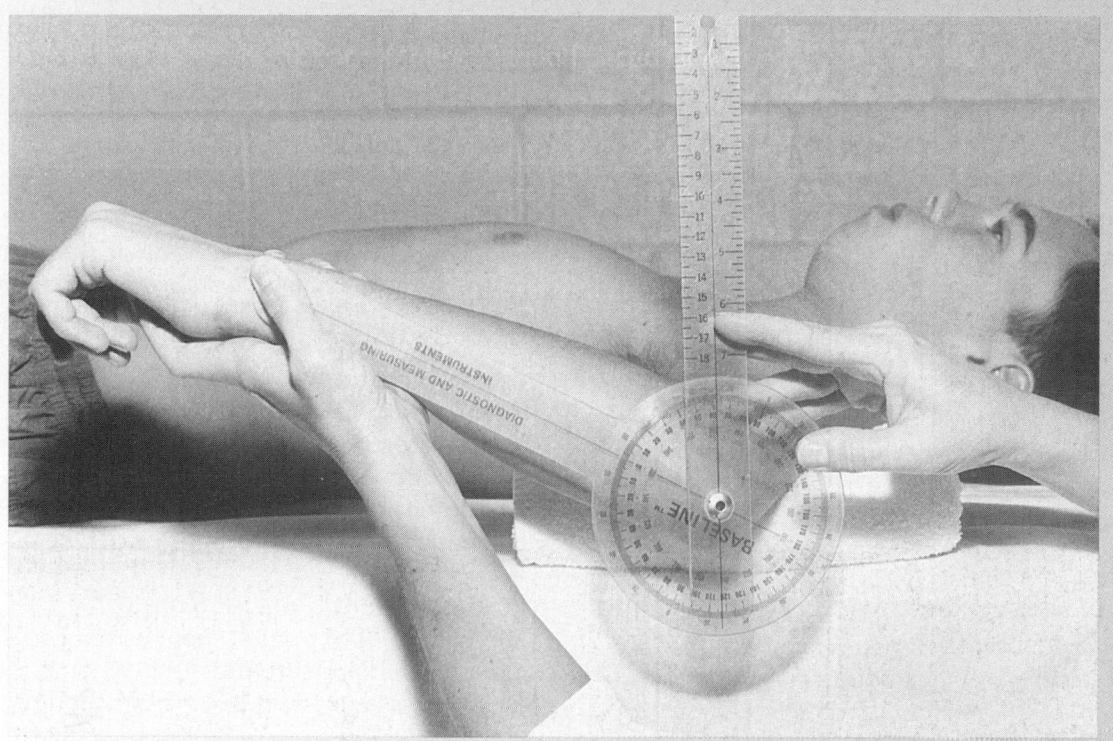

FIGURE 4.28 The alignment of the goniometer at the end of medial rotation ROM of the glenohumeral joint. The examiner uses one hand to support the subject's forearm and the distal arm of the goniometer. The examiner's other hand holds the body and the proximal arm of the goniometer.

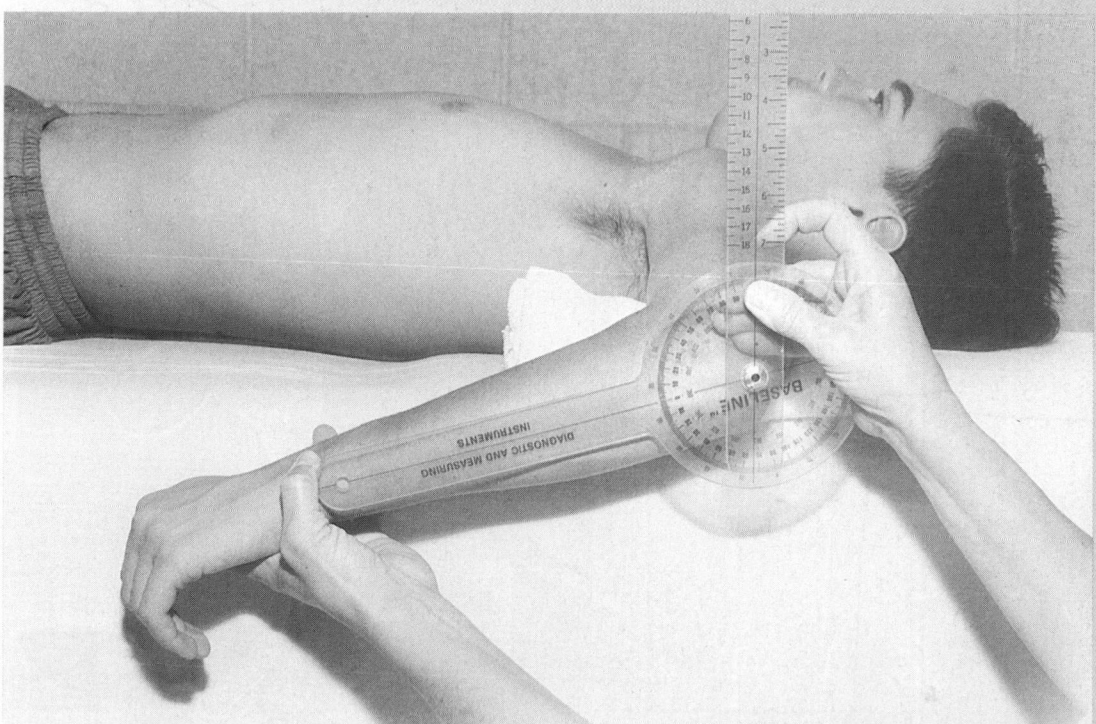

FIGURE 4.29 The alignment of the goniometer at the end medial rotation ROM of the shoulder complex.

● LATERAL (EXTERNAL) ROTATION

When the subject is in anatomical position, the motion occurs in the transverse plane around a vertical axis. When the subject is in the testing position, the motion occurs in the sagittal plane around a medial-lateral (coronal) axis. Normal shoulder complex lateral rotation for adults is 90 degrees according to the AAOS[8] and AMA[10] and 100 degrees according to Boone and Azen.[11] Normal glenohumeral medial rotation for adults is 94 degrees according to Lannan, Lehman, and Toland,[12] and for older children it is 104 degrees according to Ellenbecker[14] and 108 degrees according to Boon and Smith.[15] See Tables 4.1 to 4.4 in Research Findings for additional normal ROM values by age and gender.

Testing Position

Position the subject supine, with the arm being tested in 90 degrees of shoulder abduction. Place the forearm perpendicular to the supporting surface and in 0 degrees of supination and pronation so that the palm of the hand faces the feet. Rest the full length of the humerus on the examining table. The elbow is not supported by the examining table. Place a pad under the humerus so that the humerus is level with the acromion process.

Stabilization

Glenohumeral Lateral Rotation

At the beginning of the ROM, stabilization is often needed at the distal end of the humerus to keep the shoulder in 90 degrees of abduction. Toward the end of the ROM, the spine of the scapula is stabilized to prevent posterior tilting and retraction.

Shoulder Complex Lateral Rotation

Stabilization is often needed at the distal end of the humerus to keep the shoulder in 90 degrees of abduction. To prevent extension or rotation of the spine, the thorax may be stabilized by the weight of the subject's trunk or by the examiner's hand.

Testing Motion

Rotate the shoulder laterally by moving the forearm posteriorly, bringing the dorsal surface of the palm of the hand toward the floor. Maintain the shoulder in 90 degrees of abduction and the elbow in 90 degrees of flexion during the motion.

Glenohumeral Lateral Rotation

The end of ROM occurs when resistance to further motion is felt and attempts to overcome the resistance cause a posterior tilt or retraction of the scapula (Fig. 4.30).

Shoulder Complex Lateral Rotation

The end of ROM occurs when resistance to further motion is felt and attempts to overcome the resistance cause extension or rotation of the spine (Fig. 4.31).

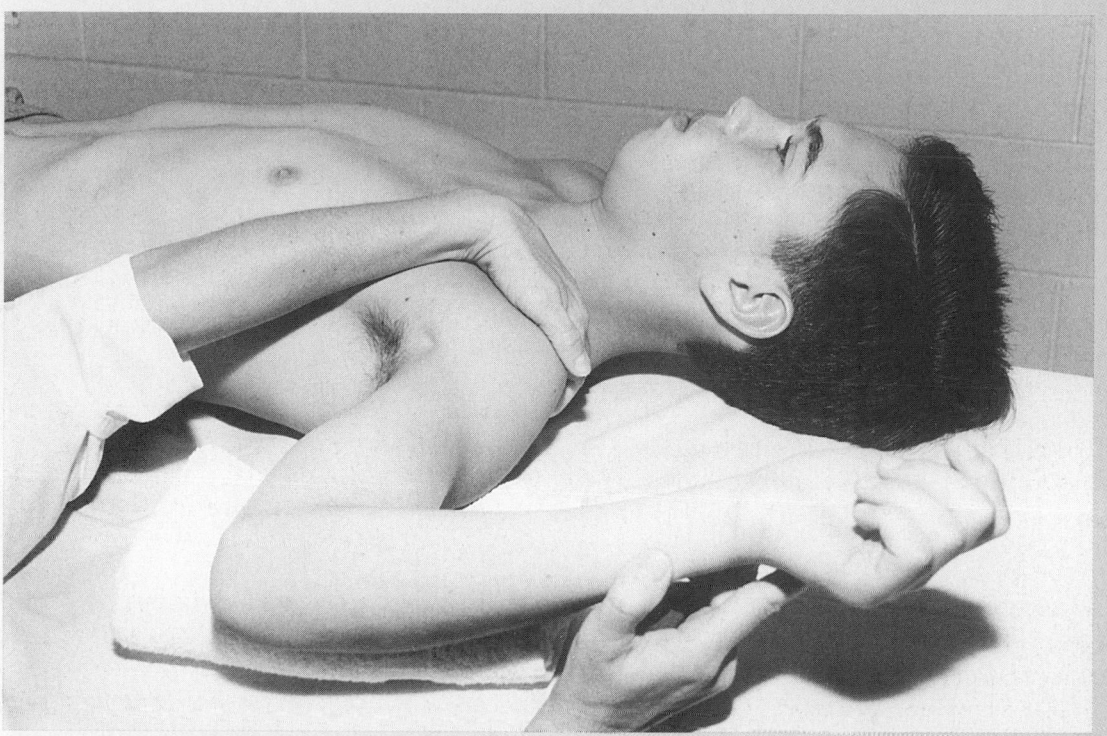

FIGURE 4.30 The end of lateral rotation ROM of the glenohumeral joint. The examiner's hand stabilizes the spine of the scapula. The end of the ROM is reached when additional motion causes the scapula to posteriorly tilt or retract and push against the examiner's hand.

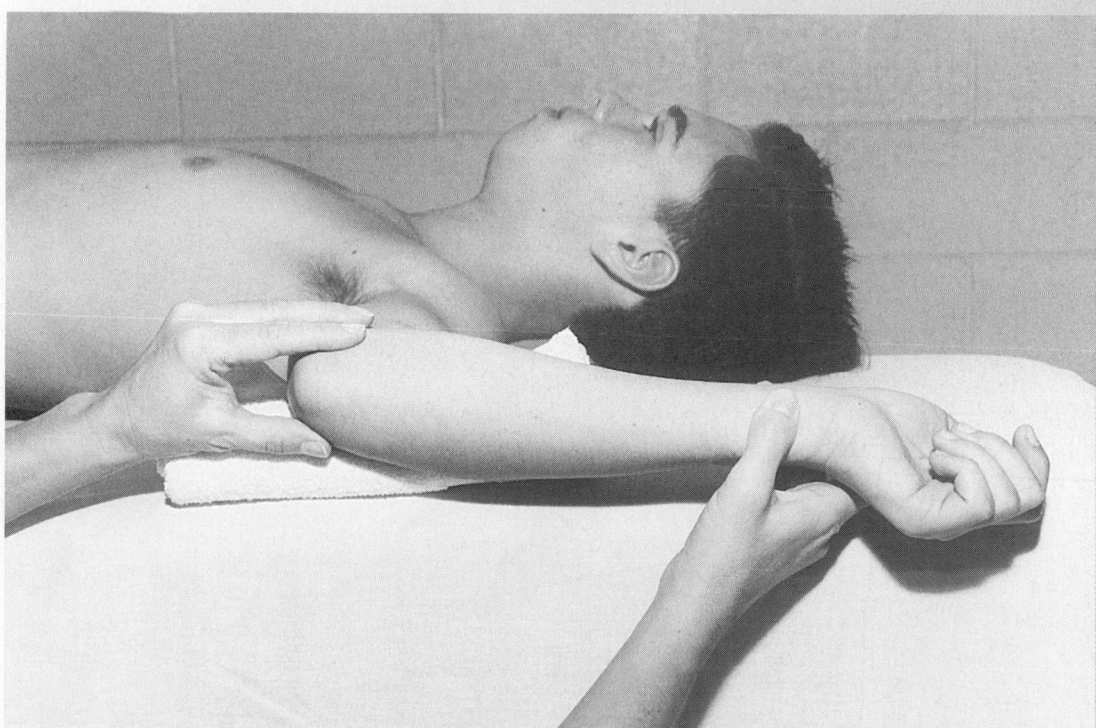

FIGURE 4.31 The end of lateral rotation ROM of the shoulder complex. The examiner stabilizes the distal humerus to prevent shoulder abduction beyond 90 degrees. The elbow is maintained in 90 degrees of flexion during the motion.

Normal End-Feel
Glenohumeral Lateral Rotation
The end-feel is firm because of tension in the anterior joint capsule; the three bands of the glenohumeral ligament; the coracohumeral ligament; and the sub-scapularis, the teres major, and the clavicular fibers of the pectoralis major muscles.

Shoulder Complex Lateral Rotation
The end-feel is firm because of tension in the SC capsule and ligaments and in the latissimus dorsi, sternocostal fibers of the pectoralis major, pectoralis minor, and serratus anterior muscles.

Goniometer Alignment
This goniometer alignment is used for measuring glenohumeral and shoulder complex lateral rotation (Figs. 4.32 to 4.34).

1. Center **fulcrum** of the goniometer over the olecranon process.
2. Align **proximal arm** so that it is either parallel to or perpendicular to the floor.
3. Align **distal arm** with the ulna, using the olecranon process and ulnar styloid for reference.

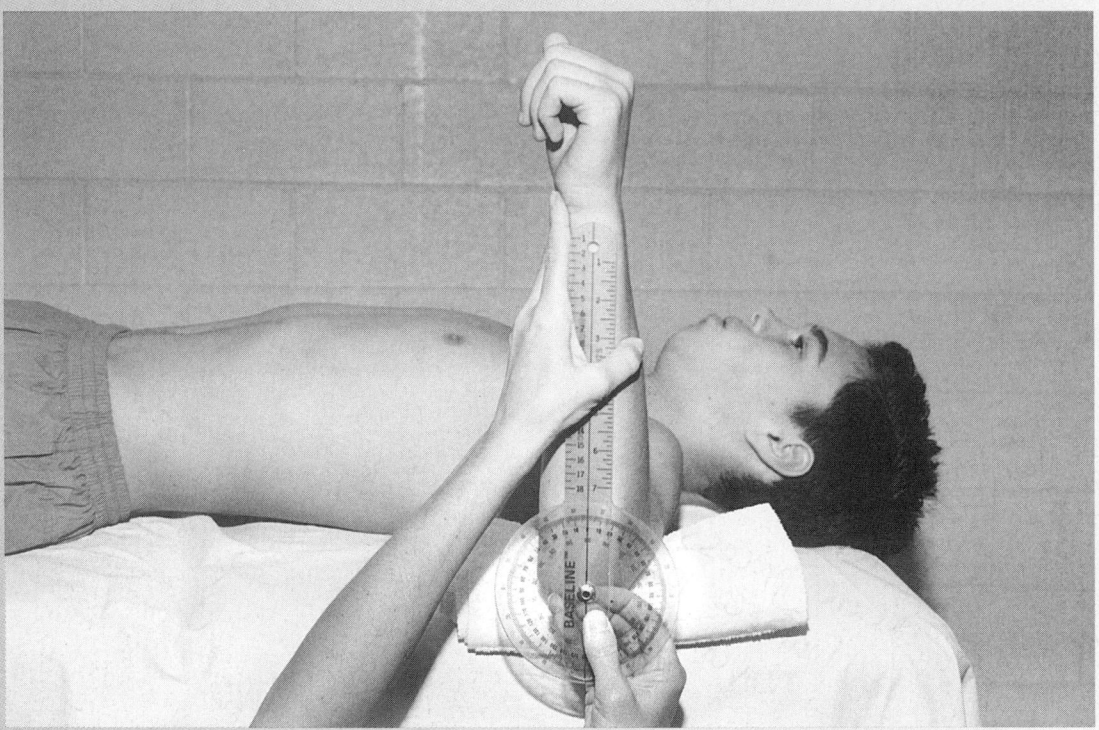

FIGURE 4.32 The alignment of the goniometer at the beginning of lateral rotation ROM of the glenohumeral joint and shoulder complex.

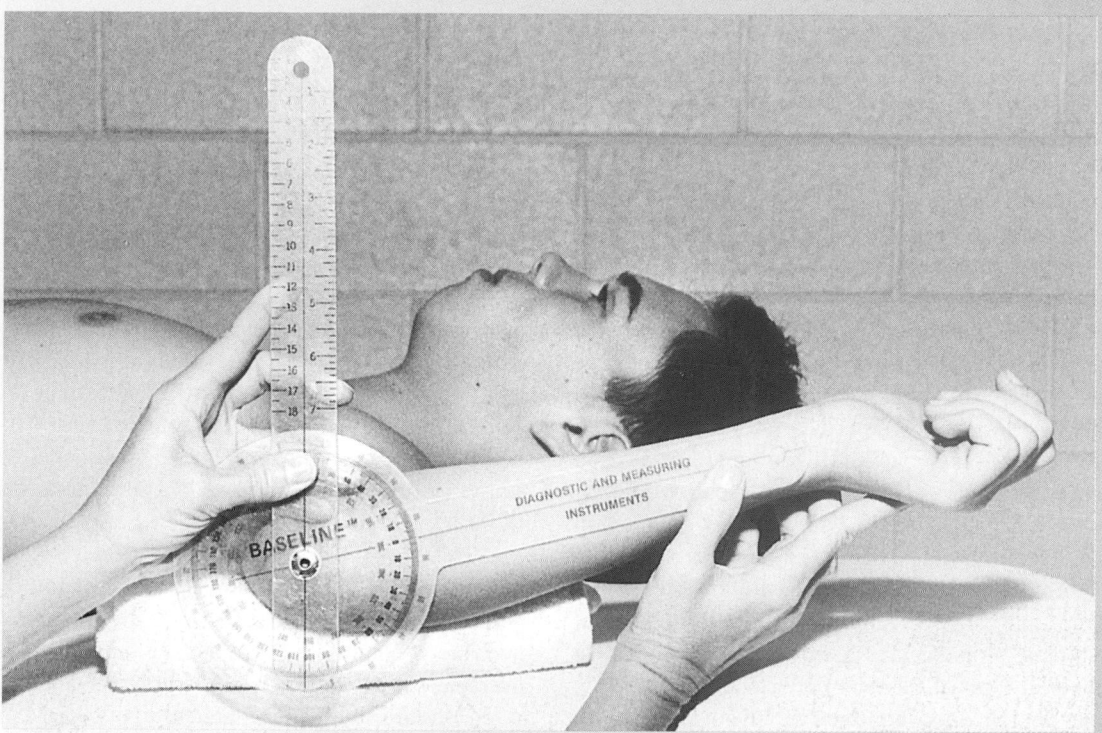

FIGURE 4.33 The alignment of the goniometer at the end of lateral rotation ROM of the glenohumeral joint. The examiner's hand supports the subject's forearm and the distal arm of the goniometer. The examiner's other hand holds the body and proximal arm of the goniometer. The placement of the examiner's hands would be reversed if the subject's right shoulder were being tested.

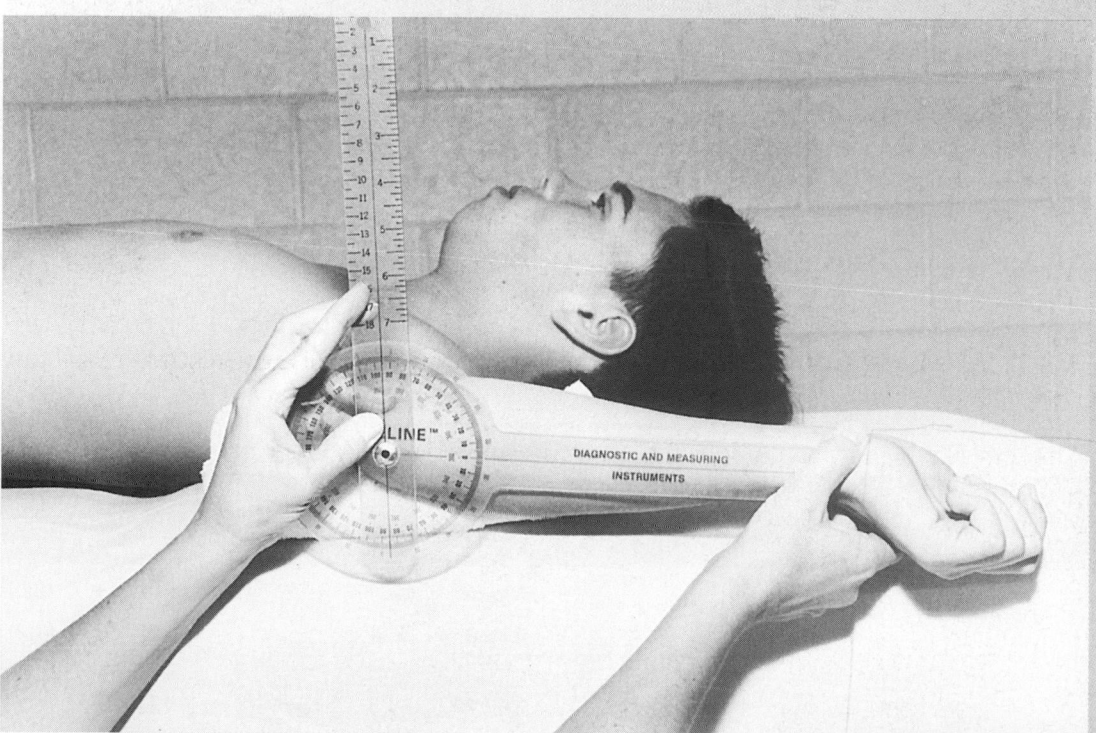

FIGURE 4.34 The alignment of the goniometer at the end of lateral rotation ROM of the shoulder complex.

⚪ Research Findings

Effects of Age, Gender, and Other Factors

Table 4.1 shows normal values of shoulder complex ROM for adults from four sources.[8,10,11,16] In general, these values range from 155 to 180 degrees for shoulder complex flexion, 50 to 60 degrees for extension, 165 to 180 degrees for abduction, 50 to 90 degrees for medial rotation, and 85 to 100 degrees for lateral rotation. The data on age, gender, and number of subjects that were measured to obtain the values reported for the AAOS[8] and AMA[10] were not reported. Information on the subjects in the studies by Boone and Azen[11] and Greene and Wolf[16] are noted in Table 4.1; both studies measured active ROM using a universal goniometer. Unless otherwise noted in this section, Research Findings, the reader should assume that shoulder ROM refers to shoulder complex ROM.

Few studies have specifically measured glenohumeral ROM using clinical tools such as a universal goniometer. In general, the overall ratio of glenohumeral to scapulothoracic motion during flexion and abduction is given as 2:1.[2,17–19] Therefore, about two-thirds of shoulder complex motion is attributed to the glenohumeral joint and one-third to the combined SC and AC joints. Table 4.2 shows normal values of glenohumeral ROM obtained from three sources.[12,14,15] These three studies used manual stabilization of the scapula and universal goniometers to obtain glenohumeral measurements. In another study of 56 healthy male and female athletes ages 13 to 18 years, Awan, Smith, and Boon[20] found mean medial rotation for the glenohumeral joint to be between 63.2 and 70.2 degrees with the scapula manually stabilized and between 60.6 and 70.7 degrees using visualized movement of the scapula to determine end range. Rundquist and coworkers[13] also provide some glenohumeral ROM data measured with electromagnetic tracking sensors on the humerus and scapula in 10 asymptomatic subjects (mean age = 51 years).

More studies are needed to establish normative values for glenohumeral ROM, especially in older adults.

Age

A review of shoulder complex ROM values presented in Table 4.3 shows very slight differences among children from birth through adolescence. Values from the study by Wanatabe and coworkers[21] were derived from measurements of passive ROM of Japanese males and females. The mean values listed from Boone[22] were derived from measurements of active ROM taken with a universal goniometer on Caucasian males. Although the values obtained from Wanatabe and coworkers[21] for infants are greater than those obtained from Boone[22] for children between the ages of 1 and 19 years, it is difficult to compare values across studies. Within one study, Boone[22] and Boone and Azen[11] found that shoulder ROM varied little in boys between 1 and 19 years of age.

There is some indication that children have greater values than adults for certain shoulder complex motions. Wanatabe and coworkers[21] found that the ROM in shoulder extension and lateral rotation was greater in Japanese infants than the average values typically reported for adults. Boone and Azen[11] found significantly greater active ROM in all shoulder motions except for abduction in male children between 1 and 19 years of age compared with male adults between 20 and 54 years of age.

Table 4.4 summarizes the effects of age on shoulder complex ROM in adults. There appears to be a trend for older adults (between 60 and 93 years of age) to have lower values than younger adults (between 20 and 39 years of age) for the motions of extension, lateral rotation, and abduction. It is interesting to note that the standard deviations for the older groups are much larger than the values reported for the younger groups. The larger standard deviations appear to indicate that ROM is more variable in the older groups than in the younger groups. However, the fact that the measurements of the two oldest groups were obtained by different investigators should be considered when drawing conclusions from this information.

| TABLE 4.1 | Shoulder Complex Motion: Normal Values for Adults in Degrees From Selected Sources |

	AAOS[8]	AMA[10]	Boone and Azen[11] 20–54 yrs n = 56 Males		Greene and Wolf[16] 18–55 yrs n = 20 Males and Females	
Motion			**Mean**	**(SD)**	**Mean**	**(SD)**
Flexion	180	180	165.0	(5.0)	155.8	(1.4)
Extension	60	50	57.3	(8.1)	—	—
Abduction	180	180	182.7	(9.0)	167.6	(1.8)
Medial rotation	70	90	67.1	(4.1)	48.7	(2.8)
Lateral rotation	90	90	99.6	(7.6)	83.6	(3.0)

TABLE 4.2 Glenohumeral Motion: Normal Values in Degrees From Selected Sources

	Lannan et al[12] 21–40 yrs n = 60 Males and Females		Boon & Smith[15] 12-18 yrs n = 50 Males and Females		Ellenbecker et al[14] 11–17 yrs n = 113 Males		Ellenbecker et al[14] 11–17 yrs n = 90 Females	
Motion	Mean	(SD)	Mean	(SD)	Mean	(SD)	Mean	(SD)
Flexion	106.2	(10.2)	—	—	—	—	—	—
Extension	20.1	(5.8)	—	—	—	—	—	—
Abduction	128.9	(9.1)	—	—	—	—	—	—
Medial rotation	49.2	(9.0)	62.8	(12.7)	50.9	(12.6)	56.3	(10.3)
Lateral rotation	94.2	(12.2)	108.1	(14.1)	102.8	(10.9)	104.6	(10.3)

TABLE 4.3 Effects of Age on Shoulder Complex Motions for Newborns Through Adolescents: Normal Values in Degrees

	Wanatabe et al[21] 0–2 yrs n = 45 Males and Females	Boone[22] 1–5 yrs n = 19 Males		6–12 yrs n = 17 Males		13–19 yrs n = 17 Males	
Motion	Range of Means	Mean	(SD)	Mean	(SD)	Mean	(SD)
Flexion	172–180	168.8	(3.7)	169.0	(3.5)	167.4	(3.9)
Extension	79–89	68.9	(6.6)	69.6	(7.0)	64.0	(9.3)
Medial rotation	72–90	71.2	(3.6)	70.0	(4.7)	70.3	(5.3)
Lateral rotation	118–134	110.0	(10.0)	107.4	(3.6)	106.3	(6.1)
Abduction	177–187	186.3	(2.6)	184.7	(3.8)	185.1	(4.3)

TABLE 4.4 Effects of Age on Shoulder Complex Motion in Adults 20 to 93 Years of Age: Normal Values in Degrees

	Boone[22] 20–29 yrs n = 19 Males		30–39 yrs n = 18 Males		40–54 yrs n = 19 Males		Walker et al[23] 60–85 yrs n = 30 Males		Downey et al[24] 61–93 yrs n = 140 Female and 60 Male Shoulders	
Motion	Mean	(SD)	Mean	(SD)	Mean	(SD)	Mean	(SD)	Mean	(SD)
Flexion	164.5	(5.9)	165.4	(3.8)	165.1	(5.2)	160.0	(11.0)	165.0	(10.7)
Extension	58.3	(8.3)	57.5	(8.5)	56.1	(7.9)	38.0	(11.0)	—	—
Medial rotation	65.9	(4.0)	67.1	(4.2)	68.3	(3.8)	59.0	(16.0)	65.0	(11.7)
Lateral rotation	100.0	(7.2)	101.5	(6.9)	97.5	(8.5)	76.0	(13.0)	80.6	(11.0)
Abduction	182.6	(9.8)	182.8	(7.7)	182.6	(9.8)	155.0	(22.0)	157.9	(17.4)

In addition to the evidence for age-related changes presented in Tables 4.3 and 4.4, West[25] Clarke and coworkers,[26] and Allander and associates[27] have also identified age-related trends. West[25] found that older subjects had between 15 and 20 degrees less shoulder complex flexion ROM and 10 degrees less extension ROM than younger subjects. Subjects ranged in age from the first decade to the eighth decade. Clarke and coworkers[26] found significant decreases with age in passive glenohumeral lateral rotation, total rotation, and abduction in a study that included 60 normal males and females ranging in age from 21 to 80 years. Mean reduction in these three glenohumeral ROMs in those aged 71 to 80 years, compared with those aged 21 to 30 years, ranged from 7 to 29 degrees. Allander and associates,[27] in a study of 517 females and 203 males aged 33 to 70 years, also found that passive shoulder complex rotation ROM significantly decreased with increasing age.

Gender

Several studies have noted that females have greater shoulder complex ROM than males. Walker and coworkers,[23] in a study of 30 men and 30 women between 60 and 84 years of age, found that women had statistically significant greater ROM than their male counterparts in all shoulder motions studied except for medial rotation. The mean differences for women were 20 degrees greater than those of males for shoulder abduction, 11 degrees greater for shoulder extension, and 9 degrees greater for shoulder flexion and lateral rotation. Allander and associates,[27] in a study of passive shoulder rotation in 208 Swedish women and 203 men aged 45 to 70 years, likewise found that women had a greater ROM in total shoulder rotation than men. Escalante, Lichenstein, and Hazuda[28] studied shoulder flexion in 687 community-dwelling adults aged 65 to 74 years and found that women had 3 degrees more flexion than men.

Gender differences have also been noted in glenohumeral ROM. Clarke and associates,[26] in a study that included 60 males and 60 females, found that females had greater glenohumeral ROM for shoulder abduction as well as lateral and total rotation. Six age groups with subjects between 20 and 40 years of age were included in the study. These gender differences were present in all age groups. Males had, on average, 92 percent of the ROM of their female counterparts, the difference being most marked in abduction. Lannan, Lehman, and Toland,[12] in a study of 40 women and 20 men aged 21 to 40 years, found that women had statistically significant greater amounts of glenohumeral flexion, extension, abduction, and medial and lateral rotation than men. The mean differences typically varied between 3 and 8 degrees. Boon and Smith,[15] in a study of 32 females and 18 males aged 12 to 18 years, reported that females had significantly more lateral and total rotation than males. The mean difference in lateral and total rotation was 4.5 and 9.1 degrees, respectively. Ellenbecker and colleagues[14] studied 113 male and 90 female elite tennis players aged 11 to 17 years (see Table 4.2). Their data seem to indicate that the females had greater ROM than males for glenohumeral medial and lateral rotation, although no statistical tests focused on the effect of gender on ROM.

Testing Position

A subject's posture and testing position have been shown to affect certain shoulder complex motions. Kebaetse, McClure, and Pratt,[29] in a study of 34 healthy adults, measured active shoulder abduction and scapula ROM while subjects were sitting in both erect and slouched trunk postures. There was significantly less active shoulder abduction ROM in the slouched than in the erect postures (mean difference = 23.6 degrees). The slouched posture also resulted in more scapula elevation during 0 to 90 degrees of abduction and less scapula posterior tilting in the interval between 90-degree and maximal abduction.

Sabari and associates[30] studied 30 adult subjects and noted greater amounts of active and passive shoulder abduction measured in the supine than in the sitting position. The mean differences in abduction ranged from 3.0 to 7.1 degrees. On visual inspection of the data there were also greater amounts of shoulder flexion in the supine versus the sitting position; however, these differences did not attain significance.

Body Mass Index

Escalante, Lichenstein, and Hazuda[28] studied shoulder complex flexion ROM in 695 community-dwelling subjects, aged 65 to 74 years, who participated in the San Antonio Longitudinal Study of Aging. They found no relationship between shoulder flexion and body mass index.

Sports

Several studies of professional and collegiate baseball players have found a significant increase in lateral rotation ROM and a decrease in medial rotation ROM of the shoulder complex in the dominant shoulder compared with the nondominant shoulder. These differences have been found in position players as well as in pitchers. Bigliani and coworkers[31] studied 148 professional baseball players (72 pitchers and 76 position players) with no history of shoulder problems. Mean lateral rotation ROM measured with the shoulder in 90 degrees of abduction was 113.5 degrees in the dominant arm and 99.9 degrees in the nondominant arm. Mean medial rotation ROM, recorded as the highest vertebral level reached behind the back and converted to a numerical value, was significantly less in the dominant arm. There were no significant differences between the dominant and the nondominant arms in shoulder flexion and shoulder lateral rotation measured with the arm at the side of the body. A study by Baltaci, Johnson, and Kohl[32] of 15 collegiate pitchers and 23 position players had similar findings. Pitchers had an average of 14 degrees more lateral rotation and 11 degrees less medial rotation in the dominant versus nondominant shoulders. Position players had an average of 8 degrees more lateral rotation and 10 degrees less medial rotation in the dominant shoulder. All measurements of rotation were taken with the shoulder in 90 degrees of abduction.

Decreases in shoulder medial rotation ROM have also been noted in the dominant (playing) compared with the nondominant (nonplaying) arms of tennis players. Chinn, Priest, and Kent,[33] in a study of 83 national and international men and women tennis players aged 14 to 50 years, found a significant decrease in active medial rotation ROM of the shoulder complex in the playing versus the nonplaying arm (mean difference = 6.8 degrees in males, 11.9 degrees in females). Men also had a significant increase in lateral rotation ROM in the playing compared with the nonplaying arm. A study by Kibler and colleagues[34] of 39 members of the U. S. Tennis Association National Tennis Team and touring professional program, found a decrease in passive glenohumeral medial rotation ROM, an increase in glenohumeral lateral rotation ROM, and a decrease in total rotation ROM in the playing versus the nonplaying arm. The differences in medial rotation ROM increased with age and years of tournament play. A study by Ellenbecker and associates[14] of 203 junior elite tennis players aged 11 to 17 years reported a significant decrease in active medial rotation ROM and total rotation ROM of the glenohumeral joint in the playing versus the nonplaying arm. The average differences in medial rotation ROM were 11 degrees in the 113 males and 8 degrees in the 90 females. There were no significant differences in glenohumeral lateral rotation ROM between playing and nonplaying arms.

Power lifters were found to have decreased ROM in shoulder complex flexion, extension, and medial and lateral rotation compared with nonlifters in a study by Chang, Buschbacker, and Edlich.[35] Ten male power lifters and 10 aged-matched male nonlifters were included in the study. The authors suggest that athletic training programs that emphasize muscle-strengthening exercise without stretching exercise may cause progressive loss of ROM.

Functional Range of Motion

Numerous activities of daily living (ADL) require adequate shoulder ROM. Tiffitt,[36] in a study of 25 patients, found a significant correlation between the amount of specific shoulder complex motions and the ability to perform activities such as combing the hair, putting on a coat, washing the back, washing the contralateral axilla, using the toilet, reaching a high shelf, lifting above the shoulder level, pulling, and sleeping on the affected side. Flexion and adduction ROM correlated best with the ability to comb the hair, whereas medial and lateral rotation ROM correlated best with the ability to wash the back.

Several studies[37–39] have examined the ROM that occurs during certain functional tasks (Table 4.5). A large amount of abduction (112 degrees) and lateral rotation is required to reach behind the head for activities such as grooming the hair (Fig 4.35), positioning a necktie, and fastening a dress zipper. Maximal flexion (148 degrees) is needed to reach a high shelf (Fig. 4.36), whereas less flexion (36 to 52 degrees) is needed for self-feeding tasks (Fig 4.37). To reach behind the back for

TABLE 4.5	Maximal Shoulder Complex Motion Necessary for Functional Activities: Mean Values in Degrees			
Activity	**Motion**	**Mean**	**(SD)**	**Source**
Eating	Flexion	52	(8)	Matsen*[37]
	Flexion	36	(14)	Safaee-Rad et al†[38]
	Abduction	22	(7)	Safaee-Rad et al
	Medial rotation	18	(10)	Safaee-Rad et al
	Horizontal adduction‡	87	(29)	Matsen
Drinking with a cup	Flexion	43	(16)	Safaee-Rad et al
	Abduction	31	(9)	Safaee-Rad et al
	Medial rotation	23	(12)	Safaee-Rad et al
Washing axilla	Flexion	52	(14)	Matsen
Combing hair	Horizontal adduction	104	(12)	Matsen
	Abduction	112	(10)	Matsen
	Horizontal adduction	54	(27)	Matsen
Maximal elevation	Flexion/abduction	148	(11)	Matsen
Maximal reaching up back	Horizontal adduction	55	(17)	Matsen
	Extension	56	(13)	Matsen
	Horizontal abduction‡	69	(11)	Matsen
Reaching perineum	Extension	38	(10)	Matsen
	Horizontal abduction	86	(13)	Matsen

* Eight normal subjects were assessed with electromagnetic sensors on the humerus.
† Ten normal male subjects were assessed with a three-dimensional video recording system.
‡ The 0-degree starting position for measuring horizontal adduction and horizontal abduction was in 90 degrees of abduction.

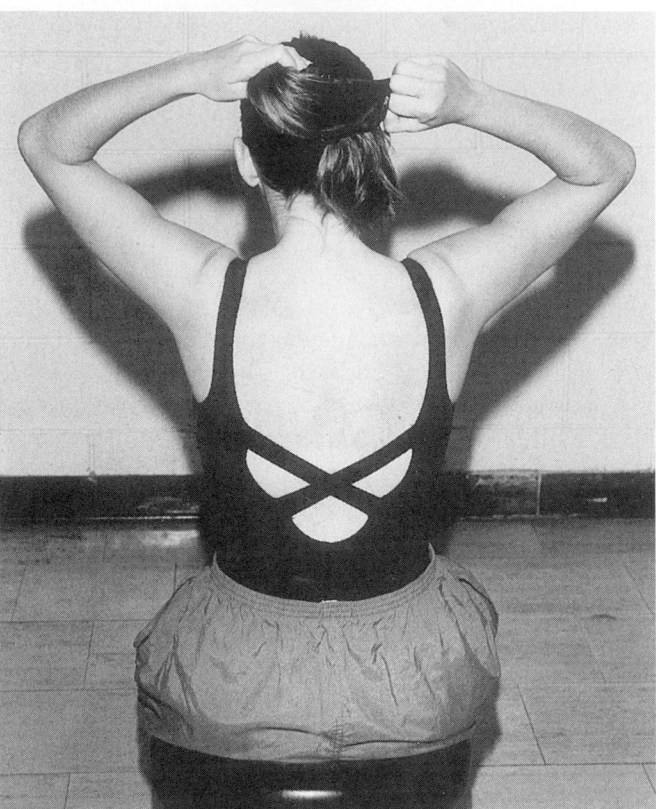

FIGURE 4.35 Reaching behind the head requires a large amount of abduction (112 degrees)[37] and lateral rotation of the shoulder.

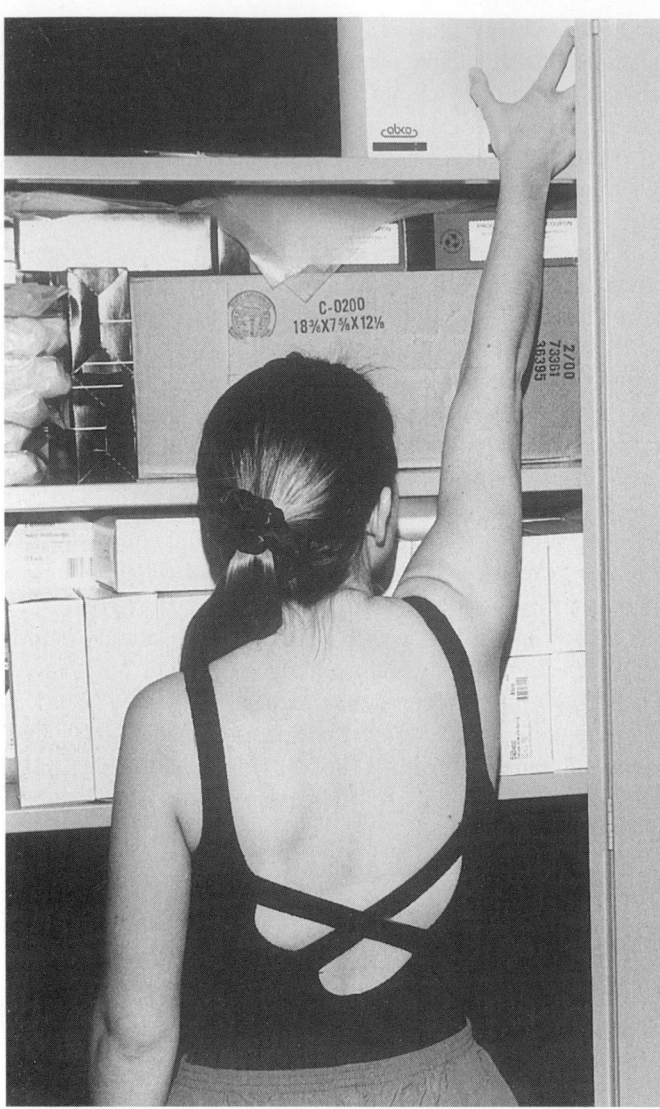

FIGURE 4.36 Reaching objects on a high shelf requires 148 degrees of shoulder flexion.[37]

tasks such as fastening a bra (Fig 4.38), tucking in a shirt, and reaching the perineum to perform hygiene activities, 38 to 56 degrees of extension and considerable medial rotation and horizontal abduction are necessary. Horizontal adduction is needed for activities performed in front of the body such as washing the contralateral axilla (104 degrees) and eating (87 degrees). If patients have difficulty performing certain functional activities, evaluation and treatment procedures need to focus on the shoulder motions necessary for the activity. Likewise, if patients have known limitations in shoulder ROM, therapists and physicians should anticipate patient difficulty in performing these tasks, and adaptations should be suggested.

Reliability and Validity

The intratester and intertester reliability of measurements of shoulder motions with a universal goniometer have been studied by many researchers. Most of these studies have presented evidence that intratester reliability is better than intertester reliability. Reliability varied according to the motion being measured. In other words, the reliability of measuring certain shoulder motions was better than the reliability of measuring other motions.

Hellebrandt, Duvall, and Moore,[40] in a study of 77 patients, found the intratester reliability of measurements of active ROM

of shoulder complex abduction and medial rotation to be less than the intratester reliability of shoulder flexion, extension, and lateral rotation. The mean difference between the repeated measurements ranged from 0.2 to 1.5 degrees. Measurements were taken with a universal goniometer and devices designed by the U.S. Army for specific joints. For most ROM measurements taken throughout the body, the universal goniometer was a more dependable tool than the special devices.

Boone and coworkers[41] examined the reliability of measuring passive ROM for lateral rotation of the shoulder complex, elbow extension–flexion, wrist ulnar deviation, hip abduction, knee extension–flexion, and foot inversion. Four physical therapists used universal goniometers to measure these motions in 12 normal males once a week for 4 weeks. Measurement of lateral rotation ROM of the shoulder was found to be more reliable than that of the other motions tested. For all motions except lateral rotation of the shoulder, intratester reliability was noted to be greater than intertester reliability. Intratester and

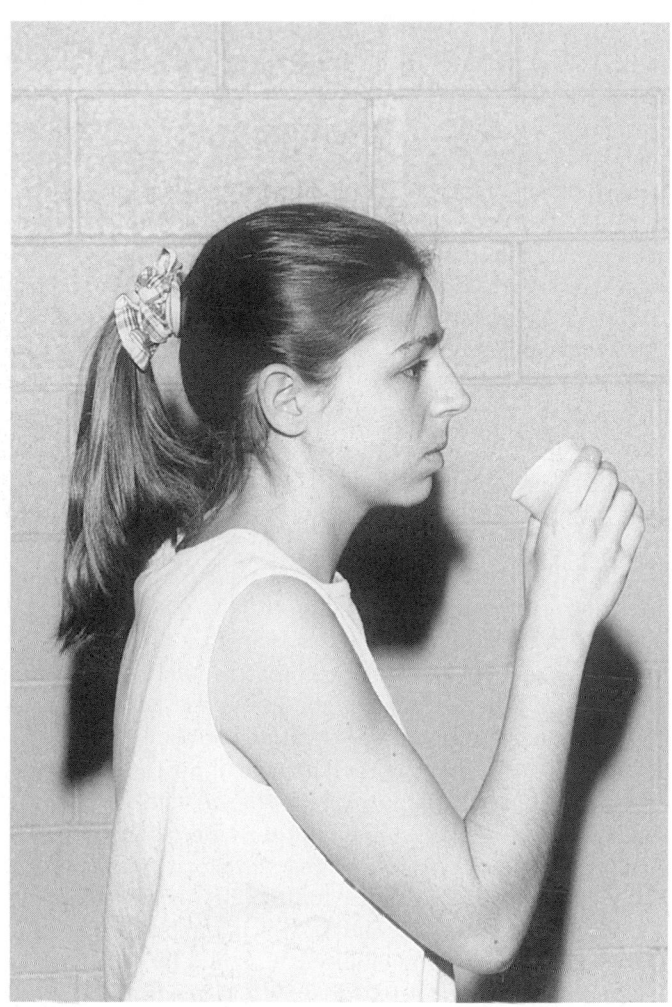

FIGURE 4.37 Feeding tasks require 36 to 52 degrees of shoulder flexion.[37,38]

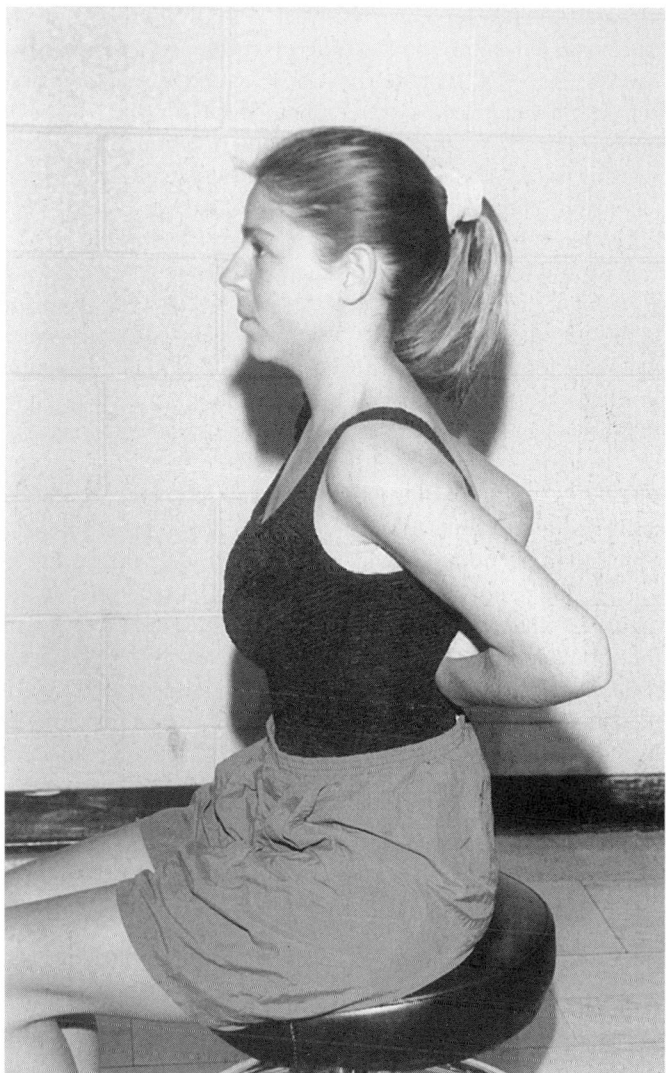

FIGURE 4.38 Reaching behind the back to fasten a bra or bathing suit requires 56 degrees of extension, 69 degrees of horizontal abduction,[37] and a large amount of medial rotation of the shoulder.

intertester reliability were similar (r = 0.96 and 0.97, respectively) for lateral rotation ROM.

Pandya and associates,[42] in a study in which five testers measured the range of shoulder complex abduction of 150 children and young adults with Duchenne muscular dystrophy, found that the intratester intraclass correlation coefficient (ICC) for measurements of shoulder abduction was 0.84. The intertester reliability for measuring shoulder abduction was lower (ICC = 0.67). In comparison with measurements of elbow and wrist extension, the measurement of shoulder abduction was less reliable.

Riddle, Rothstein, and Lamb[43] conducted a study to determine intratester and intertester reliability for passive ROM measurements of the shoulder complex. Sixteen physical therapists, assessing in pairs, used two different-sized universal goniometers (large and small) for their measurements on 50 patients. Patient position and goniometer placement during measurements were not controlled. ICC values for intratester reliability for all motions ranged from 0.87 to 0.99. ICC values for intertester reliability for flexion, abduction, and lateral rotation ranged from 0.84 to 0.90. Intertester reliability

was considerably lower for measurements of horizontal abduction, horizontal adduction, extension, and medial rotation, with ICC values ranging from 0.26 to 0.55. The authors concluded that passive ROM measurements for all shoulder motions can be reliable when taken by the same physical therapist, regardless of whether large or small goniometers are used. Measurements of flexion, abduction, and lateral rotation can be reliable when assessed by different therapists. However, because repeated measurements of horizontal abduction, horizontal adduction, extension, and medial rotation were unreliable when taken by more than one tester, these measurements should be taken by the same therapist.

Greene and Wolf[16] compared the reliability of the Ortho Ranger, an electronic pendulum goniometer, with that of a standard universal goniometer for active upper-extremity motions in 20 healthy adults. Shoulder complex motions were measured three times with each instrument during three sessions that occurred over a 2-week period. Both instruments demonstrated high intrasession correlations (ICCs ranged from 0.98 to 0.87), but correlations were higher and 95 percent confidence levels were much lower for the universal goniometer. Measurements of medial rotation and lateral rotation were less reliable than measurements of flexion, extension, abduction, and adduction. There were significant differences between measurements taken with the Ortho Ranger and the universal goniometer. Interestingly, there were significant differences in measurements between sessions for both instruments. The authors noted that the daily variations that were found might have been caused by normal fluctuation in ROM, as suggested by Boone and colleagues,[41] or by daily differences in subjects' efforts while performing active ROM.

Bovens and associates,[44] in a study of the variability and reliability of nine joint motions throughout the body, used a universal goniometer to examine active lateral rotation ROM of the shoulder complex with the arm at the side. Three physician testers and eight healthy subjects participated in the study. Intratester reliability coefficients for lateral rotation of the shoulder ranged from 0.76 to 0.83, whereas the intertester reliability coefficient was 0.63. Mean intratester standard deviations for the measurements taken on each subject ranged from 5.0 to 6.6 degrees, whereas the mean intertester standard deviation was 7.4 degrees. The measurement of lateral rotation ROM of the shoulder was more reliable than ROM measurements of the forearm and wrist. Mean standard deviations between repeated measurement of shoulder lateral rotation ROM were similar to those of the forearm and larger than those of the wrist.

Sabari and associates[30] examined intrarater reliability in the measurement of active and passive shoulder complex flexion and abduction ROM when 30 adults were positioned in supine and sitting positions. The ICCs between two trials by the same tester for each procedure ranged in value from 0.94 to 0.99, indicating high intratester reliability, regardless of whether the measurements were active or passive or whether they were taken with the subject in the supine or the sitting position. ICCs between measurements taken in supine compared with those taken in sitting positions ranged from 0.64 to 0.81. There were no significant differences between comparable flexion measurements taken in supine and sitting positions. However, significantly greater abduction ROM was found in the supine than in the sitting position.

In a study by MacDermid and colleagues,[45] two experienced physical therapists measured passive shoulder complex rotation ROM in 34 patients with a variety of shoulder pathologies. A universal goniometer was used to measure lateral rotation with the shoulder in 20 to 30 degrees of abduction. Intratester ICCs (0.88 and 0.93) and intertester ICCs (0.85 and 0.80) were high. Intratester standard errors of measurement (SEMs; 4.9 and 7.0 degrees) and intertester SEMs (7.5 and 8.0 degrees) also indicated good reliability. The SEMs indicate that differences of 5 to 7 degrees could be attributed to measurement error when the same tester repeats a measurement and about 8 degrees could be attributed to measurement error when different testers take a measurement.

Boon and Smith[15] studied 50 high school athletes to determine the reliability of measuring passive shoulder rotation ROM with and without manual stabilization of the scapula. Four experienced physical therapists working in pairs took goniometric measurements with the shoulder in 90 degrees of abduction and repeated those measurements 5 days later. Scapular stabilization, which resulted in more isolated glenohumeral motion, produced significantly smaller ROM values than when the scapula was not stabilized. According to the authors, intratester reliability for medial rotation was poor for nonstabilized motion (ICC = 0.23, SEM = 20.2 degrees) and good for stabilized motion (ICC = 0.60, SEM = 8.0). The authors state that intratester reliability for lateral rotation was good for both nonstabilized (ICC = 0.79, SEM = 5.6) and stabilized motion (ICC = 0.53, SEM = 9.1). Intertester reliability for medial rotation improved from nonstabilized motion (ICC = 0.13, SEM = 21.5) to stabilized motion (ICC = 0.38, SEM = 10.0) and was comparable for both nonstabilized and stabilized lateral rotation (ICC = 0.84, SEM = 4.9 and ICC = 0.78, SEM = 6.6), respectively.

Hayes and coworkers[46] measured the intratester reliability of active shoulder flexion, abduction, and lateral rotation ROM in nine patients using one tester, and the intertester reliability of active shoulder motion in eight patients using four testers. A universal goniometer was aligned with the humerus and various planes of motion with the subjects in sitting for flexion and abduction and in supine for lateral rotation. Intratester reliability ICC values for the universal goniometer ranged from 0.53 to 0.65, and SEM values ranged from 14 to 23 degrees. Intertester reliability ICC values for the universal goniometer ranged from 0.64 to 0.69, and SEM values ranged from 14 to 25 degrees. The reliability of using visual estimation and still photography to measure shoulder ROM was also studied and produced similar results. However, the use of a tape measure to note distance between T1 and the thumb during reaching behind the back produced even worse ICC values of 0.39 and SEM values of 6 centimeters.

The reliability of measurement devices other than a universal goniometer for assessing shoulder ROM has also been studied and is briefly mentioned here. Intratester and intertester reliability for the different motions and methods varied widely. Green and associates[47] investigated the reliability of measuring active shoulder complex ROM with a Plurimeter-V inclinometer in six patients with shoulder pain and stiffness. Tiffitt, Wildin, and Hajioff[48] studied the reliability of using an inclinometer to measure active shoulder complex motions in 36 patients with shoulder disorders. Valentine and Lewis[49] included 45 subjects with and without shoulder symptoms in a study of the intratester reliability of shoulder flexion and abduction using a gravity dependent inclinometer, lateral rotation using a tape measure, and medial rotation using visual estimation. Bower[50] and Clarke and coworkers[26] examined the reliability of measuring passive glenohumeral motions with a hydrogoniometer. Croft and colleagues[51] investigated the reliability of observing shoulder complex flexion and lateral rotation, and sketching the ROMs onto diagrams that were then measured with a protractor.

REFERENCES

1. Standring, S (ed): Gray's Anatomy, ed 39. Elsevier, New York, 2005.
2. Ludewig, PM, and Borstead, JD: The shoulder complex. In Levangie, P, and Norkin, C (eds): Joint Structure and Function: A Comprehensive Analysis, ed 4. FA Davis, Philadelphia, 2005.
3. Neumann, DA: Kinesiology of the Musculoskeletal System. Mosby, St. Louis, MO, 2002.
4. Kisner, C, and Colby, LA: Therapeutic Exercise, ed 5. FA Davis, Philadelphia, 2007.
5. Kaltenborn, FM: Manual Mobilization of the Extremity Joints, ed 5. Olaf Norlis Bokhandel, Oslo,1999.
6. Cyriax, JH, and Cyriax, PJ: Illustrated Manual of Orthopaedic Medicine. Butterworths, London, 1983.
7. Culham, E, and Peat, M: Functional anatomy of the shoulder complex. J Orthop Sports Phys Ther 18:342, 1993.
8. American Academy of Orthopaedic Surgeons: Joint Motion: Method of Measuring and Recording. AAOS, Chicago, 1965.
9. Greene, WB, and Heckman, JD: The Clinical Measurement of Joint Motion. American Academy of Orthopaedic Surgeons, Rosemont, IL, 1994.
10. Cocchiarella, L, and Andersson, GBJ: American Medical Association: Guides to the Evaluation of Permanent Impairment, ed 5. AMA, Chicago, 2001.
11. Boone, DC, and Azen, SP: Normal range of motion in male subjects. J Bone Joint Surg Am 61:756, 1979.
12. Lannan, D, Lehman, T, and Toland, M: Establishment of normative data for the range of motion of the glenohumeral joint. Master of Science Thesis, University of Massachusetts, Lowell, MA, 1996
13. Rundquist, PJ, et al: Shoulder kinematics in subjects with frozen shoulder. Arch Phys Med Rehabil 84:1473, 2003.
14. Ellenbecker, TS, et al: Glenohumeral joint internal and external rotation range of motion in elite junior tennis players. J Orthop Sports Phys Ther 24:336, 1996.
15. Boon, AJ, and Smith, J: Manual scapular stabilization: Its effect on shoulder rotational range of motion. Arch Phys Med Rehabil 81:978, 2000.
16. Greene, BL, and Wolf, SL: Upper extremity joint movement: Comparison of two measurement devices. Arch Phys Med Rehabil 70:288, 1989.
17. Soderberg, GL: Kinesiology: Application to Pathological Motion. Williams & Wilkins, Baltimore, 1986.
18. Doody, SG, Freedman, L, and Waterland, JC: Shoulder movements during abduction in the scapular plane. Arch Phys Med Rehabil 51:595, 1970.
19. Poppen, NK, and Walker, PS: Forces at the glenohumeral joint in abduction. Clin Orthop 135:165, 1978.
20. Awan, R, Smith, J, and Boon, AJ: Measuring shoulder internal rotation range of motion: A comparison of 3 techniques. Arch Phys Med Rehabil 83:1229, 2002.
21. Wanatabe, H, et al: The range of joint motions of the extremities in healthy Japanese people: The difference according to age. Nippon Seikeigeka Gakkai Zasshi 53:275, 1979. Cited by Walker, JM: Musculoskeletal development: A review. Phys Ther 71:878, 1991.
22. Boone, DC: Techniques of measurement of joint motion. (Unpublished supplement to Boone, DC, and Azen, SP: Normal range of motion in male subjects. J Bone Joint Surg Am 61:756, 1979.)
23. Walker, JM, et al: Active mobility of the extremities in older subjects. Phys Ther 64:919, 1984.
24. Downey, PA, Fiebert, I, and Stackpole-Brown, JB: Shoulder range of motion in persons aged sixty and older [abstract]. Phys Ther 71:S75, 1991.
25. West, CC: Measurement of joint motion. Arch Phys Med Rehabil 26:414, 1945.
26. Clarke, GR, et al: Preliminary studies in measuring range of motion in normal and painful stiff shoulders. Rheumatol Rehabil 14:39, 1975.
27. Allander, E, et al: Normal range of joint movement in shoulder, hip, wrist and thumb with special reference to side: A comparison between two populations. Int J Epidemiol 3:253, 1974.
28. Escalante, A, Lichenstein, MJ, and Hazuda, HP: Determinants of shoulder and elbow flexion range: Results from the San Antonio longitudinal study of aging. Arthritis Care Res 12:277, 1999.
29. Kebaetse, M, McClure, P, and Pratt, NA: Thoracic position effect on shoulder range of motion, strength, and three-dimensional scapular kinematics. Arch Phys Med Rehabil 80:945, 1999.
30. Sabari, JS, et al: Goniometric assessment of shoulder range of motion: Comparison of testing in supine and sitting positions. Arch Phys Med Rehabil 79:64, 1998.
31. Bigliani, LU, et al: Shoulder motion and laxity in the professional baseball player. Am J Sports Med 25:609, 1997.
32. Baltaci, G, Johnson, R, and Kohl H: Shoulder range of motion characteristics in collegiate baseball players. J Sports Med Phys Fitness 41:236, 2001.
33. Chinn, CJ, Priest, JD, and Kent, BA: Upper extremity range of motion, grip strength and girth in highly skilled tennis players. Phys Ther 54:474, 1974.
34. Kibler, WB, et al: Shoulder range of motion in elite tennis players: Effect of age and years of tournament play. Am J Sports Med 24:279, 1996.
35. Chang, DE, Buschbacker, LP, and Edlich, RF: Limited joint mobility in power lifters. Am J Sports Med 16:280, 1988.
36. Tiffitt, PD: The relationship between motion of the shoulder and the stated ability to perform activities of daily living. J Bone Joint Surg 80:41, 1998.
37. Matsen, FA, et al: Practical Evaluation and Management of the Shoulder. WB Saunders, Philadelphia, 1994.
38. Safaee-Rad, R, et al: Normal functional range of motion of upper limb joints during performance of three feeding activities. Arch Phys Med Rehabil 71:505, 1990.
39. Van Andel, CJ, et al: Complete 3D kinematics of upper extremity functional tasks. Gait Posture (2007), doi:10.1016/j.gaitpost 2007.03.002.
40. Hellebrandt, FA, Duvall, EN, and Moore, ML: The measurement of joint motion. Part III: Reliability of goniometry. Phys Ther Rev 29:302, 1949.
41. Boone, DC, et al: Reliability of goniometric measurements. Phys Ther 58:1355, 1978.
42. Pandya, S, et al: Reliability of goniometric measurements in patients with Duchenne muscular dystrophy. Phys Ther 65:1339, 1985.
43. Riddle, DL, Rothstein, JM, and Lamb, RL: Goniometric reliability in a clinical setting: Shoulder measurements. Phys Ther 67:668, 1987.
44. Bovens, AMP, et al: Variability and reliability of joint measurements. Am J Sports Med 18:58, 1990.
45. MacDermid, JC, et al: Intratester and intertester reliability of goniometric measurement of passive lateral shoulder rotation. J Hand Ther 12:187, 1999.
46. Hayes, K, et al: Reliability of five methods for assessing shoulder range of motion. Australian J Physiother 47:289, 2001.
47. Green, A, et al: A standardized protocol for measurement of range of movement of the shoulder using the Plurimeter-V inclinometer and assessment of its intrarater and interrater reliability. Arthritis Care Res 11:43, 1998.
48. Tiffitt, PD, Wildin, C, and Hajioff, D: The reproducibility of measurement of shoulder movement. Acta Orthop Scand 70:322, 1999.
49. Valentine, RE, and Lewis, JS: Intraobserver reliability of 4 physiologic movements of the shoulder in subjects with and without symptoms. Arch Phys Med Rehabil 87:1242, 2006.
50. Bower, KD: The hydrogoniometer and assessment of glenohumeral joint motion. Aust J Physiother 28:12, 1982.
51. Croft, P, et al: Observer variability in measuring elevation and external rotation of the shoulder. Br J Rheumatol 33:942, 1994.

The Elbow and Forearm

◯ Structure and Function

Humeroulnar and Humeroradial Joints

Anatomy

The humeroulnar and humeroradial joints between the upper arm and the forearm are considered to be a hinged compound synovial joint (Figs. 5.1 and 5.2). The proximal joint surface of the humeroulnar joint consists of the convex trochlea located on the anterior medial surface of the distal humerus. The distal joint surface is the concave trochlear notch on the proximal ulna.

The proximal joint surface of the humeroradial joint is the convex capitulum located on the anterior lateral surface of the distal humerus. The concave radial head on the proximal end of the radius is the opposing joint surface.

The joints are enclosed in a large, loose, weak joint capsule that also encloses the superior radioulnar joint. Medial and lateral collateral ligaments reinforce the sides of the capsule and help to provide medial–lateral stability (Figs. 5.3 and 5.4).[1]

When the arm is in the anatomical position of full elbow extension and supination, the long axes of the humerus and the forearm form an acute angle at the elbow. This angle is called the "carrying angle" (Fig. 5.5) and is approximately 10 to 12 degrees in men and 13 to 17 degrees in women.[2,3] The carrying angle of the dominant arm is reported to be slightly greater (1.5 degrees) than the nondominant arm and slightly greater (2 degrees) in adults than in children.[4] An angle that is greater (more acute) than average is called "cubitus valgus."[5] An angle that is less than average is called "cubitus varus."

Osteokinematics

The humeroulnar and humeroradial joints have 1 degree of freedom; flexion–extension occurs in the sagittal plane

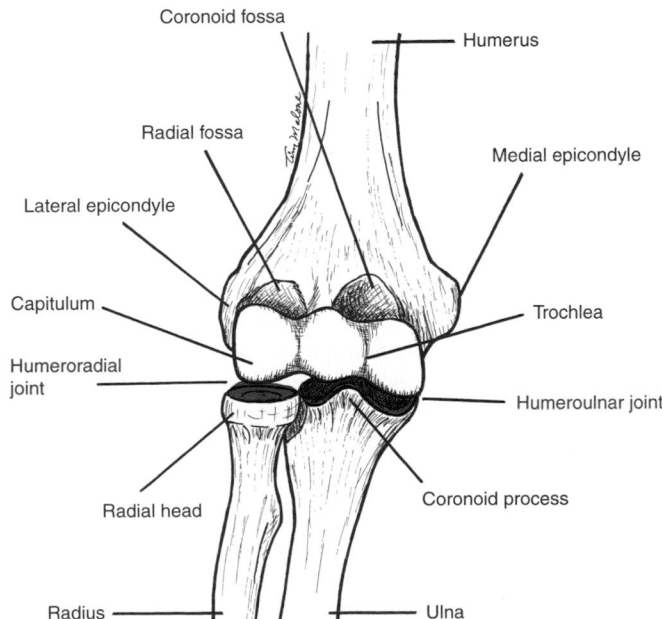

FIGURE 5.1 An anterior view of the right elbow showing the humeroulnar and humeroradial joints.

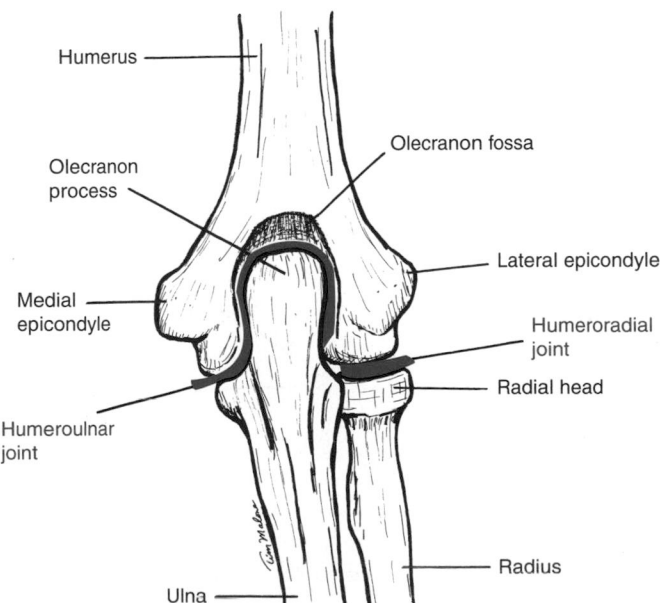

FIGURE 5.2 A posterior view of the right elbow showing the humeroulnar and humeroradial joints.

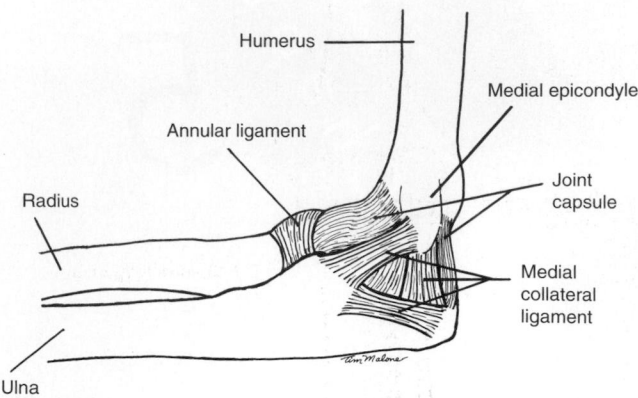

FIGURE 5.3 A medial view of the right elbow showing the medial (ulnar) collateral ligament, annular ligament, and joint capsule.

around a medial–lateral (coronal) axis. In elbow flexion and extension, the axis of rotation lies approximately through the center of the trochlea.[3]

Arthrokinematics

At the humeroulnar joint, posterior sliding of the concave trochlear notch of the ulna on the convex trochlea of the humerus continues during extension until the ulnar olecranon process enters the humeral olecranon fossa. In flexion, the ulna slides anteriorly along the humerus until the coronoid process of the ulna reaches the floor of the coronoid fossa of the humerus or until soft tissue in the anterior aspect of the elbow blocks further flexion.

At the humeroradial joint, the concave radial head slides posteriorly on the convex surface of the capitulum during extension. In flexion, the radial head slides anteriorly until the rim of the radial head enters the radial fossa of the humerus.

Capsular Pattern

Most authorities agree that the range of motion (ROM) in flexion is more limited than in extension.[7–9] Only in severe

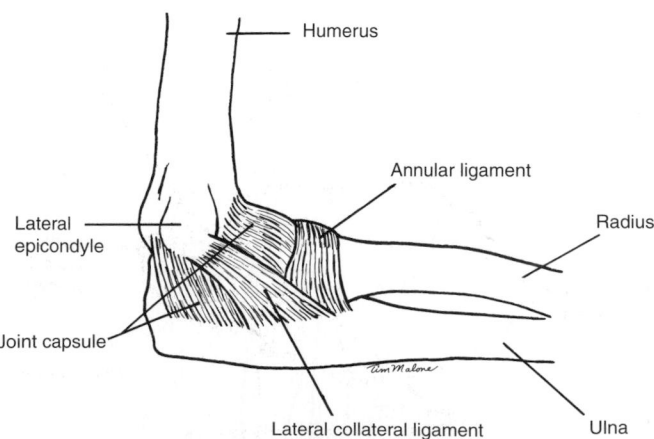

FIGURE 5.4 A lateral view of the right elbow showing the lateral (radial) collateral ligament, annular ligament, and joint capsule.

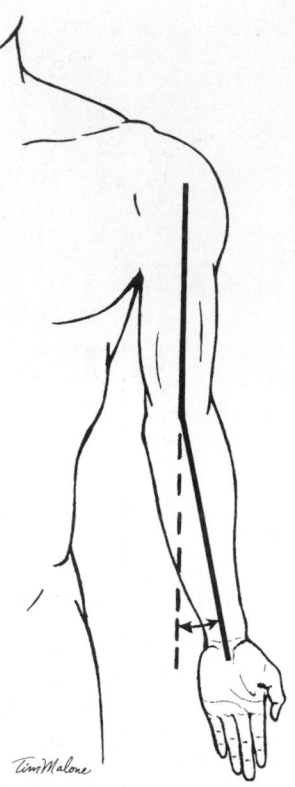

FIGURE 5.5 An anterior view of the right upper extremity showing the carrying angle between the longitudinal midline of the humerus and forearm.

cases would supination and pronation be slightly limited.[7] The literature varies as to the proportions of limitation in the capsular pattern for the elbow. For example, according to Cyriax, 30 degrees of limitation in flexion would typically correspond to about 10 degrees of limitation in extension.[7] Kaltenborn notes "that with flexion limited to 90 degrees (60-degree limitation) there is only 10 degrees of limited extension."[8]

Superior and Inferior Radioulnar Joints

Anatomy

The ulnar portion of the superior radioulnar joint includes both the radial notch located on the lateral aspect of the proximal ulna and the annular ligament (Fig. 5.6). The radial notch and the annular ligament form a concave joint surface. The radial aspect of the joint is the convex head of the radius.

The ulnar component of the inferior radioulnar joint is the convex ulnar head (see Fig. 5.6). The opposing articular surface is the ulnar notch of the radius.

The interosseous membrane, a broad sheet of collagenous tissue linking the radius and ulna, provides stability for both joints (Fig. 5.7). The following three structures provide stability for the superior radioulnar joint: the annular and quadrate ligaments and the oblique cord. Stability of

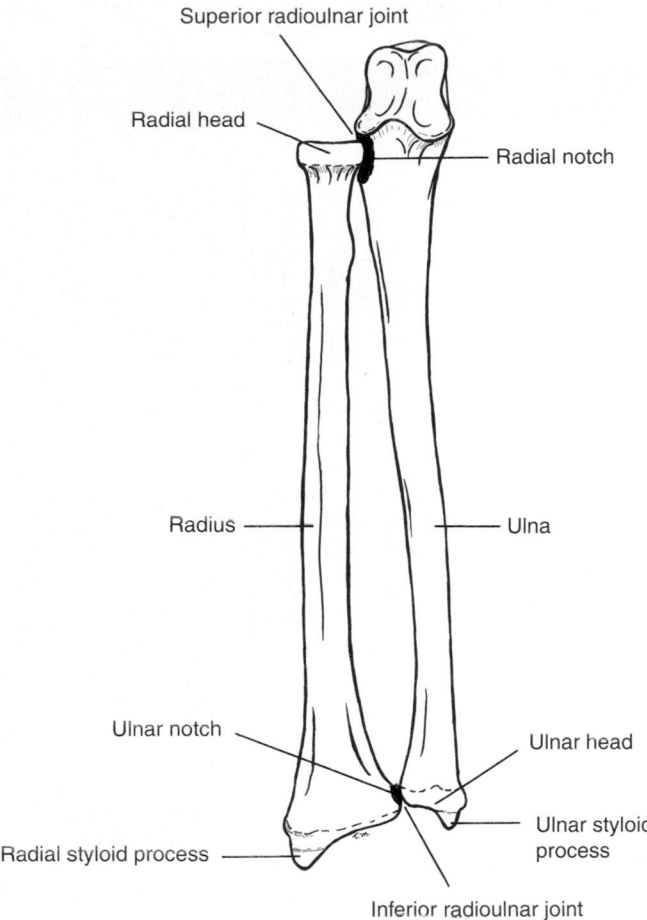

FIGURE 5.6 Anterior view of the superior and inferior radioulnar joints of the right forearm.

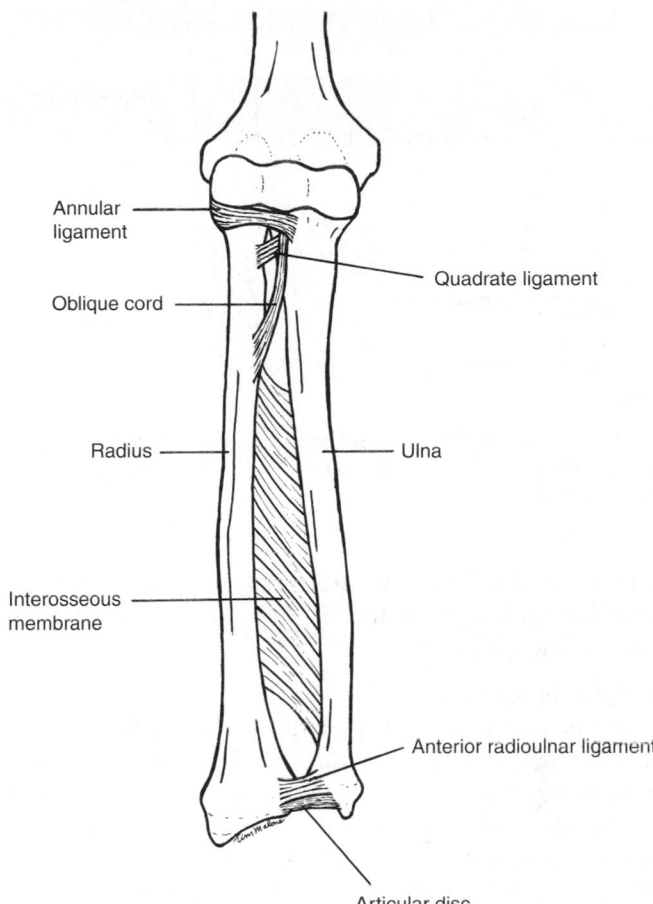

FIGURE 5.7 Anterior view of the superior and inferior radioulnar joints showing the annular ligament, quadrate ligament, oblique cord, interosseous membrane, anterior radioulnar ligament, and articular disc.

the inferior radioulnar joint is provided by the articular disc and the anterior and posterior radioulnar ligaments (Fig. 5.8).[1]

Osteokinematics

The superior and inferior radioulnar joints are mechanically linked. Therefore, motion at one joint is always accompanied by motion at the other joint. The axis for motion is a longitudinal axis extending from the radial head to the ulnar head. The mechanically linked joint is a synovial pivot joint with 1 degree of freedom. The motions permitted are pronation and supination. In pronation the radius crosses over the ulna, whereas in supination the radius and ulna lie parallel to one another.

Arthrokinematics

At the superior radioulnar joint the convex rim of the radial head spins within the annular ligament and the concave radial notch of the ulna during pronation and supination. The articular surface on the radial head spins posteriorly during pronation and anteriorly during supination.

At the inferior radioulnar joint the concave surface of the ulnar notch on the radius slides over the ulnar head. The concave articular surface of the radius slides anteriorly (in the same direction as the hand) during pronation and slides posteriorly (in the same direction as the hand) during supination.

Capsular Pattern

The capsular pattern is an equal limitation of supination and pronation according to Cyriax and Cyriax[7] and Kaltenborn.[8]

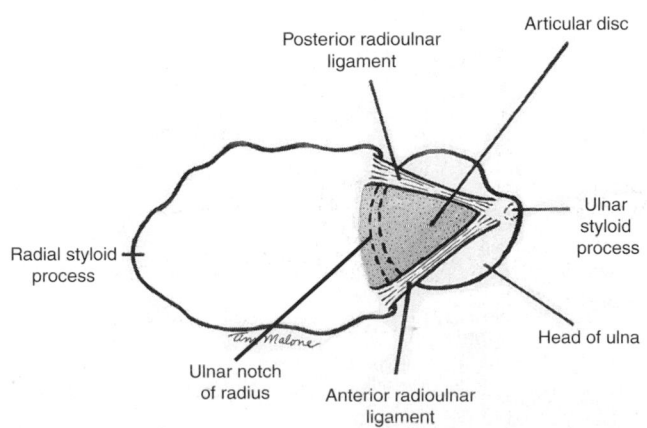

FIGURE 5.8 Distal aspect of the inferior radioulnar joint showing the articular disc and radioulnar ligaments.

RANGE OF MOTION TESTING PROCEDURES: Elbow and Forearm

Landmarks for Testing Procedures

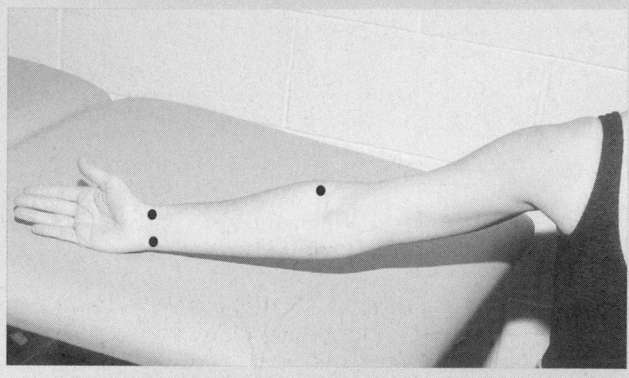

FIGURE 5.9 Anterior view of the right upper extremity showing surface anatomy landmarks for goniometer alignment during the measurement of elbow and forearm ROM.

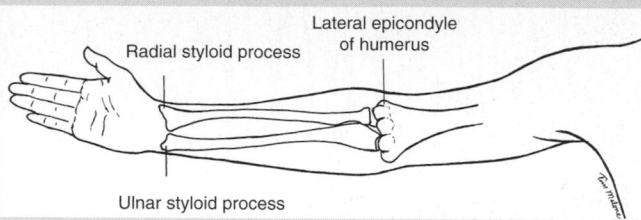

FIGURE 5.10 Anterior view of the right upper extremity showing bony anatomical landmarks for goniometer alignment during the measurement of elbow and forearm ROM.

Landmarks for Testing Procedures (continued)

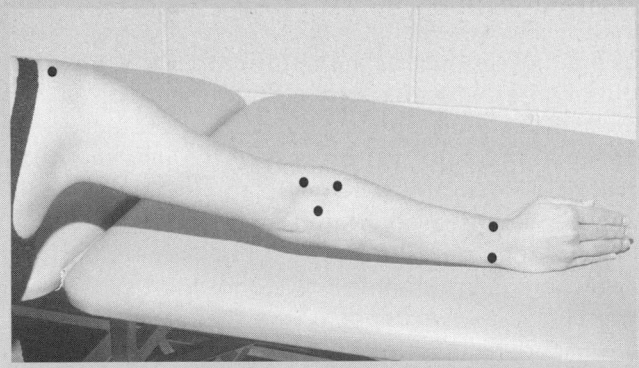

FIGURE 5.11 Posterior view of the right upper extremity showing surface anatomy landmarks for goniometer alignment during the measurement of elbow and forearm ROM.

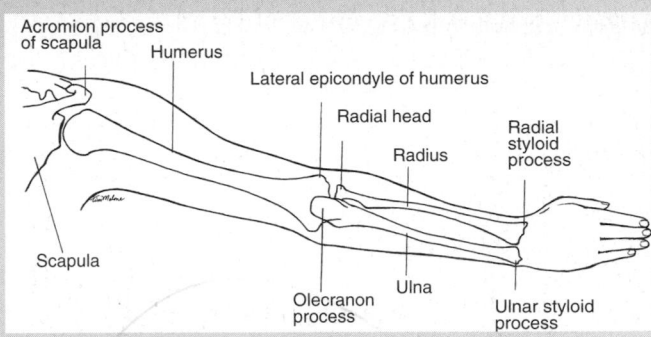

FIGURE 5.12 Posterior view of the right upper extremity showing anatomical landmarks for goniometer alignment during the measurement of elbow and forearm ROM.

take off jewlery

Range of Motion Testing Procedures/ELBOW AND FOREARM

● ELBOW FLEXION

Motion occurs in the sagittal plane around a medial–lateral axis. Normal ROM values for adults range from 140 degrees according to the American Medical Association (AMA)[12] to 150 degrees according to the American Academy of Orthopaedic Surgeons (AAOS).[10,11] See Research Findings and Tables 5.1 to 5.3 for additional normal ROM values by age and gender.

Testing Position

Position the subject supine, with the shoulder in 0 degrees of flexion, extension, and abduction so that the arm is close to the side of the body. Place a pad under the distal end of the humerus to allow full elbow extension. Position the forearm in full supination with the palm of the hand facing the ceiling.

Stabilization

Stabilize the humerus to prevent flexion of the shoulder. The pad under the distal humerus and the examining table prevent extension of the shoulder.

Testing Motion

Flex the elbow by moving the hand toward the shoulder. Maintain the forearm in supination during the motion (Fig. 5.13). The end of flexion ROM occurs when resistance to further motion is felt and attempts to overcome the resistance cause flexion of the shoulder.

Normal End-Feel

Usually the end-feel is soft because of compression of the muscle bulk of the anterior forearm with that of the anterior upper arm. If the muscle bulk is small, the end-feel may be hard because of contact between the coronoid process of the ulna and the coronoid fossa of the humerus and because of contact between the head of the radius and the radial fossa of the humerus. The end-feel may be firm because of tension in the posterior joint capsule, the lateral and medial heads of the triceps muscle, and the anconeus muscle.

Goniometer Alignment

See Figures 5.14 and 5.15.

1. Center **fulcrum** of the goniometer over the lateral epicondyle of the humerus.
2. Align **proximal arm** with the lateral midline of the humerus, using the center of the acromion process for reference.
3. Align **distal arm** with the lateral midline of the radius, using the radial head and radial styloid process for reference.

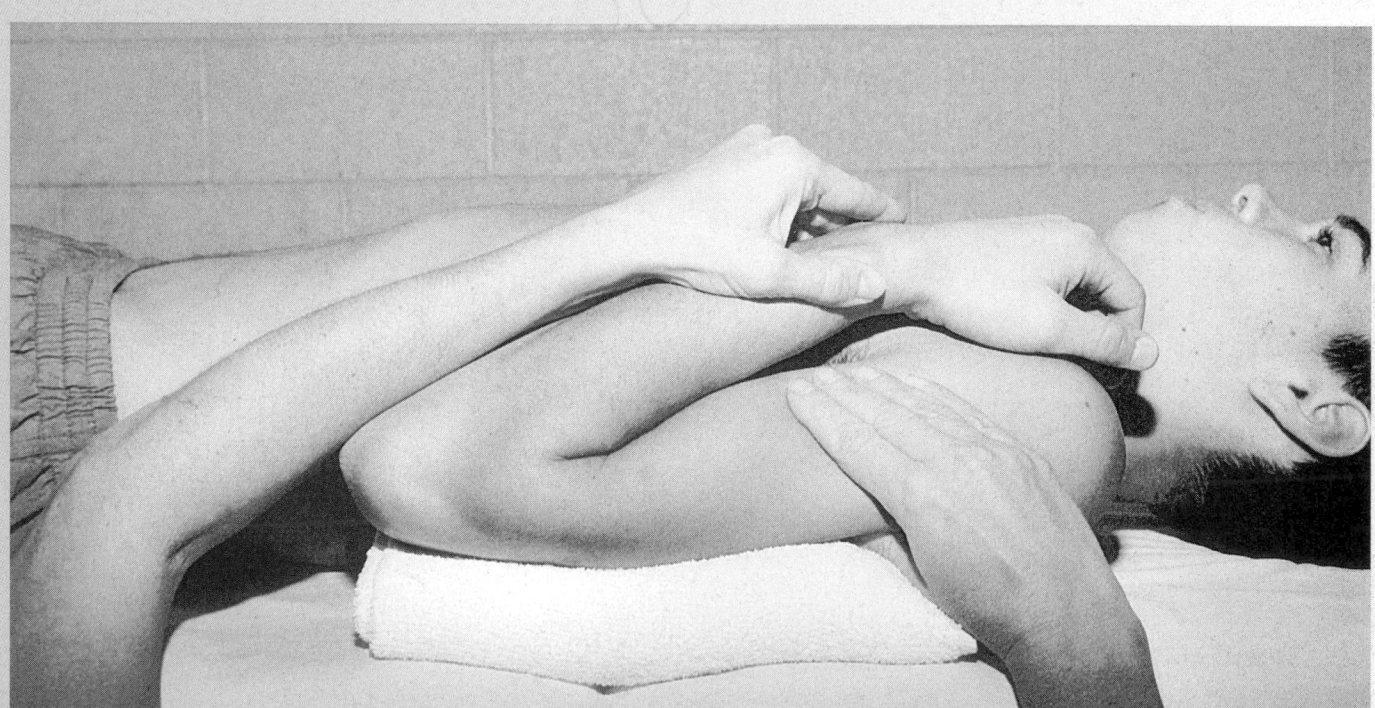

FIGURE 5.13 End of elbow flexion ROM. The examiner's hand stabilizes the humerus, but it must be positioned so it does not limit the motion.

Palm face up

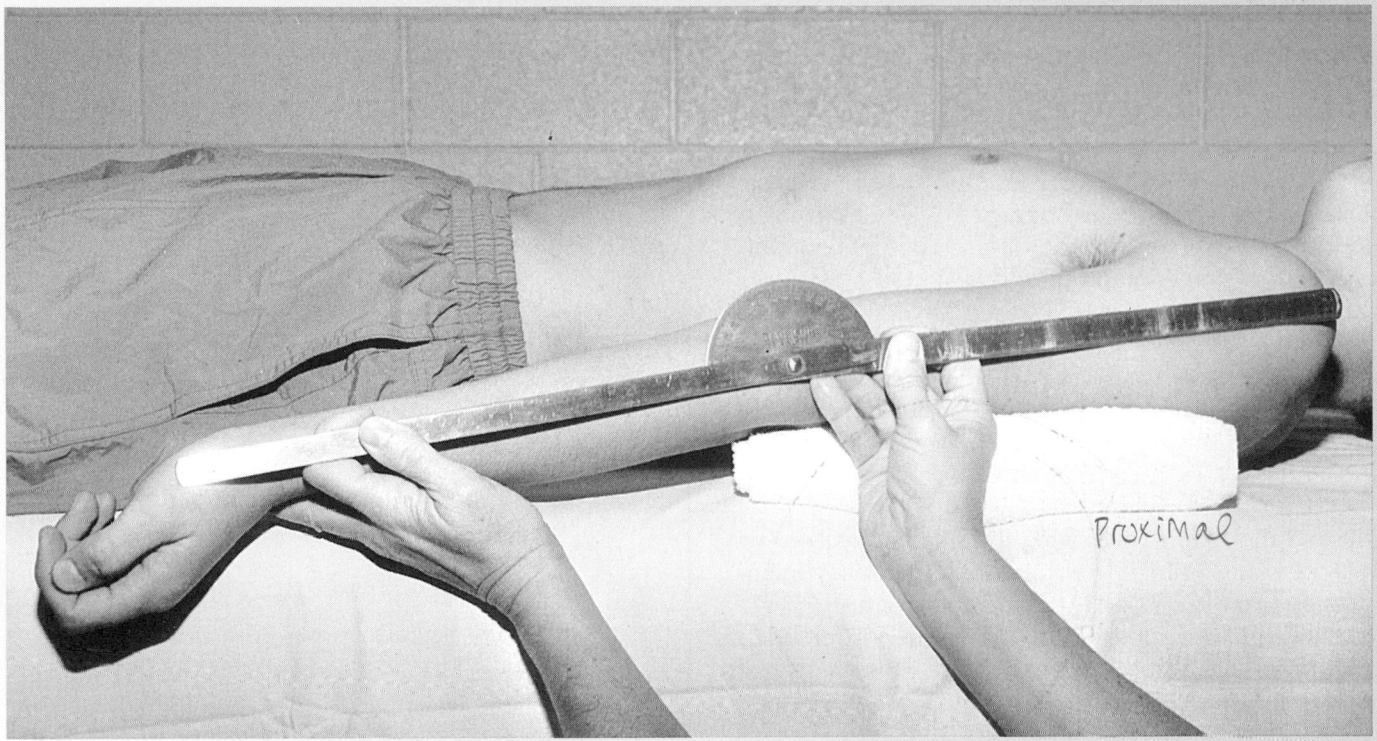

Proximal

FIGURE 5.14 Alignment of the goniometer at the beginning of elbow flexion ROM. A towel is placed under the distal humerus to ensure that the supporting surface does not prevent full elbow extension. As can be seen in this photograph, the subject's elbow is in about 5 degrees of hyperextension.

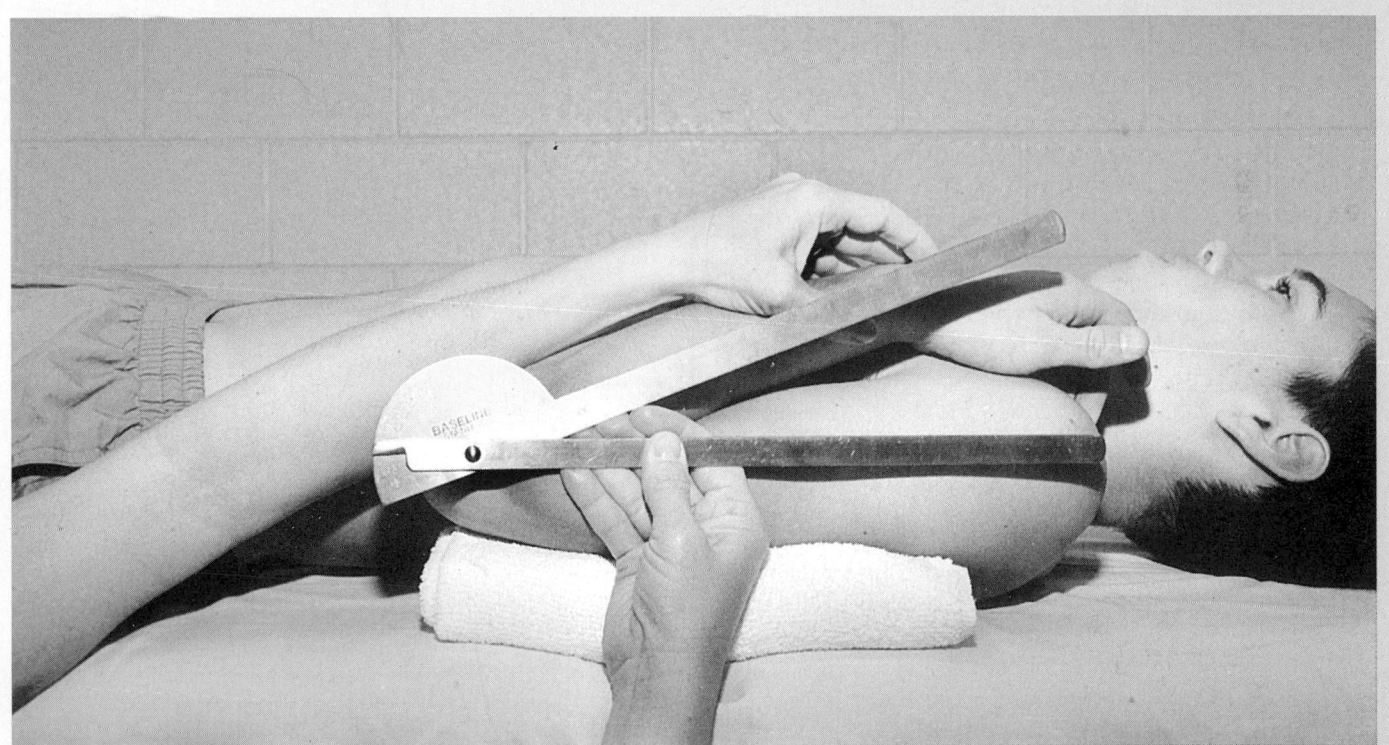

FIGURE 5.15 Alignment of the goniometer at the end of elbow flexion ROM. The proximal and distal arms of the goniometer have been switched from the starting position so that the ROM can be read from the pointer on the body of this 180-degree goniometer.

● ELBOW EXTENSION

Motion occurs in the sagittal plane around a medial–lateral axis. Elbow extension ROM is not usually measured and recorded separately because it is the return to the starting position from the end of elbow flexion ROM. If recorded, the normal extension ROM value for adults is 0 degrees.[10–12] See Research Findings and Tables 5.1 to 5.3 for additional normal ROM values by age and gender.

Testing Position, Stabilization, and Goniometer Alignment

The testing position, stabilization, and alignment are the same as those used for elbow flexion.

Testing Motion

Extend the elbow by moving the hand dorsally toward the examining table. Maintain the forearm in supination during the motion. The end of extension ROM occurs when resistance to further motion is felt and attempts to overcome the resistance cause extension of the shoulder.

Normal End-Feel

Usually the end-feel is hard because of contact between the olecranon process of the ulna and the olecranon fossa of the humerus. Sometimes the end-feel is firm because of tension in the anterior joint capsule, the collateral ligaments, and the brachialis muscle.

● FOREARM PRONATION

Motion occurs in the transverse plane around a vertical axis when the subject is in the anatomical position. When the subject is in the testing position, the motion occurs in the frontal plane around an anterior–posterior axis. Normal ROM values for adults are 76 degrees according to Boone and Azen[13] and 84 degrees according to Greene and Wolf.[14] Both the AMA[12] and the AAOS[10,11] state that normal pronation ROM is 80 degrees. See Research Findings and Tables 5.1 to 5.3 for additional normal ROM values by age and gender.

Testing Position

Position the subject sitting, with the shoulder in 0 degrees of flexion, extension, abduction, adduction, and rotation so that the upper arm is close to the side of the body. Flex the elbow to 90 degrees, and support the forearm. Initially position the forearm midway between supination and pronation so that the thumb points toward the ceiling.

Stabilization

Stabilize the distal end of the humerus to prevent medial rotation and abduction of the shoulder.

Testing Motion

Pronate the forearm by moving the distal radius in a volar direction so that the palm of the hand faces the floor. See Figure 5.16. The end of pronation ROM occurs when resistance to further motion is felt and attempts to overcome the resistance cause medial rotation and abduction of the shoulder.

Normal End-Feel

The end-feel may be hard because of contact between the ulna and the radius, or it may be firm

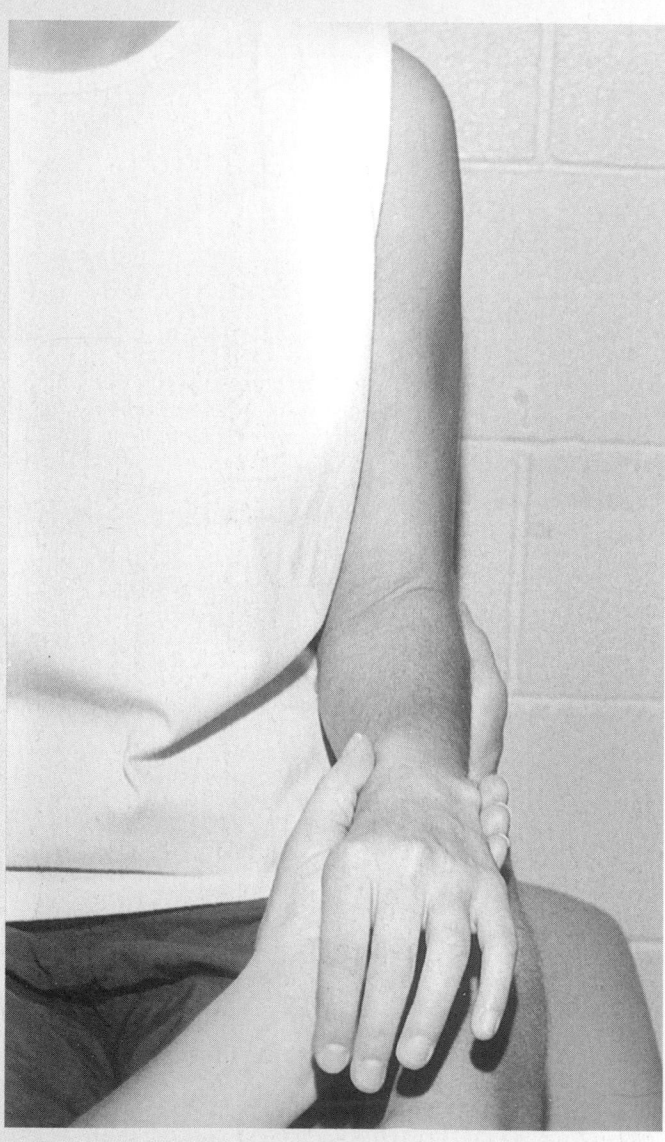

FIGURE 5.16 End of pronation ROM. The subject is sitting on the edge of a table, and the examiner is standing facing the subject. The examiner uses one hand to hold the elbow close to the subject's body and in 90 degrees of elbow flexion, helping to prevent both medial rotation and abduction of the shoulder. The examiner's other hand pushes on the radius rather than on the subject's hand. If the examiner pushes on the subject's hand, movement of the wrist may be mistaken for movement at the radioulnar joints.

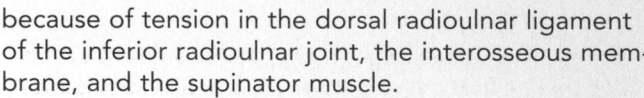
80°

because of tension in the dorsal radioulnar ligament of the inferior radioulnar joint, the interosseous membrane, and the supinator muscle.

Goniometer Alignment
See Figures 5.17 and 5.18.

1. Center **fulcrum** of the goniometer laterally and proximally to the ulnar styloid process.

2. Align **proximal** arm parallel to the anterior midline of the humerus.

3. Place **distal arm** across the dorsal aspect of the forearm, just proximal to the styloid processes of the radius and ulna, where the forearm is most level and free of muscle bulk. The distal arm of the goniometer should be parallel to the styloid processes of the radius and ulna.

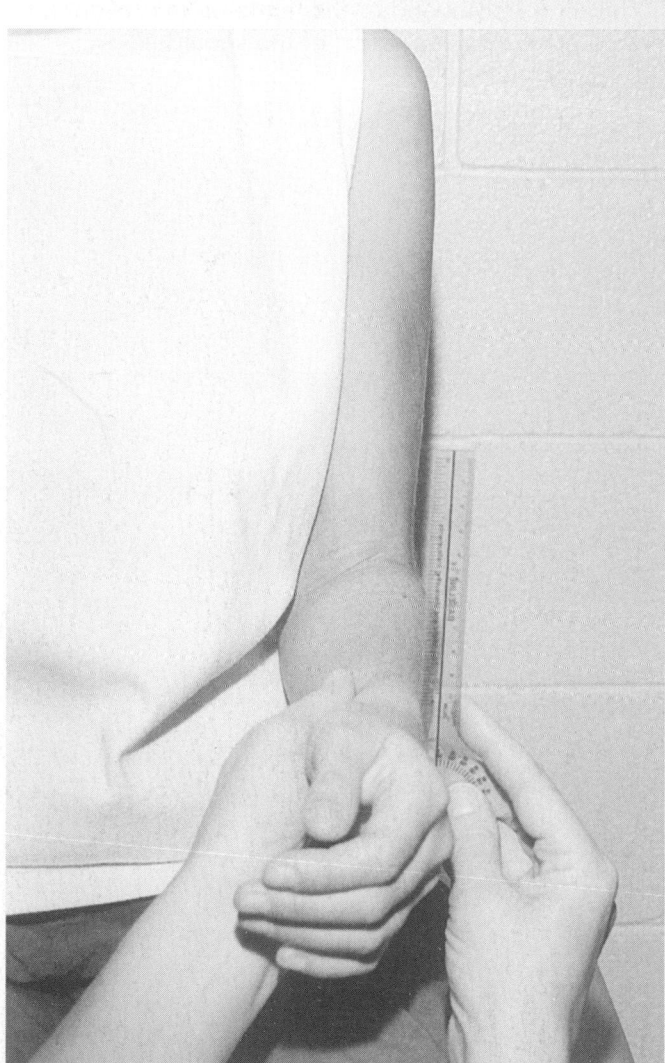

FIGURE 5.17 Alignment of the goniometer in the beginning of pronation ROM. The goniometer is placed laterally to the distal radioulnar joint. The arms of the goniometer are aligned parallel to the anterior midline of the humerus.

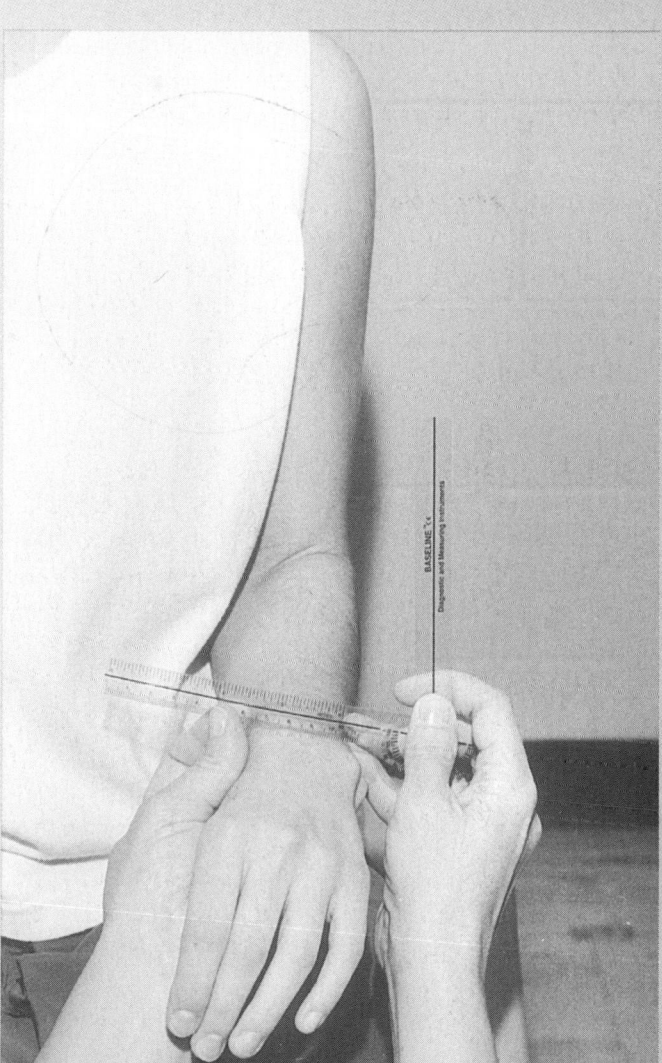

FIGURE 5.18 Alignment of the goniometer at the end of pronation ROM. The examiner uses one hand to hold the proximal arm of the goniometer parallel to the anterior midline of the humerus. The examiner's other hand supports the forearm and assists in placing the distal arm of the goniometer across the dorsum of the forearm just proximal to the radial and ulnar styloid process. The fulcrum of the goniometer is proximal and lateral to the ulnar styloid process.

● FOREARM SUPINATION

Motion occurs in the transverse plane around a longitudinal axis when the subject is in the anatomical position. When the subject is in the testing position, the motion occurs in the frontal plane around an anterior–posterior axis. Normal ROM values for adults are 92 degrees according to Gunal and coworkers,[15] 82 degrees according to Boone and Azen,[13] and 77 degrees according to Greene and Wolf.[14] Both the AMA[12] and the AAOS[10,11] state that normal supination ROM is 80 degrees. See Research Findings and Tables 5.1 to 5.3 for additional normal ROM values by age and gender.

Testing Position

Position the subject sitting, with the shoulder in 0 degrees of flexion, extension, abduction, adduction, and rotation so that the upper arm is close to the side of the body. Flex the elbow to 90 degrees, and support the forearm. Initially position the forearm midway between supination and pronation so that the thumb points toward the ceiling.

Stabilization

Stabilize the distal end of the humerus to prevent lateral rotation and adduction of the shoulder.

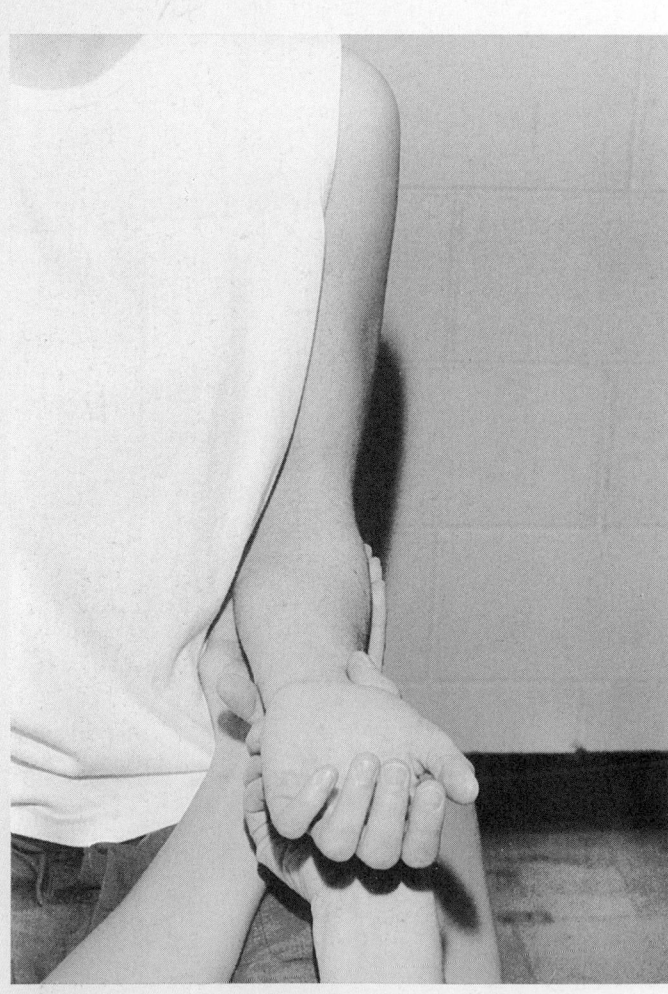

FIGURE 5.19 End of supination ROM. The examiner uses one hand to hold the elbow close to the subject's body and in 90 degrees of elbow flexion, preventing lateral rotation and adduction of the shoulder. The examiner's other hand pushes on the distal radius while supporting the forearm.

Testing Motion

Supinate the forearm by moving the distal radius in a dorsal direction so that the palm of the hand faces the ceiling. See Figure 5.19. The end of supination ROM occurs when resistance to further motion is felt and attempts to overcome the resistance cause lateral rotation and adduction of the shoulder.

Normal End-Feel

The end-feel is firm because of tension in the palmar radioulnar ligament of the inferior radioulnar joint, oblique cord, interosseous membrane, and pronator teres and pronator quadratus muscles.

Goniometer Alignment

See Figures 5.20 and 5.21.

1. Place **fulcrum** of the goniometer medially and just proximally to the ulnar styloid process.
2. Align **proximal arm** parallel to the anterior midline of the humerus.
3. Place **distal arm** across the ventral aspect of the forearm, just proximal to the styloid processes, where the forearm is most level and free of muscle bulk. The distal arm of the goniometer should be parallel to the styloid processes of the radius and ulna.

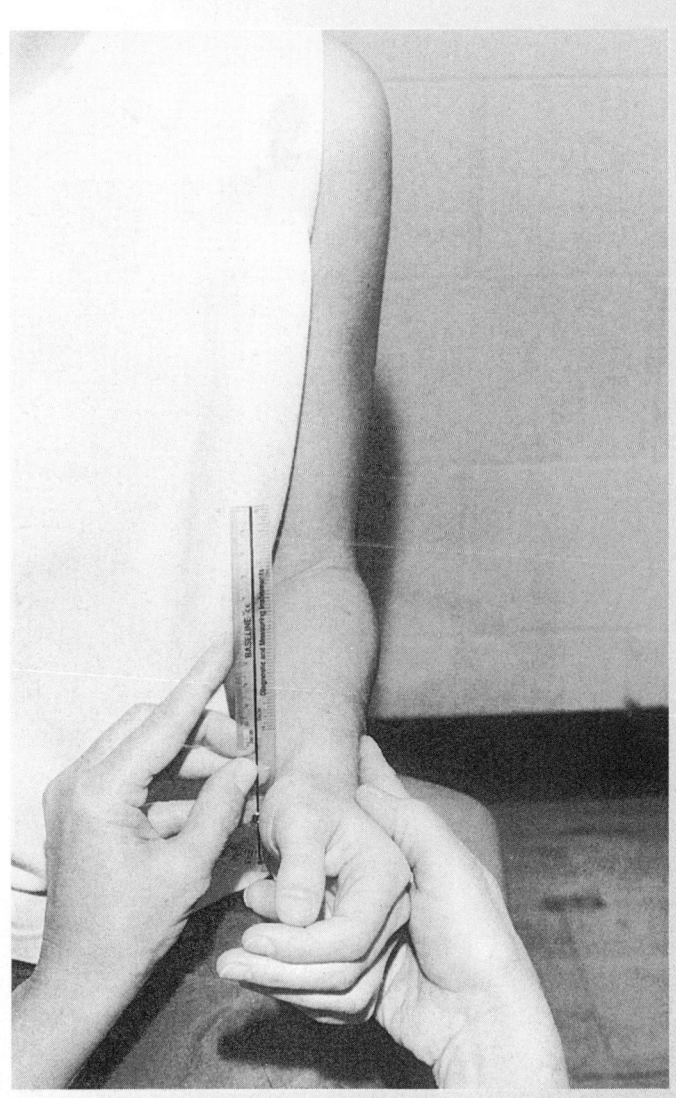

FIGURE 5.20 Alignment of the goniometer at the beginning of supination ROM. The body of the goniometer is medial to the distal radioulnar joint, and the arms of the goniometer are parallel to the anterior midline of the humerus.

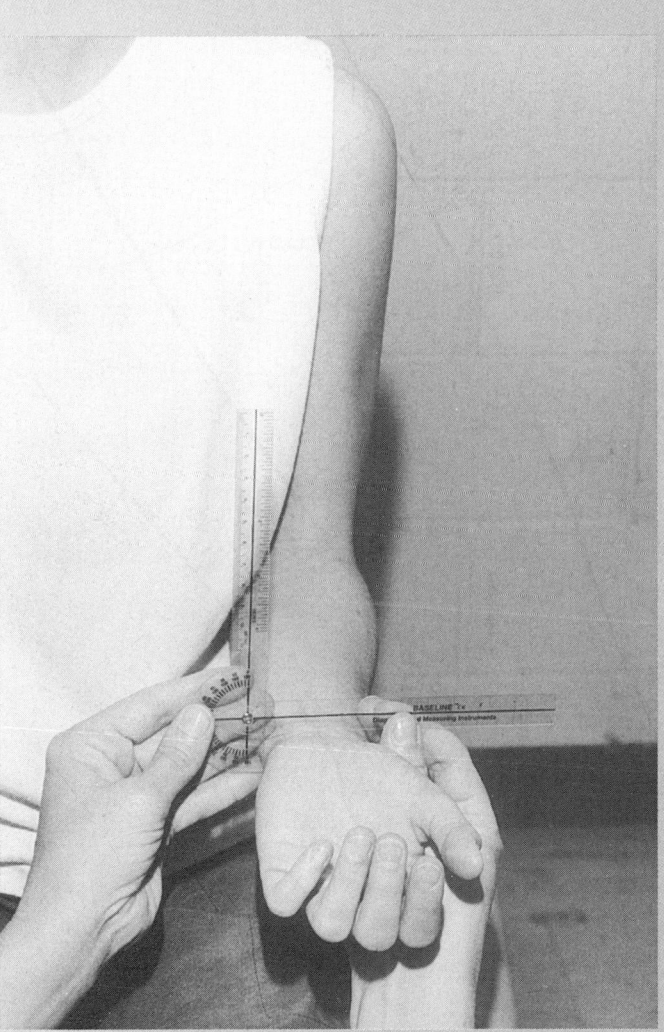

FIGURE 5.21 Alignment of the goniometer at the end of supination ROM. The examiner uses one hand to hold the proximal arm of the goniometer parallel to the anterior midline of the humerus. The examiner's other hand supports the forearm while holding the distal arm of the goniometer across the volar surface of the forearm just proximal to the radial and ulnar styloid process. The fulcrum of the goniometer is proximal and medial to the ulnar styloid process.

MUSCLE LENGTH TESTING PROCEDURES:
Elbow and Forearm

● BICEPS BRACHII

The biceps brachii muscle crosses the glenohumeral, humeroulnar, humeroradial, and superior radioulnar joints. The short head of the biceps brachii originates proximally from the coracoid process of the scapula (Fig. 5.22). The long head originates from the supraglenoid tubercle of the scapula. The biceps brachii attaches distally to the radial tuberosity.

When the biceps brachii contracts, it flexes the elbow and shoulder and supinates the forearm. The muscle is passively lengthened by placing the shoulder and elbow in full extension and the forearm in pronation. If the biceps brachii is short, it limits elbow extension when the shoulder is positioned in full extension.

If elbow extension is limited regardless of shoulder position, the limitation is caused by abnormalities of the joint surfaces, by shortening of the anterior joint capsule and collateral ligaments, or by muscles that cross only the elbow such as the brachialis and brachioradialis.

Starting Position
Position the subject supine at the edge of the examining table. See Figure 5.23. Flex the elbow and position the shoulder in full extension and 0 degrees of abduction, adduction, and rotation.

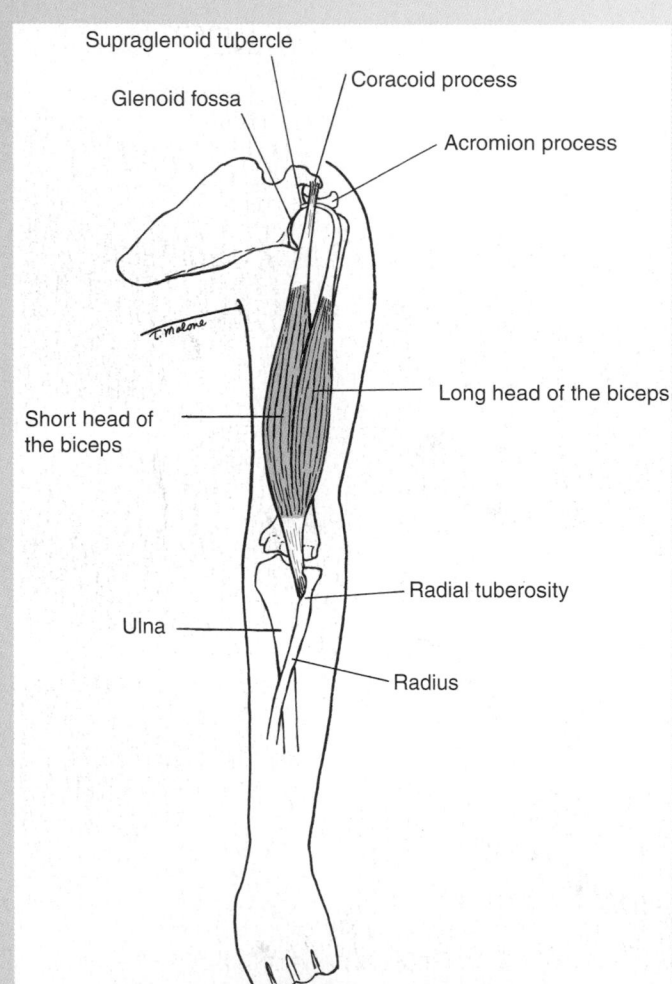

FIGURE 5.22 A lateral view of the left upper extremity showing the origins and insertion of the biceps brachii while being stretched over the glenohumeral, elbow, and superior radioulnar joints.

Labels: Supraglenoid tubercle; Glenoid fossa; Coracoid process; Acromion process; Long head of the biceps; Short head of the biceps; Radial tuberosity; Ulna; Radius

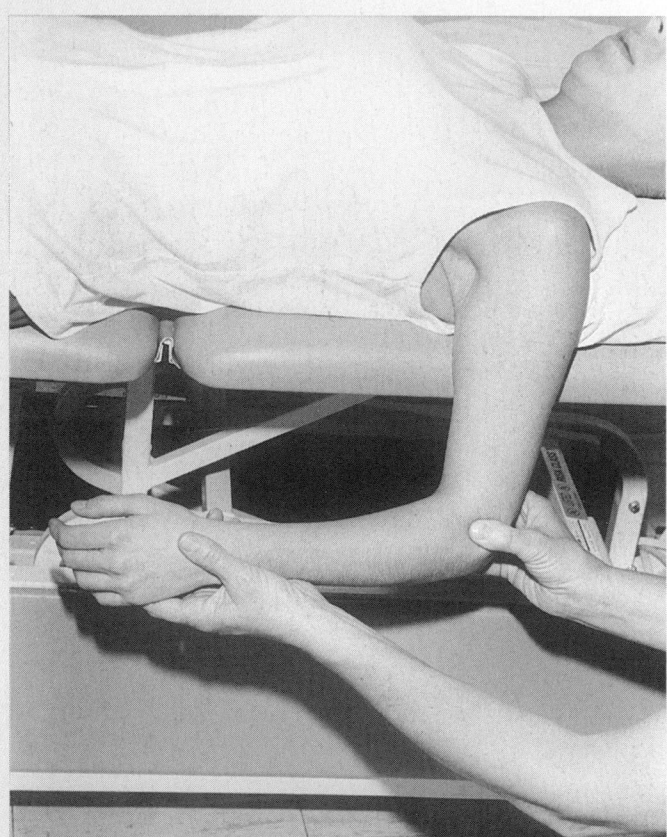

FIGURE 5.23 Starting position for testing the length of the biceps brachii.

Stabilization

The examiner stabilizes the subject's humerus. The examining table and passive tension in the serratus anterior muscle help to stabilize the scapula.

Testing Motion

Extend the elbow while holding the forearm in pronation. See Figures 5.24 and 5.22. The end of the testing motion occurs when resistance is felt and additional elbow extension causes shoulder flexion.

Normal End-Feel

The end-feel is firm because of tension in the biceps brachii muscle.

Goniometer Alignment

See Figure 5.25.

1. Center **fulcrum** of the goniometer over the lateral epicondyle of the humerus.
2. Align **proximal arm** with the lateral midline of the humerus, using the center of the acromion process for reference.
3. Align **distal arm** with the lateral midline of the ulna, using the ulna styloid process for reference.

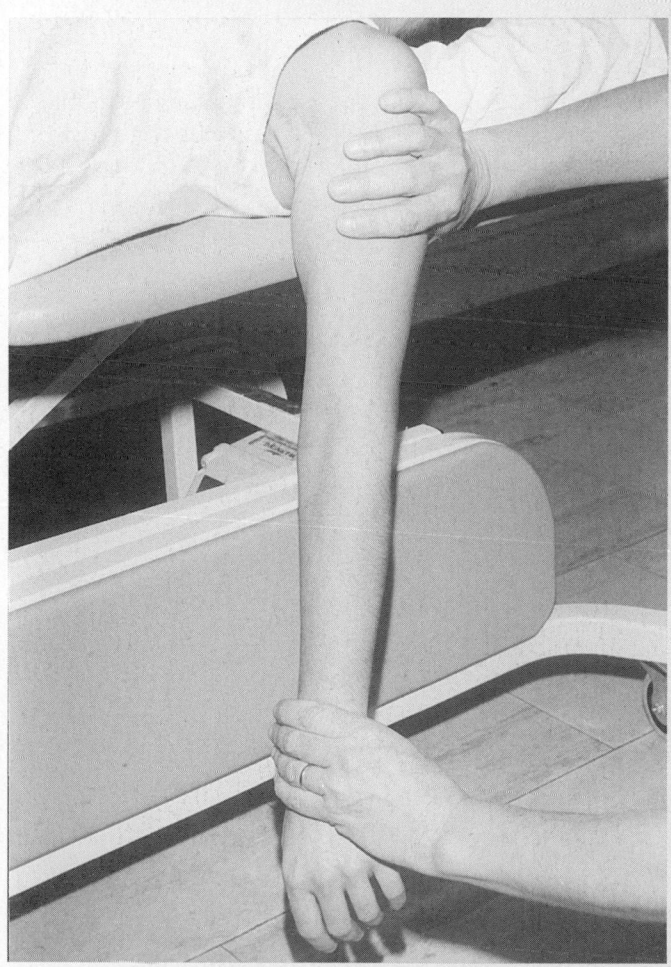

FIGURE 5.24 End of the testing motion for the length of the biceps brachii. The examiner uses one hand to stabilize the humerus in full shoulder extension while the other hand holds the forearm in pronation and moves the elbow into extension.

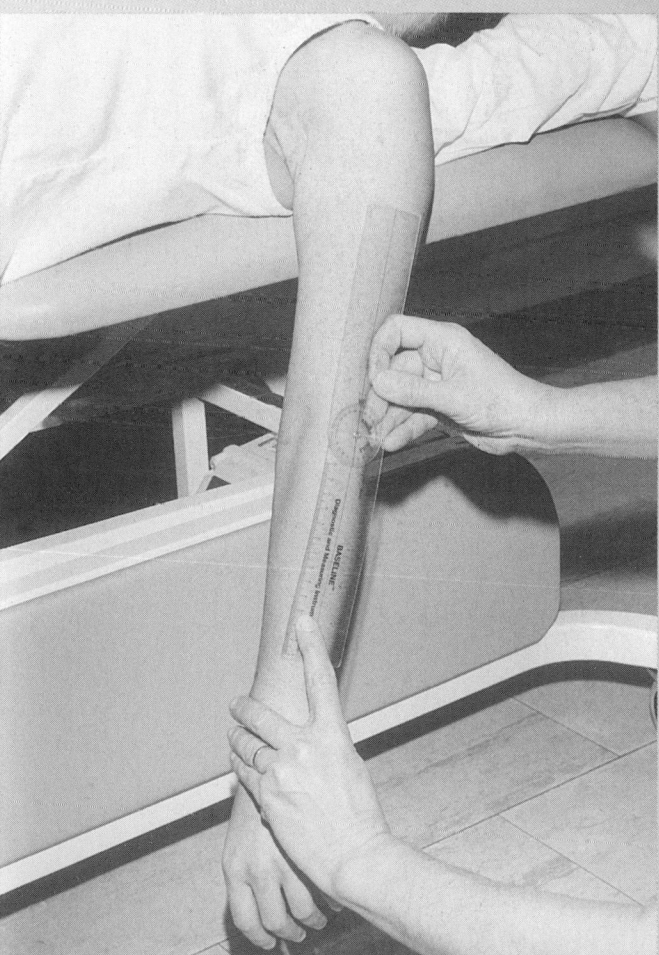

FIGURE 5.25 Alignment of the goniometer at the end of testing the length of the biceps brachii. The examiner releases the stabilization of the humerus and now uses her hand to position the goniometer.

● TRICEPS BRACHII

The triceps brachii muscle crosses the glenohumeral and humeroulnar joints. The long head of the triceps brachii muscle originates proximally from the infraglenoid tubercle of the scapula (Fig. 5.26). The lateral head of the triceps brachii originates from the posterior and lateral surfaces of the humerus, whereas the medial head originates from the posterior and medial surfaces of the humerus. All parts of the triceps brachii insert distally on the olecranon process of the ulna. When this muscle contracts, it extends the shoulder and elbow. The long head of the triceps brachii is passively lengthened by placing the shoulder and elbow in full flexion. If the long head of the triceps brachii is short, it limits elbow flexion when the shoulder is positioned in full flexion.

If elbow flexion is limited regardless of shoulder position, the limitation is due to abnormalities of the joint surfaces or shortening of the posterior capsule or muscles that cross only the elbow, such as the anconeus and the lateral and medial heads of the triceps brachii.

Starting Position

Position the subject supine, close to the edge of the examining table. Extend the elbow and position the shoulder in full flexion and 0 degrees of abduction, adduction, and rotation. Supinate the forearm (Fig. 5.27).

Stabilization

The examiner stabilizes the subject's humerus. The weight of the subject's trunk on the examining table and the passive tension in the latissumus dorsi, pectoralis minor, and rhomboid major and minor muscles help to stabilize the scapula.

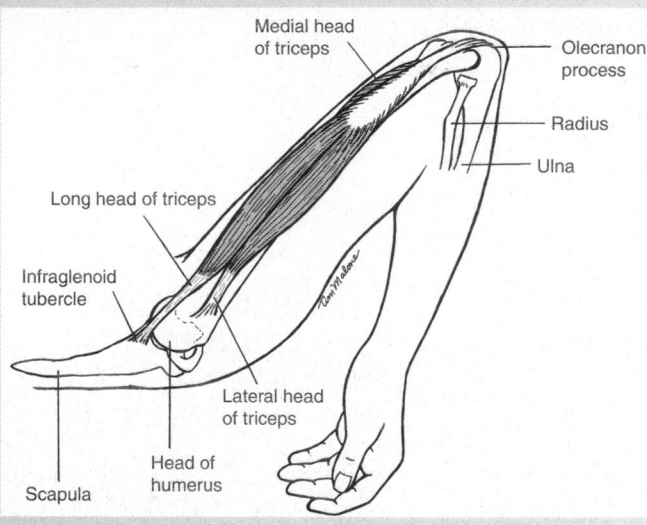

FIGURE 5.26 A lateral view of the left upper extremity showing the origins and insertions of the triceps brachii while being stretched over the glenohumeral and elbow joints.

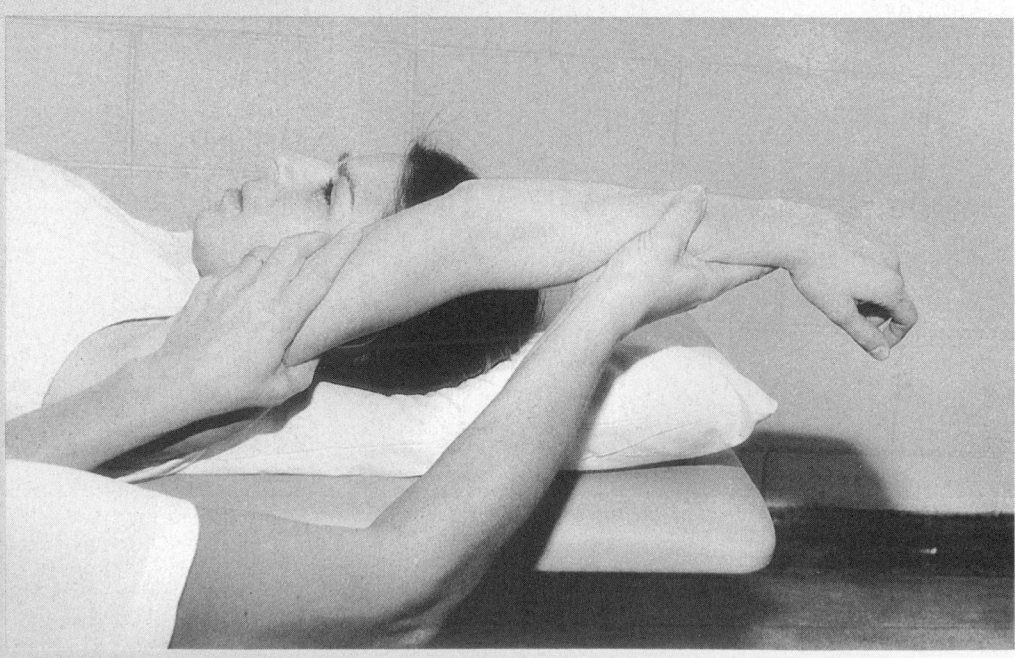

FIGURE 5.27 Starting position for testing the length of the triceps brachii.

Testing Motion

Flex the elbow by moving the hand closer to the shoulder. See Figures 5.28 and 5.26. The end of the testing motion occurs when resistance is felt and additional elbow flexion causes shoulder extension.

Normal End-Feel

The end-feel is firm because of tension in the long head of the triceps brachii muscle.

Goniometer Alignment

See Figure 5.29.

1. Center **fulcrum** of the goniometer over the lateral epicondyle of the humerus.
2. Align **proximal arm** with the lateral midline of the humerus, using the center of the acromion process for reference.
3. Align **distal arm** with the lateral midline of the radius, using the radial styloid process for reference.

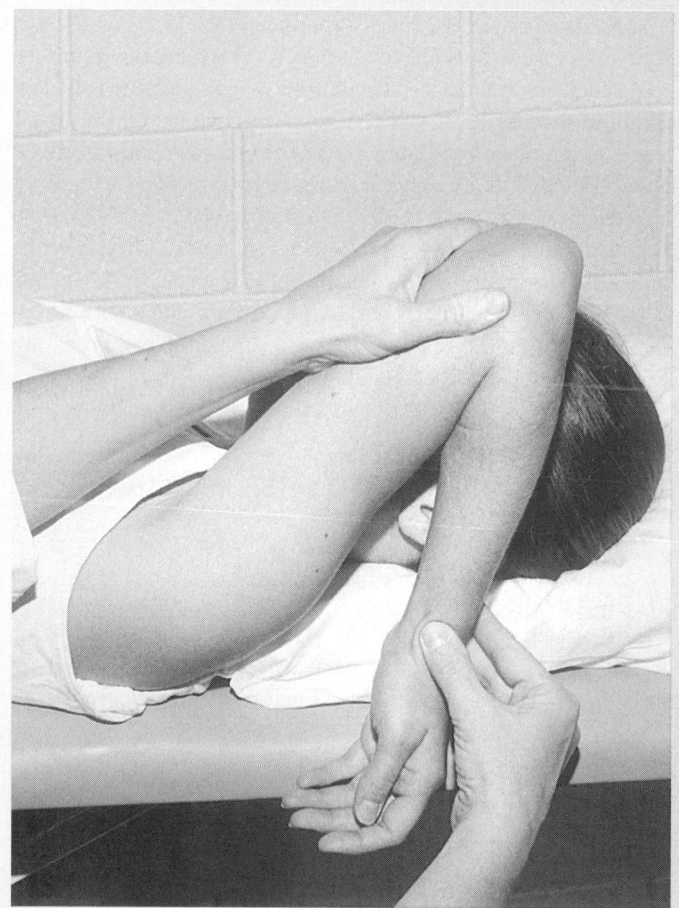

FIGURE 5.28 End of the testing motion for the length of the triceps brachii. The examiner uses one hand to stabilize the humerus in full shoulder flexion and the other hand to move the elbow into flexion.

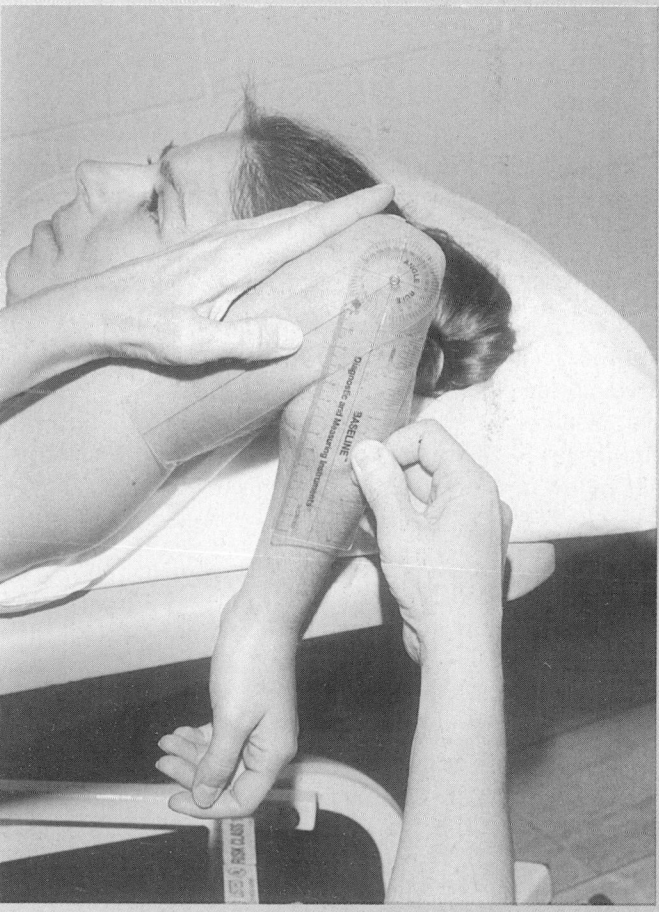

FIGURE 5.29 Alignment of the goniometer at the end of testing the length of the triceps brachii. The examiner uses one hand to continue to stabilize the humerus and align the proximal arm of the goniometer. The examiner's other hand holds the elbow in flexion and aligns the distal arm of the goniometer with the radius.

⌀ Research Findings

Effects of Age, Gender, and Other Factors

Table 5.1 provides normal elbow and forearm ROM values for adults.[10–15] In addition to the sources listed in Table 5.1, Goodwin and coworkers[16] found mean active elbow flexion to be 148.9 degrees in 23 females between 18 and 31 years of age. Petherick and associates[17] found mean active elbow flexion to be 145.8 degrees in 10 males and 20 females with a mean age of 24.0 years. Sanya and Chinyelu[18] studied 50 healthy adults (27 females and 23 males) between 20 and 71 years of age and found mean active elbow flexion to be 137.8 degrees. All of these sources used universal goniometers to obtain measurements. Fiebert, Fuhri, and New[19] measured elbow flexion and forearm motions with the Ortho Ranger (electronic inclinometer) and elbow extension with a universal goniometer in 124 men and women, 60 to 99 years of age. They found mean passive elbow flexion ROM to be 147 degrees, elbow extension –1 degree, pronation 84 degrees, and supination 85 degrees.

Age

A comparison of cross-sectional studies of normal ROM values for various age groups suggests that elbow and forearm ROM decreases slightly with increasing age. The elbow and forearm ROM values in infants reported by Wanatabe and colleagues[20] and in young male children aged 1 to 7 years reported by Hacker and coworkers[21] as noted in Table 5.2 are generally greater than the normal values for adult males found in Tables 5.1 and 5.3. However, it can be difficult to compare values obtained from various studies because subject selection and measurement methods can differ.

Within one study of 109 males ranging in age from 18 months to 54 years, Boone and Azen[13] noted a significant difference in elbow flexion and supination between subjects age 19 years or younger and those older than 19 years. Further analyses found that the group between 6 and 12 years of age had more elbow flexion and extension than other age groups. The youngest group (between 18 months and 5 years) had a significantly greater amount of pronation and supination than other age groups. However, the greatest differences between the age groups were small: 6.8 degrees of flexion, 4.4 degrees of supination, 3.9 degrees of pronation, and 2.5 degrees of extension.[22]

Older persons appear to have difficulty fully extending their elbows to 0 degrees. Walker and associates[23] found that the older men and women (between 60 and 84 years of age) in their study were unable to extend their elbows to 0 degrees to attain a neutral starting position for flexion. The mean value for the starting position was 6 degrees in men and 1 degree in women. Boone and Azen[13] also found that the oldest subjects in their study (between 40 and 54 years of age) had lost elbow extension and began flexion from a slightly flexed position. Bergstrom and colleagues,[24] in a study of 52 women and 37 men aged 79 years, found that 11 percent had flexion contractures of the right elbow greater than 5 degrees, and 7 percent had bilateral flexion contractures.

Kalscheur and associates[25] examined the effects of age in a study of 61 older women aged 63 to 83 years and the effects of age and gender in the same sample of 61 older women and 25 older men aged 66 to 86 years.[26] Depending on the linear regression models used, they found that elbow flexion declined about 0.1 to 0.2 degrees per year from age 65 to 85 years; pronation declined about 0.1 to 0.4 degrees per year, and supination declined about 0.0 to 1.0 degrees per year. It was projected that over a 20-year period elbow flexion could be expected to decline approximately 3 degrees, pronation 4 degrees, and right supination 6 degrees.[26] Only declines in right supination and pronation ROM were statistically significant.

Gender

Studies seem to concur that females have more elbow flexion and extension ROM than males, but results are unclear

| TABLE 5.1 | Normal Elbow and Forearm ROM Values for Adults in Degrees From Selected Sources |

	AAOS[10,11]	AMA[12]	Boone & Azen[13]	Greene & Wolf[14]	Gunal et al[15]
			20–54 yrs* n = 56 Males	18–55 yrs* n = 20 Males and Females	18–22 yrs† n = 1000 Males
Motion			Mean (SD)	Mean (SD)	Mean (SD)
Flexion	150	140	140.5 (4.9)	145.3 (1.2)	144.2 (5.8)
Extension	0	0	0.3 (2.7)		4.9 (11.1)
Pronation	80	80	75.0 (5.3)	84.4 (2.2)	
Supination	80	80	81.1 (4.0)	76.9 (2.1)	91.7 (9.6)

SD = standard deviation.
* Values are for active ROM measured with a universal goniometer.
† Values are for passive ROM measured with a universal goniometer. Values are extrapolated from tables.

TABLE 5.2 Effects of Age on Elbow and Forearm Motion: Normal Values in Degrees for Newborns, Children, and Adolescents

| | Wanatabe et al[20] | Hacker er al[21] | | Boone[22] | |
| | 2 wks–2 yrs*
n = 45
Males and Females | 1–7 yrs
n = 72
Males | 18 mos–5 yrs†
n = 19
Males | 6–12 yrs†
n = 17
Males | 13–19 yrs†
n = 17
Males |
Motion	Range of Means	Mean (SD)	Mean (SD)	Mean (SD)	Mean (SD)
Flexion	148–158	151.4 (1.8)	144.9 (5.7)	146.5 (4.0)	144.9 (6.0)
Extension		1.1 (3.9)	0.4 (3.4)	2.1 (3.2)	0.1 (3.8)
Pronation	90–96		78.9 (4.4)	76.9 (3.6)	74.1 (5.3)
Supination	81–93		84.5 (3.8)	82.9 (2.7)	81.8 (3.2)

SD = standard deviation.
* Values are for passive ROM.
† Values are for active ROM measured with a universal goniometer.

concerning gender effects on forearm supination and pronation ROM.

Bell and Hoshizaki,[27] using a Leighton Flexometer, studied the ROM of 124 females and 66 males between the ages of 18 and 88 years. Females had significantly more elbow flexion than males. Extrapolating from a graph, the mean differences between males and females ranged from 14 degrees in subjects aged 32 to 44 years to 2 degrees in subjects older than 75 years. Although females had greater supination–pronation ROM than males, this increase was not statistically significant.

Salter and Darcus,[28] measuring forearm supination–pronation with a specialized arthrometer in 20 males and 5 females between the ages of 16 and 29 years, found that the females had an average of 8 degrees more forearm rotation than males, although the difference was not statistically significant.

Escalante, Lichenstein, and Hazuda,[29] in a study of 695 community-dwelling older subjects between 65 and 74 years of age, found that females had an average of 4 degrees more elbow flexion than males.

Thirty older females and 30 older males, aged 60 to 84 years, were included in a study by Walker and coworkers.[23] Females had significantly more flexion ROM (1–148 degrees) than males (5–139 degrees), but males had significantly more supination (83 degrees) than females (65 degrees). Females had more pronation ROM than males, but the difference was not significant.

Kalscheru and coworkers[26] found that older women had more elbow and forearm ROM than older men in a study of a 61 women and 25 men ranging in age from 63 to 86 years. These gender differences were statistically significant for elbow flexion and pronation with mean differences of 6.2 and 4.9 degrees, respectively. There was no significant difference in supination ROM between the men and women.

Body Mass Index

Body mass index (BMI) was found by Escalante, Lichenstein, and Hazuda[29] to be inversely associated with elbow flexion in 695 older subjects. Each unit increase in BMI (kg/m^2) was

TABLE 5.3 Effects of Age on Active Elbow and Forearm Motion: Normal Values in Degrees for Adult Males 20 to 85 Years of Age

| | Boone[22] | | Walker et al[23] | |
| | 20–29 yrs
n = 19 | 30–39 yrs
n = 18 | 40–54 yrs
n = 19 | 60–85 yrs
n = 30 |
Motion	Mean (SD)	Mean (SD)	Mean (SD)	Mean (SD)
Flexion	140.1 (5.2)	141.7 (3.2)	139.0 (14.0)	139.7 (5.8)
Extension	0.7 (3.2)	0.7 (1.7)	–6.0* (5.0)	–0.4* (3.0)
Pronation	76.2 (3.9)	73.6 (4.3)	68.0 (9.0)	75.0 (7.0)
Supination	80.1 (3.7)	81.7 (4.2)	83.0 (11.0)	81.4 (4.0)

SD = standard deviation.
* The minus sign indicates flexion.

significantly associated with a 0.22 decrease in degrees of elbow flexion. Hacker and coworkers[21] also found an association between increased BMI and decreased elbow ROM in 72 healthy boys ages 1 to 7 years.

Right Versus Left Side

Studies comparing ROM between the right and left sides or between the dominant and nondominant limbs have generally found no clinically relevant differences in elbow and forearm ROM. Studies that had large numbers of subjects had the statistical power to find differences of 2 to 3 degrees to be significant. If differences were found, the left or nondominant side had more motion.

Boone and Azen[13] studied 109 males between the ages of 18 months and 54 years who were subdivided into six age groups. They found no significant differences between right and left elbow flexion, extension, supination, and pronation, except for the age group of subjects between 20 and 29 years of age, whose elbow flexion ROM was greater on the left than on the right. This one significant finding was attributed to chance. Hacker and colleagues[21] found no significant difference between sides for elbow ROM in 72 healthy boys aged 1 to 7 years. Gunal and coworkers,[15] in a study of 1000 males between 18 to 22 years of age, found significantly greater elbow flexion, extension, and supination ROM on the left as compared to the right; mean differences were 2.6 degrees, 2.0 degrees, and 2.2 degrees, respectively. Chang, Buschbacher, and Edlich[30] studied 10 power lifters and 10 age-matched non-lifters, all of whom were right handed, and found no differences between sides in elbow and forearm ROM.

Studies on older subjects have noted similar results. Escalante, Lichenstein, and Hazudal,[29] in a study of 695 older subjects, found significantly greater elbow flexion on the left than on the right, but the difference averaged only 2 degrees. Kalscheur and coworkers[25] reported no significant differences between sides for elbow flexion and pronation ROM in a study of 61 older women. A statistically significant difference between sides was noted for pronation ROM, with the left side being an average of 3.0 degrees greater than the right.

Sports

It appears that the frequent use of the upper extremities in sport activities may reduce elbow and forearm ROM. Possible causes for this association include muscle hypertrophy, muscle tightness, and joint trauma from overuse.

Chinn, Priest, and Kent,[31] in a study of 53 male and 30 female national and international tennis players, found significantly less active ROM in pronation (mean difference = 5.8 degrees) and supination (4.6 degrees) in the playing arms of all subjects. Male players also demonstrated a significant decrease (4.1 degrees) in elbow extension in the playing arm versus the nonplaying arm. Chang, Buschbacher, and Edlich[30] studied 10 power lifters and 10 age-matched nonlifters and found less active elbow flexion in the power lifters than in the nonlifters. No significant differences were found between the two groups for supination and pronation ROM. Wright and colleagues[32] noted an average decrease of 7.9 degrees for elbow extension ROM and 5.5 degrees for elbow flexion ROM in the dominant versus the nondominant arm of 33 professional pitchers. No significant differences were noted between the dominant and nondominant sides for supination and pronation ROM.

Functional Range of Motion

The amount of elbow and forearm motion that occurs during activities of daily living has been studied by several investigators. Table 5.4 has been adapted from the works of Morrey and associates,[33] Packer and colleagues,[34] and Safaee-Rad and coworkers.[35] Morrey and associates[33] used a triaxial electrogoniometer to measure elbow and forearm motion in 33 normal subjects during performance of 15 activities. They concluded that most of the activities of daily living that were studied required a total arc of about 100 degrees of elbow flexion (between 30 and 130 degrees) and 100 degrees of rotation (50 degrees of supination and 50 degrees of pronation). Using a telephone necessitated the greatest total ROM. The greatest amount of flexion was required to reach the back of the head (144 degrees), whereas feeding tasks such as drinking from a cup (Fig. 5.30) and eating with a fork required about 130 degrees of flexion. Reaching the shoes and rising from a chair (Fig. 5.31) required the greatest amount of extension. Among the tasks studied, the greatest amount of supination was needed for eating with a fork. Reading a newspaper (Fig. 5.32), pouring from a pitcher, and cutting with a knife required the most pronation.

Five healthy subjects participated in a study by Packer and colleagues,[34] which examined elbow ROM during three functional tasks. A uniaxial electrogoniometer was used to determine ROM required for using a telephone, for rising from a chair to a standing position, and for eating with a spoon. A range of 15 to 140 degrees of flexion was needed for these three activities. This ROM is slightly greater than the arc reported by Morrey and associates, but the activities that required the minimal and maximal flexion angles did not differ. The authors suggest that the height of the chair, the type of chair arms, and the positioning of the telephone could account for the different ranges found in the studies.

Safaee-Rad and coworkers[35] used a three-dimensional video system to measure ROM during three feeding activities: eating with a spoon, eating with a fork, and drinking from a handled cup. Ten healthy males participated in the study. The feeding activities required approximately 70 to 130 degrees of elbow flexion, 40 degrees of pronation, and 60 degrees of supination. Drinking with a cup required the greatest arc of elbow flexion (58 degrees) of the three activities, whereas eating with a spoon required the least (22 degrees). Eating with a fork required the greatest arc of pronation–supination (97 degrees), whereas drinking from a cup required the least (28 degrees). Maximum ROM values during feeding tasks were comparable with those reported by Morrey and associates. However, minimum values varied, possibly owing to the different chair and table heights used in the two studies.

TABLE 5.4	Elbow and Forearm Motion During Functional Activities: Mean Values in Degrees						
Activity	**Flexion**			**Pronation**	**Supination**		**Source**
	Min	*Max*	*Arc*	*Max*	*Max*	*Arc*	
Use telephone	42.8	135.6	92.8	40.9	22.6	63.5	Morrey[33]
	75	140	65				Packer[34]
Rise from chair	20.3	94.5	74.2	33.8	–9.5*	24.3	Morrey
	15	100	85				Packer
Open door	24.0	57.4	33.4	35.4	23.4	58.8	Morrey
Read newspaper	77.9	104.3	26.4	48.8	–7.3*	41.5	Morrey
Pour pitcher	35.6	58.3	22.7	42.9	21.9	64.8	Morrey
Put glass to mouth	44.8	130.0	85.2	10.1	13.4	23.5	Morrey
Drink from cup	71.5	129.2	57.7	–3.4†	31.2	27.8	Safaee-Rad[35]
Cut with knife	89.2	106.7	17.5	41.9	–26.9*	15.0	Morrey
Eat with fork	85.1	128.3	43.2	10.4	51.8	62.2	Morrey
	93.8	122.3	28.5	38.2	58.8	97.0	Safaee-Rad
Eat with spoon	101.2	123.2	22.0	22.9	58.7	81.6	Safaee-Rad
	70	115	45				Packer

* The minus sign indicates pronation.
† The minus sign indicates supination.

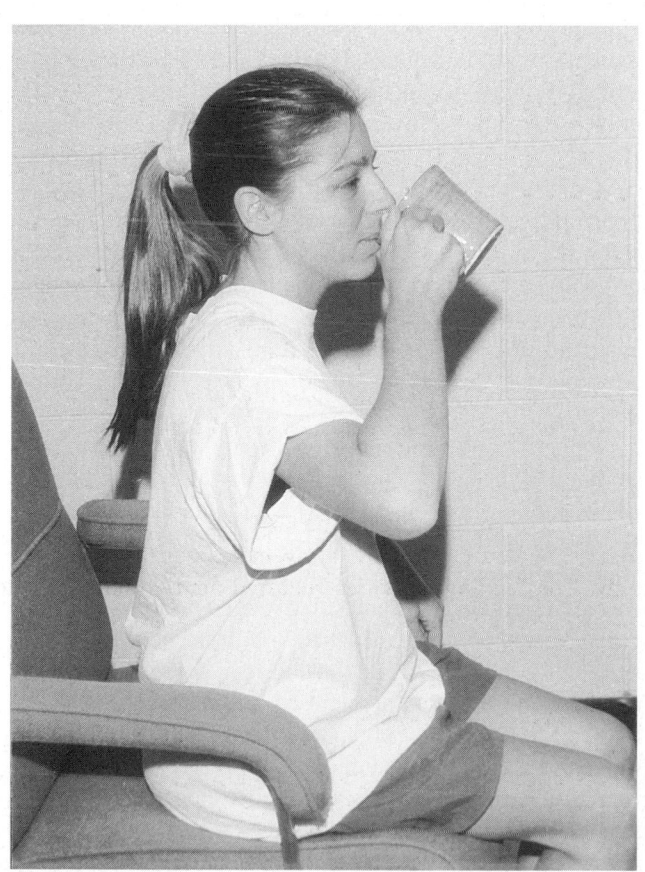

FIGURE 5.30 Drinking from a cup requires about 130 degrees of elbow flexion.

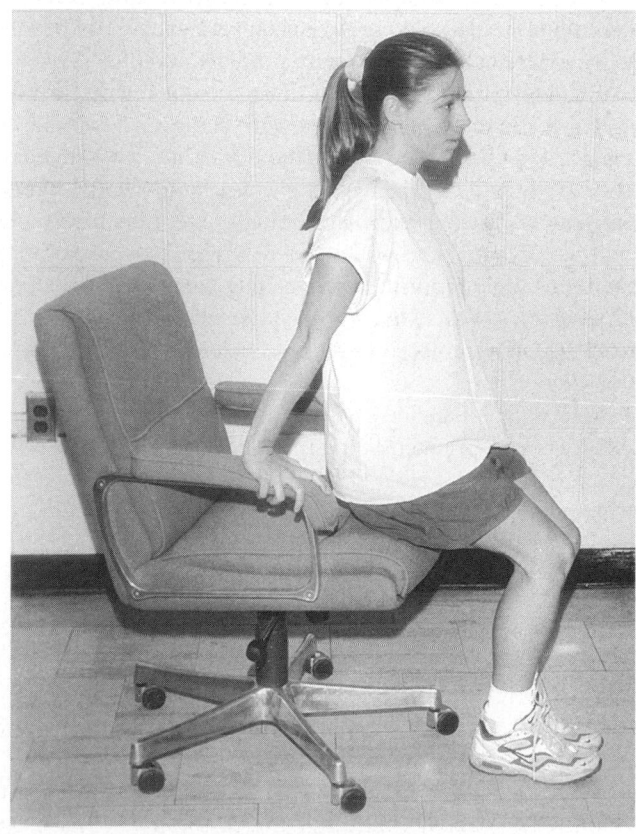

FIGURE 5.31 Studies report that rising from a chair using the upper extremities requires a large amount of elbow and wrist extension.

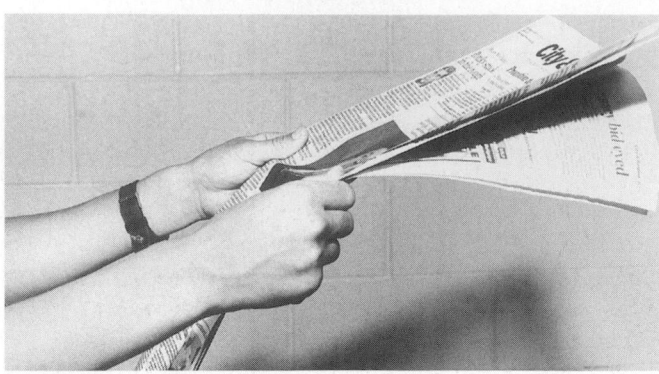

FIGURE 5.32 Approximately 50 degrees of pronation occur during the action of reading a newspaper.

Marco and coworkers[36] studied the performance of 20 activities of daily living in 10 subjects using a goniometer and torsiometer system. They concluded that eating activities required the least motion (53 to 129 degrees of elbow flexion ROM), instrument use such as writing and telephoning demanded a moderate amount of motion (44 to 130 degrees of elbow flexion ROM), and dressing activities required the greatest motion (10 to 140 degrees of elbow flexion ROM). Most instrument and dressing activities required pronation. The use of a spoon required the greatest supination (55 degrees).

Several investigators have taken a different approach in determining the amount of elbow and forearm motion needed for activities of daily living. Vasen and associates[37] studied the ability of 50 healthy adults to comfortably complete 12 activities of daily living while their elbows were restricted in an adjustable Bledsoe brace. Forty-nine subjects were able to complete all of the tasks with the elbow motion limited to between 75 and 120 degrees of flexion. Subjects used compensatory motions at adjacent normal joints to complete the activities. Cooper and colleagues[38] studied upper-extremity motion in subjects during three feeding tasks, with the elbow unrestricted and then fixed in 110 degrees of flexion with a splint. The 19 subjects were assessed with a video-based, three-dimensional motion analysis system while they were drinking with a handled cup, eating with a fork, and eating with a spoon. Compensatory motions to accommodate the fixed elbow occurred to a large extent at the shoulder and to a lesser extent at the wrist.

Reliability

A number of studies have examined the reliability of the measuring elbow and forearm ROM. Most investigators have found the intratester and intertester reliability of measuring ROM with a universal goniometer at these joints to be good to excellent. However, studies indicate that larger differences in repeated measurements are needed to detect meaningful change when examining forearm supination and pronation as compared to elbow flexion and extension. Comparisons between ROM measurements taken with different devices have also been conducted, giving some indication of the

concurrent validity of these devices with the universal goniometer. It is recommended that clinicians use the same device and alignment method to improve reliability because they are not interchangeable.

In a study published in 1949 by Hellebrandt, Duvall, and Moore,[39] one therapist repeatedly measured 13 active upper-extremity motions, including elbow flexion and extension and forearm pronation and supination, in 77 patients. The differences between the means of two trials ranged from 0.1 degrees for elbow extension to 1.5 degrees for supination. A significant difference between the measurements was noted for elbow flexion, although the difference between the means was only 1.0 degrees. Significant differences were also noted between measurements taken with a universal goniometer and those obtained by means of specialized devices, leading the author to conclude that different measuring devices could not be used interchangeably. The universal goniometer was generally found to be the more reliable device.

Boone and colleagues[40] examined the reliability of measuring six passive motions, including elbow extension–flexion. Four physical therapists used universal goniometers to measure these motions in 12 normal males weekly for 4 weeks. They found that intratester reliability (r = 0.94) was slightly higher than intertester reliability (r = 0.88).

Rothstein, Miller, and Roettger[41] found high intratester and intertester reliability for passive ROM of elbow flexion and extension. Their study involved 12 testers who used three different commonly used universal goniometers (large plastic, small plastic, and large metal) to measure 24 patients. Pearson product-moment correlation values ranged from 0.89 to 0.97 for elbow flexion and extension ROM, whereas intraclass correlation coefficient (ICC) values ranged from 0.85 to 0.95.

Grohmann,[42] in a study involving 40 testers and one subject, found that no significant differences existed between elbow measurements obtained by an over-the-joint method for goniometer alignment and the traditional lateral method. Differences between the means of the measurements were less than 2 degrees. The elbow was held in two fixed positions (an acute and an obtuse angle) by a plywood stabilizing device.

Petherick and associates,[17] in a study in which two testers measured 30 healthy subjects, found that intertester reliability for measuring active elbow ROM with a fluid-based goniometer was higher than with a universal goniometer. The Pearson product-moment correlation between the two devices was 0.83, whereas a significant difference was found between the two devices. The authors concluded that no concurrent validity existed between the fluid-based and the universal goniometers and that these instruments could not be used interchangeably.

Greene and Wolf[14] compared the reliability of the Ortho Ranger, an electronic pendulum goniometer, with the reliability of a universal goniometer for active upper-extremity motions in 20 healthy adults. Elbow flexion and extension were measured three times for each instrument during each session. The three sessions were conducted by one physical therapist during a 2-week period. Within-session reliability was higher for the universal goniometer, as indicated by ICC values and 95 percent confidence intervals. Measurements taken with the Ortho Ranger correlated poorly with those taken with the universal goniometer (r = 0.11 to 0.21), and there was a significant difference in measurements between the two devices.

Goodwin and coworkers[16] evaluated the reliability of a universal goniometer, a fluid goniometer, and an electrogoniometer for measuring active elbow ROM in 23 healthy women. Three testers took three consecutive readings using each type of goniometer, on two occasions that were 4 weeks apart. Significant differences were found between types of goniometers, testers, and replications. Measurements taken with the universal and fluid goniometers correlated the best (r = 0.90), whereas the electrogoniometer correlated poorly with the universal goniometer (r = 0.51) and fluid goniometer (r = 0.33). Intratester and intertester reliability was high during each occasion, with correlation coefficients greater than 0.98 and 0.90, respectively. Intratester reliability between occasions was highest for the universal goniometer. ICC values ranged from 0.61 to 0.92 for the universal goniometer, 0.53 to 0.85 for the fluid goniometer, and 0.00 to 0.61 for the electrogoniometer. Similar to other researchers, the authors do not advise the interchangeable use of different types of goniometers in the clinical setting.

Armstrong and associates[43] examined the intratester, intertester, and interdevice reliability of active ROM measurements of the elbow and forearm in 38 surgical patients. Five testers measured each motion twice with each of the three devices: a universal goniometer, an electrogoniometer, and a mechanical rotation measuring device. Intratester reliability was high (r values generally greater than 0.90) for all three devices and all motions. Intertester reliability was high for pronation and supination with all three devices. Intertester reliability for elbow flexion and extension was high for the electrogoniometer and moderate for the universal goniometer. Measurements taken with different devices varied widely. The authors concluded that meaningful changes in intratester ROM taken with a universal goniometer occur with 95 percent confidence if they are greater than 6 degrees for flexion, 7 degrees for extension, and 8 degrees for pronation and supination. Meaningful changes in intertester ROM taken with a universal goniometer occur if they are greater than 10 degrees for flexion, extension, and pronation and greater than 11 degrees for supination.

Two examiners measured the active ROM of several upper-extremity joints in 29 patients with reflex sympathetic dystrophy with either an inclinometer or universal goniometer in a study by Geertzen and coworkers.[44] Each examiner measured the motions of each patient once per session, and the session was repeated 30 minutes later. The smallest detectable difference, defined as the smallest amount of change in a variable that can be measured with statistical significance, for elbow flexion and extension with a universal goniometer was 9.6 and 12.1 degrees on the affected side and 7.1 and 12.1 degrees on the nonaffected side, respectively. The smallest detectable difference for supination measured with an inclinometer was 19.3 degrees on the affected side and 16.5 degrees on the nonaffected side. Correlation coefficients between repeated measurements

ranged from 0.57 to 0.84 for flexion, 0.66 to 0.92 for elbow extension, and 0.85 to 0.94 for supination. The authors concluded that random error, followed by observer and patient–observer interaction were the most important sources of variation in these patients with reflex sympathetic dystrophy.

A study by Gajdosik[45] of 31 healthy subjects compared three methods of measuring active ROM for supination and pronation. All three methods aligned the stationary arm of a universal goniometer parallel to the humerus. However, Method I aligned the movable arm of the goniometer with a pencil held in the hand. Method II placed the movable arm of the goniometer over the anterior or posterior surface of the distal forearm, and Method III aligned the movable arm of the goniometer parallel to a visualized line connecting the distal radius and ulna. There was a significant difference in values between the three methods, with Method I having the greatest amount of supination and the least amount of pronation. All methods were highly reliable with ICC values ranging from 0.81 to 0.97 for three trials by one tester in one session and from 0.86 to 0.96 for two sessions conducted 30 minutes apart. The author noted that Method I was the most reliable but was confounded during supination by movement of the fourth and fifth metacarpals. Methods II and III were recommended as reliable and more valid for clinical use but should not be used interchangeably.

Flower and associates[46] measured passive supination and pronation ROM in 30 orthopedic patients (31 wrists) with a traditional 6-inch universal goniometer aligned with the humerus and placed on the distal forearm and a new offset goniometer with a tubular handle and plumbline design. Three therapists measured each motion with each device once per session and repeated the session 20 minutes later. Intraclass correlation coefficients for supination were 0.95 for both the universal and new goniometer and 0.79 and 0.87 for pronation with the universal and new goniometer, respectively. Average standard error of the measurement for supination was 3.7 degrees for both the universal and new goniometer and 7.0 and 6.2 degrees for pronation with the universal and new goniometer, respectively. The authors stated that the difference in reliability between the two methods is probably not clinically significant.

Karagiannopoulos, Sitler, and Michlovitz[47] assessed the reliability of two methods of measuring a functional combination of active forearm and wrist rotation in 20 injured and 20 noninjured subjects. One method placed the stationary arm of a universal goniometer vertically and aligned the movable arm with a pencil held in the hand. The second method utilized an investigator-constructed tubular handle attached to a single-arm plumbline goniometer. Measurements were taken three times with each method by the two examiners during one session. Reliability was high and error was low for both methods and subject groups. Intratester and intertester ICC values ranged from 0.86 to 0.98 and from 0.91 to 0.96, respectively. Intratester SEM values ranged from 1.4 to 2.1 degrees, whereas intertester SEM values ranged from 2.2 to 3.9 degrees. To assess functional supination and pronation, the authors recommended the clinical use of the handheld pencil method over the slightly more reliable plumbline method because of the simplicity and greater availability of the equipment for the handheld pencil method.

Validity

We are unaware of any published studies that report criterion-related validity of elbow and forearm ROM measurements taken with a universal goniometer to radiographs. However, if photographic measurements are accepted as valid, then some indication of criterion-related validity may be provided by comparing goniometric and photographic measurements. In a study by Fish and Wingate,[48] 46 physical therapy students used plastic and metal universal goniometers to measure the angle of an elbow fixed in approximately 50 and 135 degrees of flexion by a splint. In some cases the landmarks were prelabeled, whereas in others the testers had to palpate and identify the landmarks for goniometer alignment. Measurements were also determined from photographs of the prelabeled, fixed elbow. In addition, passive elbow flexion ROM was measured in the unsplinted elbow. There were small but significant differences (ranging from 0.6 to 5.1 degrees) between the means of the goniometric measurements as compared to the photographic measurements, except in one case. The standard deviation of the measurements increased from a low of 0.7 to 1.1 degrees with photographic measurements to a high of 3.4 to 4.2 degrees with passive ROM. The authors proposed that small systematic errors in alignment of the goniometer, identification of bony landmarks, and variations in the amount of torque applied by the tester may account for these differences.

REFERENCES

1. Levangie, PK, and Norkin, CC: Joint Structure and Function: A Comprehensive Analysis, ed 4. FA Davis, Philadelphia, 2005.
2. Amis, AA, and Miller, JH: The elbow. Clin Rheum Dis 8:571, 1982.
3. Van Roy, P, et al: Arthro-kinematics of the elbow: Study of the carrying angle. Ergonomics 48:11, 2005.
4. Yilmaz, E, et al: Variation of carrying angle with age, sex, and special reference to side. Orthopedics 28:1360, 2005.
5. Hoppenfeld, S: Physical Examination of the Spine and Extremities. Appleton-Century-Crofts, New York, 1977.
6. Morrey, BF, and Chao, EYS: Passive motion of the elbow joint. J Bone Joint Surg Am 58:50, 1976.
7. Cyriax, JH, and Cyriax, PJ: Illustrated Manual of Orthopaedic Medicine. Butterworths, London, 1983.
8. Kaltenborn, FM: Manual Mobilization of the Extremity Joints, ed 5. Olaf Norlis Bokhandel, Oslo, 1999.
9. Magee, DJ: Orthopedic Physical Assessment, ed. 4. WB Saunders, Philadelphia, 2006.
10. American Academy of Orthopaedic Surgeons: Joint Motion: Methods of Measuring and Recording. AAOS, Chicago, 1965.
11. Green, WB, and Heckman, JD (eds): The Clinical Measurement of Joint Motion. American Academy of Orthopaedic Surgeons, Rosemont, IL, 1994.
12. American Medical Association: Guides to the Evaluation of Permanent Impairment, ed 5. Cocchiarella, L and Andersson, GBJ (eds). AMA, Chicago, 2001.
13. Boone, DC, and Azen, SP: Normal range of motion in male subjects. J Bone Joint Surg Am 61:756, 1979.
14. Greene, BL, and Wolf, SL: Upper extremity joint movement: Comparison of two measurement devices. Arch Phys Med Rehabil 70:288, 1989.
15. Gunal, I, et al: Normal range of motion of the joints of the upper extremity in male subjects, with special reference to side. J Bone Joint Surg (Am) 78(A):1401, 1996.
16. Goodwin, J, et al: Clinical methods of goniometry: A comparative study. Disabil Rehabil 14:10, 1992.
17. Petherick, M, et al: Concurrent validity and intertester reliability of universal and fluid-based goniometers for active elbow range of motion. Phys Ther 68:966, 1988.
18. Sanya, AO, and Chinyelu SO: Range of motion in selected joints of diabetic and non-diabetic subjects. African J Health Sci 6:17, 1999.
19. Fiebert, I, Fuhri, JR, and New, MD: Elbow, forearm and wrist passive range of motion in persons aged sixty and older. Phys Occup Ther Geriatr 10:17, 1992.
20. Wanatabe, H, et al: The range of joint motions of the extremities in healthy Japanese people: The difference according to age. Nippon Seikeigeka Gakkai Zasshi 53:275, 1979. (Cited in Walker, JM: Musculoskeletal development: A review. Phys Ther 71:878, 1991.)
21. Hacker, MR, Funk, SM, and Manco-Johnson, MJ: The Colorado Hemophilia Paediatric Joint Physical Examination Scale: Normal values and interrater reliability. Haemophilia 13:71, 2007.
22. Boone, DC: Techniques of measurement of joint motion. (Unpublished supplement to Boone, DC, and Azen, SP: Normal range of motion in male subjects. J Bone Joint Surg Am 61:756, 1979.)
23. Walker, JM, et al: Active mobility of the extremities in older subjects. Phys Ther 64:919, 1984.
24. Bergstrom, G, et al: Prevalence of symptoms and signs of joint impairment. Scand J Rehabil Med 17:173, 1985.
25. Kalscheur, JA, Emery, LJ, and Costello, PS: Range of motion in older women. Phys Occup Ther Geriatr 16:77, 1999.
26. Kalscheur, JA, Costello, PS, and Emery, LJ: Gender differences in range of motion in older adults. Phys Occup Ther Geriatr 22:77, 2003.
27. Bell, RD, and Hoshizaki, TB: Relationships of age and sex with range of motion of seventeen joint actions in humans. Can J Appl Spt Sci 6:202, 1981.
28. Salter, N, and Darcus, HD: The amplitude of forearm and of humeral rotation. J Anat 87:407, 1953.
29. Escalante, A, Lichenstein, MJ, and Hazuda, HP: Determinants of shoulder and elbow flexion range: Results from the San Antonio Longitudinal Study of Aging. Arthritis Care Res 12:277, 1999.
30. Chang, DE, Buschbacher, LP, and Edlich, RF: Limited joint mobility in power lifters. Am J Sports Med 16:280, 1988.
31. Chinn, CJ, Priest, JD, and Kent, BA: Upper extremity range of motion, grip strength and girth in highly skilled tennis players, Phys Ther 54:474, 1974.
32. Wright, RW, et al: Elbow range of motion in professional baseball pitchers. Am J Sports Med 34:190, 2006.
33. Morrey, BF, Askew, KN, and Chao, EYS: A biomechanical study of normal functional elbow motion. J Bone Joint Surg Am 63:872, 1981.
34. Packer, TL, et al: Examining the elbow during functional activities. Occup Ther J Res. 10:323, 1990.
35. Safaee-Rad, R, et al: Normal functional range of motion of upper limb joints during performance of three feeding activities. Arch Phys Med Rehabil 71:505, 1990.
36. Marco, SC, et al: Kinematic analysis of the elbow in the activities of daily living. Rehabilitacion 33:293, 1999.
37. Vasen, AP, et al: Functional range of motion of the elbow. J Hand Surg 20A:288, 1995.
38. Cooper, JE, et al: Elbow joint restriction: Effect on functional upper limb motion during performance of three feeding activities. Arch Phys Med Rehabil 74:805, 1993.
39. Hellebrandt, FA, Duvall, EN, and Moore, ML: The measurement of joint motion. Part III: Reliability of goniometry. Phys Ther Rev 29:302, 1949.
40. Boone, DC, et al: Reliability of goniometric measurements. Phys Ther 58:1355, 1978.
41. Rothstein, JM, Miller, PJ, and Roettger, RF: Goniometric reliability in a clinical setting: Elbow and knee measurements. Phys Ther 63:1611, 1983.
42. Grohmann, JEL: Comparison of two methods of goniometry. Phys Ther 63:922, 1983.
43. Armstrong, AD, et al: Reliability of range-of-motion measurement in the elbow and forearm. J Shoulder Elbow Surg 7:573, 1998.
44. Geertzen, JHB, et al: Variation in measurements of range of motion: A study in reflex sympathetic dystrophy patients. Clin Rehabil 12:254, 1998.
45. Gajdosik, RL: Comparison and reliability of three goniometric methods for measuring forearm supination and pronation. Percept Mot Skills 93:353, 2001.
46. Flower, KR, et al: Intrarater reliability of a new method and instrumentation for measuring passive supination and pronation: A preliminary study. J Hand Ther 14:30, 2001.
47. Karagiannopoulos, C, Sitler, M, and Michlovitz, S: Reliability of 2 functional goniometric methods for measuring forearm pronation and supination active range of motion. J Orthop Sports Phys Ther 33:523, 2003.
48. Fish, DR, and Wingate, L: Sources of goniometric error at the elbow. Phys Ther 65:1666, 1985.

The Wrist

◯ Structure and Function

Radiocarpal and Midcarpal Joints

Anatomy

The wrist is comprised of two joints, the radiocarpal and midcarpal joints, both of which are important to function. The radiocarpal joint lies closer to the forearm, whereas the midcarpal joint is closer to the hand. The proximal joint surface of the radiocarpal joint consists of the distal radius and radioulnar articular disc (Fig. 6.1; see also Fig. 5.7).[1] The disc connects the medial aspect of the distal radius to the distal ulna. The distal radius and the disc form a continuous concave surface.[2,3] The distal joint surface includes three bones from the proximal carpal row—the scaphoid, lunate, and triquetrum—which are connected by interosseous ligaments to form a

convex surface (Fig. 6.1). The radius articulates with the scaphoid and lunate, whereas the radioulnar disc articulates with the triquetrum and, to a lesser extent, the lunate. The pisiform, although found in the proximal row of carpal bones, does not participate in the radiocarpal joint. The joint is enclosed by a strong capsule and is reinforced by the palmar radiocarpal, ulnocarpal, dorsal radiocarpal, ulnar collateral, and radial collateral ligaments and numerous intercarpal ligaments (Figs. 6.2 and 6.3).

The midcarpal joint is distal to the radiocarpal joint. The predominant central and ulnar portions of the midcarpal joint consist of the concave surfaces of the scaphoid, lunate, and triquetrum proximally and the convex surfaces of the capitate and hamate distally (Fig. 6.1). On the radial side of the midcarpal joint, a smaller convex surface of the scaphoid contacts the concave surfaces of the trapezium and trapezoid. The midcarpal

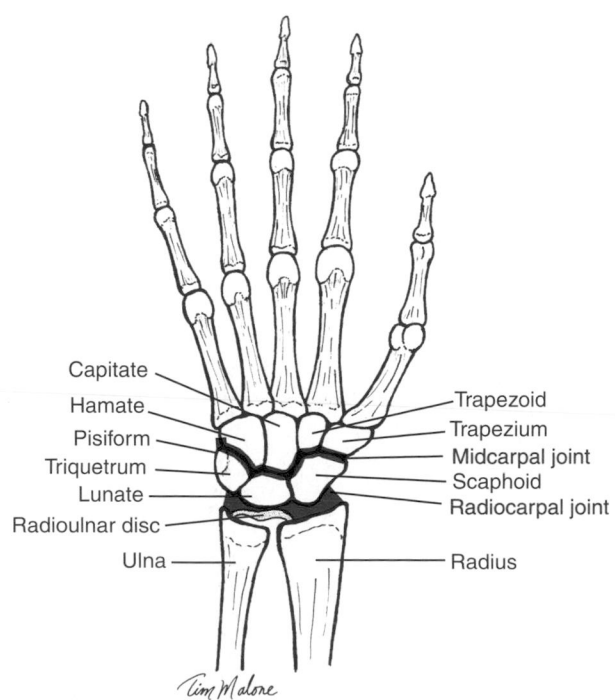

FIGURE 6.1 An anterior (palmar) view of the right wrist showing the radiocarpal and midcarpal joints.

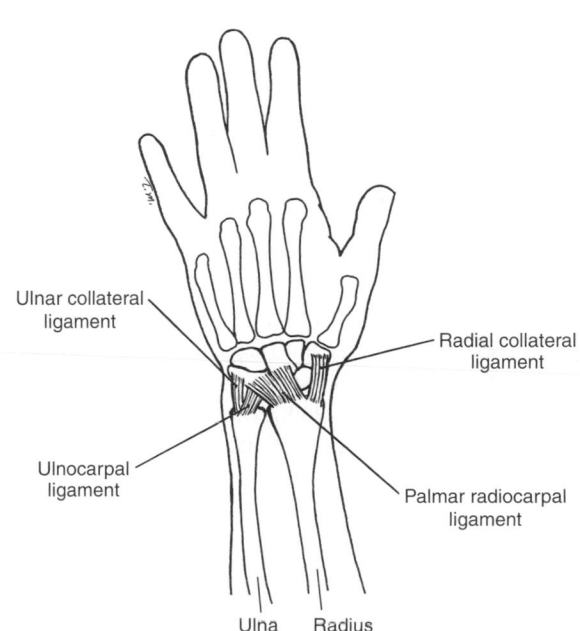

FIGURE 6.2 An anterior (palmar) view of the right wrist showing the palmar radiocarpal, ulnocarpal, and collateral ligaments.

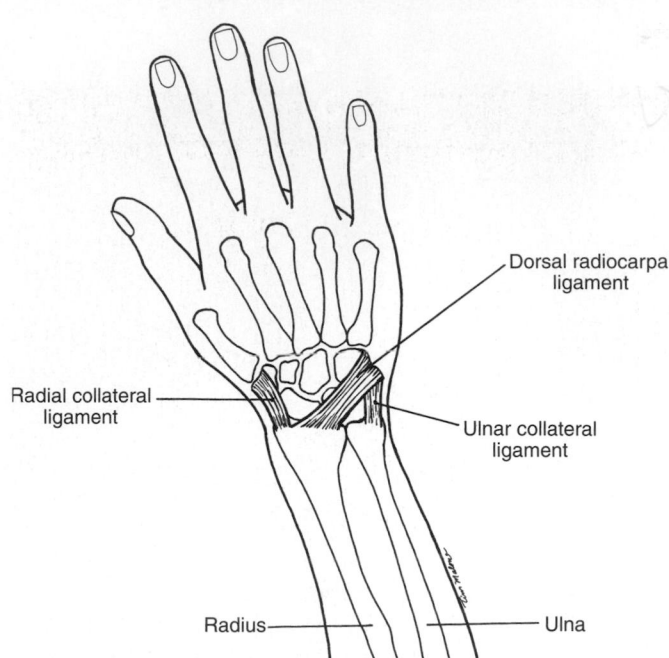

Radial collateral ligament

Dorsal radiocarpal ligament

Ulnar collateral ligament

Radius

Ulna

FIGURE 6.3 A posterior view of the right wrist showing the dorsal radiocarpal and collateral ligaments.

joint has a joint capsule that is continuous with each intercarpal joint and some carpometacarpal and intermetacarpal joints. Many of the ligaments that reinforce the radiocarpal joint also support the midcarpal joint (Figs. 6.2 and 6.3).

Osteokinematics

The radiocarpal and midcarpal joints are of the condyloid type, with 2 degrees of freedom.[2] The wrist complex (radiocarpal and midcarpal joints) permits flexion–extension in the sagittal plane around a medial–lateral axis and radial–ulnar deviation in the frontal plane around an anterior–posterior axis. Both joints contribute to these motions.[4-6] Some sources also report that a small amount of supination–pronation occurs at the wrist complex,[7] but this rotation is not usually measured in the clinical setting.

Arthrokinematics

Motion at the radiocarpal joint occurs because the convex surfaces of the proximal row of carpals roll and slide on the concave surfaces of the radius and radioulnar disc. The proximal row of carpals rolls in the same direction but slides in the opposite direction to movement of the hand.[3,8,9] The carpals slide dorsally on the radius and disc during wrist flexion and ventrally toward the palm during wrist extension. During ulnar deviation, the carpals roll in an ulnar direction and slide in a radial direction. During radial deviation, they roll in a radial direction and slide in an ulnar direction.

Motion at the midcarpal joint occurs because the distal row of carpals rolls and slides on the proximal row of carpals. The distal joint surface is predominantly convex and rolls in the same direction and slides in the opposite direction to the

osteokinematic movements of the wrist, but there is more complexity at the midcarpal joint than at the radiocarpal joint. During flexion, the large and markedly convex surfaces of the capitate and hamate roll ventrally and slide dorsally on the concave surfaces of the scaphoid, lunate, and triquetrum.[3,8,9] The smaller, shallow surfaces of the trapezium and trapezoid are slightly concave and roll and slide ventrally on the convex surface of the scaphoid with flexion. The movements during extension are opposite to that of flexion.

During radial deviation at the midcarpal joint, the convex surfaces of the capitate and hamate roll in a radial direction and slide in an ulnar direction on the concave surfaces of the scaphoid, lunate, and triquetrum. However, the concave surfaces of the trapezium and trapezoid roll and slide slightly dorsally on the scaphoid during radial deviation.[2,9,10] With ulnar deviation, the surfaces on the capitate and hamate roll in an ulnar direction and slide in a radial direction. The joint surfaces of the trapezium and trapezoid roll and slide slightly ventrally.

Capsular Pattern

Cyriax and Cyriax[11] report that the capsular pattern at the wrist is an equal limitation of flexion and extension and a slight limitation of radial and ulnar deviation. Kaltenborn[3] notes that the capsular pattern is an equal restriction in all motions.

RANGE OF MOTION TESTING PROCEDURES: Wrist

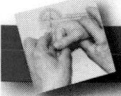

Landmarks for Testing Procedures

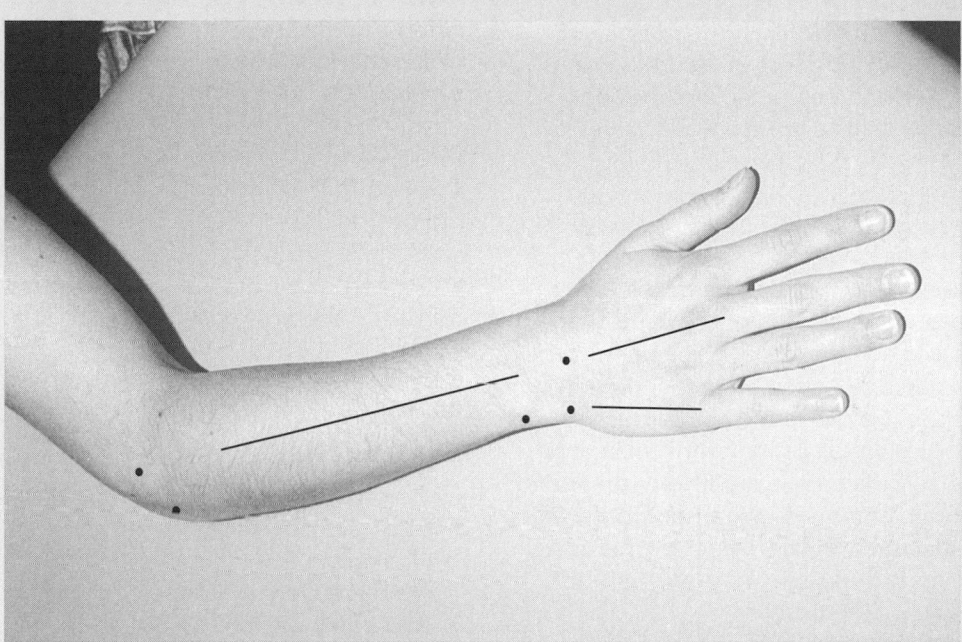

FIGURE 6.4 Posterior view of the upper extremity showing surface anatomy landmarks for goniometer alignment during the measurement of wrist ROM.

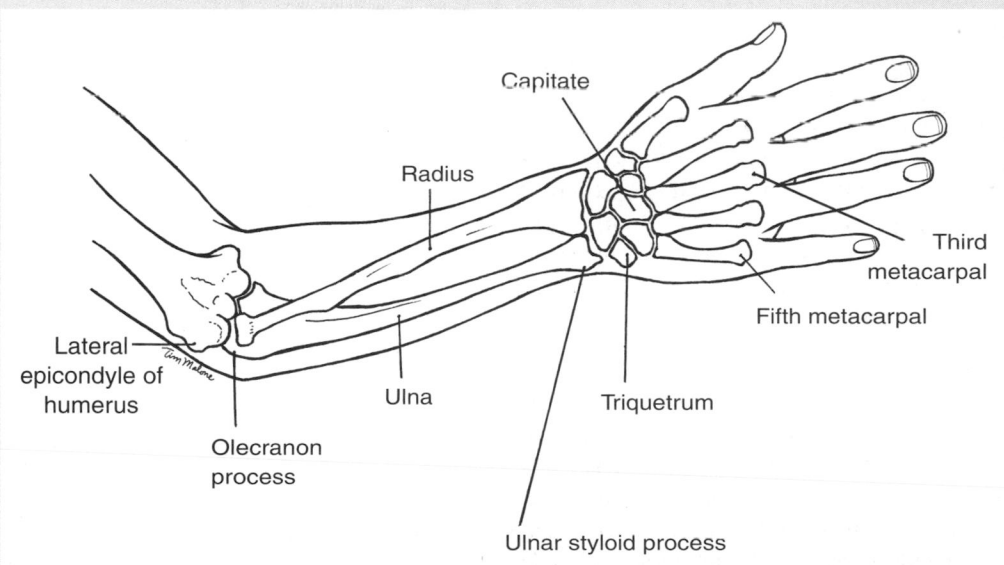

FIGURE 6.5 Posterior view of the upper extremity showing bony anatomical landmarks for goniometer alignment during the measurement of wrist ROM.

(handwritten: 80) *(handwritten: No Jewelry!)*

● Wrist Flexion

This motion occurs in the sagittal plane around a medial–lateral axis. Wrist flexion is sometimes referred to as volar or palmar flexion. Normal range of motion (ROM) values for adults are 60 degrees according to the American Medical Association (AMA),[12] 80 degrees according to the American Academy of Orthopaedic Surgeons (AAOS),[13,14] and 75 degrees according to Boone and Azen.[15] Refer to Research Findings and Tables 6.1 to 6.3 for additional normal ROM values by age and gender.

Testing Position

Position the subject sitting next to a supporting surface with the shoulder abducted to 90 degrees, the elbow flexed to 90 degrees, and the palm of the hand facing the ground. In this position the forearm will be midway between supination and pronation. Rest the forearm on the supporting surface, but leave the hand free to move. Avoid radial or ulnar deviation of the wrist and flexion of the fingers. If the fingers are flexed, tension in the extensor digitorum communis, extensor indicis, and extensor digiti minimi muscles will restrict the motion.

Stabilization

Stabilize the radius and ulna to prevent supination or pronation of the forearm and motion of the elbow.

Testing Motion

Flex the wrist by pushing on the dorsal surface of the third metacarpal, moving the hand toward the floor (Fig. 6.6). Maintain the wrist in 0 degrees of radial and ulnar deviation. The end of flexion ROM occurs when resistance to further motion is felt and attempts to overcome the resistance cause the forearm to lift off the supporting surface.

Normal End-Feel

The end-feel is firm because of tension in the dorsal radiocarpal ligament and the dorsal joint capsule. Tension in the extensor carpi radialis brevis and longus and extensor carpi ulnaris muscles may also contribute to the firm end-feel.

Goniometer Alignment

See Figures 6.7 and 6.8.

1. Center **fulcrum** on the lateral aspect of the wrist over the triquetrum. *(handwritten: –Distal to ulnar styloid process)*
2. Align **proximal arm** with the lateral midline of the ulna, using the olecranon and ulnar styloid processes for reference.
3. Align **distal arm** with the lateral midline of the fifth metacarpal. Do not use the soft tissue of the hypothenar eminence for reference.

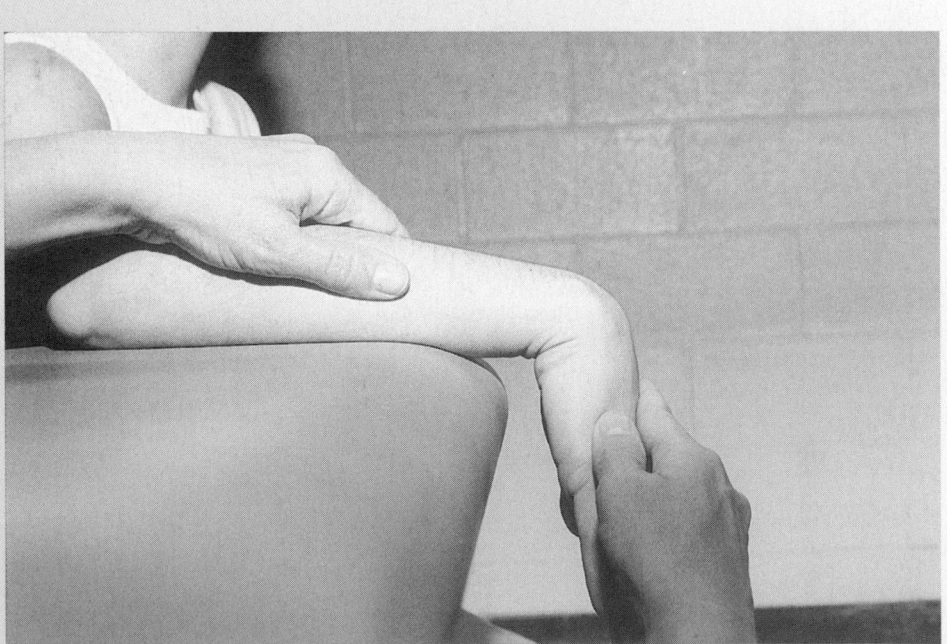

FIGURE 6.6 The end of wrist flexion ROM. Only about three-quarters of the subject's forearm is supported by the examining table so that there is sufficient space for the hand to complete the motion.

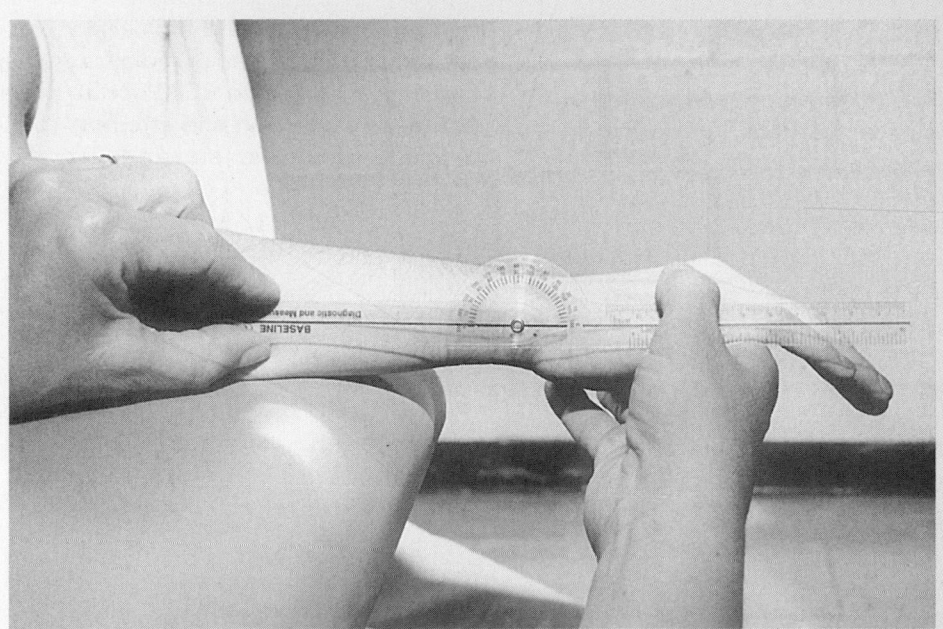

FIGURE 6.7 The alignment of the goniometer at the beginning of wrist flexion ROM.

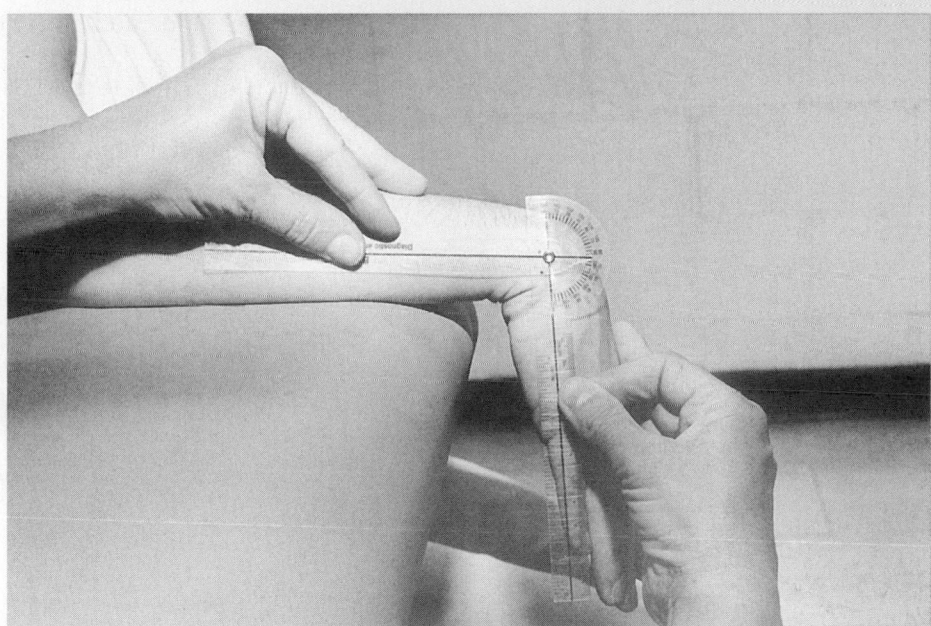

FIGURE 6.8 At the end of wrist flexion ROM the examiner uses one hand to align the distal arm of the goniometer with the fifth metacarpal while maintaining the wrist in flexion. The examiner exerts pressure on the middle of the dorsum of the subject's hand and avoids exerting pressure directly on the fifth metacarpal because such pressure will distort the goniometer alignment.

Alternative Goniometer Alignment: Dorsal Aspect

This alternative goniometer alignment is recommended by LaStoya and Wheeler,[16] although edema may make accurate alignment over the dorsal surfaces of the forearm and hand difficult. Intratester reliability is similar to lateral alignment technique (intraclass correlation coefficient [ICC] = 0.87 to 0.92).

1. Center **fulcrum** over the capitate on the dorsal aspect of the wrist joint.
2. Align **proximal arm** with the dorsal midline of the forearm.
3. Align **distal arm** with the dorsal aspect of the third metacarpal.

● Wrist Extension

Motion occurs in the sagittal plane around a medial–lateral axis. Wrist extension is sometimes referred to as dorsal flexion. Normal ROM values for adults are 60 degrees according to the AMA,[12] 70 degrees according to the AAOS,[13,14] and 74 degrees according to Boone and Azen.[15] See Research Findings and Tables 6.1 to 6.3 for additional normal ROM values by age and gender.

Testing Position
Position the subject sitting next to a supporting surface with the shoulder abducted to 90 degrees, the elbow flexed to 90 degrees, and the palm of the hand facing the ground. In this position the forearm will be midway between supination and pronation. Rest the forearm on the supporting surface, but leave the hand free to move. Avoid radial or ulnar deviation of the wrist and extension of the fingers. If the fingers are held in extension, tension in the flexor digitorum superficialis and profundus muscles will restrict the motion.

Stabilization
Stabilize the radius and ulna to prevent supination or pronation of the forearm and motion of the elbow.

Testing Motion
Extend the wrist by pushing evenly across the palmar surface of the metacarpals, moving the hand in a dorsal direction toward the ceiling (Fig. 6.9). Maintain the wrist in 0 degrees of radial and ulnar deviation. The end of extension ROM occurs when resistance to further motion is felt and attempts to overcome the resistance cause the forearm to lift off of the supporting surface.

Normal End-Feel
Usually the end-feel is firm because of tension in the palmar radiocarpal ligament, ulnocarpal ligament, and palmar joint capsule. Tension in the palmaris longus, flexor carpi radialis, and flexor carpi ulnaris muscles may also contribute to the firm end-feel. Sometimes the end-feel is hard because of contact between the radius and the carpal bones.

Goniometer Alignment
See Figures 6.10 and 6.11.

1. Center **fulcrum** on the lateral aspect of the wrist over the triquetrum.
2. Align **proximal arm** with the lateral midline of the ulna, using the olecranon and ulnar styloid process for reference.
3. Align **distal arm** with the lateral midline of the fifth metacarpal. Do not use the soft tissue of the hypothenar eminence for reference.

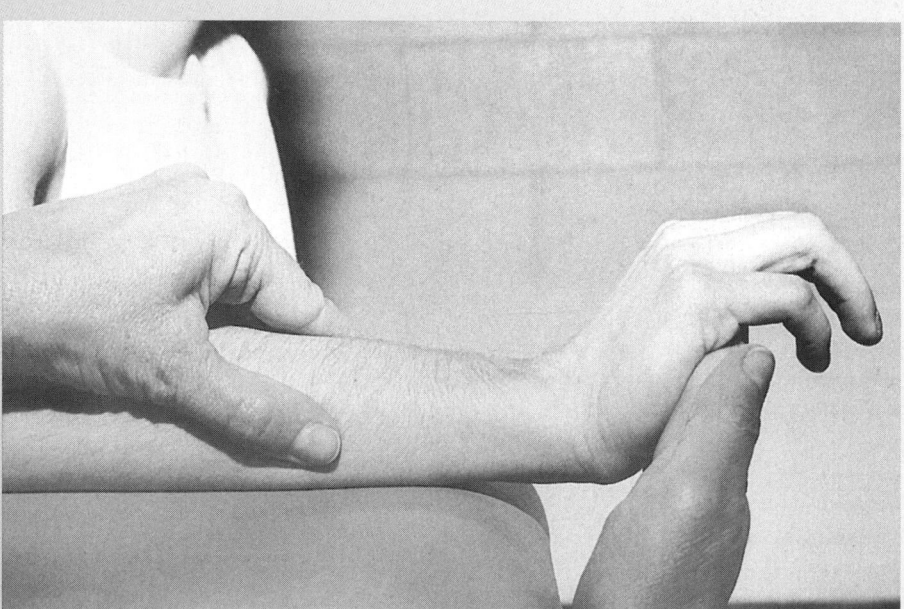

FIGURE 6.9 At the end of the wrist extension ROM, the examiner stabilizes the subject's forearm with one hand and uses her other hand to hold the subject's wrist in extension. The examiner is careful to distribute pressure equally across the subject's metacarpals.

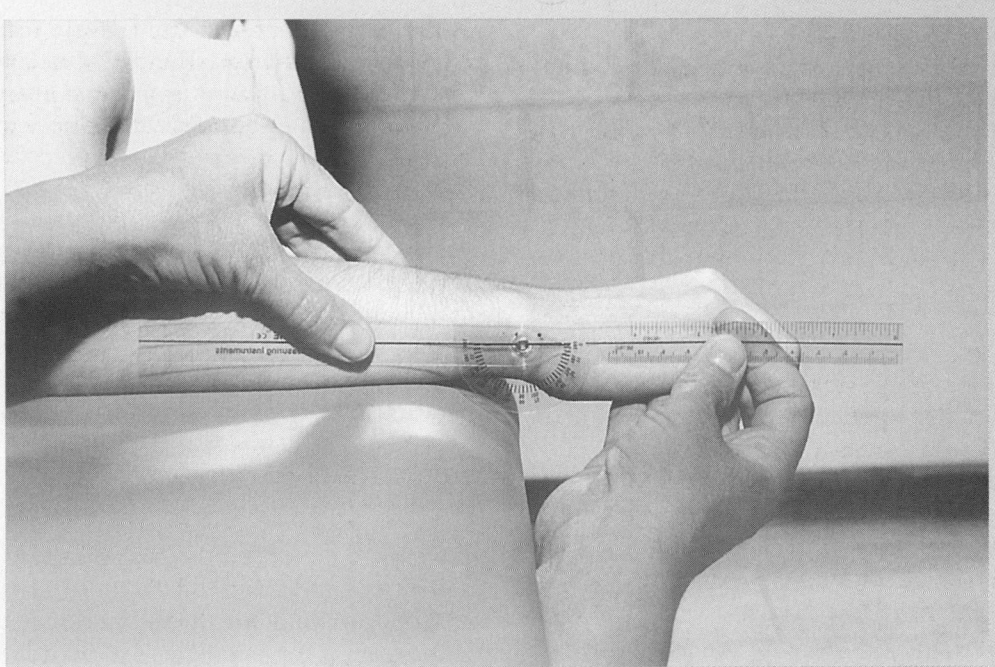

FIGURE 6.10 The alignment of the goniometer at the beginning of wrist extension ROM.

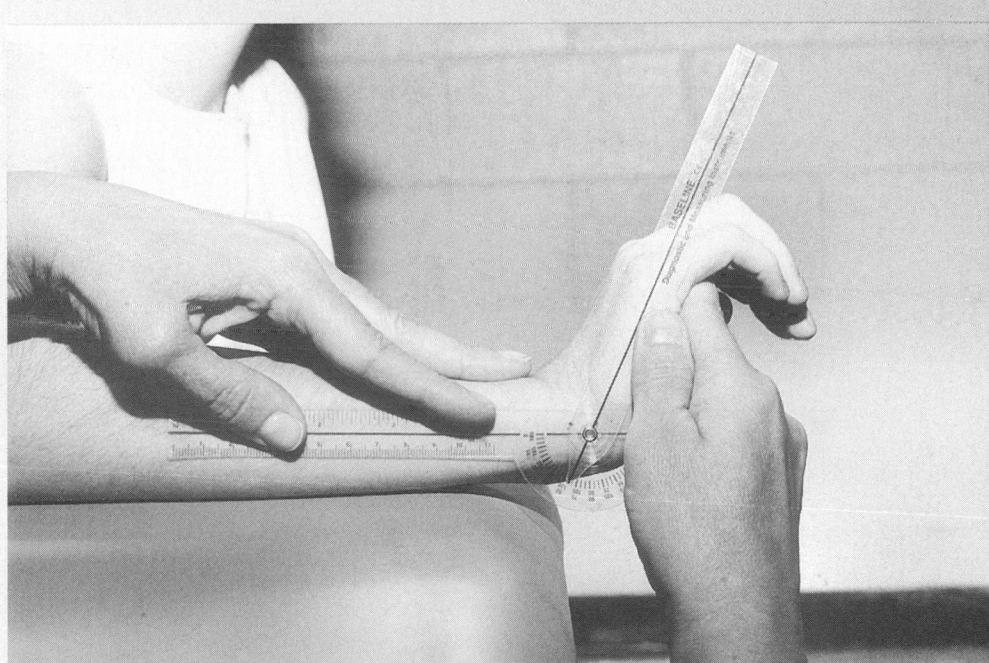

FIGURE 6.11 At the end of the ROM of wrist extension, the examiner aligns the distal goniometer arm with the fifth metacarpal while holding the wrist in extension. The examiner avoids exerting excessive pressure on the fifth metacarpal.

Alternative Goniometer Alignment: Palmar Aspect

This alternative goniometer alignment is recommended by LaStayo and Wheeler,[16] although edema may make accurate alignment over the palmar surfaces of the forearm and hand difficult. Intratester reliability is similar to lateral alignment technique (ICC = 0.80 to 0.84).

1. Center **fulcrum** on the palmar surface of the wrist joint at the level of the capitate.
2. Align **proximal arm** with the palmar midline of the forearm.
3. Align **distal arm** with the palmar midline of the third metacarpal.

● Wrist Radial Deviation

Motion occurs in the frontal plane around an anterior–posterior axis. Radial deviation is sometimes referred to as radial flexion or abduction. Normal ROM values for adults are 20 degrees according to the AMA[12] and AAOS[13,14] and 25 degrees according to Greene and Wolf.[17] See Research Findings and Tables 6.1 to 6.3 for additional normal ROM values by age and gender.

Testing Position

Position the subject sitting next to a supporting surface with the shoulder abducted to 90 degrees, the elbow flexed to 90 degrees, and the palm of the hand facing the ground. In this position the forearm will be midway between supination and pronation. Rest the forearm and hand on the supporting surface.

Stabilization

Stabilize the radius and ulna to prevent pronation or supination of the forearm and elbow flexion beyond 90 degrees.

Testing Motion

Radially deviate the wrist by moving the hand toward the thumb (Fig. 6.12). Maintain the wrist in 0 degrees of flexion and extension, and avoid rotating the hand. The end of radial deviation ROM occurs when resistance to further motion is felt and attempts to overcome the resistance cause the elbow to flex.

Normal End-Feel

Usually the end-feel is hard because of contact between the radial styloid process and the scaphoid, but it may be firm because of tension in the ulnar collateral ligament, the ulnocarpal ligament, and the ulnar portion of the joint capsule. Tension in the extensor carpi ulnaris and flexor carpi ulnaris muscles may also contribute to the firm end-feel.

Goniometer Alignment

See Figures 6.13 and 6.14.

1. Center **fulcrum** on the dorsal aspect of the wrist over the capitate. 3rd MC or flexion
2. Align **proximal arm** with the dorsal midline of the forearm. If the shoulder is in 90 degrees of abduction and the elbow is in 90 degrees of flexion, the lateral epicondyle of the humerus can be used for reference.
3. Align **distal arm** with the dorsal midline of the third metacarpal. Do not use the third phalanx for reference.

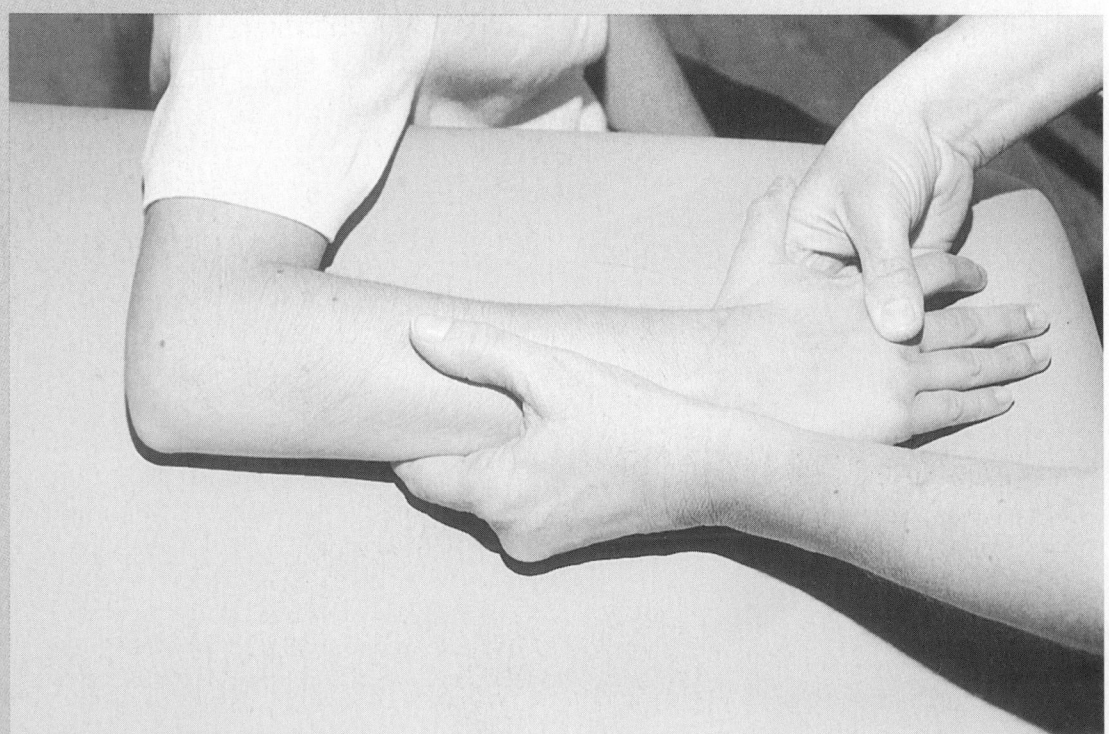

FIGURE 6.12 The examiner stabilizes the subject's forearm to prevent flexion of the elbow beyond 90 degrees when the wrist is moved into radial deviation. The examiner avoids moving the wrist into either flexion or extension.

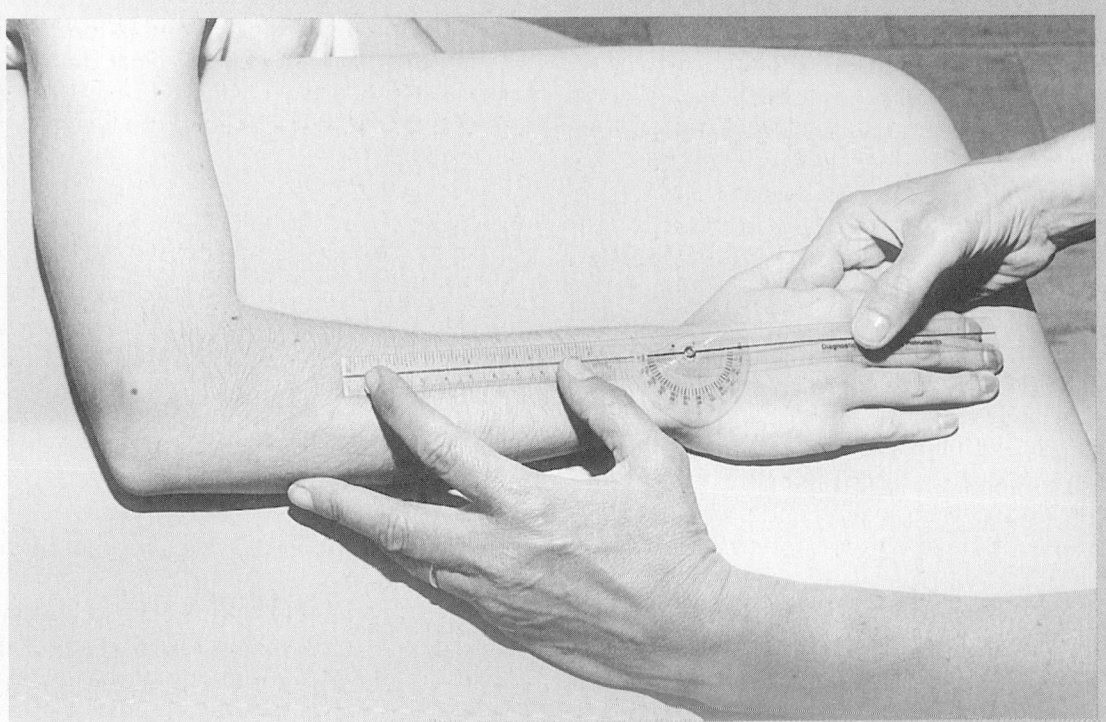

FIGURE 6.13 The alignment of the goniometer at the beginning of radial deviation ROM. The examining table can be used to support the hand.

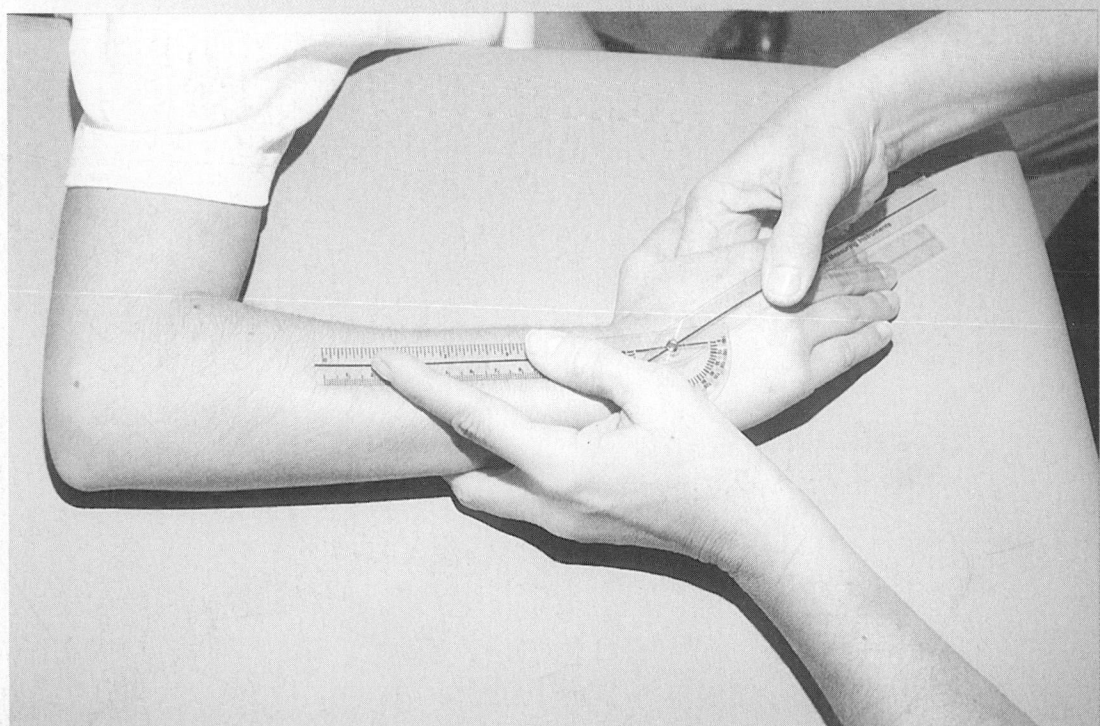

FIGURE 6.14 The alignment of the goniometer at the end of radial deviation ROM. The examiner must center the fulcrum over the dorsal surface of the capitate. If the fulcrum shifts to the ulnar side of the wrist, there will be an incorrect measurement of excessive radial deviation.

● WRIST ULNAR DEVIATION

Motion occurs in the frontal plane around an anterior–posterior axis. Ulnar deviation is sometimes referred to as ulnar flexion or adduction. Normal ROM values for adults are 30 degrees according to the AMA[12] and AAOS[13,14] and 39 degrees according to Greene and Wolf.[17] See Research Findings and Tables 6.1 to 6.3 for additional normal ROM values by age and gender.

Testing Position

Position the subject sitting next to a supporting surface with the shoulder abducted to 90 degrees, the elbow flexed to 90 degrees, and the palm of the hand facing the ground. In this position the forearm will be midway between supination and pronation. Rest the forearm and hand on the supporting surface.

Stabilization

Stabilize the radius and ulna to prevent pronation or supination of the forearm and less than 90 degrees of elbow flexion.

Testing Motion

Deviate the wrist in the ulnar direction by moving the hand toward the little finger (Fig. 6.15). Maintain the wrist in 0 degrees of flexion and extension, and avoid rotating the hand. The end of ulnar deviation ROM occurs when resistance to further motion is felt and attempts to overcome the resistance cause the elbow to extend.

Normal End-Feel

The end-feel is firm because of tension in the radial collateral ligament and the radial portion of the joint capsule. Tension in the extensor pollicis brevis and abductor pollicis longus muscles may contribute to the firm end-feel.

Goniometer Alignment

See Figures 6.16 and 6.17.

1. Center **fulcrum** on the dorsal aspect of the wrist over the capitate.
2. Align **proximal** arm with the dorsal midline of the forearm. If the shoulder is in 90 degrees of abduction and the elbow is in 90 degrees of flexion, the lateral epicondyle of the humerus can be used for reference.
3. Align **distal** arm with the dorsal midline of the third metacarpal. Do not use the third phalanx for reference.

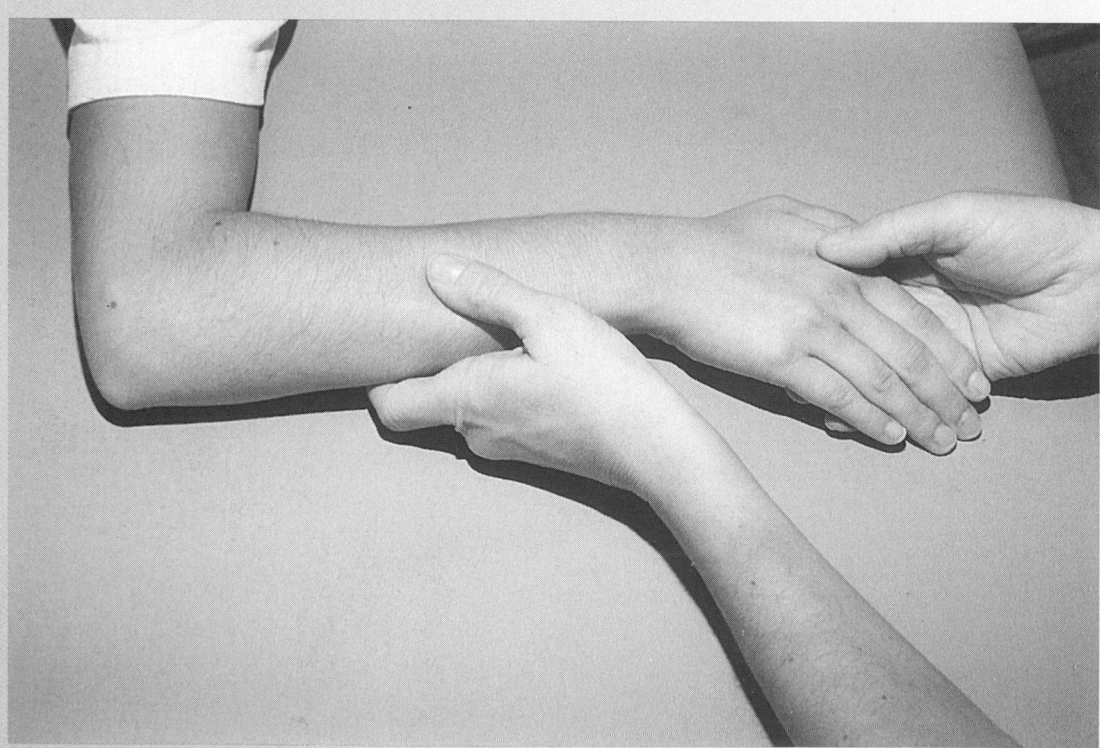

FIGURE 6.15   The examiner uses one hand to stabilize the subject's forearm and maintain the elbow in 90 degrees of flexion. The examiner's other hand moves the wrist into ulnar deviation, being careful not to flex or extend the wrist.

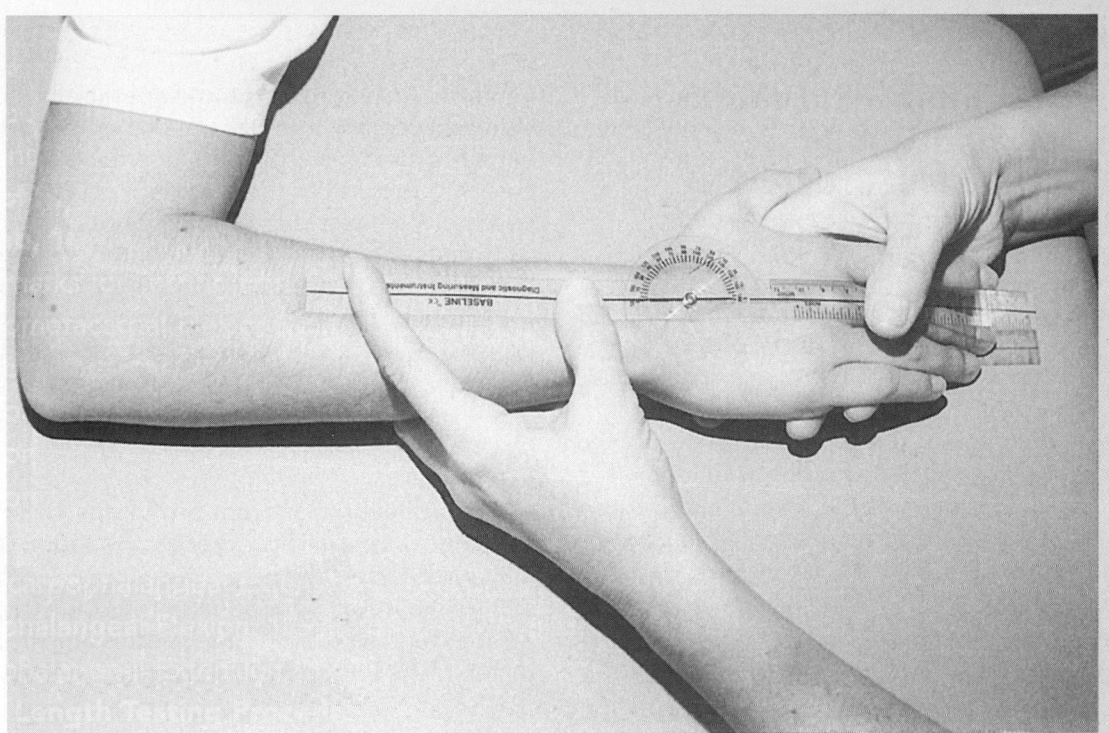

FIGURE 6.16 The alignment of the goniometer at the beginning of ulnar deviation ROM. Sometimes if a half-circle goniometer is used, the proximal and distal arms of the goniometer will have to be reversed so that the pointer remains on the body of the goniometer at the end of the ROM.

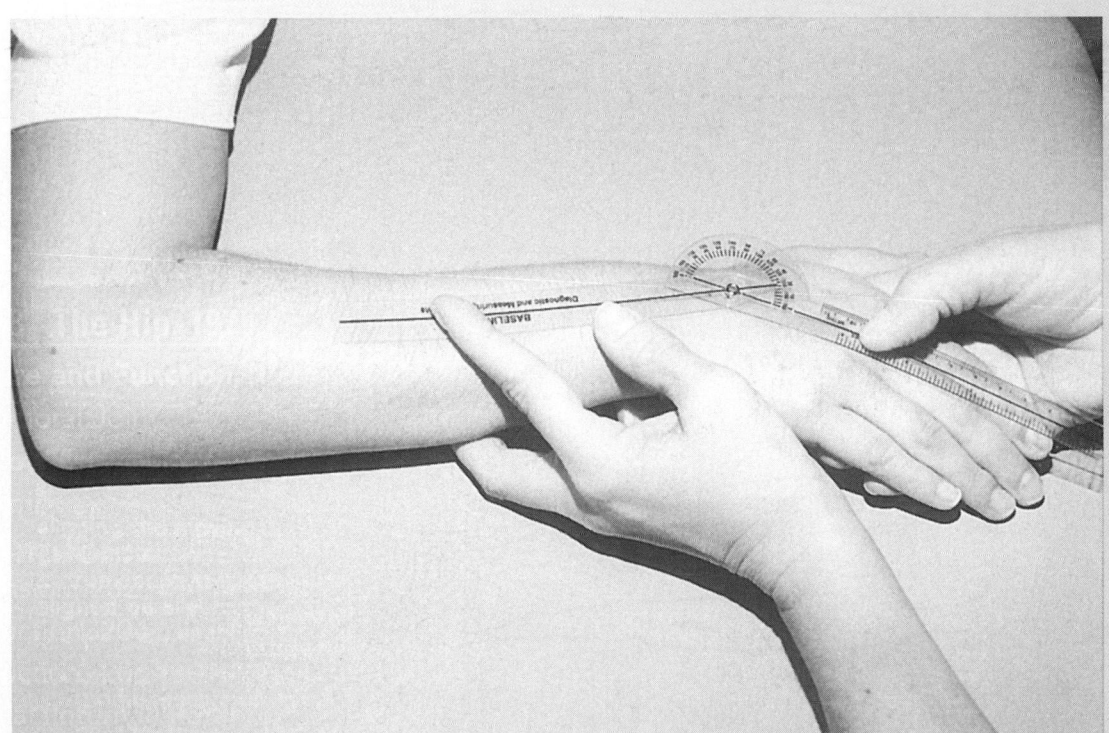

FIGURE 6.17 The alignment of the goniometer at the end of the ulnar deviation ROM. The examiner must center the fulcrum over the dorsal surface of the capitate. If the fulcrum shifts to the radial side of the wrist, there will be an incorrect measurement of excessive ulnar deviation.

MUSCLE LENGTH TESTING PROCEDURES: Wrist

● FLEXOR DIGITORUM PROFUNDUS AND FLEXOR DIGITORUM SUPERFICIALIS MUSCLE LENGTH

The flexor digitorum profundus crosses the elbow, wrist, metacarpophalangeal (MCP), proximal interphalangeal (PIP), and distal interphalangeal (DIP) joints. The flexor digitorum profundus originates proximally from the upper three-fourths of the ulna, the coronoid process of the ulna, and the interosseus membrane (Fig. 6.18). This muscle inserts distally onto the palmar surface of the bases of the distal phalanges of the fingers. When it contracts, it flexes the MCP, PIP, and DIP joints of the fingers and flexes the wrist. The flexor digitorum profundus is passively lengthened by placing the elbow, wrist, MCP, PIP, and DIP joints in extension.

The **flexor digitorum superficialis** crosses the elbow, wrist, MCP, and PIP joints. The humeroulnar head of the flexor digitorum superficialis muscle originates proximally from the medial epicondyle of the humerus, the ulnar collateral ligament, and the coronoid process of the ulna (Fig. 6.19). The radial head of the flexor digitorum superficialis muscle originates proximally from the anterior surface of the radius. It inserts distally via two slips into the sides of the bases of the middle phalanges of the fingers. When the flexor digitorum superficialis contracts, it flexes the MCP and PIP joints of the fingers and flexes the wrist. The muscle is passively lengthened by placing the elbow, wrist, MCP, and PIP joints in extension.

If the flexor digitorum profundus and flexor digitorum superficialis muscles are short, they will limit wrist extension when the elbow, MCP, PIP, and DIP joints are positioned in extension. If passive wrist extension is limited regardless of the position of the MCP, PIP, and DIP joints, the limitation is

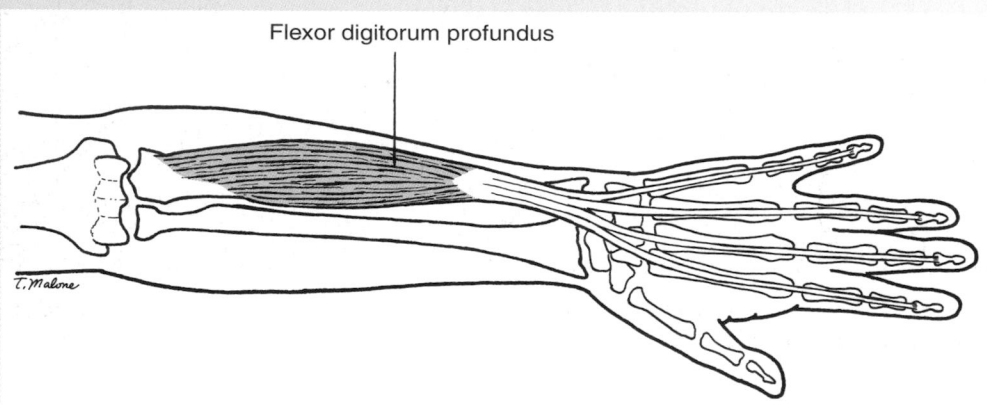

FIGURE 6.18 An anterior view of the right forearm showing the attachments of the flexor digitorum profundus muscle.

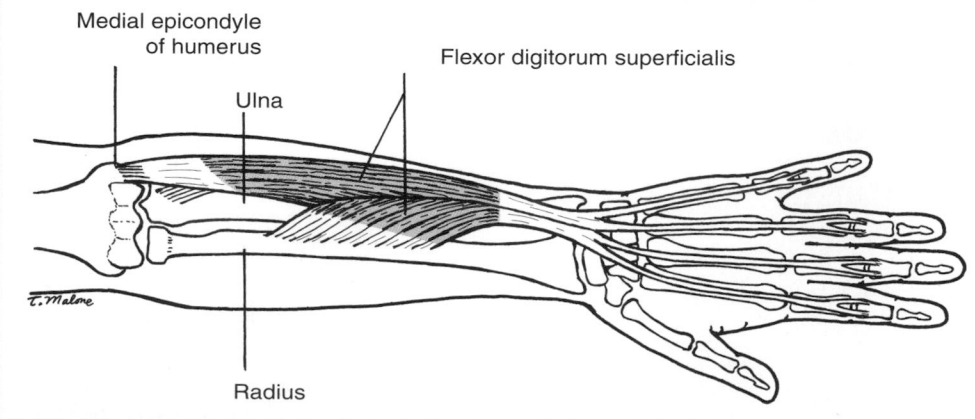

FIGURE 6.19 An anterior view of the right forearm and hand showing the attachments of the flexor digitorum superficialis muscle.

due to abnormalities of wrist joint surfaces or shortening of the palmar joint capsule, palmar radiocarpal ligament, ulnocarpal ligament, palmaris longus, flexor carpi radialis, or flexor carpi ulnaris muscles.

Starting Position

Position the subject sitting next to a supporting surface with the upper extremity resting on the surface. Place the elbow, MCP, PIP, and DIP joints in extension (Fig. 6.20). Pronate the forearm and place the wrist in neutral.

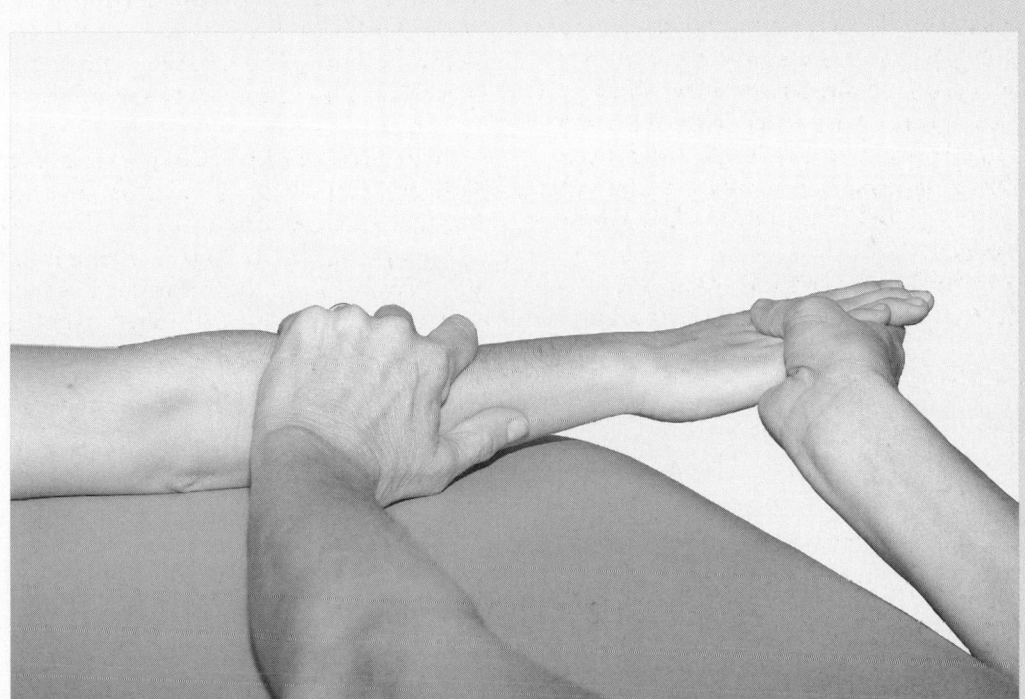

FIGURE 6.20 The starting position for testing the length of the flexor digitorum profundus and flexor digitorum superficialis muscles.

Stabilization
Stabilize the forearm to prevent elbow flexion.

Testing Motion
Hold the MCP, PIP, and DIP joints in extension while extending the wrist (Figs. 6.21 and 6.22). The end of the testing motion occurs when resistance is felt and additional wrist extension causes the fingers or elbow to flex.

End-Feel
The end-feel is firm because of tension in the flexor digitorum profundus and flexor digitorum superficialis muscles.

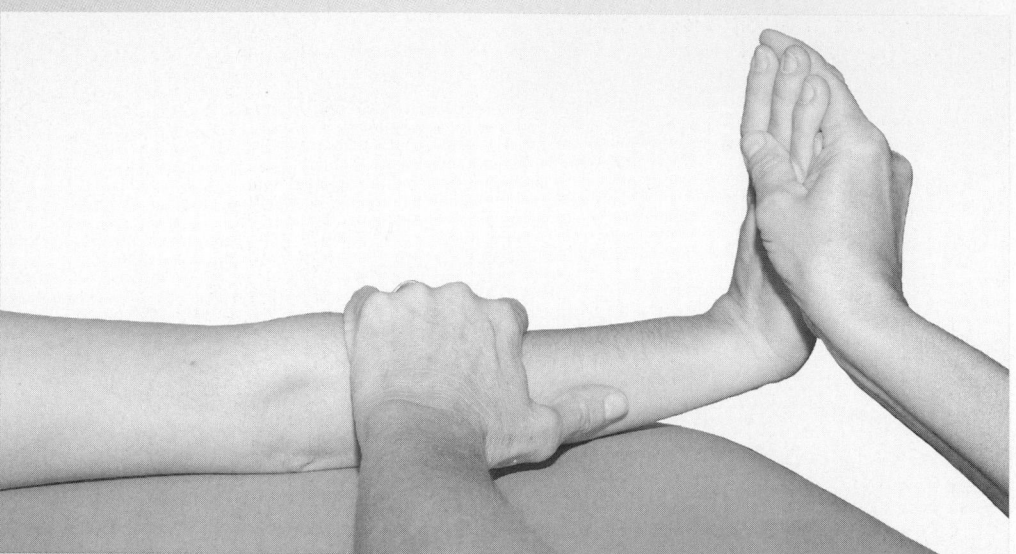

FIGURE 6.21 The end of the testing motion for the length of the flexor digitorum profundus and flexor digitorum superficialis muscles. The examiner uses one hand to stabilize the forearm, while the other hand holds the fingers in extension and moves the wrist into extension. The examiner has moved her right thumb from the dorsal surface of the fingers to allow a clearer photograph, but keeping the thumb placed on the dorsal surface would help to prevent the fingers from flexing at the PIP joints.

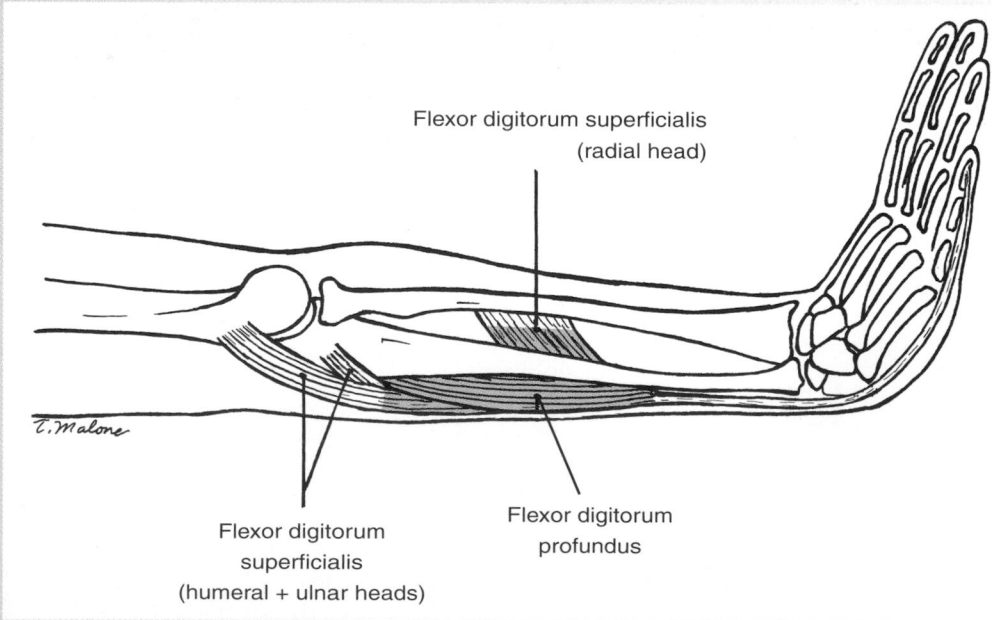

FIGURE 6.22 A lateral view of the right forearm and hand showing the flexor digitorum profundus and flexor digitorum superficialis being stretched over the elbow, wrist, MCP, PIP, and DIP joints.

Goniometer Alignment
See Figure 6.23.

1. Center **fulcrum** on the lateral aspect of the wrist over the triquetrum.
2. Align **proximal arm** with the lateral midline of the ulna, using the olecranon and ulnar styloid process for reference.
3. Align **distal arm** with the lateral midline of the fifth metacarpal. Do not use the soft tissue of the hypothenar eminence for reference.

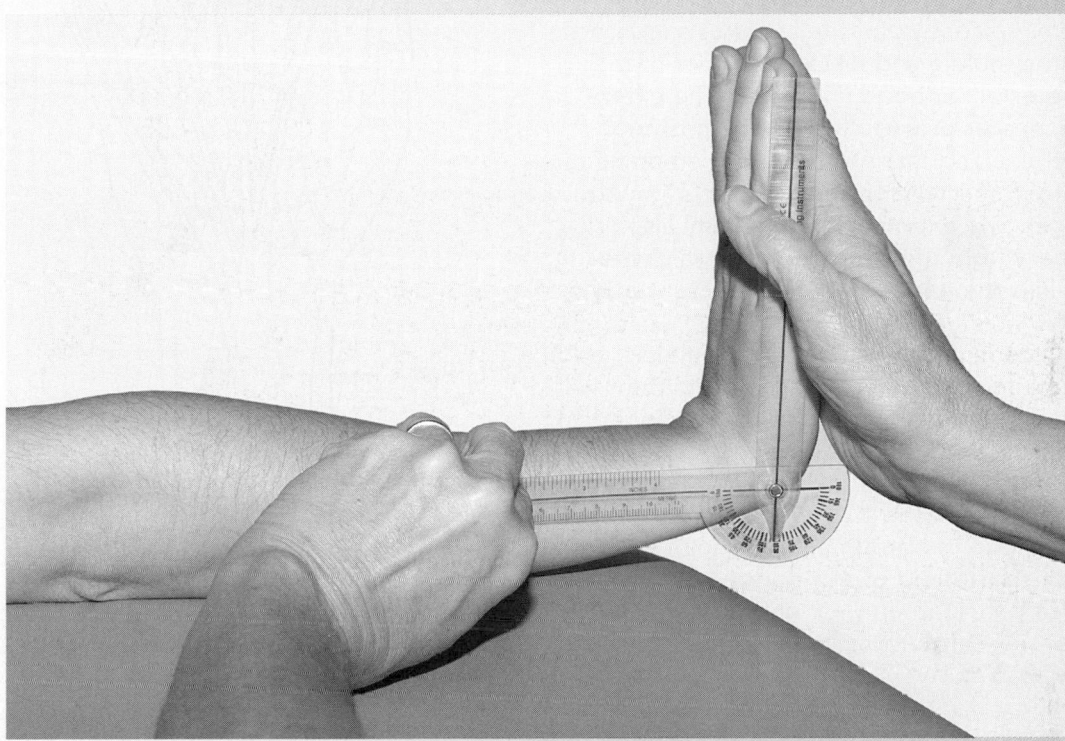

FIGURE 6.23 The alignment of the goniometer at the end of testing the length of the flexor digitorum profundus and flexor digitorum superficialis muscles.

● EXTENSOR DIGITORUM, EXTENSOR INDICIS, AND EXTENSOR DIGITI MINIMI MUSCLE LENGTH

The extensor digitorum, extensor indicis, and extensor digiti minimi muscles cross the elbow; wrist; and MCP, PIP, and DIP joints. When these muscles contract, they extend the MCP, PIP, and DIP joints of the fingers and extend the wrist. These muscles are passively lengthened by placing the elbow in extension and the wrist, MCP, PIP, and DIP joints in full flexion.

The **extensor digitorum** originates proximally from the lateral epicondyle of the humerus and inserts distally onto the middle and distal phalanges of the fingers via the extensor hood (Fig. 6.24). The **extensor indicis** originates proximally from the posterior surface of the ulna and the interosseous membrane. This muscle inserts distally onto the extensor hood of the index finger. The **extensor digiti minimi** also originates proximally from the lateral epicondyle of the humerus but inserts distally onto the extensor hood of the little finger.

If the extensor digitorum, extensor indicis, and extensor digiti minimi muscles are short, they will limit wrist flexion when the elbow is positioned in extension and the MCP, PIP, and DIP joints are positioned in full flexion. If wrist flexion is limited regardless of the position of the MCP, PIP, and DIP joints, the limitation is due to abnormalities of joint surfaces of the wrist or shortening of the dorsal joint capsule, dorsal radiocarpal ligament, extensor carpi radialis longus, extensor carpi radialis brevis, or extensor carpi ulnaris muscles.

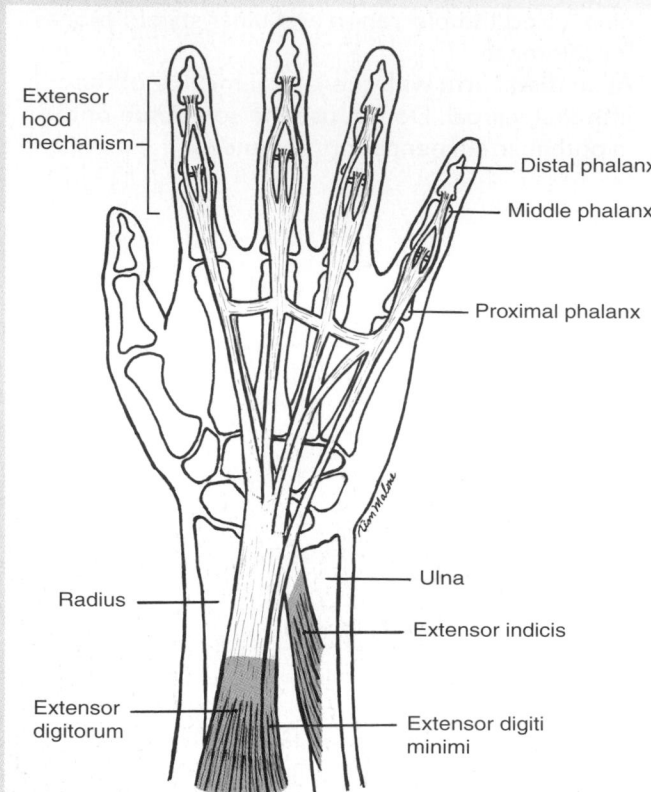

FIGURE 6.24 A posterior view of the right forearm and hand showing the distal attachments of the extensor digitorum, extensor indicis, and extensor digiti minimi muscles.

Starting Position

Position the subject sitting next to a supporting surface. The upper arm and the forearm should rest on the supporting surface, but the hand should be free to move into flexion. Place the elbow in full extension and the MCP, PIP, and DIP joints in full flexion (Fig. 6.25). Place the forearm in pronation and the wrist in neutral.

Stabilization

Stabilize the forearm to prevent elbow flexion.

Testing Motion

Hold the MCP, PIP, and DIP joints in full flexion while flexing the wrist (Figs. 6.26 and 6.27). The end of the testing motion occurs when resistance is felt and additional wrist flexion causes the fingers to extend or the elbow to flex.

Normal End-Feel

The end-feel is firm because of tension in the extensor digitorum, extensor indicis, and extensor digiti minimi muscles.

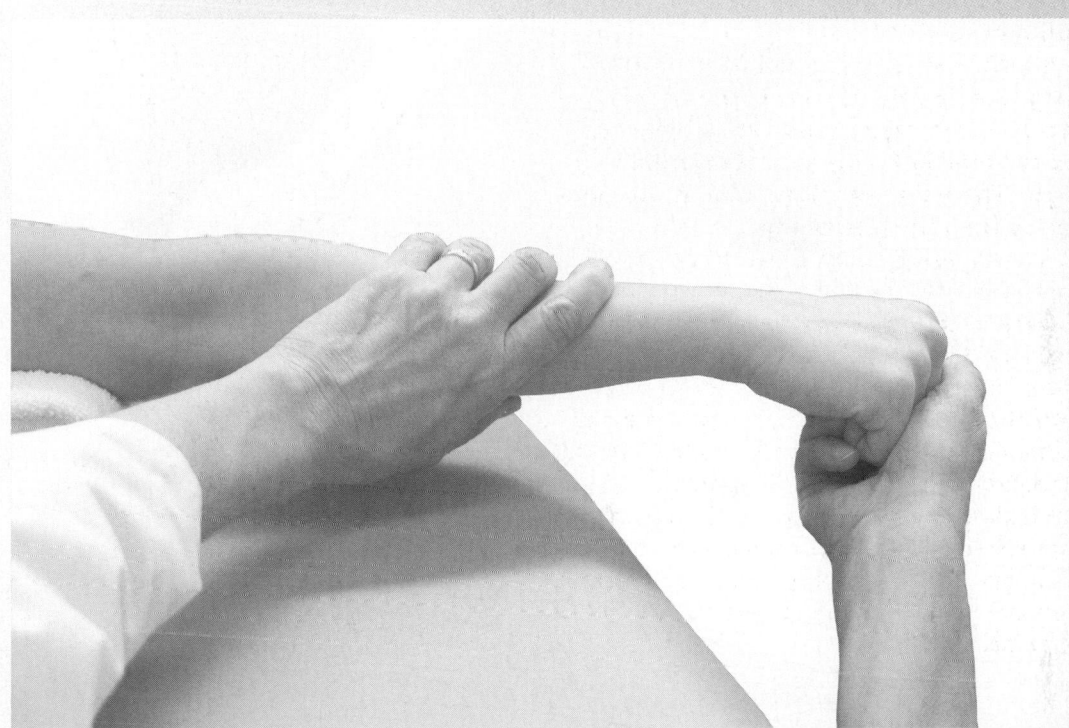

FIGURE 6.25 The starting position for testing the length of the extensor digitorum, extensor indicis, and extensor digiti minimi muscles. The hand is positioned off the end of the examining table to allow room for finger and wrist flexion.

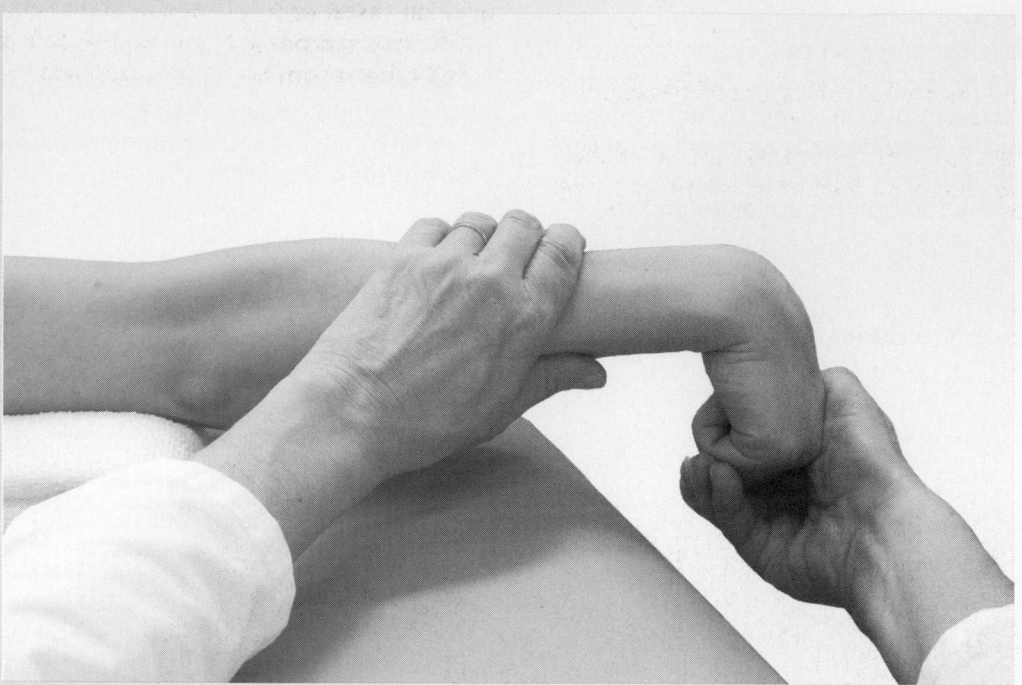

FIGURE 6.26 The end of the testing motion for the length of the extensor digitorum, extensor indicis, and extensor digiti minimi muscles. One of the examiner's hands stabilizes the forearm, while the other hand holds the fingers in full flexion and moves the wrist into flexion.

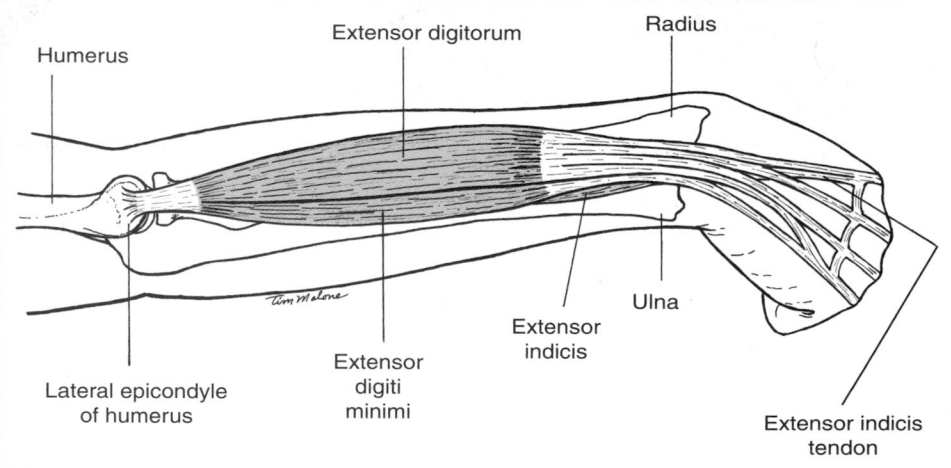

FIGURE 6.27 A posterior view of the right forearm and hand showing the extensor digitorum, extensor indicis, and extensor digiti minimi muscles stretched over the elbow, wrist, MCP, PIP, and DIP joints.

Goniometer Alignment
See Figure 6.28.

1. Center **fulcrum** on the lateral aspect of the wrist over the triquetrum.
2. Align **proximal arm** with the lateral midline of the ulna, using the olecranon and ulnar styloid process for reference.

3. Align **distal arm** with the lateral midline of the fifth metacarpal. Do not use the soft tissue of the hypothenar eminence for reference.

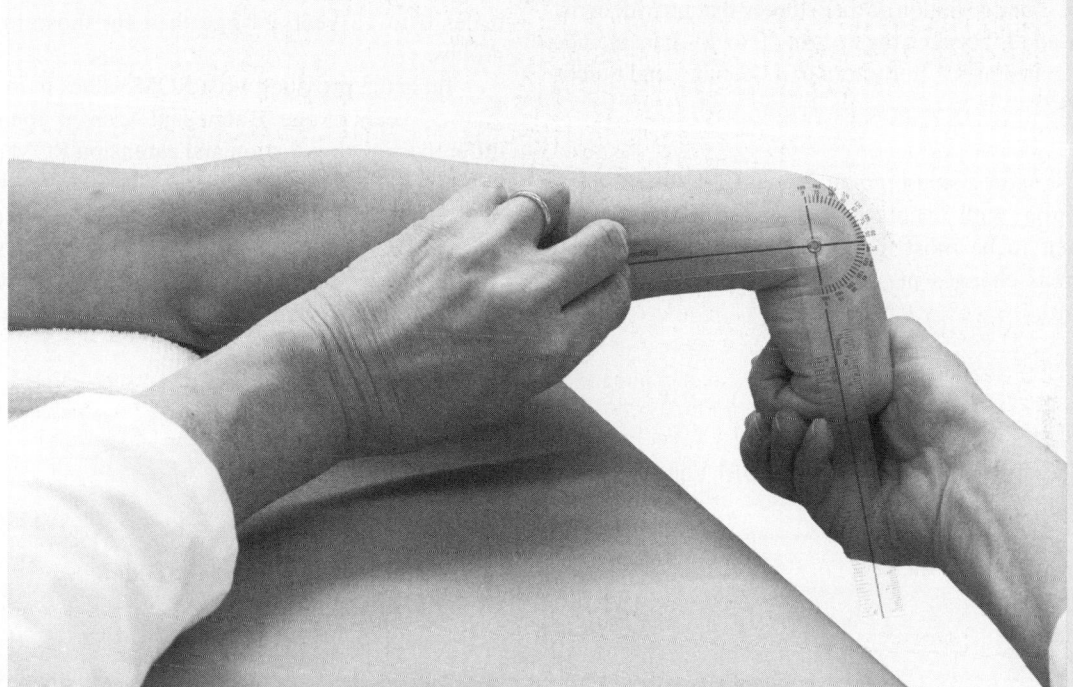

FIGURE 6.28 The alignment of the goniometer at the end of testing the length of the extensor digitorum, extensor indicis, and extensor digiti minimi muscles.

✐ Research Findings

Effects of Age, Gender, and Other Factors

Table 6.1 provides normal wrist ROM values for adults as reported by the AAOS,[12–15,17,18] AMA,[12] Boone and Azen,[15] Greene and Wolf,[17] and Ryu and associates.[18] In general, these values range from 60 to 80 degrees for flexion, 60 to 75 degrees for extension, 20 to 25 degrees for radial deviation, and 30 to 40 degrees for ulnar deviation. Other studies that provide wrist ROM data for adults between the ages of 20 to 60 years include Solgaard and colleagues,[19] Solveborn and Olerud,[20] and Stubbs and coworkers.[21]

Age

Most studies support a small, gradual decrease in the amount of wrist motion with increasing age. Age-related ROM changes appear to be most marked in young children and seniors, whereas changes in young and middle-aged adults seem minimal.

Table 6.2 provides normative wrist ROM values for newborns and children. Although caution must be used in drawing conclusions from comparisons between values obtained by different researchers, the mean flexion and extension values for infants from Wanatabe and coworkers[22] are larger than values for males aged 18 months to 19 years reported by Boone and Azen.[15,23] Within the study by Boone and Azen, wrist flexion and ulnar and radial deviation motions for the youngest age group (18 months to 5 years) were significantly larger than the values for other age groups (see Tables 6.2 and 6.3). Wrist extension values were significantly larger for males 6 to 12 years of age than for those in the other age groups.

Table 6.3 provides wrist ROM values in male adults from 20 to 54 years of age. Boone and Azen[15,23] found a significant difference in wrist flexion and extension ROM between males younger than or equal to 19 years of age and those who were older. However, the effects of age on wrist motion in adults from 20 to 54 years of age appear to be very slight. A study by Stubbs and associates[21] placed 55 male subjects between the ages of 25 and 54 years into three age groups. There was

| TABLE 6.1 | Normal Wrist ROM Values for Adults in Degrees from Selected Sources |

	AAOS[13,14]	AMA[12]	Boone and Azen[15]	Greene and Wolf[17]	Ryu et al[18]
			20–54 yrs n = 56 Males	18–55 yrs n = 20 Males and Females	n = 40 Males and Females
Motion			Mean (SD)	Mean (SD)	Mean
Flexion	80	60	74.8 (6.6)	73.3 (2.1)	79.1
Extension	70	60	74.0 (6.6)	64.9 (2.2)	59.3
Radial deviation	20	20	21.1 (4.0)	25.4 (2.0)	21.1
Ulnar deviation	30	30	35.3 (3.8)	39.2 (2.1)	37.7

| TABLE 6.2 | Effects of Age on Wrist ROM in Newborns, Children, and Adolescents: Normal Values in Degrees |

	Wanatabe et al[22]	Boone and Azen[15,23]		
	2 wks–2 yrs n = 45 Males and Females	18 mos–5 yrs n = 19 Males	6–12 yrs n = 17 Males	13–19 yrs n = 17 Males
Motion	Range of Means	Mean (SD)	Mean (SD)	Mean (SD)
Flexion	88–96	82.2 (3.8)	76.3 (5.6)	75.4 (4.5)
Extension	82–89	76.1 (4.9)	78.4 (5.9)	72.9 (6.4)
Radial deviation		24.2 (3.7)	21.3 (4.1)	19.7 (3.0)
Ulnar deviation		38.7 (3.6)	35.4 (2.4)	35.7 (4.2)

TABLE 6.3	Effects of Age on Wrist ROM in Men 20 to 54 Years Old: Normal Values in Degrees					
	Boone and Azen[15,23]			Stubbs et al[21]		
	20–29 yrs n = 19	30–39 yrs n = 18	40–54 yrs n = 19	25–34 yrs n = 15	35–44 yrs n = 20	45–54 yrs n = 20
Motion	Mean (SD)	Mean (SD)	Mean (SD)	Mean (SD)	Mean (SD)	Mean (SD)
Flexion	76.8 (5.5)	74.9 (4.0)	72.8 (8.9)	70.6 (9.3)	73.5 (10.4)	68.9 (8.4)
Extension	77.5 (5.1)	72.8 (6.9)	71.6 (6.3)	78.3 (11.8)	76.4 (10.4)	76.7 (11.7)
Radial deviation	21.4 (3.6)	20.3 (3.1)	21.6 (5.1)	23.8 (9.5)	22.5 (7.9)	18.9 (7.9)
Ulnar deviation	35.1 (3.8)	36.1 (2.9)	34.7 (4.5)	51.1 (9.0)	49.9 (7.0)	44.1 (4.3)

no significant difference among the age groups for wrist flexion, extension, and radial deviation ROM. A significant difference in ulnar deviation (7 degrees) was found between the oldest and the youngest age groups, with the oldest group having less motion.

Wrist ROM values in males 60 years of age and older are presented in Table 6.4. Flexion and extension ROM in these older adults, as presented by Walker and associates,[24] Chaparro and colleagues,[25] and Kalscheur and coworkers[26] are less than the values for the age groups presented in Table 6.3. Chaparro and colleagues[25] further subdivided the 62 male subjects in their study into four age groups: 60 to 69 years of age, 70 to 79 years of age, 80 to 89 years of age, and 90 years of age and older. They found a trend of decreasing ROM with increasing age, with the oldest group having significantly lower wrist flexion and ulnar deviation values than the two youngest groups.

Four other studies offer additional information on the effects of age on wrist motion. Hewitt,[27] in a study of 112 females between 11 and 45 years of age, found slight

differences in the average amount of active motion in various age groups, but no statistical analyses were performed. Allander and coworkers,[28] in a study of 309 Icelandic females, 208 Swedish females, and 203 Swedish males ranging in age from 33 to 70 years, found that with increasing age there was a decrease in flexion and extension ROM at both wrists. Males lost an average of 2.2 degrees of motion every 5 years. Bell and Hoshizaki[29] studied 124 females and 66 males ranging in age from 18 to 88 years. A significant negative correlation was noted between ROM and age for wrist flexion–extension and radial–ulnar deviation in females and for wrist flexion–extension in males. As age increased, wrist motions generally decreased. There was a significant difference among the five age groups of females for all wrist motions, although the difference was not significant for males. Kalscheur and associates,[30] in a study of 61 women between the ages of 63 and 85 years, found a significant linear relationship between age and right wrist flexion and extension with ROM decreasing an average of 0.4 to 0.5 degrees per year in these older women. The relationships between age and left wrist motions were not statistically significant.

Gender
The following four studies offer evidence of gender effects on the wrist joint, with most supporting the belief that women have slightly more wrist ROM than men. Cobe,[31] in a study of 100 college men and 15 women ranging in age from 20 to 30 years, found that women had a greater active ROM in all motions at the wrist than men. Allander and coworkers[28] compared wrist flexion and extension ROM in 203 Swedish men and 208 Swedish women between the ages of 45 and more than 70 years of age and noted that women had significantly greater motion than men. Both studies measured active motion with joint-specific mechanical devices. Walker and associates,[24] in a study of 30 men and 30 women aged 60 to 84 years, found that the women had more active wrist extension and flexion than the men, whereas the men had more ulnar and radial deviation than the women. These differences were statistically significant for wrist extension (4 degrees) and ulnar deviation (5 degrees). Chaparro and colleagues[25]

TABLE 6.4	Effects of Age on Wrist ROM in Men Older Than 60 Years: Normal Values in Degrees		
	Walker et al[24]	Chaparro et al[25]	Kalscheur et al[26]
	60–85 yrs n = 30	60–90+ yrs n = 62	66–86 yrs n = 25
Motion	Mean (SD)	Mean (SD)	Mean (SD)
Flexion	62.0 (12.0)	50.8 (13.8)	64.9 (8.7)
Extension	61.0 (6.0)	44.0 (9.9)	58.2 (10.9)
Radial deviation	20.0 (6.0)		
Ulnar deviation	28.0 (7.0)	35.0 (9.5)	

examined wrist flexion, extension, and ulnar deviation ROM in 62 men and 85 women from 60 to more than 90 years of age. Women had significantly greater wrist extension (6.4 degrees) and ulnar deviation (3.0 degrees) than men. Kalscheur and coworkers[26] found that women had more wrist flexion and extension ROM than men in a study of 61 women and 25 men between the ages of 63 and 86 years. These differences ranged from 1.7 to 5.3 degrees and were statistically significant for right wrist flexion (5.0 degrees) and left wrist extension (5.3 degrees).

Right Versus Left Sides

Study results vary as to whether there is a difference between left and right wrist ROM. Boone and Azen,[15] in a study of 109 normal males between 18 months and 54 years of age, found no significant difference in wrist flexion, extension, and radial and ulnar deviation between sides. Likewise, Chang, Buschbacher, and Edlich[32] found no significant difference between right and left wrist flexion and extension in the 10 power lifters and 10 nonlifters who were their subjects. Solgaard and coworkers[19] studied 8 males and 23 females aged 24 to 65 years. Right and left wrist extension and radial deviation differed significantly, but the differences were small and not significant when the total range (i.e., flexion and extension) was assessed. The authors stated that the opposite wrist could be satisfactorily used as a reference.

In contrast, several studies have found the left wrist to have greater ROM than the right wrist. Cobe[31] measured wrist motions in the positions of pronation and supination in 100 men and 15 women. He found that men had greater ROM in their left wrist than in their right for all motions except ulnar deviation measured in pronation. However, he reported that the women had greater wrist motion on the right except for extension in pronation and radial deviation in supination. No statistical tests were conducted in the 1928 study, but Allander and associates[28] reported that a recalculation of the original data collected by Cobe found a significantly greater ROM on the left in men. Cobe[31] suggests that the heavy work that men performed using their right extremities may account for the decrease in right-side motion in comparison with left-side motion. A study by Kalscheur and associates[30] found a significantly greater range of left wrist extension and right wrist flexion as compared to the contralateral side in 61 older women. The mean differences between sides were small, ranging from 3 to 5 degrees.

Allander and associates,[28] in a study subgroup of 309 Icelandic women aged 34 to 61 years, found no significant difference between the right and the left wrists. However, a subgroup of 208 women and 203 Swedish men in the study showed significantly smaller ranges of wrist flexion and extension on the right than on the left, independent of gender. The authors state that these differences may be due to a higher level of exposure to trauma of the right hand in a predominantly right-handed society. Solveborn and Olerud[20] measured wrist ROM in 16 healthy subjects in addition to 123 patients with unilateral tennis elbow. Among the healthy subjects a significantly greater ROM was found for wrist flexion and extension on the left compared with the right. However, mean differences between sides were only 2 degrees. The authors concurred with Boone and Azen[15] that a patient's healthy limb can be used to establish a norm for comparing with the affected side.

Testing Position

Several studies have reported differences in wrist ROM depending on the testing position of the forearm during measurement. These findings support the use of consistent forearm positions during wrist measurements. Cobe,[31] in a study of 100 men and 15 women, found that ulnar deviation ROM was greater in supination, whereas radial deviation was greater in pronation. It is interesting that the total amount of ulnar and radial deviation combined was similar between the two positions. Hewitt[27] measured wrist ROM in 112 females in supination and pronation and found that ulnar deviation was greater in supination, whereas radial deviation, flexion, and extension were greater in pronation. Werner and Plancher,[6] in a review article, also stated that ulnar deviation has a greater ROM when the forearm is supinated than when the forearm is pronated. They noted that radial and ulnar deviation ROMs become minimal when the wrist is fully flexed or extended. No specific references for these observations were cited.

Spilman and Pinkston[28] examined the effect of three frequently used goniometric testing positions on active wrist radial and ulnar deviation ROM in 100 subjects (63 males, 37 females). In Position One the subject's arm was at the side, with the elbow flexed to 90 degrees and the forearm fully pronated. In Position Two the shoulder was in 90 degrees of flexion, with the elbow extended and the hand prone. In Position Three the subject's shoulder was in 90 degrees of abduction, with the elbow in 90 degrees of flexion and the hand prone (in this position the forearm is in neutral pronation). Ulnar deviation and the total range of radial and ulnar deviation were significantly greater when measured in Position Three. Radial deviation was significantly greater when the subject was in Position Three or Position Two than in Position One. The differences between the means for the three positions were small—approximately 3 degrees.

Wrist ROM values have also been found to vary if different wrist positions are used during testing. It appears that the greatest ROM values are obtained with the wrist in a neutral position. Marshall, Morzall, and Shealy[34] evaluated 35 men and 19 women for wrist ROM in one plane of motion while the subjects were fixed in secondary wrist and forearm positions. For example, during the measurement of radial and ulnar deviation, the wrist was alternatively positioned in 0 degrees, 40 degrees of flexion, and 40 degrees of extension. During the measurement of flexion and extension the wrist was positioned in 0 degrees, 15 degrees radial deviation, and 25 degrees ulnar deviation. The effects of the secondary wrist and forearm postures, although statistically significant, were generally small (less than 5 degrees), with most motions having the greatest range with the wrist in neutral. However, radial deviation ROM was greatest when performed in wrist extension. The authors believed that the changes that occur in wrist ROM with positional alterations might have been due to changes in contact between articular surfaces and tautness of ligaments that span the wrist region. In a study of 10 subjects performing active circumduction, Li and associates[35] found that maximum ROM in flexion and extension occurred with the wrist near 0 degrees of radial and ulnar deviation. Likewise, maximum ROM in radial and ulnar deviation occurred with the wrist near 0 degrees of flexion and extension. Wrist deviation from the neutral position in one plane of motion reduced wrist ROM in other planes of motions.

Functional Range of Motion

Several investigators have examined the range of motion that occurs at the wrist during activities of daily living (ADLs) and during the placement of the hand on the body areas necessary for personal care. Tables 6.5 and 6.6 are adapted from the works of Brumfield and Champoux,[36] Ryu and associates,[18] Safaee-Rad and colleagues,[37] and Cooper and coworkers.[38] Differences in ROM values reported for certain functional tasks were most likely the result of variations in task definitions, measurement methods, and subject selection. However, in spite of the range of values reported, certain trends are evident.

A review of Table 6.5 shows that the majority of ADLs required wrist extension and ulnar deviation. Drinking

activities generally required the least amount of extension (6 to 24 degrees) and the smallest arc of motion (13 to 20 degrees). Using the telephone (Fig. 6.29), turning a steering wheel or a doorknob and rising from a chair (see Fig. 5.31) required the greatest amounts of extension (40 to 63 degrees) and arc of motion (43 to 85 degrees). Turning a doorknob (Fig. 6.30) involved the greatest amount of flexion (40 degrees). The greatest amounts of ulnar deviation (27 to 32 degrees) were noted while rising from a chair, turning a doorknob and steering wheel, and pouring from a pitcher.

Table 6.6 provides information on wrist position during the placement of the hand on the body areas commonly touched during personal care. The majority of positions required wrist flexion and less overall wrist motion than the ADLs presented in Table 6.5. Among the positions studied, placing the palm to the front of the chest consistently required the greatest amount of wrist flexion, whereas placing the palm to the sacrum required the greatest amount of ulnar deviation.

Brumfield and Champoux[36] used a uniaxial electrogoniometer to determine the range of wrist flexion and extension during 15 ADLs performed by 12 men and 7 women. They determined that ADLs such as eating, drinking, and using a telephone were accomplished with 5 degrees of flexion to 35 degrees of extension. Personal care activities that involved

TABLE 6.5 Wrist ROM During Functional Activities: Mean Values in Degrees

Activity	Extension*			Ulnar Deviation†			Source
	Min	Max	Arc	Min	Max	Arc	
Put glass to mouth	11.2	24.0	12.8	—	—	—	Brumfield[36]
Drink from glass	2	22	20	5	20	15	Ryu[‡18]
Drink from handled cup	−7.5*	5.9	13.4	8.3	16.1	7.8	Safaee-Rad[37]
Eat with fork	9.3	36.5	27.7	—	—	—	Brumfield
	3.3	17.7	14.4	3.2	−4.9†	8.1	Safaee-Rad
Feeding tasks: fork, spoon, cup	−6.8*	20.9	27.2	18.7	−2.4†	21.1	Cooper (males)[38]
Cut with knife	−3.5*	20.2	23.7	—	—	—	Brumfield
	−30*	−5	25	12	27	15	Ryu
Pour from pitcher	8.7	29.7	21.0	—	—	—	Brumfield
	−20*	22	42	12	32	20	Ryu
Turn doorknob	−40*	45	85	−2†	32	34	Ryu
Use telephone	−0.1*	42.6	42.7	—	—	—	Brumfield
	−15	40	55	−10†	12	22	Ryu
Turn steering wheel	−15*	45	60	−17†	27	44	Ryu
Rise from chair	0.6	63.4	62.8	—	—	—	Brumfield
	−10*	60	70	5	30	25	Ryu

*The minus sign denotes flexion.
†The minus sign denotes radial deviation.
‡Values from Ryu et al were extrapolated from graphs.

TABLE 6.6	Wrist Motions During Hand Placement Needed for Personal Care Activities: Mean Values in Degrees				
	Extension	Flexion	Ulnar Deviation	Radial Deviation	
Activity	**Mean (SD)**	**Mean (SD)**	**Mean (SD)**	**Mean (SD)**	**Source**
Hand to top of head	— —	2.3 (12.5)	— —	— —	Brumfield[36]
	— —	20.9 (13.9)	16.1 (12.7)	— —	Ryu[18]
Hand to occiput	12.7 (9.9)	— —	— —	— —	Brumfield
	— —	0.9 (17.6)	9.7 (11.9)	— —	Ryu
Hand to front of chest	— —	18.9 (8.9)	— —	— —	Brumfield
	— —	24.5 (16.7)	— —	5.1 (10.3)	Ryu
Hand to sacrum	— —	0.6 (9.8)	— —	— —	Brumfield
	— —	19.5 (19.3)	47.8 (16.8)	— —	Ryu
Hand to foot	14.2 (10.6)	— —	— —	— —	Brumfield
	0.8 (14.6)	— —	8.7 (12.2)	— —	Ryu

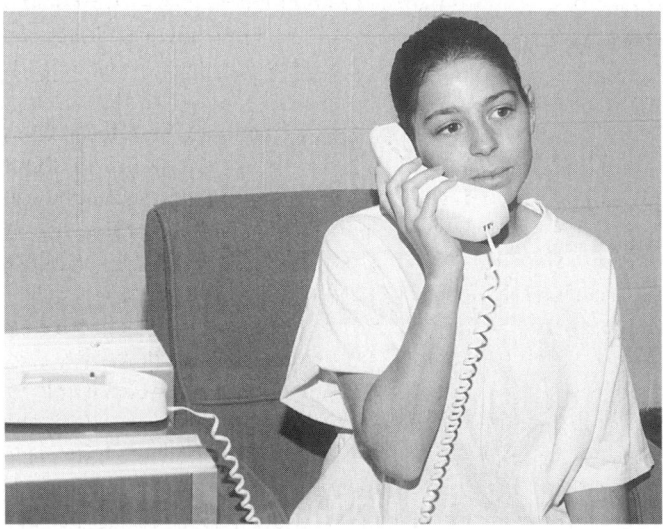

FIGURE 6.29 Using a telephone requires approximately 40 degrees of wrist extension.

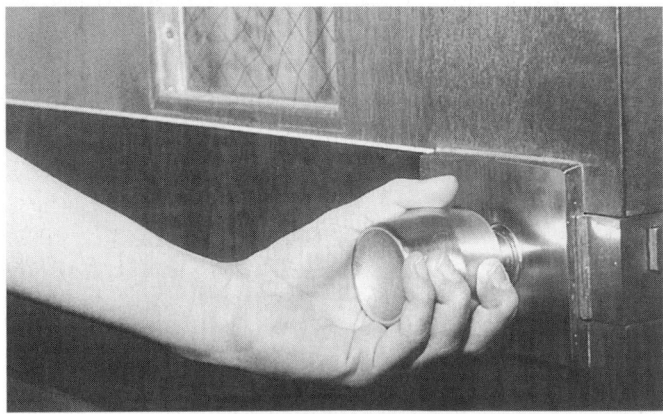

FIGURE 6.30 Turning a doorknob requires 40 degrees of wrist flexion and 45 degrees of wrist extension.

placing the hand on the body required 20 degrees of flexion to 15 degrees of extension. The authors concluded that an arc of wrist motion of 45 degrees (10 degrees of flexion to 35 degrees of extension) is sufficient to perform most of the activities studied.

Palmer and coworkers[39] used a triaxial electrogoniometer to study 10 normal subjects while they performed 52 tasks. A range of 33 degrees of flexion, 59 degrees of extension, 23 degrees of radial deviation, and 22 degrees of ulnar deviation was used in performing ADLs and personal hygiene. During these tasks the average amount of motion was about 5 degrees of flexion, 30 degrees of extension, 10 degrees of radial deviation, and 15 degrees of ulnar deviation. ROM values for individual tasks were not presented in the study.

Ryu and associates[18] found that 31 examined tasks could be performed with 54 degrees of flexion, 60 degrees of extension, 17 degrees of radial deviation, and 40 degrees of ulnar deviation. The 20 men and 20 women were evaluated with a biaxial electrogoniometer during performance of palm placement activities, personal care and hygiene, diet and food preparation, and miscellaneous ADLs.

Studies by Safaee-Rad and coworkers[37] and Cooper and coworkers[38] examined wrist ROM with a video-based three-dimensional motion analysis system during three feeding tasks: drinking from a cup, eating with a fork, and eating with a spoon. The 10 males studied by Safaee-Rad and coworkers used from 10 degrees of wrist flexion to 25 degrees of extension and from 20 degrees of ulnar deviation to 5 degrees of radial deviation during the tasks. Cooper and coworkers examined 10 males and 9 females during feeding tasks, with the elbow unrestricted and then fixed in 110 degrees of flexion. With the elbow unrestricted, males used from 7 degrees of wrist flexion to 21 degrees of extension and from 19 degrees of ulnar deviation to 2 degrees of radial deviation. Females had similar values for flexion and extension but used from

3 degrees of ulnar deviation to 18 degrees of radial deviation. Both studies found that drinking from a cup required less of an arc of wrist motion than eating with a fork or spoon.

Nelson[40] took a different approach to determining the amount of wrist motion necessary for carrying out functional tasks. He evaluated the ability of 9 males and 3 females to perform 123 ADLs with a splint on the dominant wrist that limited motion to 5 degrees of flexion, 6 degrees of extension, 7 degrees of radial deviation, and 6 degrees of ulnar deviation. All 123 activities could be completed with the splint in place, with 9 activities having a mean difficulty rating of greater than or equal to 2 (could be done with minimal difficulty or frustration and with satisfactory outcome). The most difficult activities included putting on/taking off a brassiere (Fig. 6.31), washing legs/back, writing, dusting low surfaces, cutting vegetables, handling a sharp knife, cutting meat, using a can opener, and using a manual eggbeater. It should be noted that these subjects were pain free and had normal shoulders and elbows to compensate for the restricted wrist motions. The ability to generalize these results to a patient population with pain and multiply involved joints may be limited.

Repetitive trauma disorders such as carpal tunnel syndrome and wrist/hand tendinitis have been noted to occur more frequently in performing certain types of work, sports, and artistic endeavors. To elucidate the cause of these higher incidences of injury, studies have been conducted on the wrist positions used and the amount and frequency of wrist motions required during grocery bagging,[41] grocery scanning,[42] piano playing,[43] industrial work,[44] and handrim wheelchair propulsion[45,46] and in playing sports such as basketball, baseball pitching, and golf.[6,47] The reader is advised to refer directly to these studies to gain information about the amount of wrist ROM that occurs during these activities. In general, an association has been noted between activities that require extreme wrist postures and the prevalence of hand/wrist tendinitis.[48] Tasks that involve repeated wrist flexion and extreme wrist extension, repetitive work with the hands, and repeated force applied to the base of the palm and wrist have been associated with carpal tunnel syndrome.[49]

Reliability

In early studies of wrist motion conducted by Hewitt[27] and Cobe[31] in the 1920s, both authors observed considerable differences in repeated measurements of active wrist motions. These differences were attributed to a lack of motor control on the part of the subjects in expending maximal effort. Cobe suggested that only average values have much validity and that changes in ROM should exceed 5 degrees to be considered clinically significant.

Later studies of intratester and intertester reliability were conducted by numerous researchers. The majority of these investigators found that intratester reliability was greater than intertester reliability, that reliability varied according to the motion being tested, and that different instruments should not be used interchangeably during joint measurement.

Hellebrandt, Duvall, and Moore[50] found that wrist motions measured with a universal goniometer were more reliable than those measured with a joint-specific device. Measurements of wrist flexion and extension were less reliable than measurements of radial and ulnar deviation, although mean differences between successive measurements taken with a universal goniometer by a skilled tester were 1.1 degrees for flexion and 0.9 degrees for extension. The mean differences between successive measurements increased to 5.4 degrees for flexion and 5.7 degrees for extension when successive measurements were taken with different instruments.

In a study by Low,[51] 50 testers using a universal goniometer visually estimated and then measured the author's active wrist extension and elbow flexion. Five testers also took 10 repeated measurements over the course of 5 to 10 days. Mean error improved from 12.8 degrees for visual estimates to 7.8 degrees for goniometric measurement. Intraobserver error was less than interobserver error. The measurement of wrist extension was less reliable than the measurement of elbow flexion, with mean errors of 7.8 and 5.0 degrees, respectively.

Boone et al[52] conducted a study in which four testers using a universal goniometer measured ulnar deviation on 12 male volunteers. Measurements were repeated over a period of 4 weeks. Intratester reliability was found to be

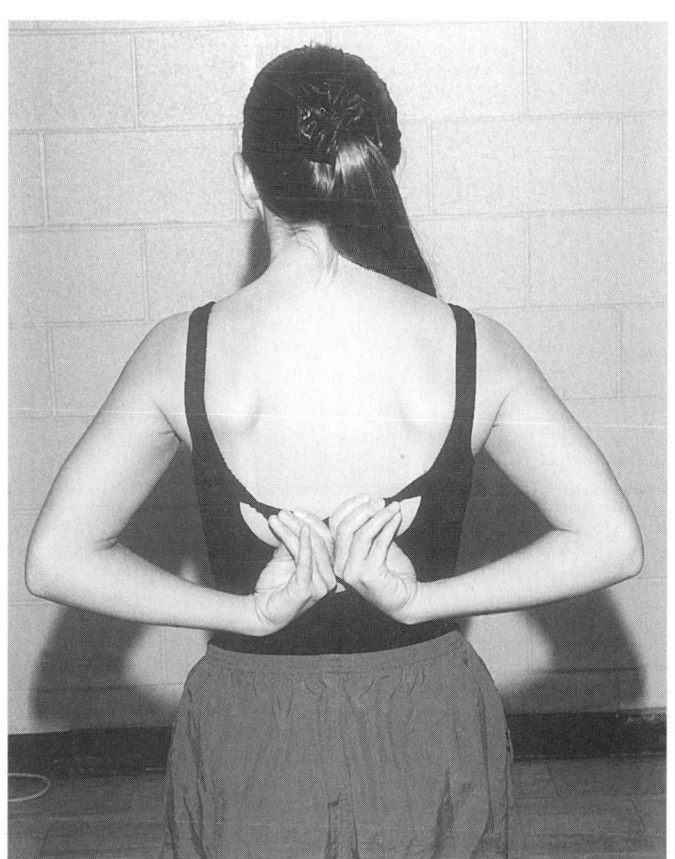

FIGURE 6.31 A large amount of wrist flexion is needed to fasten a bra or bathing suit. This is one of the most difficult activities to perform if wrist motion is limited.

better than intertester reliability. The authors concluded that to determine true change when more than one tester measures the same motion, differences in motion should exceed 5 degrees.

In a study by Bird and Stowe,[53] two observers repeatedly measured active and passive wrist ROM in three subjects. They concluded that interobserver error was greatest for extension (±8 degrees) and least for radial and ulnar deviation (±2 to 3 degrees). Error during passive ROM measurements was slightly greater than during active ROM measurements.

Greene and Wolf[17] compared the reliability of the OrthoRanger, an electronic pendulum goniometer, with a universal goniometer for active upper-extremity motions in 20 healthy adults. Wrist ROM was measured by one therapist three times with each instrument during each of three sessions over a 2-week period. There was a significant difference between instruments for wrist extension and ulnar deviation. Within-session reliability was slightly higher for the universal goniometer (ICC = 0.91 to 0.96) than for the OrthoRanger (ICC = 0.88 to 0.92). The 95 percent confidence level, which represents the variability around the mean, ranged from 7.6 to 9.3 degrees for the goniometer and from 18.2 to 25.6 degrees for the OrthoRanger. The authors concluded that the OrthoRanger provided no advantages over the universal goniometer.

Solgaard and coworkers[19] found intratester standard deviations of 5 to 8 degrees and intertester standard deviations of 6 to 10 degrees in a study of wrist and forearm motions involving 31 healthy subjects. Measurements were taken with a universal goniometer by four testers on three different occasions. The coefficients of variation (percent variation) between testers were greater for ulnar and radial deviation than for flexion, extension, pronation, and supination.

Horger[54] conducted a study in which 13 randomly paired therapists performed repeated measurements of active and passive wrist motions on 48 patients. Therapists were free to select their own method of measurement with a universal goniometer. The six specialized hand therapists used an ulnar alignment for flexion and extension, whereas the nonspecialized therapists used a radial goniometer alignment. Intratester reliability of both active and passive wrist motions were highly reliable (all ICCs higher than 0.90) for all motions. Intratester reliability was consistently higher than intertester reliability (ICC 0.66 to 0.91). Standard errors of measurements (SEM) ranged from 2.6 to 4.4 for intratester values and from 3.0 to 8.2 for intertester values. Agreement between measures was better for flexion and extension than for radial and ulnar deviation. Intertester reliability coefficients for measurements of active motion (ICC = 0.78 to 0.91) were slightly higher than were coefficients for passive motion (ICC = 0.66 to 0.86) except for radial deviation. Generally, reliability was higher for the specialized therapists than for the nonspecialized therapists. The author determined that the presence of pain reduced the reliability of both active and passive measurements, but active measurements were affected more than passive measurements.

LaStayo and Wheeler[16] studied the intratester and intertester reliability of passive ROM measurements of wrist flexion and extension in 120 patients as measured by 32 randomly paired therapists, who used three goniometric alignments (ulnar, radial, and dorsal–volar). The reliability of measuring wrist flexion ROM was consistently higher than that of measuring extension ROM. Mean intratester ICCs for wrist flexion were 0.86 for radial, 0.87 for ulnar, and 0.92 for dorsal alignment. Mean intratester ICCs for wrist extension were 0.80 for radial, 0.80 for ulnar, and 0.84 for volar alignment. The authors recommended that these three alignments, although generally having good reliability, should not be used interchangeably because there were some significant differences between the measurements taken with the three alignments. The authors suggested that the dorsal–volar alignment should be the technique of choice for measuring passive wrist flexion and extension, given its higher reliability. In an invited commentary on this study, Flower[55] suggested using the fifth metacarpal, which is easier to visualize and align with the distal arm of the goniometer in the ulnar technique, rather than the third metacarpal, which was used in the study. Flower noted that the presence and fluctuation of edema on the dorsal surface of the hand may reduce the reliability of the dorsal alignment and necessitate the use of the ulnar (fifth metacarpal) alignment in the clinical setting.

Validity

We are unaware of any published studies that report criterion-related validity of wrist ROM measurements taken with a goniometer to radiographs. However, several studies have examined construct validity between impairment measures, such as wrist ROM, and ratings of functional limitation or disability. A review of 32 published wrist outcome instruments noted that ROM was the most frequently included variable, present in 82 percent of the outcome instruments.[56]

Wagner and colleagues[57] measured passive ROM of wrist flexion, extension, radial and ulnar deviation, and the strength of the wrist extensor and flexor muscles in 18 boys with Duchenne muscular dystrophy. A highly significant negative correlation was found between difficulty performing functional hand tasks and radial deviation ROM (r = –0.76 to –0.86) and between difficulty performing functional hand tasks and wrist extensor strength (r = –0.61 to –0.83).

The relationship between wrist ROM and activity limitation, pain, and disability following wrist fractures has been examined. Tremayne and associates,[58] in a study of 20 patients with distal radius fractures, found strong, significant correlations (r = –0.51 to –0.76) between grip strength and tasks in the Jebsen Test of Hand Function (JTHF) and weaker correlations (r = –0.17 to –0.55) between wrist extenson ROM and tasks in the JTHF. In a subset of 11 patients with Colles' type fractures, there were significant correlations (r = –0.74 to –0.84) between wrist extension ROM and three of seven tasks (turning cards, stimulated feeding, and lifting large light objects) included in the JTHF.

In a study of 120 patients with distal radius fractures, MacDermid and coworkers[59] found that higher patient-rated pain and disability scores 6 months post-injury (6-month Patient-Rated Wrist Evaluation [PRWE] scores) were moderately associated ($r = -0.41$) with lower composite ROM scores. Composite ROM scores were based on wrist flexion, extension, ulnar and radial deviation, supination, pronation, and finger flexion.

Karnezis and Fragkiadakis,[60] in a study of 25 patients recovering from distal radial fractures, reported correlations between the "Function Score" of the PRWE score and grip strength ($r = 0.80$), wrist extension ROM ($r = 0.78$), pronation ($r = 0.70$), supination ($r = 0.63$), and wrist flexion ($r = 0.62$).

They concluded that grip strength, followed by wrist extension and forearm pronation, were the most sensitive clinical indicators of return of wrist function. In another report of 31 patients recovering from distal radial fracture, the same authors noted that flexion–extension and pronation–supination arcs of motion (expressed as percentages of the unaffected side) were not significantly associated with total PRWE scores in a multiple regression model that included grip strength, age, gender, presence of high-energy injury, and intra-articular fracture.[61] The possibility that some of the variables included in the regression model may be inadvertent markers for diminished ROM values may have affected the findings.

REFERENCES

1. Linscheid, RL: Kinematic considerations of the wrist. Clin Orthop 202:27, 1986.
2. Austin, NM: The Wrist and Hand Complex. In Levangie, PK, and Norkin, CC (eds): Joint Structure and Function: A Comprehensive Analysis, ed 4. FA Davis, Philadelphia, 2005.
3. Kaltenborn, FM: Manual Mobilization of the Joints, Vol 1: The Extremities, ed 5. Olaf Norlis Bokhandel, Oslo, Norway, 1999.
4. Sarrafian, SH, Melamed, JL, and Goshgarian, GM: Study of wrist motion in flexion and extension. Clin Orthop 126:153, 1977.
5. Youm, Y, et al: Kinematics of the wrist: I. An experimental study of radial–ulnar deviation and flexion–extension. J Bone Joint Surg (Am) 60:423, 1978.
6. Werner, SL, and Plancher, KD: Biomechanics of wrist injuries in sports. Clin Sports Med 17:407, 1998.
7. Ritt, M, et al: Rotational stability of the carpus relative to the forearm. J Hand Surg 20A:305, 1995.
8. Neumann, DA: Kinesiology of the Musculoskeletal System. Mosby, St. Louis, 2002.
9. Kisner, C, and Colby, LA: Therapeutic Exercise: Foundations and Techniques, ed 5. FA Davis, Philadelphia, 2007.
10. Kapandji, IA, and Kandel, MJ: The Physiology of the Joints, Vol 1, ed 5. Churchill-Livingstone, Edinburgh, 1997.
11. Cyriax, JH, and Cyriax, PJ: Illustrated Manual of Orthopaedic Medicine. Butterworths, London, 1983.
12. American Medical Association: Guides to the Evaluation of Permanent Impairment, ed 5. AMA, Chicago, 2001.
13. American Academy of Orthopaedic Surgeons: Joint Motion: Methods of Measuring and Recording. AAOS, Chicago, 1965.
14. Greene, WB, and Heckman, JD (eds):The Clinical Measurement of Joint Motion. American Academy of Orthopaedic Surgeons, Rosemont, IL, 1994.
15. Boone, DC, and Azen, SP: Normal range of motion in male subjects. J Bone Joint Surg (Am) 61:756, 1979.
16. LaStayo, PC, and Wheeler, DL: Reliability of passive wrist flexion and extension measurements: A multicenter study. Phys Ther 74:162, 1994
17. Greene, BL, and Wolf, SL: Upper extremity joint movement: Comparison of two measurement devices. Arch Phys Med Rehabil 70:288, 1989.
18. Ryu, J, et al: Functional ranges of motion of the wrist joint. J Hand Surg 16A:409, 1991.
19. Solgaard, S, et al: Reproducibility of goniometry of the wrist. Scand J Rehabil Med 18:5, 1986.
20. Solveborn, SA, and Olerud, C: Radial epicondylalgia (tennis elbow): Measurement of range of motion of the wrist and the elbow. J Orthop Sports Phys Ther 23:251, 1996.
21. Stubbs, NB, Fernandez, JE, and Glenn, WM: Normative data on joint ranges of motion of 25- to 54-year-old males. International Journal of Industrial Ergonomics 12; 265, 1993.
22. Wanatabe, H, et al: The range of joint motions of the extremities in healthy Japanese people: The difference according to age. Nippon Seikeigeka Gokkai Zasshi 53:275, 1979. (Cited in Walker, JM: Musculoskeletal development: A review. Phys Ther 71:878, 1991.)
23. Boone, DC: Techniques of measurement of joint motion. (Unpublished supplement to Boone, DC, and Azen, SP: Normal range of motion in male subjects. J Bone Joint Surg [Am] 61:756, 1979.)
24. Walker, JM, et al: Active mobility of the extremities in older subjects. Phys Ther 64:919, 1984.
25. Chaparro, A, et al: Range of motion of the wrist: Implications for designing computer input devices for the elderly. Disabil Rehabil 22:633:2000.
26. Kalscheur, JA, et al: Gender differences in range of motion in older adults. Phys Occup Ther Geriatr 22:77, 2003.
27. Hewitt, D: The range of active motion at the wrist of women. J Bone Joint Surg (Br) 26:775, 1928.
28. Allander, E, et al: Normal range of joint movements in shoulder, hip, wrist and thumb with special reference to side: A comparison between two populations. Int J Epidemiol 3:253, 1974.
29. Bell, RD, and Hoshizaki, TB: Relationships of age and sex with range of motion of seventeen joint actions in humans. Can J Appl Spt Sci 6:202, 1981.
30. Kalscheur, JA, et al: Range of motion in older women. Phys Occup Ther Geriatr 16:77, 1999.
31. Cobe, HM: The range of active motion of the wrist of white adults. J Bone Joint Surg (Br) 26:763, 1928.
32. Chang, DE, Buschbacher, LP, and Edlich, RF: Limited joint mobility in power lifters. Am J Sports Med 16:280, 1988.
33. Spilman, HW, and Pinkston, D: Relation of test positions to radial and ulnar deviation. Phys Ther 49:837, 1969.
34. Marshall, MM, Morzall, JR, and Shealy, JE: The effects of complex wrist and forearm posture on wrist range of motion. Human Factors 41:205, 1999.
35. Li, ZM, et al: Coupling between wrist flexion–extension and radial–ulnar deviation. Clin Biomech 20:177, 2005.
36. Brumfield, RH, and Champoux, JA: A biomechanical study of normal functional wrist motion. Clin Orthop 187:23, 1984.
37. Safaee-Rad, R, et al: Normal functional range of motion of upper limb joints during performance of three feeding tasks. Arch Phys Med Rehabil 71:505, 1990.
38. Cooper, JE, et al: Elbow joint restriction: Effect on functional upper limb motion during performance of three feeding tasks. Arch Phys Med Rehabil 74:805, 1993.
39. Palmer, AK, et al: Functional wrist motion: A biomechanical study. J Hand Surg 10A:39, 1985.
40. Nelson, DL: Functional wrist motion. Hand Clin 13:83, 1997.
41. Estill, CF, and Kroemer, KH: Evaluation of supermarket bagging using a wrist motion monitor. Hum Factors 40:624, 1998.
42. Marras, WS, et al: Quantification of wrist motion during scanning. Hum Factors 37:412, 1995.
43. Wagner, CH: The pianist's hand: Anthropometry and biomechanics. Ergonomics 31:97, 1998.
44. Marras, WS, and Schoenmarklin, RW: Wrist motions in industry. Ergonomics 36:341, 1995.
45. Veeger, DHEJ, et al: Wrist motion in handrim wheelchair propulsion. J Rehabil Res Dev 35:305, 1998.
46. Wei, S, et al: Wrist kinematic characterization of wheelchair propulsion in various seating positions: Implication to wrist pain. Clin Biomech 18:S46, 2003.
47. Ohinishi, N, et al: Analysis of wrist motion during basketball shooting. In Nakamura, RL, Linscheid, RL, and Miura, T (eds): Wrist Disorder: Current Concepts and Challenges. New York, Springer-Verlag, 1992.
48. Bernard, BP (ed): Musculoskeletal disorders and workplace factors. Cincinnati, Ohio: National Institute of Occupational Safety and Health. 1997.
49. Armstrong, TJ, et al: Ergonomic considerations in hand and wrist tendinitis. J Hand Surg 12A: 830, 1982.
50. Hellebrandt, FA, Duvall, EN, and Moore, ML: The measurement of joint motion. Part III: Reliability of goniometry. Phys Ther Rev 29:302, 1949.
51. Low, JL: The reliability of joint measurement. Physiotherapy 62:227, 1976.
52. Boone, DC, et al: Reliability of goniometric measurements. Phys Ther 58:1355, 1978.
53. Bird, HA, and Stowe, J: The wrist. Clin Rheum Dis 8:559, 1982.
54. Horger, MM: The reliability of goniometric measurements of active and passive wrist motions. Am J Occup Ther 44:342, 1990.
55. Flower, KR: Invited commentary. Phys Ther 74:174, 1994.
56. Bialocerkowski, AE, et al: A systematic review of the content and quality of wrist outcome instruments. Int J Qual Health Care 12:149, 2000.
57. Wagner, MB, et al: Assessment of hand function in Duchenne muscular dystrophy. Arch Phys Med Rehabil 74:801, 1993.
58. Tremayne, A, et al: Correlation of impairment and activity limitation after wrist fracture. Physiother Res Int 7:90, 2002.
59. MacDermid, JC, et al: Patient versus injury factors as predictors of pain and disability six months after a distal radius fracture. J Clin Epidemiol 55:849, 2002.
60. Karnezis, IA, and Fragkiadakis, EG: Objective clinical parameters and patient-rated wrist function. J Bone Joint Surg (Br) 85-B supplement I:7, 2003.
61. Karnezis, IA, and Fragkiadakis, EG: Association between objective clinical variables and patient-rated disability of the wrist. J Bone Joint Surg (Br) 84-B:967, 2002.

Chapter 7

The Hand

Structure and Function

Fingers: Metacarpophalangeal Joints

Anatomy

The metacarpophalangeal (MCP) joints of the fingers are composed of the convex distal end of each metacarpal and the concave base of each proximal phalanx (Fig. 7.1). The joints are enclosed in fibrous capsules (Figs. 7.2 and 7.3). The anterior portion of each capsule has a fibrocartilaginous thickening called the palmar plate (palmar ligament), which is loosely attached to the metacarpals and firmly attached to the proximal phalanx.[1,2] Ligamentous support is provided by palmar, collateral, and deep transverse metacarpal ligaments.

Osteokinematics

The MCP joints are biaxial condyloid joints that have 2 degrees of freedom, allowing flexion–extension in the sagittal plane and abduction–adduction in the frontal plane. Abduction–adduction is possible with the MCP joints positioned in extension, but it is limited with the MCP joints in flexion because of tightening of the collateral ligaments.[2] A small amount of passive axial rotation has been reported at the MCP joints,[2-4] but this motion is not usually measured in the clinical setting.

Arthrokinematics

The concave base of the phalanx slides and rolls on the convex head of the metacarpal in the same direction as movement of the shaft of the phalanx.[5] During flexion the base of the phalanx slides and rolls anteriorly toward the palm, whereas during extension the base of the phalanx slides and rolls dorsally. In

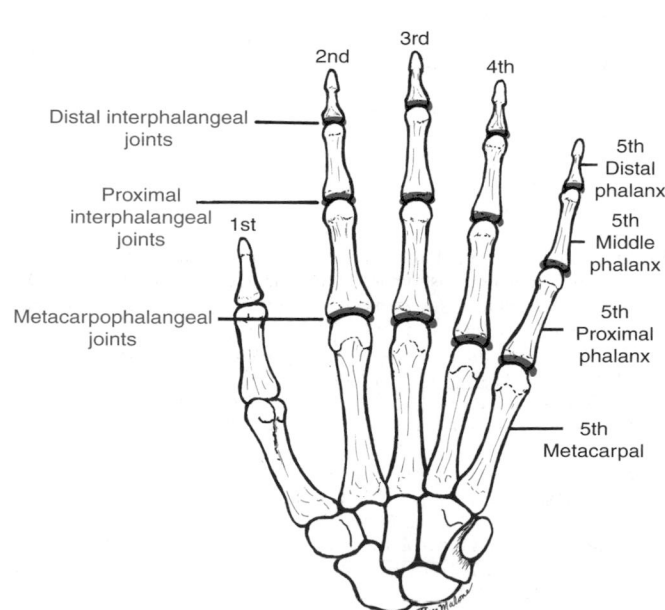

FIGURE 7.1 An anterior (palmar) view of the hand showing metacarpophalangeal, proximal interphalangeal, and distal interphalangeal joints.

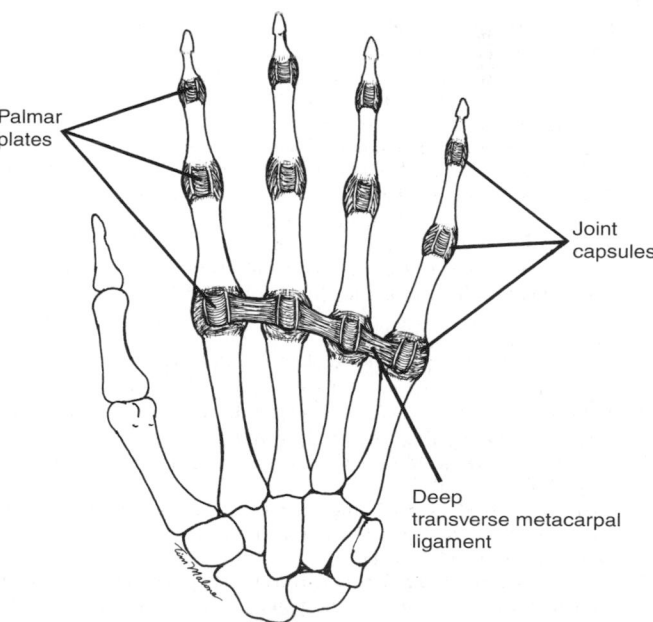

FIGURE 7.2 An anterior (palmar) view of the hand showing joint capsules and palmar plates of the metacarpophalangeal, proximal interphalangeal, and distal interphalangeal joints and the deep transverse metacarpal ligament.

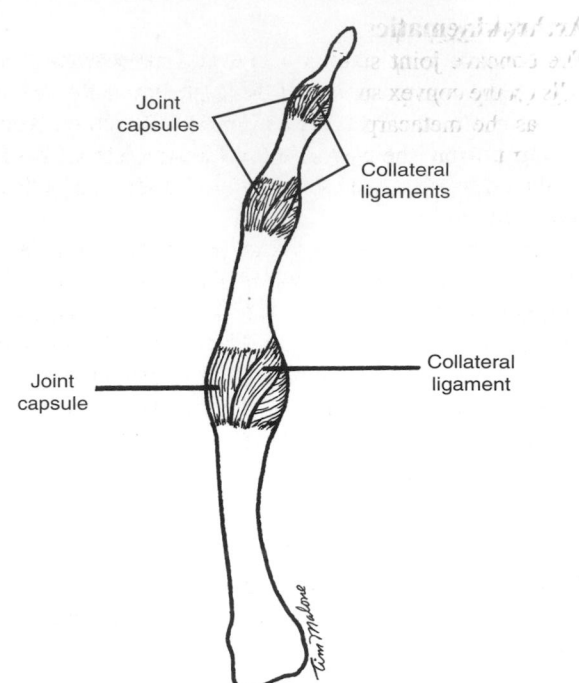

FIGURE 7.3 A lateral view of a finger showing joint capsules and collateral ligaments of the metacarpophalangeal, proximal interphalangeal, and distal interphalangeal joints.

abduction, the base of the phalanx slides and rolls in the same direction as the movement of the finger.

Capsular Pattern

Cyriax and Cyriax[6] report that the capsular pattern is an equal restriction of flexion and extension. Kaltenborn[7] notes that all motions are restricted with more limitation in flexion.

Fingers: Proximal Interphalangeal and Distal Interphalangeal Joints

Anatomy

The structure of both the proximal interphalangeal (PIP) and the distal interphalangeal (DIP) joints is very similar (see Fig. 7.1). Each phalanx has a concave base and a convex head. The joint surfaces comprise the head of the more proximal phalanx and the base of the adjacent, more distal phalanx. Each joint is supported by a joint capsule, a palmar plate, and two collateral ligaments (see Figs. 7.2 and 7.3).[1,2]

Osteokinematics

The PIP and DIP joints of the fingers are classified as synovial hinge joints with 1 degree of freedom: flexion–extension in the sagittal plane.

Arthrokinematics

Motion of the joint surfaces includes a sliding and rolling of the concave base of the more distal phalanx on the convex head of the proximal phalanx. Sliding and rolling of the base of the moving phalanx occurs in the same direction as the movement of the shaft.[5] For example, in PIP flexion the base of the middle phalanx slides and rolls toward the palm. In PIP

extension, the base of the middle phalanx slides and rolls toward the dorsum of the hand.

Capsular Pattern

The capsular pattern is an equal restriction of both flexion and extension, according to Cyriax and Cyriax.[6] Kaltenborn[7] notes that all motions are restricted with more limitation in flexion.

Thumb: Carpometacarpal Joint

Anatomy

The carpometacarpal (CMC) joint of the thumb is the articulation between the trapezium and the base of the first metacarpal (Fig. 7.4). The saddle-shaped trapezium is concave in the sagittal plane and convex in the frontal plane (Fig. 7.5).[1,5] The base of the first metacarpal has a reciprocal shape that conforms to that of the trapezium, so that the base of the metacarpal is convex in the sagittal plane and concave in the frontal plane. The joint capsule is thick but lax and is reinforced by radial, ulnar, palmar, and dorsal ligaments (Fig. 7.6).[1,2]

Osteokinematics

The first CMC joint is a saddle joint with 2 degrees of freedom: flexion–extension in the frontal plane parallel to the palm and abduction–adduction in the sagittal plane perpendicular to the palm.[1,5] These planes of movement for the CMC joint of the thumb are at right angles to the planes of movement of the fingers because the trapezium is anterior to the other carpals, effectively rotating the palmar surface of the thumb medially.[1,8] The laxity of the joint capsule also permits

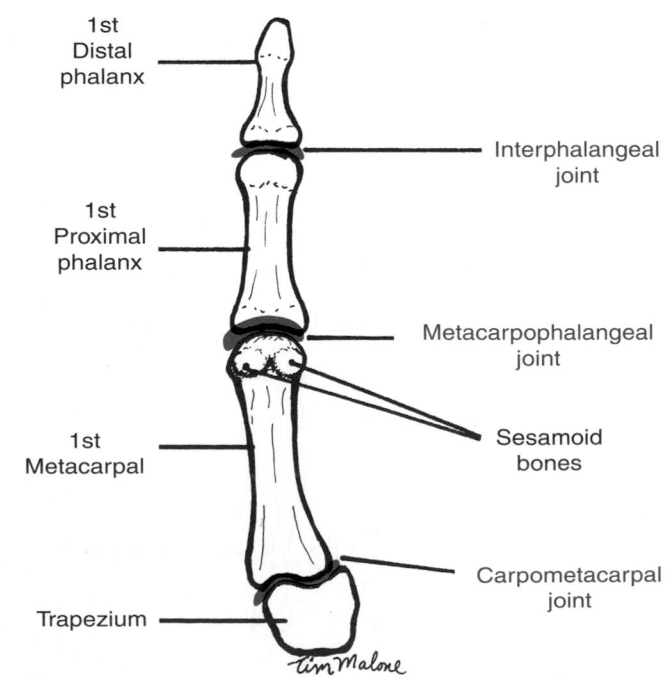

FIGURE 7.4 An anterior (palmar) view of the thumb showing carpometacarpal, metacarpophalangeal, and interphalangeal joints.

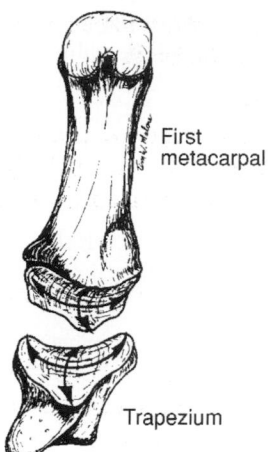

FIGURE 7.5 The saddle-shaped joint surface of the trapezium at the first carpometacarpal (CMC) joint is convex in the frontal plane (flexion–extension) and concave in the sagittal plane (abduction–adduction). The base of the metacarpal of the thumb has a shape that is reciprocal to that of the trapezium. Reproduced with permission from Levangie, PL, and Norkin, CC: Joint Structure and Function: A Comprehensive Analysis, ed 4. FA Davis, Philadelphia, 2005.

some axial rotation. This rotation allows the thumb to move into position for contact with the fingers during opposition. The sequence of motions that combines with rotation and results in opposition is as follows: abduction, flexion, medial axial rotation, and adduction.[1,5] Reposition returns the thumb to the starting position.

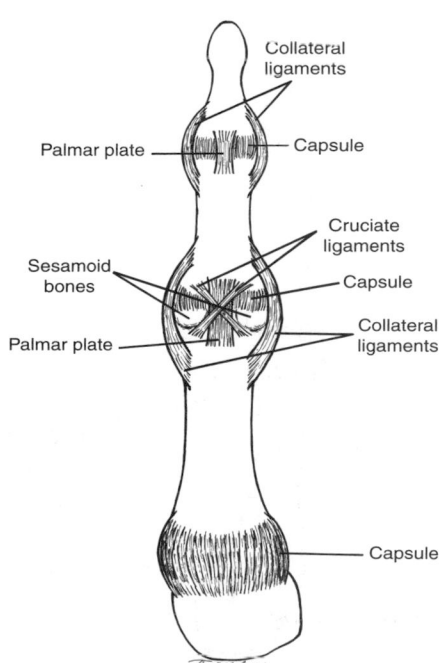

FIGURE 7.6 An anterior (palmar) view of the thumb showing joint capsules, collateral ligaments, palmar plates, and cruciate (intersesamoid) ligaments.

Arthrokinematics

The concave joint surface of the first metacarpal slides and rolls on the convex surface of the trapezium in the same direction as the metacarpal shaft to produce flexion–extension.[5,7] During flexion, the base of the metacarpal slides and rolls in an ulnar direction. During extension, it slides and rolls in a radial direction.

To produce abduction–adduction the convex joint surface of the first metacarpal slides on the concave portion of the trapezium in the opposite direction to the shaft of the metacarpal but rolls in the same direction as the shaft of the metacarpal.[5,7] Therefore, the base of the metacarpal slides toward the dorsal surface of the hand and rolls toward the palmar surface of the hand during abduction. The base of the first metacarpal slides toward the palmar surface of the hand and rolls toward the dorsal surface of the hand during adduction.

Capsular Pattern

The capsular pattern is a limitation of abduction according to Cyriax and Cyriax.[6] Kaltenborn[7] reports limitations in abduction and extension.

Thumb: Metacarpophalangeal Joint

Anatomy

The metacarpophalangeal (MCP) joint of the thumb is the articulation between the convex head of the first metacarpal and the concave base of the first proximal phalanx (see Fig. 7.4). The joint is reinforced by a joint capsule, palmar plate, two sesamoid bones on the palmar surface, two intersesamoid ligaments (cruciate ligaments), and two collateral ligaments (see Fig. 7.6).[1]

Osteokinematics

The MCP joint is a condyloid joint with 2 degrees of freedom.[1,8] The motions permitted are flexion–extension and a minimal amount of abduction–adduction. Motions at this joint are more restricted than at the MCP joints of the fingers.

Arthrokinematics

At the MCP joint the concave base of the proximal phalanx slides and rolls on the convex head of the first metacarpal in the same direction as the shaft of the phalanx.[5,7] The base of the proximal phalanx moves toward the palmar surface of the thumb in flexion and toward the dorsal surface of the thumb in extension.

Capsular Pattern

The capsular pattern for the MCP joint is a restriction of motion in all directions, but flexion is more limited than extension.[6,7]

Thumb: Interphalangeal Joint

Anatomy

The interphalangeal (IP) joint of the thumb is identical in structure to the IP joints of the fingers. The head of the proximal phalanx is convex, and the base of the distal phalanx is concave (see Fig. 7.4). The joint is supported by a joint capsule, a palmar plate, and two lateral collateral ligaments (see Fig. 7.6).

Osteokinematics

The IP joint is a synovial hinge joint with 1 degree of freedom: flexion–extension.

Arthrokinematics

At the IP joint the concave base of the distal phalanx slides and rolls on the convex head of the proximal phalanx, in the same direction as the shaft of the phalanx.[5,7] The base of the distal phalanx moves toward the palmar surface of the thumb in flexion and toward the dorsal surface of the thumb in extension.

Capsular Pattern

The capsular pattern is an equal restriction in both flexion and extension according to Cyriax.[6] Kaltenborn[7] notes that all motions are restricted with more limitation in flexion.

RANGE OF MOTION TESTING PROCEDURES:
Fingers

Included in this section are common clinical techniques for measuring joint motions of the fingers and thumb. These techniques, which often place the goniometer on the dorsal surface of the digits, are appropriate for evaluating motions in the majority of people. Groth and Ehretsman found that dorsal placement of the goniometer was preferred by 73 percent of 231 surveyed therapists.[9] However, swelling and bony deformities sometimes require that the examiner either measure the MCP and IP joints from the lateral aspect or create alternative evaluation techniques. Photocopies, photographs, and tracings of the hand at the beginning and end of the range of motion (ROM) may be helpful.

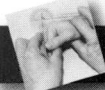 ## Landmarks for Testing Procedures

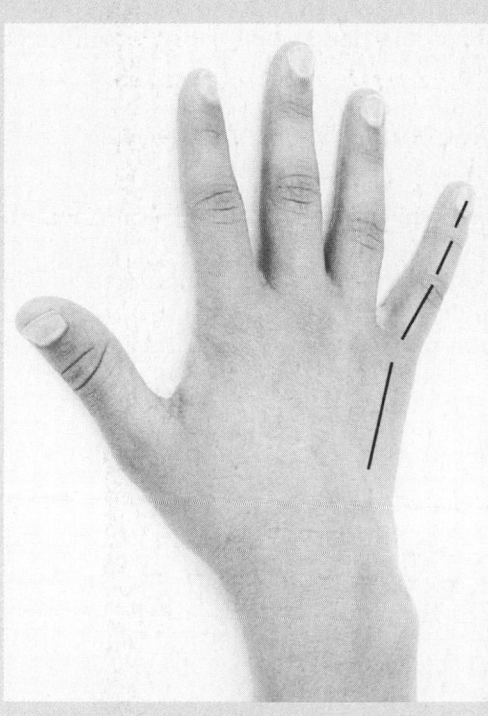

FIGURE 7.7 Posterior view of the right hand showing surface anatomy landmarks for goniometer alignment during measurement of finger range of motion.

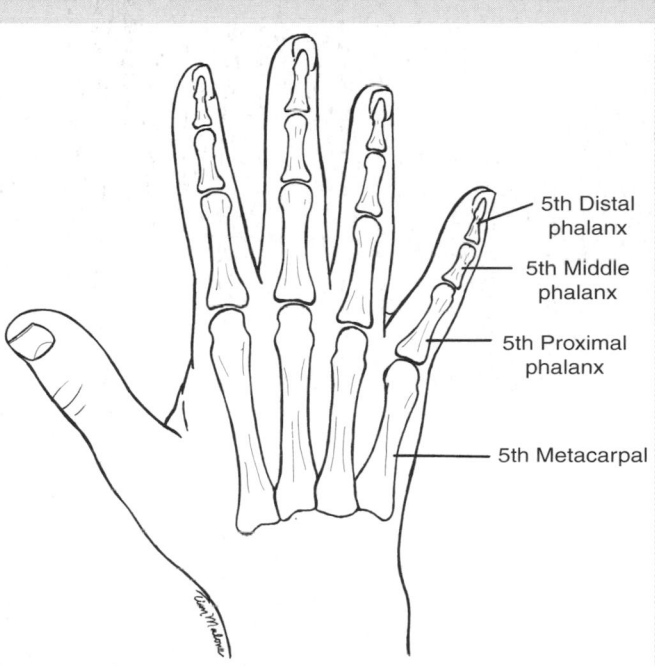

5th Distal phalanx

5th Middle phalanx

5th Proximal phalanx

5th Metacarpal

FIGURE 7.8 Posterior view of the right hand showing bony anatomical landmarks for goniometer alignment during the measurement of finger range of motion. The index, middle, ring, and little fingers each have a metacarpal and a proximal, middle, and distal phalanx.

FINGERS: METACARPOPHALANGEAL FLEXION

Motion occurs in the sagittal plane around a medial–lateral axis. Normal ROM values for adults are 90 degrees according to the American Association of Orthopaedic Surgeons (AAOS)[10] and the American Medical Association (AMA)[11] and 100 degrees according to Hume and coworkers.[12] MCP flexion appears to increase slightly in an ulnar direction from the index finger to the little finger. See Research Findings and Tables 7.1 and 7.2 for additional normal ROM values.

Testing Position

Place the subject sitting, with the forearm and hand resting on a supporting surface. Place the forearm midway between pronation and supination, the wrist in 0 degrees of flexion, extension, and radial and ulnar deviation and the MCP joint in a neutral position relative to abduction and adduction. Avoid extreme flexion of the PIP and DIP joints of the finger being examined.

Stabilization

Stabilize the metacarpal to prevent wrist motion. Do not hold the MCP joints of the other fingers in extension because tension in the transverse metacarpal ligament will restrict the motion.

Testing Motion

Flex the MCP joint by pushing on the dorsal surface of the proximal phalanx, moving the finger toward the palm (Fig. 7.9). Maintain the MCP joint in a neutral position relative to abduction and adduction. The end of flexion ROM occurs when resistance to further motion is felt and attempts to overcome the resistance cause the wrist to flex.

Normal End-Feel

The end-feel may be hard because of contact between the palmar aspect of the proximal phalanx and the metacarpal, or it may be firm because of tension in the dorsal joint capsule and the collateral ligaments.

Goniometer Alignment

See Figures 7.10 and 7.11.

1. Center **fulcrum** of the goniometer over the dorsal aspect of the MCP joint.
2. Align **proximal arm** over the dorsal midline of the metacarpal.
3. Align **distal arm** over the dorsal midline of the proximal phalanx.

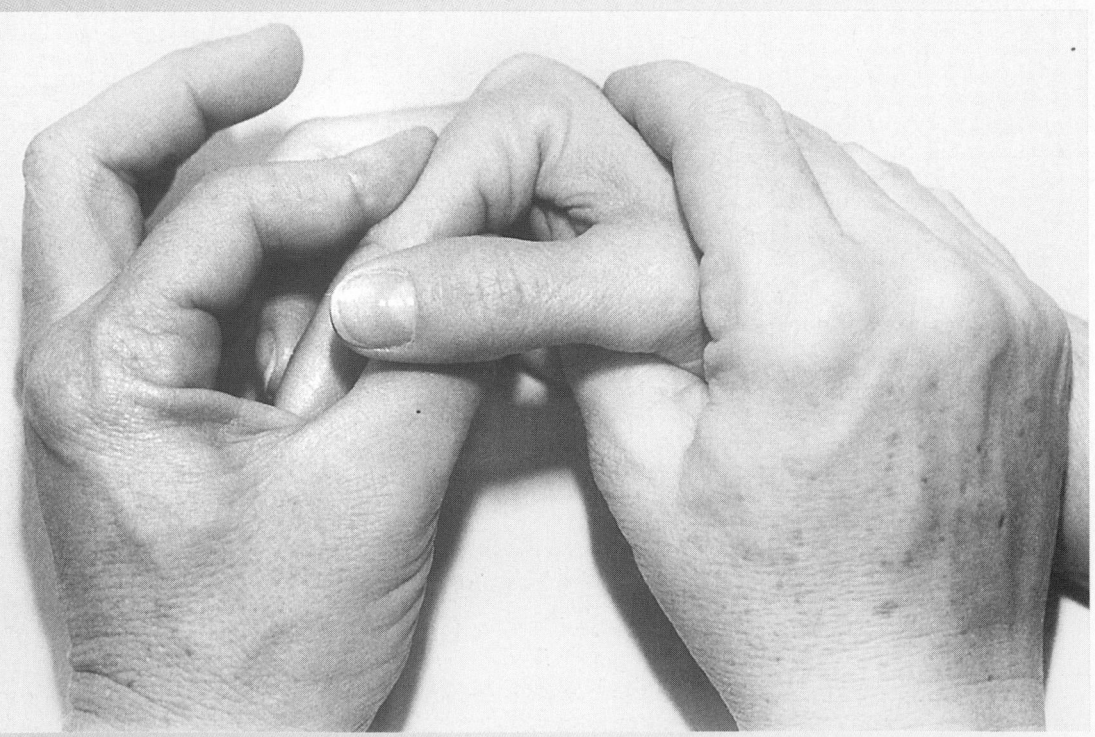

FIGURE 7.9 During flexion of the metacarpophalangeal (MCP) joint, the examiner uses one hand to stabilize the subject's metacarpal and to maintain the wrist in a neutral position. The index finger and the thumb of the examiner's other hand grasp the subject's proximal phalanx to move it into flexion.

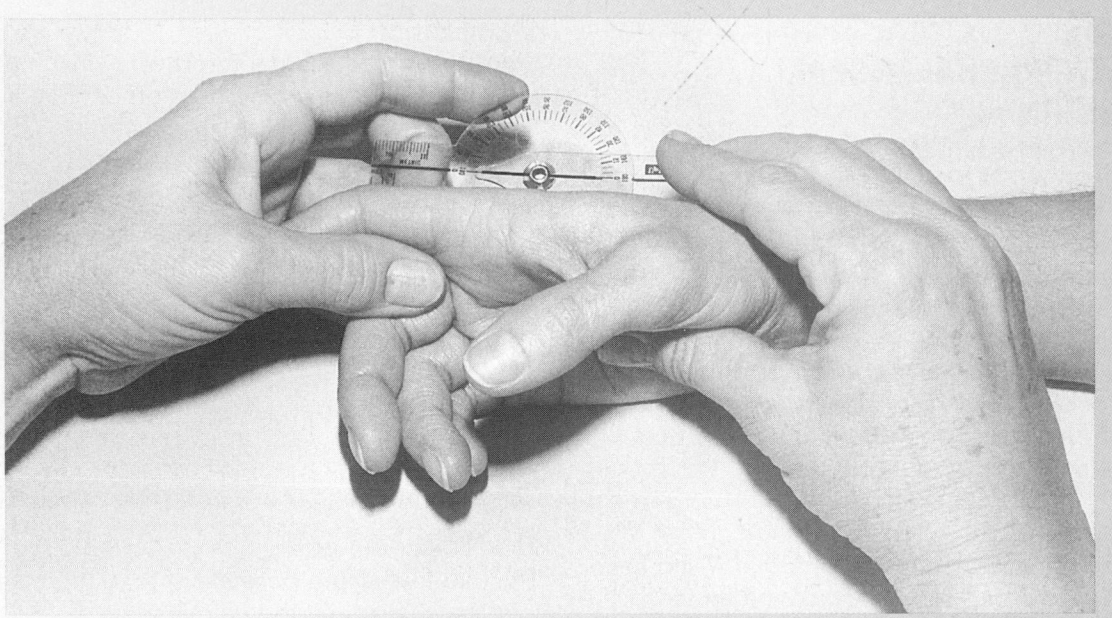

FIGURE 7.10 The alignment of the goniometer at the beginning of metacarpophalangeal (MCP) flexion range of motion. In this photograph, the examiner is using a 6-inch plastic goniometer in which the arms have been trimmed to approximately 2 inches to make it easier to align over the small joints of the hand. Most examiners use goniometers with arms that are 6 inches or shorter when measuring ROM in the hand.

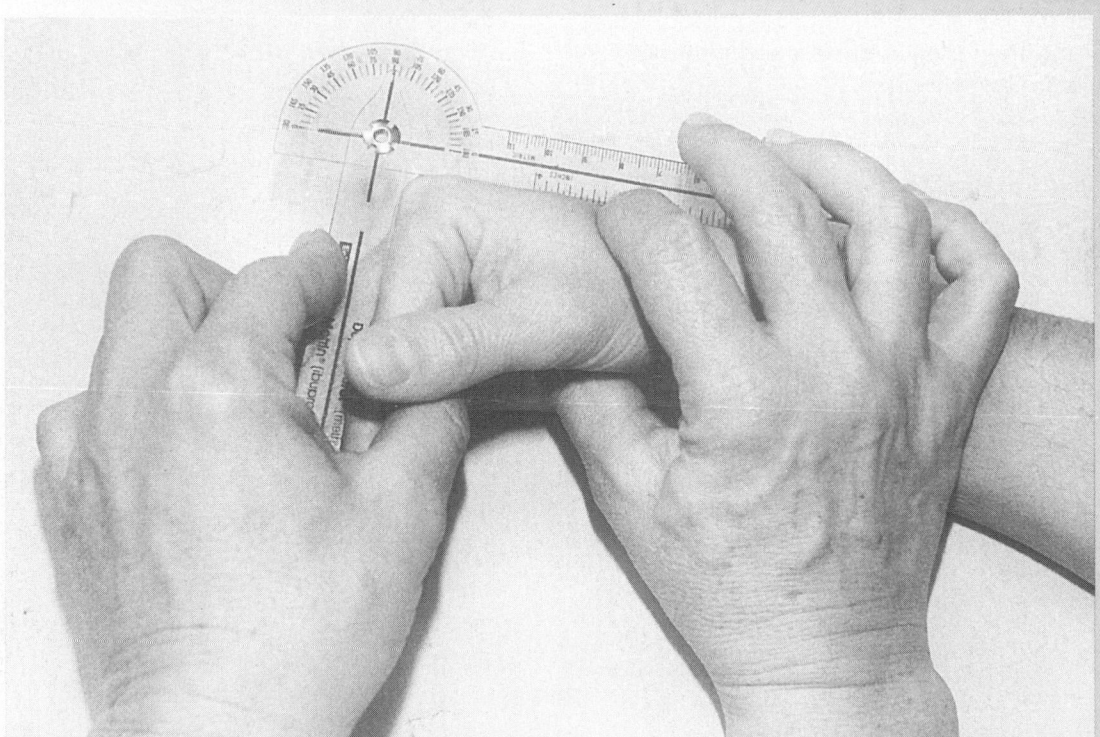

FIGURE 7.11 At the end of metacarpophalangeal (MCP) flexion range of motion, the examiner uses one hand to hold the proximal goniometer arm in alignment and to stabilize the subject's metacarpal. The examiner's other hand maintains the proximal phalanx in MCP flexion and aligns the distal goniometer arm. Note that the goniometer arms make direct contact with the dorsal surfaces of the metacarpal and proximal phalanx, causing the fulcrum of the goniometer to lie somewhat distal and dorsal to the MCP joint.

● FINGERS: METACARPOPHALANGEAL EXTENSION

Motion occurs in the sagittal plane around a medial-lateral axis. Normal ROM values for adults are 20 degrees according to the AMA[11] and 45 degrees according to the AAOS.[10] Passive MCP extension ROM is greater than active extension. Mallon, Brown, and Nunley[13] report that extension ROM at the MCP joints is equal across all fingers, whereas Skvarilova and Plevkova[14] and Smahel and Klimova[15] note that the little finger has the greatest amount of MCP extension. See Research Findings and Tables 7.1 and 7.2 for additional normal ROM values.

Testing Position
Position the subject sitting, with the forearm and hand resting on a supporting surface. Place the forearm midway between pronation and supination; the wrist in 0 degrees of flexion, extension, and radial and ulnar deviation; and the MCP joint in a neutral position relative to abduction and adduction. Avoid extension or extreme flexion of the PIP and DIP joints of the finger being tested. (If the PIP and DIP joints are positioned in extension, tension in the flexor digitorum superficialis and profundus muscles may restrict the motion. If the PIP and DIP joints are positioned in full flexion, tension in the lumbricalis and interossei muscles will restrict the motion.)

Stabilization
Stabilize the metacarpal to prevent wrist motion. Do not hold the MCP joints of the other fingers in full flexion because tension in the transverse metacarpal ligament will restrict the motion.

Testing Motion
Extend the MCP joint by pushing on the palmar surface of the proximal phalanx, moving the finger away from the palm (Fig. 7.12). Maintain the MCP joint in a neutral position relative to abduction and adduction. The end of extension ROM occurs when resistance to further motion is felt and attempts to overcome resistance cause the wrist to extend.

Normal End-Feel
The end-feel is firm because of tension in the palmar joint capsule and in the palmar plate.

Goniometer Alignment
See Figures 7.13 and 7.14 for alignment of the goniometer over the dorsal aspect of the fingers.

1. Center **fulcrum** of the goniometer over the dorsal aspect of the MCP joint.
2. Align **proximal arm** over the dorsal midline of the metacarpal.
3. Align **distal arm** over the dorsal midline of the proximal phalanx.

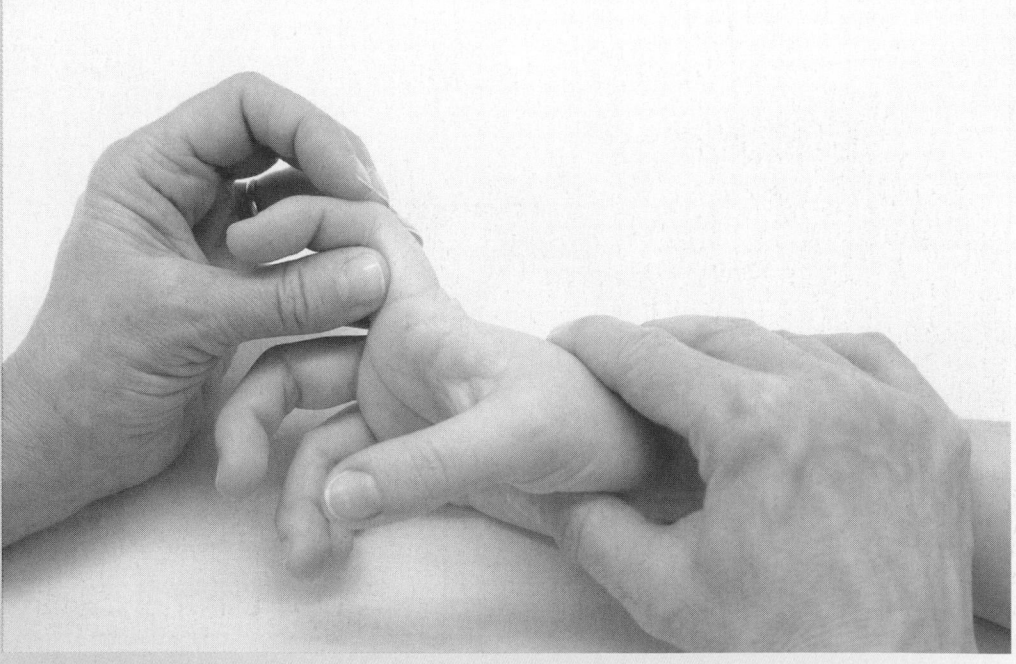

FIGURE 7.12 During metacarpophalangeal (MCP) extension, the examiner uses her index finger and thumb to grasp the subject's proximal phalanx and to move the phalanx dorsally. The examiner's other hand maintains the subject's wrist in the neutral position, stabilizing the metacarpal.

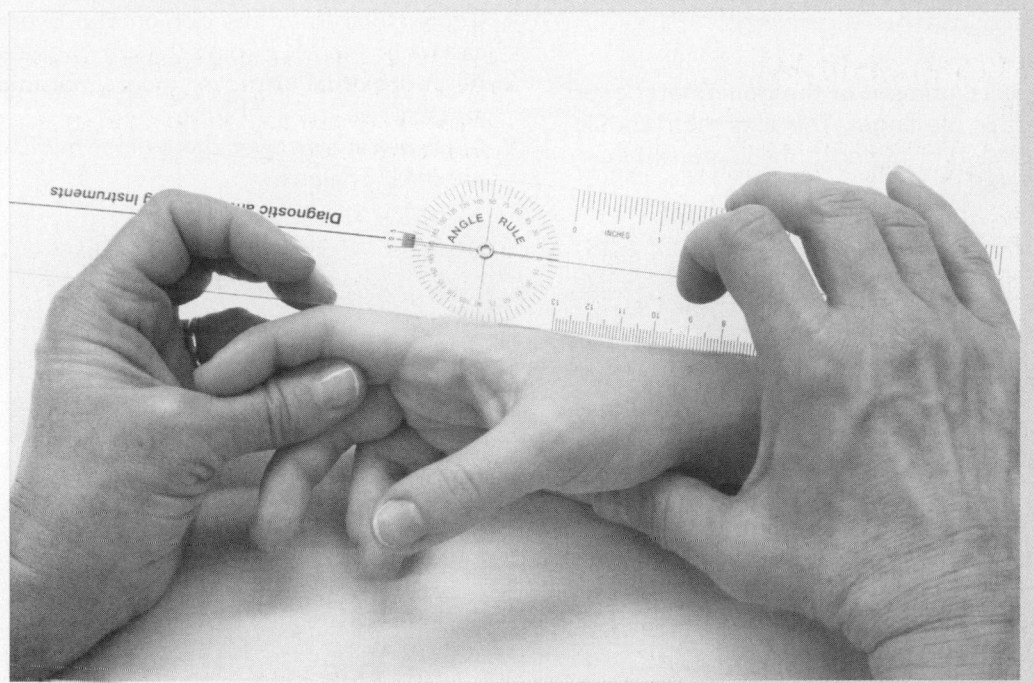

FIGURE 7.13 A full-circle, 6-inch plastic goniometer is being used to measure the beginning range of motion for metacarpophalangeal (MCP) extension. The proximal arm of the goniometer is slightly longer than necessary for optimal alignment. If a goniometer of the right size is not available, the examiner can cut the arms of a plastic model to a suitable length.

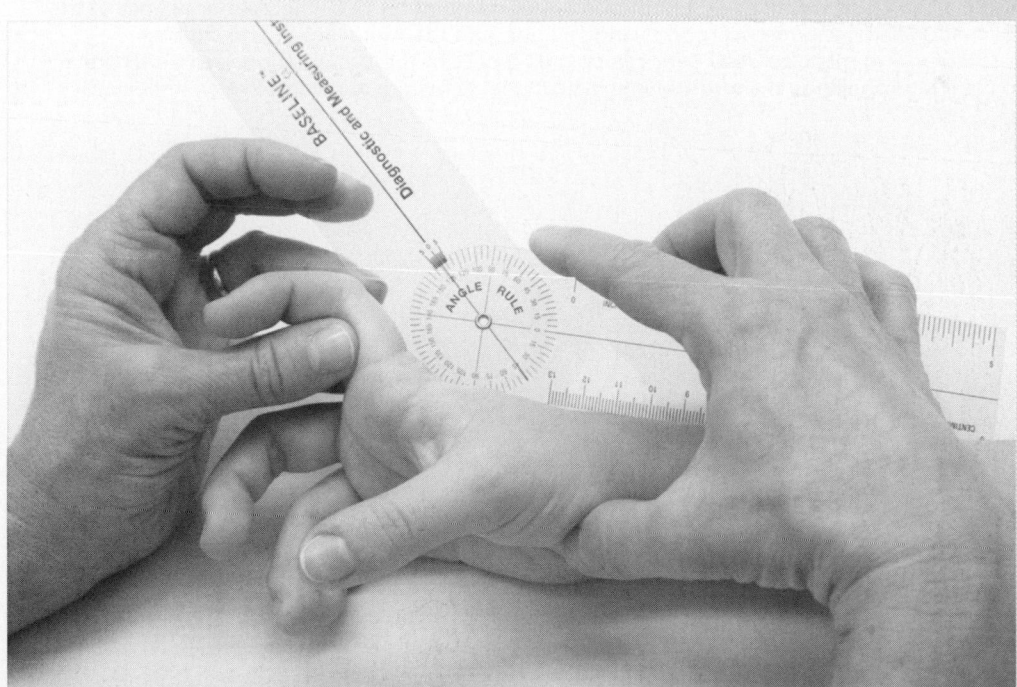

FIGURE 7.14 The alignment of the goniometer at the end of metacarpophalangeal (MCP) extension. The body of the goniometer is aligned over the dorsal aspect of the MCP joint, whereas the goniometer arms are aligned over the dorsal aspect of the metacarpal and proximal phalanx.

Alternative Goniometer Alignment: Palmar Aspect

See Figure 7.15 for alignment of the goniometer over the palmar aspect of the finger. This alignment should not be used if swelling or hypertrophy is present in the palm of the hand.

1. Center **fulcrum** of the goniometer over the palmar aspect of the MCP joint.
2. Align **proximal arm** over the palmar midline of the metacarpal.
3. Align **distal arm** over the palmar midline of the proximal phalanx.

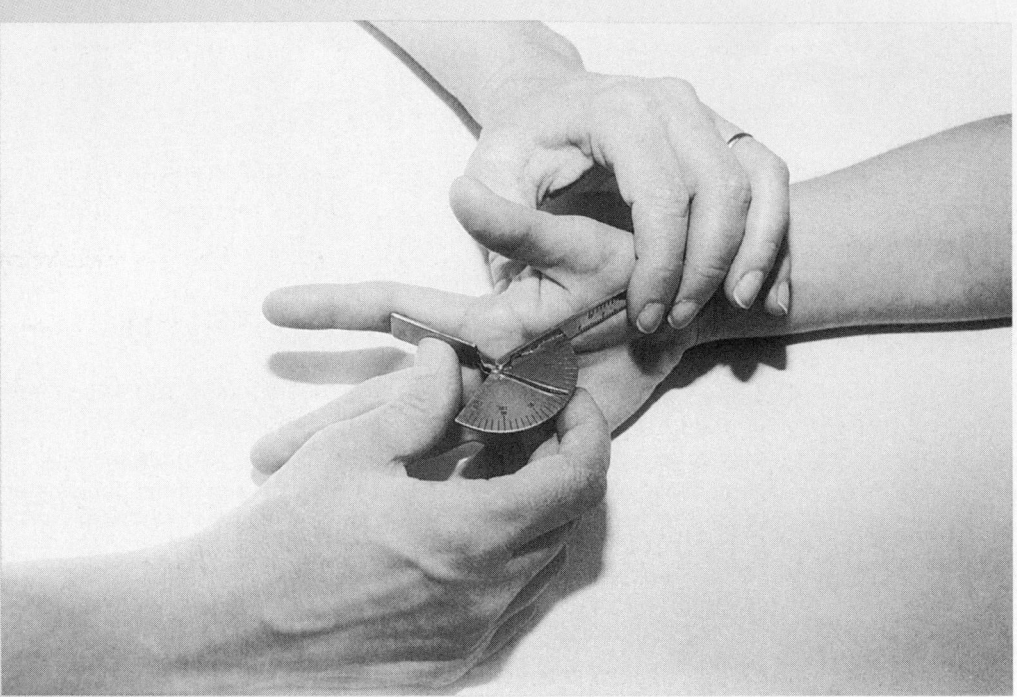

FIGURE 7.15 An alternative alignment of a finger goniometer over the palmar aspect of the proximal phalanx, the metacarpophalangeal joint, and the metacarpal. The shorter goniometer arm must be used over the palmar aspect of the proximal phalanx so that the proximal interphalangeal and distal interphalangeal joints are allowed to relax in flexion.

● FINGERS: METACARPOPHALANGEAL ABDUCTION

Motion occurs in the frontal plane around an anterior–posterior axis. No sources were found for normal abduction ROM values measured with a universal goniometer at the MCP joint. Some values have been reported for the maximal angles between adjacent fingers using tracings[15], and between fingers and the midline of the hand using a gravity-based goniometer.[16]

Testing Position
Position the subject sitting, with the forearm and hand resting on a supporting surface. Place the wrist in 0 degrees of flexion, extension, and radial and ulnar deviation; the forearm in full pronation so that the palm of the hand faces the ground; and the MCP joint in 0 degrees of flexion and extension.

Stabilization
Stabilize the metacarpal to prevent wrist motions.

Testing Motion
Abduct the MCP joint by pushing on the medial surface of the proximal phalanx, moving the finger away from the midline of the hand (Fig. 7.16). Maintain the MCP joint in a neutral position relative to flexion and extension. The end of abduction ROM occurs when resistance to further motion is felt and attempts to overcome the resistance cause the wrist to move into radial or ulnar deviation.

Normal End-Feel
The end-feel is firm because of tension in the collateral ligaments of the MCP joints, the fascia of the web space between the fingers, and the palmar interossei muscles.

Goniometer Alignment
See Figures 7.17 and 7.18.

1. Center **fulcrum** of the goniometer over the dorsal aspect of the MCP joint.
2. Align **proximal arm** over the dorsal midline of the metacarpal.
3. Align **distal arm** over the dorsal midline of the proximal phalanx.

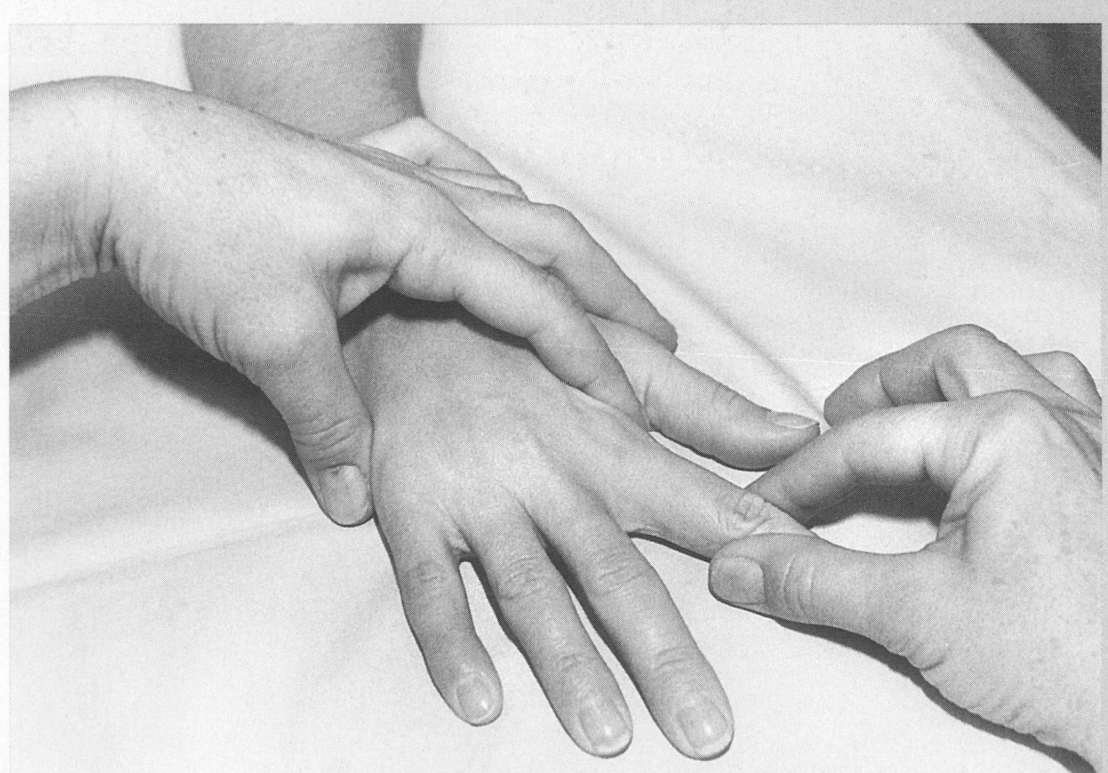

FIGURE 7.16 During metacarpophalangeal (MCP) abduction, the examiner uses the index finger of one hand to press against the subject's metacarpal and prevent radial deviation at the wrist. With the other index finger and thumb holding the distal end of the proximal phalanx, the examiner moves the subject's second MCP joint into abduction.

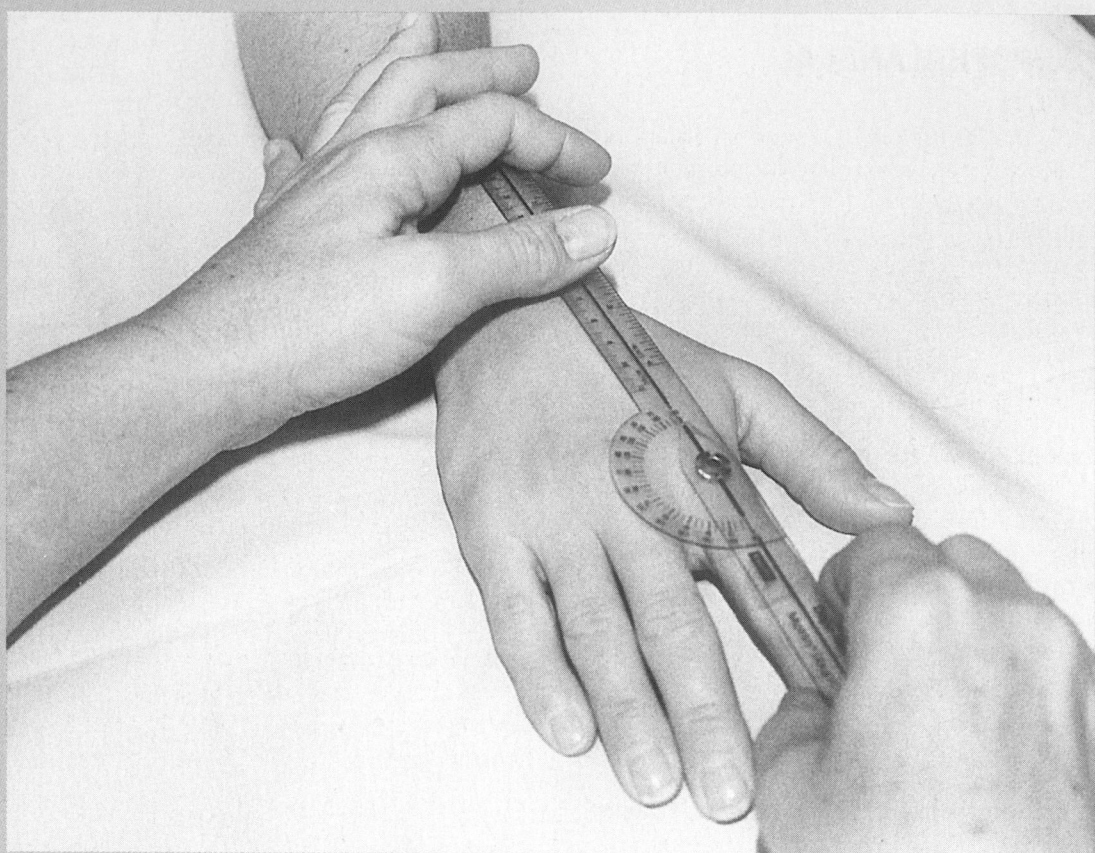

FIGURE 7.17 The alignment of the goniometer at the beginning of metacarpophalangeal abduction range of motion.

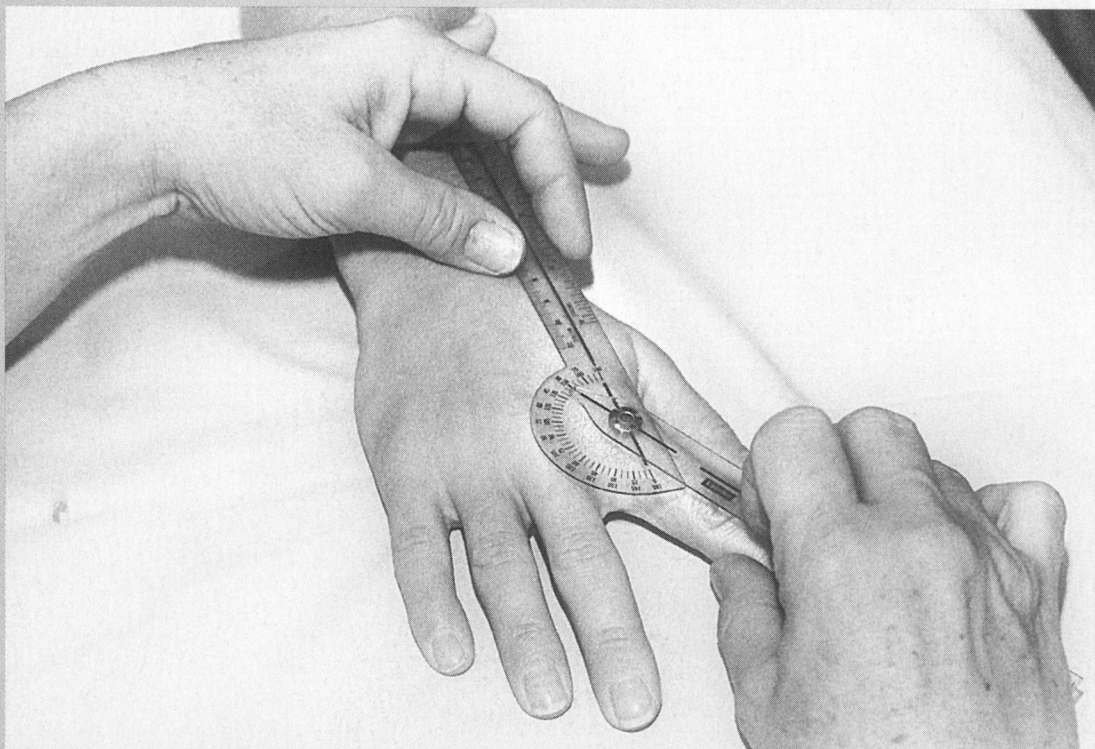

FIGURE 7.18 At the end of metacarpophalangeal (MCP) abduction, the examiner aligns the arms of the goniometer with the dorsal midline of the metacarpal and proximal phalanx rather than with the contour of the hand and finger.

⬤ FINGERS: METACARPOPHALANGEAL ADDUCTION

Motion occurs in the frontal plane around an anterior–posterior axis. MCP adduction is not usually measured and recorded because it is the return from full abduction to the 0 starting position. There is very little adduction ROM beyond the 0 starting position. No sources were found for normal MCP adduction ROM values.

⬤ FINGERS: PROXIMAL INTERPHALANGEAL FLEXION

Motion occurs in the sagittal plane around a medial–lateral axis. Normal ROM values for adults are 100 degrees according to the AAOS[10] and the AMA[11] and 105 degrees according to Hume and coworkers[12] and Mallon, Brown, and Nunley.[13] PIP flexion ROM is equal for all the fingers.[13] See Research Findings and Tables 7.1 and 7.2 for additional normal ROM values.

Testing Position

Place the subject sitting, with the forearm and hand resting on a supporting surface. Position the forearm in 0 degrees of supination and pronation; the wrist in 0 degrees of flexion, extension, and radial and ulnar deviation; and the MCP joint in 0 degrees of flexion, extension, abduction, and adduction. (If the wrist and MCP joints are positioned in full flexion, tension in the extensor digitorum communis, extensor indicis, or extensor digiti minimi muscles will restrict the motion. If the MCP joint is positioned in full extension, tension

in the lumbricalis and interossei muscles will restrict the motion.)

Stabilization

Stabilize the proximal phalanx to prevent motion of the MCP joint.

Testing Motion

Flex the PIP joint by pushing on the dorsal surface of the middle phalanx, moving the finger toward the palm (Fig. 7.19). The end of flexion ROM occurs when resistance to further motion is felt and attempts to overcome the resistance cause the MCP joint to flex.

Normal End-Feel

Usually, the end-feel is hard because of contact between the palmar aspect of the middle phalanx and the proximal phalanx. In some individuals, the end-feel may be soft because of compression of soft tissue between the palmar aspect of the middle and proximal phalanges. In other individuals, the end-feel may be firm because of tension in the dorsal joint capsule and the collateral ligaments.

Goniometer Alignment

See Figures 7.20 and 7.21.

1. Center **fulcrum** of the goniometer over the dorsal aspect of the PIP joint.
2. Align **proximal arm** over the dorsal midline of the proximal phalanx.
3. Align **distal arm** over the dorsal midline of the middle phalanx.

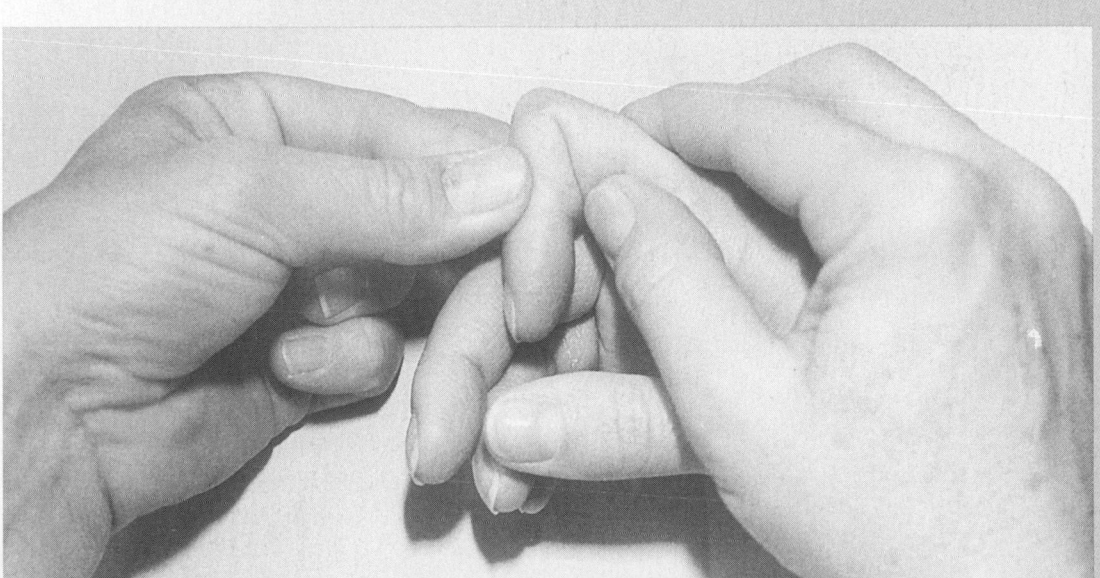

FIGURE 7.19 During proximal interphalangeal (PIP) flexion, the examiner stabilizes the subject's proximal phalanx with her thumb and index finger. The examiner uses her other thumb and index finger to move the subject's PIP joint into full flexion.

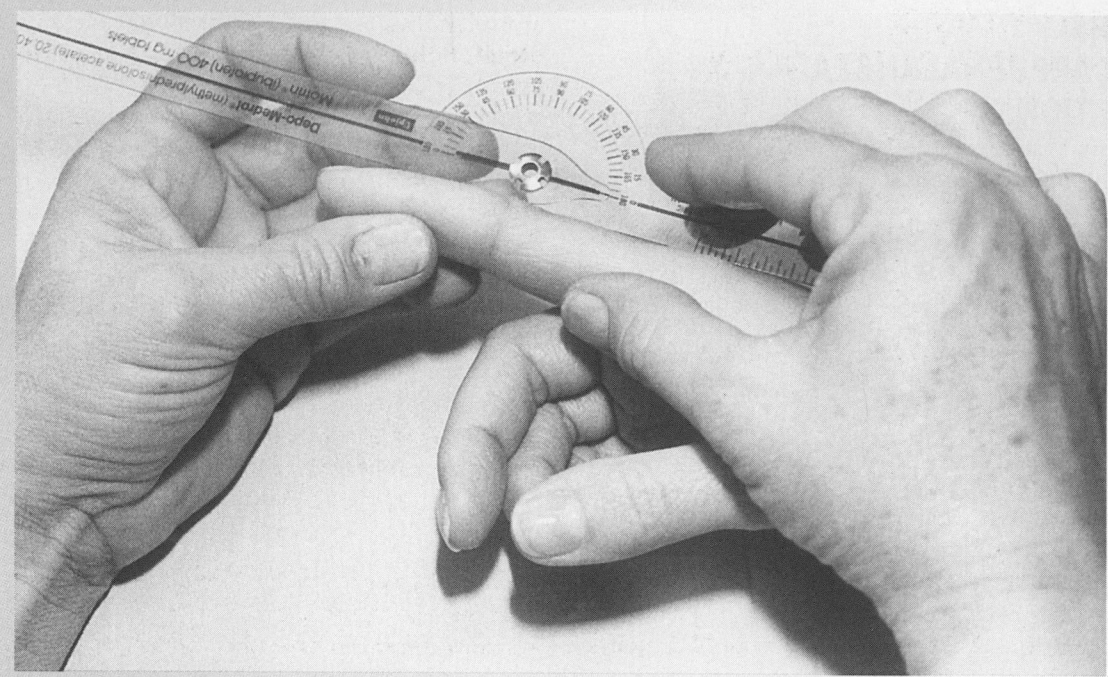

FIGURE 7.20 The alignment of the goniometer at the beginning of proximal interphalangeal (PIP) flexion range of motion.

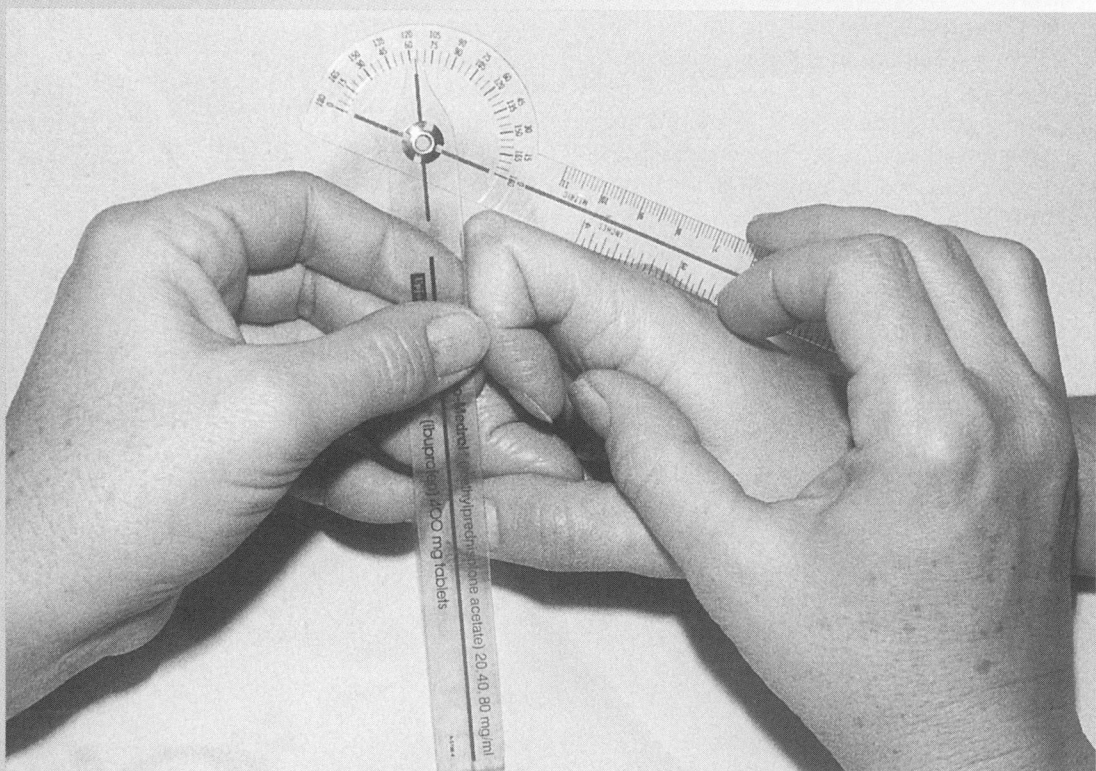

FIGURE 7.21 At the end of proximal interphalangeal (PIP) flexion, the examiner continues to stabilize and align the proximal goniometer arm over the dorsal midline of the proximal phalange with one hand. The examiner's other hand maintains the PIP joint in flexion and aligns the distal goniometer arm with the dorsal midline of the middle phalanx.

● FINGERS: PROXIMAL INTERPHALANGEAL EXTENSION

Motion occurs in the sagittal plane around a medial–lateral axis. PIP extension is usually recorded as the starting position for PIP flexion ROM. Normal ROM values for adults are 0 degrees according to the AAOS[10] and the AMA.[11] Mallon, Brown, and Nunley[13] report a mean of 7 degrees of active PIP extension and 16 degrees of passive PIP extension. PIP extension is generally equal for all fingers.[13] See Research Findings and Tables 7.1 and 7.2 for additional normal ROM values.

Testing Position

Place the subject sitting, with the forearm and hand resting on a supporting surface. Position the forearm in 0 degrees of supination and pronation; the wrist in 0 degrees of flexion, extension, and radial and ulnar deviation; and the MCP joint in 0 degrees of flexion, extension, abduction, and adduction. (If the MCP joint and wrist are extended, tension in the flexor digitorum superficialis and profundus muscles will restrict the motion.)

Stabilization

Stabilize the proximal phalanx to prevent motion of the MCP joint.

Testing Motion

Extend the PIP joint by pushing on the palmar surface of the middle phalanx, moving the finger away from the palm. The end of extension ROM occurs when resistance to further motion is felt and attempts to overcome the resistance cause the MCP joint to extend.

Normal End-Feel

The end-feel is firm because of tension in the palmar joint capsule and palmar plate (palmar ligament).

Goniometer Alignment

1. Center **fulcrum** of the goniometer over the dorsal aspect of the PIP joint.
2. Align **proximal arm** over the dorsal midline of the proximal phalanx.
3. Align **distal arm** over the dorsal midline of the middle phalanx.

● FINGERS: DISTAL INTERPHALANGEAL FLEXION

Motion occurs in the sagittal plane around a medial–lateral axis. Normal ROM values for adults range from 70 degrees according to the AMA[11] to 90 degrees according to the AAOS.[10] Hume and coworkers[12] and Skvarilova and Plevkova[14] report a mean of 85 degrees of active DIP flexion. DIP flexion ROM is generally equal for all fingers.[13] See Research Findings and Tables 7.1 and 7.2 for additional normal ROM values.

Testing Position

Position the subject sitting, with the forearm and hand resting on a supporting surface. Place the forearm in 0 degrees of supination and pronation; the wrist in 0 degrees of flexion, extension, and radial and ulnar deviation; and the MCP joint in 0 degrees of flexion, extension, abduction, and adduction. Place the PIP joint in approximately 70 to 90 degrees of flexion. (If the wrist and the MCP and PIP joints are fully flexed, tension in the extensor digitorum communis, extensor indicis, or extensor digiti minimi muscles may restrict DIP flexion. If the PIP joint is extended, tension in the oblique retinacular ligament may restrict DIP flexion.)

Stabilization

Stabilize the middle and proximal phalanx to prevent further flexion of the PIP joint.

Testing Motion

Flex the DIP joint by pushing on the dorsal surface of the distal phalanx, moving the finger toward the palm (Fig. 7.22). The end of flexion ROM occurs when resistance to further motion is felt and attempts to overcome the resistance cause the PIP joint to flex.

Normal End-Feel

The end-feel is firm because of tension in the dorsal joint capsule, collateral ligaments, and oblique retinacular ligament.

Goniometer Alignment

See Figures 7.23 to 7.25.

1. Center **fulcrum** of the goniometer over the dorsal aspect of the DIP joint.
2. Align **proximal arm** over the dorsal midline of the middle phalanx.
3. Align **distal arm** over the dorsal midline of the distal phalanx.

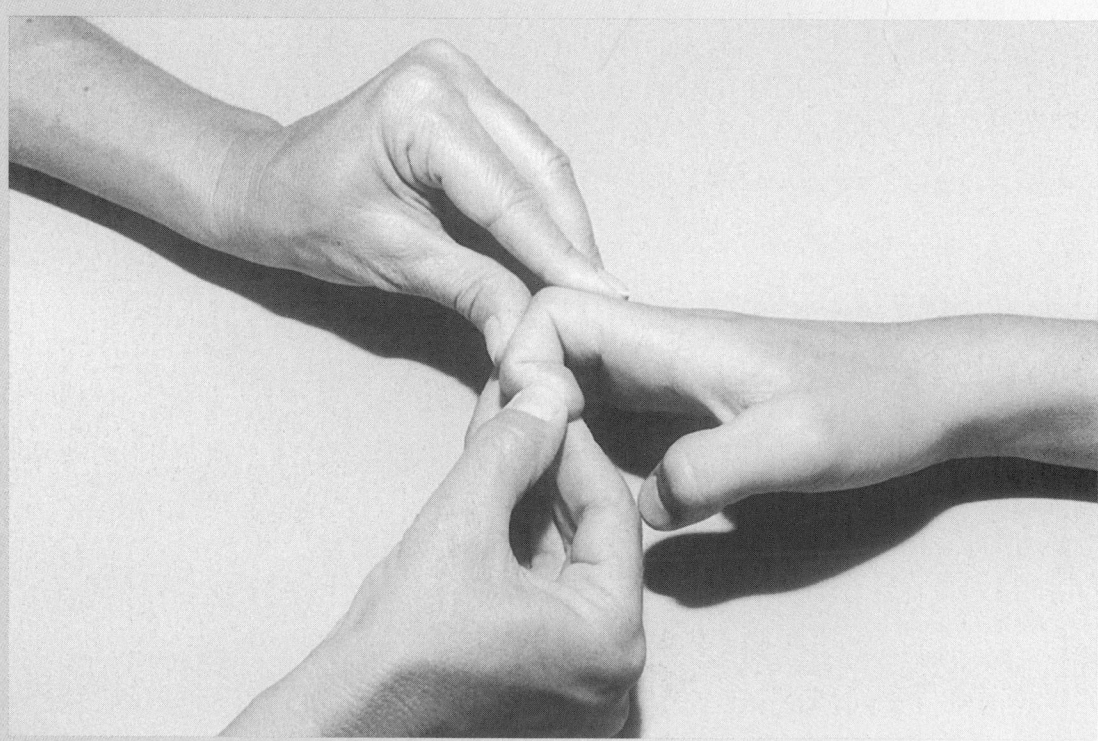

FIGURE 7.22 During distal interphalangeal (DIP) flexion, the examiner uses one hand to stabilize the middle phalanx and keep the proximal interphalangeal joint in 70 to 90 degrees of flexion. The examiner's other hand pushes on the distal phalanx to flex the DIP joint.

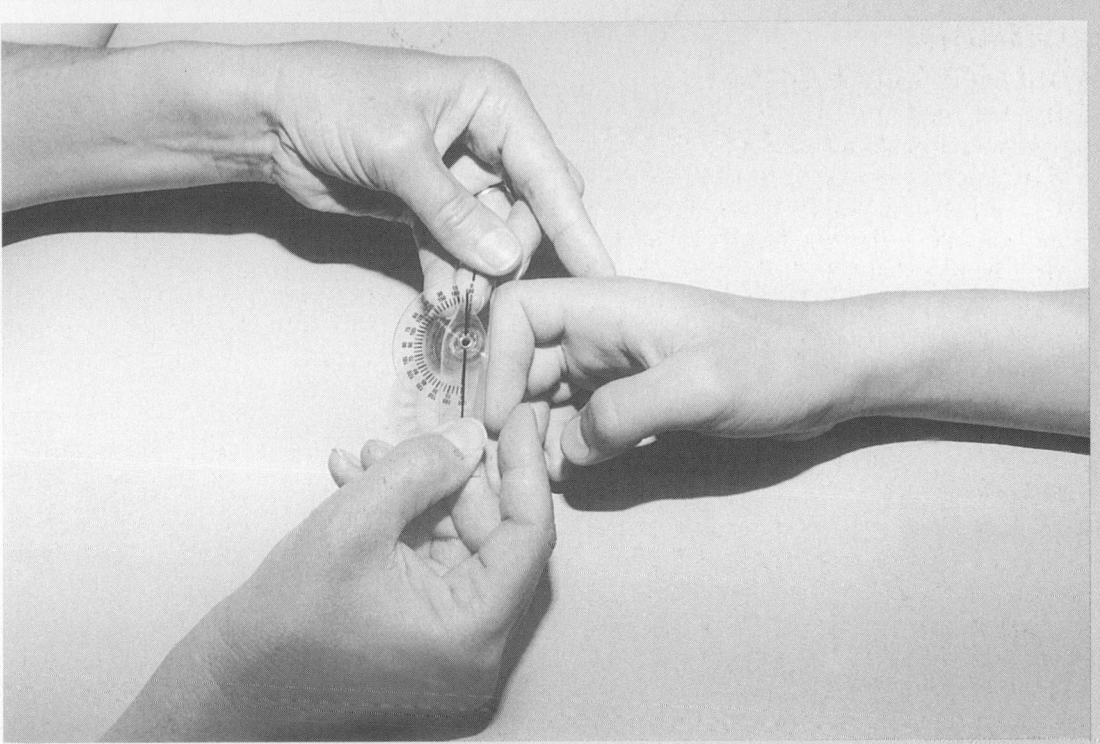

FIGURE 7.23 Measurement of the beginning of distal interphalangeal (DIP) flexion range of motion is being conducted by means of a half-circle plastic goniometer with 6-inch arms that have been trimmed to accommodate the small size of the DIP joint.

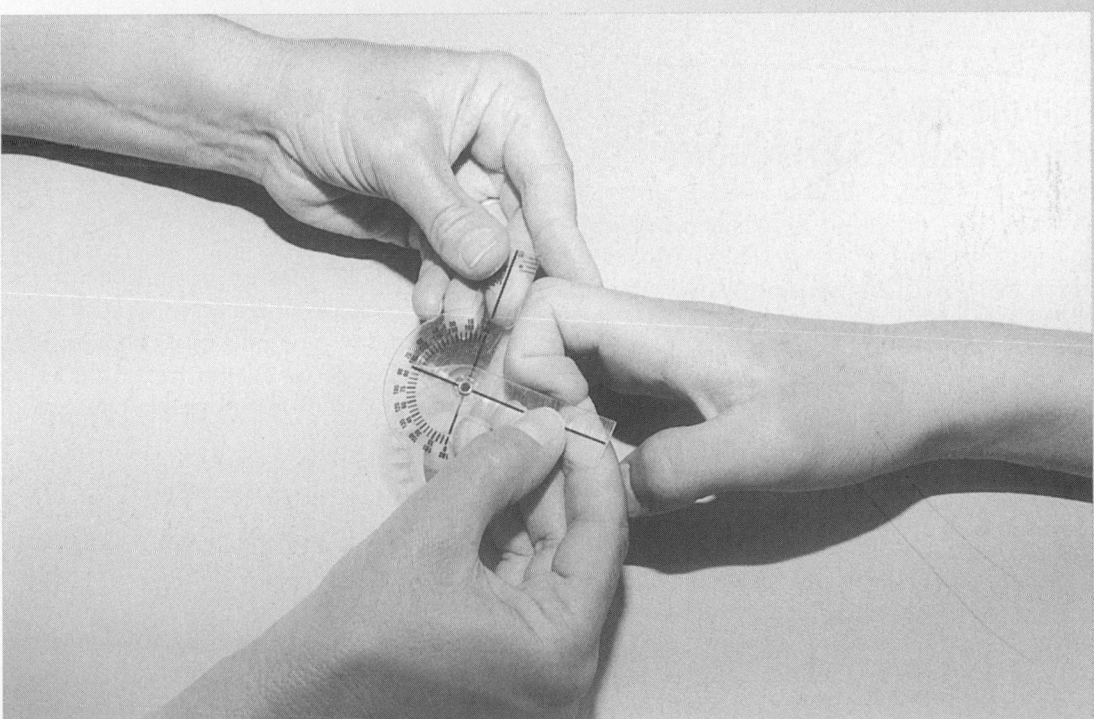

FIGURE 7.24 The alignment of the goniometer at the end of distal interphalangeal (DIP) flexion range of motion. Note that the fulcrum of the goniometer lies distal and dorsal to the proximal interphalangeal joint axis so that the arms of the goniometer stay in direct contact with the dorsal surfaces of the middle and distal phalanges.

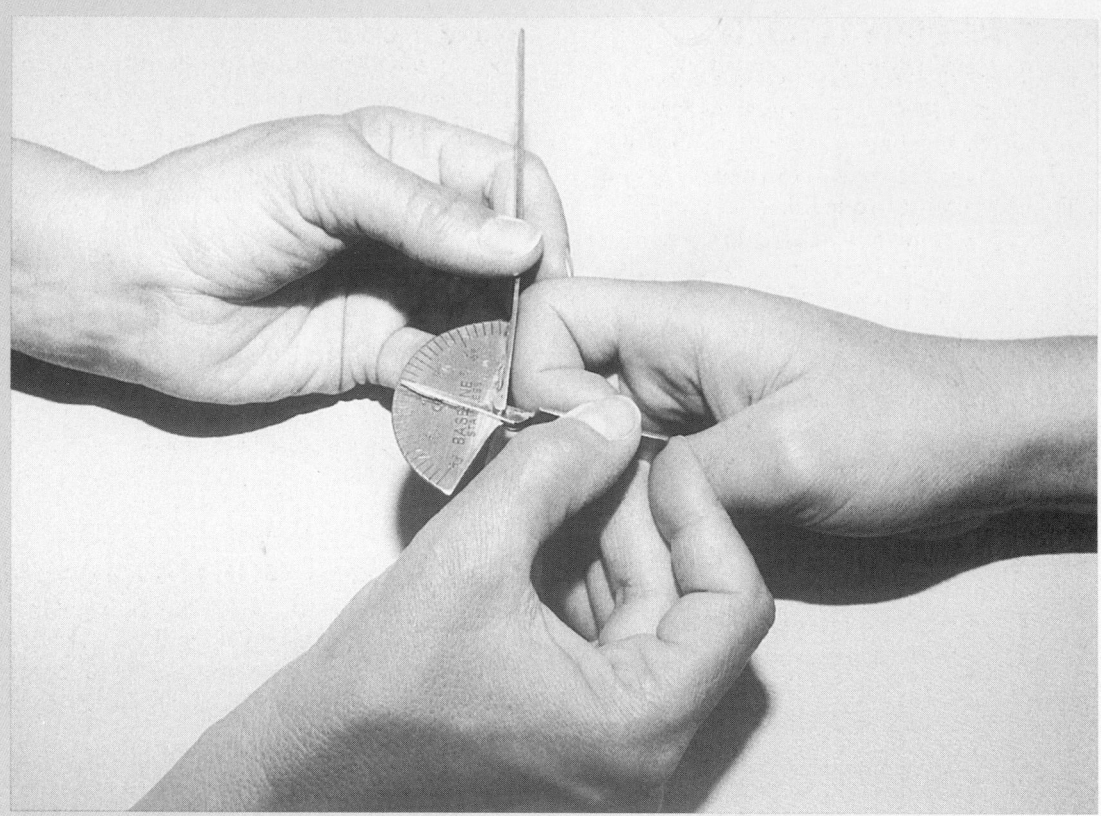

FIGURE 7.25 Distal interphalangeal flexion range of motion also can be measured by using a finger goniometer that is placed on the dorsal surface of the middle and distal phalanges. This type of goniometer is appropriate for measuring the small joints of the fingers, thumb, and toes.

● FINGERS: DISTAL INTERPHALANGEAL EXTENSION

Motion occurs in the sagittal plane around a medial–lateral axis. DIP extension is usually recorded as the starting position for DIP flexion ROM. Most references, such as the AAOS[10] and the AMA,[11] report normal ROM values to be 0 degrees. However, Mallon, Brown, and Nunley[13] report a mean of 8 degrees of active DIP extension and 20 degrees of passive DIP extension. DIP extension ROM is generally equal for all fingers.[13] See Research Findings and Tables 7.1 and 7.2 for additional normal ROM values.

Testing Position

Position the subject sitting, with the forearm and hand resting on a supporting surface. Place the forearm in 0 degrees of supination and pronation; the wrist in 0 degrees of flexion, extension, and radial and ulnar deviation; and the MCP joint in 0 degrees of flexion, extension, abduction, and adduction. Position the PIP joint in approximately 70 to 90 degrees of flexion. (If the PIP joint, MCP joint, and wrist are fully extended, tension in the flexor digitorum profundus muscle may restrict DIP extension.)

Stabilization

Stabilize the middle and proximal phalanx to prevent extension of the PIP joint.

Testing Motion

Extend the DIP joint by pushing on the palmar surface of the distal phalanx, moving the finger away from the palm. The end of extension ROM occurs when resistance to further motion is felt and attempts to overcome the resistance cause the PIP joint to extend.

Normal End-Feel

The end-feel is firm because of tension in the palmar joint capsule and the palmar plate (palmar ligament).

Goniometer Alignment

1. Center **fulcrum** of the goniometer over the dorsal aspect of the DIP joint.
2. Align **proximal arm** over the dorsal midline of the middle phalanx.
3. Align **distal arm** over the dorsal midline of the distal phalanx.

• FINGERS: COMPOSITE FLEXION OF THE MCP, PIP, AND DIP JOINTS

Composite finger flexion (CFF) is a simple method of quickly assessing multiple joints in a finger to indicate the functional ability to make a fist. However, a disadvantage of CFF is the inability to localize an impairment or response to treatment in a specific joint. Normally when the MCP, PIP, and DIP joints are maximally flexed, the distance between the fingertip and the distal palmar crease of the hand is zero. Ellis and Bruton[17] report that repeated CFF measurements fell within 5 to 6 mm 95 percent of the time when taken by the same tester and fell within 7 to 9 mm 95 percent of the time when taken by different testers.

Testing Position
Place the subject sitting, with the forearm and hand resting on a supporting surface. Position the forearm in neutral supination and pronation and the wrist in 0 degrees of flexion, extension, and radial and ulnar deviation. Alternatively, the forearm could be positioned in full supination.

Stabilization
Stabilize the metacarpals to prevent motion of the wrist.

Testing Motion
Flex the MCP, PIP, and DIP joints by pushing on the dorsal surface of the finger, moving the finger toward the palm. The end of flexion ROM occurs when resistance to further motion is felt and attempts to overcome the resistance cause the wrist to flex.

Normal End-Feel
Usually, the end-feel is soft because of contact between the palmar aspect of the proximal, middle, and distal phalanx and palm of the hand. In other individuals, the end-feel may be firm because of tension in the dorsal joint capsules and the collateral ligaments.

Measurement Method
See Figures 7.26 and 7.27. Measure the perpendicular distance between the distal palmar crease and the tip of the finger.[18,19] Alternatively, the distance between the distal palmar crease and the distal corner of the nail bed on the radial border of the finger can be measured.[17]

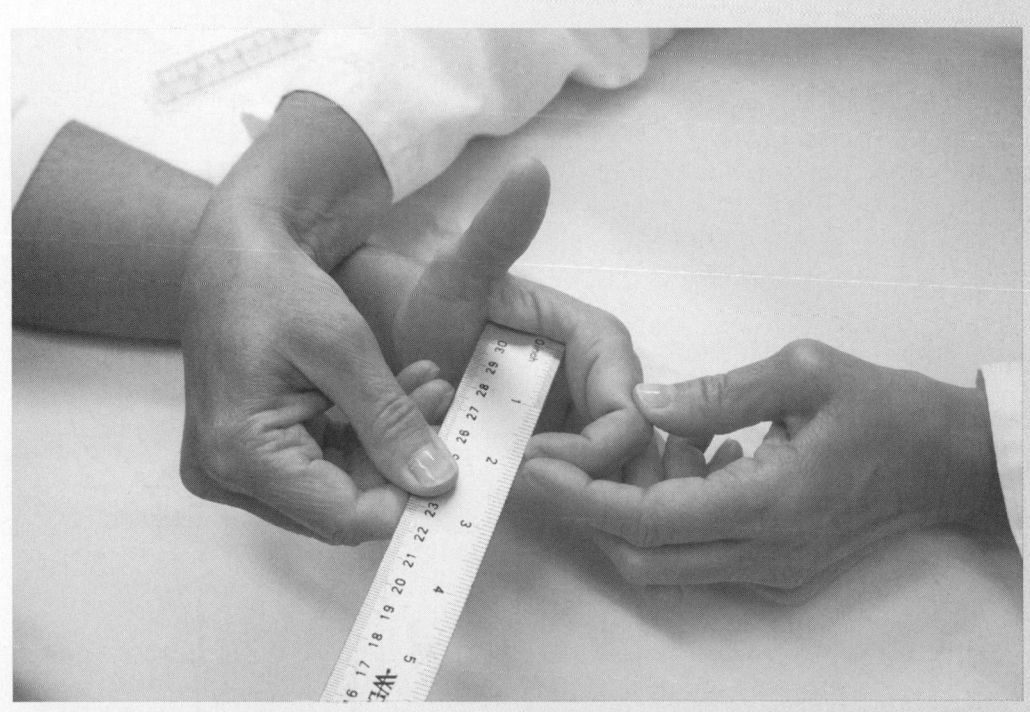

FIGURE 7.26 Composite finger flexion (CFF) is determined by measuring the distance between the distal palmar crease and the tip of the finger at the end of flexion of the MCP, PIP, and DIP joints. Normally, the tip of the finger is able to touch the palm at the distal palmar crease. This subject has limited range of motion.

RANGE OF MOTION TESTING PROCEDURES: Thumb

Landmarks for Testing Procedures

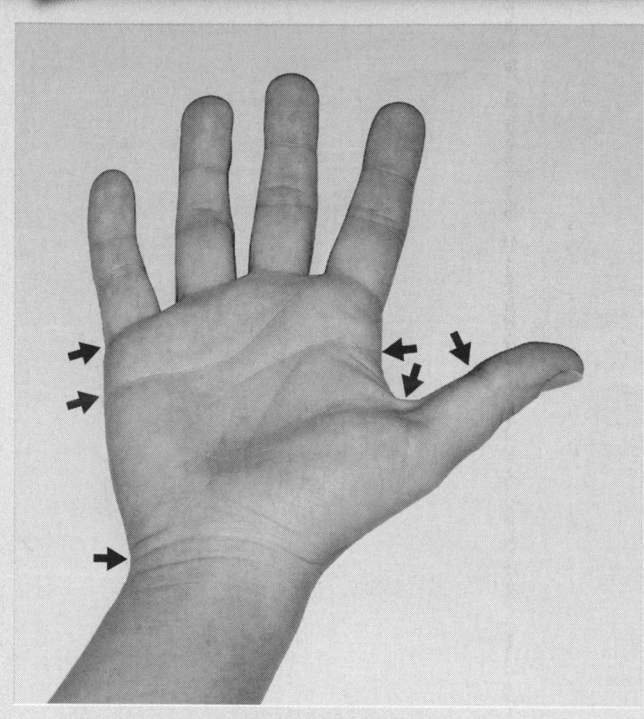
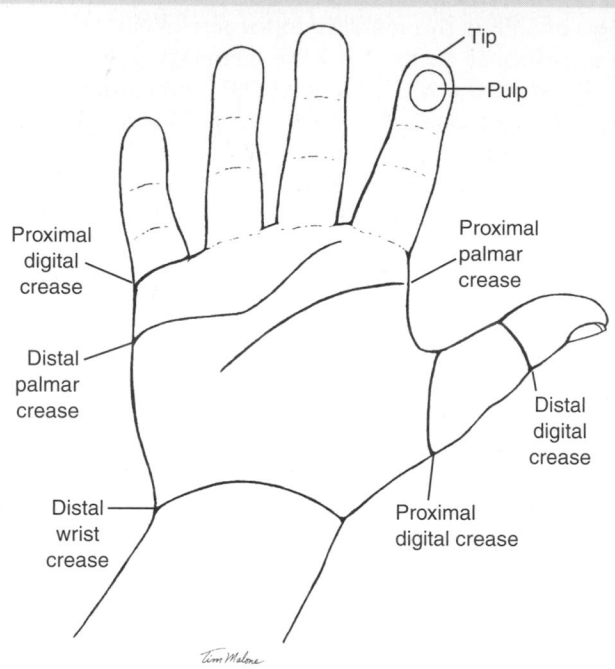

FIGURE 7.27 A, B Anterior (palmar) view of the right hand showing the digital and palmar creases used for measuring composite finger flexion and CMC opposition of the thumb.

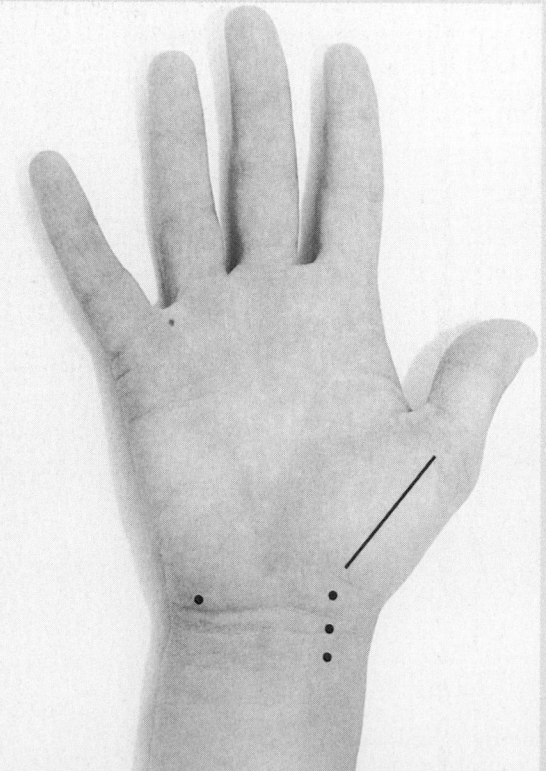
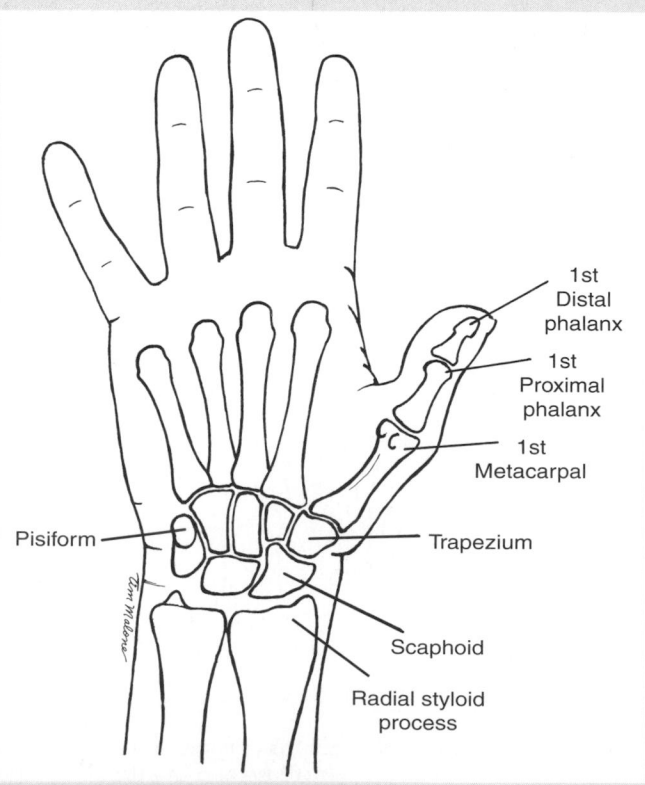

FIGURE 7.28 Anterior (palmar) view of the right hand showing surface anatomy landmarks for goniometer alignment during the measurement of thumb range of motion.

FIGURE 7.29 Anterior (palmar) view of the right hand showing bony anatomical landmarks for goniometer alignment during the measurement of thumb range of motion.

Landmarks for Testing Procedures (continued)

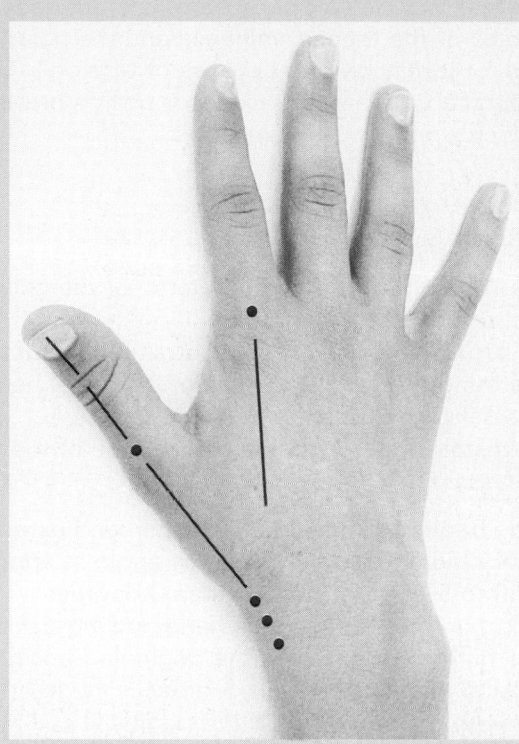

FIGURE 7.30 Posterior view of the right hand showing surface anatomy landmarks for goniometer alignment during the measurement of thumb range of motion.

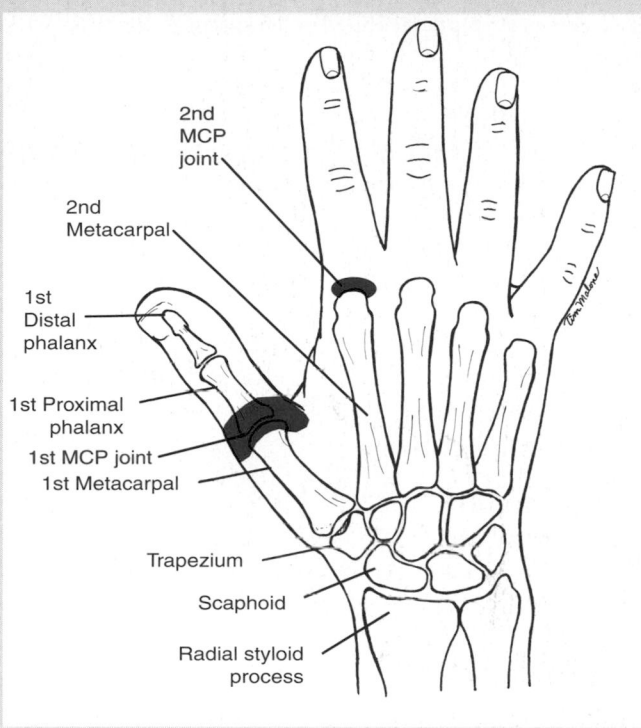

2nd MCP joint

2nd Metacarpal

1st Distal phalanx

1st Proximal phalanx

1st MCP joint

1st Metacarpal

Trapezium

Scaphoid

Radial styloid process

FIGURE 7.31 Posterior view of the right hand showing bony anatomical landmarks for goniometer alignment during the measurement of thumb range of motion.

● THUMB: CARPOMETACARPAL FLEXION

Motion occurs in the plane of the hand. When the subject is in the anatomical position, the motion occurs in the frontal plane around an anterior–posterior axis. Normal ROM is 15 degrees according to the AAOS.[10]

Testing Position

Position the subject sitting, with the forearm and hand resting on a supporting surface. Place the forearm in full supination; the wrist in 0 degrees of flexion, extension, and radial and ulnar deviation; and the CMC joint of the thumb in 0 degrees of abduction. The MCP and IP joints of the thumb are relaxed in a position of slight flexion. (If the MCP and IP joints of the thumb are positioned in full flexion, tension in the extensor pollicis longus and brevis muscles may restrict the motion.)

Stabilization

Stabilize the carpals, radius, and ulna to prevent wrist motions. Movement of the wrist will affect the accuracy of the ROM measurement.

Testing Motion

Flex the CMC joint of the thumb by pushing on the dorsal surface of the metacarpal, moving the thumb toward the ulnar aspect of the hand (Fig. 7.32). Maintain the CMC joint in 0 degrees of abduction.

The end of flexion ROM occurs when resistance to further motion is felt and attempts to overcome the resistance cause the wrist to deviate ulnarly.

Normal End-Feel

The end-feel may be soft because of contact between muscle bulk of the thenar eminence and the palm of the hand, or it may be firm because of tension in the dorsal joint capsule and the extensor pollicis brevis and abductor pollicis brevis muscles.

Goniometer Alignment

See Figures 7.33 and 7.34.

1. Center **fulcrum** of the goniometer over the palmar aspect of the first CMC joint.
2. Align **proximal arm** with the ventral midline of the radius using the ventral surface of the radial head and radial styloid process for reference.
3. Align **distal arm** with the ventral midline of the first metacarpal.

   In the beginning position for flexion and extension, the goniometer will indicate an angle of approximately 30 to 50 degrees rather than 0 degrees, depending on the shape of the hand and wrist position. The difference between the beginning-position degrees and the end-position degrees is the ROM. For example, a measurement that begins at 35 degrees and ends at 15 degrees should be recorded as 0 to 20 degrees.

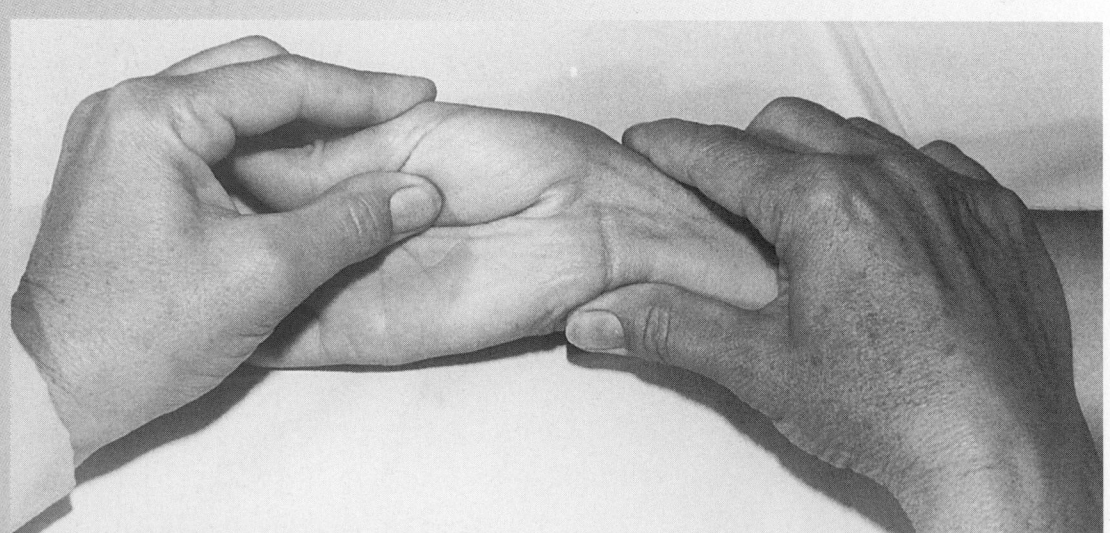

FIGURE 7.32 During carpometacarpal (CMC) flexion, the examiner uses the index finger and thumb of one hand to stabilize the carpals, radius, and ulna to prevent ulnar deviation of the wrist. The examiner's other index finger and thumb flex the CMC joint by moving the first metacarpal medially.

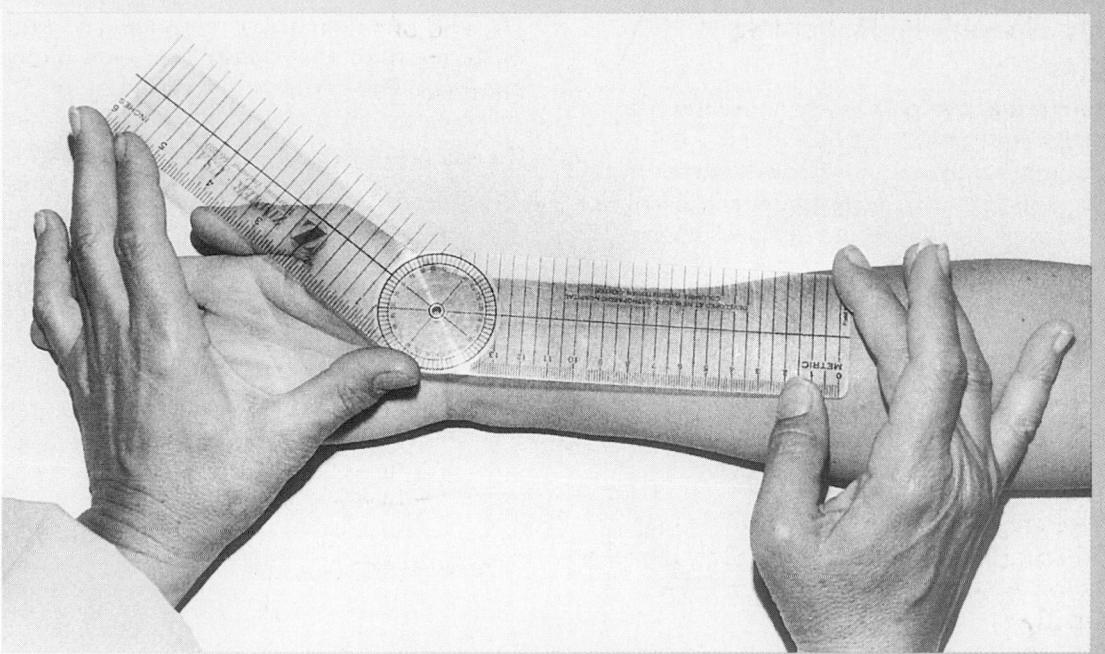

FIGURE 7.33 The alignment of the goniometer at the beginning of carpometacarpal (CMC) flexion range of motion of the thumb. Note that the goniometer does not read 0 degrees.

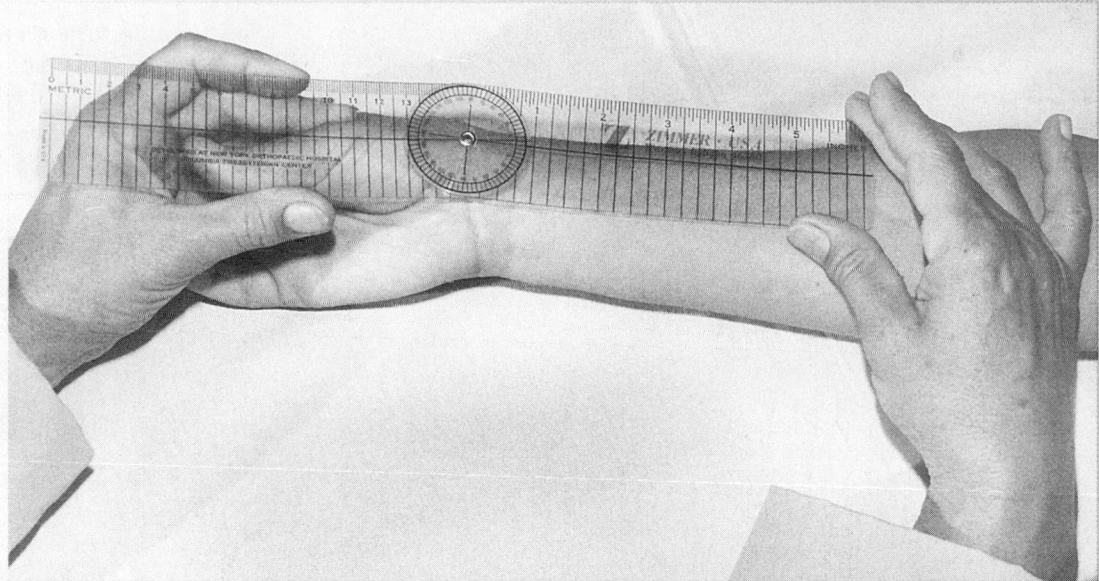

FIGURE 7.34 At the end of carpometacarpal (CMC) flexion range of motion, the examiner uses the hand that was stabilizing the wrist to align the proximal arm of the goniometer with the radius. The examiner's other hand maintains CMC flexion and aligns the distal arm of the goniometer with the first metacarpal. During the measurement, the examiner must be careful not to move the subject's wrist further into ulnar deviation or the goniometer reading will be incorrect (too high).

Alternative Goniometer Alignment
See Figures 7.35 and 7.36.

1. Center **fulcrum** of the goniometer over the palmar aspect of the first CMC joint.
2. Align **proximal arm** with an imaginary line between the palmar surfaces of the trapezium and pisiform. This line is often parallel to the distal wrist crease (refer to Figure 7.27).
3. Align **distal arm** with the ventral midline of the first metacarpal.

This alternative alignment method avoids errors in ROM measurement due to inadvertent movement of the wrist. The goniometer in the beginning position will indicate an angle of approximately 40 to 70 degrees rather than 0 degrees, depending on the shape and size of the hand. The difference between the beginning-position degrees and the end-position degrees is the ROM.

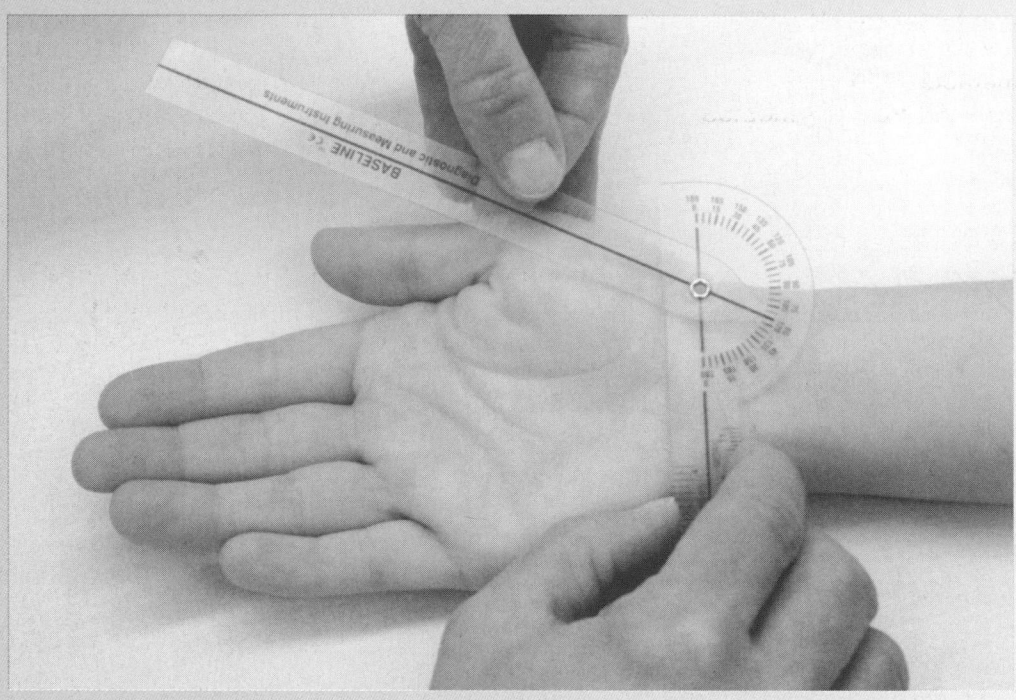

FIGURE 7.35 An alternative method of measuring the beginning of carpometacarpal (CMC) flexion aligns the proximal arm of the goniometer with the palmar surface of the trapezium and pisiform. Note that the goniometer does not read 0 degrees.

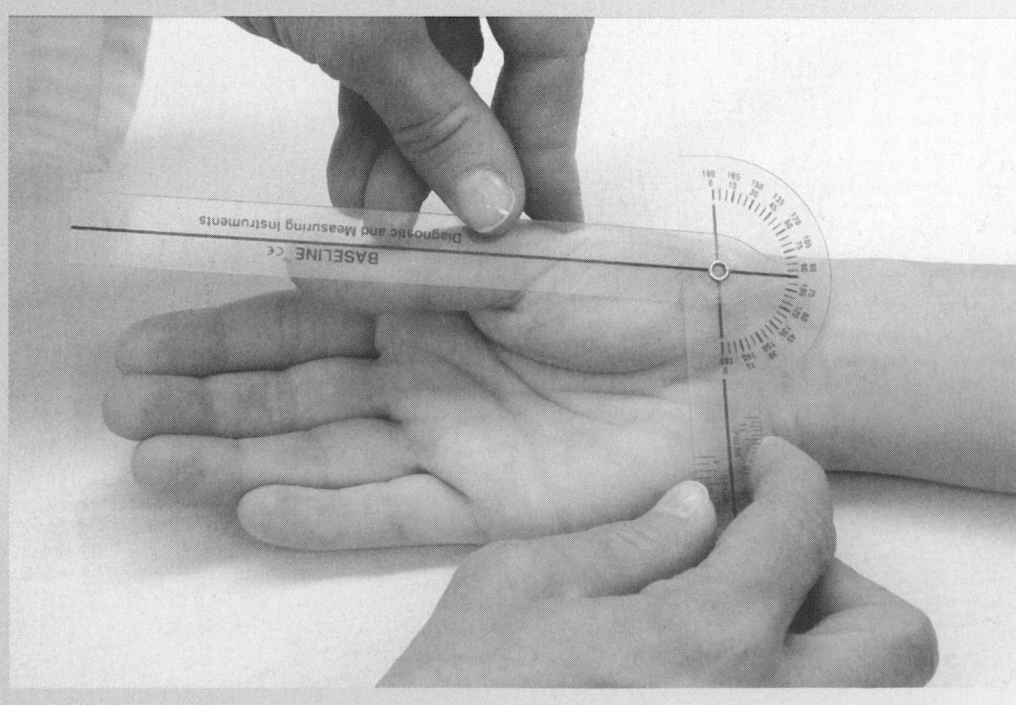

FIGURE 7.36 An alternative method of aligning the goniometer to measure the end of carpometacarpal (CMC) flexion range of motion. The difference between the degrees on the goniometer at the beginning and the end positions is the range of motion.

20-80

● THUMB: CARPOMETACARPAL EXTENSION

Motion occurs in the plane of the hand. When the subject is in the anatomical position, the motion occurs in the frontal plane around an anterior–posterior axis. This motion is sometimes called radial abduction. Reported values for CMC thumb extension ROM are 35 degrees according to the AMA[11] (this is the difference between an angle of 15 degrees of separation between the first and second metacarpal at the beginning of the motion and an angle of 50 degrees at the end of the motion), and vary from 20 degrees to 80 degrees according to the AAOS.[10,18] However, the measurement methods used by the AAOS and the AMA appear to differ from the method suggested here.

Testing Position

Position the subject sitting, with the forearm and hand resting on a supporting surface. Place the forearm in full supination; the wrist in 0 degrees of flexion, extension, and radial and ulnar deviation; and the CMC joint of the thumb in 0 degrees of abduction.

The MCP and IP joints of the thumb are relaxed in a position of slight flexion. (If the MCP and IP joints of the thumb are positioned in full extension, tension in the flexor pollicis longus muscle may restrict the motion.)

Stabilization

Stabilize the carpals, radius, and ulna to prevent wrist motions.

Testing Motion

Extend the CMC joint of the thumb by pushing on the palmar surface of the metacarpal, moving the thumb toward the radial aspect of the hand (Fig. 7.37). Maintain the CMC joint in 0 degrees of abduction. The end of extension ROM occurs when resistance to further motion is felt and attempts to overcome the resistance cause the wrist to deviate radially.

Normal End-Feel

The end-feel is firm because of tension in the anterior joint capsule and the flexor pollicis brevis, adductor pollicis, opponens pollicis, and first dorsal interossei muscles.

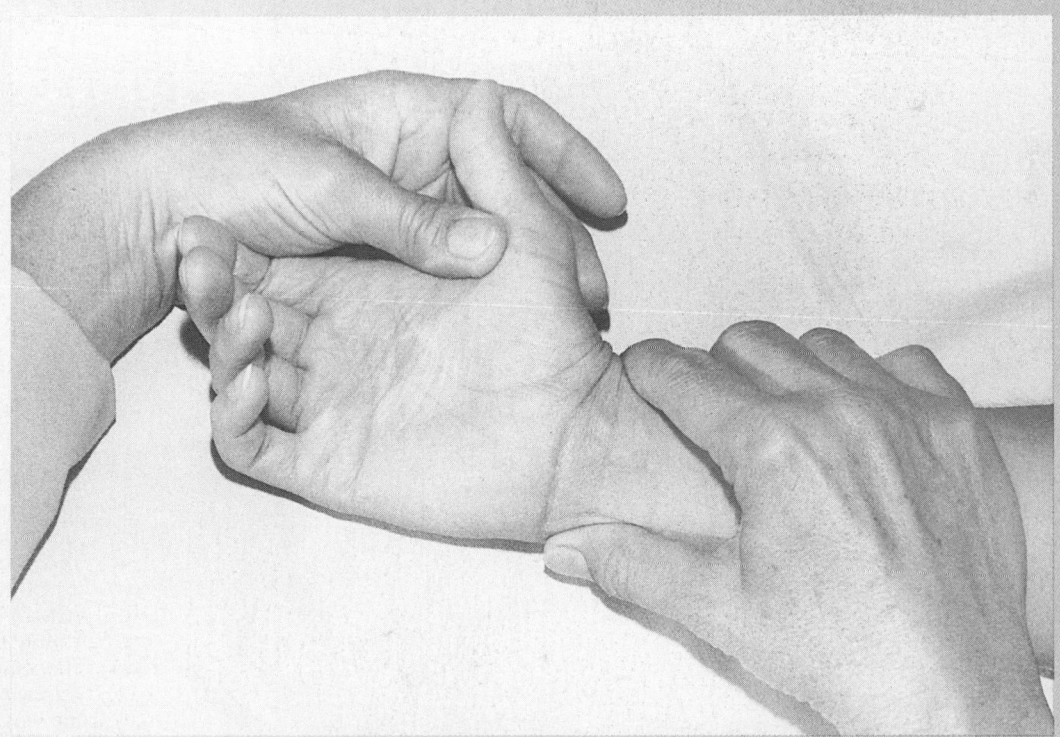

FIGURE 7.37 During carpometacarpal (CMC) extension of the thumb, the examiner uses one hand to stabilize the carpals, radius, and ulna thereby preventing radial deviation of the subject's wrist. The examiner's other hand is used to pull the first metacarpal laterally into extension.

Goniometer Alignment
See Figures 7.38 and 7.39.

1. Center **fulcrum** of the goniometer over the palmar aspect of the first CMC joint.
2. Align **proximal arm** with the ventral midline of the radius, using the ventral surface of the radial head and the radial styloid process for reference.
3. Align **distal arm** with the ventral midline of the first metacarpal.

In the beginning positions for flexion and extension, the goniometer will indicate an angle of approximately 30 to 50 degrees rather than 0 degrees, depending on the shape of the hand and wrist position. The difference between the beginning-position degrees and the end-position degrees is the ROM. For example, a measurement that begins at 35 degrees and ends at 55 degrees should be recorded as 0 to 20 degrees.

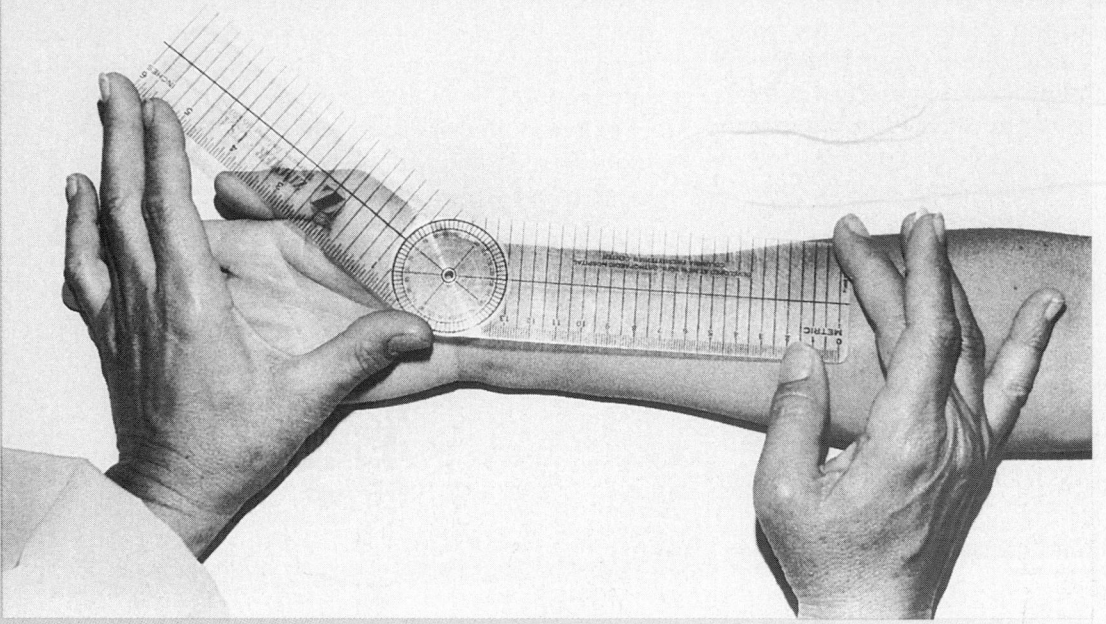

FIGURE 7.38 The goniometer alignment for measuring the beginning of carpometacarpal (CMC) extension range of motion is the same as for measuring the beginning of CMC flexion.

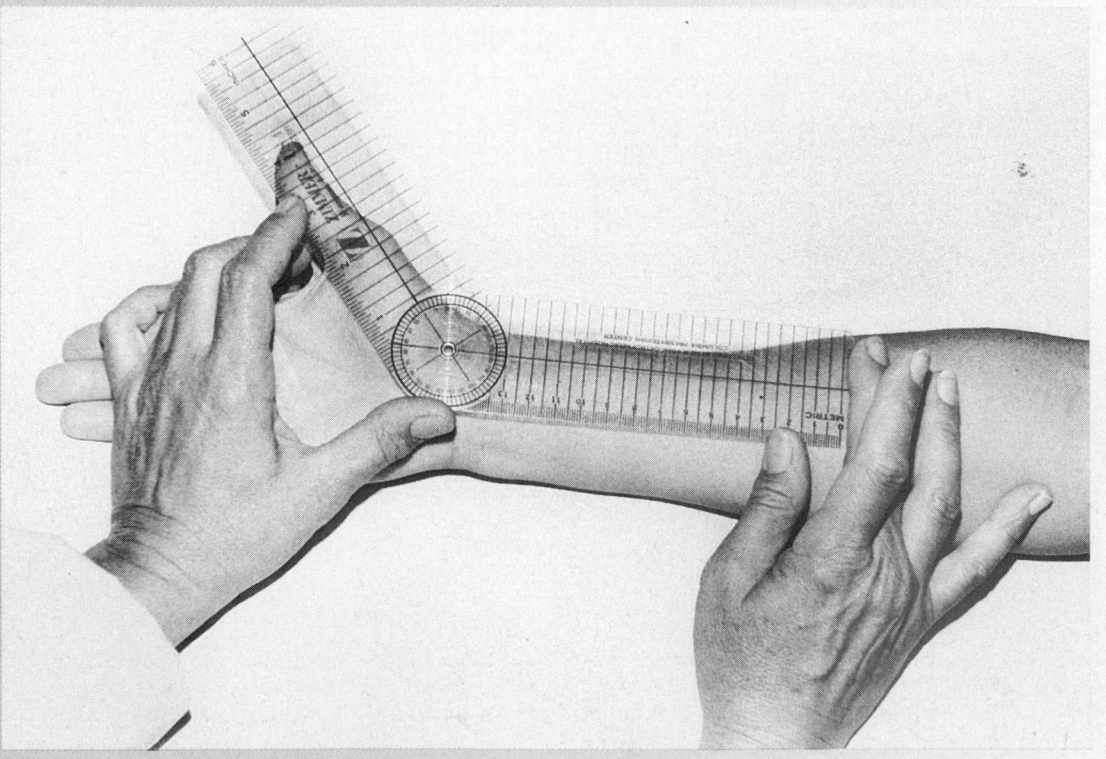

FIGURE 7.39 The alignment of the goniometer at the end of carpometacarpal (CMC) extension range of motion of the thumb. The examiner must be careful to move only the CMC joint into extension and not to change the position of the wrist during the measurement.

Alternative Goniometer Alignment
See Figures 7.40 and 7.41.

1. Center **fulcrum** of the goniometer over the palmar aspect of the first CMC joint.
2. Align **proximal arm** with an imaginary line between the palmar surface of the trapezium and pisiform. This line is often parallel to the distal wrist crease (refer to Figure 7.27).
3. Align **distal arm** with the ventral midline of the first metacarpal.

This alternative alignment method avoids errors in ROM measurement due to inadvertent movement of the wrist. The goniometer in the beginning position will indicate an angle of 40 to 70 degrees rather than 0 degrees, depending on the shape and size of the hand. The difference between the beginning and the end-position degrees is the ROM. For example, a measurement that begins at 50 degrees and ends at 30 degrees should be recorded as 0 to 20 degrees.

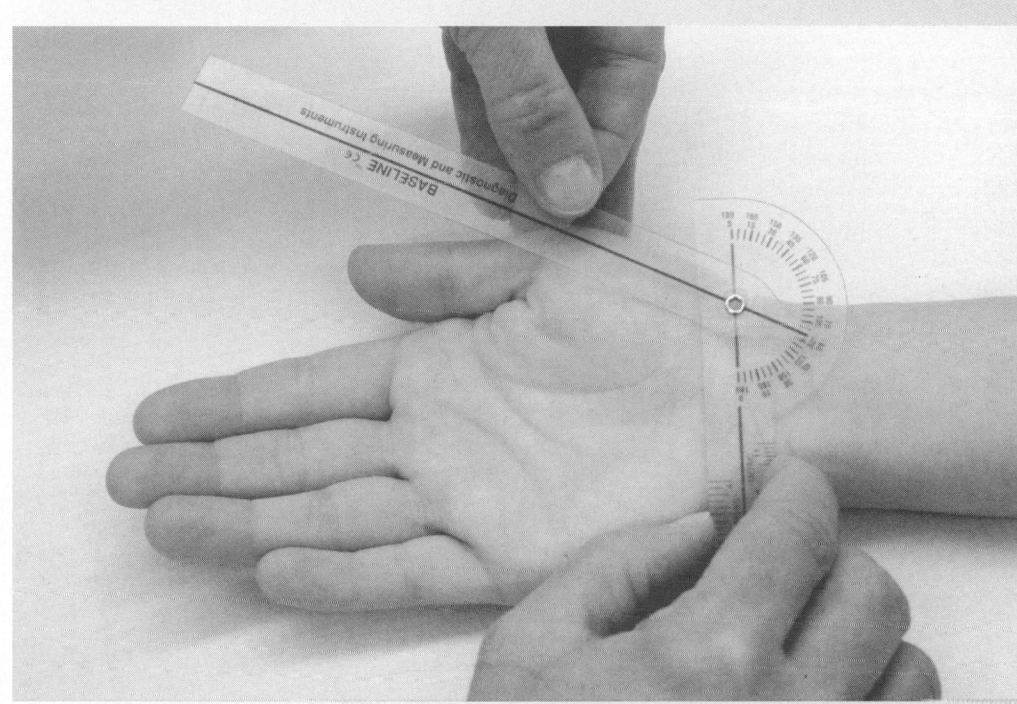

FIGURE 7.40 The alternative method of measuring the beginning of CMC extension is the same as the alternative method for measuring the beginning of CMC flexion.

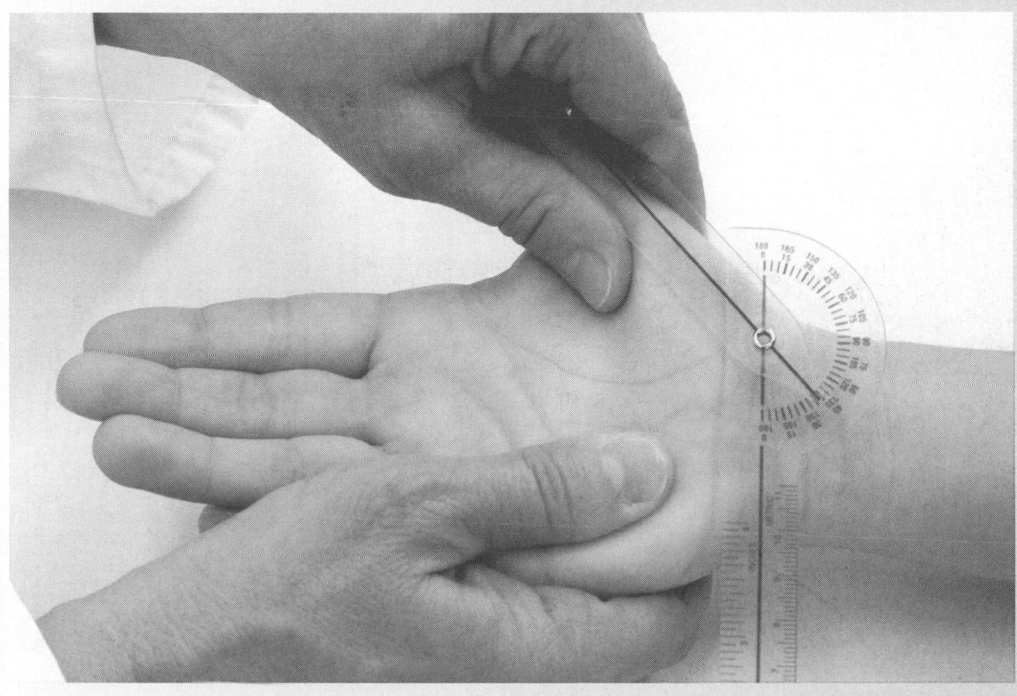

FIGURE 7.41 The alternative method of aligning the goniometer to measure the end of CMC extension ROM.

● THUMB: CARPOMETACARPAL ABDUCTION

Motion occurs at a right angle to the palm of the hand. When the subject is in the anatomical position, the motion occurs in the sagittal plane around a medial–lateral axis. This motion is sometimes called palmar abduction. Abduction ROM is 70 degrees according to the AAOS[10,18]. However, the measurement method used by the AAOS appears to differ from the method suggested here.

Testing Position

Position the subject sitting, with the forearm and hand resting on a supporting surface. Place the forearm midway between supination and pronation; the wrist in 0 degrees of flexion, extension, and radial and ulnar deviation; and the CMC, MCP, and IP joints of the thumb in 0 degrees of flexion and extension.

Stabilization

Stabilize the carpals and the second metacarpal to prevent wrist motions.

Testing Motion

Abduct the CMC joint by moving the metacarpal away from the palm of the hand (Fig. 7.42). The end of abduction ROM occurs when resistance to further motion is felt and attempts to overcome the resistance cause the wrist to flex.

Normal End-Feel

The end-feel is firm because of tension in the fascia and the skin of the web space between the thumb and the index finger. Tension in the adductor pollicis and first dorsal interossei muscles also contributes to the firm end-feel.

Goniometer Alignment

See Figures 7.43 and 7.44.

1. Center **fulcrum** of the goniometer over the lateral aspect of the radial styloid process.
2. Align **proximal arm** with the lateral midline of the second metacarpal, using the center of the second MCP joint for reference.
3. Align **distal arm** with the lateral midline of the first metacarpal, using the center of the first MCP joint for reference.

Note that the proximal surface of the first metacarpal contacts the trapezium, while the proximal surface of the second metacarpal contacts the trapezoid. Contact of the metacarpals with two

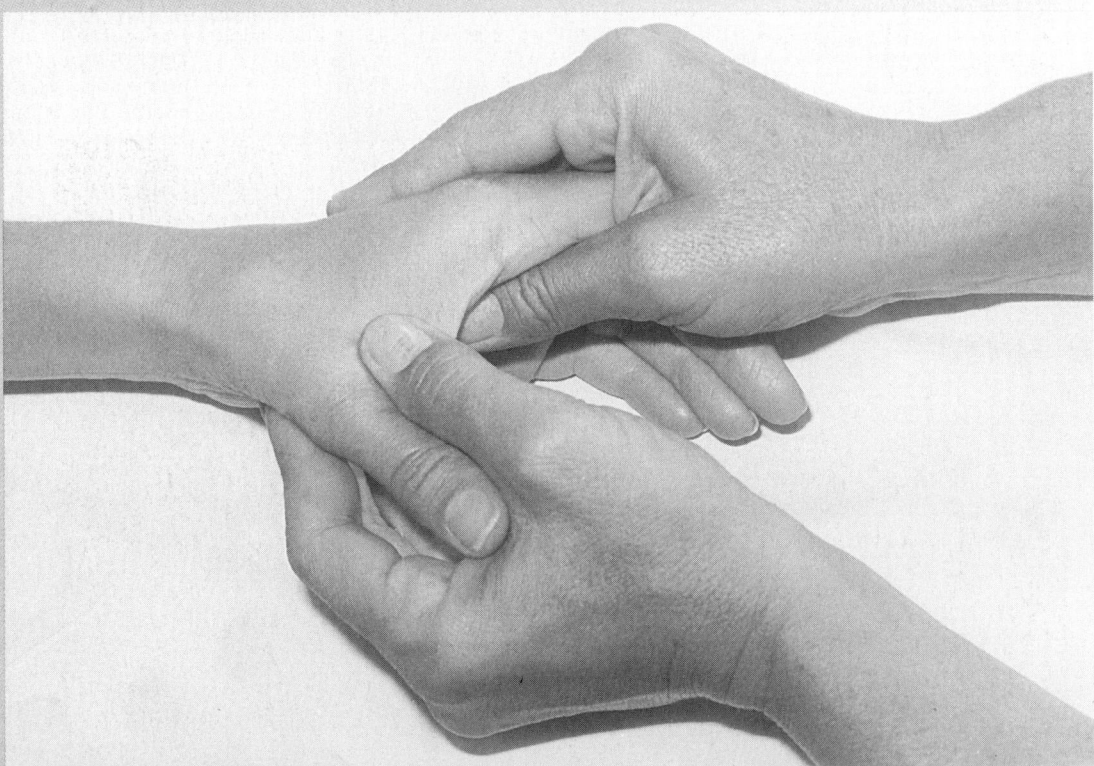

FIGURE 7.42 During carpometacarpal (CMC) abduction, the examiner uses one hand to stabilize the subject's second metacarpal. Her other hand grasps the subject's first metacarpal just proximal to the metacarpophalangeal joint to move it away from the palm and into abduction.

different carpals and the palmar position of the trapezium relative to the trapezoid create difficulties in identifying a fulcrum and alignment for the arms of the goniometer in this motion. We have chosen the radial styloid process and the first and second MCP joints as easily identifiable landmarks to indicate CMC abduction of the thumb. As the motion progresses toward the end of CMC abduction, these landmarks will be better aligned with the first and second metacarpals.

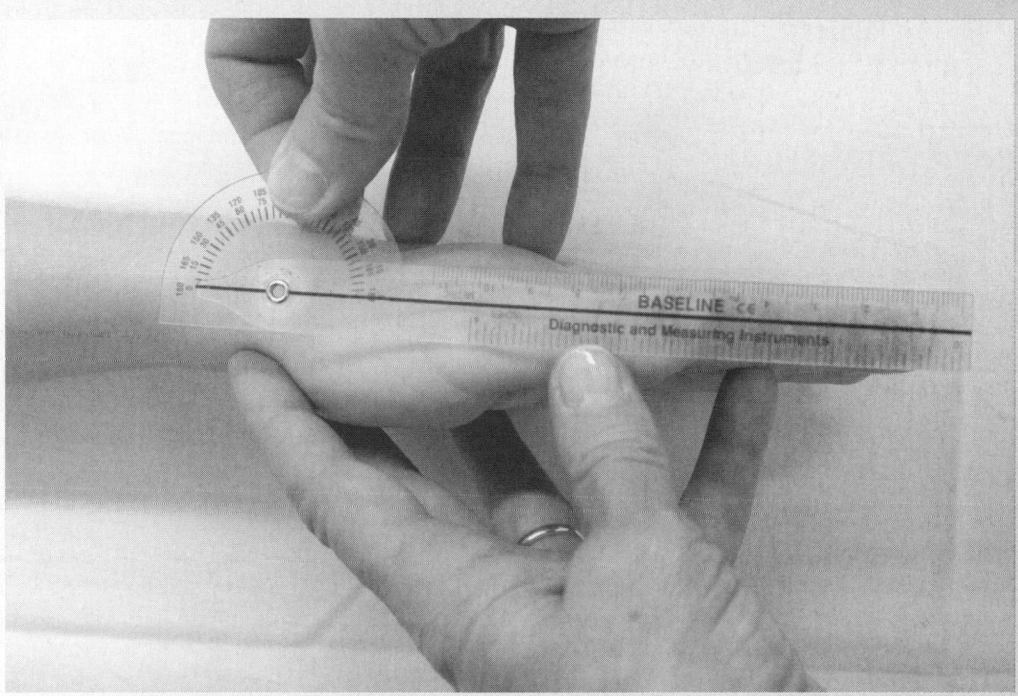

FIGURE 7.43 At the beginning of carpometacarpal (CMC) abduction range of motion, the distal end of the subject's first metacarpal of the thumb lies over the second metacarpal of the index finger.

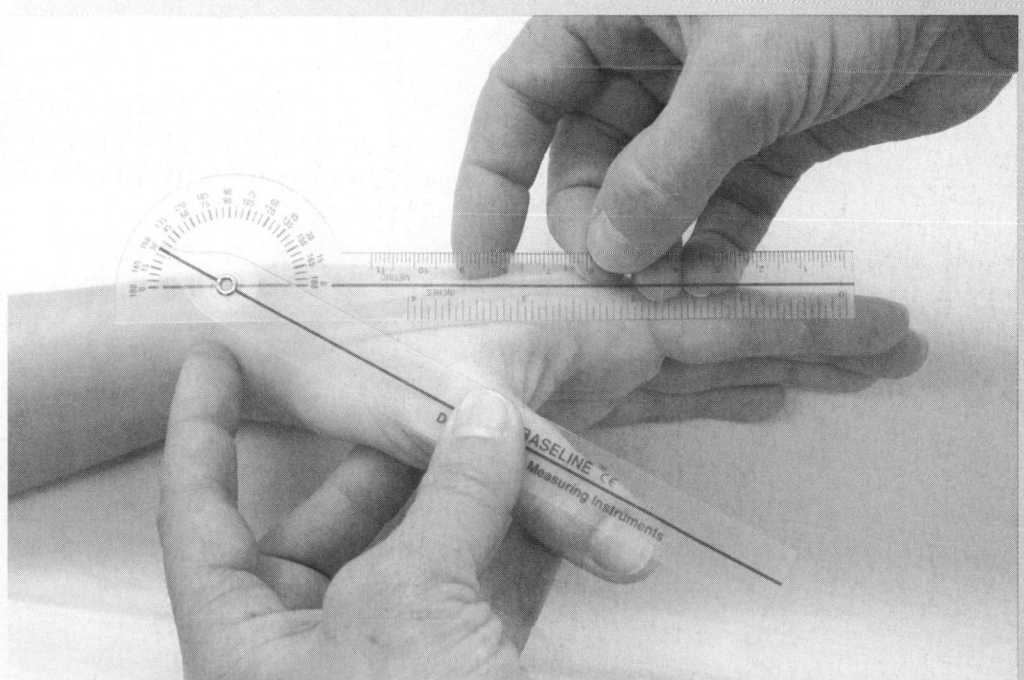

FIGURE 7.44 The alignment of the goniometer at the end of carpometacarpal (CMC) abduction range of motion.

● THUMB: CARPOMETACARPAL ADDUCTION

Motion occurs at a right angle to the palm of the hand. When the subject is in the anatomical position, the motion occurs in the sagittal plane around a medial–lateral axis. Adduction of the CMC joint of the thumb is not usually measured and recorded separately because it is the return to the 0 starting position from full abduction.

● THUMB: CARPOMETACARPAL OPPOSITION

This motion is a combination of abduction, flexion, medial axial rotation (pronation), and adduction at the CMC joints of the thumb. Contact between the tip of the thumb and the base of the little finger (proximal digital crease) is usually possible at the end of opposition ROM, providing that some flexion at the MCP and IP joints of the thumb is allowed. If no flexion of the MCP and IP joints of the thumb is allowed, there will be a distance of several centimeters between the thumb and base of the little finger at the end of opposition. Many methods of measuring CMC opposition have been suggested.[10,11,18–21] It is important to note the landmarks that are being used and the amount of motion allowed at the MCP and IP joints of the thumb so that there is consistency between repeated measurements on an individual.

Testing Position

Position the subject sitting with the forearm and hand resting on a supporting surface. Place the forearm in full supination and the wrist in 0 degrees of flexion, extension, and radial and ulnar deviation.

Stabilization

Stabilize the fifth metacarpal to prevent motion at the fifth CMC joint and wrist.

Testing Motion

Grasp the first metacarpal and move it away from the palm of the hand (abduction) and then in an ulnar direction toward the base of the little finger (flexion and adduction), allowing the first metacarpal to medially rotate (Fig. 7.45). The end of opposition ROM occurs when contact is made between the tip of the thumb and the base of the little finger, if some flexion of the MCP and IP joints of the thumb is allowed (Fig. 7.46). If no flexion is allowed at the MCP and IP joints, the end of opposition will occur when resistance to further motion is felt and attempts to overcome the resistance cause the wrist to deviate or the forearm to pronate.

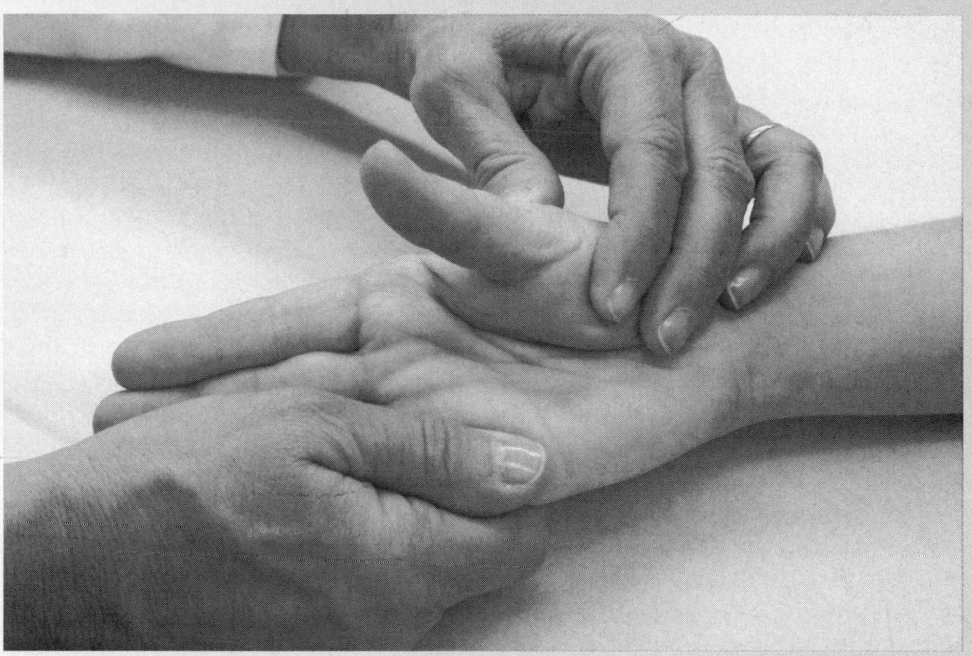

FIGURE 7.45 Midway through the range of motion of carpometacarpal (CMC) opposition, the metacarpal of the thumb is in abduction, flexion, and medial rotation. The fifth metacarpal is stabilized by the examiner.

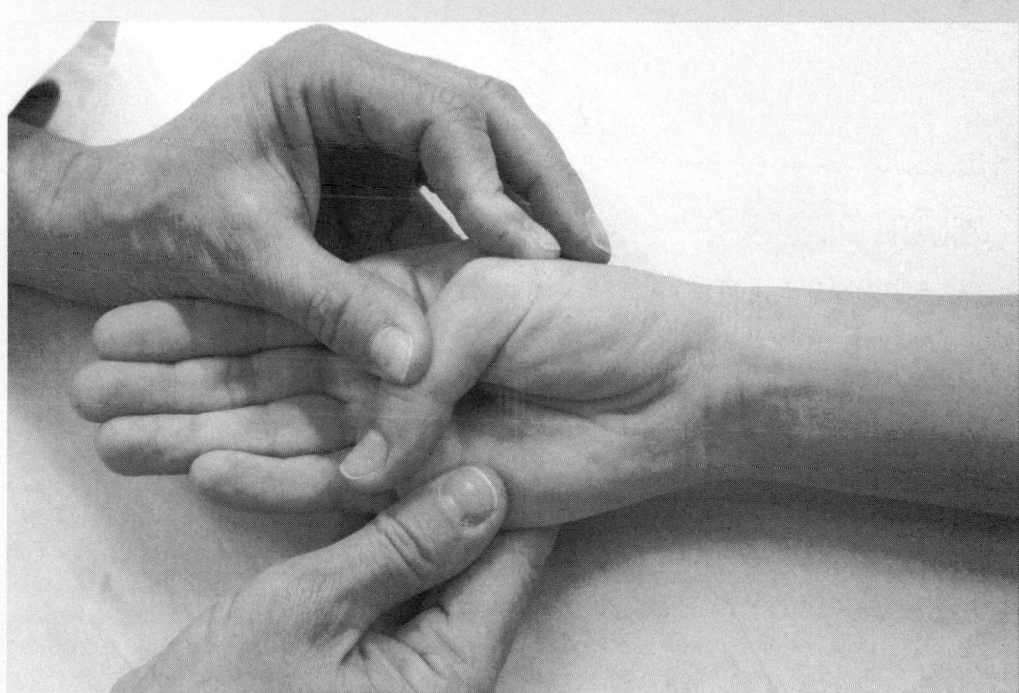

FIGURE 7.46 At the end of the range of opposition the tip of the subject's thumb is normally in contact with the base of the little finger. The thumb has moved through carpometacarpal (CMC) abduction, flexion, medial rotation, and adduction, while the metacarpophalangeal (MCP) joint is allowed to flex.

Normal End-Feel

The end-feel may be soft because of contact between the muscle bulk of the thenar eminence and the palm or between the tip of the thumb with the base of the little finger. In some individuals it may be firm because of tension in the CMC joint capsule, fascia, and skin of the web space between the thumb and the index finger and tension in the adductor pollicis, first dorsal interossei, extensor pollicis brevis, and extensor pollicis longus muscles.

Measurement Method

The goniometer is not commonly used to measure the angular range of opposition. Instead, a ruler is often used to measure the shortest distance between the **tip of the thumb** and the center of the **proximal digital crease of the little finger** at the end of opposition (Fig. 7.47).[10,18]

Alternately, the shortest distance between the center of the **proximal digital crease of the thumb** and the **distal palmar crease directly over the fifth MCP joint** can be measured (Fig. 7.48). In this manner, motion at the MCP and IP joints of the thumb will not affect the measurement of opposition.

The AMA *Guides to the Evaluation of Permanent Impairment*[11] recommends measuring the longest distance from the **flexion crease of the thumb IP joint** to the **distal palmar crease directly over the third MCP joint** (Fig. 7.49). However, this measurement method seems more consistent with the measurement of CMC abduction. A distance of less than 8 cm is considered impaired.[11]

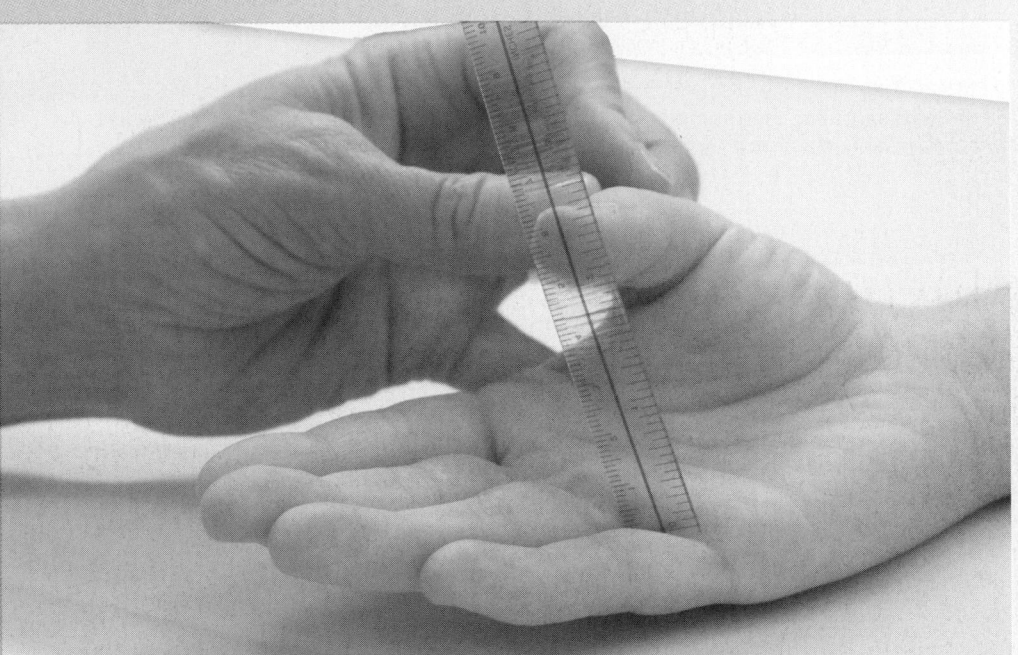

FIGURE 7.47 The range of motion (ROM) in opposition can be determined by measuring the shortest distance between the tip of the thumb and the proximal digital crease of the little finger. The examiner is using the arm of a goniometer to measure, but any ruler would suffice. This subject's hand does not have full ROM in opposition.

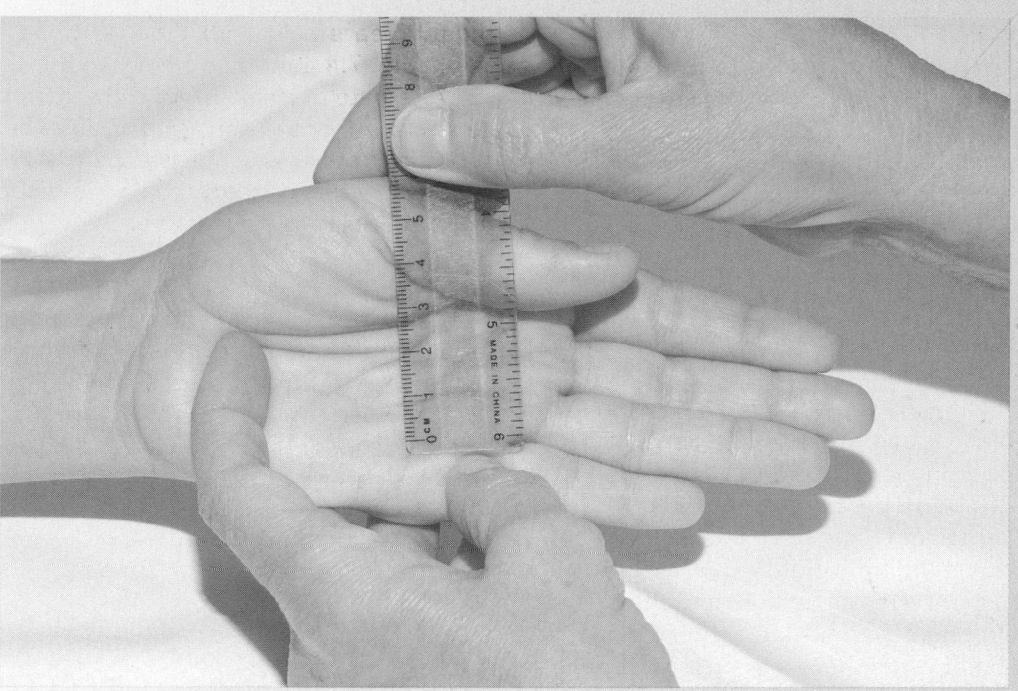

FIGURE 7.48 Another method of measuring thumb opposition is to record the distance between the proximal digital crease of the thumb and the distal palmar crease over the fifth metacarpophalangeal (MCP) joint.

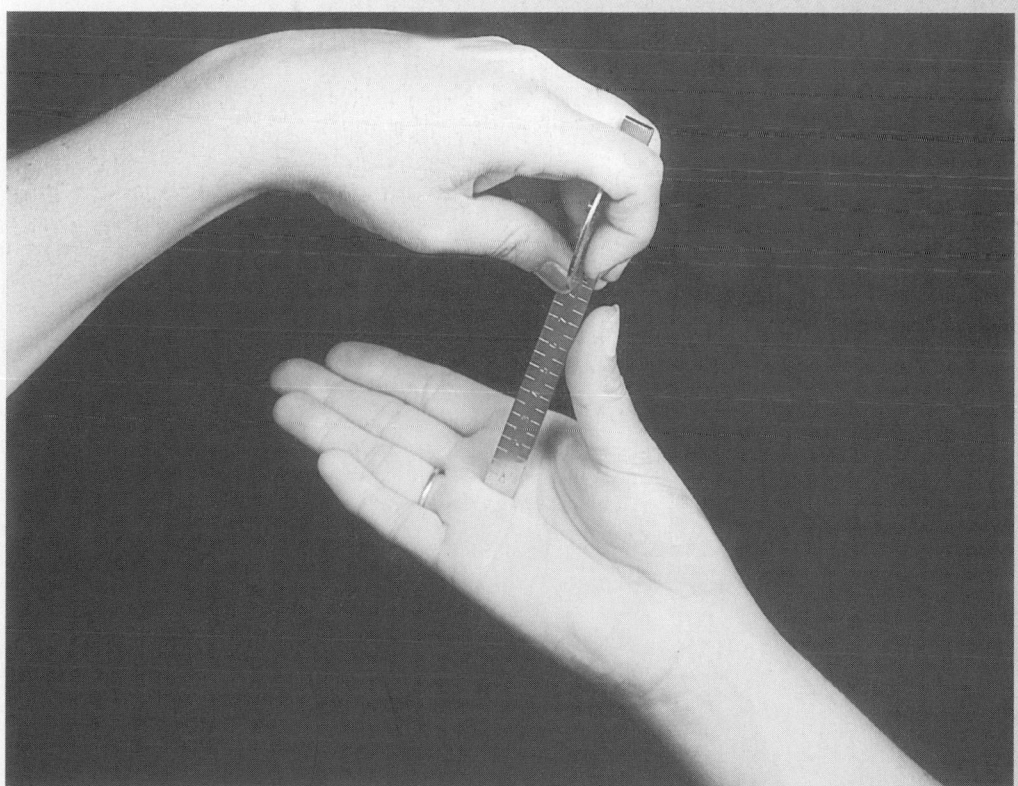

FIGURE 7.49 In an alternative method of measuring thumb opposition proposed by the American Medical Association, the examiner uses a ruler to find the longest possible distance between the distal palmar crease directly over the metacarpophalangeal joint of the middle finger and the flexion crease of the thumb interphalangeal joint. (From Stanley, BG, and Tribuzi, SM: Concepts in Hand Rehabilitation. FA Davis, Philadelphia, 1992, p 546, with permission.)

● THUMB: METACARPOPHALANGEAL FLEXION

Motion occurs in the frontal plane around an anterior–posterior axis when the subject is in the anatomical position. Normal ROM values for adults are 50 degrees according to the AAOS,[10,18] 60 degrees according to the AMA,[11] and 55 degrees according to DeSmet and colleagues.[22] See Research Findings and Table 7.3 for additional normal ROM values.

Testing Position

Position the subject sitting, with the forearm and hand resting on a supporting surface. Place the forearm in full supination; the wrist in 0 degrees of flexion, extension, and radial and ulnar deviation; the CMC joint of the thumb in 0 degrees of flexion, extension, abduction, adduction, and opposition; and the IP joint of the thumb in 0 degrees of flexion and extension. (If the wrist and IP joint of the thumb are positioned in full flexion, tension in the extensor pollicis longus muscle will restrict the motion.)

Stabilization

Stabilize the first metacarpal to prevent wrist motion and flexion of the CMC joint of the thumb.

Testing Motion

Flex the MCP joint by pushing on the dorsal aspect of the proximal phalanx, moving the thumb toward the ulnar aspect of the hand (Fig. 7.50). The end of flexion ROM occurs when resistance to further motion is felt and attempts to overcome the resistance cause the CMC joint to flex.

Normal End-Feel

The end-feel may be hard because of contact between the palmar aspect of the proximal phalanx and the first metacarpal, or it may be firm because of tension in the dorsal joint capsule, the collateral ligaments, and the extensor pollicis brevis muscle.

Goniometer Alignment

See Figures 7.51 and 7.52.

1. Center **fulcrum** of the goniometer over the dorsal aspect of the MCP joint.
2. Align **proximal arm** over the dorsal midline of the metacarpal.
3. Align **distal arm** with the dorsal midline of the proximal phalanx.

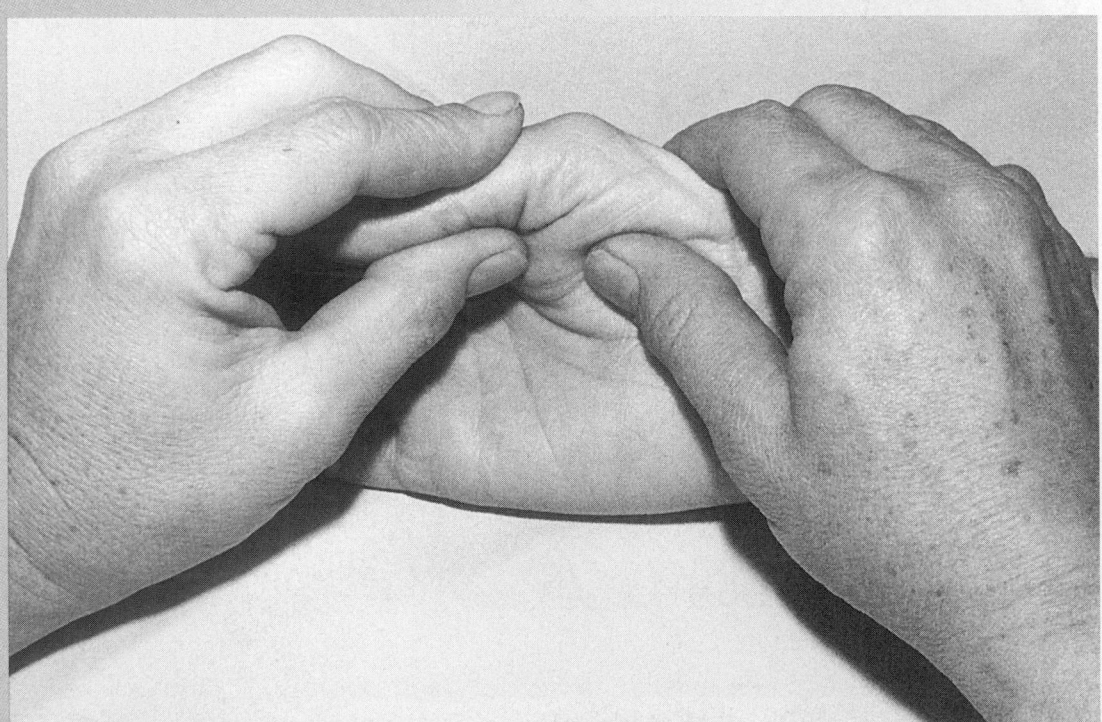

FIGURE 7.50 During metacarpophalangeal (MCP) flexion of the thumb, the examiner uses the index finger and thumb of one hand to stabilize the subject's first metacarpal and maintain the wrist in a neutral position. The examiner's other index finger and thumb grasp the subject's proximal phalanx to move it into flexion.

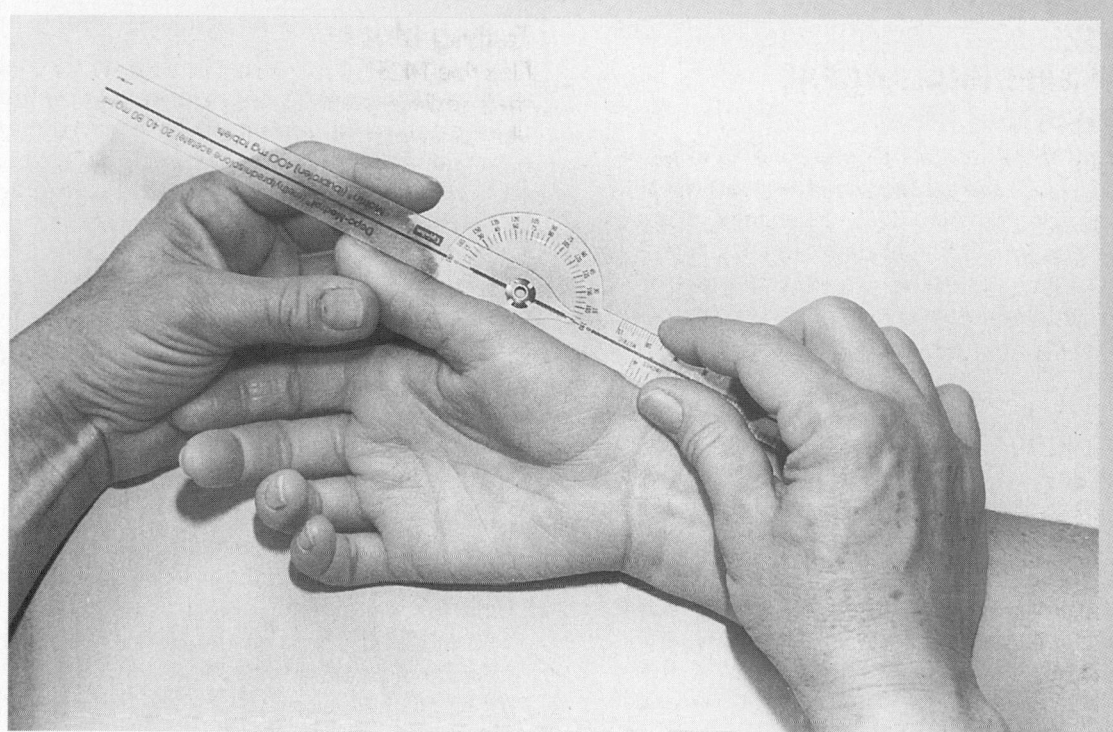

FIGURE 7.51 The alignment of the goniometer on the dorsal surfaces of the first metacarpal and proximal phalanx at the beginning of metacarpophalangeal (MCP) flexion range of motion of the thumb. If a bony deformity or swelling is present, the goniometer may be aligned with the lateral surface of these bones.

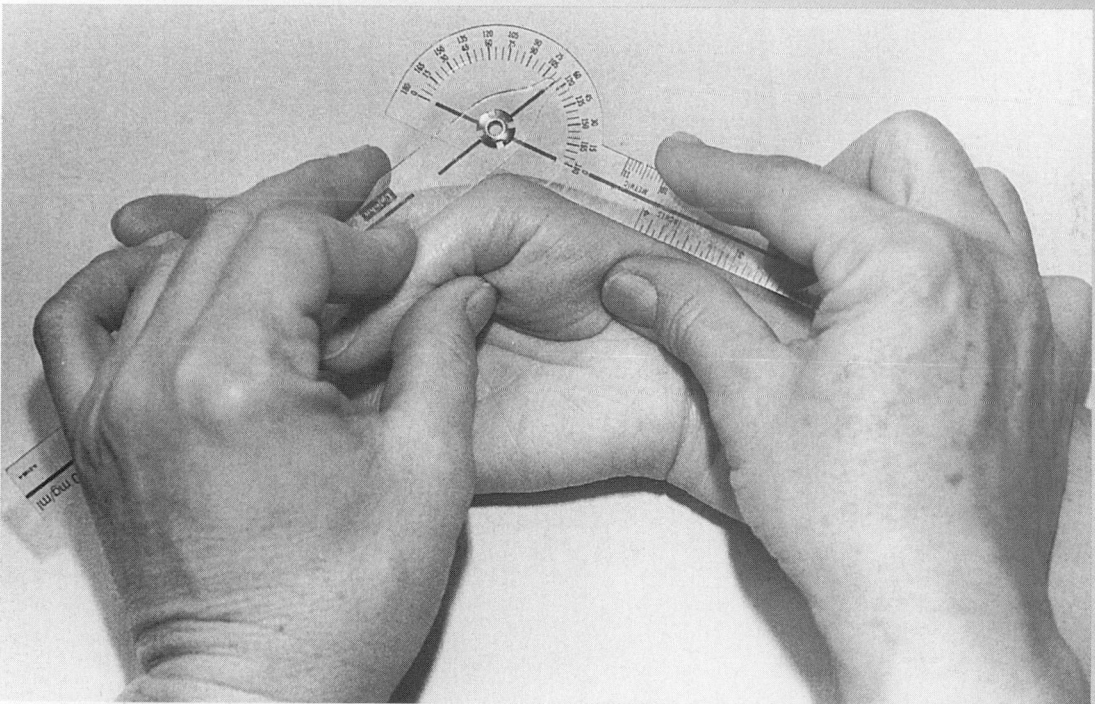

FIGURE 7.52 At the end of metacarpophalangeal (MCP) flexion, the examiner uses one hand to stabilize the subject's first metacarpal and align the proximal arm of the goniometer. The examiner uses her other hand to maintain the proximal phalanx in flexion and align the distal arm of the goniometer.

● THUMB: METACARPOPHALANGEAL EXTENSION

Motion occurs in the frontal plane around an anterior–posterior axis when the subject is in the anatomical position. Normal extension ROM values are 0 degrees according to the AAOS,[10,18] 40 degrees according to the AMA,[11] and 14 degrees (actively) and 23 degrees (passively) according to Skvarilova and Plevkova.[14] See Research Findings and Table 7.3 for additional normal ROM values.

Testing Position

Position the subject sitting, with the forearm and hand resting on a supporting surface. Place the forearm in full supination; the wrist in 0 degrees of flexion, extension, and radial and ulnar deviation; the CMC joint of the thumb in 0 degrees of flexion, extension, abduction, and opposition; and the IP joint of the thumb in 0 degrees of flexion and extension. (If the wrist and the IP joint of the thumb are positioned in full extension, tension in the flexor pollicis longus muscle may restrict the motion.)

Stabilization

Stabilize the first metacarpal to prevent motion at the wrist and at the CMC joint of the thumb.

Testing Motion

Extend the MCP joint by pushing on the palmar surface of the proximal phalanx, moving the thumb toward the radial aspect of the hand. The end of extension ROM occurs when resistance to further motion is felt and attempts to overcome the resistance cause the CMC joint to extend.

Normal End-Feel

The end-feel is firm because of tension in the palmar joint capsule, palmar plate (palmar ligament), inter-sesamoid (cruciate) ligaments, and flexor pollicis brevis muscle.

Goniometer Alignment

1. Center **fulcrum** of the goniometer over the dorsal aspect of the MCP joint.
2. Align **proximal arm** over the dorsal midline of the metacarpal.
3. Align **distal arm** with the dorsal midline of the proximal phalanx.

● THUMB: INTERPHALANGEAL FLEXION

Motion occurs in the frontal plane around an anterior–posterior axis when the subject is in the anatomical position. Normal ROM values for adults are 67 degrees according to Jenkins and associates[23] and 80 degrees according to the AAOS,[10,18] AMA,[11] DeSmet and colleagues,[22] and Skvarilova and Plevkova.[14] See Research Findings and Table 7.3 for additional normal ROM values.

Testing Position
Position the subject sitting, with the forearm and hand resting on a supporting surface. Place the forearm in full supination; the wrist in 0 degrees of flexion, extension, and radial and ulnar deviation; the CMC joint in 0 degrees of flexion, extension, abduction, and opposition; and the MCP joint of the thumb in 0 degrees of flexion and extension. (If the wrist and MCP joint of the thumb are flexed, tension in the extensor pollicis longus muscle may restrict the motion. If the MCP joint of the thumb is fully extended, tension in the abductor pollicis brevis and the oblique fibers of the adductor pollicis may restrict the motion through their insertion into the extensor mechanism.)

Stabilization
Stabilize the proximal phalanx to prevent flexion or extension of the MCP joint.

Testing Motion
Flex the IP joint by pushing on the dorsal surface of the distal phalanx, moving the tip of the thumb toward the ulnar aspect of the hand (Fig. 7.53). The end of flexion ROM occurs when resistance to further motion is felt and attempts to overcome the resistance cause the MCP joint to flex.

Normal End-Feel
Usually, the end-feel is firm because of tension in the collateral ligaments and the dorsal joint capsule. In some individuals, the end-feel may be hard because of contact between the palmar aspect of the distal phalanx, the palmar plate, and the proximal phalanx.

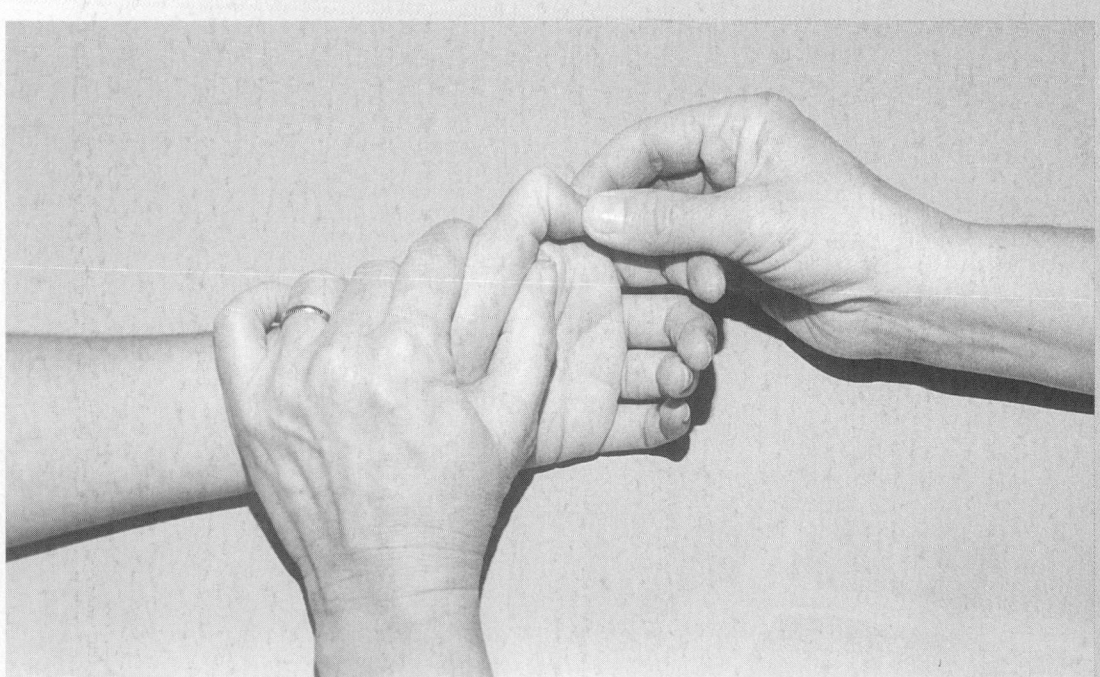

FIGURE 7.53 During interphalangeal (IP) flexion of the thumb, the examiner uses one hand to stabilize the proximal phalanx and keep the metacarpophalangeal joint in 0 degrees of flexion and the carpometacarpal joint in 0 degrees of flexion, abduction, and opposition. The examiner uses her other index finger and thumb to flex the distal phalanx.

Goniometer Alignment
See Figures 7.54 and 7.55.

1. Center **fulcrum** of the goniometer over the dorsal surface of the IP joint.
2. Align **proximal arm** with the dorsal midline of the proximal phalanx.
3. Align **distal arm** with the dorsal midline of the distal phalanx.

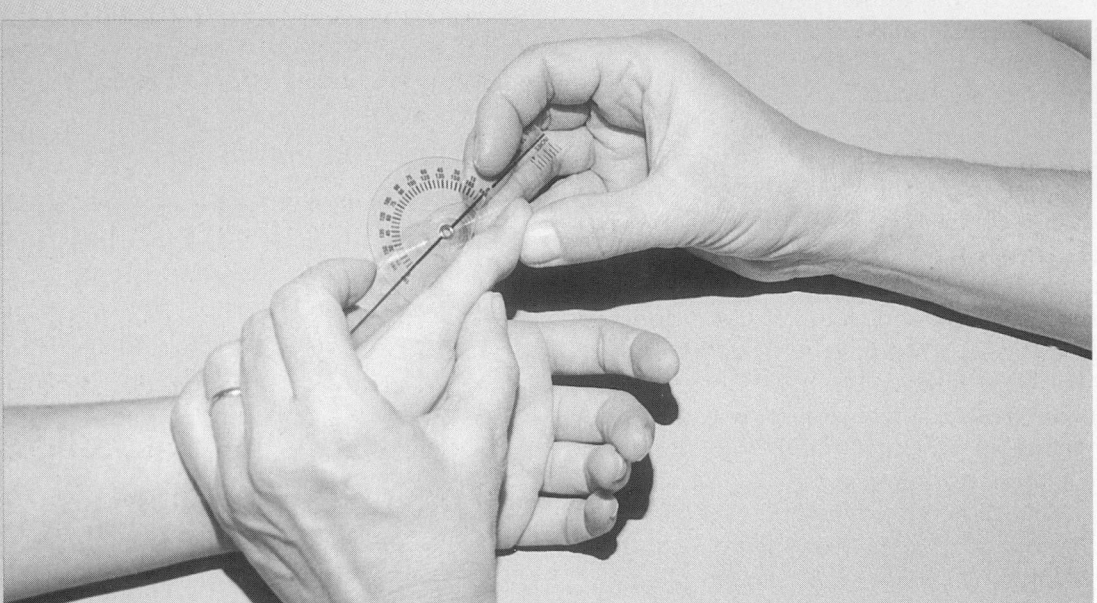

FIGURE 7.54 The alignment of the goniometer at the beginning of interphalangeal (IP) flexion range of motion. The arms of the goniometer are placed on the dorsal surfaces of the proximal and distal phalanges. However, the arms of the goniometer could instead be placed on the lateral surfaces of the proximal and distal phalanges if the nail protruded or if there was a bony prominence or swelling.

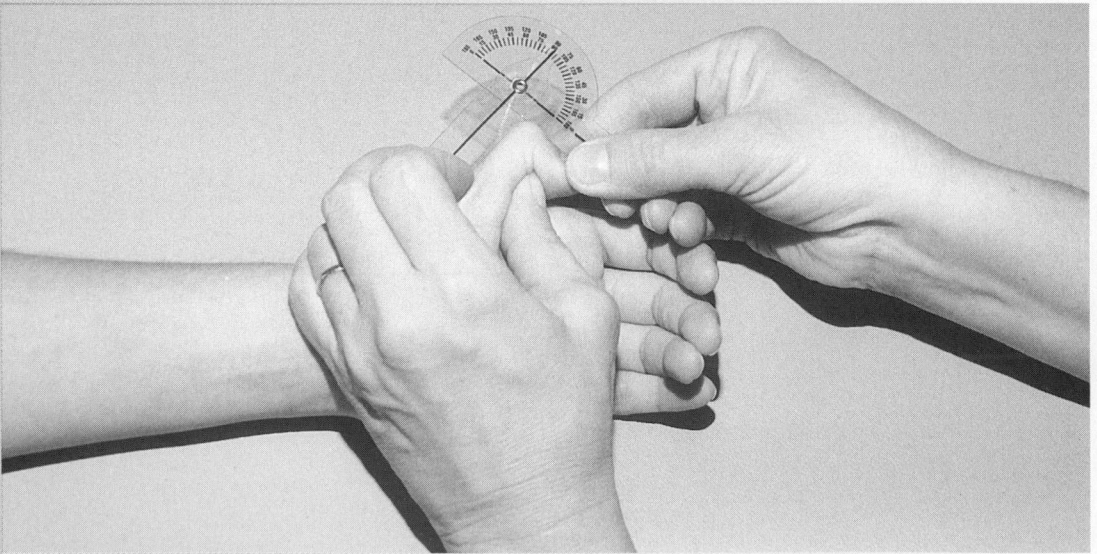

FIGURE 7.55 The alignment of the goniometer at the end of interphalangeal (IP) flexion range of motion. The examiner holds the arms of the goniometer so that they maintain close contact with the dorsal surfaces of the proximal and distal phalanges.

● THUMB: INTERPHALANGEAL EXTENSION

Motion occurs in the frontal plane around an anterior–posterior axis when the subject is in the anatomical position. Normal extension ROM at the IP joint of the thumb is 20 degrees according to the AAOS,[10] 30 degrees according to the AMA,[11] and 23 degrees (actively) and 35 degrees (passively) according to Skvarilova and Plevkova.[14] See Research Findings and Table 7.3 for additional normal ROM values.

Testing Position

Position the subject sitting, with the forearm and hand resting on a supporting surface forearm. Place the forearm in full supination; the wrist in 0 degrees of flexion, extension, and radial and ulnar deviation; the CMC joint of the thumb in 0 degrees of flexion, extension, abduction, and opposition; and the MCP joint of the thumb in 0 degrees of flexion and extension. (If the wrist and MCP joint of the thumb are extended, tension in the flexor pollicis longus muscle may restrict the motion.)

Stabilization

Stabilize the proximal phalanx to prevent extension or flexion of the MCP joint.

Testing Motion

Extend the IP joint by pushing on the palmar surface of the distal phalanx, moving the thumb toward the radial aspect of the hand. The end of extension ROM occurs when resistance to further motion is felt and attempts to overcome the resistance cause the MCP joint to extend.

Normal End-Feel

The end-feel is firm because of tension in the palmar joint capsule and the palmar plate (palmar ligament).

Goniometer Alignment

1. Center **fulcrum** of the goniometer over the dorsal surface of the IP joint.
2. Align **proximal arm** with the dorsal midline of the proximal phalanx.
3. Align **distal arm** with the dorsal midline of the distal phalanx.

MUSCLE LENGTH TESTING PROCEDURES:
Fingers

● LUMBRICALS, PALMAR INTEROSSEI, AND DORSAL INTEROSSEI

The lumbrical, palmar interossei, and dorsal interossei muscles cross the MCP, PIP, and DIP joints. The first and second lumbricals originate proximally from the radial sides of the tendons of the flexor digitorum profundus of the index and middle fingers, respectively (Fig. 7.56). The third lumbrical originates on the ulnar side of the tendon of the flexor digitorum profundus of the middle finger and the radial side of the tendon of the ring finger. The fourth lumbrical originates on the ulnar side of the tendon of the flexor digitorum profundus of the ring finger and the radial side of the tendon of the little finger. Each lumbrical passes to the radial side of the corresponding finger and inserts distally into the extensor mechanism of the extensor digitorum profundus.

The first palmar **interossei muscle** originates proximally from the ulnar side of the metacarpal of the index finger and inserts distally into the ulnar side of the proximal phalanx and the extensor mechanism of the extensor digitorum profundus of the same finger (Fig. 7.57). The second and third palmar interossei muscles originate proximally from the radial sides of the metacarpal of the ring and little fingers, respectively, and insert distally into the ulnar side of the proximal phalanx and the extensor mechanism of the extensor digitorum profundus of the same fingers.

The four **dorsal interossei** are bipenniform muscles that originate proximally from two adjacent metacarpals (Fig. 7.58): the first dorsal interossei from the metacarpals of the thumb and index finger, the second from the metacarpals of the index and middle fingers, the third from the metacarpals of the middle and ring fingers, and the fourth from the metacarpals of the ring and little fingers. The dorsal interossei insert distally into the bases of the proximal phalanges and the extensor mechanism of the extensor digitorum profundus of the same fingers.

When these muscles contract, they flex the MCP joints and extend the PIP and DIP joints. These muscles are passively lengthened by placing the MCP joints in extension and the PIP and DIP joints in full flexion. If the lumbricals and the palmar and dorsal interossei are short, they will limit MCP extension when the PIP and DIP joints are positioned in full flexion.

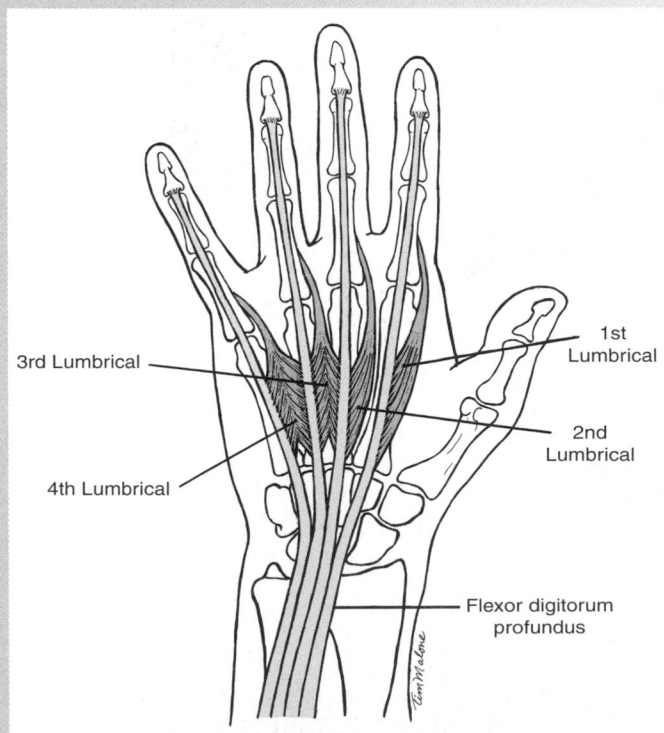

FIGURE 7.56 An anterior (palmar) view of the right hand showing the proximal attachments of the lumbricals. The lumbricals insert distally into the extensor digitorum on the posterior surface of the hand.

3rd Lumbrical

4th Lumbrical

1st Lumbrical

2nd Lumbrical

Flexor digitorum profundus

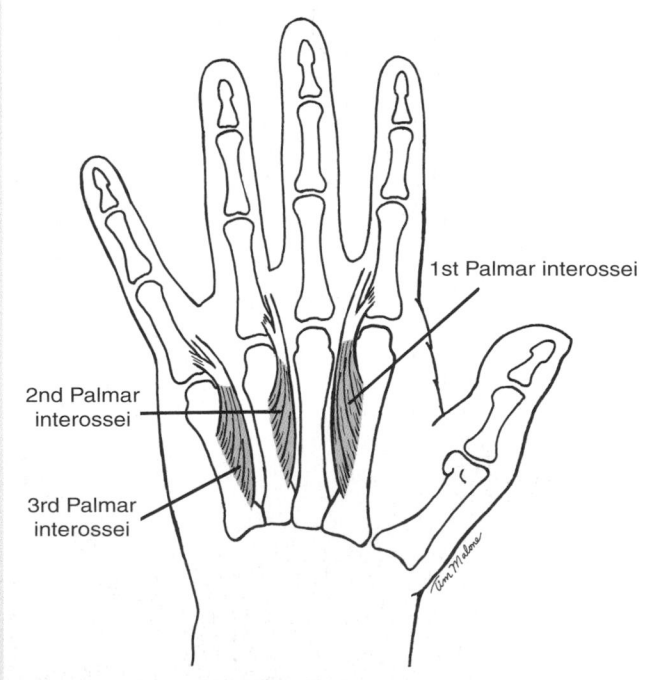

FIGURE 7.57 An anterior (palmar) view of the right hand showing the proximal and distal attachments of the palmar interossei. The palmar interossei also attach distally to the extensor digitorum on the posterior surface of the hand.

1st Palmar interossei

2nd Palmar interossei

3rd Palmar interossei

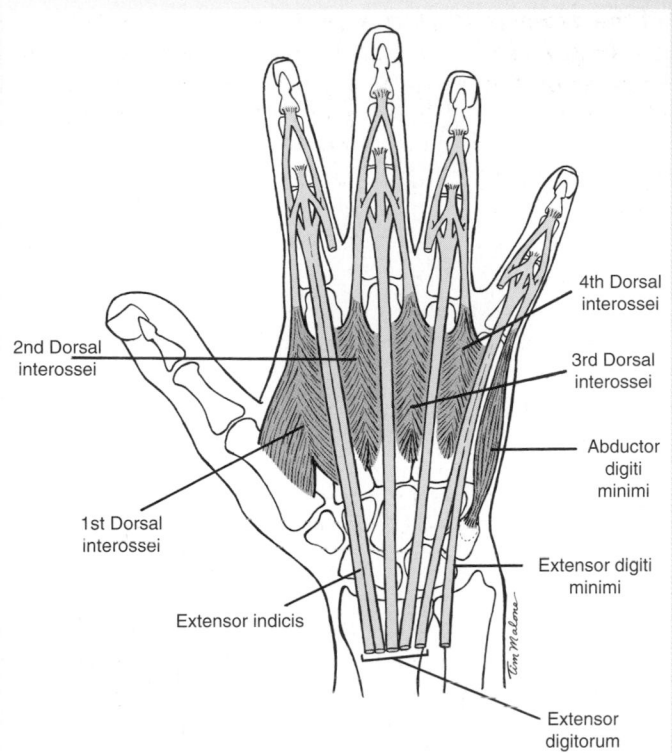

FIGURE 7.58 A posterior view of the right hand showing the proximal attachments of the dorsal interossei on the metacarpals and the distal attachments into the extensor mechanism of the extensor digitorum, extensor indicis, and extensor digiti minimi muscles.

If MCP flexion is limited regardless of the position of the PIP and DIP joints, the limitation is due to abnormalities of the joint surfaces of the MCP joint or shortening of the palmar joint capsule and the palmar plate.

Starting Position

Position the subject sitting, with the forearm and hand resting on a supporting surface. Place the forearm midway between pronation and supination and the wrist in 0 degrees of flexion, extension, and radial and ulnar deviation. Flex the MCP, PIP, and DIP joints (Fig. 7.59). The MCP joints should be in a neutral position relative to abduction and adduction.

Stabilization

Stabilize the metacarpals and the carpal bones to prevent wrist motion.

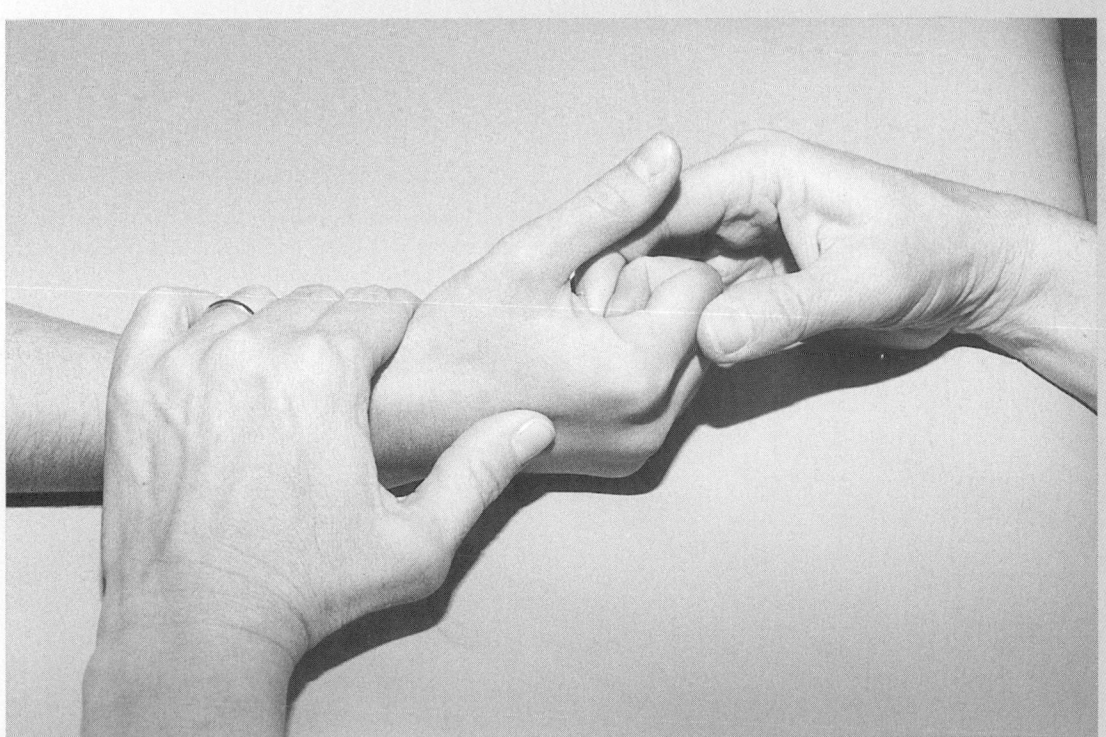

FIGURE 7.59 The starting position for testing the length of the lumbricals and the palmar and dorsal interossei. The examiner uses one hand to stabilize the subject's wrist and the other hand to position the subject's metacarpophalangeal, proximal interphalangeal, and distal interphalangeal joints in full flexion.

Testing Motion

Hold the PIP and DIP joints in full flexion while extending the MCP joint (Figs. 7.60 and 7.61). All of the fingers may be screened together, but if abnormalities are found, testing should be conducted on individual fingers. The end of flexion ROM occurs when resistance to further motion is felt and attempts to overcome the resistance cause the PIP, DIP, or wrist joints to extend.

Normal End-Feel

The end-feel is firm because of tension in the lumbrical, palmar, and dorsal interossei muscles.

Goniometer Alignment

See Figure 7.62.

1. Center **fulcrum** of the goniometer over the dorsal aspect of the MCP joint.
2. Align **proximal arm** over the dorsal midline of the metacarpal.
3. Align **distal arm** over the dorsal midline of the proximal phalanx.

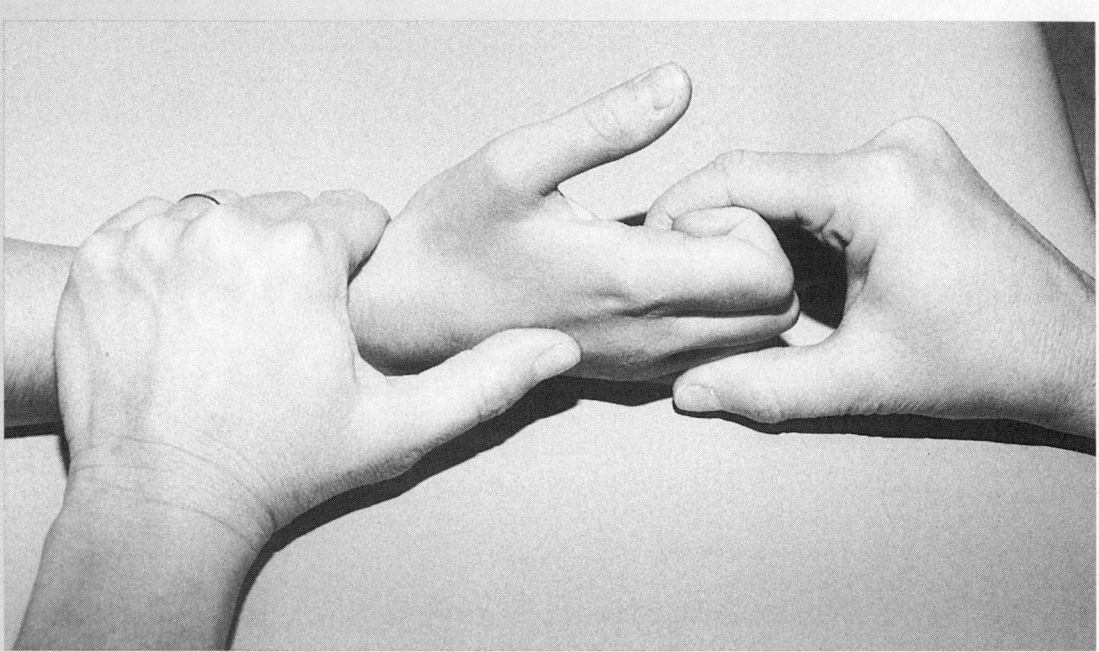

FIGURE 7.60 The end of the motion for testing the length of the lumbricals and the palmar and dorsal interossei. The examiner holds the subject's proximal interphalangeal and distal interphalangeal joints in full flexion while moving the metacarpophalangeal joint into extension.

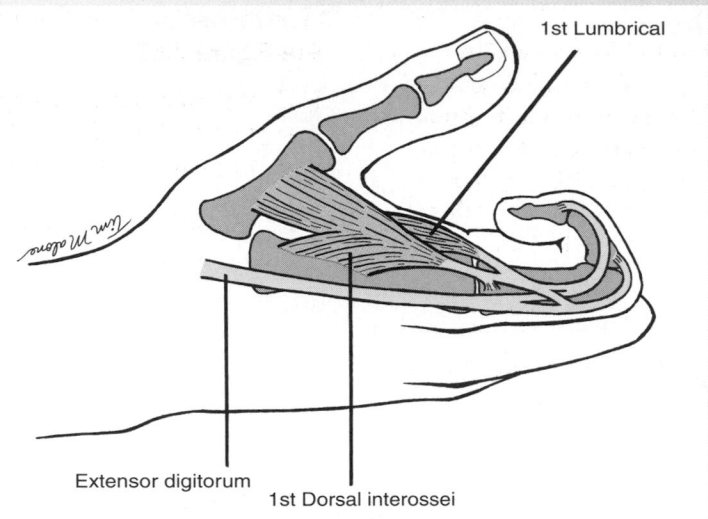

FIGURE 7.61 A lateral view of the right hand showing the first lumbrical and the first dorsal interossei muscles being stretched over the metacarpophalangeal, proximal interphalangeal, and distal interphalangeal joints.

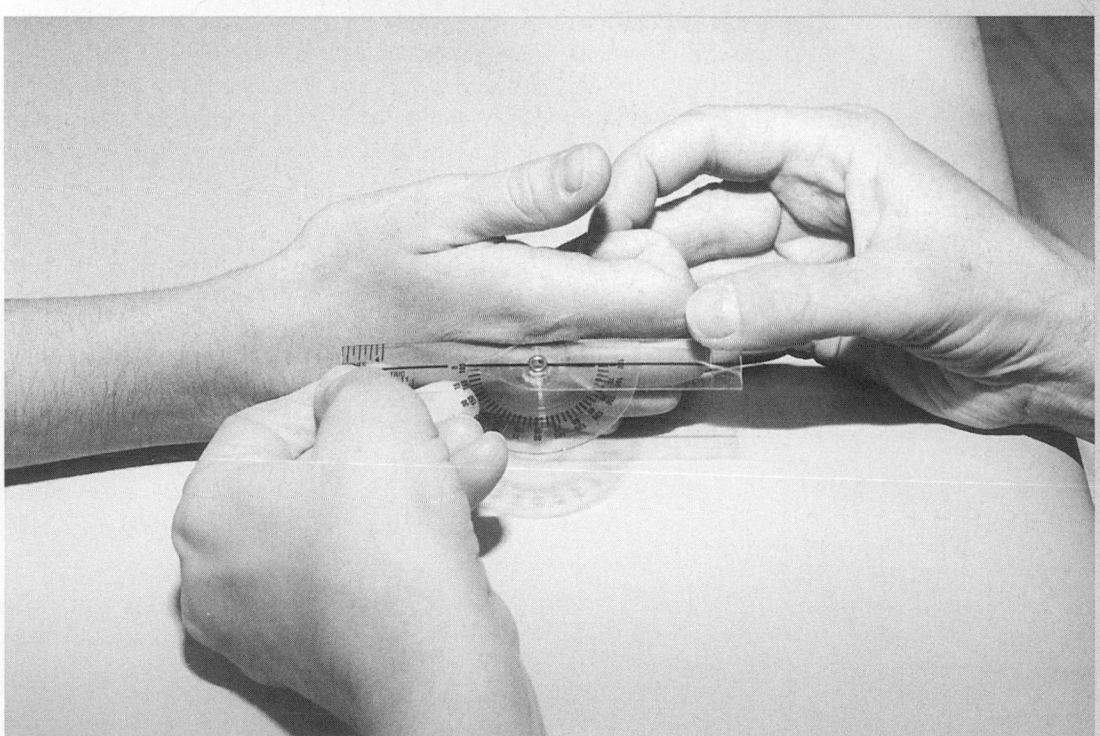

FIGURE 7.62 The alignment of the goniometer at the end of testing the length of the lumbricals and the palmar and dorsal interossei muscles. The arms of the goniometer are placed on the dorsal midline of the metacarpal and proximal phalanx of the finger being tested.

◯ Research Findings

Effects of Age, Gender, and Other Factors

Table 7.1 provides a summary of ROM values for the MCP, PIP, and DIP joints of the fingers. Certain trends are evident, although the values reported by the sources in Table 7.1 vary. The PIP joints, followed by the MCP and DIP joints, have the greatest amount of flexion. The MCP joints have the greatest amount of extension, whereas the PIP joints have the least amount of extension. Total active motion (TAM) is the sum of flexion and extension ROM of the MCP, PIP, and DIP joints of a digit. Normal TAM values range from 290 to 310 degrees for the fingers.

Mallon, Brown, and Nunley[13]; Skvarilova and Plevkova[14]; and Smahel and Klimova[15,24] also studied joint motion in individual fingers (Table 7.2). Some differences in ROM values are noted between the fingers. Flexion ROM at the MCP joints seems to increase linearly in an ulnar direction from the index finger to the little finger.[13–15] Mallon, Brown, and Nunley[13] report that extension at the MCP joints is approximately equal for all fingers. However, Skvarilova and Plevkova[14] and Smahel and Klimova[15] note that the little finger has the greatest amount of MCP extension. PIP flexion and extension and DIP flexion are generally equal for all fingers.[13] Some passive extension beyond neutral is possible at the DIP joints, with a minor increase in a radial direction from the little finger toward the index finger.[13]

Only the MCP joints of the fingers have a considerable amount of abduction–adduction. The amount of abduction–adduction varies with the position of the MCP joint. Abduction–adduction ROM is greatest in extension and least in full flexion. The collateral ligaments of the MCP joints are slack and allow full abduction in extension. However, the collateral ligaments tighten and restrict abduction in the fully flexed position.[1,3] Some authors note that the index and little fingers have a greater ROM in abduction–adduction than the middle and ring fingers,[1] whereas others report that the little finger has the greatest MCP abduction.[16]

Table 7.3 presents ROM values for the joints of the thumb. The greatest amount of flexion and extension ROM is reported at the IP joint.[10,11,14,18,22,23,25] Studies by Joseph[26] and Yoshida and coworkers[25] have identified two general anatomical shapes of the metacarpal head of the thumb. MCP joints with a round versus a flat metacarpal head had greater motion and may account for some of the variations seen in MCP values. Sauseng and coworkers[27] and Shaw and Morris[28] also present some normative data on MCP and IP flexion of the thumb. Very little data are available for normal values of motions at the CMC joint.

Age

Goniometric studies focusing on the effects of age on ROM typically exclude the joints of the fingers and thumb. However, among the limited number of studies that examined aging effects in the hand there appears to be less finger and thumb ROM with increasing age. DeSmet and colleagues[22] found a significant correlation between decreasing MCP and IP flexion of

		TABLE 7.1	**Active Finger Motion: Normal Values in Degrees from Selected Sources**			
		AAOS[10,18]	**AMA**[11]	**Hume**[12]	**Mallon***[13]	**Skvarilova†**[14]	**Smahel†**[15,24]
				26–28 yrs **n = 35 Males**	**18–35 yrs** **n = 60 Males,** **60 Females**	**20–25 yrs** **n = 100 Males,** **100 Females**	**18–28 yrs** **n = 52 Males,** **49 Females**
Joint	*Motion*			*Mean*	*Mean*	*Mean (SD)*	*Mean (SD)*
MCP	Flexion	90	90	100	95	91.0 (6.2)	91.9 (8.0)
	Extension	45	20	0	20	25.8 (6.7)	24.8 (7.2)
PIP	Flexion	100	100	105	105	107.9 (5.6)	110.7 (5.3)
	Extension	0	0	0	7	—	—
DIP	Flexion	90	70	85	68	84.5 (7.9)	81.3 (7.0)
	Extension	0	0	0	8	—	—
Total active motion		—	—	290	303	309.2 (6.6)	308.7 (6.8)

AAOS = American Association of Orthopaedic Surgeons; AMA = American Medical Association; DIP = distal interphalangeal; MCP = metacarpophalangeal; PIP = proximal interphalangeal; SD = standard deviation.
* Values were averaged from both genders and all fingers.
† Values were averaged from both genders, both hands, and all fingers and were converted from a 360-degree to a 180-degree recording system.

| TABLE 7.2 | Individual Finger Motion: Mean Values in Degrees From Selected Sources |

Finger	Joint	Motion	Mallon[13] Passive ROM 18–35 yrs		Skvarilova*[14] Passive ROM 20–25 yrs		Smahel*[15,24] Active ROM 18–28 yrs	
			Male n = 60	Female n = 60	Male n = 100	Female n = 100	Male n = 52	Female n = 49
Index	MCP	Flexion	94	95	97	97	87	87
		Extension	29	56	55	56	22	26
	PIP	Flexion	106	107	115	117	111	113
		Extension	11	19	—	—	—	—
	DIP	Flexion	75	75	87	95	78	80
		Extension	22	24	—	—	—	—
Middle	MCP	Flexion	98	100	102	104	95	94
		Extension	34	54	48	48	20	24
	PIP	Flexion	110	112	115	118	111	114
		Extension	10	20	—	—	—	—
	DIP	Flexion	80	79	87	98	84	83
		Extension	19	23	—	—	—	—
Ring	MCP	Flexion	102	103	104	102	94	93
		Extension	29	60	48	49	21	25
	PIP	Flexion	110	108	115	119	112	115
		Extension	14	20	—	—	—	—
	DIP	Flexion	74	76	83	92	80	78
		Extension	17	18	—	—	—	—
Little	MCP	Flexion	107	107	107	104	93	93
		Extension	48	62	63	65	27	32
	PIP	Flexion	111	110	111	113	104	106
		Extension	13	21	—	—	—	—
	DIP	Flexion	72	72	89	102	83	84
		Extension	15	21	—	—	—	—

DIP = distal interphalangeal; MCP = metacarpophalangeal; PIP = proximal interphalangeal.
* Values were converted from a 360-degree to a 180-degree recording system.

the thumb and increasing age. The 58 females and 43 males who were included in the study ranged in age from 16 to 83 years. Smahel and Klimova,[15,24] in studies of 101 university students, 60 senior citizens, and 52 pianists, found that the senior citizens had significantly less MCP, PIP, and DIP ranges of motion in the fingers than the university students, except for total abduction (ability to spread fingers) of the MCP joints in females. The mean age differences were 6.3 degrees for active MCP flexion, 6.1 degrees for active MCP extension, 20.4 degrees for passive MCP extension, 9.1 degrees for active PIP flexion, and 9.5 degrees for active DIP flexion. The age differences in ROM were generally greater in males than in females.

Measures of hypermobility that include motions of the thumb and little finger have shown a decrease with age. Beighton, Solomon, and Soskolne[29] used passive apposition of the thumb (with wrist flexion) to the anterior aspect of the forearm and passive hyperextension of the MCP joint of the fifth finger beyond 90 degrees as indicators of hypermobility in a study of 456 men and 625 women in an African village. They found that joint laxity decreased with age. Lamari and coworkers,[30] in a study that included similar measures of hypermobility in the thumb/wrist and little finger of 1120 healthy Brazilian children between the ages of 4 to 7 years, found that lower hypermobility scores were associated with increasing age, even within this limited age range. Overall, 76 percent of the children were able to apposition the thumb to the forearm and 53 percent were able to hyperextend the MCP joint of the little finger beyond 90 degrees. Significant age differences were present in both genders for thumb apposition but only in boys for little finger hyperextension.

| TABLE 7.3 | | Thumb Motion: Mean Values in Degrees from Selected Sources | | | | | |

Joint	Motion	AAOS[10,18]	AMA[11]	Jenkins[23] 16-72 yrs n = 50 Males, 69 Females Active Mean (SD)	DeSmet[22] 16-83 yrs n = 43 Males, 58 Females Mean (SD)	Yoshida[25] 18-63 yrs n = 51 Males, 49 Females Active Mean (SD)	Skvarilova*[14] 20-25 yrs n=100 Males, 100 Females Active Mean (SD)	Skvarilova*[14] Passive Mean (SD)
CMC	Abduction	70						
	Flexion	15						
	Extension	20, 80	35†					
MCP	Flexion	50	60	59 (11)	54.0 (13.7)	77	57.0 (10.7)	67.0 (9.0)
	Extension	0	40			35	13.7 (10.5)	22.6 (10.9)
IP	Flexion	80	80	67 (11)	79.8 (10.2)	81	79.1 (8.7)	85.8 (8.3)
	Extension	20	30			33	23.2 (13.3)	34.7 (13.3)

CMC = carpometacarpal; IP = interphalangeal; MCP = metacarpophalangeal; SD = standard deviation.
* Values were recalculated to include both thumbs for both genders and were converted from a 360-degree to a 180-degree recording system.
† The AMA reports that in this plane of motion the minimal angle of separation between the first and second metacarpal is 15 degrees, whereas the maximal angle of separation between the first and second metacarpals is 50 degrees. The ROM value of 35 degrees is the difference between these two measurements.

One study by Allander and associates[31] found that active flexion and passive extension of the MCP joint of the thumb demonstrated no consistent pattern of age-related effects in a study of 517 women and 208 men (between 33 and 70 years of age). These authors stated that the typical reduction in mobility with age resulting from degenerative arthritis found in other joints may be exceeded by an accumulation of ligamentous ruptures that reduce the stability of the first MCP joint.

Gender

Studies that examined the effect of gender on the ROM of the fingers reported varying results. Mallon, Brown, and Nunley[13] found no significant effect of gender on the amount of flexion in any joints of the fingers. However, in this study women generally had more extension at all joints of the fingers than men. Skvarilova and Plevkova[14] found that PIP flexion, DIP flexion, and MCP extension of the fingers were greater in women than in men, whereas MCP flexion of the fingers was greater in men. Smahel and Klimova[15] reported that MCP extension was significantly greater in women versus men in both groups of young and older adults, whereas no gender differences were noted in MCP flexion. In a study of PIP and DIP joint ROM of the fingers, Smahel and Klimova[24] found that women had greater PIP flexion than men, but they did not differ in DIP flexion (see Table 7.2).

Several studies have found no significant differences between males and females in the ROM of the thumb, whereas other studies have reported more mobility in females. Joseph[26] used radiographs to examine MCP and IP flexion ROM of the thumb in 90 males and 54 females; no significant differences were found between the two groups. He found two general shapes of MCP joints, round and flat, with the round MCP joints having greater range of flexion. Shaw and Morris[28] noted no differences in MCP and IP flexion ROM between 199 males and 149 females aged 16 to 86 years. Likewise, DeSmet and colleagues,[22] as well as Jenkins and associates,[23] found no differences in MCP and IP flexion of the thumb owing to gender.

Allander and associates[31] found that, in some age groups, females showed more mobility in the MCP joint of the thumb than their male counterparts. Skvarilova and Plevkova[14] noted that MCP flexion and extension of the thumb were greater in females, whereas gender differences were small and unimportant at the IP joint. Yoshida and associates,[25] in a study of 51 healthy men, 49 healthy women, and 70 cadavers, identified two general shapes of the metacarpal head: round and flat. The female gender was associated with greater MCP joint ROM and a higher prevalence of a round metacarpal head. No gender differences were noted in ROM at the IP joint. Beighton, Solomon, and Soskolne[29] in a study of 456 men and 625 women of an African village; Fairbank, Pynsett, and Phillips[32] in a study of 227 male and 219 female adolescents; and Lamari and coworkers[30] in a study of 1120 young Brazilian children measured passive apposition of the thumb toward the anterior surface of the forearm and hyperextension of the MCP joints of the fifth or middle fingers. All three studies reported an increase in laxity in females as compared with males.

Right Versus Left Sides

The studies that have compared ROM in the right and left joints of the fingers have generally found no significant difference between sides or only a small increase in motion on the left side. Mallon, Brown, and Nunley,[13] in a study in which half of the 120 subjects were right-handed and the other half left-handed, noted no difference between sides in finger motions at the MCP, PIP, and DIP joints. Skvarilova and Plevkova[14] reported only small right-left differences in the majority of the joints of the fingers and thumb in 200 subjects. Only MCP extension of the fingers and thumb and IP flexion of the thumb seemed to have greater ROM values on the left. Smahel and Klimova,[15,24] in studies of 101 university students, 60 senior citizens, and 52 pianists, found that in all three groups MCP joint ROM of the fingers was greater in the left hand. However, in most instances, ROM differences between the left and right hands were not significant for PIP and DIP joints of the fingers.

Similar to findings in studies of the fingers, most studies have reported no difference in ROM between the right and left thumbs. Joseph[26] and Shaw and Morris,[28] in a study of 144 and 248 subjects, respectively, found no significant difference between sides in MCP and IP flexion ROM of the thumb. DeSmet and colleagues[22] examined 101 healthy subjects and reported no difference between sides for the MCP and IP joints of the thumb. No difference between sides in IP flexion of the thumb was found by Jenkins and associates[23] in a study of 119 subjects. A statistically significant greater amount of MCP flexion was reported for the right thumb than for the left; however, this difference was only 2 degrees. Allander and associates[31] also found no differences attributed to side in MCP motions of the thumb in 720 subjects.

Testing Position

Mallon, Brown, and Nunley,[13] in addition to establishing normative ROM values for the fingers, also studied passive joint ROM while positioning the next most proximal joint in maximal flexion and extension. The DIP joint had significantly more flexion (18 degrees) when the PIP joint was flexed than when the PIP joint was extended. This finding has been cited as an indication of abnormal tightness of the oblique retinacular ligament (Landsmeer's ligament).[33] However, the results of Mallon, Brown, and Nunley's study[13] suggest that this finding is normal. The MCP joint had about 6 degrees more flexion when the wrist was extended than when the wrist was flexed, although this difference was not statistically significant. The extensor digitorum, extensor indicis, and extensor digiti minimi were more slack to allow greater flexion of the MCP joint when the wrist was extended than when flexed. There was no effect on PIP motion with changes in MCP joint position.

Knutson and associates[34] examined eight subjects to study the effect of seven wrist positions on the torque required to passively move the MCP joint of the index finger. The findings indicated that in many wrist positions, extrinsic tissues (those that cross more than one joint) such as the extensor digitorum, extensor indicis, flexor digitorum superficialis, and flexor digitorum profundus muscles offered greater restraint to MCP flexion and extension than intrinsic tissues (those that cross only one joint). Intrinsic tissues offered greater resistance to passive moment at the MCP joint when the wrist was flexed or extended enough to slacken the extrinsic tissues.

Functional Range of Motion

Joint motion, muscular strength and control, sensation, adequate finger length, and sufficient palm width and depth are necessary for a hand that is capable of performing functional, occupational, and recreational activities. Numerous classification systems and terms for describing functional hand patterns have been proposed.[23,35–38] Some common patterns include (1) finger-thumb prehension such as tip (Fig. 7.63), pulp, lateral, and three-point pinch (Fig. 7.64); (2) full-hand prehension, also called a power grip or cylindrical grip (Fig. 7.65); (3) nonprehension, which requires parts of the hand to be used as an extension of the upper extremity; and (4) bilateral prehension, which requires use of the palmar surfaces of both hands.[36] Texts by Stanley and Tribuzi,[39] Mackin and associates,[40] and the American Society of Hand Therapists[19] have reviewed many functional patterns and tests for the hand.

Table 7.4 summarizes the active ROM of the dominant fingers and thumb during 11 activities of daily living that

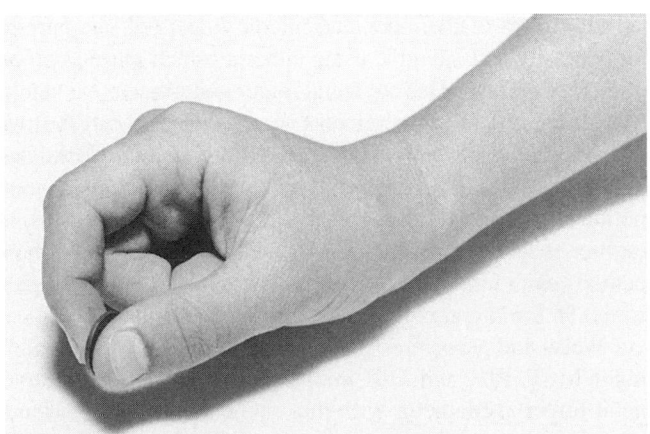

FIGURE 7.63 Picking up a coin is an example of finger–thumb prehension that requires use of the tips or pulps of the digits. In this photograph the pulp of the thumb and the tip of the index finger are being used.

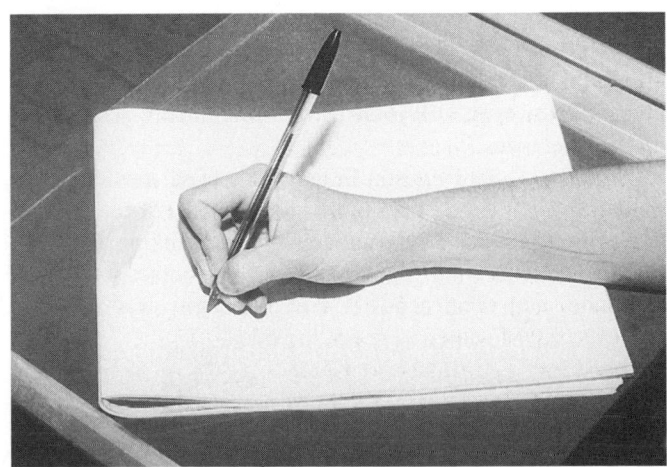

FIGURE 7.64 Writing usually requires finger–thumb prehension in the form of a three-point pinch.

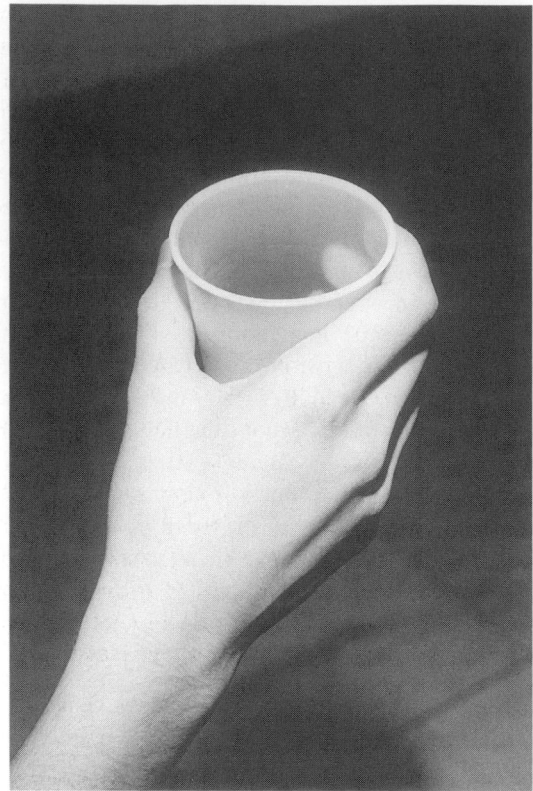

FIGURE 7.65 Holding a cylinder such as a cup requires full-hand prehension (power grip). The amount of metacarpophalangeal and proximal interphalangeal flexion varies, depending on the diameter of the cylinder.

TABLE 7.4	Finger and Thumb Motions During 11 Functional Activities: Values in Degrees[12]		
Motion	**Range**	**Mean**	**SD**
Finger MCP flexion	33–73	61	(12)
PIP flexion	36–86	60	(12)
IP flexion	20–61	39	(14)
Thumb MCP flexion	10–32	21	(5)
IP flexion	2–43	18	(5)

IP = interphalangeal; MCP = metacarpophalangeal; PIP = proximalinterphalangeal; SD = standard deviation.
The 11 functional activities include holding a telephone, can, fork, scissors, toothbrush, and hammer; using a zipper and comb; turning a key; printing with a pen; and unscrewing a jar.

require various types of finger–thumb prehension or full-hand prehension. Hume and coworkers[12] used an electrogoniometer and a universal goniometer to study 35 right-handed men aged 26 to 28 years during performance of these 11 tasks. Of the tasks that were included, holding a soda can required the least amount of finger and thumb motion, whereas holding a toothbrush required the most motion.

Lee and Rim[41] examined the amount of motion required at the joints of the fingers to grip five different-size cylinders. Data were collected from four subjects by means of markers and multi-camera photogrammetry. As cylinder diameter decreased, the amount of flexion of the MCP and PIP joints increased. However, DIP joint flexion remained constant with all cylinder sizes.

Sperling and Jacobson-Sollerman[42] used movie film in their study of the grip pattern of 15 men and 15 women aged 19 to 56 years during serving, eating, and drinking activities. The use of different digits, types of grips, contact surfaces of the hand, and relative position of the digits was reported; however, ROM values were not included.

Reliability

Several studies have been conducted to assess the reliability of goniometric measurements in the hand. Most studies found that ROM measurements of the fingers and thumb that were taken with universal goniometers and finger goniometers were highly reliable. Measurements taken over the dorsal surface of the digits appear to be similar to those taken laterally. Consistent with other regions of the body, measurements of finger and thumb ROM taken by one examiner are more reliable than measurements taken by several examiners. Research studies support the opinions of Bear-Lehman and Abreu[43] and Adams, Greene, and Topoozian,[19] which are that the margin of error is generally accepted to be 5 degrees for goniometric measurement of joints in the hand, provided that measurements are taken by the same examiner and that standardized techniques are employed.

Hamilton and Lachenbruch[44] had seven testers take measurements of MCP, PIP, and DIP flexion in one subject whose fingers were held in a fixed position. The daily measurements were taken for 4 days with three types of goniometers. These authors found intertester reliability was lower than intratester reliability. No significant differences existed between measurements taken with a dorsal (over-the-joint) finger goniometer, a universal goniometer, or a pendulum goniometer.

Groth and coworkers[45] had 39 therapists measure the PIP and DIP joints of the index and middle fingers of one patient, both dorsally and laterally, using either a 6-inch plastic universal goniometer or a DeVore metal finger goniometer. No significant difference in measurements was found between the two instruments. No differences were found between the dorsal and lateral measurement methods for seven of the eight joint motions, with mean differences ranging from 2 to 0 degrees. In a subset of six therapists, intertester reliability was high for both methods, with intraclass correlation coefficients (ICCs) ranging from 0.86 for lateral methods to 0.99 for dorsal methods.

Weiss and associates[46] compared measurements of index finger MCP, PIP, and DIP joint positions taken by a dorsal metal finger goniometer with those taken by the Exos Handmaster, a Hall-effect instrumented exoskeleton. Twelve subjects were measured with each device during one session by one examiner and again within 2 weeks of the initial session. Test-retest reliability was high for both devices, with ICCs ranging from 0.98 to 0.99. Mean differences between sessions for each instrument were statistically significant but less than 1 degree. Measurements taken by the finger goniometer and those taken by the Exos Handmaster were significantly different (mean difference = 7 degrees) but highly correlated (r = 0.89 to 0.94).

Ellis, Bruton, and Goddard[47] placed one subject in two splints while a total of 40 therapists measured the MCP, PIP, and DIP joints of the middle finger by means of a dorsal finger goniometer and a wire tracing. Each therapist measured each joint three times with each device. The goniometer consistently produced smaller ranges and smaller standard deviations than the wire tracing, indicating better reliability for the goniometer. The 95 percent confidence limit for the difference between measurements ranged from 3.8 to 9.9 degrees for the goniometer and 8.9 to 13.2 degrees for the wire tracing. Both methods had more variability when distal joints were measured, possibly because of the shorter levers used to align the goniometer or wire. Intratester reliability was always higher than intertester reliability.

Brown and colleagues[48] evaluated the ROM of the MCP, PIP, and DIP joints of two fingers in 30 patients to calculate total active motion (TAM) by means of the dorsal finger goniometer and the computerized Dexter Hand Evaluation and Treatment System. Three therapists measured each finger three times with each device during one session. Intratester and intertester reliability were high for both methods, with ICCs ranging from 0.97 to 0.99. The mean difference between methods ranged from 0.1 degrees to 2.4 degrees.

Goldsmith and Juzl[49] studied the intratester reliability of measuring active ROM of the MCP, PIP, and DIP joints of the fingers in 12 healthy subjects and intertester reliability in 12 patients with hand conditions. A universal goniometer adapted for measuring the hand (one short arm) was applied over the dorsal surface. The two therapists each took three measurements of flexion and extension at each joint in one session to assess intratester reliability and one measurement of flexion and extension at each involved joint in one session to assess intertester reliability. Both intratester and intertester reliability were high with correlation coefficients greater than 0.99. When agreement was defined as within 3 degrees, the percent agreement was 93.9 to 94.6 percent for intratester reliability and 67.7 percent for intertester reliability. When agreement was defined as within 5 degrees, the percent agreement was 99.7 percent to 100 percent for intratester reliability and 87.1 percent for intertester reliability.

Sauseng and coworkers,[27] in a study of 50 patients with type 1 diabetes mellitus and 44 healthy controls, measured active ROM of the fifth MCP joint, first MCP joint, first IP joint, wrist, ankle, and first metatarsal phalangeal joint with a pocket goniometer. Each motion was measured three times by one tester. The coefficients of variation for the measurements were between 1.3 percent and 8.2 percent. The ROM of all tested joints was significantly lower in the diabetic versus the control group except for the first IP and MTP joints.

The distance between the fingertip pulp and distal palmar crease has been suggested as a simple and quick method of estimating total finger flexion ROM at the MCP, PIP, and DIP joints.[18,19] Ellis and Bruton[17] examined the intratester and intertester reliability of composite finger flexion (CFF) and compared it to dorsal goniometric measures of PIP flexion of the index, middle, and ring fingers. One hand was splinted in three positions and measured three times by 51 therapists at 18 hospital sites with a ruler and goniometer. Intratester goniometric measurements fell within 4 to 5 degrees of each other 95 percent of the time, whereas intertester goniometric measurements fell within 7 to 9 degrees of each other 95 percent of the time. CFF measures fell within 5 to 6 mm of each other 95 percent of the time for intratester measurements and within 7 to 9 mm of each other for intertester measurements. After scaling the two methods to allow comparison, the goniometer provided better reliability than CFF for measurements taken by the same tester, but both methods were equally reliable for measurements taken by different testers. The authors suggested that CFF may be a useful alternative when multiple joint measures are needed or when goniometry is impractical.

Validity

Goniometric measurements of the fingers have been compared to radiographs, digital photographs, and disability measures in patient populations. In a study by Groth and coworkers,[45] active ROM of the PIP and DIP joints of the index and middle fingers of one patient who had sustained a crush injury with multiple fractures was measured by 39 therapists over a 3-day period. Measurements were made dorsally and laterally using either a DeVore metal finger goniometer or a 6-inch plastic universal goniometer. Prior to the goniometer measurements, radiographs were taken. In terms of concurrent validity, there were significant differences in measurements obtained from radiographs versus those from goniometers except for laterally measured index finger PIP extension and flexion. Differences between radiographic and mean goniometric measurements ranged from 1 to 2 degrees for laterally and dorsally measured index finger PIP motions to 14 degrees for laterally and dorsally measured middle finger PIP motions. The authors noted that concurrent validity was inconclusive because some of these differences may have been due to variations in the patient instructions for performing active motion, patient positioning, and patient fatigue with multiple active measurements.

Kato and coworkers[50] compared the accuracy of three therapists measuring PIP joint angles using three types of universal goniometers to lateral x-ray films in 16 fingers fixated with Kirschner wires from four cadavers. Each examiner used a 6-inch plastic goniometer with 6-inch arms, a plastic goniometer with a 3.5-inch and a 1-inch arm, and a metal goniometer with 1.5-inch arms to take measurements on the lateral and dorsal surfaces of the fingers. Intertester reliability was good with Pearson correlation coefficients ranging from 0.80 to 0.82. The mean angle discrepancies between the goniometers and x-rays ranged from 1.2 to 3.3 degrees (SD = 3.5 to 6.0 degrees) for the lateral method and from 0.5 to 2.9 degrees (SD = 3.5 to 6.4 degrees) for the dorsal method. There was no difference in angle discrepancies between types of goniometer using the lateral method. However, with two testers using the dorsal method the angle discrepancy was greater with the plastic goniometer with 6-inch arms, perhaps due to having longer arms than the other two goniometers.

In a study by Georgeu and associates,[51] one therapist measured full active flexion and extension of the MCP, PIP, and DIP joints of the little or ring finger in 20 patients. A digital camera, aligned with the MCP joint with the hand placed in a stabilizing device, was integrated with a computer to also determine ROM. There was a high correlation between the two methods (r^2 = 0.975). The photograph-computer method averaged 1 degree (95-percent confidence interval = 0 to 2 degrees, SD = 6 degrees) greater than the goniometer method but was not significantly different. The 95 percent level of agreement was –11 to 13 degrees.

Goodson and associates[52] measured ROM of the wrist, MCP and IP joints of the fingers with goniometers applied to the dorsal surface, pinch/grip strength, and pain and disability scoring (Cochin Scale) in 10 patients with rheumatoid arthritis, 10 patients with osteoarthritis, and 10 healthy control subjects. ROM and pinch/grip measurements were able to clearly discriminate between patient groups, which pain and disability scales were unable to do. Patients with rheumatoid arthritis had the greatest reduction in ROM of the MCP, followed by wrist and PIP joints. Patients with osteoarthritis had the greatest reduction in ROM at the DIP followed by the PIP joints. In the rheumatoid arthritis group, ROM of the MCP joints correlated with disability scores (R^2 = 0.31) and time since initial diagnosis (R^2 = 0.32). Wrist ROM was also related to time since diagnosis (R^2 = 0.37). The authors concluded that ROM and pinch/grip strength may more accurately reflect functional impairment associated with arthritis than pain and disability measures.

Field[53] studied 100 patients with Colles fractures of the wrist for the development of algodystrophy (complex regional pain syndrome). ROM of the PIP, DIP, and MCP joints of the fingers was measured at 1, 5, and 9 weeks on the dorsal surfaces with a finger goniometer and summed to generate a total ROM value for the hand. Pain response to pressure was assessed with a dolorimeter. Swelling was assessed using a water displacement method. Differences between the affected and unaffected hands were used in statistical tests. At 9 weeks postfracture, 24 patients were diagnosed with algodystrophy. Goniometry ROM measurements at 1 week showed a sensitivity of 96 percent and a specificity of 59 percent in predicting the development of algodystrophy. The cutoff for a positive test appeared to be about 70 degrees of ROM loss in the affected hand. The combination of dolorimetry and goniometry resulted in a sensitivity of 96 percent and improved specificity to 73 percent.

MacDermid and coworkers[54] studied the validity of using fingertip pulp-to-palm distance versus total finger flexion (also called composite finger flexion) to predict disability as measured by an upper-extremity disability score (Disabilities of the Arm, Shoulder, and Hand, or DASH). Active MCP, PIP, and DIP flexion of the most severely affected finger was measured in 50 patients by one examiner who used a dorsally placed electrogoniometer NK Hand Assessment System. A micrometer tool was used to measure pulp-to-palm distance in the same patients. The correlation between pulp-to-palm distance and total active flexion was –0.46 to –0.51, indicating that the measures were related but were not interchangeable. The relationship between DASH scores and total active flexion was stronger (r = 0.45) than the relationship between DASH scores and pulp-to-palm distances (r = 0.21 to 0.30). The authors suggested that total active motion is a more functional measure than pulp-to-palm distance and that pulp-to-palm distance "should only be used to monitor individual patient progress and not to compare outcomes between patients or groups of patients."

REFERENCES

1. Levangie, PL, and Norkin, CC: Joint Structure and Function: A Comprehensive Analysis, ed 4. FA Davis, Philadelphia, 2005.
2. Standring, S (ed): Gray's Anatomy, ed 39. Elsevier, New York, 2005.
3. Tubiana, R: Architecture and functions of the hand. In Tubiana, R, Thomine, JM, and Mackin, E (eds): Examination of the Hand and Upper Limb. WB Saunders, Philadelphia, 1984.
4. Krishnan, J, and Chipchase, L: Passive axial rotation of the metacarpophalangeal joint. J Hand Surg 22B:270, 2000.
5. Newmann, DA: Kinesiology of the Musculoskeletal System. Mosby, St. Louis, 2002.
6. Cyriax, JH, and Cyriax, PJ: Illustrated Manual of Orthopaedic Medicine. Butterworths, London, 1983.
7. Kaltenborn, FM: Manual Mobilization of the Joints: The Extremities, ed 5. Olaf Norlis Bokhandel, Oslo, Norway, 1999.
8. Ranney, D: The hand as a concept: Digital differences and their importance. Clin Anat 8:281, 1995.
9. Groth, GN, and Ehretsman, RL: Goniometry of the proximal and distal interphalangeal joints, part I: A survey of instrumentation and placement preferences. J Hand Ther 14:18, 2001.
10. American Academy of Orthopaedic Surgeons: Joint Motion: Methods of Measuring and Recording. AAOS, Chicago, 1965.
11. Cocchiarella, L, and Andersson, GBJ (eds): American Medical Association: Guides to the Evaluation of Permanent Impairment, ed 5. AMA Press, Chicago, 2001.
12. Hume, M, et al: Functional range of motion of the joints of the hand. J Hand Surg (Am) 15:240, 1990.
13. Mallon, WJ, Brown, HR, and Nunley, JA: Digital ranges of motion: Normal values in young adults. J Hand Surg (Am) 16:882, 1991.
14. Skvarilova, B, and Plevkova, A: Ranges of joint motion of the adult hand. Acta Chir Plast 38:67, 1996.
15. Smahel, Z, and Klimova, A: The influence of age and exercise on the mobility of hand joints: 1: Metacarpophalangeal joints of the three-phalangeal fingers. Acta Chirurgiae Plasticae 46:81, 2004.
16. Gurbuz, H, Mesut, R, and Turan, FN: Measurement of active abduction of metacarpophalangeal joints via electronic digital inclinometric technique. It J Anat Embryol 111:9, 2006.
17. Ellis, B, and Bruton, A: A study to compare the reliability of composite finger flexion with goniometry for measurement of range of motion in the hand. Clin Rehabil 16:562, 2002.
18. Greene, WB, and Heckman, JD (eds): The Clinical Measurement of Joint Motion. American Academy of Orthopaedic Surgeons, Rosemont, Ill., 1994.
19. Adams, LS, Greene, LW, and Topoozian, E: Range of motion. In American Society of Hand Therapists: Clinical Assessment Recommendations, ed 2. ASHT, Chicago, 1999.
20. Clarkson, HM: Joint Motion and Function Assessment. Lippincott Williams & Wilkins. Philadelphia, 2005.
21. Reese, NB, and Bandy, WD: Joint Range of Motion and Muscle Length Testing. WB Saunders, Philadelphia, 2002.
22. DeSmet, L, et al: Metacarpophalangeal and interphalangeal flexion of the thumb: Influence of sex and age, relation to ligamentous injury. Acta Orthop Belg 59:357, 1993.
23. Jenkins, M, et al: Thumb joint motion: What is normal? J Hand Surg (Br) 23:796, 1998.
24. Smahel, Z, and Klimova, A: The influence of age and exercise on the mobility of hand joints: 2: Interphalangeal joints of the three-phalangeal fingers. Acta Chirurgiae Plasticae 46:122, 2004.
25. Yoshida, R, et al: Motion and morphology of the thumb metacarpophalangeal joint. J Hand Surg 28A: 753, 2003.
26. Joseph, J: Further studies of the metacarpophalangeal and interphalangeal joints of the thumb. J Anat 85:221, 1951.
27. Sauseng, S, Kastenbauer, T, and Irsigler, K: Limited joint mobility in selected hand and foot joints in patients with type 1 diabetes mellitus: A methodology comparison. Diab Nutr Metab 15:1, 2002.
28. Shaw, SJ, and Morris, MA: The range of motion of the metacarpophalangeal joint of the thumb and its relationship to injury. J Hand Surg (Br) 17:164, 1992.
29. Beighton, P, Solomon, L, and Soskolne, CL: Articular mobility in an African population. Ann Rheum Dis 32:413, 1973.
30. Lamari, NM, Chueire, AG, and Cordeiro, JA: Analysis of joint mobility patterns among preschool children. Sao Paulo Med 123:119, 2005.
31. Allander, E, et al: Normal range of joint movements in shoulder, hip, wrist and thumb with special reference to side: A comparison between two populations. Int J Epidemiol 3:253, 1974.
32. Fairbank, JCT, Pynsett, PB, and Phillips, H: Quantitative measurements of joint mobility in adolescents. Ann Rheum Dis 43:288, 1984.
33. Nicholson, B: Clinical evaluation. In Stanley, BG, and Tribuzi, SM: Concepts in Hand Rehabilitation. FA Davis, Philadelphia, 1992.
34. Knutson, JS, et al: Intrinsic and extrinsic contributions to the passive moment at the metacarpophalangeal joint. J Biomech 33:1675, 2000.
35. Casanova, JS, and Grunert, BK: Adult prehension: Patterns and nomenclature for pinches. J Hand Ther 2:231, 1989.
36. Melvin, J: Rheumatic Disease: Occupation Therapy and Rehabilitation, ed 2. FA Davis, Philadelphia, 1982.
37. Swanson, AB: Evaluation of disabilities and record keeping. In Swanson, AB: Flexible Implant Resection Arthroplasty in the Hand and Extremities. CV Mosby, St Louis, 1973.
38. Napier, JR: Prehensile movements of the human hand. J Anat 89:564, 1955.
39. Totten, PA, and Flinn-Wagner, S: Functional evaluation of the hand. In Stanley, BG, and Tribuzi, SM (eds): Concepts in Hand Rehabilitation. FA Davis, Philadelphia, 1992.
40. Mackin, E, et al: Hunter, Mackin & Callahan's Rehabilitation of the Hand and Upper Extremity (ed 5). Elsevier, St Louis, 2002.
41. Lee, JW, and Rim, K: Measurement of finger joint angles and maximum finger forces during cylinder grip activity. J Biomed Eng 13:152, 1991.
42. Sperling, L, and Jacobson-Sollerman, C: The grip pattern of the healthy hand during eating. Scand J Rehabil Med 9:115, 1977.
43. Bear-Lehman, J, and Abreu, BC: Evaluating the hand: Issues in reliability and validity. Phys Ther 69:1025, 1989.
44. Hamilton, GF, and Lachenbruch, PA: Reliability of goniometers in assessing finger joint angle. Phys Ther 49:465, 1969.
45. Groth, G, et al: Goniometry of the proximal and distal interphalangeal joints. Part II: Placement preferences, interrater reliability, and concurrent validity. J Hand Ther 14:23, 2001.
46. Weiss, PL, et al: Using the Exos Handmaster to measure digital range of motion: Reliability and validity. Med Eng Phys 16:323, 1994.
47. Ellis, B, Bruton, A, and Goddard, JR: Joint angle measurement: A comparative study of the reliability of goniometry and wire tracing for the hand. Clin Rehabil 11:314, 1997.
48. Brown, A, et al: Validity and reliability of the Dexter Hand Evaluation and Therapy System in hand-injured patients. J Hand Ther 13:37, 2000.
49. Goldsmith, N, and Juzl, E: Inter-rater reliability of two trained raters using a goniometer for the measurement of finger joints. Br J Hand Ther 3:12, 1998.
50. Kato, M, et al: The accuracy of goniometric measurements of proximal interphalangeal joints in fresh cadavers: Comparison between methods of measurement, types of goniometers, and fingers. J Hand Ther 20:12, 2007.
51. Georgeu, GA, Mayfield, S, and Logan, AM: Lateral digital photography with computer-aided goniometry versus standard goniometry for recording finger joint angles. J Hand Surg 27B:184, 2002.
52. Goodson, A, et al: Direct, quantitative clinical assessment of hand function: Usefulness and reproducibility. Manual Ther 12:144, 2007.
53. Field, J: Measurement of finger stiffness in algodystrophy. Hand Clin 19:511, 2003.
54. MacDermid, JC, et al: Validity of pulp-to-palm distance as a measure of finger flexion. J Hand Surg 26B:432, 2001.

twp Flex /ext
IR/ER
abd / adduct

LOWER-EXTREMITY TESTING

OBJECTIVES

ON COMPLETION OF PART III, THE READER WILL BE ABLE TO:

1. **Identify:**
   - Appropriate planes and axes for each lower-extremity joint motion
   - Structures that limit the end of the range of motion
   - Expected normal end-feels

2. **Describe:**
   - Testing positions used for each lower-extremity joint motion and muscle length test
   - Goniometer alignment
   - Capsular pattern of limitation
   - Range of motion necessary for selected functional activities at each major lower-extremity joint

3. **Explain:**
   - How age, gender, and other variables may affect the range of motion
   - How sources of error in measurement may affect testing results

4. **Perform a goniometric measurement of any lower-extremity joint, including:**
   - A clear explanation of the testing procedure
   - Proper positioning of the subject

   - Adequate stabilization of the proximal joint component
   - Use of appropriate testing motion
   - Correct determination of the end of the range of motion
   - Correct identification of the end-feel
   - Palpation of the appropriate bony landmarks
   - Accurate alignment of the goniometer and correct reading and recording of goniometric measurements

5. **Plan goniometric measurements of the hip, knee, ankle, and foot that are organized by body position.**

6. **Assess the intratester and intertester reliability of goniometric measurements of the lower-extremity joints using methods described in Chapter 3.**

7. **Perform tests of muscle length at the hip, knee, and ankle, including:**
   - A clear explanation of the testing procedure
   - Proper placement of the subject in the starting position
   - Adequate stabilization
   - Use of appropriate testing motion
   - Correct identification of end-feel
   - Accurate alignment of the goniometer and correct reading and recording

---

The testing positions, stabilization techniques, testing motions, end-feels, and goniometer alignment for the joints of the lower extremities are presented in Chapters 8 through 10. The goniometric evaluation should follow the 12-step sequence that was presented in Exercise 5 in Chapter 2.

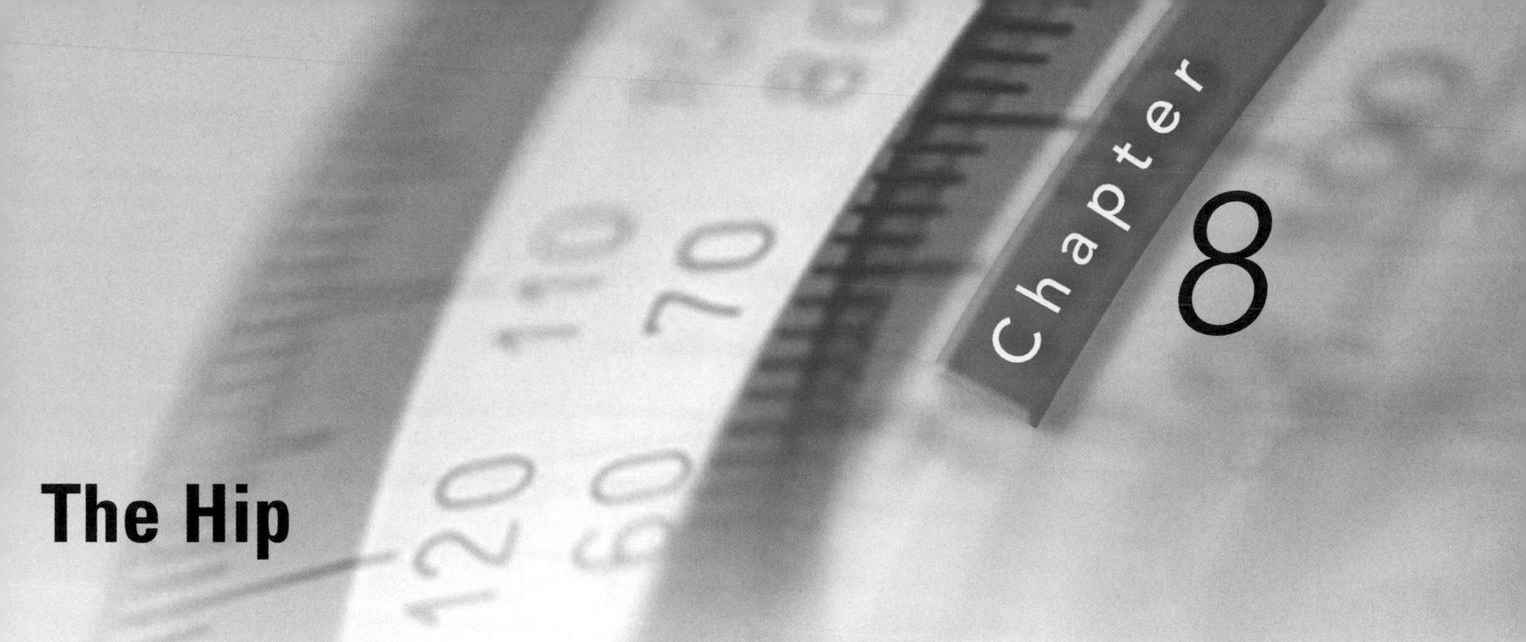

The Hip

Structure and Function

Iliofemoral Joint

Anatomy

The hip joint, or coxa, links the lower extremity with the trunk. The proximal joint surface is the acetabulum, which is formed superiorly by the ilium, posteroinferiorly by the ischium, and anteroinferiorly by the pubis (Fig. 8.1). The concave acetabulum faces laterally, inferiorly, and anteriorly and is deepened by a fibrocartilaginous acetabular labrum.[1] The distal joint surface is the convex head of the femur. The joint is enclosed by a strong, thick capsule, which is reinforced anteriorly by the iliofemoral and pubofemoral ligaments (Fig. 8.2) and posteriorly by the ischiofemoral ligament (Fig. 8.3).

Osteokinematics

The hip is a synovial ball-and-socket joint with 3 degrees of freedom. Motions permitted at the joint are flexion–extension in the sagittal plane around a medial–lateral axis, abduction–adduction in the frontal plane around an anterior–posterior axis, and medial and lateral rotation in the transverse plane around a vertical or longitudinal axis.[1] The axis of motion goes through the center of the femoral head.

Arthrokinematics

In an open kinematic (non–weight-bearing) chain, the convex femoral head rolls in the same direction and slides in the opposite direction, to movement of the shaft of the femur. In flexion, the femoral head rolls anteriorly and slides posteriorly and inferiorly on the acetabulum, whereas in extension, the femoral head rolls posteriorly and slides anteriorly and superiorly. In medial rotation, the femoral head rolls anteriorly

Ilium

Head of femur

Pubis

Hip joint

Ischium

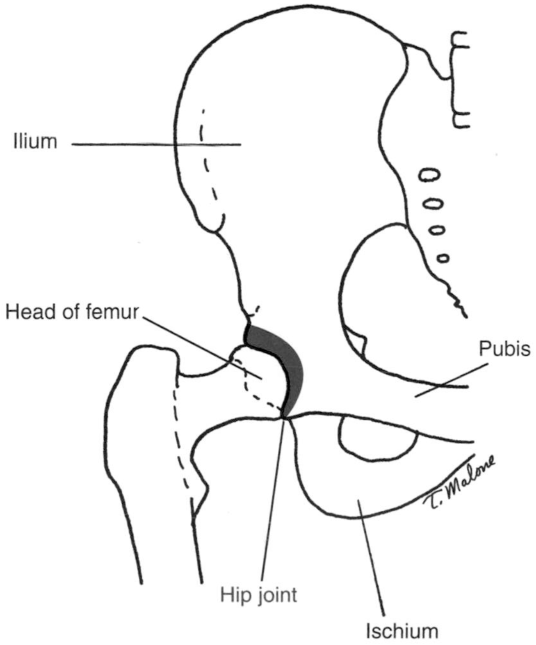

FIGURE 8.1 An anterior view of the right hip joint.

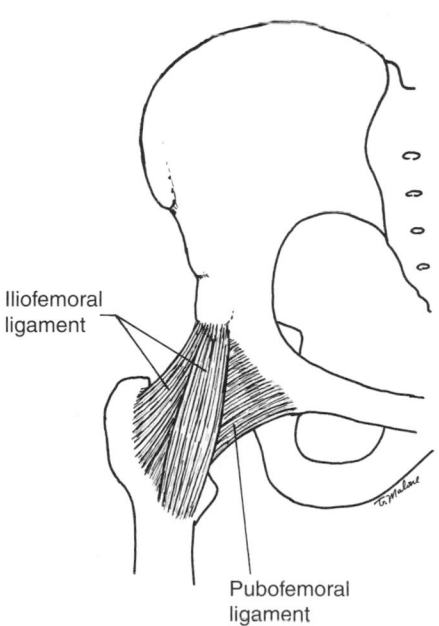

Iliofemoral ligament

Pubofemoral ligament

FIGURE 8.2 An anterior view of the right hip joint showing the iliofemoral and pubofemoral ligaments.

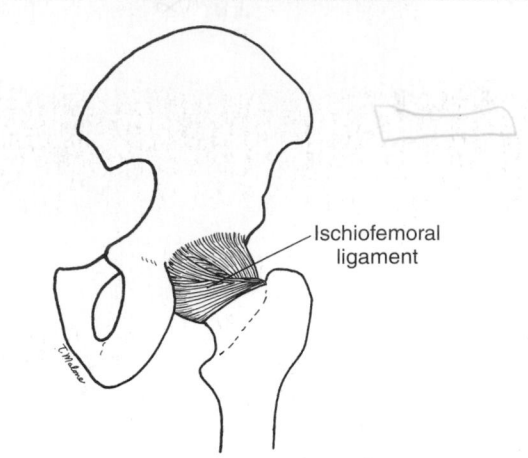

and slides posteriorly on the acetabulum. During lateral rotation, the femoral head rolls posteriorly and slides anteriorly. In abduction, the femoral head rolls superiorly and slides inferiorly, whereas in adduction, the femoral head rolls inferiorly and slides superiorly.

Capsular Pattern

The capsular pattern is characterized by a marked restriction of medial rotation accompanied by limitations in flexion and abduction. A slight limitation may be present in extension, but no limitation is present in either lateral rotation or adduction.[2]

FIGURE 8.3 A posterior view of the right hip joint showing the ischiofemoral ligament.

RANGE OF MOTION TESTING PROCEDURES: Hip

Landmarks for Testing Procedures

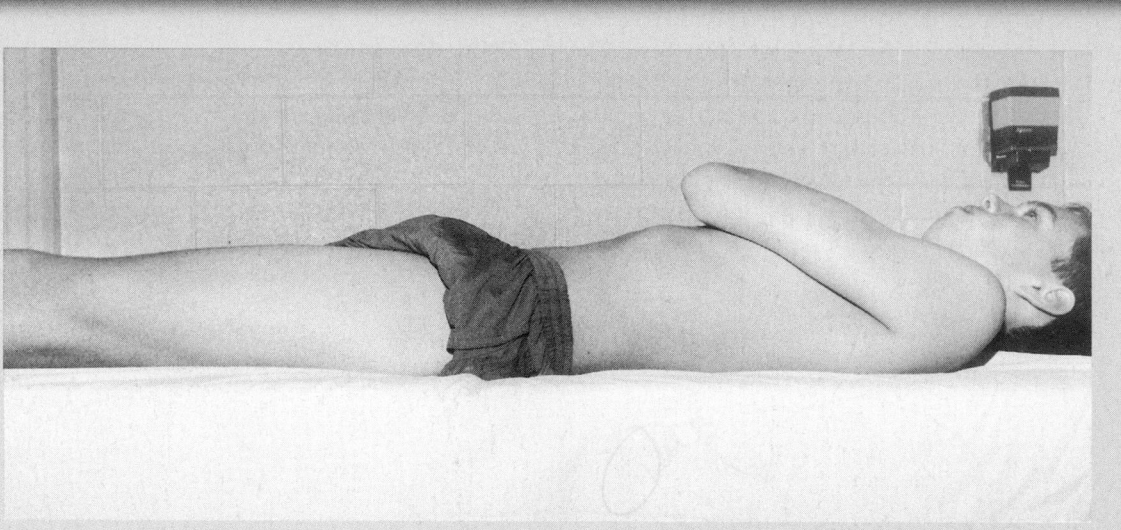

FIGURE 8.4 A lateral view of the hip showing surface anatomy landmarks for aligning the goniometer for measuring hip flexion and extension.

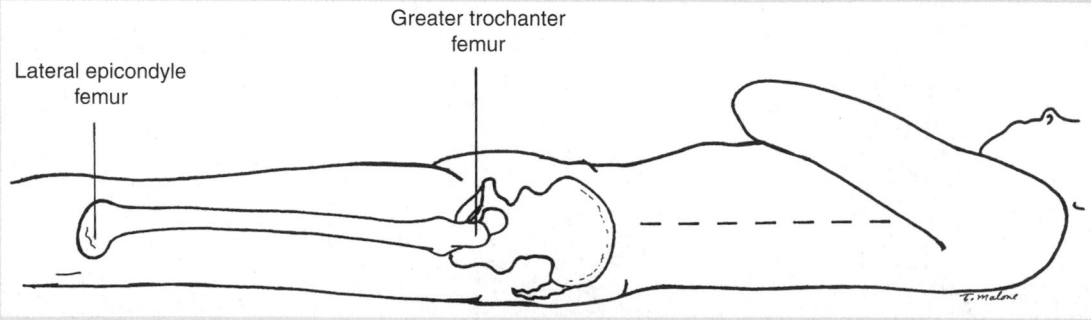

FIGURE 8.5 A lateral view of the hip showing bony anatomical landmarks for aligning the goniometer.

Landmarks for Testing Procedures (continued)

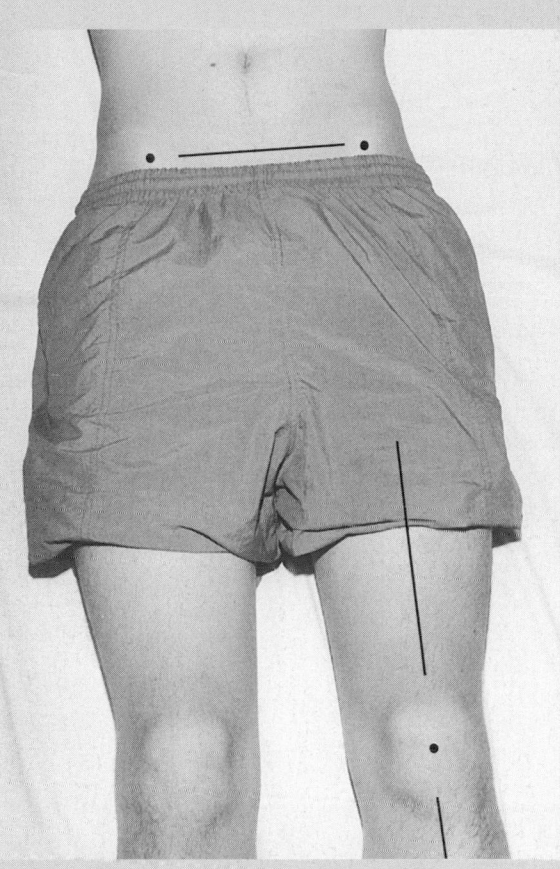

FIGURE 8.6 An anterior view of the hip showing surface anatomy landmarks for aligning the goniometer.

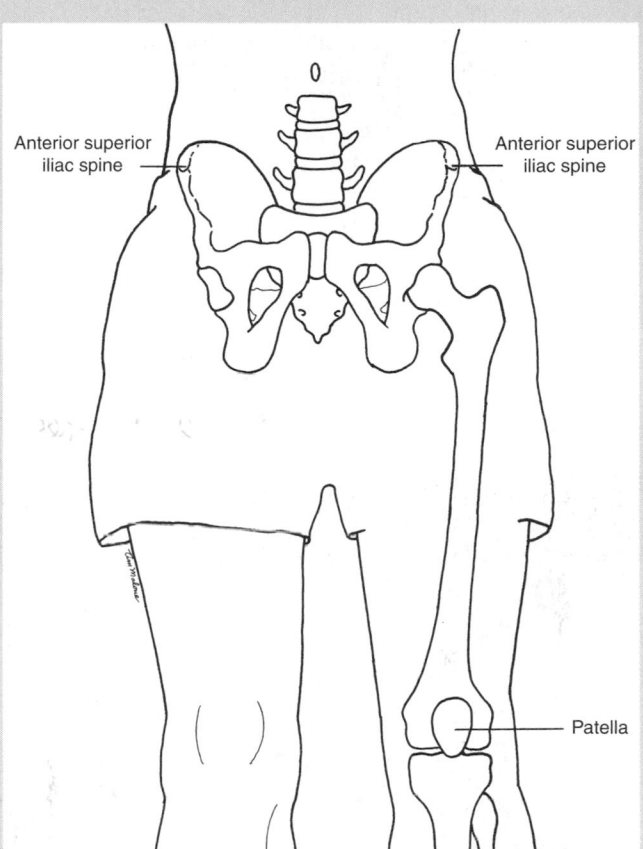

FIGURE 8.7 An anterior view of the pelvis showing the anatomical landmarks for aligning the goniometer for measuring abduction and adduction.

Anterior superior iliac spine

Anterior superior iliac spine

Patella

● HIP FLEXION

Motion occurs in the sagittal plane around a medial–lateral axis. Hip flexion range of motion (ROM) for adults is 120 degrees according to the American Academy of Orthopaedic Surgeons (AAOS)[3] and 100 degrees according to the American Medical Association (AMA).[4] The mean ROM for males and females ranges from a mean of 122 degrees for ages 25 to 39 years to 118 degrees for ages 60 to 74 years according to Roach and Miles.[5] See Tables 8.1 to 8.4 in the Research Findings section for additional normal ROM values by age and gender.

Testing Position
Place the subject in the supine position, with the knees extended and both hips in 0 degrees of abduction, adduction, and rotation.

hold femur bring hip into max flex

Stabilization
Stabilize the pelvis with one hand to prevent posterior tilting or rotation. Keep the contralateral lower extremity flat on the table in the neutral position to provide additional stabilization.

Testing Motion
Flex the hip by lifting the thigh off the table. Allow the knee to flex passively during the motion to reduce tension in the hamstring muscles. Maintain the extremity in neutral rotation and abduction and adduction throughout the motion (Fig. 8.8). The end of the ROM occurs when resistance to further motion is felt and attempts at overcoming the resistance cause posterior tilting of the pelvis.

Normal End-Feel
The end-feel is usually soft because of contact between the muscle bulk of the anterior thigh and the lower abdomen. However, the end-feel may be firm because of tension in the posterior joint capsule and the gluteus maximus muscle.

Goniometer Alignment
See Figures 8.9 and 8.10.

1. Center **fulcrum** of the goniometer over the lateral aspect of the hip joint, using the greater trochanter of the femur for reference.
2. Align **proximal arm** with the lateral midline of the pelvis.
3. Align **distal arm** with the lateral midline of the femur, using the lateral epicondyle as a reference.

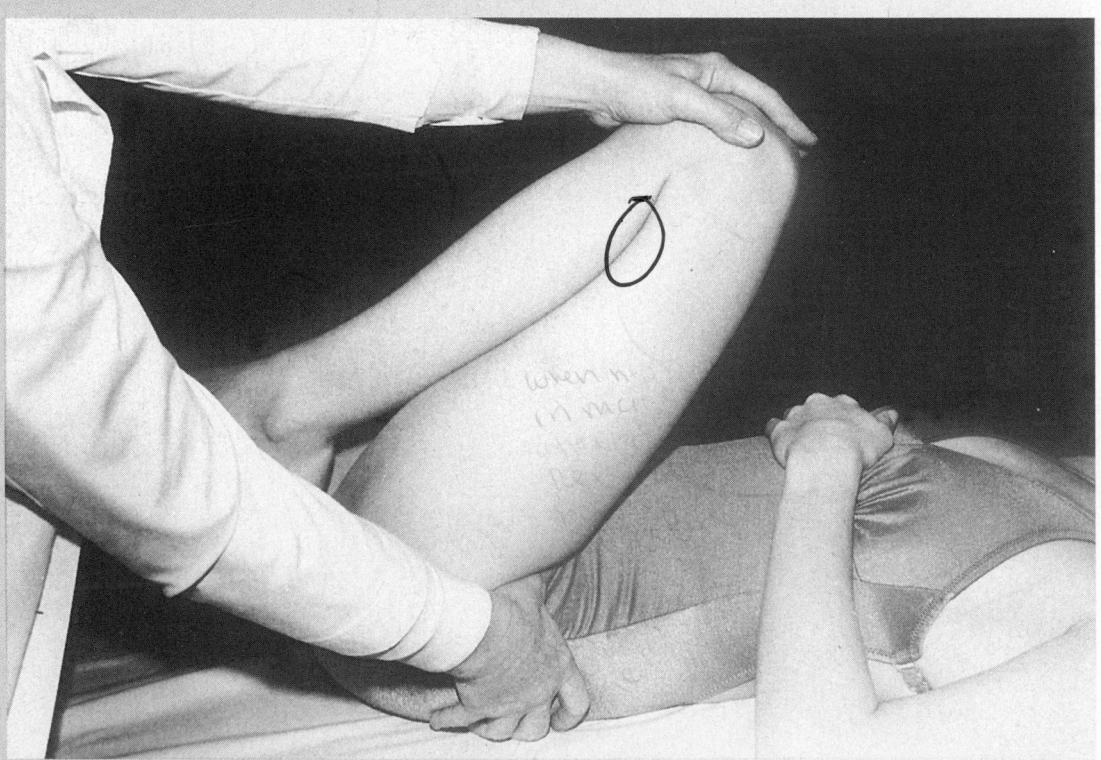

FIGURE 8.8 The end of hip flexion passive ROM. The placement of the examiner's hand on the pelvis allows the examiner to stabilize the pelvis and to detect any pelvic motion.

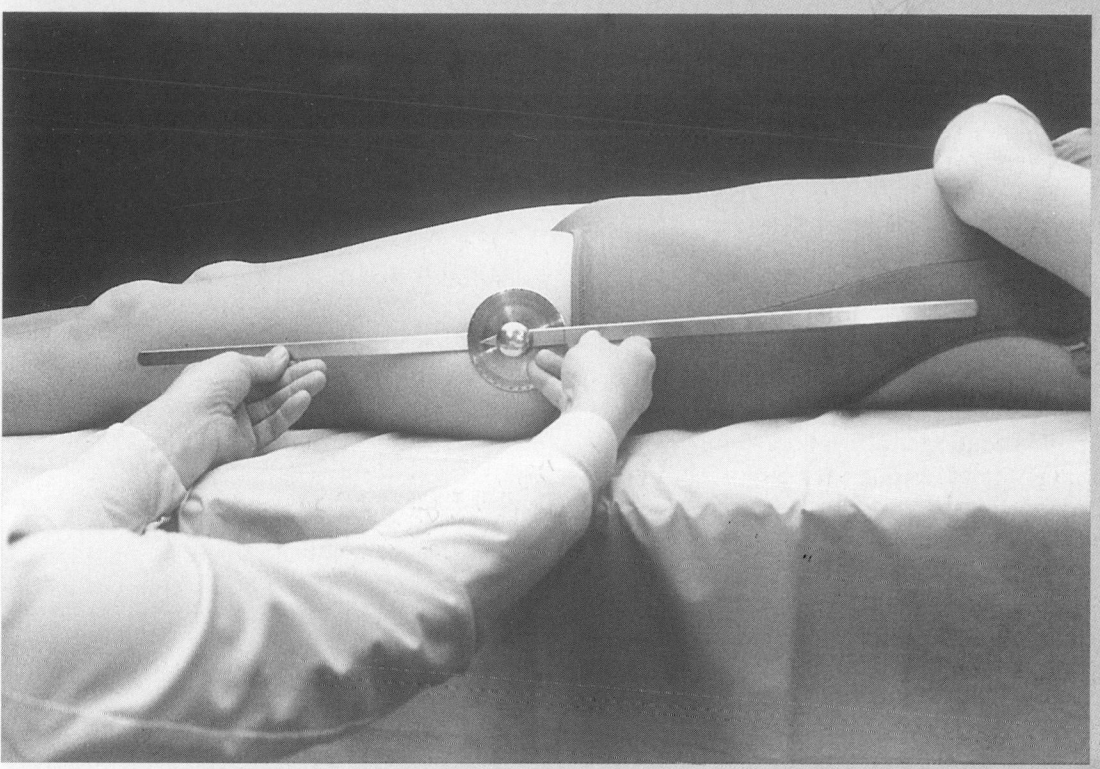

FIGURE 8.9 Goniometer alignment in the supine starting position for measuring hip flexion ROM.

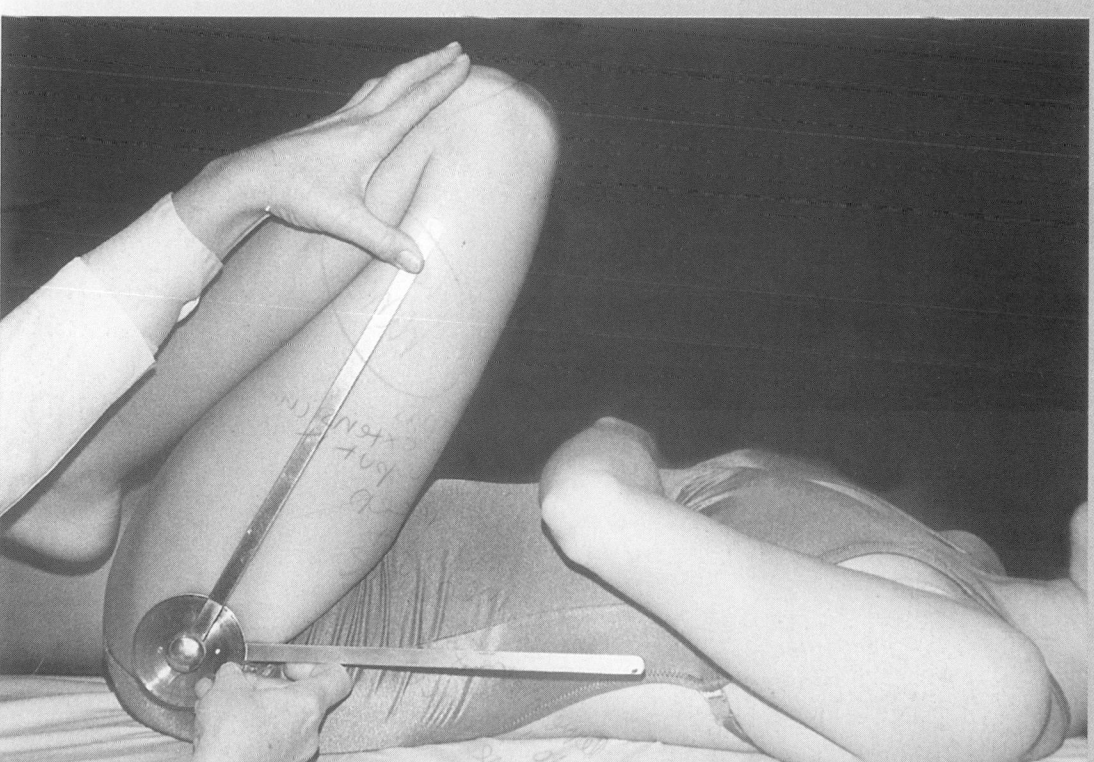

FIGURE 8.10 At the end of the left hip flexion ROM, the examiner uses one hand to align the distal goniometer arm and to maintain the hip in flexion. The examiner's other hand shifts from the pelvis to hold the proximal goniometer arm aligned with the lateral midline of the subject's pelvis.

● HIP EXTENSION

Motion occurs in a sagittal plane around a medial–lateral axis. Normal hip extension ROM is 30 degrees for adults according to the AMA[4] and 20 degrees according to the AAOS.[3] Normal hip extension ROM for adults ages 40 to 59 years is 18 degrees according to Roach and Miles.[5] See Tables 8.1 to 8.4 in the Research Findings section for additional normal ROM values by age and gender.

Testing Position

Place the subject in the prone position, with both knees extended and the hip to be tested in 0 degrees of abduction, adduction, and rotation. A pillow may be placed under the abdomen for comfort, but no pillow should be placed under the head.

Stabilization

Hold the pelvis with one hand to prevent an anterior tilt (an assistant could help stabilize the pelvis). Keep the contralateral extremity flat on the table to provide additional pelvic stabilization.

Testing Motion

Extend the hip by raising the lower extremity from the table (Fig. 8.11). Maintain the knee in extension throughout the movement to ensure that tension in the two-joint rectus femoris muscle does not limit the hip extension ROM. The end of the ROM occurs when resistance to further motion of the femur is felt and attempts at overcoming the resistance cause anterior tilting of the pelvis and/or extension of the lumbar spine.

Normal End-Feel

The end-feel is firm because of tension in the anterior joint capsule and the iliofemoral ligament and, to a lesser extent, the ischiofemoral and pubofemoral ligaments. Tension in various muscles that flex the hip, such as the iliopsoas, sartorius, tensor fasciae latae, gracilis, and adductor longus, may contribute to the firm end-feel.

Goniometer Alignment

See Figures 8.12 and 8.13.

1. Center **fulcrum** of the goniometer over the lateral aspect of the hip joint, using the greater trochanter of the femur for reference.
2. Align **proximal arm** with the lateral midline of the pelvis.
3. Align **distal arm** with the lateral midline of the femur, using the lateral epicondyle as a reference.

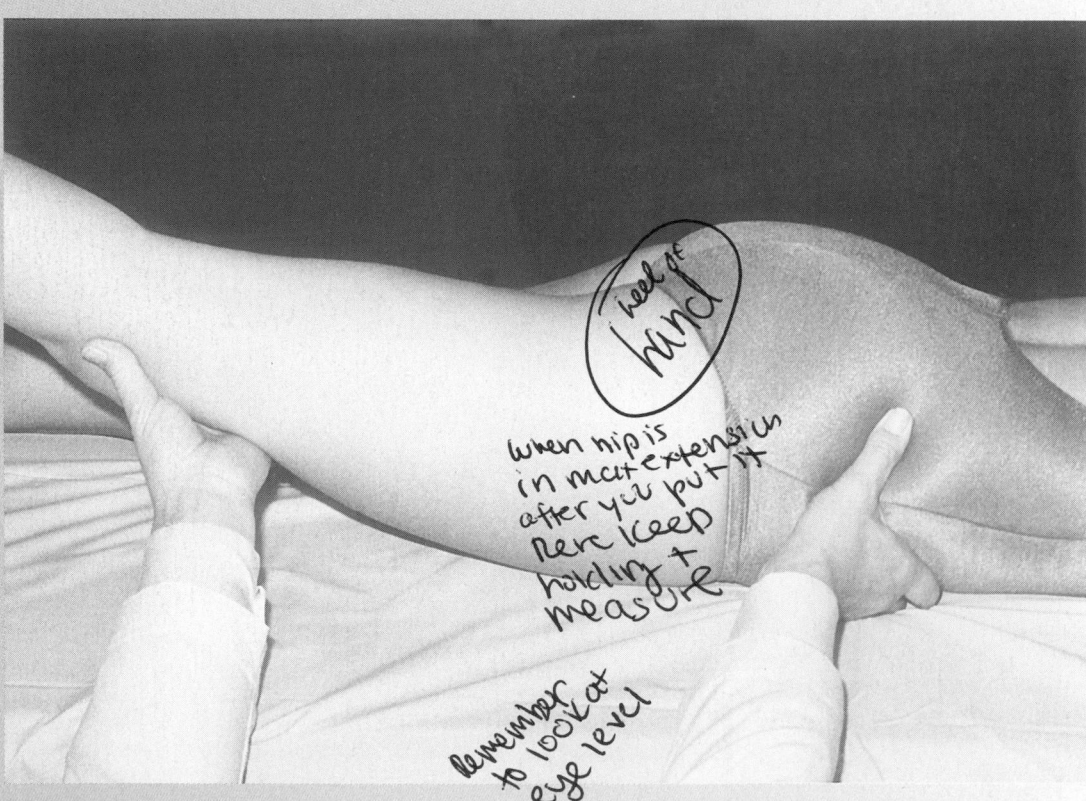

FIGURE 8.11 The subject's right lower extremity at the end of hip extension ROM. The examiner uses one hand to support the distal femur and maintain the hip in extension while her other hand grasps the pelvis at the level of the anterior superior iliac spine. Because the examiner's hand is on the subject's pelvis, the examiner is able to detect pelvic tilting.

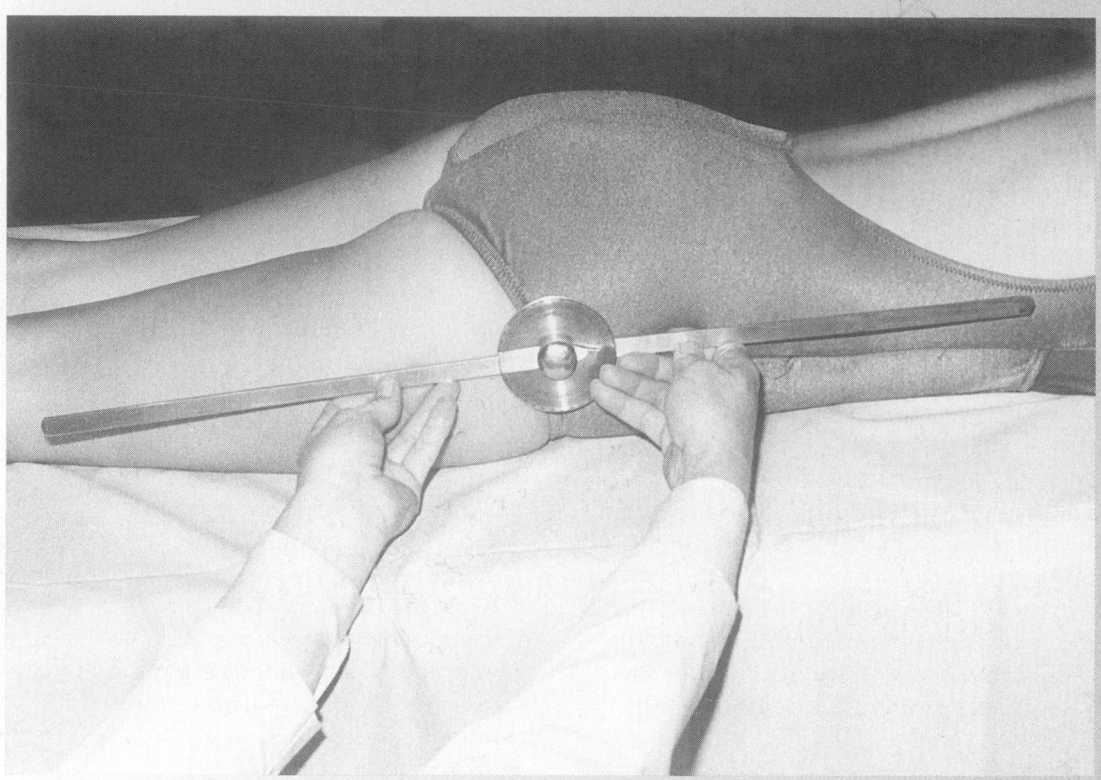

FIGURE 8.12 Goniometer alignmment in the prone starting position for measuring hip extension ROM.

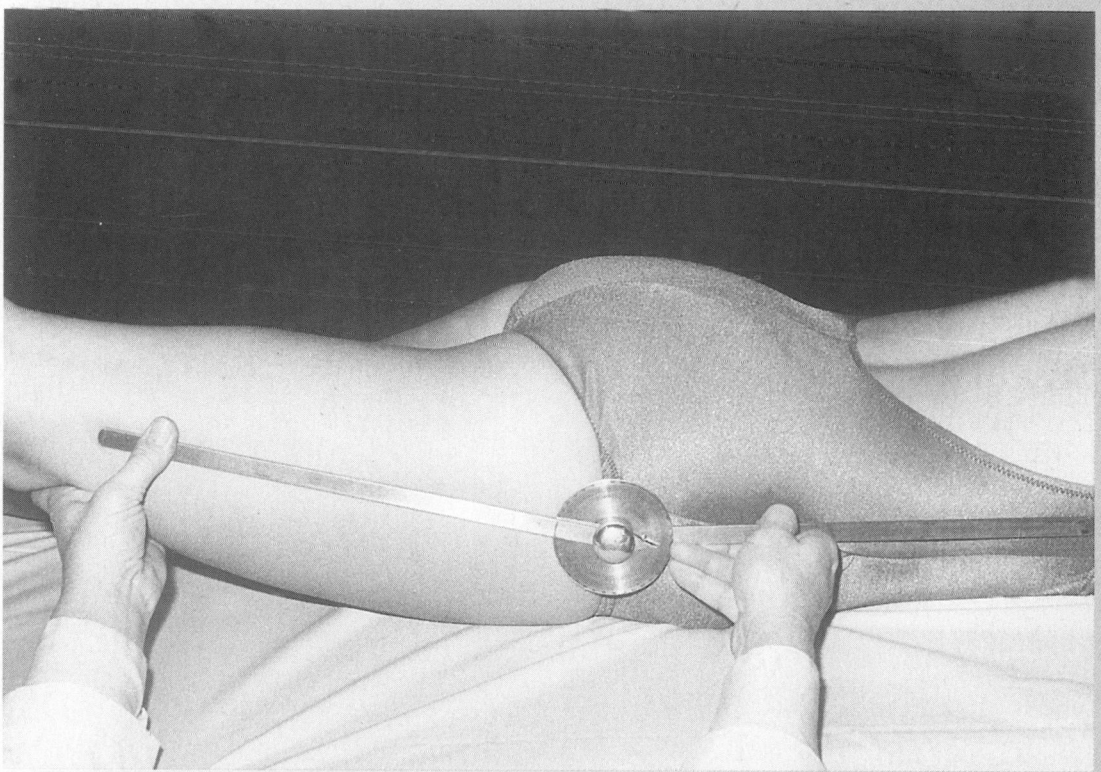

FIGURE 8.13 At the end of hip extension ROM, the examiner uses one hand to hold the proximal goniometer arm in alignment. The examiner's other hand supports the subject's femur and keeps the distal goniometer arm in alignment.

● HIP ABDUCTION

Motion occurs in the frontal plane around an anterior–posterior axis. Normal ROM in abduction is 40 degrees according to the AMA[4] and 42 degrees for adult males and females ages 40 to 59 years according to Roach and Miles.[5] See Tables 8.1 to 8.5 in the Research Findings section for additional normal ROM values by age and gender.

Testing Position

Place the subject in the supine position, with the knees extended and the hips in 0 degrees of flexion, extension, and rotation.

Stabilization

Keep a hand on the pelvis to prevent lateral tilting and rotation. Watch the trunk for lateral trunk flexion.

Testing Motion

Abduct the hip by sliding the lower extremity laterally (Fig. 8.14). Do not allow lateral rotation or flexion of the hip. The end of the ROM occurs when resistance to further motion of the femur is felt and attempts to overcome the resistance cause lateral pelvic tilting, pelvic rotation, or lateral flexion of the trunk.

Normal End-Feel

The end-feel is firm because of tension in the inferior (medial) joint capsule, pubofemoral ligament, ischiofemoral ligament, and inferior band of the iliofemoral ligament. Passive tension in the adductor magnus, adductor longus, adductor brevis, pectineus, and gracilis muscles may contribute to the firm end-feel.

Goniometer Alignment

See Figures 8.15 and 8.16.

1. Center **fulcrum** of the goniometer over the anterior superior iliac spine (ASIS) of the extremity being measured.
2. Align **proximal** arm with an imaginary horizontal line extending from one ASIS to the other.
3. Align **distal** arm with the anterior midline of the femur, using the midline of the patella for reference.

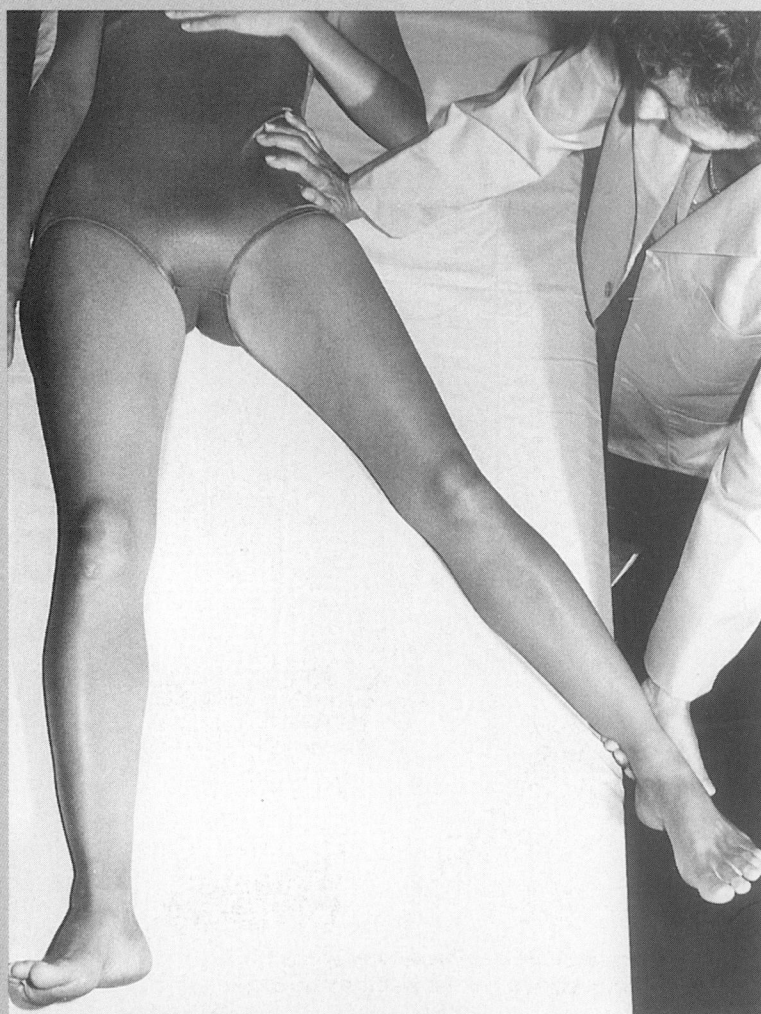

FIGURE 8.14 The left lower extremity at the end of the hip abduction ROM. The examiner uses one hand to pull the subject's leg into abduction. (The examiner's grip on the ankle is designed to prevent lateral rotation of the hip.) The examiner's other hand not only stabilizes the pelvis but also is used to detect pelvic motion.

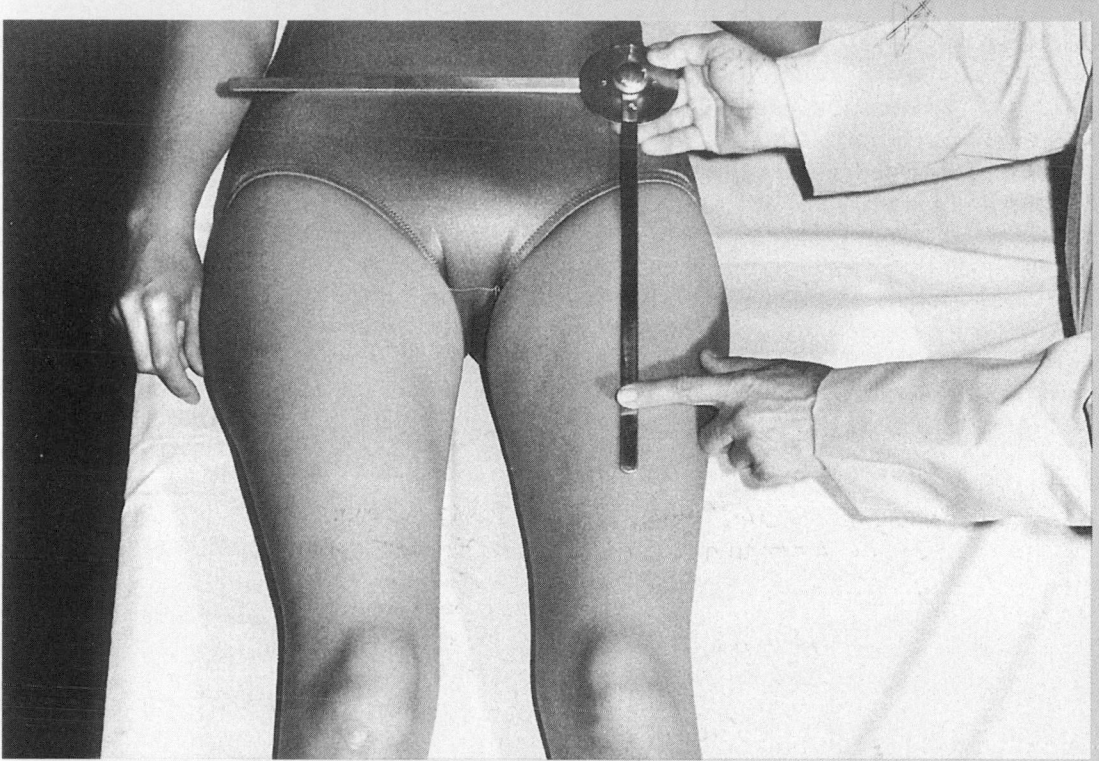

FIGURE 8.15 In the starting position for measuring hip abduction ROM, the goniometer is at 90 degrees. This position is considered to be the 0-degree starting position. Therefore, the examiner must transpose her reading from 90 degrees to 0 degrees. For example, an actual reading of 90 to 120 degrees on the goniometer is recorded as 0 - 30 degrees.

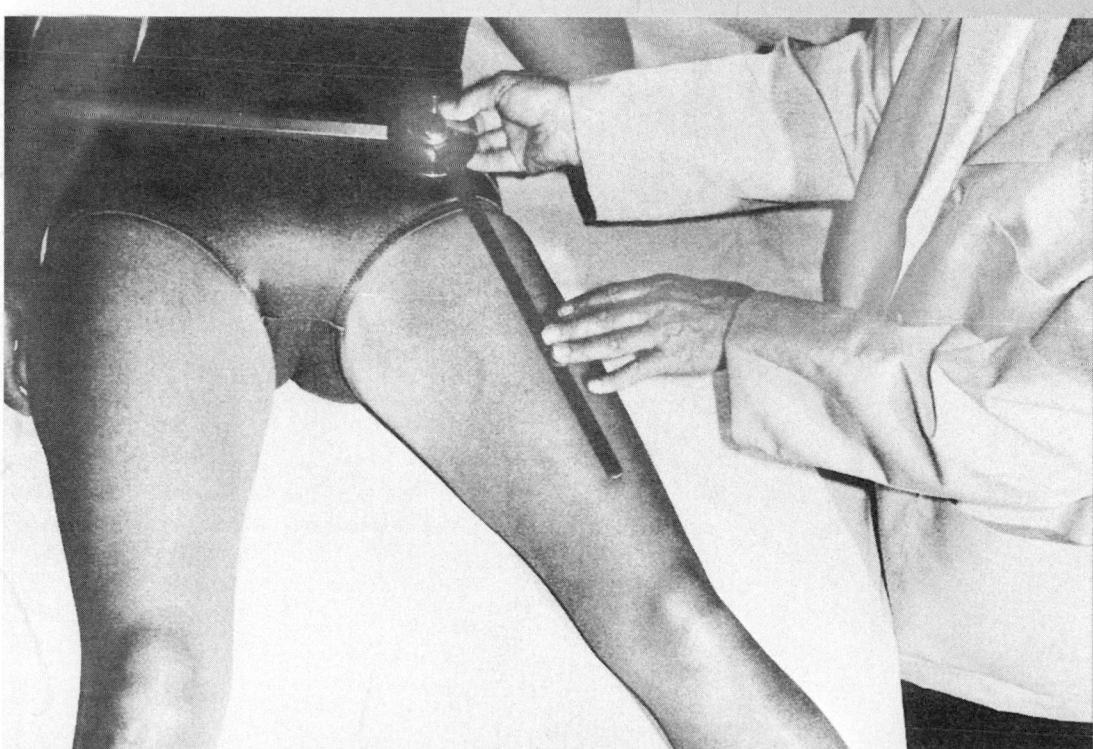

FIGURE 8.16 Goniometer alignment at the end of the abduction ROM. The examiner has determined the end-feel and has moved her right hand from stabilizing the pelvis to hold the goniometer in correct alignment.

● HIP ADDUCTION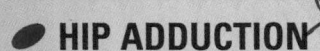

Motion occurs in a frontal plane around an anterior–posterior axis. Normal adduction ROM for adults is 20 degrees according to the AMA.[4] See Tables 8.1 to 8.5 in the Research Findings section for additional normal ROM values by age and gender.

Testing Position

Place the subject in the supine position, with both knees extended and the hip being tested in 0 degrees of flexion, extension, and rotation. Abduct the contralateral extremity to provide sufficient space to complete the full ROM in adduction.

Stabilization

Stabilize the pelvis to prevent lateral tilting.

Testing Motion

Adduct the hip by sliding the lower extremity medially toward the contralateral lower extremity (Fig. 8.17). Place one hand at the knee to move the extremity into adduction and to maintain the hip in neutral flexion and rotation. The end of the ROM occurs when resistance to further adduction is felt and attempts to overcome the resistance cause lateral pelvic tilting, pelvic rotation, and/or lateral trunk flexion.

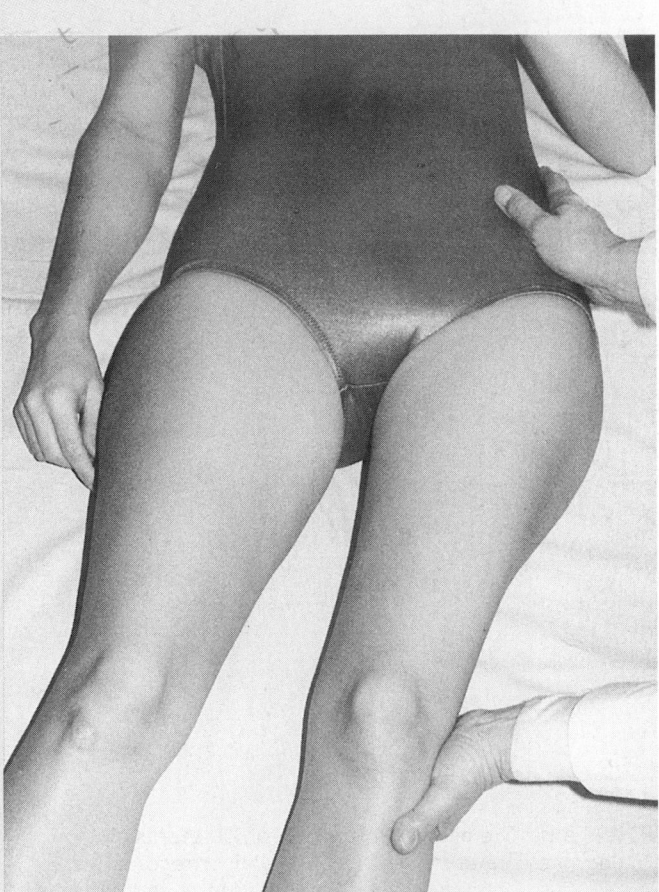

FIGURE 8.17 At the end of the hip adduction ROM, the examiner maintains the hip in adduction with one hand and stabilizes the pelvis with her other hand.

Normal End-Feel

The end-feel is firm because of tension in the superior (lateral) joint capsule and the superior band of the iliofemoral ligament. Tension in the gluteus medius and minimus and the tensor fasciae latae muscles may also contribute to the firm end-feel.

Goniometer Alignment

See Figures 8.18 and 8.19.

1. Center **fulcrum** of the goniometer over the ASIS of the extremity being measured.
2. Align **proximal arm** with an imaginary horizontal line extending from one ASIS to the other.
3. Align **distal arm** with the anterior midline of the femur, using the midline of the patella for reference.

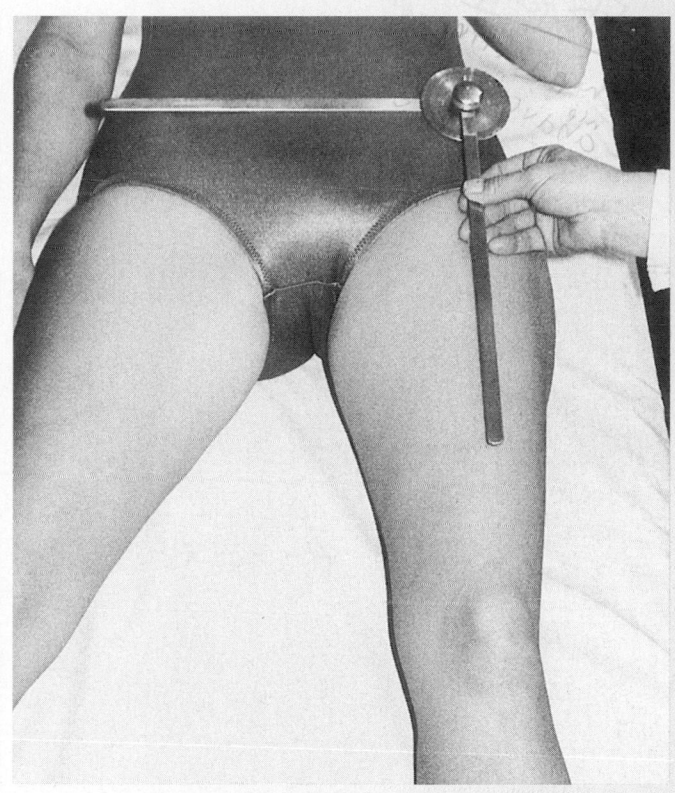

FIGURE 8.18 The alignment of the goniometer is at 90 degrees. Therefore, when the examiner records the measurement, she will have to transpose the reading so that 90 degrees is equivalent to 0 degrees. For example, an actual reading of 90 to 60 degrees is recorded as 0 - 30 degrees.

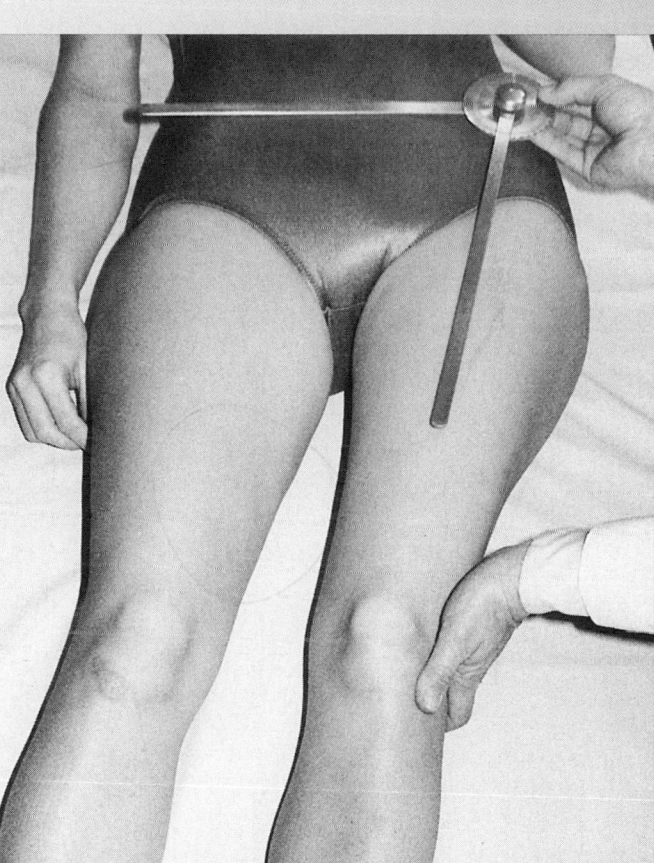

FIGURE 8.19 At the end of the hip adduction ROM, the examiner uses one hand to hold the goniometer body over the subject's anterior superior iliac spine. The examiner prevents hip rotation by maintaining a firm grasp at the subject's knee with her other hand.

Direction of femur

● HIP MEDIAL (INTERNAL) ROTATION

Motion occurs in a transverse plane around a vertical axis when the subject is in anatomical position. Normal medial rotation ROM for adults is 40 degrees according to the AMA[4] and 45 degrees according to the AAOS.[3] Normal medial rotation ROM for adults ages 40 to 59 years is 31 degrees according to Roach and Miles.[5] See Tables 8.1 to 8.5 in the Research Findings section for additional normal ROM values by age and gender.

Testing Position

Seat the subject on a supporting surface, with the knees flexed to 90 degrees over the edge of the surface. Place the hip in 0 degrees of abduction and adduction and in 90 degrees of flexion. Place a towel roll under the distal end of the femur to maintain the femur in a horizontal plane.

Stabilization

Stabilize the distal end of the femur to prevent abduction, adduction, or further flexion of the hip. Avoid rotations and lateral tilting of the pelvis.

Testing Motion

Place one hand at the distal femur to provide stabilization, and use the other hand at the distal tibia to move the lower leg laterally. The hand performing the motion also holds the lower leg in a neutral position to prevent rotation at the knee joint (Fig. 8.20). The end of the ROM occurs when attempts at resistance are felt and attempts at further motion cause tilting of the pelvis or lateral flexion of the trunk.

ER comp
- hip lifting up
- hip abduction (IR+ER)

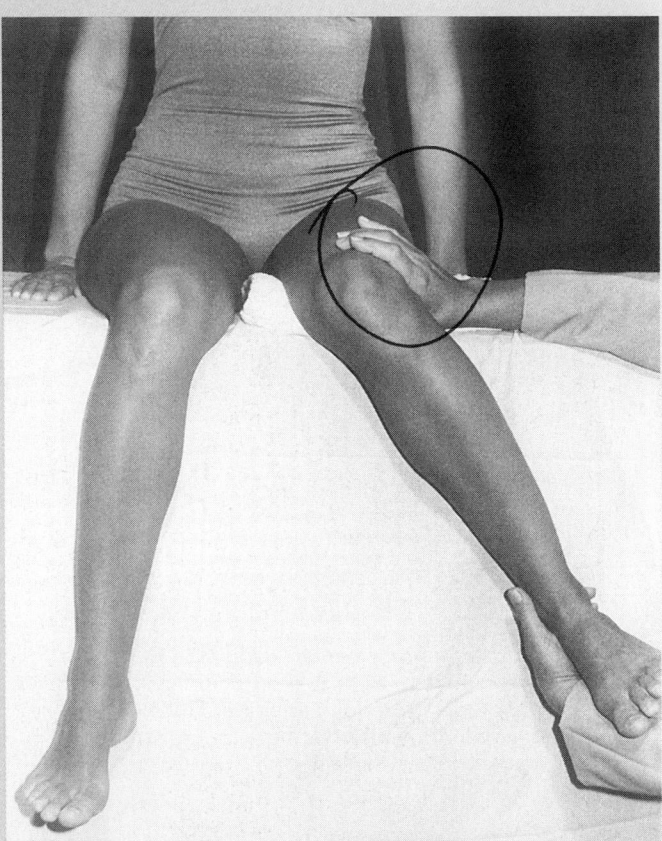

FIGURE 8.20 The left lower extremity at the end of the ROM of hip medial rotation. One of the examiner's hands is placed on the subject's distal femur to prevent hip flexion and abduction. Her other hand pulls the lower leg laterally.

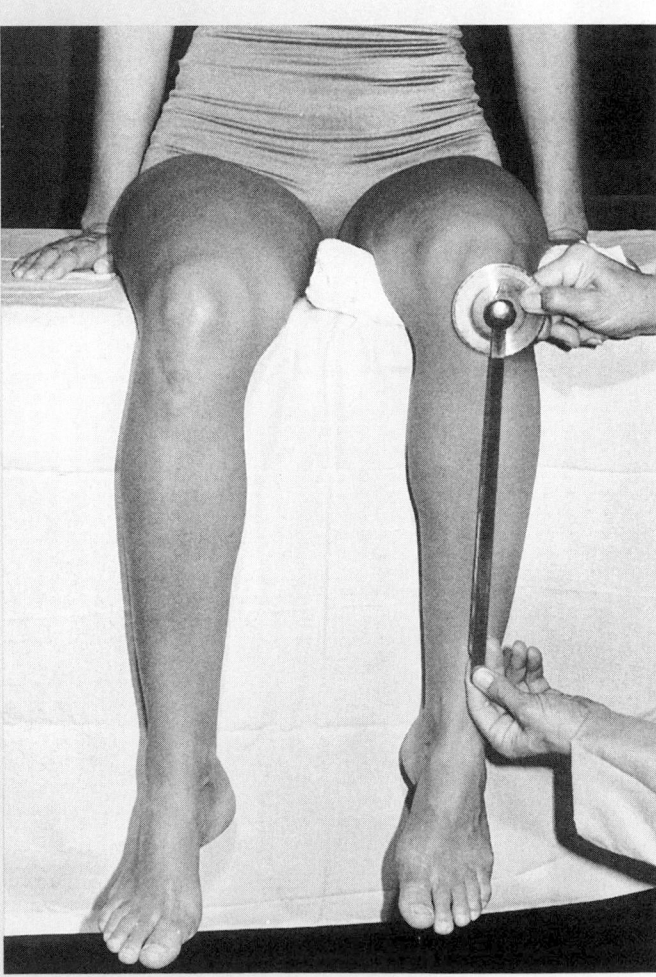

FIGURE 8.21 In the starting position for measuring hip medial rotation, the fulcrum of the goniometer is placed over the patella. Both arms of the instrument are together.

Normal End-Feel

The end-feel is firm because of tension in the posterior joint capsule and the ischiofemoral ligament. Tension in the following muscles may also contribute to the firm end-feel: piriformis, obturatorii (internus and externus), gemelli (superior and inferior), quadratus femoris, gluteus medius (posterior fibers), and gluteus maximus.

Goniometer Alignment

See Figures 8.21 and 8.22.

1. Center **fulcrum** of the goniometer over the anterior aspect of the patella.
2. Align **proximal arm** so that it is perpendicular to the floor or parallel to the supporting surface. *Stationary arm*
3. Align **distal arm** with the anterior midline of the lower leg, using the crest of the tibia and a point midway between the two malleoli for reference. *Moving arm*

Testing Position: Prone

Position subject prone with both legs extended. Flex the knee to 90 degrees in the leg to be tested. (The other leg should remain flat on the table with the knee extended.) Place a strap across the pelvis for stabilization. Goniometer alignment is the same as in the sitting position (Fig. 8.23). Note: This position should only be used if the rectus femoris is of normal length.

Prone
- same gen. alignment
- what would it mean to get diff #/ test it prone?
- friction
- muscle stretching
- more joint restriction when sitting vs. prone

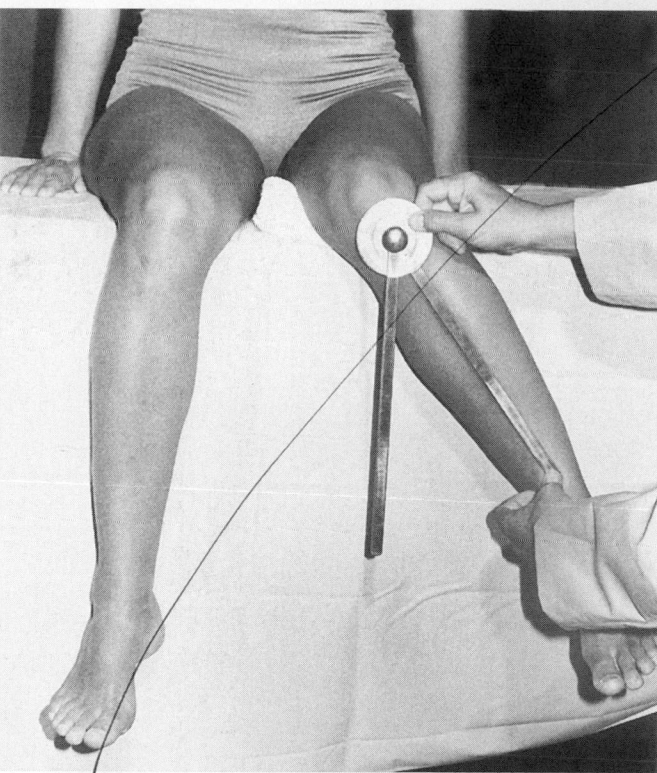

FIGURE 8.22 At the end of hip medial rotation ROM, the proximal arm of the goniometer hangs freely so that it is perpendicular to the floor.

with inclinometer
- lateral malleolus (fib)
- 0 out
- leg perp. to floor
- Don't want hip to lift up on opposite side you aren't measuring

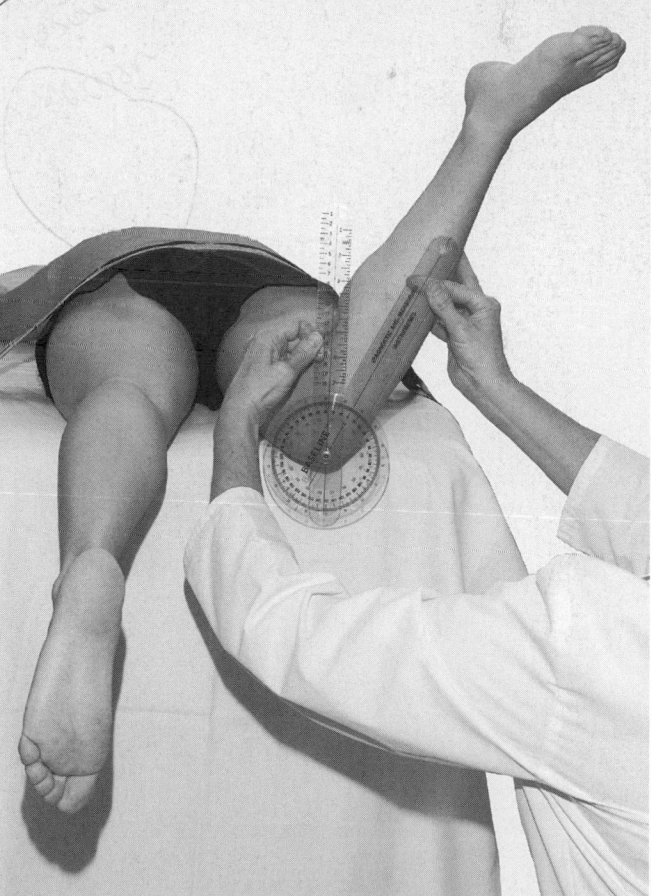

FIGURE 8.23 Hip medial rotation in the prone testing position with the goniometer aligned at the end of the motion. Note that a strap is placed across the pelvis for stabilization.

● HIP LATERAL (EXTERNAL) ROTATION

Motion occurs in a transverse plane around a longitudinal axis when the subject is in anatomical position. Normal lateral rotation ROM for adults is 50 degrees according to the AMA[4] and 45 degrees according to the AAOS.[3] The normal ROM value for lateral rotation for adults ages 40 to 59 years is 32 degrees according to Roach and Miles.[5] See Tables 8.1 to 8.5 for additional normal ROM values by age and gender.

Testing Position

Seat the subject on a supporting surface with knees flexed to 90 degrees over the edge of the surface. Place the hip in 0 degrees of abduction and adduction and in 90 degrees of flexion. Flex the contralateral knee beyond 90 degrees to allow the hip being measured to complete its full range of lateral rotation.

Stabilization

Stabilize the distal end of the femur to prevent abduction or further flexion of the hip. Avoid rotation and lateral tilting of the pelvis.

Testing Motion

Place one hand at the distal femur to provide stabilization, and place the other hand on the distal fibula to move the lower leg medially (Fig. 8.24). The hand on the fibula also prevents rotation at the knee joint. The end of the motion occurs when resistance is felt and attempts at overcoming the resistance cause tilting of the pelvis or trunk lateral flexion.

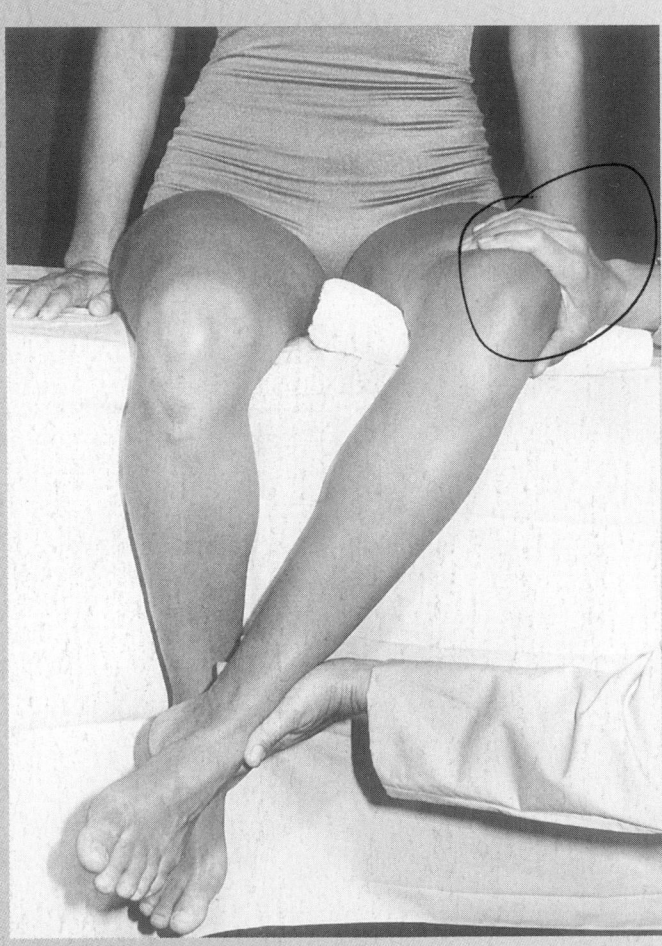

FIGURE 8.24 The left lower extremity is at the end of the ROM of hip lateral rotation. The examiner places one hand on the subject's distal femur to prevent hip flexion and hip abduction. The subject assists with stabilization by placing her hands on the supporting surface and shifting her weight over her left hip. The subject flexes her right knee to allow the left lower extremity to complete the ROM.

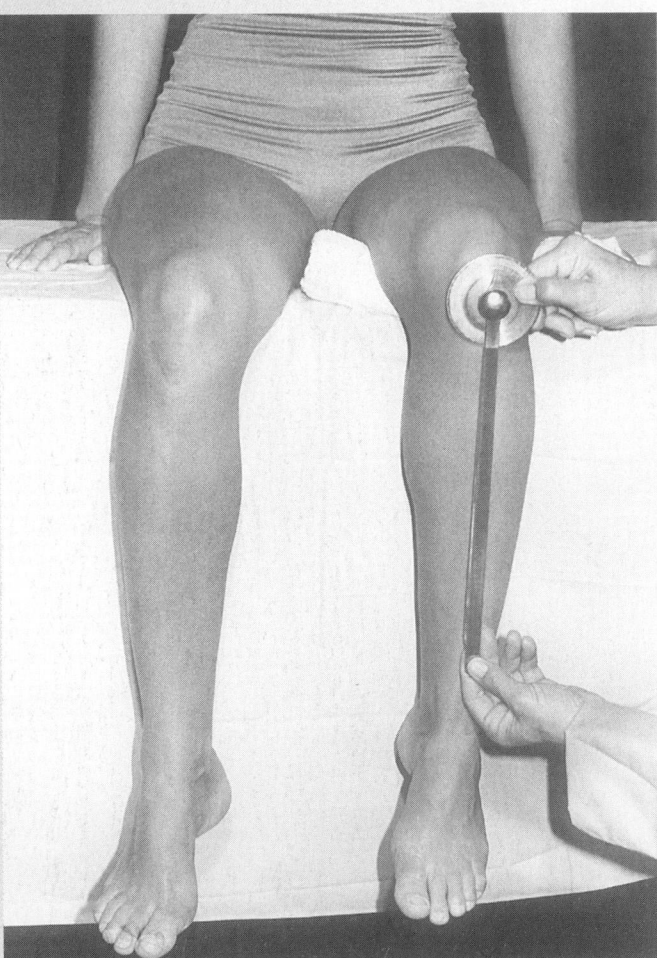

FIGURE 8.25 Goniometer alignment in the starting position for measuring hip lateral rotation.

Normal End-Feel

The end-feel is firm because of tension in the anterior joint capsule, iliofemoral ligament, and pubofemoral ligament. Tension in the anterior portion of the gluteus medius, gluteus minimus, adductor magnus, adductor longus, pectineus, and piriformis muscles also may contribute to the firm end-feel.

Goniometer Alignment

See Figures 8.25 and 8.26.

1. Center **fulcrum** of the goniometer over the anterior aspect of the patella.
2. Align **proximal arm** so that it is perpendicular to the floor or parallel to the supporting surface.
3. Align **distal arm** with the anterior midline of the lower leg, using the crest of the tibia and a point midway between the two malleoli for reference.

Testing Position: Prone

Position the subject prone with both legs extended. Flex the knee to 90 degrees in the leg to be tested. (The other leg should remain flat on the table with the knee extended.) Place a strap across the pelvis for stabilization. Goniometer alignment is the same as in the sitting position (Fig. 8.27). Note: This position should be used only if the rectus femoris is of normal length.

Substitutions
- look at hips
  - They should be parallel + equal to table
  (hip lifting up)

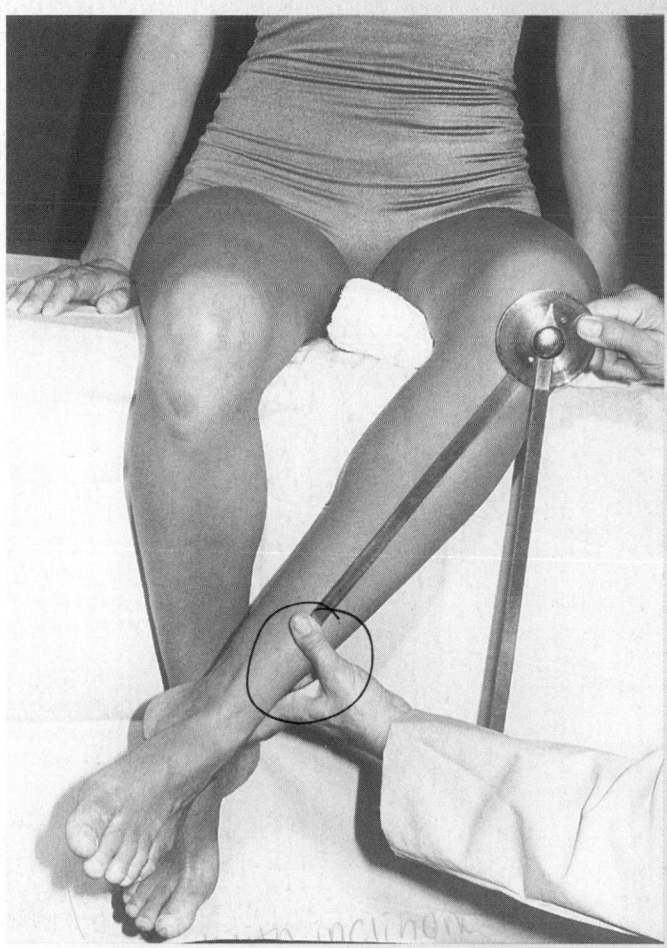

FIGURE 8.26 At the end of hip lateral rotation ROM the examiner uses one hand to support the subject's leg and to maintain alignment of the distal goniometer arm.

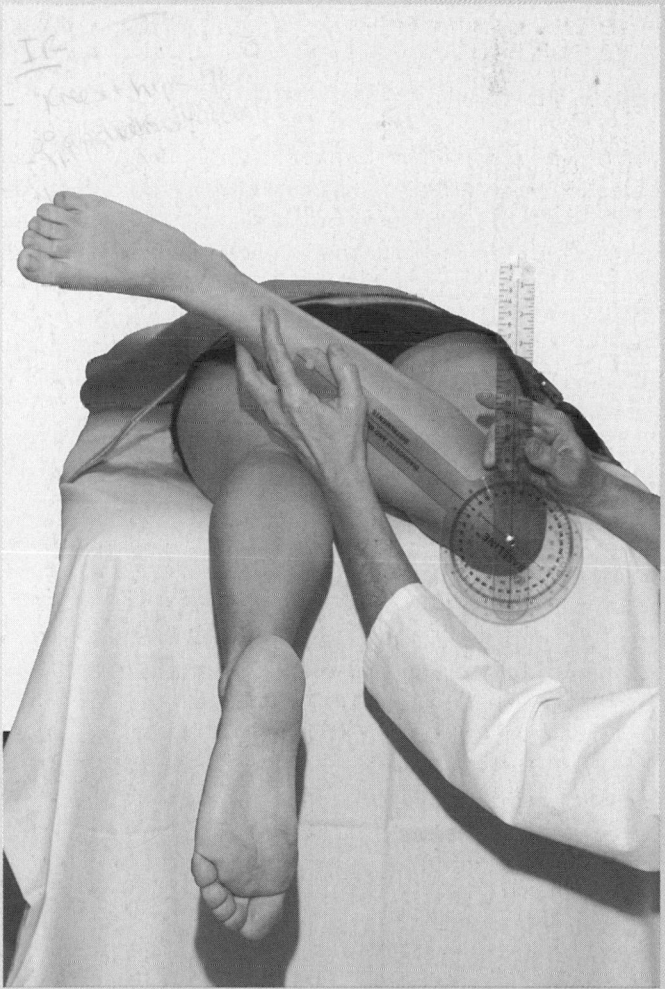

FIGURE 8.27 Hip lateral rotation in the prone testing position with the goniometer aligned at the end of the motion. Note that a strap is placed across the pelvis for stabilization.

MUSCLE LENGTH TESTING PROCEDURES: Hip

● HIP FLEXORS: THOMAS TEST

The iliacus and psoas major muscles flex the hip in the sagittal plane of motion. The rectus femoris flexes the hip in the sagittal plane but also extends the knee. Other muscles, because of their attachments, create hip flexion in combination with other motions. The sartorius flexes, abducts, and laterally rotates the hip while flexing the knee. The tensor fascia lata abducts, flexes, and medially rotates the hip and extends the knee. Several muscles that primarily adduct the hip, such as the pectineus, adductor longus, and adductor brevis, also lie anterior to the axis of the hip joint and can contribute to hip flexion. Short muscles that flex the hip limit hip extension ROM. Hip extension can also be limited by abnormalities of the joint surfaces, shortness of the anterior joint capsule, and short iliofemoral and ischiofemoral ligaments.

The anatomy of the major muscles that flex the hip is illustrated in Figure 8.28A and B. The **iliacus** originates proximally from the upper two thirds of the iliac fossa, the inner lip of the iliac crest, the lateral aspect (ala) of the sacrum, and the sacroiliac and iliolumbar ligaments. It inserts distally on the lesser trochanter of the femur. The **psoas major** originates proximally from the sides of the vertebral bodies and intervertebral discs of T12-L5 and the transverse processes of L1-L5. It inserts distally on the lesser trochanter of the femur. These two muscles are commonly referred to as the **iliopsoas.** If the iliopsoas is short, it limits hip extension without pulling the hip in another direction of motion; the thigh remains in the sagittal plane. Knee position does not affect the length of the iliopsoas muscle.

The **rectus femoris** arises proximally from two tendons: the anterior tendon from the anterior inferior iliac spine and the posterior tendon from a groove superior to the brim of the acetabulum (see Fig. 8.28B). It inserts distally into the base of the patella and into the tibial tuberosity via the patellar ligament. A short rectus femoris limits hip extension and knee flexion. If the rectus femoris is short and hip extension is attempted, the knee passively moves into extension to accommodate the shortened muscle. Sometimes, when the rectus femoris is shortened and hip extension is attempted, the knee remains flexed but hip extension is limited.

The **sartorius** (see Fig. 8.28A) arises proximally from the ASIS and the upper aspect of the iliac notch. It inserts distally into the proximal aspect of the medial tibia. If the sartorius is short, it limits hip extension, hip adduction, and knee extension. If the sartorius is short and hip extension is attempted, the hip passively moves into hip abduction and knee flexion to accommodate the short muscle.

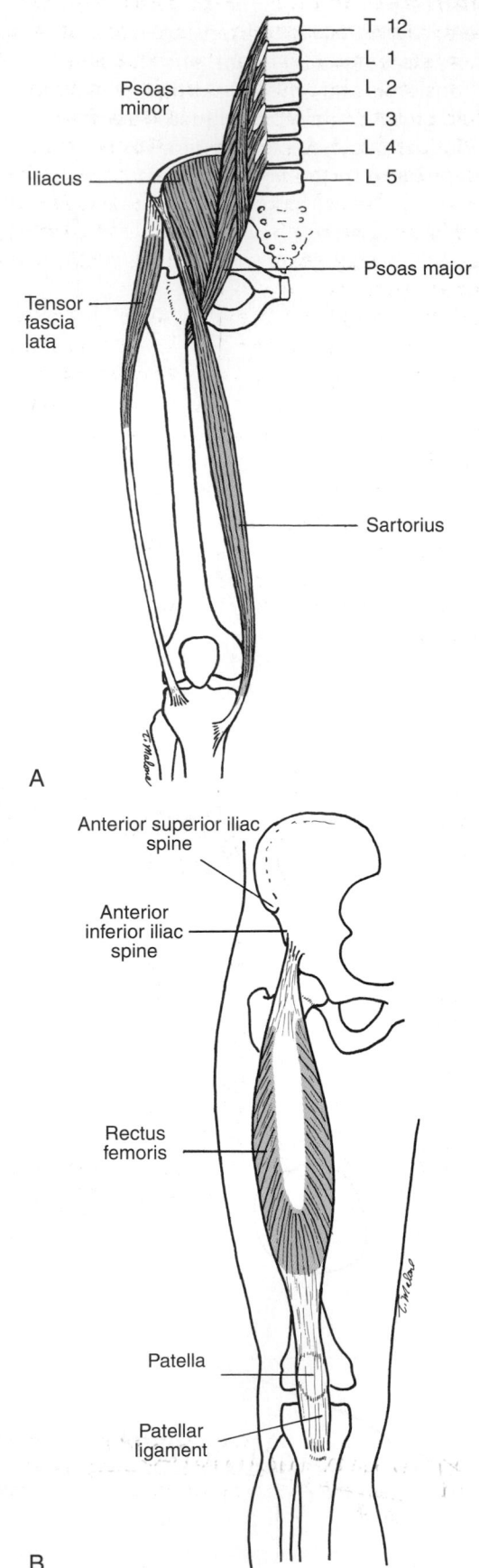

A

B

FIGURE 8.28 An anterior view of the hip flexor muscles.

The **tensor fascia lata (TFL)** arises proximally from the anterior aspect of the outer lip of the iliac crest and the lateral surface of the ASIS and iliac notch (see Fig. 8.28A). It inserts distally into the iliotibial band of the fascia lata about one-third of the distance down the thigh. The iliotibial band inserts into the lateral anterior surface of the proximal tibia. When the tensor fascia lata is short, it can limit hip adduction, extension and lateral rotation, and knee flexion. If hip extension is attempted, the hip passively moves into abduction and medial rotation to accommodate the short muscle.

The **pectineus** originates from the pectineal line of the pubis and inserts in a line from the lesser trochanter to the linea aspera of the femur. The **adductor longus** arises proximally from the anterior aspect of the pubis and inserts distally into the linea aspera of the femur. The **adductor brevis** originates from the inferior ramus of the pubis. It inserts into a line that extends from the lesser trochanter to the linea aspera and the proximal part of the linea aspera just posterior to the pectineus and proximal part of the adductor longus. Shortness of these muscles limits hip abduction and extension. If these muscles are short and hip extension is attempted,

the hip passively moves into adduction to accommodate the shortened muscles.

Starting Position

Place the subject in the sitting position at the end of the examining table, with the lower thighs, knees, and legs off the table. Assist the subject into the supine position by supporting the subject's back and flexing the hips and knees (Fig. 8.29). This sequence is used to avoid placing a strain on the subject's lower back while the starting test position is being assumed. Once the subject is supine, flex the hips by bringing the knees toward the chest just enough to flatten the low back and pelvis against the table (Fig. 8.30). In this position, the pelvis is in about 10 degrees of posterior pelvic tilt. Avoid pulling the knees too far toward the chest because this will cause the low back to go into excessive flexion and the pelvis to go into an exaggerated posterior tilt. This low back and pelvis position gives the appearance of tightness in the hip flexors when, in fact, no tightness is present.

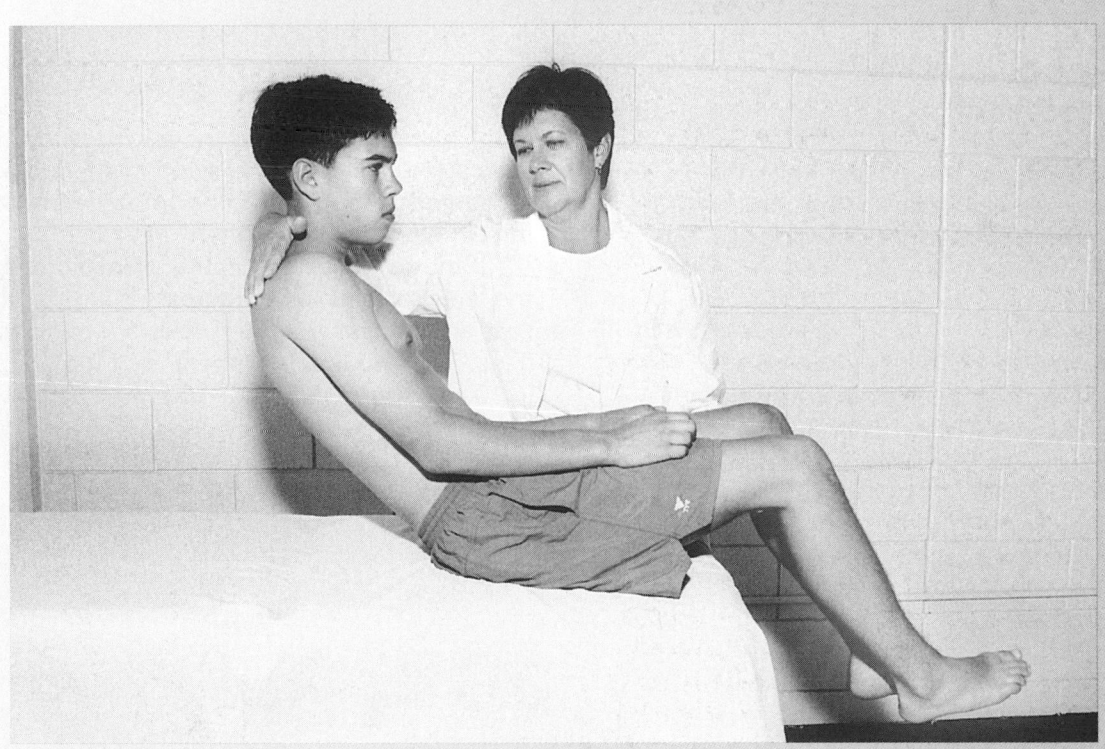

FIGURE 8.29 The examiner assists the subject into the starting position for testing the length of the hip flexors. Ordinarily the examiner stands on the same side as the hip being tested to visualize the hip region and take measurements, but the examiner is standing on the contralateral side for the photograph.

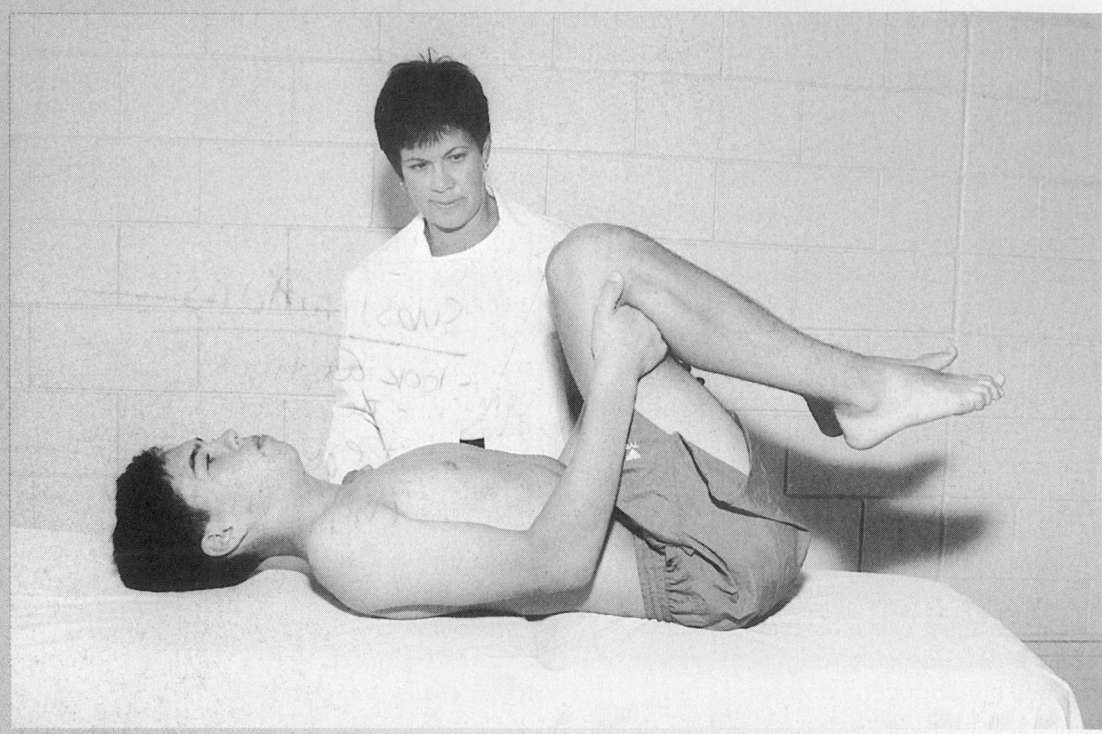

FIGURE 8.30 The starting position for testing the length of the hip flexors. Both knees and hips are flexed so that the low back and pelvis are flat on the examining table.

Stabilization

Either the examiner or the subject holds the hip not being tested in flexion (knee toward the chest) to maintain the low back and pelvis flat against the examining table.

Testing Motion

Information as to which muscles are short can be gained by varying the position of the knee and carefully observing passive motions of the hip and knee while hip extension is attempted. Extend the hip being tested by lowering the thigh toward the examining table. The knee is relaxed in approximately 80 degrees of flexion. The lower extremity should remain in the sagittal plane.

If the thigh lies flat on the examining table and the knee remains in 80 degrees of flexion, the iliopsoas and rectus femoris muscles are of normal length[6] (Figs. 8.31 and 8.32). At the end of the test, the hip is in 10 degrees of extension because the pelvis is being held in 10 degrees of posterior tilt. At this point, the test would be concluded.

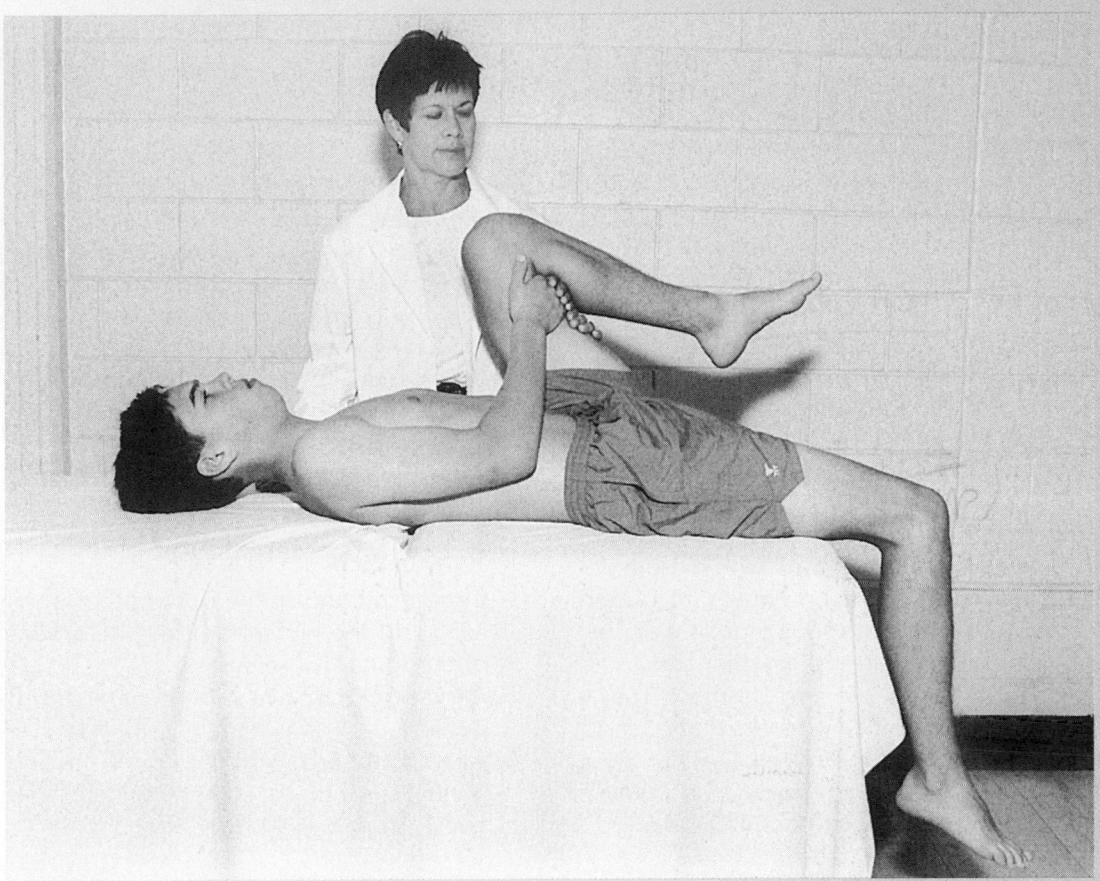

FIGURE 8.31 The end of the motion for testing the length of the hip flexors. The subject has normal length of the right hip flexors: the hip is able to extend to 10 degrees (thigh is flat on table), the knee remains in 80 degrees of flexion, and the lower extremity remains in the sagittal plane. Ordinarily the examiner would stand on the side of the hip being tested, but she has moved to the other side so that a photograph could be taken.

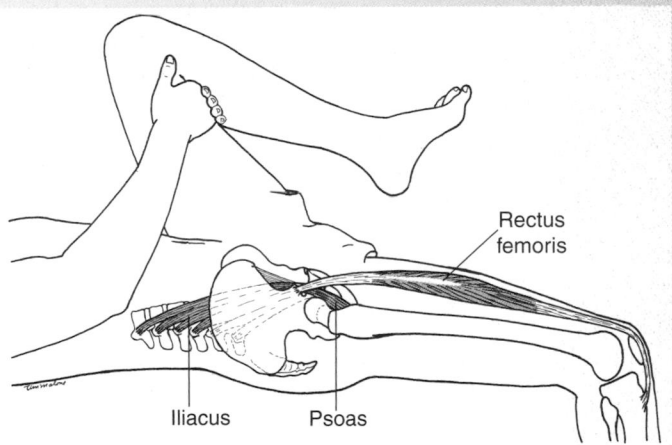

FIGURE 8.32 A lateral view of the hip showing the hip flexors at the end of the Thomas test.

If the thigh does not lie flat on the table, hip extension is limited and further testing is needed to determine the cause (Fig. 8.33). Repeat the starting portion by flexing the hips and bringing the knee toward the chest. Extend the hip by lowering the thigh toward the examining table, but this time support the knee in extension (Fig. 8.34). When the knee is held in extension, the rectus femoris is slack over the knee joint. If the hip extends with the knee held in extension so that the thigh is able to lie on the examining table, the rectus femoris can be ascertained as being short. If the hip cannot extend with the knee held in extension and the thigh does not lie on the examining table, the iliopsoas, anterior joint capsule, iliofemoral ligament, and ischiofemoral ligament may be short.

When the hip is extending toward the examining table, observe carefully to see if the lower extremity stays in the sagittal plane. If the hip moves into lateral rotation and abduction, the sartorius muscle may be short. If the hip moves into medial rotation and abduction, the tensor fascia lata may be short. The Ober test can be used specifically to check the length of the tensor fasciae latae. If the hip moves into adduction, the pectineus, adductor longus, and adductor brevis may be short. Hip abduction ROM can be measured to test more specifically for the length of the hip adductors.

Normal End-Feel

When the knee remains flexed at the end of hip extension ROM, the end-feel is firm owing to tension in the rectus femoris. When the knee is extended at the end of hip extension ROM, the end-feel is firm owing to tension in the anterior joint capsule, iliofemoral ligament, ischiofemoral ligament, and iliopsoas muscle. If one or more of the following muscles are shortened, they may also contribute to a firm end-feel: sartorius, tensor fascia lata, pectineus, adductor longus, and adductor brevis.

Goniometer Alignment
See Figure 8.35.

1. Center **fulcrum** of the goniometer over the lateral aspect of the hip joint, using the greater trochanter of the femur for reference.
2. Align **proximal arm** with the lateral midline of the pelvis.
3. Align **distal arm** with the lateral midline of the femur, using the lateral epicondyle for reference.

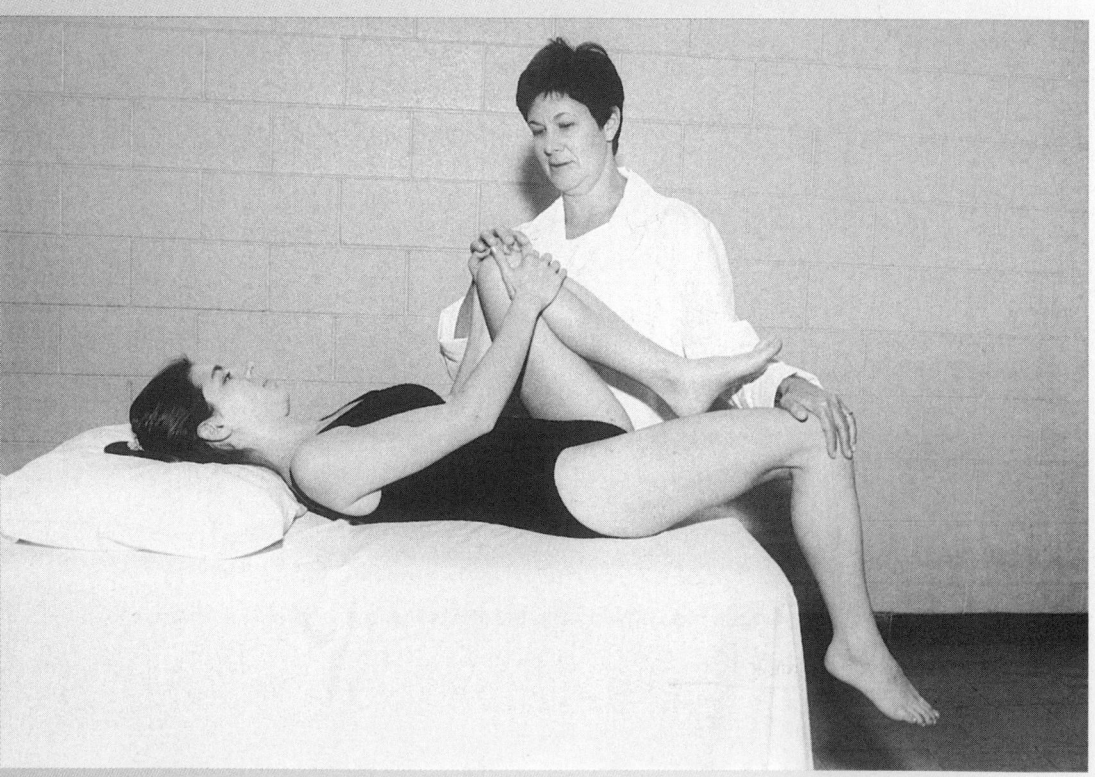

FIGURE 8.33 This subject has restricted hip extension. Her thigh is unable to lie on the table with the knee flexed to 80 degrees. Further testing is needed to determine which structures are short.

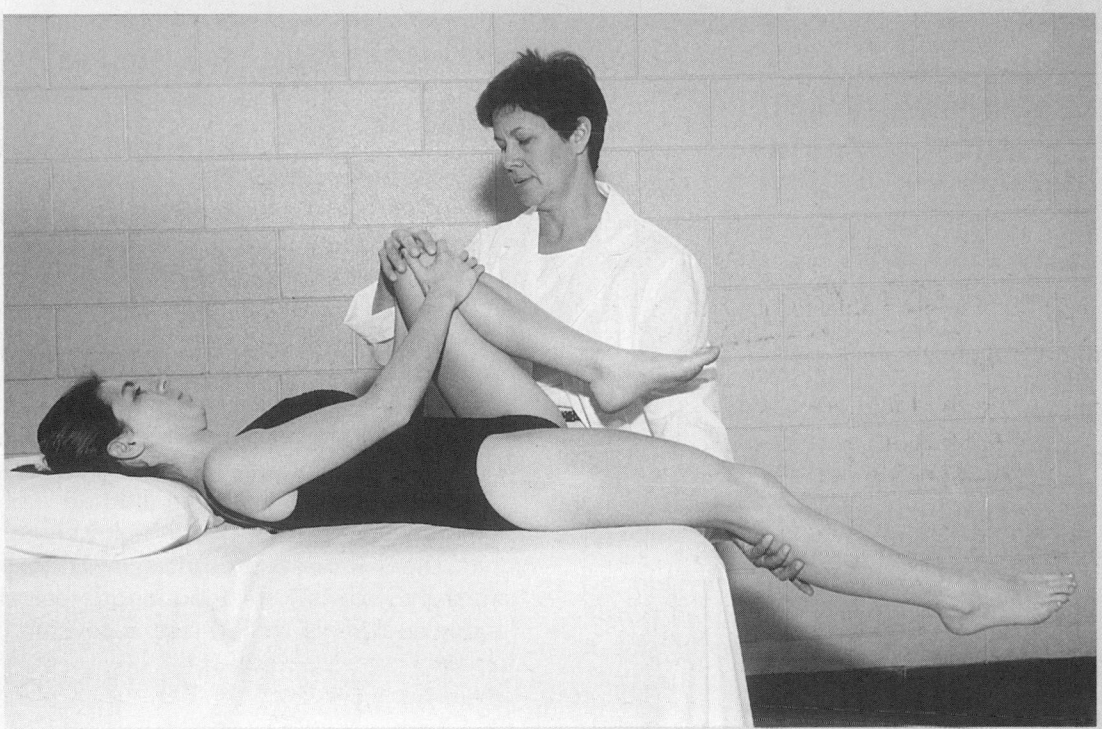

FIGURE 8.34 Because the subject had restricted hip extension at the end of the testing motion (see Fig. 8.33), the testing motion needs to be modified and repeated. This time, the knee is held in extension when the extremity is lowered toward the table. At the end of the test, the hip extends to 10 degrees, and the thigh lies flat on the table. Therefore, one may conclude that the rectus femoris is short and that the iliopsoas, anterior joint capsule, and iliofemoral and ischiofemoral ligaments are of normal length.

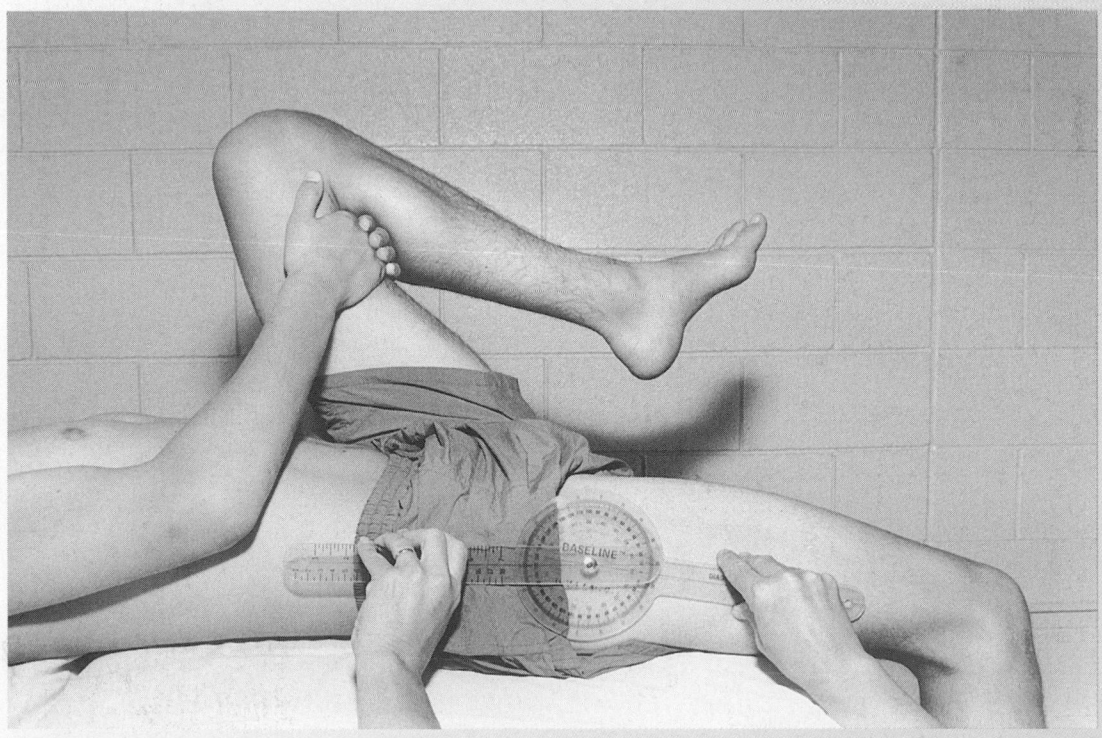

FIGURE 8.35 Goniometer alignment for measuring the length of the hip flexors.

● THE HAMSTRINGS: SEMITENDINOSUS, SEMIMEMBRANOSUS, AND BICEPS FEMORIS: STRAIGHT LEG RAISING TEST

The hamstring muscles, composed of the semitendinosus, semimembranosus, and biceps femoris, cross two joints—the hip and the knee. When they contract, they extend the hip and flex the knee. The **semitendinosus** originates proximally from the ischial tuberosity and inserts distally on the proximal aspect of the medial surface of the tibia (Fig. 8.36A). The **semimembranosus** originates from the ischial tuberosity and inserts on the posterior medial aspect of the medial condyle of the tibia (Fig. 8.36B). The long head of the **biceps femoris** originates from the ischial tuberosity and the sacrotuberous ligament, whereas the short head of the biceps femoris originates proximally from the lateral lip of the linea aspera, the lateral supracondylar line, and the lateral intermuscular septum (Fig. 8.36A). The biceps femoris inserts onto the head of the fibula with a small portion extending to the lateral condyle of the tibia and the lateral collateral ligament.

The hamstring muscles cross the hip and knee joints, and if the hamstrings are short, they can limit both hip flexion and knee extension. Hip flexion is limited when the hamstrings are short and the knee is held in full extension. However, if hip flexion is limited when the knee is flexed, abnormalities of the joint surfaces, shortness of the posterior joint capsule, or a short gluteus maximus may be present.

Hamstring length can be measured using either the straight leg raising (SLR) method, wherein the angle between the pelvis and the thigh is measured, or by the distal hamstring length method, wherein the angle between the thigh and the lower leg is measured. The SLR test is presented in the following section, and the distal hamstring length test, also called the popliteal angle (or PA) test, is covered in the knee chapter.

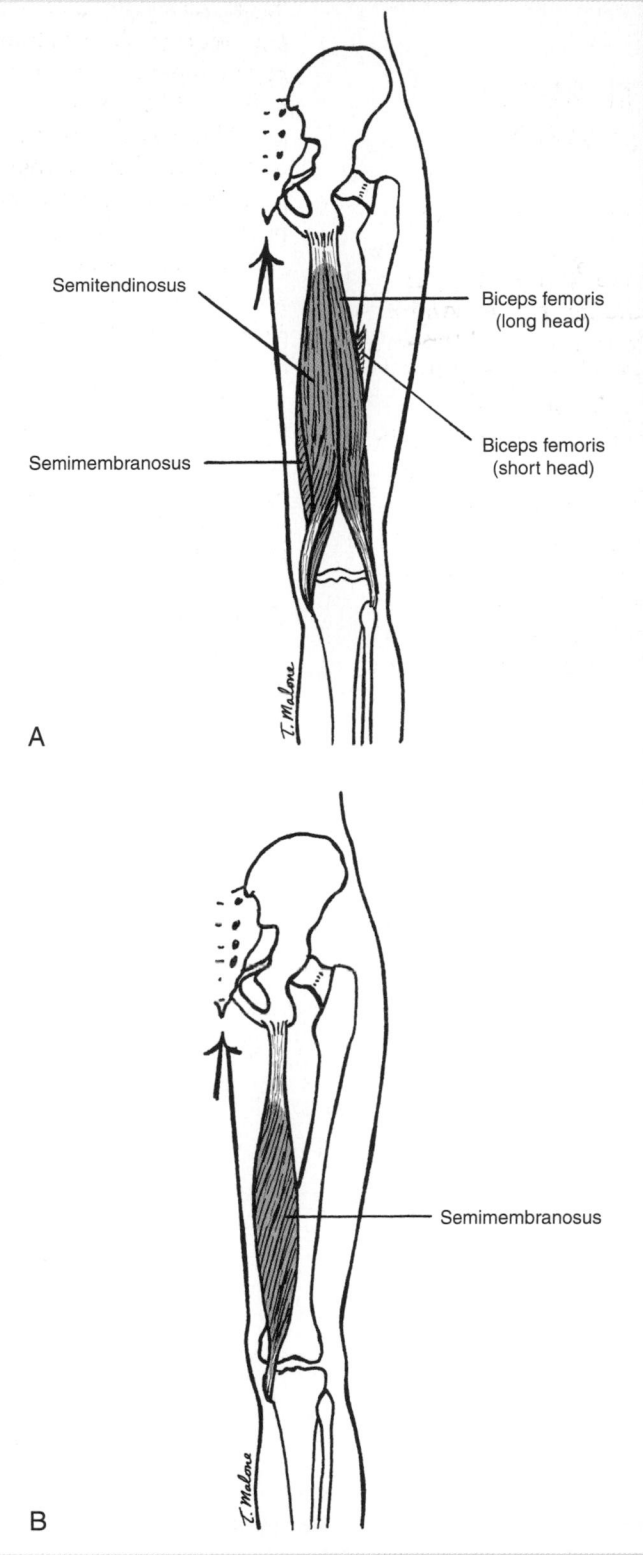

FIGURE 8.36 A posterior view of the hip showing the hamstring muscles (*A* and *B*).

Starting Position

Place the subject in the supine position, with both knees extended and hips in 0 degrees of flexion, extension, abduction, adduction, and rotation (Fig. 8.37). If possible, remove clothing covering the ilium and low back so the pelvis and lumbar spine can be observed during the test.

Stabilization

Hold the knee of the lower extremity being tested in full extension. Keep the other lower extremity flat on the examining table to stabilize the pelvis and prevent excessive amounts of posterior pelvic tilt and lumbar flexion. Usually, the weight of the lower extremity provides adequate stabilization, but a strap securing the thigh to the examining table can be added if necessary.

Testing Motion

Flex the hip by lifting the lower extremity off the table (Figs. 8.38 and 8.39). Keep the knee in full extension by applying firm pressure to the anterior thigh. As the hip flexes, the pelvis and low back should flatten against the examining table. The end of the testing motion occurs when resistance is felt from tension in the posterior thigh and further flexion of the hip causes knee flexion, posterior pelvic tilt, or lumbar flexion. If the hip can flex to between 70 and 80 degrees with the knee extended, the test indicates normal length of the hamstring muscles.[6]

In a study of 214 adults (106 men and 106 women) aged 20 to 79 years, Youdas and associates[7] measured hip flexion ROM in the SLR test and found that females had a mean hip flexion range of 76.3 (standard deviation [SD] = 9.5) degrees and males had a mean range of 68.5 (SD = 6.8) degrees.

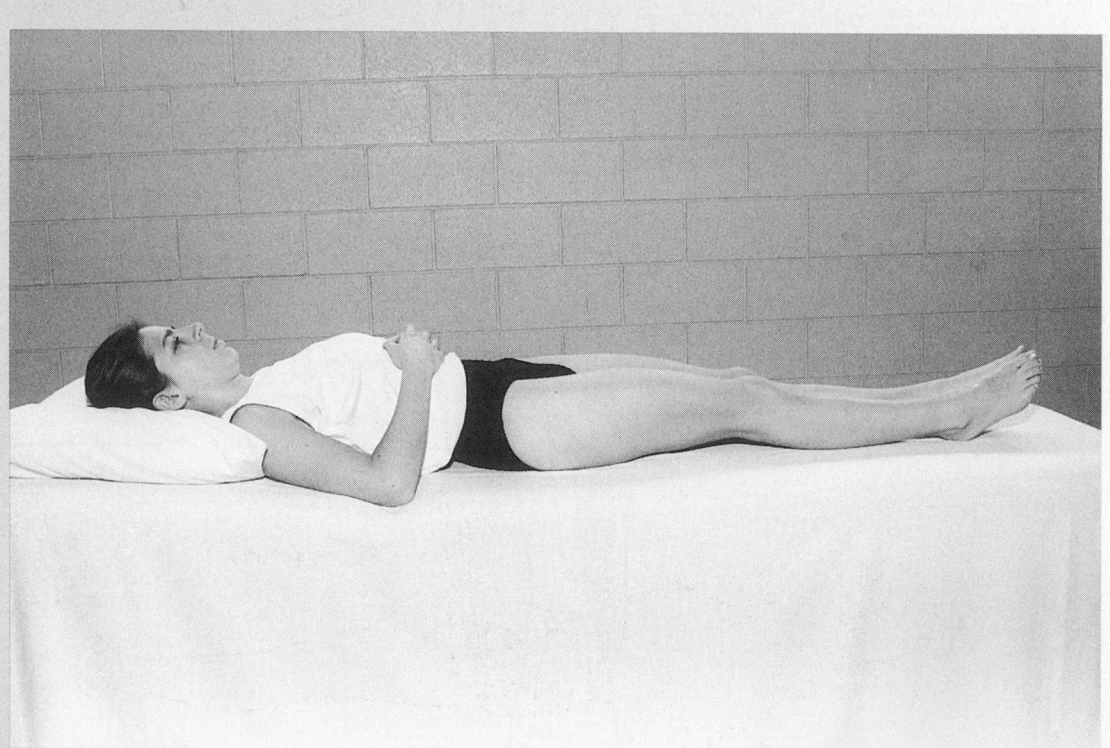

FIGURE 8.37 The starting position for testing the length of the hamstring muscles with the straight leg raising test (SLR).

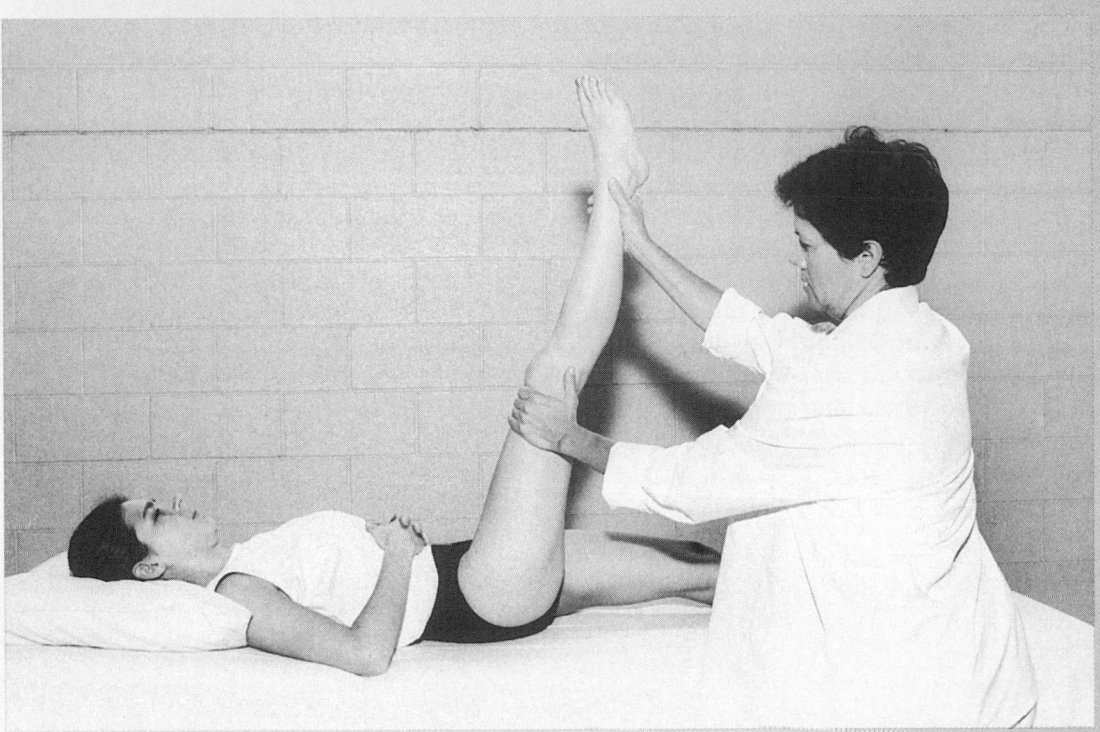

FIGURE 8.38 The end of the testing motion for the length of the hamstring muscles. The subject has normal length of the hamstrings: the hip can be passively flexed to 70 to 80 degrees with the knee held in full extension.

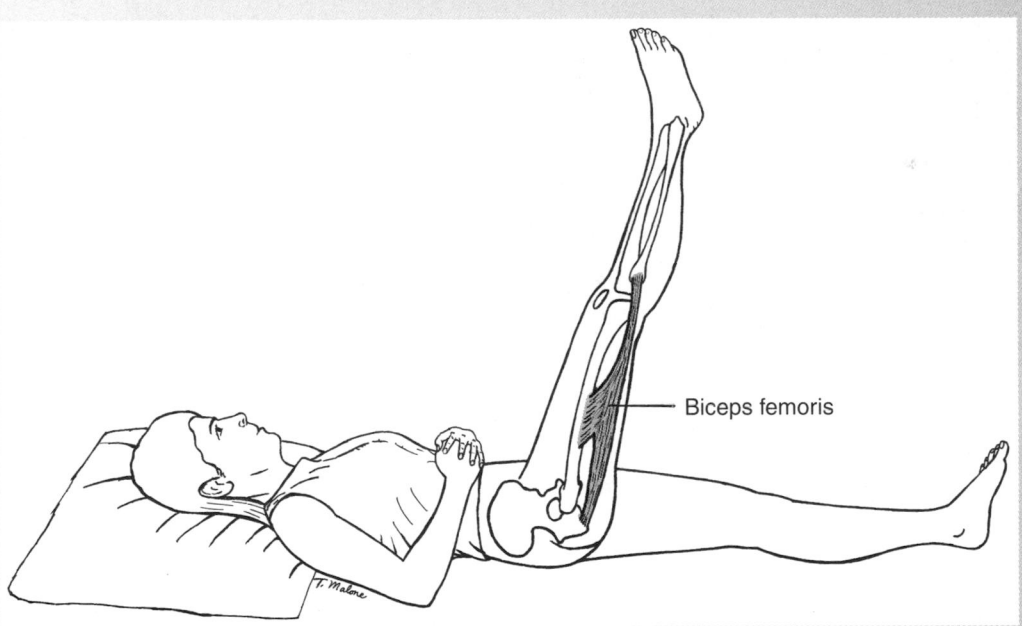

FIGURE 8.39 A lateral view of the hip showing the biceps femoris at the end of the testing motion for the length of the hamstrings.

Shortness of muscles in the hip and lumbar region influences the results of the SLR test. If the subject has short hip flexors on the side that is not being tested, the pelvis is held in an anterior tilt when that lower extremity is lying on the examining table. An anterior pelvic tilt decreases the distance that the leg being tested can lift off the examining table, thus giving the appearance of less hamstring length than is actually present. To remedy this situation, have the subject flex the hip not being tested by resting the foot on the table or by supporting the thigh with a pillow (Fig. 8.40). This position slackens the short hip flexors and allows the low back and pelvis to flatten against the examining table. Be careful to avoid an excessive amount of posterior pelvic tilt and lumbar flexion.

If the subject has short lumbar extensors, the low back has an excessive lordotic curve and the pelvis is in an anterior tilt. The distance that the leg can lift off the examining table is decreased if the pelvis is in an anterior tilt, giving the appearance of less hamstring length than is actually present. In this case, the examiner needs to carefully align the proximal arm of the goniometer with the lateral midline of the pelvis when measuring hip flexion ROM and not be misled by the height of the lower extremity from the examining table.

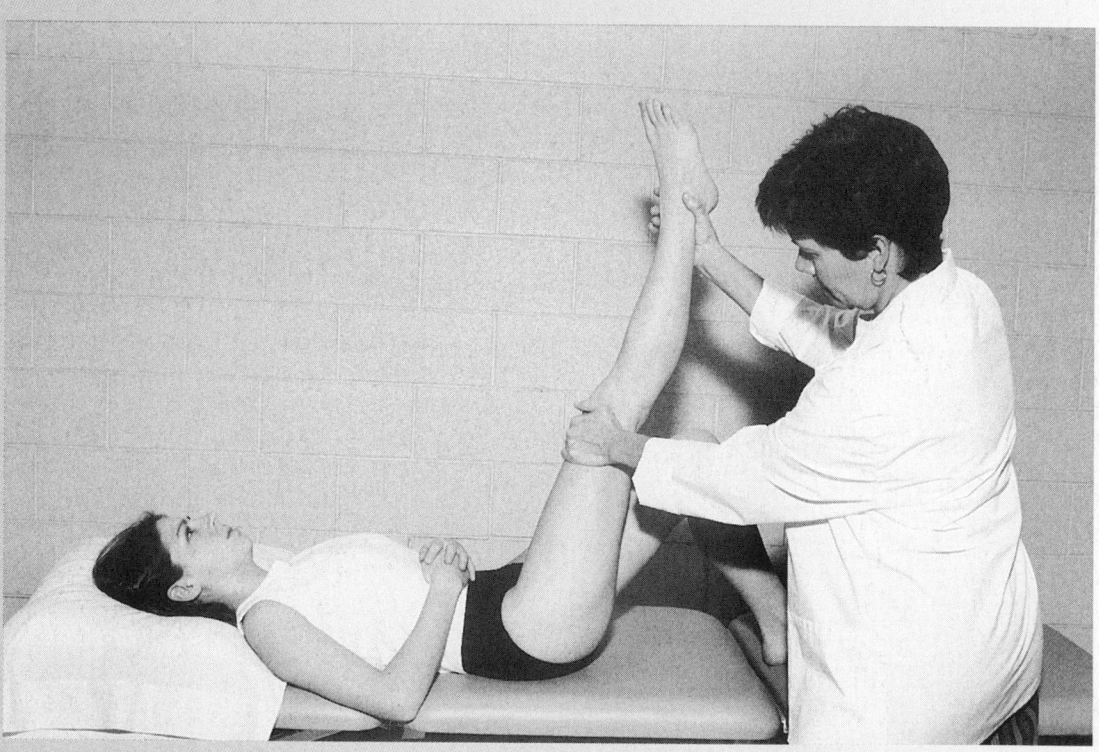

FIGURE 8.40 If the subject has shortness of the contralateral hip flexors, flex the contralateral hip to prevent an anterior pelvic tilt.

Normal End-Feel

The end-feel is firm owing to tension in the semimembranosus, semitendinosus, and biceps femoris muscles.

Goniometer Alignment

See Figure 8.41.

1. Center **fulcrum** of the goniometer over the lateral aspect of the hip joint, using the greater trochanter of the femur for reference.
2. Align **proximal arm** with the lateral midline of the pelvis.
3. Align **distal arm** with the lateral midline of the femur, using the lateral epicondyle for reference.

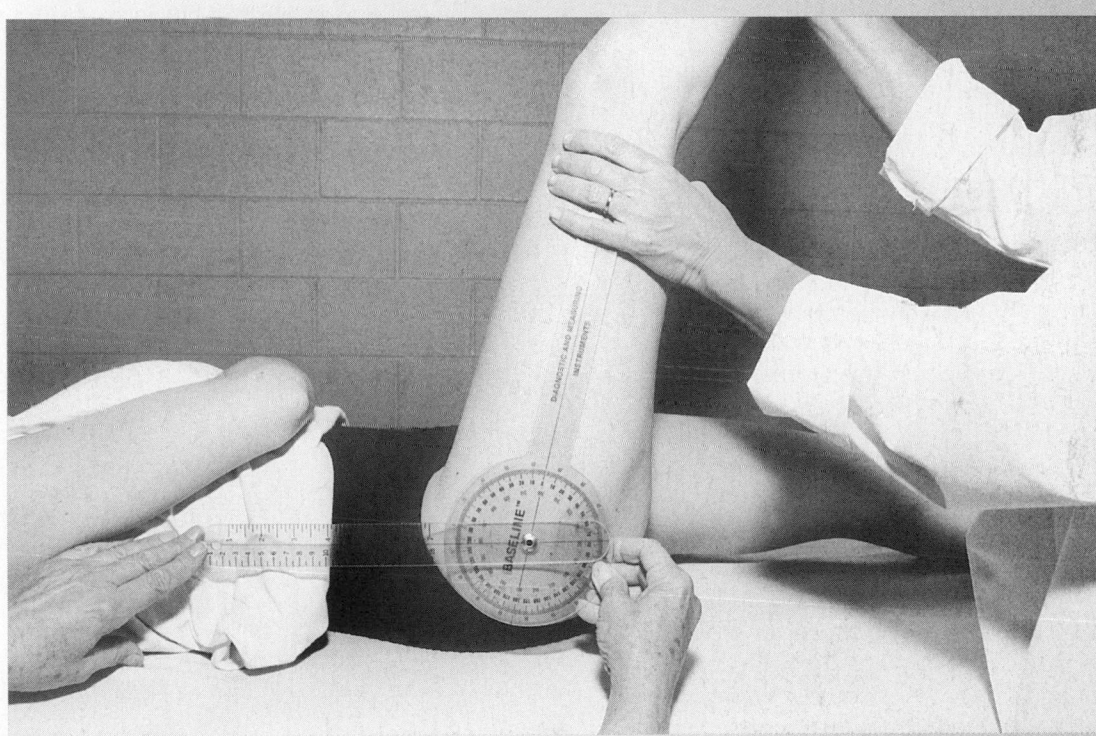

FIGURE 8.41 Goniometer alignment for measuring the length of the hamstring muscles. Another examiner will need to take the measurement while the first examiner supports the leg being tested.

• TENSOR FASCIA LATA AND ILIOTIBIAL BAND: OBER TEST

The **tensor fascia lata** crosses two joints—the hip and knee. When this muscle contracts, it abducts, flexes, and medially rotates the hip and extends the knee. The tensor fascia lata arises proximally from the anterior aspect of the outer lip of the iliac crest and the lateral surface of the ASIS and the iliac notch (Fig. 8.42). It attaches distally into the iliotibial band of the fascia lata about one-third of the way down the thigh. The **iliotibial band** inserts into the lateral tuberosity of the tibia, the head of the fibula, the lateral condyle of the femur, and the lateral patellar retinaculum. If the tensor fascia lata is short, it limits hip adduction and to a lesser extent hip extension, hip lateral rotation, and knee flexion. Shortening of this structure has been cited as a contributing cause of low-back pain,[8] iliotibial band friction syndrome,[9] and patellofemoral pain due to lateral tracking and tilting of the patella.[10]

Some authors have stated that the tensor fasciae latae is of normal length when the hip adducts to the examining table.[11,12] However, according to Kendall and colleagues,[6] stabilization of the pelvis to prevent a lateral tilt and avoidance of hip flexion and medial rotation will limit hip adduction to 10 degrees during the testing motion, which causes the thigh to drop only slightly below the horizontal position. More conservative hip adduction values have been reported as normal by Cade and associates,[13] who found that only 7 of 50 young female subjects had normal (or not short) Ober test values when the horizontal leg position or 0 degrees of adduction was used as the test parameter.

Gajdosik, Sandler, and Marr[14] used a universal goniometer centered at the ipsilateral ASIS to determine the effects of knee position and gender on Ober test values for 49 adults aged 20 to 43 years. The 26 women in the study had a range of 3 degrees of adduction to 16 degrees of abduction, whereas the 23 men had a range of 4 degrees of adduction to 15 degrees of abduction. According to Wang,[15] a normal value for 36 healthy subjects with a mean age of 24.3 years was found to be 17.8 degrees of adduction measured at the lateral femoral epicondyle at the knee with an inclinometer. Reese and Bandy[16] also used an inclinometer over the distal femur to measure the hip adduction position in 61 healthy subjects with a mean age of 24 years. The authors obtained a mean value of 18.9 degrees of adduction (SD = 7.6 degrees), which is similar to the value obtained by Wang.

Starting Position

Place the subject in the sidelying position, with the hip being tested uppermost. Position the subject near the edge of the examining table, so that the examiner can stand directly behind the subject. Initially, extend the uppermost knee and place the hip in 0 degrees of flexion, extension, adduction, abduction, and rotation. The patient flexes the bottom hip and knee to stabilize the trunk, flatten the lumbar curve, and keep the pelvis in a slight posterior tilt.

Stabilization

Place one hand on the iliac crest to stabilize the pelvis. Firm pressure is usually required to prevent the pelvis from laterally tilting during the testing motion. Having the patient flex the bottom hip and knee can also help to stabilize the trunk and pelvis.

Testing Motion

Support the leg being tested by holding the medial aspect of the knee and the lower leg. Flex the hip and the knee to 90 degrees (Fig. 8.43). Keep the knee flexed and move the hip into abduction and extension to position the tensor fascia lata over the greater trochanter of the femur (Fig. 8.44). Test the length of the tensor fascia lata and iliotibial

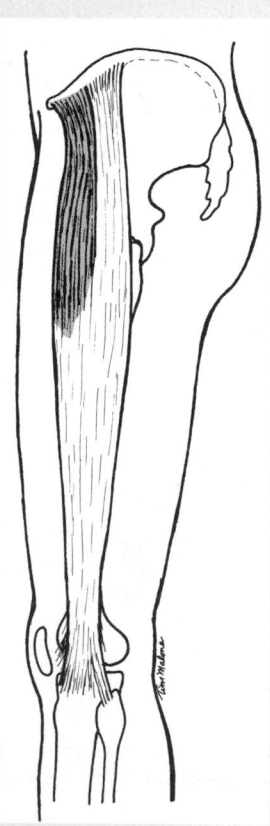

FIGURE 8.42 A lateral view of the left hip showing the tensor fascia lata muscle (in red) and the iliotibial band.

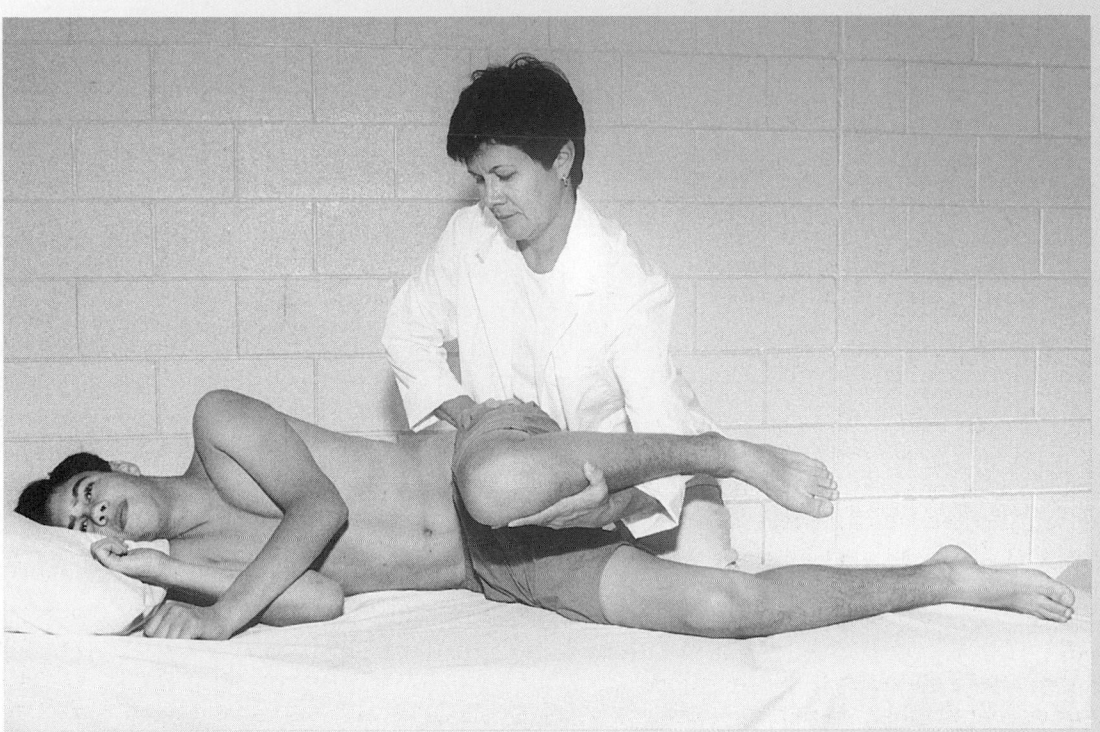

FIGURE 8.43 The first step in the testing motion for the length of the tensor fascia lata and iliotibial band is to flex the hip and knee.

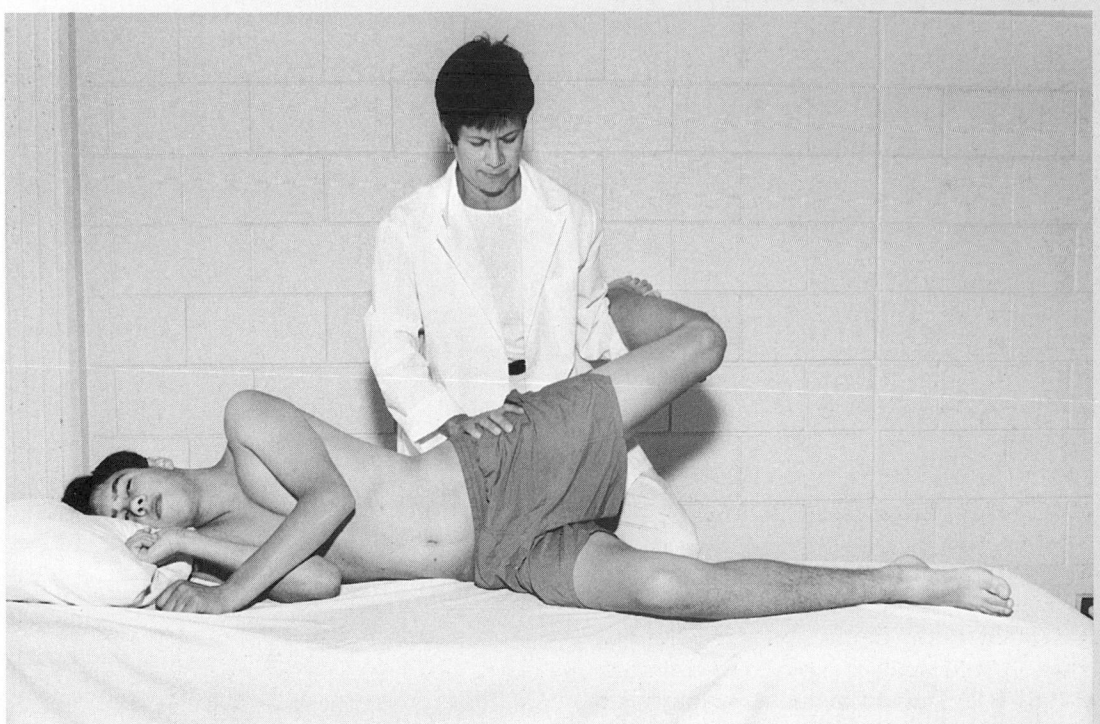

FIGURE 8.44 The next step in the testing motion for the length of the tensor fascia lata and iliotibial band is to abduct and extend the hip.

band by lowering the leg into hip adduction and bringing it down toward the examining table (Figs. 8.45 and 8.46). Do not allow the pelvis to tilt laterally or the hip to flex because these motions slacken the muscle. Keep the knee flexed to control medial rotation of the hip and to maintain the stretch of the muscle. If the thigh drops to slightly below horizontal (10 degrees of hip adduction), the test is negative and the tensor fascia lata and iliotibial band are of normal length.[6] If the thigh remains above horizontal in hip abduction, the tensor fasciae latae and iliotibial band may be tight.

Normal End-Feel

The end-feel is firm owing to tension in the tensor fascia lata.

Goniometer Alignment
See Figure 8.47.

1. Center **fulcrum** of the goniometer over the ASIS of the extremity being measured.
2. Align **proximal arm** with an imaginary line extending from one ASIS to the other.
3. Align **distal arm** with the anterior midline of the femur, using the midline of the patella for reference.

Note that at least 0 degrees of hip extension is needed to perform length testing of the tensor fascia lata and iliotibial band. If the iliopsoas is tight, it prevents the proper positioning of the tensor fascia lata over the greater trochanter. If the rectus femoris is short, the knee may be extended during the test,[6] but extreme care must be taken to avoid medial rotation of the hip as the leg is lowered into adduction. This change in test position is called a Modified Ober test.

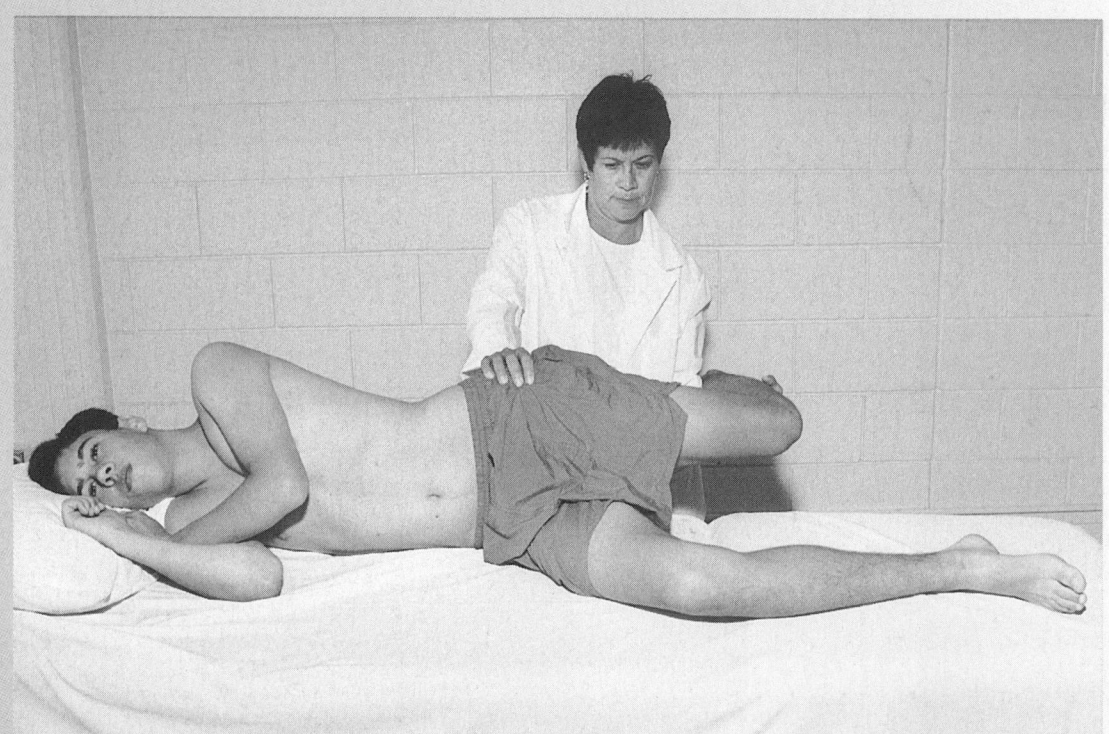

FIGURE 8.45 The end of the testing motion for the length of the tensor fascia lata and iliotibial band. The examiner is firmly holding the iliac crest to prevent a lateral tilt of the pelvis while the hip is lowered into adduction. No flexion or medial rotation of the hip is allowed. The subject has a normal length of the tensor fascia lata and iliotibial band; the thigh drops to slightly below horizontal.

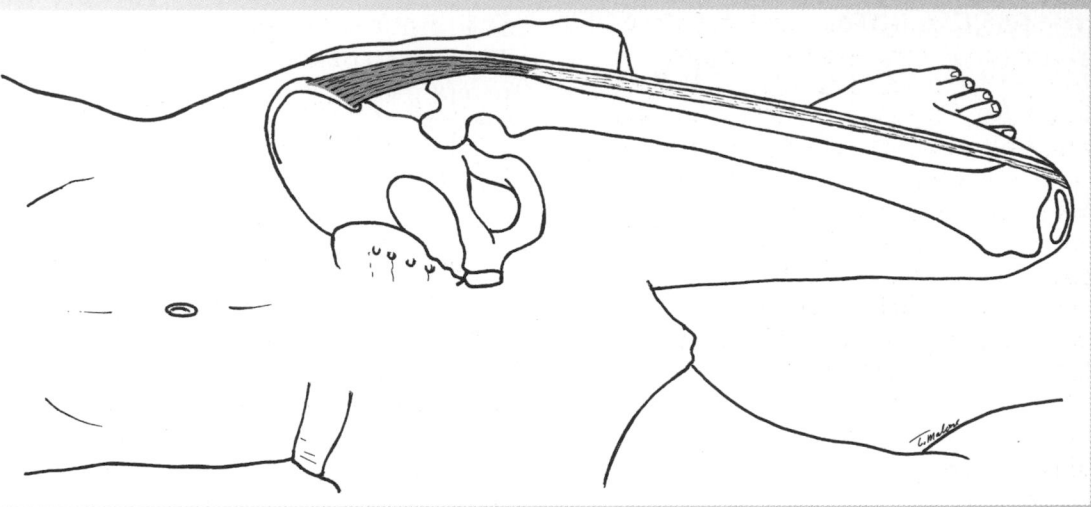

FIGURE 8.46 An anterior view of the hip showing the tensor fascia lata and iliotibial band at the end of the Ober test.

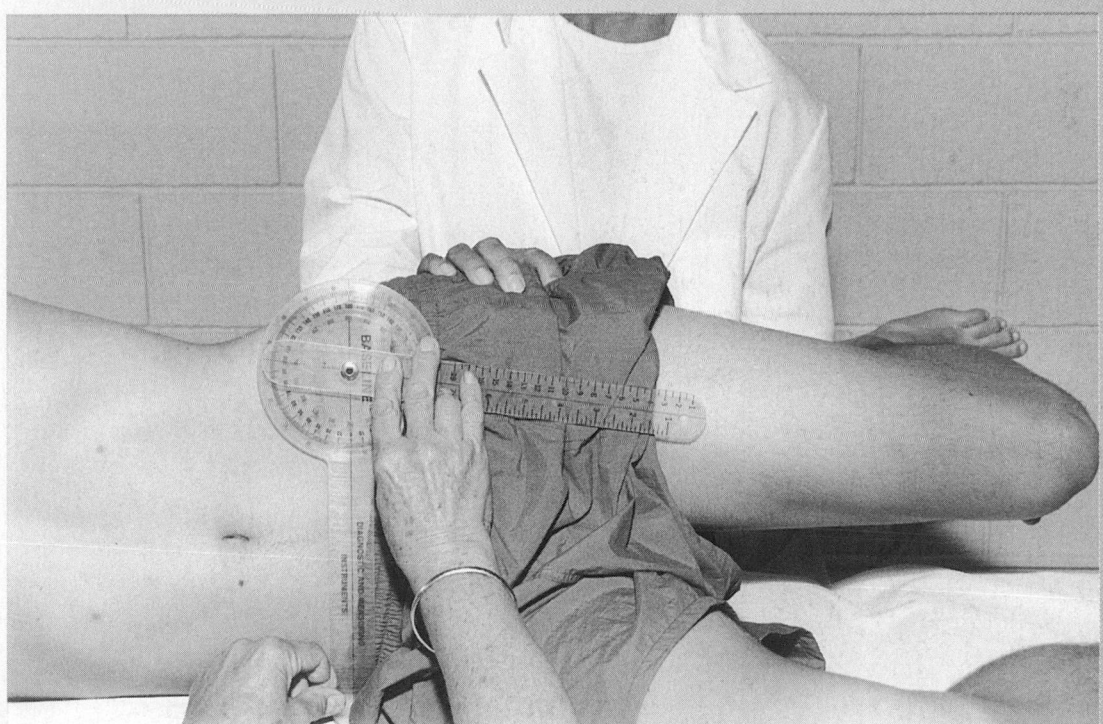

FIGURE 8.47 Goniometer alignment for measuring the length of the tensor fascia lata and iliotibial band. The examiner stabilizes the pelvis and positions the leg being tested while another examiner takes the measurement. If another examiner is not available, a visual estimate will have to be made.

● TENSOR FASCIA LATA AND ILIOTIBIAL BAND: MODIFIED OBER TEST

The Modified Ober test was first proposed by the Kendalls in 1952 to reduce strain in the medial aspect of the knee joint, to reduce tension on the patella, and to reduce the influence of a tight two-joint rectus femoris muscle.[6] Gajdosik, Sandler, and Marr[14] suggest that the two tests yield different results and should not be used interchangeably. The results of the authors' study using a universal goniometer showed that there was a difference between men and women, with men having a range of 20 degrees of adduction to 3 degrees of abduction, whereas women had a range of 11 degrees of adduction to 5 degrees of abduction. Reese and Bandy[16] determined that the hip adduction position measured with an inclinometer over the lateral femoral epicondyle was 23.4 degrees (SD = 7.0 degrees) in the Modified Ober test.

Starting Position

The starting position is the same as for the Ober test except that the knee is held in extension throughout the test.

Stabilization

Stabilization is essentially the same as in the Ober test, but a second person may be needed to assist in either holding the extended leg or in stabilizing the pelvis.

Testing Motion

The testing motion is the same as for the Ober test, but medial rotation may be more of a concern and must be prevented. The end of the test occurs when the pelvis begins to tilt laterally or the leg stops dropping.

Goniometer Alignment

Goniometer alignment is the same as in the Ober test (Fig. 8.48).

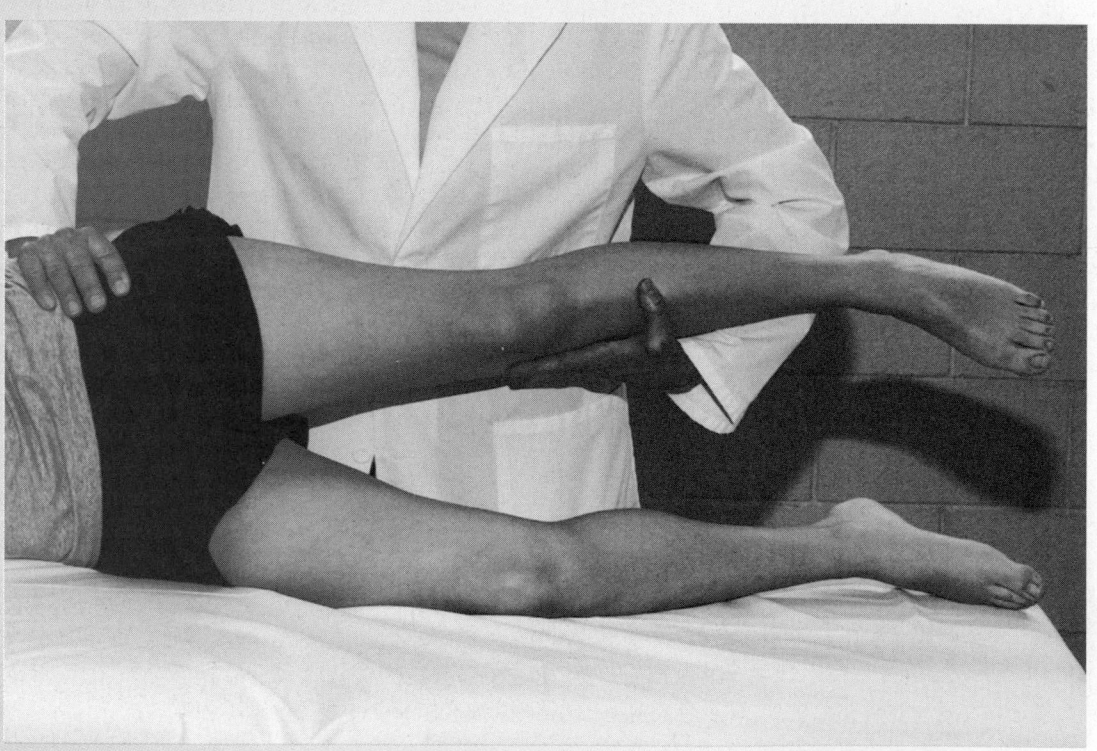

FIGURE 8.48 The extended position of the knee is shown at the end of the Modified Ober test.

⟳ Research Findings

Effects of Age, Gender, and Other Factors

Table 8.1 shows nomal hip range of motion (ROM) values from various sources. The age, gender, measurement instrument used, and number of subjects measured to obtain the AAOS[3] and AMA[4] values were not reported. In Table 8.1, the 9.8 degrees of hip extension motion reported by Boone and Azen[17] is much smaller than the degrees listed by the other authors.[3–5,18] This finding is most likely due to the fact that very young children who often have limitations in hip extension were included in Boone and Azen's study.

Age

Researchers tend to agree that age affects hip ROM[19–25] and that the effects are motion specific in neonates, infants, children, and adults. In neonates some motions are larger than in other age groups and some motions are considerably smaller. Table 8.2 shows passive ROM values for neonates as reported in five studies.[19–23] All values presented in Table 8.2 were obtained by means of a universal goniometer. A comparison of the neonates' passive ROM values shown in Table 8.2 with the values of older children and adults shown in Table 8.1 reveals that the neonates studied have larger passive ROM in most hip motions except for extension, which is limited. The neonates' ROM in hip lateral and medial rotation and abduction is much larger than the ROM values of adults and older children for the same motions. Also, the relationship between hip lateral and medial rotation appears to differ from that found in a majority of older children and adults. Hip lateral rotation values for the neonates are considerably greater than the values for medial rotation, whereas in children and adults the lateral rotation values are either about the same or less than the values for medial rotation.[25]

Kozic and colleagues,[26] in a study of passive lateral and medial rotation in 1140 children aged 8 to 9 years, found that 90 percent of the children had less than 10 degrees difference between lateral and medial rotation. Ellison and coworkers,[27] in a study of 100 healthy adults and 50 patients with back problems, found that only 27 percent of healthy subjects compared with 48 percent of patients had greater lateral rotation than medial rotation. The large number of patients who had greater lateral than medial rotation suggests a rotational imbalance that may be related to back problems.

However, as seen in Table 8.2 and Table 8.3, the most dramatic effect of age is on hip extension ROM in newborns and infants because they are unable to extend the hip from full flexion to the neutral position (returning to 0 degrees from the end of the flexion ROM).[15–22] Waugh and associates[19] found that all 40 infants tested lacked complete hip extension, with limitations ranging from 21.7 degrees to 68.3 degrees. Forero, Okamura, and Larson[25] found that all 60 healthy, full-term neonates studied had hip extension limitations that ranged from 17 to 39 degrees, with a mean range of 30 degrees. Schwarze and Denton[20] found mean limitations of 19 degrees for boys and 21 degrees for girls, and Broughton, Wright, and Menelaus[21] found a mean hip extension limitation of 34.1 degrees in 57 boys and girls.

Limitations in hip extension found in the very young are considered to be normal and to decrease with age, as seen in Table 8.3. The term "physiological limitation of motion" has been used by Waugh and associates[19] and Walker[29] to describe the normal hip extension limitation of motion in infants. According to Walker,[29] movement into extension evolves without the need for intervention and should not be considered pathological in newborns and infants. The extension limitation has been attributed to the increased flexor tone that is present in neonates and infants and to the flexed position of the hip in the womb. Usually, a return from flexion to the neutral position is attained in children by 2 years of age, and

TABLE 8.1	Hip Motion: Normal Values in Degrees						
	AAOS[3]	AMA[4]	Boone and Azen[17] 18 mos – 54 yrs Males n = 109	Svenningsen et al[18] 23 yrs Males n = 102	Svenningsen et al[18] 23 yrs Females n = 104	Roach and Miles[5] 25 – 47yrs Males and Females n = 1683	
Motion			Mean (SD)	Mean	Mean	Mean (SD)	
Flexion	120	100	122.3 (6.1)	137	141	121.0 (13.0)	
Extension	20	30	9.8 (6.8)	23	26	19.0 (8.0)	
Abduction		40	45.9 (9.3)	40	42	42.0 (11.0)	
Adduction		20	26.9 (4.1)	29	30		
Medial rotation	45	40*	47.3 (6.0)	38	52	32.0 (8.0)	
Lateral rotation	45	50*	47.2 (6.3)	43	41	32.0 (9.0)	

SD = standard deviation.
* Measurements taken with subjects in the supine position.

| TABLE 8.2 | Age Effects on Hip Motion in Neonates 6 Hours to 4 Weeks of Age: Normal Values in Degrees |

	Waugh et al[19]	Drews et al[22]	Schwarze and Denton[20]	Broughton et al[21]	Wanatabe et al[23]	Forero et al[25]
	6 – 65 hrs n = 40	12 hrs – 6 days n = 54	1 – 3 days n = 1000	1 – 7 days n = 57	4 wks n = 62	1 – 3 days n = 60
Motion	*Mean (SD)*	*Mean (SD)*	*Mean*	*Mean (SD)*	*Mean*	*Mean (SD)*
Flexion	—	—	—	—	138.0	127.5 (4.8)
Extension*	46.3 (8.2)[†]	28.3 (6.0)[‡]	20.0	34.1 (6.3)	12.0	29.9 (4.0)
Abduction	—	55.5 (9.5)[†]	78.0[†]	—	51.0	38.9 (5.1)
Adduction	—	6.4 (3.9)[†]	15.0[†]	—	—	17.3 (3.5)
Medial rotation	—	79.8 (9.3)[†]	58.0	—	24.0	76.0 (5.6)
Lateral rotation	—	113.7 (10.4)[†]	80.0	—	66.0	91.9 (3.0)

SD = standard deviation.
* All values in this row represent the magnitude of the extension limitation.
[†] Tested with subjects in the supine position.
[‡] Tested with subjects in the side-lying position.

extension ROM beginning at the neutral position usually approaches adult values by early adolescence.

Broughton, Wright, and Menelaus[21] found that by 6 months of age, mean hip extension limitations in infants had decreased to 7.5 degrees, and 27 of 57 subjects had no limitation. However, Phelps, Smith, and Hallum[24] found that 100 percent of the 9- and 12-month-old infants tested (n = 50) had some degree of hip extension limitation. At 18 months of age, 89 percent of infants had limitations, and at 24 months, 72 percent still had limitations.

In Table 8.4, very little difference is evident between the ROM values for hip flexion and hip abduction across the life span of 4 to 74 years in contrast to hip medial and lateral rotation, which have the greatest decrease in ROM. Roach and Miles[5] have suggested that differences in active ROM representing less than 10 percent of the arc of motion are of little clinical significance and that any substantial loss of mobility in individuals between 25 and 74 years of age should

be viewed as abnormal and not attributable to aging. In the data from Roach and Miles,[5] hip extension was the only motion in which the difference between the youngest and the oldest groups constituted a decrease of more than 20 percent of the available arc of motion.

Although Svenningsen and associates[18] studied hip ROM in fairly young subjects (761 males and females aged 4 to 28 years), these authors found that even in this limited age span, the ROM for most hip motions showed a decrease with increasing age. However, the reductions in ROM varied according to the motion. Decreases in flexion, abduction, medial rotation, and total rotation were greater than decreases in extension, adduction, and lateral rotation.

Nonaka and associates,[30] in a study of 77 healthy male volunteers aged 15 to 73 years, found that passive hip ROM decreased progressively with increasing age, but no change was observed in knee ROM in the same population. The authors suggested that most activities of daily living can be

| TABLE 8.3 | Hip Extension Limitations in Infants and Young Children 4 Weeks to 5 Years of Age: Values in Degrees |

Wanatabe et al[23]	Broughton et al[21]	Phelps et al[24]		Boone[28]	
4–8 mos n = 54	3 mos n = 57	6 mos n = 57	9 mos n = 25	18 mos n = 18	1–5 yrs n = 19
Mean (SD)	*Mean (SD)*	*Mean (SD)*	*Mean (SD)*	*Mean (SD)*	*Mean (SD)*
4.0	18.9 (6.0)	7.5 (5.7)	10.0 (2.6)	4.0 (3.2)	0.8 (3.4)

SD = standard deviation.

TABLE 8.4	Age Effects on Hip Motion in Individuals 4 to 74 Years of Age: Normal Values in Degrees						

	Svenningsen[18]		Boone[28]		Roach and Miles[5]		
	Female 4 yrs n = 52	Male 4 yrs n = 51	Males		Males and Females		
			6–12 yrs n = 17	13–19 yrs n = 17	25–39 yrs n = 433	40–59 yrs n = 727	60–74 yrs n = 523
Motion	**Mean**	**Mean**	**Mean (SD)**	**Mean (SD)**	**Mean (SD)**	**Mean (SD)**	**Mean (SD)**
Flexion	151	149	124.4 (5.9)	122.6 (5.2)	122.0 (12)	120.0 (14)	118.0 (13)
Extension	29	28	10.4 (7.5)	11.6 (5.0)	22.0 (8)	18.0 (7)	17.0 (8)
Abduction	55	53	48.1 (6.3)	46.8 (6.0)	44.0 (11)	42.0 (11)	39.0 (12)
Adduction	30	30	27.6 (3.8)	26.3 (2.9)	—	—	—
Medial rotation	60	51	48.4 (4.8)	47.1 (5.2)	33.0 (7)	31.0 (8)	30.0 (7)
Lateral rotation	44	48	47.5 (3.2)	47.4 (5.2)	34.0 (8)	32.0 (8)	29.0 (9)

SD = standard deviation.

performed without maximal lengthening of hip joint muscles. Therefore, loss of hip ROM with increasing age may result from shortening of muscles or connective tissue due to reduced compliance of joint structures and degenerative changes in spinal alignment as a result of a decrease in physical activities that stretch the musculature surrounding the hip.

A number of other researchers have investigated age or gender effects on hip ROM.[31–34] Allander and colleagues[31] measured hip ROM in a population of 517 females and 203 males between 33 and 70 years of age. These authors found that older groups had significantly less hip rotation ROM than younger groups.

Walker and colleagues[32] measured all active hip motions in 30 women and 30 men ranging from 60 to 84 years of age. Although Walker and colleagues[32] found no differences in hip ROM between the group aged 60 to 69 years and the group aged 75 to 84 years, both age groups demonstrated a reduced ability to attain a neutral starting position for hip flexion. The mean starting position for both groups for measurements of flexion ROM was 11 degrees instead of 0 degrees. The mean ROM values obtained for both age groups for hip rotation, abduction, and adduction were 14 to 25 degrees less than the average values published by the AAOS.[3] This finding appears to provide support for the use of age-appropriate norms.

James and Parker[34] measured active and passive ROM at the hip, knee, and ankle in 80 healthy men and women ranging from 70 years to 92 years of age. Measurements of hip abduction ROM were taken with a universal goniometer. All other measurements were taken with a Leighton flexometer. Systematic decreases in both active and passive ROM were found in subjects between 70 and 92 years of age. Hip abduction decreased the most with age and was 33.4 percent less in the oldest group of men and women (those aged 85 to 92 years) compared with the youngest group (those aged 70 to 74 years). Medial and lateral rotation also decreased considerably, but the decrease was not as great as that seen in abduction. In contrast, hip flexion with the knee either extended or flexed was least affected by age, with a significant reduction occurring only in those older than 85 years of age. Passive ROM was greater than active ROM for all joint motions tested, with the largest difference (7 degrees) occurring in hip flexion with the knee flexed.

In a large study by Steinberg and colleagues,[35] passive hip ROM was compared in 1320 female dancers aged 8 to 16 years and 223 nondancers of similar age. Hip flexion and medial and lateral rotation decreased in both groups with increasing age, whereas hip abduction decreased significantly with increasing age only in the dancers. Hip extension ROM was found to increase with age in both groups, but the increase was only significant in the dancer group.

Gender

The effects of gender on hip ROM are usually age and motion specific and account for only a relatively small amount of total variance in measurement. Gender effects have been found in both children and adults, but these effects have not been found in neonates and infants. Phelps, Smith, and Hallum[24] found no gender differences in hip rotation in 86 infants and young children (aged 9 to 24 months). Forero, Okamura, and Larson[25] found no significant gender differences in any of six hip motions in 60 neonates (26 females and 34 males).

Some studies have found that female children and adults have greater hip flexion ROM than males.[18,33,34] Boone and coworkers[33] found significant differences for most hip motions when gender comparisons were made for three age groupings of males and females. These findings were age and motion specific. Female children (1 to 9 years of age), young adult females (21 to 29 years of age), and older adult females (61 to 69 years of age) had significantly more hip flexion than their male counterparts. However, female children and young adult females had less hip adduction and lateral rotation than males in comparison groups.

Both young adult females and older adult females had less hip extension ROM than males.

Svenningson and associates[18] measured the passive ROM of 1552 hips in 761 healthy females and males between 4 and 28 years of age. Females of all age groups had greater passive ROM than males for total passive ROM, total rotation, medial rotation, and abduction. The following two findings agreed with Boone's findings: female children in the 11- and 15-year-old age groups and female adults had greater passive ROM in hip flexion than males in the same age groups, and females in the 4- and 6-year-old groups and female adults had less hip lateral rotation than males in the same age groups. However, females had more hip adduction than males, which is opposite to Boone's findings.

Allander and colleagues[31] determined that in five of eight age groups tested, females had a greater amount of hip rotation than males. Walker and colleagues[32] found that 30 females aged 60 to 84 years had 14 degrees more ROM in hip medial rotation than their male counterparts. Simoneau and coworkers[36] discovered that females (with a mean age of 21.8 years) had higher mean values in both medial and lateral rotation than age-matched male subjects. The authors used a universal metal goniometer to measure active ROM of hip rotation in 39 females and 21 males.

James and Parker[34] found that women were significantly more mobile than men in 7 of the 10 motions tested at the hip, knee, and ankle. At the hip, women had greater mobility than men in all hip motions except abduction. Men and women had similar mean values in hip flexion ROM, both with the knee flexed and with the knee extended, in the group aged 70 to 74 years, but in the group between 70 and 85-plus years of age, men had an approximate 25 percent decrease in ROM, whereas women had a decrease of only about 11 percent.

In a study by Youdas and colleagues,[7] two testers used a 360-degree goniometer to measure hamstring length by two methods (straight leg raising and popliteal angle) in 214 adults (108 women and 106 men) aged 20 to 79 years. A significant gender effect was found in both testing methods, with women having approximately 8 degrees more motion than men in the SLR test and 11 degrees more motion than men in the popliteal angle test.

In contrast to the previously mentioned studies, Hu and associates,[37] using a photographic method, found no significant gender differences in all six hip motions in 51 male and 54 female healthy Chinese subjects between the ages of 65 and 85 years living in Beijing, China.

Sanya and Obi[38] found no significant gender differences between 50 male and female patients with diabetes and a control group of 50 healthy subjects. Both groups ranged in age from 21 to 71 years.

Body Mass Index

Increases in body mass index (BMI) seem to decrease the ROM at the hip. Kettunen and colleagues[39] found that former elite athletes with a high BMI had lower total amounts of hip passive ROM compared with former elite athletes with a low BMI. Subjects in the study included 117 former elite athletes between the ages of 45 and 68 years. Measurements were taken by means of a Myrin inclinometer with the subjects in the prone position.

Escalante and coworkers[40] determined that there was a loss of at least 1 degree of passive range of motion in hip flexion for each unit increase in BMI in a group of 687 community-dwelling elders (those who were 65 to 78 years of age). Subjects who were severely obese had an average of 18 degrees less hip flexion than nonobese subjects as measured in the supine position with an inclinometer. BMI explained a higher proportion of the variance in hip flexion ROM than any other variable examined by the authors.

Lichtenstein and associates[41] studied interrelationships among the variables in the study by Escalante and coworkers[40] and concluded that BMI could be considered a primary direct determinant of hip flexion passive ROM. However, Bennell and associates[42] found no effect of BMI on active ROM in hip rotation in a study comparing 77 novice ballet dancers and 49 age-matched controls between the ages of 8 and 11 years. The control subjects, who had a higher BMI than the dancers, also had a significantly greater range of lateral and medial hip rotation.

Testing Position

Simoneau and coworkers[36] found that measurement position (sitting versus prone) had little effect on active hip medial rotation ROM in 60 healthy male and female college students (aged 18 to 21 years), but position had a significant effect on lateral rotation ROM. Lateral rotation measured in the sitting position was statistically less (mean = 36 degrees) than it was when measured on subjects in the prone position (mean = 45 degrees). Bierma-Zeinstra and associates[43] found that both lateral and medial rotation ROMs were significantly less when measured in two males and seven females aged 21 to 43 years in the sitting and supine positions compared to measurements taken in the prone position (Table 8.5). However, Schwarze and Denton[20] found no difference in passive ROM measurements of hip medial and lateral rotation with neonates in the prone position compared to measurements of the 1000 neonates taken in the supine position.

Van Dillen and coworkers[44] compared the effects of knee and hip position on passive hip extension ROM in 10 patients (mean age = 33 years) with low-back pain and 35 healthy subjects (mean age = 31 years). Both groups had less hip extension when the hip was in neutral abduction than when the hip was fully abducted. Both groups also displayed less hip extension ROM when the knee was flexed to 80 degrees than when the knee was fully extended. This finding lends support for Kendall and colleagues,[6] who maintain that changing the knee joint angle during the Thomas test for hip flexor length can affect the passive ROM in hip extension.

Gajdosik, Sandler, and Marr[14] found that changing the position from knee flexion in the Ober test to knee extension in the Modified Ober test changed the angle of hip adduction in 49 subjects (26 women and 23 men). The knee flexed position limited hip adduction more than the knee extended position.

TABLE 8.5	Effects of Position on Hip ROM: Normal Values in Degrees				

Author	Motion	Position		
		Seated	**Prone**	**Supine**
		Mean (SD)	*Mean (SD)*	*Mean*
Simoneau et al[36]	Lateral rotation*	36 (7)	45 (10)	—
	Medial rotation*	33 (7)	36 (9)	—
	Total rotation*	69 (9)	81 (12)	—
Bierma-Zeinstra et al[43]	Lateral rotation*	33.9	47.0	33.1
	Medial rotation*	33.6	46.3	36.0
	Lateral rotation†	37.6	51.9	34.2
	Medial rotation†	38.8	53.2	39.9

SD = standard deviation.
* Active ROM measured with a universal goniometer.
† Passive ROM measured with a universal goniometer.

Arts and Sports

A sampling of articles related to the effects of ballet and other forms of dance, ice hockey, and running on ROM are presented in the following paragraphs. As expected, the effects of the activity on ROM vary with the activity and involve motions that are specific to the particular activity.

Gilbert, Gross, and Klug[45] conducted a study of 20 female ballet dancers (aged 11 to 14 years) to determine the relationship between the dancer's ROM in hip lateral rotation and the turnout angle. An ideal turnout angle is a position in which the longitudinal axes of the feet are rotated 180 degrees from each other. The authors found that turnout angles were significantly greater (between 13 and 17 degrees) than measurements of hip lateral rotation ROM. This finding indicated that the dancers were using excessive movements at the knee and ankle to attain an acceptable degree of turnout. According to the authors, the use of compensatory motions at the knee and ankle predisposes the dancers to injury. The dancers had had 3 years of classical ballet training and still had not been able to attain the degree of hip lateral rotation that would give a 180-degree turnout angle. Consequently, the authors suggest that hip ROM may be genetically determined.

Bennell and associates[42] determined that age-matched control subjects had significantly greater active ROM in hip lateral and medial rotation than a group of 77 ballet dancers (aged 8 to 11 years), although there was no significant difference in the degree of turnout between the two groups. The amount of non-hip lateral rotation was 40 percent in the dancers compared to 20 percent in the control subjects. Non-hip lateral rotation increases torsional forces on the medial aspect of the knee, ankle, and foot in the young dancers and puts this group at high risk of injury. Similar to the findings of Gilbert, Gross, and Klug,[45] the authors found no relationship between number of years of training and lateral rotation ROM, which again suggests a genetic component of ROM.

The authors hypothesized that a shortening of the hip extensors (resulting from constant use) and the dancers' avoidance of full hip medial rotation might account for the fact that the dancers had less hip medial rotation than the control subjects.

Tyler and colleagues[46] found that a group of 25 professional male ice hockey players had about 10 degrees less hip extension ROM than a group of 25 matched control subjects. The authors postulated that the loss of hip extension in the hockey players was probably due to tight anterior hip capsule structures and tight iliopsoas muscles. The flexed hip and knee posture assumed by the players during skating probably contributed to the muscle shortness and loss of hip extension ROM.

Van Mechelen and colleagues[47] used goniometry to measure hip ROM in 16 male runners who had sustained running injuries during the year but who were fit at the time of the study. No right–left differences in hip ROM were found either in the previously injured group or in a control group of runners who had not sustained an injury. However, hip ROM in the injured group was on average 59.4 degrees, or about 10 degrees less than the average ROM of 68.1 degrees in runners without injuries.

Disability

Steultjens and associates[48] used a universal goniometer to measure bilateral active assistive ROM at the hip and knee in 198 patients with osteoarthritis (OA) of the hip or knee. Generally a decrease in hip ROM was associated with an increase in disability, but that association was motion specific. Hip flexion contractures were present in 15 percent of the patients, whereas contractures at the knee were found in 31.5 percent of the patients. Twenty-five percent of the variation in disability levels was accounted for by differences in ROM.

Mollinger and Steffan,[49] in a study of 111 nursing home residents, found a mean hip extension of only 4 degrees.

Beissner, Collins, and Holmes,[50] in a study of 22 men and 58 women with an average age of 81 years, concluded that lower-extremity passive ROM and upper-extremity muscle force were important predictors of function for elderly individuals living in assisted living residences or skilled nursing facilities. Conversely, upper-extremity ROM and age were the strongest predictors of function in elderly individuals residing in independent living situations.

Sanya and Obi[38] measured the hip flexion and extension ROM in 50 diabetic and 50 non-diabetic age-matched control subjects aged 21 to 72 years. The men and women with diabetes had less right (mean = 92.1 degrees) and left hip flexion (mean = 91.7 degrees) than control subjects, whose mean right hip flexion was 110.4 degrees and left hip flexion was 111.0 degrees. Hip extension ROM was also less in the group with diabetes, but the differences were not as large as the differences in hip flexion ROM. The authors suggested that the decreased mobility in this group of patients may affect their ability to perform normal activities of daily living and that people involved in their care should be aware that patients with diabetes may have decreases in ROM that go unnoticed.

Functional Range of Motion

Table 8.6 shows the hip flexion ROM necessary for selected functional activities as reported in several sources. An adequate ROM at the hip is important for meeting mobility demands such as walking, climbing stairs (Fig. 8.49), and performing many activities of daily living that require sitting and bending. According to Magee,[51] ideal functional ranges are 120 degrees of flexion, 0 degrees of abduction, and 20 degrees of lateral rotation. However, as can be seen in Table 8.6, considerably less ROM is necessary for gait on level surfaces.[52]

Livingston, Stevenson, and Olney[53] studied ascent and descent on stairs of different dimensions, using 15 female subjects between 19 and 26 years of age. McFayden and Winter[54] also studied stairclimbing; however, these authors used eight repeated trials of one subject.

Protopapadaki and colleagues [55] compared the ROM required for stair ascent and descent in 33 healthy young individuals using a Vicon Motion Analysis System. No significant difference in hip ROM was found between right and left

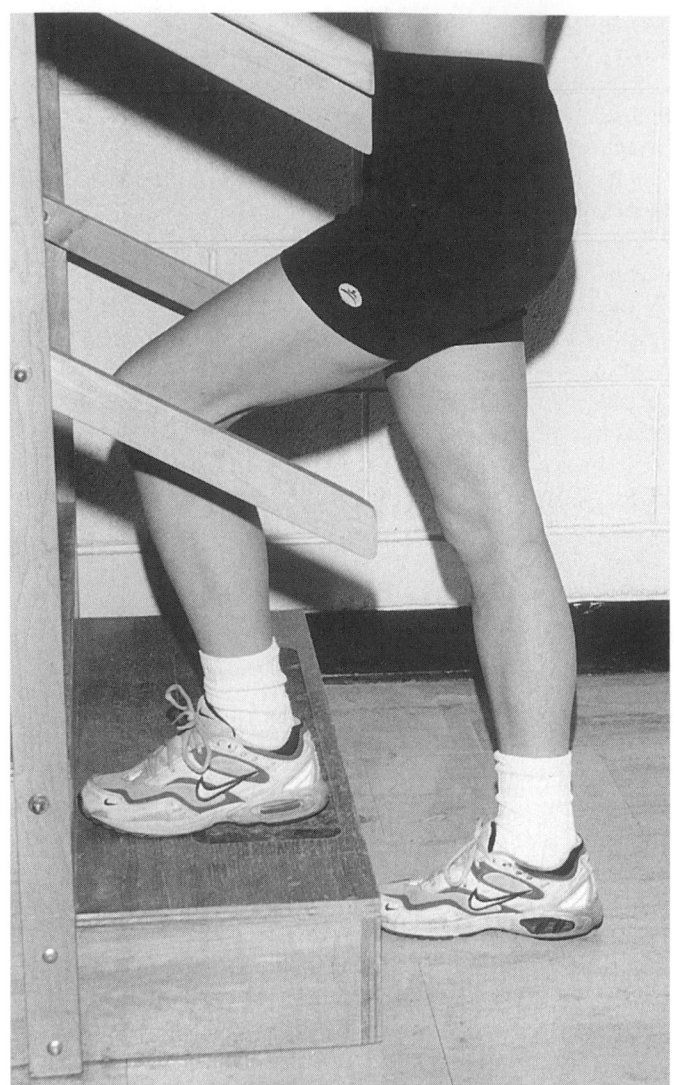

FIGURE 8.49 Ascending stairs requires between 47 and 66 degrees of hip flexion, depending on stair dimensions.[53]

TABLE 8.6	Hip Flexion Range of Motion Required for Functional Activities: Normal Values in Degrees From Selected Sources			
	Livingston, et al[53]	Ranchos Los Amigos Medical Center[39]	McFayden and Winter[54]	Protopapadaki et al[55]
Activity	Range	Range	Mean (SD)	Mean (SD)
Walking on level surfaces	0–30	0–30	44 (4.5)	—
Ascending stairs	1–0–66	—	60	65.1 (7.1)
Descending stairs	1–0–45	—	66 (0.1)	49.0 (7.8)

legs in the 16 males and 17 females (aged 18 to 39 years). The mean hip flexion ROM of 65.1 degrees required for stair ascent was greater than the hip flexion ROM of 40.0 degrees required for descent on stairs with 18-cm risers and a tread length of 28.5 cm.

In a study to determine the effects of age-related ROM on functional activity, Oberg, Krazinia, and Oberg[56] measured hip and knee active ROM with an electrogoniometer during gait in 240 healthy male and female individuals aged 10 to 79 years of age. Age-related changes were slightly more pronounced at slow gait speeds than at fast speeds, but the rate of changes was less than 1 degree per decade, and no distinct pattern was evident, except that hip flexion–extension appeared to be affected less than other motions.

Other functional and self-care activities require a larger ROM at the hip. For example, sitting requires at least 90 to 112 degrees of hip flexion with the knees flexed (Fig. 8.50). Additional hip flexion ROM (120 degrees) is necessary for putting on socks (Fig. 8.51), squatting (115 degrees), and stooping (125 degrees).[54]

The daily activities of various cultures may require a different set of functional ROM values. Hemmerich and coworkers[57] used a Fastrak electromagnetic tracking system to assess

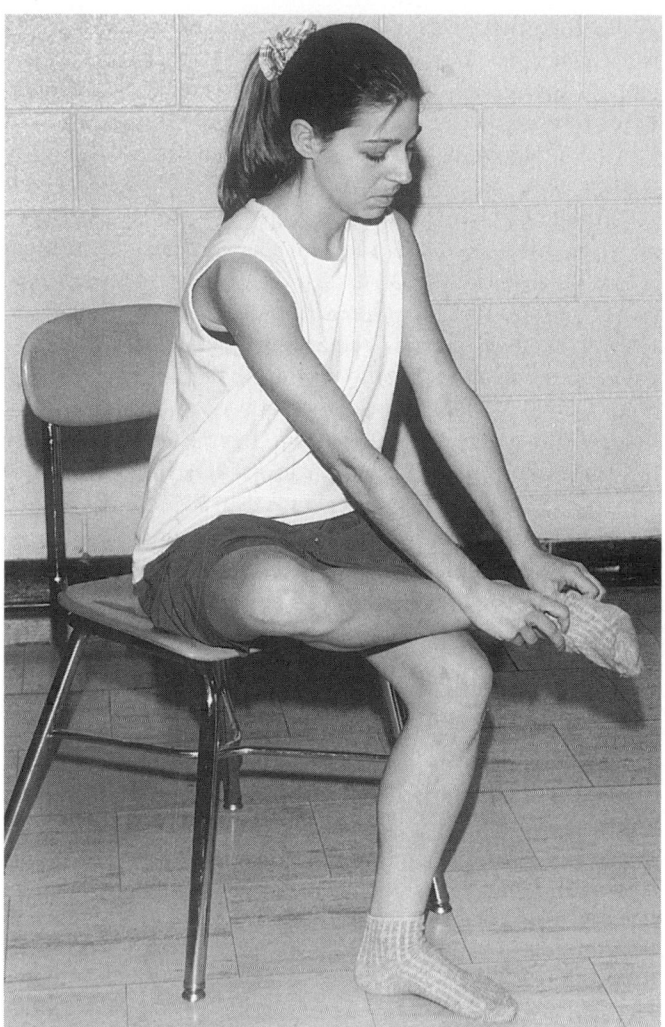

FIGURE 8.51 Putting on socks requires 120 degrees of flexion, 20 degrees of abduction, and 20 degrees of lateral rotation.[51]

hip, knee, and ankle ROM in 30 healthy Indian subjects (10 women and 20 men) with an average age of 48 years. The daily activities of this group of subjects included squatting with heels up or down, kneeling with ankles either dorsiflexed or plantarflexed, and sitting cross-legged on the floor. The mean maximum amount of hip flexion for squatting with the heels down was 95.4 degrees. Sitting cross-legged required a mean maximal angle of hip flexion of 83.5 degrees, a mean maximal angle of hip abduction of 34 degrees, and a mean maximal angle of hip lateral rotation of 37 degrees. The authors suggested that the prayer positions of Muslims and customs of other cultures may involve additional ROM at the hips, knees, and ankles.

Reliability and Validity

Studies of the reliability of hip measurements have included both active and passive motion and different types of measuring instruments. Also, reliability has been assessed in different age and patient populations.[58–63] Therefore, comparisons among studies are difficult. Boone and associates[64] and Clapper and

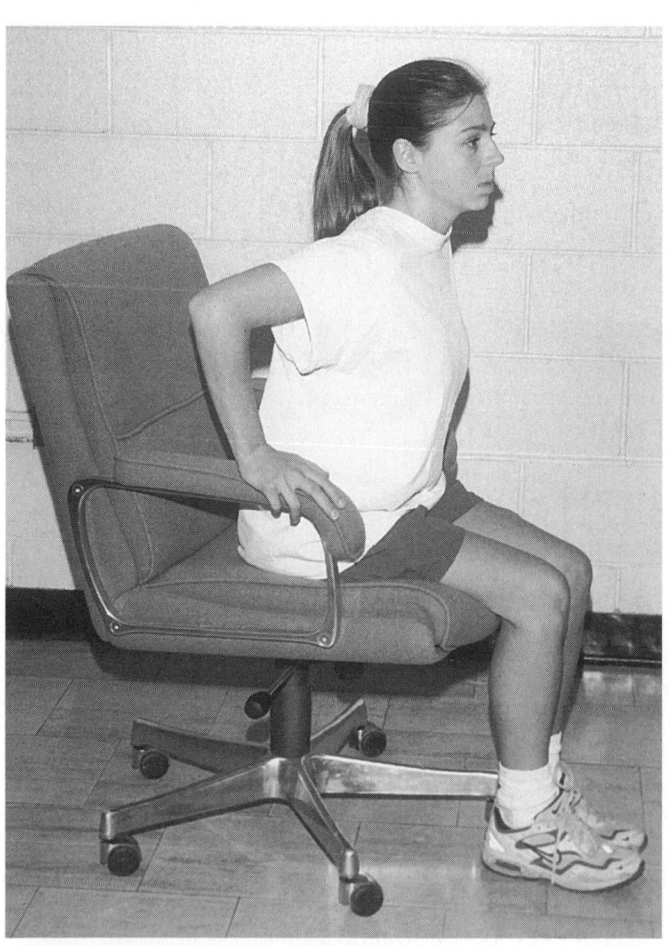

FIGURE 8.50 Sitting in a chair with an average seat height requires 112 degrees of hip flexion.[51]

Wolf[65] investigated the reliability of measurements of active ROM, whereas other researchers[27,44,47,60,61,66–68] studied passive motion. Bierma-Zeinstra and associates[43] studied the reliability of both active and passive ROM. Table 8.7 and Table 8.8 provide a sampling of intratester and intertester reliability studies.

Boone and associates[64] conducted a study in which four physical therapists used a universal goniometer to measure active hip abduction ROM in 12 healthy male volunteers aged 26 to 54 years. Three measurements were taken by each tester at each of four sessions scheduled on a weekly basis for 4 weeks. Intratester reliability for hip abduction was r = 0.75, with a total standard deviation between measurements of 4 degrees taken by the same testers. Intertester reliability for hip abduction was r = 0.55, with a total standard deviation of 5.2 degrees between measurements taken by different testers.

Clapper and Wolf[65] compared the reliability of the Ortho-Ranger (Orthotronics, Daytona Beach, Fla.), an electronic computed pendulum goniometer, with that of the universal goniometer in a study of active hip motion involving 10 males and 10 healthy females between the ages of 23 and 40 years. The authors found that the universal goniometer showed significantly less variation within sessions than the Ortho-Ranger, except for measurements of hip adduction and lateral rotation. The authors concluded that the universal goniometer was a more reliable instrument than the OrthoRanger, and, due to the poor correlation between the two instruments, the authors cautioned that the instruments should not be used interchangeably

Ekstrand and associates[66] measured the passive ROM of hip flexion, extension, and abduction in 22 healthy men aged 20 to 30 years in two testing series. In the first series, the testing procedures were not controlled. In the second series, procedures were standardized and anatomical landmarks were indicated. The intratester coefficient of variation was lower than the intertester coefficient of variation for both series, but standardization of procedures improved reliability considerably.

Ellison and coworkers[27] compared passive ROM measurements of hip rotation taken with an inclinometer and a universal goniometer and found no significant differences between the means. Both instruments were found to be reliable, but the authors preferred the inclinometer because it was easier to use.

Bierma-Zeinstra and associates[43] compared the reliability of hip ROM measurements taken with an electronic inclinometer with those taken by a universal goniometer. The two instruments showed equal intratester reliability for both active and passive hip ROM in general and passive hip flexion and passive extension ROM. The intratester reliability of the inclinometer was higher than that of the goniometer for passive hip lateral rotation and sitting medial rotation. The goniometer had higher reliability for active and passive medial rotation in the prone position. The authors concluded that because the inclinometer and goniometer do not result in the same ROM values, the instruments should not be used interchangeably.

Gajdosik, Sandler, and Marr[14] assessed the intratester reliability of measurements of hip abduction or adduction during both the Ober and Modified Ober tests. One therapist administered all of the tests, and an assistant positioned and

TABLE 8.7   Intratester Reliability

Author	n	Sample	Position	Motion	ICC	
Van Dillen et al[44]	35	Healthy subjects	Supine: Hip in neutral and knee in 80 degrees flexion	Extension	Right hip	0.70
					Left hip	0.89
			Hip in neutral and knee in full extension	Extension	Right hip	0.72
					Left hip	0.76
			Hip in full abduction and knee in 80 degrees flexion	Extension	Right hip	0.87
					Left hip	0.76
			Hip in full abduction flexion and knee in full extension	Extension	Right hip	0.96
					Left hip	0.90
Ellison et al[27]	22	Healthy subjects	Prone: hip in neutral position and knee flexed to 90 degrees	Medial rotation	Right hip	0.99
				Lateral rotation	Right hip	0.96
Cadenhead et al[68]	6	Adults with cerebral palsy	Supine	Abduction	Right hip	0.99
			Prone	Extension	Right hip	0.98
			Supine	Lateral rotation	Right hip	0.79

ICC = intraclass correlation coefficient.

TABLE 8.8 Intertester Reliability

Author	n	Sample	Position	Motion	ICC
Simoneau et al[36]	60	Healthy subjects (18–27 yrs)	Prone	Medial rotation	0.82, 0.96, 0.97
			Seated	Medial rotation	0.89, 0.85, 0.93
			Prone	Lateral rotation	0.89, 0.79, 0.98
			Seated	Lateral rotation	0.90, 0.76, 0.95
Ellison et al[27]	22	Healthy subjects (20–41 yrs)	Prone	Left medial rotation	0.98
			Prone	Left lateral rotation	0.97
			Prone	Right medial rotation	0.99
			Prone	Right lateral rotation	0.96
	15	Adults with back pain (23–61 yrs)	Prone	Left medial rotation	0.97
			Prone	Left lateral rotation	0.95
			Prone	Right medial rotation	0.96
			Prone	Right lateral rotation	0.95

ICC = intraclass correlation coefficient.

read the universal goniometer. The intraclass correlation coefficients (ICCs) among three trials for women were 0.87 for the Ober test and 0.92 for the Modified Ober test. The ICCs for men were slightly lower, with an ICC of 0.83 for the Ober test and an ICC of 0.82 for the Modified Ober test.

Reese and Bandy,[16] in a study involving 61 healthy subjects with a mean age of 24 years, used an inclinometer to determine the intratester reliability of the repeated measurements of the Ober and Modified Ober tests. Intertester reliability was greater than an ICC of 0.90 for both tests using the inclinometer. T tests showed a significant difference in hip adduction ROM between the Ober test (18.9 degrees) and the Modified Ober test (23.4 degrees), but the actual difference between the two tests was 4.5 degrees.

Youdas and associates[7] had two experienced testers measure hamstring length with a 360-degree goniometer using the passive SLR test in 214 adults (108 women and 106 men between the ages of 20 and 79 years. ICCs were 0.97 for the right side and 0.98 for the left side.

Piva and colleagues[69] determined the intertester reliability of measurements of the length of the hamstrings, tensor fasciae latae, and the quadriceps. Two pairs of testers took the measurements with an inclinometer in 30 subjects with a mean age of 28.1 years. All ICCs were higher than 0.80. (Hamstring length ICC = 0.92 and tensor fascia latae ICC = 0.97).

Steinberg and associates[35] calculated intratester reliability coefficients on test-retest ROM measurements on 20 subjects. Intratester Pearson values ranged from r = 0.90 for hip medial rotation to r = 0.96 for both hip abduction and hip flexion. Predictably, intertester reliability r values were lower, ranging from 0.74 to 0.95.

In a study by Pandya and colleagues,[60] five physical therapists using universal goniometers measured passive joint motions including hip extension in 105 children and adolescents, aged 1 to 20 years, who had Duchenne muscular dystrophy. The intratester reliability for measurements of hip extension was good (ICC = 0.85), and the intertester reliability for measurements of hip extension was fair (ICC = 0.74). The results indicated the need for the same examiner to take measurements for long-term follow-up and to assess the results of therapeutic intervention.

McWhirk and Glanzman[58] employed two therapists (one with 10 years of experience and one with 1 year of experience) to measure abduction and extension ROM in both hips of 25 children aged 2 to 18 years with spastic cerebral palsy. To achieve the standarized positioning recommended by Norkin and White, the therapists assisted each other to help support and stabilize the limbs. Hip extension was measured using the Thomas test and was the least reliable intertester measurement with ICC = 0.58 (95 percent confidence interval (CI) for mean absolute difference = 3.96 ± 1.87 degrees), but intertester reliability for hip abduction ROM had an ICC of 0.91 (95 percent CI for mean absolute difference = 3.47 ± 1.47 degrees). The authors demonstrated that therapists with differing levels of pediatric experience can achieve moderate to high levels of intertester reliability. The effect of a strict protocol and the use of a second person to either stabilize or help hold the test limb in patients with cerebral palsy appeared to contribute to the high level of reliability.

Kilgour, McNair, and Stott[62] conducted a study in which three testers used a pediatric plastic goniometer with 10-cm moveable arms to measure straight leg raise, popliteal angle, prone hip extension, and hip extension in supine in the Thomas test and other joints in 25 children with spastic cerebral palsy aged 6 to 17 years and 25 age- and sex-matched healthy controls. The ICCs for intrasessional measures for straight leg raise (hip flexion) and for the popliteal angle were 0.95 and higher in both groups. The ICCs for the Thomas tests were poor for both groups, although there were low median absolute differences. Intersessional variation in both groups was high, indicating that the measurement variability was not influenced by the presence of spasticity. Measurement of a fixed joint by the three physical therapists was very reliable, with a maximum difference of 5 degrees and a between-sessions difference of 6.5 degrees. Therefore, the authors concluded that a major source of error in the study was difficulty in determining the correct end-range joint positioning.

Mutlu and associates [63] conducted a study in which passive range of motion was measured in 38 patients aged 18 to 108 months with spastic cerebral palsy. Three physical therapists used a 360-degree goniometer to measure each child's hip ROM once in each session on two different occasions 1 week apart. The highest intertester reliability (ICC = 0.95) was for hip extension using the Thomas test, and the lowest (ICC = 0.61) was for hip abduction. Intrareliability and interreliability was also high for hip flexion with the knee flexed and the opposite leg extended.

Croft and associates [61] had six clinicians use a fluid-filled inclinometer called a Plurimeter to take passive hip flexion and rotation ROM measurements of both hips in six patients with osteoarthritis involving only one hip joint. The results showed that the degree of agreement among testers was greatest for measurements of hip flexion.

Cibulka and colleagues, [67] in a study of passive ROM in medial and lateral hip rotation in 100 patients with low-back pain, determined that for this group of patients, measurements of rotation taken in the prone position were more reliable than those taken in the sitting position.

Holm and associates [59] compared the reliability of goniometric and visual measurements in 25 patients with hip osteoarthritis symptoms and a mean age of 64 years. Two teams consisting of two therapists each and one team consisting of a single experienced therapist took passive standardized goniometric measurements using a half-circle metal goniometer. The fourth team was an orthopedic surgeon who made visual estimates. Each team took measurements on two occasions with a week between sessions. There were highly significant differences in degrees between measurements made by the single persons when compared to measurements made by two people working together, except for internal rotation. The authors concluded that to obtain the most accurate results, measurements should be performed by two people working together. No significant differences were found between goniometric measurements and visual estimates or between measurements from the first and second sessions for the same team with the exception of hip abduction. Reproducibility of meaurements was best for hip flexion.

Cliborne and associates [70] determined the ROM and intra-tester reliability of hip flexion in 22 patients with osteoarthritis of the knee (mean age = 61.2 years) and 17 subjects without symptoms. Intratester reliability for hip flexion for two pairs of testers using an inclinometer was an ICC of 0.94 (95% CI = 0.89–0.97).

Owen and colleagues [71] followed the goniometric protocols used by the AAOS to measure 82 children aged 4 to 10 years with femoral shaft fractures at 15 and 24 months post-fracture. Hip abduction and adduction were measured in the supine position, and hip rotation was measured in the prone position. Active hip extension was measured using the Thomas test. The most reliable measure was for hip flexion ROM, but that was low with an ICC of 0.48 (95% CI = 0.29–0.63). The authors concluded that standarized protocols for hip ROM in this population had low reliability because only when differences in rotation exceeded at least 30 degrees and ROM in flexion–extension exceeded 50 degrees could clinicians conclude that true change has occurred.

In a reliability and validity study by Sprigle and associates, [72] radiographs were taken as 10 healthy male subjects sat in erect, anterior, and posterior postures. An electromagnetic tracking device (Flock of Birds) was used to digitize the anterior and posterior superior iliac spines as a 6 degree of freedom sensor was mounted on the thigh and sacrum. The variables were pelvic tilt and hip thigh flexion angle. Intratester reliability was calculated using nine radiographs and two testers. Intertester reliability was calculated from 30 radiographs and two testers. The ICCs for both intratester and intertester reliability were 0.98 or higher. Validity was determined by comparison of Flock of Birds measurements with radiographic measurements.

REFERENCES

1. Levangie, PK, and Norkin, CC: Joint Structure and Function: A Comprehensive Analysis, ed 4. FA Davis, Philadelphia, 2005.

2. Cyriax, JH, and Cyriax, PJ: Illustrated Manual of Orthopaedic Medicine. Butterworths, London, 1983.

3. Greene, WB, and Heckman, JD (eds): American Academy of Orthopaedic Surgeons: The Clinical Measurement of Joint Motion. AAOS, Chicago, 1994.

4. American Medical Association: Guides to the Evaluation of Permanent Impairment, ed 5. Cocchiarella, L and Andersson, GBL (eds). AMA, Chicago, 2000.

5. Roach, KE, and Miles, TP: Normal hip and knee active range of motion: The relationship to age. Phys Ther 71:656, 1991.

6. Kendall, FP, et al: Muscles: Testing and Function with Posture and Pain, ed 5. Lippincott Williams and Wilkins, Baltimore, 2005.

7. Youdas, JW, et al:The influence of gender and age on hamstring length in healthy adults. J Orthop Sports Phys Ther 35:246, 2005.

8. Ober, FR: The role of the iliotibial band and fascia lata as a factor in the causation of low-back disabilities and sciatica. J Bone Joint Surg 18:105, 1936.

9. Noble, HB, Hajek, MR, and Porter, M: Diagnosis and treatment of iliotibial band tightness in runners. Phys Sports Med 10:67, 1982.

10. McConnell, J: The physical therapist's approach to patellofemoral disorders. Clin Sports Med 21:363, 2002.

11. Hoppenfeld, S: Physical Examination of the Spine and Extremities. Appleton-Century-Crofts, New York, 1976, p 167.

12. Gose, JC, and Schweizer, P: Iliotibial band tightness. J Orthop Sports Phys Ther 10:399, 1989.

13. Cade, DL, et al: Indirectly measuring length of the iliotibial band and related hip structures: A correlational analysis of four adduction tests. Abstract Platform Presentation at APTA Mid-Winter. Tex J Orthop Sports Phys Ther 31:A22, 2001.

14. Gajdosik, RL, Sandler, MM, and Marr, HL: Influence of knee position and gender on the Ober test for length of the iliotibial band. Clin Biomech 18:77, 2003.

15. Wang, T-G, et al: Assessment of stretching of the iliotibial tract with Ober and Modified Ober Tests: An Ultrasonographic study. Arch Phys Med Rehabil 87:1407-1410, 2006.

16. Reese, NB, and Bandy, WD: Use of an inclinometer to measure flexibility of the iliotibial band using the Ober Test and the Modified Ober Test: Differences in magnitude and reliability of measurement. J Orthop Sports Phys Ther 33:326, 2003.

17. Boone, DC, and Azen, SP: Normal range of motion of joints in male subjects. J Bone Joint Surg Am 61:756, 1979.

18. Svenningsen, S, et al: Hip motion related to age and sex. Acta Orthop Scand 60:97, 1989.

19. Waugh, KG, et al: Measurement of selected hip, knee and ankle joint motions in newborns. Phys Ther 63:1616, 1983.

20. Schwarze, DJ, and Denton, JR: Normal values of neonatal limbs: An evaluation of 1000 neonates. J Pediatr Orthop 13:758, 1993.

21. Broughton, NS, Wright, J, and Menelaus, MB: Range of knee motion in normal neonates. J Pediatr Orthop 13:263, 1993.

22. Drews, JE, Vraciu, JK, and Pellino, G: Range of motion of the joints of the lower extremities of newborns. Phys Occup Ther Pediatr 4:49, 1984.

23. Wanatabe, H, et al: The range of joint motions of the extremities in healthy Japanese people: The difference according to age. Cited in Walker, JM: Musculoskeletal development: A review. Phys Ther 71:878, 1991.

24. Phelps, E, Smith, LJ, and Hallum, A: Normal range of hip motion of infants between 9 and 24 months of age. Dev Med Child Neurol 27:785, 1985.

25. Forero, N, Okamura, LA, and Larson, MA: Normal ranges of hip motion in neonates. J Pediatr Orthop 9:391, 1989.

26. Kozic, S, et al: Femoral anteversion related to side differences in hip rotation. Passive rotation in 1140 children aged 8-9 years. Acta Orthop Scand 68:533, 1997.

27. Ellison, JB, Rose, SJ, and Sahrman, SA: Patterns of hip rotation: A comparison between healthy subjects and patients with low back pain. Phys Ther 70:537, 1990.

28. Boone, DC: Techniques of measurement of joint motion. (Unpublished supplement to Boone, DC, and Azen, SP: Normal range of motion in male subjects. J Bone Joint Surg Am 61:756, 1979.)

29. Walker, JM: Musculoskeletal development: A review. Phys Ther 71:878, 1991.

30. Nonaka, H, et al: Age-related changes in the interactive mobility of the hip and knee joints: A geometrical analysis. Gait Posture 15:236, 2002.

31. Allander, E, et al: Normal range of joint movements in shoulder, hip, wrist and thumb with special reference to side: A comparison between two populations. Int J Epidemiol 3:253, 1974.

32. Walker, JM, et al: Active mobility of the extremities in older subjects. Phys Ther 64:919, 1984.

33. Boone, DC, Walker, JM, and Perry, J: Age and sex differences in lower extremity joint motion. Presented at the National Conference of the American Physical Therapy Association, Washington, DC, 1981.

34. James, B, and Parker, AW: Active and passive mobility of lower limb joints in elderly men and women. Am J Phys Med Rehabil 68:162, 1989.

35. Steinberg, N, et al: Range of movement in female dancers and non-dancers aged 8–16 years. Am J Sports Med 34:814, 2006.

36. Simoneau, GG, et al: Influence of hip position and gender on active hip internal and external rotation. J Orthop Sports Phys Ther 28:158, 1998.

37. Hu, H, et al: Measurements of voluntary joint range of motion of the Chinese elderly living in Beijing area by a photographic method. Intern J Indust Ergonomics 36: 861, 2006.

38. Sanya, AO, and Obi, CS: Range of motion in selected joints of diabetic and non-diabetic subjects. Afr J Health Sci 6:17, 1999.

39. Kettunen, J, et al: Factors associated with hip joint rotation in former elite athletes. Br J Sports Med 34:44, 2000.

40. Escalante, A, et al: Determinants of hip and knee flexion range: Results from the San Antonio Longitudinal Study of Aging. Arthritis Care Res 12:8, 1999.

41. Lichtenstein, MJ, et al: Modeling impairment: Using the disablement process as a framework to evaluate determinants of hip and knee flexion. Aging (Milan) 12:208, 2000.

42. Bennell, K, et al: Hip and ankle range of motion and hip muscle strength in young novice female ballet dancers and controls. Br J Sports Med 33:340, 1999.

43. Bierma-Zeinstra, SMA, et al: Comparison between two devices for measuring hip joint motions. Clin Rehabil 12:497, 1998.

44. Van Dillen, LR, et al: Effect of knee and hip position on hip extension range of motion in individuals with and without low back pain. J Orthop Sports Phys Ther 30:307, 2000.

45. Gilbert, CB, Gross, MT, and Klug, KB: Relationship between hip external rotation and turnout angle for the five classical ballet positions. J Orthop Sports Phys Ther 27:339, 1998.

46. Tyler, T, et al: A new pelvic tilt detection device: Roentgenographic validation and application to assessment of hip motion in professional hockey players. J Orthop Sports Phys Ther 24:303, 1996.

47. Van Mechelen, W, et al: Is range of motion of the hip and ankle joint related to running injuries? A case control study. Int J Sports Med 13:606, 1992.

48. Steultjens, MPM, et al: Range of motion and disability in patients with osteoarthritis of the knee or hip. Rheumatology 39:955, 2000.

49. Mollinger, LA, and Steffan, TM: Knee flexion contractures in institutionalized elderly: Prevalence, severity, stability and related variables. Phys Ther 73:437, 1993.

50. Beissner, KL, Collins, JE, and Holmes, H: Muscle force and range of motion as predictors of function in older adults. Phys Ther 80:556, 2000.

51. Magee, DJ: Orthopedic Physical Assessment, ed 4. WB Saunders, Philadelphia, 2002.

52. The Pathokinesiology Service and the Physical Therapy Department: Observational Gait Analysis Handbook. Ranchos Los Amigos Medical Center, Downey, Cal., 1989.

53. Livingston, LA, Stevenson, JM, and Olney, SJ: Stairclimbing kinematics on stairs of differing dimensions. Arch Phys Med Rehabil 72:398, 1991.

54. McFayden, BJ, and Winter, DA: An integrated biomechanical analysis of normal stair ascent and descent. J Biomech 21:733, 1988.

55. Protopapadaki, A, Drechsler, WI, Cramp, MC, et al: Hip knee and ankle kinematics and kinetics during stair ascent and descent in healthy young individuals. Clin Biomech 22:203, 2007.

56. Oberg, T, Krazinia, A, and Oberg, K: Joint angle parameters in gait: Reference data for normal subjects 10–79 years of age. J Rehabil Res Dev 31:199, 1994.

57. Hemmerich, A, Brown, H, Smith, S, et al: Hip, knee and ankle kinematics of high range of motion activities of daily living. J Orthop Res 24:770, 2006.

58. McWhirk, LB, and Glanzman, AM: Within-session inter-rater reliability of goniometeric measures in patients with spastic cerebral palsy. Pediatr Phys Ther 18:262, 2006.

59. Holm, I, et al: Reliability of goniometric measurements and visual estimates of hip ROM in patients with osteoarthrosis. Physiother Res Int 5:242, 2000.

60. Pandya, S, et al: Reliability of goniometric measurements in patients with Duchenne muscular dystrophy. Phys Ther 65:1339, 1985.

61. Croft, PR, et al: Interobserver reliability in measuring flexion, internal rotation and external rotation of the hip using a pleurimeter. Ann Rheum Dis 55:320, 1996.

62. Kilgour, G, McNair, P and Stott, NS: Intrarater reliability of lower limb sagittal range of motion measures in children with spastic cerebral palsy. Develop Med Child Neurol 45:391, 2003.

63. Mutlu, A, Livanelioglu A, and Gunel, MK: Reliability of goniometric measurements in children with spastic cerebral palsy. Med Sci Monit 13:CR323, 2007.

64. Boone, DC, et al: Reliability of goniometric measurements. Phys Ther 58:1355, 1978.

65. Clapper, MP, and Wolf, SL: Comparison of the reliability of the Orthoranger and the standard goniometer for assessing active lower extremity range of motion. Phys Ther 68:214, 1988.

66. Ekstrand, J, et al: Lower extremity goniometric measurements: A study to determine their reliability. Arch Phys Med Rehabil 63:171, 1982.

67. Cibulka, MT, et al: Unilateral hip rotation range of motion asymmetry in patients with sacroiliac joint regional pain. Spine 23:1009, 1998.

68. Cadenhead, SL, McEwen, IR, and Thompson, DM: Effect of passive range of motion exercises on lower extremity goniometric measurements of adults with cerebral palsy: A single subject study design. Phys Ther 82:658, 2002.

69. Piva, SR, et al: Reliability of measures of impairments associated with patellofemoral pain syndrome. BMC Musculoskelet Disord 7:33, 2006.

70. Cliborne, AV, et al: Clinical hip tests and a functional squat test in patients with knee osteoarthritis: Reliability, prevalence of positive test findings, and short-term response to hip mobilization. J Orthop Sports Phys Ther 234:676, 2004.

71. Owen, J, Stephens, D, and Wright, JG: Reliability of hip range of motion using goniometry in pediatric femur shaft fractures. Can J Surg 50:251, 2007.

72. Sprigle, S, et al: Development of a noninvasive measure of pelvic and hip angles in seated posture. Arch Phys Med Rehabil 83:1597, 2002.

Chapter 9

The Knee

Structure and Function

Tibiofemoral and Patellofemoral Joints

Anatomy

The knee is composed of two distinct articulations enclosed within a single joint capsule: the tibiofemoral joint and the patellofemoral joint. At the tibiofemoral joint, the proximal joint surfaces are the convex medial and the lateral condyles of the distal femur (Fig. 9.1). Posteriorly and inferiorly, the longer medial condyle is separated from the lateral condyle by a deep groove called the intercondylar notch. Anteriorly, the condyles are separated by a shallow area of bone called the femoral patellar surface. The distal articulating surfaces are the two shallow concave medial and lateral condyles on the proximal end of the tibia. Two bony spines called the intercondylar tubercles separate the medial condyle from the lateral condyle. Two joint discs called menisci are attached to the articulating surfaces on the tibial condyles (Fig. 9.2). At the patellofemoral joint, the articulating surfaces are the posterior surface of the patella and the femoral patellar surface (Fig. 9.3).

The joint capsule that encloses both joints is large, loose, and reinforced by tendons and expansions from the surrounding muscles and ligaments. The quadriceps tendon, patellar ligament, and expansions from the extensor muscles provide anterior stability (see Fig. 9.3). The lateral and medial collateral ligaments, iliotibial band, and pes anserinus help to provide medial–lateral stability, and the knee flexors help to

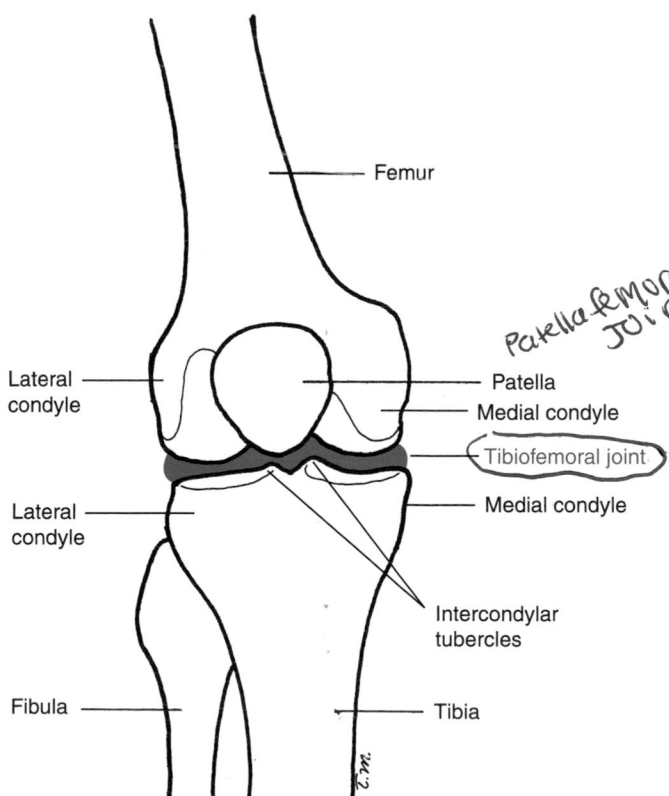

Patellafemoral joint – sliding medial fat, inferior/superior
flex, extend

Tibiofemoral joint

FIGURE 9.1 An anterior view of a right knee showing the tibiofemoral joint.

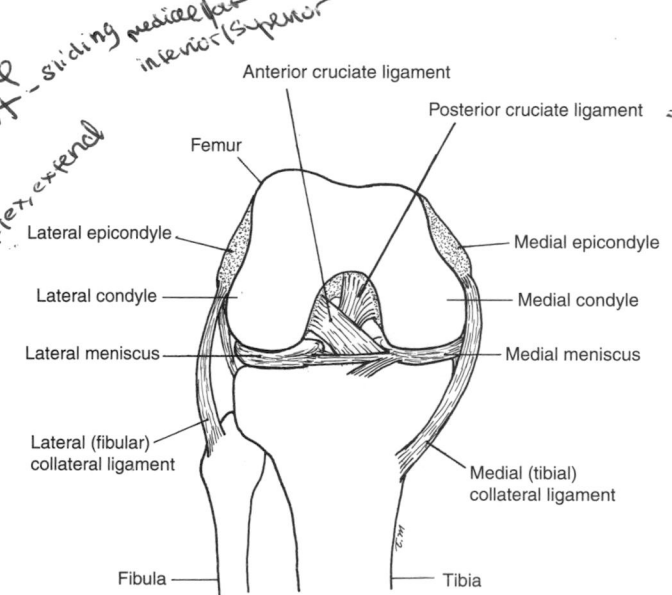

FIGURE 9.2 An anterior view of a right knee in the flexed position showing femoral and tibial condyles, medial and lateral menisci, and cruciate and collateral ligaments.

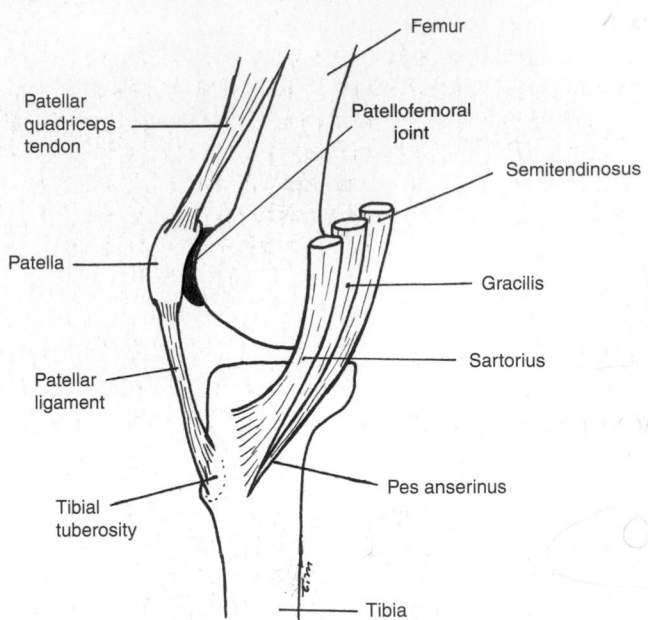

Labels on figure:
- Femur
- Patellar quadriceps tendon
- Patellofemoral joint
- Semitendinosus
- Patella
- Gracilis
- Sartorius
- Patellar ligament
- Pes anserinus
- Tibial tuberosity
- Tibia

FIGURE 9.3 A view of a right knee showing the medial aspect, where the cut tendons of the three muscles that insert into the anteromedial aspect of the tibia make up the pes anserinus. Also included are the patellofemoral joint, the patellar ligament, and the patellar tendon.

provide posterior stability. In addition, the tibiofemoral joint is reinforced by the anterior and posterior cruciate ligaments, which are located within the joint (see Fig. 9.2).

Osteokinematics

The tibiofemoral joint is a double condyloid joint with 2 degrees of freedom. Flexion–extension occurs in the sagittal plane around a medial–lateral axis; rotation occurs in the transverse plane around a vertical (longitudinal) axis.[1] The incongruence and asymmetry of the tibiofemoral joint surfaces combined with muscle activity and ligamentous restraints produce an automatic rotation. This automatic rotation is involuntary and occurs primarily toward the end of extension when motion stops on the shorter lateral femoral condyle but continues on the longer medial condylar surface. During the last portion of active extension range of motion (ROM) automatic rotation produces what is referred to as either the screw-home mechanism, or "locking," of the knee. For example, during non–weight-bearing active knee extension with the tibia moving on the femur, the tibia laterally rotates during the last 10 to 15 degrees of extension to lock the knee.[2] Therefore, in the fully extended position of the knee, the tibia is laterally rotated in relation to the femur. To unlock the knee, either the tibia has to rotate medially or the femur has to rotate laterally to unlock the knee. This rotation is not under voluntary control and should not be confused with the voluntary rotation movement possible at the joint when the knee is flexed.

Passive ROM in flexion is generally considered to be between 130 and 140 degrees. The range of extension beyond 0 degrees is about 5 to 10 degrees in young children, whereas 0 degrees is considered to be within normal limits for adults.[3]

The greatest range of voluntary knee rotation occurs at 90 degrees of flexion; at this point, about 45 degrees of lateral rotation and 15 degrees of medial rotation are possible.

Arthrokinematics

In non–weight-bearing active motion, the concave tibial articulating surfaces slide on the convex femoral condyles in the same direction as the movement of the shaft of the tibia. The tibial condyles slide posteriorly on the femoral condyles during flexion, and the tibial condyles slide anteriorly on the femoral condyles during extension.

The incongruence of the tibiofemoral joint and the fact that the femoral articulating surfaces are larger than the tibial articulating surfaces dictate that when the femoral condyles are moving on the tibial condyles (in a weight-bearing situation) the femoral condyles must roll and slide to remain on the tibia. In weight-bearing flexion, the femoral condyles roll posteriorly and slide anteriorly. The menisci follow the roll of the condyles by distorting posteriorly in flexion. In extension, the femoral condyles roll anteriorly and slide posteriorly.[1] In the last portion of extension, motion stops at the lateral femoral condyle, but sliding continues on the medial femoral condyle to produce locking of the knee.

The patella slides superiorly in extension and inferiorly in flexion. Some patellar rotation and tilting accompany the sliding during flexion and extension.[1]

Capsular Pattern

The capsular pattern at the knee is characterized by a smaller limitation of extension than of flexion and no restriction of rotations.[4,5] Fritz and associates[6] found that patients with a capsular pattern, defined as a ratio of extension loss to flexion loss between 0.03 and 0.50, were 3.2 times more likely to have arthritis or arthroses of the knee. Hayes reported a mean ratio of extension loss to flexion loss of 0.40 in a study of 79 patients with osteoarthritis.[7,8]

RANGE OF MOTION TESTING PROCEDURES: Knee

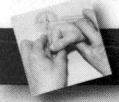

Landmarks for Testing Procedures

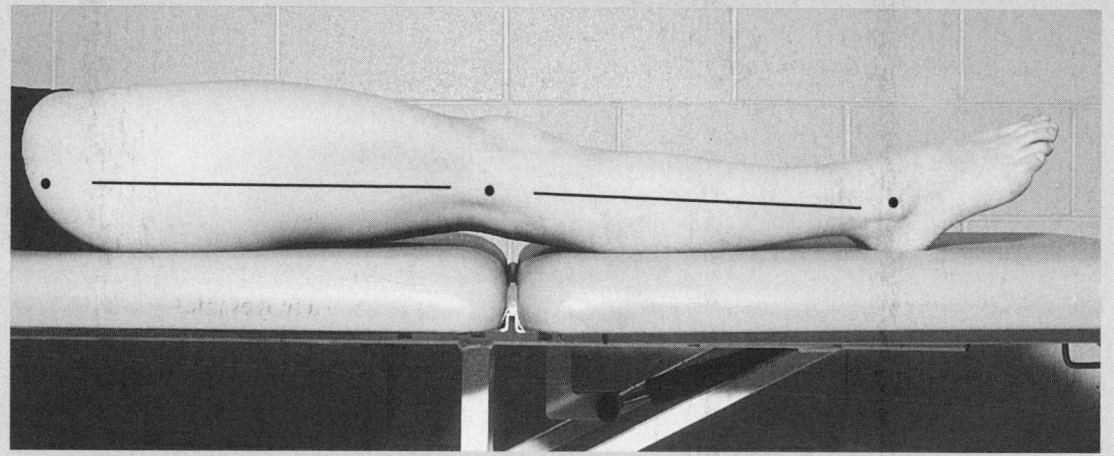

FIGURE 9.4 A lateral view of the subject's right lower extremity showing surface anatomy landmarks for goniometer alignment.

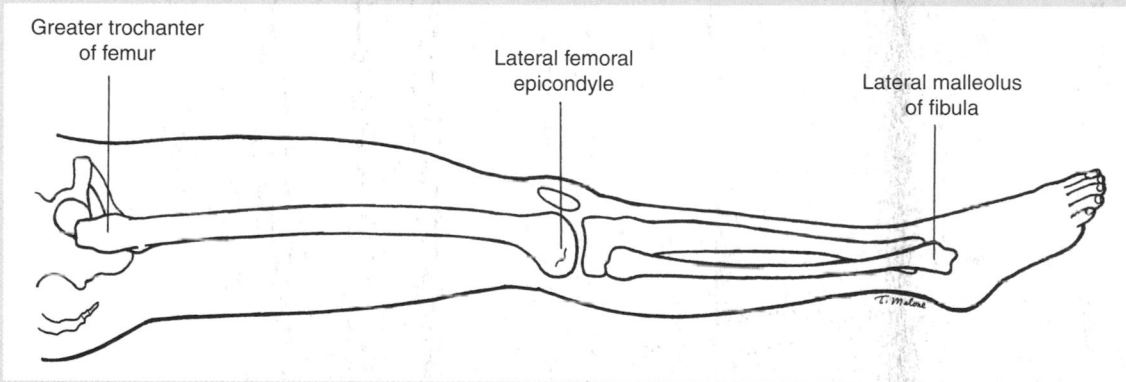

Greater trochanter
of femur

Lateral femoral
epicondyle

Lateral malleolus
of fibula

T. Malone

FIGURE 9.5 A lateral view of the subject's right lower extremity showing bony anatomical landmarks for goniometer alignment for measuring knee flexion ROM.

● KNEE FLEXION

135

Motion occurs in the sagittal plane around a medial–lateral axis. According to the American Medical Association (AMA),[9] the normal flexion ROM for adults is 150 degrees. According to Boone and Azen,[10] the mean flexion ROM for males age 18 months to 54 years is 142.5 degrees. Roach and Miles[11] found a mean knee flexion range of 132.0 degrees for males and females 25 to 74 years of age. Please refer to Tables 9.1 through 9.4 in the Research Findings section for additional normal ROM values by age and gender.

Testing Position
Place the subject supine, with the knee in extension. Position the hip in 0 degrees of extension, abduction, and adduction. Place a towel roll under the ankle to allow the knee to extend as much as possible.

Stabilization
Stabilize the femur to prevent rotation, abduction, and adduction of the hip.

Testing Motion
Hold the subject's ankle in one hand and the posterior thigh with the other hand. Move the subject's thigh to approximately 90 degrees of hip flexion and move the knee into flexion (Fig. 9.6). Stabilize the thigh to

prevent further motion and guide the lower leg into knee flexion. The end of the range of knee flexion occurs when resistance is felt and attempts to overcome the resistance cause additional hip flexion.

Normal End-Feel
Usually, the end-feel is soft because of contact between the muscle bulk of the posterior calf and the thigh or between the heel and the buttocks. The end-feel may be firm because of tension in the vastus medialis, vastus lateralis, and vastus intermedialis muscles.

Goniometer Alignment
See Figures 9.7 and 9.8.

1. Center **fulcrum** of the goniometer over the lateral epicondyle of the femur.
2. Align **proximal arm** with the lateral midline of the femur, using the greater trochanter for reference.
3. Align **distal arm** with the lateral midline of the fibula, using the lateral malleolus and fibular head for reference.

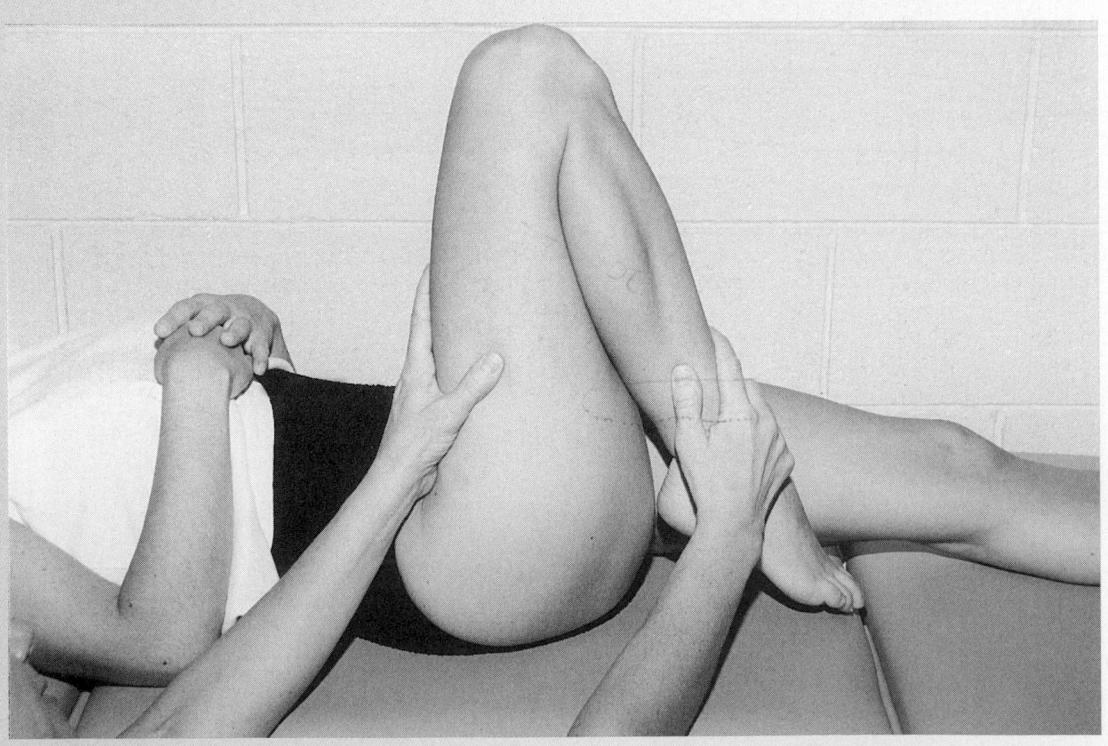

FIGURE 9.6 The right lower extremity at the end of knee flexion ROM. The examiner uses one hand to move the subject's thigh to approximately 90 degrees of hip flexion and then stabilizes the femur to prevent further flexion. The examiner's other hand guides the subject's lower leg through full knee flexion ROM.

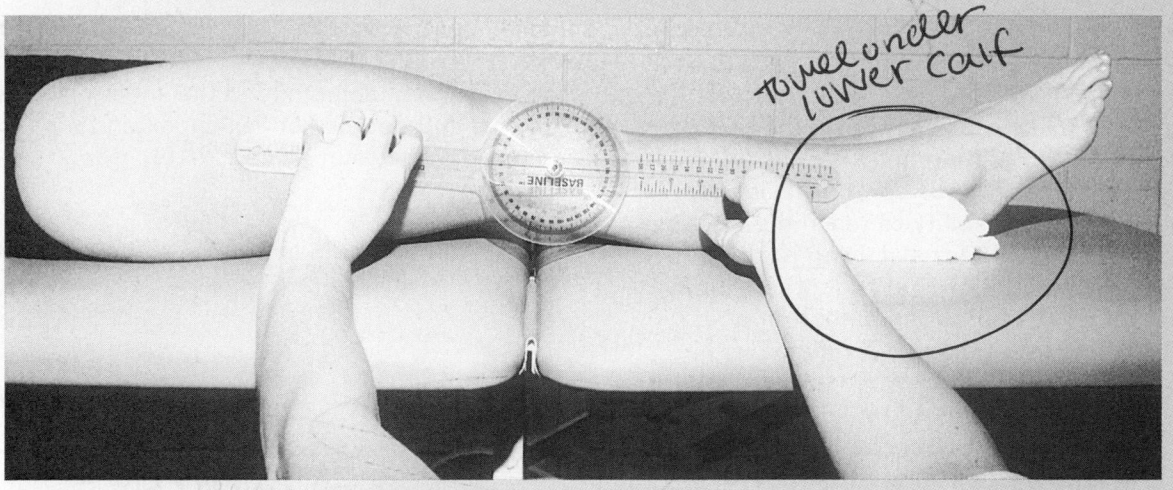

towel under lower calf

FIGURE 9.7 In the starting position for measuring knee flexion ROM, the subject is supine with the upper thigh exposed so that the greater trochanter can be visualized and palpated. The examiner either kneels or sits on a stool to align and read the goniometer at eye level.

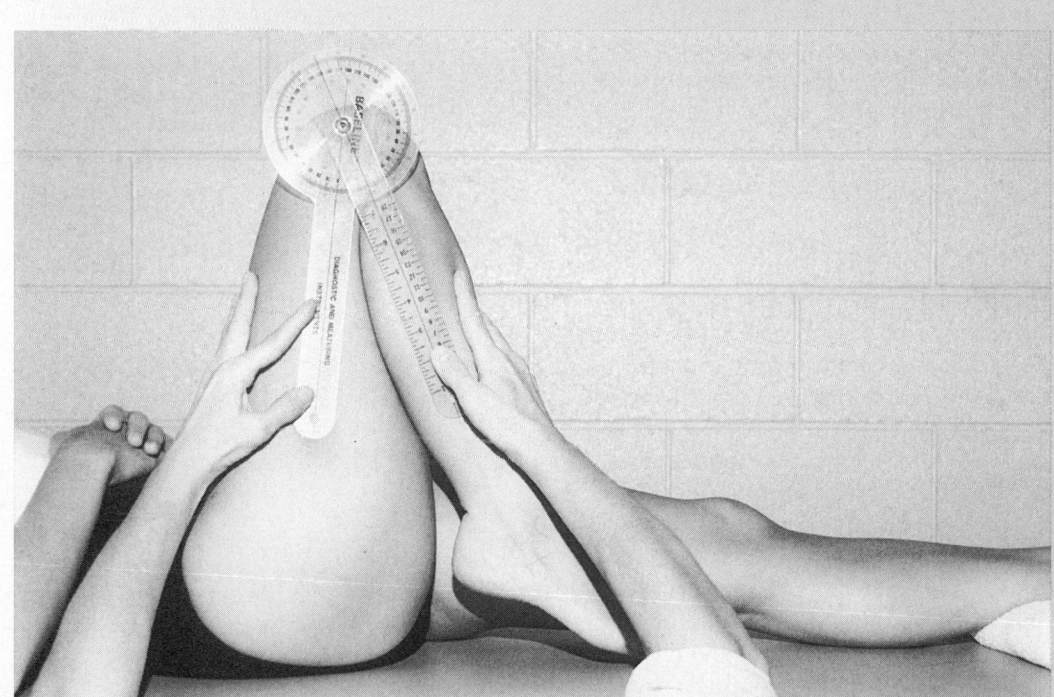

FIGURE 9.8 At the end of the knee flexion ROM, the examiner uses one hand to maintain knee flexion and also to keep the distal arm of the goniometer aligned with the lateral midline of the leg.

DOCUMENTATION

1) Ⓡ Knee 5-0-140
   = 5° hyperextension
   = 140° flexion
   - think of it as number line

2) 5° hyperextension - 140°

3) 5-140°
   = lacking 5° to 140°

4) 0-5-140
   = lacking 5 degrees to 140°

● KNEE EXTENSION

Extension occurs in the sagittal plane around a medial–lateral axis and may be described as a return to the 0 starting position from the end of the knee flexion ROM. Knee extension is usually recorded as the starting position for flexion. An extension limitation (inability to reach the 0 starting position) is present when the starting position for flexion ROM does not begin at 0 degrees but in some amount of flexion. When extension goes beyond the 0 starting position, it may be within normal limits in children, but when it exceeds 5 or more degrees in the adult, it is called **hyperextension** or **genu recurvatum**. See Table 9.2 in the Research Findings section for normal extension limitations in neonates, and see Table 9.3 for normal extension beyond 0 in children 0 to 12 years of age.

Normal End-Feel

The end-feel is firm because of tension in the posterior joint capsule, the oblique and arcuate popliteal ligaments, the collateral ligaments, and the anterior and posterior cruciate ligaments.

MUSCLE LENGTH TESTING PROCEDURES: Knee

● RECTUS FEMORIS: ELY TEST

The rectus femoris is one of the four muscles that make up the muscle group called the quadriceps femoris. The rectus femoris is the only one of the four muscles that crosses both the hip and the knee joints. The muscle arises proximally from two tendons: an anterior tendon from the anterior inferior iliac spine and a posterior tendon from a groove superior to the brim of the acetabulum. Distally, the muscle attaches to the base of the patella by way of the thick, flat quadriceps tendon and attaches to the tibial tuberosity by way of the patellar ligament (Fig. 9.9).

When the rectus femoris muscle contracts, it flexes the hip and extends the knee. If the rectus femoris is short, knee flexion is limited when the hip is maintained in a neutral position. If knee flexion is limited when the hip is in a flexed position, the limitation is not due to a short rectus femoris muscle but to abnormalities of joint structures or short one-joint knee extensor muscles. In a study by Piva and associates, the mean of four tester's measurements of the length of the rectus femoris in 30 patients with patellofemoral pain syndrome aged 14 to 47 years was 138.5 degrees, with a standard deviation (SD) of 12.3 degrees.[12]

Starting Position

Place the subject prone, with both feet off the end of the examining table. Extend the knees and position the hips in 0 degrees of flexion, extension, abduction, adduction, and rotation (Fig. 9.10).

Stabilization

Stabilize the hip to maintain the neutral position. Do not allow the hip to flex.

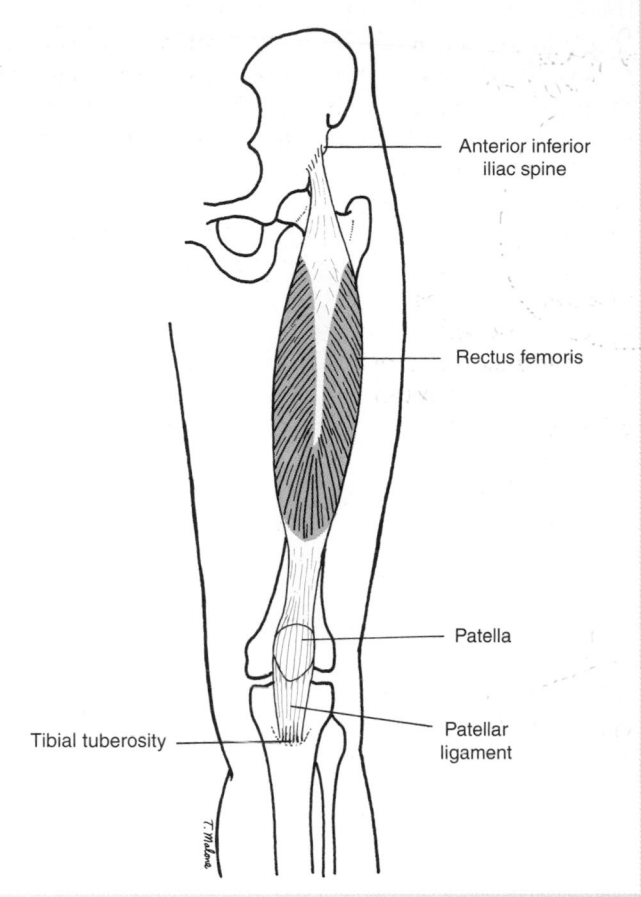

FIGURE 9.9 An anterior view of the left lower extremity showing the attachments of the rectus femoris muscle.

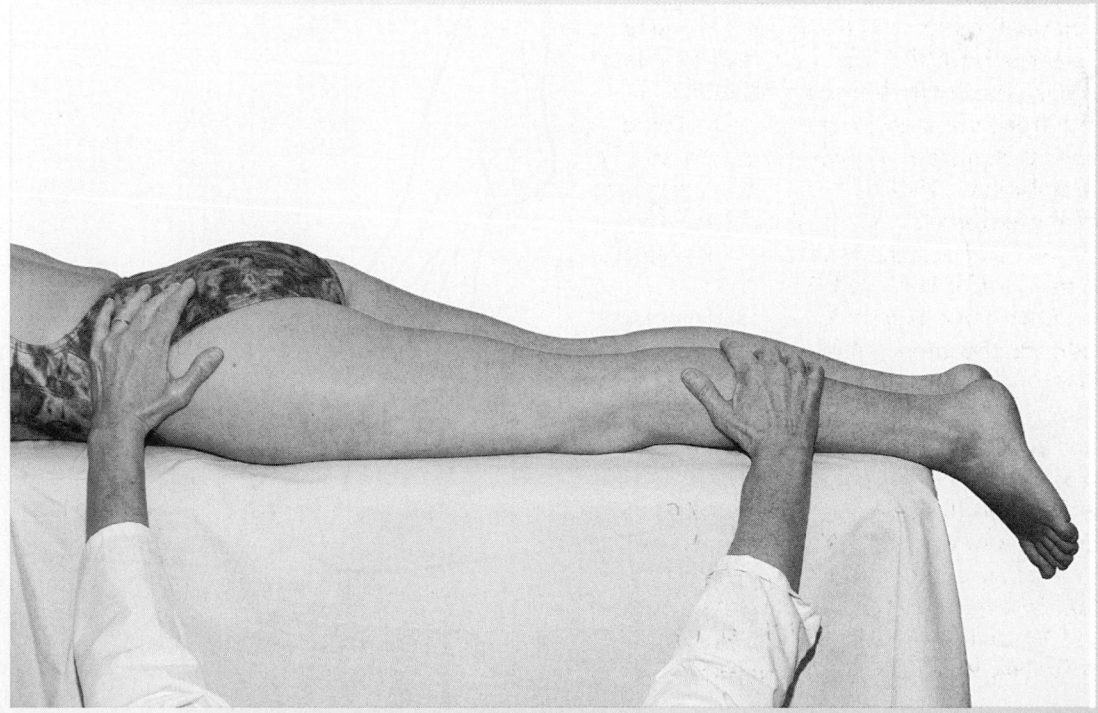

FIGURE 9.10 The subject is shown in the prone starting position for testing the length of the rectus femoris muscle.

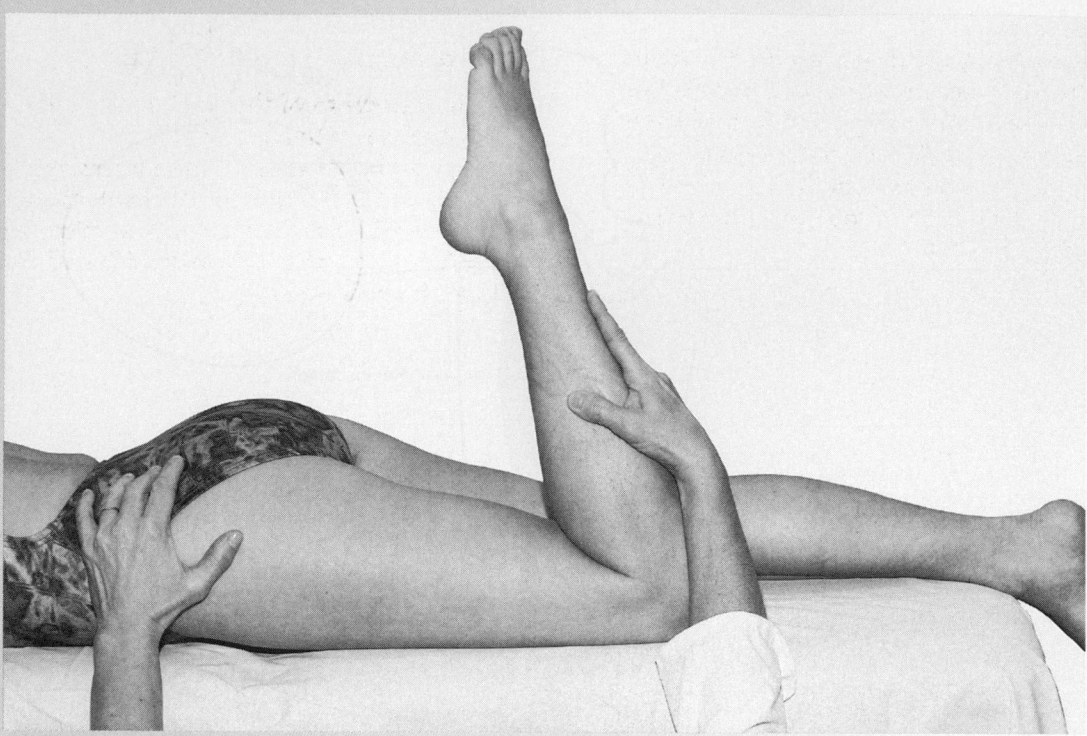

FIGURE 9.11 A lateral view of the subject at the end of the testing motion for the length of the left rectus femoris muscle.

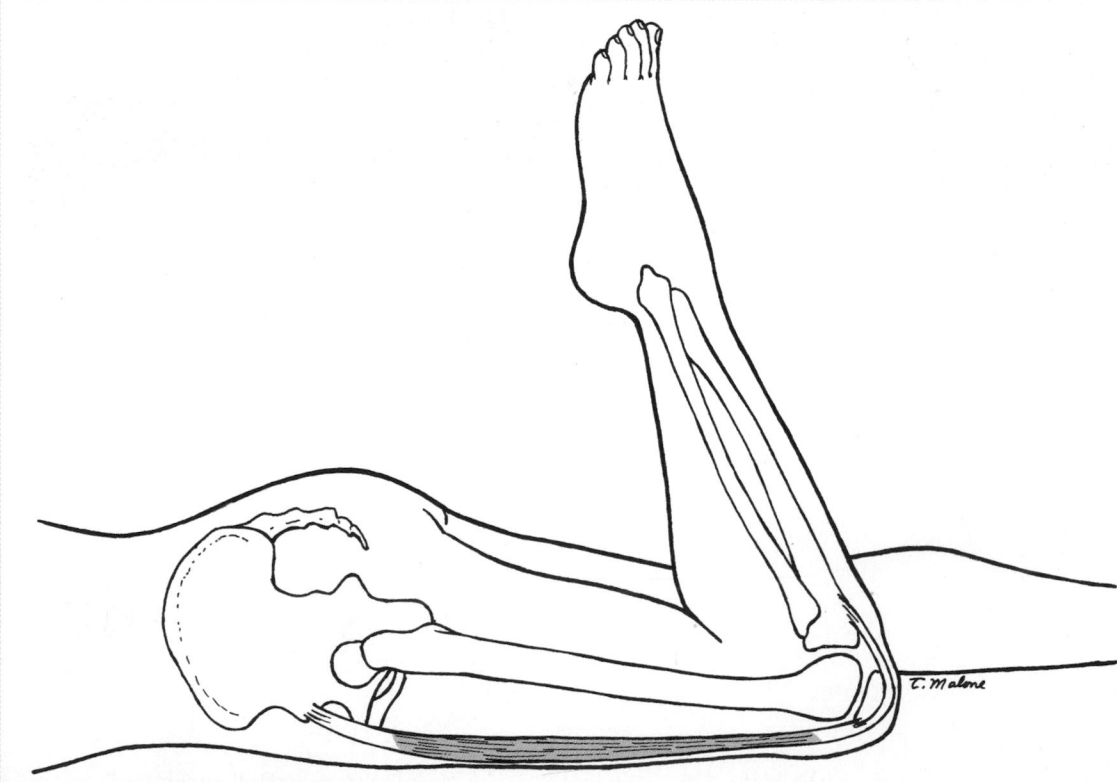

FIGURE 9.12 A lateral view of the left rectus femoris muscle being stretched over the hip and knee joints at the end of the testing motion.

Testing Motion

Flex the knee by lifting the lower leg off the table. The end of the ROM occurs when resistance is felt from tension in the anterior thigh and further knee flexion causes the hip to flex. If the knee can be flexed to at least 90 degrees with the hip in the neutral position, the length of the rectus femoris is normal (Figs. 9.11 and 9.12).

Goniometer Alignment

See Figure 9.13.

1. Center **fulcrum** of the goniometer over the lateral epicondyle of the femur.
2. Align **proximal arm** with the lateral midline of the femur, using the greater trochanter as a reference.
3. Align **distal arm** with the lateral midline of the fibula, using the lateral malleolus and the fibular head for reference.

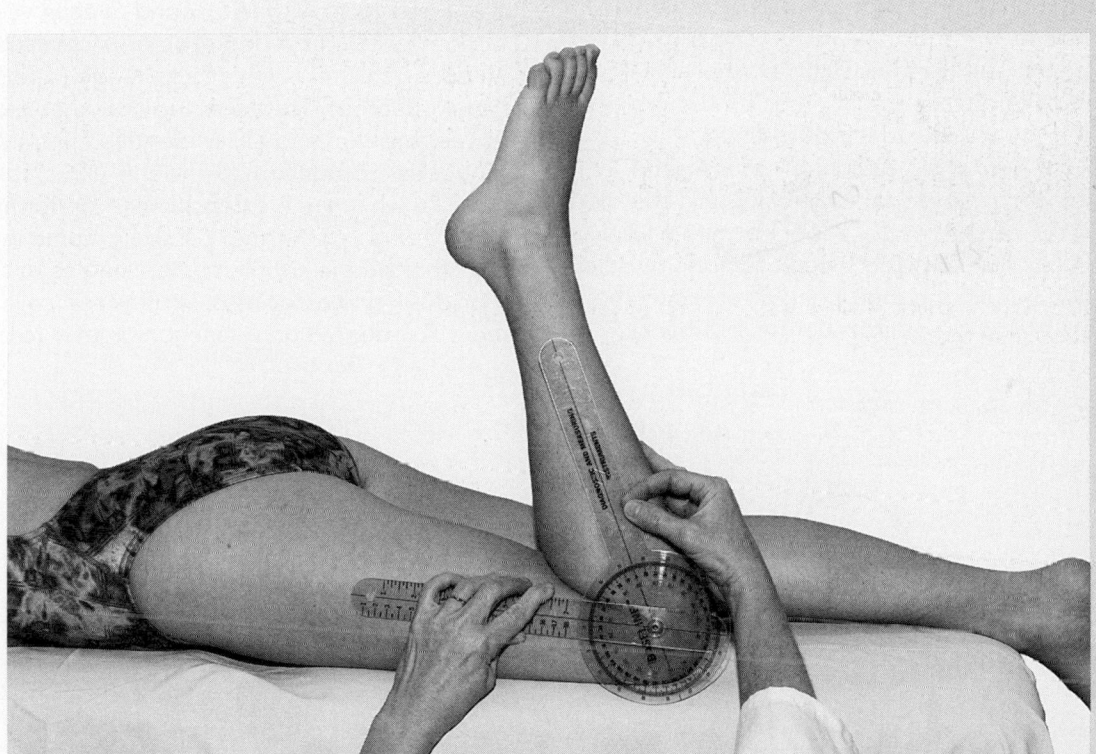

FIGURE 9.13 Goniometer alignment for measuring the position of the knee.

[Handwritten notes:]

No standard normative ROM but probably less than supine.

Prone = Rectus femoris stretches over knee + hip
- Probably less ROM here
- Shortened Rectus fem = less ROM here too

- use this for after surgery + patients w/ knee replacement

HAMSTRING MUSCLES: SEMITENDINOSUS, SEMIMEMBRANOSUS, AND BICEPS FEMORIS: DISTAL HAMSTRING LENGTH TEST OR POPLITEAL ANGLE TEST

The distal hamstring length test is also called the popliteal angle (PA) test because the angle that is being measured is the popliteal angle between the femur and the lower leg. The hamstring muscles are composed of the semitendinosus, semimembranosus, and biceps femoris. The semitendinosus, semimembranosus, and the long head of the biceps femoris cross both the hip and the knee joints. The proximal attachment of the **semitendinosus** is on the ischial tuberosity, and the distal attachment is on the proximal aspect of the medial surface of the tibia (Fig. 9.14A). The proximal attachment of the **semimembranosus** is on the ischial tuberosity, and the distal attachment is on the medial aspect of the medial tibial condyle (Fig. 9.14B). The **biceps femoris** muscle arises from two heads; the long head attaches to the ischial tuberosity and the sacrotuberous ligament,

whereas the short head attaches along the lateral lip linear aspera, the lateral supracondylar line, and the lateral intermuscular septum. The distal attachments of the biceps femoris are on the head of the fibula, with a small portion attaching to the lateral tibial condyle and the lateral collateral ligament (see Fig. 9.14A).

When the hamstring muscles contract, they extend the hip and flex the knee. In the following test, the hip is maintained in 90 degrees of flexion while the knee is extended to determine whether the muscles are of normal length. If the hamstrings are short, the muscles limit knee extension ROM when the hip is positioned at 90 degrees of flexion.

Gajdosik and associates,[13] in a study of 30 healthy males aged 18 to 40 years, found a mean value of 31 degrees (SD = 7.5 degrees) for passive knee extension during this test with a large range of values from 17 to 45 degrees. Testers noted that knee extension end-feel was firm and easily identified. Intrarater reliability intraclass correlation coefficients (ICCs) for the test were 0.86 when knee extension was performed actively and 0.90 when performed passively. Some researchers have reported the supplementary angles to those noted by Gajdosik and associates. Youdas and colleagues[14] used a 360-degree universal goniometer to measure the

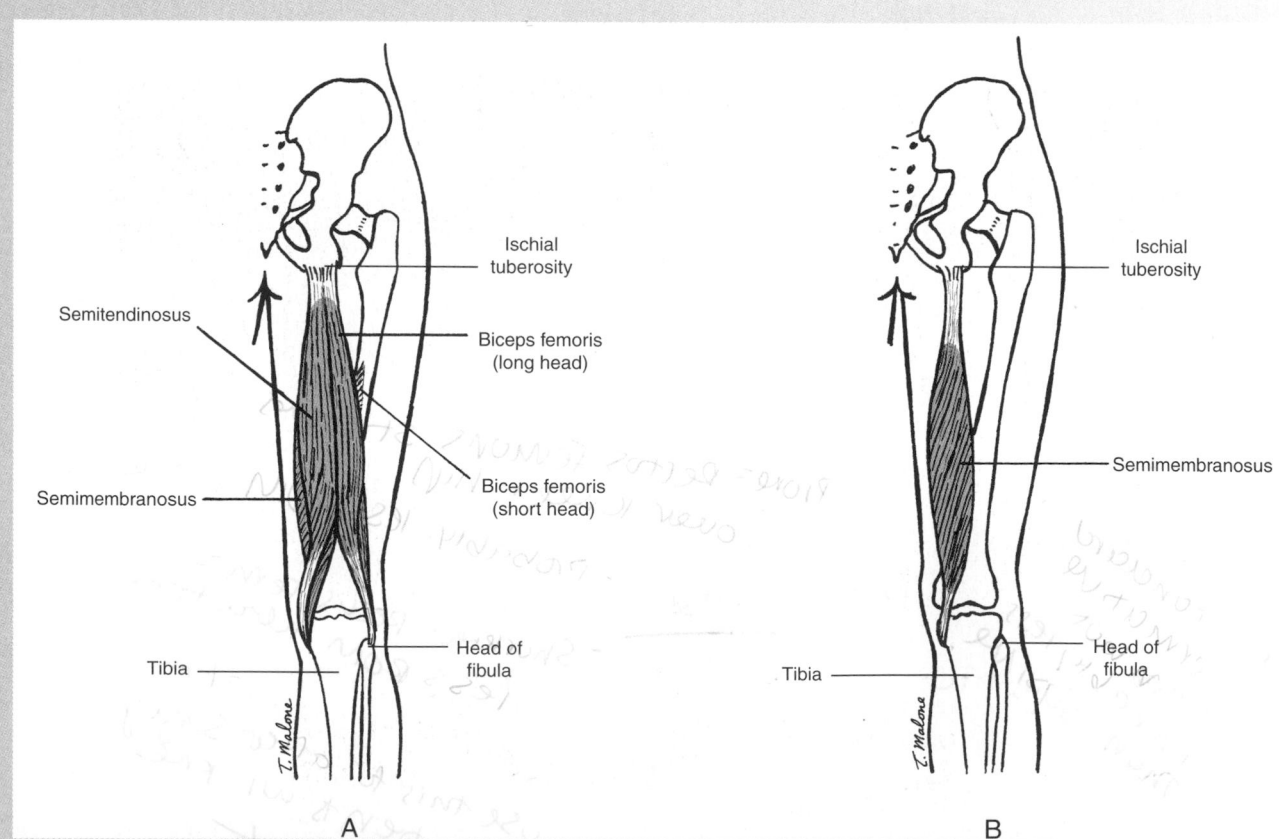

FIGURE 9.14 A: A posterior view of the thigh showing the attachments of the semitendinosus and the biceps femoris muscles. **B:** A posterior view of the thigh showing the attachments of the semimembranosus muscle, which lies under the two hamstring muscles shown in A.

PA in 214 subjects (108 women and 106 men) between the ages of 20 and 79 years. The mean value for the women of 152.0 degrees (SD = 10.6 degrees) was greater than the mean value for men of 141.4 degrees (SD = 8.1 degrees). The supplementary angles of these values for women and men are 28.0 and 38.6 degrees respectively, which is generally consistent with the values noted by Gajdosik and associates.

Two testers in a study by Fredriksen and colleagues[15] found that passive knee extension angle measurements for a single female subject tested 16 times per side ranged from 153 to 159 degrees for the left leg and from 154 to 165 degrees for the right leg. The supplementary angles of these values range from 27 to 21 degrees for the left leg and from 26 to 15 degrees for the right leg. A standardized force using a dynamometer was used to extend the knee, and the pelvis was stabilized by a belt. The hip was positioned in 120 degrees of flexion, which is a considerably larger angle of flexion than the 90 degrees of hip flexion used by both Youdas and associates[14] and Gadjosik and associates.[13]

Starting Position
Position the subject supine with the hip on the side being tested in 90 degrees of flexion and 0 degrees of abduction, adduction, and rotation (Fig. 9.15). Initially, the knee being tested is allowed to relax in flexion. The lower extremity that is not being tested rests on the examining table with the knee fully extended and the hip in 0 degrees of flexion, extension, abduction, adduction, and rotation.

Stabilization
Stabilize the femur to prevent rotation, abduction, and adduction at the hip and to maintain the hip in 90 degrees of flexion.

Testing Motion
Extend the knee to the end of the ROM. The end of the testing motion occurs when resistance is felt from tension in the posterior thigh and further knee extension causes the hip to move toward extension (Figs. 9.16 and 9.17).

Normal End-Feel
The end-feel is firm owing to tension in the semimembranosus, semitendinosus, and biceps femoris muscles.

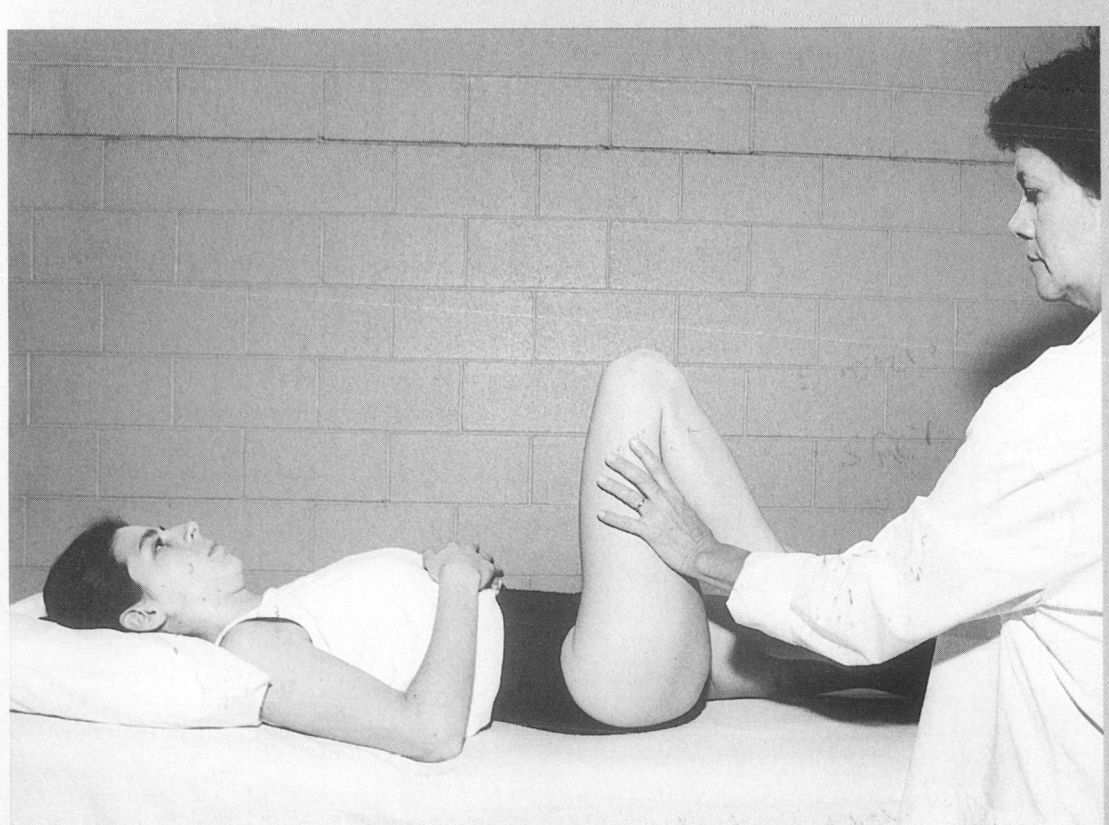

FIGURE 9.15 Starting position for measuring the length of the hamstring muscles.

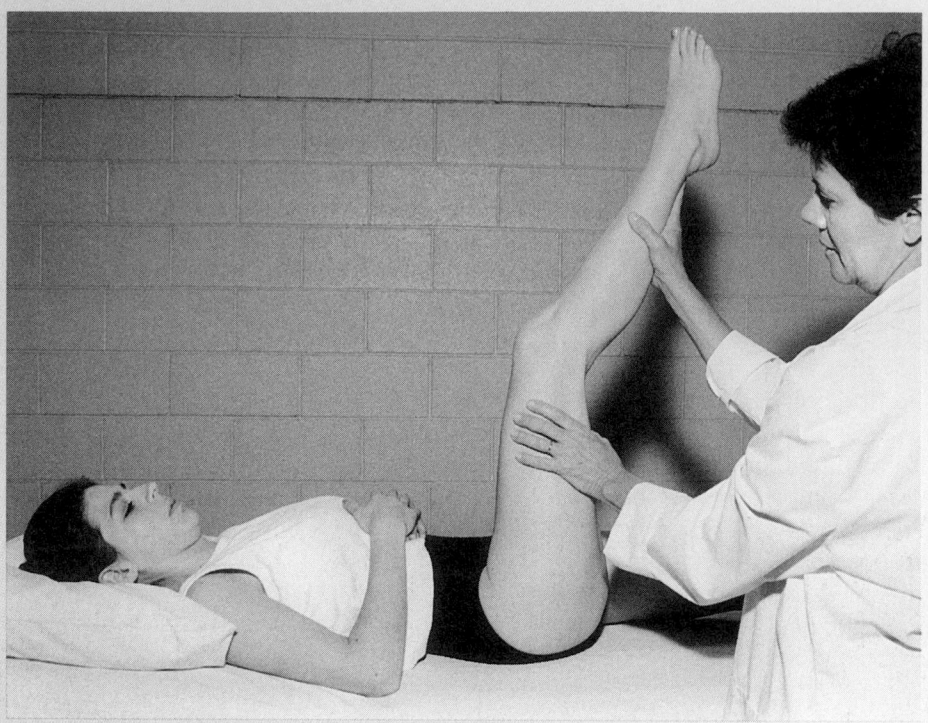

FIGURE 9.16 End of the testing motion for the length of the right hamstring muscles.

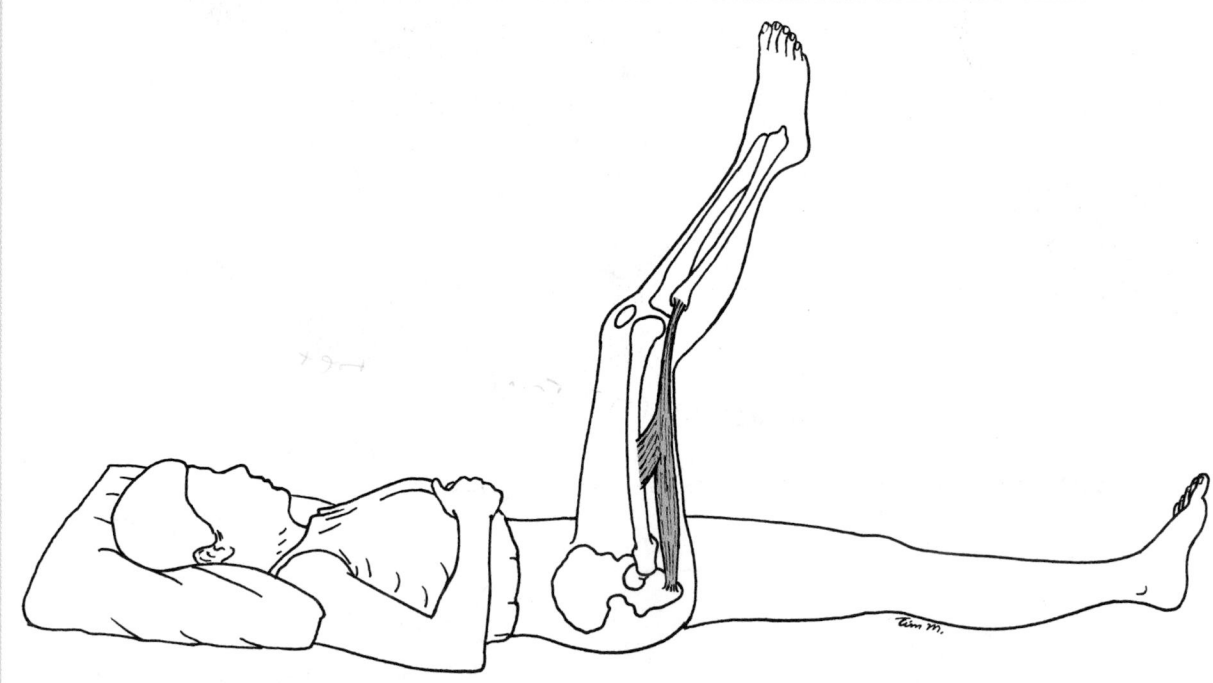

FIGURE 9.17 A lateral view of the right lower extremity shows the hamstring muscles being stretched over the hip and knee joints at the end of the testing motion.

Goniometer Alignment
See Figure 9.18.

1. Center **fulcrum** of the goniometer over the lateral epicondyle of the femur.
2. Align **proximal arm** with the lateral midline of the femur, using the greater trochanter for a reference.
3. Align **distal arm** with the lateral midline of the fibula, using the lateral malleolus and fibular head for reference.

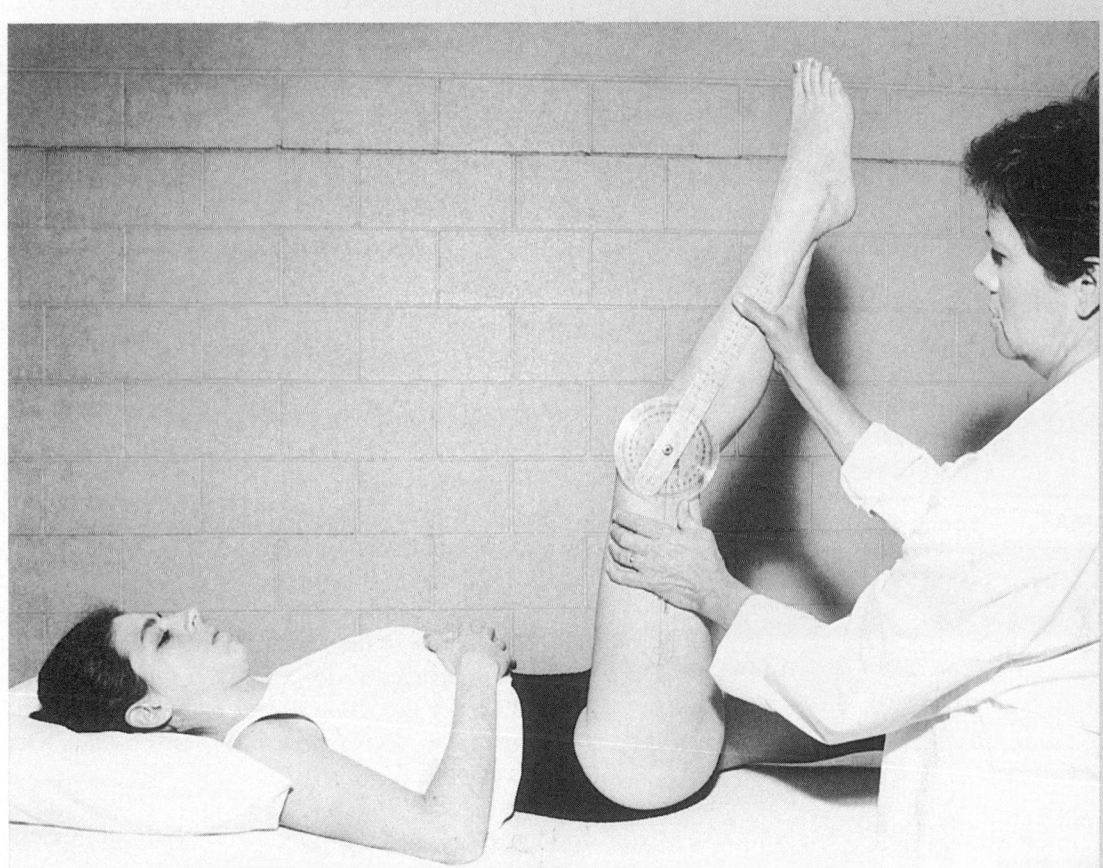

FIGURE 9.18 Goniometer alignment for measuring knee position.

⟋ Research Findings

This section of the chapter includes not only age and gender effects on knee ROM but also the effects of body mass. Also included is the range of functional knee ROM required for stairs and other activities of daily living followed by a sampling of reliability and validity studies in normal and patient populations. Table 9.1 provides knee ROM values from selected sources.[9-11] See Tables 9.2 to 9.4 for additional ROM values by age and gender.

Effects of Age, Gender, and Other Factors

Age
Knee extension limitations at birth are normal and similar to extension limitations found at the hip joint at birth. The term "extension limitation" is used rather than "flexion contracture" because contracture refers to an abnormal condition caused by fixed muscle shortness, which may be permanent.[16] Knee extension limitations in the neonate gradually disappear, and extension, instead of being limited, may become excessive in the toddler. Waugh and colleagues[17] and Drews and coworkers[18] found that newborns lacked approximately 15 to 20 degrees of knee extension. Schwarze and Denton,[19] in a study of 1000 neonates (527 girls and 473 boys) in the first 3 days of life, found a mean extension limitation of 15 degrees. These findings agree with the findings of Wanatabe and associates,[20] who found that newborns lacked 14 degrees of knee extension. The extension limitation gradually disappears, as shown by comparing Tables 9.2 and 9.3.

Broughton, Wright, and Menelaus[21] measured extension limitations in normal neonates at birth and again at 3 months and 6 months. At birth, 53 of the 57 (93 percent) neonates had extension limitations of 15 degrees or greater, whereas only 30 of 57 (53 percent) infants had extension limitations at 6 months of age. The mean reduction in extension limitations was 3.5 degrees per month from birth to 3 months and 2.8 degrees between 3 and 6 months (see Table 9.3). The 2 year olds in the study conducted by Wanatabe and associates[20] (see Table 9.3) had no evidence of a knee extension limitation.

Knee extension beyond 0 degrees (often referred to as hyperextension) is considered to be a normal finding in young children but is not usually observed in adults,[3] who may have slightly less than full knee extension. Wanatabe and associates[20] found that the 2 year olds had up to 5 degrees of extension beyond 0. This finding is similar to the mean of 5.4 degrees of extension beyond 0 noted by Boone[22] for the group of children between 1 year and 5 years of age. Beighton, Solomon, and Soskolne,[23] in a study of joint laxity in 1081 males and females, found that joint laxity decreased rapidly throughout childhood in both genders and decreased at a slower rate during adulthood. The authors used a ROM of greater than 10 degrees of knee extension beyond 0 as one of the criteria of joint laxity. Cheng and colleagues,[24] in a study of 2360 Chinese children, found that the average of 16 degrees of knee extension beyond 0 in children of 3 years of age decreased to 7 degrees by the time the children reached 9 years of age. A comparison of the knee extension beyond 0 mean values for the group aged 13 to 19 years in Table 9.4 with the extension values for the group aged 1 to 5 years in Table 9.3, demonstrates the decrease in extension beyond 0 that occurs in childhood.

TABLE 9.1	Knee Flexion Range of Motion: Normal Values in Degrees	
	AMA[9]	Boone[10]	Roach and Miles[11]
		Males 18 mos–54 yrs n = 109	Males and Females 25–74 yrs n = 1683
Motion		Mean (SD)	Mean (SD)
Flexion	150	142.5 (5.4)	132.0 (10.0)

(SD) = standard deviation.

TABLE 9.2	Knee Extension Limitations in Neonates 6 Hours to 7 Days of Age: Normal Values in Degrees			
	Waugh et al[17]	Drews et al[18]	Schwarze and Denton[19]	Broughton et al[21]
	6–65 hrs n = 40	12 hrs–6 days n = 54	1–3 days n = 1000	1–7 days n = 57
Motion	Mean (SD)	Mean (SD)	Mean	Mean (SD)
Extension limitation	15.3 (9.9)	20.4 (6.7)	15.0	21.4 (7.7)

(SD) = standard deviation.
All values were obtained from passive range of motion measurements with use of a universal goniometer.

| TABLE 9.3 | Knee Range of Motion in Infants and Young Children 0 to 12 Years of Age: Normal Values in Degrees | | | | |

	Broughton et al[21]		Wanatabe et al[20]	Boone[22]	
	3 mos n = 57	6 mos n = 57	0–2 yrs n = 109	1–5 yrs n = 19	6–12 yrs n = 17
Motion	Mean (SD)	Mean (SD)	Range of means	Mean (SD)	Mean (SD)
Flexion	145.5 (5.3)	141.7 (6.3)	148–159	141.7 (6.2)	147.1 (3.5)
Extension	10.7 (5.1)*	3.3 (4.3)*		5.4 (3.1)†	0.4 (0.9)

(SD) = standard deviation.
* Indicates extension limitations.
† Indicates extension beyond 0 degrees.

In Table 9.4 the mean values obtained by Boone[22] are from male subjects, whereas the values obtained by Roach and Miles[11] are from both genders. If values presented for the oldest groups (those aged 40 to 74 years) in both studies are compared with the values for the youngest group (those aged 13 to 19 years), it can be seen that the oldest groups have smaller mean values of flexion. However, with a SD of 11 degrees in the oldest groups, the difference between the youngest and the oldest groups is not more than 1 SD. Roach and Miles[11] concluded that, at least in individuals up to 74 years of age, any substantial loss (greater than 10 percent of the arc of motion) in joint mobility should be viewed as abnormal and not attributable to the aging process. The flexion values obtained by these authors were considerably smaller than the 150-degree average value published by the AMA.[9]

Walker and colleagues[25] studied active ROM of the extremity joints in 30 men and 30 women (ranging in age from 60 to 84 years) from recreational centers. No differences were found in knee ROM between subjects aged 60 to 69 years and subjects aged 75 to 84 years. However, average values indicated that the subjects had an extension limitation (inability to attain a neutral 0-degree starting position). This finding was similar to the loss of extension noted at the hip, elbow, and first metatarsophalangeal (MTP) joints. The 2-degree extension limitation found at the knee was much smaller than that found at the hip joint. According to the American Association of Orthopaedic Surgeons (AAOS) handbook,[3] extension limitations of 2 degrees are considered to be normal in adults. Extension limitations greater than 5 degrees in adults may be considered as knee flexion contractures. These contractures often occur in the elderly because of disease, sedentary lifestyles, and the effects of the aging process on connective tissues.

Mollinger and Steffan[26] used a universal goniometer (UG) to assess knee ROM among 112 nursing home residents with an average age of 83 years. The authors found that only 13 percent of the subjects had full (0 degrees) passive knee extension bilaterally. Thirty-seven of the 112 subjects (33 percent) had bilateral knee extension limitations of 5 degrees or less bilaterally, which the AAOS considers to be normal in older adults. Forty-seven subjects (42 percent) had greater than 10 degrees of limitations in extension (flexion contractures). Residents with a 30-degree loss of knee extension had an increase in resistance to passive motion and a loss of ambulation.

Steultjens and coworkers[27] found knee flexion contractures in 31.5 percent of 198 patients with osteoarthritis of the knee or hip. (It should be noted that these authors considered knee flexion contractures as an inability to attain the horizontal 0 position

| TABLE 9.4 | Age Effects on Knee Motion in Individuals 13 to 74 Years of Age: Mean Values in Degrees | | | | |

	Boone[22]			Roach and Miles[11]	
	13–19 yrs n = 17	20–29 yrs n = 19	40–45 yrs n = 19	40–59 yrs n = 727	60–74 yrs n = 523
Motion	Mean (SD)	Mean (SD)	Mean (SD)	Mean (SD)	Mean (SD)
Flexion	142.9 (3.7)	140.2 (5.2)	142.6 (5.6)	132.0 (11.0)	131.0 (11.0)
Extension	0.0 (0.0)	0.4 (0.9)	1.6 (2.4)		

(SD) = standard deviation.

starting position for measuring flexion.) Flexion contractures of the knee or hip or both were found in 73 percent of patients. Generally, a decrease in active assistive ROM was associated with an increase in disability but was motion specific. The motions that had the strongest relationship with disability were knee flexion, hip extension, and lateral rotation. Ersoz and Ergun[28] found that in a group of 44- to 76-year-old patients with primary knee osteoarthritis, 33 out of the 40 knees tested (82.5 percent) had extension limitations ranging from 1 to 14 degrees.

Despite the knee flexion contractures found in the elderly by Mollinger and Steffan,[26] many elderly individuals appear to have at least a functional flexion ROM. Escalante and coworkers[29] used a universal goniometer (UG) to measure knee flexion passive ROM in 687 community-dwelling elderly subjects between the ages of 65 and 79 years. More than 90 degrees of knee flexion was found in 619 (90.1 percent) of the subjects. The authors used a cutoff value of 124 degrees of flexion as being within normal limits. Subjects who failed to reach 124 degrees of flexion were classified as having an abnormal ROM. Using this criterion, 76 (11 percent) right knees and 63 (9 percent) left knees were below this value and thus had abnormal (limited) passive ROM in flexion.

Nonaka and colleagues[30] examined age-related changes at the hip and knee in 77 healthy male volunteers aged 15 to 73 years. The authors found that passive range of motion (PROM) of the hip joint decreased with increasing age but the knee joint PROM remained unchanged. However, interactive motion of the hip and knee showed an age-related reduction, which the authors attributed to shortening of muscle and connective tissue.

Gender

Beighton, Solomon, and Soskolne[23] defined more than 10 degrees of knee extension beyond 0 as hyperextension and included this criterion in a study of joint laxity in 1081 males and females. Females in the study had more joint laxity than males at any age. Loudon, Goist, and Loudon[31] operationally defined knee hyperextension (genu recurvatum) as more than 5 degrees of extension beyond the 0 position. Clinically, the authors had observed that not only was hyperextension more common in females than males, but that the condition might be associated with functional deficits in muscle strength, instability, and poor proprioceptive control of terminal knee extension. The authors cautioned that the female athlete with hyperextended knees may be at risk for anterior cruciate ligament injury. Hall and colleagues[32] found that 10 female patients diagnosed with hypermobility syndrome had alterations in proprioceptive acuity at the knee compared with an age-matched and gender-matched control group.

James and Parker[33] studied knee flexion ROM in 80 men and women who ranged in age from 70 years to older than 85 years. Women in this group had greater ROM in both active and passive knee flexion than men. Overall knee flexion values were lower than expected for both genders, possibly owing to the fact that the subjects were measured in the prone position, where the two-joint rectus femoris muscle may have limited the ROM.

In contrast to the findings of James and Parker,[33] Escalante and coworkers[29] found that female subjects had reduced passive knee flexion ROM compared with males of the same age. However, the women had on average only 2 degrees less knee flexion than men. The women also had a higher body mass index (BMI) than the men, which may have contributed to their reduced knee flexion.

Schwarze and Denton[19] observed no differences owing to gender in a study of 527 girls and 473 boys aged 1 to 3 days. Likewise, Cleffken and colleagues[34] found no gender differences in active and passive knee flexion and extension ROM in 23 male and 19 female healthy volunteers aged 19 to 27 years.

Body Mass Index

Lichtenstein and associates[35] found that among 647 community-dwelling elderly subjects (aged 64 to 78 years), those with high BMI had lower knee ROM than their counterparts with low BMI. Elderly subjects who were severely obese had an average loss of 13 degrees of knee flexion ROM compared with their counterparts who were not obese. The authors determined that a loss of knee ROM of at least 1 degree occurred for each unit increase in BMI. Escalante and coworkers[29] found that obesity was significantly associated with a decreased passive knee flexion ROM. Knees of subjects who were overweight had a flexion ROM that was 5 degrees less than subjects who were not obese. Sobti and colleagues[36] found that obesity was significantly associated with the risk of pain or stiffness at the knee or hip in a survey of 5042 Post Office pensioners. Knees of subjects who were overweight had a knee flexion ROM that was 5 degrees less than subjects who were not obese.

Functional Range of Motion

Table 9.5 provides knee ROM values required for various functional activities. Figures 9.19 to 9.21 show a variety of functional activities requiring different amounts of knee flexion. Of the activities measured by Jevsevar and coworkers[37] (stair ascent and descent, gait, and rising from a chair), stair ascent required the greatest range of knee motion.

Livingston and associates[38] used three testing staircases with different dimensions. Shorter subjects had a greater maximum mean knee flexion range (92 to 105 degrees) for stair ascent in comparison with taller subjects (83 to 96 degrees). Laubenthal, Smidt, and Kettlekamp[39] used an electrogoniometric method to measure knee motion in three planes (sagittal, coronal, and transverse). Stair dimensions used by McFayden and Winter[40] were 22 cm for stair height and 28 cm for stair tread. Similar dimension stairs were used by Protopapadaki and associates,[41] who used a rise height of 18 cm and a stair tread length of 28.5 cm to determine the knee motion during stair ascent and descent of 33 young healthy male and female subjects ranging in age from 18 to 39 years. The mean knee flexion

TABLE 9.5	Knee Flexion Range of Motion Necessary for Functional Activities: Normal Values in Degrees				
	Jevsevar et al*[37]	Livingston et al[38]	Laubenthal et al[39]	McFayden and Winter[40]	Rowe et al[42]
	Healthy Subjects (6M, 5F) Mean = 53 yrs n = 11	Healthy Women Range 19-26 yrs n = 15	Healthy Men Mean = 25 yrs n = 30	Healthy Male* n = 1	Normal Elderly Mean = 67 yrs n = 20
Motion	Mean (SD)	Mean range	Mean range (SD)	Mean range	Mean (SD)
Walk on level surfaces	63.1 (7.7)				64.5 (5.9)
Ascend stairs	92.9 (9.4)	2–105.0	0–83.0 (8.4)	10–100.0	80.3 (8.1)
Descend stairs	86.9 (5.7)	1–107.0	0–83.0 (8.2)	20–100.0	77.8 (8.3)
Rise from chair	90.1 (9.8)				89.8 (9.4)
Sit in chair			0–93.0 (10.3)		91.0 (11.8)
Tie shoes			0–106.0 (9.3)		
Lift object from floor			0–117.0 (13.1)		

(SD) = standard deviation.
* Sample consisted of one subject measured during eight trials.

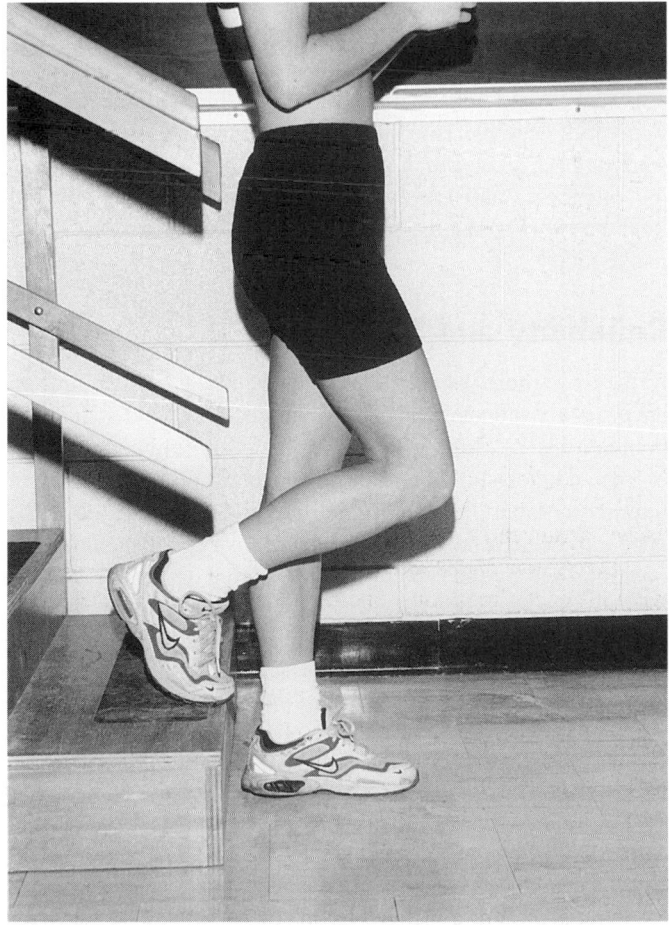

FIGURE 9.19 Descending stairs requires between 86.9[37] and 107[38] degrees of knee flexion depending on the stair dimensions.

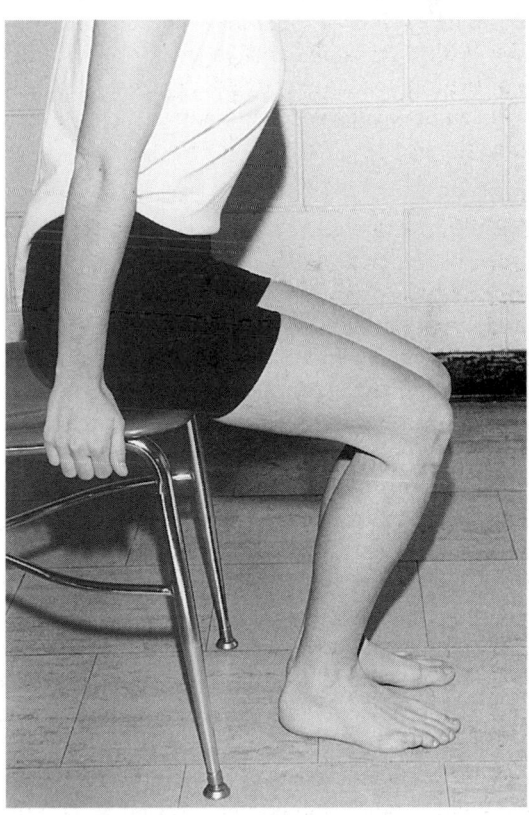

FIGURE 9.20 Rising from a chair requires a mean range of knee flexion of 90.1[37] to 95.0 degrees.[41]

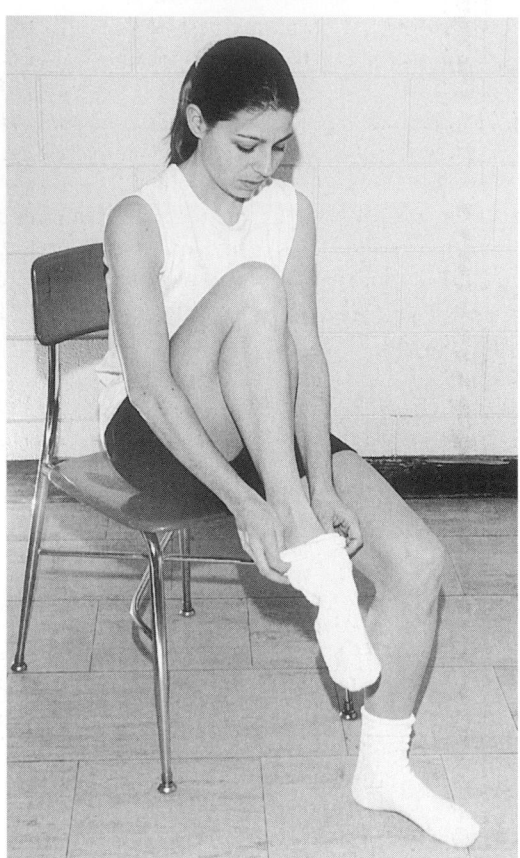

FIGURE 9.21 Putting on socks requires approximately 117 degrees of knee flexion.[39]

angles were 93.9 degrees for stair ascent and 90.5 degrees for stair descent.

Rowe and associates[42] used a flexible electrogoniometer to measure knee joint motion in gait, stairs, and getting in and out of a chair and a bath. Walking required the least amount of knee flexion for the 20 elderly subjects (aged 54 to 90 years) in the study, whereas getting in and out of a bath required the most knee flexion (135 degrees). The authors suggested that a clinical guideline of at least 110 degrees of flexion is necessary to allow patients to be able to walk, negotiate stairs, and get in and out of chairs. A goal of 90 degrees of knee flexion is not adequate to allow patients to carry out normal activities.

Lark and colleagues[43] compared knee ROM in stair descent in six healthy elderly males (mean age = 64 years) and six height- and weight-matched young males (mean age = 25 years). Knee flexion ROM was 12 percent less in the elderly group than in the younger group, but there was no difference between the groups in knee extension. However, the elderly group used 80 percent to 100 percent of their passive knee ROM, whereas the younger males used only 70 percent to 80 percent.

Oberg, Karsznia, and Oberg[44] used electrogoniometers to measure knee joint motion in midstance and swing phases of gait in 233 healthy males and females aged 10 to 79 years.

Only minor changes were attributable to age, and the authors determined that an increase in knee angle of about 0.5 degrees per decade occurred at midstance and a decrease of 0.5 to 0.8 degrees in knee angle occurred in swing phase. According to Rancho Los Amigos Medical Center,[45] the mean range of values for knee motion in gait on level surfaces is 5 to 60 degrees; however, the age, sex, and health status of the population used to obtain these values is unknown.

Mullholland and Wyss[46] reviewed the literature on the functional range of knee motions that are required in non-Western cultures for normal activities of daily living. The review revealed that in many parts of Asia, chairs were not commonly used and floor sitting, squatting, kneeling, or sitting cross-legged were the preferred positions. Hemmerich and colleagues[47] used an electrogoniometry motion tracking device to determine the range of motion needed to perform some of the activities identified by Mullholland and Wyss.[46] Thirty healthy Indian subjects (10 women and 20 men) with an average age of 48.2 years performed squatting with the heels up and down, cross-legged sitting, and kneeling with ankles dorsiflexed and plantarflexed. The authors found that medial rotation at the knee accompanied hip flexion in all activities. The greatest mean maximum knee medial rotation (33 degrees) was necessary for sitting cross-legged. Mean maximum knee flexion angles reached values greater than 150 degrees for both types of squatting and for kneeling with the ankles dorsiflexed. The maximal angle of knee flexion needed for kneeling with ankles plantarflexed was 144.4 degrees, whereas the mean maximum angle of knee flexion for squatting with the heels up was 156.9 degrees. The ranges of motion results found in this study are far greater than can be accommodated by any existing prostheses and are many degrees more than the clinical guideline of 110 degrees of knee flexion suggested by Rowe and associates.[42]

Reliability and Validity

Reliability studies of active and passive range of knee motion have been conducted in healthy subjects[48–52] and in patient populations.[53–59] Similar to findings at other joints, the results of knee studies show that intratester reliability is higher than intertester reliability.[48,55] Reliability and ROM values also appear to be affected by measurement instruments and testing positions and by the type of motion (active or passive) tested. Factors that have been shown to improve reliability include training of testers, use of more than one person to assist with stabilization (especially in the presence of spasticity), holding of heavy extremities, and marking of landmarks.

Reliability: Universal Goniometer in Healthy Populations

Boone and associates[48] had four testers use UGs to measure active knee flexion and extension ROM at four weekly sessions. Intratester reliability was higher than intertester reliability, and the total intratester SD for measurements at the knee was 4 degrees, whereas the intertester SD was 5.9 degrees. The authors recommended that when more than one tester measures the range of knee motion, changes in ROM should exceed 6 degrees to show that a real change has occurred.

Rheault and coworkers[50] found good intertester reliability for the UG (Table 9.6) and the fluid-based inclinometer ($r = 0.83$) for measurements of active knee flexion. However, significant differences in the ROM values were found between the instruments. Therefore, the authors concluded that, although the universal and fluid-based goniometers each appeared to have good reliability, they should not be used interchangeably in the clinical setting.

Bartholomy, Chandler, and Kaplan[51] had similar findings. These authors compared measurements of passive knee flexion ROM taken with a UG with measurements taken with a fluid-based inclinometer and an Optotrak motion analysis system. Eighty subjects aged 22 to 43 years were measured. Individually, the UG and the inclinometer were found to be reliable instruments for measuring passive knee flexion. ICCs for the UG were 0.97, and ICCs for the fluid inclinometer were 0.98. However, there were significant differences in the ROM values obtained among the three devices used, and the authors caution that these instruments should not be used interchangeably.

Mollinger and Steffan[26] collected intratester reliability data on measurement of knee extension made by two testers using a UG. ICCs for repeated measurements of knee extension were high (see Table 9.6), with differences between measurements averaging 1 degree.

Brosseau and associates[60] used a UG and a parallel goniometer (PG) to measure two flexion-angle positions in the right knees of 60 healthy subjects (44 females and 16 males). Intratester reliability of the smaller-angle (about 20 degrees) and larger-angle (about 100 degrees) positions

TABLE 9.6	Intratester and Intertester Reliability: Knee Range of Motion Measured with a Universal Goniometer						
Author	n	Sample	Motion	Intra ICC	Inter ICC	Intra r	Inter r
Boone et al [48]	12	Healthy adult males (25–54 yrs)	AROM Flexion	0.87	0.50		
Brosseau et al[60]	60	Healthy adults (mean age 20.6 yrs)	Flexion fixed angles	0.86–0.97	0.91–0.94		
Rheault et al [50]	20	Healthy adults (mean age 24.8 yrs)	AROM Flexion				0.87
Gogia et al [49]	30	Healthy adults (20–60 yrs)	PROM Flexion		0.99		0.98
Drews et al [18]	9	Healthy infants (12 hrs–6 days)	PROM Flexion				0.69 left 0.89 right
Rothstein et al [53]	12	Patients (ages not reported)	PROM Flexion Extension	0.97–0.99 0.91–0.97	0.84–0.99 0.59–0.80	0.97–0.99 0.91–0.96	0.83–0.92 0.57–0.79
Watkins et al [54]	43	Patients (mean age 39.5 yrs)	PROM Flexion Extension	0.99 0.98	0.90 0.86		
Pandya et al [55]	150* 21†	Duchenne muscular dystrophy (<1 yr–20 yrs)	PROM Extension	0.93	0.73		
Mollinger and Steffan [26]	10	Nursing home residents	Extension	0.99	0.97		
Beissner et al [56]	10	Nursing home and Independent living residents (mean age 81.0 yrs)	PROM Flexion Extension			0.70–0.93 0.70–0.93	

AROM = active range of motion; ICC = intraclass correlation coefficient; PROM = passive range of motion; r = pearson product moment correlation coefficient.
*150 subjects were used to calculate intratester ICC.
†21 subjects were used to calculate intertester ICC.

were good to excellent for the UG and good for the PG. Intertester reliability was lower than intratester reliability for both positions and goniometers, however, the smaller angle had lower intertester reliability compared to the large angle (see Table 9.6).

Reliability: Universal Goniometer in Patient Populations

Rothstein, Miller, and Roettger[53] investigated intratester, intertester, and interdevice reliability in a study involving 12 patients referred to physical therapy for their knee. Intratester reliability for passive ROM measurements for knee flexion and extension was high. Intertester reliability also was high among the 12 testers for passive ROM measurements for flexion but was lower for knee extension measurements (see Table 9.6). Intertester reliability was not improved by repeated measurements but was improved when testers used the same patient positioning. Interdevice reliability was high for all measurements. Neither the composition of the UG (metal or plastic) nor the size (large or small) had a significant effect on the measurements.

Watkins and associates[54] compared passive ROM measurements of the knees of 43 patients made by 14 physical therapists who used a UG and visual estimates. These authors found that intratester reliability with the UG was high for both knee flexion and knee extension. Intertester reliability for goniometric measurements also was high for knee flexion but only good for knee extension (see Table 9.6). Both intratester and intertester reliability were lower for visual estimation than for goniometric measurement. The authors suggested that therapists should not substitute visual estimates for goniometric measurements when assessing a patient's range of knee motion because of the additional error that is introduced with use of visual estimation.

Pandya and colleagues[55] studied intratester and intertester reliability of passive knee extension measurements in 150 children aged 1 to 20 years who had a diagnosis of Duchenne muscular dystrophy. Intratester reliability with use of the UG was high, but intertester reliability was only fair (see Table 9.6).

McWhirk and Glanzman[57] had two physical therapists measure the knee ROM and the popliteal angle in 46 knees in 25 children (aged 2 to 18 years) with spastic cerebral palsy. The intertester reliability of knee extension measurements was an ICC of 0.78 with a 95% confidence interval (CI) = ±1.75, and the popliteal angle measurement had an ICC of 0.93 with a 95% CI = ±1.47. The therapists helped each other during the measurements by having one or the other either provide support for the test leg or stabilize the other extremity.

In a study by Lessen and associates,[58] two physical therapists used a long arm UG to measure active and passive knee flexion and extension in 30 patients within the first 4 days after total knee arthoplasty. Measurements were taken with the patients supine in a hospital bed and in the sitting position on an examination table. The highest levels of agreement between the testers were found for passive flexion and extension in the sitting position. The lowest level of agreement was found for passive flexion in the supine position with 16.2 to 19.0 degrees difference between the two testers. ICC values for intertester reliability were highest for active and passive flexion while sitting.

Kilgour, McNair, and Stott[59] had three pediatric physical therapists measure bilateral knee extension in 25 children with spastic cerebral palsy ranging in age from 6 to 17 years and 25 age- and sex-matched controls. Intrasessional absolute differences ranged from 0 to 2.7 degrees in the control group and 0 to 2.4 degrees in the cerebral palsy (CP) group. Intrasessional ICCs were good in the control group (ICC = 0.79 to 0.87) and excellent in the CP group (ICC = 0.97 to 0.99). Intersessional ICCs were lower for both the control and CP group, but only the control group had unacceptable ICCs (0.34 to 0.67) compared to an ICC of 0.89 to 0.92 for the CP group. The authors concluded that sagittal plane ROM measures have similar levels of reliability in children with spastic CP compared with healthy controls both within and between sessions.

Reliability: Electronic Digital Inclinometer (CYBEX EDI320)

Cleffken and associates[34] conducted a study to determine both intratester and intertester reproducibility for measurements of active and passive knee flexion and extension in 42 healthy volunteers. Each motion was measured by two testers three times in four measurements sessions. Measurements of passive maximum flexion of the knee resulted in a smaller detectable difference (SDD = 0 ± 6.4 degrees) than active knee flexion (SDD = 0 ± 7.4 degrees) for intertester comparisons. Intratester reliability showed better reproducibility with SDDs reduced by 0.4 to 1.9 degrees over intertester values.

Reliability: Electrogoniometer

Piriyaprasarth and colleagues[61] assessed intratester and intertester reliability of measurements using a flexible electrogoniometer of two different fixed flexion angles (45 and 75 degrees) in sitting, supine, and standing positions Thirty-seven healthy volunteers (mean age 31 years) participated in the intratester study, and 35 healthy volunteers (mean age 30 years) participated in the intertester reliability study. Ten repetitions of joint angles were taken by two testers. Intratester reliability of measurements ranged from fair for supine (ICC = 0.75 to 0.76), good in sitting (ICC = 0.86 to 0.87), to very good in standing (ICC = 0.87 to 0.88). Intertester reliability was poor to fair for supine (ICC = 0.58 to 0.71), poor to fair for sitting (ICC = 0.68 to 0.79), and poor to good for standing (ICC = 0.57 to 0.80). The sitting position had larger ICCs and lower standard errors of measurement (SEMs) for both intratester and intertester reliability compared to the supine position. One drawback of the study was that only angles less than 90 degrees were measured. The SEM was less than 1.7 degrees when the same tester repeated the measurements.

Reliability: Inclinometer

The mean knee flexion ROM for the Ely test was 138.5 degrees for four testers using an inclinometer in a study by Piva and associates.[12] Measurements were taken of 30 patients with patellofemoral pain syndrome ranging in age from 14 to 47 years. The intertester reliability ICC was 0.91.

Validity: Universal Goniometer

Gogia and colleagues[49] measured knee joint angles between 0 and 120 degrees of flexion. These measurements were immediately followed by radiographs. Intertester reliability was high (Table 9.6). The ICC for validity also was high (0.99). The authors concluded that the knee angle measurements taken with a UG were both reliable and valid.

Enwemeka[52] compared the measurements of six knee joint positions (0, 15, 30, 45, 60, and 90 degrees) taken with a UG with bone angle measurements provided by radiographs. The measurements were taken on 10 healthy adult volunteers (four women and six men) between 21 and 35 years of age. The mean differences ranged from 0.52 to 3.81 degrees between goniometric and radiographic measurements taken between 30 and 90 degrees of flexion. However, mean differences were higher (4.59 degrees) between goniometric and radiographic measurements of the smaller angles between 0 and 15 degrees.

Ersoz and Ergun[28] used a UG with 25-cm arms and 1-degree increments to measure the ROM in both knees of 20 patients with bilateral knee osteoarthritis. Radiographs were taken of tibiofemoral, lateral tibiofemoral, and patellofemoral compartments of the same knees. The authors found a clear relationship between knee ROM measurements of flexion, extension, and medial and lateral rotation taken with a UG and radiographs. For example, limitations in internal rotation ROM provided a prediction of advanced disease in the lateral knee compartment. The authors concluded that measurements of joint ROM were helpful in the determination of the compartment or compartments that were affected by the disease process.

Brousseau and associates[60] measured active knee flexion in two positions in 60 healthy university students (44 females and 16 males) with a mean age of 21 years. Two trained testers alternately used either a universal (UG) or a pendulum (PG) goniometer for the measurements. Eight measurements were taken with the knee flexed in the supine position and eight with the knee in the first 20 degrees of flexion in the supine position. A radiograph was taken of each subject in each knee position. Criterion validity was determined by calculating Pearson product moment correlation coefficients between each goniometric and radiologic measurement. Results showed that both the PGs and UGs had higher validity when measuring the larger fixed knee flexion angle compared to the smaller angle when using radiographs as the gold standard.

Rheault and coworkers[50] investigated the concurrent validity of a UG and an inclinometer for measurements of active knee flexion. Each instrument had good validity, but instruments could not be used interchangeably.

REFERENCES

1. Levangie, PK, and Norkin, CC: Joint Structure and Function: A Comprehensive Analysis, ed 4. FA Davis, Philadelphia, 2005.
2. Williams, PL (ed): Gray's Anatomy, ed 38. Churchill Livingstone, New York, 1995.
3. Greene, WB, and Heckman, JD (eds): The Clinical Measurement of Joint Motion. American Academy of Orthopaedic Surgeons, Chicago, 1994.
4. Kaltenborn, FM: Mobilization of the Extremity Joints, ed 5. Olaf Norlis Bokhandel, Oslo, 1999.
5. Cyriax, JH, and Cyriax, PJ: Illustrated Manual of Orthopaedic Medicine. Butterworths, London, 1983.
6. Fritz, JM, et al: An examination of the selective tissue tension scheme, with evidence for the concept of a capsular pattern of the knee. Phys Ther 78:1046, 1998.
7. Hayes, KW: Invited commentary. Phys Ther 78:1057, 1998.
8. Hayes KW, Petersen C, and Falcone, J: An examination of Cyriax's passive motion tests with patients having osteoarthritis of the knee. Phys Ther 74:697, 1994.
9. American Medical Association: Guides to the Evaluation of Permanent Impairment, ed 3 (revised). AMA, Chicago, 1990.
10. Boone, DC, and Azen, SP: Normal range of motion of joints in male subjects. J Bone Joint Surg Am 61:756, 1979.
11. Roach, KE, and Miles, TP: Normal hip and knee active range of motion: The relationship to age. Phys Ther 71:656, 1991.
12. Piva, SR, et al: Reliability of measures of impairments associated with patellofemoral pain syndrome. BMC Musculoskelet Disord 7:33, 2006.
13. Gajdosik, RL, et al: Comparison of four clinical tests for assessing hamstring muscle length. J Orthop Sport Phys Ther 18:614, 1993.
14. Youdas, JW, et al: The influence of gender and age on hamstring muscle length in healthy adults. J Orthop Sports Phys Ther 35:246–252, 2005.
15. Fredriksen, H, et al: Passive knee extension test to measure hamstring muscle tightness. Scand J Med Sci Sports 7:279–282, 1997.
16. Rothstein, JM, Roy, SH, and Wolf, SL: The Rehabilitation Specialist's Handbook, ed 2. FA Davis, Philadelphia, 1998.
17. Waugh, KG, et al: Measurement of selected hip, knee, and ankle joint motions in newborns. Phys Ther 63:1616, 1983.
18. Drews, JE, Vraciu, JK, and Pellino, G: Range of motion of the lower extremities of newborns. Phys Occup Ther Pediatr 4:49, 1984.
19. Schwarze, DJ, and Denton, JR: Normal values of neonatal limbs: An evaluation of 1000 neonates. J Pediatr Orthop 13:758, 1993.
20. Wanatabe, H, et al: The range of joint motions of the extremities in healthy Japanese people: The difference according to age. Nippon Seikeigeka Gakkai Zasshi 53:275, 1979 (Cited by Walker, JM: Musculoskeletal development: A review. Phys Ther 71:878, 1991.)
21. Broughton NS, Wright J, and Menelaus, MB: Range of knee motion in normal neonates. J Pediatr Orthop 13:263, 1993.
22. Boone, DC: Techniques of measurement of joint motion. (Unpublished supplement to Boone, DC, and Azen, SP: Normal range of motion in male subjects. J Bone Joint Surg Am 61:756, 1979.)
23. Beighton, P, Solomon, L, and Soskolne, CL: Articular mobility in an African population. Ann Rheum Dis 32:23, 1973.
24. Cheng, JC, Chan, PS, and Hui, PW: Joint laxity in children. J Pediatr Orthop 11:752, 1991.
25. Walker, JM, et al: Active mobility of the extremities in older subjects. Phys Ther 64:919, 1984.
26. Mollinger, LA, and Steffan, TM: Knee flexion contractures in institutionalized elderly: Prevalence, severity, stability and related variables. Phys Ther 73:437, 1993.
27. Steultjens, MPM, et al: Range of motion and disability in patients with osteoarthritis of the knee or hip. Rheumatology 39:955, 2000.
28. Ersoz, M, and Ergun, S: Relationship between knee range of motion and Kellgren-Lawrence radiographic scores in knee osteoarthritis. Am J Phys Med Rehabil 82:110–115, 2003.
29. Escalante, A, et al: Determinants of hip and knee flexion range: Results from the San Antonio Longitudinal Study of Aging. Arthritis Care Res 12:8, 1999.
30. Nonaka, H, Mita, K, Watakabe, M et al: Age-related changes in the interactive mobility of the hip and knee joints: A geometrical analysis. Gait Posture 15:236–243, 2002.
31. Loudon, JK, Goist, HL, and Loudon, KL: Genu recurvatum syndrome. J Orthop Sports Phys Ther 27:361, 1998.
32. Hall, MG, et al: The effect of hypermobility syndrome on knee joint proprioception. Br J Rheumatol 34:121, 1995.
33. James, B, and Parker, AW: Active and passive mobility of the lower limb joints in elderly men and women. Am J Phys Med Rehab 68:162, 1989.
34. Cleffken, B, van Breukelen, G, Brink, P, et al: Digital goniometric measurement of knee joint motion. Evaluation of usefulness for research settings and clinical practice. Knee 14:385–389, 2007
35. Lichtenstein, MJ, et al: Modeling impairment: Using the disablement process as a framework to evaluate determinants of hip and knee flexion. Aging (Milano) 12:208, 2000.
36. Sobti, A, et al: Occupational physical activity and long term risk of musculoskeletal symptoms: A national survey of post office pensioners. Am J Indust Med 32:76, 1997.
37. Jevsevar, DS, et al: Knee kinematics and kinetics during locomotor activities of daily living in subjects with knee arthroplasty and in healthy control subjects. Phys Ther 73:229, 1993.
38. Livingston, LA, Stevenson, JM, and Olney, SJ: Stairclimbing kinematics on stairs of differing dimensions. Arch Phys Med Rehabil 72:398, 1991.
39. Laubenthal, KN, Smidt, GL, and Kettlekamp, DB: A quantitative analysis of knee motion during activities of daily living. Phys Ther 52:34, 1972.
40. McFayden, BJ, and Winter, DA: An integrated biomechanical analysis of normal stair ascent and descent. J Biomech 21:733, 1988.
41. Protopapadaki, A, Drechsler, WI, Cramp, MC, et al: Hip, knee and ankle kinematics and kinetics during stair ascent and descent in healthy young individuals. Clin Biomech 22:203–210, 2007.
42. Rowe, PJ, et al: Knee joint kinematics in gait and other functional activities measured using flexible electrogoniometry: How much knee motion is sufficient for a normal daily life? Gait Posture 12:143–155, 2000.
43. Lark, SD, et al: Knee and ankle range of motion during stepping down in elderly compared to young men. Eur J Appl Physiol 9:287–295, 2004.
44. Oberg, T, Karsznia, A, and Oberg, K: Joint angle parameters in gait: Reference data for normal subjects, 10–79 years of age. J Rehabil Res Dev 31:199, 1994.
45. The Pathokinesiology Service and Physical Therapy Department: Observational Gait Analysis, ed. 4. Los Amigos Research and Education Institute, Inc. Rancho Los Amigos National Rehabilitation Center, Downey, CA, 2001.
46. Mulholland, SJ, Wyss, UP: Activities of daily living in non-Western cultures: range of motion requirements for hip and knee joints. Int J Rehabil Res 24:191–198, 2001.
47. Hemmerich, A, Brown, H, Smith, S, et al: Hip, knee and ankle kinematics of high range of motion activities of daily living. J Orthop Res 24:770–781, 2006.
48. Boone, DC, et al: Reliability of goniometric measurements. Phys Ther 58:1355, 1978.
49. Gogia, PP, et al: Reliability and validity of goniometric measurements at the knee. Phys Ther 67:192, 1987.
50. Rheault, W, et al: Intertester reliability and concurrent validity of fluid-based and universal goniometers for active knee flexion. Phys Ther 68:1676, 1988.
51. Bartholomy, JK, Chandler, RF, and Kaplan, SE: Validity analysis of fluid goniometer measurements of knee flexion. [Abstr] Phys Ther 80:S46, 2000.
52. Enwemeka, CS: Radiographic verification of knee goniometry. Scand J Rehabil Med 18:47, 1986.
53. Rothstein, JM, Miller, PJ, and Roettger, RF: Goniometric reliability in a clinical setting. Phys Ther 63:1611, 1983.
54. Watkins, MA, et al: Reliability of goniometric measurements and visual estimates of knee range of motion obtained in a clinical setting. Phys Ther 71:90, 1991.
55. Pandya, S, et al: Reliability of goniometric measurements in patients with Duchenne muscular dystrophy. Phys Ther 65:1339, 1985.
56. Beissner K, Collins JE, and Holmes H: Muscle force and range of motion as predictors of function in older adults. Phys Ther 80:556, 2000.
57. McWhirk, LB, Glanzman, AM: Within-session inter-rater reliability of goniometric measures in patients with spastic cerebral palsy. Paedtr Phys Ther 18:262–265, 2006.
58. Lessen, AF, van Dam, EM, Crijns, YH, et al: Reproducibility of goniometric measurement of the knee in the in-hospital phase following total knee arthroplasty. BMC Musculoskeletal Disord 8:83, 2007.
59. Kilgour, G, McNair, PM, Stott, NS: Intrarater reliability of lower limb sagittal range-of-motion measures in children with spastic diplegia. Dev Med Child Neurol 45:391–399, 2003.
60. Brosseau, L, Tousignant, M, Budd, J, et al: Intratester and intertester reliability and criterion validity of the parallelogram and universal goniometers for active knee flexion in healthy adults. Physiother Res Int 2:150–166, 1997.
61. Piriyaprasarth, P, et al: The reliability of knee joint position testing using electrogoniometry. BMC Musculoskelet Disord 9:6, 2008.

The Ankle and Foot

⟠ Structure and Function

Proximal and Distal Tibiofibular Joints

Anatomy

The proximal tibiofibular joint is formed by a slightly convex tibial facet and a slightly concave fibular facet and is surrounded by a joint capsule that is reinforced by anterior and posterior ligaments. The distal tibiofibular joint is formed by a fibrous union between a concave facet on the lateral aspect of the distal tibia and a convex facet on the distal fibula (Fig. 10.1A). Both joints are supported by the interosseous membrane, which is located between the tibia and the fibula (Fig. 10.1B). The distal joint does not have a joint capsule but is supported by anterior and posterior ligaments and the crural interosseous tibiofibular ligament (Fig. 10.1C).

Osteokinematics

The proximal and distal tibiofibular joints are anatomically distinct from the talocrural joint but function to serve the ankle. The proximal joint is a plane synovial joint that allows a small amount of superior and inferior sliding of the fibula on the tibia and a slight amount of rotation. The distal joint is a syndesmosis, or fibrous union, but it also allows a small amount of motion.

Arthrokinematics

During dorsiflexion of the ankle, the fibula moves proximally and slightly posteriorly (lateral rotation) away from the tibia. During plantarflexion, the fibula glides distally and slightly anteriorly toward the tibia.

Capsular Pattern

The capsular pattern is not defined for the tibiofibular joints.

Talocrural Joint

Anatomy

The talocrural joint comprises the articulations between the talus and the distal tibia and fibula. Proximally, the joint is formed by the concave surfaces of the distal tibia and the tibial and fibular malleoli. Distally, the joint surface is the convex dome of the talus. The joint capsule is thin and weak anteriorly and posteriorly, and the joint is reinforced by lateral and medial ligaments. Anterior and posterior talofibular ligaments and the calcaneofibular ligament provide lateral support for the capsule and joint (Fig. 10.2A and B). The deltoid ligament provides medial support (Fig. 10.3).

Osteokinematics

The talocrural joint is a synovial hinge joint with 1 degree of freedom. The motions available are dorsiflexion and plantarflexion. These motions occur around an oblique axis and thus do not occur purely in the sagittal plane. The motions cross three planes and therefore are considered to be triplanar. Dorsiflexion of the ankle brings the foot up and slightly lateral, whereas plantarflexion brings the foot down and slightly medial. The ankle is considered to be in the 0-degree neutral position when the foot is at a right angle to the tibia.

Arthrokinematics

During dorsiflexion in the non–weight-bearing position, the talus moves posteriorly. During plantarflexion, the talus moves anteriorly. During dorsiflexion, in the weight-bearing position, the tibia moves anteriorly. During plantarflexion, the tibia moves posteriorly.

Capsular Pattern

The pattern is a greater limitation in plantarflexion than in dorsiflexion.

Subtalar Joint

Anatomy

The subtalar (talocalcaneal) joint is composed of three separate plane articulations: the posterior, anterior, and middle articulations between the talus and the calcaneus. The posterior articulation, which is the largest, includes a concave facet on the inferior surface of the talus and a convex facet on the body of the calcaneus. The anterior and middle articulations are formed by two convex facets on the talus and two concave facets on the calcaneus. The anterior and middle articulations share a joint capsule with the talonavicular joint; the posterior articulation has its own capsule. The subtalar joint is

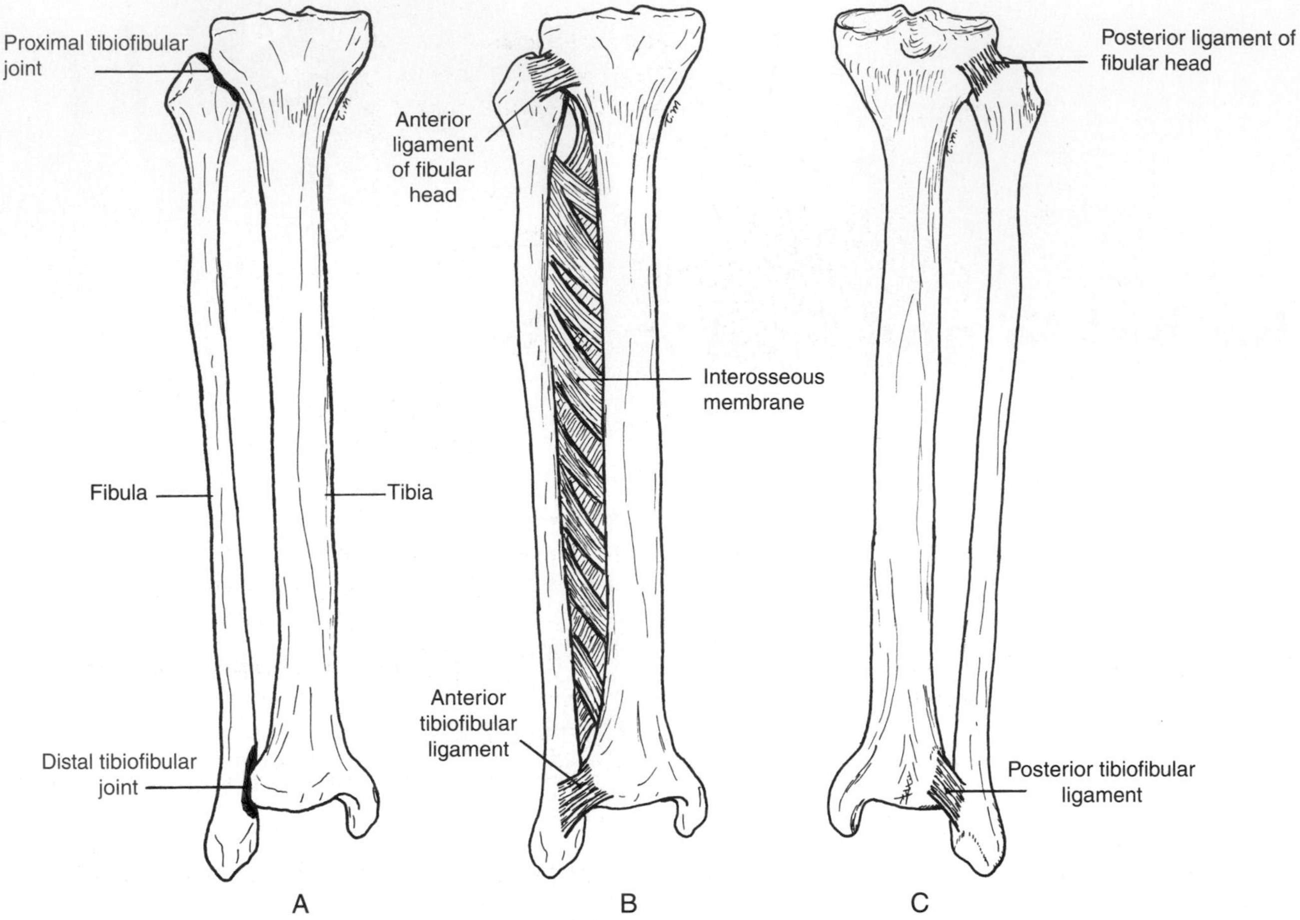

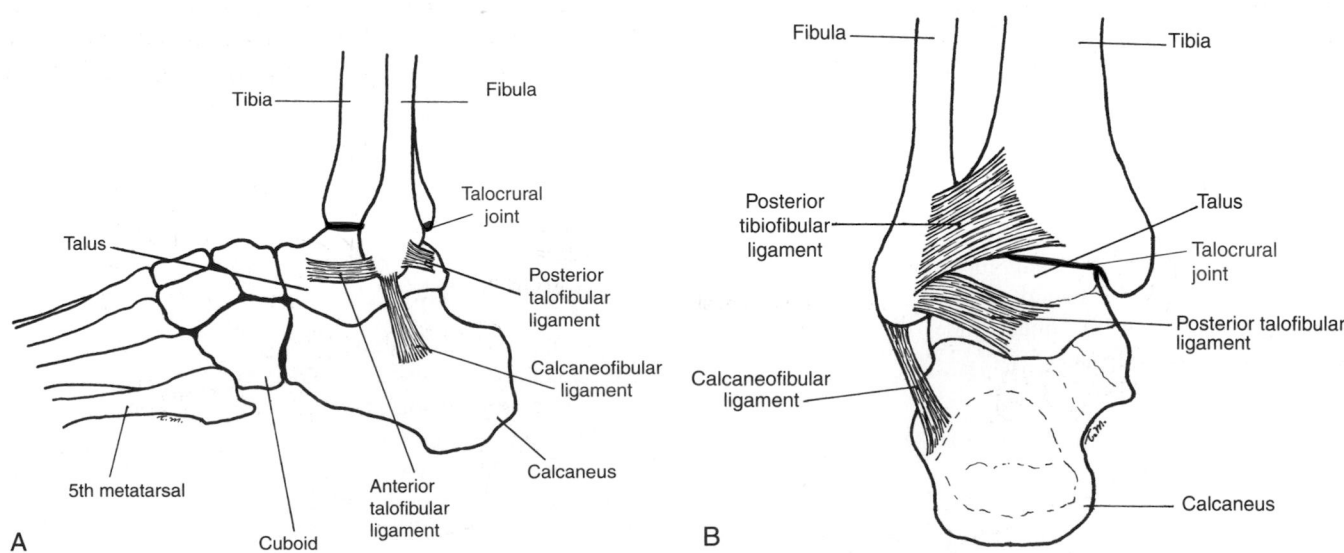

FIGURE 10.1 A: The anterior aspect of the proximal and distal tibiofibular joints of a right lower extremity. **B:** The anterior tibiofibular ligaments and the interosseous membrane. **C:** The posterior aspect of the tibiofibular joints and the posterior tibiofibular ligaments of a right lower extremity.

FIGURE 10.2 A: A lateral view of a left talocrural joint with the anterior and posterior talofibular ligaments and the calcaneofibular ligament. **B:** A posterior view of a left talocrural joint shows the posterior talofibular ligament and the calcaneofibular ligament.

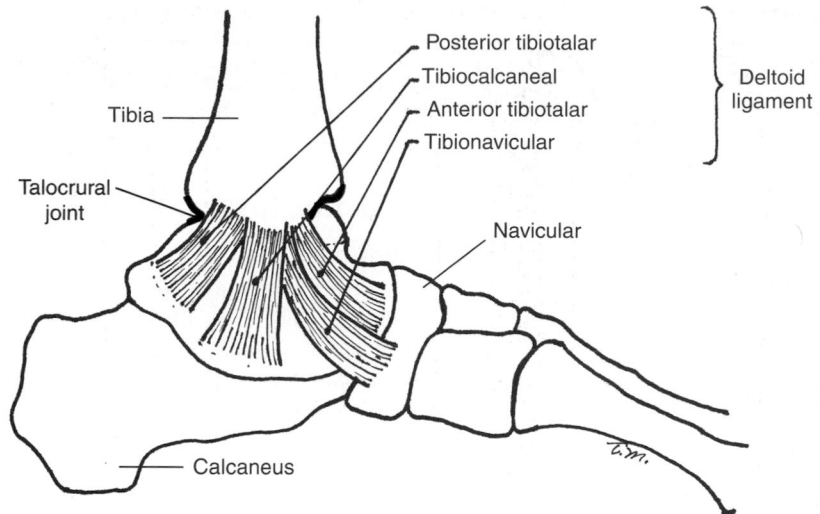

FIGURE 10.3 The deltoid ligament in a medial view of a left talocrural joint.

reinforced by anterior, posterior, lateral, and medial talocalcaneal ligaments and the interosseus talocalcaneal ligament (Figs. 10.4 and 10.5).

Osteokinematics

The motions permitted at the joint are inversion and eversion, which occur around an oblique axis. These motions are composite motions consisting of abduction–adduction, flexion–extension, and supination–pronation.[1] During non–weight-bearing inversion, the calcaneus adducts around an anterior–posterior axis, supinates around a longitudinal axis, and plantarflexes around a medial–lateral axis. During eversion, the calcaneus abducts, pronates, and dorsiflexes.

Arthrokinematics

The alternating convex and concave facets limit mobility and create a twisting motion of the calcaneus on the talus. During inversion of the foot, the calcaneus slides laterally on a fixed talus. During eversion, the calcaneus slides medially on the talus.

Capsular Pattern

The capsular pattern consists of a greater limitation in inversion.[2]

Transverse Tarsal (Midtarsal) Joint

Anatomy

The transverse tarsal, or midtarsal, joint is a compound joint formed by the talonavicular and calcaneocuboid joints (Fig. 10.6A). The talonavicular joint is composed of the large convex head of the talus and the concave posterior portion of the navicular bone. The concavity is enlarged by the plantar calcaneonavicular ligament (spring ligament). The joint shares a capsule with the anterior and middle portions of the subtalar joint and is reinforced by the spring, bifurcate

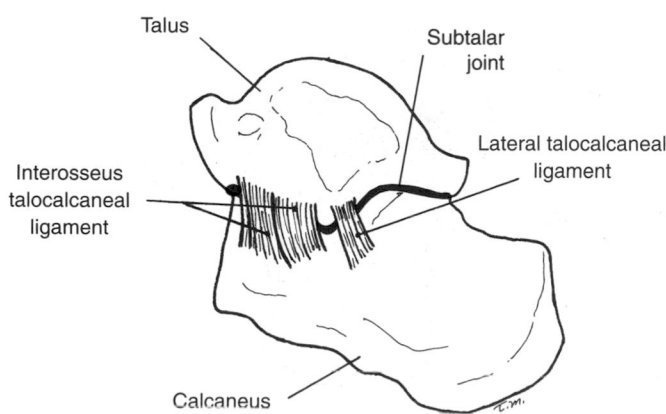

FIGURE 10.4 The interosseus talocalcaneal and lateral talocalcaneal ligaments in a lateral view of a left subtalar joint.

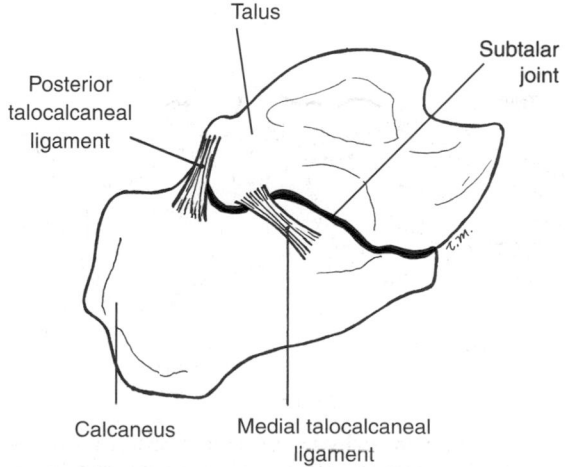

FIGURE 10.5 The medial and posterior talocalcaneal ligaments in a medial view of a left subtalar joint.

(calcaneocuboid and calcaneonavicular), and dorsal talonavicular ligaments (Fig. 10.6B).

The calcaneocuboid joint is composed of the shallow convex–concave surfaces on the anterior calcaneus and the convex–concave surfaces on the posterior cuboid. The joint is enclosed in a capsule that is reinforced by the bifurcate (calcaneocuboid and calcaneonavicular), dorsal calcaneocuboid, plantar calcaneocuboid, and long plantar ligaments (Fig. 10.6C).

Osteokinematics
The joint is considered to have two axes, one longitudinal and one oblique. Motions around both axes are triplanar and consist of inversion and eversion. The transverse tarsal joint is the transitional link between the hindfoot and the forefoot.

Arthrokinematics
During inversion in a non-weight-bearing position, the concave navicular slides medially and dorsally on the convex talus. The cuboid slides medially and toward the plantar surface on the calcaneus. During eversion, the navicular slides laterally and toward the plantar surface; the cuboid slides laterally and toward the dorsal surface.

Capsular Pattern
The capsular pattern consists of a limitation in inversion (adduction and supination). Other motions are full.

Tarsometatarsal Joints

Anatomy
The five tarsometatarsal (TMT) joints link the distal tarsals with the bases of the five metatarsals (Fig. 10.7). The concave base of the first metatarsal articulates with the convex surface of the medial cuneiform. The base of the second metatarsal articulates with the mortise formed by the intermediate cuneiform and the sides of the medial and lateral cuneiforms. The base of the third metatarsal articulates with the lateral cuneiform, and the base of the fourth metatarsal articulates with the lateral cunieform and the cuboid. The fifth metatarsal articulates with the cuboid. The first joint has its own capsule,

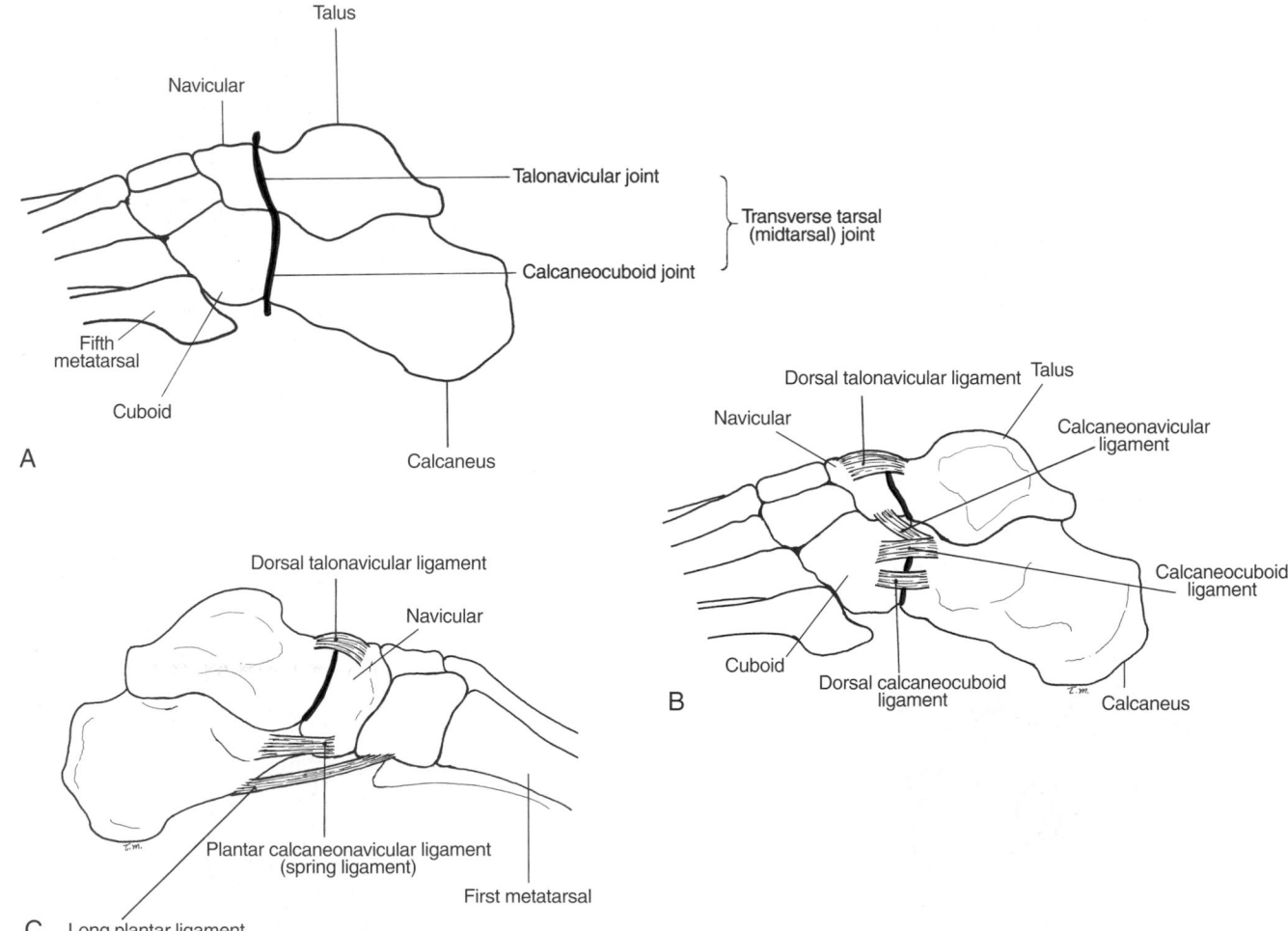

FIGURE 10.6 **A:** The two joints that make up the transverse tarsal joint are shown in a lateral view of a left ankle. **B:** The dorsal talonavicular ligament, the bifurcate ligament (calcaneonavicular and calcaneocuboid ligaments), and the dorsal calcaneocuboid ligament in a lateral view of a left ankle. **C:** The long plantar ligament, the plantar calcaneonavicular ligament, and the dorsal talonavicular ligament in a medial view.

whereas the second and third joints and the fourth and fifth joints share capsules. Each joint is reinforced by numerous dorsal, plantar, and interosseous ligaments.

Osteokinematics

The TMT joints are plane synovial joints that permit gliding motions, including flexion–extension, a minimal amount of abduction–adduction, and rotation. The type and amount of motion vary at each joint. For example, at the third TMT joint, the predominant motion is flexion–extension. The combination of motions at the various joints contributes to the hollowing and flattening of the foot, which helps the foot conform to a supporting surface.

Arthrokinematics

The distal joint surfaces glide in the same direction as the shafts of the metatarsals.

Metatarsophalangeal Joints

Anatomy

The five metatarsophalangeal (MTP) joints are formed proximally by the convex heads of the five metatarsals and distally by the concave bases of the proximal phalanges (Fig. 10.8A). The first MTP joint has two sesamoid bones that lie in two grooves on the plantar surface of the distal metatarsal. The four lesser toes are interconnected on the plantar surface by the

deep transverse metatarsal ligament (Fig. 10.8B). The plantar aponeurosis helps to provide stability and limits extension.

Osteokinematics

The five MTP joints are condyloid synovial joints with 2 degrees of freedom, permitting flexion–extension and abduction–adduction. The axis for flexion–extension is oblique and is referred to as the metatarsal break. The range of motion (ROM) in extension is greater than in flexion, but the total ROM varies according to the relative lengths of the metatarsals and the weight-bearing status.

Arthrokinematics

In flexion, the bases of the phalanges slide in a plantar direction on the heads of the metatarsals. In abduction, the concave bases of the phalanges slide on the convex heads of the

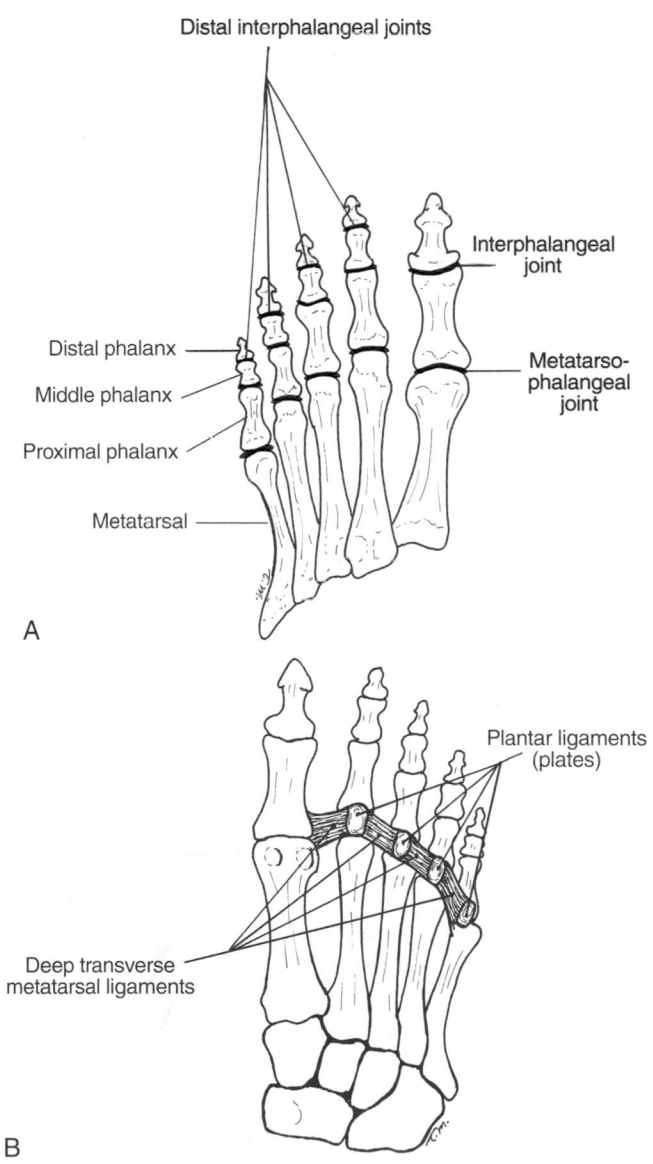

A

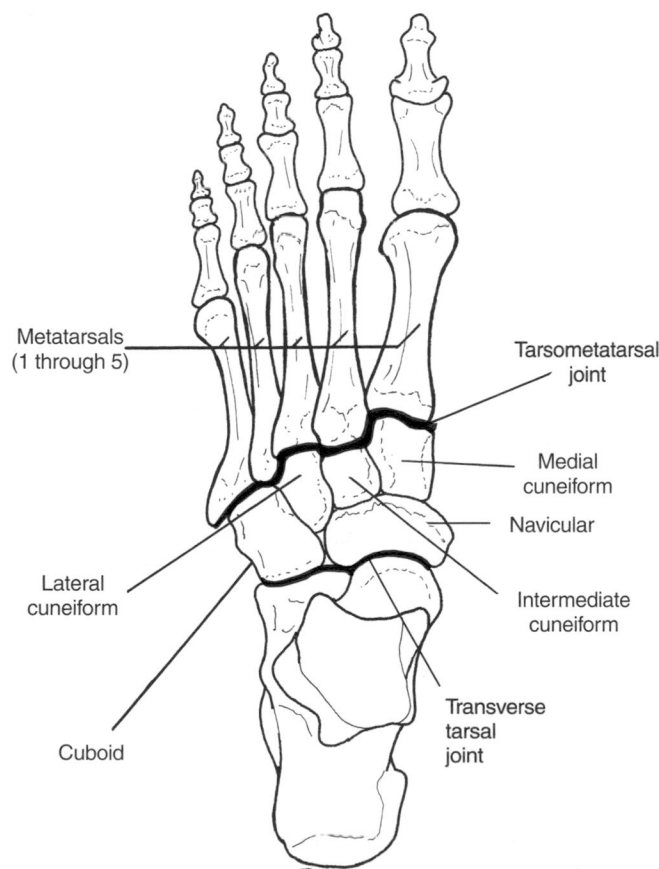

FIGURE 10.7 The tarsometatarsal joints and transverse tarsal joint in a dorsal view of a left foot.

B

FIGURE 10.8 A: The metatarsophalangeal, interphalangeal, and distal interphalangeal joints in a dorsal view of a left foot. **B:** The deep transverse metatarsal ligaments and the plantar plates in a plantar view of a left foot.

metatarsals in a lateral direction away from the second toe. In adduction, the bases of the phalanges slide in a medial direction toward the second toe.

Capsular Pattern

The pattern at the first MTP joint is gross limitation of extension and slight limitation of flexion. At the other joints (second to fifth), the limitation is more restriction of flexion than extension.[2]

Interphalangeal Joints

Anatomy

The structure of the interphalangeal (IP) joints of the feet is identical to that of the IP joints of the fingers. Each IP joint is composed of the concave base of a distal phalanx and the convex head of a proximal phalanx (see Fig. 10.8A).

Osteokinematics

The IP joints are synovial hinge joints with 1 degree of freedom. The motions permitted are flexion and extension in the sagittal plane. Each joint is enclosed in a capsule and reinforced with collateral ligaments.

Arthrokinematics

The concave base of the distal phalanx slides on the convex head of the proximal phalanx in the same direction as the shaft of the distal bone. The concave base slides toward the plantar surface of the foot during flexion and toward the dorsum of the foot during extension.

RANGE OF MOTION TESTING PROCEDURES: Ankle and Foot

Landmarks for Testing Procedures: Talocrural Joint

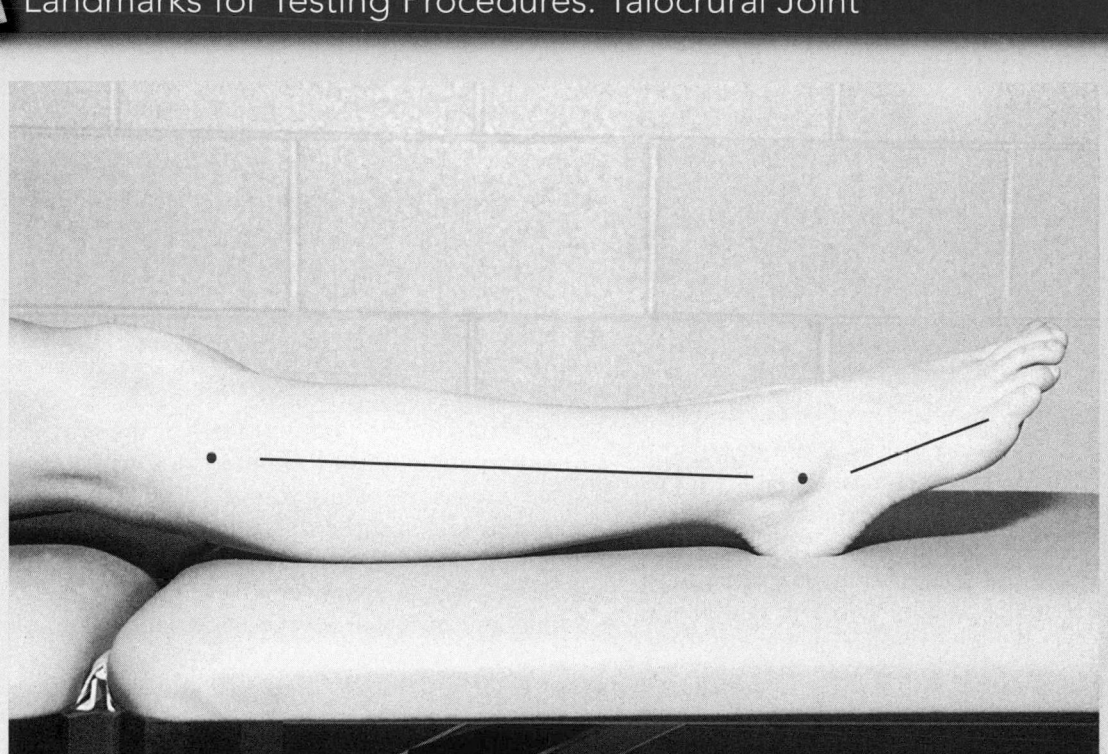

FIGURE 10.9 The subject's right lower extremity showing surface anatomy landmarks for goniometer alignment in measurement of dorsiflexion and plantarflexion range of motion.

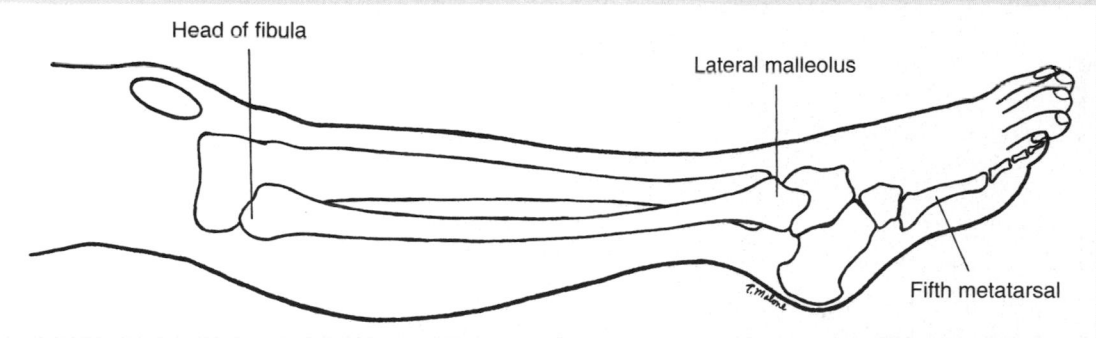

FIGURE 10.10 The subject's right lower extremity shows the bony anatomical landmarks for goniometer alignment for measurement of dorsiflexion and plantarflexion range of motion.

have patient seated not 14ur b/c gasnos in way

● DORSIFLEXION: TALOCRURAL JOINT

Motion occurs in the sagittal plane around a medial–lateral axis. The mean dorsiflexion ROM in adults according to both the American Academy of Orthopaedic Surgeons (AAOS)[3,4] and the American Medical Association (AMA)[5] is 20 degrees. The mean active dorsiflexion ROM in the non–weight-bearing position is 12.6 degrees according to Boone and Azen.[6] Refer to Tables 10.1 through 10.7 in the Research Findings section for additional normal ROM values by age and gender.

Dorsiflexion ROM is affected by the testing position (knee flexed or extended) and by whether the measurement is taken in either a weight-bearing or non–weight-bearing position. Dorsiflexion ROM measured with the knee flexed is usually greater than that measured with the knee extended. Knee flexion slackens the gastrocnemius muscles, so passive tension in the muscle does not limit dorsiflexion ROM. Knee extension stretches the gastrocnemius muscle, and ROM measured in this position represents the length of the muscle. Weight-bearing dorsiflexion ROM is usually greater than non–weight-bearing measurements, and these positions should not be used interchangeably.

Testing Position

Place the subject sitting, with the knee flexed to 90 degrees. The foot should be in 0 degrees of inversion and eversion.

Stabilization

Stabilize the tibia and fibula to prevent knee motion and hip rotation.

Testing Motion

Use one hand to move the foot into dorsiflexion by pushing on the bottom of the foot (Fig. 10.11). Avoid pressure on the lateral border of the foot under the fifth metatarsal and the toes. A considerable amount of force is necessary to overcome the passive tension in the soleus and Achilles musculotendinous unit. Often, a comparison of the active and passive ROMs for a particular individual helps to determine the amount of upward force necessary to complete the

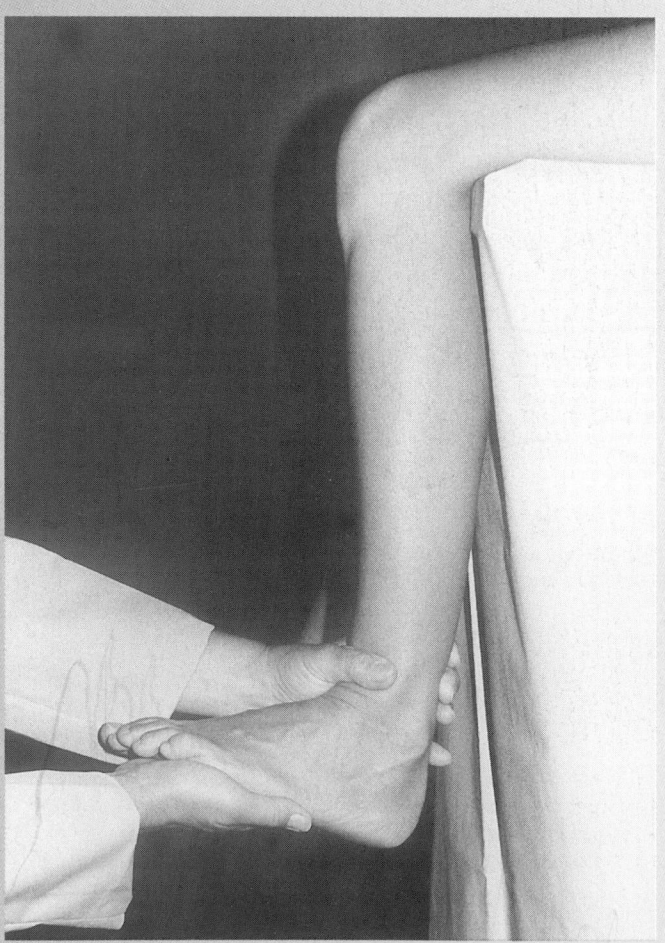

FIGURE 10.11 The subject's left ankle at the end of dorsiflexion range of motion. The examiner holds the distal portion of the lower leg with one hand to prevent knee motion and uses her other hand to push on the palmar surface of the foot to maintain dorsiflexion.

passive ROM in dorsiflexion. The end of the ROM occurs when resistance to further motion is felt and attempts to produce additional motion cause knee extension.

Normal End-Feel

The end-feel is firm because of tension in the posterior joint capsule, the soleus muscle, the Achilles tendon, the posterior portion of the deltoid ligament, the posterior talofibular ligament, and the calcaneofibular ligament.

Goniometer Alignment

Red #S

See Figures 10.12 and 10.13.

1. Center **fulcrum** of the goniometer over the lateral aspect of the lateral malleolus.

2. Align **proximal arm** with the lateral midline of the fibula, using the head of the fibula for reference.

3. Align **distal arm** parallel to the lateral aspect of the fifth metatarsal. Although it is usually easier to palpate and align the distal arm parallel to the fifth metatarsal, an alternative method is to align the distal arm parallel to the inferior aspect of the calcaneus. However, if the latter landmark is used, the full cycle ROM in the sagittal plane (dorsiflexion plus plantarflexion) may be similar to the total ROM of the preferred technique, but the separate ROM values for dorsiflexion and plantarflexion will differ considerably.

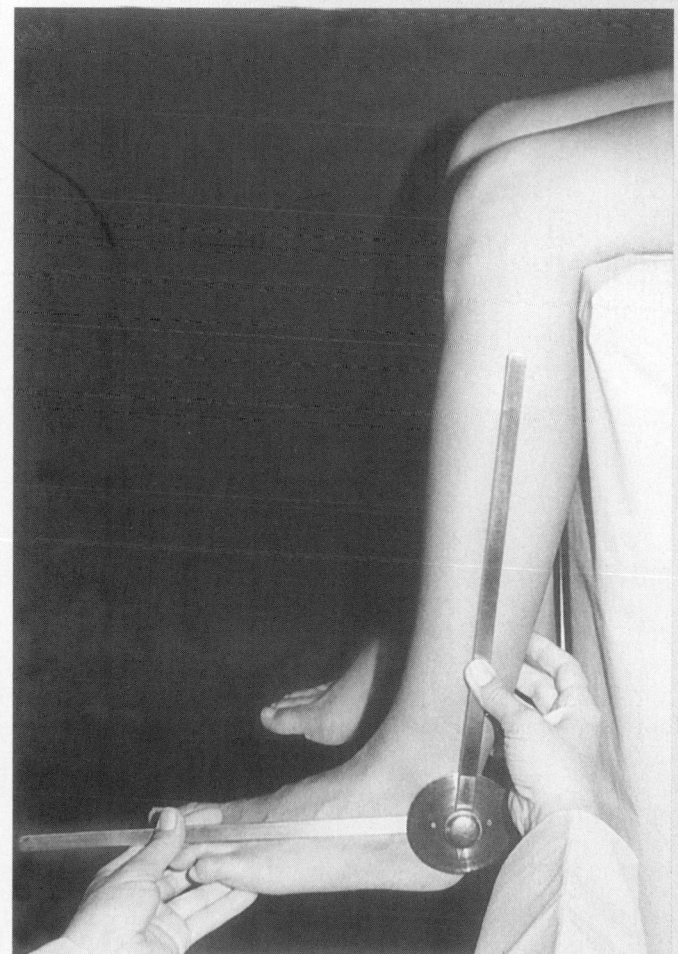

FIGURE 10.12 In the starting position for measuring dorsiflexion range of motion the ankle is positioned so that the goniometer is at 90 degrees. This goniometer reading is transposed and recorded as 0 degrees. The examiner sits on a stool or kneels in order to align the goniometer and perform the readings at eye level.

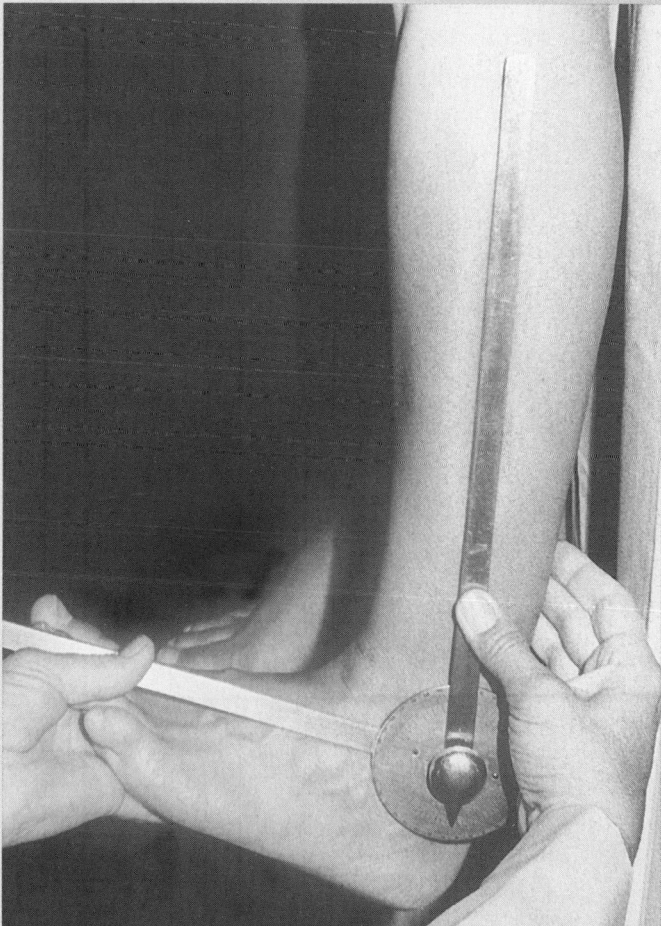

FIGURE 10.13 At the end of dorsiflexion range of motion, the examiner uses one hand to align the proximal goniometer arm while the other hand maintains dorsiflexion and alignment of the distal goniometer arm.

Non–Weight-Bearing Dorsiflexion ROM: Supine Position (Knee Flexed)

Place the subject supine with the knee flexed to 30 degrees and supported by a pillow. Goniometer alignment is the same as that for the seated position.

Non–Weight-Bearing Dorsiflexion ROM: Prone Position

Position the subject prone with the knee on the side being tested flexed to 90 degrees. Position the foot in 0 degrees of inversion, eversion, and plantarflexion (Fig.10.14). Goniometer alignment is the same as that for the seated position.

Weight-Bearing Dorsiflexion ROM: Standing (Knee Flexed)

Usually measurements taken in the standing position are considerably larger than measurements taken in non–weight-bearing positions; therefore, the two positions should not be used interchangeably. Weight-bearing measurements may be able to provide the examiner with information that is relevant to the performance of functional activities such as walking. However, it may be difficult to control substitute motions of the hindfoot and forefoot in the weight-bearing position. Also, some subjects may not have the strength and balance necessary to assume the weight-bearing position.

Position the subject standing with all his or her weight on the leg to be tested. The knee of the test leg should be flexed as far as possible while maintaining the foot flat on the floor. The end of the motion occurs when additional motion causes the heel to raise from the floor (Fig. 10.15). Goniometer alignment is the same as that for the seated position.

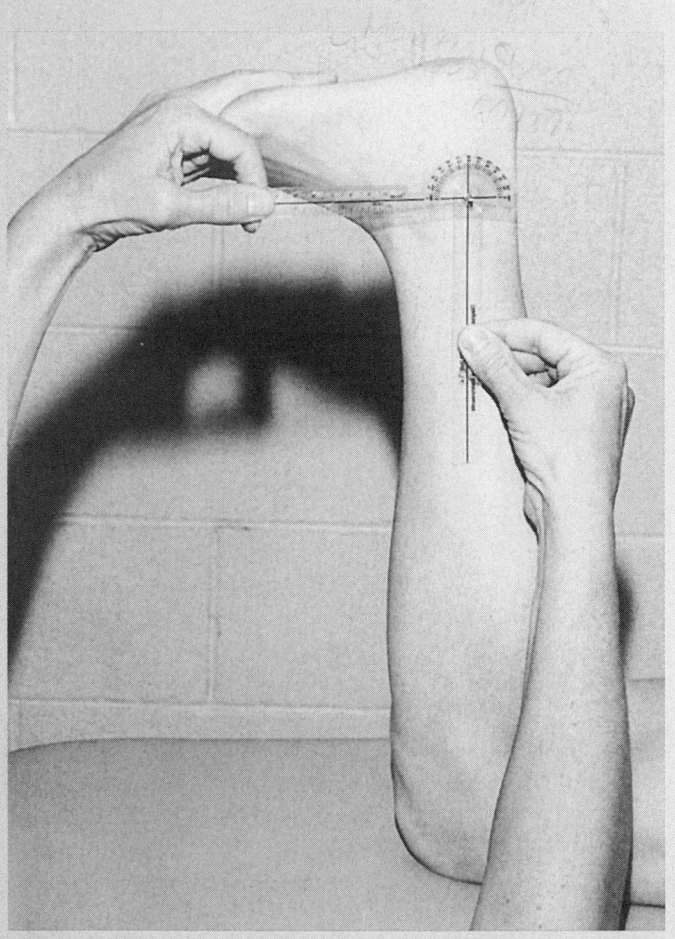

FIGURE 10.14 Goniometer alignment at the end of dorsiflexion range of motion. The subject is in an alternative prone position with the knee flexed to 90 degrees.

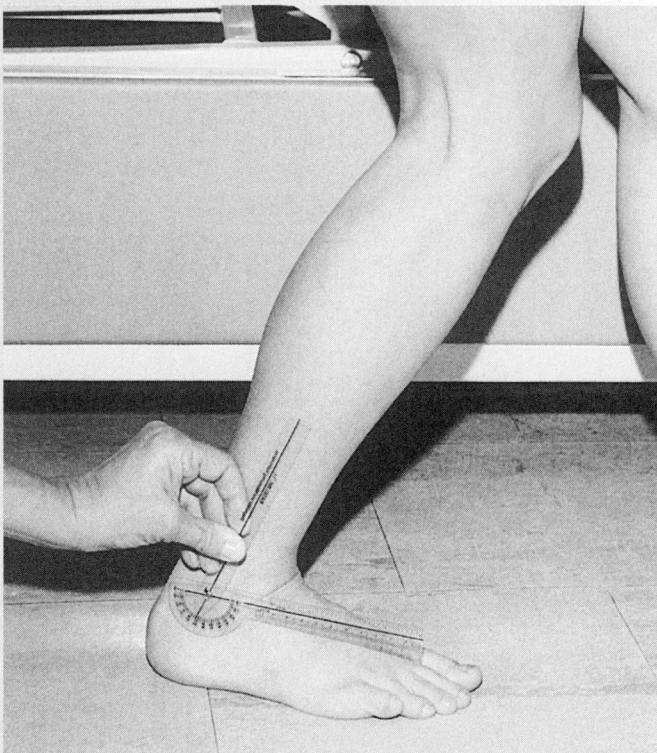

FIGURE 10.15 Goniometer alignment at the end of dorsiflexion range of motion. The subject is in an alternative weight-bearing position with the knee flexed.

● PLANTARFLEXION: TALOCRURAL JOINT

Motion occurs in the sagittal plane around a medial–lateral axis. The ROM is 50 degrees for adults according to the AAOS,[3,4] 40 degrees for adults according to the AMA,[5] and 56.1 degrees for males ages 1 to 54 years according to Boone and Azen.[6] Refer to Tables 10.1 through 10.4 in the Research Findings section for additional normal ROM values by age and gender.

Testing Position

Place the subject sitting with the knee flexed to 90 degrees. Position the foot in 0 degrees of inversion and eversion. Alternatively, it is possible to place the subject in the supine position.

Stabilization

Stabilize the tibia and fibula to prevent knee flexion and hip rotation.

Testing Motion

Push downward with one hand on the dorsum of the subject's foot to produce plantarflexion (Fig. 10.16). Do not exert any force on the subject's toes, and be careful to avoid pushing the ankle into inversion or eversion. The end of the ROM is reached when resistance is felt and attempts to produce additional plantarflexion result in knee flexion.

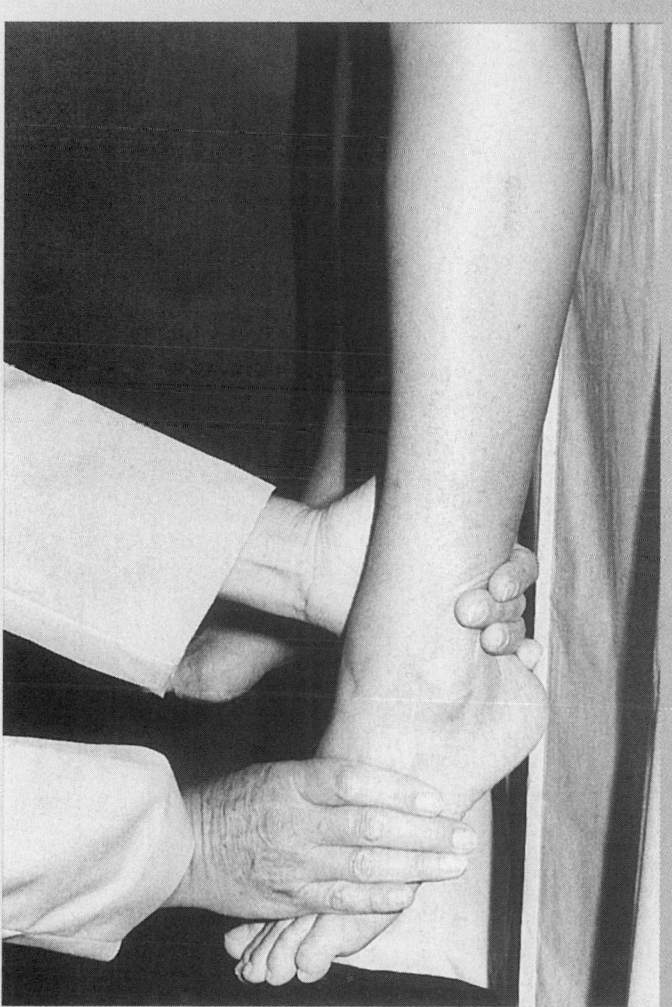

FIGURE 10.16 The subject's left ankle at the end of plantarflexion range of motion.

Normal End-Feel

Usually, the end-feel is firm because of tension in the anterior joint capsule; the anterior portion of the deltoid ligament; the anterior talofibular ligament; and the tibialis anterior, extensor hallucis longus, and extensor digitorum longus muscles. The end-feel may be hard because of contact between the posterior tubercles of the talus and the posterior margin of the tibia.

Goniometer Alignment

See Figures 10.17 and 10.18.

1. Center **fulcrum** of the goniometer over the lateral aspect of the lateral malleolus.
2. Align **proximal arm** with the lateral midline of the fibula, using the head of the fibula for reference.

3. Align **distal arm** parallel to the lateral aspect of the fifth metatarsal. Although it is usually easier to palpate and align the distal arm parallel to the fifth metatarsal, as an alternative, the distal arm can be aligned parallel to the inferior aspect of the calcaneus. If the alternative landmark is used, full cycle ROM in the sagittal plane (dorsiflexion plus plantarflexion) may be similar to full cycle ROM measurement using the fifth metatarsal as a landmark, but the single cycle ROM values for dorsiflexion and plantarflexion will differ considerably. Measurements taken with the alternative landmark should not be used interchangeably with those taken using the fifth metatarsal landmark.

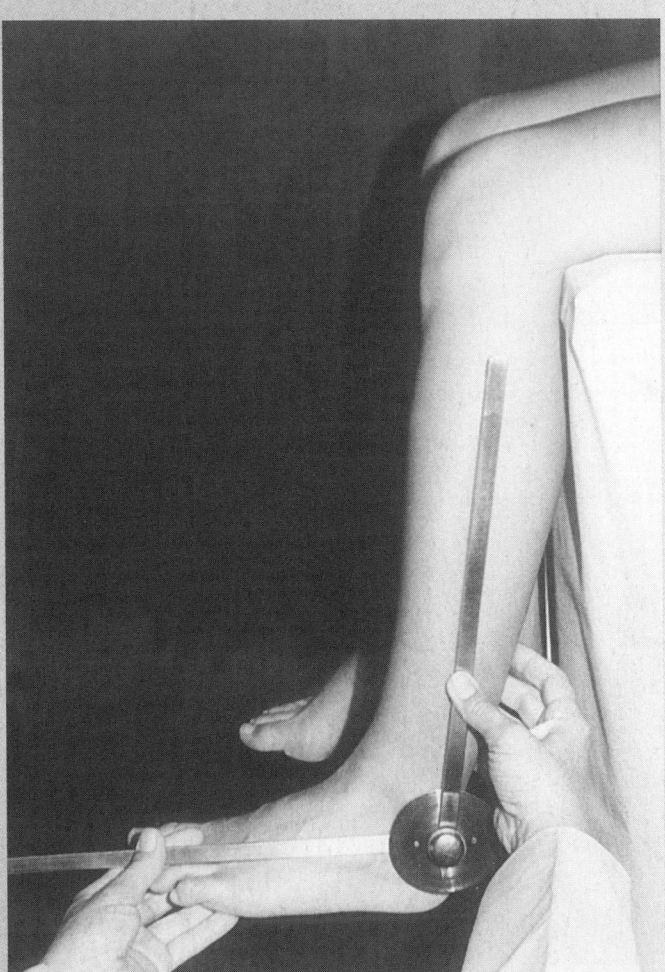

FIGURE 10.17 Goniometer alignment in the starting position for measuring plantarflexion range of motion.

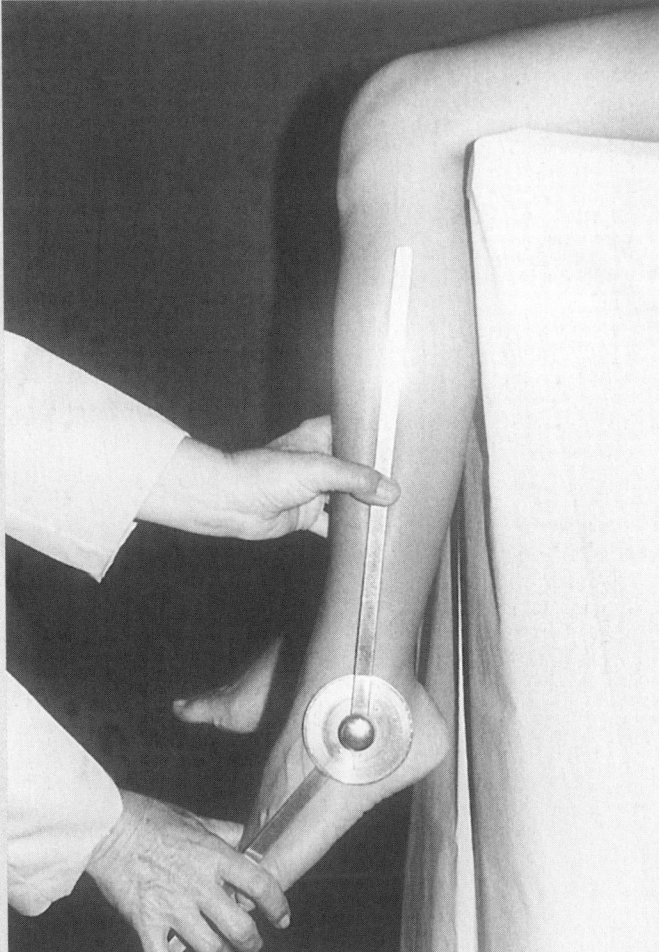

FIGURE 10.18 At the end of the plantarflexion range of motion, the examiner uses one hand to maintain plantarflexion and to align the distal goniometer arm. The examiner holds the dorsum and sides of the subject's foot to avoid exerting pressure on the toes. She uses her other hand to stabilize the tibia and align the proximal arm of the goniometer.

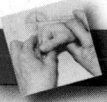

Landmarks for Testing Procedures: Tarsal Joints

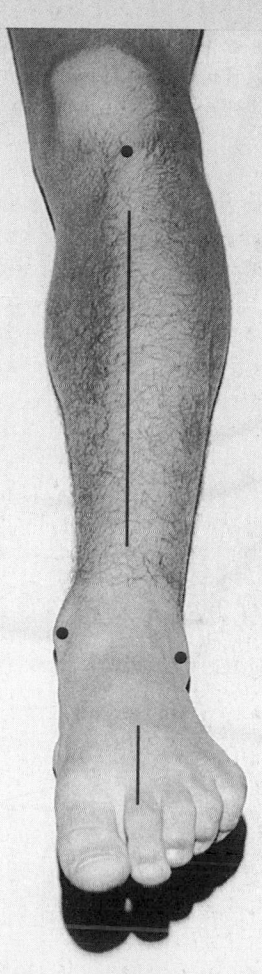

FIGURE 10.19 An anterior view of the subject's left ankle with surface anatomy landmarks to indicate goniometer alignment for measuring inversion and eversion range of motion.

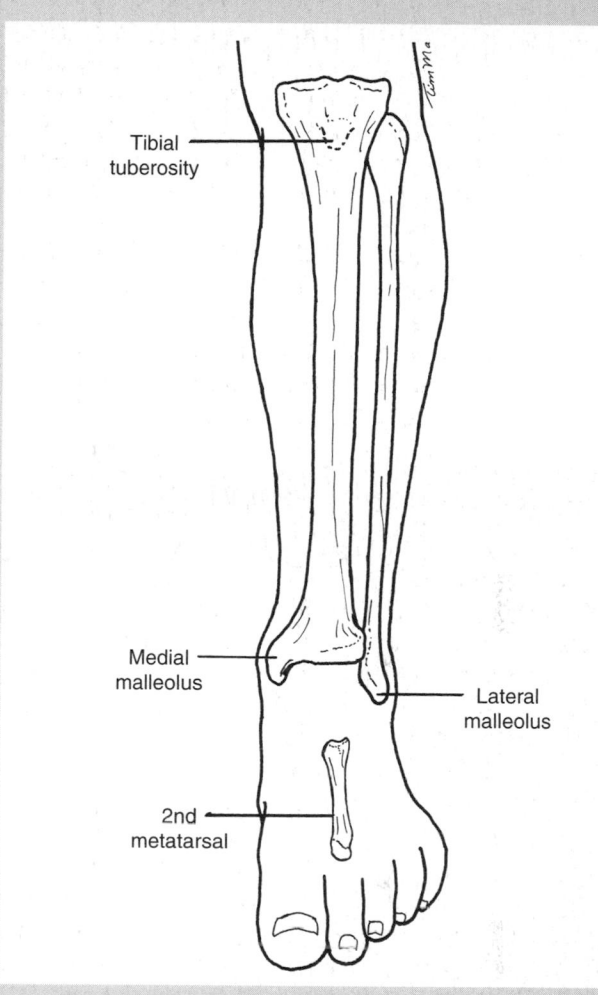

Tibial tuberosity

Medial malleolus

Lateral malleolus

2nd metatarsal

FIGURE 10.20 An anterior view of the subject's left ankle with bony anatomical landmarks to indicate goniometer alignment for measuring inversion and eversion range of motion.

● INVERSION: TARSAL JOINTS

Inversion is a combination of supination, adduction, and plantarflexion occurring in varying degrees at the subtalar, transverse tarsal (talocalcaneonavicular and calcaneocuboid), cuboideonavicular, cuneonavicular, intercuneiform, cuneocuboid, tarsometarsal (TMT), and intermetatarsal joints. The functional ability of the foot to adapt to the ground and to absorb contact forces depends on the combined movement of all of these joints. Because of the uniaxial limitations of the goniometer, inversion is measured in the frontal plane around an anterior–posterior axis.

Menadue and colleagues measured active inversion in both ankles in 30 male and female subjects with a mean age of 35 years. Mean values obtained with a universal goniometer ranged from 30 degrees to 35.0 degrees.[7]

Testing Position
Place the subject in the sitting position, with the knee flexed to 90 degrees and the lower leg over the edge of the supporting surface. Position the hip in 0 degrees of rotation, adduction, and abduction. Alternatively, it is possible to place the subject in the supine position, with the foot over the edge of the supporting surface.

Stabilization
Stabilize the tibia and the fibula to prevent medial rotation and extension of the knee and lateral rotation and abduction of the hip.

Testing Motion
Push the forefoot downward into plantarflexion, medially into adduction, and turn the sole of the foot medially into supination to produce inversion (Fig. 10.21). The end of the ROM occurs when resistance is felt and attempts at further motion produce medial rotation of the knee and/or lateral rotation and abduction at the hip.

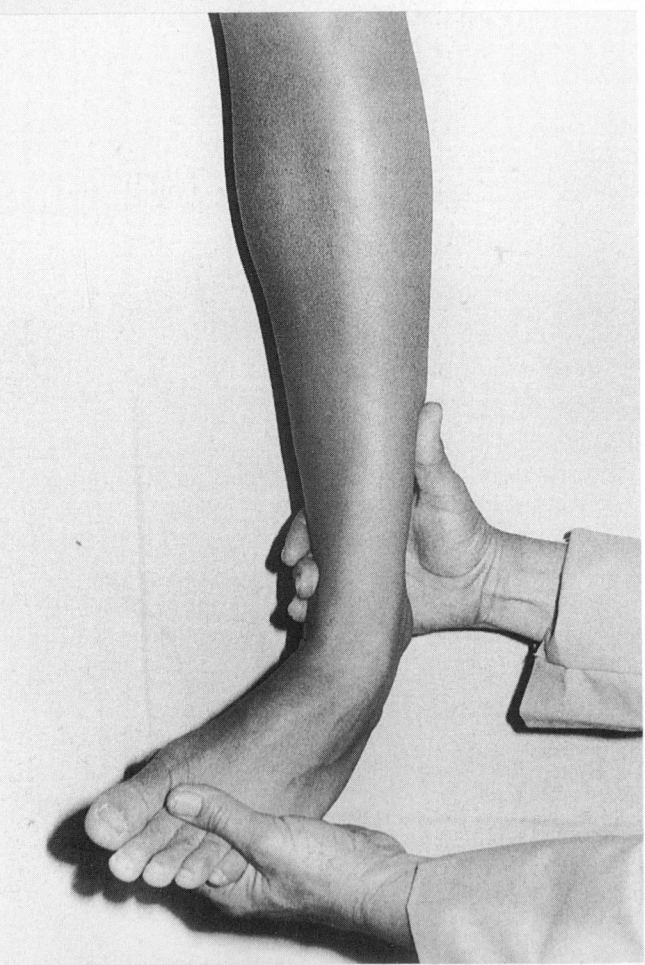

FIGURE 10.21 The subject's left foot and ankle at the end of inversion range of motion. The examiner uses one hand on the subject's distal lower leg to prevent knee and hip motion while her other hand maintains inversion.

Normal End-Feel

The end-feel is firm because of tension in the joint capsules; the anterior and posterior talofibular ligament; the calcaneofibular ligament; the anterior, posterior, lateral, and interosseous talocalcaneal ligaments; the dorsal calcaneal ligaments; the dorsal calcaneocuboid ligament; the dorsal talonavicular ligament; the lateral band of the bifurcate ligament; the transverse metatarsal ligament; and various dorsal, plantar, and interosseous ligaments of the cuboideonavicular, cuneonavicular, intercuneiform, cuneocuboid, TMT, and intermetatarsal joints; and the peroneus longus and brevis muscles.

Goniometer Alignment

See Figures 10.22 and 10.23.

1. Center **fulcrum** of the goniometer over the anterior aspect of the ankle midway between the malleoli. (The flexibility of a plastic goniometer makes this instrument easier to use for measuring inversion than a metal goniometer.)
2. Align **proximal arm** of the goniometer with the anterior midline of the lower leg, using the tibial tuberosity for reference.
3. Align **distal arm** with the anterior midline of the second metatarsal.

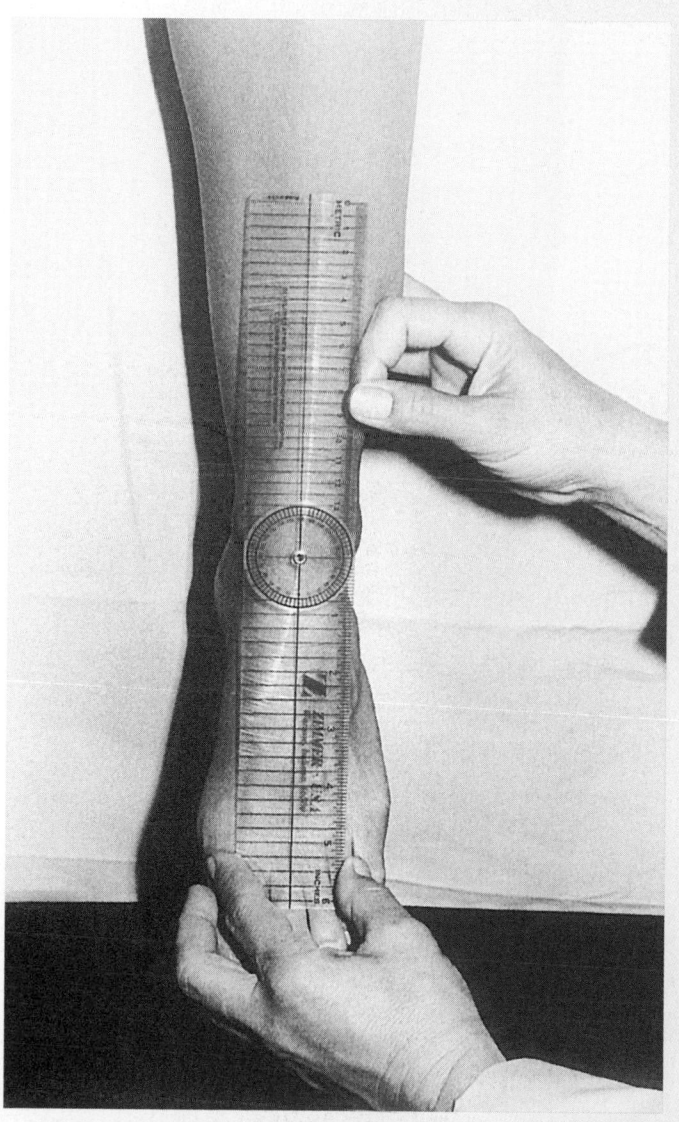

FIGURE 10.22 Goniometer alignment in the starting position for measuring inversion range of motion.

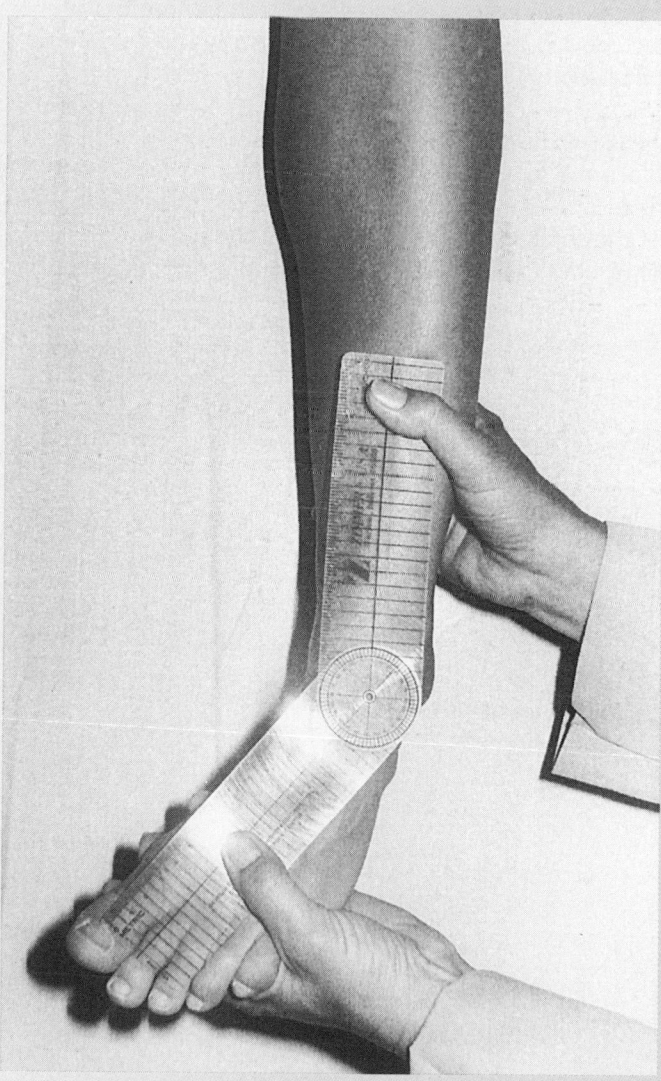

FIGURE 10.23 At the end of the range of motion, the examiner uses her one hand to maintain inversion and to align the distal goniometer arm.

● Eversion: Tarsal Joints

Eversion is a combination of pronation, abduction, and dorsiflexion occurring in varying degrees at the subtalar, transverse tarsal (talocalcaneonavicular and calcaneocuboid), cuboideonavicular, cuneonavicular, intercuneiform, cuneocuboid, TMT, and intermetatarsal joints. The functional ability of the foot to adapt to the ground and to absorb contact forces depends on the combined movement of all of these joints. Because of the uniaxial limitations of the goniometer, this motion is measured in the frontal plane around an anterior–posterior axis. Menadue and colleagues[7] measured active eversion in both ankles in 30 male and female subjects with a mean age of 35 years. Mean values obtained with a universal goniometer ranged from 11.0 degrees to 12.0 degrees.[7] (Methods for measuring eversion isolated to the rearfoot and the forefoot are included in the sections on the subtalar and transverse tarsal joints.)

Testing Position

Place the subject in the sitting position, with the knee flexed to 90 degrees and the lower leg over the edge of the supporting surface. Position the hip in 0 degrees of rotation, adduction, and abduction. Alternatively, it is possible to place the subject in the supine position, with the foot over the edge of the supporting surface.

Stabilization

Stabilize the tibia and fibula to prevent lateral rotation and flexion of the knee and medial rotation and adduction of the hip.

Testing Motion

Pull the forefoot laterally into abduction and upward into dorsiflexion, turning the forefoot into pronation so that the lateral side of the foot is higher than the medial side to produce eversion (Fig. 10.24). The end of the

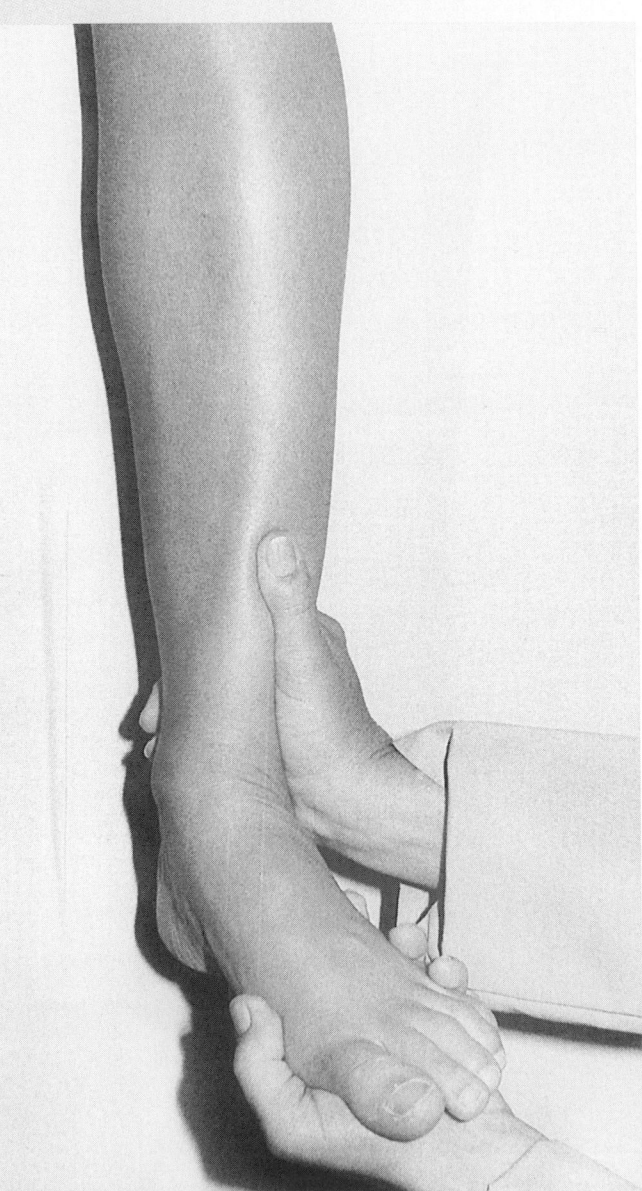

FIGURE 10.24 The left ankle and foot at the end of the range of motion in eversion. The examiner uses one hand on the subject's distal lower leg to prevent knee flexion and lateral rotation. The examiner's other hand maintains eversion.

ROM occurs when resistance is felt and attempts at further motion cause lateral rotation at the knee and/or medial rotation and adduction at the hip.

Normal End-Feel

The end-feel may be hard because of contact between the calcaneus and the floor of the sinus tarsi. In some cases, the end-feel may be firm because of tension in the joint capsules; the deltoid ligament; the medial talocalcaneal ligament; the plantar calcaneonavicular and calcaneocuboid ligaments; the dorsal talonavicular ligament; the medial band of the bifurcated ligament; the transverse metatarsal ligament; various dorsal, plantar, and interosseous ligaments of the cuboideonavicular, cuneonavicular, intercuneiform, cuneocuboid, TMT, and intermetatarsal joints; and the tibialis posterior muscle.

Goniometer Alignment
See Figures 10.25 and 10.26.

1. Center the **fulcrum** of the goniometer over the anterior aspect of the ankle midway between the malleoli. (The flexibility of a plastic goniometer makes this instrument easier to use than a metal goniometer for measuring inversion.)
2. Align **proximal arm** of the goniometer with the anterior midline of the lower leg, using the tibial tuberosity for reference.
3. Align **distal arm** with the anterior midline of the second metatarsal.

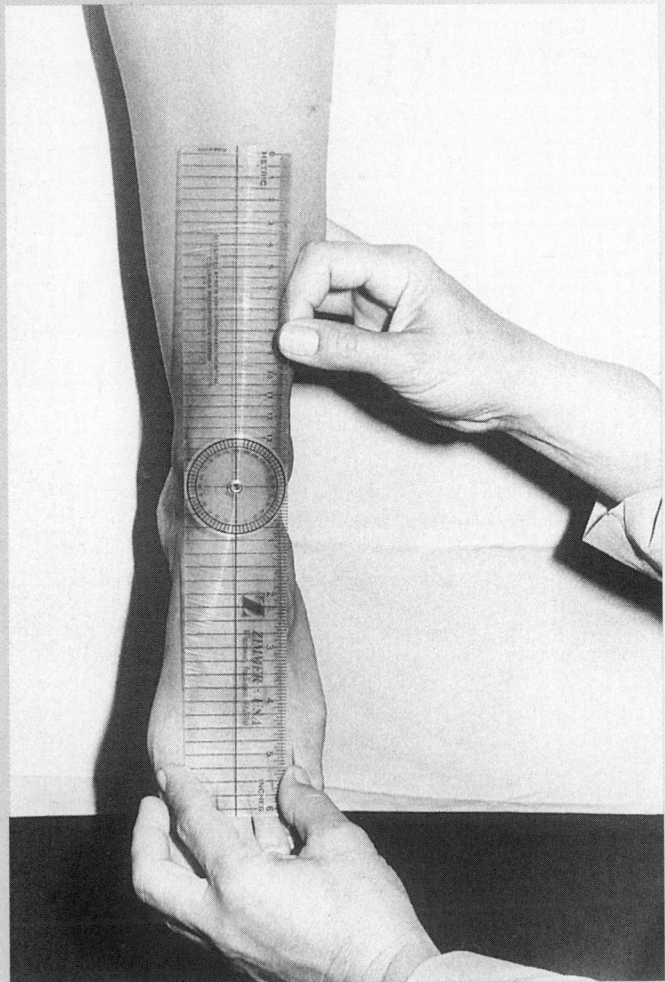

FIGURE 10.25 Goniometer alignment in the starting position for measuring eversion range of motion.

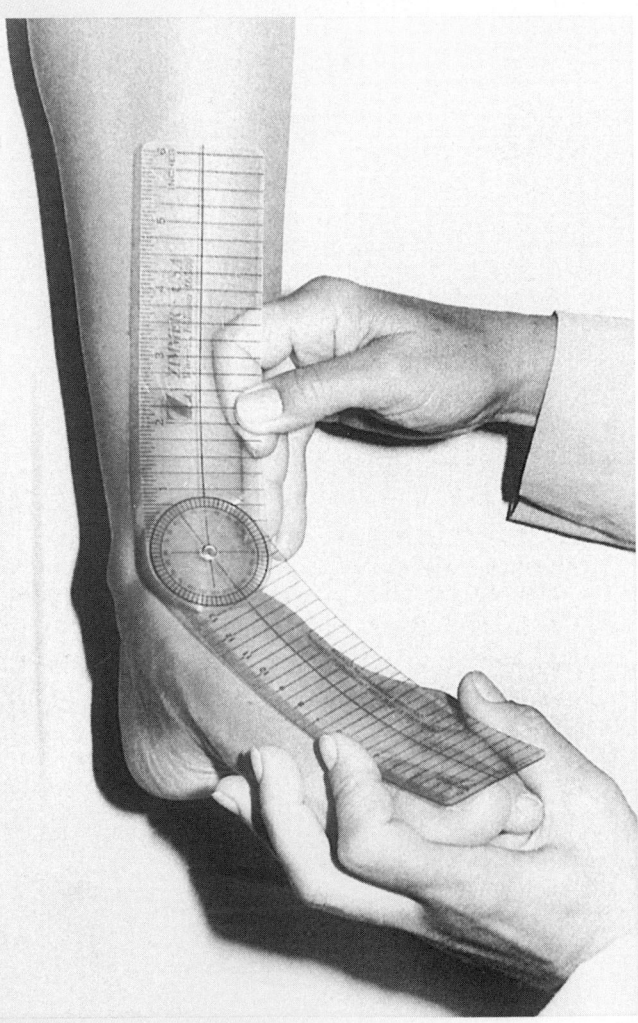

FIGURE 10.26 At the end of the eversion range of motion, the examiner's left hand maintains eversion and keeps the distal goniometer arm aligned with the subject's second metatarsal.

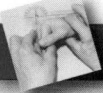

Landmarks for Testing Procedures: Subtalar Joint (Rearfoot)

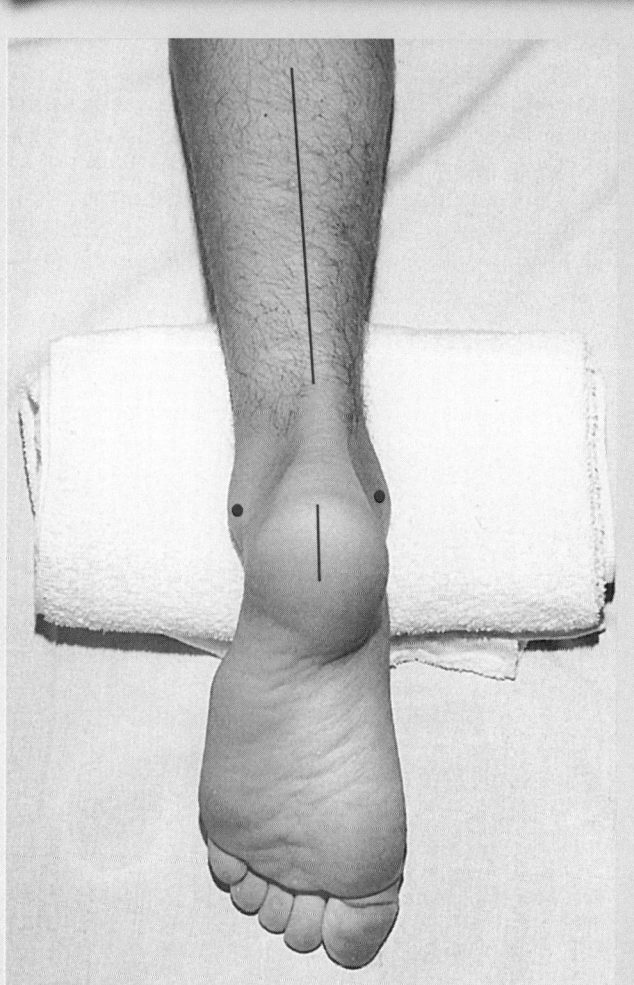

FIGURE 10.27 Surface anatomy landmarks indicate goniometer alignment for measuring rearfoot inversion and eversion range of motion in a posterior view of a subject's left lower leg and foot.

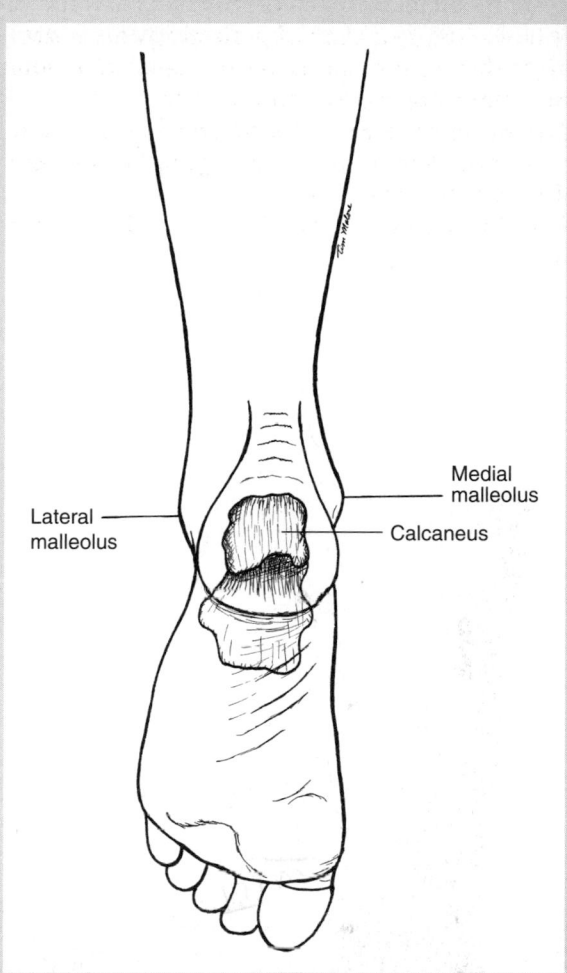

FIGURE 10.28 Bony anatomical landmarks for measuring subtalar (rearfoot) inversion and eversion range of motion in a posterior view of the subject's left lower leg and foot.

Labels: Lateral malleolus, Medial malleolus, Calcaneus

⬤ INVERSION: SUBTALAR JOINT (REARFOOT)

Inversion is a combination of supination, adduction, and plantarflexion. Because of the uniaxial limitations of the goniometer, inversion of the subtalar joint is measured in the frontal plane around an anterior–posterior axis. The ROM is about 5 degrees according to the AAOS [3] and a mean ROM of 15 degrees according to Menadue and colleagues,[7] who measured active inversion in 60 ankles in the prone position.

Testing Position

Place the subject in the prone position, with the hip in 0 degrees of flexion, extension, abduction, adduction, and rotation. Position the knee in 0 degrees of flexion and extension. Position the foot over the edge of the supporting surface.

Stablization

Stabilize the tibia and fibula to prevent lateral hip and knee rotation and hip adduction.

Testing Motion

Hold the subject's lower leg with one hand and use the other hand to pull the subject's calcaneus medially into adduction and to rotate it into supination, thereby producing rearfoot subtalar inversion (Fig. 10.29). Avoid pushing on the forefoot. The end of the ROM is reached when resistance to further motion is felt and attempts at overcoming the resistance produce lateral rotation at the hip or knee.

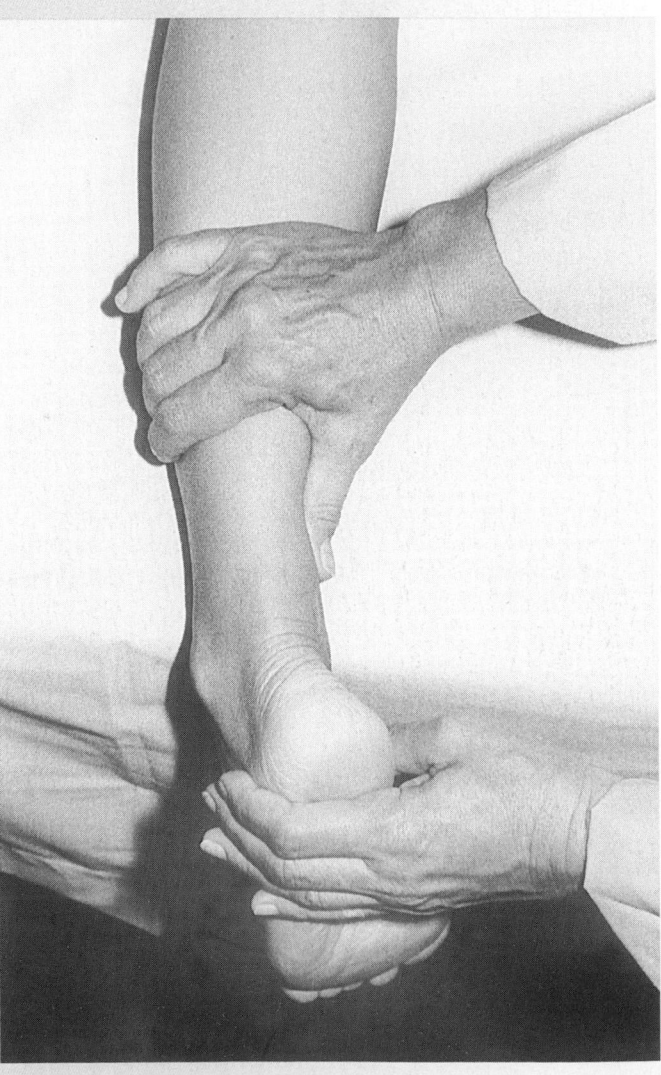

FIGURE 10.29 The left lower extremity at the end of subtalar (rearfoot) inversion range of motion.

Normal End-Feel

The end-feel is firm because of tension in the lateral joint capsule; the anterior and posterior talofibular ligaments; the calcaneofibular ligament; and the lateral, posterior, anterior, and interosseous talocalcaneal ligaments.

Goniometer Alignment

See Figures 10.30 and 10.31.

1. Center **fulcrum** of the goniometer over the posterior aspect of the ankle midway between the malleoli.
2. Align **proximal arm** with the posterior midline of the lower leg.
3. Align **distal arm** with the posterior midline of the calcaneus.

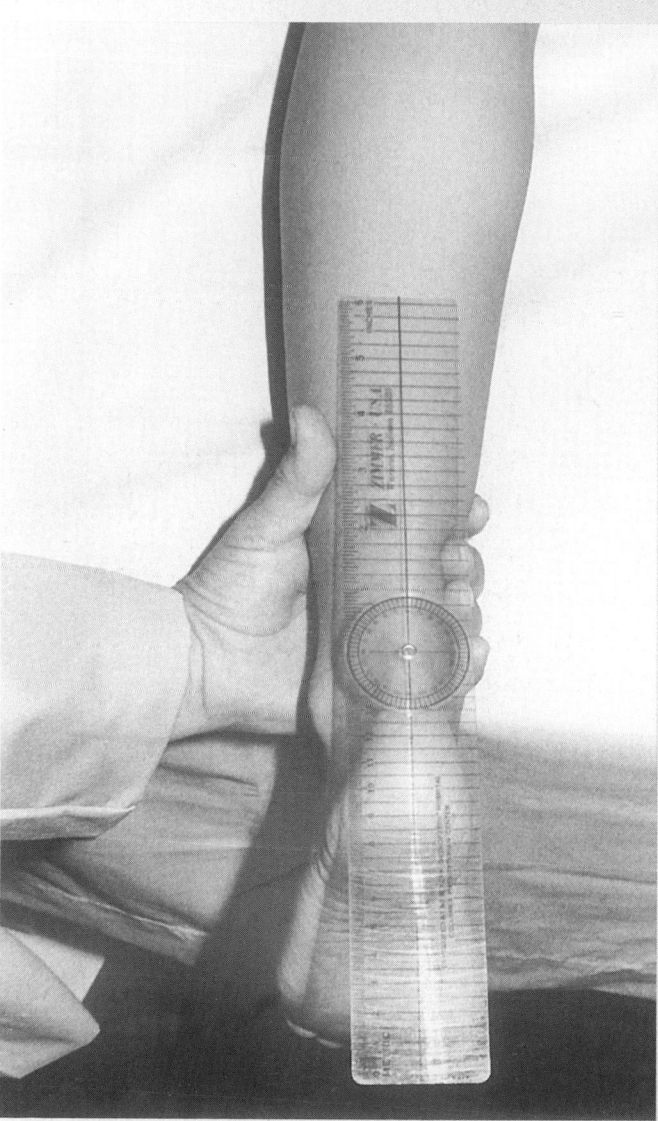

FIGURE 10.30 Goniometer alignment in the starting position for measuring subtalar (rearfoot) inversion range of motion. Normally, the examiner's hand would be holding the distal goniometer arm, but for the purpose of this photograph, she has removed her hand.

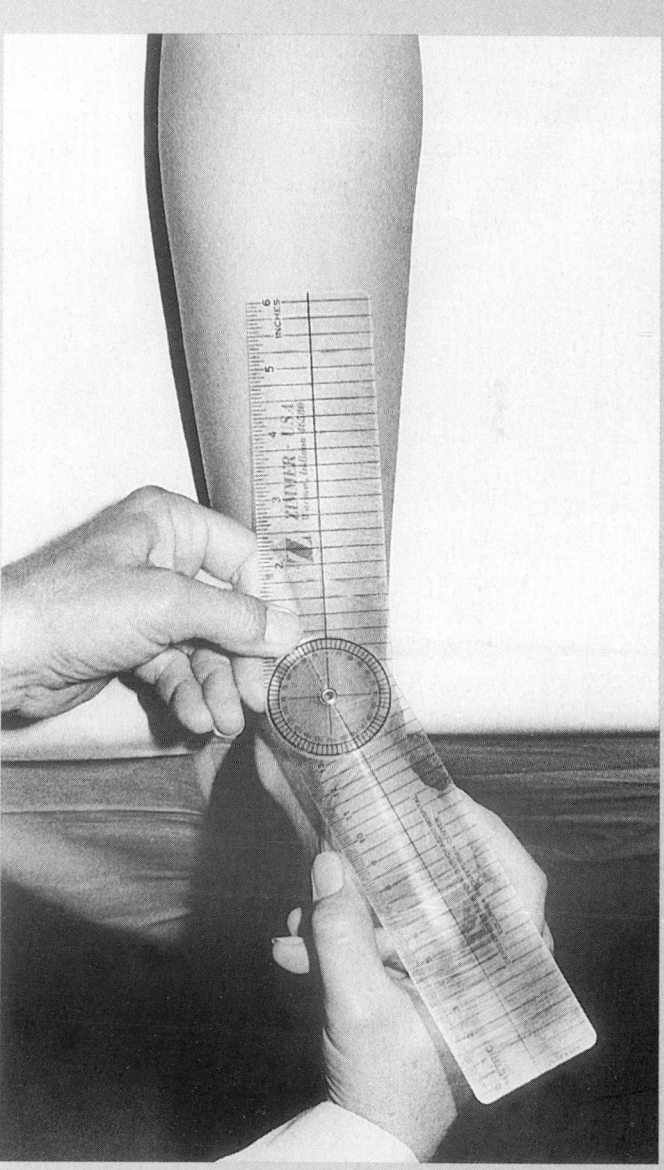

FIGURE 10.31 At the end of subtalar (rearfoot) inversion, the examiner's hand maintains inversion and keeps the distal goniometer arm in alignment.

● EVERSION: SUBTALAR JOINT (REARFOOT)

Eversion is a combination of pronation, abduction, and dorsiflexion. Because of the uniaxial limitations of the goniometer, eversion of the subtalar joint is measured in the frontal plane around an anterior–posterior axis. The ROM is about 5 degrees according to the AAOS[3] and between 8 and 9 degrees for active eversion according to Menadue and colleagues.[7]

Testing Position
Place the subject prone, with the hip in 0 degrees of flexion, extension, abduction, adduction, and rotation. Position the knee in 0 degrees of flexion and extension. Place the foot over the edge of the supporting surface.

Stabilization
Stabilize the tibia and fibula to prevent medial hip and knee rotation and hip abduction.

Testing Motion
Pull the calcaneus laterally into abduction and rotate it into pronation to produce subtalar eversion (Fig. 10.32). The end of the ROM occurs when resistance to further

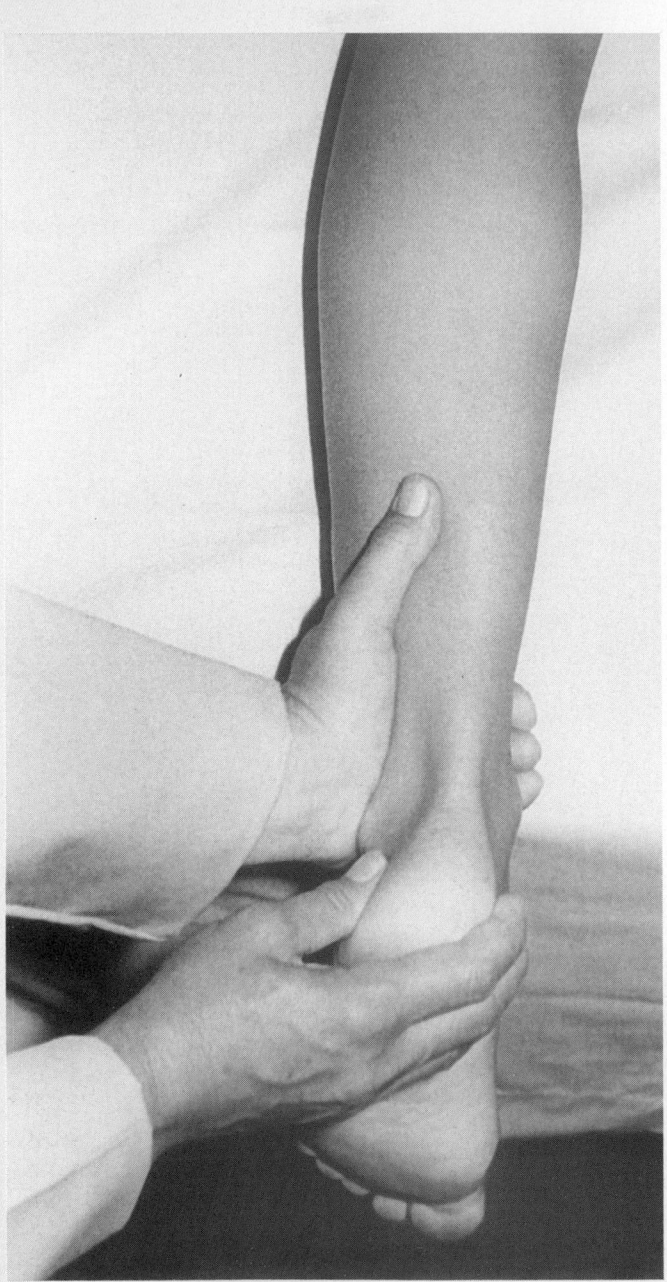

FIGURE 10.32 The left lower extremity at the end of subtalar (rearfoot) eversion range of motion. One can observe that this subject's eversion is quite limited. The examiner's hand maintains subtalar eversion by pulling the calcaneus laterally.

movement is felt and additional attempts to move the calcaneus result in medial hip or knee rotation.

Normal End-Feel

The end-feel may be hard because of contact between the calcaneus and the floor of the sinus tarsi, or it may be firm because of tension in the deltoid ligament, the medial talocalcaneal ligament, and the tibialis posterior muscle.

Goniometer Alignment

See Figures 10.33 and 10.34.

1. Center **fulcrum** of the goniometer over the posterior aspect of the ankle midway between the malleoli.
2. Align **proximal arm** with the posterior midline of the lower leg.
3. Align **distal arm** with the posterior midline of the calcaneus.

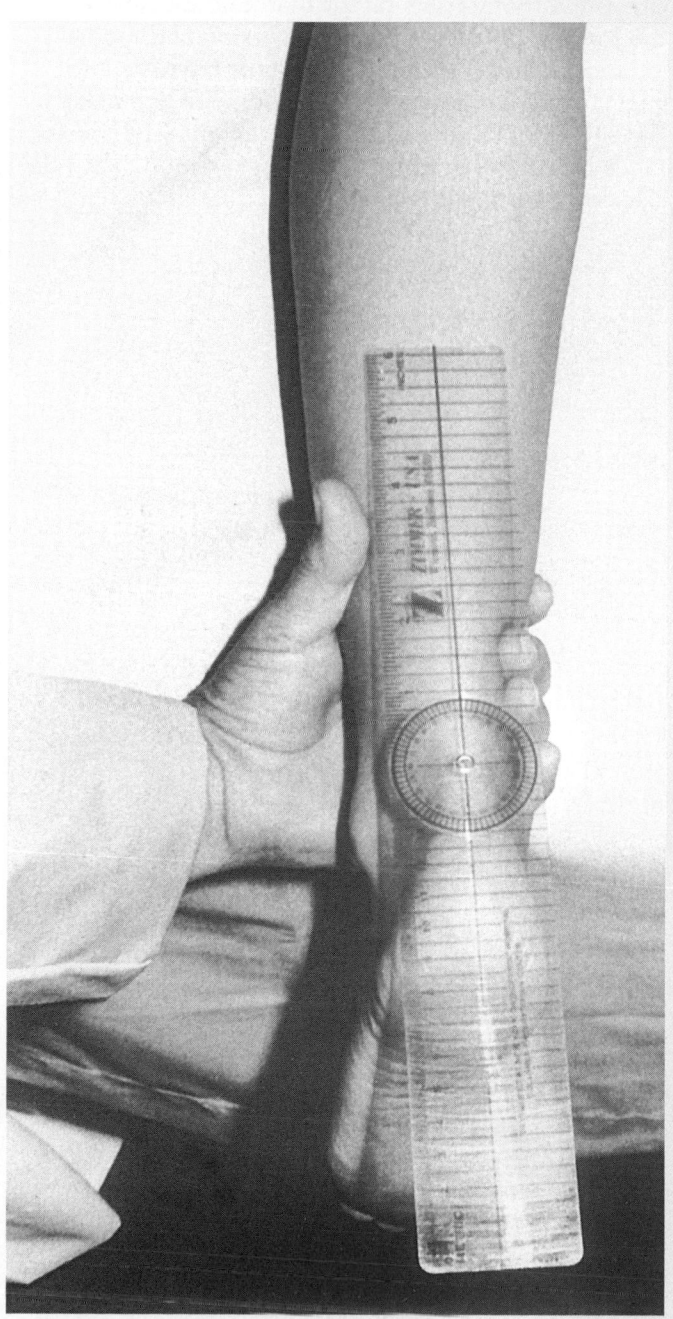

FIGURE 10.33 Goniometer alignment in the starting position for measuring subtalar (rearfoot) eversion.

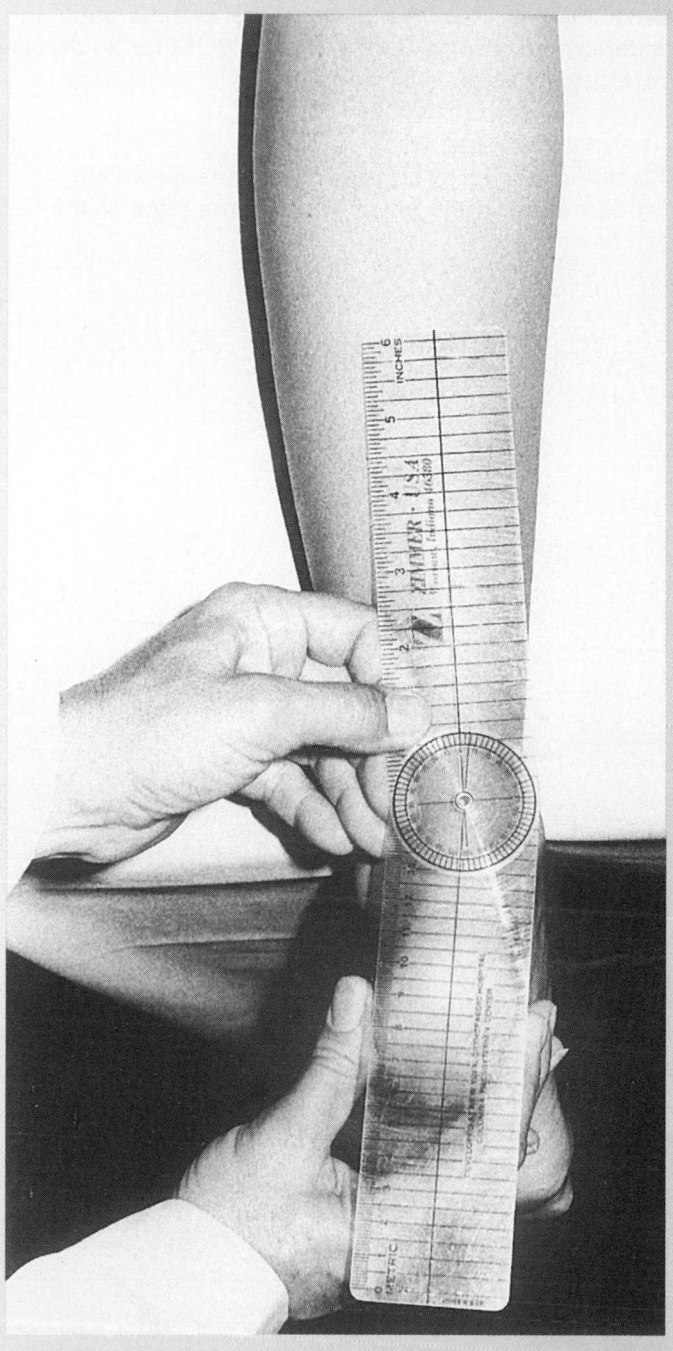

FIGURE 10.34 At the end of subtalar eversion, the examiner's hand maintains eversion and keeps the distal goniometer arm aligned.

● INVERSION: TRANSVERSE TARSAL JOINT

Most of the motion in the midfoot and forefoot occurs at the transverse tarsal joint which comprises the talonavicular and calcaneocuboid joints. Some additional motion occurs at the cuboideonavicular, cuneonavicular, intercuneiform, cuneocuboid, and TMT joints.

Inversion is a combination of supination, adduction, and plantarflexion. Because of the uniaxial limitation of the goniometer, inversion of the transverse tarsal joint is measured in the frontal plane around an anterior–posterior axis. The normal ROM for adults for forefoot inversion is 35 degrees.[3,6]

Testing Position

Place the subject sitting, with the knee flexed to 90 degrees and the lower leg over the edge of the supporting surface. The hip is in 0 degrees of rotation, adduction, and abduction, and the subtalar joint is placed in the 0 starting position. Alternatively, it is possible to place the subject in the supine position, with the foot over the edge of the supporting surface.

Stabilization

Stabilize the calcaneus to prevent dorsiflexion of the ankle and inversion of the subtalar joint.

Testing Motion

Grasp the metatarsals rather than the toes and push the forefoot slightly into plantarflexion and medially into adduction. Turn the sole of foot medially into supination, being careful not to dorsiflex the ankle (Fig. 10.35). The end of the ROM occurs when resistance is felt and attempts at further motion cause dorsiflexion and/or subtalar eversion.

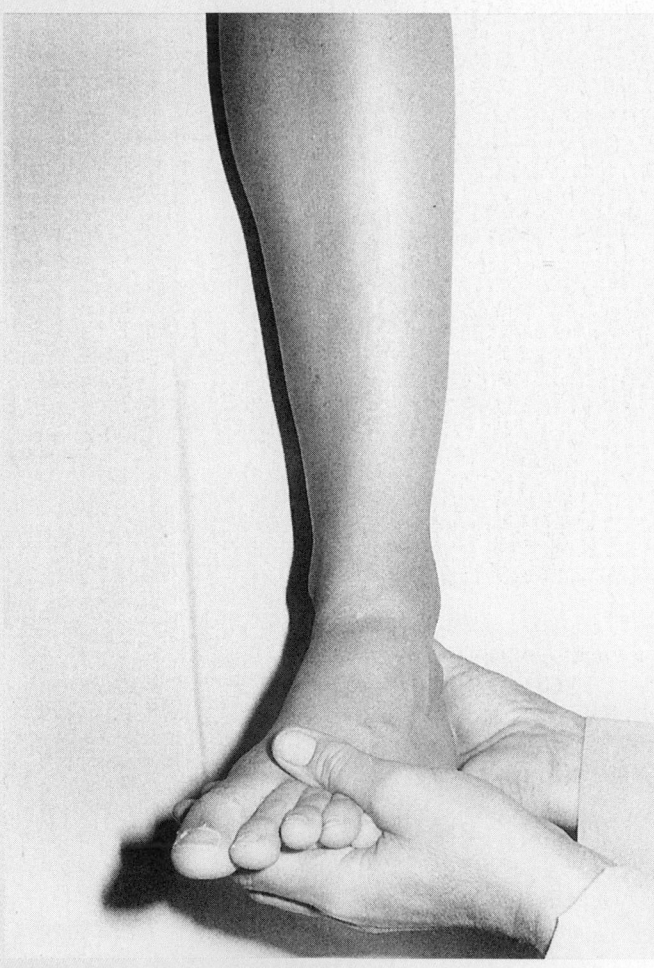

FIGURE 10.35 The left lower extremity at the end of transverse tarsal inversion range of motion (ROM). The examiner's hand stabilizes the calcaneus to prevent subtalar inversion. Notice that the ROM for the transverse tarsal joint is less than that of all of the tarsal joints combined.

Normal End-Feel

The end-feel is firm because of tension in the joint capsules; the dorsal calcaneocuboid ligament; the dorsal talonavicular ligament; the lateral band of the bifurcated ligament; the transverse metatarsal ligament; various dorsal, plantar, and interosseous ligaments of the cuboideonavicular, cuneonavicular, intercuneiform, cuneocuboid, TMT, and intermetatarsal joints; and the peroneus longus and brevis muscles.

Goniometer Alignment

See Figures 10.36 and 10.37.

1. Center **fulcrum** of the goniometer over the anterior aspect of the ankle slightly distal to a point midway between the malleoli.
2. Align **proximal** arm with the anterior midline of the lower leg, using the tibial tuberosity for reference.
3. Align **distal arm** with the anterior midline of the second metatarsal.

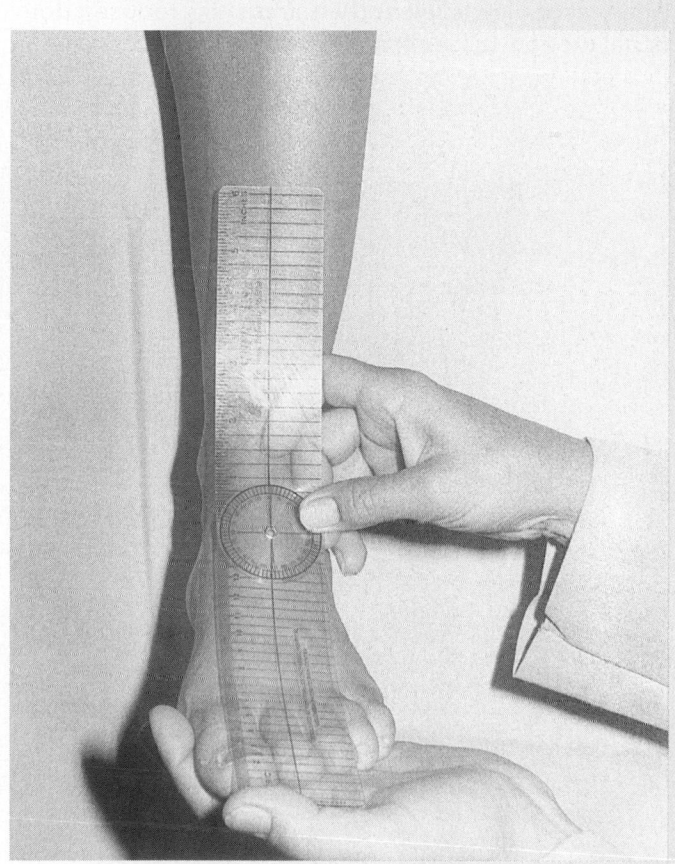

FIGURE 10.36 Goniometer alignment in the starting position for measuring transverse tarsal inversion.

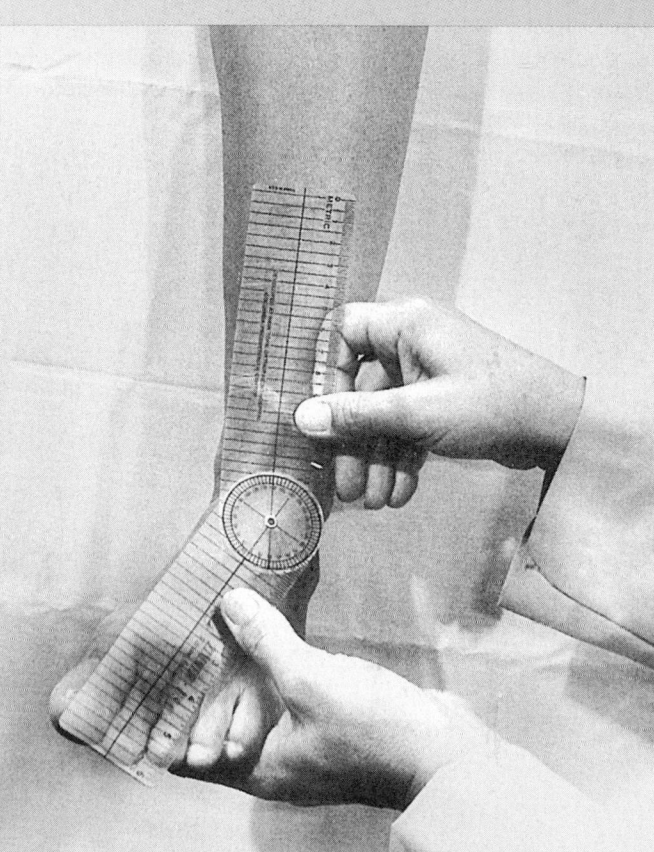

FIGURE 10.37 At the end of transverse tarsal inversion, one of the examiner's hands releases the calcaneus and aligns the proximal goniometer arm with the lower leg. The examiner's other hand maintains inversion and holds the distal goniometer arm aligned with the second metatarsal.

● EVERSION: TRANSVERSE TARSAL JOINT

Eversion is a combination of pronation, abduction, and dorsiflexion. Because of the uniaxial limitations of the goniometer, eversion of the transverse tarsal joint is measured in the frontal plane around an anterior–posterior axis. The normal ROM for forefoot eversion ranges from 15 to 21 degrees.[5,6]

Testing Position

Place the subject sitting, with the knee flexed to 90 degrees and the lower leg over the edge of the supporting surface. Position the hip in 0 degrees of rotation, adduction, and abduction and the subtalar joint in the 0 starting position. Alternatively, it is possible to place the subject in the supine position, with the foot over the edge of the supporting surface.

Stabilization

Stabilize the calcaneus and talus to prevent plantarflexion of the ankle and eversion of the subtalar joint.

Testing Motion

Pull the forefoot laterally into abduction and upward into dorsiflexion. Turn the forefoot into pronation so that the lateral side of the foot is higher than the medial side (Fig. 10.38). The end of the ROM occurs when resistance is felt and attempts to produce additional motion cause plantarflexion and/or subtalar eversion.

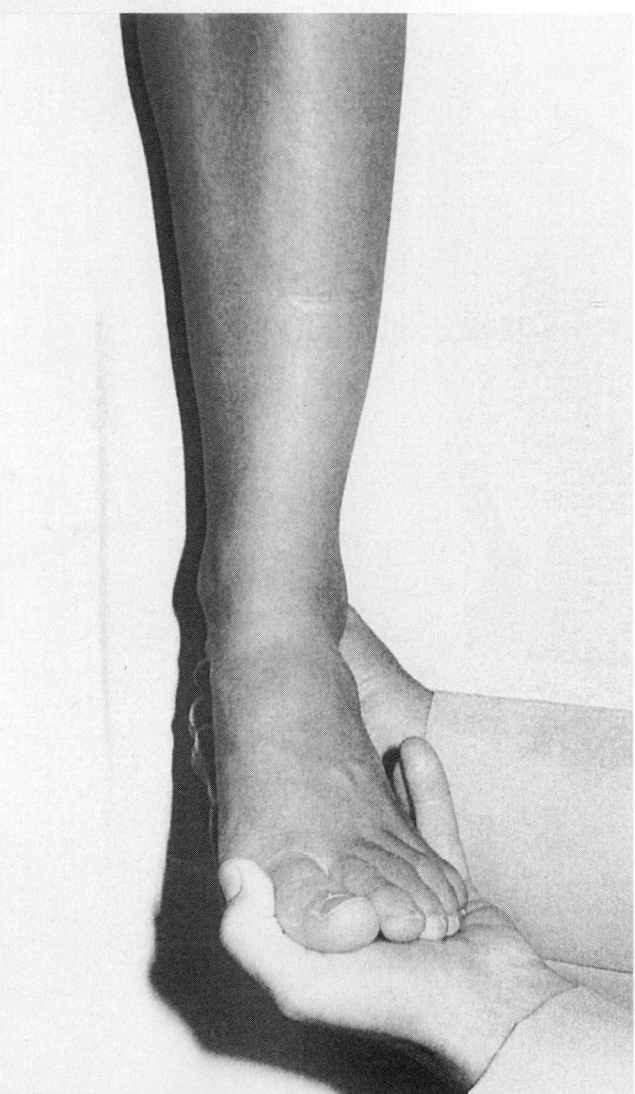

FIGURE 10.38 The end of transverse tarsal eversion range of motion. The examiner's hand stabilizes the calcaneus to prevent subtalar eversion. As can be seen in the photograph, only a small amount of motion is available at the transverse tarsal joint in this subject.

Normal End-Feel

The end-feel is firm because of tension in the joint capsules; the deltoid ligament; the plantar calcaneo-navicular and calcaneocuboid ligaments; the dorsal talonavicular ligament; the medial band of the bifur-cated ligament; the transverse metatarsal ligament; various dorsal, plantar, and interosseous ligaments of the cuboideonavicular, cuneonavicular, intercuneiform, cuneocuboid, TMT, and intermetatarsal joints; and the tibialis posterior muscle.

Goniometer Alignment

See Figures 10.39 and 10.40.

1. Center **fulcrum** of the goniometer over the anterior aspect of the ankle slightly distal to a point midway between the malleoli.
2. Align **proximal arm** with the anterior midline of the lower leg, using the tibial tuberosity for reference.
3. Align **distal arm** with the anterior midline of the second metatarsal.

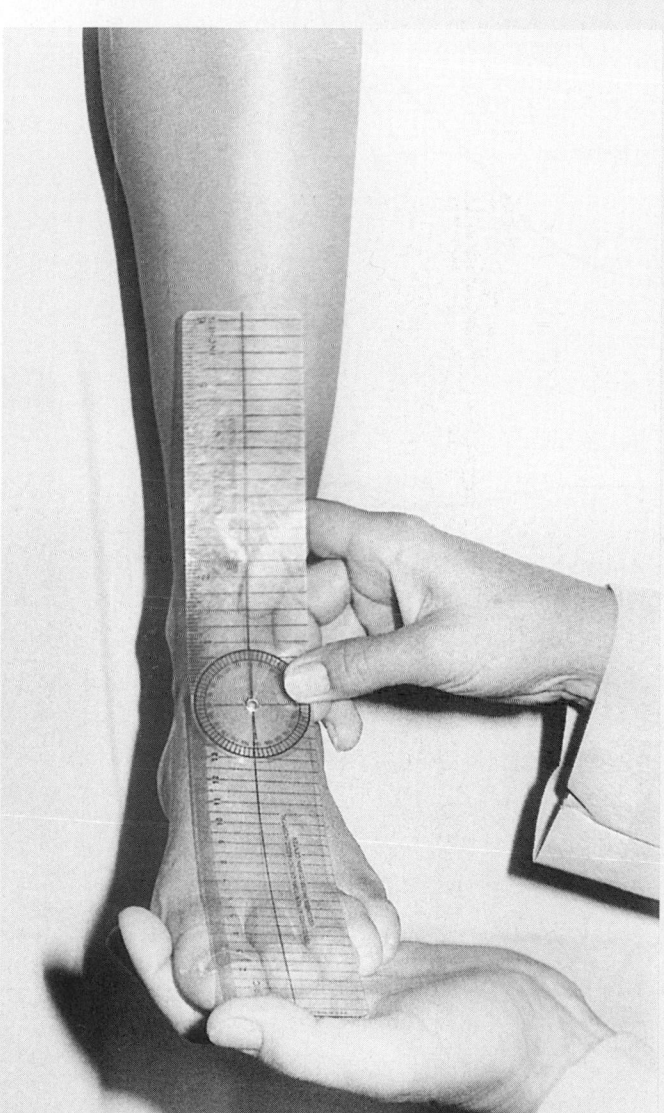

FIGURE 10.39 Goniometer alignment in the starting position for measuring transverse tarsal eversion range of motion.

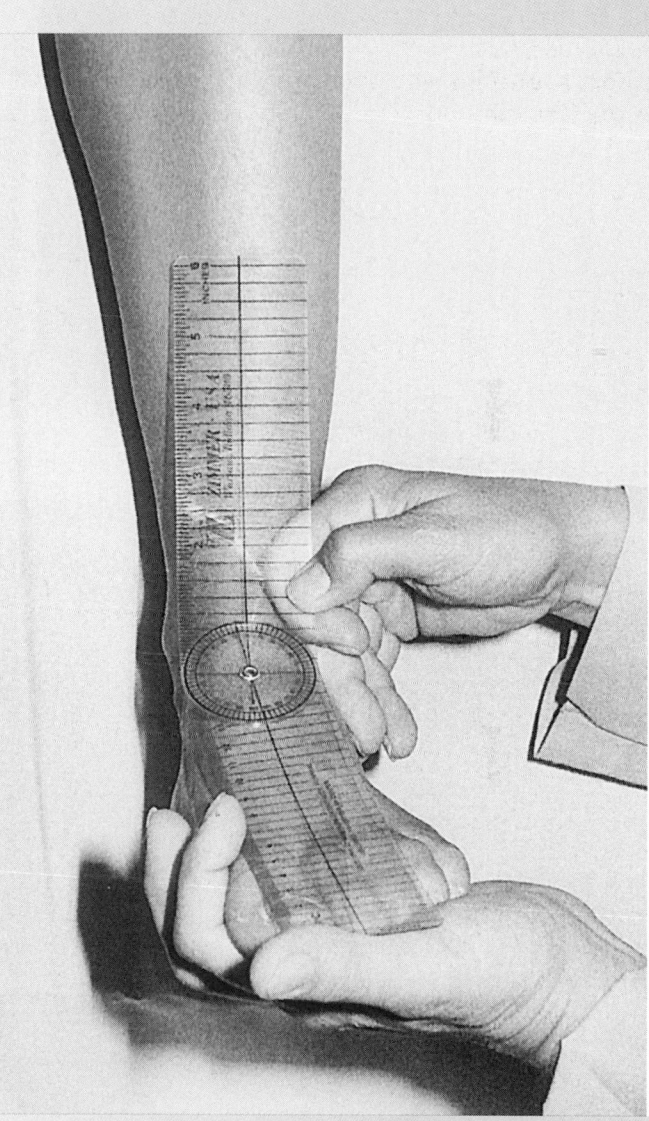

FIGURE 10.40 At the end of the transverse tarsal eversion range of motion, one of the examiner's hands releases the calcaneus and aligns the proximal goniometer arm with the lower leg. The examiner's other hand maintains eversion and alignment of the distal goniometer arm.

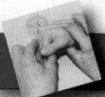

Landmarks for Testing Procedures: Metarsophalangeal Joint

See Figures 10.41 A and B and 10.42 A and B.

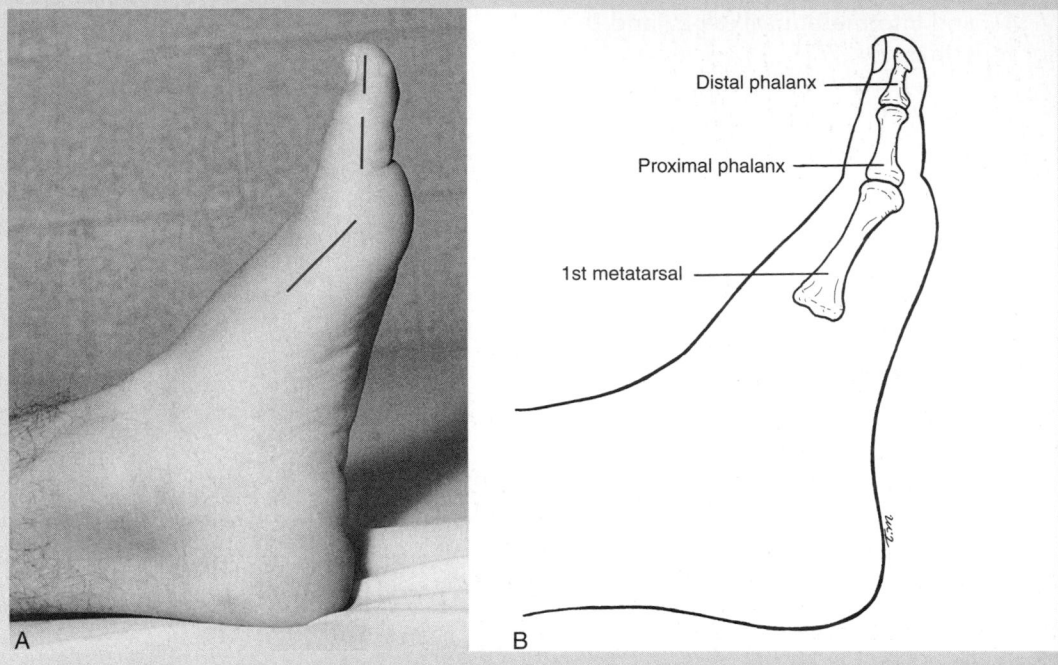

FIGURE 10.41 A: Surface anatomy landmarks for measuring flexion and extension at the first metatarsophalangeal (MTP) joint and first interphalangeal (IP) joint in a medial view of the subject's left foot. **B:** Bony anatomical landmarks for measuring flexion and extension at the first MTP and IP joints.

Landmarks for Testing Procedures: Metarsophalangeal Joint (continued)

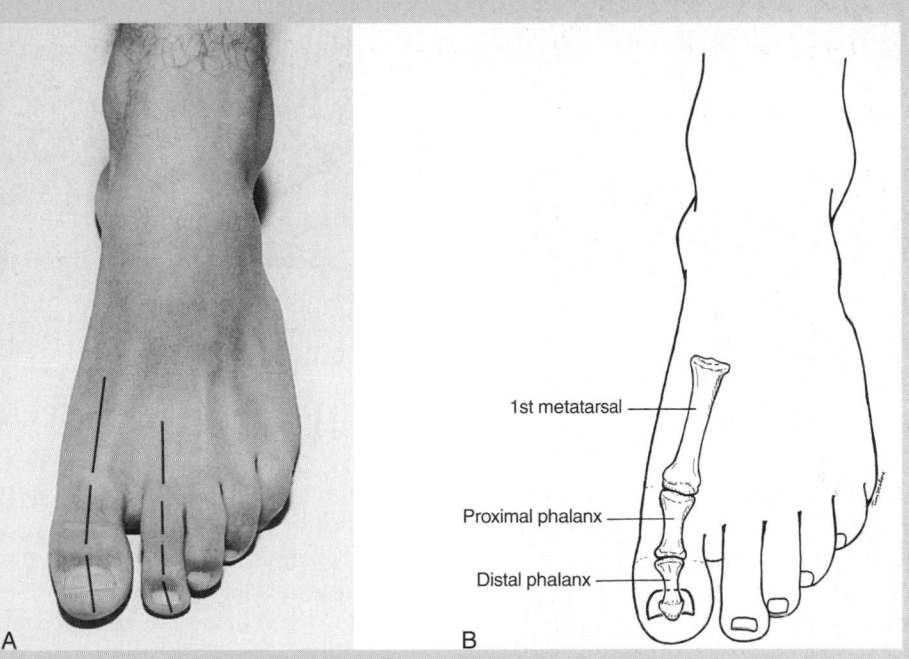

1st metatarsal

Proximal phalanx

Distal phalanx

A   B

FIGURE 10.42 A: Surface anatomy landmarks for goniometer alignment for measuring flexion and extension range of motion at the first and second MTP and IP joints and abduction and adduction at the first MTP joint. **B:** Bony anatomical landmarks for flexion and extension at the first and second MTP and IP joints and abduction and adduction at the first MTP joint.

● FLEXION: METATARSOPHALANGEAL JOINT

Motion occurs in the sagittal plane around a medial–lateral axis. Flexion ROM at the fist MTP joint ranges between 30 degrees[5] and 45 degrees.[3]

Testing Position

Place the subject in the supine or sitting position, with the ankle and foot in 0 degrees of dorsiflexion, plantarflexion, inversion, and eversion. Position the MTP joint in 0 degrees of abduction and adduction and the IP joints in 0 degrees of flexion and extension. (If the ankle is plantarflexed and the IP joints of the toe being tested are flexed, tension in the extensor hallucis longus or extensor digitorum longus muscle will restrict the motion.)

Stabilization

Stabilize the metatarsal to prevent plantarflexion of the ankle and inversion or eversion of the foot. Do not hold the MTP joints of the other toes in extension because tension in the transverse metatarsal ligament will restrict the motion.

Testing Motion

Pull the great toe downward toward the plantar surface into flexion (Fig. 10.43). Avoid pushing on the distal phalanx and causing interphalangeal flexion. The end of the ROM is reached when resistance is felt and attempts at further motion cause plantarflexion at the ankle.

Normal End-Feel

The end-feel is firm because of tension in the dorsal joint capsule and the collateral ligaments. Tension in the extensor digitorum brevis muscle may contribute to the firm end-feel.

Goniometer Alignment

See Figures 10.44 and 10.45.

1. Center **fulcrum** of the goniometer over the dorsal aspect of the MTP joint.
2. Align **proximal arm** over the dorsal midline of the metatarsal.
3. Align **distal arm** over the dorsal midline of the proximal phalanx.

Alternative Goniometer Alignment for First Metatarsophalangeal Joint

1. Center **fulcrum** of the goniometer over the medial aspect of the first MTP joint.
2. Align **proximal arm** with the medial midline of the first metatarsal.
3. Align **distal arm** with the medial midline of the proximal phalanx of the first toe.

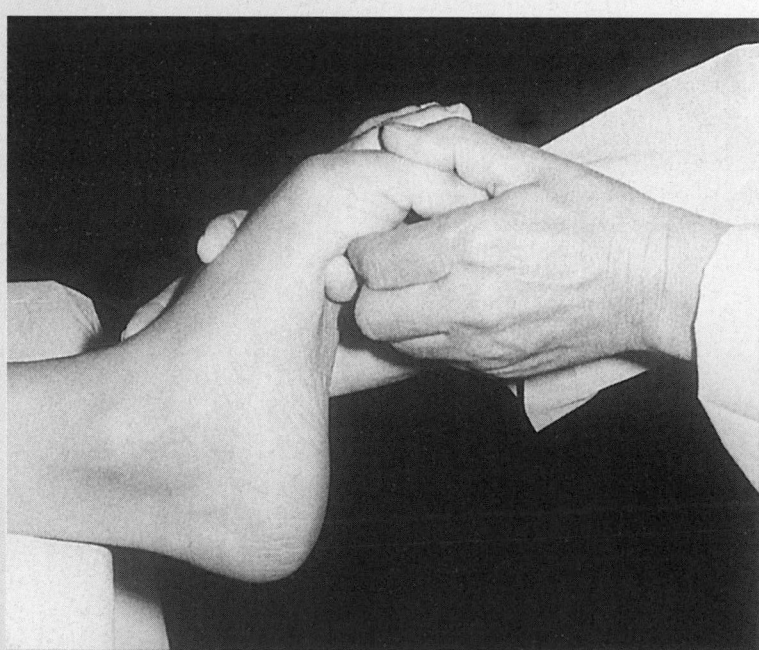

FIGURE 10.43 The left first metatarsophalangeal (MTP) joint at the end of the flexion range of motion. The subject is supine, with her foot and ankle placed over the edge of the supporting surface. However, the subject's foot could rest on the supporting surface. The examiner uses her thumb across the metatarsals to prevent ankle plantarflexion. The examiner's other hand maintains the first MTP joint in flexion.

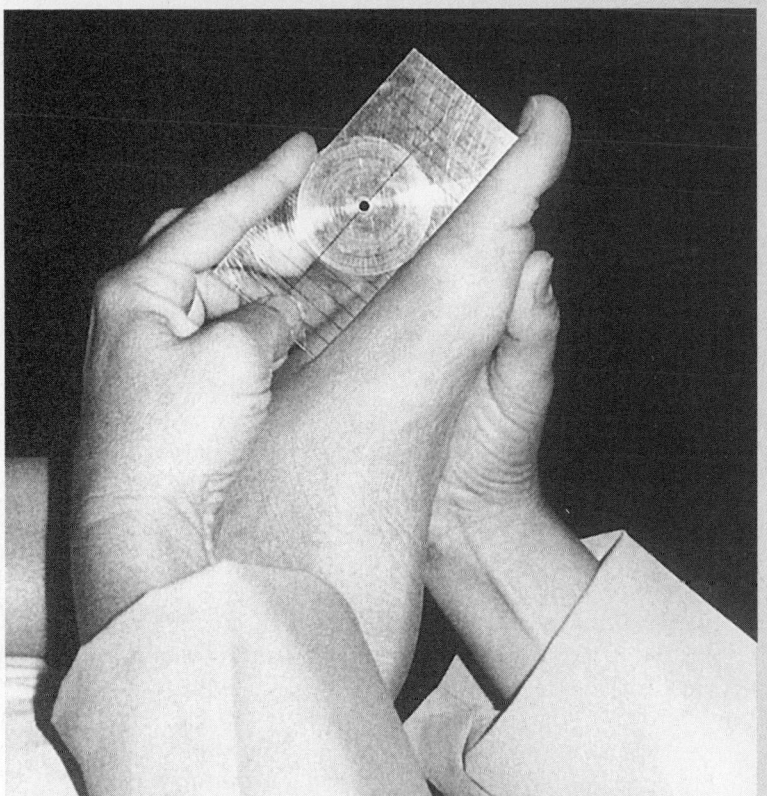

FIGURE 10.44 Goniometer alignment in the starting position for measuring metatarsophalangeal flexion range of motion. The arms of this goniometer have been cut short to accommodate the relative shortness of the proximal and distal joint segments.

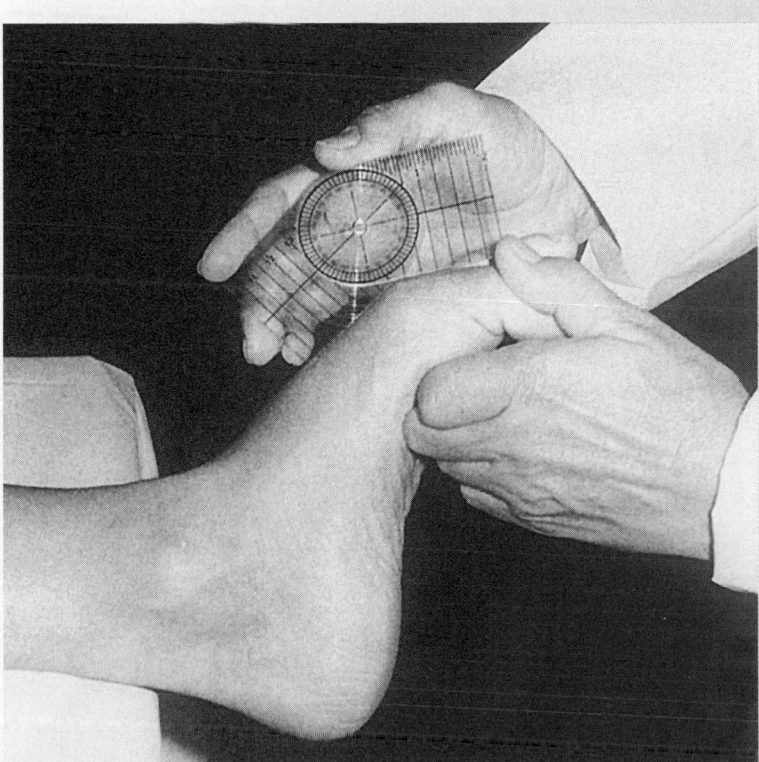

FIGURE 10.45 At the end of the range of motion, the examiner uses one hand to align the goniometer while her other hand maintains metatarsophalangeal flexion.

● EXTENSION:
METATARSOPHALANGEAL JOINT

Motion occurs in the sagittal plane around a medial–lateral axis. The ROM ranges between 50 degrees[5] and 70 degrees.[3]

Testing Position

The testing position is the same as that for measuring flexion of the MTP joint. (If the ankle is dorsiflexed and the IP joints of the toe being tested are extended, tension in the flexor hallucis longus or flexor digitorum longus muscle will restrict the motion. If the IP joints of the toe being tested are in extreme flexion, tension in the lumbricalis and interosseus muscles may restrict the motion.)

Stabilization

Stabilize the metatarsal to prevent dorsiflexion of the ankle and inversion or eversion of the foot. Do not hold the MTP joints of the other toes in extreme flexion because tension in the transverse metatarsal ligament will restrict the motion.

Testing Motion

Push the proximal phalanx toward the dorsum of the foot, moving the MTP joint into extension (Fig. 10.46). Avoid pushing on the distal phalanx, which causes IP extension. The end of the motion occurs when

resistance is felt and attempts at further motion cause dorsiflexion at the ankle.

Normal End-Feel

The end-feel is firm because of tension in the plantar joint capsule; the plantar pad (plantar fibrocartilaginous plate); and the flexor hallucis brevis, flexor digitorum brevis, and flexor digiti minimi muscles.

Goniometer Alignment

See Figures 10.47 and 10.48.

1. Center **fulcrum** of the goniometer over the dorsal aspect of the MTP joint.
2. Align **proximal arm** over the dorsal midline of the metatarsal.
3. Align **distal arm** over the dorsal midline of the proximal phalanx.

Alternative Goniometer Alignment for First Metatarsophalangeal Joint

1. Center **fulcrum** of the goniometer over the medial aspect of the first MTP joint.
2. Align **proximal arm** with the medial midline of the first metatarsal.
3. Align **distal arm** with the medial midline of the proximal phalanx of the first toe.

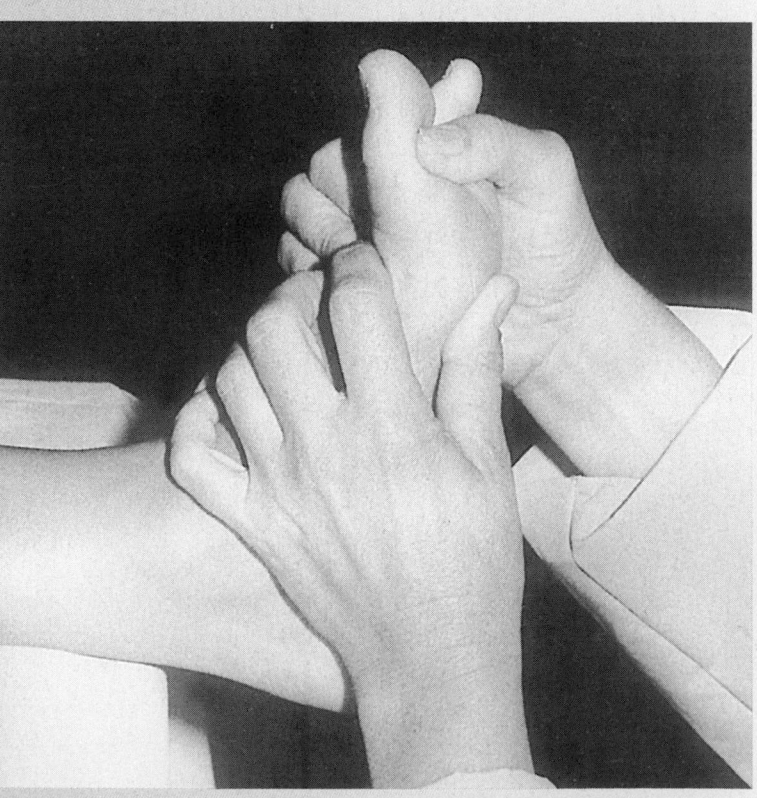

FIGURE 10.46 The left first metatarsophalangeal joint at the end of extension range of motion. The examiner places her digits on the dorsum of the subject's foot to prevent dorsiflexion and uses the thumb on her other hand to push the proximal phalanx into extension.

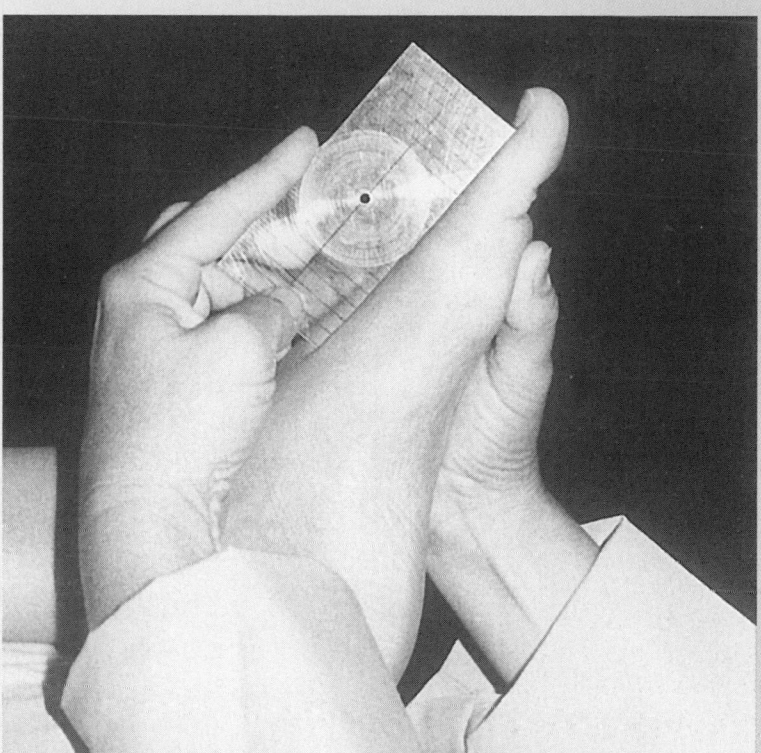

FIGURE 10.47 Goniometer alignment in the starting position for measuring extension at the first metatarsophalangeal joint.

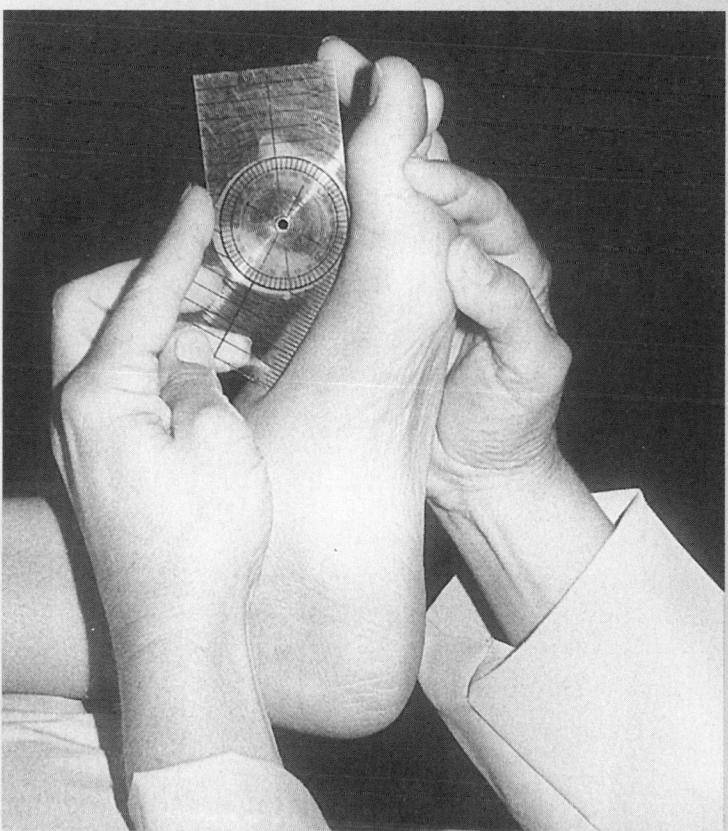

FIGURE 10.48 At the end of metatarsophalangeal extension, the examiner maintains goniometer alignment with one hand while using the index finger of her other hand to maintain extension.

• ABDUCTION: METATARSOPHALANGEAL JOINT

Motion occurs in the transverse plane around a vertical axis when the subject is in anatomical position.

Testing Position

Place the subject supine or sitting, with the foot in 0 degrees of inversion and eversion. Position the MTP and IP joints in 0 degrees of flexion and extension. Stabilize the metatarsal to prevent inversion or eversion of the foot.

Stabilization

Stabilize the metatarsal to prevent inversion or eversion of the foot.

Testing Motion

Pull the proximal phalanx of the toe laterally away from the midline of the foot into abduction (Fig. 10.49). Avoid pushing on the distal phalanx, which places a strain on the IP joint. The end of the ROM occurs when resistance is felt and attempts at further motion cause either inversion or eversion of the foot.

Normal End-Feel

The end-feel is firm because of tension in the joint capsule, the collateral ligaments, the fascia of the web space between the toes, and the adductor hallucis and plantar interosseus muscles.

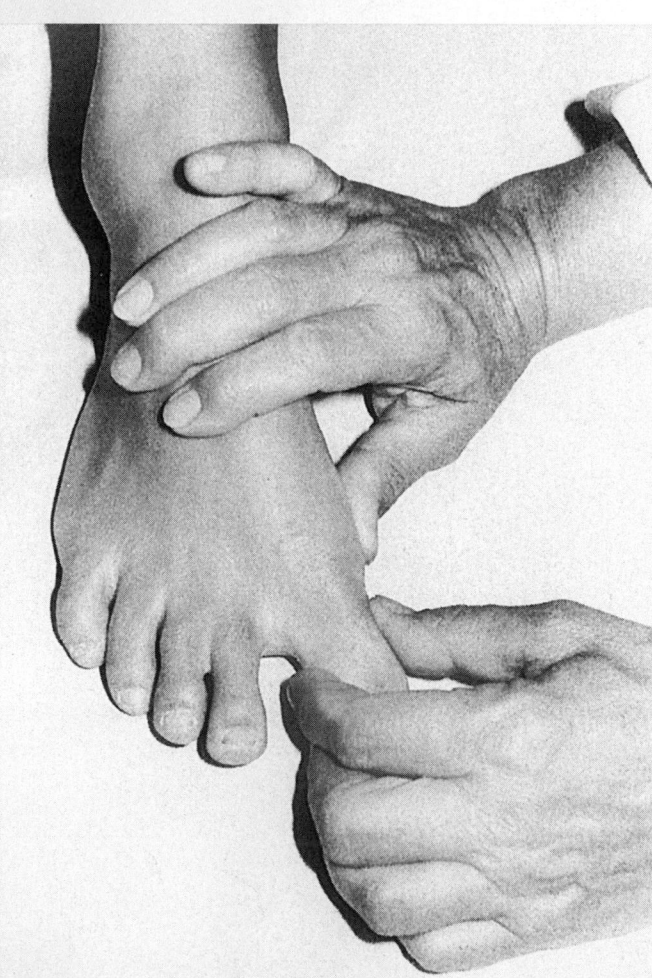

FIGURE 10.49 The subject's right first toe at the end of abduction range of motion. The examiner uses one thumb to prevent transverse tarsal inversion. She uses the index finger and thumb of her other hand to pull the proximal phalanx into abduction.

Goniometer Alignment
See Figures 10.50 and 10.51.

1. Center **fulcrum** of the goniometer over the dorsal aspect of the MTP joint.

2. Align **proximal arm** with the dorsal midline of the metatarsal.

3. Align **distal arm** with the dorsal midline of the proximal phalanx.

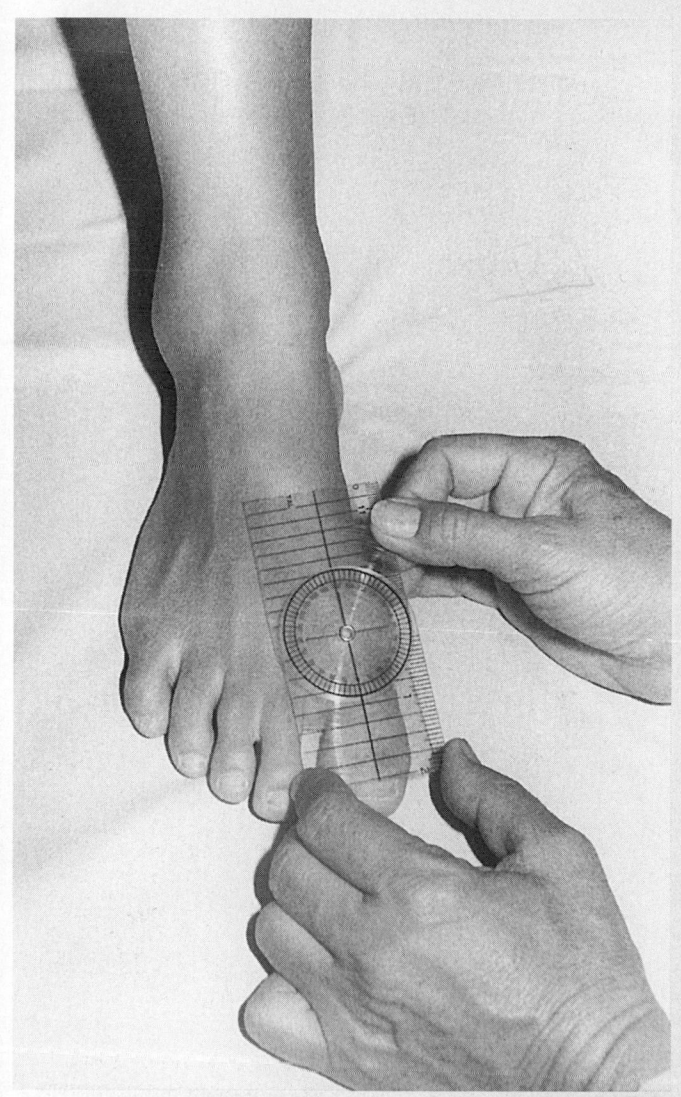

FIGURE 10.50 Goniometer alignment in the starting position for measuring metatarsophalangeal abduction range of motion.

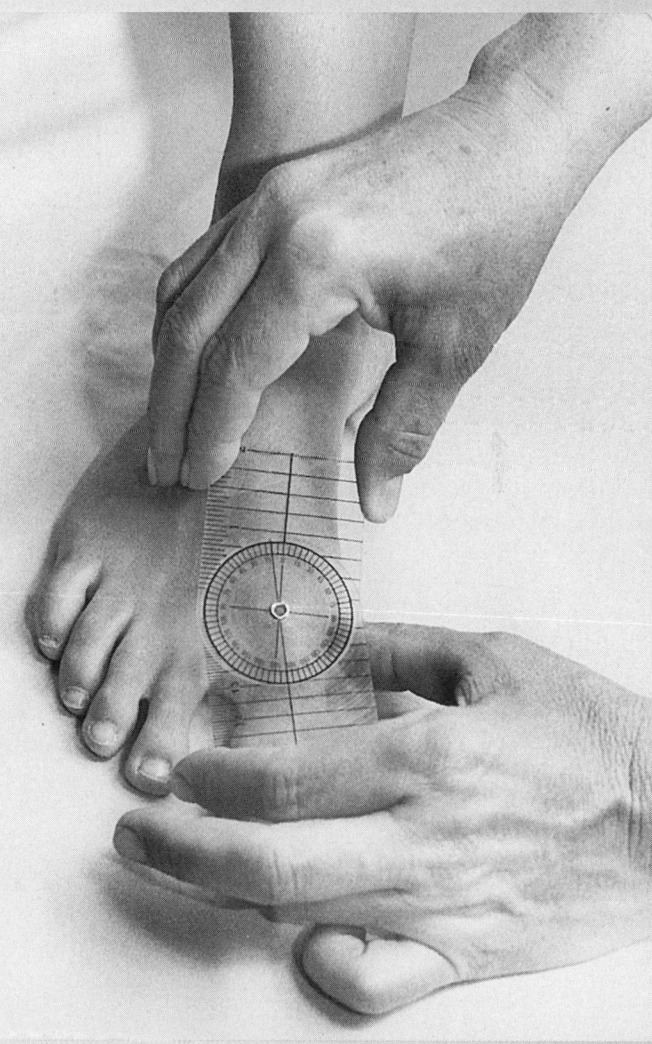

FIGURE 10.51 At the end of metatarsophalangeal (MTP) abduction, the examiner's hand maintains alignment of the distal goniometer arm while keeping the MTP in abduction.

● ADDUCTION: METATARSOPHALANGEAL JOINT

Motion occurs in the transverse plane around a vertical axis when the subject is in anatomical position. Adduction is the return from abduction to the 0 starting position and is not usually measured.

● FLEXION: INTERPHALANGEAL JOINT OF THE FIRST TOE AND PROXIMAL INTERPHALANGEAL JOINTS OF THE FOUR LESSER TOES

Motion occurs in the sagittal plane around a medial–lateral axis. The ROM is between 30 degrees[5] and 90 degrees for the first toe.[3] See Table 10.2 in the Research Findings section for normal ROM values for the four lesser toes.

Testing Position

Place the subject supine or sitting, with the ankle and foot in 0 degrees of dorsiflexion, plantarflexion, inversion, and eversion. Position the MTP joint in 0 degrees of flexion, extension, abduction, and adduction. (If the ankle is positioned in plantarflexion and the MTP joint is flexed, tension in the extensor hallucis longus or extensor digitorum longus muscles will restrict the motion. If the MTP joint is positioned in full extension, tension in the lumbricalis and interosseus muscles may restrict the motion.)

Stabilization

Stabilize the metatarsal and proximal phalanx to prevent dorsiflexion or plantarflexion of the ankle and inversion or eversion of the foot. Avoid flexion and extension of the MTP joint.

Testing Motion

Pull the distal phalanx of the first toe or the middle phalanx of the lesser toes down toward the plantar surface of the foot. The end of the ROM occurs when resistance is felt and attempts at further flexion cause plantarflexion of the ankle or flexion at the MTP joint.

Normal End-Feel

The end-feel for flexion of the IP joint of the big toe and the proximal interphalangeal (PIP) joints of the smaller toes may be soft because of compression of soft tissues between the plantar surfaces of the phalanges. Sometimes, the end-feel is firm because of tension in the dorsal joint capsule and the collateral ligaments.

Goniometer Alignment

1. Center **fulcrum** of the goniometer over the dorsal aspect of the interphalangeal joint being tested.
2. Align **proximal arm** over the dorsal midline of the proximal phalanx.
3. Align **distal arm** over the dorsal midline of the phalanx distal to the joint being tested.

● EXTENSION: INTERPHALANGEAL JOINT OF THE FIRST TOE AND PROXIMAL INTERPHALANGEAL JOINTS OF THE FOUR LESSER TOES

Motion occurs in the sagittal plane around a medial–lateral axis. Usually this motion is not measured because it is a return from flexion to the 0 starting position.

● FLEXION: DISTAL INTERPHALANGEAL JOINTS OF THE FOUR LESSER TOES

Motion occurs in the sagittal plane around a medial–lateral axis. Flexion ROM is 0 to 30 degrees.[4]

Testing Position

Place the subject supine or sitting, with the ankle and foot in 0 degrees of dorsiflexion, plantarflexion, inversion, and eversion. Position the MTP and PIP joints in 0 degrees of flexion, extension, abduction, and adduction.

Stabilization

Stabilize the metatarsal, proximal, and middle phalanx to prevent dorsiflexion or plantarflexion of the ankle and inversion or eversion of the foot. Avoid flexion and extension of the MTP and PIP joints of the toe being tested.

Testing Motion

Push the distal phalanx toward the plantar surface of the foot. The end of the motion occurs when resistance is felt and attempts to produce further flexion cause flexion at the MTP and PIP joints and/or plantarflexion of the ankle.

Normal End-Feel

The end-feel is firm because of tension in the dorsal joint capsule, the collateral ligaments, and the oblique retinacular ligament.

Goniometer Alignment

1. Center **fulcrum** of the goniometer over the dorsal aspect of the distal interphalangeal (DIP) joint.
2. Align **proximal arm** over the dorsal midline of the middle phalanx.
3. Align **distal arm** over the dorsal midline of the distal phalanx.

● EXTENSION: DISTAL INTERPHALANGEAL JOINTS OF THE FOUR LESSER TOES

Motion occurs in the sagittal plane around a medial–lateral axis. Usually this motion is not measured because it is a return from flexion to the 0 starting position.

MUSCLE LENGTH TESTING PROCEDURES:
The Ankle and Foot

● GASTROCNEMIUS

The gastrocnemius muscle is a two-joint muscle that crosses both the ankle and knee. The medial head of the gastrocnemius originates proximally from the posterior aspect of the medial condyle of the femur, whereas the lateral head of the gastrocnemius originates from the posterior lateral aspect of the lateral condyle (Fig. 10.52). Both heads join with the tendon of the soleus muscle to form the tendocalcaneus (Achilles) tendon, which inserts distally into the posterior surface of the calcaneus. When the gastrocnemius contracts, it plantarflexes the ankle and flexes the knee.

A short gastrocnemius can limit ankle dorsiflexion and knee extension. During the test for the length of the gastrocnemius the knee is held in full extension. A short gastrocnemius results in a decrease in ankle dorsiflexion ROM when the knee is extended. If, however, ankle dorsiflexion ROM is decreased with the knee in a flexed position, the dorsiflexion limitation is due to shortness of the one-joint soleus muscle or other joint structures.

Normal values for dorsiflexion of the ankle with the knee in extension vary. See Tables 10.6 and 10.7 in the Research Findings section for normal ROM values by age and gender.

Starting Position
Place the subject supine, with the knee extended and the foot in 0 degrees of inversion and eversion.

Stabilization
Hold the knee in full extension. Usually, the weight of the limb and hand pressure on the anterior leg can maintain an extended knee position.

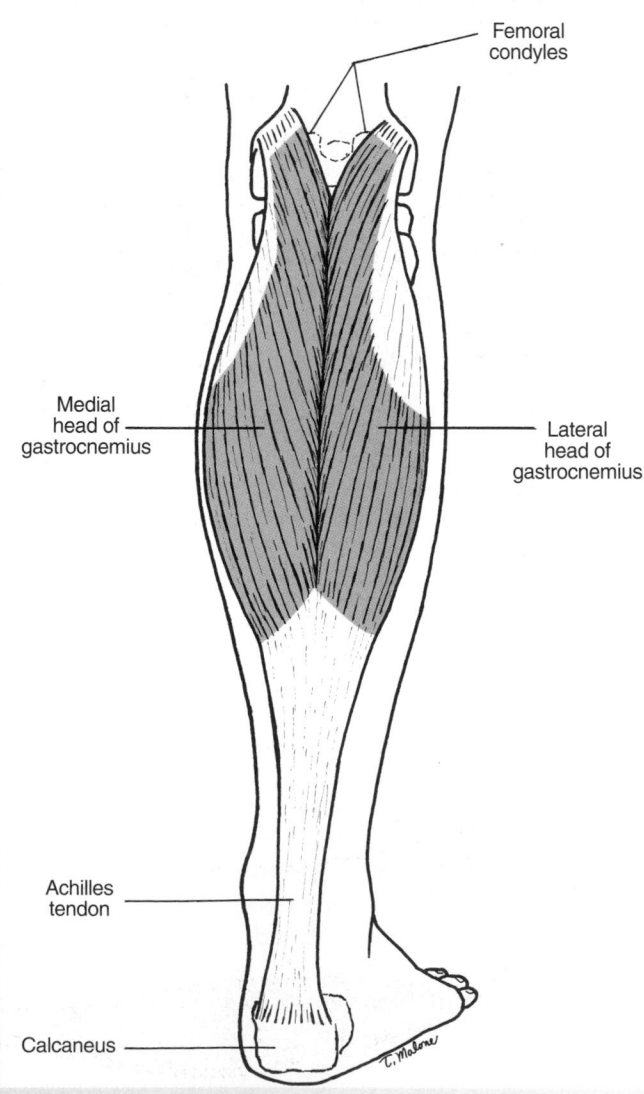

FIGURE 10.52 A posterior view of a right lower extremity shows the attachments of the gastrocnemius muscle.

Testing Motion

Dorsiflex the ankle to the end of the ROM by pushing upward across the plantar surface of the metatarsal heads (Fig. 10.53 and Fig. 10.54). Do not allow the foot to rotate and move into inversion or eversion. The end of the testing motion occurs when considerable resistance is felt from tension in the posterior calf and knee and further ankle dorsiflexion causes the knee to flex.

Normal End-Feel

The end-feel is firm owing to tension in the gastrocnemius muscle.

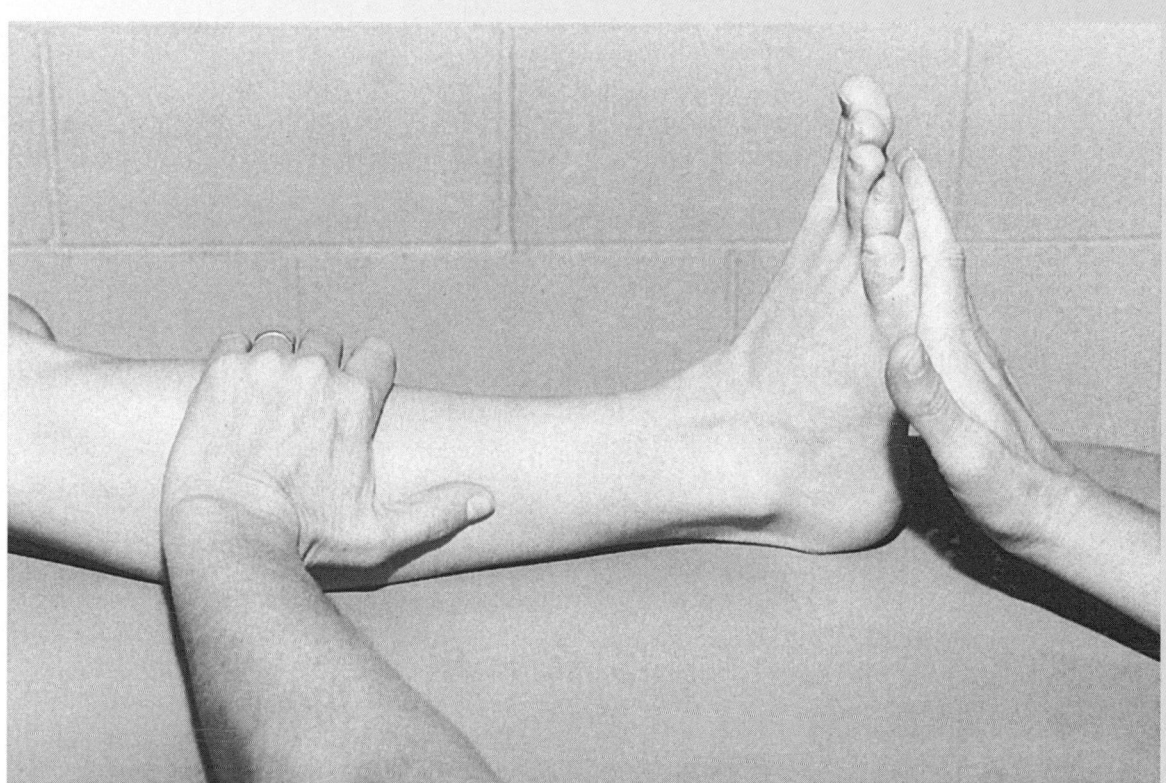

FIGURE 10.53 The subject's right ankle at the end of the testing motion for the length of the gastrocnemius muscle.

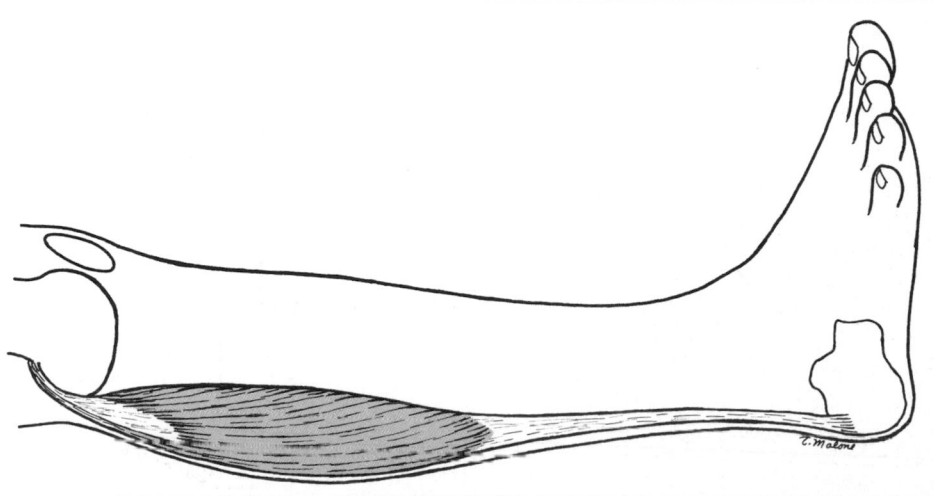

FIGURE 10.54 The gastrocnemius muscle is stretched over the extended knee and dorsiflexed ankle.

Goniometer Alignment
See Figure 10.55.

1. Center **fulcrum** of the goniometer over the lateral aspect of the lateral malleolus.
2. Align **proximal arm** with the lateral midline of the fibula, using the head of the fibula for reference.
3. Align **distal arm** parallel to the lateral aspect of the fifth metatarsal.

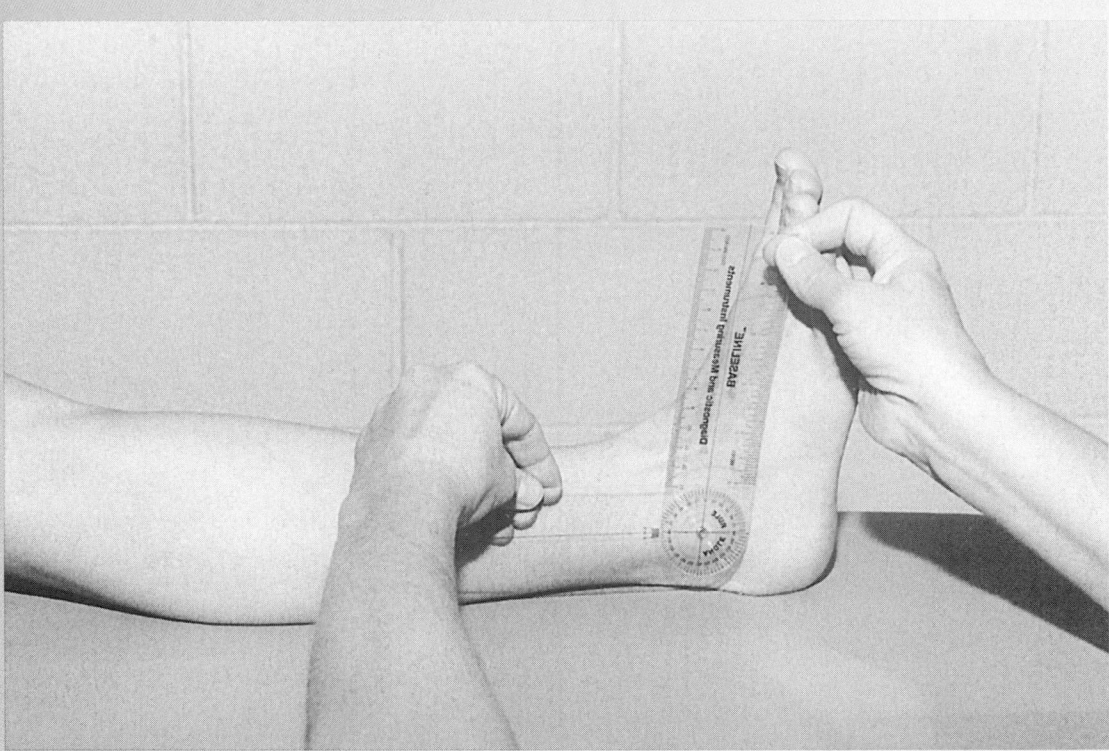

FIGURE 10.55 Goniometer alignment at the end of the testing motion for the length of the gastrocnemius muscle.

● GASTROCNEMIUS LENGTH TESTING POSITION: STANDING

Place the subject in the standing position, with the knee extended and the foot in 0 degrees of inversion and eversion. The foot is in line (sagittal plane) with the lower leg and knee. The subject stands facing a wall or examining table, which can be used for balance and support.

Stabilization
Maintain the knee in full extension, and ensure the heel remains in total contact with the floor. The examiner may hold the heel in contact with the floor.

Testing Motion
The patient dorsiflexes the ankle by leaning the body forward (Fig. 10.56). The end of the testing motion occurs when the patient feels tension in the posterior calf and knee and further ankle dorsiflexion causes the knee to flex.

Goniometer Alignment
See Figure 10.57.

1. Center **fulcrum** of the goniometer over the lateral aspect of the lateral malleolus.
2. Align **proximal arm** with the lateral midline of the fibula, using the head of the fibula for reference.
3. Align **distal arm** parallel to the lateral aspect of the fifth metatarsal.

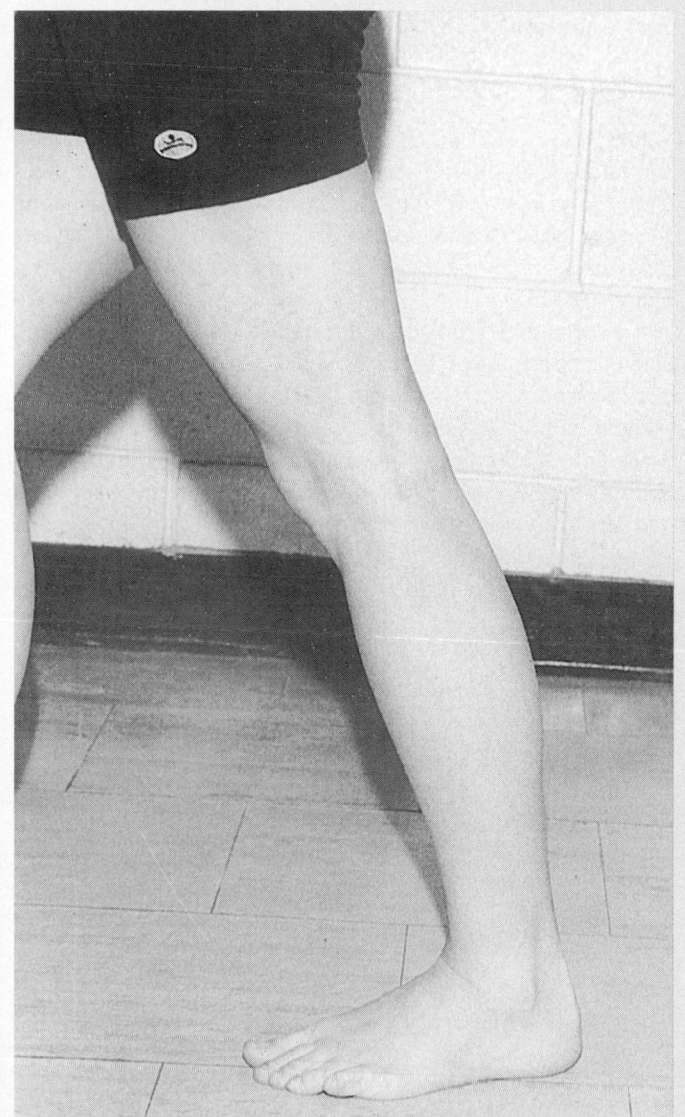

FIGURE 10.56 The subject's left ankle at the end of the weight-bearing testing motion for the length of the gastrocnemius muscle.

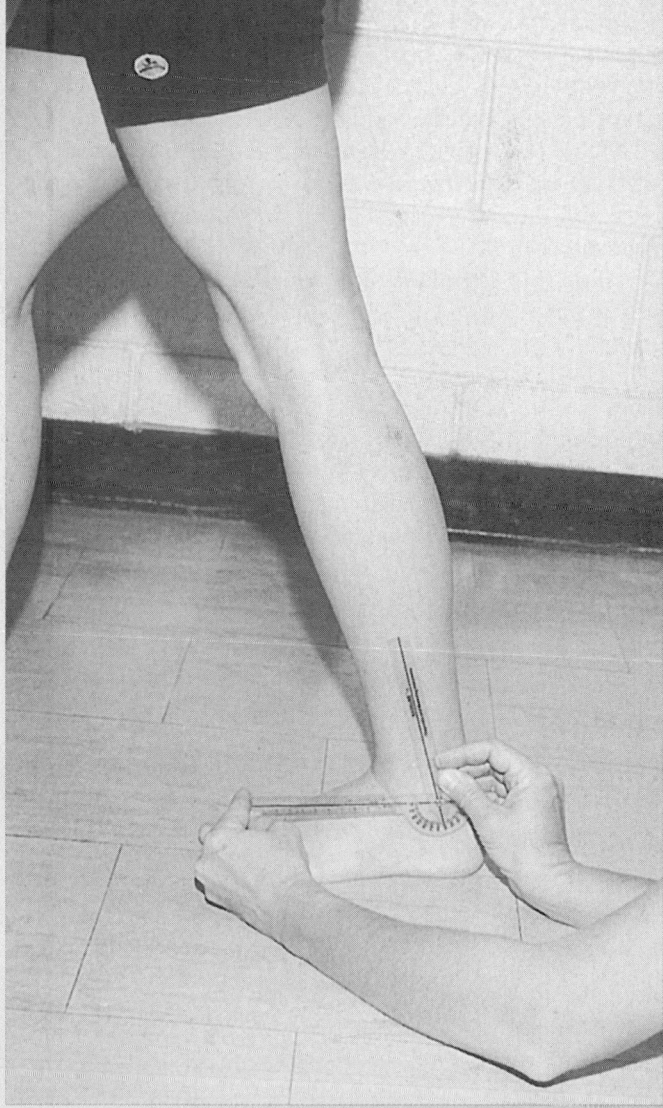

FIGURE 10.57 Goniometer alignment in the alternative testing position.

Research Findings

Tables 10.1 and 10.2 provide ankle and toe ROM values from various sources. The 1994 AAOS[4] edition includes ROM values from various research studies, including the same values from Boone and Azen[6] that are found in Table 10.1, and a few values from the 1965 edition. Boone and Azen,[6] using a universal goniometer, measured active ROM on male subjects.

Effects of Age, Gender, and Other Factors

Age

Table 10.3 shows that newborns, infants, and 2 year olds have a larger dorsiflexion ROM than older children. The mean values for dorsiflexion in the youngest age groups are more than double the average adult values presented in Tables 10.1 and 10.4. However, between 1 and 5 years of age, dorsiflexion values show a decrease (Table 10.3). Plantarflexion ROM in newborns is smaller compared to adults, but newborns attain adult values in the first few weeks of life. According to Walker,[11] the persistence in infants of a limited ROM in plantarflexion may indicate pathology.

Table 10.4 provides evidence that decreases in both dorsiflexion and plantarflexion ROM occur with increases in age. However, the difference between dorsiflexion values in the youngest and oldest groups constitutes less than 1 standard deviation (SD). Plantarflexion values in the oldest group are slightly more than 1 SD less than values for the youngest group.

Alanen and colleagues[13] found a wide variation in maximum passive ROM measurements of dorsiflexion and plantarflexion in 245 boys and girls with a mean age of 10 years and an age range of 7 to 14 years. ROM values varied from 5 to 50 degrees for maximum dorsiflexion with the knee extended in the prone position and from 21 to 61 degrees with the knee flexed in the weight-bearing position. Plantarflexion

values also varied widely, ranging from 30 to 80 degrees. Intraindividual differences of greater than 5 to 10 degrees were found between children's right and left ankles, leading the authors to caution testers about using the ROM in one ankle as a normal ROM for the opposite ankle in this young age group.

Saxena and Kim[14] tested dorsiflexion ROM in 40 high school athletes ages 14 to 17 years. An experienced tester used a goniometer to measure ankle dorsiflexion in the supine position in both ankles with the knees extended and flexed. In contrast to the findings of Alenan and colleagues,[13] no significant differences were found between measurements of right and left ankles or between girls and boys. However, the age groups are considerably different between the two studies. Ankle dorsiflexion in this group of adolescent athletes was

TABLE 10.2   Toe Motion: Values in Degrees from Selected Sources

Joint	Extension		Flexion	
	AMA[5]	AAOS[3]	AMA[5]	AAOS[3]
MTP 1	50	70	30	45
2	40	40	30	40
3	30	40	20	40
4	20	40	10	40
5	10	40	10	40
IP 1	—	—	30	90
PIP 2–5	—	—	—	35
DIP 2–5	—	—	—	60

AMA = American Medical Association; AAOS = American Associaion of Orthopaedic Surgeons; DIP = distal interphalangeal; IP = interphalangeal; MTP = metatarsophalangeal; PIP = proximal interphalangeal.

TABLE 10.1   Ankle Motion: Values in Degrees from Selected Sources

	AAOS[3]	AAOS[4]	AMA[5]	Boone and Azen[*6]
Motion				Mean (SD)
Dorsiflexion	20	20	20	12.6 (4.4)
Plantarflexion	50	50	40	56.2 (6.1)
Inversion	35	—	30	36.8 (4.5)
Eversion	15	—	20	20.7 (5.0)
Subtalar inversion	5	—	—	— —
Subtalar eversion	5	—	—	— —

AMA = American Medical Association; AAOS = American Association of Orthopaedic Surgeons; SD = standard deviation.
* Subjects were 109 males 1 to 54 years of age.

TABLE 10.3 Effects of Age on Ankle Motion in Newborns and Children Aged 6 to 12 Years: Mean Values in Degrees

	Waugh et al[8]	Wanatabe et al[9]			Boone[10]	
	6–72 hrs n = 40	2–4 wks n = 57	4–8 mos n = 54	2 yrs n = 57	1–5 yrs n = 19	6–12 yrs n = 17
Motion	*Mean (SD)*	*Mean range*			*Mean (SD)*	*Mean (SD)*
Dorsiflexion	58.9 (7.9)	0–53.0	0–51.0	0–41.0	14.5 (5.0)	13.8 (4.4)
Plantarflexion	25.7 (6.3)	0–58.0	0–60.0	0–62.0	59.7 (5.4)	59.6 (4.7)

SD = standard deviation.

found to be 0.35 (SD = 2.2) degrees with the knees extended and just less than 5 degrees with the knees flexed. These values for dorsiflexion are below the normal values and less than the 10 degrees needed for normal gait. The authors did not offer any explanation for the limited ROM, but it is possible that it is related to either developmental changes in this group of adolescents or athletic activities that decreased the extensibility of the gastrocnemius and soleus muscles.

James and Parker[15] found a consistent reduction in both active and passive ROM with increasing age in all ankle joint motions in a group of 80 active men and women ranging in age from 70 to 92 years. The most rapid reduction in ROM occurred for individuals in the ninth decade. Ankle dorsiflexion measured with the knee extended (a test of the length of the gastrocnemius muscle) showed the most marked change. The investigators suggested that the decrease in extensibility of the plantarflexor muscle-tendon unit was due to connective tissue changes associated with the aging process. In another study that examined the effects of aging on dorsiflexion ROM, Gajdosik, VanderLinden, and Williams[16] used an isokinetic dynamometer to passively stretch the calf muscles in 74 females (aged 20 to 84 years). The older women (aged 60 to 84 years) had a significantly smaller mean dorsiflexion angle of 15.4 degrees than the younger women (aged 20 to 39 years), who had a mean of 25.8 degrees, and the middle-aged women, who had a mean of 22.8 degrees. The decrease

in dorsiflexion in the older women was associated with a decrease in plantarflexor muscle-tendon unit extensibility.

In a subsequent study, Gajdosik and colleagues[17] compared the passive stretch and release characteristics of the calf muscles of 15 healthy older women with a mean age of 79 years with that of 15 healthy young women with a mean age of 24 years. The right ankles of all subjects were stretched from plantarflexion to maximal dorsiflexion and then released into plantarflexion. Older women had less calf muscle length extensibility, less passive resistive force, less stored passive-elastic energy, and less mean maximum passive dorsiflexion ROM (10.3 degrees) compared to younger women (28.0 degrees).

Nigg and associates[18] found that age-related changes in ankle ROM were motion specific and differed between males and females. The authors measured active ROM in 121 subjects (61 males and 60 females) between the ages of 20 and 79 years. For the entire group of subjects, decreases in active ROM with increases in age occurred in plantarflexion, inversion, abduction, and adduction but not in eversion and dorsiflexion (tested in the sitting position with the knee flexed). Plantarflexion decreased about 8 degrees from the youngest to the oldest group.

Gender

Gender effects on ROM are joint specific and motion specific and are often related to age. Nigg and associates[18] found gender differences in ankle motion but determined that the differences

TABLE 10.4 Effects of Age on Active Ankle Motion for Individuals 13 to 69 Years of Age: Normal Values in Degrees

	Boone[10]				Boone et al[11]
	13–19 yrs n = 17	20–29 yrs n = 19	30–39 yrs n = 18	40–54 yrs n = 19	61–69 yrs n = 10
Motion	*Mean (SD)*	*Mean (SD)*	*Mean (SD)*	*Mean (SD)*	*Mean (SD)*
Dorsiflexion	10.6 (3.7)	12.1 (3.4)	12.2 (4.3)	12.4 (4.7)	8.2 (4.6)
Plantarflexion	55.5 (5.7)	55.4 (3.6)	54.6 (6.0)	52.9 (7.6)	46.2 (7.7)

SD = standard deviation.

changed with increasing age. Only in the oldest group did women have more (8 degrees) plantarflexion than men. The only gender differences noted by Boone, Walker, and Perry[12] were that females in the 1-year-old to 9-year-old group and those in the 61-year-old to 69-year-old group had significantly more ROM in plantarflexion than their male counterparts. Four other studies also found that females had more plantarflexion than males.[13,15,19,20] Alanen and colleagues,[13] in a study of ankle joint mobility in 245 children ages 7 to 14 years (mean age 10 years), found that girls had a significantly greater range of passive plantarflexion compared to the boys in the study. However, according to the authors, the differences were small and probably not of clinical inportance.

Bell and Hoshizaki[19] studied 17 joint motions in 124 females and 66 males ranging in age from 18 to 88 years. Females between 17 and 30 years of age had a greater ROM in plantarflexion and dorsiflexion than males in the same age groups. Walker and colleagues[20] studied active ROM in 30 men and 30 women ranging in age from 60 to 84 years. Women had 11 degrees more ankle plantarflexion than men.

James and Parker[15] found that the only motion that showed a significant difference between the genders was plantarflexion measured with the knee extended. Women and men had similar mean values in the group between 70 and 74 years of age, but the reduction in active and passive ROM over the entire age range was greater for men (25.2 percent) than for women (11.3 percent). High-heeled shoe wear has been proposed by Nigg and associates[18] as one reason why women have a greater ROM in plantarflexion than men.

In contrast to the findings that women have greater ROM in plantarflexion than men, a few investigators have found that females have less active and passive dorsiflexion ROM than males.[18,20,21] In a study by Nigg and associates,[18] males in the oldest group had a greater active ROM in dorsiflexion (8 degrees) measured with the knee flexed than females in the same age group (Table 10.5). Females showed a significant decrease in active dorsiflexion ROM with increasing age, from 26.0 degrees in the youngest group to 18.5 degrees in the oldest group. Females also showed a significant decrease in eversion of 5.8 degrees with increasing age. Males, however, had little or no change in either active dorsiflexion or eversion ROM from the youngest to the oldest group. Vandervoort and coworkers[21] experienced similar findings in a study measuring passive dorsiflexion ROM with the knee flexed. The end of the ROM was defined as the maximum degree of dorsiflexion possible before muscle contraction occurred, or when the subject felt discomfort, or when the heel lifted from a floor plate. Females in the study showed a decrease in passive dorsiflexion ROM, from a high of 19.3 degrees in the youngest group (aged 55 to 60 years) to a low of 12.1 degrees in the oldest group (aged 81 to 85 years; Table 10.5). In comparison, male subjects showed a decrease of only 2.3 degrees in dorsiflexion from the youngest group (mean = 15.4 degrees) to the oldest group (mean = 13.1 degrees). Males had greater passive elastic stiffness than females, with 10 degrees of dorsiflexion.

In a study conducted by Baggett and Young[22] of 18 to 66 year olds, males compared to females had less dorsiflexion ROM in non–weight-bearing and a greater ROM in weight-bearing. However the differences in ROM were small between the genders and probably not of clinical importance.

Grimston and associates[23] measured active ROM in 120 subjects (58 males and 62 females) ranging in age from 9 to 20 years. These authors found that females generally had a greater ROM in all ankle motions than males. Both males and females showed a consistent trend toward decreasing ROM with increasing age, but females had a larger decrease than males.

In contrast to the findings of the previously mentioned studies, Saxena and Kim[14] found no differences in dorsiflexion ROM values between 24 boys and 16 girls ages 14 to 17 years. However, the age range in this study was relatively small compared to Grimston's[23] study.

Testing Position

A variety of positions are used to measure dorsiflexion ROM, including sitting with the knee flexed, supine with the knee either flexed or extended, prone with the knee either flexed or extended, and standing with the knee either flexed or extended. Positions in which the knee is flexed bring the distal and proximal attachments of the gastrocnemius muscle closer together and result in relaxing the muscle so that its effect on dorsiflexion ROM is reduced. Positions in which the knee is extended generally are used for testing the length of the gastrocnemius muscle (Tables 10.6 and 10.7). Dorsiflexion measurements taken in the weight-bearing position are usually greater than measurements taken in non–weight-bearing positions.[22]

McPoil and Cornwall[28] compared dorsiflexion ROM measurements taken with the knee flexed with measurements taken with the knee extended in 27 healthy young adults. As might be expected, the mean dorsiflexion ROM (16.2 degrees) with the knee flexed was greater than the mean (10.1 degrees) with the knee extended (Table 10.7). In a study of dorsiflexion ROM in 7 to 14 year olds, Alanen and colleagues[13] found that dorsiflexion measurements taken with the knee flexed to 90 degrees were 10 to 19 degrees greater than measurements taken with the knee extended.

Riemann and coworkers[29] measured the resistance to passive dorsiflexion from 23 degrees of plantarflexion to 13 degrees of dorsiflexion in 12 physically active men (mean age 22 years) and 12 women (mean age 20 years). Passive movements at a constant angular velocity were applied using a Biodex System 2 Isokinetic Dynamometer in passive mode. Significantly higher stiffness values were found in the knee extended position compared with the knee flexed position. The stiffness values in the gastrocnemius increased significantly as the ankle moved from plantarflexion toward dorsiflexion. Stiffness was defined by the authors as representing the amount of deformation proportional to the load applied.

Moseley, Crosbie, and Adams[24] quantified the passive dorsiflexion ROM resulting from a 12-Nm torque applied by a dynamometer to the soles of both feet of 300 healthy male and

TABLE 10.5 Effects of Age and Gender on Dorsiflexion Range of Motion in Males and Females Aged 40 to 85 Years: Normal Values in Degrees

Nigg et al*[18]				Vandervoort et al†[21]			
40–59 yrs		70–79 yrs		55–60 yrs		81–85 yrs	
Males n = 15	Females n = 15	Males n = 15	Females n = 15	Males n = 20	Females n = 16	Males n = 18	Females n = 17
Mean (SD)	Mean (SD)	Mean (SD)	Mean (SD)	Mean (SD)	Mean (SD)	Mean (SD)	Mean (SD)
25.0 (7.0)	26.0 (6.4)	26.4 (4.7)	18.5 (4.8)	15.4 (4.3)	19.3 (3.2)	13.1 (3.5)	12.1 (5.5)

ROM = range of motion; SD = standard deviation.
* A laboratory coordinate system ROM instrument was used to measure active ROM in subjects sitting with the knee flexed.
† An electric computer-controlled torque motor system was used to produce passive ROM in subjects positioned prone with the knee flexed.

TABLE 10.6 Dorsiflexion Range of Motion Measured in Non–Weight-Bearing Positions with the Knee Extended in Male and Female Subjects Aged 20 to 85 Years: Normal Values in Degrees

Gajdosik et al*[16]			Moseley et al†[24]	Jonson and Gross‡[25]	Vandervoort et al§[21]	
20–24 yrs n = 24	40–59 yrs n = 24	60–84 yrs n = 33	15–34 yrs n = 298	18–30 yrs n = 57	55–60 yrs n = 36	80–85 yrs n = 35
Mean (SD)	Mean (SD)	Mean (SD)	Mean (SD)	Mean (SD)	Mean (SD)	Mean (SD)
25.83 (5.5)	22.8 (4.4)	15.4 (5.8)	18.1 (6.9)	16.2 (3.7)	20.3 (4.6)	11.8 (5.2)

ROM = range of motion; SD = standard deviation.
* All measurements are of passive ROM in female subjects taken in the supine position with a universal goniometer.
† All measurements are of passive ROM in both genders taken in the prone position with use of a protractor and with the application of 12.0 Nm of torque.
‡ All measurements are of active assistive ROM in the prone position.
§ All measurements are of active ROM in the prone position with use of a footplate and a potentiometer.

TABLE 10.7 Comparison Between Dorsiflexion Range of Motion Measurements Taken With the Knee Flexed and Extended in Subjects Aged 8 to 87 Years: Normal Values in Degrees

	Bennell et al*[26]		Ekstrand et al†[27]		McPoil and Cornwall‡[23]	Mecagni et al§[24]
	8–11 yrs n = 77	8.2–11 yrs n = 49	20–25 yrs n = 10	22–30 yrs n = 12	Mean 26.1 yrs n = 56 feet	64–87 yrs n = 34
	Mean (SD)	Mean (SD)	Mean (SD)	Mean (SD)	Mean (SD)	Mean (SD)
Knee flexed	31.9 (6.8)	29.2 (6.4)	26.6 (2.5)	24.9 (0.8)	16.2 (3.2)	10.9 (4.2)
Knee extended	25.0 (7.6)	25.4 (8.5)	22.9 (2.5)	22.5 (0.7)	10.1 (2.2)	8.5 (3.1)

ROM = range of motion; SD = standard deviation.
* All measurements were taken in weight-bearing positions with use of an inclinometer.
† All measurements were taken in weight-bearing positions with use of a Leighton Floxometer (a type of gravity inclinometer). The flexed-knee testing position was greater than 90 degrees.
‡ All measurements were taken by one tester using a masked goniometer. The testing position was not reported, but in the flexed-knee position, the knee was flexed to 90 degrees.
§ All measurements were taken in non–weight-bearing positions with use of an active assistive ROM technique.

female subjects who were in the supine position with the knee extended. Based on the results, the authors proposed a scheme in which application of the same Nm torque would classify passive dorsiflexion ROM less than 4 degrees as hypomobile, 11.2 to 25 degrees as normal, and 32 degrees as hypermobile.

Baggett and Young[22] compared measurements of dorsiflexion ROM taken in the non–weight-bearing supine position with those taken in the standing weight-bearing position in 10 males and 20 female patients aged 18 to 66 years. Both supine and standing measurements were taken with the knees extended. The average dorsiflexion ROM in the supine position was 8.3 degrees, whereas the average dorsiflexion ROM in the standing position was 20.9 degrees. Little correlation was found between measurements taken in the non–weight-bearing position with those taken in the weight-bearing position. Consequently, the authors recommended to examiners that the non–weight-bearing and weight-bearing positions should not be used interchangeably and that the weight-bearing position might be more clinically relevant.

Bohannon, Tiberio, and Waters,[30] in a study involving 11 males and 11 females aged 21 to 43 years, investigated passive ROM for ankle dorsiflexion by means of different goniometer alignments. In one alignment, the arms of the goniometer were arranged parallel with the fibula and the heel. The second alignment used the fibula and a line parallel to the fifth metatarsal. These authors found that passive ROM measurements for dorsiflexion differed significantly according to which landmarks were used.

Menadue and colleagues[7] compared measurements of inversion and eversion in both ankles of 60 male and female patients between the ages of 21 and 59 years. Some of the patients had a past history of a variety of orthopedic ankle conditions. Three testers used universal goniometers to perform the measurements in the sitting and prone positions. Full cycle (inversion-eversion) ROM was 43.1 degrees in the sitting position and 24.2 degrees in the prone position. Naturally, the two positions should not be used interchangeably.

Lattanza, Gray, and Kanter[31] measured subtalar joint eversion in weight-bearing and non–weight-bearing postures in 15 females and 2 males. Measurements of subtalar joint eversion in a weight-bearing posture were found to be significantly greater than those in a non–weight-bearing posture. The authors advocated measurement in both positions.

Nawoczenski, Baumjauer, and Umberger[32] measured active and passive extension ROM of the MTP joint of the first toe in different positions in 14 women and 19 men between the ages of 20 and 54 years. Active and passive toe extension measurements were taken with the subject standing on a platform with toes extending over the edge. Passive measurements were taken in the non–weight-bearing seated position and during heel rise in standing. Mean values in the weight-bearing position were 37.0 degrees for passive MTP extension and 44.0 degrees for active extension, compared with a mean value of 57.0 degrees obtained in the non–weight-bearing seated position and 58 degrees during heel rise in the standing position. Similar to the effects of different testing positions on ankle ROM, the results showed that the positions could not be used interchangeably, with the exception of the heel rise and seated non–weight-bearing positions.

Injury/Disease

Wilson and Gansneder[33] measured physical impairments (loss of passive ankle dorsiflexion, plantarflexion ROM, and swelling), functional limitations, and disability duration in 21 athletes with acute ankle sprains. ROM loss was obtained by subtracting the passive ROM total of the affected ankle from the passive ROM measurements taken on the unaffected ankle. The authors found that the combination of ROM loss and swelling predicted an acceptable estimate of disability duration, accounting for one third of the variance. Functional limitation measures alone provided a better estimate of disability duration, accounting for 67 percent of the variance in the number of days the athletes were unable to work after the acute ankle sprain.

Morrison and Kaminski[34] reviewed the literature for the years 1965 to 2005 for information that identified the risk factors for acute and chronic ankle inversion injuries and for the role that the foot played in these types of injuries. The authors found that the most commonly identified risk factors were a high longitudal arch, large foot width, cavovarus foot deformity, open chain large calcaneal eversion ROM in women, subtalar joint instability, and a large ROM in MTP extension. However, the authors suggested that a great deal of research was necessary to adequately evaluate these risk factors.

Kaufman and associates[35] tracked 449 trainees at a Naval Special Warfare Training Center to determine whether an association existed between foot structure and the development of musculoskeletal overuse injuries of the lower extremities. Restricted dorsiflexion ROM was one of the five risk factors associated with overuse injury.

Chesworth and Vandervoort[36] measured dorsiflexion ROM after ankle fractures due to snowboarding accidents. They found that large differences occurred in the maximum passive dorsiflexion ROM between fractured ankles and the contralateral uninvolved ankles. Maximum passive dorsiflexion was defined as that point just prior to the initiation of muscle activity in the plantarflexor muscles. The authors hypothesized that the reflex length-tension relationship was altered in the fractured ankles and that this reflex activity acted as a protective mechanism to prevent overstretching of the fragile plantarflexors after a period of immobilization.

Reynolds and colleagues[37] found that in rats, 6 weeks of immobilization of a healthy hind limb resulted in a significant (70 percent) loss of dorsiflexion ROM when a fixed torque was applied. The authors suggested that loss of extensibility of the musculotendinous unit was probably caused by tissue remodeling that occurred during extended immobilization.

Hastings and coworkers[38] studied a single patient with diabetes mellitus who had received a tendo-achilles lengthening procedure. The operation resulted in an increase in dorsiflexion ROM with the knee extended from a preoperative level of 0 degrees to a 7-month postoperative level of 18 degrees. Plantar pressure during gait was considerably reduced by 55 percent when the patient was wearing shoes, and the patient's scores on the performance of a number of functional tasks was improved by 24 percent.

Salsich, Mueller, and Sahrmann[39] found that patients with diabetes mellitus and peripheral neuropathy demonstrated less dorsiflexion ROM (extensibility of the musculotendinous unit) than a group of age-matched control subjects. Salsich, Brown, and Mueller[40] determined that there was a positive relationship between body size and passive plantar flexor muscle stiffness.

Rao and colleagues[41] compared ankle ROM and stiffness in 25 individuals with diabetes mellitus (mean age 54 years) and 64 people without diabetes who were similar in age and gender. Significantly lower peak dorsiflexion ROM and higher passive ankle stiffness were found in the group with diabetes compared to the controls. Peak dorsiflexion with the knee extended was 13 degrees in the group with diabetes and 21 degrees in the controls. Peak dorsiflexion with the knee flexed was 20 degrees in the group with diabetes and 28 degrees in controls. The authors suggested that the resistance to passive elongation may be attributed to change in the properties of the contractile and elastic elements of the plantarflexors in people with diabetes.

Functional Range of Motion

An adequate ROM at the ankle, foot, and toes is necessary for normal gait. At least 10[42,43] to 15[44] degrees of dorsiflexion is necessary in the stance phase of gait so that the tibia can advance over the foot (Table 10.8), and 15 degrees of plantarflexion is necessary in preswing phase of gait.[42] Five degrees of eversion is necessary at loading response to unlock the midtarsal joint for shock absorption.[42] When the midtarsal joint is unlocked, the foot is able to accommodate to various surfaces by tilting medially and laterally. In normal walking the first toe extends at every step, and it has been estimated that this MTP extension occurs about 900 times in walking a mile.[45] About 30 degrees of extension is required at the MTP joints in the terminal stance phase of gait. In preswing, extension at the MTP joints reaches a maximum of approximately 60 degrees when the toes maintain contact with the floor after heel rise. The subject standing on her toes in Figure 10.58 has

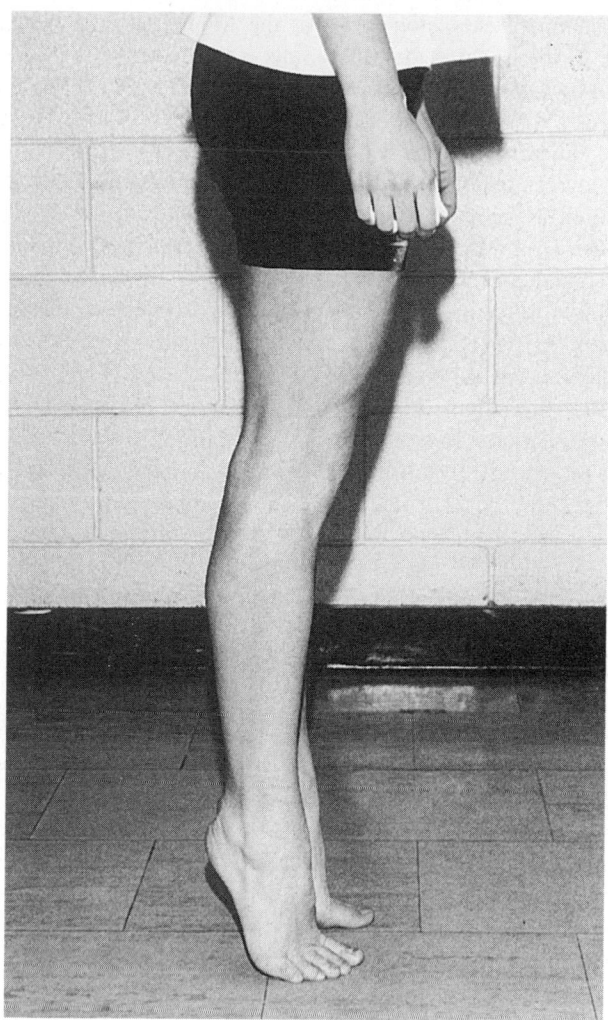

FIGURE 10.58 Standing on tiptoe requires a full range of motion in plantarflexion and 58 to 60 degrees of extension[32] at the first metatarsophalangeal joint.

TABLE 10.8	Range of Ankle Motion Necessary for Functional Locomotor Activities: Values in Degrees		
	Gait Level Surfaces	**Stair Ascent**	**Stair Descent**
Dorsiflexion	0–10 (Murray) [43]	14–27 (Livingston et al)* [48]	21–36 (Livingston et al)* [48]
	0–10 (Rancho Los Amigos) [42]	15–25 (McFayden and Winter)* [47]	21.1 (Protopadaki et al) †[49]
	0–15 (Ostrosky et al) [44]	11.2 (Protopadaki et al) † [49]	
Plantarflexion	15–30 (Murray)* [43]	23–30 (Livingston et al)*[48]	24–31 (Livingston et al)* [48]
	0–15 (Rancho Los Amigos) [42]	15–25 (McFayden and Winter)* [47]	40.1 (Protopadaki et al) †[49]
	0–31 (Ostrosky et al) [44]	31.3 (Protopadaki et al)†[49]	

* Range of maximum mean angles observed during the activity.
† Mean maximum angle observed during the activity.

an adequate extension ROM at the MTP joints for normal gait. If the ROM at the MTP joints is limited, it will interfere with forward progression, and the step length of the contralateral leg will be decreased.[42]

Running requires 0 to 20 degrees of dorsiflexion and 0 to 30 degrees of plantarflexion.[46] These ROMs are similar to the amount of motion required for stair ascent and descent, as shown in Table 10.8. Ascending stairs requires between 11 and 27 degrees of dorsiflexion,[47] whereas descending stairs requires a maximum of between 21 and 36 degrees of dorsiflexion[48] (Fig. 10.59) and between 24 and 40 degrees of plantarflexion.[49] The height of the stair risers will affect the amount of ROM required. Another activity requiring maximum dorsiflexion is rising from a chair (Fig. 10.60).

In a study by Lark and associates,[50] six elderly and six young subjects performed a stepping-down task from a range of stair heights. At all stair heights, the maximum dorsiflexion angle during descent was significantly greater in the elderly than in the younger subjects. The authors determined that the elderly used 200 percent of their passive dorsiflexion ROM so that they could spend more time in foot flat to increase their stability.

Mecagni and colleagues[51] suggested that decreases in dorsiflexion ROM constituted a risk factor for decreased balance and alteration of movement patterns. Hastings and coworkers[38] identified limited dorsiflexion ROM as a risk factor for increased plantar pressures during walking and decreased functional performance in patients with diabetes mellitus.

Torburn, Perry, and Gronley[52] found that when subjects assumed a relaxed, one-legged standing position in three trials, they stood with the rearfoot in approximately the same everted position (mean of 9.8 degrees). This position of the rearfoot during one-legged standing could be used as an indication of the maximum eversion ROM needed for the single support phase of gait. Garbalosa and associates[53] measured forefoot–rearfoot frontal plane relationships in 234 feet (120 healthy males and females with a mean age of 28.1 years).

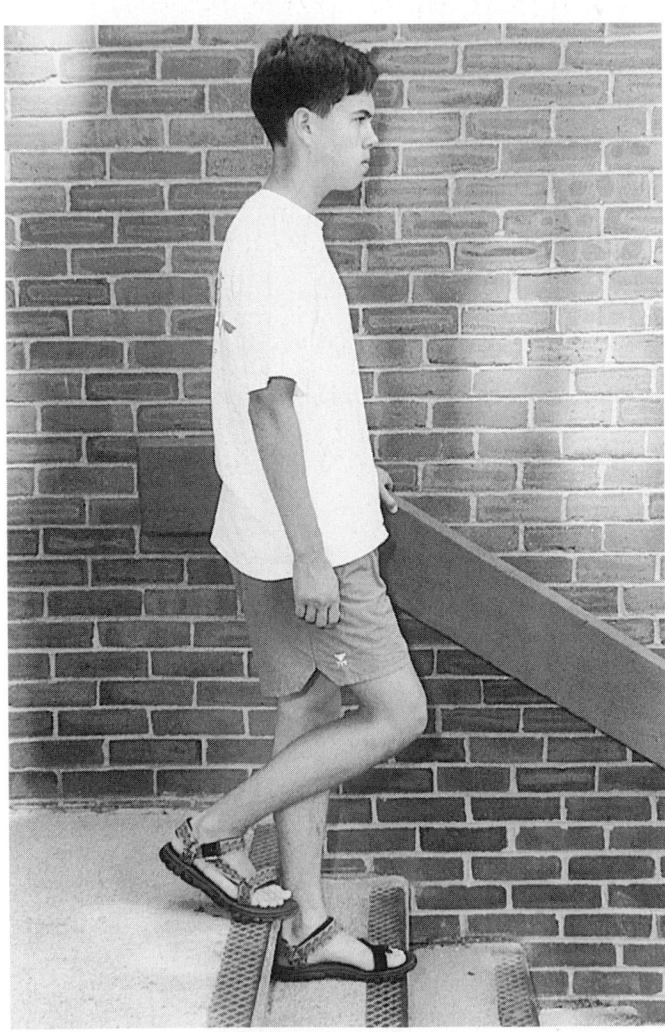

FIGURE 10.59 Descending stairs requires an average of 21 to 36 degrees of dorsiflexion.[48]

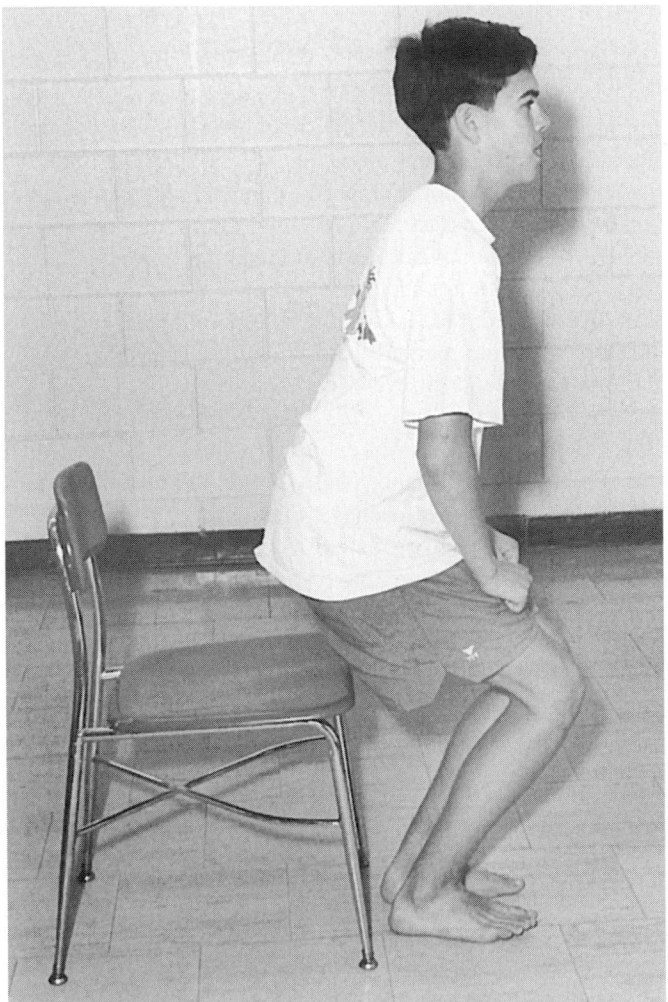

FIGURE 10.60 Getting out of a chair may require a full dorsiflexion range of motion (ROM), depending on the height of the chair seat. The lower the seat, the greater the ROM required.

Approximately 87 percent of the measured feet had forefoot varus, 8.8 percent had forefoot valgus, and 4.6 percent had a neutral forefoot–rearfoot relationship.

Hemmerich and associates,[54] in a study of activities of daily living in a non-Western culture, found that the largest mean dorsiflexion angle required by 30 Indian subjects was 39.7 degrees for kneeling with the ankles dorsiflexed. Squatting with the heels down required 38.5 degrees of dorsiflexion. These amounts of dorsiflexion are much larger than required for many activities of daily living in Western cultures, such as getting in and out of a chair or bed or walking up and down stairs. Cross-legged sitting on the floor is another common posture assumed in non–Western cultures, and that activity was found to require a maximum angle of 17 degrees of eversion. Because health-care workers are apt to encounter people of many different cultures, it is important that they are aware that other cultures may require different ROM goals for rehabilitation.

Reliability and Validity

Reliability studies involving one or more motions at the ankle have been conducted on healthy subjects[13,56–60] and on patient populations.[66–68] Also, motions of the subtalar joint, the subtalar joint neutral position, and the forefoot position have been investigated.

In 2004 Martin and McPoil[55] reviewed the existing ankle literature and found ample evidence for intratester reliability for dorsiflexion and plantarflexion ROM, some evidence for intertester reliability of dorsiflexion, but little evidence of intertester reliability for plantarflexion ROM. The authors also determined that subject diagnosis, with the exception of cerebral palsy, did not appear to affect intratester reliability. Training sessions prior to measurement appeared to have a positive effect on intrarater reliability. However, the authors concluded that on the basis of the literature review, the responsiveness of ankle measurements was uncertain.

Reliability: Dorsiflexion and Plantarflexion in Healthy Populations

Some joints and motions can be measured more reliably than others. Boone and associates[56] found that intratester reliability for selected motions at the ankle was better than that obtained for hip and wrist motions, but it was not as good as that obtained for selected motions at the shoulder, elbow, and knee.

Clapper and Wolf[57] found that both the universal goniometer and the OrthoRanger (Orthotronics, Daytona Beach, FL) were reliable instruments for measuring dorsiflexion and plantarflexion but that the intraclass correlation coefficients (ICCs) were higher for the universal goniometer. The ICC for measurements of active dorsiflexion for the universal goniometer was 0.92, in comparison with 0.80 for the OrthoRanger. The ICC for the universal goniometer for plantarflexion was 0.96, whereas the ICC for the OrthoRanger was 0.93.

Bennell and colleagues[58] determined intertester and intratester reliability using the weight-bearing lunge method for measuring dorsiflexion. Four examiners used an inclinometer to measure the angle between the anterior border and the vertical border of the tibia and a tape measure to determine the distance of the lunging toe from the wall. Intratester and intertester reliability was extremely high (ICC = 0.97 to 0.99) for the four examiners with both methods of assessment (Table 10.9).

Three testers in a study by Evans and Scutter[60] used visual estimation to assess dorsiflexion ROM in 29 healthy children ages 4 to 6 years. The estimates were made with children in the prone position with the knee both flexed and extended. Intertester reliability of measures in both positions was very poor and highly variable between testers.

Alanen and colleagues[13] used a universal goniometer to assess the ROM of the ankle in 245 healthy children ages 7 to 14 years. Passive dorsiflexion was measured in the prone position with the knee extended and flexed. Plantarflexion was measured in the supine position. Dorsiflexion in the weight-bearing position was measured from photographs. The range of ICCs varied from a low of 0.51 for right eversion to 0.88 for weight-bearing dorsiflexion measurements.

Reliability: Dorsiflexion and Plantarflexion in Patient Populations

Allington, Leroy, and Doneux[61] had two testers follow a strict protocol to assess intratester and intertester reliability and reproducibility of ankle ROM in 24 children ages 3 to 14 years with cerebral palsy. Pearson's correlation coefficients for intratester and intertester reliability for both the universal goniometer and visual estimates were excellent (r >90) for dorsiflexion with the knee flexed and extended. The Pearson's correlation coefficients for intratester and intertester reliability for plantarflexion for both goniometric and visual estimates were in the good category (r >0.80) and in the fair to good category for inversion and eversion. The SEM for dorsiflexion and plantarflexion was 4 to 5 degrees; the SEM for eversion was 6 to 9 degrees; and the SEM for inversion was 5 to 9 degrees. Even though both goniometric and visual estimates were reliable, the mean measurement error of 5 degrees plus the standard deviation of 5 degrees produced a 0- to 10.degree error that would have to be taken into account in clinical decision-making.

McWhirk and Glanzman[62] assessed intertester reliability of measurements of ankle dorsiflexion in 25 children (ages 2 to 18 years) with spastic cerebral palsy. The two therapists who took the measurements succesively on the same day helped each other hold the limbs at end range. Intertester reliability was very good, with an ICC = 0.87 and a mean absolute difference of 3.6 degrees. The 95 percent confidence interval around the mean absolute difference was ±1.2 degrees.

Mutlu, Livanelioglu, and Gunel[63] assessed the intratester and intertester reliability of goniometric measurements of ankle dorsiflexion that were taken by three therapists in 38 children (ages 18 to 108 months) with spastic cerebral palsy. The therapists used a 360-degree universal goniometer to measure dorsiflexion once in two different sessions a week apart. Intratester reliability was determined using Pearson's

TABLE 10.9 Intratester and Intertester Reliability: Dorsiflexion

Authors	n	Sample	Position	Intra ICC	Inter ICC	SEM
Bennell et al[58]	13	Healthy adults (mean age 18.8 yrs)	Weight bearing lunge with knee flexed	0.98	0.97	1.1° (Intra) 1.4° (Inter)
Clapper and Wolfe[56]	20	Healthy adults (20–36 yrs)		0.92		
McPoil and Cornwall[28]	27	Healthy adults (mean age 26.1 yrs)	Knee flexed to 90° Knee extended	0.97 0.98		
Jonson and Gross[25]	18	Healthy adults (18–30 yrs)	Knee extended— prone position	0.74	0.65	
Salsich et al[39]	34	One-half healthy/ one-half with diabetes mellitus (59–63 yrs)	Knee extended— prone position	0.95		
Elveru et al[64]	43	Patients with orthopedic or neurological problems (12–81 yrs)	Passive ROM— no standard position used	0.90	0.50	
Youdas et al[65]	38	Patients with orthopedic problems (13–71 yrs)	Active ROM— no standard position used*	0.64–0.96 Median 0.83	0.28	

ICC = Intertester or intertester correlation coefficient, as noted; ROM = range of motion;
  SEM = standard error of the measurement.
* Knee was extended in 87.7 percent of measurement sessions.

reliability coefficient (r) and ICCs. The r values ranged from 0.65 to 0.81, and ICCs ranged from 0.81 to 0.90, with the most experienced tester obtaining the highest reliability. Intertester reliability r values ranged from 0.65 to 0.75, and the ICC value was very good (0.88). Based on the findings of this study and the previous study, it appears to be possible to obtain reliable goniometric measurements in this population of children with spastic cerebral palsy. The authors suggested that this study needs to be followed with a validity study.

Elveru and associates[64] employed 12 physical therapists using universal goniometers to measure the passive ankle ROM in 43 patients with either neurological or orthopedic problems. The ICCs for intratester reliability for inversion and eversion were 0.74 and 0.75, respectively, and intertester reliability was poor (see Tables 10.9, 10.10, and 10.11). Intertester reliability also was poor for dorsiflexion, and patient diagnosis affected the reliability of dorsiflexion measurements. Sources of error were identified as variable amounts of force being exerted by the therapist, resistance to

movement in neurological patients, and difficulties encountered by the examiner in maintaining the foot and ankle in the desired position while holding the goniometer. It would appear that the latter problem could be solved by having another person either maintain the foot and ankle in position or hold the goniometer.

Youdas, Bogard, and Suman[65] used 10 examiners in a study to determine the intratester and intertester reliability for active ROM in dorsiflexion and plantarflexion. The authors compared measurements made by a universal goniometer with visual estimates on 38 patients with orthopedic problems. Fair to excellent reliability was noted when repeated measurements were made by the same therapist using a goniometer. Reliability was higher using the mean of two repeated measurements than using one measurement. A considerable measurement error was found to exist when two or more therapists made either repeated goniometric or visual estimates of the ankle ROM on the same patient (see Tables 10.9 and 10.10). Therapists used various patient

TABLE 10.10 Intratester and Intertester Reliability: Plantarflexion

Author	n	Sample	Type of Motion	Intra ICC	Inter ICC
Clapper and Wolf[57]	20	Healthy adults (20–36 yrs)	Active ROM	0.96	—
Elveru et al[64]	43	Patients with orthopedic or neurological problems (12–81 yrs)	Passive ROM	0.86	0.72
Youdas et al[65]	38	Patients with orthopedic problems (13–71 yrs)	Active ROM	0.47–0.98 Median 0.87	0.25

ICC = intertester or intratester coefficient, as noted.; ROM = range of motion

positions and goniometer alignment methods. The authors suggested that the same therapist should make two goniometric measurements and record the average value when making repeated measurements of ankle ROM.

Reliability: Eversion and Inversion

The subtalar joint neutral position, which has been the subject of numerous studies, is not the same as the 0 starting position for the subtalar joint as used in this book and many others, including those of the AAOS,[3,4] the AMA,[5] and Clarkson.[66] The subtalar joint neutral position is defined as one in which the calcaneus inverts twice as many degrees as it everts. According to Elveru and associates,[67] this position can be found when the head of the talus either cannot be palpated or is equally extended at the medial and lateral borders of the talonavicular joint. This is the position usually used in the casting of foot orthotics, but it also has been used for measurement of joint motion. However, Elveru, Rothstein, and Lamb[64] found that referencing passive ROM measurements for inversion and eversion to the subtalar joint neutral position consis-

tently reduced reliability (see Table 10.11). Based on the study of Elveru, Rothstein, and Lamb[64] and information from the following studies, we have decided not to use the subtalar neutral position as defined by Elveru and associates[67] in this text.

Bailey, Perillo, and Forman[68] used tomography to study the subtalar joint neutral position in 2 female and 13 male volunteers aged 20 to 30 years. These authors found that the neutral subtalar joint position was quite variable in relation to the total ROM and that it was not always found at one third of the total ROM from the maximally everted position. Furthermore, the neutral position varied not only from subject to subject but also between right and left sides of each subject.

Picciano, Rowlands, and Worrell[69] conducted a study to determine the intratester and intertester reliability of measurements of open-chain and closed-chain subtalar joint neutral positions. Both ankles of 15 volunteer subjects (with a mean age of 27 years) were measured by two inexperienced physical therapy students. The students had a 2-hour training session using a universal goniometer prior to data collection. The method of taking measurements was based on the work of Elveru and

TABLE 10.11 Intratester and Intertester Reliability: Inversion and Eversion

Author	n	Sample	Motion	Intra ICC	Inter ICC
McPoil and Cornwall[28]	27	Healthy adults (mean age 26.1 yrs)	Inversion Eversion	0.95 0.96	—
Torburn et al[52]	42	—	Inversion Eversion	—	0.37 0.39
Menadue et al[7]	60 ankles	Nonacute ankle conditions in 11 of the 30 subjects (ages 21–59 years)	Inversion in sitting Eversion in sitting Inversion prone Eversion prone	0.92, 0.91, 0.96 0.90, 0.82, 0.93 0.94, 0.94, 0.94 0.94, 0.83, 0.88	0.73 (0.61–0.82) 0.62 (0.49–0.74) 0.54 (0.33–0.70) 0.41 (0.25–0.56)
Elveru et al[64]	43	Patients with orthopedic and neurological problems	Inversion Eversion	0.62* 0.74 0.59* 0.75	0.15* 0.32 0.12* 0.17

ICC = Intertester and intratester correlation coefficient as noted.
* Referenced to subtalar joint neutral.

associates.[67] Intratester reliability of open-chain measurements of the subtalar joint neutral position was an ICC of 0.27 for one tester and ICC of 0.06 for the other tester. Intertester reliability was 0.00. Intratester and intertester reliability also were poor for closed-kinematic-chain measurements. The authors[69] concluded that subtalar joint neutral measurements taken by inexperienced testers were unreliable; they recommended that clinicians should practice taking measurements and performing repeated measurements to determine their own reliability for these measurements. However, Torburn, Perry, and Gronley[52] suggested that inaccuracy of measurement technique with use of a universal goniometer, rather than the ability of examiners to position the subtalar joint in the neutral position, might be responsible for poor reliability findings for subtalar joint neutral positioning. The ICC for intertester reliability for three examiners was an ICC of 0.76 for positioning the subtalar joint in the neutral position. In this study, the examiners palpated the head of the talus in 10 subjects lying in the prone position while an electrogoniometer was used to record the position (see Table 10.11). already inserted Table 10.11

Keenan, App, and Bach[70] used a prone measurement position system described by Elveru et al[67] to assess the non–weight-bearing subtalar neutral position and subtalar inversion and eversion in 24 healthy subjects. Static and dynamic measurements were made on two different occasions by four experienced clinicians using a universal goniometer. Intertester reliability was poor and so was test-retest reliability for static measurements. Reliability was also poor for visual assessments of dynamic measurements. The most experienced clinician had the highest overall reliability, whereas the clinician with only a year's experience had the lowest reliability. However, the same trend was not evident in static measurements.

In contrast to the low reliability found in the aforementioned studies, McPoil and Cornwall[46] found high intratester reliability for both subtalar inversion and eversion ROM measurements taken by two testers (see Table 10.11).

Menadue and colleagues[7] assessed active inversion and eversion ROM in the prone lying position with the ankle over the edge of the table. The 30 subjects in the study had both ankles measured by three testers using a blinded universal goniometer. Test and retest measurements were made 2 weeks apart. Within-session intratester reliability for inversion was excellent (ICC = 0.94) for all testers, whereas intratester reliability for eversion was slightly lower and ranged from good (ICC = 0.83) to excellent (ICC = 0.96) among the three testers. Intertester reliability ranged from poor (ICC = 0.33) to fair (ICC = 0.70) for inversion and was unacceptable for eversion. Between-sessions measurement error ranged from 4 degrees to 8 degrees. (See Table 10.11 for additional information.)

Validity: Eversion, Inversion, Dorsiflexion, and Plantarflexion

We are unaware of any studies that compared ankle and foot ROM values measured with a universal goniometer to values measured with radiographs. However, eversion and inversion values measured with a universal goniometer have been compared to values taken with another device. Menadue and colleagues[7] found low correlations between full-cycle active inversion and eversion measurements taken with the 3Space Fastrak electromagnetic tracking system and the universal goniometer. Only 18 percent of the variance in Fastrak measurements could be explained by the goniometric measurements. The discrepancy between the goniometric and Fastrak measurements may be partially explained by the fact that the Fastrak system records motion in all planes, whereas the universal goniometer measures motion in one plane.

Ankle ROM values have been compared to functional assessment measures. Mecagni and coworkers[51] assessed active assistive and passive ankle ROM and balance performance using the Performance Oriented Mobility Assessment (POMA) in 34 healthy elderly women ages 64 to 87 years. Correlations between the POMA gait subtest indicated that all ankle motions contributed to the maintenance of balance during gait: inversion (r = 0.50), dorsiflexion with knee flexed (r = 0.44), plantarflexion (r = 0.42), and eversion (r = 0.32). Active assistive ROM had higher correlations compared to passive ROM. The highest correlation was between active assistive ROM and the POMA gait subtest (r = 0.63).

Reliability: Metatarsophalangeal Extension

Hopson, McPoil, and Cornwall[71] conducted four static clinical tests to measure extension ROM of the first MTP joint in 20 healthy adult subjects between 21 and 45 years of age. All measurement techniques were found to be reliable but not interchangeable. Approximately 65 degrees of first MTP extension was required for normal walking as determined from video recordings. The values from the four clinical tests of first MTP extension ROM exceeded the amount required for walking.

Validity: Metatarsophalangeal Extension

No studies were noted that examined the concurrent validity of MTP motions measured with a universal goniometer to radiographs. Construct validity of clinical measures of first MTP extension ROM to indicate ROM during gait have been initally explored.[71,32] Nawoczenski, Baumjauer, and Umberger[32] used four clinical tests to measure the first MTP joint extension: active and passive ROM and heel rise in the weight-bearing position, and passive ROM in the non–weight-bearing position. Test values were compared with measurements of MTP extension during normal walking. Active ROM in the weight-bearing position (44 degrees) and extension measured during heel rise (58 degrees) had the strongest correlations with motion of the MTP joint (42 degrees) during normal walking (r = 0.80 and 0.87, respectively).

REFERENCES

1. Levangie, PK, and Norkin, CC: Joint Structure and Function: A Comprehensive Analysis, ed 4. FA Davis, Philadelphia, 2005.
2. Cyriax, JM, and Cyriax, PJ: Illustrated Manual of Orthopaedic Medicine. Butterworths, London, 1983.
3. American Academy of Orthopaedic Surgeons: Joint Motion: Method of Measuring and Recording. AAOS, Chicago, 1965
4. Greene, WB, and Heckman, JD (eds): The Clinical Measurement of Joint Motion: American Academy of Orthopaedic Surgeons, Chicago, 1994.
5. American Medical Association: Guides to the Evaluation of Permanent Impairment, ed 3 (revised). AMA, Chicago, 1988.
6. Boone, DC, and Azen, SP: Normal range of motion of joints in male subjects. J Bone Joint Surg Am 61:756, 1979.
7. Menadue, C, et al: Reliabililty of two goniometric methods of measuring active inversion and eversion range of motion at the ankle. BMC Musculoskelet Diord 7:60, 2006.
8. Waugh, KG, et al: Measurement of selected hip, knee and ankle joint motions in newborns. Phys Ther 63:1616, 1983.
9. Wanatabe, H, et al: The range of joint motion of the extremities in healthy Japanese people: The differences according to age. Nippon Seikeigeka Gakkai Zasshi 53:275, 1979. (Cited in Walker, JM: Musculoskeletal development: A review. Phys Ther 71:878, 1991.)
10. Boone, DC: Techniques of measurement of joint motion. (Unpublished supplement to Boone, DC, and Azen, SP: Normal range of motion in male subjects. J Bone Joint Surg Am 61:756, 1979.)
11. Walker, JM: Musculoskeletal development: A review. Phys Ther 71:878, 1991.
12. Boone, DC, Walker, JM, and Perry, J: Age and sex differences in lower extremity joint motion. Presented at the National Conference, American Physical Therapy Association, Washington, DC, 1981.
13. Alancn, JT, et al: Ankle joint complex mobility of children 7-14 years old. J Pediatr Orthop 21:731, 2001.
14. Saxena, A, and Kim, W: Ankle dorsiflexion in the adolescent. J Am Podiatr Med Assoc 93:312, 2003.
15. James, B, and Parker, AW: Active and passive mobility of lower limb joints in elderly men and women. Am J Phys Med Rehabil 68:162, 1989.
16. Gajdosik, RL, VanderLinden, DW, and Williams, AK: Influence of age on length and passive elastic stiffness: Characteristics of the calf muscletendon unit of women. Phys Ther 79:827, 1999.
17. Gajdosik, RL, et al: Slow passive stretch and release characteristics of the calf muscles of older women with limited dorsiflexion range of motion. Clin Biomech 19:398, 2004.
18. Nigg, BM, et al: Range of motion of the foot as a function of age. Foot Ankle 613:336, 1992.
19. Bell, RD, and Hoshizaki, TB: Relationships of age and sex with range of motion of seventeen joint actions in humans. Can J Appl Sport Sci 6:202, 1981.
20. Walker, JM, et al: Active mobility of the extremities of older subjects. Phys Ther 64:919, 1984.
21. Vandervoort, AA, et al: Age and sex effects on the mobility of the human ankle. J Gerontol 476:M17, 1992.
22. Baggett, BD, and Young, G: Ankle joint dorsiflexion. Establishment of a normal range. J Am Podiatr Med Assoc 83:251, 1993.
23. Grimston, SK, et al: Differences in ankle joint complex range of motion as a function of age. Foot Ankle 14:215, 1993.
24. Moseley, AN, Crosbie, J, and Adams, R: Normative data for passive plantarflexion-dorsiflexion flexibility. Clin Biomech (Bristol, Avon) 16:514, 2001.
25. Jonson, SR, and Gross, MT: Intraexaminer reliability, interexaminer reliability and mean values for nine lower extremity skeletal measures in healthy midshipmen. J Orthop Sports Phys Ther 25:253, 1997.
26. Bennell, K, et al: Hip and ankle range of motion and hip muscle strength in young female ballet dancers and controls. Br J Sports Med 33:340, 1999.
27. Ekstrand, MD, et al: Lower extremity goniometric measurements: A study to determine their reliability. Arch Phys Med Rehabil 63:171, 1982.
28. McPoil, TG, and Cornwall, MW: The relationship between static lower extremity measurements and rearfoot motion during walking. J Orthop Sports Phys Ther 24: 309, 1996.
29. Riemann, BL, et al: The effects of sex, joint angle, and the gastrocnemius muscle on passive ankle joint complex stiffness. J Athl Train 93:312, 2003.
30. Bohannon, RW, Tiberio, D, and Waters, G: Motion measured from forefoot and hindfoot landmarks during passive ankle dorsiflexion range of motion. J Orthop Sports Phys Ther 13:20, 1991.
31. Lattanza, L, Gray, GW, and Kanter, RM: Closed versus open kinematic chain measurements of subtalar joint eversion: Implications for clinical practice. J Orthop Sports Phys Ther 9:310, 1988.
32. Nawoczenski, DA, Baumhauer, JF, and Umberger, BR: Relationship between clinical measurements and motion of the first metatarsophalangeal joint during gait. J Bone Joint Surg 81:370, 1999.
33. Wilson, RW, and Gansneder, BM: Measures of functional limitation as predictors of disablement in athletes with acute ankle sprains. J Orthop Sports Phys Ther 30:528, 2000.
34. Morrison, KE, and Kaminski, TW: Foot characteristics in association with inversion ankle injury. J Athl Train 42:135, 2007.
35. Kaufman, KR, et al: The effect of foot structure and range of motion on musculoskeletal overuse injuries. Am J Sports Med 27:585, 1999.
36. Chesworth, BM, and Vandervoort, AA: Comparison of passive stiffness variables and range of motion in uninvolved and involved ankle joints of patients following ankle fractures. Phys Ther 75:253, 1995.
37. Reynolds, CA, et al: The effect of nontraumatic immobilization on ankle dorsiflexion stiffness in rats. J Orthop Sports Phys Ther 23: 27, 1996.
38. Hastings, MK, et al: Effects of a tendo-achilles lengthening procedure on muscle function and gait characteristics in a patient with diabetes mellitus. J Orthop Sports Phys Ther 30:85, 2000.
39. Salsich, GB, Mueller, MJ, and Sahrmann, SA: Passive ankle stiffness in subjects with diabetes and peripheral neuropathy versus an age matched comparison group. Phys Ther 80:352, 2000.
40. Salsich, GB, Brown, M, and Mueller, MJ: Relationship between plantarflexor muscle stiffness, strength and range of motion in subjects with diabetes; peripheral neuropathy compared to age-matched controls. J Orthop Sports Phys Ther 30: 473, 2000.
41. Rao, SR, et al: Increased passive ankle stiffness and reduced dorsiflexion range of motion in individuals with diabetes mellitus. Foot Ankle Int 27:617, 2006.
42. Pathokinesiology Service and Physical Therapy Dept: Observational Gait Analysis, ed 4. LAREI, Rancho Los Amigos National Rehabilitation Center, Downey, CA, 2001.
43. Murray, MP: Gait as a total pattern of movement. Am J Phys Med Rehabil 46:290, 1967.
44. Ostrosky, KM: A comparison of gait characteristics in young and old subjects. Phys Ther 74:637, 1994.
45. Cailliet, R: Foot and Ankle, ed 3. FA Davis, Philadelphia, 1997.
46. McPoil, TG, and Cornwall, MW: Applied sports biomechanics in rehabilitation running. In Zachazewski, JE, Magee, DJ, and Quillen, WS (eds): Athletic Injuries and Rehabilitation. WB Saunders, Philadelphia, 1996.
47. McFayden, BJ, and Winter, DA: An integrated biomechanical analysis of normal stair ascent and descent. J Biomech 21:733, 1988.
48. Livingston, LA, Stevenson, JM, and Olney, SJ: Stairclimbing kinematics on stairs of differing dimensions. Arch Phys Med Rehabil 72:398, 1991.
49. Protopapadaki, A, et al: Hip, knee, ankle kinematics and kinetics during stair ascent and descent in healthy young individuals. Clin Biomech 22:203, 2007.
50. Lark, SD, et al: Knee and ankle range of motion during stepping down in elderly compared to young men. Eur J Appl Physiol 91:287, 2004.
51. Mecagni, C, et al: Balance and ankle range of motion in community-dwelling women aged 64–87 years: A correlational study. Phys Ther 80:1004, 2000.
52. Torburn, L, Perry, J, and Gronley, J-AK: Assessment of rearfoot motion: Passive positioning, one-legged standing, gait. Foot Ankle Int 19:688, 1998.
53. Garbalosa, JC, et al: The frontal plane relationship of the forefoot to the rearfoot in an asymptomatic population. J Orthop Sports Phys Ther 20:200, 1994.
54. Hemmerich, A, Brown, H, Smith, S: Hip, knee and ankle kinematics of high range of motion activities of daily living. J Orthop Res 24:770, 2006.
55. Martin, RRL, McPoil, TG: Reliability of ankle goniometric measurements: A literature review. J Am Podiatr Med Assoc 95:564, 2005.
56. Boone, DC, et al: Reliability of goniometric measurements. Phys Ther 68:1355, 1978.
57. Clapper, MP, and Wolf, SL: Comparison of the reliability of the Orthoranger and the standard goniometer for assessing active lower extremity range of motion. Phys Ther 68:214, 1988.

58. Bennell, K, et al: Interrater and intrarater reliability of a weight-bearing lunge measure of ankle dorsiflexion. Aust Physiother 44:175, 1998.
59. Rome, K, and Cowieson, F: A reliability study of the universal goniometer, fluid goniometer, and electrogoniometer for the measurement of ankle dorsiflexion. Foot Ankle Int 17:28, 1996.
60. Evans, AM, and Scutter, SD: Sagittal plane range of motion of the pediatric ankle joint. Am Podiatr Med Assoc 96:418, 2006.
61. Allington, NJ, Leroy, N, Doneux, C: Ankle joint range of motion measurements in spastic cerebral palsy children: Intraobserver and Interobserver reliability and reproducibility of goniometry and visual estimation. J Pediatr Orthop 11:2236, 2002.
62. McWhirk, LB, and Glanzman, AM: Within-session inter-rater reliability of goniometric measures in patients with spastic cerebral palsy. Pediatr Phys Ther 18:262, 2006.
63. Mutlu, A, Livanelioglu, A, and Gunel, MK: Reliability of goniometric measurements in children with spastic cerebral palsy. Med Sci Monit 23:CR323, 2007.
64. Elveru, RA, Rothstein, J, and Lamb, RL: Goniometric reliability in a clinical setting: Subtalar and ankle joint measurements. Phys Ther 68:672, 1988.
65. Youdas, JW, Bogard, CL, and Suman, VJ: Reliability of goniometric measurements and visual estimates of ankle joint range of motion obtained in a clinical setting. Arch Phys Med Rehabil 74:1113, 1993.
66. Clarkson, HM: Musculoskeletal Assessment: Joint Range of Motion and Manual Muscle Strength, ed. 2. Lippincott Williams & Wilkins, Philadelphia, 2000.
67. Elveru, RA, et al: Methods for taking subtalar joint measurements: A clinical report. Phys Ther 68:678, 1988.
68. Bailey, DS, Perillo, JT, and Forman, M: Subtalar joint neutral: A study using tomography. J Am Podiatr Assoc 74:59, 1984.
69. Picciano, AM, Rowlands, MS, and Worrell, T: Reliability of open and closed kinetic chain subtalar joint neutral positions and navicular drop test. J Orthop Sports Phys Ther 18:553, 1993.
70. Keenan, A-M, and Bach, TM: Clinician's assessment of the hindfoot: A study of reliability. Foot Ankle Int 27:451, 2006.
71. Hopson, MM, McPoil, TG, and Cornwall, MW: Motion of the first metatarsophalangeal joint. Reliability and validity of four measurement techniques. J Am Podiatr Med Assoc 85:198, 1995.

TESTING OF THE SPINE AND TEMPOROMANDIBULAR JOINT

OBJECTIVES

ON COMPLETION OF PART IV, THE READER WILL BE ABLE TO:

1. **Identify:**
   - Appropriate planes and axes for each spinal and jaw motion
   - Expected normal end-feels
   - Structures (contractile and noncontractile) that have the potential to limit the end of the range of motion

2. **Describe:**
   - Testing positions for motions of the spine and jaw
   - Goniometer, tape measure, and inclinometer alignments
   - Capsular patterns of restrictions
   - Range of motion necessary for functional tasks

3. **Explain:**
   - How age, gender, and other factors may affect the range of motion
   - How sources of error in measurement may affect testing results

4. **Perform a range of motion assessment of the cervical spine** using the universal goniometer, tape measure, inclinometers (double and single), and cervical range of motion (CROM) device.

Perform a range of motion assessment of the thoracic and lumbar spines using the universal goniometer, tape measure, and inclinometers. Please include the following in your assessment:
- A clear explanation of the testing procedure
- Placement of the subject in the appropriate testing position
- Adequate stabilization of the proximal joint component
- Correct determination of the end of the range of motion
- Correct identification of the end-feel
- Palpation and marking of the correct bony landmarks
- Accurate alignment of the goniometer
- Correct reading and recording

5. **Perform a range of motion assessment of the temporomandibular joint** using a ruler.

6. **Assess the intratester and intertester reliability** of measurements of the spine and temporomandibular joint.

7. **Discuss the reliability and validity of range of motion measurements** using the universal goniometer, tape measure, inclinometers, CROM device, and ruler.

Chapters 11 through 13 present common clinical techniques for measuring gross motions of the cervical, thoracic, and lumbar spine and the temporomandibular joint. Evaluation of the range of motion and end-feels of individual facet joints of the spine are not included.

The Cervical Spine

Structure and Function

Atlanto-Occipital and Atlantoaxial Joints

Anatomy

The atlanto-occipital joint is composed of the right and left deep concave superior facets of the atlas (C1) that articulate with the right and left convex occipital condyles of the skull (Fig. 11.1).

The atlantoaxial joint is composed of three separate articulations: the median atlantoaxial and two lateral joints. The median atlantoaxial joint consists of an anterior facet on the dens (the odontoid process of C2) that articulates with a facet on the internal surface of the atlas (C1). The two lateral joints are composed of the right and left superior facets of the axis (C2) that articulate with the right and left slightly convex inferior facets on the atlas (C1) (Fig. 11.2).

The atlanto-occipital and atlantoaxial joints are reinforced anteriorly by the anterior-occipital and atlantoaxial membranes (Fig.11.3A) and posteriorly by the posterior atlanto-occipital, atlantoaxial, and tectorial membranes (Fig.11.3B).

Osteokinematics

The atlanto-occipital joint is a condylar synovial joint that permits active flexion–extension as a nodding motion.[1] However, a very limited amount of axial rotation and lateral flexion may be produced passively.[1] Flexion–extension takes place in the sagittal plane around a medial–lateral axis. Extremes of flexion are limited by osseous contact of the anterior ring of the foramen magnum with the dens. Normally flexion is limited by tension in the posterior neck muscles and tectorial membrane and by impaction of the submandibular tissues against the throat. Extension is limited by the occiput compressing the suboccipital muscles.[1] Combined flexion–extension is reported to be between 20 degrees[2] and 30 degrees[3] and is usually described as the amount of motion that occurs during nodding of the head. However, according to Cailliet,[4] the range of motion (ROM) in flexion is 10 degrees and the range in extension is 30 degrees. Maximum rotation at the atlanto-occipital joint is between approximately 2.5 percent and 5 percent of the total cervical spine rotation.[5] Lateral flexion is approximately 10 degrees.[2]

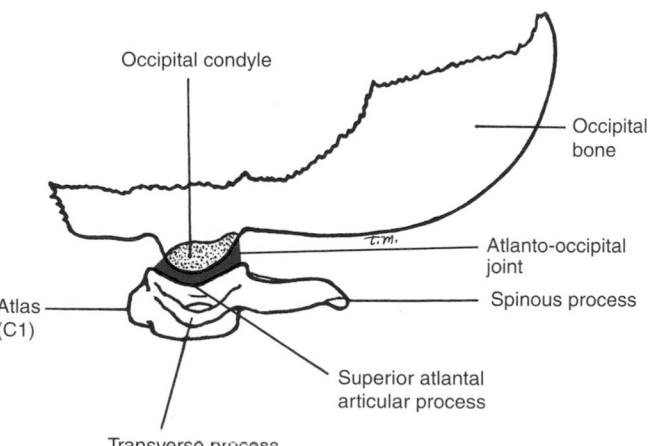

FIGURE 11.1 A lateral view of a portion of the atlanto-occipital joint shows the superior atlantal articular process of the atlas (C1) and the corresponding occipital condyle. The joint space has been widened to show the articular processes.

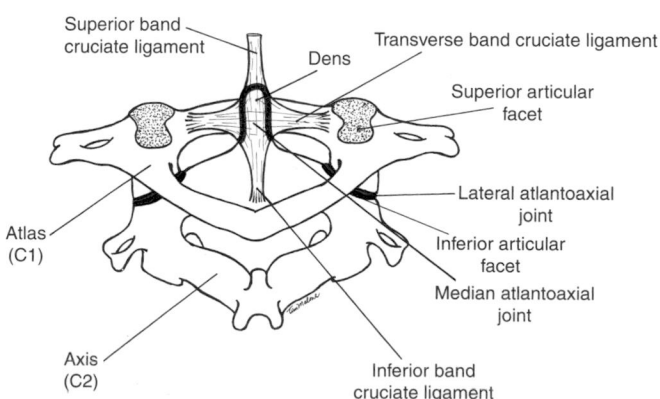

FIGURE 11.2 A posterior view of the atlantoaxial joint and the superior, inferior, and transverse bands of the cruciate ligament.

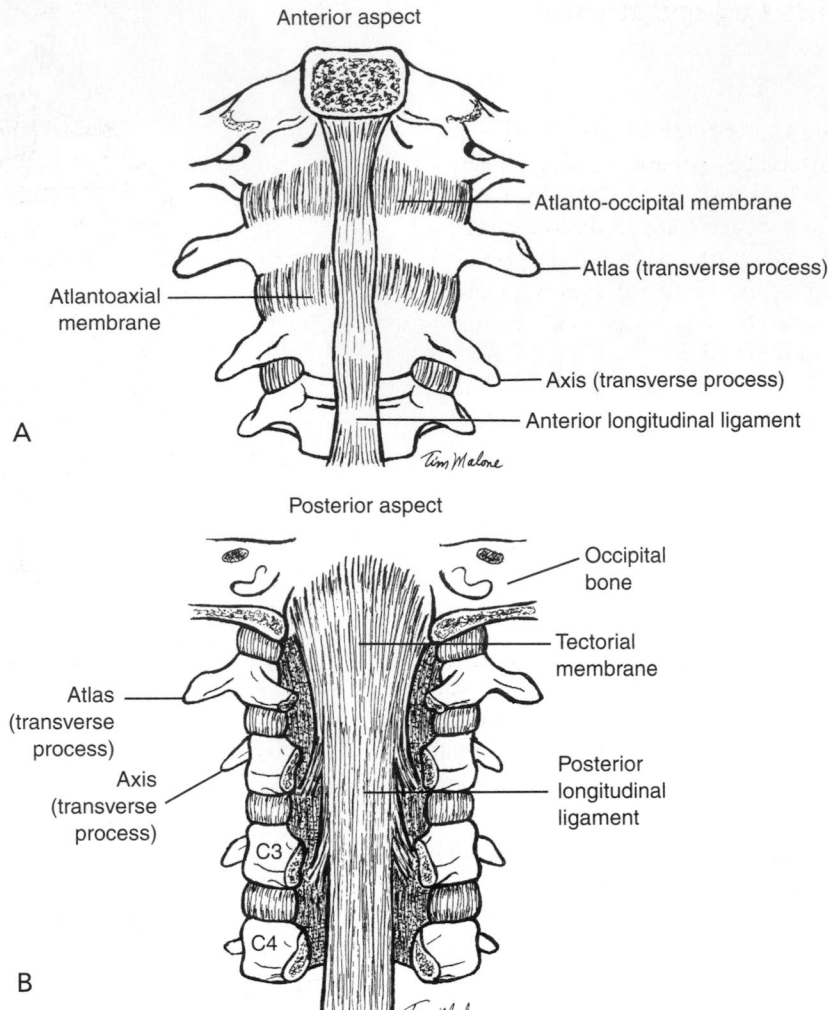

Anterior aspect

Atlanto-occipital membrane

Atlas (transverse process)

Atlantoaxial membrane

Axis (transverse process)

Anterior longitudinal ligament

A

Posterior aspect

Occipital bone

Tectorial membrane

Atlas (transverse process)

Axis (transverse process)

Posterior longitudinal ligament

C3

C4

B

FIGURE 11.3 A: The anterior atlanto-occipital and atlantoaxial membranes help to support the anterior aspect of the atlanto-occipital and atlantoaxial joints. **B:** The posterior atlanto-occipital, atlantoaxial, and tectorial membranes help to support the posterior aspect of the atlanto-occipital and atlantoaxial joints. The tectorial membrane is an extension of the posterior longitudinal ligament.

The two lateral atlantoaxial joints are plane synovial joints that allow flexion–extension, lateral flexion, and rotation. The median atlantoaxial joint is a synovial trochoid (pivot) joint that permits rotation. Approximately 55 percent of the total cervical range of rotation occurs at the atlantoaxial joint. Rotation at the median atlantoaxial joint is limited primarily by the two alar ligaments, with minor restraint being provided by the capsules of the lateral atlantoaxial joints.[1] About 45 degrees of rotation to the right and left sides are available. The motions permitted at the three atlantoaxial articulations are flexion–extension, lateral flexion, and rotation.[6]

Arthrokinematics

At the atlanto-occipital joint when the head moves on the atlas (convex surfaces moving on concave surfaces), the occipital condyles roll in the same direction as the top of the head and glide in the direction opposite to the movement of the top of the head. For example, in flexion, the occipital condyles roll anteriorly and glide posteriorly on the concave articular surfaces of the atlas. In extension, the occipital condyles roll posteriorly and glide anteriorly on the atlas and the back of the head moves posteriorly.[1]

At the lateral atlantoaxial joints the inferior zygapophyseal articular facets of the atlas are convex and articulate with the superior concave articular facets of the axis. At the median joint the atlas forms a ring with the transverse ligament (band) of the cruciate ligament, and this ring rotates around the dens (odontoid process), which serves as a pivot for rotation. The dens articulates with a small facet in the central area of the anterior arch of the atlas.

Capsular Pattern

The capsular pattern for the atlanto-occipital joint is an equal restriction of extension and lateral flexion. Rotation and flexion are not affected.[2]

Intervertebral and Zygapophyseal Joints

Anatomy

The intervertebral joints are composed of the superior and inferior surfaces of the vertebral bodies and the adjacent intervertebral discs (Fig. 11.4). The joints are reinforced anteriorly by the anterior longitudinal ligament, which limits extension (Fig. 11.5), and posteriorly by the posterior longitudinal ligament, ligamentum nuchae, ligamentum flavum, supraspinous and interspinous ligaments (Fig. 11.6), and the back extensors, which help to limit flexion.

The zygapophyseal joints are formed by the right and left superior articular facets (processes) of one vertebra and the right and left inferior articular facets of an adjacent superior vertebra (Fig. 11.7). Each joint has its own capsule and capsular ligaments, which are lax and permit a relatively large ROM. The ligamentum flavum helps to reinforce the joint capsules.

Osteokinematics

According to White and Punjabi,[7] one vertebra can move in relation to an adjacent vertebra in six different directions (three translations and three rotations) along and around three axes. The compound effects of sliding and tilting at a series of vertebrae produce a large ROM for the column as a whole, including flexion–extension, lateral flexion, and rotation. Some motions in the vertebral column are coupled with other motions; this coupling varies from region to region. A coupled motion is one in which one motion around one axis is consistently associated with another motion or motions around a different axis or axes. For example, left lateral

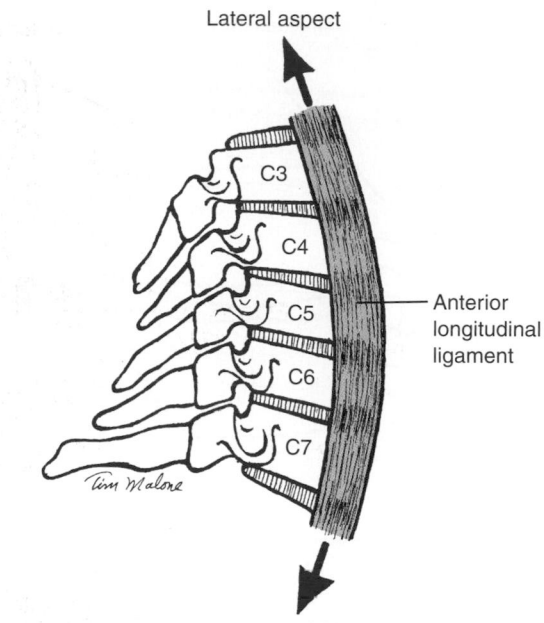

FIGURE 11.5 The anterior longitudinal ligament reinforces the anterior portion of the discs and helps to prevent extremes of extension.

flexion from C2 to C5 is accompanied by rotation to the left (spinous processes move to the right) and forward flexion. In the cervical region from C2 to C7, flexion and extension are the only motions that are not coupled.[7]

The intervertebral joints are cartilaginous joints of the symphysis type. The zygapophyseal joints are synovial plane joints. In the cervical region, the facets are oriented at 45 degrees to the transverse plane. The inferior facets of the

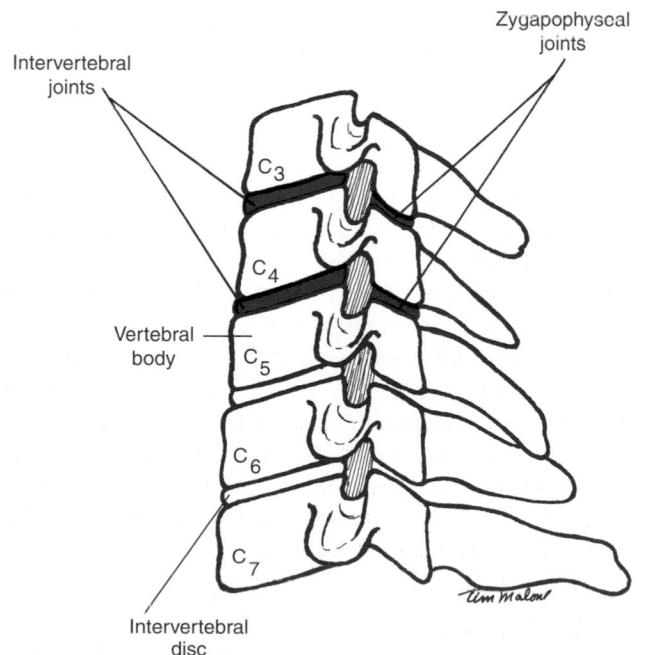

FIGURE 11.4 The lateral view of the cervical spine shows the intervertebral and zygapophyseal joints from C3 to C7.

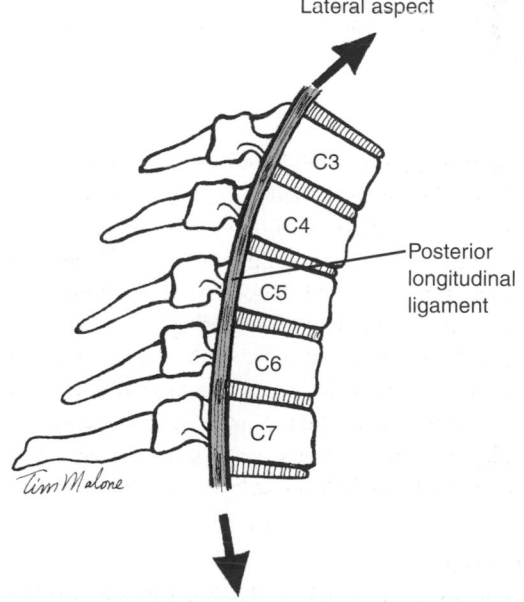

FIGURE 11.6 The posterior longitudinal ligament reinforces the posterior portion of the discs and helps to prevent extremes of forward flexion.

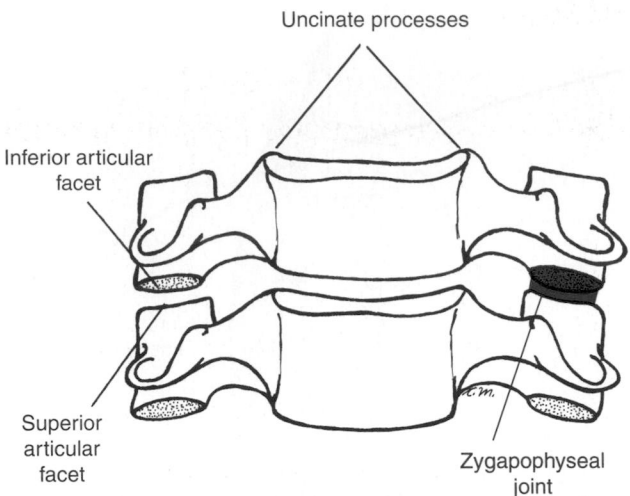

Uncinate processes

Inferior articular facet

Superior articular facet

Zygapophyseal joint

FIGURE 11.7 An anterior view of the right and left zygapophyseal joints between two cervical vertebrae. The vertebrae have been separated to provide a clear view of the inferior articular facets of the superior vertebra and the superior articular facets of the adjacent inferior vertebra.

superior vertebrae face anteriorly and inferiorly. The superior facets of the inferior vertebrae face posteriorly and superiorly. The orientation of the articular facets, which varies from region to region, determines the direction of the tilting and sliding of the vertebra, whereas the size of the disc determines the amount of motion. In addition, passive tension in a number of soft tissues and bony contacts controls and limits motions of the vertebral column. In general, although regional variations exist, the soft tissues that control and limit extremes of motion in forward flexion include the supraspinous and interspinous ligaments, zygapophyseal joint capsules, ligamentum flavum, posterior longitudinal ligament, posterior fibers of the annulus fibrosus of the intervertebral disc, and back extensors.

Extension is limited by bony contact of the spinous processes and by passive tension in the zygapophyseal joint capsules, anterior fibers of the annulus fibrosus, anterior longitudinal ligament, and anterior trunk muscles. Lateral flexion is limited by the intertransverse ligaments, by passive tension in the annulus fibrosus on the side opposite the motion on the convexity of the curve, and by the uncinate processes. Rotation is limited by fibers of the annulus fibrosus.

Arthrokinematics

The intervertebral joints permit a small amount of sliding and tilting of one vertebra on another. In all of the motions at the intervertebral joints, the nucleus pulposus of the intervertebral disc acts as a pivot for the tilting and sliding motions of the vertebrae. Flexion is a result of anterior sliding and tilting of a superior vertebra on the interposed disc of an adjacent inferior vertebra. Extension is the result of posterior sliding and tilting.

The zygapophyseal joints permit small amounts of sliding of the right and left inferior facets on the right and left superior facets of an adjacent inferior vertebra. In flexion, the inferior facets of the superior vertebrae slide anteriorly and superiorly on the superior facets of the inferior vertebrae. In extension, the inferior facets of the superior vertebrae slide posteriorly and inferiorly on the superior facets of the inferior vertebrae. In lateral flexion and rotation, one inferior facet of the superior vertebra slides inferiorly and posteriorly on the superior facet of the inferior vertebra on the side to which the spine is laterally flexed. The opposite inferior facet of the superior vertebra slides superiorly and anteriorly on the superior facet of the adjacent inferior vertebra.

Capsular Pattern

The capsular pattern for C2 to C7 is recognizable by pain and equal limitation of all motions except flexion, which is usually minimally restricted. The capsular pattern for unilateral facet involvement is a greater restriction of movement in lateral flexion to the opposite side and in rotation to the same side. For example, if the right articular facet joint capsule is involved, lateral flexion to the left and rotation to the right are the motions most restricted.[8]

Measurement of the cervical spine ROM is complicated by the region's multiple joint structure, lack of well-defined and standardized landmarks, lack of an accurate and workable definition of the neutral position, and lack of a standardized method of stabilization to isolate cervical motion from thoracic spine motion. The search for instruments and methods that are capable of providing accurate and affordable measurements of the cervical spine ROM is ongoing. Tables 11.1 through 11.4 in the Research Findings Section provide normal cervical spine ROM values from various sources and with use of a variety of methods. Additional tables and text in the Research Findings section provide ROM values by age and gender. This information is followed by functional ranges of motion and a review of research studies on the reliability and validity of the various instruments used to measure cervical range of motion.

RANGE OF MOTION TESTING PROCEDURES: Cervical Spine

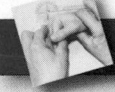 Landmarks for Testing Procedures

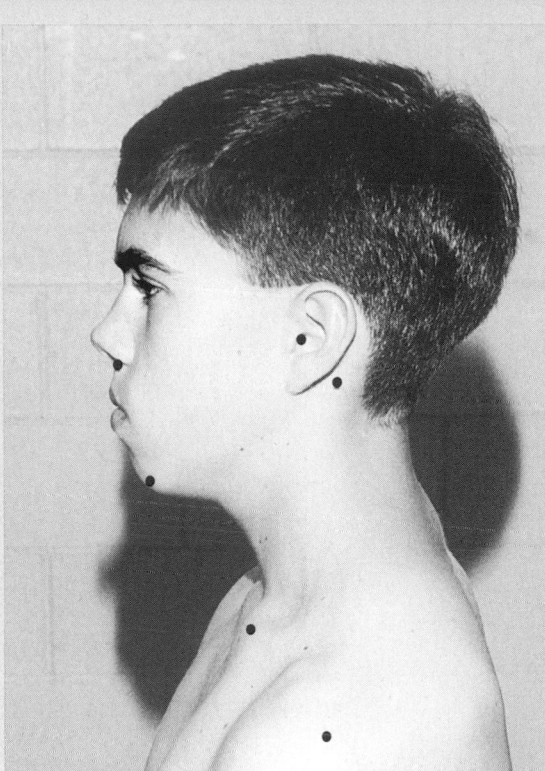

FIGURE 11.8 Surface anatomy landmarks for goniometer alignment and tape measure alignment for measuring cervical motions.

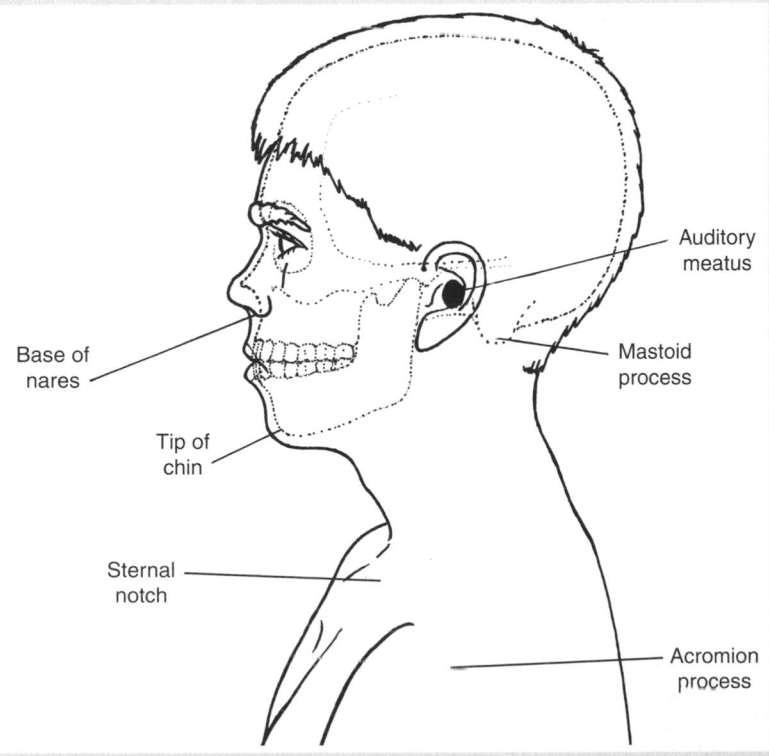

Auditory meatus

Base of nares

Mastoid process

Tip of chin

Sternal notch

Acromion process

FIGURE 11.9 Bony anatomical landmarks for goniometer alignment for measuring cervical flexion and extension.

Landmarks for Testing Procedures (continued)

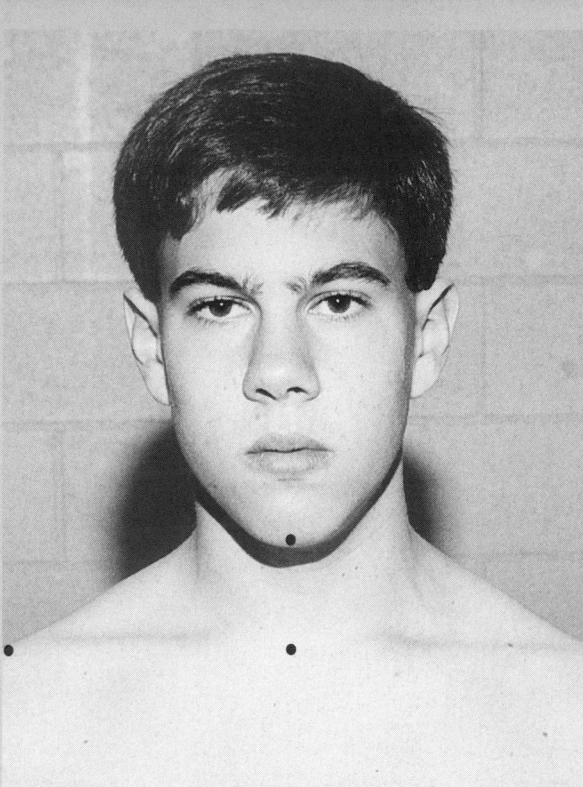

FIGURE 11.10 Surface anatomy landmarks used to measure cervical motion with a tape measure: tip of the chin, sternal notch, and acromion process. The mastoid process, which is used to measure lateral flexion, is included in Figure 11.8.

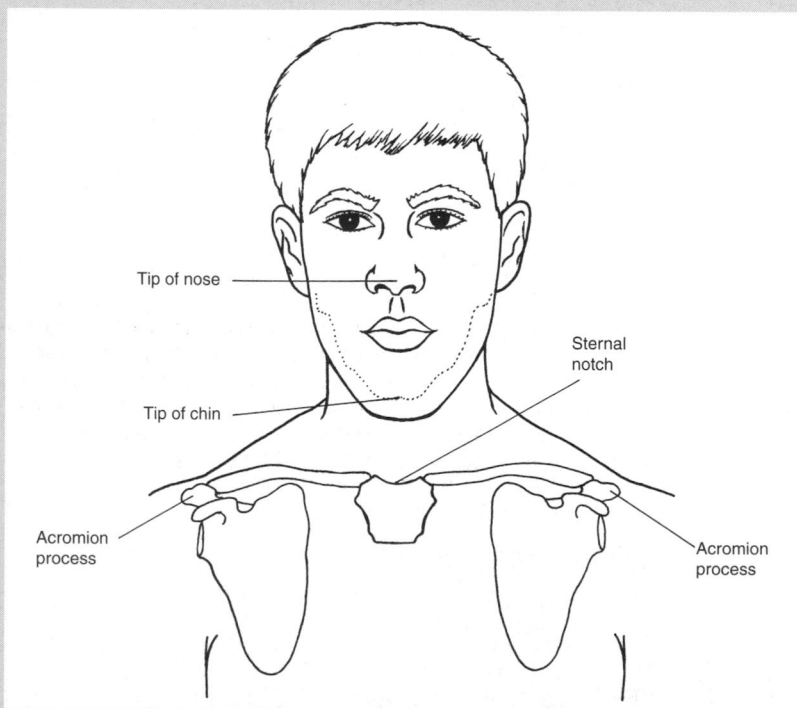

Tip of nose

Sternal notch

Tip of chin

Acromion process

Acromion process

FIGURE 11.11 Bony anatomical landmarks for measuring cervical spine range of motion with a tape measure and universal goniometer.

Landmarks for Testing Procedures (continued)

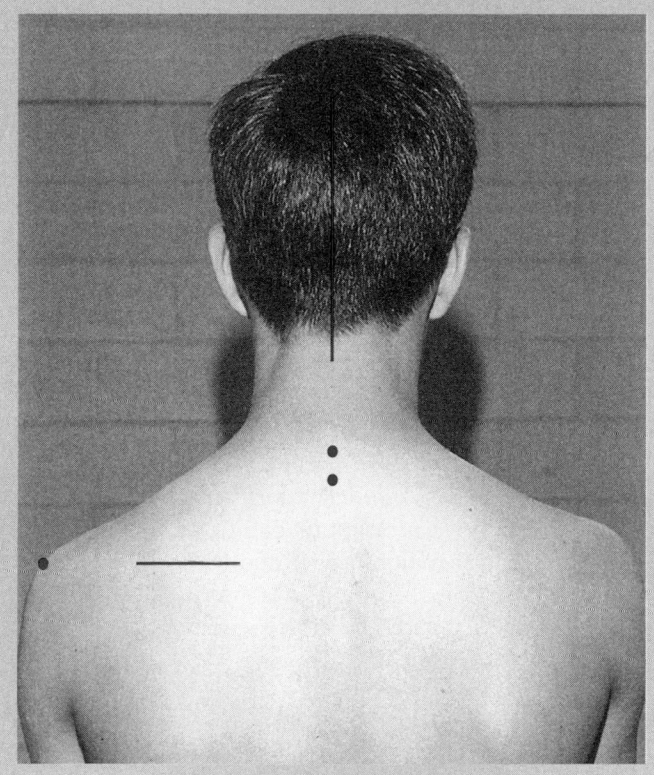

FIGURE 11.12 A posterior view of the subject's head and cervical spine shows the surface anatomy landmarks used for measuring lateral flexion with a goniometer and flexion and extension with dual inclinometers.

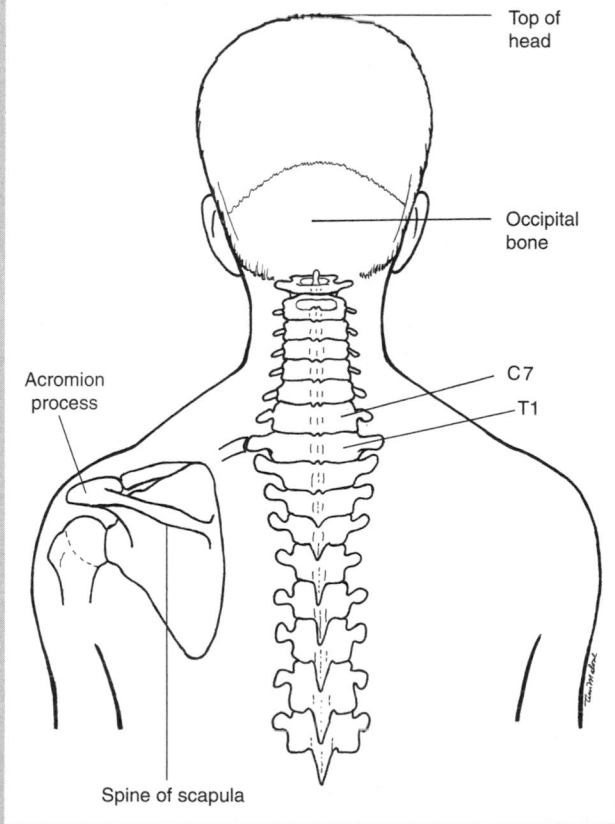

Top of head

Occipital bone

Acromion process

C7

T1

Spine of scapula

FIGURE 11.13 Bony anatomical landmarks used to align the goniometer, inclinometers, and cervical range of motion device. The goniometer uses the spinous process of the seventh cervical vertebra as a landmark for the measurement of at least one cervical motion. The inclinometers use the spinous process of the T1 vertebra.

● CERVICAL FLEXION: UNIVERSAL GONIOMETER

Motion occurs in the sagittal plane around a medial–lateral axis. The mean cervical flexion ROM measured with a universal goniometer is 40 degrees (standard deviation [SD] = 12 degrees) in adults.[9] See Youdas, Carey, and Garrett[9] in Table 11.1 in the Research Findings section for additional normal ROM values by age and gender.

Testing Position

Place the subject in the sitting position, with the thoracic and lumbar spine well supported by the back of a chair. Position the head in 0 degrees of rotation and lateral flexion.

Stabilization

Stabilize the shoulder girdle and chest by using a strap because the examiner's hands are involved in the measurement. Have the subject place his or her hands on their knees.

Testing Motion

Put one hand on the back of the subject's head and, with the other hand, hold the subject's chin. Push gently but firmly on the back of the subject's head to move the head anteriorly. Pull the subject's chin in toward the chest to move the subject through flexion ROM (Fig. 11.14). The end of the ROM occurs when resistance to further motion is felt and further attempts at flexion cause forward flexion of the trunk.

Normal End-Feel

The normal end-feel is firm owing to stretching of the posterior ligaments (supraspinous, infraspinous, ligamentum flavum, and ligamentum nuchae), posterior fibers of the annulus fibrosus in the intervertebral disks, and the zygapophyseal joint capsules and because of impaction of the submandibular tissues against the throat and passive tension in the following muscles: iliocostalis cervicis, longissimus capitis, longissimus cervicis, obliquus capitis superior, rectus capitis posterior major, rectus capitis posterior minor, semispinalis capitis, semispinalis cervicis, splenius cervicis, splenius capitis, spinalis capitis, spinalis cervicis, and upper trapezius.

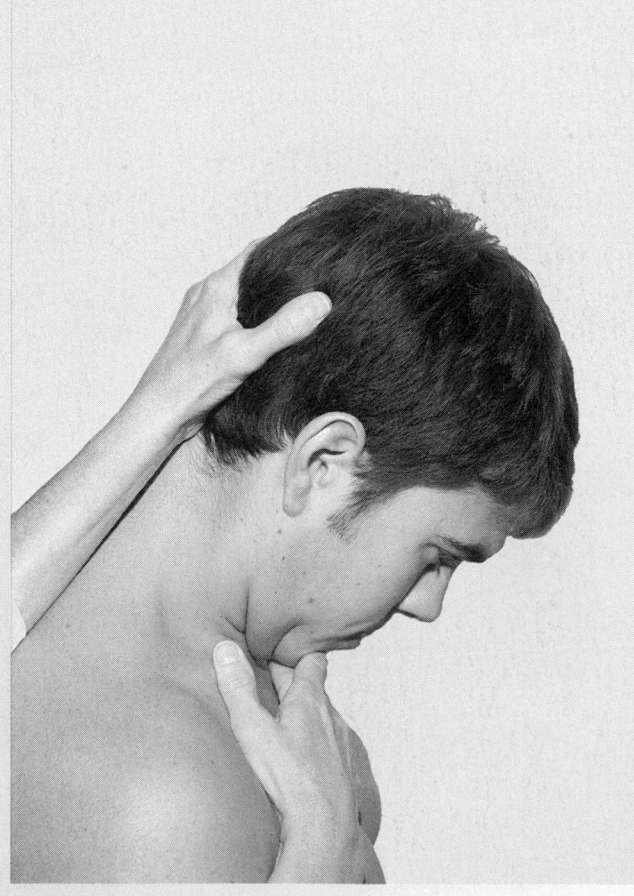

FIGURE 11.14 The subject at the end of cervical flexion range of motion.

Goniometer Alignment
See Figures 11.15 and 11.16.

1. Center **fulcrum** of the goniometer over the external auditory meatus.
2. Align **proximal arm** so that it is either perpendicular or parallel to the ground.
3. Align **distal arm** with the base of the nares. If a tongue depressor is used, align the arm of the goniometer parallel to the longitudinal axis of the tongue depressor.

▶ **NOTE: The same testing position, testing motion, and stabilization described for measuring flexion using a goniometer are to be used for all of the following alternative methods.**

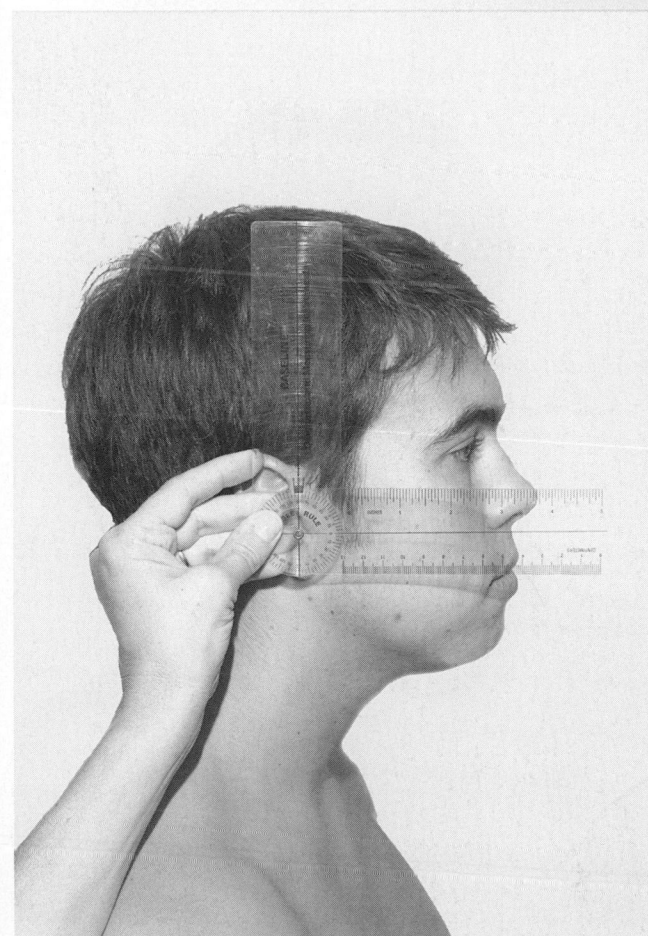

FIGURE 11.15 In the 0 starting position for measuring cervical flexion range of motion, the goniometer reads 90 degrees. This reading should be transposed and recorded as 0 degrees.

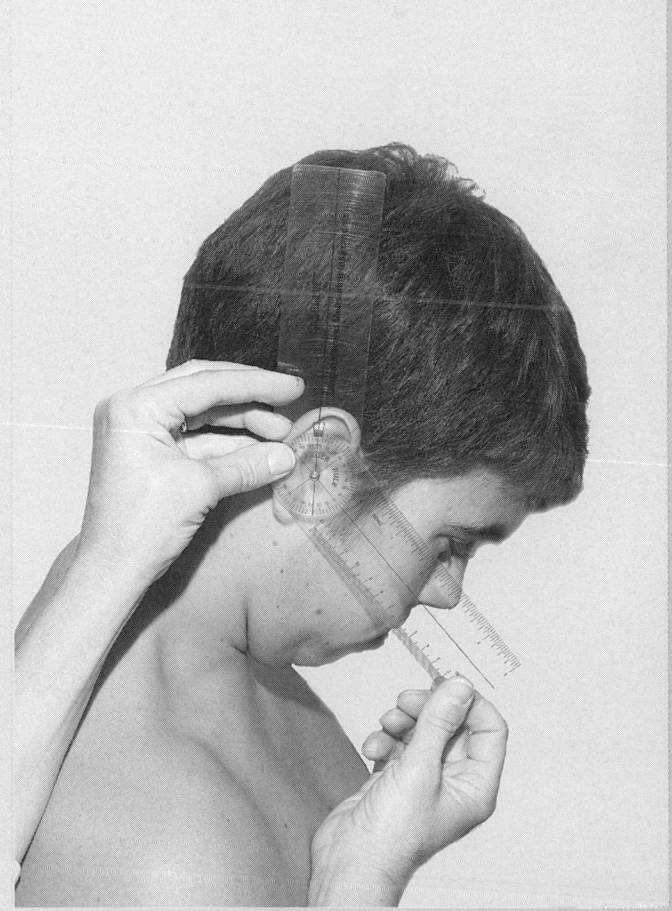

FIGURE 11.16 The goniometer reads 135 degrees at the end of the range of motion (ROM) but the ROM should be recorded as 0-45 degrees.

● CERVICAL FLEXION: TAPE MEASURE

The mean cervical flexion ROM obtained with a tape measure ranges from 1.0 to 4.3 cm[10,11] for ages 14 to 31 years. See Table 11.2 in the Research Findings section for normal values, but remember that you need to check that the landmarks that are being used by the researchers are the same as the ones that you are using.

Alignment

Use a skin marking pencil to place marks on the following landmarks: the lower edge of the sternal notch and the middle of the tip of the chin. Ask the subject to tuck his or her chin in and bend his or her head as far forward as possible without moving the trunk.

Measure the distance between the mark on the tip of the chin and the mark at the lower edge of the sternal notch at the end of the ROM. Make sure that the subject's mouth remains closed during the motion (Fig. 11.17).

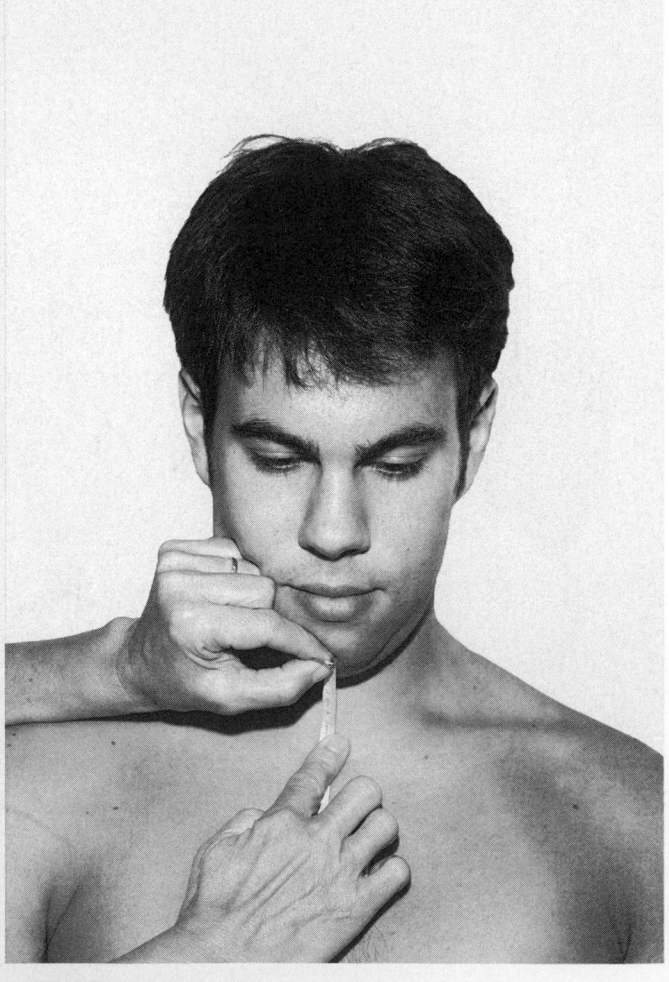

FIGURE 11.17 The examiner uses a tape measure for cervical flexion by determining the distance from the tip of the chin to the sternal notch.

● CERVICAL FLEXION: DOUBLE INCLINOMETERS

The double inclinometer method is included because the fifth edition of the *Guides to Evaluation of Permanent Impairment*[12] published by the American Medical Assocation (AMA) requires the use of double inclinometers for measurements of the spine. However, not enough studies have been done to establish the reliability and validity of this method of measurement and hence to provide normative data.

Both inclinometers must be zeroed after they are positioned on the subject and prior to the beginning of the measurement. To zero the inclinometer, adjust the rotating dial so the bubble or pointer is at 0 degrees on the scale.

Inclinometer Alignment

1. Place **one inclinometer** directly over the spinous process of the T-1 vertebra, making sure that the inclinometer is adjusted to 0 degrees.
2. Place the **second inclinometer** firmly on the top of the head, making sure that the inclinometer is adjusted to 0 degrees (Fig. 11.18).

Testing Motion

Instruct the subject to bring the head forward into flexion while keeping the trunk straight (Fig. 11.19). (Note that active ROM [AROM] is being measured.) At the end of the motion, read and record the degrees on the dials of each inclinometer. The ROM is the difference between the readings of the two instruments.

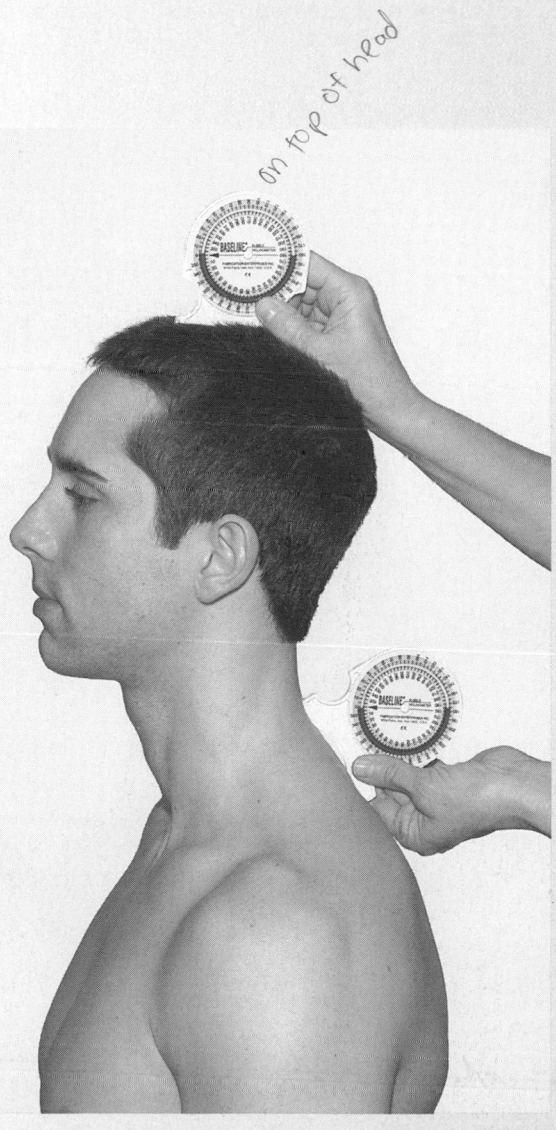

FIGURE 11.18 Inclinometer alignment in the starting position for measuring cervical flexion range of motion.

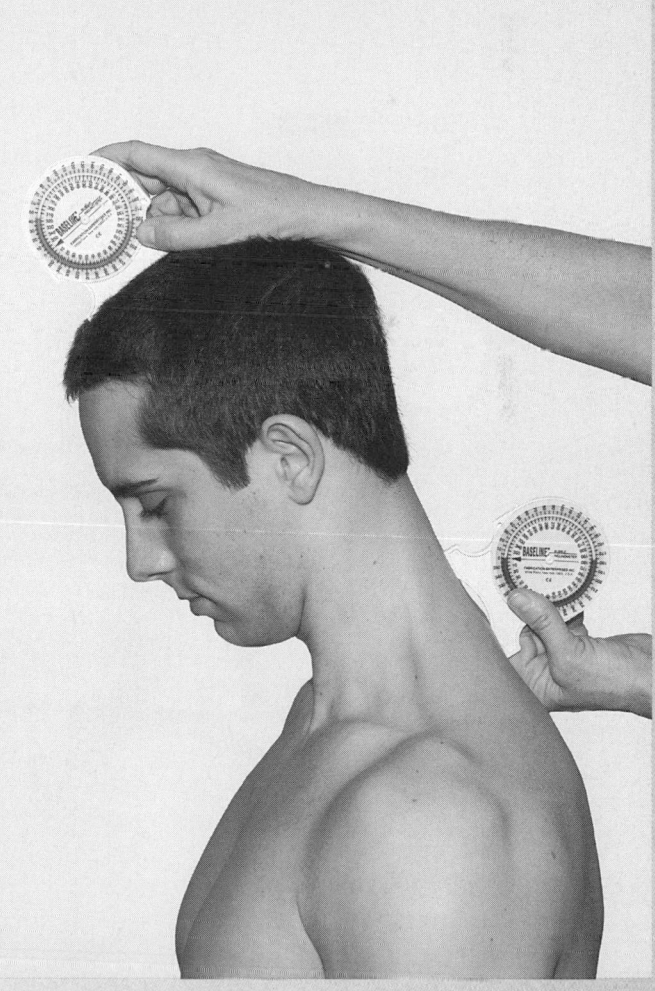

FIGURE 11.19 Inclinometer alignment at the end of cervical flexion range of motion.

● CERVICAL FLEXION: CERVICAL RANGE OF MOTION (CROM) DEVICE

The mean flexion ROM for the CROM device ranges from 64 degrees in subjects aged 11 to 19 years to 40 degrees in subjects aged 80 to 89 years.[13] For additional ROM values by age and gender, refer to Capuano-Pucci[14] and Tousignant[15] in Table 11.1 in the Research Findings section; to Nilsson[16] in Tables 11.5, 11.6, and 11.7; and to Youdas[13] in Tables 11.4, 11.8, and 11.9.

Familiarize yourself with the CROM device prior to beginning the measurement. The CROM device consists of a headpiece that supports two gravity inclinometers and a compass inclinometer. One gravity inclinometer is located on the side of the head in the sagittal plane and is used to measure flexion and extension. The other gravity inclinometer is located over the forehead in the frontal plane and is used to measure lateral flexion. The compass inclinometer has a gravity needle and is situated over the top of the head in the transverse plane and is used to measure rotation. A neckpiece containing two strong magnets is placed around the subject's neck to ensure the accuracy of the compass inclinometer.

The CROM device should fit comfortably over the bridge of the subject's nose. A Velcro strap that goes around the back of the head can be adjusted to make a snug fit. One size instrument fits all, and it is relatively easy for an examiner to fit the device to a subject.[17] Remember to stabilize the subject's trunk to prevent thoracic motion.

CROM Device Alignment[17]

1. Place the CROM device carefully on the subject's head so that the nosepiece is on the bridge of the nose and the Velcro strap fits snugly across the back of the subject's head (Fig. 11.20).
2. Position the subject's head so that the inclinometer on the side of the head reads 0 degrees.

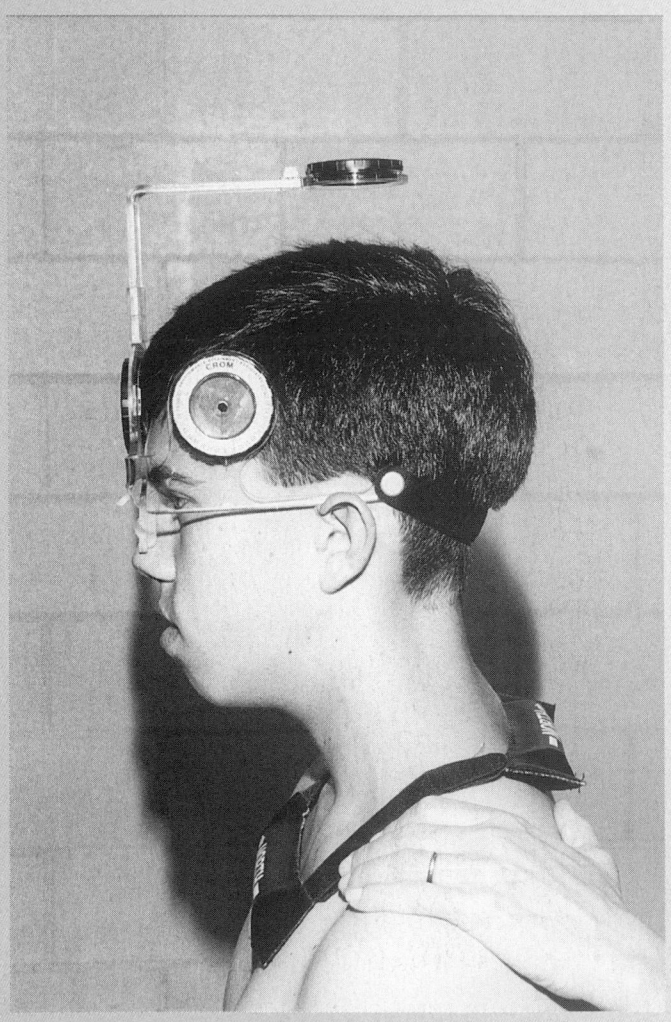

FIGURE 11.20 The CROM device positioned on the subject's head in the starting position for measuring cervical flexion range of motion. The dial on the gravity inclinometer located on the side of the subjects head is at 0 degrees.

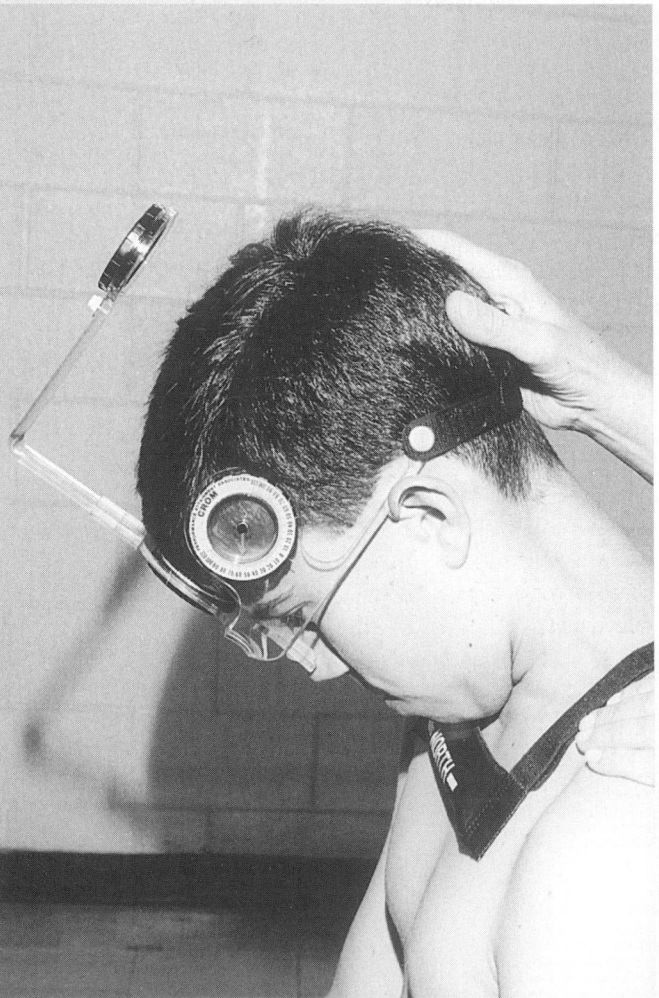

FIGURE 11.21 The examiner is shown stabilizing the trunk with one hand and maintaining the end of the flexion range of motion with her other hand.

Testing Motion

Push gently but firmly on the back of the subject's head to move it anteriorly and inferiorly through flexion ROM (Fig. 11.21). At the end of the motion, read the dial on the inclinometer on the side of the head and record the reading.

● CERVICAL EXTENSION: UNIVERSAL GONIOMETER

Motion occurs in the sagittal plane around a medial–lateral axis. Mean cervical extension ROM measured with a universal goniometer is 50 degrees (SD = 14 degrees)[9] in adults. Refer to Youdas et al[9] in Table 11.1 in the Research Findings section for additional normal ROM values by age and gender.

Testing Position

Place the subject in the sitting position, with the thoracic and lumbar spine well supported by the back of a chair. Position the cervical spine in 0 degrees of rotation and lateral flexion. A tongue depressor can be held between the teeth for reference.

Stabilization

Stabilize the shoulder girdle and chest to prevent extension of the thoracic and lumbar spine. Usually, the stabilization is achieved through the cooperation of the patient and support from the back of the chair. A strap placed around the chest and the back of the chair also may be used.

Testing Motion

Put one hand on the back of the subject's head and, with the other hand, hold the subject's chin. Push gently but firmly upward and posteriorly on the chin to move the head through the ROM in extension (Fig. 11.22). The end of the ROM occurs when resistance to further motion is felt and further attempts at extension cause extension of the trunk.

Normal End-Feel

The normal end-feel is firm owing to the passive tension developed by stretching of the anterior longitudinal ligament, anterior fibers of the annulus fibrosus, zygapophyseal joint capsules, and the following muscles: sternocleidomastoid, longus capitis, longus colli, rectus capitis anterior, and scalenus anterior. Extremes of extension may be limited by contact between the spinous processes.

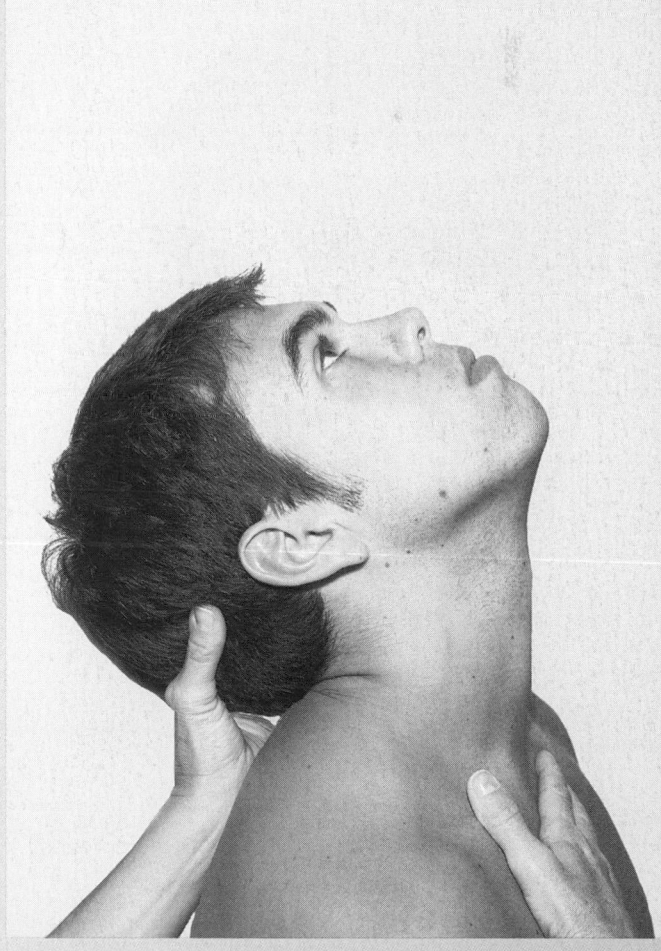

FIGURE 11.22 The end of cervical extension ROM. The examiner helps to prevent cervical rotation and lateral flexion by holding the back of the subject's head. Ideally the examiner's other hand should be on the subject's chin in order to move the head into extension.

Goniometer Alignment
See Figures 11.23 and 11.24.

1. Center **fulcrum** of the goniometer over the external auditory meatus.
2. Align **proximal arm** so that it is either perpendicular or parallel to the ground.

3. Align **distal arm** with the base of the nares. If a tongue depressor is used, align the arm of the goniometer parallel to the longitudinal axis of the tongue depressor.

▶ **NOTE: The same testing position, testing motions, and stabilization decribed for measuring extension with a goniometer should be used for all of the following alternative measurement methods.**

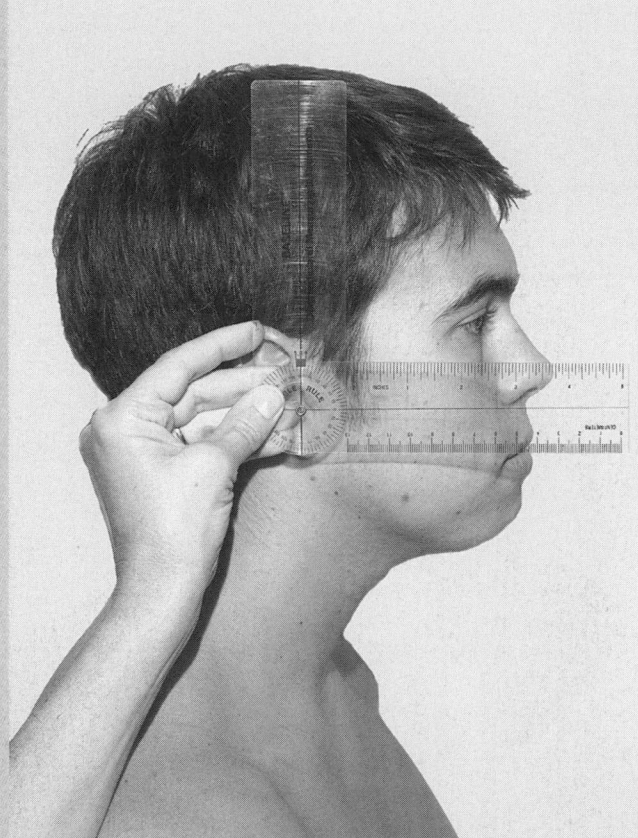

FIGURE 11.23 In the 0 starting position for measuring cervical extension range of motion the goniometer reads 90 degrees. This reading should be transposed and recorded as 0 degrees.

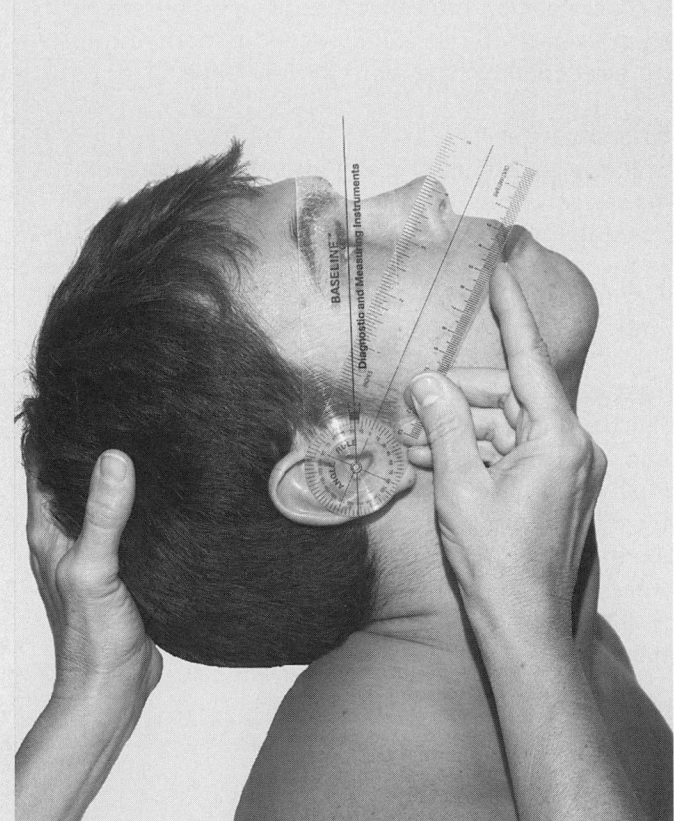

FIGURE 11.24 At the end of cervical extension, the examiner maintains the perpendicular alignment of the proximal goniometer arm and keeps the distal arm aligned with the base of the nares.

● CERVICAL EXTENSION: TAPE MEASURE

The mean cervical extension ROM measured with a tape measure ranges from 18.5 to 22.4 cm[10,11] in adults. See Table 11.2 in the Research Findings section for additional normal ROM values by age and gender.

Use a skin marking pencil to place a mark at the lower edge of the sternal notch and on the tip of the chin. Ask the subject to look straight ahead and then move his or her head posteriorly as far as possible, being careful not to extend the trunk. Measure the distance between the mark at the sternal notch and the mark on the tip of the chin at the end of cervical extension ROM (Fig. 11.25). The distance between the two points of reference is recorded in centimeters. Be sure that the subject's mouth remains closed during the measurement.

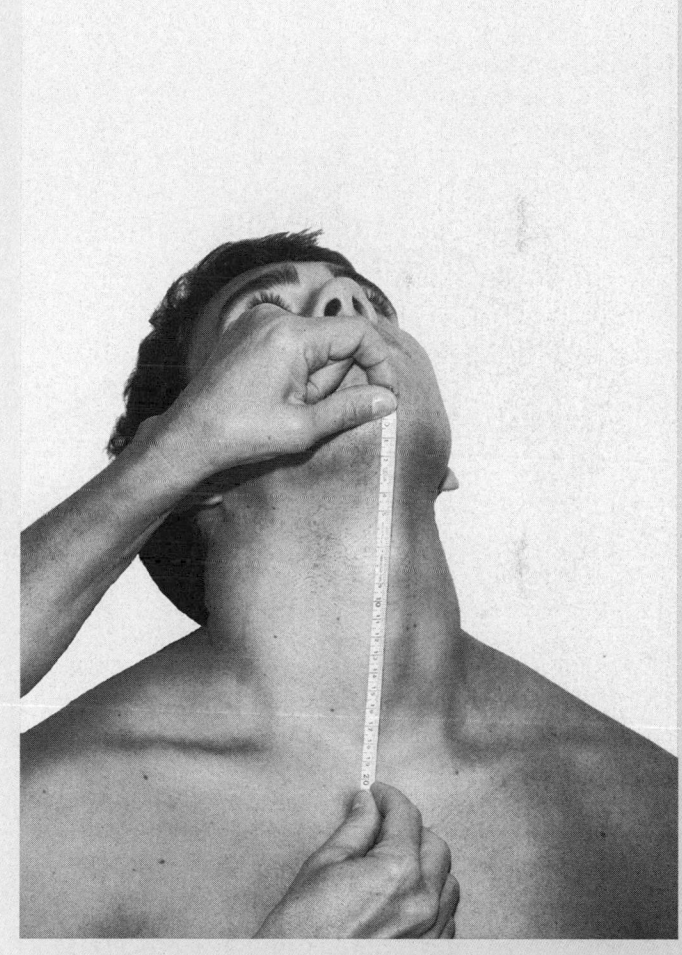

FIGURE 11.25 In the tape measure method for measuring cervical extension one end of the tape measure is placed on the tip of the subject's chin; the other end is placed at the subject's sternal notch.

● CERVICAL EXTENSION: DOUBLE INCLINOMETERS

Inclinometer Alignment

1. Place **one inclinometer** directly over the spine of the scapula. Adjust the dial of the inclinometer so that it reads 0 degrees. (If the inclinometer is placed over the first thoracic vertebra, it may contact the back of the head in full extension.)

2. Place the **second inclinometer** firmly on the top of the head, making sure that the inclinometer reads 0 degrees (Fig. 11.26).

Testing Motion

Instruct the subject to move the head into extension while keeping the trunk straight (Fig. 11.27). (Note that AROM is being measured.) At the end of the motion, read and record the information on the dials of each inclinometer. The ROM is the difference between the readings of the two instruments.

Extension same position as flexion

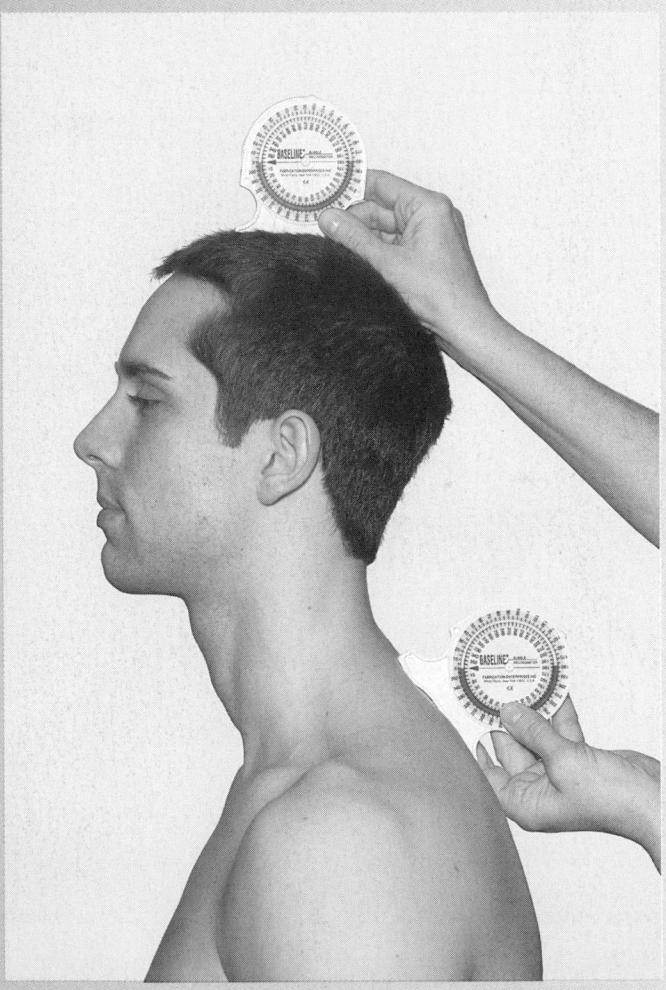

FIGURE 11.26 Inclinometer alignment in the starting position for measuring cervical extension range of motion. The examiner has zeroed both inclinometers prior to beginning the motion.

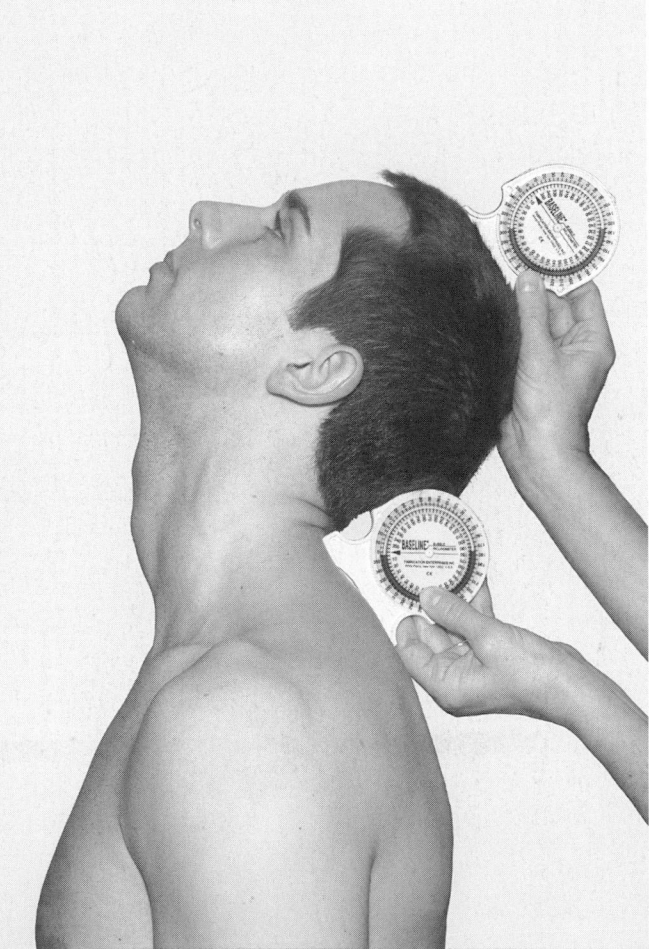

FIGURE 11.27 Inclinometer alignment at the end of cervical extension range of motion.

● CERVICAL EXTENSION: CROM DEVICE

The mean cervical ROM in extension measured with the CROM device ranges from 86 degrees in males aged 11 to 19 years and to 49 degrees in males aged 80 to 89 years.[13] For additional normal ROM values by age and gender, refer to ROM values listed under Capuano-Pucci[14] and Tousignant[15] in Table 11.1; to Nilsson[16] in Tables 11.5, 11.6, and 11.7; and to Youdas[13] in Tables 11.8 and 11.9 in the Research Findings section.

CROM Device Alignment

1. Place the CROM device carefully on the subject's head so that the nosepiece is on the bridge of the nose and the Velcro strap fits snugly across the back of the subject's head (Fig. 11.28).
2. Position the subject's head so that the gravity inclinometer on the side of the head reads 0 degrees.

Testing Motion

Guide the subject's head posteriorly and inferiorly through extension ROM (Fig. 11.29). At the end of the motion read the dial on the inclinometer on the side of the head.

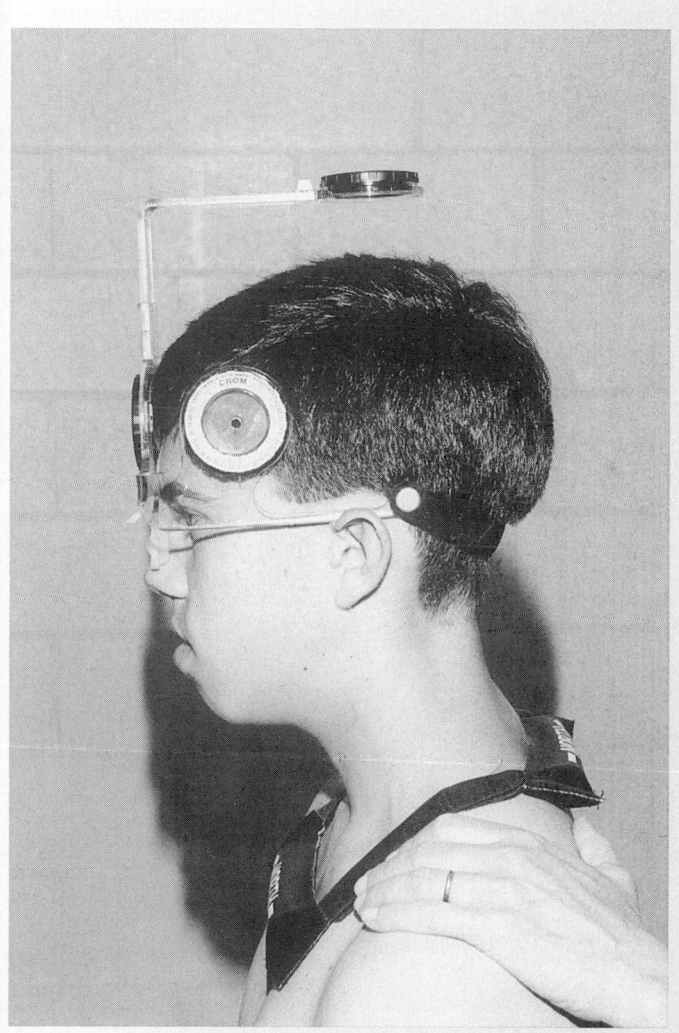

FIGURE 11.28 The subject is positioned in the starting position with the CROM device in place. The gravity inclinometer located at the side of the subject's head is at 0 degrees prior to beginning the motion.

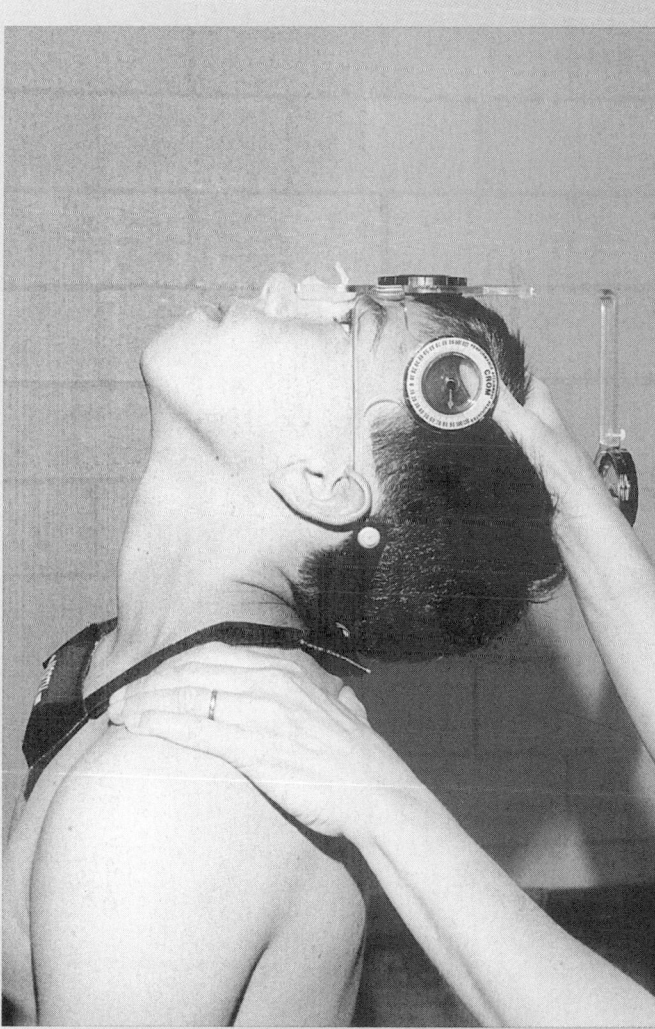

FIGURE 11.29 At the end of cervical extension range of motion (ROM), the examiner is stabilizing the trunk with one hand and maintaining the end of the ROM with her other hand on top of the subject's head.

• CERVICAL LATERAL FLEXION: UNIVERSAL GONIOMETER

Motion occurs in the frontal plane around an anterior–posterior axis. The mean cervical lateral flexion ROM to one side, measured with a universal goniometer, is 22 degrees (SD = 7 to 8 degrees) in adults.[9] See Youdas[9] in Table 11.1 in the Research Findings section for additional normal ROM values by age and gender.

Testing Position
Place the subject sitting with the cervical spine in 0 degrees of flexion, extension, and rotation.

Stabilization
Stabilize the shoulder girdle and chest to prevent lateral flexion of the thoracic and lumbar spine.

Testing Motion
Grasp the subject's head at the top and side (opposite to the direction of the motion). Pull the head toward the shoulder. Do not allow the head to rotate, forward flex, or extend during the motion (Fig. 11.30). The end of the motion occurs when resistance to motion is felt and attempts to produce additional motion cause lateral trunk flexion.

Normal End-Feel
The normal end-feel is firm owing to the passive tension developed in the intertransverse ligaments, the lateral annulus fibrosus fibers, and the following contralateral

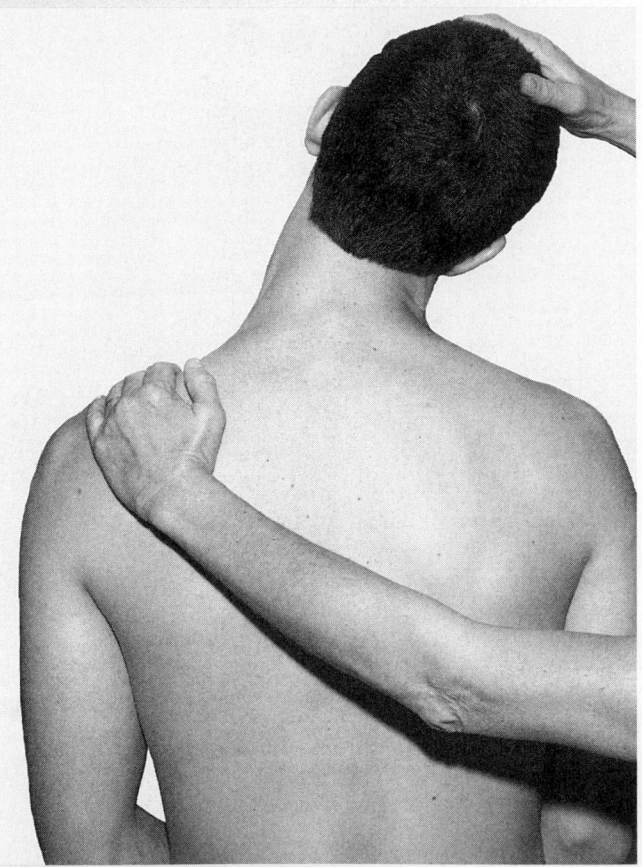

FIGURE 11.30 The end of the cervical lateral flexion range of motion. The examiner's hand holds the subject's left shoulder to prevent lateral flexion of the thoracic and lumbar spine. The examiner's other hand maintains cervical lateral flexion by pulling the subject's head laterally.

muscles: longus capitis, longus colli, scalenus anterior, and sternocleidomastoid.

Goniometer Alignment
See Figures 11.31 and 11.32.

1. Center **fulcrum** of the goniometer over the spinous process of the C7 vertebra.
2. Align **proximal arm** with the spinous processes of the thoracic vertebrae so that the arm is perpendicular to the ground.
3. Align **distal arm** with the dorsal midline of the head, using the occipital protuberance for reference.

▶ NOTE: The same testing position, testing motion, and stabilization decribed for measuring lateral flexion with a goniometer should be used for all of the following lateral flexion measurement methods.

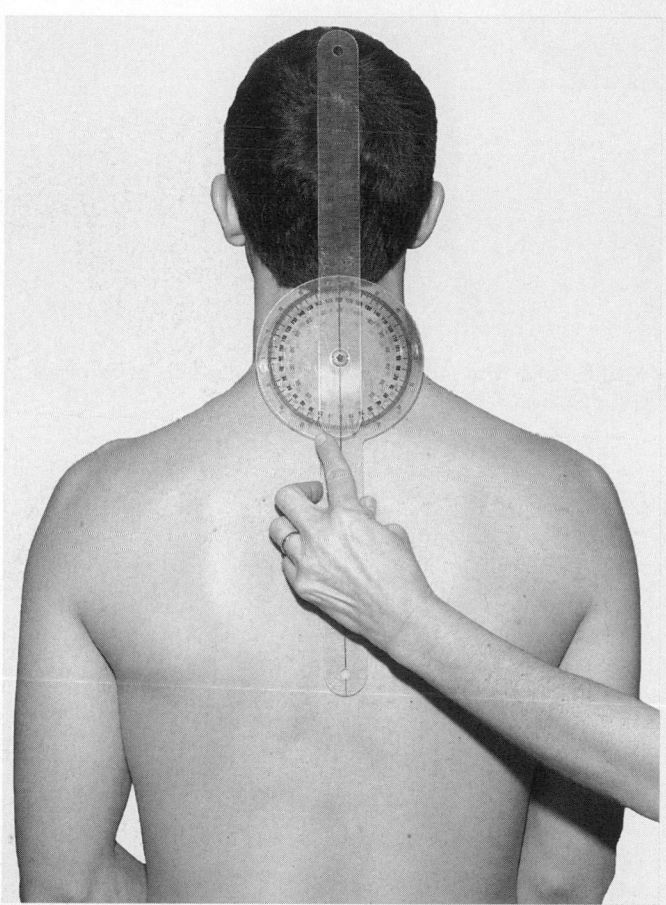

FIGURE 11.31 In the starting position for measuring cervical lateral flexion range of motion, the proximal goniometer arm is perpendicular to the floor.

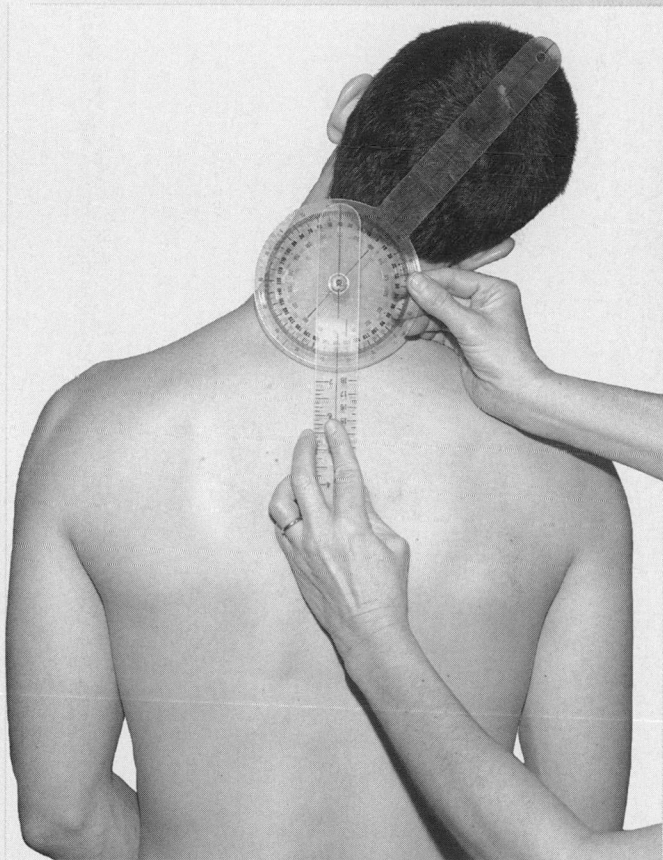

FIGURE 11.32 At the end of cervical lateral flexion ROM, the examiner maintains alignment of the proximal goniometer arm. In practice, the examiner would have one hand on the subject's head to maintain lateral flexion.

● CERVICAL LATERAL FLEXION: TAPE MEASURE

The mean cervical lateral flexion ROM measured with a tape measure ranges from 10.7 to 12.9 cm for subjects 14 to 31 years of age. Refer to Table 11.2 in the Research Findings section for additional normal ROM values by age and gender.

Use a skin marking pencil to place marks on the subject's mastoid process and on the lateral tip of the acromial process. Measure the distance between the two marks at the end of cervical lateral flexion ROM (Fig. 11.33).

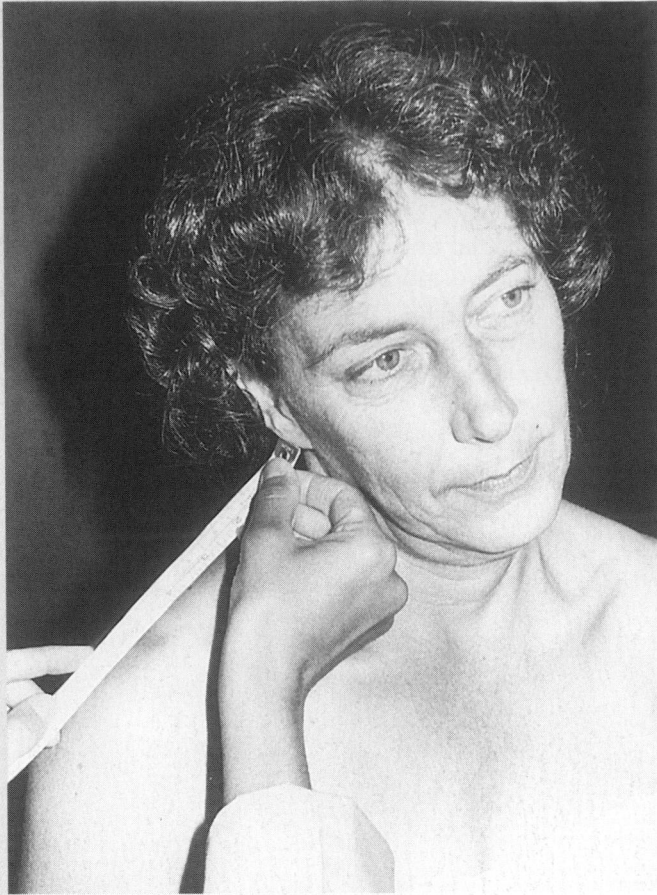

FIGURE 11.33 The subject is shown at the end of cervical lateral flexion range of motion.

CERVICAL LATERAL FLEXION: DOUBLE INCLINOMETERS

Inclinometer Alignment

1. Position **one inclinometer** directly over the spinous process of the T1 vertebra. Adjust the rotating dial so that the bubble is at 0 on the scale.
2. Place the **second inclinometer** firmly on the top of the subject's head and adjust the dial so that it reads 0 (Fig. 11.34).

Testing Motion

Instruct the subject to move the head into lateral flexion while keeping the trunk straight (Fig. 11.35). (Note that AROM is being measured.) The ROM is the difference between the two instruments.

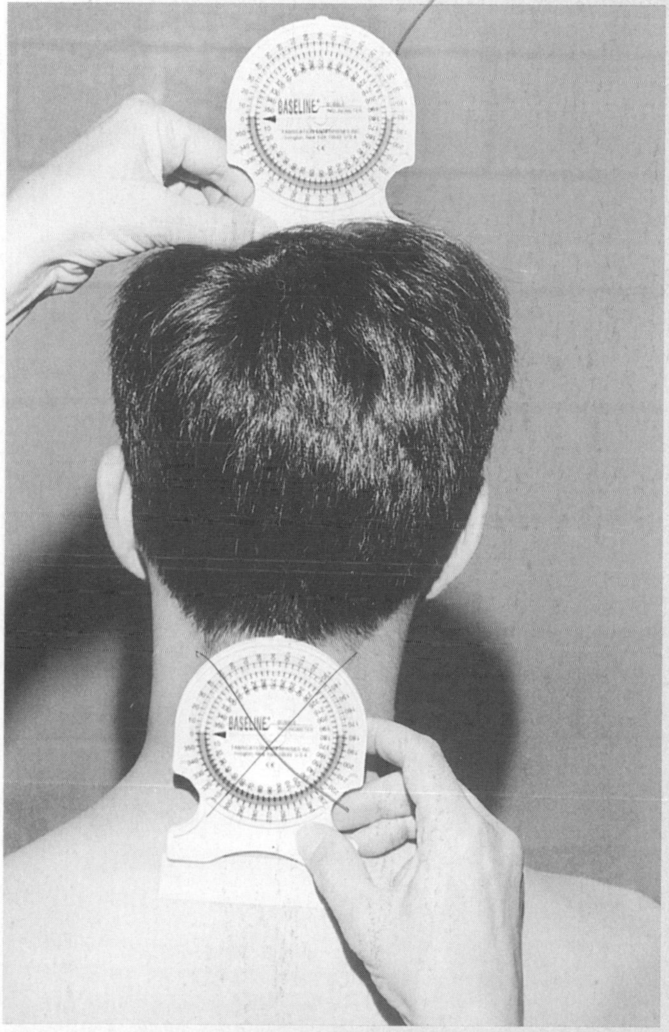

FIGURE 11.34 In the starting position for measuring cervical lateral flexion range of motion, one inclinometer is positioned at the level of the spinous process of the first thoracic vertebra. A piece of tape has been placed at that level to help align the inclinometer. The examiner has zeroed both inclinometers prior to beginning the motion.

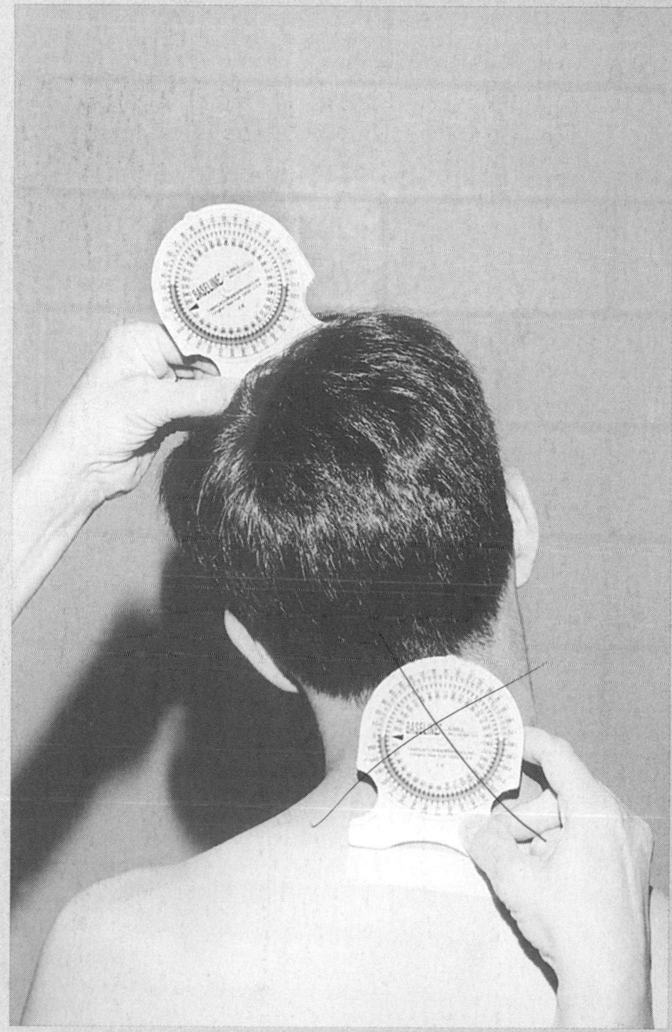

FIGURE 11.35 Inclinometer alignment at the end of lateral flexion range of motion. At the end of the motion, the examiner reads and records the information on the dials of each inclinometer. The range of motion is the difference between the readings of the two instruments.

● CERVICAL LATERAL FLEXION: CROM DEVICE

The ROM in lateral flexion using the CROM device ranges from a mean of 45 degrees in subjects aged 11 to 19 years to a mean of 24 in male subjects and 26 degrees in female subjects aged 80 to 89 years.[13] For additional normal ROM values by age and gender, see Capuano-Pucci[14] and Tousignant[15] in Table 11.1; and Nilsson[16] in Tables 11.4, 11.5, and 11.6; and Youdas[13] in Tables 11.7 and 11.8 in the Research Findings section.

CROM Device Alignment[17]

1. Place the CROM device on the subject's head so that the nosepiece is on the bridge of the nose and the band fits snugly across the back of the subject's head.
2. Position the subject in the testing position so that the gravity inclinometer on the front of the CROM device reads 0 degrees (Fig. 11.36).

Testing Motion

Guide the subject's head into lateral flexion (Fig.11.37). At the end of the motion, read the dial located in front of the forehead and record the number of degrees.

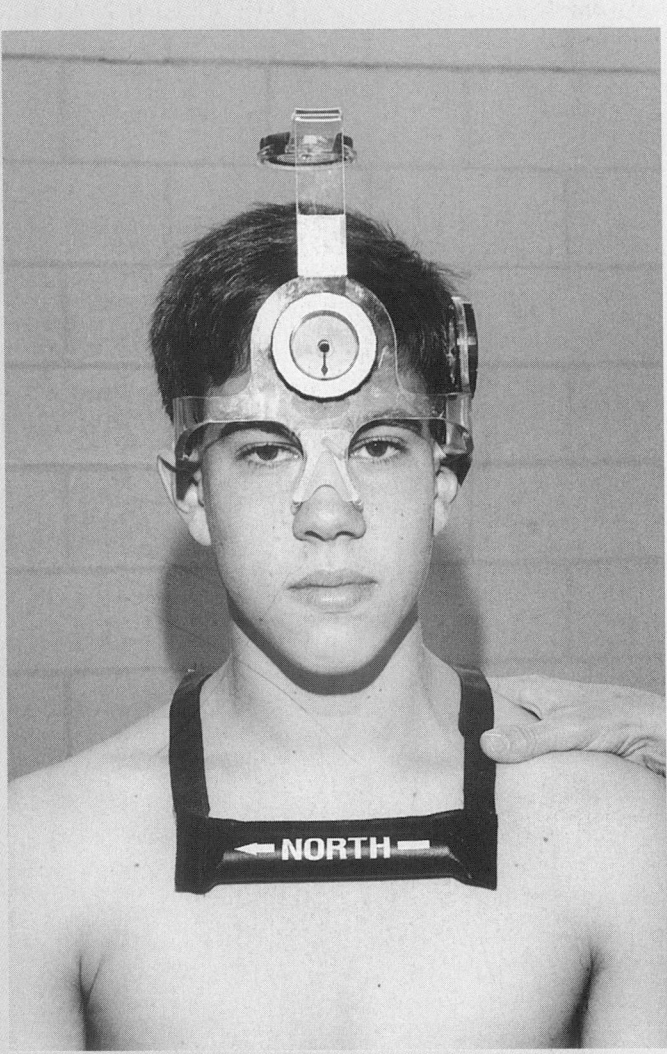

FIGURE 11.36 The subject is placed in the starting position for measuring cervical lateral flexion range of motion so that the inclinometer located in front of the subject's forehead is zeroed before starting the motion.

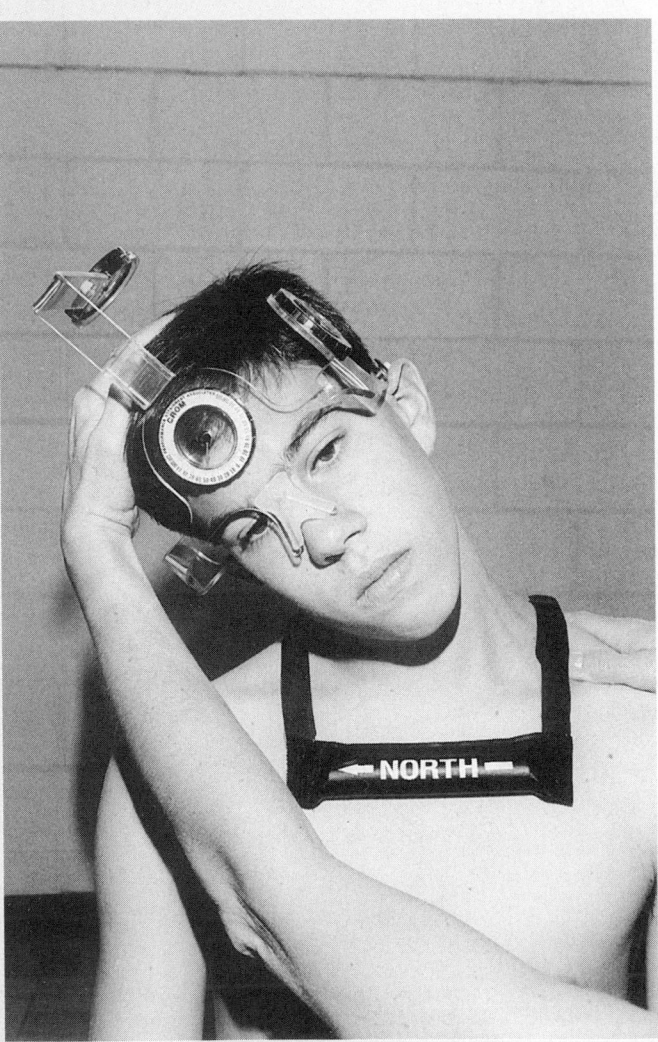

FIGURE 11.37 At the end of lateral flexion range of motion (ROM), the examiner is stabilizing the subject's shoulder with one hand and maintaining the end of the ROM with her other hand on the subject's head.

● CERVICAL ROTATION: UNIVERSAL GONIOMETER

Motion occurs in the transverse plane around a vertical axis. The mean cervical ROM in rotation measured with a universal goniometer is 49 degrees to the left (SD = 9 degrees) and 51 degrees to the right (SD = 11 degrees) in adults.[9] See Youdas[9] in Table 11.1 in the Research Findings section for additional normal ROM values by age and gender. Magee[2] reports that the ROM in rotation is between 70 and 90 degrees but cautions that cervical rotation past 50 degrees may lead to kinking of the contralateral vertebral artery. The ipsilateral artery may kink at 45 degrees of rotation.[2]

Testing Position
Place the subject sitting, with the thoracic and lumbar spine well supported by the back of the chair. Position the cervical spine in 0 degrees of flexion, extension, and lateral flexion. The subject may hold a tongue depressor between the front teeth for reference.

Stabilization
Stabilize the shoulder girdle and chest to prevent rotation of the thoracic and lumbar spine. A strap across the chest may be used to keep the trunk from rotating.

Testing Motion
Grasp the subject's chin and rotate the head by moving the head toward the shoulder, as shown in Figure 11.38. The end of the ROM occurs when resistance to movement is felt and further movement causes rotation of the trunk.

Normal End-Feel
The normal end-feel is firm owing to stretching of the alar ligament, the fibers of the zygapophyseal joint capsules, and the following contralateral muscles: longus capitis, longus colli, and scalenus anterior. Passive tension in the ipsilateral sternocleidomastoid may limit extremes of rotation.

Goniometer Alignment
See Figures 11.39 and 11.40.

1. Center **fulcrum** of the goniometer over the center of the cranial aspect of the head.
2. Align **proximal arm** parallel to an imaginary line between the two acromial processes.
3. Align **distal arm** with the tip of the nose. If a tongue depressor is used, align the arm of the goniometer parallel to the longitudinal axis of the tongue depressor.

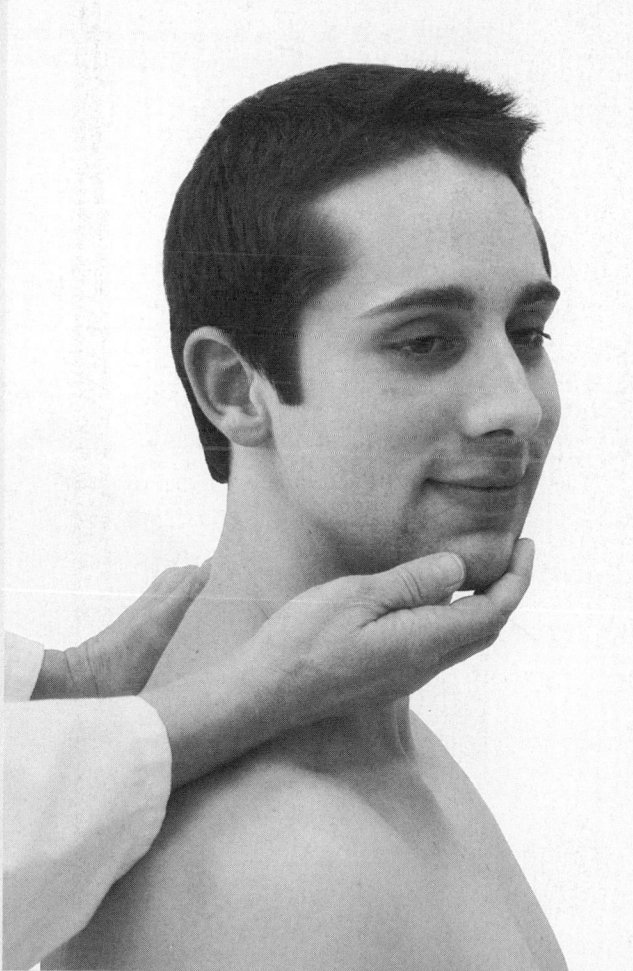

FIGURE 11.38 The end of the cervical rotation range of motion. One of the examiner's hands maintains rotation and prevents cervical flexion and extension. The examiner's other hand is placed on the subject's left shoulder to prevent rotation of the thoracic and lumbar spine.

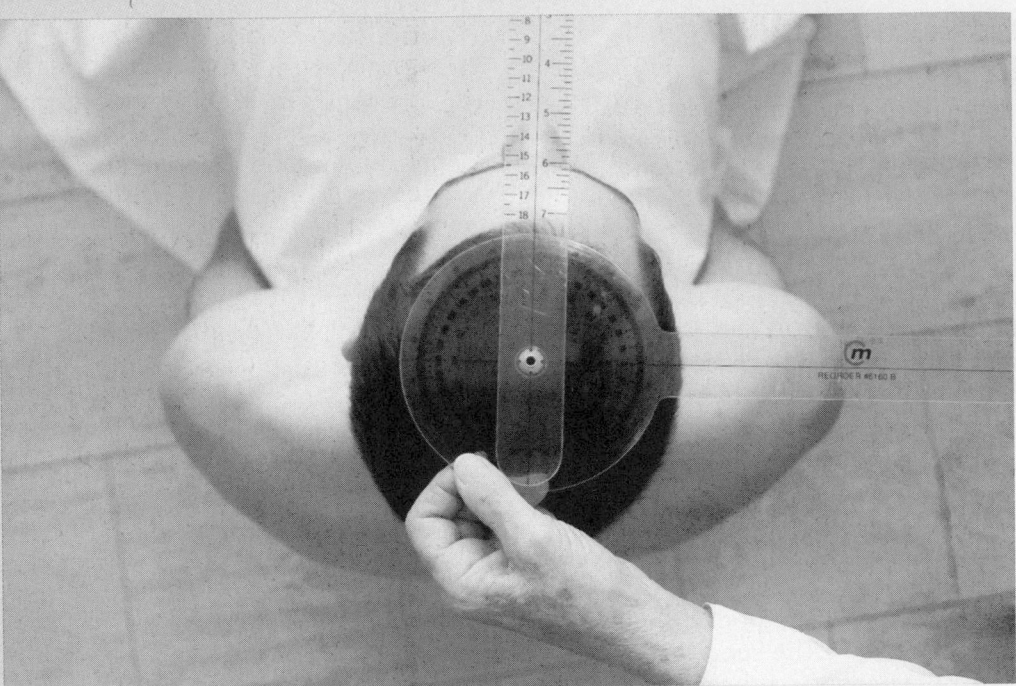

FIGURE 11.39 To align the goniometer at the starting position for measuring cervical rotation range of motion, the examiner stands in back of the subject, who is seated in a low chair.

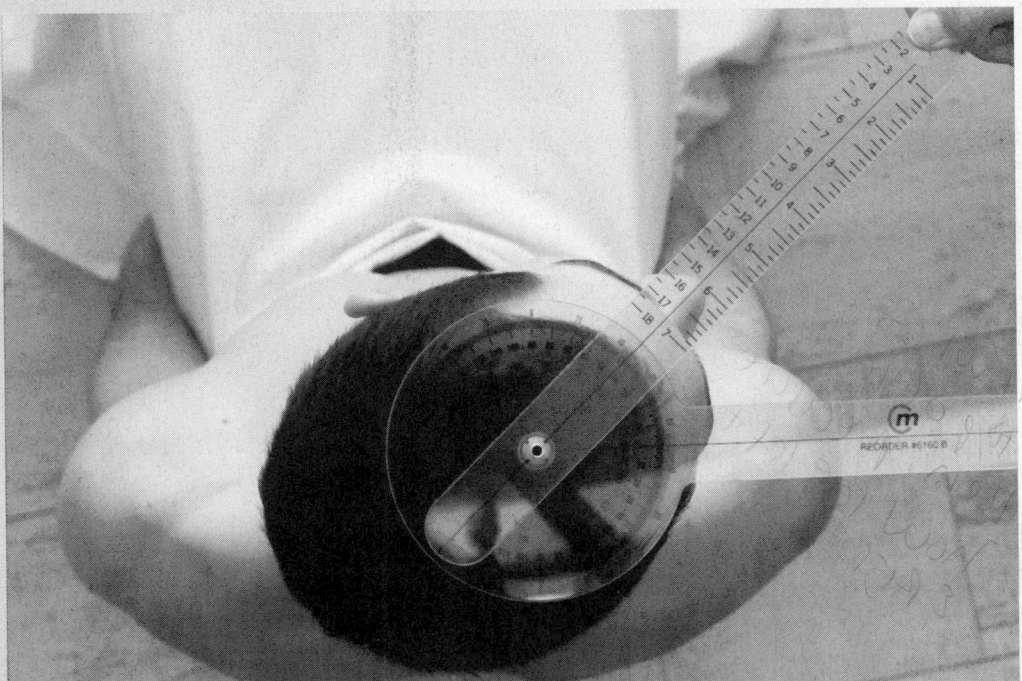

FIGURE 11.40 At the end of the range of right cervical rotation, one of the the examiner's hands maintains alignment of the distal goniometer arm with the tip of the subject's nose. The examiner's other hand keeps the proximal arm aligned parallel to the imaginary line between the acromial processes.

● CERVICAL ROTATION: TAPE MEASURE

The mean cervical rotation ROM to the left measured with a tape measure ranges from 11.0 to 13.2 cm[10,11] in 14 to 31 year olds. See Table 11.2 in the Research Findings section for additional normal ROM values by age and gender.

Use a skin marking pencil to place marks on the tip of the chin and the acromial process. Have the subject look straight ahead and then turn his or her head to the right as far as possible without rotating the trunk. Measure the distance between the two marks at the end of the motion (Fig. 11.41). Have the subject return his or her head to the neutral starting position and then turn the head as far to the left as possible wihtout rotating the trunk.

● CERVICAL ROTATION: INCLINOMETER

The normal ROM for rotation using an inclinometer is 80 degrees to each side, according to the AMA.[12]

Testing Position
Place the subject supine with the head in neutral rotation, lateral flexion, flexion, and extension.

Inclinometer Alignment
1. Place the inclinometer in the middle of the subject's forehead, and zero the inclinometer (Fig. 11.42).
2. Hold the inclinometer firmly while the subject's head moves through rotation ROM (Fig. 11.43).

Testing Motion
Instruct the subject to roll the head into rotation. The ROM can be read on the inclinometer at the end of the ROM.

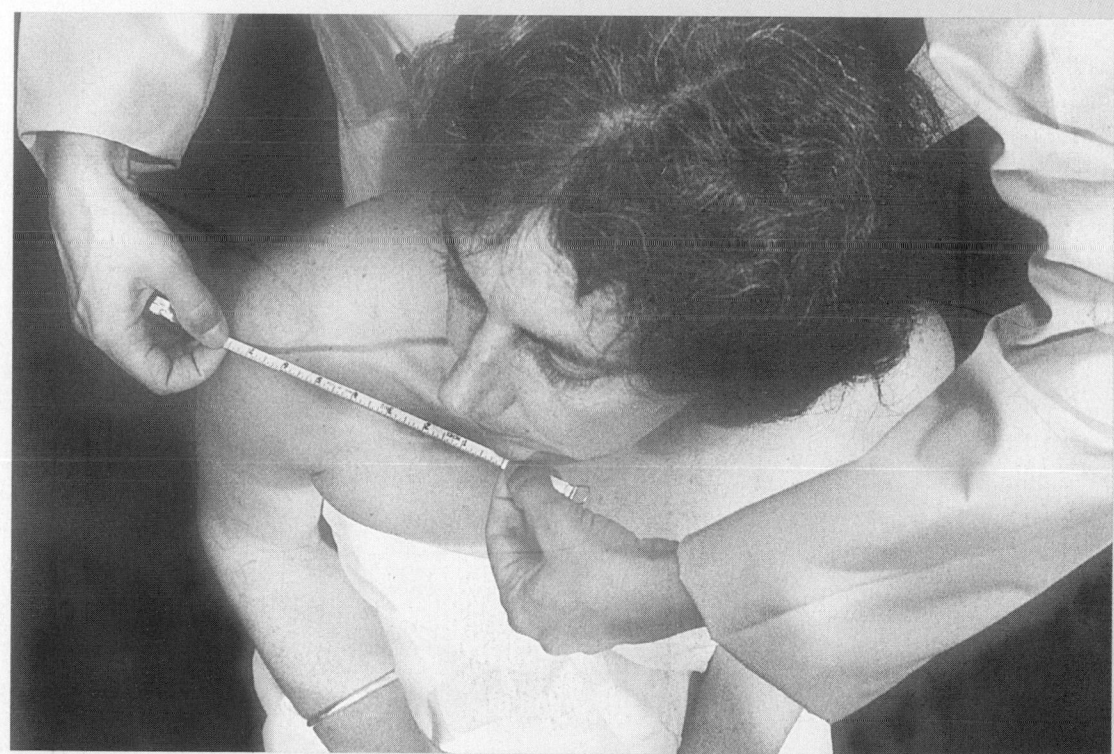

FIGURE 11.41 At the end of the right cervical range of motion, the examiner is using a tape measure to determine the distance between the tip of the subject's chin and her right acromial process.

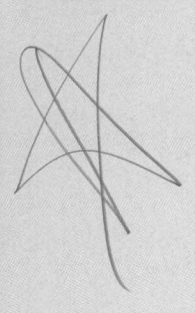

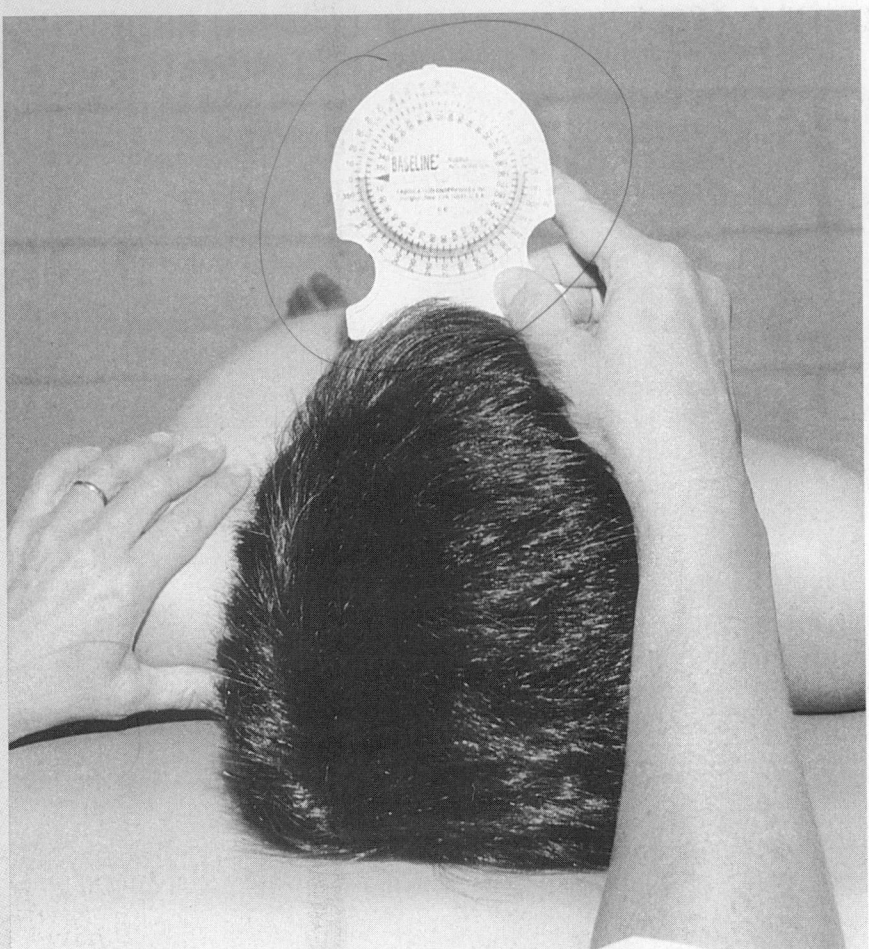

FIGURE 11.42 Inclinometer alignment in the starting position for measuring cervical rotation range of motion. Only one inclinometer is used for this measurement.

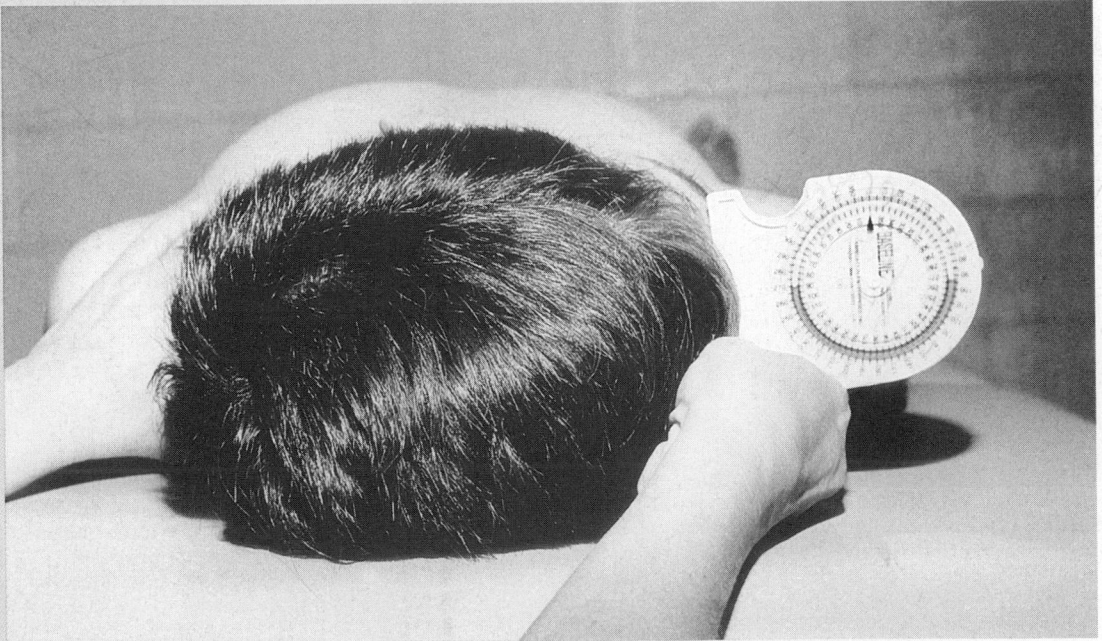

FIGURE 11.43 Inclinometer alignment at the end of cervical rotation range of motion (ROM). The number of degrees on the dial of the inclinometer equals the ROM in rotation.

● CERVICAL ROTATION: CROM DEVICE

The mean ROM in right rotation with use of the CROM device varies from 75 degrees in female subjects aged 11 to 19 years to 46 degrees in male subjects aged 80 years.[13] For additional ROM values by age and gender, refer to Capuano-Pucci[14] and Tousignant[15] in Table 11.1; to Nilsson[16] in Tables 11.4, 11.5, and 11.6; and to Youdas[13] in Tables 11.7 and 11.8 in the Research Findings section.

CROM Device Alignment[17]

1. Place the CROM device on the subject's head so that the nosepiece is on the bridge of the nose and the band fits snugly across the back of the subject's head. The arrow on the magnetic yoke should be pointing north (Fig. 11.44).
2. To ensure that the compass inclinometer is level, adjust the position of the subject's head so that both gravity inclinometers read 0 degrees (Fig. 11.45).
3. After leveling the compass inclinometer, turn the rotation meter on the compass inclinometer until the pointer is at 0 degrees.

Testing Motion

Guide the subject's head into rotation and read the inclinometer at the end of the ROM.

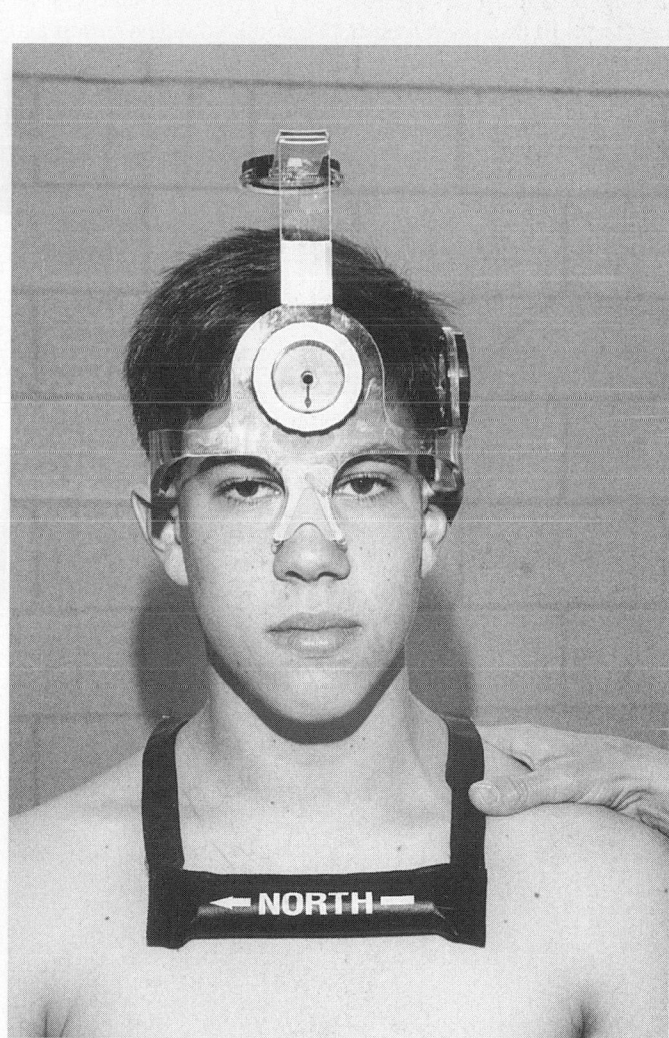

FIGURE 11.44 The compass inclinometer on the top of the CROM device has been leveled so that the examiner is able to zero it prior to the beginning of the motion.

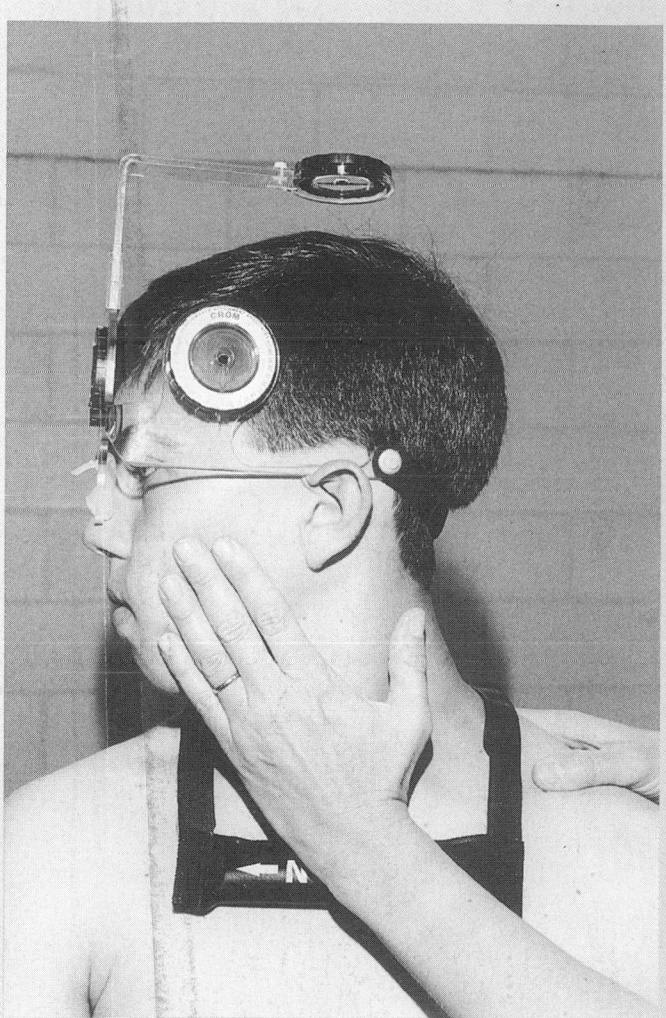

FIGURE 11.45 At the end of right rotation range of motion (ROM), the examiner is stabilizing the subject's shoulder with one hand and maintaining the end of rotation ROM with the other hand. The examiner will read the dial of the inclinometer on the top of the CROM device. Rotation ROM will be the number of degrees on the dial at the end of the ROM.

Research Findings

Measurement of the cervical spine ROM is complicated by the region's multiple joint structure and lack of well-defined landmarks, a workable definition of the neutral position, and a standardized method of stabilization to isolate cervical motion from thoracic motion. The search for instruments and methods capable of providing accurate and affordable measurements of the cervical spine is ongoing. At this time the universal goniometer appears to be the most commonly used instrument in the clinic, although relatively few research studies are available to provide normative data and to attest to the goniometer's reliability and validity. ROM values from one study are presented in Table 11.1. The tape measure also is used in the clinical setting and ROM values can be found in Table 11.2. Single inclinometer values are found in Table 11.3.

Effects of Age, Gender, and Other Factors on Cervical Range of Motion Measurements

Age

A large number of researchers have investigated the effects of age on active cervical ROM,[13,16,20–36] but differences between the populations tested and the wide variety of instruments and procedures employed in these studies make it difficult to compare results. Generally, most researchers agree that in adults a tendency exists for cervical ROM to decrease with increasing age. The only exception that has been found by some authors is that axial rotation (occurring primarily at the atlantoaxial joint) has been shown either to stay the same or to increase with increasing age to compensate for an age-related decrease in rotation in the lower cervical spine.[22,29] Age may not account for a large amount of the variance in cervical ROM, but age appears to have a stronger effect than gender.

O'Driscoll and Tomenson[20] studied cervical ROM across age groups using a type of inclinometer. They measured 79 females and 80 males ranging in age from 0 to 79 years and found that ROM decreased with increasing age and differences existed between males and females. In another study that included a relatively large number of subjects (250) and a large age range (from 14 to 70 years), Feipel and colleagues[28] found a significant decrease in all cervical motions with increasing age. Kulman[30] compared the range of motion of 42 subjects aged 70 to 90 years and 31 subjects aged 20 to 30 years and found that the elderly group had significantly less motion than the younger group for all motions measured, including rotation. Sforza and coworkers,[35] who studied the effects of age on ROM in 20 male adolescents (mean age 16 years), 30 young adult males (mean age 23 years), and 20 middle-aged men (mean age 37 years) also found that all cervical AROMs decreased between the youngest group and the oldest group.

Pellachia and Bohannon[26] found that the mean values for lateral flexion in subjects younger than 30 years of age exceeded 42 degrees, whereas mean values for lateral flexion in subjects older than 79 years of age were less than 25 degrees. Nilsson, Hartvigsen, and Christensen,[16] in a study of 90 healthy men and women aged 20 to 60 years, concluded that the decrease in half cycle cervical passive range of motion (PROM) with increasing age could be explained by using a simple linear regression of ROM as a function of age. Chen and colleagues,[27] in a detailed review of the literature regarding the effects of aging on cervical spine ROM, concluded that active cervical ROM decreased by 4 degrees per decade. This finding is very close to the 5-degree decrease found by Youdas and associates.[13]

TABLE 11.1 Cervical Spine Range of Motion: Normal Values in Degrees

	Lantz, Chen, and Buch[34]	AMA[†12]	Capuano-Pucci et al[14]	Youdas et al[9]	Tousignant et al[15]
	CA-6000 Spine Motion Analyzer Ages 20–39 yrs n = 63	Inclinometer	CROM Mean age = 23.5 yrs n = 20	Universal Goniometer Mean age = 59.1 yrs n = 20	CROM Mean age = 51.5 yrs n = 55
Motion	Mean (SD)		Mean (SD)	Mean (SD)	Mean (SD)
Flexion	60 (8)	50	51 (9)	40 (12)	47 (11)
Extension	56 (11)	60	70 (9)	50 (14)	50 (14)
Right lateral flexion	43 (8)	45	—	22 (8)	30 (9)
Left lateral flexion	41 (7)	45	44 (8)	22 (7)	33 (9)
Right rotation	72 (7)	80	—	51 (11)	56 (10)
Left rotation	73 (6)	80	71 (5)	49 (9)	56 (12)

CROM = cervical range of motion device; ROM = range of motion; SD = standard deviation.

TABLE 11.2 Cervical Spine Range of Motion Measured With a Tape Measure: Normal Values in Centimeters

	Hsieh and Yeung*[10]		Balogun et al[†11]
	Ages 14–31 yrs		Ages 18–26 yrs
	Tester 1 n = 17	Tester 2 n = 17	n = 21
Motion	Mean (SD)	Mean (SD)	Mean (SD)
Flexion	1.0 (1.7)	1.8 (1.6)	4.3 (2.0)
Extension	22.4 (1.6)	20.8 (2.4)	18.5 (2.0)
Right lateral flexion	11.0 (1.9)	11.5 (2.1)	12.9 (2.4)
Left lateral flexion	10.7 (1.9)	11.1 (2.1)	12.8 (2.5)
Right rotation	11.6 (1.7)	12.6 (2.5)	11.0 (2.5)
Left rotation	11.2 (1.9)	13.2 (2.4)	11.0 (2.5)

CI = confidence interval; r = Pearson product moment correlation coefficient; SD = standard deviation.
* 99% CI of measurement error ranged from 1.4 cm to 2.6 cm for tester 1 (experienced). CI ranged from 1.9 cm to 3.3 cm for tester 2 (inexperienced).
† r values ranged from 0.26 to 0.88 for intratester reliability and from 0.30 to 0.92 for intertester reliability.

In Table 11.4 the mean values for active neck flexion in the two oldest groups of males and females ages 80 to 90 years have about 20 degrees less motion than the youngest group of 1 to 19 year olds. Both men and women were measured using the CROM device; therefore, the values presented in the table should be used for reference only if the examiners are using the CROM as their measuring instrument. Ideally, the examiner should use norms that are appropriate to the method of measurement and the age and gender of the individuals being examined.

Hole, Cook, and Bolton[33] determined that the loss of cervical mobility equals to approximately 4 percent per decade in flexion and lateral flexion and 6 to 7 percent for extension. The decrease in extension, lateral flexion, and rotation occurred between 20 and 29 year olds and 30 and 39 year olds in their study of 84 asymptomatic men and women. Demaille-Wlodyka,[32] in a study of 232 healthy volunteers ranging in age from 15 to 65 years of age or older, found that all cervical motions decreased after age 25 and that the age effect was significant. Nilsson and associates[16] measured PROM using the CROM device in 90 healthy men and women with a mean age of 39 years and an age range of 21 to 60 years. The authors determined that the decrease in PROM as age increases could be described by a simple linear regression. See Tables 11.5, 11.6, and 11.7.

Other investigators have postulated that the effects of age on ROM may be motion specific and age specific; however,

TABLE 11.3 Cervical Spine ROM Measured With the Myrin Single Inclinometer: Normal Values in Degrees

| | Balogen et al[11] | Malstrom et al[18] | Alaranta et al[19] |
| | Healthy young people Mean age = 22 yrs n = 21 | Healthy men and women Ages 22–58 yrs n = 60 | White and blue collar employees Ages 35–54 yrs n = 508 |
Motions	Mean (SD)	Mean (SD)	Mean (SD)
Extension	64 (17)	67 (12)	120* (16)
Flexion	32 (13)	65 (8)	—
Left lateral flexion	41 (9)	41 (7)	37† (6)
Right lateral flexion	42 (9)	42 (7)	—
Left rotation	64 (17)	76 (8)	75 (7)
Right rotation	68 (15)	76 (9)	—

* Full cycle (flexion plus extension)
† Mean of two measurements

TABLE 11.4 Age Effects on Active Cervical Flexion ROM in Males and Females Aged 11 to 89 Years: Normal Values in Degrees Using the CROM Device

11–19 yrs n = 40	20–29 yrs n = 42	30–39 yrs n = 41	40–49yrs n = 42	50–59 yrs n = 40	60–69 yrs n = 40	70–79 yrs n = 40	80–89 yrs n = 38
Mean (SD)	Mean (SD)	Mean (SD)	Mean (SD)	Mean (SD)	Mean (SD)	Mean (SD)	Mean (SD)
64 (9)	54 (9)	47 (10)	50 (11)	46 (9)	41 (8)	39 (9)	40 (9)

SD = standard deviation; CROM = cervical range of motion device.
Adapted from Youdas, JW, et al[13]: Reprinted from Physical Therapy with the permission of the American Physical Therapy Association.

the evidence appears to be somewhat controversial. Trott and colleagues[25] found a significant decrease in the means of all motions (flexion–extension, lateral flexion, and axial rotation) with increasing age, but they determined that most coupled motions were not affected by age. In contrast to Trott's findings, Damaille-Wlodyka[32] found that lateral flexion, which was always coupled with axial rotation, decreased with increasing age, whereas axial rotation increased. In fact, these authors found that coupled motions showed a tendency to decrease with age in all three planes.

Pearson and Walmsley[23] and Walmsley, Kimber, and Culham[24] were the only authors to include the cervical spine motions of retraction and protraction in their studies. Pearson and Walmsley[23] found that the older age groups had less ROM in retraction but that they showed no age difference in the neutral resting position. In contrast to Pearson and Walmsley's[23] findings, Walmsley, Kimber, and Culham[24] found age-related decreases in both protraction and retraction.

Lantz, Chen, and Buch,[34] in a study of 52 matched males and females, found a significant age effect, with subjects in the third decade having greater ROM in rotation and flexion–extension than subjects in the fourth decade. Dvorak and associates[22] determined that the most dramatic decrease in ROM in 150 healthy men and women (aged 20 to 60 years and older) occurred between the 30-year-old group and the 40-year-old group. A somewhat similar result was found by Peolsson and colleagues,[36] who investigated the age effects on cervical motion in 101 volunteers including 51 men ages 25 to 63 years and 50 women ages 25 to 60 years. These authors found that AROM in all planes decreased by about 30 degrees from the 25- to 34-year-old group to the 55- to 64-year-old group. The decrease in AROM was statistically significant in all planes but was most pronounced in extension and least evident in flexion (0.3 degrees/year).

In contrast to the findings of Dvorak and associates[22] and Peolsson and colleagues,[36] Trott and colleagues[25] found that

TABLE 11.5 Age and Gender Effects on Cervical Lateral Flexion ROM: Normal Values in Degrees*

	Nilsson et al[†16]	Dvorak et al[‡22]	Castro et al[§29]	Nilsson et al[16]	Dvorak et al[22]	Castro et al[29]
	Males n = 31	Males n = 86	Males n = 71	Females n = 59	Females n = 64	Females n = 86
Age Groups	Mean (SD)	Mean (SD)	Mean (SD)	Mean (SD)	Mean (SD)	Mean (SD)
20–29 yrs	122 (4)	101 (13)	92 (14)	116 (18)	100 (9)	90 (13)
30–39 yrs	111 (12)	95 (10)	89 (23)	108 (14)	106 (18)	86 (18)
40–49 yrs	102 (15)	84 (14)	74 (15)	99 (11)	88 (16)	77 (12)
50–59 yrs	104 (12)	88 (29)	70 (12)	97 (7)	76 (10)	69 (15)
60–69 yrs	—	74 (14)	65 (14)	—	80 (18)	68 (12)
70–79 yrs	—	—	47 (12)	—	—	70 (14)
80+ yrs	—	—	—	—	—	50 (18)

SD =standard deviation.
* The values in this table represent the combined total of right and left lateral flexion range of motion.
† Nilsson et al used the cervical range of motion (CROM) device to measure passive range of motion.
‡ Dvorak et al used the CA-6000 Spine Motion Analyzer to measure passive range of motion.
§ Castro et al used an ultasound-based coordinate measuring system, the CMS 50, to measure active range of motion.

TABLE 11.6 Age and Gender Effects on Cervical Flexion–Extension ROM: Normal Values in Degrees*

	Nilsson et al[†16]	Dvorak et al[‡22]	Castro et al[§29]	Nilsson et al[16]	Dvorak et al[22]	Castro et al[29]
	Males n = 31	Males n = 86	Males n = 71	Females n = 59	Females n = 64	Females n = 86
Age Groups	Mean (SD)	Mean (SD)	Mean (SD)	Mean (SD)	Mean (SD)	Mean (SD)
20–29 yrs	129 (6)	153 (20)	149 (18)	128 (12)	149 (12)	152 (15)
30–39 yrs	120 (8)	141 (11)	135 (26)	120 (12)	156 (23)	141 (12)
40–49 yrs	110 (6)	131 (19)	129 (21)	114 (10)	140 (13)	125 (13)
50–59 yrs	111 (8)	136 (16)	116 (14)	117 (19)	127 (15)	124 (24)
60–69 yrs	—	116 (19)	110 (16)	—	133 (8)	117 (15)
70–79 yrs	—	—	102 (13)	—	—	121 (21)
80+ yrs	—	—	—	—	—	98 (11)

SD = standard deviation.
* The values in this table represent the combined total of flexion and extension range of motion.
† Nilsson et al used the cervical range of motion device (CROM) to measure passive range of motion.
‡ Dvorak et al used the CA-6000 Spine Motion Analyzer to measure passive ROM.
§ Castro et al used an ultasound-based coordinate measuring system, the CMS 50, to measure active range of motion.

the greatest decrease in flexion–extension ROM in 60 healthy men and women (aged 20 to 59 years) occurred between the 20-year-old group and the 30-year-old group. The decrease in ROM as one ages after adulthood appears to be different in young children. Arbogast[31] found that in 67 young children AROM in cervical flexion and right and left rotation measured by the CROM device actually increased slightly between 3 and 12 years of age.

Gender

Many of the same researchers who looked at the effects of age on cervical ROM also studied the effects of gender, but the results of these studies appear to be more inconsistent and controversial than the results of the age studies. In some studies, the trend for women to have a greater ROM than men was apparent, although differences were small and generally not significant. Also, in some instances, the effects of gender

TABLE 11.7 Age and Gender Effects on Cervical Rotation ROM: Normal Values in Degrees*

	Nilsson et al[†16]	Dvorak et al[‡22]	Castro et al[§29]	Nilsson et al[16]	Dvorak et al[22]	Castro et al[29]
	Males n = 31	Males n = 86	Males n = 71	Females n = 59	Females n = 64	Females n = 86
Age Groups	Mean (SD)	Mean (SD)	Mean (SD)	Mean (SD)	Mean (SD)	Mean (SD)
20–29 yrs	174 (13)	184 (12)	161 (16)	174 (13)	182 (10)	160 (14)
30–39 yrs	166 (12)	175 (10)	156 (32)	167 (13)	186 (10)	150 (15)
40–49 yrs	161 (21)	157 (20)	141 (15)	170 (10)	169 (14)	142 (15)
50–59 yrs	158 (10)	166 (14)	145 (11)	163 (12)	152 (16)	139 (19)
60–69 yrs	—	146 (13)	136 (18)	—	154 (15)	126 (14)
70–79 yrs	—	—	121 (14)	—	—	135 (16)
80+ yrs	—	—	—	—	—	113 (21)

SD = standard deviation.
* The values in this table represent the combined total of right and left rotation range of motion.
† Nilsson et al used the cervical range of motion device (CROM) to measure passive range of motion.
‡ Dvorak et al used the CA-6000 Spine Motion Analyzer to measure passive ROM.
§ Castro et al used an ultasound-based coordinate measuring system, the CMS 50, to measure active range of motion.

appeared to be motion specific and age specific in that some motions at some ages were affected more than others.

Castro[29] was one of the authors who found significant gender differences in cervical ROM, but this author noted that the differences occurred primarily in the motions of lateral flexion and flexion–extension in subjects between the ages of 70 and 79 years (see Tables 11.5, 11.6, and 11.7). Women older than 70 years of age were on the average more mobile in flexion–extension than men of the same age. Nilsson, Hartvigsen, and Christensen[16] found a significant difference between genders in lateral flexion ROM, but, in this study, males were more mobile than females, as seen in Table 11.6. Lantz, Chen, and Buch[34] studied a total of 56 healthy men and women aged 20 to 39 years. The authors found no difference between genders in total combined left and right lateral flexion, but women had greater ranges of active and passive axial rotation and flexion–extension than men of the same age. Women had an average of 12.7 degrees more active flexion–extension and an average of 6.50 degrees more active axial rotation than men of the same age. Women also had greater passive ROM in all cervical motions. Dvorak and associates[22] found that women between 40 and 49 years of age had greater ROM in all motions than men in the same age group. However, within each of the other age groups—20 to 29 years, 60 to 69 years, 70 to 79 years, and 80 to 89 years—no differences in cervical ROM were found between genders. Tables 11.8 and 11.9 contain information from a study by Youdas and associates[13] that shows that females in almost all age groups appear to have greater mean values for active cervical motion than males. Ferrario and associates[37] used a digital optoelectronic instrument to measure cervical motion in 30 women and 30 men and found that the women had greater ROM in all motions than the men. More support for a gender difference comes from Demaille-Wlodyka,[32] who found that of 232 healthy subjects aged 15 to 79 years, females had greater range of motion in flexion–extension and lateral flexion than males but not in axial rotation.

Youdas and associates[13] found a significant gender effect in all motions except flexion and determined that both males and females lose about 5 degrees of active extension and 3 degrees of active lateral flexion and rotation with each 10-year increase in age. If the measurements using the CROM device are valid, one can expect to find approximately 15 degrees to 20 degrees less active neck extension in a healthy 60-year-old individual compared with a healthy 20-year-old individual of the same gender.

In contrast to the preceding studies, a number of investigators concluded that gender had no effect on cervical ROM.[24,25,27,28,33] Ordway and associates[38] found a nonsignificant gender effect, and Pellachia and Bohannon,[26] in a study of 135 subjects aged 15 to 95 years with a history of neck pain, concluded that neither neck pain nor gender had any effect on ROM. Arbogast and coworkers[31] also found no effects of gender in the 67 children tested between the ages of 3 and 12. Hole, Cook, and Bolton[33] determined that gender had no significant effect on cervical range of motion in a group of 84 healthy men and women 20 to 69 years of age. Mannion[39] also found no effects of gender in 10 men and women whose AROM was measured in all cervical motions.

Active Versus Passive ROM

The AMA's fifth edition of the *Guides to the Evaluation of Permanent Impairment* recommends that AROM be performed.[12] The authors of the *Guides* are aware that a number of factors may affect a person's performance of AROM, such as pain, fear of injury, and motivation; therefore, they stress that a patient must be encouraged to put forth a maximal effort. They also state that AROM is probably much closer than PROM to the type of motion that a patient would use functionally and therefore is more relevant to impairment. Furthermore, PROM is dependent on the amount of force applied by the examiner, and a patient could be at risk of injury. Also, if a patient can perform a full ROM actively, then there is no reason to perform PROM.[12]

Other reasons for using AROM rather than PROM have been investigated by the following researchers, who have found that AROM is more reliably measured than PROM and has less variability. Assink and coworkers[40] determined that the intraclass correlation coefficients (ICCs) of AROM measurements were higher than the ICCs of PROM measurements in 30 symptomatic and 30 unsymptomatic volunteers. In asymptomatic subjects, PROM was generally larger than in AROM. In symptomatic subjects, the percentage of paired observations within 5 degrees varied from a low of 17 percent for PROM in extension to a high of 60 percent for AROM in rotation.

Nilsson[41] used the CROM device to measure half cycle PROM in 14 asymptomatic volunteers (seven men and seven women between the ages of 23 and 45 years). All motions were measured by two testers from neutral 0, and intratester reliability was found to be acceptable to the author, ranging from an r of 0.61 for right lateral flexion to an r of 0.85 for extension. Intertester reliability was unacceptable because the correlation coefficients fell below 0.60 in four out of the six directions, ranging from an r of 0.29 for left rotation to an r of 0.71 for flexion.

Nilsson, Christensen, and Hartvigsen[42] conducted a study to correct any problems with the previous study. More extensive training was arranged for the testers, and the number of subjects was increased from 14 to 35 (17 men and 18 women) who ranged in age from 20 to 28 years. Intertester reliability still was unacceptable for half cycle PROM because three out of six measurements fell below an r of 0.60. Intertester reliability for full cycle PROM was much better with r values in three planes ranging from 0.61 to 0.88. It appears as if the half cycle motions may be contributing more than the passive range of motion to the poor intertester reliability.

Bergman and associates[43] found that the highest variation in both 58 subjects in the symptomatic group and the 48 men and women in the asymptomatic group occurred in PROM testing versus AROM testing. The variation over a 12-week period ranged from 20.4 degrees for passive lateral flexion in

TABLE 11.8 Age and Gender Effects on Half Cycle Active Cervical Spine Motion in Males and Females Aged 11 to 49 Years: Normal Values in Degrees Using the CROM Device

| | Ages 11–19 yrs | | Ages 20–29 yrs | | Ages 30–39 yrs | | Ages 40–49 yrs | |
| | Males n = 20 | Females n = 20 | Males n = 20 | Females n = 20 | Males n = 20 | Females n = 21 | Males n = 20 | Females n = 22 |
Motion	Mean (SD)	Mean (SD)	Mean (SD)	Mean (SD)	Mean (SD)	Mean (SD)	Mean (SD)	Mean (SD)
Extension	86 (12)	84 (15)	77 (13)	86 (11)	68 (13)	78 (14)	63 (12)	78 (13)
Right lateral flexion	45 (8)	49 (7)	45 (7)	46 (7)	43 (9)	47 (8)	38 (11)	42 (9)
Left lateral flexion	46 (7)	47 (7)	41 (7)	43 (5)	41 (10)	44 (8)	36 (8)	41 (9)
Right rotation	74 (8)	75 (10)	70 (6)	75 (6)	67 (7)	72 (6)	65 (10)	70 (7)
Left rotation	72 (7)	71 (10)	69 (7)	72 (6)	65 (9)	66 (8)	62 (8)	64 (8)

SD = standard deviation; CROM = cervical range of motion device.
Adapted from Youdas, JW, et al[13]: Reprinted from *Physical Therapy* with the permission of the American Physical Therapy Association.

TABLE 11.9 Age and Gender on Half Cycle Active Cervical Spine Motion in Subjects Aged 50 to 89 Years: Mean Values in Degrees Using the CROM Device

| | Ages 50–59 yrs | | Ages 60–69 yrs | | Ages 70–79 yrs | | Ages 80–89 yrs | |
| | Males n = 20 | Females n = 20 | Males n = 20 | Females n = 20 | Males n = 20 | Females n = 20 | Males n = 20 | Females n = 18 |
Motion	Mean (SD)	Mean (SD)	Mean (SD)	Mean (SD)	Mean (SD)	Mean (SD)	Mean (SD)	Mean (SD)
Extension	60 (10)	65 (16)	57 (11)	65 (13)	54 (14)	55 (10)	49 (11)	50 (15)
Right lateral flexion	36 (5)	37 (7)	30 (5)	33 (10)	26 (7)	28 (7)	24 (6)	26 (6)
Left lateral flexion	35 (7)	35 (6)	30 (5)	34 (8)	25 (8)	27 (7)	24 (7)	23 (7)
Right rotation	61 (8)	61 (9)	54 (7)	65 (10)	50 (10)	53 (9)	46 (8)	53 (11)
Left rotation	58 (9)	63 (8)	57 (7)	60 (9)	50 (9)	53 (9)	47 (9)	51 (11)

SD = standard deviation; CROM = cervical range of motion device.
Adapted from Youdas, JW, et al[13]: Reprinted from *Physical Therapy* with the permission of the American Physical Therapy Association.

the asymptomatic group to 85.2 degrees for passive rotation in the symptomatic group. The fact that a substantial amount of variation occurred in PROM measurement prompted the authors to question whether PROM should be used as an outcome measure in intervention studies. Demaille-Wlodyka and colleagues[32] recommended that PROM should not be used because it overestimates a subject's mobility.

Testing Position

The lack of a well-defined neutral cervical spine position is thought to be responsible for the lower reliability of cervical spine motions starting in the neutral position (**half cycle motions**) compared with those starting at the end of one ROM and continuing to the end of another ROM (**full cycle motions**). An example of a half cycle motion is flexion, whereas an example of a full cycle motion is flexion-extension.

Studies that have attempted to better define the neutral position have used either radiographs[38,44] or motion analysis systems.[45,46] In the radiographic study conducted by Ordway and associates,[38] the authors determined that when the cervical spine is in the neutral position, the upper segments are in flexion and the lower segments have progressively less flexion; therefore, at C6 to C7, the spine is in a considerable amount of extension. Miller, Polissar, and Haas,[44] in the other radiographic study, found that the cervical spine is in the neutral position when the hard palate is in the horizontal plane. Although these findings are of considerable interest, they provide little help to the average clinician, who does not have access to radiographs for patient positioning.

Two studies that are more clinically relevant used the CA-6000 Spine Motion Analyzer.[45,46] This motion analysis system is capable of giving the location of neutral 0 position as coordinates in three dimensions corresponding to the three planes of motion. Christensen and Nilsson[45] found that the ability of 38 young (20 to 30 years of age) subjects to reproduce the neutral spine position with eyes and mouth closed was very good. The mean difference from neutral 0 in three motion planes was 2.7 degrees in the sagittal plane, 1.0 degrees in the horizontal plane, and 0.65 degrees in the frontal plane. Possibly, patients may be able to find the neutral position on their own, but the subjects in this study were healthy individuals, and the ability of patients to reproduce the neutral position is unknown. Solinger, Chen, and Lantz[46] attempted to standardize a neutral head position when measuring cervical motion in 20 subjects. For flexion and extension, the authors described a neutral position as one in which the corner of the eye was aligned with the upper angle of the ear, at the point where it meets the scalp. For lateral flexion, neutral was defined as the point at which the axis of the head was perceived to be vertically aligned. Compared with data collected using a less stringent head positioning, Solinger, Chen, and Lantz[46] demonstrated that by standardizing head position they obtained increases in reliability of 3 percent to 15 percent for rotation and lateral flexion but showed a decrease in reliability of up to 14 percent for flexion–extension.

Demaille-Wlodyka and colleagues[32] determined that neither age nor gender affected the 232 healthy volunteers'

ability to return their heads to a self-defined neutral position after performing a cervical ROM. However, Owens,[47] who used a computer interface electrogoniometer to measure head position in 48 students (36 males and 12 females) with a mean age of 28 years, found that active contractions of the posterior neck muscles caused subjects to undershoot their target neutral position by 2.1 degrees. This finding demonstrated that a recent history of cervical paraspinal muscle contraction can influence head repositioning in flexion–extension.

In a study using the 3Space Isotrak System, Pearson and Walmsley[23] found a significant difference in the neutral resting position (it became more retracted) after repeated neck retractions performed by 30 healthy subjects, but no statistically significant difference was found in the neck retraction ROM.

Another potential positional problem that testers need to be aware of has been identified by Lantz, Chen, and Buch.[34] These authors found that ROM measurements of the cervical spine taken in the seated position were consistently about 2.6 degrees greater than measurements taken in the standing position in all planes of motion. Greater differences occurred between seated and standing positions when flexion and extension were measured as half cycle motions starting in the neutral 0 position as opposed to measurement of full cycle motions. For axial rotation there was no significant difference in half cycle motions between sitting and standing.

Body Size

Castro[29] found that patients who were obese were not as mobile as patients who were not obese. Mean values for motions in all planes decreased with increasing body weight. Chibnall, Duckro, and Baumer,[48] in a study of 42 male and female subjects, found that body size reflected by distances between specific anatomical landmarks (e.g., between the chin and the acromial process) influenced ROM measurements taken with a tape measure. Any variation in body size among subjects resulted in an underestimation of ROM for subjects with large distances between landmarks and an overestimation of ROM for subjects with small distances between landmarks. The authors concluded that the use of **proportion of distance** (POD) should be used when comparing testing results among subjects. The use of POD (calculated by dividing the distance between the at-rest value and the end-of-range value by the at-rest value) helps to eliminate the effect of body size on ROM values obtained with a tape measure. Obviously, calculation of POD is not necessary if the progress of only one subject is measured. Peolsson and colleagues[36] found no significant correlation between body mass index (BMI) and AROM, with the exception of extension for both men and women and flexion for men.

Functional Range of Motion

Motion of the cervical spine is necessary for most activities of daily living and for most recreational and occupational activities. Bennett and asssociates[49] used the CROM device to determine the range of cervical motion required for 13 daily tasks performed by 28 college students. The greatest amount of motion was required by the following activities: backing up a car, tying shoes, and crossing the street. Relatively small amounts of flexion, extension, and rotation are required for eating, reading, writing, and using a computer. Drinking requires more cervical extension ROM than eating, and stargazing or simply looking up at the ceiling requires a full ROM in extension (Fig. 11.46). Using a telephone requires lateral flexion and rotation. Bathing and grooming require a considerable amount of motion.[49]

Sports activities such as serving a tennis ball, catching or batting a baseball, canoeing, and kayaking may require a full ROM in all planes. Different types of sports activities may have effects on ROM. For example, Guth[50] compared cervical rotation ROM in a group of 40 swimmers with that in 40 nonathletic volunteers. The swimmers, aged 14 to 17 years, had a mean total rotation ROM that was 9 degrees greater than the ROM of those aged 14 to 17 years in the control group. Certain occupational activities such as house painting or wallpapering require a full range of cervical extension and, possibly, a full range of flexion. A full ROM in cervical rotation is essential for safe driving of cars or trucks (Fig. 11.47).

Reliability and Validity

An article by Jordan[51] provides an excellent review of reliability studies and the instruments and methods used to evaluate cervical range of motion. The author identifies a number of problems with studies, including among others, the lack of an adequate sample size, appropriate statistical methods, and standardized protocols for measurement and for performance of the motions. These deficits make it difficult to compare studies and to be able to use the data that they generate.

Many different methods and instruments have been employed to assess motion of the head and neck. Similar to other areas of the body, intratester reliability generally is better than intertester reliability, no matter what instrument is used. Also, some motions seems to be more reliably measured than others. For example, the full cycle motions such as flexion–extension and right–left lateral flexion measured from one extreme of the range to the other appear to be more reliably measured than half cycle motions such as flexion measured from the neutral position.[18,32,40–43,52] This finding may be owed to the variability of the neutral position and the lack of a standardized method that an examiner can use for placing a subject's head in the neutral position. However, the problem with only measuring full cycle motions is that full cycle measurements do not provide any information about where unilateral limitations in motion occur.

Nilsson[41] found that intratester reliability was good when measuring half cycle motions, but intertester reliability was poor. Nilsson, Christensen, and Hartvigsen[42] found that the intertester reliability of passive range of motion measurements of half cycle motions was poor (r = 0.39 to 0.70), but the intertester reliability of passive range of motion measurements of full cycle motions was acceptable (r = 0.61 to 0.70). Jordan and colleagues,[52] who used the three-dimensional Fastrak system to measure cervical ROM, also found that the intertester reliability of full cycle motions (intraclass correlation coefficients [ICCs] = 0.81 to 0.89) was better than the reliability of half cycle motions (ICCs = 0.61 to 0.80) in 40 healthy subjects with two testers. The same was true for intratester reliability in which the ICCs for full cycle motions ranged from 0.76 to 0.82, whereas the ICCs for half cycle motions ranged from 0.54 to 0.70 in 32 healthy subjects with one tester on three occasions.

Malstrom and colleagues,[18] using both the Zebris ultrasonic system and the Myrin inclinometer, found that the full cycle motions showed less variability than the half cycle motions in 60 healthy volunteers (25 men and 35 women) 22 to 58 years of age. The ICCs ranged from 0.92 to 0.97 for full cycle motions and from 0.88 to 0.93 for half cycle motions. The full cycle motions also showed better concurrent validity with the Zebris than did half cycle measurements.

Damaille-Wlodyka,[32] in a study of 232 subjects, determined that full cycle motions had better validity than half cycle motions but half cycle motions allow for better assessment of unilateral limitations. Piva and associates,[53] using a

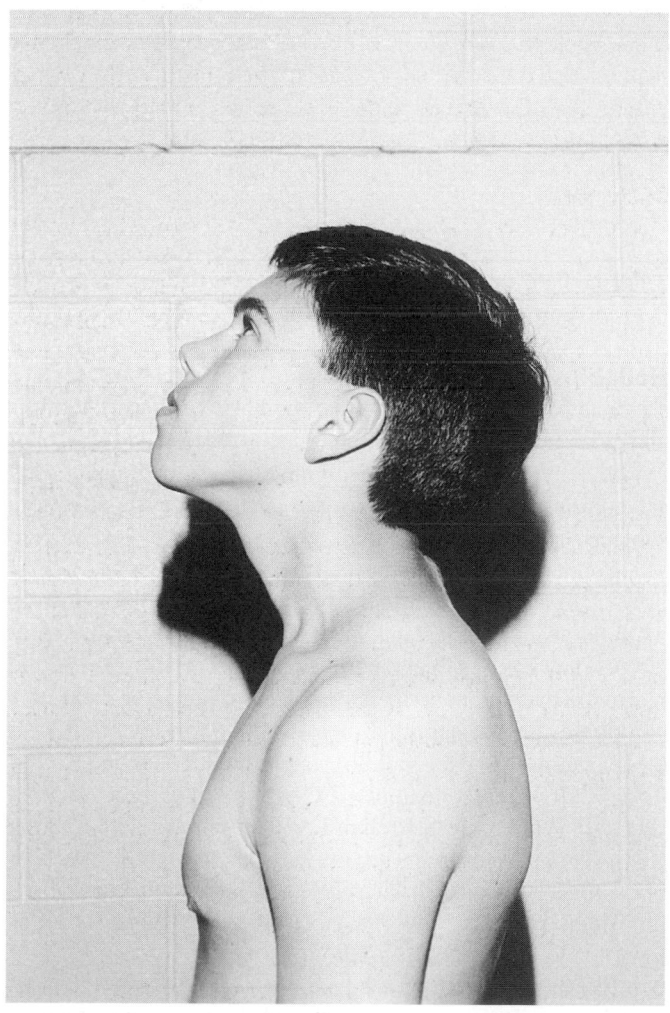

FIGURE 11.46 One needs at least 40 to 50 degrees of cervical extension range of motion (ROM) to look up at the ceiling.[2] If cervical extension ROM is limited, the person must extend the entire spine in an effort to place the head in a position whereby the eyes can look up at the ceiling.

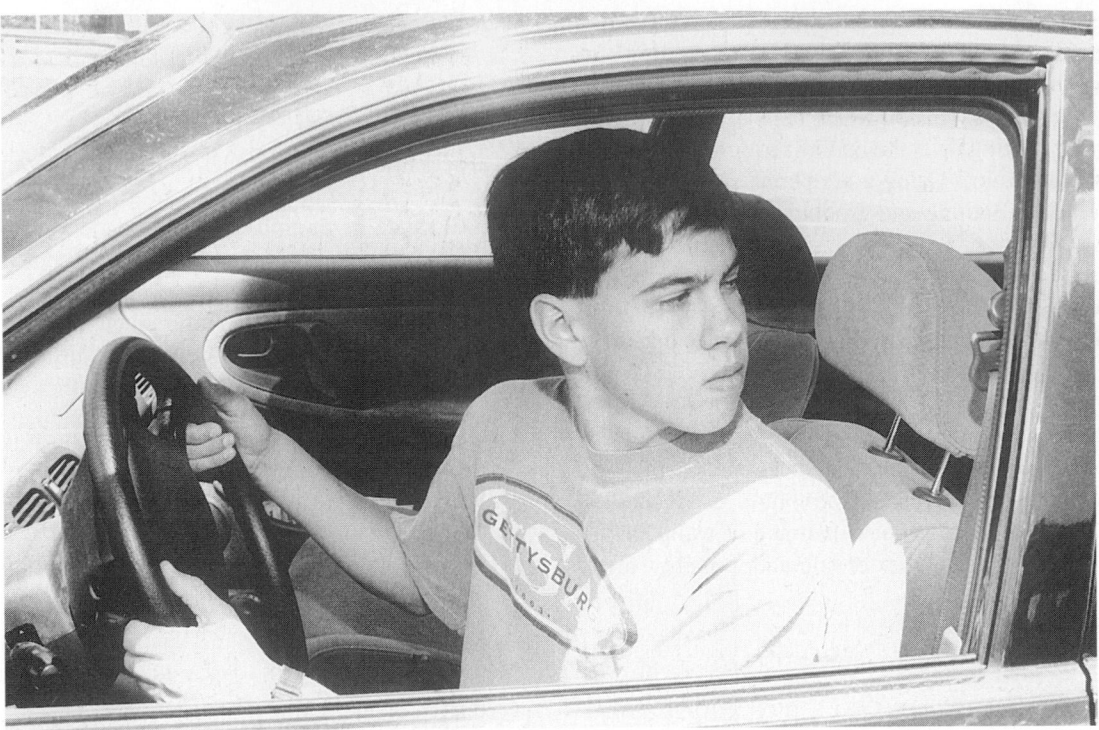

FIGURE 11.47 One needs a minimum of 60 to 70 degrees of cervical rotation to look over the shoulder.[2] If cervical rotation range of motion is limited, the person has to rotate the entire trunk to position the head to check for oncoming traffic.

single gravity goniometer to measure half cycle motions in 30 patients with neck pain, found that the standard error of measurement (SEM) ranged from 3.7 degrees for right lateral flexion to 5.6 degrees for extension. ICCs ranged from 0.78 for flexion to 0.91 for axial rotation, and intertester reliability was moderate to substantial for measuring active ROM in the sagittal and transverse planes of motion.

According to Chen and colleagues,[27] it is not possible to obtain a true validation of cervical ROM measurements because radiographic measurement has not been subjected to reliability and validity studies. Therefore, no valid gold standard exists. The only option available for investigators at the present time is to conduct concurrent validity studies to obtain agreement between instruments and procedures.[27] However, many researchers still consider radiographic measurement to be the gold standard.

Some of the studies that have been conducted to assess reliability or validity (or both) of the various instruments and methods are reviewed in the following section. The terms high, good, fair, poor, and unacceptable are used to designate different degrees of reliability. High reliability refers to ICCs of 90 to 99, good reliability refers to ICCs of 80 to 89, fair reliability refers to ICCs of 70 to 79, low or poor reliability is an ICC of 60 to 69, and unacceptable reliability is an ICC of less than 0.60. These definitions of reliability appear to be the most commonly used terms in the following studies, although a few authors have used the interpretation by Portney and Watkins[54] in which correlation coefficients higher than 0.75 indicate good reliability and coefficients of less than 0.75 indicate poor to moderate reliability.

Reliability: Universal Goniometer

Tucci and coworkers[55] found that the ICCs for intertester reliability of cervical spine motion ranged from –0.08 for flexion to 0.82 for extension for measurements taken with the universal goniometer by two experienced testers on 10 volunteer subjects.

Youdas, Carey, and Garrett[9] measured half cycle AROM in 60 patients with orthopedic problems ranging in age from 21 to 84 years. The patients were divided into three groups of 20 people. Each subject performed five repetitions of the motion in each plane to increase the compliance of the neck's soft tissues. Intratester reliability was good for flexion (ICC = 0.83), extension (ICC = 0.86), right lateral flexion (ICC = 0.85), left lateral flexion (ICC=0.84 and right rotation (ICC=0.90). Intratester reliability was fair for left rotation (ICC=0.78). Intertester reliability was fair (ICC=0.72 to 0.79) for extension, left lateral flexion, and right lateral flexion. Intertester reliability was poor (ICC = 0.54 to 0.62) for flexion and left and right rotation.

Pile and associates[56] used a universal goniometer to measure half cycle lateral flexion and flexion and extension in 10 patients with ankylosing spondylitis with minimal disease activity and ranging from 28 to 73 years of age. The testers included a rheumatologist, a rheumatology registrar, and three physical therapists. For intratester reliability each tester measured one patient four times. The authors did not present intratester reliability coefficients. The intertester reliability coefficient for right lateral flexion was 0.74; for left lateral flexion it was 0.68. The landmarks used for the lateral flexion measurement were the sternal notch as the axis and a line through the nose and forehead for the proximal arm. Flexion and extension were measured in the same way as the goniometer is used in this text. The intertester reliability coefficient for flexion was unacceptable (0.21), whereas the coefficient for extension was somewhat better (0.59).

Maksymowych and colleagues[57] measured full cycle rotation AROM using a plastic universal goniometer in 44 patients with ankylosing spondylitis with a mean age of 42.7 years. All measurements were taken by two testers (a trained clinical nurse and a rheumatologist) in mid-morning to avoid the effects of early morning stiffness. Intratester reliability was high for two testers (ICC = 0.98 and 0.97), and intertester reliability also was high (ICC = 0.95).

Validity: Universal Goniometer

In a search of the literature, no validity studies were found for the universal goniometer in which radiographs were used as the gold standard.

Reliability: Tape Measure

The fact that the landmarks used to obtain the measurements varied from study to study diminishes the usefulness of some of the following information. Landmarks and methods need to be standardized to make valid comparisons. The landmarks and results of studies by the authors[10,11] in Table 11.2 and by others are described in the following paragraphs.

Hsieh and Young[10] used two testers (one experienced and one inexperienced) to measure half cycle AROM in 34 healthy volunteers (27 men and 7 women) with an average age of 18 years. The landmarks used in the study for flexion and extension were the sternal notch and the chin. The landmarks for rotation were the acromial process and the chin, and the landmarks for lateral flexion were the acromion process and the lowest point of the earlobe. One tester measured 17 subjects, and the other tester measured a different group of 17 subjects. Intratester reliability coefficents (Pearson's r) ranged from 0.80 to 0.95 for the experienced tester and from 0.78 to 0.91 for the inexperienced tester. Measurement error for the experienced tester at the 99 percent confidence interval (CI) was approximately ±1 cm for sagittal motions and ± 2 cm for other motions. The inexperienced tester had a higher measurement error of approximately ±2 to 3 cm for sagittal motions and ±3 cm for other motions.

Balogen and associates[11] employed three physical therapists to measure half cycle AROM in 21 physical therapy students. The test-retest interval ranged from 4 to 110 days. The landmarks used to measure cervical flexion were the tip of the chin and the sternal notch. Landmarks for measuring lateral flexion were the anterior dimples in the shoulder to the lowest point of the earlobe. For rotation, the landmarks were the tip of the chin and the anterior dimples in the shoulder. Intratester reliability coefficients (r) for measuring neck flexion was poor

for all three therapists. Intratester reliability for extension was very good for two therapists and fair for one therapist. The intratester values for left and right rotation ranged from an r of 0.58 to 0.86. The fact that the interval between the first and second sessions was so long may have had an adverse effect on the intratester values. Intertester values ranged from an r of 0.35 to 0.90 in Session I and from an r of 0.47 for left lateral flexion to an r of 0.92 for extension in Session II.

Haywood and associates[58] used a plastic tape measure for measuring half cycle AROM in 159 patients with ankylosing spondylitis. The authors used the tip of the nose and the acromioclavicular joint as landmarks to measure right and left cervical rotation. The ROM was the difference between the tape measurement in the neutral position and the measurement in maximal ipsilateral rotation. Fifty-five patients participated in the reliability study. The intratester reliability (test-retest at 2-week interval) was high (ICC >0.90), but intertester reliability was unacceptable for the neutral starting position.

Maksymowych and coworkers[57] measured full cycle rotation AROM on 263 patients with ankylosing spondylitis from three different countries. Forty-four of the patients were involved in the reliability study. Landmarks used for measuring rotation were the tragus of the right ear and the suprasternal notch. Measurements were taken with a tape-based tool at full right rotation (D1) and at full left rotation (D2). Full cycle rotation was defined as the distance between the two measurements (D1-D2). Intratester reliability was good for the two testers (ICC = 0.80 and 0.89); intertester reliability also was good (ICC = 0.82).

Viitanen and associates[59] measured cervical lateral flexion and rotation in a series of 52 male patients with idiopathic ankylosing spondylitis with a mean age of 45 years. Testing was done by two physical therapists. Intratester aand intertester reliability coefficients for tape measurements were excellent for cervical lateral flexion (ICCs = 0.96 and ICC = 0.97, respectively) and for rotation (ICC = 0.98 and ICC = 0.97, respectively).

Validity: Tape Measure

Balogun and associates[11] compared measurements taken with a tape measure with measurements taken with a Myrin Reference Goniometer (Inclinometer). The r values of each of the three testers were higher for the tape measuring method than for the inclinometer method. Therefore, the authors recommended that the tape measure method be used more widely.

Viitanen and associates[59] compared cervical rotation and lateral flexion tape measurements with radiologic changes such as changes in the apophyseal joints, calcification of discs, and ossification of spinal ligaments. Cervical rotation and lateral flexion measurements correlated significantly with cervical radiologic changes and, therefore, according to the authors, the tape measure was an appropriate method for assessing disease severity and progression.

Maksymowych and coworkers[57] compared measurements of cervical AROM taken with a tape measure with measurements of cervical rotation AROM taken with a plastic universal goniometer. The authors found that the tape measure approach was comparable to the universal goniometer, which the authors used as the gold standard.

Reliability: Inclinometer

Viitanen and associates[59] used the Myrin Gravity Reference Goniometer to measure AROM in 52 male patients with ankylosing spondylitis with a mean age of 44.7 years. Two physical therapists measured patients on successive days. Both intratester reliability and intertester reliability were high with ICCs of 0.89 to 0.98.

Balogun and coworkers[11] employed three testers to use the Myrin Gravity Reference Goniometer to measure the AROM of half cycle motions. Twenty-one healthy students were measured over a period of several days (between 4 and 110). Intratester reliability coefficients (r) values for all motions ranged from unacceptable (r = 0.31) for flexion to good (r = 0.86) for extension. Intertester reliability coefficients across two testing sessions ranged from unacceptable (r = 0.26) for left rotation to good (r = 0.84) for extension.

Alaranta and associates[19] used a liquid single inclinometer, the MIE (Medical Research Ltd, London), which they attached by Velcro to a cloth helmet to the top of the subject's head to measure half cycle AROM flexion and extension and lateral flexion. A gravitational inclinometer was attached to the helmet, and the subject was placed in a supine position to measure rotation. Ninety-nine subjects participated in the intratester reliability part of the study in which one physiotherapist measured all subjects twice at an interval of 1 year. The correlation coefficient values for half cycle motions were an r of 0.68 for flexion and extension, r of 0.61 for lateral flexion, and unacceptable (r = 0.37) for rotation. Forty-eight subjects participated in the intertester reliability study in which two physiotherapists did the testing at a 1-week interval. The values for full cycle motions ranged from an r of 0.69 for flexion-extension to an r of 0.86 for left-right rotation.

Hole, Cook, and Bolton[33] also had two testers use an MIE single inclinometer to measure AROM in 30 healthy volunteers ages 20 to 69 years. Intratester reliability for flexion-extension, right lateral flexion, and right rotation was high (ICC = 0.93 to 0.94) and intratester reliability for left lateral flexion and left rotation was good (ICC = 0.84 to 0.88). Intertester reliability was good (ICC = 0.81 to 0.86) for flexion-extension, both right and left lateral flexion as well as left rotation. However, intertester reliability was only fair for right rotation (ICC = 0.76).

Hoving and associates[60] used a Cybex Electronic Digital Inclinometer-320 (EDI-320) to measure full cycle AROM in 32 patients 18 to 70 years of age with neck pain, neck stiffness, or both. Intratester reliability was high for motions in three planes, with values ranging from an ICC of 0.93 for lateral flexion for both raters to an ICC of 0.97 for flexion–extension for one rater. Intertester reliability was good to high with ICCs of 0.89 and higher. The smallest detectable differences (SDDs) based upon intratester agreement results for one of the testers were 11.1 degrees for flexion–extension, 10.4 degrees for lateral flexion, and 13.5 degrees for rotation.

Therefore, only changes greater than these values can be detected beyond measurement error when a single therapist performs the measurements. The SDD values were higher if two different raters performed the measurements.

Piva and coworkers[53] measured half cycle AROM with a gravity goniometer (MIE) in 30 patients ages 18 to 75 years of age who had symptoms in their neck, scapula, or head. ICC values ranged from fair to high (ICC = 0.78 to ICC = 0.91). The minimal detectable change (MDC) the authors considered to be adequate for clinical use ranged from 9 degrees for left rotation in flexion to 16 degrees for the motions of flexion and extension. The SEM was as follows: extension = 5.6 degrees, flexion = 5.8 degrees, left lateral flexion = 4.2 degrees, right lateral flexion = 3.7 degrees, left rotation = 4.1 degrees, and right rotation = 4.8 degrees.

Malstrom and associates[18] used the Myrin Gravity Reference Goniometer to measure both full and half cycle AROM in 60 "neck healthy" volunteers (35 women and 25 men) ranging in age from 22 to 58 years of age (Table 11.10). Intratester reliability was high, with ICCs of 0.90 and higher for full cycle flexion–extension, lateral flexion, and rotation. Intratester reliability was lower for half cycle motions, with the ICC ranging from 0.69 for left rotation to 0.89 for extension.

Bush and associates[61] evaluated the reliability of the following inclinometers: a single inclinometer, double inclinometers, and a single inclinometer with stabilization. Six Gerhardts Uni-Level pendulum inclinometers were used by 34 practicing physical therapists to take half cycle measurements of AROM of neck motions in three healthy models. The reliability between the three methods was unacceptable, with ICC values of 0.13 for extension, 0.31 for right lateral flexion, and 0.20 for left lateral flexion.

Validity: Inclinometer

Herrmann[62] took radiographic measurements of passive ROM of neck flexion–extension in 16 individuals aged 2 to 68 years. The radiographic measurements were compared with those obtained by means of a pendulum goniometer (inclinometer). ICCs of 0.98 indicated a good agreement between the two methods.

Lanz, Chen, and Buch[34] compared the double inclinometer Dualer digital dual inclinometer and the CA-6000 electrogoniometer. Simultaneous measurements by the two instruments were performed twice over a 1-week interval. Concurrent validity of the two instruments showed almost identical mean values for flexion, extension, and lateral flexion. The ICC for between-instrument comparison in the same session was high.

Malstrom and associates[18] compared the Myrin Gravity Reference Goniometer with a three-dimensional ultrasound motion device—the Zebris, CMS 30/70P system (Zebris Medizintechnik GmbH, Isny, Germany). Both instruments were used to measure full cycle AROM in 60 healthy volunteers (35 women and 25 men) ranging in age from 22 to 58 years of age. The test and retest ICC was high, greater than 0.90 for intradevice reliability. The ICC was greater than 0.93 for concurrent validity. The authors concluded that their research supports the continued use of the Myrin in routine clinical work.

TABLE 11.10 Cervical Range of Motion (CROM) Device: Intratester and Intertester Reliability

Author	Tester n	Subject n	Mean Age	Sample	Motions	Intra ICC	Inter ICC	Intra r	Inter r	SEM
Cupuano-Pucci et al[14]	2	20	23.5 yrs	Healthy	Flexion					
					Tester 1			0.63		
					Tester 2			0.91		
					Extension					
					Tester 1			0.90		
					Tester 2			0.82		
					Right lateral flexion					
					Tester 1			0.79	0.84	
					Tester 2			0.89		
					Right rotation					
					Tester 1			0.85	0.84	
					Tester 2			0.62		
Youdas et al[13]	5	6 (Intratester)	27.2 yrs	Healthy	Flexion	0.88	0.83			
		20 (Intertester)	33.0 yrs		Extension	0.94	0.90			
					Right lateral flexion	0.88	0.87			
					Right rotation	0.82	0.82			
Nilsson[41]	2	14	20–45 yrs	Healthy	Flexion			0.76	0.71	6°*
					Extension			0.85	0.47	5°
					Right lateral flexion			0.61	0.58	5°
					Right rotation			0.75	0.66	6°
Nilsson et al*[42]	2	35	20–28 yrs	Healthy	Flexion		0.65		0.70	
					Extension		0.54		0.55	
					Right lateral flexion		0.64		0.70	
					Right rotation		0.41		0.41	
					Flexion–extension		0.60		0.61	
					Right-left lateral flexion		0.69		0.71	
					Right-left rotation		0.88		0.88	

Continued

TABLE 11.10 Cervical Range of Motion (CROM) Device: Intratester and Intertester Reliability—cont'd

Author	Tester n	Subject n	Mean Age	Sample	Motions	Intra ICC	Inter ICC	Intra r	Inter r	SEM
Rheault et al[63]		22	37.4 yrs	Hx of cervical spine pathology	Flexion		0.76			
					Extension		0.98			
					Right lateral flexion		0.87			
					Right rotation		0.81			
Peolsson et al[36]	2	31	32.3 yrs	Healthy	Flexion-extension	0.91	0.90			2°
					Right and Left lateral flexion	0.94	0.90			3°
Olson et al[72]	4	12	21-47 yrs	Healthy	Flexion	0.88	0.58			4°†
					Extension	0.99	0.97			3°
					Right lateral flexion	0.98	0.96			2°
					Right rotation	0.99	0.96			3°
Youdas et al[9]	11	20	55.9 yrs	Orthopedic disorders	Flexion	0.95	0.86			
					Extension	0.90	0.86			
		20	60.7 yrs		Right lateral flexion	0.92	0.88			
		20	60.8 yrs		Left lateral flexion	0.93	0.92			

ICC = intraclass correlation coefficient; r = Pearson product moment correlation coefficient; SEM = standard error of measurement.
* 95% confidence interval for single subject measurement.
† Represents intertester SEM.

Bush and associates[61] compared three methods of inclinometry measurements of sagittal and frontal plane cervical motion with radiographic measurements. Transverse plane motion measurements were compared with computed tomography scan measurements. The authors defined validity as those inclinometry measurements that fell within ±5 degrees of radiographic measurements. Using this standard, only the single and double inclinometer methods were valid for measuring flexion; only the single and single stabilization methods were valid for measuring extension. No methods were valid for measuring either lateral flexion or rotation. The single inclinometer method had the highest validity among the three methods.

Reliability: CROM Device

Capuano-Pucci[14] in 1981 conducted one of the earliest studies on the CROM device in which two testers took measurements of each half cycle AROM performed by 20 subjects (16 women and 4 men) with a mean age of 23.5 years. The author found good intratester reliability for four out of six half cycle motions for one tester and for five out six motions for the second tester. All correlation coefficients were greater than 0.80 for intertester reliability, which was slightly higher than intratester reliability. This unusual finding was attributed to the fact that the time interval between testers was only minutes, whereas the time interval between the first and second trials by one tester was 2 days. More detailed information about this study and other studies in the section can be found in Table 11.10.

In the 1991 study by Youdas, Carey, and Garrett,[9] 11 volunteer physical therapists were given a 1-hour training session on the CROM device prior to measuring half cycle AROM in 60 patients (39 women and 21 men) with orthopedic disorders. The patients, ranging in age from 21 to 84 years, were divided into groups of 20 and were tested twice by two therapists. The results of the testing showed high intratester reliability and good intertester reliability for both flexion and extension. Intratester reliability was good for left neck lateral flexion (ICC = 0.84) and was high for right lateral flexion (ICC = 0.92). Intertester reliability was fair for left lateral flexion and good for right lateral flexion. Intratester reliability was high for both left and right rotation, and intertester reliability for rotation ranged from good for left rotation to high for right rotation.

Youdas and associates[13] used five testers to measure half cycle AROM in 337 healthy subjects (171 women and 166 men) who were 11 to 97 years of age. Each subject performed three repetitions of each motion, and each subject was tested by three testers within minutes of each other. Intratester reliability was low for flexion (ICC = 0.76), high for extension (ICC = 0.94), and good for left and right lateral flexion. Intratester reliability for rotation also was good, with ICCs of 0.84 for left rotation and 0.80 for right rotation. The intertester reliability of all half cycle neck motion measurements was good except for left rotation, which was poor (ICC = 0.66).

Nilsson[41] measured half cycle PROM on 14 volunteers 23 to 45 years of age. Each subject was measured three times at 20-minute intervals. Intratester reliability was considered to be acceptable (r = 0.61 to 0.86). Intertester reliability was unacceptable (r = 0.29 to 0.66) based on the mean of five repeated measures and the fact that in four out of six motions the r was less than 0.60.

Hole, Cook, and Bolton[33] selected 30 of 84 asymptomatic subjects for the reliability portion of a study of full cycle AROM. Intratester reliability was high (ICC = 0.96) for the full cycle combined motion of flexion and extension, and intertester reliability was good (ICC = 0.88). Intratester reliability was high (ICC = 0.96) for full cycle right-left lateral flexion, and intertester reliability was good (ICC = 0.84). Both intratester and intertester reliability were high (ICC = 0.92) for the full cycle motion of left-right rotation.

Nilsson, Christiansen, and Hartvigsen[42] measured half and full cycle PROM on 17 males and 18 females 20 to 28 years of age. Subjects were asked to close their eyes and position their heads in neutral while the dials on the CROM device were set to 0. Intertester reliability was acceptable (r = 0.61 to 0.88) for full cycle motions, but intertester reliability for measuring single cycle motions was an r of 0.39 to 0.70. Rheault and colleagues[63] found only small mean differences ranging from 0.5 degrees to 3.6 degrees between two testers who measured half cycle extension AROM with the CROM device.

Lindell, Eriksson, and Strender[64] compared the performance of a medically untrained tester with an experienced physical therapist using the therapist as the gold standard. The untrained tester received 4 hours of training and practice in 10 tests including measurements of half cycle cervical flexion and extension and rotation taken with the CROM device. The subjects in the study included 30 patients with neck and back pain and 20 healthy subjects. In the interrater reliability study, all 50 subjects were tested once by each tester. In the intertester study, each tester measured neck motions twice in 10 of the 20 healthy subjects. Intratester reliability for the therapist was good for flexion (ICC = 0.86) and high for extension (ICC = 0.98), with an SEM of 2 degrees for each measurement. The ICCs for intratester reliability for the other tester were 0.62 for flexion and 0.80 for extension. The ICC for the therapist for right rotation was high; for left rotation the ICC was good. The other tester had good ICCs for both right and left rotation and slightly higher SEMs compared to the therapist. Cervical flexion and extension had poor intertester reliability, which the authors attributed to the need for manual stabilization. Other tests that required manual stabilization also had poor intertester reliability, but overall, the medically untrained tester was able to perform acceptably in 7 out of 10 tests.

Validity: CROM Device

Ordway and coworkers[65] simultaneously measured full cycle AROM of combined flexion-extension with the CROM device, 3Space system, and radiographs in 20 healthy volunteers (11 women and 9 men) between 20 and 49 years of age. The authors found no significant difference between CROM device measurements and the radiographic angle between the occipital line and the vertical body, nor between the 3Space system and radiographic angle between the occipital line and the C7 vertebral body. However, there was a significant difference between flexion and extension measurements taken with the CROM device and the 3Space system. Therefore, these methods could not be used interchangeably. The authors determined that full cycle flexion–extension could be reliably measured by all three methods but that standardization of positioning was required to minimize upper thoracic motion with the CROM device. Protraction and retraction measured with the 3Space system were in agreement with the radiographic measurements but differed significantly from the measurements taken with the CROM device The CROM device's advantages over the 3Space system were lower cost and ease of use.

Tousignant[66] used radiographs to determine the criterion validity of the CROM device for measuring half cycle flexion and extension on 31 healthy participants who were 18 to 25 years of age. CROM measurements were highly correlated with measurements obtained by the radiographic method for extension (r = 0.98, P <0.001) and flexion (r = 0.97, P <0.001) so that the validity of the CROM device for measuring flexion and extension was supported.

Tousignant and associates[67] determined that the CROM measurements of half cycle AROM of lateral flexion demonstrated a very good linear relationship with radiographic measurements. A physiotherapist who had received 4 hours of instruction in using the CROM device measured right and left lateral flexion in 24 patients with neck pain. The measurements of left lateral flexion and right lateral flexion were compared with radiographic measurements as the gold standard. The correlation between the CROM device and radiographic measurements was good for both left (r = 0.82) and right (r = 0.84) lateral flexion. Therefore, the criterion validity of the CROM device for measuring lateral flexion was supported.

Tousignant and associates,[15] in another criterion validity study, compared half cycle AROM measurements taken with the CROM device with measurements taken with the Optotrak (an optoelectronic system). Subjects in the study included 34 women (21 to 85 years of age) and 21 men (19 to 80 years of age) recruited from the community. The results showed a very strong linear relationship between cervical rotation measured with the CROM device and the values obtained with the Optotrak. Pearson correlation coefficients (r) between CROM values and Optotrak values were good to excellent for rotation and for all other cervical motions. Based on their findings, the authors concluded that the validity of the CROM device was supported for the measurement of half cycle rotation in healthy individuals.

Hole, Cook, and Bolton[33] compared measurements of full cycle AROM taken with the CROM device to measurements taken with a single gravity inclinometer (MIE) to determine the reliability and concurrent validity of the two instruments for measuring cervical motion. Eighty-four asymptomatic subjects were included in the study. There was good agreement between the two instruments when measuring AROM in the sagittal and coronal planes, and concurrent validity was supported for flexion–extension and for right–left lateral flexion, but there was no agreement when measuring rotation in the transverse plane because, according to the authors, motion was consistently overestimated by the MIE.

Reliability: CA-6000 Electrogoniometer

Lantz, Chen, and Buch[34] measured active and passive half cycle motions in healthy students with the CA-6000. Intratester reliability ICC ranged from fair (0.76) to high (0.97) for AROM for full cycle motions and from poor (0.58) to high (0.95) for PROM for full cycle motions. Intertester ICCs for full cycle AROM were higher, ranging from good (0.84) to high (0.91), compared to ICCs for full cycle PROM, which were fair (0.74) to good (0.86).

Solinger, Chen, and Lantz[46] measured half and full cycle AROM in 20 healthy volunteer subjects (9 men and 11 women) ranging in age from 20 to 40 years. Each subject's ROM was measured twice by two experienced testers. Intertester and intratester reliability for full cycle motions of rotation and lateral flexion had high ICCs, ranging from 0.93 to 0.97, whereas intertester and intratester reliability ICCs for half cycle motions ranged from good (0.83) to high (0.95). Reliability values were consistently lower for measurements beginning in the neutral position compared with full cycle motions. The ICCs indicated that the electrogoniometer performed very reliably for rotation and lateral flexion but only at an acceptable level for flexion–extension (0.75 to 0.93). Flexion from the neutral position was the least reliable measurement even when taken by a single tester.

Christensen and Nilsson[68] found good intratester and intertester reliability for measurements of AROM in 40 individuals tested by two testers. Intratester reliability was also good for PROM, but intertester reliability was good only for full cycle motions.

Validity: CA-6000 Spine Motion Analyzer Electrogoniometer

Mannion and associates[39] compared cervical CROM measurements taken with the CA-6000 Spine Motion Analyzer with measurements taken with a three-dimensional ultrasound motion device called the Zebris CMS System. Initial measurements by both systems were taken in 19 healthy volunteers, and the same measurements were taken 3 days later. Test-retest reliability was good for each instrument, but a small significant difference (1 to 10 percent) between the values obtained by each instrument occurred.

Petersen and coworkers[69] determined that there was a large difference between the measurements obtained with the CA-6000 Spine Motion Analyzer and radiographs.

Reliability: Visual Estimation

The reliability of visual estimates has been studied by Viikari-Juntura[71] in a neurological patient population and by Youdas, Carey, and Garrett[9] in an orthopedic patient population. In the study by Viikari-Juntura,[71] the subjects were 52 male and female neurological patients ranging in age from 13 to 66 years who had been referred for cervical myelography. Intertester reliability between two testers of visual estimates of cervical ROM was determined by the authors to be fair. The weighted kappa reliability coefficient for intratester agreement in categories of normal, limited, or markedly limited ROM ranged from 0.50 to 0.56.

In the study by Youdas, Carey, and Garrett,[9] the subjects were 60 orthopedic patients ranging in age from 21 to 84 years. Intertester reliability for visual estimates of both active flexion and extension was poor (ICC = 0.42). Intertester reliability for visual estimates of active neck lateral flexion ROM was fair. The ICC for left lateral flexion was 0.63; for right lateral flexion it was 0.70. The intertester reliability for visual estimates of rotation was poor for left rotation (ICC = 0.69) and good for right rotation (ICC = 0.82).

Summary

Each of the techniques for measuring cervical ROM discussed in this chapter has certain advantages and disadvantages. The universal goniometer and tape measure are the least inexpensive and easiest to obtain, transport, and use, and therefore may be more acceptable clinically than other instruments. Generally, intratester reliability is better than intertester reliability. Therefore, if these methods are used to determine a patient's progress, repeated measurements should be taken by a single therapist. However, both the universal goniometer and tape measure require more extensive research to validate their continued use in the clinic.

In consideration of the cost and availability of the various instruments for measuring cervical ROM, and because of the fact that the intratester reliability of the universal goniometer and tape measure appears comparable with that of measurements taken with other instruments, we have retained the universal goniometer and tape measure methods in this edition, but we added methods using the double inclinometer and the CROM device. We included the double inclinometer because this method is advocated for measuring the cervical spine by the American Medical Association, although research on the reliability and validity of this method is lacking. The reliability and validity of the CROM device has been very well researched, as presented in this section. If the tape measure is being used to compare ROM among subjects, calculation of proportion of distance (POD) should help to eliminate the effects of different body sizes on measurements (refer to Body Size in the Research Findings section).[48]

REFERENCES

1. Bogduk, N, and Mercer, S: Biomechanics of the cervical spine, I: Normal kinematics. Clin Biomech 15:633, 2000.
2. Magee, DJ: Orthopedic Physical Assessment, ed 4. WB Saunders, Elsevier Science USA, Philadelphia, 2002.
3. Goel, VK: Moment-rotation relationships of the ligamentous occipito-atlanto-axial complex. J Biomech 8:673, 1988.
4. Cailliet, R: Soft Tissue Pain and Disability, ed 3. FA Davis, Philadelphia, 1991.
5. Crisco, JJ, Panjabi, MM, and Dvorak, J: A model of the alar ligaments of the upper cervical spine in axial rotation. J Biomech 24:607, 1991.
6. Dumas, JL, et al: Rotation of the cervical spinal column. A computed tomography in vivo study. Surg Radiol Anat 15:33, 1993.
7. White, AA, and Punjabi, MM: Clinical Biomechanics of the Spine, ed 2. JB Lippincott, Philadelphia, 1990.
8. Hertling, D, and Kessler, RM: Management of Common Musculoskeletal Disorders, ed 3. JB Lippincott, Philadelphia, 1996.
9. Youdas, JW, Carey, JR, and Garrett, TR: Reliability of measurements of cervical spine range of motion: Comparison of three methods. Phys Ther 71:2, 1991.
10. Hsieh, C-Y, and Yeung, BW: Active neck motion measurements with a tape measure. J Orthop Sports Phys Ther 8:88, 1986.
11. Balogun, JA, et al: Inter- and intratester reliability of measuring neck motions with tape measure and Myrin gravity-reference goniometer. J Orthop Sports Phys Ther 10:248, 1989.
12. American Medical Association: Guides to the Evaluation of Permanent Impairment, ed 5. AMA, Chicago, 2000.
13. Youdas, JW, et al: Normal range of motion of the cervical spine: An initial goniometric study. Phys Ther 72:770, 1992.
14. Capuano-Pucci, D, et al: Intratester and intertester reliability of the cervical range of motion device. Arch Phys Med Rehabil 72:338, 1991.
15. Tousignant M, et al: Criterion validity study of the Cervical Range of Motion (CROM) Device for rotational range of motion on healthy adults. J Orthop Sports Phys Ther 36:242, 2006.
16. Nilsson, N, Hartvigsen, J, and Christensen, HW: Normal ranges of passive cervical motion for women and men 20–60 years old. J Manipulative Physiol Ther 19:306, 1996.
17. CROM Procedure Manual: Procedure for Measuring Neck Motion with the CROM. Performance Attainment Association, St Paul, MN.
18. Malstrom, EM, et al: Zebris versus Myrin: A comparative study between a three-dimensional ultrasound movement analysis and an inclinometer/compass method: Interdevice reliability, concurrent validity, intertester comparison, intertester reliability, and intraindividual variability. Spine 28:E433, 2003.
19. Alaranta, H, et al: Flexibility of the spine: Normative values of goniometric and tape measurements. Scand J Rehab Med 26:147, 1994.
20. O'Driscoll, SL, and Tomenson, J: The cervical spine. Clin Rheum Dis 8:617, 1982.
21. Keske, J, Johnson, G, and Ellingham, C: A reliability study of cervical range of motion of young and elderly subjects using an electromagnetic range of motion system (ENROM) (abstract). Phys Ther 71:S94, 1991.
22. Dvorak, J, et al: Age and gender related normal motion of the cervical spine. Spine 17:S-393, 1992.
23. Pearson, ND, and Walmsley, RP: Trial into the effects of repeated neck retractions in normal subjects. Spine 20:1245, 1995.
24. Walmsley, RP, Kimber, P, and Culham, E: The effect of initial head position on active cervical axial rotation range of motion in two age populations. Spine 21:2435, 1996
25. Trott, PH, et al: Three dimensional analysis of active cervical motion: The effect of age and gender. Clin Biomech 11:201, 1996.
26. Pellachia, GL, and Bohannon, RW: Active lateral neck flexion range of motion measurements obtained with a modified goniometer: Reliability and estimates of normal. J Manipulative Physiol Ther 21:443, 1998.
27. Chen, J, et al: Meta-analysis of normative cervical motion. Spine 24:1571, 1999.
28. Feipel, V, et al: Normal global motion of the cervical spine: An electro-goniometric study. Clin Biomech (Bristol, Avon) 14:462, 1999.
29. Castro, WHM: Noninvasive three-dimensional analysis of cervical spine motion in normal subjects in relation to age and sex. Spine 25:445, 2000.
30. Kulman KA: Cervical range of motion in the elderly. Arch Phys Med Rehabil 74:1071, 1993.
31. Arbogast KB, et al: Normal cervical range of motion in children 3–12 years old. Spine 12:E309, 2007

32. Demaille-Wlodyka S, et al: Cervical range of motion and cephalic kinesthesis: Ultrasonographic analysis by age and sex. Spine 32:E254, 2007.
33. Hole DE, Cook JM, and Bolton JE: Reliability and concurrent validity of two instruments for measuring cervical range of motion: Effects of age and gender. Manual Therapy 1:36, 1995.
34. Lantz, CA, Chen, J, and Buch, D: Clinical validity and stability of active and passive cervical range of motion with regard to total and unilateral uniplanar motion. Spine 11:1082, 1999.
35. Sforza, C, et al:Three dimensional analyses of active head and cervical spine range of motion: Effect of age in healthy male subjects. Clin Biomech 17:611, 2002.
36. Peolsson, A, et al: Intra- and inter-tester reliability and range of motion of the neck. Physiother Canada Summer:233, 2000
37. Ferrario VF, et al: Active motion of the head and cervical spine: A three-dimensional investigation in healthy young adults. J Othop Res 20:122, 2002.
38. Ordway, NR, et al: Cervical flexion, extension, protrusion and retraction. A radiographic segmental analysis. Spine 24:240, 1999.
39. Mannion, AF, et al: Range of global motion of the cervical spine: Intraindividual reliability and the influence of measurement device. Eur Spine J 9:379, 2000.
40. Assink N, et al: Interobserver reliability of neck-mobility measurements by means of the flock of birds electromagnetic tracking system. J Manipulative Physiol Ther 28:408, 2005.
41. Nilsson N: Measuring passive cervical motion: A study of reliability. J Manipulative Physiol Ther 18:293, 1995
42. Nilsson N, Christensen, HW, and Hartvigsen, J: The interexaminer reliability of measuring passive cervical range of motion. J Manipulative Physiol Ther 19:302, 1996.
43. Bergman GJ, et al: Variation in the cervical range of motion over time measured by the "flock of birds" electromagnetic tracking system. Spine 30:650, 2005.
44. Miller, JS, Polissar, NL, and Haas, M: A radiographic comparison of neutral cervical posture with cervical flexion and extension ranges of motion. J Manipulative Physiol Ther 19:296, 1996.
45. Christiansen, HW, and Nilsson, N: The ability to reproduce the neutral zero position of the head. J Manipulative Physiol Ther 22:26, 1999.
46. Solinger, AB, Chen, J, and Lantz, CA: Standardized initial head position in cervical range-of-motion assessment: Reliability and error analysis. J Manipulative Physiol 23:20, 2000.
47. Owens, EF, et al: Head repositioning erors in normal student volunteers: A possible tool to assess the neck's neuromuscular system. Chirop Osteopat 14:5, 2006.
48. Chibnall, JT, Duckro, PN, and Baumer, K. The influence of body size on linear measurements used to reflect cervical range of motion. Phys Ther 74:1134, 1994.
49. Bennett, SE, Schenk, RJ, Simmons, ED: Active range of motion utilized in the cervical spine to perform daily functional tastks. J Spinal Disord Tech 15:307, 2002.
50. Guth, EH: A comparison of cervical rotation in age-matched adolescent competitive swimmers and healthy males. J Orthop Sports Phys Ther 21:21, 1995.
51. Jordan, K: Assessment of published reliability studies for cervical range of motion measurement tools. J Manipulative Physiol Ther 23:180, 2000.
52. Jordan K, et al: The reliability of the three-dimensional FASTRAK measurement system in measuring cervical spine and shoulder range of motion in healthy subjects. Rheumatol 39:382, 2000.
53. Piva SR, et al: Inter-tester reliability of passive intervertebral and active movements of the cervical spine. Man Ther 11:321, 2006.
54. Portney, L and Watkins, M: Foundations of Clinical Research: Applicaions to Practice, ed 2. Prentice-Hall, Upper Saddle River, NJ, 2000.
55. Tucci, SM, et al: Cervical motion assessment: A new, simple and accurate method. Arch Phys Med Rehabil 67:225, 1986.
56. Pile, K,D, et al: Clinical assessment of ankylosing spondylitis: A study of observer variation in spinal measurements. Br J Rheumatol 30:29,1991.
57. Maksymowych WP, et al: Development and validation of a simple tape-based measurement tool for recording cervical rotation in patients with ankylosing spondylitis: Comparison with a goniometer-based approach. J Rheumatol 33:2242, 2006.
58. Haywood KL, et al: Spinal mobility in ankylosing spondylitis: reliability, validity and responsiveness, Rheumatology (Oxford) 43:750, 2004.
59. Viitanen JV, et al: Clinical assessment of spinal mobility measurements in ankylosing spondylitis: A compact set for follow-up trials? Clin Rheumatol 19:131, 2000.

60. Hoving JL, et al.: Reproducibility of cervical range of motion in patients with neck pain. BMC Musculoskelet Dis 6:59, 2005.

61. Bush, KW, et al: Validity and intertester reliability of cervical range of motion using inclinometer measurements. J Manual Manipul Ther 8:52, 2000.

62. Herrmann, DB: Validity study of head and neck flexion-extension motion comparing measurements of a pendulum goniometer and roentgenograms. J Orthop Sports Phys Ther 11:414, 1990.

63. Rheault, W, et al: Intertester reliability of the flexible ruler for the cervical spine. J Orthop Sports Phys Ther Jan:254, 1989.

64. Lindell O, Eriksson L, and Strender L-E: The reliability of a 10-test package for patients with prolonged back and neck pain: could an examiner without formal medical education be used without loss of quality? A methodological study. BMC Musculoskelet Dis 8:31, 2007.

65. Ordway, NR, et al: Cervical sagittal range of motion. Analysis using three methods: Cervical range-of-motion device. 3. Space and radiography. Spine 22:501, 1997.

66. Tousignant, MA: Criterion validity of the cervical range of motion (CROM) goniometer for cervical flexion and extension. Spine 25:324, 2000.

67. Tousignant M, et al: Validity study for the Cervical Range of Motion Device used for lateral flexion in patients with neck pain. Spine 27:812, 2002.

68. Christensen, HW, and Nilsson, N: The reliability of measuring active and passive cervical range of motion: An observer blinded and randomized repeated measures design. J Manipulative Physiol Ther 21:341, 1998.

69. Petersen CM, et al: Agreement of measures obtained radiographically and by the OSI CA-8000 Spine Motion Analyzer for cervical spine motion. Man Ther 13:200, 2008.

70. Defibaugh, JJ: Measurement of head motion. Part II: An experimental study of head motion in adult males. Phys Ther 44:163, 1964.

71. Viikari-Juntura, E: Interexaminer reliability of observations in physical examination of the neck. Phys Ther 67:1526, 1987.

72. Olson, SL, et al: Tender point sensitivity, range of motion, and perceived disability in subjects with neck pain. J Ortho Sports Phys Ther 30:13, 2000.

Palpation - Thoracolumbar

- Sternum
- xiphoid process
- ribs
- spinous process of T+L

- L4 is b/w PSISs under middle to iliac crest

- ASIS - roll hands up + down anterior pelvis to find bony prominence

- Sacro iliac joint - prone - find PSIS

- sacral angle (inferior lateral angle)

- Greater trochanter - IR/ER - you'll feel bump raise + cover

~~look~~ look for symmetry
   - ASIS - maybe one pelvic bone rotates more

Thoracic flexion - sitting

- patient sit
- ask to bend (slump down)
   - "make hole in chest")
- measure quantitative

Standing

- find T12
- count 5 down from inferior border of scap (T7)
- put inclinometer on
- have patient bend

Extend

- sit up after sitting
- you can put towel roll behind thoracic
- can have patient lift up elbows
- chair is stabilizer

Extension Stand

- hips on "back packet"
- patients extends back

Chapter 12

The Thoracic and Lumbar Spine

Structure and Function

Thoracic Spine

Anatomy of the Vertebrae

The 12 vertebrae of the thoracic spine form a curve that is convex posteriorly (Fig. 12.1A). These vertebrae have a number of unique features. Spinous processes slope inferiorly from T1 to T10 and overlap from T5 to T8, whereas the spinous processes of T11 and T12 take on the horizontal orientation of the lumbar region's spinous processes. The transverse processes from T1 to T10 are large, with thickened ends that support paired costal facets for articulation with the ribs. Paired demifacets (superior and inferior costovertebral facets), also for articulation with the ribs, are located on the posterolateral corners of the vertebral bodies from T2 to T9.

Anatomy of the Joints

The intervertebral and zygapophyseal joints in the thoracic region have essentially the same structure as described for the cervical region, except that the superior articular zygapophyseal facets face posteriorly, somewhat laterally, and cranially. The superior articular facet surfaces are slightly convex, whereas the inferior articular facet surfaces are slightly concave. The inferior articular facets face anteriorly and slightly medially and caudally. In addition, the joint capsules are tighter than those in the cervical region.

The costovertebral joints are formed by slightly convex costal superior and inferior demifacets (costovertebral facets) on the head of a rib and corresponding demifacets on the vertebral bodies of a superior and an inferior vertebra (Fig. 12.1B). From T2 to T8, the costovertebral facets articulate with concave demifacets located on the inferior body of one vertebra and on the superior aspect of the adjacent inferior vertebral body. Some of the costovertebral facets also articulate with the interposed intervertebral disc, whereas the 1st, 11th, and 12th ribs articulate with only one vertebra. A thin, fibrous capsule, which is strengthened by radiate ligaments (see Fig. 12.1B) and the posterior longitudinal ligament, surrounds the costovertebral joints. An intra-articular ligament lies within the capsule and holds the head of the rib to the annulus pulposus.

The costotransverse joints are the articulations between the costal tubercles of the 1st to the 10th ribs and the costal facets on the transverse processes of the 1st to the 10th thoracic vertebrae. The costal tubercles of the 1st to the 7th ribs are slightly convex, and the costal facets on the corresponding transverse processes are slightly concave. The articular surfaces of the costal and vertebral facets are quite flat from about T7 to T10. The costotransverse joint capsules are strengthened by the medial, lateral, and superior costotransverse ligaments.

Osteokinematics

The zygapophyseal articular facets lie in the frontal plane from T1 to T6 and therefore limit flexion and extension in this region. The articular facets in the lower thoracic region are oriented more in the sagittal plane and thus permit somewhat more flexion and extension. The ribs and costal joints restrict lateral flexion in the upper and middle thoracic region, but in the lower thoracic segments, lateral flexion and rotation are relatively free because these segments are not limited by the ribs. In general, the thoracic region is less flexible than the cervical spine because of the limitations on movement imposed by the overlapping spinous processes, the tighter joint capsules, and the rib cage.

Arthrokinematics

In flexion, the body of the superior thoracic vertebra tilts anteriorly, translates anteriorly, and rotates slightly on the adjacent inferior vertebra. At the zygapophyseal joints, the inferior articular facets of the superior vertebra slide upwards on the superior articular facets of the adjacent inferior vertebra. In extension, the opposite motions occur: the superior vertebra tilts and translates posteriorly and the inferior articular facets glide downward on the superior articular facets of the adjacent inferior vertebra.

In lateral flexion to the right, the right inferior articular facets of the superior vertebra glide downward on the right superior articular facets of the inferior vertebra. On the

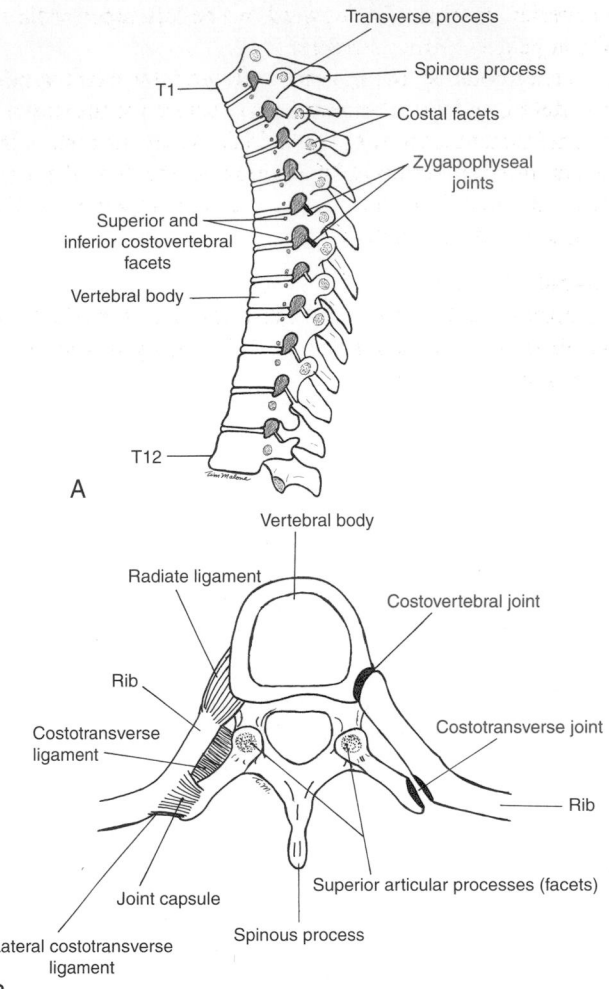

FIGURE 12.1 A: A lateral view of the thoracic spine shows the costal facets on the enlarged ends of the transverse processes from T1 to T10 and the costovertebral facets on the lateral edges of the superior and inferior aspects of the vertebral bodies. The zygapophyseal joints are shown between the inferior articular facets of the superior vertebrae and the superior articular facets of the adjacent inferior vertebra.
B: A superior view of a thoracic vertebra shows the articulations between the vertebra and the ribs: the left and right costovertebral joints, the costotransverse joints between the costal facets on the left and right transverse processes, and the costal tubercles on the corresponding ribs.

contralateral side, the left inferior articular facets of the superior vertebra glide upward on the left superior articular facets of the adjacent inferior vertebra.

In axial rotation, the superior vertebra rotates on the inferior vertebra, and the inferior articular surfaces of the superior vertebra impact on the superior articular surfaces of the adjacent inferior vertebra. For example, in rotation to the left, the right inferior articular facet impacts on the right superior articular facet of the adjacent inferior vertebra. Rotation and gliding motions occur between the ribs and the vertebral bodies at the costovertebral joints. A slight amount of rotation is possible between the joint surfaces of the ribs and the transverse processes at the upper costotransverse joints, and more

rotation is allowed in the gliding that occurs at the lower joints (T7 to T10). The movements at the costal joints are primarily for ventilation of the lungs but also allow some flexibility of the thoracic region.

Capsular Pattern

The capsular pattern for the thoracic spine is a greater limitation of extension, lateral flexion, and rotation than of forward flexion.[1]

Lumbar Spine

Anatomy of the Vertebrae

The bodies of the five lumbar vertebrae are more massive than those in the other regions of the spine in order to support the weight of the trunk. Spinous processes are broad and thick and extend almost horizontally (Fig. 12.2A). The fifth lumbar vertebra differs from the other four vertebrae in having a wedge-shaped body, with the anterior height greater than the posterior height. The inferior articular facets of the fifth vertebra are widely spaced for articulation with the sacrum.

Anatomy of the Joints

The surfaces of the superior articular facets at the zygapophyseal joints are concave and face medially and posteriorly. The inferior articular facet surfaces are convex and face laterally and anteriorly. Joint capsules are strong and ligaments of the region are essentially the same as those for the thoracic region, except for the addition of the iliolumbar ligament and thoracolumbar fascia and the fact that the posterior longitudinal ligament is not well developed in the lumbar area. The supraspinous ligament is well developed only in the upper lumbar spine. However, the intertransverse ligament is well developed in the lumbar area, and the anterior longitudinal ligament is strongest in this area (Fig. 12.2B). The interspinous ligaments connect one spinous process to another, and the iliolumbar ligament helps to stabilize the lumbosacral joint and prevent anterior displacement.

Osteokinematics

The zygapophyseal articular facets of L1 to L4 lie primarily in the sagittal plane, which favors flexion and extension and limits lateral flexion and rotation. However, flexion is more limited than extension. During combined flexion and extension, the greatest mobility takes place between L4 and L5, whereas the greatest amount of flexion takes place at the lumbosacral joint, L5-S1. Lateral flexion and rotation are greatest in the upper lumbar region, and little or no lateral flexion is present at the lumbosacral joint because of the orientation of the facets.

Arthrokinematics

According to Bogduk,[2] flexion at the lumbar intervertebral joints consistently involves a combination of 8 to 13 degrees of anterior rotation (tilting), 1 to 3 mm of anterior translation (sliding), and some axial rotation. The superior vertebral body rotates, tilts, and translates (slides) anteriorly on the adjacent inferior vertebral body. During flexion at the zygapophyseal

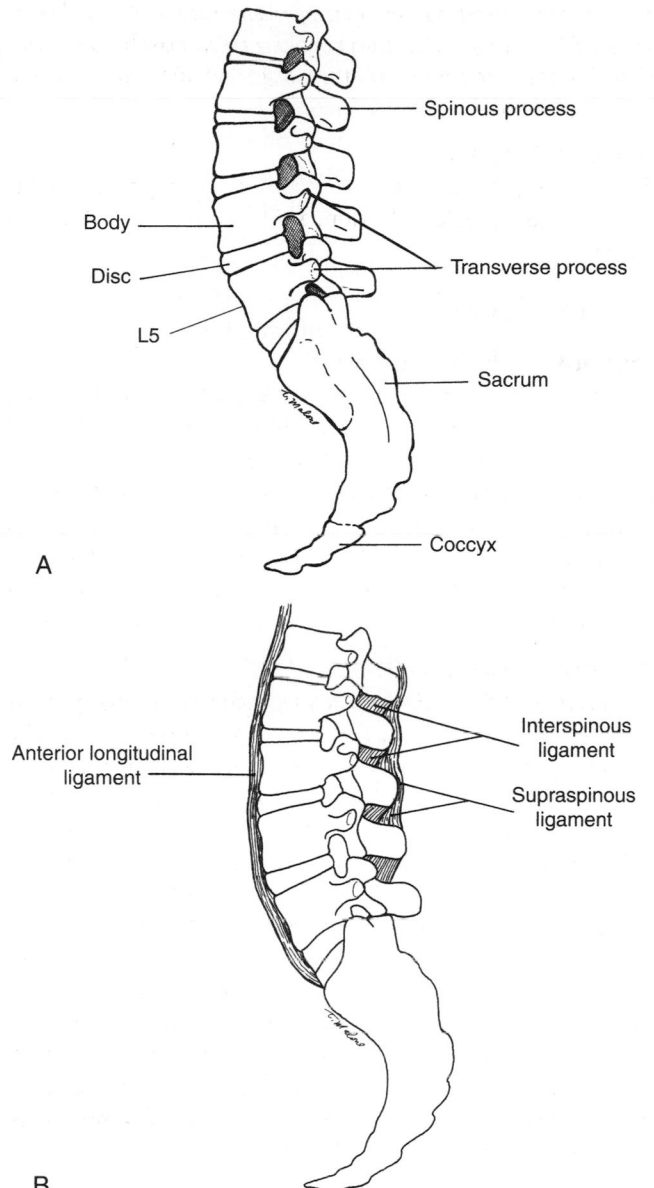

Spinous process

Body

Disc

L5

Transverse process

Sacrum

Coccyx

A

Anterior longitudinal ligament

Interspinous ligament

Supraspinous ligament

B

FIGURE 12.2 A: A lateral view of the lumbar spine shows the broad, thick, horizontally oriented spinous processes and large vertebral bodies. **B:** A lateral view of the lumbar spine shows the anterior longitudinal, supraspinous, and interspinous ligaments.

the superior vertebra slide upward on the left superior facets of the adjacent inferior vertebra.

In axial rotation, the superior vertebra rotates on the inferior vertebra, and the inferior articular surfaces of the superior vertebra impact on the superior articular facet surfaces of the adjacent inferior vertebra. In rotation to the left, the right inferior articular facet impacts on the right superior facet of the adjacent inferior vertebra.

Capsular Pattern

The capsular pattern for the lumbar spine is a marked and equal restriction of lateral flexion followed by restriction of flexion and extension.[1]

joints, the inferior articular facets of the superior vertebra slide upward on the superior articular facets of the adjacent inferior vertebra. In extension, the opposite motions occur: the vertebral body of the superior vertebra tilts and slides posteriorly on the adjacent inferior vertebra, and the inferior articular facets of the superior vertebra slide downward on the superior articular facets of the adjacent inferior vertebra.

In lateral flexion, the superior vertebra tilts and translates laterally on the adjacent vertebra below. In lateral flexion to the right side, the right inferior articular facets of the superior vertebra slide downward on the right superior facets of the adjacent inferior vertebra. The left inferior articular facets of

RANGE OF MOTION TESTING PROCEDURES

Measurement of the thoracic and lumbar spines is complicated by the regions' multiple joint structure, lack of well-defined landmarks, and difficulty separating thoracic and lumbar motion from hip motion. These difficulties have given rise to the variety of different methods used to measure ROM. The testing procedures presented in this section include the tape measure method, the Modified Schober technique (MST) as described by Macrae and Wright,[3] the Modified–Modified Schober Test (MMST), the universal goniometer (UG) method, and the double inclinometer method. The first four methods were selected because they are inexpensive, are relatively easy to use, and have acceptable reliability. The double inclinometer method has been included in this edition because the fifth edition of the American Medical Association's (AMA) *Guides to the*

Evaluation of Permanent Impairment[4] requires that this method be used to obtain reliable spinal mobility measurements for disability determination. According to the *Guides*, full ROM is interpreted as no impairment, and restriction of movement in one or more directions is interpreted as a degree of impairment.

Normal thoracic and lumbar spine ROM values using a variety of instruments are located in the Research Findings section, where Tables 12.1 to 12.5 provide information about the effects of age and gender on thoracic and lumber ROM. This information is followed by functional ranges of motion and a review of research studies on the reliability and validity of the various instruments and methods used to measure thoracic and lumbar ROM (see Tables 12.6 to 12.8 in the Research Findings section). Note that in the following testing procedures we are measuring active range of motion (AROM).

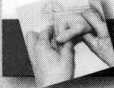 ## Landmarks for Testing Procedures

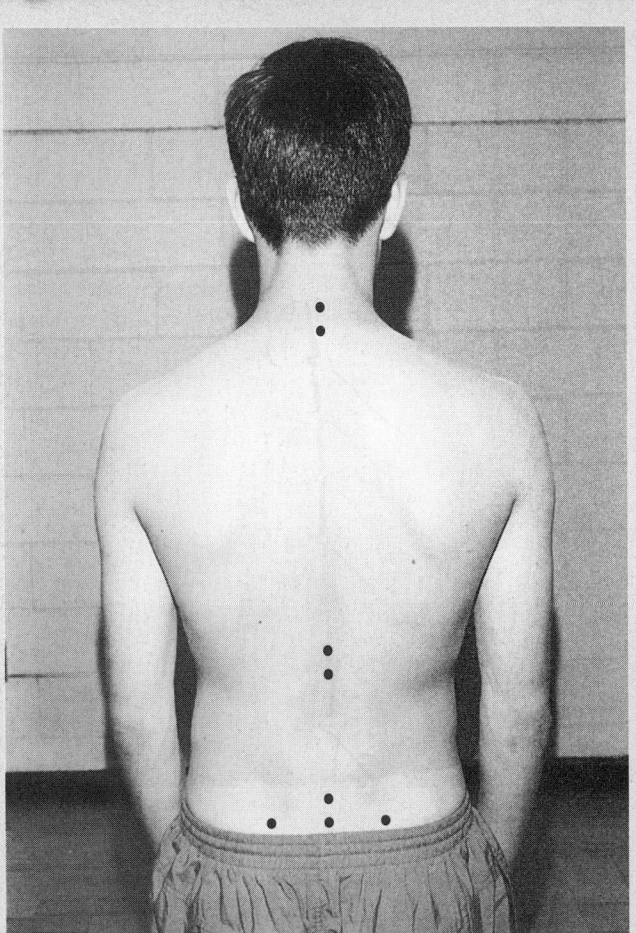

FIGURE 12.3 Surface anatomy landmarks for tape measure, universal goniometer, and inclinometer alignment for measuring the thoracolumbar spine motion. The dots are located over spinous processes of C7, T1, T12, L1, L5, and S2 and over the right and left posterior superior iliac spines (PSIS).

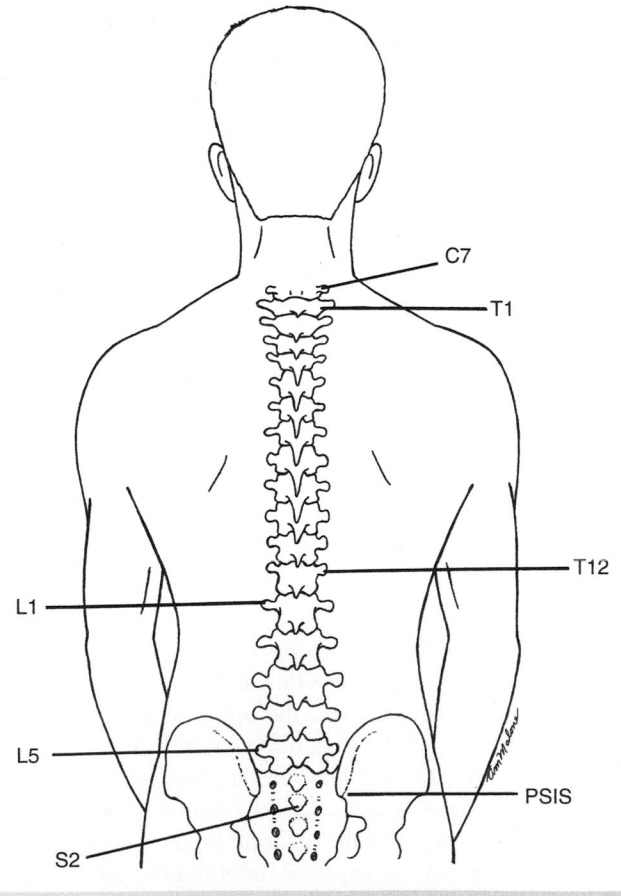

FIGURE 12.4 Bony anatomical landmarks for tape measure, universal goniometer, and inclinometer alignment for measuring thoracolumbar spine motion.

● THORACOLUMBAR FLEXION

Motion occurs in the sagittal plane around a medial–lateral axis.

Testing Position

Place the subject standing with feet shoulder width apart and with the cervical, thoracic, and lumbar spine in 0 degrees of lateral flexion and rotation.

Stabilization

Stabilize the pelvis to prevent anterior tilting.

Testing Motion

Direct the subject to bend forward gradually while keeping the arms relaxed (Fig. 12.5) and the knees straight. The end of the motion occurs when resistance to additional flexion is experienced by the subject and the examiner feels the pelvis start to tilt anteriorly.

Normal End-Feel

The normal end-feel is firm owing to the stretching of the posterior longitudinal ligament (in the thoracic region), the ligamentum flavum, the supraspinous and interspinous ligaments, and the posterior fibers of the annulus pulposus of the intervertebral discs and the zygapophyseal joint capsules. Passive tension in the thoracolumbar fascia and the following muscles may contribute to the end-feel: spinalis thoracis, semispinalis thoracis, iliocostalis lumborum and iliocostalis thoracis, interspinales, intertransversarii, longissimus thoracis, and multifidus. The orientation of the zygapophyseal facets from T1 to T6 restricts flexion in the upper thoracic spine.

▶ **NOTE: Use the same testing position, stabilization, testing motion, and normal end-feel described in the Thoracolumbar Flexion section above for the following flexion measurement methods unless changes are noted.**

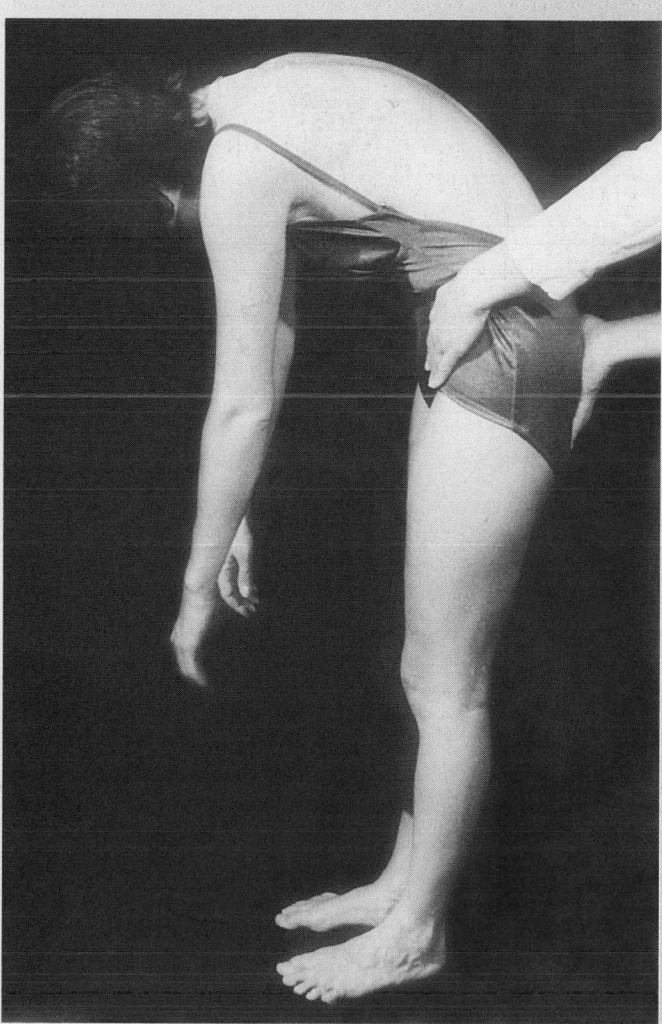

FIGURE 12.5 The subject is shown at the end of thoracolumbar flexion ROM. The examiner is shown stabilizing the subject's pelvis to prevent anterior pelvic tilting.

● THORACOLUMBAR FLEXION: TAPE MEASURE

Four inches (10 cm) is considered to be an average measurement for healthy adults.[5]

Procedure

1. Mark the spinous processes of the C7 and S2 vertebrae using a skin marking pencil, with the subject in the standing position. The spinous process of S2 is on a horizontal level with the posterior superior iliac spines [PSIS]. We have chosen to use the spinous process of S2 for a landmark as it is easier to

identify than the spinous process of S1, and there is no motion between S1 and S2.

2. Align the tape measure between the two spinous processes and record the distance at the starting of the ROM (Fig. 12.6).
3. Hold the tape measure in place as the subject performs flexion ROM. (Allow the tape measure to unwind and accommodate the motion.)
4. Record the distance at the end of the ROM (Fig. 12.7). The difference between the first and the second measurements indicates the amount of thoracolumbar flexion ROM.

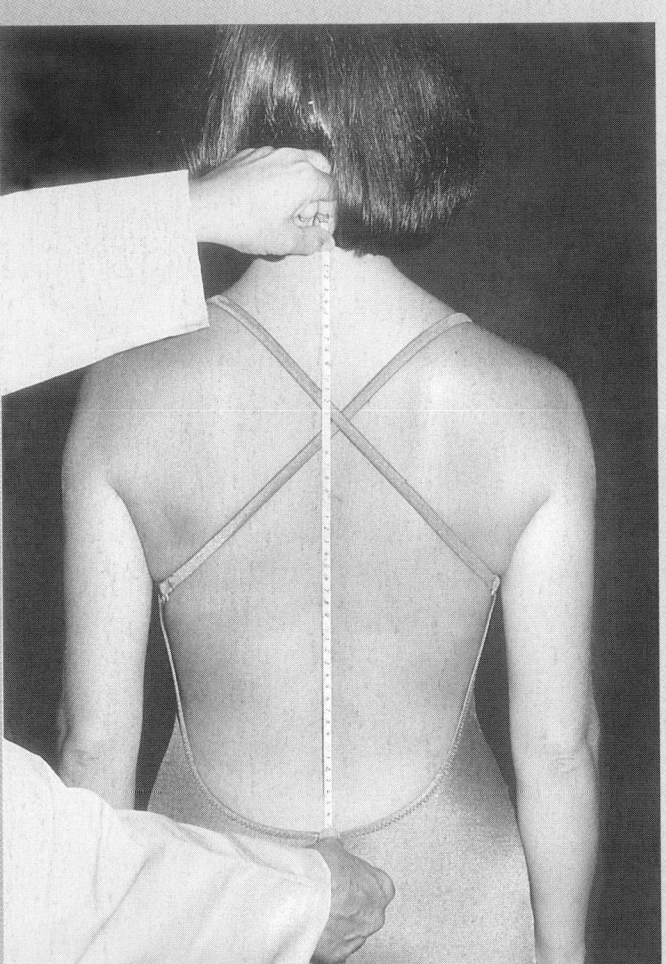

FIGURE 12.6 Tape measure alignment in the starting position for measuring thoracolumbar flexion ROM.

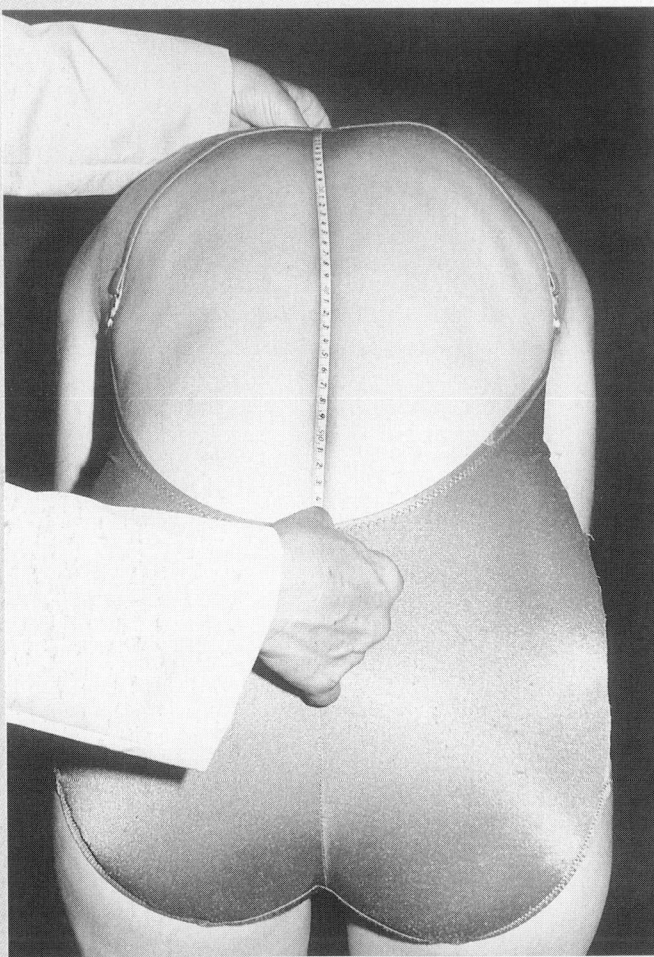

FIGURE 12.7 Tape measure alignment at the end of thoracolumbar flexion ROM. The metal tape measure case (not visible in the photo) is in the examiner's right hand.

THORACOLUMBAR FLEXION: FINGERTIP-TO-FLOOR

In a study by Quack and associates, the fingertip-to-floor distance was 0.1 cm for 70 healthy females with a mean age of 53 years.[8] In another study the ROM was 2.2 cm for 6 males and 14 females ranging in age from 22 to 55 years.[9]

According to Perret and associates,[10] this test has excellent intratester and intertester reliability (intraclass correlation coefficient [ICC] = 0.99) and validity. However, this test only can be used to assess general body flexibility[11–13] because it combines spinal and hip flexion, making it impossible to isolate either motion.

Procedure

1. Ask the subject to slowly bend forward as far as possible in an attempt to touch the floor with the fingers while keeping the knees extended and feet together.
2. No stabilization is provided by the examiner.
3. At the end of the motion, measure the perpendicular distance between the tip of the subject's middle finger and the floor either with a tape measure or ruler (Fig.12.8).

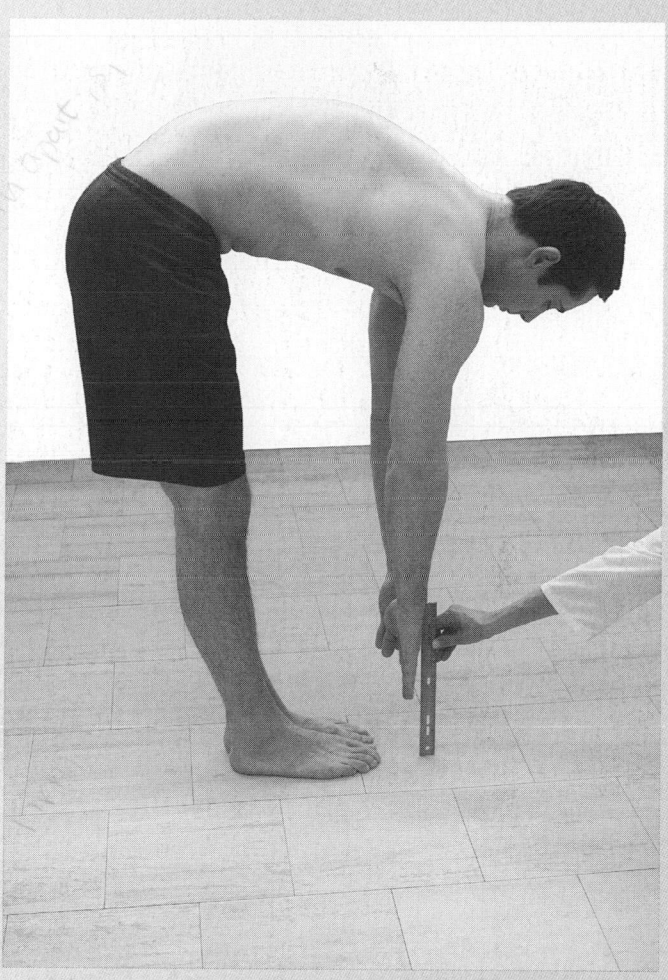

FIGURE 12.8 At the end of trunk and hip flexion the examiner measures the distance between the tip of the subject's middle finger and the floor with either a centimeter ruler or a tape measure.

THORACOLUMBAR FLEXION: DOUBLE INCLINOMETER

Procedure

1. Use a skin marking pencil to mark the spinous process of the T1 vertebra and the spinous process of the S2 vertebra (which is on a level with the posterior superior iliac spines [PSIS]), with the subject in the standing position.
2. Position **one inclinometer** over the spinous process of T1 and the **second inclinometer** over the sacrum at the level of S2. Then **zero** both inclinometers (Fig. 12.9).
3. At the end of the motion, read and record the values on both inclinometers (Fig. 12.10). The difference between the two inclinometers indicates the amount of thoracolumbar flexion ROM.

measures lumbar but if Lower thoracic is problem it will affect

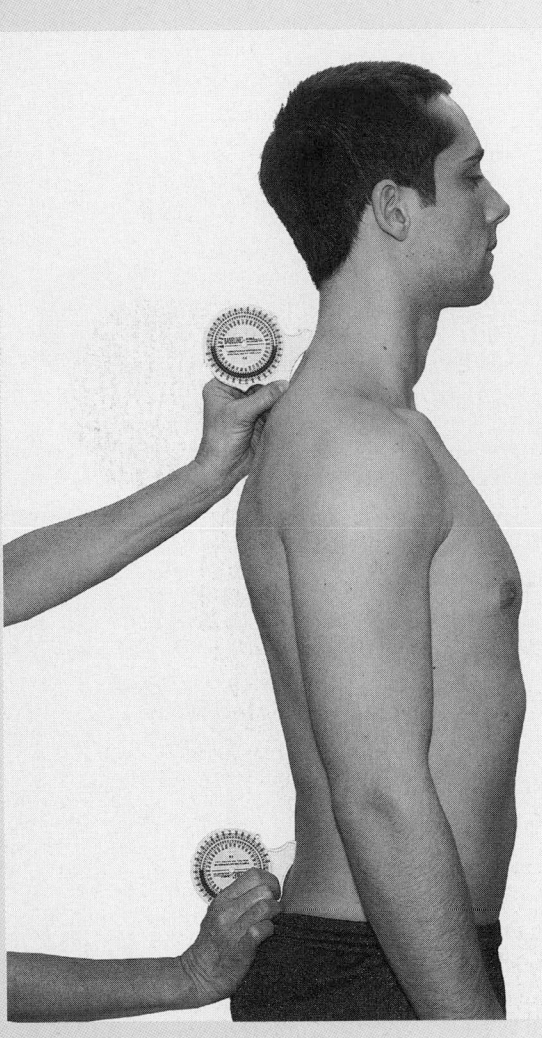

FIGURE 12.9 The starting position for measuring thoracolumbar flexion with both inclinometers aligned and zeroed.

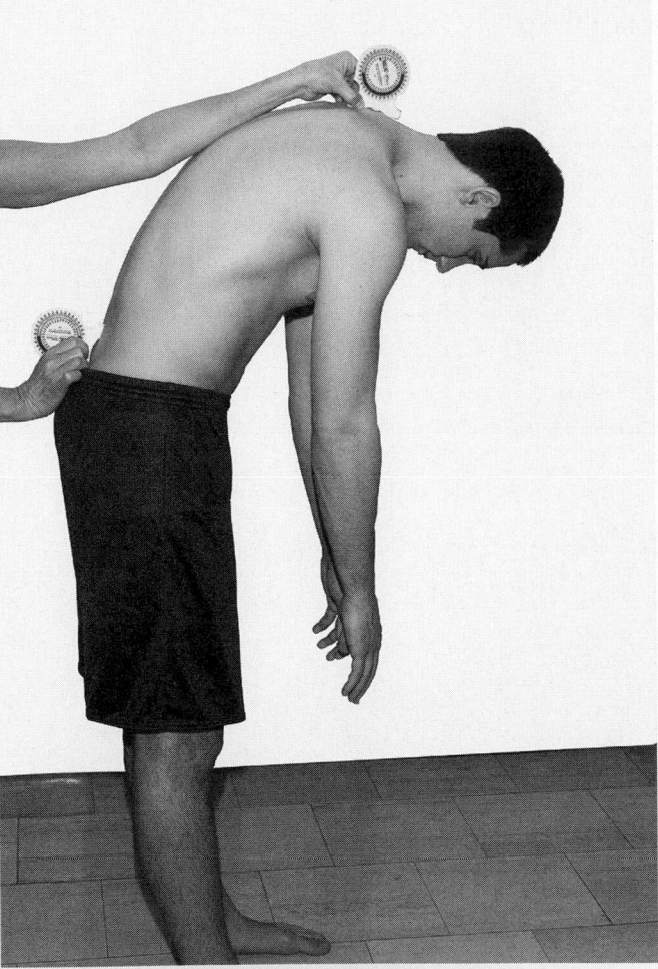

FIGURE 12.10 Inclinometer alignment at the end of thoracolumbar flexion ROM.

● THORACOLUMBAR EXTENSION

Motion occurs in the sagittal plane around a medial–lateral axis.

Testing Position

Place the subject standing with feet shoulder width apart and with the cervical, thoracic, and lumbar spine in 0 degrees of lateral flexion and rotation.

Stabilization

Stabilize the pelvis to prevent posterior tilting.

Testing Motion

Ask the subject to extend the spine as far as possible (Fig. 12.11). The end of the extension ROM occurs when the pelvis begins to tilt posteriorly.

Normal End-Feel

The end-feel is firm owing to stretching of the zygapophyseal joint capsules, anterior fibers of the annulus fibrosus, anterior longitudinal ligament, rectus abdominis, and external and internal oblique abdominals. The end-feel also may be hard owing to contact by the spinous processes and the zygapophyseal facets.

▶ **NOTE: Use the same testing position, stabilization, testing motion, and normal end-feel described in the Thoracolumbar Extension section above for the following extension measurement methods unless changes are noted.**

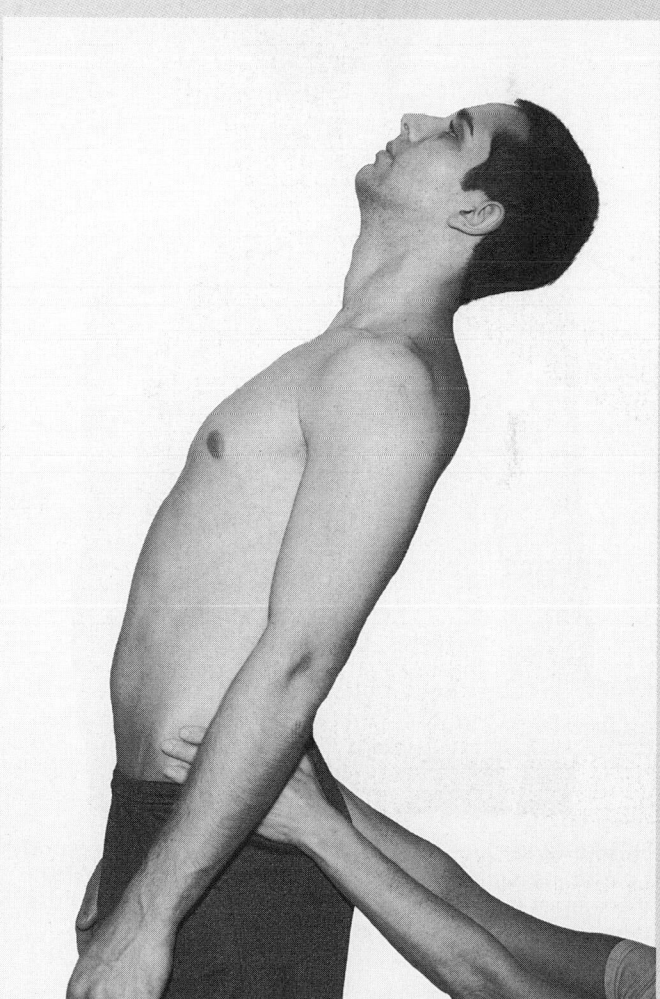

FIGURE 12.11 At the end of thoracolumbar extension ROM, the examiner uses her hands on the subject's iliac crests to prevent posterior pelvic tilting. If the subject has balance problems or muscle weakness in the lower extremities, the measurement can be taken in either the prone or side-lying position.

● THORACOLUMBAR EXTENSION: TAPE MEASURE

Procedure

1. Mark the spinous processes of the C7 and S2 vertebrae using a skin marking pencil, with the subject in the standing positon.
2. Align the tape measure between the two spinous processes and record the measurement (Fig. 12.12).

3. Keep the tape measure aligned during the motion and record the measurement at the end of the ROM (Fig. 12.13). The difference between the measurement taken at the beginning of the motion and that taken at the end indicates the amount of thoracic and lumbar extension.

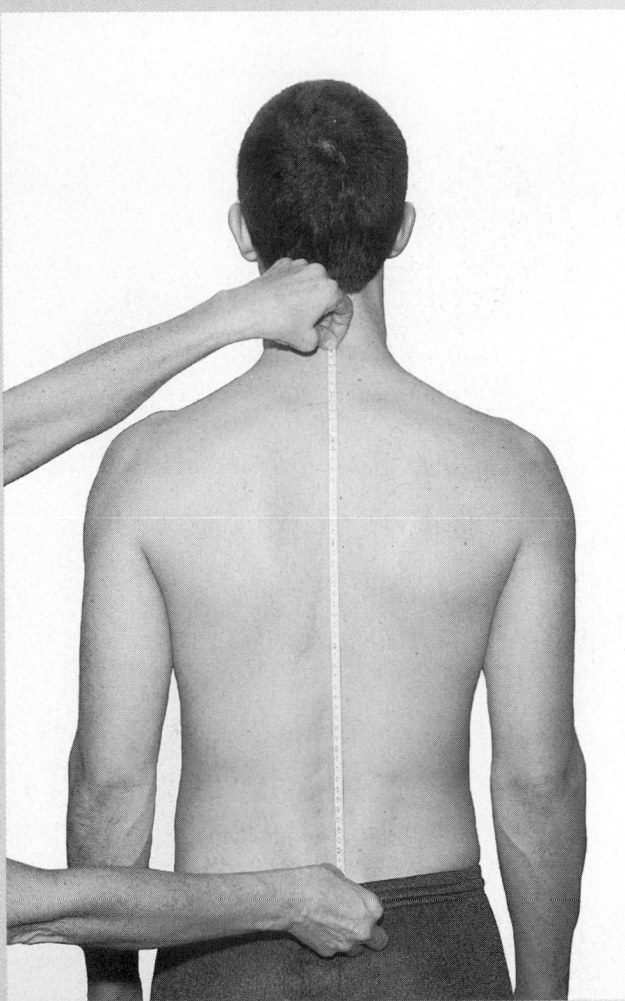

FIGURE 12.12 Tape measure alignment in the starting position for measurement of thoracolumbar extension. When the subject moves into extension, the tape slides into the tape measure case in the examiner's hand.

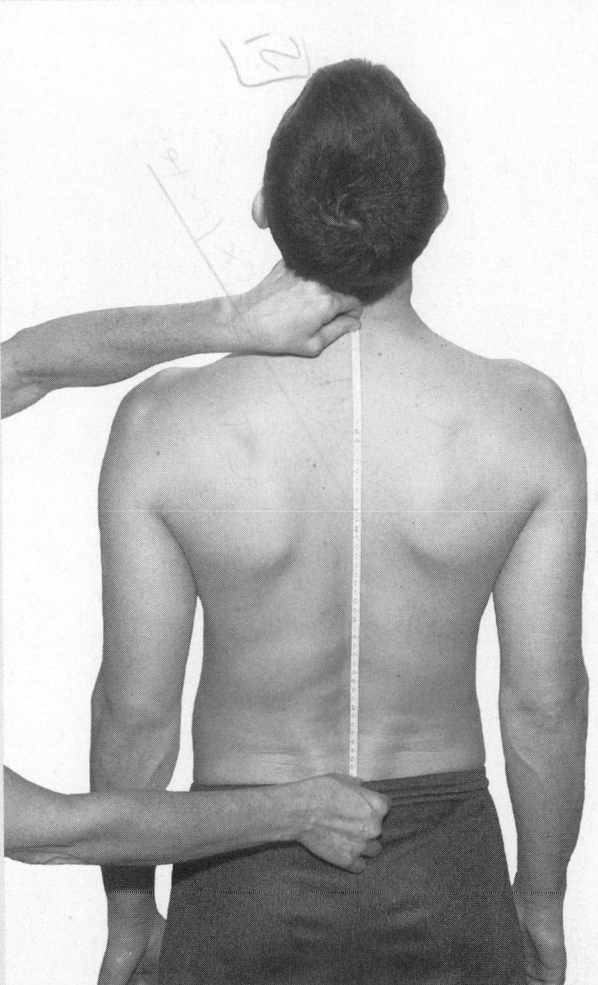

FIGURE 12.13 At the end of thoracolumbar extension ROM, the distance between the two landmarks is less than it was in the starting position.

THORACOLUMBAR EXTENSION: DOUBLE INCLINOMETERS

Procedure

1. Mark the spinous processes of the T1 and S2 vertebrae using a skin marking pencil, with the subject in the standing position.
2. Position **one inclinometer** over the spinous process of T1 and the second **inclinometer** over the sacrum at the level of S2. Then **zero** both inclinometers. (Fig. 12.14).

3. At the end of the motion, read and record the values on both inclinometers (Fig. 12.15). The difference between the two inclinometers indicates the amount of thoracolumbar extension ROM.

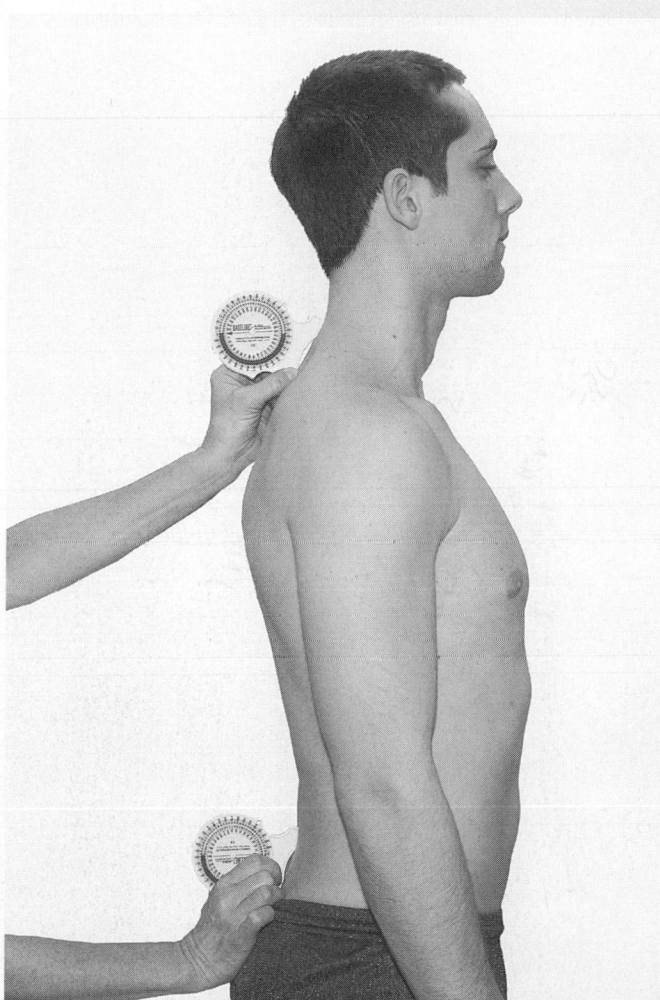

FIGURE 12.14 The starting position for measuring thoracolumbar extension with both inclinometers aligned and zeroed.

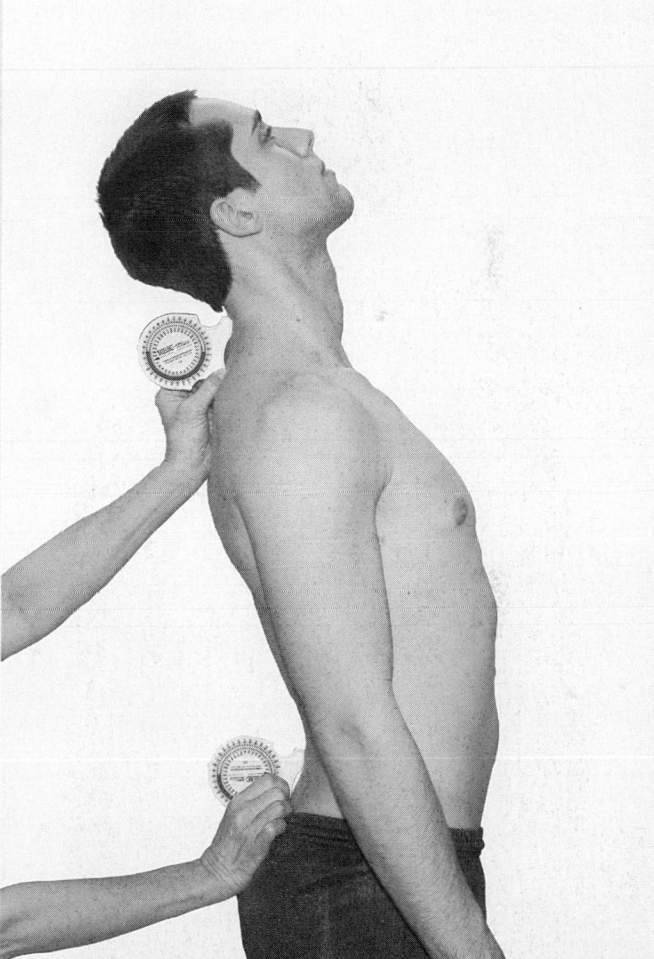

FIGURE 12.15 Inclinometer alignment at the end of thoracolumbar extension.

● THORACOLUMBAR LATERAL FLEXION

Testing Position

Place the subject standing with the feet shoulder width apart and the cervical, thoracic, and lumbar spine in 0 degrees of flexion, extension, and rotation.

Stabilization

Stabilize the pelvis to prevent lateral tilting.

Testing Motion

Ask the subject to bend the trunk to one side while keeping the arms in a relaxed position at the sides of the body. Keep both feet flat on the floor with the knees extended (Fig. 12.16). The end of the motion

occurs when the heel begins to rise on the foot opposite to the side of the motion and the pelvis begins to tilt laterally.

Normal End-Feel

The end-feel is firm owing to the stretching of the contralateral fibers of the annulus fibrosus, zygapophyseal joint capsules, intertransverse ligaments, thoracolumbar fascia, and the following muscles: external and oblique abdominals, longissimus thoracis, iliocostalis lumborum and thoracis lumborum, quadratus lumborum, multifidus, spinalis thoracis, and serratus posterior inferior. The end-feel may also be hard owing to impact of the ipsilateral zygapophyseal facets (right facets when

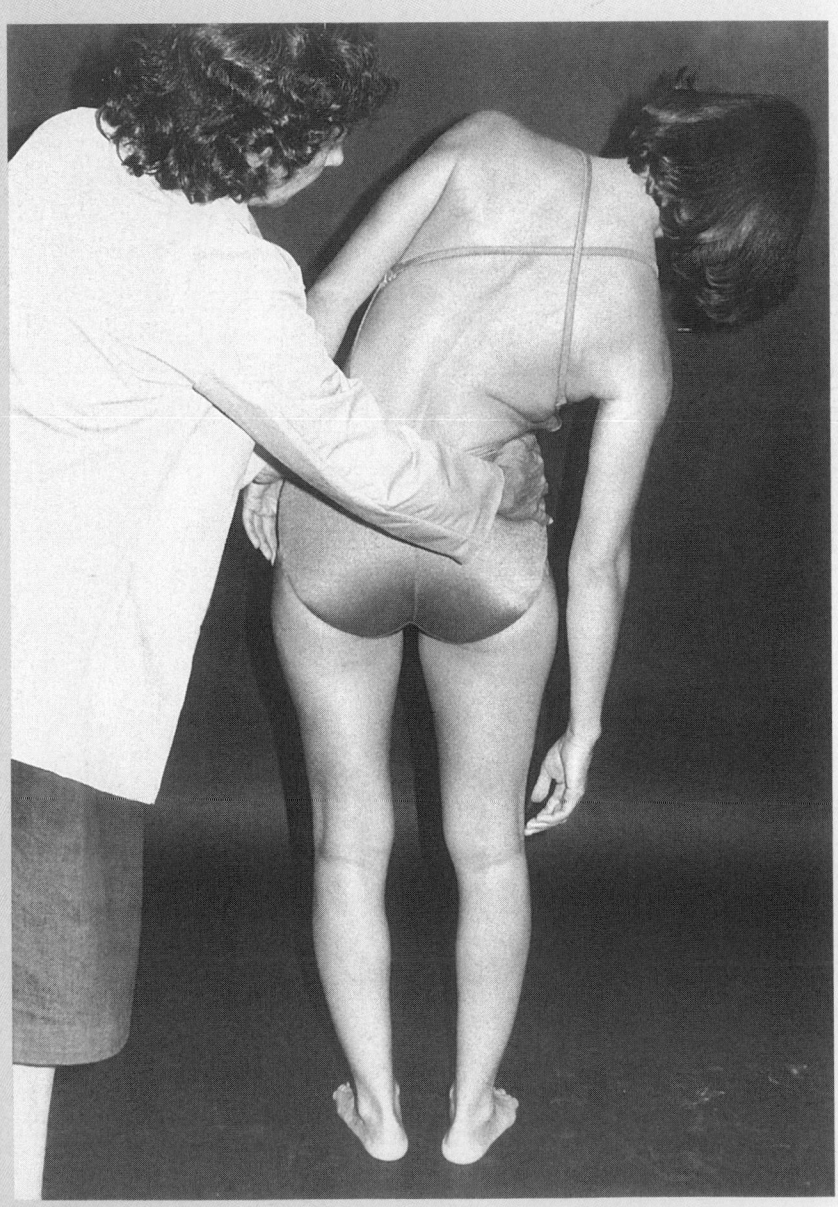

FIGURE 12.16 The end of thoracolumbar lateral flexion ROM. The examiner places both hands on the subject's pelvis to prevent lateral pelvic tilting.

bending to the right) and the restrictions imposed by the ribs and costal joints in the upper thoracic spine.

♦ NOTE: Use the same testing position, stabilization, testing motion, and normal end-feel described in the Thoracolumbar Lateral Flexion section above for the following lateral flexion measurement methods unless changes are noted.

● THORACOLUMBAR LATERAL FLEXION: UNIVERSAL GONIOMETER

According to the American Academy of Orthopaedic Surgeons (AAOS),[6] the ROM is 35 degrees to each side (see Table 12.1 in the Research Findings section). Fitzgerald and associates[14] found that normal values ranged from a mean of 37.6 degrees (in a group of 20 to 29 year olds) to 18.0 degrees (in a group of 70 to 79 year olds). See Table 12.2 in the Research Findings section for additional information.[14] According to Sahrmann,[15] more than three-fourths of thoracic and lumbar lateral flexion ROM takes place in the thoracic spine.

Procedure

1. Mark the spinous processes of C7 and S2 vertebrae using a skin marking pencil.
2. Center **fulcrum** of the goniometer over the posterior aspect of the spinous process of S2 (Fig. 12.17).
3. Align **proximal arm** so that it is perpendicular to the ground.
4. Align **distal arm** with the posterior aspect of the spinous process of C7 (Fig. 12.18).

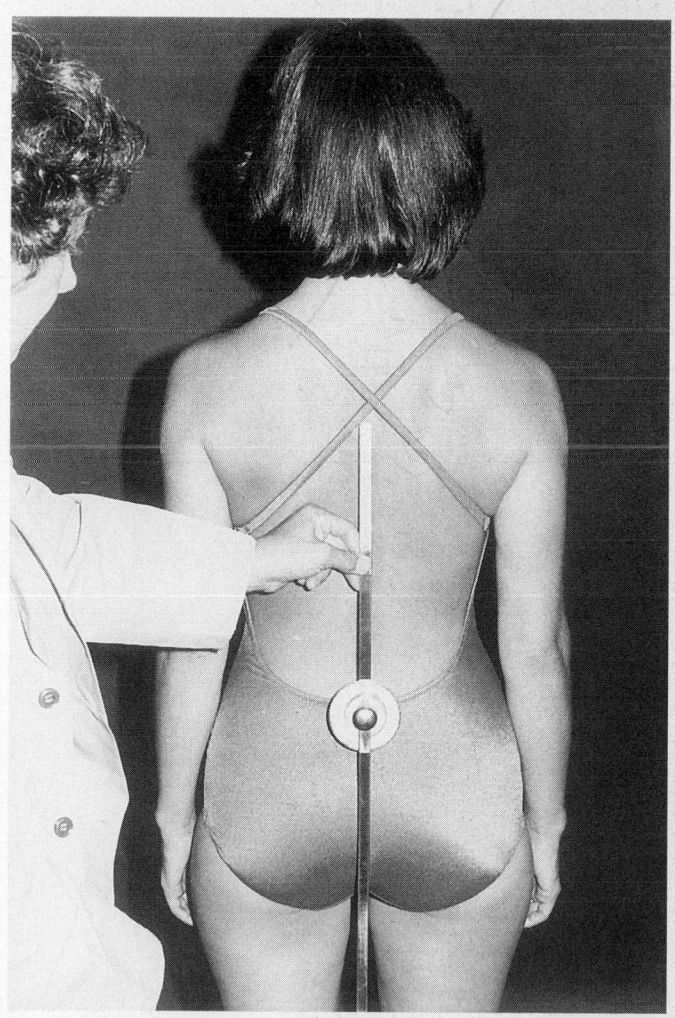

FIGURE 12.17 The subject is shown with the goniometer aligned in the starting position for measurement of thoracolumbar lateral flexion.

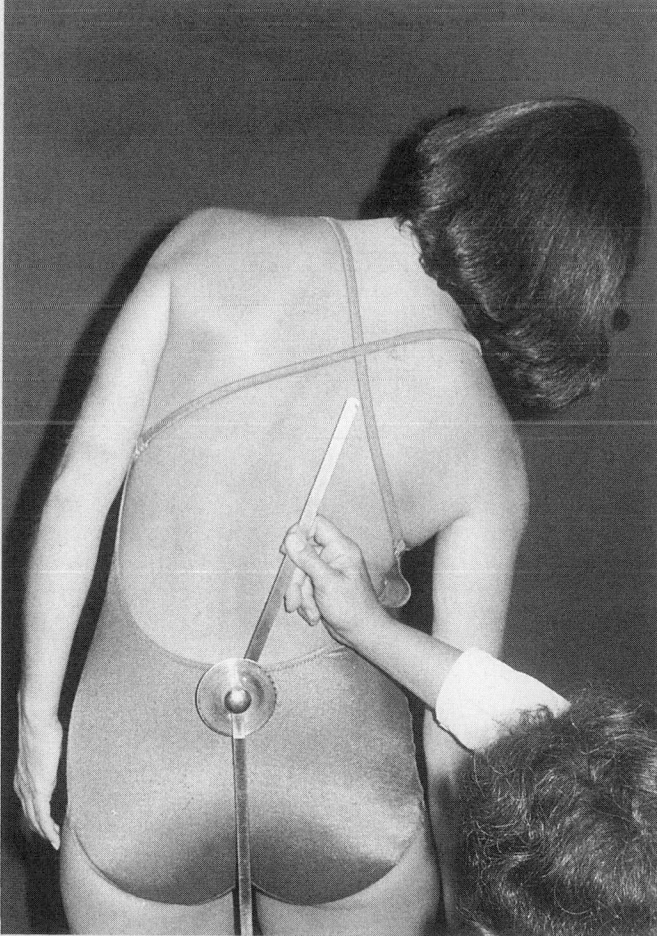

FIGURE 12.18 At the end of thoracolumbar lateral flexion, the examiner keeps the distal goniometer arm aligned with the subject's C7 vertebra. The examiner makes no attempt to align the distal arm with the subject's vertebral column. As can be seen in the photograph, the lower thoracic and upper lumbar spine become convex to the left during right lateral flexion.

● THORACOLUMBAR LATERAL FLEXION: FINGERTIP-TO-FLOOR

The normal values for females with a mean age of 53 years was determined to be 15.9 cm for right lateral flexion and 16.9 cm for left lateral flexion.[8] One problem with this method is that it will be affected by the subject's body proportions. Therefore, it should be used only to compare repeated measurements for a single subject and not for comparing one subject with another subject.

Procedure

1. Have the subject stand with feet shoulder width apart and arms hanging freely at the sides of the body. Ask the subject to bend to the side as far as possible while keeping both feet flat on the ground with knees extended.
2. At the end of the ROM, make a mark on the leg level with the tip of the middle finger and use a tape measure or ruler to measure the distance between the mark on the leg and the floor (Fig. 12.19).

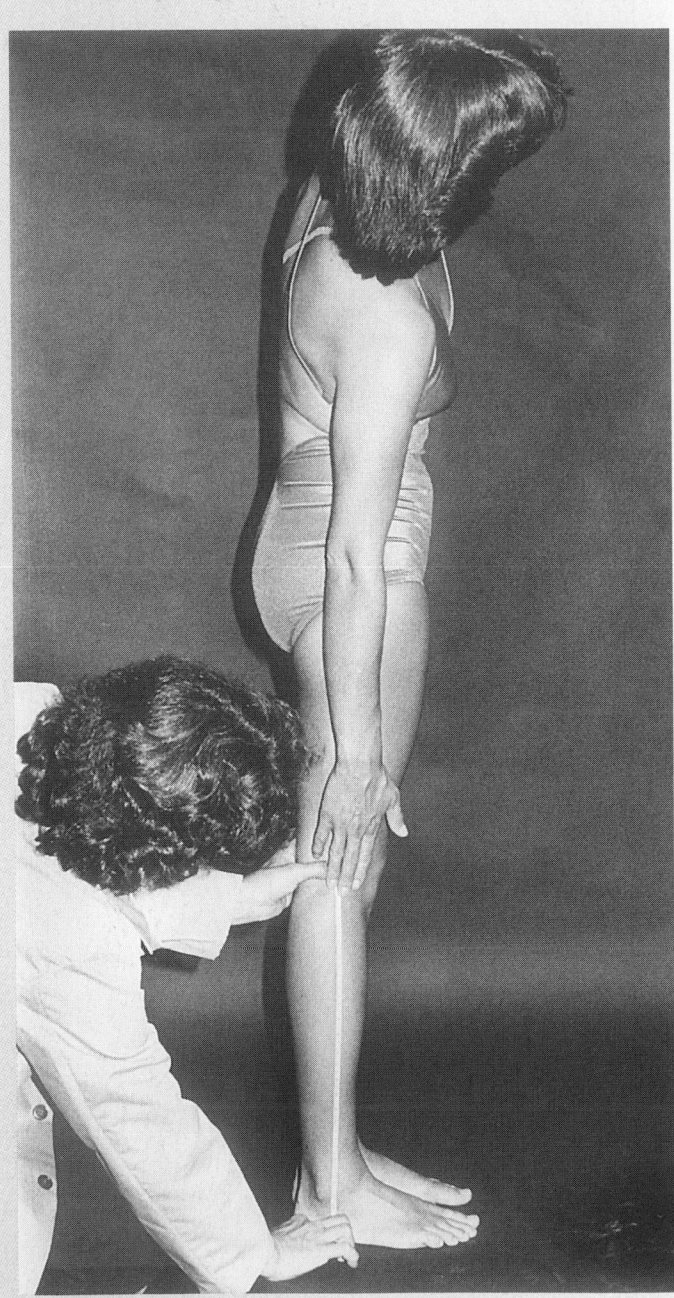

FIGURE 12.19 At the end of thoracolumbar lateral flexion range of motion, the examiner is using a tape measure to determine the distance from the tip of the subject's third finger to the floor. Lateral pelvic tilting should be avoided.

● THORACOLUMBAR LATERAL FLEXON: FINGERTIP-TO-THIGH

This method is a variation of the fingertip-to-floor method, designed to account for differences in body size.[16] The normal ROM values for children ages 11 to 16 years were 21.0 cm for both right and left lateral flexion.[17] ROM values derived from 39 healthy adults were 21.6 cm.[16] Lindell and associates[9] found similar values for 20 healthy adults ages 22 to 55 years. Right lateral flexion was 21.2 cm, and left lateral flexion was 21.0 cm. Alaranta and colleagues,[18] in a study of 119 blue and white collar workers ages 35 to 59 years, found a mean value of 19.1 cm. See Table 12.7 in the Research Findings section for reliability information on this procedure.

Procedure

1. Have the subject stand with his or her back against the wall with feet shoulder width apart and arms hanging freely at the sides of the body.
2. Place a mark on the thigh where the tip of the subject's third finger rests (Fig. 12.20).
3. Ask the subject to bend to the side as far as possible while keeping the back and shoulders against the wall and both feet flat on the ground with knees extended.
4. At the end of the ROM, make a second mark on the leg level with the tip of the middle finger (Fig. 12.21).
5. Use a tape measure or ruler to measure the distance between the first mark on the leg and the second mark on the leg (Fig. 12.22). The distance between the two marks is the value for thoracolumbar lateral flexion ROM.

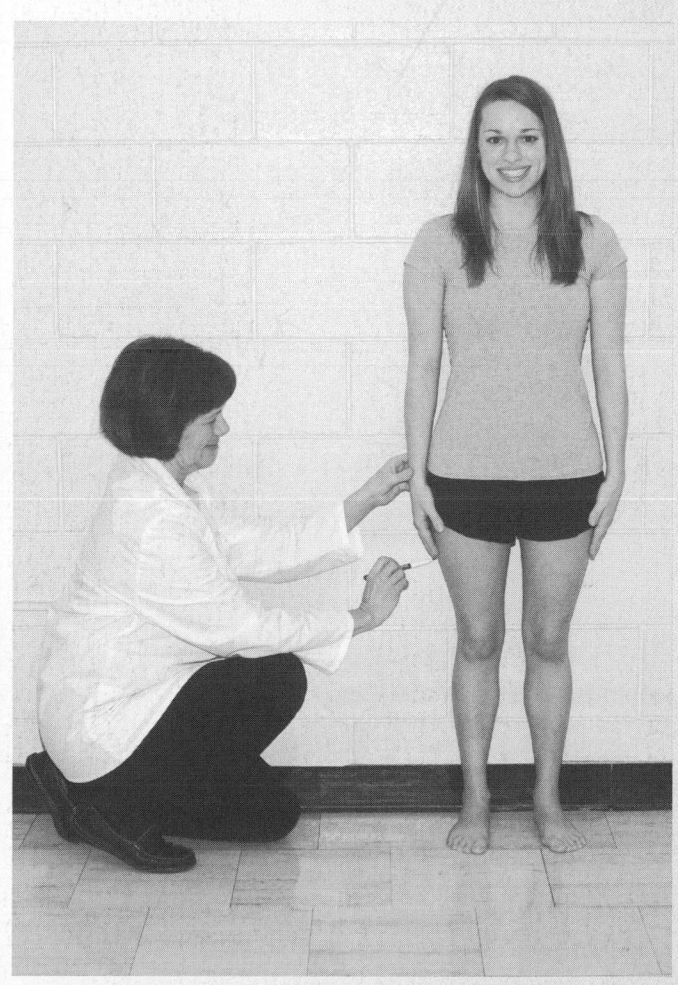

FIGURE 12.20 In the starting position for measuring thoracolumbar lateral flexion the examiner marks the thigh at the level of the tip of the subject's middle finger.

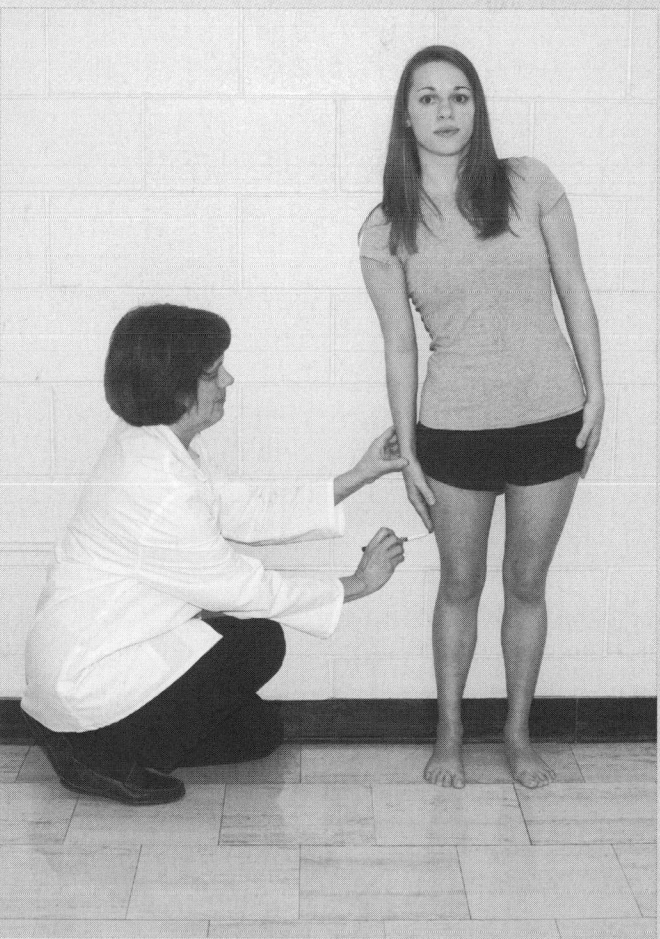

FIGURE 12.21 At the end of thoracolumbar lateral flexion the examiner places a second mark on the thigh on a level with the new position of the tip of the subject's middle finger.

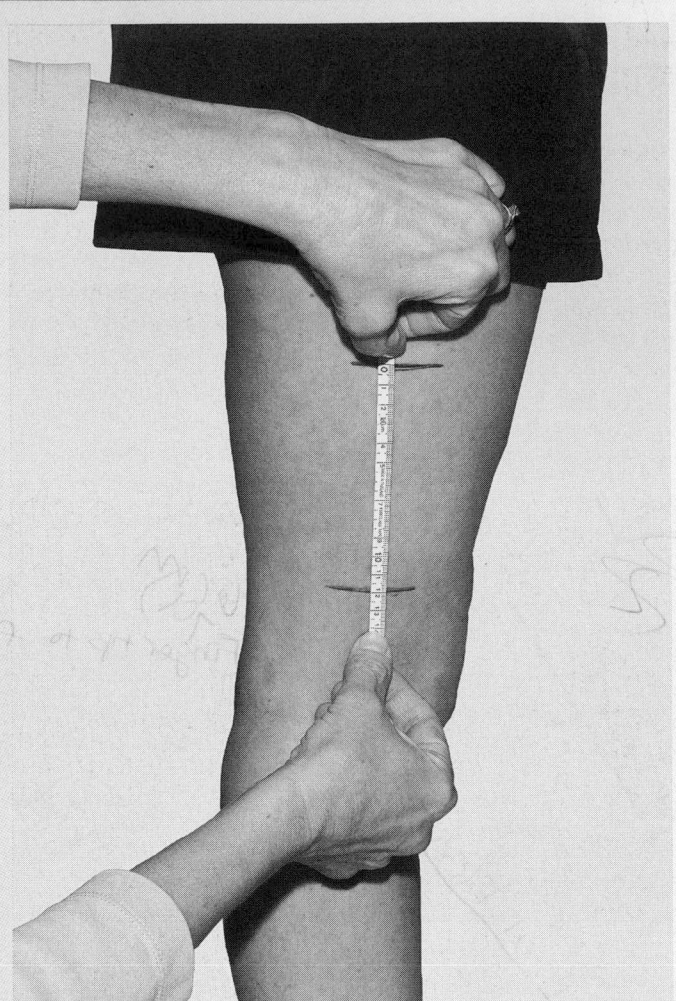

FIGURE 12.22 The examiner uses a tape measure or ruler to measure the distance between the two thigh marks to obtain the ROM.

● THORACOLUMBAR LATERAL FLEXION: DOUBLE INCLINOMETER

Procedure

1. Mark the spinous processes of the T1 and S2 vertebrae using a skin marking pencil, with the subject in the standing position.
2. Place **one inclinometer** over the T1 spinous process and the **second inclinometer** over the sacrum at the level of S2. Then **zero** both inclinometers (Fig. 12.23).

3. Ask the subject to bend to the side as far as possible while keeping both knees straight and both feet firmly on the ground (Fig. 12.24).
4. At the end of the ROM, read and record the information on both inclinometers. Subtract the degrees on the sacral inclinometer from the degrees on the thoracic inclinometer to obtain the lateral flexion ROM.
5. Repeat the measurement process to measure lateral flexion ROM on the other side.

Center of inclinometer at T12

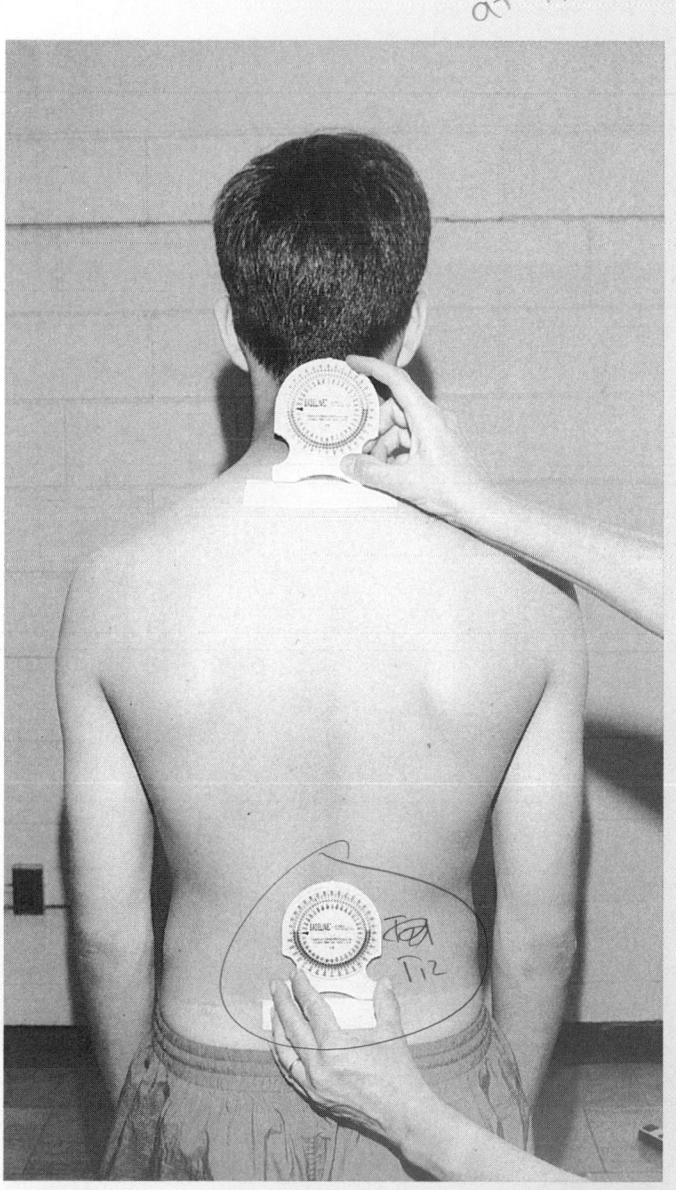

FIGURE 12.23 The subject is in the starting position for measurement of thoracolumbar lateral flexion with both inclinometers aligned and zeroed.

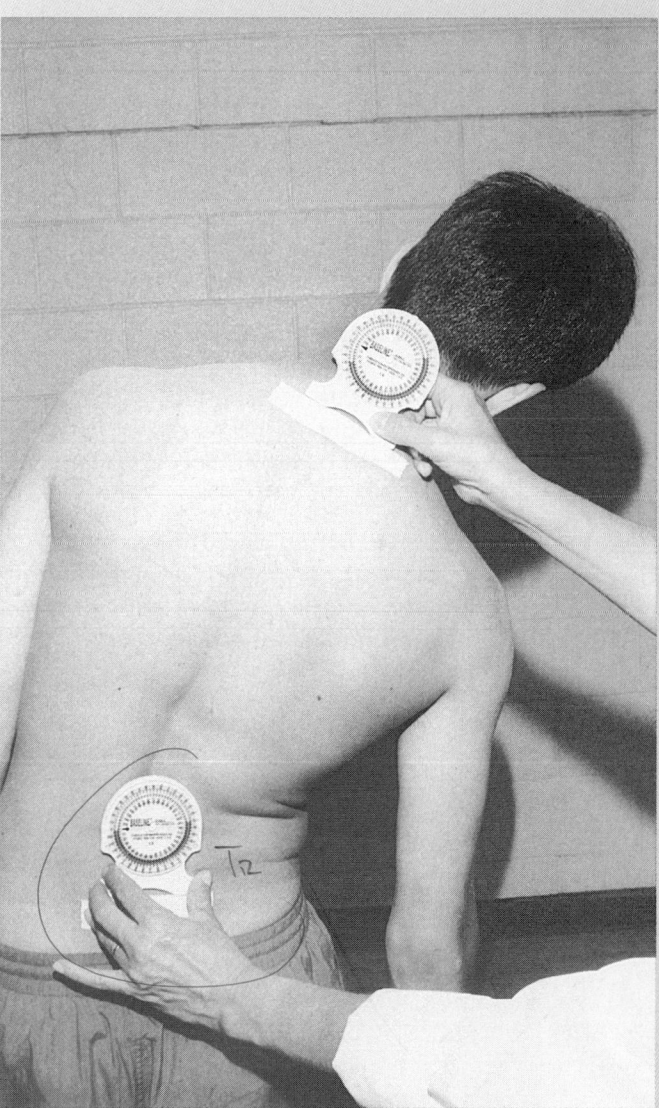

FIGURE 12.24 Inclinometer alignment at the end of thoracolumbar lateral flexion ROM.

● THORACOLUMBAR ROTATION

Motion occurs in the transverse plane around a vertical axis.

Testing Position

Place the subject sitting, with the feet on the floor to help stabilize the pelvis. A seat without a back support is preferred so that rotation of the spine can occur freely. The cervical, thoracic, and lumbar spine are in 0 degrees of flexion, -extension, and lateral flexion.

Stabilization

Stabilize the pelvis to prevent rotation. Avoid flexion, extension, and lateral flexion of the spine.

Testing Motion

Ask the subject to turn his or her body to one side as far as possible, keeping the trunk erect and feet flat on the floor (Fig. 12.25). The end of the motion occurs when the examiner feels the pelvis start to rotate.

Normal End-Feel

The end-feel is firm owing to stretching of the fibers of the contralateral annulus fibrosus and zygapophyseal joint capsules; costotransverse and costovertebral joint capsules; supraspinous, interspinous, and iliolumbar ligaments; and the following muscles: rectus abdominis, external and internal obliques and multifidus, and semispinalis thoracis and rotatores. The end-feel may also be hard owing to contact between the zygapophyseal facets.

▶ **NOTE: Use the same testing position, stabilization, testing motion, and normal end-feel described in the Thoracolumbar Rotation section above for the following rotation measurement methods unless changes are noted.**

● THORACOLUMBAR ROTATION: UNIVERSAL GONIOMETER

According to the AMA, the normal ROM value for thoracolumbar rotation using the universal goniometer is 45 degrees.[6] See Figures 12.26 and 12.27.

Procedure

1. Center **fulcrum** of the goniometer over the center of the cranial aspect of the subject's head.
2. Align **proximal arm** parallel to an imaginary line between the two prominent tubercles on the iliac crests.
3. Align **distal arm** with an imaginary line between the two acromial processes.

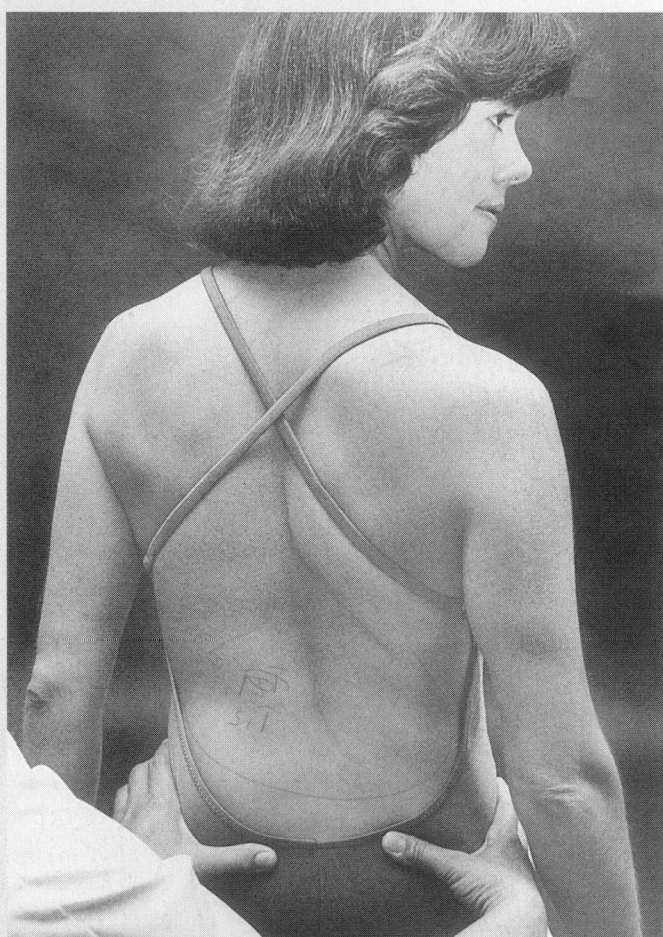

FIGURE 12.25 The subject is shown at the end of the thoracolumbar rotation ROM. The subject is seated on a low stool without a back rest so that spinal movement can occur without interference. The examiner positions her hands on the subject's iliac crests to prevent pelvic rotation.

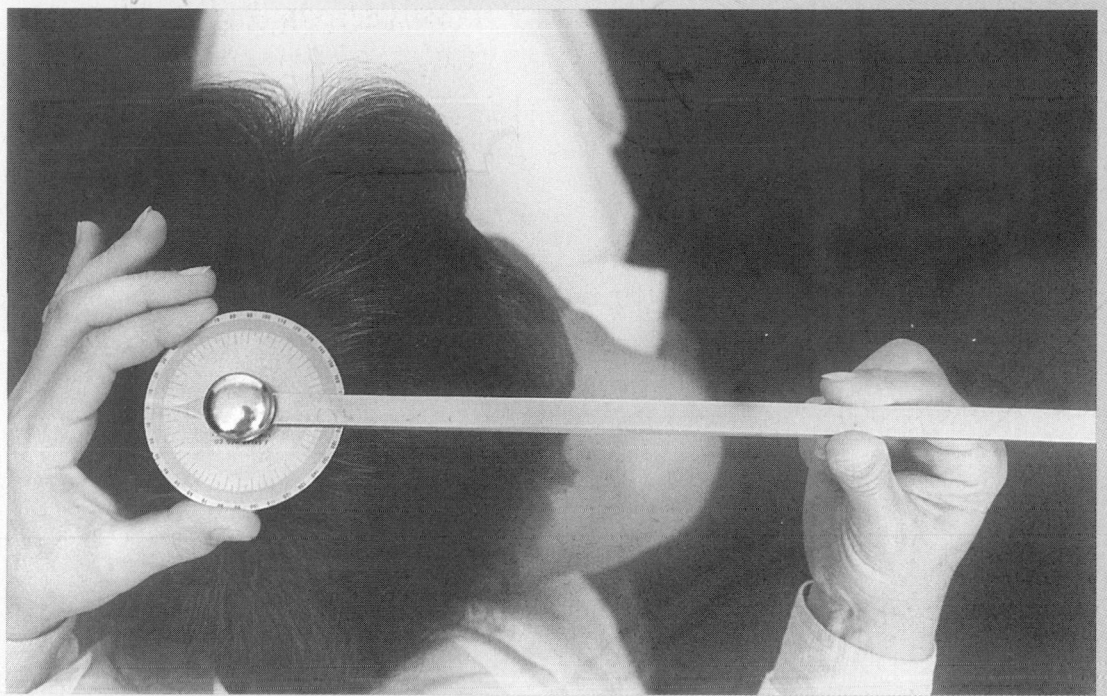

FIGURE 12.26 In the starting position for measurement of rotation range of motion, the examiner stands behind the seated subject. The examiner positions the fulcrum of the goniometer on the superior aspect of the subject's head. One of the examiner's hands is holding both arms of the goniometer aligned with the subject's acromion processes. The subject should be positioned so that the acromion processes are aligned directly over the iliac tubercles.

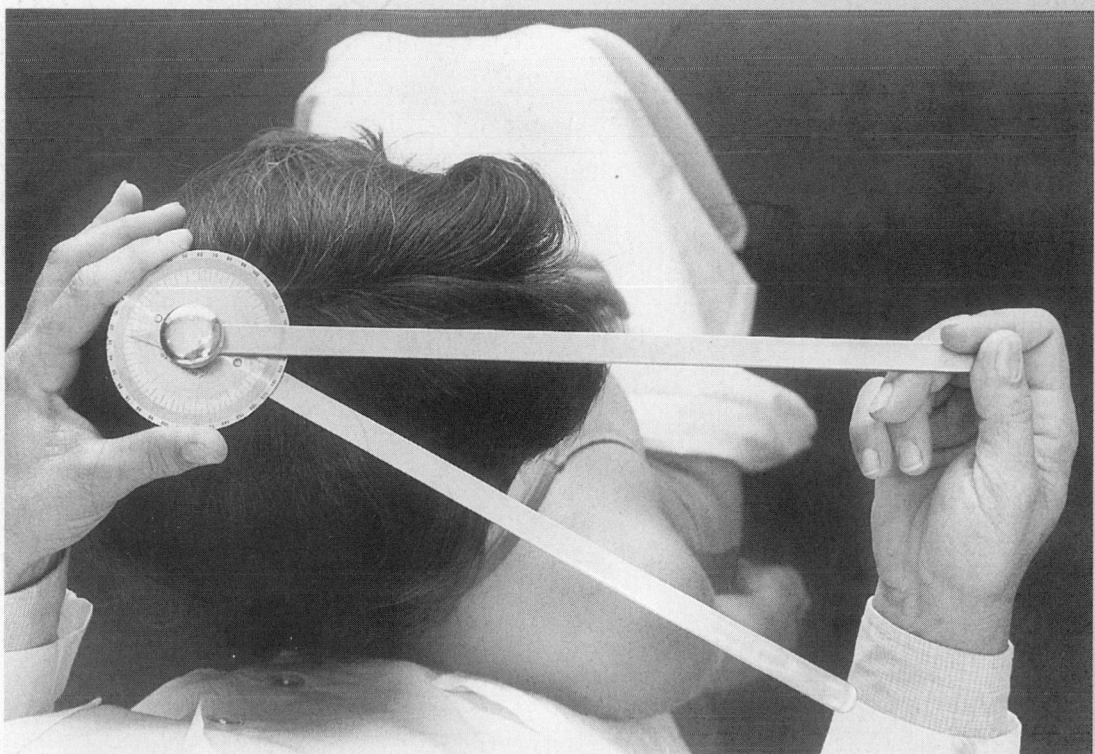

FIGURE 12.27 At the end of rotation, one of the examiner's hands keeps the proximal goniometer arm aligned with the subject's iliac tubercles while keeping the distal goniometer arm aligned with the subject's right acromion process.

● THORACOLUMBAR ROTATION: DOUBLE INCLINOMETER

Procedure

1. Mark the spinous processes of the T1 and S2 vertebrae using a skin marking pencil
2. Place the subject in a forward flexed standing position so that the subject's back is parallel to the floor.
3. Place **one inclinometer** over the spinous process of T1 and the **second inclinometer** over the sacrum at the level of S2. Then **zero** both inclinometers (Fig. 12.28).

4. Ask the subject to rotate the trunk as far as possible without moving into extension (Fig. 12.29). The examiner needs to hold the inclinometers firmly against the subject's back during the motion.
5. Note the degrees shown on the inclinometers at the end of the motion. The difference between inclinometer readings is the rotation ROM.

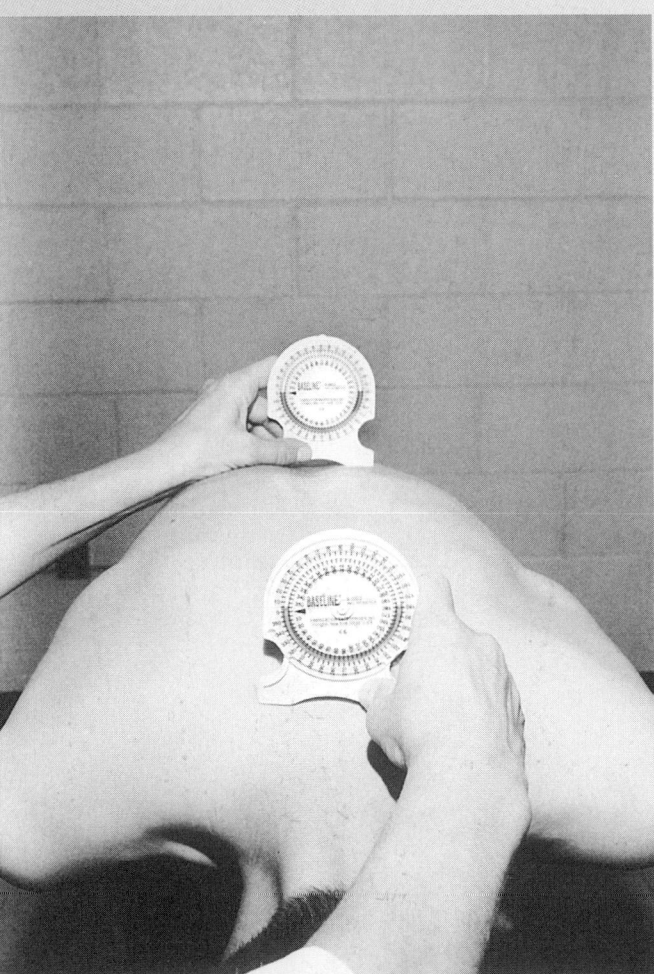

FIGURE 12.28 The subject is in the starting position for measurement of thoracolumbar rotation with inclinometers aligned and zeroed.

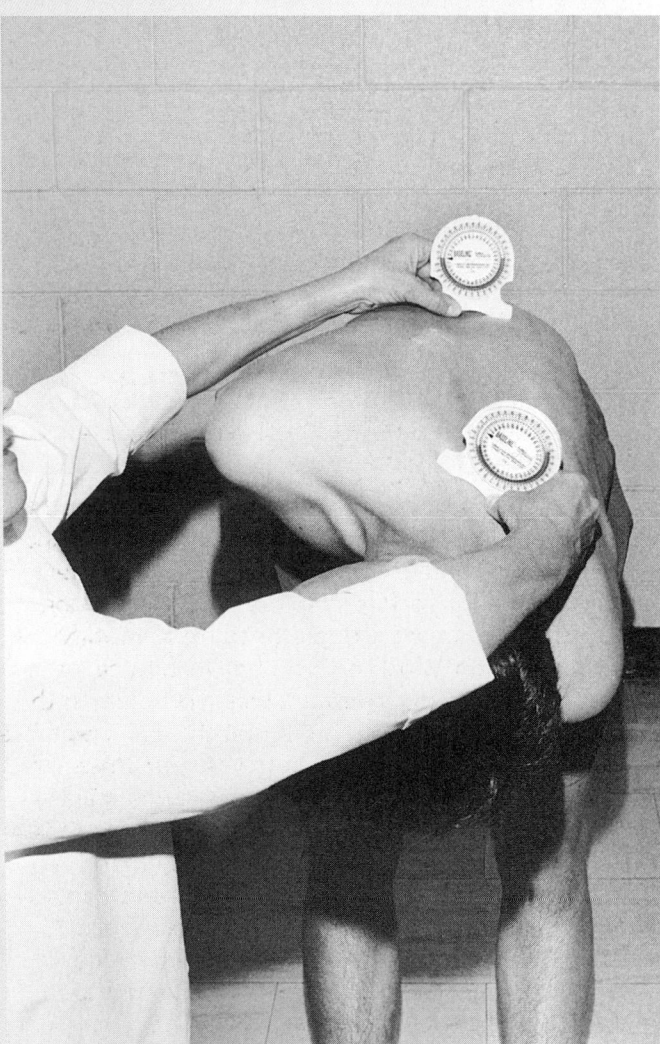

FIGURE 12.29 The subject is shown with the inclinometers aligned at the end of thoracolumbar range of motion.

LUMBAR FLEXION

Testing Position

Place the subject standing, with the cervical, thoracic, and lumbar spine in 0 degrees of lateral flexion and rotation.

Stabilization

Stabilize the pelvis to prevent anterior tilting.

Testing Motion

Ask the subject to bend forward as far as possible while keeping the knees straight.

Normal End-Feel

The end-feel is firm owing to stretching of the ligamentum flavum; posterior fibers of the annulus fibrosus and zygapophyseal joint capsules; thoracolumbar fascia; illiolumbar ligaments; and the multifidus, quadratus lumborum, and iliocostalis lumborum muscles. The location of the following muscles suggests that they may limit flexion, but the actual actions of the interspinales and intertransversaii mediales and laterales are unknown.[2]

LUMBAR FLEXION: MODIFIED–MODIFIED SCHOBER TEST[19,20] OR SIMPLIFIED SKIN DISTRACTION TEST[21]

In the original Schober method, the examiner made only two marks on the subject's back. The first mark was made at the lumbosacral junction, and the second mark was made 10 cm above the first mark on the spine. Macrae and Wright[3] decided to modify the Schober method (Modified Schober test) because they found that skin movement was a problem in the original method. They believed that the skin was more firmly attached in the region below the lumbosacral junction and therefore decided to use three marks—the first mark at the lumbosacral junction, the second mark 10 cm above the first mark, and the third mark 5 cm below the lumbosacral junction. The tape measurement is placed between the most superior and the most inferior marks. However, difficulty in correctly identifying the lumbosacral junction led to another modification of the original Schober test, called the Modified–Modified Schober Test (or MMST), which was proposed by van Adrichem and van der Korst.[20] The MMST is sometimes referred to as the simplified skin distraction test[21] and is described in the next paragraph.

The MMST uses two marks: one over the sacral spine on a line connecting the two PSISs and the other mark over the spine 15 cm superior to the first mark. Because the PSISs are much easier to identify than the lumbosacral junction, van Adrichem and van der Korst[20]

were able to eliminate one potential source of error in the original Schober and Modified Schober tests.

Normal values for the MMST for subjects between 15 and 18 years of age are 6.7 cm for males and 5.8 cm for females in the same age group.[20] Jones and associates[17] found a slightly larger normal value of 7.7 cm in a study of 89 healthy children between the ages of 11 and 16 years.

Procedure

1. Use a ruler to locate and place a **first mark** at a midline point on the sacrum that is level with the posterior superior iliac spines (this mark will be over the spinous process of S2). Make a **second mark** 15 cm above the midline sacral mark (Fig. 12.30).
2. Align the tape measure between the superior and inferior marks (Fig. 12.31). Ask the subject to bend forward as far as possible while keeping the knees straight. Maintain the tape measure against the subject's back during the motion, but allow the tape measure to unwind to accommodate the motion.
3. At the end of flexion ROM, note the distance between the two marks (Fig. 12.32). The ROM is the difference between 15 cm and length measured at the end of the motion.

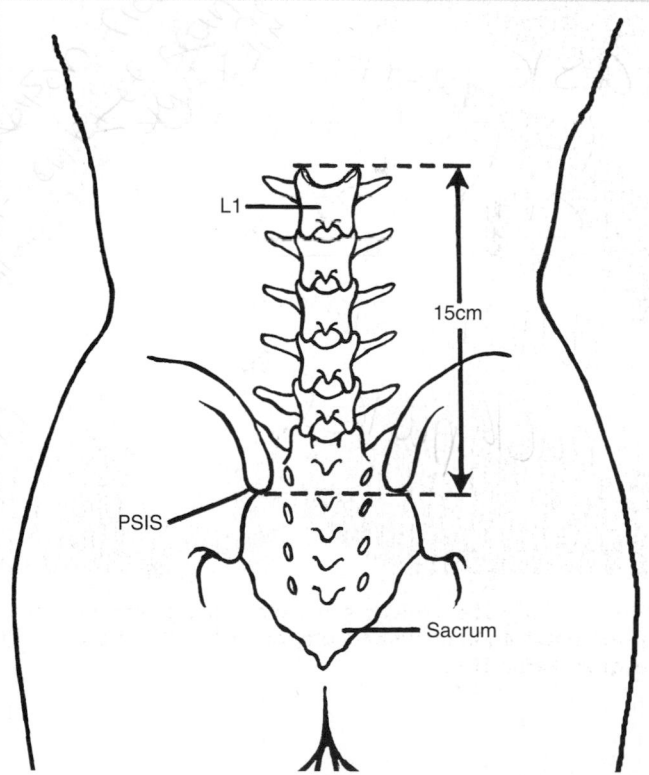

FIGURE 12.30 A line is drawn between the two posterior superior iliac spines and the point at which the lower end of the tape measure should be positioned. The location of the 15-cm mark shows that all five of the lumbar vertebrae in this subject are included.

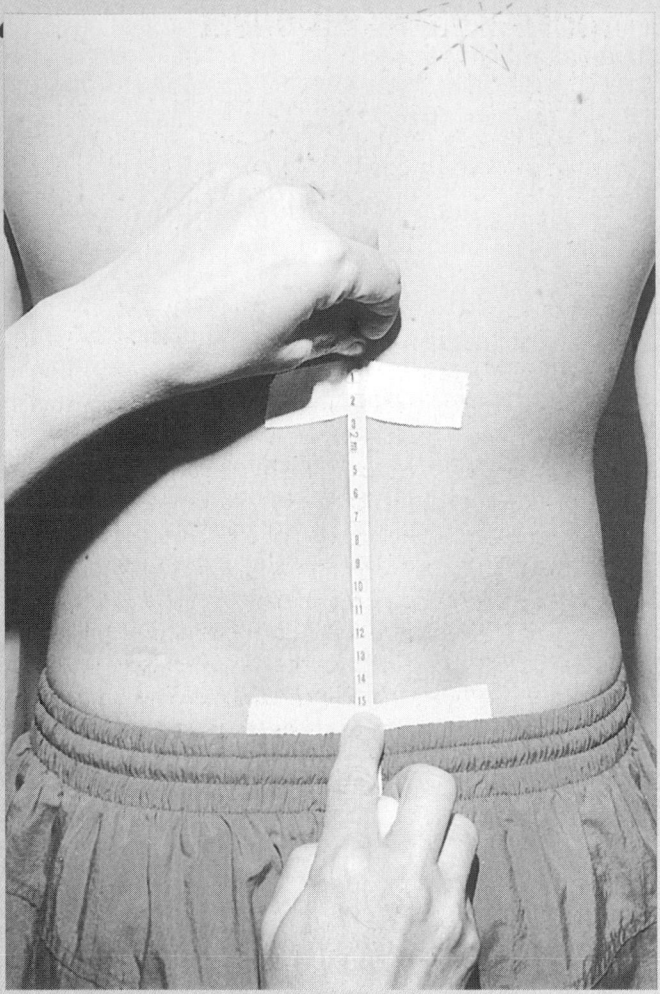

FIGURE 12.31 The tape measure is aligned between the upper and the lower landmarks at the beginning of lumbar flexion range of motion. Paper tape was placed over the skin marking pencil dots to improve visibility of landmarks for the photograph.

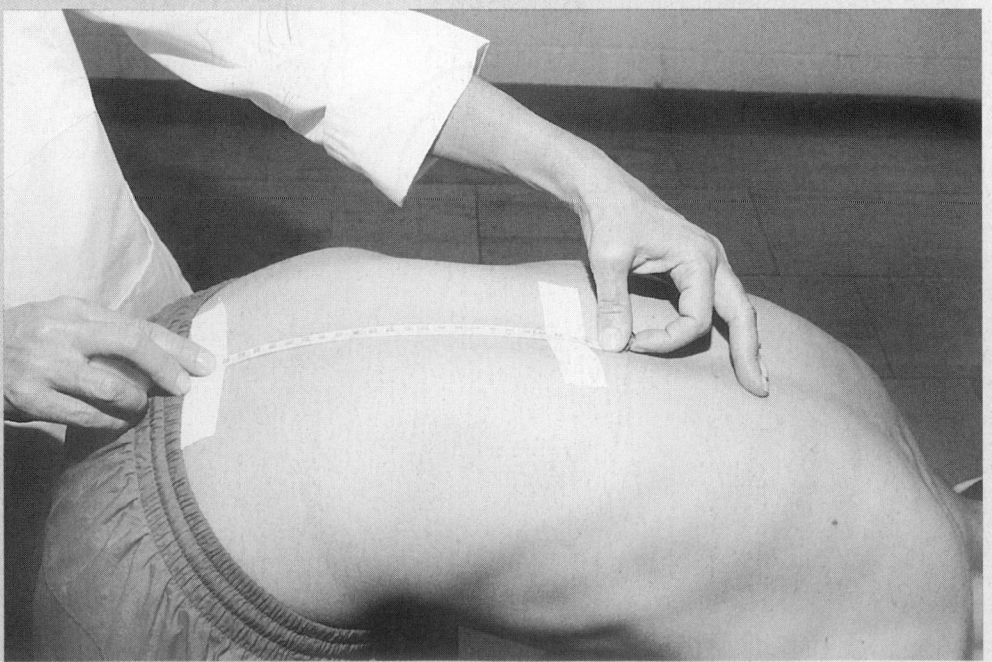

FIGURE 12.32 The tape measure is stretched between the upper and the lower landmarks at the end of lumbar flexion range of motion.

● LUMBAR FLEXION:MODIFIED SCHOBER TEST

Macrae and Wright[3] found an average of 6.3 cm of flexion in healthy adults, and Battie and coworkers[22] found an average of 6.9 cm in a similar group of subjects.

Procedure

1. Place the **first mark** at the lumbosacral junction with a skin marking pencil. Place a **second mark** 10 cm above the first mark. Place a **third mark** 5 cm below the first mark at the lumbosacral junction.
2. Align the tape measure between the most superior and the most inferior marks. Ask the subject to bend forward as far as possible while keeping the knees straight.
3. Maintain the tape measure against the subject's back during the movement, and note the distance between the most superior and the most inferior marks at the end of the ROM. The ROM is the difference between 15 cm and the length measured at the end of the motion.

● LUMBAR FLEXION: DOUBLE INCLINOMETER

The normal adult ROM is 60 degrees according to the AMA[4,6] and 0 to 66 degrees (for males 15 to 30 years of age) according to Loebl.[23] Ng and associates[24] found a mean value of 52 degrees for 35 healthy men with a mean age of 29 years.

Procedure

1. Mark the spinous processes of the T12 and S2 vertebrae using a skin marking pencil, with the subject in the standing position.
2. Place **one inclinometer** over the spinous process of T12 and the **second inclinometer** over the sacrum at the level of S2. **Zero** both inclinometers (Fig. 12.33).
3. Ask the subject to bend forward as far as possible while keeping the knees straight. Maintain the inclinometers firmly against the spine during the motion.
4. Note the information on the inclinometers at the end of flexion ROM (Fig. 12.34). Calculate the ROM by subtracting the degrees on the sacral inclinometer from the degrees on T12 inclinometer. The degrees on the sacral inclinometer are supposed to represent hip flexion ROM, and that is why they are subtracted.[21]

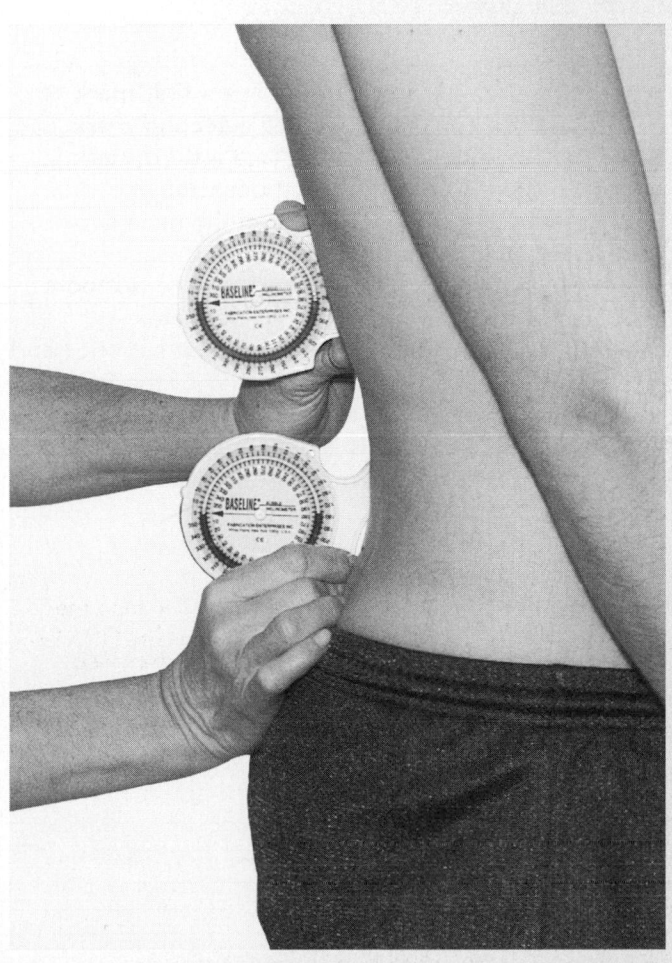

FIGURE 12.33 The starting position for measurement of lumbar flexion range of motion, with inclinometers aligned and zeroed.

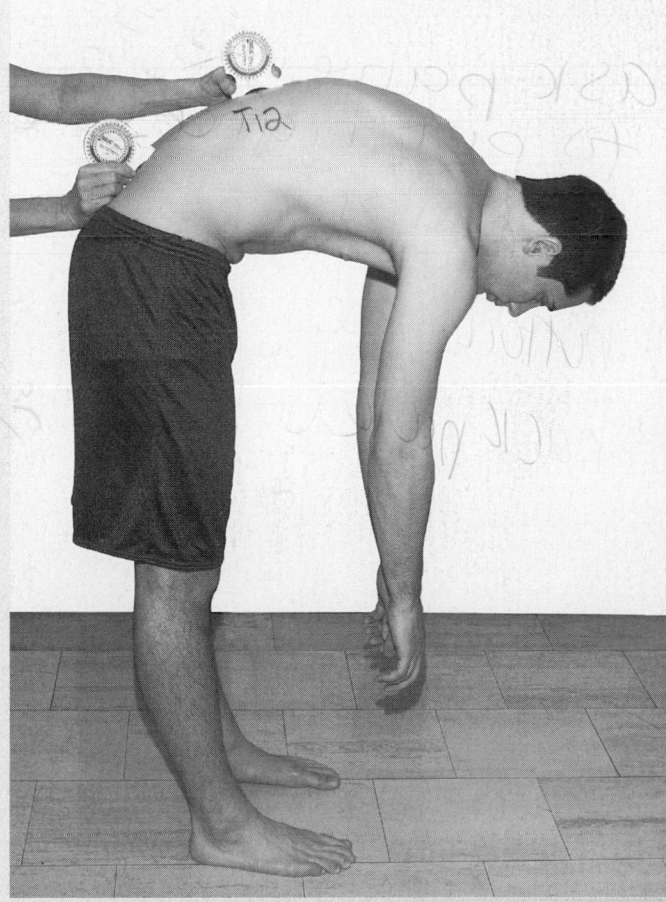

FIGURE 12.34 The end of lumbar flexion range of motion, with inclinometers aligned over the spinous processes of T12 and S2.

● LUMBAR EXTENSION

Testing Position

Place the subject standing, with the cervical, thoracic, and lumbar spine in 0 degrees of lateral flexion and rotation.

Stabilization

Stabilize the pelvis to prevent posterior tilting.

Testing Motion

Ask the subject to extend the spine as far as possible. The end of the extension ROM occurs when the pelvis begins to tilt posteriorly.

Normal End-Feel

The end-feel is firm owing to stretching of the anterior longitudinal ligament, anterior fibers of the annulus fibrosus, zygapophyseal joint capsules, rectus abdominis, and external and internal oblique muscles. The end-feel may also be hard owing to contact between the spinous processes.

▶ NOTE: Use the same testing position, stabilization, testing motion, and normal end-feel described in the Lumbar Extension section above for the following extension measurement methods unless changes are noted.

● LUMBAR EXTENSION: SIMPLIFIED SKIN ATTRACTION TEST MODIFIED-MODIFIED SCHOBER TEST (MMST)

Procedure[21]

1. Hold a ruler between two posterior superior iliac spines (PSIS) and place a **first mark** on a midline point of the sacrum that is on a level with the PSIS; this will be over the spinous process of S2. A second mark should be made on the lumbar spine that is 15 cm above the first mark.
2. Align the tape measure between the first and **second marks** on the spine (Fig. 12.35), and ask the subject to bend backward as far as possible.
3. At the end of the ROM, note the distance between the superior and the inferior marks (Fig. 12.36). The ROM is the difference between 15 cm and the length measured at the end of the motion.

● LUMBAR EXTENSION: MODIFIED SCHOBER TEST

Battie and coworkers[22] found a normal value of 1.6 cm in 100 healthy adults.

Procedure

1. Use a skin-marking pencil to place a **first mark** at the lumbosacral junction. Place a **second mark** 10 cm above the first mark. Place a **third mark** 5 cm below the first mark (lumbosacral junction).
2. Align the tape measure between the most superior and the most inferior marks.
3. Ask the subject to put the hands on the buttocks and to bend backward as far as possible.
4. Note the distance between the most superior and the most inferior marks at the end of the ROM, and subtract the final measurement from the initial 15 cm. The ROM is the difference between 15 cm and the length measured at the end of the motion.

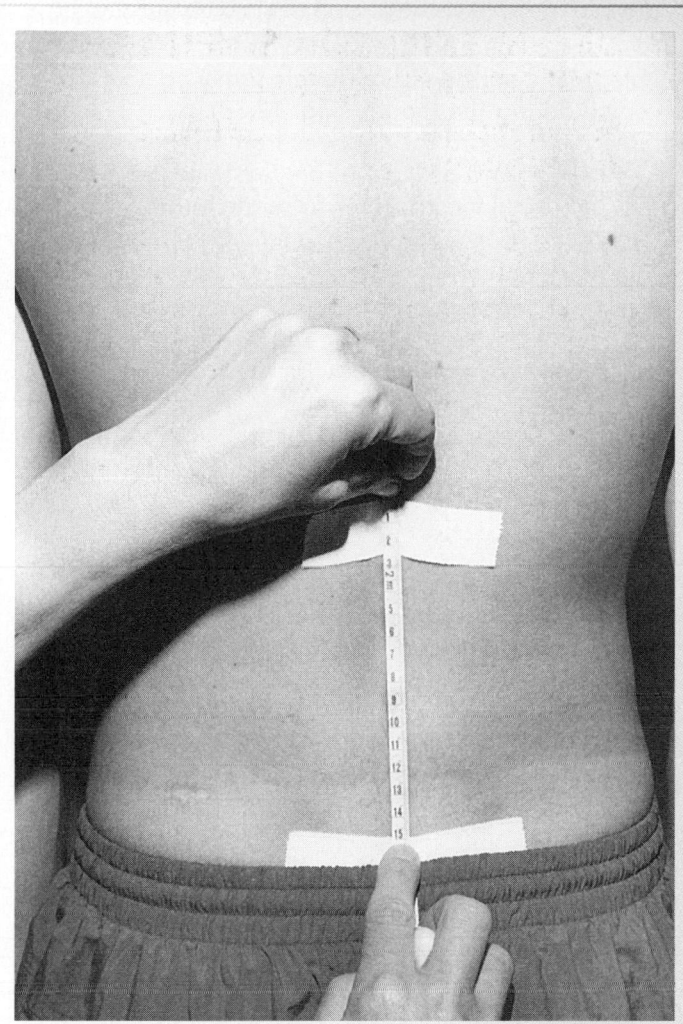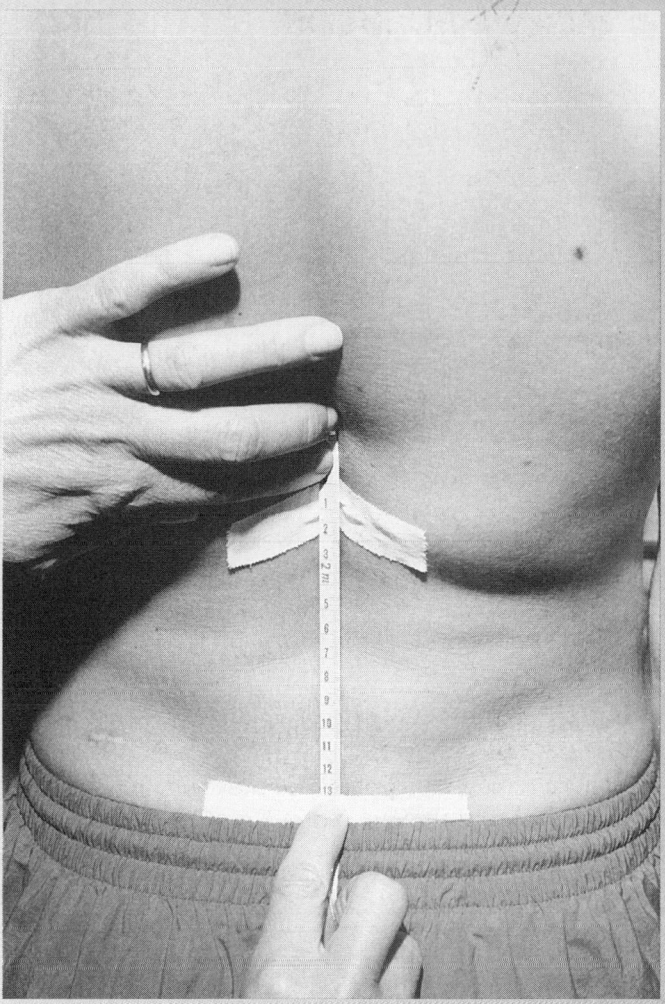

FIGURE 12.35 Tape measure alignment in the starting position for measurement of lumbar extension range of motion with use of the simplified skin distraction method (modified–modified Schober method).

FIGURE 12.36 Tape measure alignment at the end of lumbar extension range of motion, with use of the simplified skin distraction method.

● LUMBAR EXTENSION: DOUBLE INCLINOMETER

The normal ROM values for young-adult males (15 to 30 years) is 38 degrees, whereas the value for middle-age males (31 to 60 years) is 35 degrees. In males older than age 60 years the ROM is 33 degrees. In young-adult females the ROM is 42 degrees, in middle-aged females the ROM is 40 degrees, and in females older than 60 years the ROM is 36 degrees.[23] According to the AMA,[6] the normal ROM for adults is from 20[7] to 25[4] degrees; both of these values are considerably less than the values that were found by Loebl.[23]

Procedure

1. Mark the spinous processes of the T12 and S2 vertebrae using a skin marking pencil, with the subject in the standing position.
2. Place **one inclinometer** over the spinous process of T12 and the **second inclinometer** over the midline of the sacrum at S2. Then **zero** both inclinometers (Fig 12.37).

3. Ask the subject to bend backward as far as possible. Maintain the inclinometers firmly against the spine during the motion (Fig. 12.38).
4. Read and record the degrees from both inclinometers at the end of the motion. Subtract the degrees on the sacral inclinometer from the degrees on the T12 inclinometer to obtain the lumbar extension ROM.

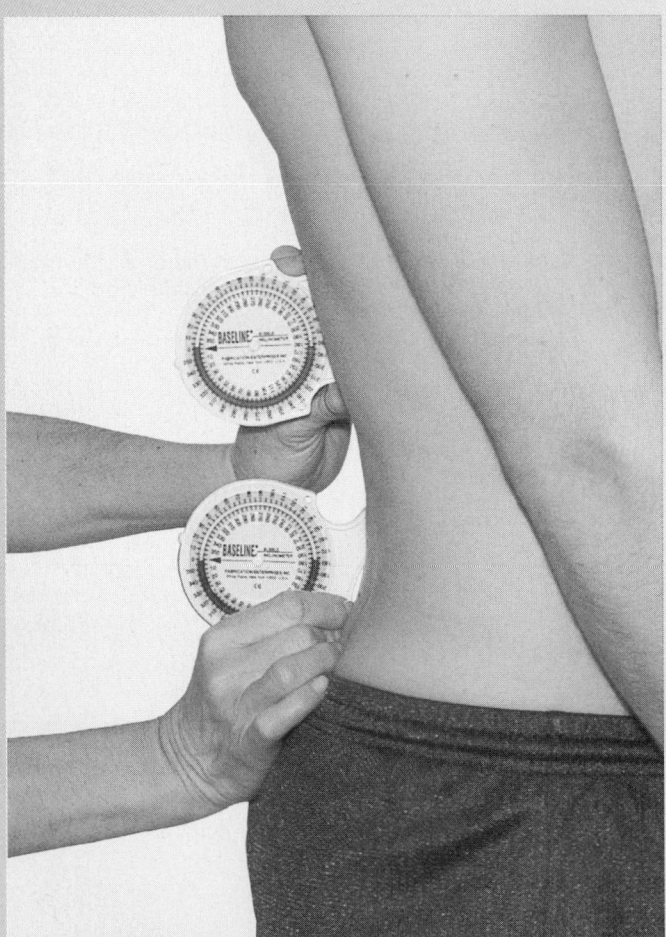

FIGURE 12.37 Starting position for measuring lumbar extension range of motion with double inclinometers placed over the T12 and S2 spinous processes.

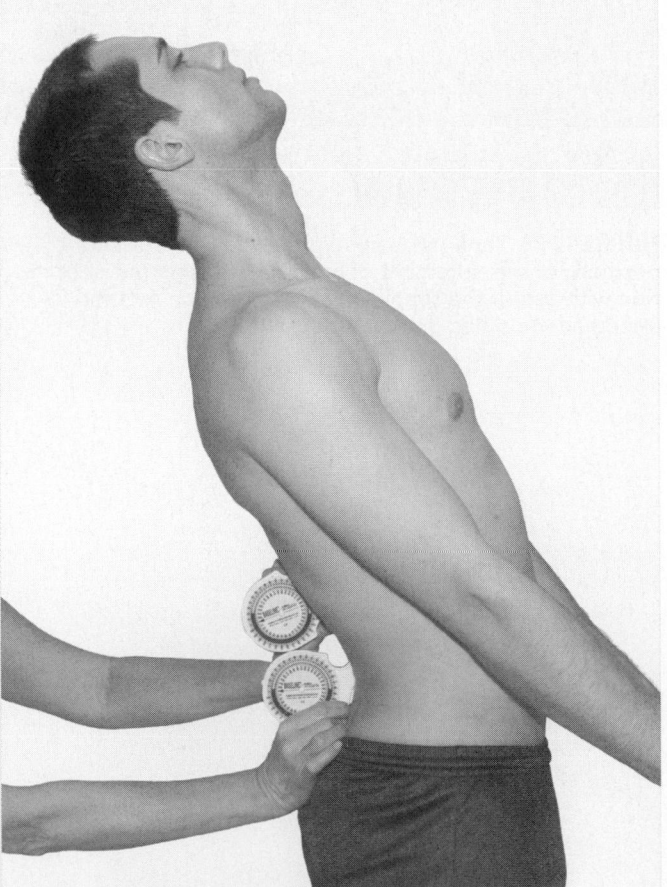

FIGURE 12.38 At the end of the lumbar extension range of motion (ROM), read and record the degrees on both inclinometers. Subtract the degrees on the sacral inclinometer from the T12 reading to obtain the ROM.

● LUMBAR LATERAL FLEXION

Testing Position

Place the subject standing with the feet shoulder width apart and the cervical, thoracic, and lumbar spine in 0 degrees of lateral flexion and rotation.

Stabilization

Stabilize the pelvis to prevent lateral tilting.

Testing Motion

Ask the subject to bend to the side as far as possible. The end of the lateral flexion ROM occurs when the pelvis begins to tilt laterally.

Normal End-Feel

The end-feel is firm owing to stretching of the contralateral band of the iliolumbar ligament, contralateral thoracolumbar fascia, contralateral fibers of the annulus fibrosus, and zygapophyseal joint capsules. The following contralateral muscles may contract eccentrically to control and resist lateral flexion when gravity begins to affect the motion: quadratus lumborum, interspinales, and iliocostales lumborum. The end-feel could be hard due to contact of the ipsilateral apophyseal joints.

▶ NOTE: **Use the same testing position, stabilization, testing motion and normal end-feel described in the Lumbar Lateral Flexion section above for the following lateral flexion measurement methods unless changes are noted.**

● LUMBAR LATERAL FLEXION: DOUBLE INCLINOMETER

According to the AMA, the ROM value is 25 to 30 degrees to each side.[4,7]

Procedure

1. Mark the spinous processes of the T12 and S2 vertebrae using a skin marking pencil, with the subject in the standing position.
2. Position **one inclinometer** over the T12 spinous process and the **second inclinometer** over the sacrum at the level of S2. Then, **zero** both inclinometers (Fig. 12.39).
3. Ask the subject to bend the trunk laterally while keeping both feet flat on the ground and the knees straight (Fig. 12.40).
4. Read and record the degrees on both inclinometers. Subtract the degrees on the sacral inclinometer from the degrees on the T12 inclinometer to obtain the lumbar lateral flexion ROM to one side.
5. Repeat the measurement process to measure lumbar lateral flexion ROM on the other side.

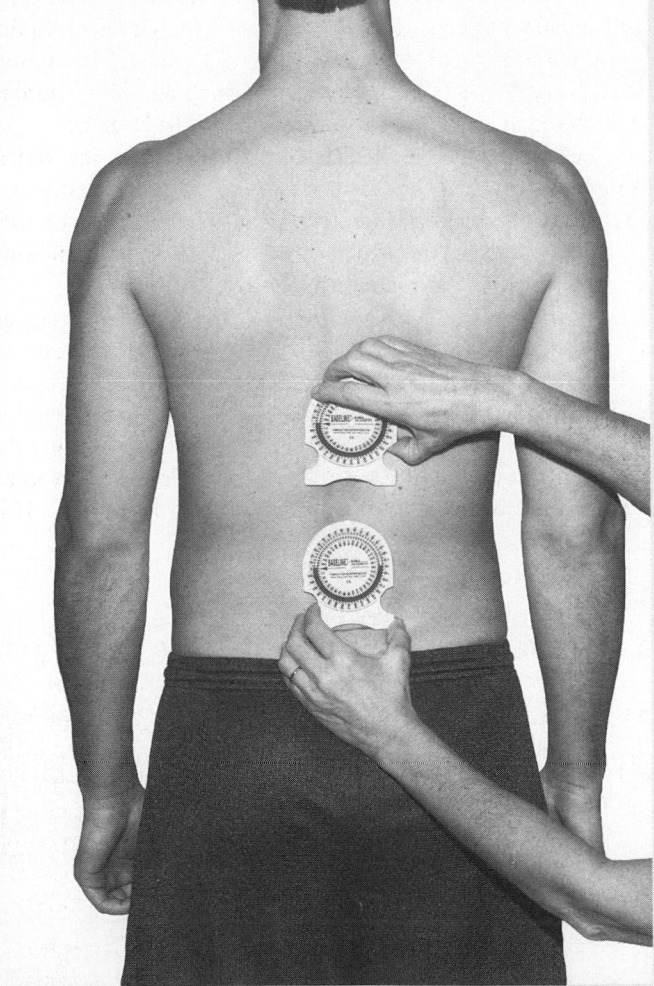

FIGURE 12.39 Starting position for measuring lumbar lateral flexion range of motion with double inclinometers placed over the spinous processes of T12 and S2.

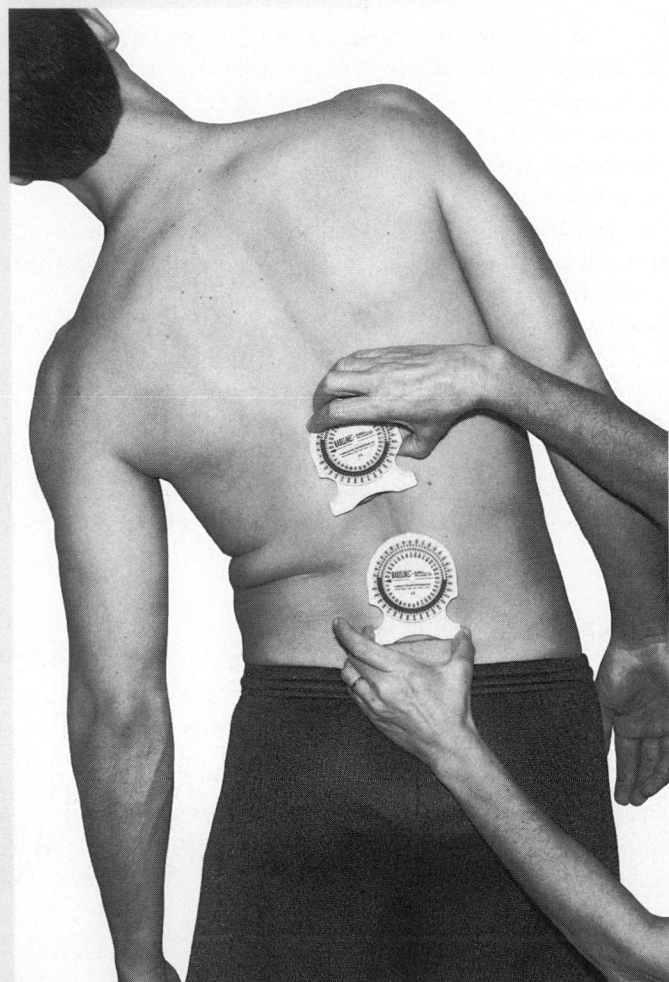

FIGURE 12.40 At the end of lumbar lateral flexion range of motion (ROM), read and record the degrees on each inclinometer. Subtract the degrees on the sacral inclinometer from the T12 reading to obtain the ROM.

Research Findings

Table 12.1 shows thoracolumbar spine ROM values from the AAOS and lumbar spine ROM values from the AMA.

Effects of Age, Gender, and Other Factors

Age

Many instruments and methods have been used to determine the range of thoracic, thoracolumbar, and lumbar motion. Therefore, comparisons between studies are difficult. As is true for other regions of the body, conflicting evidence exists regarding the effects of age on ROM. However, the majority of studies appear to indicate that age-related decreases in spinal ROM occur and that these changes may affect certain motions more than others at the same joint or region.[3,18,23–33]

The following two studies with relatively large numbers of subjects and extended age ranges arrived at similar conclusions regarding the motions that showed the greatest and least decrease in ROM with increasing age. Extension was one of the motions that showed the greatest decrease, and axial rotation showed the least decrease.

McGregor, McCarthy, and Hughes[29] found that, although age had a significant effect on all planes of motion, the effect varied for each motion, and age accounted for only a small portion of the variability seen in the 203 normal subjects studied. Maximum extension was the most affected motion, with significant decreases between each decade. Lateral flexion decreased after age 40 and each decade thereafter. Flexion decreased initially after age 30 years but stayed the same until an additional decrease after age 50 years. No similar decreases or trends were found in axial rotation.

The findings of Troke and associates[31,32] were similar in that these authors found no change in lumbar axial rotation in 405 asymptomatic subjects (196 females and 209 males) ages 16 to 90 years. Likewise, lumbar extension showed the greatest decline in ROM (approximately 76 percent). Male and female lumbar spine flexion range of motion declined considerably less, by about 40 percent over the age span, and right and left lateral flexion each declined about 43 percent. These authors used the CA-6000 Spine Motion Analyzer to measure half cycle motions at different times of the day to account for diurnal variations.

In another fairly large study, Moll and Wright[26] used skin markings and a plumb line to measure the range of lumbar extension in a study involving 237 subjects (119 men and 118 women) aged 20 to 90 years. These authors found a wide variation in normal values but detected a gradual decrease in lumbar extension in subjects between 35 and 90 years of age.

Van Herp and associates,[33] in a study of 100 healthy male and female subjects 20 to 77 years of age, used the 3Space System to measure lumbar ROM from T12 to S1. The authors found a constant decrease with increasing age in all lumbar motions except for flexion in 50- to 59-year-old males.

Fitzgerald and associates[14] determined that the oldest group had considerably less motion than the youngest group in all motions except for flexion. Also, the coefficients of variation (CV) indicated that a greater amount of variability existed in the ROM in the oldest groups (Table 12.2).

Alaranta and coworkers[18] used both a tape measure and an inclinometer to assess lumbar ROM in 508 males and females 35 to 45 years of age. Some of these subjects had either neck or back pain, but all were actively employed. Lumbar flexion showed more than a 10 percent decrease when comparing the youngest to the oldest subjects, but lateral flexion showed an even greater decrease (19 percent) with increasing age. This

TABLE 12.1	Thoracolumbar and Lumbar Spine Motion: Normal Values for Adults in Inches and Degrees From Selected Sources				
Instrument	**Tape Measure & Goniometer**	**Double Inclinometers**	**BROM II**	**3Space isotrak system**	**Inclinometer**
Motion **Authors** **Sample**	**Thoracolumbar** **AAOS*[5]**	**Lumbar** **AMA†[6]**	**Lumbar** **Breum et al[70]** **18–38 years**	**Lumbar** **VanHerp et al[33]** **20–29 years**	**Lumbar** **Ng et al[24]** **30 yrs**
Motion			*Mean (SD)*	*Mean (SD)*	*Mean (SD)*
Flexion	4 inches	60 degrees	56.3 (1.3) degrees	56.4 (7.1) degrees	52 (90) degrees
Extension	20–30 degrees	25 degrees	21.5 (8.2) degrees	22.5 (7.8) degrees	19 (9) degrees
Right lateral flexion	35 degrees	25 degrees	33.3 (5.9) degrees	26.2 (8.4) degrees	31 (6) degrees
Left lateral flexion	35 degrees	25 degrees	33.6 (6.2) degrees	25.8 (7.8) degrees	30 (6) degrees
Right rotation	45 degrees			14.4 (5.1) degrees	33 (9) degrees

AAOS = American Association of Orthopaedic Surgeons; AMA = American Medical Association.
* Flexion measurement in inches was obtained with a tape measure with use of the spinous processes of C7 and S1 as reference points. The remaining motions were measured with a universal goniometer and are in degrees.
† Lumbar motion was measured from sacrum (S1) to T12.

TABLE 12.2 Age Effects on Lumbar and Thoracolumbar Spine Motion in 20- to 79-Year-Old Adults: Normal Values in Centimeters and Degrees

Sample	20–29 yrs n = 31	30–39 yrs n = 42	40–49 yrs n = 16	50–59 yrs n = 43	60–69 yrs n = 26	70–79 yrs n = 9
Motion	*Mean (SD)*	*Mean (SD)*	*Mean (SD)*	*Mean (SD)*	*Mean (SD)*	*Mean (SD)*
Flexion*	3.7 (0.7)	3.9 (1.0)	3.1 (0.8)	3.0 (1.1)	2.4 (0.7)	2.2 (0.6)
Extension	41.2 (9.6)	40.0 (8.8)	31.1 (8.9)	27.4 (8.0)	17.4 (7.5)	16.6 (8.8)
Right lateral flexion	37.6 (5.8)	35.3 (6.5)	27.1 (6.5)	25.3 (6.2)	20.2 (4.8)	18.0 (4.7)
Left lateral flexion	38.7 (5.7)	36.5 (6.0)	28.5 (5.2)	26.8 (6.4)	20.3 (5.3)	18.9 (6.0)

SD = standard deviation.
* Flexion measurements were obtained with use of the Schober method and are reported in centimeters.
All other measurements were obtained with use of a universal goniometer and are reported in degrees.
Adapted from Fitzgerald, GK, et al: Objective assessment with establishment of normal values for lumbar
  spine range of motion. Phys Ther 63:1776, 1983.[14] With the permission of the American Physical Therapy Association.

decrease in lateral flexion is similar to the findings of McGregor, McCarthy, and Hughes,[29] who found that lateral flexion showed a slightly higher decrease in ROM (43 percent) than the decrease in forward flexion (40 percent).

In other studies the authors reported that both flexion and extension ROM were found to decline with increasing age, but in some of the studies the motions were full cycle motions, so it is difficult to tell whether the decrease was in flexion or in extension.

In one of the earlier studies, in 1967 Loebl[23] used an inclinometer to measure active sagittal plane ROM of the thoracic and lumbar spine of 126 males and females between 15 and 84 years of age. He found age-related effects for both males and females and concluded that both genders should expect a loss of about 8 degrees of spinal ROM per decade with increases in age.

In a more recent study, Sullivan, Dickinson, and Troup[25] used double inclinometers to measure sagittal plane lumbar motion in 1126 healthy male and female subjects. These authors found that when gender was controlled, flexion and extension decreased with increasing age. The authors suggested that the ROM thresholds that determine impairment ratings should take age into consideration.

In 1969 Macrae and Wright[3] used a modification of the Schober technique to measure forward lumbar flexion in 195 women and 147 men (18 to 71 years of age). The authors found that active flexion ROM decreased with age.

Anderson and Sweetman[27] used a device that combined a flexible rule and a hydrogoniometer to measure the ROM of 432 working men aged 20 to 59 years. Increasing age was associated with a lower total lumbar spine ROM (flexion and extension) in this group of subjects.

The preceding studies are fairly consistent in concluding that both thoracolumbar and lumbar ROM decreases with increasing age, and that extension and lateral flexion may be affected more than flexion. Axial rotation was not measured in the majority of studies, but when it was measured, no age-related changes in ROM were found.

The following two studies investigated segmental mobility. Gracovetsky and associates[28] found a significant difference between young and old in a group of 40 subjects aged 19 to 64 years. Older subjects had decreased segmental mobility in the lower lumbar spine compared with younger subjects. To compensate for the decrease in mobility, the older subjects increased the contribution of the pelvis to flexion and extension.

Wong and colleagues[35] assessed intervertebral lumbar flexion and extension in 100 healthy volunteers (50 males and 50 females) ages 20 to 76 years. The results showed that all segmental lumbar spinal motion profiles within the ROM of 10 degrees of extension to 40 degrees of flexion did not change as age increased until subjects were 51 years of age or older. Subjects in the oldest age group had a decrease in maximum flexion and extension ROM, but an increase in the slopes of the intervertebral flexion-extension curves at each lumbar segment.

Gender

Investigations of the effects of gender on lumbar spine ROM indicate that the effects may be motion specific and possibly age specific, but controversy still exists concerning which motions are affected, and some authors report that gender has no effects. The fact that investigators used different instruments and methods makes comparisons between studies difficult. However, the following five studies appear to agree that the ROM in flexion is greater in males than in females, at least in subjects 15 to 65 years of age. This difference in flexion ROM between males and females is apparent even in children between the ages of 5 to 11 years.[30] At the other end of the age spectrum, this difference between the genders in flexion ROM may have evened out by the time men and women were in their 80s.[31,32]

Macrae and Wright[3] found that females had significantly less forward flexion than males across all age groups. Sullivan, Dickinson, and Troup[25] also found that when age was controlled, mean flexion ROM was greater in males. However, mean extension ROM and total ROM were significantly greater in females. Subjects in the study were 1126 healthy male and female volunteers aged 15 to 65 years. The authors noted that, although female total ROM was significantly greater than male total ROM, the difference of 1.5 degrees was not clinically relevant. Age and gender combined accounted for only 14 percent of the variance in flexion, 25 percent in extension, and 20 percent of the variance in total ROM (Table 12.3). Alaranta and associates,[18] in a study of 508 males and females ages 35 to 45 years, also determined that men had greater flexion ROM than women. However, these authors found no difference between the sexes in extension ROM. Kondratek and associates,[30] in a study of 116 girls and 109 boys aged 5 to 11 years of age, found a statistically significant difference between the youngest and oldest subjects in active lumbar flexion in girls and active lumbar lateral flexion and rotation in both girls and boys. The older girls, aged 11 years, consistently demonstrated less motion in forward flexion and right and left lateral flexion than the boys. Extension varied very little in either gender. Troke and colleagues[31,32] found that men had greater ROM in flexion at 16 years than women, but in the final decade (80 to 90 years) men and women were equal.

Moll and Wright's[26] findings are directly opposite to the findings of the previous three studies in that Moll and Wright determined that male mobility in extension significantly exceeded female mobility by 7 percent. Differences in findings between studies may have resulted from the fact that Moll and Wright[26] did not control for age. These authors measured the range of lumbar extension in a study involving 237 subjects (119 males and 118 females) aged 15 to 90 years, who were clinically and radiologically normal relatives of patients with psoriatic arthritis (Tables 12.4 and 12.5).

Van Herp and associates,[33] in an investigation of lumbar range of motion in 100 subjects (50 male and 50 female) 20 to 77 years of age, found that females consistently showed greater flexibility than males in lumbar flexion–extension, lateral flexion, and axial rotation throughout the age range. Because flexion was not separated from extension, it is difficult to know which motion was responsible for the increase.

In contrast to the preceding authors, the following three studies reported no significant effects for gender on lumbar spine ROM. Loebl[23] found no significant gender differences between the 126 males and females aged 15 to 84 years of age for measurements of lumbar flexion and extension. Bookstein and associates[34] used a tape measure to measure the lumbar extension ROM in 75 elementary school children aged 6 to 11 years. The authors found no differences for age or gender, but they found a significant difference for age–gender interaction in the 6-year-old group. Girls aged 6 years had a mean range of extension of 4.1 cm, in contrast to the 6-year-old boys, who had a mean range of extension of 2.1 cm. Wong and colleagues[35] used an electrogoniometer and videofluoroscopy to assess the flexion–extension profile of the lumbar spine in different genders and age groups. A total of 100 healthy volunteers (50 females and 50 males) ages 21 to 51 years and older participated in the study, but no statistically significant differences in the pattern of motion were found between the genders.

Diurnal Effects

Ensink and coworkers[36] determined that the average increase in height in the morning after 8 hours of bed rest was 2 mm, with 40 percent of the increase occurring in the lumbar spine. The increase in height was due to the hydration of the discs that occurred during bed rest. Lumbar spine ROM in flexion was decreased in the morning but increased during the day as water was squeezed out of the discs. ROM in extension was not affected. Consequently, examiners should try to test and retest lumbar flexion ROM during the same time of day.

Occupation and Lifestyle

Researchers have investigated the following factors among others in relation to their effects on lumbar ROM: occupation,[37] lifestyle,[29,37–39] time of day,[36] and disability.[25,40–44] Similar to the findings related to age and gender, the results have been controversial.

Sughara and colleagues,[37] using a device called a spinometer, studied age-related and occupation-related changes in thoracolumbar active ROM in 1071 men and 1243 women aged 20 to 60 years. Subjects were selected from three occupational groups: fishermen, farmers, and industrial workers. Although both flexion and extension were found to decrease with increasing age, decreases in the extension ROM were

TABLE 12.3	Age and Gender Effects on Lumbar Motion in Individuals 15 to 65 Years Old: Normal Values in Degrees Using a Fluid-Filled Inclinometer					
Sample	16-24 yrs Male n = 122	15–24 yrs Female n = 161	25–34 yrs Male n = 295	25–34 yrs Female n = 143	35–65 yrs Male n = 269	35–65 yrs Female n = 136
Motion	*Mean (SD)*	*Mean (SD)*	*Mean (SD)*	*Mean (SD)*	*Mean (SD)*	*Mean (SD)*
Flexion	33 (9)	26 (9)	31 (8)	24 (8)	27 (8)	22 (8)
Extension	54 (10)	63 (9)	52 (9)	60 (10)	47 (9)	53 (9)

SD = standard deviation.
Adapted from Sullivan, MS, Dickinson, CE, and Troup, JDG: The influence of age and gender on lumbar spine sagittal plane range of motion: A study of 1126 healthy subjects. Spine 19:682, 1994.[40]

TABLE 12.4	Age and Gender Effects on Lumbar and Thoracolumbar Motion in Individuals Ages 15 to 44 Years: Normal Values in Centimeters					
Sample	15–24 yrs		25–34 yrs		35–44 yrs	
	Male n = 21	Female n = 10	Male n = 13	Female n = 16	Male n = 14	Female n = 18
Motion	Mean (SD)	Mean (SD)	Mean (SD)	Mean (SD)	Mean (SD)	Mean (SD)
Flexion*	7.23 (0.92)	6.66 (1.03)	7.48 (0.82)	6.69 (1.09)	6.88 (0.88)	6.29 (1.04)
Extension*	4.21 (1.64)	4.34 (1.52)	5.05 (1.41)	4.76 (1.53)	3.73 (1.47)	3.09 (1.31)
Right lateral flexion†	5.43 (1.30)	6.85 (1.46)	5.34 (1.06)	6.32 (1.93)	4.83 (1.34)	5.30 (1.61)
Left lateral flexion†	5.06 (1.40)	7.20 (1.66)	5.93 (1.07)	6.13 (1.42)	4.83 (0.99)	5.48 (1.30)

Adapted from Moll, JMH, and Wright, V: Normal range of spinal mobility: An objective clinical study. Ann Rheum Dis 30:381, 1971.[26] The authors used skin markings and a plumb line on the thorax for lateral flexion.
SD = standard deviation.
*Lumbar motion.
†Thoracolumbar motion.

greater than decreases in flexion. Decreases in active extension ROM were less in fishermen and their wives than in the other occupational groups in the study. The researchers concluded that because both fishermen and their wives had more extension than other groups, other variables than the physical demands of fishing were affecting the maintenance of extension ROM.

Sjolie[39] compared low-back strength and low-back and hip mobility between a group of 38 adolescents living in a community without access to pedestrian roads and a group of 50 adolescents with excellent access to pedestrian roads. Low-back mobility was measured by means of the modified Schober technique. The results showed that adolescents living in rural areas without easy access to pedestrian roads had less low-back extension and hamstring flexibility than their counterparts in urban areas. The hypothesis that negative associations would

exist between school bus use and physical performance was confirmed. The distance traveled by the school bus was inversely associated with hamstring flexibility and other hip motions but not with low-back flexion. Walking or bicycling to leisure activities was positively associated with low-back strength, low-back extension ROM, and hip flexion and extension.

Freidrich and colleagues[38] conducted a comprehensive examination of spinal posture during stooped walking in 22 male sewer workers aged 24 to 49 years. Working in a stooped posture has been identified as one of the risk factors associated with spinal disorders. Five posture levels corresponding to standardized sewer heights ranging in decreasing size from 150 to 105 cm were taped by a video-based motion analysis system. The results showed that the lumbar spine abruptly changed from the usual lordotic position in normal

TABLE 12.5	Age and Gender Effects on Lumbar and Thoracolumbar Motion in Individuals Ages 45 to 74 Years: Normal Values in Centimeters					
Sample	45–54 yrs		55–64 yrs		65–74 yrs	
	Male n = 19	Female n = 23	Male n = 34	Female n = 30	Male n = 14	Female n = 14
Motion	Mean (SD)	Mean (SD)	Mean (SD)	Mean (SD)	Mean (SD)	Mean (SD)
Flexion*	7.17 (1.20)	6.02 (1.32)	6.87 (0.89)	6.08 (1.32)	5.67 (1.31)	4.93 (0.90)
Extension*	3.88 (1.19)	3.12 (1.36)	3.56 (1.28)	3.57 (1.32)	3.41 (1.56)	2.72 (0.95)
Right lateral flexion†	4.71 (1.35)	5.37 (1.54)	5.05 (1.30)	5.10 (1.85)	4.44 (1.03)	5.56 (2.04)
Left lateral flexion†	4.55 (0.94)	5.14 (1.54)	4.94 (1.22)	4.88 (1.61)	4.38 (0.98)	5.55 (2.16)

Adapted from Moll, JMH, and Wright, V: Normal range of spinal mobility: An objective clinical study. Ann Rheum Dis 30:381, 1971.[26] The authors used skin markings and a plumb line on the thorax for lateral flexion.
SD = standard deviation.
*Lumbar motion.
†Thoracolumbar motion.

upright walking to a kyphotic position in mild, 150-cm head-room restriction. As ceiling height decreased, the neck progressively assumed a more extended lordotic position; the thoracic spine extended and flattened, becoming less kyphotic; and the lumbar spine became more kyphotic. As expected, the older workers showed decreased segmental mobility in the lumbar spine and an increase in cervical lordosis with decreasing ceiling height.

Disability

The relationship between ROM findings and disability is a topic of considerable interest and importance to health professionals. Researchers have reported conflicting results, so that there appears to be no clear relationship between range of motion and disability at the present time.

Sullivan, Dickinson, and Troup[25] used dual inclinometers to measure lumbar spine sagittal motion in 1126 healthy individuals. The authors found a large variation in measurements and suggested that detection of ROM impairments might be difficult because 95% confidence intervals yielded up to a 36-degree spread in normal ROM values. Sullivan, Shoaf, and Riddle[40] examined the relationship between impairment of active lumbar flexion ROM and disability. The authors used normative data to determine when an impairment in flexion ROM was present and used the judgment of physical therapists to determine whether flexion ROM impairment was relevant to the patient's disability. Low correlations between lumbar ROM and disability were found, and the authors concluded that active lumbar ROM measurements should not be used as treatment goals.

Nattrass and associates[43] used a long-arm goniometer to measure thoracolumbar ROM and dual inclinometers to measure low-back ROM in 34 patients aged 20 to 65 years with chronic low-back pain. ROM for all subjects was compared with ratings on commonly used impairment and disability indexes. Only flexion measured with the goniometer demonstrated greater than 50 percent of the variance in common with one of the disability measues. The authors concluded that lumbar ROM alone is not enough to represent impairment and, therefore, the AMA *Guides to the Evaluation of Permanent Impairment* should not limit impairment ratings to ROM because ROM seems to represent only one aspect of impairment.

However, Lundberg and Gerdle,[41] who investigated spinal and peripheral joint mobility and spinal posture in 607 female home care employees (mean age 40.5 years), found that lumbar sagittal hypomobility alone was associated with higher disability, and a combination of positive pain provocation tests and lumbar sagittal hypomobility was associated with particularly high disability levels. Peripheral joint mobility, spinal sagittal posture, and thoracic sagittal mobility showed low correlations with disability.

Kujala and coworkers[42] conducted a 3-year longitudinal study of lumbar mobility and occurrence of low-back pain in 98 adolescents. The subjects included 33 nonathletes (16 males and 17 females), 34 male athletes, and 31 female athletes. Participation in sports and low maximal lumbar flexion predicted low-back pain during the follow-up in males, but accounted for only 16 percent of the variance between groups with and without low-back pain. A decreased ROM in the lower lumbar segments, low maximal ROM in extension, and high body weight were predictive of low-back pain in females and accounted for 31 percent of the variability between groups.

Alaranta and associates,[18] in a study of 508 male and female white and blue collar employees ages 35 to 54 years, found that the strongest connections were between trunk lateral flexion ROM and low-back pain during the preceding year.

Functional Range of Motion

Hsieh and Pringle[45] used a CA-6000 Spinal Motion Analyzer (Orthopedic Systems, Inc., Hayward, CA) to measure the amount of lumbar motion required for selected activities of daily living performed by 48 healthy subjects with a mean age of 26.5 years. Activities included stand to sit, sit to stand, putting on socks, and picking up an object from the floor. The individual's peak flexion angles for the activities were normalized to the subject's own peak flexion angle in erect standing. Stand to sit and sit to stand (Fig. 12.41) required approximately 56 percent to 66 percent of lumbar flexion. The mean was 34.6 degrees for sit to stand and 41.8 degrees for stand to sit. Putting on socks (Fig. 12.42) required 90 percent of lumbar flexion ROM (mean 56.4 degrees), and picking up an object from the floor (Fig. 12.43) required 95 percent of lumbar flexion (mean 60.4 degrees). In view of these findings, one can understand how limitations in lumbar ROM may

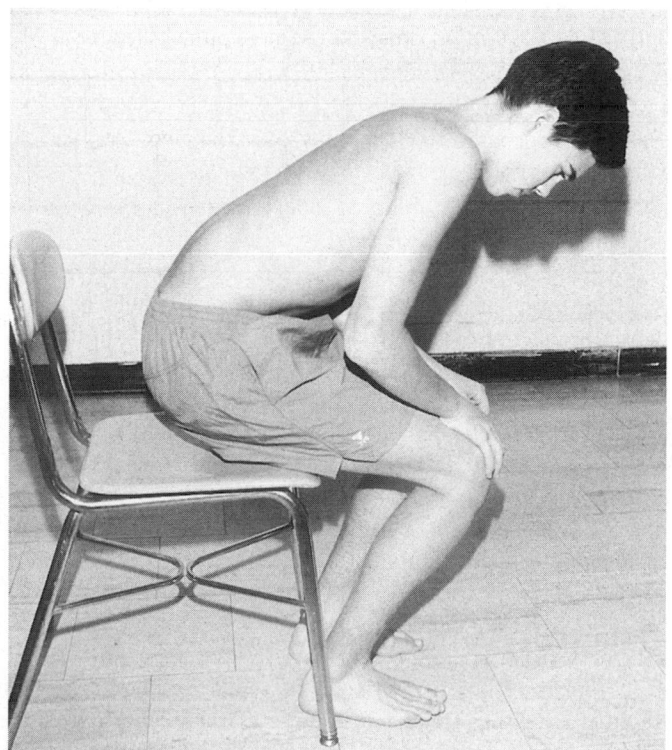

FIGURE 12.41 Sit to stand requires an average of 35 degrees of lumbar flexion.[45]

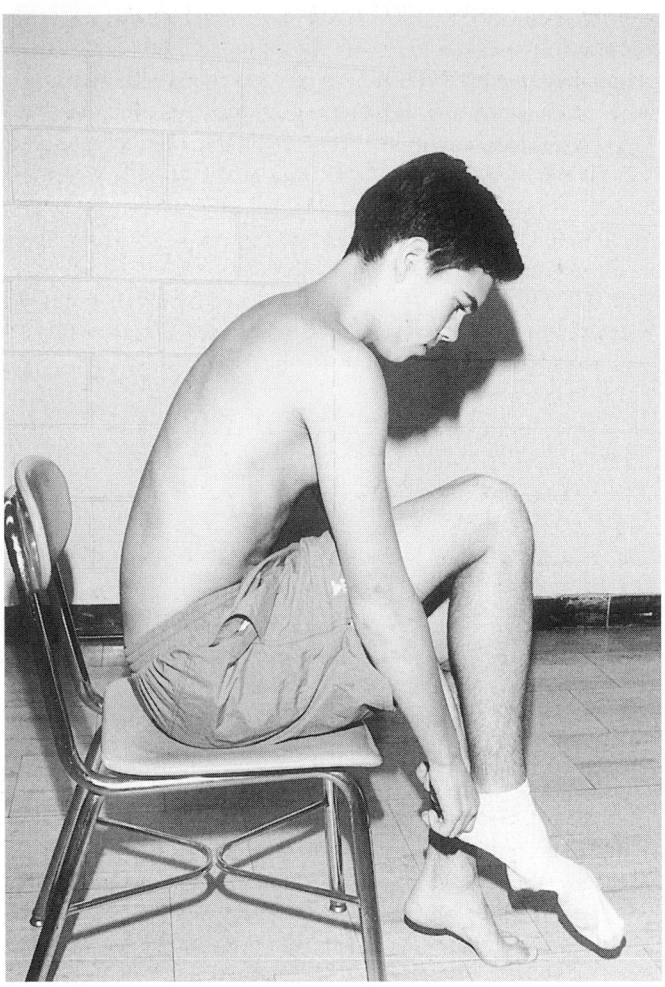

FIGURE 12.42 Putting on socks requires an average of 56 degrees of lumbar flexion.[45]

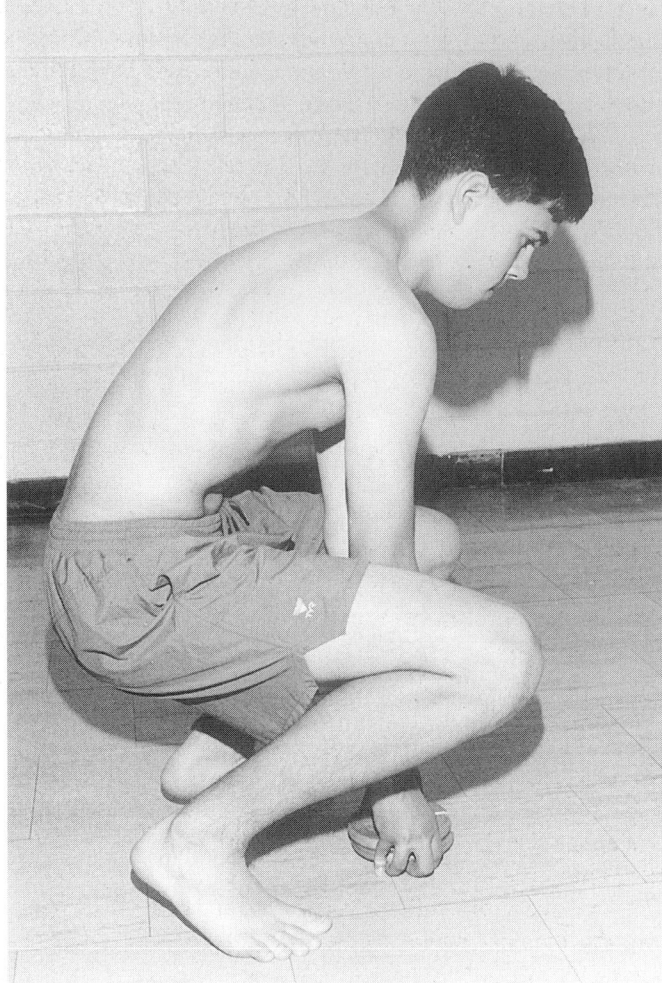

FIGURE 12.43 Picking up an object from the floor requires an average of 60 degrees of lumbar flexion.[45]

affect an individual's ability to independently carry out dressing and other activities of daily living.

Levine and associates[46] conducted a study with 20 healthy women (mean age 23.4 years) from a university student population to determine changes in lumbar spine motion in standing, walking, and running on a treadmill at three different gradients. According to results obtained from the Vicon Motion Analysis System, total lumbar spine ROM was greater during running than during walking, and greater walking downhill than walking uphill or on a level surface. However, the maximum amount of lumbar extension (anterior pelvic tilt) was found in standing at the three gradients.

Reliability and Validity

The following section on reliability and validity has been divided according to the instruments and methods used to obtain the measurements. However, some overlap occurs between the sections because several investigators have compared different methods and instruments within one study.

Littlewood and May[47] conducted a systematic review of 86 ROM studies to determine what low tech measurement methods were valid for measuring lumbar spine ROM. Only four studies—those by Samo and colleagues,[48] Saur and colleagues,[49] Williams and colleagues,[19] and Tousignant and colleagues[50]—were found to meet the criteria of English language only, evaluated validity by comparison to radiographs, included adult subjects with non-specific low back pain, and included measurement accuracy to enable judgement on validity. All failed to meet the criteria of blinding the examiners. Double inclinometers were used in three of the four studies, and the Modified-Modified-Schober Test (MMST) was used in the other study. Littlewood and May[4] performed a qualitative analysis but did not perform a meta-analysis. In regard to the double inclinometer method, they concluded that there was only limited positive supporting evidence for the validity of measuring total lumbar ROM in comparison to radiographic analysis; there was conflicting evidence for the validity of measuring lumbar flexion ROM; and there was limited positive evidence for the lack of validity of measuring lumbar extension. In regard to the

MMST they determined that there was limited positive evidence for the lack of validity for measuring lumbar flexion ROM. The authors concluded that there is a need for scientific evidence on the validity of these measurement procedures.

In another review, Essendrop and colleagues[51] screened databases from 1980 to 1999 for reliability studies regarding the measurement of low-back ROM, strength, and endurance. Seventy-nine studies were located, 6 of which met the predetermined criteria for a quality study and focused on the measurement of low back ROM. Noting the difficulty in making definite conclusions based on these limited studies, the authors reported that the tape measure was the most reliable instrument for flexion measurements. Reliable extension measurements were difficult to achieve with any of the reviewed instruments. The tape measure and Cybex EDI 320 goniometer were reliable for trunk lateral flexion when comparing groups but not individuals. Trunk rotation measurements were the most unreliable for all instruments including the double inclinometer, Myrin inclinometer, tape measure, and universal goniometer.

Reliability:Inclinometer

The AMA *Guides to the Evaluation of Permanent Impairment*[4] states that "measurement techniques using inclinometers are necessary to obtain reliable spinal mobility measurements." However, in a study by Williams and coworkers[19] that compared the measurements of the inclinometer with those of the tape measure, the authors found that the double inclinometer technique had questionable intertester reliability (Table 12.6). Reliability problems with the use of double inclinometers are often related to difficulty in identifying landmarks and in holding the inclinometers correctly. Other problems include too long a time period between test and retest and lack of sufficient practice to familiarize the examiner with the instruments.

Loebl[23] has stated that the only reliable technique for measuring lumbar spine motion is radiography. However, radiography is expensive and may pose a health risk to the subject; moreover, the validity of radiographic assessment of ROM is unreported. Loebl[23] used an inclinometer to measure flexion and extension in nine subjects. He found that in five repeated active measurements, the ROM varied by 5 degrees in the most consistent subject and by 23 degrees in the most inconsistent subject. Variability decreased when measurements were taken on an hourly basis rather than on a daily basis. Patel,[52] who used the double inclinometer method to measure lumbar flexion on 25 subjects aged 21 to 37 years, found intratester reliability to be high (r = 0.91), but intertester reliability was considerably lower (r = 0.68).

Mayer and associates[53] compared repeated measurements of lumbar ROM of 18 healthy subjects taken by 14 different examiners using three different instruments: a fluid-filled inclinometer, the kyphometer, and the electrical inclinometer. The three instruments were found to be equally reliable, but significant differences were found between examiners. Poor intertester reliability was the most significant source of variance. The authors identified sources of error as being caused by differences in instrument placement among examiners and inability to locate the necessary landmarks.

Saur and colleagues[49] used Pleurimeter V inclinometers to measure lumbar ROM in 54 patients with chronic low-back pain who were between 18 and 60 years of age. Measurements were taken with and without radiographic verification of the T12 and S1 landmarks used for positioning the inclinometers. Intertester reliability of the inclinometry technique for full cycle flexion–extension in a subgroup of 48 patients was high (r = 0.94) and half cycle flexion was good (r = 0.88), but half cycle extension was poor (r = 0.42). The authors concluded that the Pleurimeter V was a reliable and valid method for measuring lumbar ROM and that with use of this instrument it was possible to differentiate lumbar spine movements from hip movements.

Chen and associates[54] investigated intertester and intratester reliability using three health professionals to measure lumbar ROM using a Pleurimeter V (double inclinometer), a carpenter's double inclinometer, and a computed single-sensor inclinometer. Intertester reliability was poor, with all ICCs less than 0.75; with a single exception, intratester reliability was less than 0.90. The authors determined that the largest source of measurement error was attributable to the examiners and associated factors and concluded that these three surface methods had only limited clinical usefulness.

Mayer and colleagues[55] used a Cybex EDI-320 (Lumex, Ronkonkoma, NY), a computed inclinometer with a single sensor, to measure lumbar ROM in 38 healthy individuals. Full cycle sagittal ROM was the most accurate measurement, and extension was the least accurate. Clinical utility of lumbar sagittal plane ROM measurement appeared to be highly sensitive to the training of the test administrator in aspects of the process such as locating bony landmarks of T12 and S1 and maintaining inclinometer placement without rocking on the sacrum. Device error was negligible relative to the error associated with the test process itself. The authors found that practice was the most significant factor in eliminating the largest source of error when inexperienced examiners were used.

Nitschke and colleagues[56] compared the following measurement methods in a study involving 34 male and female subjects with chronic low-back pain and two examiners: dual inclinometers for lumbar spine ROM (flexion, extension, and lateral flexion) and a plastic long-arm goniometer for thoracolumbar ROM (flexion, extension, lateral flexion, and rotation). Intertester reliability was poor for all measurements except for flexion taken with the long-arm goniometer (Table 12.6). The dual inclinometer method had no systematic error, but there was a large random error for all measurements. The authors concluded that the standard error of measurement might be a better indicator of reliability than the ICC.

Reynolds[57] compared intratester and intertester reliability with use of a spondylometer, a plumb line and skin distraction, and an inclinometer. Intertester error was calculated by comparing the results of two testers taking 10 repeated measurements of lumbar flexion, extension, and lateral flexion on 30 volunteers with a mean age of 38.1 years. Highly significant positive correlations were found between flexion–extension

TABLE 12.6 Intratester and Intertester Reliability for Thoracolumbar and Lumbar ROM

Author	Subject n	Sample	Instrument	Motions	Intra ICC	Inter ICC	Intra r	Inter r
Fitzgerald[14]	17	Healthy adults	Tape measure* (Schober)	Flexion				1.0
			Universal goniometer+	Extension				0.88
				R. lat. flexion				0.76
				L. lat. flexion				0.91
Nitschke et al[56]	34	Patients with back pain 20–65 yrs	Universal goniometer+ +	Flexion	0.92	0.84		
				Extension	0.81	0.63		
				R. lat. flexion	0.76	0.62		
				Flexion	0.90	0.52		
			Dual inclinometers*	Extension	0.70	0.35		
				R. lat. flexion	0.90	0.18		
Williams et al[19]	15	Patients with CLBP	Dual inclinometers*	Flexion		0.60		0.13 – 0.87
				Extension		0.48		0.28 – 0.66
Madson et al[67]	40	Healthy adults 20–40 yrs	BROM*	Flexion	0.67			
				Extension	0.78			
				R. lat. flexion	0.95			
				R. rotation	0.93			
Kachingwe and Phillips[68]	91	Healthy adults mean age = 28 yrs	BROM*	Lat. flexion	0.83 – 0.85			
				Flexion	0.79 – 0.84			
Kondratek et al[30]	15	Healthy Children 5–11 yrs	BROM II*	Flexion	0.53 – 0.71			
				Extension	0.82 – 0.94			
Petersen et al[70]	21	Healthy subjects 10–79 yrs	OSI CA-6000+ +	Flexion	0.90	0.85		
				Extension	0.96	0.96		
				R. lat. flexion	0.89	0.85		
				R. rotation	0.95	0.90		

BROM = Back Range of Motion Device; OSI CA-6000 = Spine Motion Analyzer.
* Lumbar ROM.
+ Thoracolumbar ROM.

ROM measured with the inclinometer and that measured with the spondylometer. The inclinometer had acceptable intertester reliability, with the highest reliability for measurement of lateral flexion to the right.

Validity: Double Inclinometers

Saur and colleagues[49] found that the correlation of radiographic ROM measurements with inclinometer ROM measurements demonstrated an almost linear correlation for flexion (r = 0.98) and total lumbar flexion–extension ROM (r = 0.97), but extension did not correlate as well (r = 0.75).

In contrast to the findings of Saur and colleagues,[49] Samo and coworkers[48] reported poor criterion validity with the use of inclinometers. Samo and coworkers[48] compared radiographic measurements of lumbar ROM in 30 subjects with measurements taken with the following three instruments: a Pleurimeter V (double inclinometer), a carpenter's double inclinometer, and a computed single-sensor inclinometer. All ICCs between radiographs and each method were less than the 0.90 established by the authors as the criterion. Therefore, the authors judged that each method had poor validity.

Reliability: Universal Goniometer

Nitschke and colleagues[56] compared lumbar spine ROM measurements taken with the universal goniometer and the double inclinometer in a study involving 34 males and females with low-back pain. The goniometer was used to measure all ranges of lumbar spine motion. Intertester reliability was poor for all measurements for both instruments except for flexion using the goniometers (see Table 12.6).

Fitztgerald and associates[14] used the universal goniometer to measure thoracolumbar lateral flexion and extension. Two testers measured half cycle motions in 17 volunteers who were physical therapy students. The intertester reliability was high for left lateral flexion (r = 0.91), good for extension (r = 0.88), and fair for right lateral flexion (r = 0.76).

Validity: Universal Goniometer

Nattrass and coworkers[43] compared measurements of the thoracolumbar spine taken with the universal goniometer and measurements of the lumbar spine with the Dualer Electric Inclinometer with three measures of impairment. Thirty-four patients between 20 and 65 years of age with chronic low-back pain were the subjects for the study. The results showed that only flexion ROM measured with the goniometer demonstrated greater than 50 percent of the variance in common with one of the disability measures.

Reliability: Schober Test

Fitzgerald and associates[14] used the Schober technique to measure lumbar flexion and the universal goniometer to measure thoracolumbar lateral flexion and extension. Intertester reliability was calculated from measurements taken by two testers on 17 volunteers who were physical therapy students. Pearson reliability coefficients were calculated on paired results of the two testers (see Table 12.6). Intertester reliability using the Schober Test was excellent with an r value of +1.0.

Reliability: Modified Schober Test

Many of the following reliability studies were conducted on patient populations that usually have lower reliability scores than healthy populations. However, one can see by looking at Table 12.7 that some of the intrareliability and interreliability coefficients for the modified Schober test (MST) are in the good to excellent category for patient populations.

Haywood and colleagues[58] used the MST to evaluate the measurement properties of spinal mobility in 159 patients with ankylosing spondylitis (133 males and 26 females, 20 to 74 years of age). Fifty-one patients participated in the reliability study in which both intratester (ICC = 0.94) and intertester (ICC = 0.90) reliability were high. Also, the MST had a strong relationship with all mobility measures.

Viitanen and associates[59] employed two physical therapists to use the MST to measure lumbar flexion ROM in 52 patients with ankylosing spondylitis with a mean age of 45 years. Repeat tests were performed within 72 hours from entry on successive days at the same time of day. Intratester

reliability was excellent (ICC = 0.94) and so was intertester reliability (ICC = 0.96).

Jones and associates[17] conducted a repeated measures study of 119 children aged 11 to 16 years to assess the measurement error associated with spinal mobility measures. Thirty children in the sample reported recurrent low-back pain, and 89 children were asymptomatic (Table 12.8). The correlation coefficient for lumbar flexion using the MST was 0.99 for the asymptomatic group and 0.93 for the symptomatic group. Little systematic error was present, but the 95 percent limits of agreement showed that all measures exhibited random error, which was greater in the symptomatic group and could affect the reliability of spinal mobility tests in children with back pain.

Reynolds[57] calculated intertester error by comparing the results of two testers taking 10 repeated measurements of lumbar flexion and extension on 30 volunteers with a mean age of 38.1 years. The MST had acceptable intertester reliability only for extension.

Pile and colleagues[60] had five testers (three physical therapists, a rheumatologist, and a rheumatology registrar) use the MST to measure lumbar flexion twice in each of 10 patients with ankylosing spondylitis. Intertester reliability was fair (r = 0.78).

Lindell and coworkers[9] conducted a study with one medically trained physiotherapist and one medically untrained tester (research assistant) using the MST to measure lumbar flexion in 50 subjects (30 patients with low-back or neck pain, and 20 healthy participants). The intratester reliability was an ICC of 0.87 with a standard error of the measurement (SEM) of 0.3 cm for the medically trained tester, and an ICC of 0.79 with a SEM of 0.7 cm for the other tester. Intertester reliability ranged from an ICC of 0.94 (SEM=0.4 cm) when testing patients to an ICC of 0.22 (SEM=1.0 cm) when testing healthy participants. The intertester ICC for all subjects was 0.79 (SEM=0.7 cm). The authors concluded that reliable measurements could be taken by medically untrained testers using tests like the MST, forward bending fingertip-to-floor test, and lateral bending fingertip-to-thigh test that did not require manual stabilization.

Gill and coworkers[37] compared the reliability of four methods of measurement including fingertip-to-floor distance, the Modified Schober technique, the two-inclinometer method, and a photometric technique. The subjects of the study were 10 volunteers (5 men and 5 women) aged 24 to 34 years. Repeatability of the fingertip-to-floor method was poor (coefficient of variation (CV) = 14.1 percent). Repeatability of the inclinometer for the measurement of full flexion was also poor (CV = 33.9 percent). The MST yielded a CV of 0.9 percent for full flexion and a CV of 2.8 percent for extension.

Validity: Schober and Modified Schober Tests

Macrae and Wright[3] tested the validity of both the original two-mark Schober technique and a three-mark modification of the Schober technique (modified Schober). The authors

TABLE 12.7   Reliability of Schober Tests: Modified Schober Test (MST) and Modified–Modified Schober Test (MMST)

Test Author	MST Lindell et al[9]		MST Haywood et al[58]		MST Jones et al[17]		MST Pile et al[60]	MMST Williams et al[19]		MMST Tousignant et al[50]	
Sample	20 healthy and 30 patients with back/neck pain		Patients with ankylosing spondylitis (AS)		89 healthy and 30 patients with LBP		Patients with AS	Patients with CLBP		Patients with LBP	
	20–63 yrs		18–75 yrs		11–16 yrs		26–73 yrs	25–53 yrs		Mean age = 44 yrs	
	n = 20	n = 50	n = 26	n = 51	n = 30	n = 89	n = 10	n = 15		n = 31	
Motion	Intra ICC	Inter ICC	Intra ICC	Inter ICC	Inter r	Inter r	Inter	Intra r	Inter ICC	Intra ICC	Inter ICC
Flexion	0.87	0.79	0.90	0.94	0.94	0.94	0.78	0.78 - 0.89	0.72	0.95	0.91
Extension								0.69 - 0.91	0.76		

CLBP = chronic low-back pain; LBP = low-back pain. ICC = intraclass correlation coefficient; r = pearson product moment correlation coefficient; Intra = intratester reliability; Inter = intertester reliability.

found a linear relationship between measurements of lumbar flexion obtained by these methods and radiographic measurements. The correlation coefficient was 0.90 between the Schober technique and radiographs (x-rays), with an SE of 6.2 degrees. The correlation coefficient was 0.97 between the modified Schober measurement and the radiographic measurements, with an SE of 3.25 degrees. Clinical identification of the lumbosacral junction was not easy, and faulty placement of skin marks seriously impaired the accuracy of the unmodified Schober technique. Placement of marks 2 cm too low led to an overestimate of 14 degrees. Marks placed 2 cm too high led to an underestimate of 15 degrees. In the MST, the same errors in placement led to overestimates and underestimates of 5 and 3 degrees, respectively.

TABLE 12.8   Reliability of Thoracolumbar Lateral Flexion ROM: Tape Measure

Test Author	Fingertip-to-Thigh Alaranta et al[18]		Fingertip-to-Thigh Lindell et al[9]		Fingertip-to-Thigh Jones et al[17]		Fingertip-to-Floor Haywood et al[58]		Fingertip-to-Floor Pile et al[60]
Sample	508 employed workers*		20 healthy and 30 patients with back/neck pain		89 healthy and 30 patients with LBP		Patients with AS		Patients with AS†
	35–45 yrs		22–55 yrs		11–16 yrs		18–75 yrs		28–73 yrs
	n = 34	n = 93	n = 20	n = 30	n = 89	n = 30	n=26	n=51	n= 10
Motion	Intra r	Inter r	Intra ICC	Inter ICC	Intra r	Intra r	Intra ICC	Inter ICC	Inter
Right and Left	0.81	0.91							
Right			0.99	0.93	0.99	0.93	0.98	0.98	0.83
Left			0.94	0.95	0.99	0.95	0.95	0.95	0.79

AS = ankylosing spondylitis; ICC = intraclass correlation coefficient; LBP = low-back pain; r = Pearson product moment correlation coefficient; Intra = intratester reliability;   Inter = intertester reliability.
* Some workers had back or neck pain, and some had no pain.

Viitanen and associates[59] found that the MST, thoracolumbar lateral flexion, and fingertip-to-floor test using a tape measure had the most significant correlations with thoracolumbar changes seen on x-ray (calcifications of discs, ossification of liagments, and changes in the apophyseal joints).

In contrast to the preceding studies, the following two studies did not find good evidence for the validity of the Schober and the MST. Portek and colleagues[63] compared the MST and two other clinical methods with each other and with radiographs. These authors found little correlation either among the measurements obtained by two testers using three clinical techniques to measure lumbar flexion in 11 subjects or among the three clinical techniques and radiographs. A Pearson's reliability coefficient of 0.43 was found between the MST and the radiographic measurement. The intertester error for the MST for lumbar flexion showed significant differences between testers according to paired t-tests. However, intertester error was calculated between 10 measurements on 10 different days, and the authors attributed the error to difficulties in reestablishing a neutral starting position and the mobility of the skin over the landmarks.

Quack and colleagues,[8] in a study involving 112 female subjects with a mean age of 53 years, compared the MST with magnetic resonance imaging (MRI) findings. The authors did not find any statistically significant findings between the MST and MRI findings. Therefore, the validity for the MST with respect to segmental lumbar degeneration was questioned.

Reliability: Modified–Modified Schober Test

Williams and coworkers[19] measured flexion and extension on 15 patient volunteers with a mean age of 36 years who had chronic low-back pain. The authors compared the MMST,[20] which is also referred to as the simplified skin distraction method,[21] with the double inclinometer method. Intratester Pearson correlation coefficients for the MMST were an r of 0.89 for tester 1, an r of 0.78 for tester 2, and an r of 0.83 for tester 3. Intertester Pearson correlation coefficients between the three physical therapist testers were an r of 0.72 for flexion and an r of 0.77 for extension with use of the MMST. The therapists underwent training in the use of standardized procedures for each method prior to testing. According to the testers, the MMST was easier and quicker to use than the double inclinometer method. The only disadvantage to using the MMST method is that norms have not been established for all age groups.

Tousignant and associates[50] used the MMST to obtain lumbar flexion ROM measurements in 31 patients with low-back pain. The authors found excellent intratester reliability (ICC = 0.95) and very good intertester reliability (ICC = 0.91).

Validity: Modified–Modified Schober Test

The ease of finding landmarks for measuring lumbar flexion and extension with the MMST appears to make this method a better choice over the Schober and MST; however, more studies need to be performed to confirm its validity. Tousignant and associates[50] used the MMST to obtain lumbar flexion ROM measurements in 31 patients with low-back pain. The authors compared these measurements with measurements calculated on x-rays as the gold standard. The comparison showed that the MMST had moderate validity (r = 0.67; 95% confidence interval = 0.44 to 0.84). The minimum metrically detectable change (MMDC) of 1 cm was determined to be excellent in this group of patients, but because of the moderate validity finding, the authors suggest that further studies need to be perfomed to establish the test's validity.

Reliability: Prone Press-Up (for Extension)

Bandy and Reese[64] compared the reliability of the prone press-up to measure lumbar extension under two conditions: with and without a strap to control pelvic motion. Sixty-three unimpaired individuals with a mean age of 26 years participated as subjects in the study. Measurements of extension ROM were taken by an experienced group and a student group using a tape measure. Intratester reliability was excellent for the experienced group in both the strapped (ICC − 0.91) and unstrapped (ICC = 0.90) conditions and good for the student group. Intertester reliability for both the strapped and unstrapped conditions was good (ICC = 0.87 and ICC = 0.85, respectively).

Reliability and Validity: Fingertip-to-Floor Test (for Forward Flexion)

Perret and colleagues[10] included 32 patients with low-back pain with a mean age of 52 years in a reliability study. Intratester and intertester reliability were excellent (ICC = 0.99). Ten patients with low-back pain (mean age of 42 years) participated in the validity study. Two lateral radiographs were taken: one of the dorsal spine with the patients in the neutral standing position and one taken in full trunk flexion. Spearman's correlation coefficient for this validity test of trunk flexion was excellent (r = 0.96). Seventy-two patients with low-back pain participated in the responsiveness study. High values were found for responsiveness for the fingertip-to-floor method, which showed that the fingertip test has very good sensitivity to change.

Haywood and colleagues[58] also assessed reliability, validity, and responsiveness of the fingertip-to-floor forward flexion test in 77 patients with ankylosing spondylitis. The authors found both intratester and intertester reliability to be excellent, with ICCs between 0.94 and 0.99. Also, the test was the most responsive to self-perceived changes in health at 6 months. Authors recommended this test for clinical practice and research.

Viitanen and associates[59] found that the fingertip-to-floor test had significant correlations with thoracolumbar changes seen on x-ray (calcifications of disc, ossification of ligaments, and changes in apophyseal joints).

Pile and associates[60] found that the sagittal plane fingertip-to-floor test had an excellent intertester reliability (ICC = 0.95) in a study in which three physical therapists, a rheumatologist, and a rheumatology registrar measured 10 patients twice.

Lindell and coworkers[9], in a study of 50 subjects (30 patients with low-back or neck pain, and 20 healthy participants), found intratester reliability to be excellent with an ICC = 0.95 and SEM=0.9 cm for both an experienced physiotherapist and a medically untrained research assistant. Intertester reliability was also excellent with ICC values greater than 0.95 and SEM values ranging from 0.9 to 1.2 cm.

Gauvin, Riddle, and Rothstein[65] used a modified version of the fingertip-to-floor test by placing subjects on a stool and then measuring the distance from the tip of the subject's middle finger to the stool. Seventy-three patients with low-back pain participated in the study, and both intratester (ICC = 0.98) and intertester (ICC = 0.95) reliability were excellent. The modified version of the test is supposed to account for the fact that many people can reach the floor, and in this study 27 percent of the subjects were able to reach the top of the stool or beyond the top.

In contrast to the preceding studies, the following study did not find acceptable retest reliability. Gill and coworkers[61] compared the reliability of four methods of measurement including fingertip-to-floor distance, the Modified Schober technique, the two-inclinometer method, and a photometric technique. The subjects of the study were 10 volunteers (5 men and 5 women) aged 24 to 34 years. Repeatability of the fingertip-to-floor method was poor (CV = 14.1 percent). Repeatability of the inclinometer for the measurement of full flexion was also poor (CV = 33.9 percent).

Reliability: Fingertip-to-Thigh Test (for Lateral Flexion)

Alaranta and associates,[18] in a study involving 508 white and blue collar workers between the ages of 35 and 54 years, found that the intertester reliability was high at an interval of 1 week for the fingertip-to-thigh method of assessing thoracolumbar lateral flexion. Intratester reliability at the interval of 1 year was remarkably good for the large time interval between tests (see Table 12.8).

Jones and colleagues,[17] in a study of 119 children ages 11 to 16 years (30 children with low-back pain and 89 asymptomatic children), found excellent correlation coefficients for right and left lateral flexion in the low-back pain group (r = 0.93 to 0.95) and in the asymptomatic group (r = 0.99). Limits of agreement, expressed as the mean difference between test and retest ± 1.96 × SD of the difference between test and retest, were 0.16 mm ± 6.78 for right lateral flexion for the asymptomatic children but much larger for the symptomatic group (0.50 mm ± 16.93 mm). The authors concluded that there was very little systematic bias but all measures exhibited random error, which was larger in the symptomatic group (see Table 12.8).

Lindell and coworkers[9] conducted a study of 50 subjects (30 patients with low-back or neck pain, and 20 healthy subjects) who were tested by two examiners. The intratester reliability for the fingertip-to-thigh test for lateral bending was excellent for the experienced physiotherapist (ICC = 0.94-0.99, SEM = 0.5-1.0 cm) and fair for the medically untrained tester (ICC = 0.73-0.86, SEM = 1.4-1.6 cm). Intertester reliability was fair to excellent depending on the group and side tested, with ICCs ranging from 0.79 to 0.98 and SEMs ranging from 0.9 to 1.5 cm.

Reliability: Back Range of Motion Device

Reliability results are inconclusive, and it appears that additional research needs to be done on this method of measurement to warrant the expenditure involved in purchasing the back range of motion (BROM) device. The BROM II device (Performance Attainment Associates, Roseville, MN) is a revised and improved version of the original BROM. Two groups of researchers investigating the reliability of the BROM II device agreed that the instrument had high reliability for measuring lumbar lateral flexion and low reliability for measuring extension. However, the two groups differed regarding the reliability of the BROM II device for measuring flexion and rotation. Breum, Wiberg, and Bolton[66] concluded that the BROM II device could measure flexion and rotation reliably, whereas Madson, Youdas, and Suman[67] determined that rotation but not flexion could be reliably measured (see Table 12.6). Potential sources of error identified by the authors[67] included slippage of the device over the sacrum during flexion and extension and variations in the identification of landmarks from one measurement to another.

Kondratek and colleagues[30] used the BROM II to conduct one of the few studies on lumbar ROM in children. The subjects were 225 normally developing children ages 5 to 11 years of age. Two physical therapists experienced working with children were trained in the use of the BROM II. Intrarater reliability on 15 children was good to excellent for one tester for all half cycle motions except for flexion, which was unacceptable (ICC = 0.53). The intratester reliability for the second tester ranged from an ICC of 0.71 for flexion and an ICC of 0.76 for right lateral flexion, to an ICC of 0.91 for right rotation.

Kachingwe and Phillips[68] employed two testers to use the BROM to measure lumbar motions in 91 healthy men and women with a mean age of 28 years. Intratester reliability for lateral flexion was good (ICC = 0.85 to 0.83), forward flexion was good to fair (ICC = 0.84 to 0.79), and extension and rotation was fair to poor (ICC = 0.76 to 0.58). Intertester reliability was fair to poor for all lumbar motions and for pelvic inclination (ICC = 0.76 to 0.58).

Reliability: Motion Analysis Systems

A number of researchers have investigated the reliability of motion analysis systems including, among others, the CA-6000 Spine Motion Analyzer,[14,29] the SPINETRAK,[71] and the FASTRAK (Polhemus, Colchester, VT).[69] Two research groups found that intratester reliability for measuring lumbar flexion was very high with use of the CA-6000.[29,45] In one of the studies, both intratester and intertester reliability ranged from good to high for lumbar forward flexion and extension, but intratester and intertester reliability were poor for rotation.[29]

In a study using the SPINETRAK,[72] ICCs were 0.89 or greater for intratester reliability. ICCs for intertester reliability ranged from 0.77 for thoracolumbar flexion to 0.95 for thoracolumbopelvic flexion. Steffan and colleagues[69] used the FASTRAK system to measure segmental motion in forward lumbar flexion by tracking sensors attached to Kirschner wires that had been inserted into the spinous processes of L3 and L4 in 16 healthy men. Segmental forward flexion showed large intersubject variation.

Van Herp and associates[33] used the Polhemus Navigation Sciences 3 Space System to measure ROM in 100 healthy subjects (50 male and 50 female subjects) ranging in age from 20 to 77 years of age. Recorded ranges of motion including flexion, extension, lateral flexion and rotation showed a level of agreement with x-ray data indicating good concurrent validity.

Summary

The sampling of studies reviewed in this chapter reflects the amount of effort that has been directed toward finding reliable and valid methods for measuring spinal motion. Each method reviewed has advantages and disadvantages, and clinicians should select a method that appears to be appropriate for their particular clinical situation.

REFERENCES

1. Cyriax, JH, and Cyriax, P: Illustrated Manual of Orthopaedic Medicine. Butterworths, London, 1983.
2. Bogduk, N: Clinical Anatomy of the Lumbar Spine and Sacrum, ed 3. Churchill Livingstone, New York, 1997.
3. Macrae, IF, and Wright, V: Measurement of back movement. Ann Rheum Dis 28:584, 1969.
4. American Medical Association: Guides to the Evaluation of Permanent Impairment, ed 5. Cocchiarella, L, and Andersson, GBJ (eds). AMA, Chicago, 2000.
5. American Academy of Orthopaedic Surgeons: Joint Motion: Method of Measuring and Recording. AAOS, Chicago, 1965.
6. American Medical Association: Guides to the Evaluation of Permanent Impairment, ed 3. Chicago, 1988.
7. Gerhardt, J, Cocchiarella, L, and Lea, R: The Practical Guide to Range of Motion Assessment. AMA, Chicago, 2002.
8. Quack, C, et al: Do MRI findings correlate with mobility tests? An explorative analysis of the test validity with regard to structure. Eur Spine J 16:803, 2007.
9. Lindell, O, Eriksson, L, and Strender, L-E: The reliability of a 10-test package for patients with prolonged back and neck pain: Could an examiner without formal medical education be used without loss of quality? A methodological study. BMC Musculoskelet Dis 8:31, 2007.
10. Perret, C, et al: Validity, reliability, and responsiveness of the fingertip-to-floor test. Arch Phys Med Rehabil 82:1566, 2001.
11. Kraus, H, and Hirschland, RP: Minimum muscular fitness tests in school children. Res Q Exerc Sport 25:178, 1954.
12. Nicholas, JA: Risk factors, sports medicine and the orthopedic system: An overview. J Sports Med 3:243, 1975.
13. Brodie, DA, Bird, HA and Wright,V: Joint laxity in selected athletic populations. Med Sci Sports Exerc 14:190, 1982.
14. Fitzgerald, GK, et al: Objective assessment with establishment of normal values for lumbar spine range of motion. Phys Ther 63:1776, 1983.
15. Sahrmann, SA: Diagnosis and Treatment of Movement Impairment Syndromes. Mosby, St. Louis, 2002.
16. Mellin, GP: Accuracy of measuring lateral flexion of the spine with a tape measure. Clin Biomech 1:85, 1986.
17. Jones, MA, et al: Measurement error associated with spinal mobility measures in children with and without low-back pain. Acta Paediatr 91:1339, 2002.
18. Alaranta, H, et al: Flexibility of the spine: Normative values of goniometric and tape measurements. Scand J Rehab Med 26:147, 1994.
19. Williams, R, et al: Reliability of the modified–modified Schober and double inclinometer methods for measuring lumbar flexion and extension. Phys Ther 73:26, 1993.
20. Van Adrichem, JAM, and van der Korst, JK: Assessment of the flexibility of the lumbar spine. A pilot study in children and adolescents. Scand J Rheumatol 2:87, 1973.
21. Greene, WB, and Heckman, JD (eds): The Clinical Measurement of Joint Motion. American Academy of Orthopaedic Surgeons. Rosemont, IL, 1994.
22. Battie, MC, et al: The role of spinal flexibility in back pain complaints in industry. A prospective study. Spine 15:768, 1990.
23. Loebl, WY: Measurement of spinal posture and range of spinal movement. Ann Phys Med 9:103, 1967.
24. Ng, JK, et al: Range of motion and lordosis of the lumbar spine: Reliability of measurement and normative values. Spine 26:53, 2001.
25. Sullivan, MS, Dickinson, CE and Troup, JDG: The influence of age and gender on lumbar spine range of motion. A study of 1126 healthy subjects. Spine 19:682, 1994.
26. Moll, JMH, and Wright, V: Normal range of spinal mobility: An objective clinical study. Ann Rheum Dis 30:381, 1971.
27. Anderson, JAD, and Sweetman, BJ: A combined flexi-rule hydrogoniometer for measurement of lumbar spine and its sagittal movement. Rheumatol Rehabil 14:173, 1975.
28. Gracovetsky, S, et al: A database for estimating normal spinal motion derived from non-invasive measurements. Spine 20:1036, 1995.
29. McGregor, AH, McCarthy, D and Hughes, SP: Motion characteristics of the lumbar spine in the normal population. Spine 20:2421, 1995.
30. Kondratek, M, et al: Normative values for active lumbar range of motion in children. Pediatr Phys Ther 19:236, 2007.
31. Troke, M, et al: A normative database of lumbar ranges of motion. Man Ther 10: 198, 2005.
32. Troke, M, et al: A new comprehensive normative database of lumbar spine ranges of motion. Clin Rehabil 15:371, 2001.
33. Van Herp, G, et al: Three dimensional lumbar spine kinematics: a study of range of movement in 100 healthy subjects aged 20 to 60+ years. Rheumatology 39:1337, 2000.
34. Bookstein, NA, et al: Lumbar extension range of motion in elementary school children. Abstr Phys Ther 72:S35, 1992.
35. Wong, KWN, et al: The flexion–extension profile of lumbar spine in 100 healthy volunteers. Spine 29:1636, 2004.
36. Ensink, FB, et al: Lumbar range of motion. Influence of time of day and individuals factors on measurements. Spine 21:1339, 1996.
37. Sughara, M, et al: Epidemiological study on the change of mobility of the thoraco-lumbar spine and body height with age as indices for senility. J Hum Ergol (Tokyo) 10:49, 1981.
38. Freidrich, M, et al: Spinal posture during stooped walking under vertical space constraints. Spine 25:1118, 2000.
39. Sjolie, AN: Access to pedestrian roads, daily activities and physical performance of adolescents. Spine 25:1965, 2000.
40. Sullivan, MS, Shoaf, LD, and Riddle, DL: The relationship of lumbar flexion to disability in patients with low back pain. Phys Ther 80:240, 2000.
41. Lundberg, G, and Gerdle, B: Correlations between joint and spinal mobility, spinal sagittal configuration, segmental mobility, segmental pain symptoms and disabilities in female homecare personnel. Scand J Rehab Med 32:124, 2000.
42. Kujala UM, et al: Lumbar mobility and low back pain during adolescence. A longitudinal three-year follow-up study in athletes and controls. Am J Sports Med 25:363, 1997.
43. Nattrass, CL, et al: Lumbar spine range of motion as a measure of physical and functional impairment: An investigation of validity (abstract). Clin Rehabil 13:211, 1999.
44. Shirley, FR, et al: Comparison of lumbar range of motion using three measurement devices in patients with chronic low back pain. Spine 19:779, 1994.
45. Hsieh, CY, and Pringle, RK: Range of motion of the lumbar spine required for four activities of daily living. J Manipulative Physiol Ther 17:353, 1994.
46. Levine, D, et al: Sagittal lumbar spine position during standing, walking and running at various gradients. J Athlet Train 42:29, 2007.
47. Littlewood, C, and May, S: Measurement of range of movement in the lumbar spine: What methods are valid? A systematic review. Physiother 93:201, 2007.
48. Samo, DG, et al: Validity of three lumbar sagittal motion measurement methods: Surface inclinometers compared with radiographs. J Occup Environ Med 39:209, 1997.
49. Saur, PMM, et al: Lumbar range of motion: Reliability and validity of the inclinometer technique in the clinical measurement of trunk flexibility. Spine 21:1332, 1996.
50. Tousignant, M, et al: The Modified-Modified Schober test for range of motion assessment of lumbar flexion in patients with low back pain: A study of criterion validity, intra-and inter-rater reliability and minimum metrically detectable change. Disabil Rehabil 27:553, 2005.
51. Essendrop, M, et al: Measures of low back function: A review of reproducibility studies. Clin Biomech 17:235, 2002.
52. Patel, RS: Intratester and intertester reliability of the inclinometer in measuring lumbar flexion. Phys Ther 72:S44, 1992.
53. Mayer, RS, et al: Variance in the measurement of sagittal lumbar range of motion among examiners, subjects, and instruments. Spine 20:1489, 1995.
54. Chen, SP, et al: Reliability of the lumbar sagittal motion measurement methods: Surface inclinometers. J Occup Environ Med 39:217, 1997.
55. Mayer, TG, et al: Spinal range of motion. Accuracy and sources of error with inclinometric measurement. Spine 22:1976, 1997.
56. Nitschkje, JE, et al: Reliability of the American Medical Association Guides' Model for Measuring Spinal Range of Motion. Its implication for whole-person impairment ratings. Spine 24:262, 1999.
57. Reynolds, PMG: Measurement of spinal mobility: A comparison of three methods. Rheumatol Rehabil 14:180, 1975.
58. Haywood, KL, et al: Spinal mobility in ankylosing spondylitis: Reliability, validity and responsivenesss. Rheumatol 43:750, 2004.
59. Viitanen, JV, et al: Clinical assessment of spinal mobility measurements in ankylosing spondylitis: A compact set for follow-up and trials? Clin Rheumatol 19:131, 2000.
60. Pile, KD, et al: Clinical assessment of ankylosing spondylitis: A study of observer variatioin in spinal measurements. Br J Rheumatol 30:29, 1991.

61. Gill, K, et al: Repeatability of four clinical methods for assessment of lumbar spinal motion. Spine 13:50, 1988.
62. Miller, MH, et al: Measurement of spinal mobility in the sagittal plane: New skin distraction technique compared with established methods. J Rheumatol 11:4, 1984.
63. Portek, I, et al: Correlation between radiographic and clinical measurement of lumbar spine movement. Br J Rheumatol 22:197, 1983.
64. Bandy, WD, and Reese, NB: Strapped versus unstrapped technique of the prone press-up for measurement of lumbar extension using a tape measure: Differences in magnitude and reliability of measurements. Arch Phys Med Rehabil 85:99, 2004.
65. Gauvin, MG, Riddle, DL, and Rothstein, JM: Reliability of clinical measurements of forward bending using the modified fingertip-to-floor method. Phys Ther 70:443, 2000.
66. Breum, J, Wiberg, J, and Bolton, JE: Reliability and concurrent validity of the BROM II for measuring lumbar mobility. J Manipulative Physiol Ther 18:497, 1995.
67. Madson, TJ, Youdas, JW and Suman, VJ: Reproducibility of lumbar spine range of motion measurements using the back range of motion device. J Orthop Sports Phys Ther 29:470, 1999.
68. Kachingwe, AF, and Phillips, BJ: Inter and Intrarater reliability of a back range of motion instrument. Arch Phys Med Rehabil 86:2347, 2005.
69. Steffan, T, et al: A new technique for measuring lumbar segmental motion in vivo: Method, accuracy and preliminary results. Spine 22:156, 1997.
70. Petersen, CM, et al: Intraobserver and interobserver reliability of asymptomatic subject's thoracolumbar range of motion using the OSI CA-6000 Spine Motion Analyzer. J Orthop Sports Phys Ther 220:207, 1997.
71. Robinson, ME, et al: Intrasubject reliability of spinal range of motion and velocity determined by video motion analysis. Phys Ther 73:626, 1993.

Chapter 13

The Temporomandibular Joint

⦾ Structure and Function

Temporomandibular Joint

Anatomy

The temporomandibular joint (TMJ) is the articulation between the mandible, the articular disc, and the temporal bone of the skull (Fig. 13.1A, B). The disc divides the joint into two distinct parts, which are referred to as the upper and lower joints. The larger upper joint is formed by the convex articular eminence, concave mandibular fossa of the temporal bone, and the superior surface of the disc. The lower joint consists of the convex surface of the mandibular condyle and the concave inferior surface of the disc.[1–3] The articular disc helps the convex mandible conform to the convex articular surface of the temporal bone.[2]

The TMJ capsule is described as being thin and loose above the disc but taut below the disc in the lower joint. Short capsular fibers surround the joint and extend between the mandibular condyle and the articular disc and between the disc and the temporal eminence.[3] Longer capsular fibers extend from the temporal bone to the mandible.

The primary ligament associated with the TMJ is the temporomandibular ligament. The stylomandibular and the sphenomandibular ligaments (Fig. 13.2) are considered to be accessory ligaments.[4,5] The muscles associated with the TMJ are the medial and lateral pterygoids, temporalis, masseter, digastric, stylohyoid, mylohyoid, and geniohyoid.

Osteokinematics

The upper joint is an amphiarthrodial gliding joint, and the lower joint is a hinge joint. The TMJ as a whole allows motions in three planes around three axes. All of the motions except mouth closing begin from the resting position of the joint in which the teeth are slightly separated (freeway space).[3,6] The amount of freeway space, which usually varies from 2 mm to 4 mm, allows free anterior, posterior, and lateral movement of the mandible.

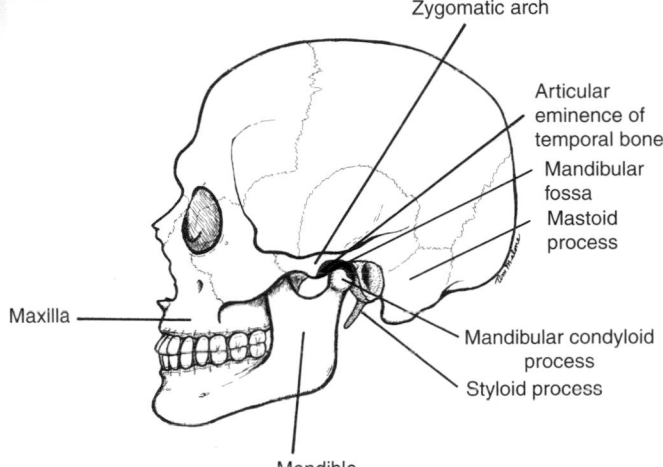

A

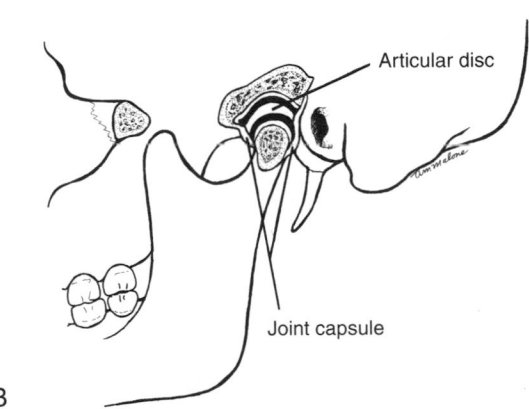

B

FIGURE 13.1 A: Lateral view of the skull showing the temporomandibular joint (TMJ) and surrounding structures. **B:** A lateral view of the TMJ showing the articular disc and a portion of the joint capsule.

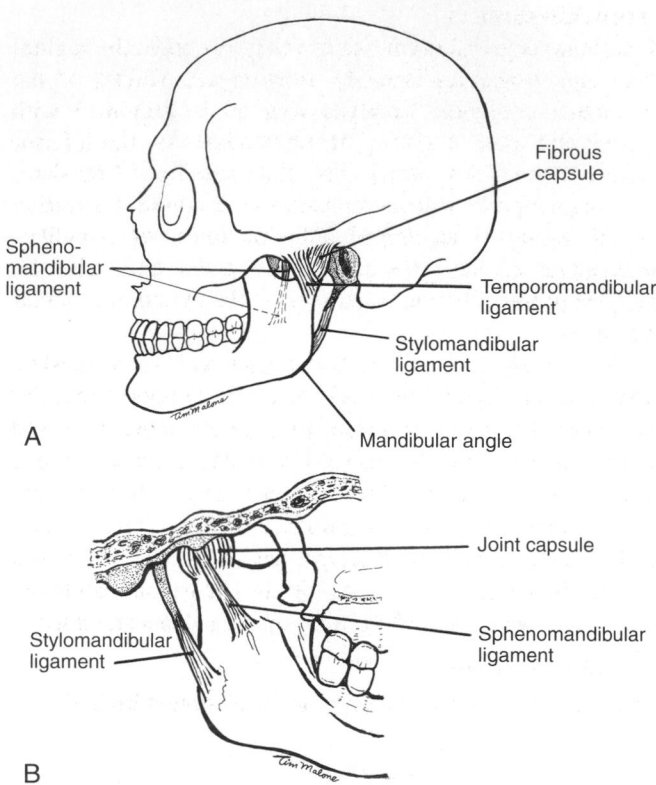

A

B

FIGURE 13.2 A: A lateral view of the temporomandibular joint showing the oblique fibers of the temporomandibular ligament and the stylomandibular and sphenomandibular ligaments. **B:** A medial view of the temporomandibular joint showing the medial portion of the joint capsule and the stylomandibular and sphenomandibular ligaments.

The functional motions permitted are mandibular depression (mouth opening), mandibular elevation (mouth closing), protrusion (anterior translation; Fig.13.3) and retrusion (posterior translation; Fig.13.4), and right and left lateral excursion or laterotrusion (lateral deviation; Fig. 13.5). Maximal contact of the teeth in mouth closing is called centric occlusion.

Reinforcement of the TMJ is provided primarily by the temporomandibular ligament, which limits mouth opening, retrusion, and lateral excursion. The functions of the stylomandibular and sphenomandibular ligaments are somewhat controversial, but these ligaments appear to help suspend the mandible from the cranium.[4] According to Magee,[7] the ligaments keep the condyle, disc, and temporal bone in close approximation. These ligaments also may prevent excessive protrusion, but their exact function has not been verified.

The inferior head of the lateral pterygoid muscles and the digastric muscles produce mandibular depression (mouth opening),[1,3–7] whereas the mylohyoid and geniohyoid muscles assist in the motion, especially against resistance.[3,7] Mandibular elevation (mouth closing) is produced by bilateral contractions of the temporalis, masseter, and medial pterygoid muscles.[1,3–7] Mandibular protrusion is a result of bilateral action of the masseter,[1,7] medial,[1,3,7] and lateral[3–8] pterygoid muscles, which may be assisted by the mylohyoid, stylohyoid, and digastric muscles.[7] Retrusion is brought about by bilateral action of the posterior fibers of the temporalis muscles[1,3–7]; by the digastric,[1,3–7] middle, and deep fibers of the masseter[3,7]; and by the stylohyoid, mylohyoid,[1,7] and geniohyoid[1,3,7] muscles. Mandibular lateral excursion is produced by a unilateral contraction of the medial and lateral pterygoid muscles,[1–7] which produce contralateral motion, whereas a unilateral contraction of the temporalis muscle causes lateral motion to the same side.

Cervical spine muscles may be activated in conjunction with TMJ muscles because of the close functional relationship that exists between the head and the neck.[1,4–11] Extension of the head and neck has been found to occur simultaneously with mouth opening, whereas flexion of the head and neck accompanies mouth closing. These coordinated and parallel movements at the TMJ and cervical spine joints have been observed in studies, and researchers suggest that preprogrammed neural commands may simultaneously activate both jaw and neck muscles.[9–11]

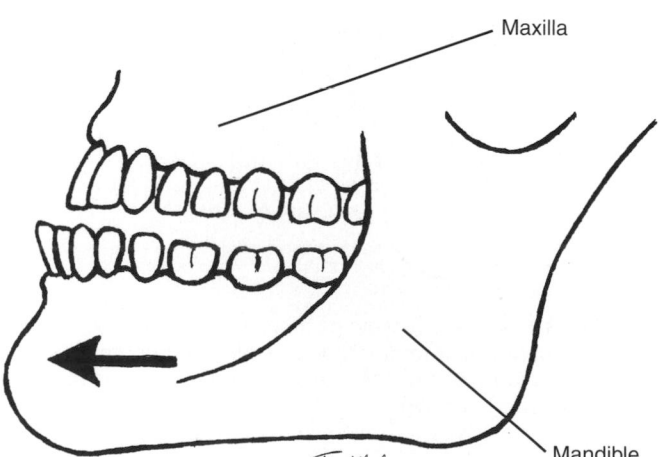

FIGURE 13.3 Protrusion is an anterior motion of the mandible in relation to the maxilla.

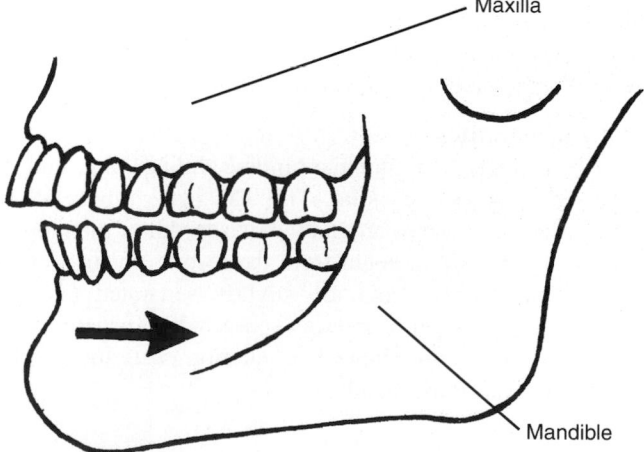

FIGURE 13.4 Retrusion is a posterior motion of the mandible in relation to the maxilla.

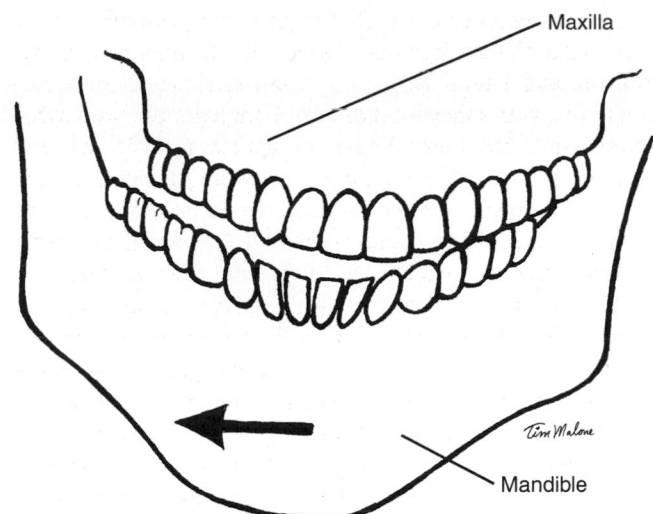

Maxilla

Mandible

FIGURE 13.5 Lateral excursion is a lateral motion of the mandible to either side.

Arthrokinematics

Mandibular depression (mouth opening) occurs in the sagittal plane and is accomplished by rotation and sliding of the mandibular condyles. Condylar rotation is combined with anterior and inferior sliding of the condyles on the inferior surface of the discs, which also slide anteriorly (translate) along the temporal articular eminences. Mandibular elevation (mouth closing) is accomplished by rotation of the mandibular condyles on the discs and sliding of the discs with the condyles posteriorly and superiorly on the temporal articular eminences.

In protrusion, the bilateral condyles and discs translate together anteriorly and inferiorly along the temporal articular eminences. The movement takes place at the upper joint, and no rotation occurs during this motion. In lateral excursion, one mandibular condyle and disc slide inferiorly, anteriorly, and medially along the articular eminence. The other mandibular condyle rotates about a vertical axis and slides medially within the mandibular fossa. For example, in left lateral excursion, the left condyle spins and the right condyle slides anteriorly.

Capsular Pattern

In the capsular pattern, mandibular depression is limited.[7]

RANGE OF MOTION TESTING PROCEDURES: Temporomandibular Joint

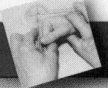

Landmarks for Testing Procedures

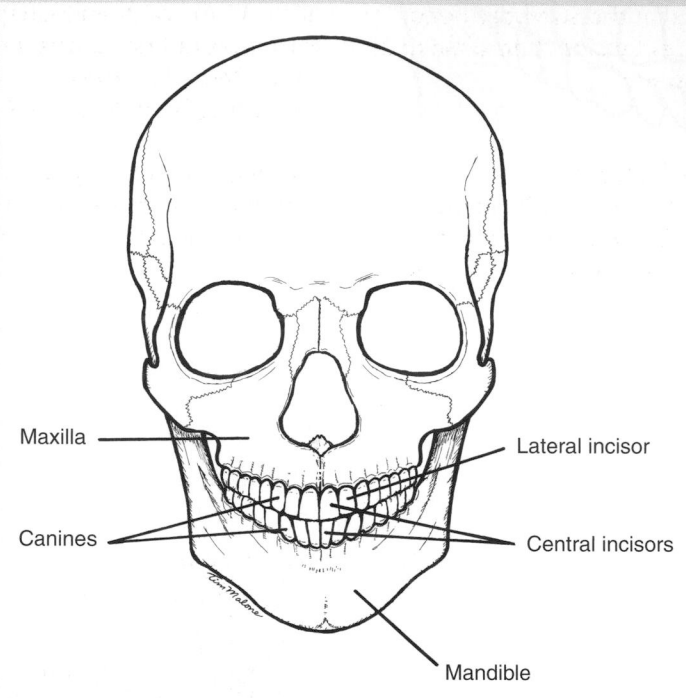

FIGURE 13.6 The adult has between 28 and 32 permanent teeth, including 8 incisors, 4 canines, 8 premolars, and 8 to 12 molars. The central incisors serve as landmarks for ruler placement.

● DEPRESSION OF THE MANDIBLE (MOUTH OPENING)

Motion occurs in the sagittal plane around a medial–lateral axis. Functionally, the mandible is able to depress approximately 35 mm to 50 mm so that the subject's three fingers or two knuckles can be placed between the upper and the lower central incisor teeth.[7] According to the consensus judgments of the Permanent Impairment Conference in 1995, the normal range of motion (ROM) for mouth opening ranges between 40 mm and 50 mm.[12] See Table 13.1 in the Research Findings section for additional normal values. The mean ROM for depression of the mandible in Table 13.1 ranges from 41 mm to 58.6 mm.

The Research Diagnostic Criteria for Temporomandibular Disorders (RDC/TMD) recommends that the examiner observe pain-free active mouth opening and describe fully any deviations of the mandible that take place during the motion.[13] The observation of active mouth opening should be followed with measurements of maximal active mouth opening and passive mouth opening.

Testing Position

Place the subject sitting, with the cervical spine in 0 degrees of flexion, extension, lateral flexion, and rotation.

Stabilization

Stabilize the posterior aspect of the subject's head and neck to prevent flexion, extension, lateral flexion, and rotation of the cervical spine.

Testing Motions

Active Pain Free Mouth Opening

Ask the subject to open his or her mouth slowly and as far as possible without pain. Observe the motion for any lateral excursion of the mandible. In normal active movement, no lateral mandibular motion occurs during mandibular depression (Fig. 13.7). If lateral excursion does occur, it may take the form of either a C-shaped or an S-shaped curve. With a C-shaped curve, the lateral excursion is to one side and should be noted on the recording form (Fig. 13.8). With an S-shaped curve, the lateral excursion occurs first to one side and then to the opposite side.[7] Include a description of the deviation on the recording form (Fig. 13.9).

Active Mouth Opening

Ask the subject to make an effort to open his or her mouth as wide as possible even if pain is present.

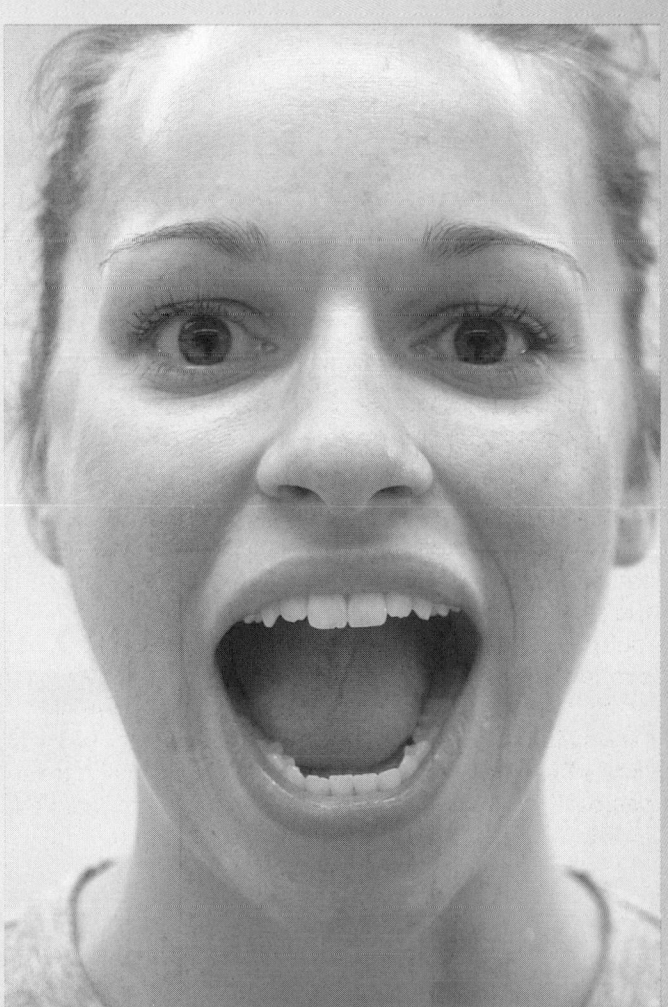

FIGURE 13.7 Normal maximal active mouth opening.

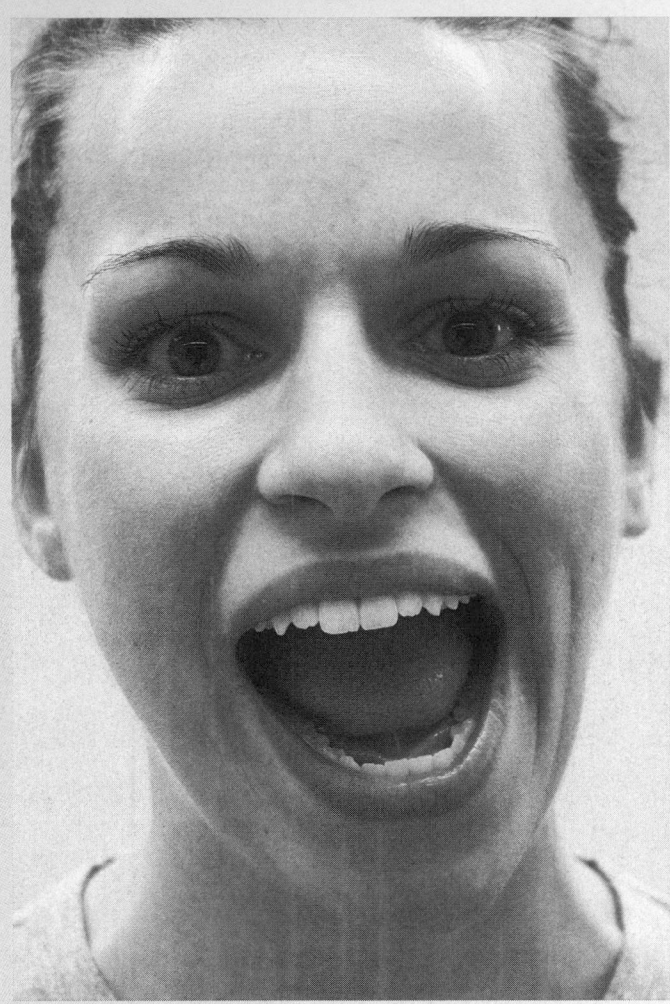

FIGURE 13.8   Abnormal mouth opening with lateral deviation to the left.

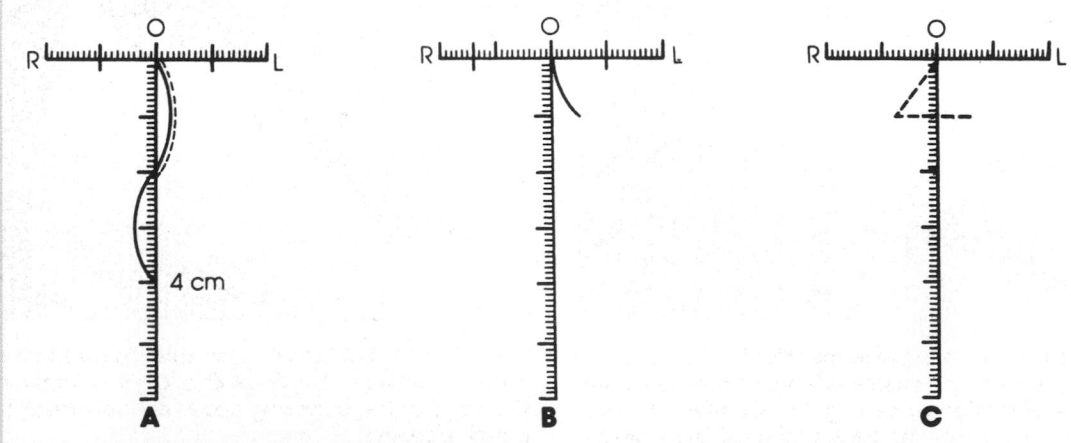

FIGURE 13.9   Examples of recording temporomandibular motions. **A:** Lateral deviation R and L on opening, maximal opening is 4 cm; lateral excursions are equal and 1 cm in each direction; protrusion on functional opening (dashed line). **B:** Opening limited to 1 cm; deviation to the left on opening; lateral excursion greater to the R than to L. **C:** Protrusion is 1 cm; lateral deviation to R on protrusion (indicates weak pterygoid on opposite side). Adapted from Magee, DJ: Orthopedic Physical Assessment, ed 3. WB Saunders, Philadelphia, 1997, p. 165, with permission.

Testing Motions

Passive Mouth Opening

Grasp the mandible so that it fits between the thumb and the index finger, and pull the mandible inferiorly (Fig. 13.10). The subject may assist with the motion by opening the mouth as far as possible. The end of the motion occurs when resistance is felt and attempts to produce additional motion cause the head to nod forward (cervical flexion).

Normal End-Feel

The end-feel is firm owing to stretching of the joint capsule; retrodiscal tissue; the temporomandibular ligament; and the masseter, temporalis, and medial pterygoid muscles.[6,7]

Measurement Method

Use a millimeter ruler to measure the vertical distance between the edge of the upper central incisor and the corresponding edge of the lower central incisor. The correct ruler placement is shown in Figure 13.11.

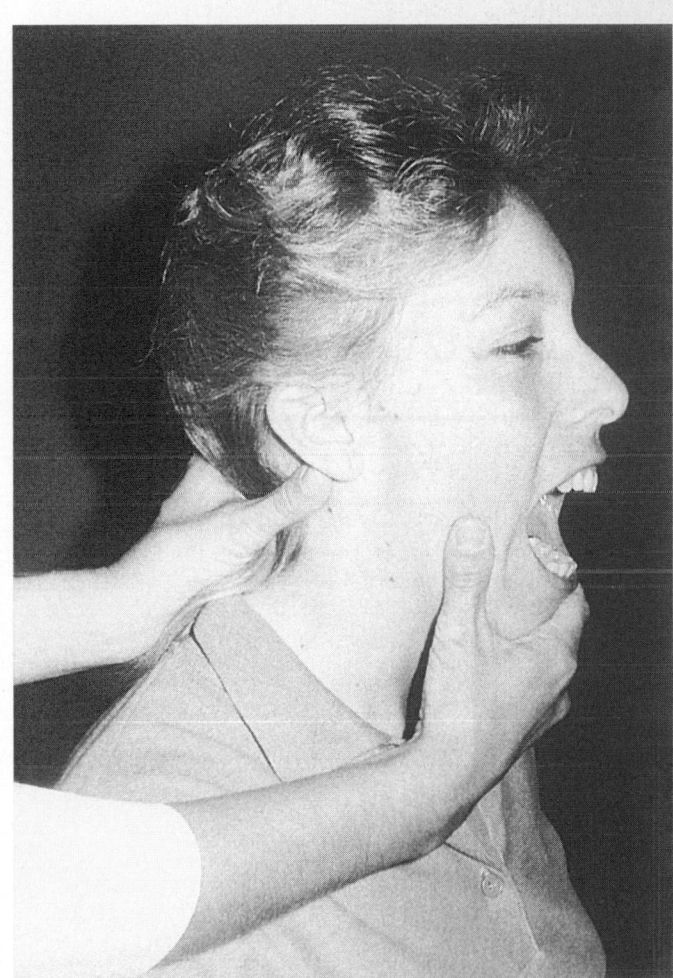

FIGURE 13.10 At the end of passive mandibular depression (mouth opening), one of the examiner's hands maintains the end of the range of motion by pulling the jaw inferiorly. The examiner's other hand holds the back of the subject's head to prevent cervical motion.

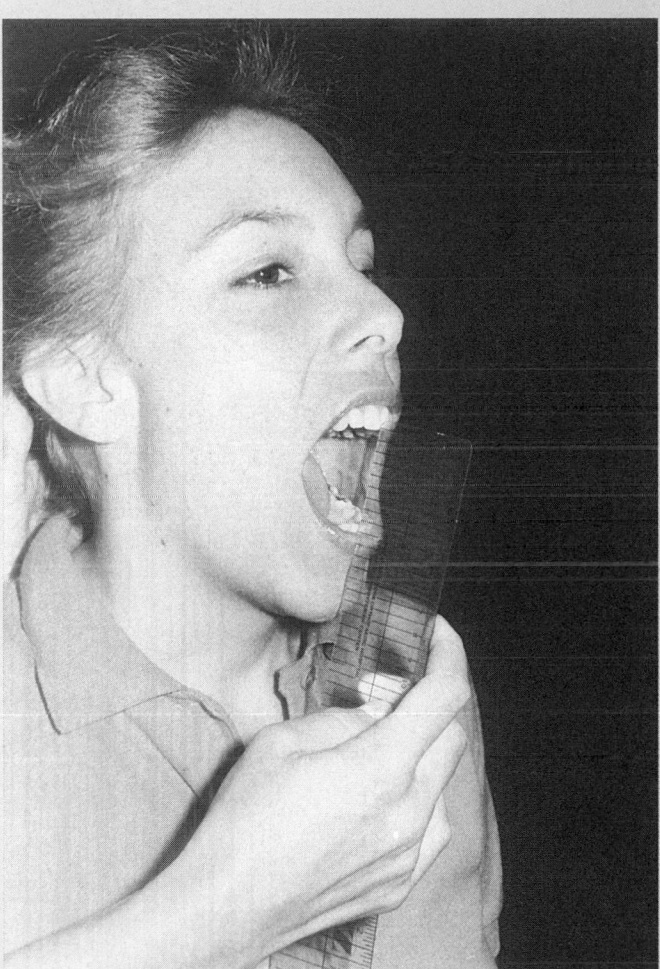

FIGURE 13.11 Use a millimeter ruler to measure the vertical distance between the edge of a lower central incisor and the edge of the opposing upper central incisor to measure mouth opening.

● OVERBITE

Overbite, which is the amount that the upper teeth extend over the lower teeth when the mouth is closed, is usually added to the mouth opening measurements. This addition provides a more accurate measurement of mouth opening ROM, especially in persons with a large overbite. Most normal values published from research studies add the amount of overbite to mouth opening values as recommended by the RDC/TMD criteria.

Measurement Method

When the person's mouth is closed, use a nontoxic marking pencil to make a horizontal line on the lower central incisors at the bottom edge of the overlapping upper central incisors[14] (Fig.13.12). After the line is drawn and the person's mouth is opened, measure the amount of overbite between the horizontal line and upper edge of the mandibular central incisors (Fig.13.13).

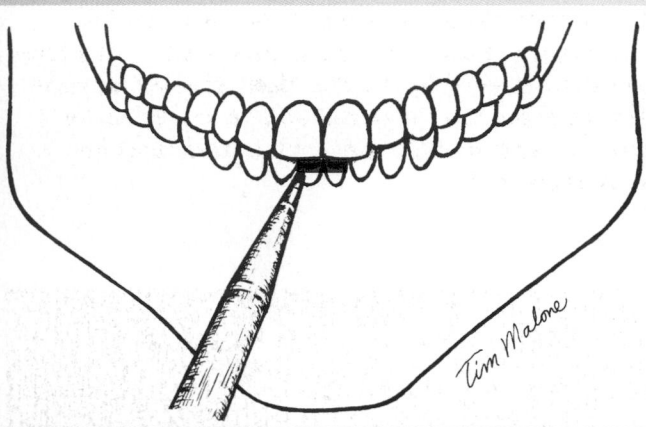

FIGURE 13.12 To measure the amount of overbite that is present use a nontoxic marking pencil to draw a horizontal line across the lower central incisors where the upper central incisors overlap when the mouth is closed.

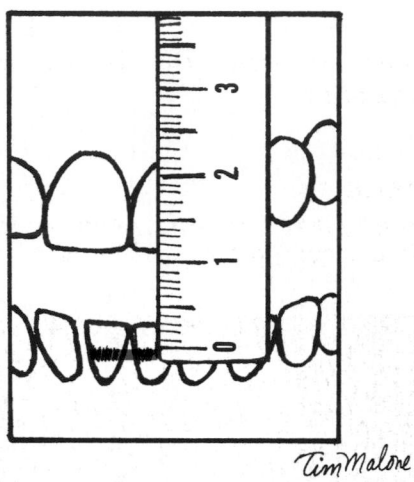

FIGURE 13.13 Ask the subject to open the mouth slightly so that it is possible to measure the amount of overbite as the distance from the horizontal line drawn on the lower central incisors to the top edge of the lower incisors.

● PROTRUSION OF THE MANDIBLE

Protrusion of the mandible is a translatory motion that occurs in the transverse plane. Normally, the lower central incisor teeth are able to protrude 6 mm to 9 mm beyond the upper central incisor teeth. However, the normal ROM for adults may range from 3 mm[7] to 10 mm.[6] See Table 13.2 in the Research Findings section for additional normal values and the effects of age and gender on ROM.

Testing Position
Place the subject sitting, with the cervical spine in 0 degrees of flexion, extension, lateral flexion, and rotation. The TMJ is opened slightly.

Stabilization
Stabilize the posterior aspect of the head and neck to prevent flexion, extension, lateral flexion, and rotation of the cervical spine.

Testing Motion
Active Protrusion
Have the subject push the lower jaw as far forward as possible without moving the head forward.

Passive Protrusion
Grasp the mandible between the thumb and the fingers from underneath the chin. The subject may assist with the movement by pushing the chin anteriorly as far as possible. The end of the motion occurs when resistance is felt and attempts at additional motion cause anterior motion of the head (Fig. 13.14).

Normal End-Feel
The end-feel is firm owing to stretching of the joint capsule; stylomandibular and sphenomandibular ligaments; and the temporalis, masseter, digastric, stylohyoid, mylohyoid, and geniohyoid muscles.[3,7]

Measurement Method
Measure the distance between the lower central incisor and the upper central incisor teeth with a tape measure or ruler (Fig. 13.15). Alternatively, two vertical lines drawn on the upper and lower canines or lateral incisors may be used as the landmarks for measurement.[14]

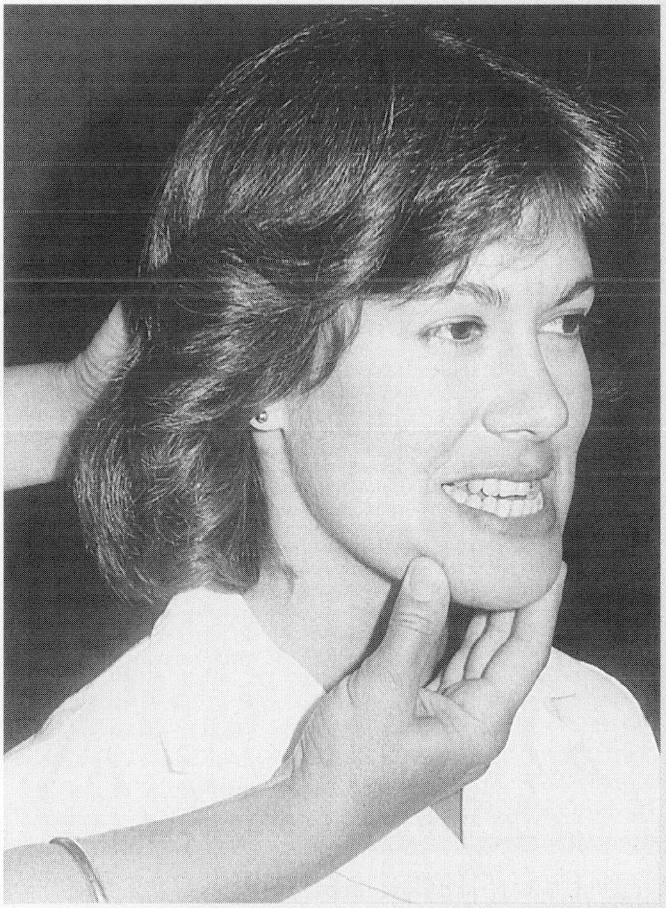

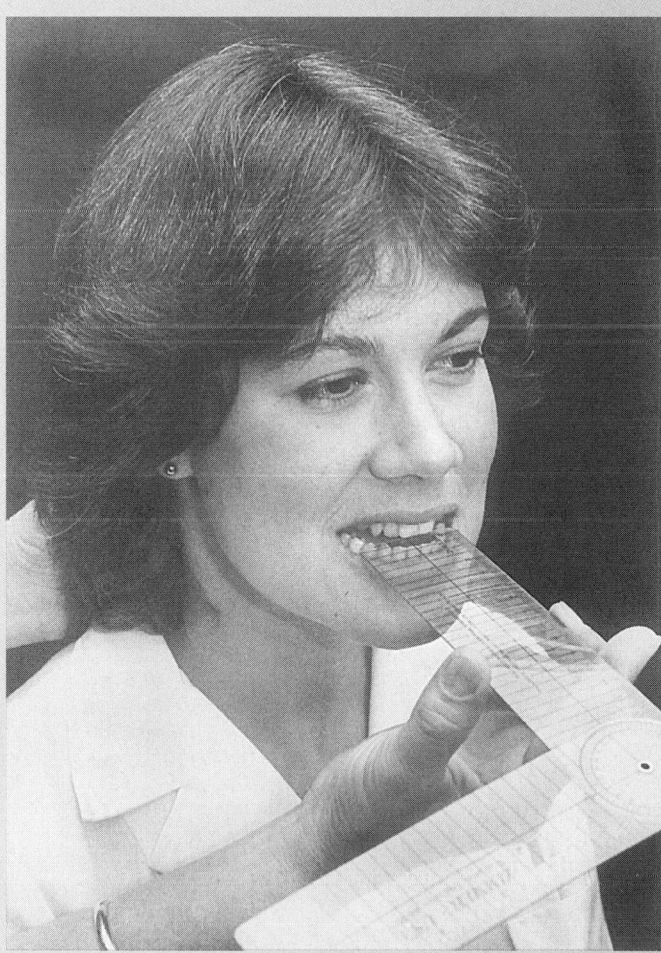

FIGURE 13.14 At the end of passive mandibular protrusion range of motion, the examiner uses one hand to stabilize the posterior aspect of the subject's head while her other hand moves the mandible into protrusion.

FIGURE 13.15 At the end of mandibular protrusion range of motion, the examiner uses the end of a plastic goniometer to measure the distance between the subject's upper and lower central incisors. The subject maintains the position.

● LATERAL EXCURSION OF THE MANDIBLE

This translatory motion occurs in the transverse plane. The amount of lateral movement to the right and left sides is not usually symmetrical, and there is some evidence that movement to the left is greater than to the right.[15] The normal ROM for adults is between 10 mm and 12 mm[2] but may range from 10 mm to 15 mm.[7] According to the consensus judgment of the Permanent Impairment Conference, the normal ROM is between 8 mm and 12 mm.[12] See Table 13.2 in the Research Findings section for additional normal values and the effects of age and gender on ROM.

Testing Position

Place the subject sitting, with the cervical spine in 0 degrees of flexion, extension, lateral flexion, and rotation. The TMJ is opened slightly so that the subject's upper and lower teeth are not touching prior to the start of the motion.

Stabilization

Stabilize the posterior aspect of the head and neck to prevent flexion, extension, lateral flexion, and rotation of the cervical spine.

Testing Motion

Active Lateral Excursion

Have the subject slide his or her lower jaw as far to the right as possible. Have the subject move the lower jaw as far to the left as possible.

Passive Lateral Excursion

Grasp the mandible between the fingers and the thumb and move it to the side. The end of the motion occurs when resistance is felt and attempts to produce additional motion causes lateral cervical flexion (be careful to avoid depression, elevation, and protrusion and retrusion during the movement; Fig. 13.16).

Normal End-Feel

The normal end-feel is firm owing to stretching of the joint capsule; the temporomandibular ligaments; and the temporalis, medial, and lateral pterygoid muscles.

Measurement Method

Measure the lateral distance between the center of the lower incisors and the center of the upper central incisors with a millimeter ruler (Fig. 13.17). The distance that the mandible has moved laterally in relation to the maxilla is evident by comparing the position of the upper and lower central incisors in Figures 13.17 and 13.18.

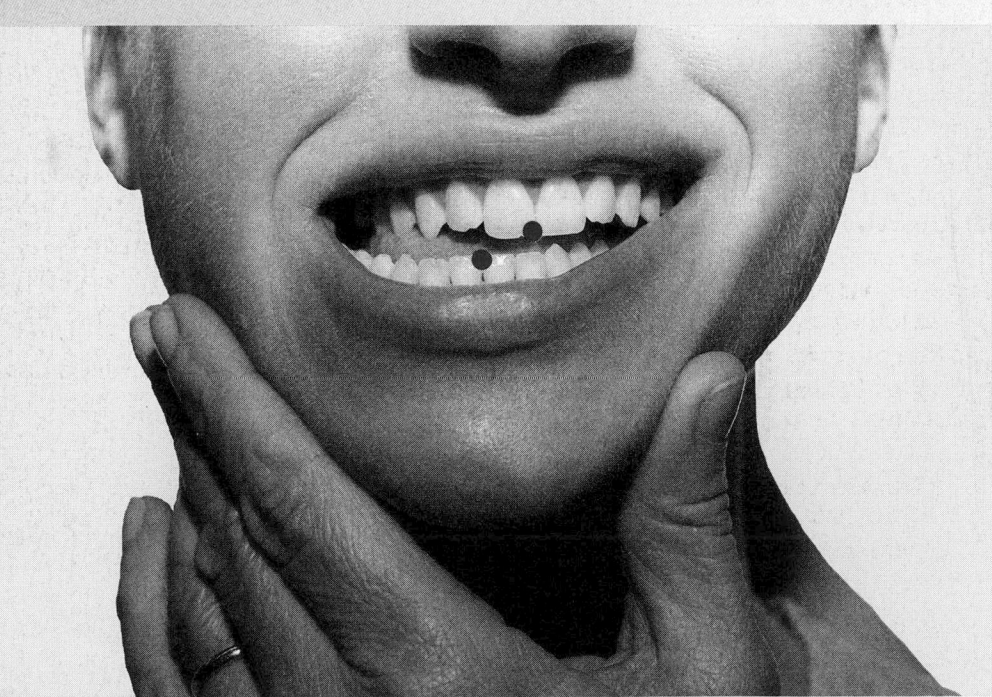

FIGURE 13.16 At the end of passive mandibular lateral excursion range of motion, the examiner uses one hand to prevent cervical motion and the other hand to maintain a lateral pull on the mandible.

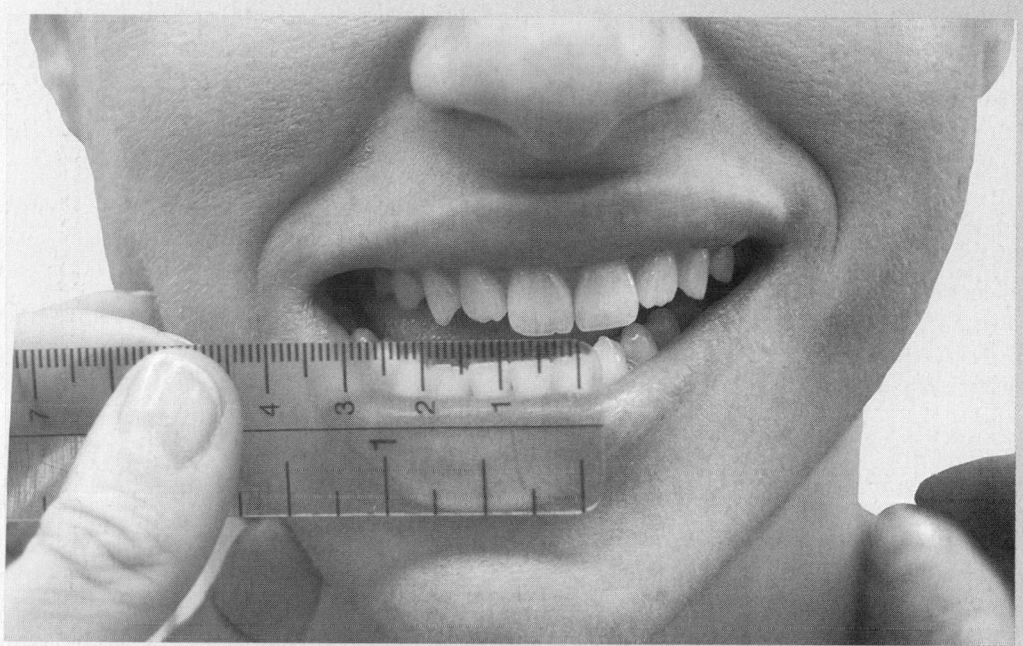

FIGURE 13.17 The examiner uses a millimeter ruler to measure the lateral distance between the center of the two upper incisors and the center of the two low incisors. Align the ruler with the upper incisors first as these teeth have not moved during the motion.

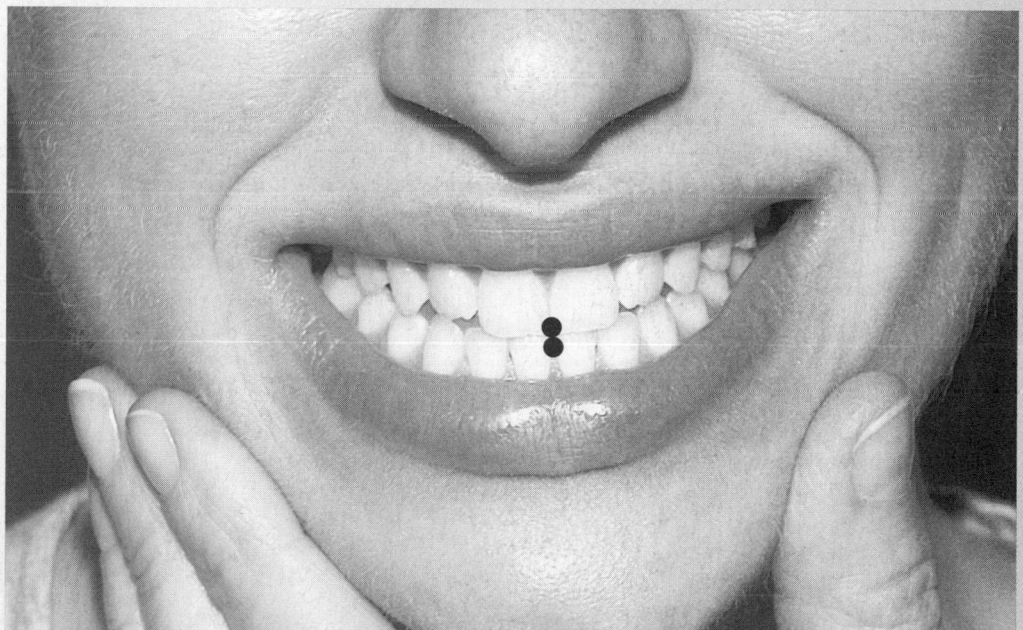

FIGURE 13.18 Note the difference between the alignment of the lower and upper central incisors in the neutral position compared to alignment of these incisors at the end of lateral excursion as shown in Figs. 3.16 and 3.17.

◯ Research Findings

The search for normative ROM values for TMJ joint motions is ongoing and includes various age groups of males and females in different populations and ethnic groups. A sampling of these studies is included in this section and in the sections that follow on the effects of age and gender on TMJ ROM.

In one of the few studies conducted to determine reference values for children, Cortese, Oliver, and Biondi[16] found that the normal range of mouth opening in boys and girls with a mean age of 4.6 years was 38.6 mm. For children in the study with a mean age of 6.9 years, the ROM was found to be 42.0 mm.[16] Hirsch and colleagues,[17] in a study involving children and adolescents 10 to 17 years old, found that the mean ROM for mouth opening was 50.6 mm.

Functional mouth opening is a distance sufficient for the subject to place two or three flexed proximal interphalangeal joints within the opening. That distance in adults may range from 35 mm to 50 mm, although an opening of only 25 mm to 35 mm is needed for normal activities.[7] A slightly more restricted normal range of adult values (40 to 50 mm) was arrived at by consensus judgments made at a 1995 Permanent Impairment Conference by representatives of all major societies and academies whose members treat TMJ disorders.[12] Similar normative mean values for adult mouth opening, from a low of 41 mm to a high of 58.6 mm, are presented in Table 13.1. Normal mean values for the ROM in protrusion and lateral excursive motions are presented from four sources in Table 13.2.

Dijkstra and coworkers[18] investigated the relationship between vertical and horizontal mandibular ROM in 91 healthy subjects (59 women and 32 men) with a mean age of 27.2 years. A mean ratio was found ranging from 6.0:1 to 6.6:1 between vertical and horizontal ROM. Therefore, based on the results of this study, the authors concluded that the 4:1 ratio between vertical and horizontal ROM that has been used as a standard in the past[19] should be replaced by the approximately 6:1 ratio found in this study. However, the authors found that the ratio has poor predictive value.

Effects of Age, Gender, and Other Factors

Age

Temporomandibular joint ROM in children tends to show an increase in ROM as age increases between the ages of 3 and 17 years.[16,17] Similar to other areas of the body, the ROM in adults tends to decrease rather than increase as age increases from ages 16 or 17 years onward. Also, like other areas of the body, some TMJ motions appear to be affected by age more than other TMJ motions in both adults and children.

Cortese, Oliver, and Biondi[16] determined ROM values in a sample of 212 boys and girls ages 3 to 11 years of age. The ROM in mouth opening and lateral excursion was found to be smaller in young children (3 to 4 years) compared to slightly older children (11 years), but no change in protrusion ROM was observed.

In a population-based study involving 1011 German male and female children and adolescents between the ages of 10 and 17 years, Hirsch and colleagues[17] also found an increase in the ROM of some motions as age increased. A significant difference occurred between maximum active mouth opening in the 10- to 13-year-old group and in the 14- to 17-year-old group, with the older adolescent group having a greater range of mouth opening. The authors determined that maximal unassisted mouth opening increased by 0.4 mm per year of age. Lateral excursion and protrusion also were influenced by age, with lateral excursion

| TABLE 13.1 | Maximum Active Mouth Opening ROM in Subjects 10 to 99 Years of Age: Normal Linear Distance in Millimeters* | | | | | | | |

Author	Hirsch et al[17]	Marklund and Wunman[20]	Goulet et al[21]	Celic et al[22]	Gallagher et al[23]		Turp et al[15]	
Sample	Male and female German school children	Male and female Swedish dental students	Male and female volunteers	Male Croatian dental students	Males and females from population in Ireland		Male and female German dental students and staff	
			Mean age				Mean age	
	10–17 yrs	18–48 yrs	29 yrs	19–28 yrs	16–99 yrs		26.1 yrs	
					Males	Females	Males	Females
	n = 1011	n = 371	n = 36	n = 60	n = 657	n = 856	n = 58	n = 83
	Mean (SD)	Mean (SD)	Mean (SD)	Mean (SD)	Mean	Mean	Mean (SD)	Mean (SD)
ROM	50.6 (6.4)	55.3 (6.1)	52.6 (6.3)	50.8 (5.0)	43	41	58.6 (7.1)	54.6 (7.9)

SD = standard deviation;.

* All measurements were obtained with a millimeter ruler, and all measurements include the amount of overbite except for measurements taken by Gallagher et al.

TABLE 13.2 Mandibular Protrusion and Lateral Excursion Range of Motion: Normal Linear Distance in Millimeters*

Author	Hirsch et al[17]		Celic et al[22]		Walker et al[14]		Turp et al[15]	
Sample	486 male and 525 female students 10–17 yrs n = 1011		Males and females 19–28 yrs n = 60		3 males and 12 females 21–61 yrs n = 15		Male and female students and staff Mean age = 26.1 yrs n = 141	
							Male	Female
Motion	Mean (SD)	Range	Mean (SD)	Range	Mean (SD)	Range	Mean (SD)	Mean (SD)
Protrusion	8.2 (2.5)	1–22	7.9 (2.5)	3–13	7.1 (2.3)	4–11	—	
Left lateral excursion	10.6 (2.3)	3–21	10.1 (3.0)	3–15	8.6 (2.1)	5–12	12.1 (2.3)	11.5 (2.4)
Right lateral excursion	10.2 (2.2)	3–17	10.0 (2.8)	4–15	9.2 (2.6)	6–14	11.0 (2.6)	10.9 (2.1)

SD = standard deviation.
* All measurements were obtained with a millimeter ruler.

increasing 0.1 mm per year of age and protrusion decreasing 0.1 mm per year of age.

Gallagher and coworkers[23] conducted a population-based study of mouth opening in 1513 Irish adults ages 16 to 99 years. Maximum mouth opening showed a decrease in ROM from 45 mm in the 16- to 24-year-old group of males to 41 mm in the 65- to 99-year-old group of males. A similar decrease in mouth opening ROM occurred in females from the youngest to the oldest group. Thurnwald[24] also found that mouth opening decreased with increasing age. The decrease was about 5 mm from a mean of 59.4 mm in the 17-year-old group to 54.3 mm in the 65-year-old group. In fact, active ROM in all TMJ motions except for retrusion decreased with increasing age in the 100 subjects in the study.

In contrast to the preceding studies Hassel, Rammelsberg, and Schmitter,[25] in a comparison of ROM between a group of 44 young adults ages 18 to 45 years and a group of 43 elderly patients ages 68 to 96 years, found that mouth opening ROM did not decrease from the youngest to the oldest groups. However, the ROM in protrusion and lateral excursion followed the normal pattern and decreased from the youngest to the oldest group.

Gender

A definite gender difference appears to be present in adults 16 to 99 years of age, with males having larger ROM in mouth opening than females.[23,24,26] Studies also have found that male adults have a larger ROM in lateral excursion than females.[15,24] Furthermore, Hirsch and colleagues[17] detected a gender effect in 10 to 17 year olds, with males having a significantly larger (1.8 mm) ROM in maximum active mouth opening than females. However, according to Cortese, Oliver, and Biondi,[16] the gender effect on mouth opening does not appear to be present in young children 3 to 11 years of age.

Gallagher and coworkers,[23] in a study of mouth opening in 1513 Irish males and females, determined that the 657 males 16 to 99 years of age had greater maximum active mouth opening ROM compared to the 856 females in the study.

Thurnwald[24] found that the subject's gender significantly affected both mouth opening and lateral excursion. The 50 males in this study had a greater mean range of mouth opening (59.4 mm) than the 50 females (54.0 mm). The males also had a greater mean ROM in right lateral excursion, but the difference between genders in this instance was small. The healthy 26-year-old males in a study by Turp, Alpaslan, and Gerds[15] had significantly larger maximum ROM in mouth opening and in both right and left lateral excursion in comparison to healthy females of the same age (see Table 13.1). Lewis, Buschang, and Throckmorton[26] determined that males had significantly greater mouth opening ROM (mean = 52.1 mm) than females (mean = 46.0 mm).

However, when mouth opening was measured as the angular displacement of the mandible in relation to the cranium (angle of mouth opening), Westling and Helkimo[27] found that maximal jaw opening in adolescents was slightly larger in females than in males. This finding might have been influenced by the fact that females generally reach adult ROM values by 10 years of age, whereas males do not reach adult ROM values until 15 years of age.[28]

Mandibular Length

The ROM in mouth opening appears to be related to the length of the mandible. Dijkstra and colleagues,[29] in a study of mouth opening in 13 females and 15 males, found that the linear distance between the upper and the lower incisors during mandibular depression was significantly influenced by mandibular length. In a subsequent study, Dijkstra and associates[30] investigated the relationship between incisor distances, mandibular length, and angle of mouth opening in 91 healthy subjects (59 women and 32 men) ranging from 13 to 56 years of age (mean 27.2 years). Mouth opening was influenced by both mandibular length and angle of mouth opening. Therefore, it is possible that subjects with the same mouth opening distance may differ from each other in regard to TMJ mobility. Lewis, Buschang, and Throckmorton[26] found that mandibular length accounted for some of the gender differences in mouth opening and for most of the gender differences in condylar translation in mouth opening. Westling and Helkimo[27] found that passive mouth opening ROM was strongly correlated to mandibular length.

To adjust for mandibular length, Miller and coworkers[31] developed a "mouth opening index," called the temporomandibular opening index (TOI), which was determined by using the following formula: TOI = (PO − MVO/PO + MVO) × 100. PO is passive opening, and MVO refers to maximal voluntary opening. In a subsequent study, Miller and associates[32] compared the TOI in patients with a temporomandibular disorder (TMD) with the TOI in a control group of individuals without TMDs. Based on the results of the study, the authors concluded that the TOI appeared to be independent of age, gender, and mandibular length. Moipolai, Karic, and Miller,[33] in a study of 42 asymptomatic patients, used analysis of covariance to assess the association between the TOI and age, gender, ramus length, and gonial angle. No relationship between the variables and the TOI was found. In a more recent study, Miller[34] found that the TOI was able to distinquish between two groups of patients with myogenous TMD, a finding that should make the TOI valuable as a diagnostic tool.

Head and Neck Positions and Motions

Head and neck positions and motions are closely linked with mouth opening and closing movements. Also, the ROM of mouth opening is affected by the static position of the head and neck, so examiners need to be aware of the subject's head and neck position during measurements of the TMJ. According to Zafar,[9,10] there is a functional linkage between the temporomandibular and craniocervical regions, with head and neck extension movements being an integral part of natural active mouth opening and head and neck flexion being an integral part of mouth closing.

Higbie and associates[35] investigated the effects of static head positions (forward, neutral, and retracted) on mouth opening in 20 healthy males and 20 healthy females between 18 and 54 years of age. Mouth opening ROM measured with a millimeter ruler was significantly different among the three positions. Mouth opening was greatest (mean = 44.5 mm, standard deviation [SD] = 5.3) in the forward head position, which includes extension of the upper cervical region; it was less in the neutral head position (mean = 41.5 mm, SD = 4.8); and it was least (mean = 36.2 mm, SD = 4.5) in the retracted head position, which includes cervical flexion. Day-to-day reliability was found to vary from an r value of 0.90 to 0.97, depending on head position, and the standard error of measurement (SEM) ranged from 0.77 to 1.69 mm, also depending on head position. As a result of the findings, the authors concluded that the head position should be controlled when mouth opening measurements are taken. However, the authors found that an error of 1 mm to 2 mm occurred regardless of the position in which the head was placed.

Temporomandibular Disorders (TMDs)

The structure of the TMJs and the fact that these joints get so much use predisposes the joints, associated ligaments, and

musculature to injury, mechanical problems, and degenerative changes. For example, the articular disc may become entrapped, deformed, or torn; the capsule may become thickened; the ligaments may become shortened or lengthened; and the muscles may become inflamed, contracted, and hypertrophied. These problems may give rise to a variety of symptoms and signs that are included in the TMD classification.

Restricted mouth opening ROM is considered to be one of the important signs of TMD.[36] Popping or clicking noises (or both) in the joint during mouth opening and/or closing and deviation of the mandible during mouth opening and closing may be present.[36–39] Other signs and symptoms include facial pain; muscular pain[36]; tenderness in the region of the TMJ, either unilaterally or bilaterally; headaches; and stiffness of the neck. TMDs appear to be more prevalent in females of all ages after puberty, although the actual percentages of women affected varies among investigators.[36,39–43]

A number of studies have investigated TMJ disorders in populations of children, adolescents, and elderly individuals.[17,20,22,25,39,44–46] Celic and colleagues[22] investigated the range of mandibular movements in a young male population of 180 patients with TMD disorders and 60 control subjects. A significant difference was found in maximal active mouth opening and active lateral excursion and protrusion between the controls and patients with TMD, but the authors concluded that it was not possible to discriminate among the following three patient groups: myogenous, disc, and combined myogenous and disc.

Cooper and Kleinberg[47] reviewed the records of 4528 men, women, and children patients between the ages of 11 and 70 years and found that the prevalence of TMDs was highest between the ages of 21 and 50 years of age. The authors also found a gender difference in that 77 percent of the patients were females.

In a study of 114 males and 194 female university students with a mean age of 23 years, Marklund and Wanman[20] found that the persistence of signs and symptoms over the period of a year was higher in female students. However, the 1-year incidence of TMJ signs and symptoms (12 percent) was not significantly different between men and women.

Possible reasons for a gender preference have been attributed to a number of factors including, among others, greater stress levels in women,[42] hormonal influences,[43] and habits of adolescent girls that are extremely harmful to the temporomandibular joints (e.g., intensive gum chewing, continuous arm leaning, ice crushing, nail biting, biting foreign objects, jaw play, clenching, and bruxism).[37,38]

Reliability and Validity

As is the case in other areas of the body, some TMJ motions appear to be more reliably measured than other motions in both asymptomatic and symptomatic subjects. Mouth opening (active and passive) measured with a millimeter ruler as the vertical distance between the upper and lower central incisors has consistently demonstrated good to excellent reliability (see Table 13.3).[14,35,47-50] Measurements of protrusion have also shown good reliability, but lateral excursion has consistently shown poor to good reliability.[25,48,50-53]

Walker, Bohannon, and Cameron[14] determined that all six TMJ motions measured with a millimeter ruler were reliable. Measurements were taken by two testers at three sessions, each of which were separated by a week. The 30 subjects who were measured included 15 patients with a TMJ disorder (13 females and 2 males with a mean age of 35.2 years) and 15 subjects without a TMJ disorder (12 females and 3 males with a mean age of 42.9 years). The intratester reliability intraclass correlation coefficients (ICCs) for tester 1 ranged from 0.82 to 0.99, and the intratester reliability for tester 2 ranged from 0.70 to 0.90. However, only mouth opening measurements had construct validity and were useful for discriminating between subjects with and without TMJ disorders. The technical error of measurement (difference between measurements that would have to be exceeded if the measurements were to be truly different) was 2.5 mm for mouth opening measurement in subjects without a TMJ disorder.

Higbie and associates[35] also found that ROM measurements of mouth opening were highly reliable with the use of a millimeter ruler. Twenty males and 20 females with a mean age of 32.9 years were measured by two examiners. Intratester, intertester, and test-retest reliability ICCs ranged from 0.90 to 0.97, depending on head position. SEM values indicated that an error of 1 mm to 2 mm existed for the measurement technique used in the study.

Kropmans and colleagues[48] found similar high reliability in a study of mouth opening involving 5 male and 20 female patients with painfully restricted TMJs. Intratester, intertester,

and test-retest reliability varied between 0.90 and 0.96. However, in contrast to the findings of Walker, Bohannon, and Cameron[14] and those of Higbie and associates,[35] the authors found that the smallest detectable difference of maximal mouth opening in this group of subjects varied from 9 mm to 6 mm. Based on these results, a clinician would have to measure at least 9 mm of improvement in maximal mouth opening in this group of patients to say that improvement had occurred.

Reliability appears to be improved when examiners participate in a calibration training program in which examiners are calibrated to a standarized set of examination procedures and criteria, as described by the RDC/TMD. Lobbezoo and colleagues[52] found that calibration training resulted in good to excellent interexaminer reliability of both active and passive mouth opening measurements and protrusion ROM. Only lateral excursion ROM measurements had fair interexaminer reliability.

In a study by Leher and colleagues,[51] no significant difference was found in the reliability of ROM measurements between inexperienced dental students and experienced practitioners who had participated in a calibration program. The authors concluded that calibration training was more important than experience. However, both groups had unacceptable reliability scores for lateral excursive motions. Lausten, Glaros, and Williams[53] compared nonexpert and expert examiners' ability to measure TMJ ROM following calibration training. The nonexperts were able to measure maximum active mouth opening ROM with a high degree of reliability, but, similar to Leher's results, neither group was able to measure lateral excursive motions reliably.

TABLE 13.3 Intertester Reliability of Mandibular Measurements Using a Millimeter Ruler

Author	Goulet et al[21]	Walker et al[14]	Walker et al[14]	John et al[50]
Testers Sample	5 experienced 10 males and 62 females; 36 patients with TMD and 36 without TMD Mean age 29 yrs n = 72	2 experienced 2 male and 13 female patients with TMD 20–52 yrs n = 15	2 experienced 3 males and 12 females without TMD 21–61 yrs n = 15	4 experienced 11 patients with TMD and 25 without TMD 17–71 yrs n = 36
	ICC	ICC	ICC	ICC
Mouth opening	0.87	0.99	0.98	0.93
Right lateral excursion	0.59	0.96	0.90	0.73
Left lateral excursion	0.68	0.94	0.95	0.79
Protrusion	—	0.98	0.95	0.91

ICC = intraclass correlation coefficient; TMD = temporomandibular disorder.

REFERENCES

1. Hoover, D, and Ritzline, P: The temporomandibular joint. In Levangie, PK, and Norkin, CC (eds): Joint Structure and Function: A Comprehensive Analysis, ed 4. FA Davis, Philadelphia, 2005.
2. Iglarsh, ZA, and Synder-Mackler, L: The temporomandibular joint and the cervical spine. In Richardson, JK, and Iglarsh, ZA (eds): Clinical Orthopaedic Physical Therapy. WB Saunders, Philadelphia, 1994.
3. Williams, PL: Gray's Anatomy, ed 38. Churchill Livingstone, New York, 1995.
4. Neumann, DA: Kinesiology of the Musculoskeletal System: Foundations for Physical Rehabilitation. Mosby, Inc., St. Louis, 2002.
5. Otis, CA: Kinesiology: The Mechanics and Pathomechanics of Human Movement. Lippincott William and Wilkins, Philadelphia, 2004.
6. Harrison, AL: The temporomandibular joint. In Malone, TR, McPoil, T, and Nitz, AJ (eds): Orthopedic and Sports Physical Therapy, ed 3. CV Mosby, St. Louis, 1997.
7. Magee, DJ: Orthopedic Physical Assessment, ed 3. WB Saunders, Philadelphia, 1997.
8. Cailliet, R: Soft Tissue Pain and Disability, ed 3. FA Davis, Philadelphia, 1996.
9. Zafar, H, Nordh, E, and Eriksson, PO: Temporal coordination between mandibular and head-neck movements during jaw opening-closing tasks in man. Arch Oral Biol 45:675, 2000.
10. Zafar, H: Integrated jaw and neck function in man. Studies of mandibular and head-neck movements during jaw opening-closing tasks. Swed Dent J 143(Suppl):1, 2000.
11. Eriksson, PO, et al: Co-ordinated mandibular and head-neck movements during rhythmic jaw activities in man. J Dent Res 79:1378, 2000.
12. Phillips, DJ, et al: Guide to evaluation of permanent impairment of the temporomandibular joint. J Craniomandibular Pract 15:170, 1997.
13. Dworkin, SF, and Le Resche, L: Research diagnostic criteria for temporomandibular disorders. J Craniomandib Disord 6:301,1992.
14. Walker, N, Bohannon, RW, and Cameron, D: Discriminant validity of temporomandibular joint range of motion measurements obtained with a ruler. J Orthop Sports Phys Ther 30:484, 2000.
15. Turp, JC, Alpaslan, C, and Gerds,T: Is there a greater mandibular movement capacity towards the left? Verification of an observation from 1921. J Oral Rehabil 32:242, 2005.
16. Cortese, SG, Oliver, LM, and Biondi, AM: Determination of mandibular movements in children without temporomandibular disorders. J Craniomandibular Practice 25:200, 2007.
17. Hirsch,C, et al: Mandibular jaw movement capacity in 10–17-yr-old children and adolescents: Normative values and the influence of gender, age, and temporomandibular disorders. Eur J Oral Sci 114:465, 2006.
18. Dijkstra, PU, et al: Ratio between vertical and horizontal mandibular range of motion. J Oral Rehabil 25:353, 1998.
19. Hockstedler, JL, Allen, JD, and Follmar, MA: Temporomandibular joint range of motion: a ratio of intercisal opening to excursive movement in a healthy population. Cranio 14:296, 1996.
20. Marklund, S, and Wanman, A: Incidence and prevalence of temporomandibular joint pain and dysfunction. A one-year prospective study of university students. Acta Odontologica Scandanavia 65:119, 2007.
21. Goulet, J-P, et al: The reproducibility of muscle and joint tenderness detection methods and maxumum mandibular movement measurement for the temporomandibular system. J Orofacial Pain 12:17, 1998.
22. Celic, R, et al: Measurement of mandibular movement in patients with temporomandibular disorders and in asymptomatic subjects. Coll Antropol Suppl 2:43, 2003.
23. Gallagher, C, et al: The normal range of mouth opening in an Irish population. J Oral Rehabil 31:110, 2004.
24. Thurnwald, PA: The effect of age and gender on normal temporomandibular joint motion. Physiother Theory Pract 7:209, 1991.
25. Hassel AJ, Rammelsberg, P, and Schmitter, M: Inter-examiner reliability in the clinical examination of temporomandibular disorders: Influence of age. Community Dent Oral Epidemiol 34:41, 2006.
26. Lewis, RP, Buschang, PH, and Throckmorton, GS: Sex differences in mandibular movements during opening and closing. Am J Orthod Dentofacial Orthop 120:294, 2001.
27. Westling, L, and Helkimo, E: Maximum jaw opening capacity in adolescents in relation to general joint mobility. 19:485, 1992.
28. Wright, DM, and Moffat, BC, Jr: The postnatal development of the human temporomandibular joint. Am J Anat 141:235, 1974.
29. Dijkstra, PU, et al: Temporomandibular joint mobility assessment: A comparison between four methods. J Oral Rehabil 22:439, 1995.
30. Dijkstra, PU, et al: Influence of mandibular length on mouth opening. J Oral Rehabil 26:117, 1999.
31. Miller, VJ, et al: A mouth opening index for patients with temporomandibular disorders. J Oral Rehabil 26:534, 1999.
32. Miller, VJ, et al: The temporomandibular opening index (TOI) in patients with closed lock and a control group with no temporomandibular disorders (TMD): An initial study. J Oral Rehabil 27:815, 2000.
33. Moipolai, P, Karic, VV, and Miller, VJ: The effect of gonial angle, ramus length, age and gender on temporomandibular opening index. J Oral Rehabil 30:1195, 2003.
34. Miller, VJ, Karic, VV, and Myers, SL: Differences in initial symptom scores between myogenous TMD patients with high and low TOI scores. J Craniomandib Pract 24:25, 2006.
35. Higbie, EJ, et al: Effect of head position on vertical mandibular opening. J Orthop Sports Phys Ther 29:127, 1999.
36. Esposito, CJ, Panucci, PJ, and Farman, AG: Associations in 425 patients having temporomandibular disorders. J Kentucky Med Assoc 98:213, 2001.
37. Gavish, A, et al: Oral habits and their association with signs and symptoms of temporomandibular disorders in adolescent girls. J Oral Rehabil 27:22, 2000.
38. Winocur, E, et al: Oral habits among adolescent girls and their association with symptoms of temporomandibular disorders. J Oral Rehabil 28:624, 2001.
39. Rauhala, K, et al: Facial pain and temporomandibular disorders: An epidemiological study of the northern Finland 1966 birth cohort. J Craniomandib Pract 18:40, 2000.
40. Hiltunen, K, et al: Prevalence of signs of temporomandibular disorders among elderly inhabitants of Helsinki, Finland. Acta Odontol Scand 53:20, 1995.
41. La Resche, L: Epidemiology of temporormandibular disorders: Implications for the investigation of etiologic factors. Crit Rev Oral Biol Med 8:291, 1997.
42. Kutilla, M, et al: TMD treatment need in relation to age, gender, stress and diagnostic subgroup. J Orofac Pain 12:67, 1998.
43. Warren, MP, and Fried, JL: Temporomandibular disorders and hormones in women. Cells Tissues Organs 169:187, 2000.
44. Sonmez, H, et al: Prevalence of temporomandibular dysfunction in Turkish children with mixed and permanent dentition. J Oral Rehabil 28:280, 2001.
45. Alamoudi, N, et al: Temporomandibular disorders among school children. J Clin Pediatr Dent 22:323, 1998.
46. Nilsson, IM: Reliability, validity, incidence and impact of temporomandibular pain disorders in adolescents. Swed Dent J Suppl 183:7, 2007.
47. Cooper, BC, and Kleinberg, I: Examination of a large patient population for the presence of symptoms and signs of temporomandibular disorders. J Craniomandibular Pract 25:115, 2007.
48. Kropmans, T, et al: Smallest detectable difference of maximal mouth opening in patients with painfully restricted temporomandibular joint function. Eur J Oral Sci 108:9, 2000.
49. List, T, et al: Recalibration improves inter-examiner reliability of TMD examination. Acta Odontologica Scandinavia 64:146, 2006.
50. John, MT, and Zwignenberg, AJ: Interobserver variables in assessment of signs of TMD. Intl J Prosthodontics 14:265, 2001.
51. Leher, A, et al: Is there a difference in the reliable measurement of temporomandibular disorder signs between experienced and inexperienced examiners ? J Orofac Pain 19:58, 2005.
52. Lobbezoo, F, et al:Use of the research diagnostic criteria for temporomandibular disorders for multinational research: Translation efforts and reliability assessments in the Netherlands. J Orofac Pain 19:301, 2005.
53. Lausten, LL, Glaros, AC, and Williams, K: Inter-examiner reliability of physical assessment methods for assessing temporomandibular disorders. Gen Dent 52:509, 2004.

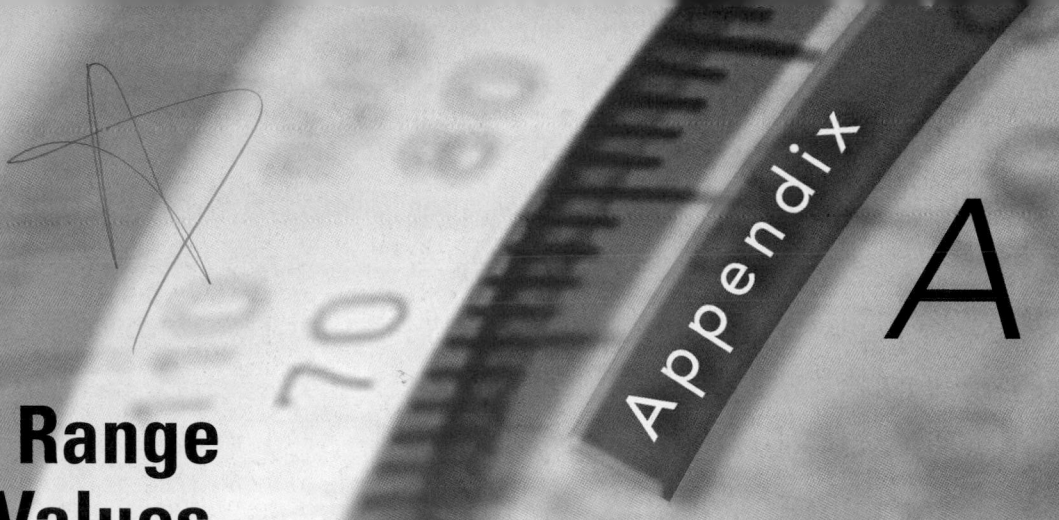

Normative Range of Motion Values

TABLE A.1	Shoulder, Elbow, Forearm, and Wrist Motion: Mean Values in Degrees

Motion	Wanatabe et al*[1] 0–2 yrs n = 45	Boone and Azen[2] 1–54 yrs n = 109 (M)	Green and Wolf[3] 18–55 yrs n = 20 (10 M, 10 F)	Walker et al[4] 65–85yrs n = 60 (30 M, 30 F)	Downey et al[5] 61–93 yrs n = 106 (60 M, 140 F shoulders)	AAOS[6]	AMA[7]
Shoulder Complex							
Flexion	172–180	167	156	165	165	180	180
Extension	78–89	62	—	44	—	60	50
Abduction	177–187	184	168	165	158	180	180
Medial rotation	72–90	69	49	62	65	70	90
Lateral rotation	118–134	104	84	81	81	90	90
Elbow and Forearm							
Flexion	148–158	143	145	143	—	150	140
Extension	—	1	0	4[†]	—	0	0
Pronation	90–96	76	84	71	—	80	80
Supination	81–93	82	77	74	—	80	80
Wrist							
Flexion	88–96	76	73	64	—	80	60
Extension	82–89	75	65	63	—	70	60
Radial deviation	—	22	25	19	—	20	20
Ulnar deviation	—	36	39	26	—	30	30

AAOS = American Association of Orthopaedic Surgeons; AMA = American Medical Association;
  M = males; F = females.
All values obtained with a universal goniometer.
* Values in this column represent a range of means.
† Value refers to extension limitation.

TABLE A.2 Glenohumeral Motion: Mean Values in Degrees

Author	Ellenbecker et al[8]	Ellenbecker et al[8]	Boon & Smith[9]	Lannan et al[10]
	11–17 yrs n = 113	11–17 yrs n = 90	12–18 yrs n = 50	21–40 yrs n = 60
Motion	*(M)*	*(F)*	*(18 M, 32 F)*	*(20 M, 40 F)*
Glenohumeral				
Flexion	—	—	—	106
Extension	—	—	—	20
Abduction	—	—	—	129
Medial rotation	51	56	63	49
Lateral rotation	103	105	108	94

M = males; F = females.
Values obtained with a universal goniometer.

TABLE A.3 Finger Motions: Mean Values in Degrees

Author	Skarilova & Plevkova*,[11]	Mallon et al‡,[12]	Smahel & Klimova*,[13,14]	Hume et al†,[15]	AAOS[6]	AMA[7]
	20–25 yrs n = 200	18–35 yrs n = 120	18–28 yrs n = 101	26–28 yrs n = 35		
Motion	*(100 M, 100 F)*	*(60 M, 60 F)*	*(52 M, 49 F)*	*(M)*		
Finger MCP						
Flexion	91	95	92	100	90	90
Extension	26	20	25	—	45	20
Finger PIP						
Flexion	108	105	111	105	100	100
Extension	—	7	—	0	0	0
Finger DIP						
Flexion	85	68	81	85	90	70
Extension	—	8	—	0	0	0

CMC = carpometacarpal; IP = interphalangeal; MCP = metacarpophalangeal; AAOS = American Association
of Orthopaedic Surgeons; AMA = American Medical Association; F = females ; M = males.
* Values obtained with a metallic slide goniometer on dorsal aspect.
† Values obtained with a computerized Greenleaf goniometer.
‡ Values obtained with a gonimeter applied to the dorsal aspect.

TABLE A.4 Thumb Motions: Mean Values in Degrees

Author	Skarilova and Plevkova*,11	Skarilova and Plevkova*,11	Jenkins et al†,16	DeSmet et al‡,17	AAOS6	AMA7
	20–25 yrs n = 200 (100 M, 100 F)	20–25 yrs n = 200 (100 M, 100 F)	16–72 yrs n = 119 (50 M, 69 F)	16–83 yrs n = 101 (43 M, 58 F)		
Motion	*Active*	*Passive*	*Active*			
Thumb CMC						
Abduction	—	—	—	—	70	—
Flexion	—	—	—	—	15	—
Extension	—	—	—	—	20, 80	35§
Thumb MCP						
Flexion	57	67	59	54	50	60
Extension	14	23	—	—	0	40
Thumb IP						
Flexion	79	86	67	80	80	80
Extension	23	35	—	—	20	30

DIP = Distal interphalangeal; MCP = metacarpophalangeal; PIP = proximal interphalangeal;
AAOS = American Association of Orthopaedic Surgeons; AMA = American Medical Association; M = Males; F = females.
* Values obtained with a metallic slide goniometer on dorsal aspect.
† Values obtained with a universal goniometer on lateral aspect.
‡ Values obtained with a digital goniometer on dorsal aspect.
§ Range of motion value of 35 degrees is the difference between the minimal angle (15 degrees)
   of separation between first and second metacarpals and the maximal angle (50 degrees) of separation.

TABLE A.5 Hip and Knee Motions: Mean Values in Degrees

Author	Waugh et al18	Drews et al 19	Schwarze and Denton20	Wanatabe et al1	Phelps et al21	Boone and Azen2	Roach and Miles22	AAOS6	AMA7
	6–65 hrs n = 40	12 hrs– 6 days n = 54	1–3 days n = 1000	4 weeks n = 62	9 mos n = 25	1–54 yrs n = 109	25–74 yrs n = 1683		
Motion		(26 M, 28 F)	(473 M, 527 F)		(M and F)	(109 M)	(821 M, 862 F)		
Hip									
Flexion	—	—	—	138	—	122	121	120	100
Extension	46*	28*†	20*	12*	10*	10	19	20	30
Abduction	—	55‡	78‡	51	—	46	42		40
Adduction	—	6‡	15‡	—	—	27	—		20
Medial rotation	—	80‡	58	24	52	47	32	45	50
Lateral rotation	—	114‡	80	66	47	47	32	45	50
Knee									
Flexion	—	—	150	—	—	142	132	135	150
Extension	15*	20*	15*	—	—	—	—	10	—

AAOS = American Association of Orthopaedic Surgeons; AMA = American Medical Association;
  M = males; F = females.
* Values refer to extension limitations.
† Tested wiith subjects in sidelying position
‡ Tested with subjects in supine position

TABLE A.6 — Ankle and Foot Motions: Mean Values in Degrees

Author	Waugh et al[18]	Wanatabe et al[1]	Boone and Azen[2]	McPoil and Cornwall[25]	Mecagni et al[24]	AAOS[6]	AMA[7]
	6–65 hrs n = 40	4–8 mos n = 54	1–54 yrs n = 109	26.1 yrs n = 27 (54 feet)	64–87 yrs n = 34		
Motion	*(18 M, 22 F)*		*(M)*	*(9 M, 18 F)*	*(F)*		
Ankle							
Dorsiflexion	59	51	13	16	11	20	20
Plantar flexion	26	60	56	—	64	50	40
Inversion	—	—	37	19 (Subtalar)	26	35	30
Eversion	—	—	21	12 (Subtalar)	17	15	20
First MTP							
Flexion	—	—	—	—	—	45	30
Extension	—	—	—	86	—	70	50

AAOS = American Association of Orthopaedic Surgeons; AMA = American Medical Association; M =males; F = females.
All range of motion values in the table obtained with a universal goniometer.

TABLE A.7 — Cervical Spine Motions: Mean Values in Centimeters and Degrees

Author	Youdas et al[*,26]						Lantz et al[†,27]		Hsieh and Young[‡,28]	Balogun et al[§,29]		AAOS[6]	AMA[7]
	11–19 yrs n = 40 (20M, 20F)		30–39 yrs n = 41 (20 M, 21 F)		70–79 yrs n = 40 (20 M, 20 F)		20–39 yrs n = 63		14–31 yrs n = 34 (27 M, 7 F)	18–26 yrs n = 21 (15 M, 6 F)		26–39 yrs n = 63	
Motion	M	F	M	F	M	F	Active	Passive					
Flexion	64	—	47	—	39	—	60	74	1.0 cm	4.3 cm	32	45	50
Extension	86	84	68	78	54	55	56	53	22 cm	19 cm	64	45	60
Right lateral flexion	45	49	43	47	26	28	43	48	11 cm	13 cm	41	45	45
Right rotation	74	75	67	72	50	53	72	79	12 cm	11 cm	64	60	80

AAOS = American Association of Orthopaedic Surgeons; AMA = American Medical Association; F = female; M = male.
* Values in degrees were obtained for active range of motion using the cervical range of motion (CROM) instrument.
† Values in degrees were obtained for active and passive range of motion with use of the OSI CA-6000 Spinal Motion Analyzer.
‡ Values in centimeters were obtained with a tape measure.
§ Values in centimeters obtained with a tape measure appear in the last column, whereas values in degrees obtained with a Myrin gravity-referenced goniometer appear in the second column.
NB: AMA values in degrees were obtained with use of a universal goniometer, and AAOS values in degrees were obtained with use of an inclinometer.

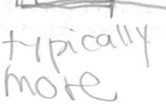
typically more

TABLE A.8 — Thoracic and Lumbar Spine Motions: Mean Values in Centimeters and Degrees

Author	Haley et al*,[30]	Moll and Wright*,[31]	Van Adrichem and van der Korst†,[32]		Breum et al‡,[33]		McGregor et al§,[34]		Fitzgerald et al¶,[35]	AAOS[6]		AMA[7]
	5–9 yrs n = 282 (140 M, 142 F)	15–75 yrs n = 237 (119 M, 118 F)	15–18 yrs n = 66 (34 M, 32 F)		18–38 yrs n = 47 (27 M, 20 F)		50–59 yrs n = 41 (21 M, 20 F)		20–82 yrs n = 172 (168 M, 4 F)			
Motion			M	F	M	F	M	F		M		F
Flexion	6–7 cm	5–7 cm	7 cm	6 cm	56	54	55	60	—	80		60
Extension	—	—	—	—	22	21	21	18	16–41	25		25
Right lateral flexion	—	—	—	—	33	31	30	30	18–38	35		25
Right rotation	—	—	—	—	8	8	26	26	—	45		30

AAOS = American Association of Orthopaedic Surgeons; AMA = American Medical Association; F = female; M = male.
* Lumbar values obtained with use of the Modified Schober method.
† Lumbar values obtained using the Modified–Modified Schober (simplified skin distraction) method.
‡ Lumbar values in the first column were obtained with the BROM II. Lumbar values in the second column were obtained with double inclinometers.
§ Lumbar values obtained with the OSI CA-6000.
¶ Range of motion (ROM) values for thoracolumbar extension and lateral flexion were obtained with a universal goniometer. Lower values are for ages 70–79 years and higher values are for ages 20–29 years.
NB: AAOS values for thoracolumbar motions were obtained with a universal goniometer. AMA values were obtained with use of the two-inclinometer method for lumbar motions of flexion, extension, and lateral flexion. The AMA value for rotation is for the thoracic spine.

TABLE A.9 — Tempomandibular Motions: Mean Values in Millimeters

Author	Walker et al*,[36]	Hirsch et al*,[37]		Thurnwald†,[38]			
	21–61 yrs n = 15 (3 M, 12 F)	10–17yrs n = 1011 (486 M, 525 F)		17–25 yrs n = 50 (25 M, 25 F)		50–65 yrs n = 50 (25 M, 25 F)	
Motion		M	F	M	F	M	F
Opening	43	51	51	61	55	58	51
Left lateral excursion	9	11	10	9	8	8	6
Right lateral excursion	9	10	10	10	9	7	9
Protrusion	7	8	8	5	5	5	4

* Values were obtained for active range of motion (ROM) with an 11-cm plastic ruler marked in millimeters.
† Values were obtained for active ROM with Vernier calipers as the measuring instrument.

REFERENCES

1. Wanatabe, H, et al: The range of joint motion of the extremities in healthy Japanese people: The differences according to age. (Cited in Walker, JM: Musculoskeletal development: A review. Phys Ther 71:878, 1991.)
2. Boone, DC, and Azen, SP: Normal range of motion of joints in male subjects. J Bone Joint Surg 61:756, 1979.
3. Greene, BL, and Wolf, SL: Upper extremity joint movement: Comparison of two measurement devices. Arch Phys Med Rehabil 70:288, 1989.
4. Walker, JM, et al: Active mobility of the extremities in older subjects. Phys Ther 4:919, 1984.
5. Downey, PA, Fiebert, I, and Stackpole-Brown, JB: Shoulder range of motion in persons aged sixty and older. (abstract). Phys Ther 71:S75, 1991.
6. American Academy of Orthopaedic Surgeons: Joint Motion: Method of measuring and recording. American Academy of Orthopaedic Surgeons, Chicago, 1965.
7. Cocchiarella, L and Andersson, GBJ (eds) American Medical Association: Guides to the Evaluation of Permanent Impairment, ed 5. AMA, Chicago 2001.
8. Ellenbecker, TS, et al: Glenohumeral joint internal and external rotation range of motion in elite junior tennis players. J Orthop Sports Phys Ther 24:336, 1996.
9. Boon, AJ, and Smith, J: Manual scapular stabilization: Its effect on shoulder rotational range of motion. Arch Phys Med Rehabil 81:978, 2000.
10. Lannan, D, Lehman, T, and Toland, M: Establishment of normative data for the range of motion of the glenohumeral joint. Master of Science thesis, University of Massachusetts, Lowell, 1996.
11. Skarilova, B, and Plevkova, A: Ranges of joint motion of the adult hand. Acta Chir Plast 38:67, 1996.
12. Mallon, WJ, Brown, HR, and Nunley, JA: Digital ranges of motion: Normal values in joung adults. J Hand Surg 16A:882, 1991.
13. Smahel, Z and Klimova, A: The influence of age and exercise on the mobility of hand joints 1: metacarpophalangeal joint of the three-phalangeal fingers. Acta Chirurgiae Plasticae 46:81, 2004.
14. Smahel, Z and Klimova, A: The influence of age and exercise on the mobility of hand joints 2: interphalangeal joints of the three-phalangeal fingers. Acta Chirurgiae Plasticae 46:122, 2004.
15. Hume, M, et al: Functional range of motion of the joints of the hand. J Hand Surg 15A:240, 1990.
16. Jenkins, M, et al: Thumb joint motion: What is normal? J Hand Surg 23B:796, 1998.
17. DeSmett, L, et al: Metacarpophalangeal and interphalangeal flexion of the thumb: Influence of sex and age, relation to ligamentous injury. Acta Orhtop Belg 59:37, 1993.
18. Waugh, KG, et al: Measurement of selected hip, knee and ankle joint motions in newborns. Phys Ther 63:1616, 1983.
19. Drews, JE, Vraciu, JK, and Pellino, G: Range of motion of the lower extremities of newborns. Phys Occup Ther Pediatr 4:49, 1884.
20. Schwarze, DJ, and Denton, JR: normal values of neonatal limbs: An evaluation of 1000 neonates. J Pediatr Orthop 13:758, 1993.
21. Phelps, E, Smith, LJ, and Hallum, A: Normal ranges of hip motion of infants between 9 and 24 months of age. Dev Med Child Neurol 27:785, 1985.
22. Roach, KE, and Miles, TP: Normal hip and knee active range of motion: The relationship of age. Phys Ther 71: 656, 1991.
23. Greene, WB, and Heckman, JD (eds): The Clinical Measurement of Joint Motion. American Academy of Orthopaedic Surgeons, Rosemont, Ill. 1994.
24. Mecagni, C, et al: Balance and ankle range of motion in community dwelling women aged 64–87 years: A correlational study. Phys Ther 80:1004, 2000.
25. McPoil, TG, and Cornwall, MW: The relationship between static lower extremity measurements and rearfoot motion during walking. Phys Ther 24:309, 1996.
26. Youdas, J, et al: Normal range of motion of the cervical spine: An initial goniometric study. Phys Ther 72:770, 1992.
27. Lantz, CA, Chen, J, and Buch, D: Clinical validity and stability of active and passive cervical range of motion with regard to total and uniplanar motion. Spine 24:1082, 1999.
28. Hsieh, C-Y and Yeung, BW: Active neck motion measurements with a tape measure. J Orthop Sports Phys Ther 8:88, 1986.
29. Balogun, JA, et al: Inter-and intratester reliability of measuring neck motions with tape measure and Myrin Gravity-Reference Goniometer. J Orthop Sports Phys Ther 9:248, 1989.
30. Haley, SM, Tada, WL, Carmichael, EM: Spinal mobility in young children. Phys Ther 66:1697, 1986.
31. Moll, JMH, and Wright, V: Normal range of spinal mobility: An objective clinical study. Ann Rheum Dis 30:381, 1971.
32. van Adrichem, JAM, and van der Korst, JK: Assessment of flexibility of the lumbar spine. A pilot study in children and adolescents. Scand J Rheumatol 2:87, 1973.
33. Breum, J, Wiberg, J, and Bolton, JE: Reliability and concurrent validity of the BROM II for measuring lumbar mobility. J Manipulative Physiol Ther 18:497, 1995.
34. Mcgregor, AH, MacCarthy, ID, and Hughes, SP: Motion characteristics of the lumbar spine in the normal population. Spine 20:2421, 1995.
35. Fitzgerald, GK, et al: Objective assessment with establishment of normal values for lumbar spine range of motion. Phys Ther 63:1776, 1983.
36. Walker, N, Bohannon, RW, Cameron, D: Validity of temporomandibular joint range of motion measurements obtained with a ruler. J Orthop Sports Phys Ther 30:484, 2000.
37. Hirsch,C, John, MT, Lautenschlager,C, List, T: Mandibular jaw movement capacity in 10-17-yr-old children and adolescents;normative values and the influence of gender,age, and temporomandibular disorders. Eur. J Oral Sci 114:465-470, 2006.
38. Thurnwald, PA: The effect of age and gender on normal temporomandibular joint movement. Physiother Theory Pract 7:209, 1991.

Joint Measurements by Body Position

	Prone	Supine	Sitting	Standing
Shoulder	Extension	Flexion Abduction Medial rotation Lateral rotation		
Elbow		Flexion		
Forearm			Pronation Supination	
Wrist			Flexion Extension Radial deviation Ulnar deviation	
Hand			All motions	
Hip	Extension Medial rotation[††] Lateral rotation[††]	Flexion Abduction Adduction	Medial rotation Lateral rotation	
Knee		Flexion		
Ankle and foot	Subtalar inversion Subtalar eversion	Dorsiflexion Plantar flexion Inversion Eversion Midtarsal inversion Midtarsal eversion	Dorsiflexion Plantar flexion Inversion Eversion Midtarsal inversion Midtarsal eversion	
Toes		All motions	All motions	
Cervical spine		Rotation*	Flexion Extension Lateral flexion Rotation[†]	
Thoracic and lumbar spine			Rotation	Flexion Extension Lateral flexion
Temporomandibular joint			Depression (opening) Protrusion Lateral excursion Overbite	

* Measurement position using single inclinometer.
[†] Measurement position using universal goniometer, tape measure, and cervical range of motion device (CROM).
[††] Alternative position.

Numerical Recording Forms

	Left		Range of Motion—Temporomandibular Joint and Spine	Right		
			Patient's Name: _____ **Date of Birth** _____			
			Date			
			Examiner's Initials			
			Temporomandibular Joint			
			Depression (opening)			
			Protrusion			
			Lateral Excursion			
			Overbite			
			Comments:			
			Cervical Spine			
			Flexion			
			Extension			
			Lateral Flexion			
			Rotation			
			Comments:			
			Thoracolumbar Spine			
			Flexion			
			Extension			
			Lateral Flexion			
			Rotation			
			Comments:			
			Lumbar Spine			
			Flexion			
			Extension			
			Lateral Flexion			
			Comments:			

Range of Motion—Upper Extremity

Patient's Name:_____ Date of Birth _____

Left				Right		
			Date			
			Examiner's Initials			
			Shoulder Complex			
			Flexion			
			Extension			
			Abduction			
			Medial Rotation			
			Lateral Rotation			
			Comments:			
			Glenohumeral			
			Flexion			
			Extension			
			Abduction			
			Medial Rotation			
			Lateral Rotation			
			Comments:			
			Elbow and Forearm			
			Flexion			
			Supination			
			Pronation			
			Comments:			
			Wrist			
			Flexion			
			Extension			
			Ulnar Deviation			
			Radial Deviation			
			Comments:			

			Range of Motion—Hand			
Patient's Name:				Date of Birth		
Left					**Right**	
			Date			
			Examiner's Initials			
			Thumb			
			CMC Flexion			
			CMC Extension			
			CMC Abduction			
			CMC Opposition			
			MCP Flexion			
			IP Flexion			
			IP Extension			
			Index Finger			
			MCP Flexion			
			MCP Extension			
			MCP Abduction			
			PIP Flexion			
			DIP Flexion			
			Middle Finger			
			MCP Flexion			
			MCP Extension			
			MCP Radial Abduction			
			MCP Ulnar Abduction			
			PIP Flexion			
			DIP Flexion			
			Ring Finger			
			MCP Flexion			
			MCP Extension			
			MCP Abduction			
			PIP Flexion			
			DIP Flexion			
			Little Finger			
			MCP Flexion			
			MCP Extension			
			MCP Abduction			
			PIP Flexion			
			DIP Flexion			
			Comments:			

Left			Range of Motion—Lower Extremity	Right		
			Date			
			Examiner's Initials			
			Hip			
			Flexion			
			Extension			
			Abduction			
			Adduction			
			Medial Rotation			
			Lateral Rotation			
			Knee			
			Flexion			
			Ankle			
			Dorsiflexion			
			Plantarflexion			
			Inversion—Tarsal			
			Eversion—Tarsal			
			Inversion—Subtalar			
			Eversion—Subtalar			
			Inversion—Midtarsal			
			Eversion—Midtarsal			
			Great Toe			
			MTP Flexion			
			MTP Extension			
			MTP Abduction			
			IP Flexion			
			Toe _____			
			MTP Flexion			
			MTP Extension			
			MTP Abduction			
			PIP Flexion			
			DIP Flexion			
			Comments:			

Patient's Name: _____ **Date of Birth** _____

			Muscle Length			

Patient's Name: _____ **Date of Birth** _____

Left				Right		
			Date			
			Examiner's Initials			
			Upper Extremity			
			Biceps Brachii			
			Triceps Brachii			
			Flexor Digitorum Profundus and Superficialis			
			Extensor Digitorum, Indicis, and Digiti Minimi			
			Lumbricals, Palmar and Dorsal Interossei			
			Comments:			
			Lower Extremity			
			Hip Flexors—Thomas Test			
			Rectus Femoris—Ely Test			
			Hamstrings—SLR			
			Hamstrings—Distal Hamstring Length Test			
			Tensor Fascia Lata—Ober Test			
			Gastrocnemius			
			Comments:			

Index

10) Hypertensive Crisis

Assign a code from category I16, Hypertensive crisis, for documented hypertensive urgency, hypertensive emergency or unspecified hypertensive crisis. Code also any identified hypertensive disease (I10-I15). The sequencing is based on the reason for the encounter.

b. Atherosclerotic coronary artery disease and angina

ICD-10-CM has combination codes for atherosclerotic heart disease with angina pectoris. The subcategories for these codes are I25.11, Atherosclerotic heart disease of native coronary artery with angina pectoris and I25.7, Atherosclerosis of coronary artery bypass graft(s) and coronary artery of transplanted heart with angina pectoris.

When using one of these combination codes it is not necessary to use an additional code for angina pectoris. A causal relationship can be assumed in a patient with both atherosclerosis and angina pectoris, unless the documentation indicates the angina is due to something other than the atherosclerosis.

If a patient with coronary artery disease is admitted due to an acute myocardial infarction (AMI), the AMI should be sequenced before the coronary artery disease.

See Section I.C.9. Acute myocardial infarction (AMI)

> Patient is being seen for spastic angina pectoris. She also has a documented history of progressive coronary artery disease of the native vessels.
>
> **I25.111**   **Atherosclerotic heart disease of native coronary artery with angina pectoris with documented spasm**
>
> *Explanation*: Report the combination code for atherosclerotic heart disease (coronary artery disease) with angina pectoris. A causal relationship is assumed in a patient with both atherosclerosis and angina pectoris, unless the documentation indicates the angina is due to something other than the atherosclerosis. When using one of these combination codes, it is not necessary to use an additional code for angina pectoris.

c. Intraoperative and postprocedural cerebrovascular accident

Medical record documentation should clearly specify the cause- and- effect relationship between the medical intervention and the cerebrovascular accident in order to assign a code for intraoperative or postprocedural cerebrovascular accident.

Proper code assignment depends on whether it was an infarction or hemorrhage and whether it occurred intraoperatively or postoperatively. If it was a cerebral hemorrhage, code assignment depends on the type of procedure performed.

> Embolic cerebral infarction of the right middle cerebral artery that occurred during hip replacement surgery. The surgeon documented as due to the surgery.
>
> **I97.811**   **Intraoperative cerebrovascular infarction during other surgery**
>
> **I63.411**   **Cerebral infarction due to embolism of right middle cerebral artery**
>
> *Explanation*: Code assignment for intraoperative or postprocedural cerebrovascular accident is based on the provider's documentation of a cause-and-effect relationship between the condition and the procedure. Proper code assignment also depends on whether the cerebrovascular accident was an infarction or hemorrhage, occurred intraoperatively or postoperatively, and the type of procedure performed.

d. Sequelae of cerebrovascular disease

1) Category I69, Sequelae of cerebrovascular disease

Category I69 is used to indicate conditions classifiable to categories I60-I67 as the causes of sequela (neurologic deficits), themselves classified elsewhere. These "late effects" include neurologic deficits that persist after initial onset of conditions classifiable to categories I60-I67. The neurologic deficits caused by cerebrovascular disease may be present from the onset or may arise at any time after the onset of the condition classifiable to categories I60-I67.

Codes from category I69, Sequelae of cerebrovascular disease, that specify hemiplegia, hemiparesis and monoplegia identify whether the dominant or nondominant side is affected. Should the affected side be documented, but not specified as dominant or nondominant, and the classification system does not indicate a default, code selection is as follows:

- For ambidextrous patients, the default should be dominant.
- If the left side is affected, the default is non-dominant.
- If the right side is affected, the default is dominant.

2) Codes from category I69 with codes from I60–I67

Codes from category I69 may be assigned on a health care record with codes from I60-I67, if the patient has a current cerebrovascular disease and deficits from an old cerebrovascular disease.

3) Codes from category I69 and personal history of transient ischemic attack (TIA) and cerebral infarction (Z86.73)

Codes from category I69 should not be assigned if the patient does not have neurologic deficits.

See Section I.C.21. 4. History (of) for use of personal history codes

e. Acute myocardial infarction (AMI)

1) ST elevation myocardial infarction (STEMI) and non ST elevation myocardial infarction (NSTEMI)

The ICD-10-CM codes for acute myocardial infarction (AMI) identify the site, such as anterolateral wall or true posterior wall. Subcategories I21.0-I21.2 and code I21.3 are used for ST elevation myocardial infarction (STEMI). Code I21.4, Non-ST elevation (NSTEMI) myocardial infarction, is used for non ST elevation myocardial infarction (NSTEMI) and nontransmural MIs.

If NSTEMI evolves to STEMI, assign the STEMI code. If STEMI converts to NSTEMI due to thrombolytic therapy, it is still coded as STEMI.

> Acute inferior NSTEMI evolved into STEMI
>
> **I21.19**   **ST elevation (STEMI) myocardial infarction involving other coronary artery of inferior wall**
>
> *Explanation*: If an NSTEMI converts to a STEMI, report only the STEMI code.

For encounters occurring while the myocardial infarction is equal to, or less than, four weeks old, including transfers to another acute setting or a postacute setting, and the myocardial infarction **meets the definition for "other diagnoses" (see Section III, Reporting Additional Diagnoses)**, codes from category I21 may continue to be reported. For encounters after the 4 week time frame and the patient is still receiving care related to the myocardial infarction, the appropriate aftercare code should be assigned, rather than a code from category I21. For old or healed myocardial infarctions not requiring further care, code I25.2, Old myocardial infarction, may be assigned.

2) Acute myocardial infarction, unspecified

Code I21.3, ST elevation (STEMI) myocardial infarction of unspecified site, is the default for unspecified acute myocardial infarction. If only STEMI or transmural MI without the site is documented, assign code I21.3.

3) AMI documented as nontransmural or subendocardial but site provided

If an AMI is documented as nontransmural or subendocardial, but the site is provided, it is still coded as a subendocardial AMI.

See Section I.C.21.3 for information on coding status post administration of tPA in a different facility within the last 24 hours.

> Acute inferior subendocardial myocardial infarction (NSTEMI)
>
> **I21.4**   **Non-ST elevation (NSTEMI) myocardial infarction**
>
> *Explanation*: An AMI documented as subendocardial or nontransmural is coded as such (I21.4, I22.2), even if the site of infarction is specified.

4) Subsequent acute myocardial infarction

A code from category I22, Subsequent ST elevation (STEMI) and non ST elevation (NSTEMI) myocardial infarction, is to be used when a patient who has suffered an AMI has a new AMI within the 4 week time frame of the initial AMI. A code from category I22 must be used in conjunction with a code from category I21. The sequencing of the I22 and I21 codes depends on the circumstances of the encounter.

> Acute inferior STEMI status post acute NSTEMI two weeks ago.
>
> **I22.1**   **Subsequent ST elevation (STEMI) infarction of inferior wall**
>
> **I21.4**   **Non-ST elevation (NSTEMI) myocardial infarction**
>
> *Explanation*: A code from I22 must be used in conjunction with a code from I21 when a patient who has suffered an AMI has a new AMI within four weeks of the initial one. Category I22 is never reported alone. The guidelines for assigning the correct I22 code are the same as those for reporting the initial MI (I21). Sequencing is determined by the circumstances of the encounter.

Chapter 9. Diseases of the Circulatory System *(sidebar)*

Chapter 9. Diseases of the Circulatory System (I00-I99)

EXCLUDES 2   certain conditions originating in the perinatal period (P04-P96)
certain infectious and parasitic diseases (A00-B99)
complications of pregnancy, childbirth and the puerperium (O00-O9A)
congenital malformations, deformations, and chromosomal abnormalities (Q00-Q99)
endocrine, nutritional and metabolic diseases (E00-E88)
injury, poisoning and certain other consequences of external causes (S00-T88)
neoplasms (C00-D49)
symptoms, signs and abnormal clinical and laboratory findings, not elsewhere classified (R00-R94)
systemic connective tissue disorders (M30-M36)
transient cerebral ischemic attacks and related syndromes (G45.-)

This chapter contains the following blocks:

I00-I02   Acute rheumatic fever
I05-I09   Chronic rheumatic heart diseases
▶I10-I16◀   Hypertensive diseases
I20-I25   Ischemic heart diseases
I26-I28   Pulmonary heart disease and diseases of pulmonary circulation
I30-I52   Other forms of heart disease
I60-I69   Cerebrovascular diseases
I70-I79   Diseases of arteries, arterioles and capillaries
I80-I89   Diseases of veins, lymphatic vessels and lymph nodes, not elsewhere classified
I95-I99   Other and unspecified disorders of the circulatory system

Acute rheumatic fever (I00-I02)

I00   Rheumatic fever without heart involvement
   INCLUDES   arthritis, rheumatic, acute or subacute
   EXCLUDES 1   rheumatic fever with heart involvement (I01.0-I01.9)

✓4ᵗʰ **I01   Rheumatic fever with heart involvement**
   EXCLUDES 1   chronic diseases of rheumatic origin (I05-I09) unless rheumatic fever is also present or there is evidence of reactivation or activity of the rheumatic process

   I01.0   Acute rheumatic pericarditis
     Any condition in I00 with pericarditis
     Rheumatic pericarditis (acute)
     EXCLUDES 1   acute pericarditis not specified as rheumatic (I30.-)

   I01.1   Acute rheumatic endocarditis
     Any condition in I00 with endocarditis or valvulitis
     Acute rheumatic valvulitis

   I01.2   Acute rheumatic myocarditis
     Any condition in I00 with myocarditis

   I01.8   Other acute rheumatic heart disease
     Any condition in I00 with other or multiple types of heart involvement
     Acute rheumatic pancarditis

   I01.9   Acute rheumatic heart disease, unspecified   ▽
     Any condition in I00 with unspecified type of heart involvement
     Rheumatic carditis, acute
     Rheumatic heart disease, active or acute

✓4ᵗʰ **I02   Rheumatic chorea**
   INCLUDES   Sydenham's chorea
   EXCLUDES 1   chorea NOS (G25.5)
       Huntington's chorea (G10)

   I02.0   Rheumatic chorea with heart involvement
     Chorea NOS with heart involvement
     Rheumatic chorea with heart involvement of any type classifiable under I01.-

   I02.9   Rheumatic chorea without heart involvement
     Rheumatic chorea NOS

Chronic rheumatic heart diseases (I05-I09)

✓4ᵗʰ **I05   Rheumatic mitral valve diseases**
   INCLUDES   conditions classifiable to both I05.0 and I05.2-I05.9, whether specified as rheumatic or not
   EXCLUDES 1   mitral valve disease specified as nonrheumatic (I34.-)
     mitral valve disease with aortic and/or tricuspid valve involvement (I08.-)

   I05.0   Rheumatic mitral stenosis
     Mitral (valve) obstruction (rheumatic)

   I05.1   Rheumatic mitral insufficiency
     Rheumatic mitral incompetence
     Rheumatic mitral regurgitation
     EXCLUDES 1   mitral insufficiency not specified as rheumatic (I34.0)

   I05.2   Rheumatic mitral stenosis with insufficiency
     Rheumatic mitral stenosis with incompetence or regurgitation

   I05.8   Other rheumatic mitral valve diseases
     Rheumatic mitral (valve) failure

   I05.9   Rheumatic mitral valve disease, unspecified   ▽
     Rheumatic mitral (valve) disorder (chronic) NOS

✓4ᵗʰ **I06   Rheumatic aortic valve diseases**
   EXCLUDES 1   aortic valve disease not specified as rheumatic (I35.-)
     aortic valve disease with mitral and/or tricuspid valve involvement (I08.-)

   I06.0   Rheumatic aortic stenosis
     Rheumatic aortic (valve) obstruction

   I06.1   Rheumatic aortic insufficiency
     Rheumatic aortic incompetence
     Rheumatic aortic regurgitation

   I06.2   Rheumatic aortic stenosis with insufficiency
     Rheumatic aortic stenosis with incompetence or regurgitation

   I06.8   Other rheumatic aortic valve diseases

   I06.9   Rheumatic aortic valve disease, unspecified   ▽
     Rheumatic aortic (valve) disease NOS

✓4ᵗʰ **I07   Rheumatic tricuspid valve diseases**
   INCLUDES   rheumatic tricuspid valve diseases specified as rheumatic or unspecified
   EXCLUDES 1   tricuspid valve disease specified as nonrheumatic (I36.-)
     tricuspid valve disease with aortic and/or mitral valve involvement (I08.-)

   I07.0   Rheumatic tricuspid stenosis
     Tricuspid (valve) stenosis (rheumatic)

   I07.1   Rheumatic tricuspid insufficiency
     Tricuspid (valve) insufficiency (rheumatic)

   I07.2   Rheumatic tricuspid stenosis and insufficiency

   I07.8   Other rheumatic tricuspid valve diseases

   I07.9   Rheumatic tricuspid valve disease, unspecified   ▽
     Rheumatic tricuspid valve disorder NOS

✓4ᵗʰ **I08   Multiple valve diseases**
   INCLUDES   multiple valve diseases specified as rheumatic or unspecified
   EXCLUDES 1   endocarditis, valve unspecified (I38)
     multiple valve disease specified a nonrheumatic (I34.-, I35.-, I36.-, I37.-, I38.-, Q22.-, Q23.-, Q24.8-)
     rheumatic valve disease NOS (I09.1)

   I08.0   Rheumatic disorders of both mitral and aortic valves
     Involvement of both mitral and aortic valves specified as rheumatic or unspecified

   I08.1   Rheumatic disorders of both mitral and tricuspid valves

   I08.2   Rheumatic disorders of both aortic and tricuspid valves

   I08.3   Combined rheumatic disorders of mitral, aortic and tricuspid valves

   I08.8   Other rheumatic multiple valve diseases

   I08.9   Rheumatic multiple valve disease, unspecified   ▽

✓4ᵗʰ **I09   Other rheumatic heart diseases**

   I09.0   Rheumatic myocarditis
     EXCLUDES 1   myocarditis not specified as rheumatic (I51.4)

   I09.1   Rheumatic diseases of endocardium, valve unspecified   ▽
     Rheumatic endocarditis (chronic)
     Rheumatic valvulitis (chronic)
     EXCLUDES 1   endocarditis, valve unspecified (I38)

   I09.2   Chronic rheumatic pericarditis
     Adherent pericardium, rheumatic
     Chronic rheumatic mediastinopericarditis
     Chronic rheumatic myopericarditis
     EXCLUDES 1   chronic pericarditis not specified as rheumatic (I31.-)

✓5ᵗʰ **I09.8   Other specified rheumatic heart diseases**

     I09.81   Rheumatic heart failure
       Use additional code to identify type of heart failure (I50.-)
       DEF: Decreased cardiac output, edema, and hypertension; due to rheumatic heart disease.

     I09.89   Other specified rheumatic heart diseases
       Rheumatic disease of pulmonary valve

   I09.9   Rheumatic heart disease, unspecified   ▽
     Rheumatic carditis
     EXCLUDES 1   rheumatoid carditis (M05.31)

EXCLUDES 1 Not coded here   **EXCLUDES 2** Not included here   **N** Newborn Age : 0   **P** Pediatric Age : 0-17   **M** Maternity Age : 12-55   **A** Adult Age : 15-124

Hypertensive diseases ▶(I10-I16)◀

Use additional code to identify:
  exposure to environmental tobacco smoke (Z77.22)
  ▶history of tobacco dependence (Z87.891)◀
  occupational exposure to environmental tobacco smoke (Z57.31)
  tobacco dependence (F17.-)
  tobacco use (Z72.0)
  EXCLUDES 1   neonatal hypertension (P29.2)
      primary pulmonary hypertension (I27.0)
  EXCLUDES 2 ▶hypertensive disease complicating pregnancy, childbirth and the
      puerperium (O10-O11, O13-O16)◀

I10 Essential (primary) hypertension
  INCLUDES high blood pressure
      hypertension (arterial) (benign) (essential) (malignant)
        (primary) (systemic)
  EXCLUDES 1 hypertensive disease complicating pregnancy, childbirth and
      the puerperium (O10-O11, O13-O16)
  EXCLUDES 2 essential (primary) hypertension involving vessels of brain
      (I60-I69)
      essential (primary) hypertension involving vessels of eye
      (H35.0-)

✓4ᵗʰ I11 Hypertensive heart disease
  INCLUDES any condition in I51.4-I51.9 due to hypertension

I11.0 Hypertensive heart disease with heart failure
  Hypertensive heart failure
  Use additional code to identify type of heart failure (I50.-)

I11.9 Hypertensive heart disease without heart failure   ▽
  Hypertensive heart disease NOS

✓4ᵗʰ I12 Hypertensive chronic kidney disease
  INCLUDES any condition in N18 and N26 - due to hypertension
      arteriosclerosis of kidney
      arteriosclerotic nephritis (chronic) (interstitial)
      hypertensive nephropathy
      nephrosclerosis
  EXCLUDES 1 hypertension due to kidney disease (I15.0, I15.1)
      renovascular hypertension (I15.0)
      secondary hypertension (I15.-)
  EXCLUDES 2 acute kidney failure (N17.-)

I12.0 Hypertensive chronic kidney disease with stage 5 chronic
  kidney disease or end stage renal disease
    Use additional code to identify the stage of chronic kidney
      disease (N18.5, N18.6)

I12.9 Hypertensive chronic kidney disease with stage 1   ▽
  through stage 4 chronic kidney disease, or unspecified
  chronic kidney disease
    Hypertensive chronic kidney disease NOS
    Hypertensive renal disease NOS
    Use additional code to identify the stage of chronic kidney
      disease (N18.1-N18.4, N18.9)

✓4ᵗʰ I13 Hypertensive heart and chronic kidney disease
  INCLUDES any condition in I11.- with any condition in I12.-
      cardiorenal disease
      cardiovascular renal disease

I13.0 Hypertensive heart and chronic kidney disease with heart
  failure and stage 1 through stage 4 chronic kidney disease,
  or unspecified chronic kidney disease
    Use additional code to identify type of heart failure (I50.-)
    Use additional code to identify stage of chronic kidney disease
      (N18.1-N18.4, N18.9)

✓5ᵗʰ I13.1 Hypertensive heart and chronic kidney disease without heart
  failure

  I13.10 Hypertensive heart and chronic kidney   ▽
    disease without heart failure, with stage 1
    through stage 4 chronic kidney disease, or
    unspecified chronic kidney disease
      Hypertensive heart disease and hypertensive chronic
        kidney disease NOS
      Use additional code to identify the stage of chronic
        kidney disease (N18.1-N18.4, N18.9)

  I13.11 Hypertensive heart and chronic kidney disease
    without heart failure, with stage 5 chronic kidney
    disease, or end stage renal disease
      Use additional code to identify the stage of chronic
        kidney disease (N18.5, N18.6)

I13.2 Hypertensive heart and chronic kidney disease with heart
  failure and with stage 5 chronic kidney disease, or end stage
  renal disease
    Use additional code to identify type of heart failure (I50.-)
    Use additional code to identify the stage of chronic kidney
      disease (N18.5, N18.6)

✓4ᵗʰ I15 Secondary hypertension
  Code also underlying condition
  EXCLUDES 1 postprocedural hypertension (I97.3)
  EXCLUDES 2 secondary hypertension involving vessels of brain (I60-I69)
      secondary hypertension involving vessels of eye (H35.0-)

I15.0 Renovascular hypertension
I15.1 Hypertension secondary to other renal disorders
I15.2 Hypertension secondary to endocrine disorders
I15.8 Other secondary hypertension
I15.9 Secondary hypertension, unspecified   ▽

● ✓4ᵗʰ I16 Hypertensive crisis
  Code also any identified hypertensive disease (I10-I15)
 ● **I16.0** Hypertensive urgency
 ● **I16.1** Hypertensive emergency
 ● **I16.9** Hypertensive crisis, unspecified   ▽

Ischemic heart diseases (I20-I25)

Use additional code to identify presence of hypertension ▶ (I10-I16)◀

✓4ᵗʰ I20 Angina pectoris
  Use additional code to identify:
  exposure to environmental tobacco smoke (Z77.22)
  ▶history of tobacco dependence (Z87.891)◀
  occupational exposure to environmental tobacco smoke (Z57.31)
  tobacco dependence (F17.-)
  tobacco use (Z72.0)
  EXCLUDES 1 angina pectoris with atherosclerotic heart disease of native
      coronary arteries (I25.1-)
      atherosclerosis of coronary artery bypass graft(s) and coronary
      artery of transplanted heart with angina pectoris (I25.7-)
      postinfarction angina (I23.7)

I20.0 Unstable angina
  Accelerated angina
  Crescendo angina
  De novo effort angina
  Intermediate coronary syndrome
  Preinfarction syndrome
  Worsening effort angina
  DEF: A condition representing an intermediate stage between
  angina of effort and acute myocardial infarction.

I20.1 Angina pectoris with documented spasm
  Angiospastic angina
  Prinzmetal angina
  Spasm-induced angina
  Variant angina

I20.8 Other forms of angina pectoris
  Angina equivalent
  Angina of effort
  Coronary slow flow syndrome
  ▶Stable angina◀
  Stenocardia
  Use additional code(s) for symptoms associated with angina
    equivalent

I20.9 Angina pectoris, unspecified   ▽
  Angina NOS
  Anginal syndrome
  Cardiac angina
  Ischemic chest pain

☑ Additional Character Required   ✓x7ᵗʰ Placeholder Alert   Manifestation Dx   ▽ Unspecified Dx   ▶◀ Revised Text   ● New Code   ▲ Revised Code Title

ICD-10-CM 2017   **607**

✓4th I21 ST elevation (STEMI) and non-ST elevation (NSTEMI) myocardial infarction

INCLUDES cardiac infarction
coronary (artery) embolism
coronary (artery) occlusion
coronary (artery) rupture
coronary (artery) thrombosis
infarction of heart, myocardium, or ventricle
myocardial infarction specified as acute or with a stated duration of 4 weeks (28 days) or less from onset

Use additional code, if applicable, to identify:
exposure to environmental tobacco smoke (Z77.22)
► history of tobacco dependence (Z87.891)◄
occupational exposure to environmental tobacco smoke (Z57.31)
status post administration of tPA (rtPA) in a different facility within the last 24 hours prior to admission to current facility (Z92.82)
tobacco dependence (F17.-)
tobacco use (Z72.0)

EXCLUDES 2 *old myocardial infarction (I25.2)*
postmyocardial infarction syndrome (I24.1)
subsequent myocardial infarction (I22.-)

AHA: 2015,2Q,16; 2013,1Q,25; 2012,4Q,96,102-103

✓5th I21.0 ST elevation (STEMI) myocardial infarction of anterior wall

I21.01 ST elevation (STEMI) myocardial infarction involving left main coronary artery

I21.02 ST elevation (STEMI) myocardial infarction involving left anterior descending coronary artery
ST elevation (STEMI) myocardial infarction involving diagonal coronary artery
AHA: 2013,1Q,25

I21.09 ST elevation (STEMI) myocardial infarction involving other coronary artery of anterior wall
Acute transmural myocardial infarction of anterior wall
Anteroapical transmural (Q wave) infarction (acute)
Anterolateral transmural (Q wave) infarction (acute)
Anteroseptal transmural (Q wave) infarction (acute)
Transmural (Q wave) infarction (acute) (of) anterior (wall) NOS
AHA: 2012,4Q,102-103

✓5th I21.1 ST elevation (STEMI) myocardial infarction of inferior wall

I21.11 ST elevation (STEMI) myocardial infarction involving right coronary artery
Inferoposterior transmural (Q wave) infarction (acute)

I21.19 ST elevation (STEMI) myocardial infarction involving other coronary artery of inferior wall
Acute transmural myocardial infarction of inferior wall
Inferolateral transmural (Q wave) infarction (acute)
Transmural (Q wave) infarction (acute) (of) diaphragmatic wall
Transmural (Q wave) infarction (acute) (of) inferior (wall) NOS
EXCLUDES 2 *ST elevation (STEMI) myocardial infarction involving left circumflex coronary artery (I21.21)*
AHA: 2012,4Q,96

✓5th I21.2 ST elevation (STEMI) myocardial infarction of other sites

I21.21 ST elevation (STEMI) myocardial infarction involving left circumflex coronary artery
ST elevation (STEMI) myocardial infarction involving oblique marginal coronary artery

I21.29 ST elevation (STEMI) myocardial infarction involving other sites
Acute transmural myocardial infarction of other sites
Apical-lateral transmural (Q wave) infarction (acute)
Basal-lateral transmural (Q wave) infarction (acute)
High lateral transmural (Q wave) infarction (acute)
Lateral (wall) NOS transmural (Q wave) infarction (acute)
Posterior (true) transmural (Q wave) infarction (acute)
Posterobasal transmural (Q wave) infarction (acute)
Posterolateral transmural (Q wave) infarction (acute)
Posteroseptal transmural (Q wave) infarction (acute)
Septal transmural (Q wave) infarction (acute) NOS

I21.3 ST elevation (STEMI) myocardial infarction of unspecified site ▽
Acute transmural myocardial infarction of unspecified site
Myocardial infarction (acute) NOS
Transmural (Q wave) myocardial infarction NOS

I21.4 Non-ST elevation (NSTEMI) myocardial infarction
Acute subendocardial myocardial infarction
Non-Q wave myocardial infarction NOS
Nontransmural myocardial infarction NOS

✓4th I22 Subsequent ST elevation (STEMI) and non-ST elevation (NSTEMI) myocardial infarction

INCLUDES acute myocardial infarction occurring within four weeks (28 days) of a previous acute myocardial infarction, regardless of site
cardiac infarction
coronary (artery) embolism
coronary (artery) occlusion
coronary (artery) rupture
coronary (artery) thrombosis
infarction of heart, myocardium, or ventricle
recurrent myocardial infarction
reinfarction of myocardium
rupture of heart, myocardium, or ventricle

Use additional code, if applicable, to identify:
exposure to environmental tobacco smoke (Z77.22)
► history of tobacco dependence (Z87.891)◄
occupational exposure to environmental tobacco smoke (Z57.31)
status post administration of tPA (rtPA) in a different facility within the last 24 hours prior to admission to current facility (Z92.82)
tobacco dependence (F17.-)
tobacco use (Z72.0)

AHA: 2013,1Q,25; 2012,4Q,97,102-103

I22.0 Subsequent ST elevation (STEMI) myocardial infarction of anterior wall
Subsequent acute transmural myocardial infarction of anterior wall
Subsequent transmural (Q wave) infarction (acute)(of) anterior (wall) NOS
Subsequent anteroapical transmural (Q wave) infarction (acute)
Subsequent anterolateral transmural (Q wave) infarction (acute)
Subsequent anteroseptal transmural (Q wave) infarction (acute)

I22.1 Subsequent ST elevation (STEMI) myocardial infarction of inferior wall
Subsequent acute transmural myocardial infarction of inferior wall
Subsequent transmural (Q wave) infarction (acute)(of) diaphragmatic wall
Subsequent transmural (Q wave) infarction (acute)(of) inferior (wall) NOS
Subsequent inferolateral transmural (Q wave) infarction (acute)
Subsequent inferoposterior transmural (Q wave) infarction (acute)
AHA: 2012,4Q,102

I22.2 Subsequent non-ST elevation (NSTEMI) myocardial infarction
Subsequent acute subendocardial myocardial infarction
Subsequent non-Q wave myocardial infarction NOS
Subsequent nontransmural myocardial infarction NOS

EXCLUDES 1 Not coded here   EXCLUDES 2 Not included here   N Newborn Age : 0   P Pediatric Age : 0-17   M Maternity Age : 12-55   A Adult Age : 15-124

I22.8 Subsequent ST elevation (STEMI) myocardial infarction of other sites
Subsequent acute transmural myocardial infarction of other sites
Subsequent apical-lateral transmural (Q wave) myocardial infarction (acute)
Subsequent basal-lateral transmural (Q wave) myocardial infarction (acute)
Subsequent high lateral transmural (Q wave) myocardial infarction (acute)
Subsequent transmural (Q wave) myocardial infarction (acute)(of) lateral (wall) NOS
Subsequent posterior (true)transmural (Q wave) myocardial infarction (acute)
Subsequent posterobasal transmural (Q wave) myocardial infarction (acute)
Subsequent posterolateral transmural (Q wave) myocardial infarction (acute)
Subsequent posteroseptal transmural (Q wave) myocardial infarction (acute)
Subsequent septal NOS transmural (Q wave) myocardial infarction (acute)

I22.9 Subsequent ST elevation (STEMI) myocardial infarction of unspecified site ▽
Subsequent acute myocardial infarction of unspecified site
Subsequent myocardial infarction (acute) NOS

✓4ᵗʰ **I23 Certain current complications following ST elevation (STEMI) and non-ST elevation (NSTEMI) myocardial infarction (within the 28 day period)**

I23.0 Hemopericardium as current complication following acute myocardial infarction Ⓐ
EXCLUDES 1 hemopericardium not specified as current complication following acute myocardial infarction (I31.2)

I23.1 Atrial septal defect as current complication following acute myocardial infarction Ⓐ
EXCLUDES 1 acquired atrial septal defect not specified as current complication following acute myocardial infarction (I51.0)

I23.2 Ventricular septal defect as current complication following acute myocardial infarction Ⓐ
EXCLUDES 1 acquired ventricular septal defect not specified as current complication following acute myocardial infarction (I51.0)

I23.3 Rupture of cardiac wall without hemopericardium as current complication following acute myocardial infarction Ⓐ

I23.4 Rupture of chordae tendineae as current complication following acute myocardial infarction Ⓐ
EXCLUDES 1 rupture of chordae tendineae not specified as current complication following acute myocardial infarction (I51.1)

I23.5 Rupture of papillary muscle as current complication following acute myocardial infarction Ⓐ
EXCLUDES 1 rupture of papillary muscle not specified as current complication following acute myocardial infarction (I51.2)

I23.6 Thrombosis of atrium, auricular appendage, and ventricle as current complications following acute myocardial infarction Ⓐ
EXCLUDES 1 thrombosis of atrium, auricular appendage, and ventricle not specified as current complication following acute myocardial infarction (I51.3)

I23.7 Postinfarction angina Ⓐ
AHA: 2015,2Q,16

I23.8 Other current complications following acute myocardial infarction Ⓐ

✓4ᵗʰ **I24 Other acute ischemic heart diseases**
EXCLUDES 1 angina pectoris (I20.-)
transient myocardial ischemia in newborn (P29.4)

I24.0 Acute coronary thrombosis not resulting in myocardial infarction
Acute coronary (artery) (vein) embolism not resulting in myocardial infarction
Acute coronary (artery) (vein) occlusion not resulting in myocardial infarction
Acute coronary (artery) (vein) thromboembolism not resulting in myocardial infarction
EXCLUDES 1 atherosclerotic heart disease (I25.1-)
AHA: 2013,1Q,24

I24.1 Dressler's syndrome
Postmyocardial infarction syndrome
EXCLUDES 1 postinfarction angina (I23.7)

I24.8 Other forms of acute ischemic heart disease

I24.9 Acute ischemic heart disease, unspecified ▽
EXCLUDES 1 ischemic heart disease (chronic) NOS (I25.9)

✓4ᵗʰ **I25 Chronic ischemic heart disease**
Use additional code to identify:
chronic total occlusion of coronary artery (I25.82)
exposure to environmental tobacco smoke (Z77.22)
▶history of tobacco dependence (Z87.891)◀
occupational exposure to environmental tobacco smoke (Z57.31)
tobacco dependence (F17.-)
tobacco use (Z72.0)

Atheromas

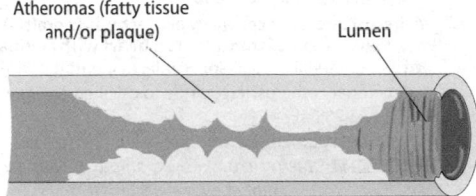

Atheromas (fatty tissue and/or plaque)   Lumen

✓5ᵗʰ **I25.1 Atherosclerotic heart disease of native coronary artery**
Atherosclerotic cardiovascular disease
Coronary (artery) atheroma
Coronary (artery) atherosclerosis
Coronary (artery) disease
Coronary (artery) sclerosis
Use additional code, if applicable, to identify:
coronary atherosclerosis due to calcified coronary lesion (I25.84)
coronary atherosclerosis due to lipid rich plaque (I25.83)
EXCLUDES 2 atheroembolism (I75.-)
atherosclerosis of coronary artery bypass graft(s) and transplanted heart (I25.7-)

I25.10 Atherosclerotic heart disease of native coronary artery without angina pectoris Ⓐ ▽
Atherosclerotic heart disease NOS
AHA: 2015,2Q,16; 2012,4Q,92

✓6ᵗʰ **I25.11 Atherosclerotic heart disease of native coronary artery with angina pectoris**
I25.110 Atherosclerotic heart disease of native coronary artery with unstable angina pectoris Ⓐ
EXCLUDES 1 unstable angina without atherosclerotic heart disease (I20.0)

I25.111 Atherosclerotic heart disease of native coronary artery with angina pectoris with documented spasm Ⓐ
EXCLUDES 1 angina pectoris with documented spasm without atherosclerotic heart disease (I20.1)

I25.118 Atherosclerotic heart disease of native coronary artery with other forms of angina pectoris Ⓐ
EXCLUDES 1 other forms of angina pectoris without atherosclerotic heart disease (I20.8)
AHA: 2015,2Q,16

☑ Additional Character Required   ✓x7ᵗʰ Placeholder Alert   Manifestation Dx   ▽ Unspecified Dx   ▶◀ Revised Text   ● New Code   ▲ Revised Code Title

ICD-10-CM 2017   609

Chapter 9. Diseases of the Circulatory System

I25.119   **Atherosclerotic heart disease of native coronary artery with unspecified angina pectoris**   A ▽

Atherosclerotic heart disease with angina NOS

Atherosclerotic heart disease with ischemic chest pain

EXCLUDES 1   *unspecified angina pectoris without atherosclerotic heart disease (I20.9)*

I25.2   **Old myocardial infarction**

Healed myocardial infarction

Past myocardial infarction diagnosed by ECG or other investigation, but currently presenting no symptoms

I25.3   **Aneurysm of heart**

Mural aneurysm

Ventricular aneurysm

✓5th **I25.4**   **Coronary artery aneurysm and dissection**

I25.41   **Coronary artery aneurysm**

Coronary arteriovenous fistula, acquired

EXCLUDES 1   *congenital coronary (artery) aneurysm (Q24.5)*

I25.42   **Coronary artery dissection**

DEF: A tear in the intimal arterial wall of a coronary artery resulting in the sudden intrusion of blood within the layers of the wall.

I25.5   **Ischemic cardiomyopathy**

EXCLUDES 2   *coronary atherosclerosis (I25.1-, I25.7-)*

I25.6   **Silent myocardial ischemia**

✓5th **I25.7**   **Atherosclerosis of coronary artery bypass graft(s) and coronary artery of transplanted heart with angina pectoris**

Use additional code, if applicable, to identify:

coronary atherosclerosis due to calcified coronary lesion (I25.84)

coronary atherosclerosis due to lipid rich plaque (I25.83)

EXCLUDES 1   *atherosclerosis of bypass graft(s) of transplanted heart without angina pectoris (I25.812)*

atherosclerosis of coronary artery bypass graft(s) without angina pectoris (I25.810)

atherosclerosis of native coronary artery of transplanted heart without angina pectoris (I25.811)

embolism or thrombus of coronary artery bypass graft(s) (T82.8-)

✓6th **I25.70**   **Atherosclerosis of coronary artery bypass graft(s), unspecified, with angina pectoris**

I25.700   **Atherosclerosis of coronary artery bypass graft(s), unspecified, with unstable angina pectoris**   A ▽

EXCLUDES 1   *unstable angina pectoris without atherosclerosis of coronary artery bypass graft (I20.0)*

I25.701   **Atherosclerosis of coronary artery bypass graft(s), unspecified, with angina pectoris with documented spasm**   A ▽

EXCLUDES 1   *angina pectoris with documented spasm without atherosclerosis of coronary artery bypass graft (I20.1)*

I25.708   **Atherosclerosis of coronary artery bypass graft(s), unspecified, with other forms of angina pectoris**   A ▽

EXCLUDES 1   *other forms of angina pectoris without atherosclerosis of coronary artery bypass graft (I20.8)*

I25.709   **Atherosclerosis of coronary artery bypass graft(s), unspecified, with unspecified angina pectoris**   A ▽

EXCLUDES 1   *unspecified angina pectoris without atherosclerosis of coronary artery bypass graft (I20.9)*

✓6th **I25.71**   **Atherosclerosis of autologous vein coronary artery bypass graft(s) with angina pectoris**

I25.710   **Atherosclerosis of autologous vein coronary artery bypass graft(s) with unstable angina pectoris**   A

EXCLUDES 1   *unstable angina without atherosclerosis of autologous vein coronary artery bypass graft(s) (I20.0)*

I25.711   **Atherosclerosis of autologous vein coronary artery bypass graft(s) with angina pectoris with documented spasm**   A

EXCLUDES 1   *angina pectoris with documented spasm without atherosclerosis of autologous vein coronary artery bypass graft(s) (I20.1)*

I25.718   **Atherosclerosis of autologous vein coronary artery bypass graft(s) with other forms of angina pectoris**   A

EXCLUDES 1   *other forms of angina pectoris without atherosclerosis of autologous vein coronary artery bypass graft(s) (I20.8)*

I25.719   **Atherosclerosis of autologous vein coronary artery bypass graft(s) with unspecified angina pectoris**   A ▽

EXCLUDES 1   *unspecified angina pectoris without atherosclerosis of autologous vein coronary artery bypass graft(s) (I20.9)*

✓6th **I25.72**   **Atherosclerosis of autologous artery coronary artery bypass graft(s) with angina pectoris**

Atherosclerosis of internal mammary artery graft with angina pectoris

I25.720   **Atherosclerosis of autologous artery coronary artery bypass graft(s) with unstable angina pectoris**   A

EXCLUDES 1   *unstable angina without atherosclerosis of autologous artery coronary artery bypass graft(s) (I20.0)*

I25.721   **Atherosclerosis of autologous artery coronary artery bypass graft(s) with angina pectoris with documented spasm**   A

EXCLUDES 1   *angina pectoris with documented spasm without atherosclerosis of autologous artery coronary artery bypass graft(s) (I20.1)*

I25.728   **Atherosclerosis of autologous artery coronary artery bypass graft(s) with other forms of angina pectoris**   A

EXCLUDES 1   *other forms of angina pectoris without atherosclerosis of autologous artery coronary artery bypass graft(s) (I20.8)*

I25.729   **Atherosclerosis of autologous artery coronary artery bypass graft(s) with unspecified angina pectoris**   A ▽

EXCLUDES 1   *unspecified angina pectoris without atherosclerosis of autologous artery coronary artery bypass graft(s) (I20.9)*

✓6th **I25.73**   **Atherosclerosis of nonautologous biological coronary artery bypass graft(s) with angina pectoris**

I25.730   **Atherosclerosis of nonautologous biological coronary artery bypass graft(s) with unstable angina pectoris**   A

EXCLUDES 1   *unstable angina without atherosclerosis of nonautologous biological coronary artery bypass graft(s) (I20.0)*

EXCLUDES 1   Not coded here   EXCLUDES 2   Not included here   N Newborn Age : 0   P Pediatric Age : 0-17   M Maternity Age : 12-55   A Adult Age : 15-124

610

ICD-10-CM 2017

I25.731   **Atherosclerosis of nonautologous biological coronary artery bypass graft(s) with angina pectoris with documented spasm** ▢A

     EXCLUDES 1   *angina pectoris with documented spasm without atherosclerosis of nonautologous biological coronary artery bypass graft(s) (I20.1)*

I25.738   **Atherosclerosis of nonautologous biological coronary artery bypass graft(s) with other forms of angina pectoris** ▢A

     EXCLUDES 1   *other forms of angina pectoris without atherosclerosis of nonautologous biological coronary artery bypass graft(s) (I20.8)*

I25.739   **Atherosclerosis of nonautologous biological coronary artery bypass graft(s) with unspecified angina pectoris** ▢A ▽

     EXCLUDES 1   *unspecified angina pectoris without atherosclerosis of nonautologous biological coronary artery bypass graft(s) (I20.9)*

✓6ᵗʰ   **I25.75**   **Atherosclerosis of native coronary artery of transplanted heart with angina pectoris**

     EXCLUDES 1   *atherosclerosis of native coronary artery of transplanted heart without angina pectoris (I25.811)*

I25.750   **Atherosclerosis of native coronary artery of transplanted heart with unstable angina**

I25.751   **Atherosclerosis of native coronary artery of transplanted heart with angina pectoris with documented spasm**

I25.758   **Atherosclerosis of native coronary artery of transplanted heart with other forms of angina pectoris**

I25.759   **Atherosclerosis of native coronary artery of transplanted heart with unspecified angina pectoris** ▽

✓6ᵗʰ   **I25.76**   **Atherosclerosis of bypass graft of coronary artery of transplanted heart with angina pectoris**

     EXCLUDES 1   *atherosclerosis of bypass graft of coronary artery of transplanted heart without angina pectoris (I25.812)*

I25.760   **Atherosclerosis of bypass graft of coronary artery of transplanted heart with unstable angina** ▢A

I25.761   **Atherosclerosis of bypass graft of coronary artery of transplanted heart with angina pectoris with documented spasm** ▢A

I25.768   **Atherosclerosis of bypass graft of coronary artery of transplanted heart with other forms of angina pectoris** ▢A

I25.769   **Atherosclerosis of bypass graft of coronary artery of transplanted heart with unspecified angina pectoris** ▢A ▽

✓6ᵗʰ   **I25.79**   **Atherosclerosis of other coronary artery bypass graft(s) with angina pectoris**

I25.790   **Atherosclerosis of other coronary artery bypass graft(s) with unstable angina pectoris** ▢A

     EXCLUDES 1   *unstable angina without atherosclerosis of other coronary artery bypass graft(s) (I20.0)*

I25.791   **Atherosclerosis of other coronary artery bypass graft(s) with angina pectoris with documented spasm** ▢A

     EXCLUDES 1   *angina pectoris with documented spasm without atherosclerosis of other coronary artery bypass graft(s) (I20.1)*

I25.798   **Atherosclerosis of other coronary artery bypass graft(s) with other forms of angina pectoris** ▢A

     EXCLUDES 1   *other forms of angina pectoris without atherosclerosis of other coronary artery bypass graft(s) (I20.8)*

I25.799   **Atherosclerosis of other coronary artery bypass graft(s) with unspecified angina pectoris** ▢A ▽

     EXCLUDES 1   *unspecified angina pectoris without atherosclerosis of other coronary artery bypass graft(s) (I20.9)*

✓5ᵗʰ   **I25.8**   **Other forms of chronic ischemic heart disease**

✓6ᵗʰ   **I25.81**   **Atherosclerosis of other coronary vessels without angina pectoris**

     Use additional code, if applicable, to identify:

        coronary atherosclerosis due to calcified coronary lesion (I25.84)

        coronary atherosclerosis due to lipid rich plaque (I25.83)

     EXCLUDES 1   *atherosclerotic heart disease of native coronary artery without angina pectoris (I25.10)*

I25.810   **Atherosclerosis of coronary artery bypass graft(s) without angina pectoris** ▢A

     Atherosclerosis of coronary artery bypass graft NOS

     EXCLUDES 1   *atherosclerosis of coronary bypass graft(s) with angina (I25.70-I25.73-, I25.79-)*

I25.811   **Atherosclerosis of native coronary artery of transplanted heart without angina pectoris**

     Atherosclerosis of native coronary artery of transplanted heart NOS

     EXCLUDES 1   *atherosclerosis of native coronary artery of transplanted heart with angina pectoris (I25.75-)*

I25.812   **Atherosclerosis of bypass graft of coronary artery of transplanted heart without angina pectoris** ▢A

     Atherosclerosis of bypass graft of transplanted heart NOS

     EXCLUDES 1   *atherosclerosis of bypass graft of transplanted heart with angina pectoris (I25.76)*

I25.82   **Chronic total occlusion of coronary artery**

     Complete occlusion of coronary artery

     Total occlusion of coronary artery

     Code first coronary atherosclerosis (I25.1-, I25.7-, I25.81-)

     EXCLUDES 1   *acute coronary occlusion with myocardial infarction (I21.-, I22.-)*

        acute coronary occlusion without myocardial infarction (I24.0)

I25.83   **Coronary atherosclerosis due to lipid rich plaque** ▢A

     Code first coronary atherosclerosis (I25.1-, I25.7-, I25.81-)

I25.84   **Coronary atherosclerosis due to calcified coronary lesion**

     Coronary atherosclerosis due to severely calcified coronary lesion

     Code first coronary atherosclerosis (I25.1-, I25.7-, I25.81-)

I25.89   **Other forms of chronic ischemic heart disease**

I25.9   **Chronic ischemic heart disease, unspecified** ▽

     Ischemic heart disease (chronic) NOS

☑ Additional Character Required   ✓x7ᵗʰ Placeholder Alert   Manifestation Dx   ▽ Unspecified Dx   ▶◀ Revised Text   ● New Code   ▲ Revised Code Title

ICD-10-CM 2017   611

Pulmonary heart disease and diseases of pulmonary circulation (I26-I28)

✓4th I26 Pulmonary embolism

> INCLUDES pulmonary (acute)(artery)(vein) infarction
> pulmonary (acute) (artery)(vein) thromboembolism
> pulmonary (acute)(artery)(vein) thrombosis
>
> EXCLUDES 2 chronic pulmonary embolism (I27.82)
> personal history of pulmonary embolism (Z86.711)
> pulmonary embolism complicating abortion, ectopic or molar pregnancy (O00-O07, O08.2)
> pulmonary embolism complicating pregnancy, childbirth and the puerperium (O88.-)
> pulmonary embolism due to complications of surgical and medical care (T80.0, T81.7-, T82.8-)
> pulmonary embolism due to trauma (T79.0, T79.1)
> septic (non-pulmonary) arterial embolism (I76)

✓5th I26.0 Pulmonary embolism with acute cor pulmonale

I26.01 Septic pulmonary embolism with acute cor pulmonale
Code first underlying infection

I26.02 Saddle embolus of pulmonary artery with acute cor pulmonale

I26.09 Other pulmonary embolism with acute cor pulmonale
Acute cor pulmonale NOS
AHA: 2014,4Q,21

✓5th I26.9 Pulmonary embolism without acute cor pulmonale

I26.90 Septic pulmonary embolism without acute cor pulmonale
Code first underlying infection

I26.92 Saddle embolus of pulmonary artery without acute cor pulmonale

I26.99 Other pulmonary embolism without acute cor pulmonale
Acute pulmonary embolism NOS
Pulmonary embolism NOS

✓4th I27 Other pulmonary heart diseases

I27.0 Primary pulmonary hypertension
> EXCLUDES 1 pulmonary hypertension NOS (I27.2)
> secondary pulmonary hypertension (I27.2)

I27.1 Kyphoscoliotic heart disease

I27.2 Other secondary pulmonary hypertension
Pulmonary hypertension NOS
Code also associated underlying condition
AHA: 2016,2Q,8; 2014,4Q,21

✓5th I27.8 Other specified pulmonary heart diseases

I27.81 Cor pulmonale (chronic)
Cor pulmonale NOS
> EXCLUDES 1 acute cor pulmonale (I26.0-)
AHA: 2014,4Q,21

I27.82 Chronic pulmonary embolism
Use additional code, if applicable, for associated long-term (current) use of anticoagulants (Z79.01)
> EXCLUDES 1 personal history of pulmonary embolism (Z86.711)

I27.89 Other specified pulmonary heart diseases
Eisenmenger's complex
Eisenmenger's syndrome
> EXCLUDES 1 Eisenmenger's defect (Q21.8)

I27.9 Pulmonary heart disease, unspecified ▽
Chronic cardiopulmonary disease

✓4th I28 Other diseases of pulmonary vessels

I28.0 Arteriovenous fistula of pulmonary vessels
> EXCLUDES 1 congenital arteriovenous fistula (Q25.72)

I28.1 Aneurysm of pulmonary artery
> EXCLUDES 1 congenital aneurysm (Q25.79)
> congenital arteriovenous aneurysm (Q25.72)

I28.8 Other diseases of pulmonary vessels
Pulmonary arteritis
Pulmonary endarteritis
Rupture of pulmonary vessels
Stenosis of pulmonary vessels
Stricture of pulmonary vessels

I28.9 Disease of pulmonary vessels, unspecified ▽

Other forms of heart disease (I30-I52)

✓4th I30 Acute pericarditis

> INCLUDES acute mediastinopericarditis
> acute myopericarditis
> acute pericardial effusion
> acute pleuropericarditis
> acute pneumopericarditis
>
> EXCLUDES 1 Dressler's syndrome (I24.1)
> rheumatic pericarditis (acute) (I01.0)

Cardiac Tamponade

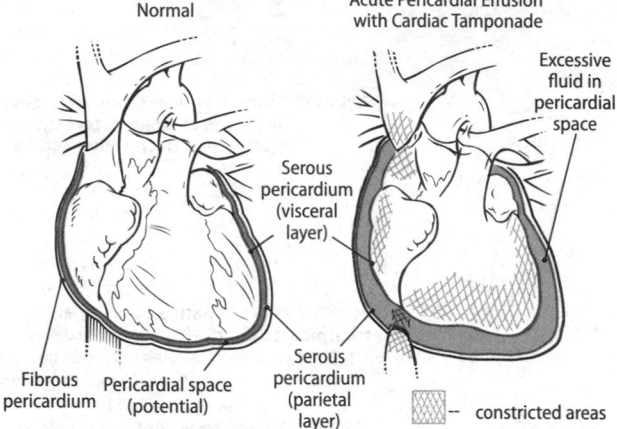

Normal   Acute Pericardial Effusion with Cardiac Tamponade

Excessive fluid in pericardial space

Serous pericardium (visceral layer)

Fibrous pericardium   Pericardial space (potential)

Serous pericardium (parietal layer)

▨ -- constricted areas

I30.0 Acute nonspecific idiopathic pericarditis

I30.1 Infective pericarditis
Pneumococcal pericarditis
Pneumopyopericardium
Purulent pericarditis
Pyopericarditis
Pyopericardium
Pyopneumopericardium
Staphylococcal pericarditis
Streptococcal pericarditis
Suppurative pericarditis
Viral pericarditis
Use additional code (B95-B97) to identify infectious agent

I30.8 Other forms of acute pericarditis

I30.9 Acute pericarditis, unspecified ▽

✓4th I31 Other diseases of pericardium

> EXCLUDES 1 diseases of pericardium specified as rheumatic (I09.2)
> postcardiotomy syndrome (I97.0)
> traumatic injury to pericardium (S26.-)

I31.0 Chronic adhesive pericarditis
Accretio cordis
Adherent pericardium
Adhesive mediastinopericarditis

I31.1 Chronic constrictive pericarditis
Concretio cordis
Pericardial calcification

I31.2 Hemopericardium, not elsewhere classified
> EXCLUDES 1 hemopericardium as current complication following acute myocardial infarction (I23.0)

I31.3 Pericardial effusion (noninflammatory)
Chylopericardium
> EXCLUDES 1 acute pericardial effusion (I30.9)

I31.4 Cardiac tamponade
Code first underlying cause

I31.8 Other specified diseases of pericardium
Epicardial plaques
Focal pericardial adhesions

I31.9 Disease of pericardium, unspecified ▽
Pericarditis (chronic) NOS

EXCLUDES 1 Not coded here   EXCLUDES 2 Not included here   N Newborn Age : 0   P Pediatric Age : 0-17   M Maternity Age : 12-55   A Adult Age : 15-124

I32   *Pericarditis in diseases classified elsewhere*
Code first underlying disease
EXCLUDES 1   pericarditis (in):
     coxsackie (virus) (B33.23)
     gonococcal (A54.83)
     meningococcal (A39.53)
     rheumatoid (arthritis) (M05.31)
     syphilitic (A52.06)
     systemic lupus erythematosus (M32.12)
     tuberculosis (A18.84)

✓4ᵗʰ   **I33**   **Acute and subacute endocarditis**
EXCLUDES 1   acute rheumatic endocarditis (I01.1)
     endocarditis NOS (I38)

I33.0   **Acute and subacute infective endocarditis**
Bacterial endocarditis (acute) (subacute)
Infective endocarditis (acute) (subacute) NOS
Endocarditis lenta (acute) (subacute)
Malignant endocarditis (acute) (subacute)
Purulent endocarditis (acute) (subacute)
Septic endocarditis (acute) (subacute)
Ulcerative endocarditis (acute) (subacute)
Vegetative endocarditis (acute) (subacute)
Use additional code (B95-B97) to identify infectious agent

I33.9   **Acute and subacute endocarditis, unspecified**   ▽
Acute endocarditis NOS
Acute myoendocarditis NOS
Acute periendocarditis NOS
Subacute endocarditis NOS
Subacute myoendocarditis NOS
Subacute periendocarditis NOS

✓4ᵗʰ   **I34**   **Nonrheumatic mitral valve disorders**
EXCLUDES 1   mitral valve disease (I05.9)
     mitral valve failure (I05.8)
     mitral valve stenosis (I05.0)
     mitral valve disorder of unspecified cause with diseases of aortic
       and/or tricuspid valve(s) (I08.-)
     mitral valve disorder of unspecified cause with mitral stenosis
       or obstruction (I05.0)
     mitral valve disorder specified as congenital (Q23.2, Q23.3)
     mitral valve disorder specified as rheumatic (I05.-)

I34.0   **Nonrheumatic mitral (valve) insufficiency**
Nonrheumatic mitral (valve) incompetence NOS
Nonrheumatic mitral (valve) regurgitation NOS

I34.1   **Nonrheumatic mitral (valve) prolapse**
Floppy nonrheumatic mitral valve syndrome
EXCLUDES 1   Marfan's syndrome (Q87.4-)

I34.2   **Nonrheumatic mitral (valve) stenosis**
I34.8   **Other nonrheumatic mitral valve disorders**
I34.9   **Nonrheumatic mitral valve disorder, unspecified**   ▽

✓4ᵗʰ   **I35**   **Nonrheumatic aortic valve disorders**
EXCLUDES 1   aortic valve disorder of unspecified cause but with diseases of
       mitral and/or tricuspid valve(s) (I08.-)
     aortic valve disorder specified as congenital (Q23.0, Q23.1)
     aortic valve disorder specified as rheumatic (I06.-)
     hypertrophic subaortic stenosis (I42.1)

I35.0   **Nonrheumatic aortic (valve) stenosis**
I35.1   **Nonrheumatic aortic (valve) insufficiency**
Nonrheumatic aortic (valve) incompetence NOS
Nonrheumatic aortic (valve) regurgitation NOS
I35.2   **Nonrheumatic aortic (valve) stenosis with insufficiency**
I35.8   **Other nonrheumatic aortic valve disorders**
I35.9   **Nonrheumatic aortic valve disorder, unspecified**   ▽

✓4ᵗʰ   **I36**   **Nonrheumatic tricuspid valve disorders**
EXCLUDES 1   tricuspid valve disorders of unspecified cause (I07.-)
     tricuspid valve disorders specified as congenital (Q22.4, Q22.8,
       Q22.9)
     tricuspid valve disorders specified as rheumatic (I07.-)
     tricuspid valve disorders with aortic and/or mitral valve
       involvement (I08.-)

I36.0   **Nonrheumatic tricuspid (valve) stenosis**
I36.1   **Nonrheumatic tricuspid (valve) insufficiency**
Nonrheumatic tricuspid (valve) incompetence
Nonrheumatic tricuspid (valve) regurgitation
I36.2   **Nonrheumatic tricuspid (valve) stenosis with insufficiency**
I36.8   **Other nonrheumatic tricuspid valve disorders**

I36.9   **Nonrheumatic tricuspid valve disorder, unspecified**   ▽

✓4ᵗʰ   **I37**   **Nonrheumatic pulmonary valve disorders**
EXCLUDES 1   pulmonary valve disorder specified as congenital (Q22.1, Q22.2,
       Q22.3)
     pulmonary valve disorder specified as rheumatic (I09.89)

I37.0   **Nonrheumatic pulmonary valve stenosis**
I37.1   **Nonrheumatic pulmonary valve insufficiency**
Nonrheumatic pulmonary valve incompetence
Nonrheumatic pulmonary valve regurgitation
I37.2   **Nonrheumatic pulmonary valve stenosis with insufficiency**
I37.8   **Other nonrheumatic pulmonary valve disorders**
I37.9   **Nonrheumatic pulmonary valve disorder, unspecified**   ▽

I38   **Endocarditis, valve unspecified**   ▽
INCLUDES   endocarditis (chronic) NOS
     valvular incompetence NOS
     valvular insufficiency NOS
     valvular regurgitation NOS
     valvular stenosis NOS
     valvulitis (chronic) NOS
EXCLUDES 1   congenital insufficiency of cardiac valve NOS (Q24.8)
     congenital stenosis of cardiac valve NOS (Q24.8)
     endocardial fibroelastosis (I42.4)
     endocarditis specified as rheumatic (I09.1)

I39   *Endocarditis and heart valve disorders in diseases classified elsewhere*
Code first underlying disease, such as:
    Q fever (A78)
EXCLUDES 1   endocardial involvement in:
     candidiasis (B37.6)
     gonococcal infection (A54.83)
     Libman-Sacks disease (M32.11)
     listerosis (A32.82)
     meningococcal infection (A39.51)
     rheumatoid arthritis (M05.31)
     syphilis (A52.03)
     tuberculosis (A18.84)
     typhoid fever (A01.02)

✓4ᵗʰ   **I40**   **Acute myocarditis**
INCLUDES   subacute myocarditis
EXCLUDES 1   acute rheumatic myocarditis (I01.2)

I40.0   **Infective myocarditis**
Septic myocarditis
Use additional code (B95-B97) to identify infectious agent
I40.1   **Isolated myocarditis**
Fiedler's myocarditis
Giant cell myocarditis
Idiopathic myocarditis
I40.8   **Other acute myocarditis**
I40.9   **Acute myocarditis, unspecified**   ▽

I41   *Myocarditis in diseases classified elsewhere*
Code first underlying disease, such as:
    typhus (A75.0-A75.9)
EXCLUDES 1   myocarditis (in):
     Chagas' disease (chronic) (B57.2)
     acute (B57.0)
     coxsackie (virus) infection (B33.22)
     diphtheritic (A36.81)
     gonococcal (A54.83)
     influenzal (J09.X9, J10.82, J11.82)
     meningococcal (A39.52)
     mumps (B26.82)
     rheumatoid arthritis (M05.31)
     sarcoid (D86.85)
     syphilis (A52.06)
     toxoplasmosis (B58.81)
     tuberculous (A18.84)

✓4ᵗʰ   **I42**   **Cardiomyopathy**
INCLUDES   myocardiopathy
Code first pre-existing cardiomyopathy complicating pregnancy and
    puerperium (O99.4)
EXCLUDES 2   ▶ischemic cardiomyopathy (I25.5)◀
     ▶peripartum cardiomyopathy (O90.3)◀
     ventricular hypertrophy (I51.7)

I42.0   **Dilated cardiomyopathy**
Congestive cardiomyopathy

I42.1 **Obstructive hypertrophic cardiomyopathy**
Hypertrophic subaortic stenosis (idiopathic)

I42.2 **Other hypertrophic cardiomyopathy**
Nonobstructive hypertrophic cardiomyopathy

I42.3 **Endomyocardial (eosinophilic) disease**
Endomyocardial (tropical) fibrosis
Löffler's endocarditis

I42.4 **Endocardial fibroelastosis**
Congenital cardiomyopathy
Elastomyofibrosis

I42.5 **Other restrictive cardiomyopathy**
Constrictive cardiomyopathy NOS

I42.6 **Alcoholic cardiomyopathy**
Code also presence of alcoholism (F10.-)

I42.7 **Cardiomyopathy due to drug and external agent**
Code first poisoning due to drug or toxin, if applicable (T36-T65 with fifth or sixth character 1-4 or 6)
Use additional code for adverse effect, if applicable, to identify drug (T36-T50 with fifth or sixth character 5)

I42.8 **Other cardiomyopathies**

I42.9 **Cardiomyopathy, unspecified** ▽
Cardiomyopathy (primary) (secondary) NOS

I43 *Cardiomyopathy in diseases classified elsewhere*
Code first underlying disease, such as:
amyloidosis (E85.-)
glycogen storage disease (E74.0)
gout (M10.0-)
thyrotoxicosis (E05.0-E05.9-)
EXCLUDES 1 *cardiomyopathy (in):*
coxsackie (virus) (B33.24)
diphtheria (A36.81)
sarcoidosis (D86.85)
tuberculosis (A18.84)

☑4ᵗʰ **I44** **Atrioventricular and left bundle-branch block**

I44.0 **Atrioventricular block, first degree**

I44.1 **Atrioventricular block, second degree**
Atrioventricular block, type I and II
Möbitz block, type I and II
Second degree block, type I and II
Wenckebach's block

I44.2 **Atrioventricular block, complete**
Complete heart block NOS
Third degree block

☑5ᵗʰ **I44.3** **Other and unspecified atrioventricular block**
Atrioventricular block NOS

I44.30 **Unspecified atrioventricular block** ▽

I44.39 **Other atrioventricular block**

I44.4 **Left anterior fascicular block**

I44.5 **Left posterior fascicular block**

☑5ᵗʰ **I44.6** **Other and unspecified fascicular block**

I44.60 **Unspecified fascicular block** ▽
Left bundle-branch hemiblock NOS

I44.69 **Other fascicular block**

I44.7 **Left bundle-branch block, unspecified** ▽

Conduction Disorders

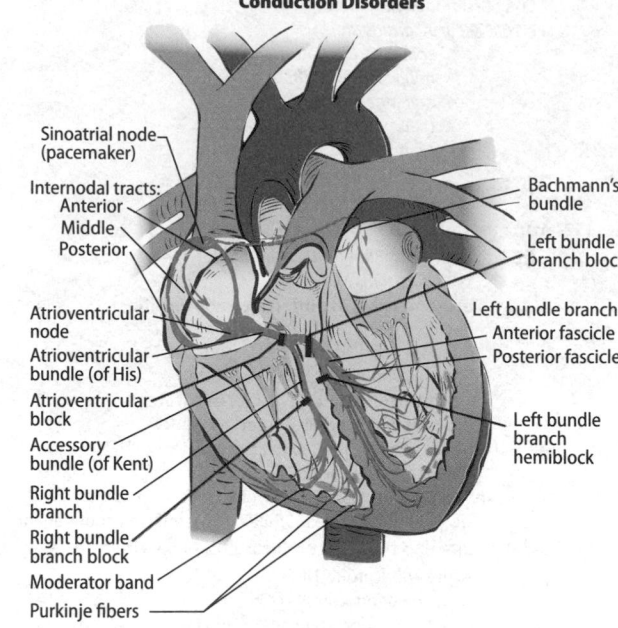

☑4ᵗʰ **I45** **Other conduction disorders**

I45.0 **Right fascicular block**

☑5ᵗʰ **I45.1** **Other and unspecified right bundle-branch block**

I45.10 **Unspecified right bundle-branch block** ▽
Right bundle-branch block NOS

I45.19 **Other right bundle-branch block**

I45.2 **Bifascicular block**

I45.3 **Trifascicular block**

I45.4 **Nonspecific intraventricular block**
Bundle-branch block NOS

I45.5 **Other specified heart block**
Sinoatrial block
Sinoauricular block
EXCLUDES 1 *heart block NOS (I45.9)*

I45.6 **Pre-excitation syndrome**
Accelerated atrioventricular conduction
Accessory atrioventricular conduction
Anomalous atrioventricular excitation
Lown-Ganong-Levine syndrome
Pre-excitation atrioventricular conduction
Wolff-Parkinson-White syndrome

☑5ᵗʰ **I45.8** **Other specified conduction disorders**

I45.81 **Long QT syndrome**
DEF: Condition characterized by recurrent syncope, malignant arrhythmias, and sudden death; characteristic prolonged Q-T interval on electrocardiogram.

I45.89 **Other specified conduction disorders**
Atrioventricular [AV] dissociation
Interference dissociation
Isorhythmic dissociation
Nonparoxysmal AV nodal tachycardia
AHA: 2013,2Q,31

I45.9 **Conduction disorder, unspecified** ▽
Heart block NOS
Stokes-Adams syndrome

☑4ᵗʰ **I46** **Cardiac arrest**
EXCLUDES 1 *cardiogenic shock (R57.0)*

I46.2 **Cardiac arrest due to underlying cardiac condition**
Code first underlying cardiac condition

I46.8 **Cardiac arrest due to other underlying condition**
Code first underlying condition

I46.9 **Cardiac arrest, cause unspecified** ▽

EXCLUDES 1 Not coded here   **EXCLUDES 2** Not included here   **N** Newborn Age : 0   **P** Pediatric Age : 0-17   **M** Maternity Age : 12-55   **A** Adult Age : 15-124

614

ICD-10-CM 2017

☑️4ᵗʰ **I47 Paroxysmal tachycardia**

Code first tachycardia complicating:
abortion or ectopic or molar pregnancy (O00–O07, O08.8)
obstetric surgery and procedures (O75.4)

EXCLUDES 1   *tachycardia NOS (R00.0)*
sinoauricular tachycardia NOS (R00.0)
sinus [sinusal] tachycardia NOS (R00.0)

I47.0   Re-entry ventricular arrhythmia

I47.1   Supraventricular tachycardia

Atrial (paroxysmal) tachycardia
Atrioventricular [AV] (paroxysmal) tachycardia
Atrioventricular re-entrant (nodal) tachycardia [AVNRT] [AVRT]
Junctional (paroxysmal) tachycardia
Nodal (paroxysmal) tachycardia

I47.2   Ventricular tachycardia

AHA: 2013,3Q,23

I47.9   Paroxysmal tachycardia, unspecified   ▽

Bouveret (-Hoffman) syndrome

☑️4ᵗʰ **I48 Atrial fibrillation and flutter**

I48.0   Paroxysmal atrial fibrillation

I48.1   Persistent atrial fibrillation

I48.2   Chronic atrial fibrillation

Permanent atrial fibrillation

I48.3   Typical atrial flutter

Type I atrial flutter

I48.4   Atypical atrial flutter

Type II atrial flutter

☑️5ᵗʰ **I48.9   Unspecified atrial fibrillation and atrial flutter**

I48.91   Unspecified atrial fibrillation   ▽

I48.92   Unspecified atrial flutter   ▽

☑️4ᵗʰ **I49 Other cardiac arrhythmias**

Code first cardiac arrhythmia complicating:
abortion or ectopic or molar pregnancy (O00–O07, O08.8)
obstetric surgery and procedures (O75.4)

EXCLUDES 1   *bradycardia NOS (R00.1)*
neonatal dysrhythmia (P29.1-)
sinoatrial bradycardia (R00.1)
sinus bradycardia (R00.1)
vagal bradycardia (R00.1)

☑️5ᵗʰ **I49.0   Ventricular fibrillation and flutter**

I49.01   Ventricular fibrillation

I49.02   Ventricular flutter

I49.1   Atrial premature depolarization

Atrial premature beats

I49.2   Junctional premature depolarization

I49.3   Ventricular premature depolarization

☑️5ᵗʰ **I49.4   Other and unspecified premature depolarization**

I49.40   Unspecified premature depolarization   ▽

Premature beats NOS

I49.49   Other premature depolarization

Ectopic beats
Extrasystoles
Extrasystolic arrhythmias
Premature contractions

I49.5   Sick sinus syndrome

Tachycardia-bradycardia syndrome

I49.8   Other specified cardiac arrhythmias

Coronary sinus rhythm disorder
Ectopic rhythm disorder
Nodal rhythm disorder

I49.9   Cardiac arrhythmia, unspecified   ▽

Arrhythmia (cardiac) NOS

☑️4ᵗʰ **I50 Heart failure**

Code first:
heart failure complicating abortion or ectopic or molar pregnancy (O00–O07, O08.8)
heart failure due to hypertension (I11.0)
heart failure due to hypertension with chronic kidney disease (I13.-)
heart failure following surgery (I97.13-)
obstetric surgery and procedures (O75.4)
rheumatic heart failure (I09.81)

EXCLUDES 1   *neonatal cardiac failure (P29.0)*

EXCLUDES 2   ▶*cardiac arrest (I46.-)*◀

AHA: 2014,1Q,25; 2013,2Q,33

I50.1   Left ventricular failure

Cardiac asthma
Edema of lung with heart disease NOS
Edema of lung with heart failure
Left heart failure
Pulmonary edema with heart disease NOS
Pulmonary edema with heart failure

EXCLUDES 1   *edema of lung without heart disease or heart failure (J81.-)*
pulmonary edema without heart disease or failure (J81.-)

☑️5ᵗʰ **I50.2   Systolic (congestive) heart failure**

EXCLUDES 1   *combined systolic (congestive) and diastolic (congestive) heart failure (I50.4-)*

AHA: 2016,1Q,10

I50.20   Unspecified systolic (congestive) heart failure   ▽

I50.21   Acute systolic (congestive) heart failure

I50.22   Chronic systolic (congestive) heart failure

I50.23   Acute on chronic systolic (congestive) heart failure

☑️5ᵗʰ **I50.3   Diastolic (congestive) heart failure**

EXCLUDES 1   *combined systolic (congestive) and diastolic (congestive) heart failure (I50.4-)*

AHA: 2016,1Q,10

I50.30   Unspecified diastolic (congestive) heart failure   ▽

I50.31   Acute diastolic (congestive) heart failure

I50.32   Chronic diastolic (congestive) heart failure

I50.33   Acute on chronic diastolic (congestive) heart failure

☑️5ᵗʰ **I50.4   Combined systolic (congestive) and diastolic (congestive) heart failure**

AHA: 2016,1Q,10

I50.40   Unspecified combined systolic (congestive) and diastolic (congestive) heart failure   ▽

I50.41   Acute combined systolic (congestive) and diastolic (congestive) heart failure

I50.42   Chronic combined systolic (congestive) and diastolic (congestive) heart failure

I50.43   Acute on chronic combined systolic (congestive) and diastolic (congestive) heart failure

I50.9   Heart failure, unspecified   ▽

Biventricular (heart) failure NOS
Cardiac, heart or myocardial failure NOS
Congestive heart disease
Congestive heart failure NOS
Right ventricular failure (secondary to left heart failure)

EXCLUDES 2   ▶*fluid overload (E87.70)*◀

AHA: 2014,4Q,21; 2012,4Q,92

☑️4ᵗʰ **I51 Complications and ill-defined descriptions of heart disease**

EXCLUDES 1   *any condition in I51.4-I51.9 due to hypertension (I11.-)*
any condition in I51.4-I51.9 due to hypertension and chronic kidney disease (I13.-)
heart disease specified as rheumatic (I00-I09)

I51.0   Cardiac septal defect, acquired   🅐

Acquired septal atrial defect (old)
Acquired septal auricular defect (old)
Acquired septal ventricular defect (old)

EXCLUDES 1   *cardiac septal defect as current complication following acute myocardial infarction (I23.1, I23.2)*

I51.1   Rupture of chordae tendineae, not elsewhere classified

EXCLUDES 1   *rupture of chordae tendineae as current complication following acute myocardial infarction (I23.4)*

I51.2   Rupture of papillary muscle, not elsewhere classified

EXCLUDES 1   *rupture of papillary muscle as current complication following acute myocardial infarction (I23.5)*

☑️ Additional Character Required   ✓ˣ7ᵗʰ Placeholder Alert   Manifestation Dx   ▽ Unspecified Dx   ▶◀ Revised Text   ● New Code   ▲ Revised Code Title

ICD-10-CM 2017   615

Chapter 9. Diseases of the Circulatory System

I51.3   Intracardiac thrombosis, not elsewhere classified
Apical thrombosis (old)
Atrial thrombosis (old)
Auricular thrombosis (old)
Mural thrombosis (old)
Ventricular thrombosis (old)
> *EXCLUDES 1*   intracardiac thrombosis as current complication following acute myocardial infarction (I23.6)

AHA: 2013,1Q,24

I51.4   Myocarditis, unspecified   ▽
Chronic (interstitial) myocarditis
Myocardial fibrosis
Myocarditis NOS
> *EXCLUDES 1*   acute or subacute myocarditis (I40.-)

I51.5   Myocardial degeneration
Fatty degeneration of heart or myocardium
Myocardial disease
Senile degeneration of heart or myocardium

I51.7   Cardiomegaly
Cardiac dilatation
Cardiac hypertrophy
Ventricular dilatation

✓5th **I51.8   Other ill-defined heart diseases**

     I51.81   Takotsubo syndrome
Reversible left ventricular dysfunction following sudden emotional stress
Stress induced cardiomyopathy
Takotsubo cardiomyopathy
Transient left ventricular apical ballooning syndrome

     I51.89   Other ill-defined heart diseases
Carditis (acute)(chronic)
Pancarditis (acute)(chronic)

I51.9   Heart disease, unspecified   ▽

I52   *Other heart disorders in diseases classified elsewhere*
Code first underlying disease, such as:
congenital syphilis (A50.5)
mucopolysaccharidosis (E76.3)
schistosomiasis (B65.0-B65.9)
> *EXCLUDES 1*   heart disease (in):
> gonococcal infection (A54.83)
> meningococcal infection (A39.50)
> rheumatoid arthritis (M05.31)
> syphilis (A52.06)

Cerebrovascular diseases (I60-I69)

Use additional code to identify presence of:
alcohol abuse and dependence (F10.-)
exposure to environmental tobacco smoke (Z77.22)
▶history of tobacco dependence (Z87.891)◀
hypertension (I10-I15)
occupational exposure to environmental tobacco smoke (Z57.31)
tobacco dependence (F17.-)
tobacco use (Z72.0)
> *EXCLUDES 1*   transient cerebral ischemic attacks and related syndromes (G45.-)
> traumatic intracranial hemorrhage (S06.-)

AHA: 2014,3Q,5; 2012,4Q,91-92

✓4th **I60   Nontraumatic subarachnoid hemorrhage**
> *INCLUDES*   ruptured cerebral aneurysm
> *EXCLUDES 1*   syphilitic ruptured cerebral aneurysm (A52.05)
> *EXCLUDES 2*   ▶sequelae of subarachnoid hemorrhage (I69.0-)◀

✓5th **I60.0   Nontraumatic subarachnoid hemorrhage from carotid siphon and bifurcation**

     I60.00   Nontraumatic subarachnoid hemorrhage from unspecified carotid siphon and bifurcation   ▽

     I60.01   Nontraumatic subarachnoid hemorrhage from right carotid siphon and bifurcation

     I60.02   Nontraumatic subarachnoid hemorrhage from left carotid siphon and bifurcation

✓5th **I60.1   Nontraumatic subarachnoid hemorrhage from middle cerebral artery**

     I60.10   Nontraumatic subarachnoid hemorrhage from unspecified middle cerebral artery   ▽

     I60.11   Nontraumatic subarachnoid hemorrhage from right middle cerebral artery

     I60.12   Nontraumatic subarachnoid hemorrhage from left middle cerebral artery

I60.2   Nontraumatic subarachnoid hemorrhage from anterior communicating artery

✓5th **I60.3   Nontraumatic subarachnoid hemorrhage from posterior communicating artery**

     I60.30   Nontraumatic subarachnoid hemorrhage from unspecified posterior communicating artery   ▽

     I60.31   Nontraumatic subarachnoid hemorrhage from right posterior communicating artery

     I60.32   Nontraumatic subarachnoid hemorrhage from left posterior communicating artery

I60.4   Nontraumatic subarachnoid hemorrhage from basilar artery

✓5th **I60.5   Nontraumatic subarachnoid hemorrhage from vertebral artery**

     I60.50   Nontraumatic subarachnoid hemorrhage from unspecified vertebral artery   ▽

     I60.51   Nontraumatic subarachnoid hemorrhage from right vertebral artery

     I60.52   Nontraumatic subarachnoid hemorrhage from left vertebral artery

I60.6   Nontraumatic subarachnoid hemorrhage from other intracranial arteries

I60.7   Nontraumatic subarachnoid hemorrhage from unspecified intracranial artery   ▽
Ruptured (congenital) berry aneurysm
Ruptured (congenital) cerebral aneurysm
Subarachnoid hemorrhage (nontraumatic) from cerebral artery NOS
Subarachnoid hemorrhage (nontraumatic) from communicating artery NOS
> *EXCLUDES 1*   berry aneurysm, nonruptured (I67.1)

I60.8   Other nontraumatic subarachnoid hemorrhage
Meningeal hemorrhage
Rupture of cerebral arteriovenous malformation

I60.9   Nontraumatic subarachnoid hemorrhage, unspecified   ▽

✓4th **I61   Nontraumatic intracerebral hemorrhage**
> *EXCLUDES 2*   ▶sequelae of intracerebral hemorrhage (I69.1-)◀

I61.0   Nontraumatic intracerebral hemorrhage in hemisphere, subcortical
Deep intracerebral hemorrhage (nontraumatic)

I61.1   Nontraumatic intracerebral hemorrhage in hemisphere, cortical
Cerebral lobe hemorrhage (nontraumatic)
Superficial intracerebral hemorrhage (nontraumatic)

I61.2   Nontraumatic intracerebral hemorrhage in hemisphere, unspecified   ▽

I61.3   Nontraumatic intracerebral hemorrhage in brain stem

I61.4   Nontraumatic intracerebral hemorrhage in cerebellum

I61.5   Nontraumatic intracerebral hemorrhage, intraventricular

I61.6   Nontraumatic intracerebral hemorrhage, multiple localized

I61.8   Other nontraumatic intracerebral hemorrhage

I61.9   Nontraumatic intracerebral hemorrhage, unspecified   ▽

✓4th **I62   Other and unspecified nontraumatic intracranial hemorrhage**
> *EXCLUDES 2*   ▶sequelae of intracranial hemorrhage (I69.2)◀

✓5th **I62.0   Nontraumatic subdural hemorrhage**

     I62.00   Nontraumatic subdural hemorrhage, unspecified   ▽

     I62.01   Nontraumatic acute subdural hemorrhage

     I62.02   Nontraumatic subacute subdural hemorrhage

     I62.03   Nontraumatic chronic subdural hemorrhage

I62.1   Nontraumatic extradural hemorrhage
Nontraumatic epidural hemorrhage

I62.9   Nontraumatic intracranial hemorrhage, unspecified   ▽

✓4th **I63   Cerebral infarction**
> *INCLUDES*   occlusion and stenosis of cerebral and precerebral arteries, resulting in cerebral infarction

Use additional code, if applicable, to identify status post administration of tPA (rtPA) in a different facility within the last 24 hours prior to admission to current facility (Z92.82)
▶Use additional code, if known, to indicate National Institutes of Health Stroke Scale (NIHSS) score (R29.7-)◀
> *EXCLUDES 2*   ▶sequelae of cerebral infarction (I69.3-)◀

AHA: 2014,1Q,23

✓5th **I63.0   Cerebral infarction due to thrombosis of precerebral arteries**

     I63.00   Cerebral infarction due to thrombosis of unspecified precerebral artery   ▽

EXCLUDES 1 Not coded here   *EXCLUDES 2* Not included here   N Newborn Age : 0   P Pediatric Age : 0-17   M Maternity Age : 12-55   A Adult Age : 15-124

616   **ICD-10-CM 2017**

√6ᵗʰ **I63.01** **Cerebral infarction due to thrombosis of** vertebral artery

    I63.011 **Cerebral infarction due to thrombosis of** right vertebral artery

    I63.012 **Cerebral infarction due to thrombosis of** left vertebral artery

    I63.013 **Cerebral infarction due to thrombosis of** bilateral vertebral arteries

    I63.019 **Cerebral infarction due to thrombosis of unspecified vertebral artery** ▽

I63.02 **Cerebral infarction due to thrombosis of** basilar artery

√6ᵗʰ **I63.03** **Cerebral infarction due to thrombosis of** carotid artery

    I63.031 **Cerebral infarction due to thrombosis of** right carotid artery

    I63.032 **Cerebral infarction due to thrombosis of** left carotid artery

    I63.033 **Cerebral infarction due to thrombosis of** bilateral carotid arteries

    I63.039 **Cerebral infarction due to thrombosis of unspecified carotid artery** ▽

I63.09 **Cerebral infarction due to thrombosis of other precerebral artery**

√5ᵗʰ **I63.1** **Cerebral infarction due to** embolism of precerebral arteries

I63.10 **Cerebral infarction due to embolism of unspecified precerebral artery** ▽

√6ᵗʰ **I63.11** **Cerebral infarction due to embolism of** vertebral artery

    I63.111 **Cerebral infarction due to embolism of** right vertebral artery

    I63.112 **Cerebral infarction due to embolism of** left vertebral artery

    I63.113 **Cerebral infarction due to embolism of** bilateral vertebral arteries

    I63.119 **Cerebral infarction due to embolism of unspecified vertebral artery** ▽

I63.12 **Cerebral infarction due to embolism of** basilar artery

√6ᵗʰ **I63.13** **Cerebral infarction due to embolism of** carotid artery

    I63.131 **Cerebral infarction due to embolism of** right carotid artery

    I63.132 **Cerebral infarction due to embolism of** left carotid artery

    I63.133 **Cerebral infarction due to embolism of** bilateral carotid arteries

    I63.139 **Cerebral infarction due to embolism of unspecified carotid artery** ▽

I63.19 **Cerebral infarction due to embolism of other precerebral artery**

√5ᵗʰ **I63.2** **Cerebral infarction due to unspecified** occlusion or stenosis of precerebral arteries

I63.20 **Cerebral infarction due to unspecified occlusion or stenosis of unspecified precerebral arteries** ▽

√6ᵗʰ **I63.21** **Cerebral infarction due to unspecified occlusion or stenosis of** vertebral arteries

    I63.211 **Cerebral infarction due to unspecified occlusion or stenosis of** right **vertebral arteries**

    I63.212 **Cerebral infarction due to unspecified occlusion or stenosis of** left **vertebral arteries**

    I63.213 **Cerebral infarction due to unspecified occlusion or stenosis of** bilateral **vertebral arteries**

    I63.219 **Cerebral infarction due to unspecified occlusion or stenosis of unspecified vertebral arteries** ▽

I63.22 **Cerebral infarction due to unspecified occlusion or stenosis of** basilar **arteries**

√6ᵗʰ **I63.23** **Cerebral infarction due to unspecified occlusion or stenosis of** carotid arteries

    I63.231 **Cerebral infarction due to unspecified occlusion or stenosis of** right **carotid arteries**

    I63.232 **Cerebral infarction due to unspecified occlusion or stenosis of** left **carotid arteries**

    I63.233 **Cerebral infarction due to unspecified occlusion or stenosis of** bilateral **carotid arteries**

    I63.239 **Cerebral infarction due to unspecified occlusion or stenosis of unspecified carotid arteries** ▽

I63.29 **Cerebral infarction due to unspecified occlusion or stenosis of other precerebral arteries**

√5ᵗʰ **I63.3** **Cerebral infarction due to** thrombosis of cerebral arteries

I63.30 **Cerebral infarction due to thrombosis of unspecified cerebral artery** ▽

√6ᵗʰ **I63.31** **Cerebral infarction due to thrombosis of** middle cerebral artery

    I63.311 **Cerebral infarction due to thrombosis of** right **middle cerebral artery**

    I63.312 **Cerebral infarction due to thrombosis of** left **middle cerebral artery**

    I63.313 **Cerebral infarction due to thrombosis of** bilateral **middle cerebral arteries**

    I63.319 **Cerebral infarction due to thrombosis of unspecified middle cerebral artery** ▽

√6ᵗʰ **I63.32** **Cerebral infarction due to thrombosis of** anterior cerebral artery

    I63.321 **Cerebral infarction due to thrombosis of** right **anterior cerebral artery**

    I63.322 **Cerebral infarction due to thrombosis of** left **anterior cerebral artery**

    I63.323 **Cerebral infarction due to thrombosis of** bilateral **anterior arteries**

    I63.329 **Cerebral infarction due to thrombosis of unspecified anterior cerebral artery** ▽

√6ᵗʰ **I63.33** **Cerebral infarction due to thrombosis of** posterior cerebral artery

    I63.331 **Cerebral infarction due to thrombosis of** right **posterior cerebral artery**

    I63.332 **Cerebral infarction due to thrombosis of** left **posterior cerebral artery**

    I63.333 **Cerebral infarction to thrombosis of** bilateral **posterior arteries**

    I63.339 **Cerebral infarction due to thrombosis of unspecified posterior cerebral artery** ▽

√6ᵗʰ **I63.34** **Cerebral infarction due to thrombosis of** cerebellar artery

    I63.341 **Cerebral infarction due to thrombosis of** right **cerebellar artery**

    I63.342 **Cerebral infarction due to thrombosis of** left **cerebellar artery**

    I63.343 **Cerebral infarction to thrombosis of** bilateral **cerebellar arteries**

    I63.349 **Cerebral infarction due to thrombosis of unspecified cerebellar artery** ▽

I63.39 **Cerebral infarction due to thrombosis of other cerebral artery**

√5ᵗʰ **I63.4** **Cerebral infarction due to** embolism of cerebral arteries

I63.40 **Cerebral infarction due to embolism of unspecified cerebral artery** ▽

√6ᵗʰ **I63.41** **Cerebral infarction due to embolism of** middle cerebral artery

    I63.411 **Cerebral infarction due to embolism of** right **middle cerebral artery**

    I63.412 **Cerebral infarction due to embolism of** left **middle cerebral artery**

    I63.413 **Cerebral infarction due to embolism of** bilateral **middle cerebral arteries**

    I63.419 **Cerebral infarction due to embolism of unspecified middle cerebral artery** ▽

√6ᵗʰ **I63.42** **Cerebral infarction due to embolism of** anterior cerebral artery

    I63.421 **Cerebral infarction due to embolism of** right **anterior cerebral artery**

    I63.422 **Cerebral infarction due to embolism of** left **anterior cerebral artery**

    I63.423 **Cerebral infarction due to embolism of** bilateral **anterior cerebral arteries**

    I63.429 **Cerebral infarction due to embolism of unspecified anterior cerebral artery** ▽

☑ Additional Character Required   ▢x7ᵗʰ Placeholder Alert   Manifestation Dx   ▽ Unspecified Dx   ▶◀ Revised Text   ● New Code   ▲ Revised Code Title

Chapter 9. Diseases of the Circulatory System

√6ᵗʰ **I63.43**   **Cerebral infarction due to embolism of** posterior cerebral artery
- **I63.431**   Cerebral infarction due to embolism of right posterior cerebral artery
- **I63.432**   Cerebral infarction due to embolism of left posterior cerebral artery
- **I63.433**   Cerebral infarction due to embolism of bilateral posterior cerebral arteries
- **I63.439**   Cerebral infarction due to embolism of unspecified posterior cerebral artery ▽

√6ᵗʰ **I63.44**   **Cerebral infarction due to embolism of** cerebellar artery
- **I63.441**   Cerebral infarction due to embolism of right cerebellar artery
- **I63.442**   Cerebral infarction due to embolism of left cerebellar artery
- **I63.443**   Cerebral infarction due to embolism of bilateral cerebellar arteries
- **I63.449**   Cerebral infarction due to embolism of unspecified cerebellar artery ▽

I63.49   **Cerebral infarction due to embolism of other cerebral artery**

√5ᵗʰ **I63.5**   **Cerebral infarction due to unspecified** occlusion or stenosis of cerebral arteries
- **I63.50**   Cerebral infarction due to unspecified occlusion or stenosis of unspecified cerebral artery ▽

√6ᵗʰ **I63.51**   **Cerebral infarction due to unspecified occlusion or stenosis of** middle cerebral artery
- **I63.511**   Cerebral infarction due to unspecified occlusion or stenosis of right middle cerebral artery
- **I63.512**   Cerebral infarction due to unspecified occlusion or stenosis of left middle cerebral artery
- **I63.513**   Cerebral infarction due to unspecified occlusion or stenosis of bilateral middle arteries
- **I63.519**   Cerebral infarction due to unspecified occlusion or stenosis of unspecified middle cerebral artery ▽

√6ᵗʰ **I63.52**   **Cerebral infarction due to unspecified occlusion or stenosis of** anterior cerebral artery
- **I63.521**   Cerebral infarction due to unspecified occlusion or stenosis of right anterior cerebral artery
- **I63.522**   Cerebral infarction due to unspecified occlusion or stenosis of left anterior cerebral artery
- **I63.523**   Cerebral infarction due to unspecified occlusion or stenosis of bilateral anterior arteries
- **I63.529**   Cerebral infarction due to unspecified occlusion or stenosis of unspecified anterior cerebral artery ▽

√6ᵗʰ **I63.53**   **Cerebral infarction due to unspecified occlusion or stenosis of** posterior cerebral artery
- **I63.531**   Cerebral infarction due to unspecified occlusion or stenosis of right posterior cerebral artery
- **I63.532**   Cerebral infarction due to unspecified occlusion or stenosis of left posterior cerebral artery
- **I63.533**   Cerebral infarction due to unspecified occlusion or stenosis of bilateral posterior arteries
- **I63.539**   Cerebral infarction due to unspecified occlusion or stenosis of unspecified posterior cerebral artery ▽

√6ᵗʰ **I63.54**   **Cerebral infarction due to unspecified occlusion or stenosis of** cerebellar artery
- **I63.541**   Cerebral infarction due to unspecified occlusion or stenosis of right cerebellar artery
- **I63.542**   Cerebral infarction due to unspecified occlusion or stenosis of left cerebellar artery
- **I63.543**   Cerebral infarction due to unspecified occlusion or stenosis of bilateral cerebellar arteries

- **I63.549**   Cerebral infarction due to unspecified occlusion or stenosis of unspecified cerebellar artery ▽

I63.59   **Cerebral infarction due to unspecified occlusion or stenosis of other cerebral artery**

I63.6   **Cerebral infarction due to** cerebral venous thrombosis, nonpyogenic

I63.8   **Other cerebral infarction**

I63.9   **Cerebral infarction, unspecified** ▽
    Stroke NOS
    AHA: 2015,1Q,25

√4ᵗʰ **I65**   **Occlusion and stenosis of** precerebral **arteries, not resulting in cerebral infarction**
    INCLUDES   embolism of precerebral artery
       narrowing of precerebral artery
       obstruction (complete) (partial) of precerebral artery
       thrombosis of precerebral artery
    EXCLUDES 1   *insufficiency, NOS, of precerebral artery (G45.-)*
       insufficiency of precerebral arteries causing cerebral infarction (I63.0-I63.2)

√5ᵗʰ **I65.0**   **Occlusion and stenosis of** vertebral **artery**
- **I65.01**   Occlusion and stenosis of right vertebral artery
- **I65.02**   Occlusion and stenosis of left vertebral artery
- **I65.03**   Occlusion and stenosis of bilateral vertebral arteries
- **I65.09**   Occlusion and stenosis of unspecified vertebral artery ▽

I65.1   **Occlusion and stenosis of** basilar **artery**

√5ᵗʰ **I65.2**   **Occlusion and stenosis of** carotid **artery**
- **I65.21**   Occlusion and stenosis of right carotid artery
- **I65.22**   Occlusion and stenosis of left carotid artery
- **I65.23**   Occlusion and stenosis of bilateral carotid arteries
- **I65.29**   Occlusion and stenosis of unspecified carotid artery ▽

I65.8   **Occlusion and stenosis of other precerebral arteries**

I65.9   **Occlusion and stenosis of unspecified precerebral artery** ▽
    Occlusion and stenosis of precerebral artery NOS

√4ᵗʰ **I66**   **Occlusion and stenosis of** cerebral **arteries, not resulting in cerebral infarction**
    INCLUDES   embolism of cerebral artery
       narrowing of cerebral artery
       obstruction (complete) (partial) of cerebral artery
       thrombosis of cerebral artery
    EXCLUDES 1   *occlusion and stenosis of cerebral artery causing cerebral infarction (I63.3-I63.5)*

√5ᵗʰ **I66.0**   **Occlusion and stenosis of** middle **cerebral artery**
- **I66.01**   Occlusion and stenosis of right middle cerebral artery
- **I66.02**   Occlusion and stenosis of left middle cerebral artery
- **I66.03**   Occlusion and stenosis of bilateral middle cerebral arteries
- **I66.09**   Occlusion and stenosis of unspecified middle cerebral artery ▽

√5ᵗʰ **I66.1**   **Occlusion and stenosis of** anterior **cerebral artery**
- **I66.11**   Occlusion and stenosis of right anterior cerebral artery
- **I66.12**   Occlusion and stenosis of left anterior cerebral artery
- **I66.13**   Occlusion and stenosis of bilateral anterior cerebral arteries
- **I66.19**   Occlusion and stenosis of unspecified anterior cerebral artery ▽

√5ᵗʰ **I66.2**   **Occlusion and stenosis of** posterior **cerebral artery**
- **I66.21**   Occlusion and stenosis of right posterior cerebral artery
- **I66.22**   Occlusion and stenosis of left posterior cerebral artery
- **I66.23**   Occlusion and stenosis of bilateral posterior cerebral arteries
- **I66.29**   Occlusion and stenosis of unspecified posterior cerebral artery ▽

I66.3   **Occlusion and stenosis of** cerebellar **arteries**

I66.8   **Occlusion and stenosis of** other **cerebral arteries**
    Occlusion and stenosis of perforating arteries

I66.9   **Occlusion and stenosis of unspecified cerebral artery** ▽

EXCLUDES 1 Not coded here   **EXCLUDES 2** Not included here   N Newborn Age : 0   P Pediatric Age : 0-17   M Maternity Age : 12-55   A Adult Age : 15-124

618   ICD-10-CM 2017

✓4ᵗʰ I67 Other cerebrovascular diseases

EXCLUDES 2 ▶*sequelae of the listed conditions (I69.8)*◀

Berry Aneurysm

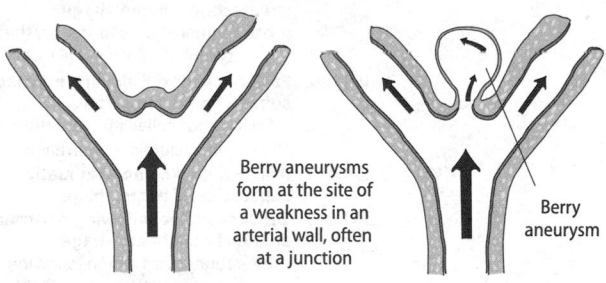

Berry aneurysms form at the site of a weakness in an arterial wall, often at a junction

Berry aneurysm

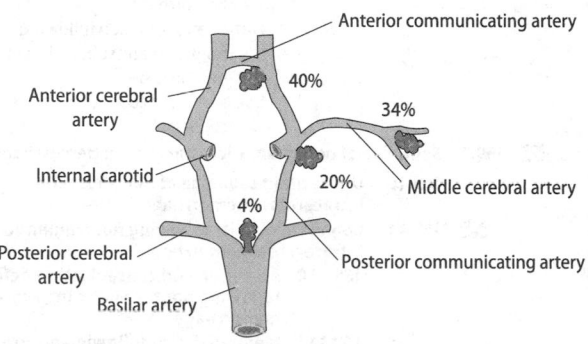

Anterior communicating artery

Anterior cerebral artery

40%

34%

Internal carotid

20%

Middle cerebral artery

4%

Posterior cerebral artery

Posterior communicating artery

Basilar artery

Common sites of berry aneurysms in the circle of Willis arteries

I67.0 Dissection of cerebral arteries, nonruptured
EXCLUDES 1 *ruptured cerebral arteries (I60.7)*

I67.1 Cerebral aneurysm, nonruptured
Cerebral aneurysm NOS
Cerebral arteriovenous fistula, acquired
Internal carotid artery aneurysm, intracranial portion
Internal carotid artery aneurysm, NOS
EXCLUDES 1 *congenital cerebral aneurysm, nonruptured (Q28.-)*
ruptured cerebral aneurysm (I60.7)

I67.2 Cerebral atherosclerosis   🄰
Atheroma of cerebral and precerebral arteries

I67.3 Progressive vascular leukoencephalopathy
Binswanger's disease

I67.4 Hypertensive encephalopathy

I67.5 Moyamoya disease
DEF: Cerebrovascular ischemia; vessels occlude and rupture, causing tiny hemorrhages at base of brain; affects predominantly Japanese people.

I67.6 Nonpyogenic thrombosis of intracranial venous system
Nonpyogenic thrombosis of cerebral vein
Nonpyogenic thrombosis of intracranial venous sinus
EXCLUDES 1 *nonpyogenic thrombosis of intracranial venous system causing infarction (I63.6)*

I67.7 Cerebral arteritis, not elsewhere classified
Granulomatous angiitis of the nervous system
EXCLUDES 1 *allergic granulomatous angiitis (M30.1)*

✓5ᵗʰ I67.8 Other specified cerebrovascular diseases

I67.81 Acute cerebrovascular insufficiency
Acute cerebrovascular insufficiency unspecified as to location or reversibility

I67.82 Cerebral ischemia
Chronic cerebral ischemia

I67.83 Posterior reversible encephalopathy syndrome
PRES

✓6ᵗʰ I67.84 Cerebral vasospasm and vasoconstriction

I67.841 Reversible cerebrovascular vasoconstriction syndrome
Call-Fleming syndrome
Code first underlying condition, if applicable, such as eclampsia (O15.00-O15.9)

I67.848 Other cerebrovascular vasospasm and vasoconstriction

I67.89 Other cerebrovascular disease

I67.9 Cerebrovascular disease, unspecified   ▽

✓4ᵗʰ I68 Cerebrovascular disorders in diseases classified elsewhere

I68.0 *Cerebral amyloid angiopathy*
Code first underlying amyloidosis (E85.-)

I68.2 *Cerebral arteritis in other diseases classified elsewhere*
Code first underlying disease
EXCLUDES 1 *cerebral arteritis (in):*
listerosis (A32.89)
syphilis (A52.04)
systemic lupus erythematosus (M32.19)
tuberculosis (A18.89)

I68.8 *Other cerebrovascular disorders in diseases classified elsewhere*
Code first underlying disease
EXCLUDES 1 *syphilitic cerebral aneurysm (A52.05)*

✓4ᵗʰ I69 Sequelae of cerebrovascular disease

NOTE   Category I69 is to be used to indicate conditions in I60-I67 as the cause of sequelae. The "sequelae" include conditions specified as such or as residuals which may occur at any time after the onset of the causal condition

EXCLUDES 1 *personal history of cerebral infarction without residual deficit (Z86.73)*
personal history of prolonged reversible ischemic neurologic deficit (PRIND) (Z86.73)
personal history of reversible ischemic neurolgcial deficit (RIND) (Z86.73)
sequelae of traumatic intracranial injury (S06.-)
transient ischemic attack (TIA) (G45.9)

AHA: 2012,4Q,106

✓5ᵗʰ I69.0 Sequelae of nontraumatic subarachnoid hemorrhage

I69.00 Unspecified sequelae of nontraumatic subarachnoid hemorrhage   ▽

✓6ᵗʰ I69.01 Cognitive deficits following nontraumatic subarachnoid hemorrhage

I69.010 Attention and concentration deficit following nontraumatic subarachnoid hemorrhage

I69.011 Memory deficit following nontraumatic subarachnoid hemorrhage

I69.012 Visuospatial deficit and spatial neglect following nontraumatic subarachnoid hemorrhage

I69.013 Psychomotor deficit following nontraumatic subarachnoid hemorrhage

I69.014 Frontal lobe and executive function deficit following nontraumatic subarachnoid hemorrhage

I69.015 Cognitive social or emotional deficit following nontraumatic subarachnoid hemorrhage

I69.018 Other symptoms and signs involving cognitive functions following nontraumatic subarachnoid hemorrhage

I69.019 Unspecified symptoms and signs involving cognitive functions following nontraumatic subarachnoid hemorrhage   ▽

✓6ᵗʰ I69.02 Speech and language deficits following nontraumatic subarachnoid hemorrhage

I69.020 Aphasia following nontraumatic subarachnoid hemorrhage

I69.021 Dysphasia following nontraumatic subarachnoid hemorrhage

I69.022 Dysarthria following nontraumatic subarachnoid hemorrhage

I69.023 Fluency disorder following nontraumatic subarachnoid hemorrhage
Stuttering following nontraumatic subarachnoid hemorrhage

I69.028 Other speech and language deficits following nontraumatic subarachnoid hemorrhage

✓6ᵗʰ I69.03 Monoplegia of upper limb following nontraumatic subarachnoid hemorrhage

I69.031 Monoplegia of upper limb following nontraumatic subarachnoid hemorrhage affecting right dominant side

✓ Additional Character Required   √x7ᵗʰ Placeholder Alert   Manifestation Dx   ▽ Unspecified Dx   ▶◀ Revised Text   ● New Code   ▲ Revised Code Title

ICD-10-CM 2017   619

Chapter 9. Diseases of the Circulatory System

I67–I69.031

I69.032 Monoplegia of upper limb following nontraumatic subarachnoid hemorrhage affecting left dominant side

I69.033 Monoplegia of upper limb following nontraumatic subarachnoid hemorrhage affecting right non-dominant side

I69.034 Monoplegia of upper limb following nontraumatic subarachnoid hemorrhage affecting left non-dominant side

I69.039 Monoplegia of upper limb following nontraumatic subarachnoid hemorrhage affecting unspecified side ▽

✓6ᵗʰ **I69.04** Monoplegia of lower limb following nontraumatic subarachnoid hemorrhage

I69.041 Monoplegia of lower limb following nontraumatic subarachnoid hemorrhage affecting right dominant side

I69.042 Monoplegia of lower limb following nontraumatic subarachnoid hemorrhage affecting left dominant side

I69.043 Monoplegia of lower limb following nontraumatic subarachnoid hemorrhage affecting right non-dominant side

I69.044 Monoplegia of lower limb following nontraumatic subarachnoid hemorrhage affecting left non-dominant side

I69.049 Monoplegia of lower limb following nontraumatic subarachnoid hemorrhage affecting unspecified side ▽

✓6ᵗʰ **I69.05** Hemiplegia and hemiparesis following nontraumatic subarachnoid hemorrhage •
AHA: 2015,1Q,25

I69.051 Hemiplegia and hemiparesis following nontraumatic subarachnoid hemorrhage affecting right dominant side •

I69.052 Hemiplegia and hemiparesis following nontraumatic subarachnoid hemorrhage affecting left dominant side •

I69.053 Hemiplegia and hemiparesis following nontraumatic subarachnoid hemorrhage affecting right non-dominant side •

I69.054 Hemiplegia and hemiparesis following nontraumatic subarachnoid hemorrhage affecting left non-dominant side •

I69.059 Hemiplegia and hemiparesis following nontraumatic subarachnoid hemorrhage affecting unspecified side ▽ •

✓6ᵗʰ **I69.06** Other paralytic syndrome following nontraumatic subarachnoid hemorrhage •
Use additional code to identify type of paralytic syndrome, such as:
locked-in state (G83.5)
quadriplegia (G82.5-)
EXCLUDES 1 hemiplegia/hemiparesis following nontraumatic subarachnoid hemorrhage (I69.05-)
monoplegia of lower limb following nontraumatic subarachnoid hemorrhage (I69.04-)
monoplegia of upper limb following nontraumatic subarachnoid hemorrhage (I69.03-)

I69.061 Other paralytic syndrome following nontraumatic subarachnoid hemorrhage affecting right dominant side

I69.062 Other paralytic syndrome following nontraumatic subarachnoid hemorrhage affecting left dominant side

I69.063 Other paralytic syndrome following nontraumatic subarachnoid hemorrhage affecting right non-dominant side

I69.064 Other paralytic syndrome following nontraumatic subarachnoid hemorrhage affecting left non-dominant side

I69.065 Other paralytic syndrome following nontraumatic subarachnoid hemorrhage, bilateral

I69.069 Other paralytic syndrome following nontraumatic subarachnoid hemorrhage affecting unspecified side ▽

✓6ᵗʰ **I69.09** Other sequelae of nontraumatic subarachnoid hemorrhage

I69.090 Apraxia following nontraumatic subarachnoid hemorrhage

I69.091 Dysphagia following nontraumatic subarachnoid hemorrhage
Use additional code to identify the type of dysphagia, if known (R13.1-)

I69.092 Facial weakness following nontraumatic subarachnoid hemorrhage
Facial droop following nontraumatic subarachnoid hemorrhage

I69.093 Ataxia following nontraumatic subarachnoid hemorrhage

I69.098 Other sequelae following nontraumatic subarachnoid hemorrhage
Alterations of sensation following nontraumatic subarachnoid hemorrhage
Disturbance of vision following nontraumatic subarachnoid hemorrhage
Use additional code to identify the sequelae

✓5ᵗʰ **I69.1** Sequelae of nontraumatic intracerebral hemorrhage

I69.10 Unspecified sequelae of nontraumatic intracerebral hemorrhage ▽

✓6ᵗʰ **I69.11** Cognitive deficits following nontraumatic intracerebral hemorrhage

I69.110 Attention and concentration deficit following nontraumatic intracerebral hemorrhage

I69.111 Memory deficit following nontraumatic intracerebral hemorrhage

I69.112 Visuospatial deficit and spatial neglect following nontraumatic intracerebral hemorrhage

I69.113 Psychomotor deficit following nontraumatic intracerebral hemorrhage

I69.114 Frontal lobe and executive function deficit following nontraumatic intracerebral hemorrhage

I69.115 Cognitive social or emotional deficit following nontraumatic intracerebral hemorrhage

I69.118 Other symptoms and signs involving cognitive functions following nontraumatic intracerebral hemorrhage

I69.119 Unspecified symptoms and signs involving cognitive functions following nontraumatic intracerebral hemorrhage ▽

✓6ᵗʰ **I69.12** Speech and language deficits following nontraumatic intracerebral hemorrhage

I69.120 Aphasia following nontraumatic intracerebral hemorrhage

I69.121 Dysphasia following nontraumatic intracerebral hemorrhage

I69.122 Dysarthria following nontraumatic intracerebral hemorrhage

I69.123 Fluency disorder following nontraumatic intracerebral hemorrhage
▶Stuttering following nontraumatic intracerebral hemorrhage◀

I69.128 Other speech and language deficits following nontraumatic intracerebral hemorrhage

✓6ᵗʰ **I69.13** Monoplegia of upper limb following nontraumatic intracerebral hemorrhage

I69.131 Monoplegia of upper limb following nontraumatic intracerebral hemorrhage affecting right dominant side

I69.132 Monoplegia of upper limb following nontraumatic intracerebral hemorrhage affecting left dominant side

I69.133 Monoplegia of upper limb following nontraumatic intracerebral hemorrhage affecting right non-dominant side

I69.134 Monoplegia of upper limb following nontraumatic intracerebral hemorrhage affecting left non-dominant side

       I69.139   **Monoplegia of upper limb following nontraumatic intracerebral hemorrhage affecting unspecified side**   ▽

✓6ᵗʰ   **I69.14**   **Monoplegia of lower limb following nontraumatic intracerebral hemorrhage**

       I69.141   **Monoplegia of lower limb following nontraumatic intracerebral hemorrhage affecting right dominant side**

       I69.142   **Monoplegia of lower limb following nontraumatic intracerebral hemorrhage affecting left dominant side**

       I69.143   **Monoplegia of lower limb following nontraumatic intracerebral hemorrhage affecting right non-dominant side**

       I69.144   **Monoplegia of lower limb following nontraumatic intracerebral hemorrhage affecting left non-dominant side**

       I69.149   **Monoplegia of lower limb following nontraumatic intracerebral hemorrhage affecting unspecified side**   ▽

✓6ᵗʰ   **I69.15**   **Hemiplegia and hemiparesis following nontraumatic intracerebral hemorrhage**
       AHA: 2015,1Q,25

       I69.151   **Hemiplegia and hemiparesis following nontraumatic intracerebral hemorrhage affecting right dominant side**

       I69.152   **Hemiplegia and hemiparesis following nontraumatic intracerebral hemorrhage affecting left dominant side**

       I69.153   **Hemiplegia and hemiparesis following nontraumatic intracerebral hemorrhage affecting right non-dominant side**

       I69.154   **Hemiplegia and hemiparesis following nontraumatic intracerebral hemorrhage affecting left non-dominant side**

       I69.159   **Hemiplegia and hemiparesis following nontraumatic intracerebral hemorrhage affecting unspecified side**   ▽

✓6ᵗʰ   **I69.16**   **Other paralytic syndrome following nontraumatic intracerebral hemorrhage**
       Use additional code to identify type of paralytic syndrome, such as:
       locked-in state (G83.5)
       quadriplegia (G82.5-)
       EXCLUDES 1   *hemiplegia/hemiparesis following nontraumatic intracerebral hemorrhage (I69.15-)*
       monoplegia of lower limb following nontraumatic intracerebral hemorrhage (I69.14-)
       monoplegia of upper limb following nontraumatic intracerebral hemorrhage (I69.13-)

       I69.161   **Other paralytic syndrome following nontraumatic intracerebral hemorrhage affecting right dominant side**

       I69.162   **Other paralytic syndrome following nontraumatic intracerebral hemorrhage affecting left dominant side**

       I69.163   **Other paralytic syndrome following nontraumatic intracerebral hemorrhage affecting right non-dominant side**

       I69.164   **Other paralytic syndrome following nontraumatic intracerebral hemorrhage affecting left non-dominant side**

       I69.165   **Other paralytic syndrome following nontraumatic intracerebral hemorrhage, bilateral**

       I69.169   **Other paralytic syndrome following nontraumatic intracerebral hemorrhage affecting unspecified side**   ▽

✓6ᵗʰ   **I69.19**   **Other sequelae of nontraumatic intracerebral hemorrhage**

       I69.190   **Apraxia following nontraumatic intracerebral hemorrhage**

       I69.191   **Dysphagia following nontraumatic intracerebral hemorrhage**
       Use additional code to identify the type of dysphagia, if known (R13.1-)

       I69.192   **Facial weakness following nontraumatic intracerebral hemorrhage**
       Facial droop following nontraumatic intracerebral hemorrhage

       I69.193   **Ataxia following nontraumatic intracerebral hemorrhage**

       I69.198   **Other sequelae of nontraumatic intracerebral hemorrhage**
       Alteration of sensations following nontraumatic intracerebral hemorrhage
       Disturbance of vision following nontraumatic intracerebral hemorrhage
       Use additional code to identify the sequelae

✓5ᵗʰ   **I69.2**   **Sequelae of other nontraumatic intracranial hemorrhage**

       I69.20   **Unspecified sequelae of other nontraumatic intracranial hemorrhage**   ▽

✓6ᵗʰ   **I69.21**   **Cognitive deficits following other nontraumatic intracranial hemorrhage**

       ●   **I69.210**   **Attention and concentration deficit following other nontraumatic intracranial hemorrhage**

       ●   **I69.211**   **Memory deficit following other nontraumatic intracranial hemorrhage**

       ●   **I69.212**   **Visuospatial deficit and spatial neglect following other nontraumatic intracranial hemorrhage**

       ●   **I69.213**   **Psychomotor deficit following other nontraumatic intracranial hemorrhage**

       ●   **I69.214**   **Frontal lobe and executive function deficit following other nontraumatic intracranial hemorrhage**

       ●   **I69.215**   **Cognitive social or emotional deficit following other nontraumatic intracranial hemorrhage**

       ●   **I69.218**   **Other symptoms and signs involving cognitive functions following other nontraumatic intracranial hemorrhage**

       ●   **I69.219**   **Unspecified symptoms and signs involving cognitive functions following other nontraumatic intracranial hemorrhage**   ▽

✓6ᵗʰ   **I69.22**   **Speech and language deficits following other nontraumatic intracranial hemorrhage**

       I69.220   **Aphasia following other nontraumatic intracranial hemorrhage**

       I69.221   **Dysphasia following other nontraumatic intracranial hemorrhage**

       I69.222   **Dysarthria following other nontraumatic intracranial hemorrhage**

       I69.223   **Fluency disorder following other nontraumatic intracranial hemorrhage**
       ► Stuttering following other nontraumatic intracranial hemorrhage ◄

       I69.228   **Other speech and language deficits following other nontraumatic intracranial hemorrhage**

✓6ᵗʰ   **I69.23**   **Monoplegia of upper limb following other nontraumatic intracranial hemorrhage**

       I69.231   **Monoplegia of upper limb following other nontraumatic intracranial hemorrhage affecting right dominant side**

       I69.232   **Monoplegia of upper limb following other nontraumatic intracranial hemorrhage affecting left dominant side**

       I69.233   **Monoplegia of upper limb following other nontraumatic intracranial hemorrhage affecting right non-dominant side**

       I69.234   **Monoplegia of upper limb following other nontraumatic intracranial hemorrhage affecting left non-dominant side**

       I69.239   **Monoplegia of upper limb following other nontraumatic intracranial hemorrhage affecting unspecified side**   ▽

✓ Additional Character Required   ✓x7ᵗʰ Placeholder Alert   Manifestation Dx   ▽ Unspecified Dx   ►◄ Revised Text   ● New Code   ▲ Revised Code Title

✓6ᵗʰ **I69.24 Monoplegia of lower limb following other nontraumatic intracranial hemorrhage**

- **I69.241 Monoplegia of lower limb following other nontraumatic intracranial hemorrhage affecting right dominant side**
- **I69.242 Monoplegia of lower limb following other nontraumatic intracranial hemorrhage affecting left dominant side**
- **I69.243 Monoplegia of lower limb following other nontraumatic intracranial hemorrhage affecting right non-dominant side**
- **I69.244 Monoplegia of lower limb following other nontraumatic intracranial hemorrhage affecting left non-dominant side**
- **I69.249 Monoplegia of lower limb** ▽ **following other nontraumatic intracranial hemorrhage affecting unspecified side**

✓6ᵗʰ **I69.25 Hemiplegia and hemiparesis following other nontraumatic intracranial hemorrhage**
    AHA: 2015,1Q,25

- **I69.251 Hemiplegia and hemiparesis following other nontraumatic intracranial hemorrhage affecting right dominant side**
- **I69.252 Hemiplegia and hemiparesis following other nontraumatic intracranial hemorrhage affecting left dominant side**
- **I69.253 Hemiplegia and hemiparesis following other nontraumatic intracranial hemorrhage affecting right non-dominant side**
- **I69.254 Hemiplegia and hemiparesis following other nontraumatic intracranial hemorrhage affecting left non-dominant side**
- **I69.259 Hemiplegia and hemiparesis** ▽ **following other nontraumatic intracranial hemorrhage affecting unspecified side**

✓6ᵗʰ **I69.26 Other paralytic syndrome following other nontraumatic intracranial hemorrhage**
    Use additional code to identify type of paralytic syndrome, such as:
    locked-in state (G83.5)
    quadriplegia (G82.5-)
    EXCLUDES 1   *hemiplegia/hemiparesis following other nontraumatic intracranial hemorrhage (I69.25-)*
        monoplegia of lower limb following other nontraumatic intracranial hemorrhage (I69.24-)
        monoplegia of upper limb following other nontraumatic intracranial hemorrhage (I69.23-)

- **I69.261 Other paralytic syndrome following other nontraumatic intracranial hemorrhage affecting right dominant side**
- **I69.262 Other paralytic syndrome following other nontraumatic intracranial hemorrhage affecting left dominant side**
- **I69.263 Other paralytic syndrome following other nontraumatic intracranial hemorrhage affecting right non-dominant side**
- **I69.264 Other paralytic syndrome following other nontraumatic intracranial hemorrhage affecting left non-dominant side**
- **I69.265 Other paralytic syndrome following other nontraumatic intracranial hemorrhage, bilateral**
- **I69.269 Other paralytic syndrome** ▽ **following other nontraumatic intracranial hemorrhage affecting unspecified side**

✓6ᵗʰ **I69.29 Other sequelae of other nontraumatic intracranial hemorrhage**

- **I69.290 Apraxia following other nontraumatic intracranial hemorrhage**
- **I69.291 Dysphagia following other nontraumatic intracranial hemorrhage**
    Use additional code to identify the type of dysphagia, if known (R13.1-)

- **I69.292 Facial weakness following other nontraumatic intracranial hemorrhage**
    Facial droop following other nontraumatic intracranial hemorrhage
- **I69.293 Ataxia following other nontraumatic intracranial hemorrhage**
- **I69.298 Other sequelae of other nontraumatic intracranial hemorrhage**
    Alteration of sensation following other nontraumatic intracranial hemorrhage
    Disturbance of vision following other nontraumatic intracranial hemorrhage
    Use additional code to identify the sequelae

✓5ᵗʰ **I69.3 Sequelae of cerebral infarction**
    Sequelae of stroke NOS
    AHA: 2013,4Q,127-128; 2012,4Q,92,94

I69.30 Unspecified sequelae of cerebral infarction ▽

✓6ᵗʰ **I69.31 Cognitive deficits following cerebral infarction**

- ● **I69.310 Attention and concentration deficit following cerebral infarction**
- ● **I69.311 Memory deficit following cerebral infarction**
- ● **I69.312 Visuospatial deficit and spatial neglect following cerebral infarction**
- ● **I69.313 Psychomotor deficit following cerebral infarction**
- ● **I69.314 Frontal lobe and executive function deficit following cerebral infarction**
- ● **I69.315 Cognitive social or emotional deficit following cerebral infarction**
- ● **I69.318 Other symptoms and signs involving cognitive functions following cerebral infarction**
- ● **I69.319 Unspecified symptoms and signs** ▽ **involving cognitive functions following cerebral infarction**

✓6ᵗʰ **I69.32 Speech and language deficits following cerebral infarction**

- **I69.320 Aphasia following cerebral infarction**
- **I69.321 Dysphasia following cerebral infarction**
    AHA: 2012,4Q,91
- **I69.322 Dysarthria following cerebral infarction**
- **I69.323 Fluency disorder following cerebral infarction**
    ▶Stuttering following cerebral infarction◀
- **I69.328 Other speech and language deficits following cerebral infarction**

✓6ᵗʰ **I69.33 Monoplegia of upper limb following cerebral infarction**

- **I69.331 Monoplegia of upper limb following cerebral infarction affecting right dominant side**
- **I69.332 Monoplegia of upper limb following cerebral infarction affecting left dominant side**
- **I69.333 Monoplegia of upper limb following cerebral infarction affecting right non-dominant side**
- **I69.334 Monoplegia of upper limb following cerebral infarction affecting left non-dominant side**
- **I69.339 Monoplegia of upper limb** ▽ **following cerebral infarction affecting unspecified side**

✓6ᵗʰ **I69.34 Monoplegia of lower limb following cerebral infarction**

- **I69.341 Monoplegia of lower limb following cerebral infarction affecting right dominant side**
- **I69.342 Monoplegia of lower limb following cerebral infarction affecting left dominant side**
- **I69.343 Monoplegia of lower limb following cerebral infarction affecting right non-dominant side**
- **I69.344 Monoplegia of lower limb following cerebral infarction affecting left non-dominant side**

I69.349   **Monoplegia of lower limb following cerebral infarction affecting unspecified side** ▽

✓6ᵗʰ I69.35   **Hemiplegia and hemiparesis following cerebral infarction**
     AHA: 2015,1Q,25

I69.351   **Hemiplegia and hemiparesis following cerebral infarction affecting right dominant side**

I69.352   **Hemiplegia and hemiparesis following cerebral infarction affecting left dominant side**

I69.353   **Hemiplegia and hemiparesis following cerebral infarction affecting right non-dominant side**

I69.354   **Hemiplegia and hemiparesis following cerebral infarction affecting left non-dominant side**
     AHA: 2012,4Q,91

I69.359   **Hemiplegia and hemiparesis following cerebral infarction affecting unspecified side** ▽

✓6ᵗʰ I69.36   **Other paralytic syndrome following cerebral infarction**
     Use additional code to identify type of paralytic syndrome, such as:
     locked-in state (G83.5)
     quadriplegia (G82.5-)
     EXCLUDES 1   *hemiplegia/hemiparesis following cerebral infarction (I69.35-)*
         monoplegia of lower limb following cerebral infarction (I69.34-)
         monoplegia of upper limb following cerebral infarction (I69.33-)

I69.361   **Other paralytic syndrome following cerebral infarction affecting right dominant side**

I69.362   **Other paralytic syndrome following cerebral infarction affecting left dominant side**

I69.363   **Other paralytic syndrome following cerebral infarction affecting right non-dominant side**

I69.364   **Other paralytic syndrome following cerebral infarction affecting left non-dominant side**

I69.365   **Other paralytic syndrome following cerebral infarction, bilateral**

I69.369   **Other paralytic syndrome following cerebral infarction affecting unspecified side** ▽

✓6ᵗʰ I69.39   **Other sequelae of cerebral infarction**

I69.390   **Apraxia following cerebral infarction**

I69.391   **Dysphagia following cerebral infarction**
     Use additional code to identify the type of dysphagia, if known (R13.1-)

I69.392   **Facial weakness following cerebral infarction**
     Facial droop following cerebral infarction

I69.393   **Ataxia following cerebral infarction**

I69.398   **Other sequelae of cerebral infarction**
     Alteration of sensation following cerebral infarction
     Disturbance of vision following cerebral infarction
     Use additional code to identify the sequelae

✓5ᵗʰ I69.8   **Sequelae of other cerebrovascular diseases**
     EXCLUDES 1   *sequelae of traumatic intracranial injury (S06.-)*

I69.80   **Unspecified sequelae of other cerebrovascular disease** ▽

✓6ᵗʰ I69.81   **Cognitive deficits following other cerebrovascular disease**

●   I69.810   **Attention and concentration deficit following other cerebrovascular disease**

●   I69.811   **Memory deficit following other cerebrovascular disease**

●   I69.812   **Visuospatial deficit and spatial neglect following other cerebrovascular disease**

●   I69.813   **Psychomotor deficit following other cerebrovascular disease**

●   I69.814   **Frontal lobe and executive function deficit following other cerebrovascular disease**

●   I69.815   **Cognitive social or emotional deficit following other cerebrovascular disease**

●   I69.818   **Other symptoms and signs involving cognitive functions following other cerebrovascular disease**

●   I69.819   **Unspecified symptoms and signs involving cognitive functions following other cerebrovascular disease** ▽

✓6ᵗʰ I69.82   **Speech and language deficits following other cerebrovascular disease**

I69.820   **Aphasia following other cerebrovascular disease**

I69.821   **Dysphasia following other cerebrovascular disease**

I69.822   **Dysarthria following other cerebrovascular disease**

I69.823   **Fluency disorder following other cerebrovascular disease**
     ▶Stuttering following other cerebrovascular disease◀

I69.828   **Other speech and language deficits following other cerebrovascular disease**

✓6ᵗʰ I69.83   **Monoplegia of upper limb following other cerebrovascular disease**

I69.831   **Monoplegia of upper limb following other cerebrovascular disease affecting right dominant side**

I69.832   **Monoplegia of upper limb following other cerebrovascular disease affecting left dominant side**

I69.833   **Monoplegia of upper limb following other cerebrovascular disease affecting right non-dominant side**

I69.834   **Monoplegia of upper limb following other cerebrovascular disease affecting left non-dominant side**

I69.839   **Monoplegia of upper limb following other cerebrovascular disease affecting unspecified side** ▽

✓6ᵗʰ I69.84   **Monoplegia of lower limb following other cerebrovascular disease**

I69.841   **Monoplegia of lower limb following other cerebrovascular disease affecting right dominant side**

I69.842   **Monoplegia of lower limb following other cerebrovascular disease affecting left dominant side**

I69.843   **Monoplegia of lower limb following other cerebrovascular disease affecting right non-dominant side**

I69.844   **Monoplegia of lower limb following other cerebrovascular disease affecting left non-dominant side**

I69.849   **Monoplegia of lower limb following other cerebrovascular disease affecting unspecified side** ▽

✓6ᵗʰ I69.85   **Hemiplegia and hemiparesis following other cerebrovascular disease**
     AHA: 2015,1Q,25

I69.851   **Hemiplegia and hemiparesis following other cerebrovascular disease affecting right dominant side**

I69.852   **Hemiplegia and hemiparesis following other cerebrovascular disease affecting left dominant side**

I69.853   **Hemiplegia and hemiparesis following other cerebrovascular disease affecting right non-dominant side**

I69.854   **Hemiplegia and hemiparesis following other cerebrovascular disease affecting left non-dominant side**

I69.859   **Hemiplegia and hemiparesis following other cerebrovascular disease affecting unspecified side** ▽

Chapter 9. Diseases of the Circulatory System

I69.349–I69.859

✓6th **I69.86** **Other paralytic syndrome following other cerebrovascular disease**
Use additional code to identify type of paralytic syndrome, such as:
  locked-in state (G83.5)
  quadriplegia (G82.5-)
EXCLUDES 1 *hemiplegia/hemiparesis following other cerebrovascular disease (I69.85-)*
  monoplegia of lower limb following other cerebrovascular disease (I69.84-)
  monoplegia of upper limb following other cerebrovascular disease (I69.83-)

I69.861 **Other paralytic syndrome following other cerebrovascular disease affecting right dominant side**

I69.862 **Other paralytic syndrome following other cerebrovascular disease affecting left dominant side**

I69.863 **Other paralytic syndrome following other cerebrovascular disease affecting right non-dominant side**

I69.864 **Other paralytic syndrome following other cerebrovascular disease affecting left non-dominant side**

I69.865 **Other paralytic syndrome following other cerebrovascular disease, bilateral**

I69.869 **Other paralytic syndrome following other cerebrovascular disease affecting unspecified side** ▽

✓6th **I69.89** **Other sequelae of other cerebrovascular disease**

I69.890 **Apraxia following other cerebrovascular disease**

I69.891 **Dysphagia following other cerebrovascular disease**
Use additional code to identify the type of dysphagia, if known (R13.1-)

I69.892 **Facial weakness following other cerebrovascular disease**
Facial droop following other cerebrovascular disease

I69.893 **Ataxia following other cerebrovascular disease**

I69.898 **Other sequelae of other cerebrovascular disease**
Alteration of sensation following other cerebrovascular disease
Disturbance of vision following other cerebrovascular disease
Use additional code to identify the sequelae

✓5th **I69.9** **Sequelae of unspecified cerebrovascular diseases**
EXCLUDES 1 *sequelae of stroke (I69.3)*
  sequelae of traumatic intracranial injury (S06.-)

I69.90 **Unspecified sequelae of unspecified cerebrovascular disease** ▽

✓6th **I69.91** **Cognitive deficits following unspecified cerebrovascular disease**

● **I69.910** **Attention and concentration deficit following unspecified cerebrovascular disease**

● **I69.911** **Memory deficit following unspecified cerebrovascular disease**

● **I69.912** **Visuospatial deficit and spatial neglect following unspecified cerebrovascular disease**

● **I69.913** **Psychomotor deficit following unspecified cerebrovascular disease**

● **I69.914** **Frontal lobe and executive function deficit following unspecified cerebrovascular disease**

● **I69.915** **Cognitive social or emotional deficit following unspecified cerebrovascular disease**

● **I69.918** **Other symptoms and signs involving cognitive functions following unspecified cerebrovascular disease**

● **I69.919** **Unspecified symptoms and signs involving cognitive functions following unspecified cerebrovascular disease** ▽

✓6th **I69.92** **Speech and language deficits following unspecified cerebrovascular disease**

I69.920 **Aphasia following unspecified cerebrovascular disease** ▽

I69.921 **Dysphasia following unspecified cerebrovascular disease** ▽

I69.922 **Dysarthria following unspecified cerebrovascular disease** ▽

I69.923 **Fluency disorder following unspecified cerebrovascular disease** ▽
  ▶Stuttering following unspecified cerebrovascular disease◀

I69.928 **Other speech and language deficits following unspecified cerebrovascular disease** ▽

✓6th **I69.93** **Monoplegia of upper limb following unspecified cerebrovascular disease**

I69.931 **Monoplegia of upper limb following unspecified cerebrovascular disease affecting right dominant side** ▽

I69.932 **Monoplegia of upper limb following unspecified cerebrovascular disease affecting left dominant side** ▽

I69.933 **Monoplegia of upper limb following unspecified cerebrovascular disease affecting right non-dominant side** ▽

I69.934 **Monoplegia of upper limb following unspecified cerebrovascular disease affecting left non-dominant side** ▽

I69.939 **Monoplegia of upper limb following unspecified cerebrovascular disease affecting unspecified side** ▽

✓6th **I69.94** **Monoplegia of lower limb following unspecified cerebrovascular disease**

I69.941 **Monoplegia of lower limb following unspecified cerebrovascular disease affecting right dominant side** ▽

I69.942 **Monoplegia of lower limb following unspecified cerebrovascular disease affecting left dominant side** ▽

I69.943 **Monoplegia of lower limb following unspecified cerebrovascular disease affecting right non-dominant side** ▽

I69.944 **Monoplegia of lower limb following unspecified cerebrovascular disease affecting left non-dominant side** ▽

I69.949 **Monoplegia of lower limb following unspecified cerebrovascular disease affecting unspecified side** ▽

✓6th **I69.95** **Hemiplegia and hemiparesis following unspecified cerebrovascular disease**
AHA: 2015,1Q,25

I69.951 **Hemiplegia and hemiparesis following unspecified cerebrovascular disease affecting right dominant side** ▽

I69.952 **Hemiplegia and hemiparesis following unspecified cerebrovascular disease affecting left dominant side** ▽

I69.953 **Hemiplegia and hemiparesis following unspecified cerebrovascular disease affecting right non-dominant side** ▽

I69.954 **Hemiplegia and hemiparesis following unspecified cerebrovascular disease affecting left non-dominant side** ▽

I69.959 **Hemiplegia and hemiparesis following unspecified cerebrovascular disease affecting unspecified side** ▽

√6ᵗʰ **I69.96 Other paralytic syndrome following unspecified cerebrovascular disease**

Use additional code to identify type of paralytic syndrome, such as:

locked-in state (G83.5)

quadriplegia (G82.5-)

EXCLUDES 1   *hemiplegia/hemiparesis following unspecified cerebrovascular disease (I69.95-)*

monoplegia of lower limb following unspecified cerebrovascular disease (I69.94-)

monoplegia of upper limb following unspecified cerebrovascular disease (I69.93-)

I69.961 Other paralytic syndrome following unspecified cerebrovascular disease affecting right dominant side ▽

I69.962 Other paralytic syndrome following unspecified cerebrovascular disease affecting left dominant side ▽

I69.963 Other paralytic syndrome following unspecified cerebrovascular disease affecting right non-dominant side ▽

I69.964 Other paralytic syndrome following unspecified cerebrovascular disease affecting left non-dominant side ▽

I69.965 Other paralytic syndrome following unspecified cerebrovascular disease, bilateral ▽

I69.969 Other paralytic syndrome following unspecified cerebrovascular disease affecting unspecified side ▽

√6ᵗʰ **I69.99 Other sequelae of unspecified cerebrovascular disease**

I69.990 Apraxia following unspecified cerebrovascular disease ▽

I69.991 Dysphagia following unspecified cerebrovascular disease ▽

Use additional code to identify the type of dysphagia, if known (R13.1-)

I69.992 Facial weakness following unspecified cerebrovascular disease ▽

Facial droop following unspecified cerebrovascular disease

I69.993 Ataxia following unspecified cerebrovascular disease ▽

I69.998 Other sequelae following unspecified cerebrovascular disease ▽

Alteration in sensation following unspecified cerebrovascular disease

Disturbance of vision following unspecified cerebrovascular disease

Use additional code to identify the sequelae

Diseases of arteries, arterioles and capillaries (I70-I79)

√4ᵗʰ **I70 Atherosclerosis**

INCLUDES   arterial degeneration

arteriolosclerosis

arteriosclerosis

arteriosclerotic vascular disease

arteriovascular degeneration

atheroma

endarteritis deformans or obliterans

senile arteritis

senile endarteritis

vascular degeneration

Use additional code to identify:

exposure to environmental tobacco smoke (Z77.22)

▶history of tobacco dependence (Z87.891)◀

occupational exposure to environmental tobacco smoke (Z57.31)

tobacco dependence (F17.-)

tobacco use (Z72.0)

EXCLUDES 2   *arteriosclerotic cardiovascular disease (I25.1-)*

arteriosclerotic heart disease (I25.1-)

atheroembolism (I75.-)

cerebral atherosclerosis (I67.2)

coronary atherosclerosis (I25.1-)

mesenteric atherosclerosis (K55.1)

precerebral atherosclerosis (I67.2)

primary pulmonary atherosclerosis (I27.0)

I70.0 Atherosclerosis of aorta Ⓐ

I70.1 Atherosclerosis of renal artery Ⓐ

Goldblatt's kidney

EXCLUDES 2   *atherosclerosis of renal arterioles (I12.-)*

√5ᵗʰ **I70.2 Atherosclerosis of native arteries of the extremities**

Mönckeberg's (medial) sclerosis

Use additional code, if applicable, to identify chronic total occlusion of artery of extremity (I70.92)

EXCLUDES 2   *atherosclerosis of bypass graft of extremities (I70.30-I70.79)*

√6ᵗʰ **I70.20 Unspecified atherosclerosis of native arteries of extremities**

I70.201 Unspecified atherosclerosis of native arteries of extremities, right leg Ⓐ ▽

I70.202 Unspecified atherosclerosis of native arteries of extremities, left leg Ⓐ ▽

I70.203 Unspecified atherosclerosis of native arteries of extremities, bilateral legs Ⓐ ▽

I70.208 Unspecified atherosclerosis of native arteries of extremities, other extremity Ⓐ ▽

I70.209 Unspecified atherosclerosis of native arteries of extremities, unspecified extremity Ⓐ ▽

√6ᵗʰ **I70.21 Atherosclerosis of native arteries of extremities with intermittent claudication**

I70.211 Atherosclerosis of native arteries of extremities with intermittent claudication, right leg Ⓐ

I70.212 Atherosclerosis of native arteries of extremities with intermittent claudication, left leg Ⓐ

I70.213 Atherosclerosis of native arteries of extremities with intermittent claudication, bilateral legs Ⓐ

I70.218 Atherosclerosis of native arteries of extremities with intermittent claudication, other extremity Ⓐ

I70.219 Atherosclerosis of native arteries of extremities with intermittent claudication, unspecified extremity Ⓐ ▽

√6ᵗʰ **I70.22 Atherosclerosis of native arteries of extremities with rest pain**

INCLUDES   any condition classifiable to I70.21-

I70.221 Atherosclerosis of native arteries of extremities with rest pain, right leg Ⓐ

☑ Additional Character Required   √x7ᵗʰ Placeholder Alert   Manifestation Dx   ▽ Unspecified Dx   ▶◀ Revised Text   ● New Code   ▲ Revised Code Title

ICD-10-CM 2017   625

I70.222 Atherosclerosis of native arteries of extremities with rest pain, left leg   Ⓐ

I70.223 Atherosclerosis of native arteries of extremities with rest pain, bilateral legs   Ⓐ

I70.228 Atherosclerosis of native arteries of extremities with rest pain, other extremity   Ⓐ

I70.229 Atherosclerosis of native arteries of extremities with rest pain, unspecified extremity   Ⓐ ▽

✓6ᵗʰ **I70.23 Atherosclerosis of native arteries of right leg with ulceration**

    INCLUDES   any condition classifiable to I70.211 and I70.221

    Use additional code to identify severity of ulcer (L97.-)

I70.231 Atherosclerosis of native arteries of right leg with ulceration of thigh   Ⓐ

I70.232 Atherosclerosis of native arteries of right leg with ulceration of calf   Ⓐ

I70.233 Atherosclerosis of native arteries of right leg with ulceration of ankle   Ⓐ

I70.234 Atherosclerosis of native arteries of right leg with ulceration of heel and midfoot   Ⓐ

    Atherosclerosis of native arteries of right leg with ulceration of plantar surface of midfoot

I70.235 Atherosclerosis of native arteries of right leg with ulceration of other part of foot   Ⓐ

    Atherosclerosis of native arteries of right leg extremities with ulceration of toe

I70.238 Atherosclerosis of native arteries of right leg with ulceration of other part of lower right leg   Ⓐ

I70.239 Atherosclerosis of native arteries of right leg with ulceration of unspecified site   Ⓐ ▽

✓6ᵗʰ **I70.24 Atherosclerosis of native arteries of left leg with ulceration**

    INCLUDES   any condition classifiable to I70.212 and I70.222

    Use additional code to identify severity of ulcer (L97.-)

I70.241 Atherosclerosis of native arteries of left leg with ulceration of thigh   Ⓐ

I70.242 Atherosclerosis of native arteries of left leg with ulceration of calf   Ⓐ

I70.243 Atherosclerosis of native arteries of left leg with ulceration of ankle   Ⓐ

I70.244 Atherosclerosis of native arteries of left leg with ulceration of heel and midfoot   Ⓐ

    Atherosclerosis of native arteries of left leg with ulceration of plantar surface of midfoot

I70.245 Atherosclerosis of native arteries of left leg with ulceration of other part of foot   Ⓐ

    Atherosclerosis of native arteries of left leg extremities with ulceration of toe

I70.248 Atherosclerosis of native arteries of left leg with ulceration of other part of lower left leg   Ⓐ

I70.249 Atherosclerosis of native arteries of left leg with ulceration of unspecified site   Ⓐ ▽

I70.25 Atherosclerosis of native arteries of other extremities with ulceration   Ⓐ

    INCLUDES   any condition classifiable to I70.218 and I70.228

    Use additional code to identify the severity of the ulcer (L98.49-)

✓6ᵗʰ **I70.26 Atherosclerosis of native arteries of extremities with gangrene**

    INCLUDES   any condition classifiable to I70.21-, I70.22-, I70.23-, I70.24-, and I70.25-

    Use additional code to identify the severity of any ulcer (L97.-, L98.49-), if applicable

I70.261 Atherosclerosis of native arteries of extremities with gangrene, right leg   Ⓐ

I70.262 Atherosclerosis of native arteries of extremities with gangrene, left leg   Ⓐ

I70.263 Atherosclerosis of native arteries of extremities with gangrene, bilateral legs   Ⓐ

I70.268 Atherosclerosis of native arteries of extremities with gangrene, other extremity   Ⓐ

I70.269 Atherosclerosis of native arteries of extremities with gangrene, unspecified extremity   Ⓐ ▽

✓6ᵗʰ **I70.29 Other atherosclerosis of native arteries of extremities**

I70.291 Other atherosclerosis of native arteries of extremities, right leg   Ⓐ

I70.292 Other atherosclerosis of native arteries of extremities, left leg   Ⓐ

I70.293 Other atherosclerosis of native arteries of extremities, bilateral legs   Ⓐ

I70.298 Other atherosclerosis of native arteries of extremities, other extremity   Ⓐ

I70.299 Other atherosclerosis of native arteries of extremities, unspecified extremity   Ⓐ ▽

✓5ᵗʰ **I70.3 Atherosclerosis of unspecified type of bypass graft(s) of the extremities**

    Use additional code, if applicable, to identify chronic total occlusion of artery of extremity (I70.92)

    EXCLUDES 1   *embolism or thrombus of bypass graft(s) of extremities (T82.8-)*

✓6ᵗʰ **I70.30 Unspecified atherosclerosis of unspecified type of bypass graft(s) of the extremities**

I70.301 Unspecified atherosclerosis of unspecified type of bypass graft(s) of the extremities, right leg   Ⓐ ▽

I70.302 Unspecified atherosclerosis of unspecified type of bypass graft(s) of the extremities, left leg   Ⓐ ▽

I70.303 Unspecified atherosclerosis of unspecified type of bypass graft(s) of the extremities, bilateral legs   Ⓐ ▽

I70.308 Unspecified atherosclerosis of unspecified type of bypass graft(s) of the extremities, other extremity   Ⓐ ▽

I70.309 Unspecified atherosclerosis of unspecified type of bypass graft(s) of the extremities, unspecified extremity   Ⓐ ▽

✓6ᵗʰ **I70.31 Atherosclerosis of unspecified type of bypass graft(s) of the extremities with intermittent claudication**

I70.311 Atherosclerosis of unspecified type of bypass graft(s) of the extremities with intermittent claudication, right leg   Ⓐ

I70.312 Atherosclerosis of unspecified type of bypass graft(s) of the extremities with intermittent claudication, left leg   Ⓐ

I70.313 Atherosclerosis of unspecified type of bypass graft(s) of the extremities with intermittent claudication, bilateral legs   Ⓐ

I70.318 Atherosclerosis of unspecified type of bypass graft(s) of the extremities with intermittent claudication, other extremity   Ⓐ

I70.319 Atherosclerosis of unspecified type of bypass graft(s) of the extremities with intermittent claudication, unspecified extremity   Ⓐ ▽

✓6ᵗʰ **I70.32 Atherosclerosis of unspecified type of bypass graft(s) of the extremities with rest pain**

    INCLUDES   any condition classifiable to I70.31-

I70.321 Atherosclerosis of unspecified type of bypass graft(s) of the extremities with rest pain, right leg   Ⓐ

EXCLUDES 1   Not coded here   EXCLUDES 2   Not included here   Ⓝ Newborn Age : 0   Ⓟ Pediatric Age : 0-17   Ⓜ Maternity Age : 12-55   Ⓐ Adult Age : 15-124

626   ICD-10-CM 2017

I70.322 Atherosclerosis of unspecified type of bypass graft(s) of the extremities with rest pain, **left leg** Ⓐ

I70.323 Atherosclerosis of unspecified type of bypass graft(s) of the extremities with rest pain, **bilateral legs** Ⓐ

I70.328 Atherosclerosis of unspecified type of bypass graft(s) of the extremities with rest pain, other extremity Ⓐ

I70.329 Atherosclerosis of unspecified type of bypass graft(s) of the extremities with rest pain, unspecified extremity Ⓐ ▽

✓6ᵗʰ **I70.33** Atherosclerosis of unspecified type of bypass graft(s) of the **right leg** with **ulceration**

INCLUDES any condition classifiable to I70.311 and I70.321

Use additional code to identify severity of ulcer (L97.-)

I70.331 Atherosclerosis of unspecified type of bypass graft(s) of the right leg with ulceration of **thigh** Ⓐ

I70.332 Atherosclerosis of unspecified type of bypass graft(s) of the right leg with ulceration of **calf** Ⓐ

I70.333 Atherosclerosis of unspecified type of bypass graft(s) of the right leg with ulceration of **ankle** Ⓐ

I70.334 Atherosclerosis of unspecified type of bypass graft(s) of the right leg with ulceration of **heel and midfoot** Ⓐ
    Atherosclerosis of unspecified type of bypass graft(s) of right leg with ulceration of plantar surface of midfoot

I70.335 Atherosclerosis of unspecified type of bypass graft(s) of the right leg with ulceration of **other part of foot** Ⓐ
    Atherosclerosis of unspecified type of bypass graft(s) of the right leg with ulceration of toe

I70.338 Atherosclerosis of unspecified type of bypass graft(s) of the right leg with ulceration of other part of lower leg Ⓐ

I70.339 Atherosclerosis of unspecified type of bypass graft(s) of the right leg with ulceration of unspecified site Ⓐ ▽

✓6ᵗʰ **I70.34** Atherosclerosis of unspecified type of bypass graft(s) of the **left leg** with **ulceration**

INCLUDES any condition classifiable to I70.312 and I70.322

Use additional code to identify severity of ulcer (L97.-)

I70.341 Atherosclerosis of unspecified type of bypass graft(s) of the left leg with ulceration of **thigh** Ⓐ

I70.342 Atherosclerosis of unspecified type of bypass graft(s) of the left leg with ulceration of **calf** Ⓐ

I70.343 Atherosclerosis of unspecified type of bypass graft(s) of the left leg with ulceration of **ankle** Ⓐ

I70.344 Atherosclerosis of unspecified type of bypass graft(s) of the left leg with ulceration of **heel and midfoot** Ⓐ
    Atherosclerosis of unspecified type of bypass graft(s) of left leg with ulceration of plantar surface of midfoot

I70.345 Atherosclerosis of unspecified type of bypass graft(s) of the left leg with ulceration of **other part of foot** Ⓐ
    Atherosclerosis of unspecified type of bypass graft(s) of the left leg with ulceration of toe

I70.348 Atherosclerosis of unspecified type of bypass graft(s) of the left leg with ulceration of other part of lower leg Ⓐ

I70.349 Atherosclerosis of unspecified type of bypass graft(s) of the left leg with ulceration of unspecified site Ⓐ ▽

I70.35 Atherosclerosis of unspecified type of bypass graft(s) of other extremity with ulceration Ⓐ
    INCLUDES any condition classifiable to I70.318 and I70.328
    Use additional code to identify severity of ulcer (L98.49-)

✓6ᵗʰ **I70.36** Atherosclerosis of unspecified type of bypass graft(s) of the extremities with **gangrene** Ⓐ
    INCLUDES any condition classifiable to I70.31-, I70.32-, I70.33-, I70.34-, I70.35
    Use additional code to identify the severity of any ulcer (L97.-, L98.49-), if applicable

I70.361 Atherosclerosis of unspecified type of bypass graft(s) of the extremities with gangrene, **right leg** Ⓐ

I70.362 Atherosclerosis of unspecified type of bypass graft(s) of the extremities with gangrene, **left leg** Ⓐ

I70.363 Atherosclerosis of unspecified type of bypass graft(s) of the extremities with gangrene, **bilateral legs** Ⓐ

I70.368 Atherosclerosis of unspecified type of bypass graft(s) of the extremities with gangrene, other extremity Ⓐ

I70.369 Atherosclerosis of unspecified type of bypass graft(s) of the extremities with gangrene, unspecified extremity Ⓐ ▽

✓6ᵗʰ **I70.39** Other atherosclerosis of unspecified type of bypass graft(s) of the extremities

I70.391 Other atherosclerosis of unspecified type of bypass graft(s) of the extremities, **right leg** Ⓐ

I70.392 Other atherosclerosis of unspecified type of bypass graft(s) of the extremities, **left leg** Ⓐ

I70.393 Other atherosclerosis of unspecified type of bypass graft(s) of the extremities, **bilateral legs** Ⓐ

I70.398 Other atherosclerosis of unspecified type of bypass graft(s) of the extremities, other extremity Ⓐ

I70.399 Other atherosclerosis of unspecified type of bypass graft(s) of the extremities, unspecified extremity Ⓐ ▽

✓5ᵗʰ **I70.4** Atherosclerosis of **autologous vein bypass graft(s)** of the extremities
    Use additional code, if applicable, to identify chronic total occlusion of artery of extremity (I70.92)

✓6ᵗʰ **I70.40** Unspecified atherosclerosis of autologous vein bypass graft(s) of the extremities

I70.401 Unspecified atherosclerosis of autologous vein bypass graft(s) of the extremities, **right leg** Ⓐ ▽

I70.402 Unspecified atherosclerosis of autologous vein bypass graft(s) of the extremities, **left leg** Ⓐ ▽

I70.403 Unspecified atherosclerosis of autologous vein bypass graft(s) of the extremities, **bilateral legs** Ⓐ ▽

I70.408 Unspecified atherosclerosis of autologous vein bypass graft(s) of the extremities, other extremity Ⓐ ▽

I70.409 Unspecified atherosclerosis of autologous vein bypass graft(s) of the extremities, unspecified extremity Ⓐ ▽

✓6ᵗʰ **I70.41** Atherosclerosis of autologous vein bypass graft(s) of the extremities with **intermittent claudication**

I70.411 Atherosclerosis of autologous vein bypass graft(s) of the extremities with intermittent claudication, **right leg** Ⓐ

✓ Additional Character Required   ✓x7ᵗʰ Placeholder Alert   Manifestation Dx   ▽ Unspecified Dx   ►◄ Revised Text   ● New Code   ▲ Revised Code Title

Chapter 9. Diseases of the Circulatory System

I70.412–I70.503

I70.412 Atherosclerosis of autologous vein bypass graft(s) of the extremities with intermittent claudication, left leg ▪A▪

I70.413 Atherosclerosis of autologous vein bypass graft(s) of the extremities with intermittent claudication, bilateral legs ▪A▪

I70.418 Atherosclerosis of autologous vein bypass graft(s) of the extremities with intermittent claudication, other extremity ▪A▪

I70.419 Atherosclerosis of autologous vein bypass graft(s) of the extremities with intermittent claudication, unspecified extremity ▪A▪ ▽

✓6ᵗʰ **I70.42** Atherosclerosis of autologous vein bypass graft(s) of the extremities with rest pain

     INCLUDES any condition classifiable to I70.41-

I70.421 Atherosclerosis of autologous vein bypass graft(s) of the extremities with rest pain, right leg ▪A▪

I70.422 Atherosclerosis of autologous vein bypass graft(s) of the extremities with rest pain, left leg ▪A▪

I70.423 Atherosclerosis of autologous vein bypass graft(s) of the extremities with rest pain, bilateral legs ▪A▪

I70.428 Atherosclerosis of autologous vein bypass graft(s) of the extremities with rest pain, other extremity ▪A▪

I70.429 Atherosclerosis of autologous vein bypass graft(s) of the extremities with rest pain, unspecified extremity ▪A▪ ▽

✓6ᵗʰ **I70.43** Atherosclerosis of autologous vein bypass graft(s) of the right leg with ulceration

     INCLUDES any condition classifiable to I70.411 and I70.421

     Use additional code to identify severity of ulcer (L97.-)

I70.431 Atherosclerosis of autologous vein bypass graft(s) of the right leg with ulceration of thigh ▪A▪

I70.432 Atherosclerosis of autologous vein bypass graft(s) of the right leg with ulceration of calf ▪A▪

I70.433 Atherosclerosis of autologous vein bypass graft(s) of the right leg with ulceration of ankle ▪A▪

I70.434 Atherosclerosis of autologous vein bypass graft(s) of the right leg with ulceration of heel and midfoot ▪A▪

     Atherosclerosis of autologous vein bypass graft(s) of right leg with ulceration of plantar surface of midfoot

I70.435 Atherosclerosis of autologous vein bypass graft(s) of the right leg with ulceration of other part of foot ▪A▪

     Atherosclerosis of autologous vein bypass graft(s) of right leg with ulceration of toe

I70.438 Atherosclerosis of autologous vein bypass graft(s) of the right leg with ulceration of other part of lower leg ▪A▪

I70.439 Atherosclerosis of autologous vein bypass graft(s) of the right leg with ulceration of unspecified site ▪A▪ ▽

✓6ᵗʰ **I70.44** Atherosclerosis of autologous vein bypass graft(s) of the left leg with ulceration

     INCLUDES any condition classifiable to I70.412 and I70.422

     Use additional code to identify severity of ulcer (L97.-)

I70.441 Atherosclerosis of autologous vein bypass graft(s) of the left leg with ulceration of thigh ▪A▪

I70.442 Atherosclerosis of autologous vein bypass graft(s) of the left leg with ulceration of calf ▪A▪

I70.443 Atherosclerosis of autologous vein bypass graft(s) of the left leg with ulceration of ankle ▪A▪

I70.444 Atherosclerosis of autologous vein bypass graft(s) of the left leg with ulceration of heel and midfoot ▪A▪

     Atherosclerosis of autologous vein bypass graft(s) of left leg with ulceration of plantar surface of midfoot

I70.445 Atherosclerosis of autologous vein bypass graft(s) of the left leg with ulceration of other part of foot ▪A▪

     Atherosclerosis of autologous vein bypass graft(s) of left leg with ulceration of toe

I70.448 Atherosclerosis of autologous vein bypass graft(s) of the left leg with ulceration of other part of lower leg ▪A▪

I70.449 Atherosclerosis of autologous vein bypass graft(s) of the left leg with ulceration of unspecified site ▪A▪ ▽

I70.45 Atherosclerosis of autologous vein bypass graft(s) of other extremity with ulceration ▪A▪

     INCLUDES any condition classifiable to I70.418, I70.428, and I70.438

     Use additional code to identify severity of ulcer (L98.49)

✓6ᵗʰ **I70.46** Atherosclerosis of autologous vein bypass graft(s) of the extremities with gangrene

     INCLUDES any condition classifiable to I70.41-, I70.42-, and I70.43-, I70.44-, I70.45

     Use additional code to identify the severity of any ulcer (L97.-, L98.49-), if applicable

I70.461 Atherosclerosis of autologous vein bypass graft(s) of the extremities with gangrene, right leg ▪A▪

I70.462 Atherosclerosis of autologous vein bypass graft(s) of the extremities with gangrene, left leg ▪A▪

I70.463 Atherosclerosis of autologous vein bypass graft(s) of the extremities with gangrene, bilateral legs ▪A▪

I70.468 Atherosclerosis of autologous vein bypass graft(s) of the extremities with gangrene, other extremity ▪A▪

I70.469 Atherosclerosis of autologous vein bypass graft(s) of the extremities with gangrene, unspecified extremity ▪A▪ ▽

✓6ᵗʰ **I70.49** Other atherosclerosis of autologous vein bypass graft(s) of the extremities

I70.491 Other atherosclerosis of autologous vein bypass graft(s) of the extremities, right leg ▪A▪

I70.492 Other atherosclerosis of autologous vein bypass graft(s) of the extremities, left leg ▪A▪

I70.493 Other atherosclerosis of autologous vein bypass graft(s) of the extremities, bilateral legs ▪A▪

I70.498 Other atherosclerosis of autologous vein bypass graft(s) of the extremities, other extremity ▪A▪

I70.499 Other atherosclerosis of autologous vein bypass graft(s) of the extremities, unspecified extremity ▪A▪ ▽

✓5ᵗʰ **I70.5** Atherosclerosis of nonautologous biological bypass graft(s) of the extremities

     Use additional code, if applicable, to identify chronic total occlusion of artery of extremity (I70.92)

✓6ᵗʰ **I70.50** Unspecified atherosclerosis of nonautologous biological bypass graft(s) of the extremities

I70.501 Unspecified atherosclerosis of nonautologous biological bypass graft(s) of the extremities, right leg ▪A▪ ▽

I70.502 Unspecified atherosclerosis of nonautologous biological bypass graft(s) of the extremities, left leg ▪A▪ ▽

I70.503 Unspecified atherosclerosis of nonautologous biological bypass graft(s) of the extremities, bilateral legs ▪A▪ ▽

EXCLUDES 1 Not coded here   *EXCLUDES 2* Not included here   **N** Newborn Age : 0   **P** Pediatric Age : 0-17   **M** Maternity Age : 12-55   **A** Adult Age : 15-124

628   ICD-10-CM 2017

I70.508 Unspecified atherosclerosis of nonautologous biological bypass graft(s) of the extremities, other extremity ▲ ▽

I70.509 Unspecified atherosclerosis of nonautologous biological bypass graft(s) of the extremities, unspecified extremity ▲ ▽

✓6ᵗʰ **I70.51** Atherosclerosis of nonautologous biological bypass graft(s) of the extremities intermittent claudication

    I70.511 Atherosclerosis of nonautologous biological bypass graft(s) of the extremities with intermittent claudication, right leg ▲

    I70.512 Atherosclerosis of nonautologous biological bypass graft(s) of the extremities with intermittent claudication, left leg ▲

    I70.513 Atherosclerosis of nonautologous biological bypass graft(s) of the extremities with intermittent claudication, bilateral legs ▲

    I70.518 Atherosclerosis of nonautologous biological bypass graft(s) of the extremities with intermittent claudication, other extremity ▲

    I70.519 Atherosclerosis of nonautologous biological bypass graft(s) of the extremities with intermittent claudication, unspecified extremity ▲ ▽

✓6ᵗʰ **I70.52** Atherosclerosis of nonautologous biological bypass graft(s) of the extremities with rest pain
    INCLUDES any condition classifiable to I70.51-

    I70.521 Atherosclerosis of nonautologous biological bypass graft(s) of the extremities with rest pain, right leg ▲

    I70.522 Atherosclerosis of nonautologous biological bypass graft(s) of the extremities with rest pain, left leg ▲

    I70.523 Atherosclerosis of nonautologous biological bypass graft(s) of the extremities with rest pain, bilateral legs ▲

    I70.528 Atherosclerosis of nonautologous biological bypass graft(s) of the extremities with rest pain, other extremity ▲

    I70.529 Atherosclerosis of nonautologous biological bypass graft(s) of the extremities with rest pain, unspecified extremity ▲ ▽

✓6ᵗʰ **I70.53** Atherosclerosis of nonautologous biological bypass graft(s) of the right leg with ulceration
    INCLUDES any condition classifiable to I70.511 and I70.521
    Use additional code to identify severity of ulcer (L97.-)

    I70.531 Atherosclerosis of nonautologous biological bypass graft(s) of the right leg with ulceration of thigh ▲

    I70.532 Atherosclerosis of nonautologous biological bypass graft(s) of the right leg with ulceration of calf ▲

    I70.533 Atherosclerosis of nonautologous biological bypass graft(s) of the right leg with ulceration of ankle ▲

    I70.534 Atherosclerosis of nonautologous biological bypass graft(s) of the right leg with ulceration of heel and midfoot ▲
        Atherosclerosis of nonautologous biological bypass graft(s) of right leg with ulceration of plantar surface of midfoot

    I70.535 Atherosclerosis of nonautologous biological bypass graft(s) of the right leg with ulceration of other part of foot ▲
        Atherosclerosis of nonautologous biological bypass graft(s) of the right leg with ulceration of toe

I70.538 Atherosclerosis of nonautologous biological bypass graft(s) of the right leg with ulceration of other part of lower leg ▲

I70.539 Atherosclerosis of nonautologous biological bypass graft(s) of the right leg with ulceration of unspecified site ▲ ▽

✓6ᵗʰ **I70.54** Atherosclerosis of nonautologous biological bypass graft(s) of the left leg with ulceration
    INCLUDES any condition classifiable to I70.512 and I70.522
    Use additional code to identify severity of ulcer (L97.-)

    I70.541 Atherosclerosis of nonautologous biological bypass graft(s) of the left leg with ulceration of thigh ▲

    I70.542 Atherosclerosis of nonautologous biological bypass graft(s) of the left leg with ulceration of calf ▲

    I70.543 Atherosclerosis of nonautologous biological bypass graft(s) of the left leg with ulceration of ankle ▲

    I70.544 Atherosclerosis of nonautologous biological bypass graft(s) of the left leg with ulceration of heel and midfoot ▲
        Atherosclerosis of nonautologous biological bypass graft(s) of left leg with ulceration of plantar surface of midfoot

    I70.545 Atherosclerosis of nonautologous biological bypass graft(s) of the left leg with ulceration of other part of foot ▲
        Atherosclerosis of nonautologous biological bypass graft(s) of the left leg with ulceration of toe

    I70.548 Atherosclerosis of nonautologous biological bypass graft(s) of the left leg with ulceration of other part of lower leg ▲

    I70.549 Atherosclerosis of nonautologous biological bypass graft(s) of the left leg with ulceration of unspecified site ▲ ▽

I70.55 Atherosclerosis of nonautologous biological bypass graft(s) of other extremity with ulceration ▲
    INCLUDES any condition classifiable to I70.518, I70.528, and I70.538
    Use additional code to identify severity of ulcer (L98.49)

✓6ᵗʰ **I70.56** Atherosclerosis of nonautologous biological bypass graft(s) of the extremities with gangrene
    INCLUDES any condition classifiable to I70.51-, I70.52-, and I70.53-, I70.54-, I70.55
    Use additional code to identify the severity of any ulcer (L97.-, L98.49-), if applicable

    I70.561 Atherosclerosis of nonautologous biological bypass graft(s) of the extremities with gangrene, right leg ▲

    I70.562 Atherosclerosis of nonautologous biological bypass graft(s) of the extremities with gangrene, left leg ▲

    I70.563 Atherosclerosis of nonautologous biological bypass graft(s) of the extremities with gangrene, bilateral legs ▲

    I70.568 Atherosclerosis of nonautologous biological bypass graft(s) of the extremities with gangrene, other extremity ▲

    I70.569 Atherosclerosis of nonautologous biological bypass graft(s) of the extremities with gangrene, unspecified extremity ▲ ▽

✓6ᵗʰ **I70.59** Other atherosclerosis of nonautologous biological bypass graft(s) of the extremities

    I70.591 Other atherosclerosis of nonautologous biological bypass graft(s) of the extremities, right leg ▲

✔ Additional Character Required   ✓x7ᵗʰ Placeholder Alert   Manifestation Dx   ▽ Unspecified Dx   ▶◀ Revised Text   ● New Code   ▲ Revised Code Title

ICD-10-CM 2017   629

I70.592   Other atherosclerosis of nonautologous biological bypass graft(s) of the extremities, left leg   A

I70.593   Other atherosclerosis of nonautologous biological bypass graft(s) of the extremities, bilateral legs   A

I70.598   Other atherosclerosis of nonautologous biological bypass graft(s) of the extremities, other extremity   A

I70.599   Other atherosclerosis of nonautologous biological bypass graft(s) of the extremities, unspecified extremity   A ▽

√5th **I70.6**   **Atherosclerosis of nonbiological bypass graft(s) of the extremities**
> Use additional code, if applicable, to identify chronic total occlusion of artery of extremity (I70.92)

√6th **I70.60**   **Unspecified atherosclerosis of nonbiological bypass graft(s) of the extremities**

I70.601   Unspecified atherosclerosis of nonbiological bypass graft(s) of the extremities, right leg   A ▽

I70.602   Unspecified atherosclerosis of nonbiological bypass graft(s) of the extremities, left leg   A ▽

I70.603   Unspecified atherosclerosis of nonbiological bypass graft(s) of the extremities, bilateral legs   A ▽

I70.608   Unspecified atherosclerosis of nonbiological bypass graft(s) of the extremities, other extremity   A ▽

I70.609   Unspecified atherosclerosis of nonbiological bypass graft(s) of the extremities, unspecified extremity   A ▽

√6th **I70.61**   **Atherosclerosis of nonbiological bypass graft(s) of the extremities with intermittent claudication**

I70.611   Atherosclerosis of nonbiological bypass graft(s) of the extremities with intermittent claudication, right leg   A

I70.612   Atherosclerosis of nonbiological bypass graft(s) of the extremities with intermittent claudication, left leg   A

I70.613   Atherosclerosis of nonbiological bypass graft(s) of the extremities with intermittent claudication, bilateral legs   A

I70.618   Atherosclerosis of nonbiological bypass graft(s) of the extremities with intermittent claudication, other extremity   A

I70.619   Atherosclerosis of nonbiological bypass graft(s) of the extremities with intermittent claudication, unspecified extremity   A ▽

√6th **I70.62**   **Atherosclerosis of nonbiological bypass graft(s) of the extremities with rest pain**
> INCLUDES   any condition classifiable to I70.61-

I70.621   Atherosclerosis of nonbiological bypass graft(s) of the extremities with rest pain, right leg   A

I70.622   Atherosclerosis of nonbiological bypass graft(s) of the extremities with rest pain, left leg   A

I70.623   Atherosclerosis of nonbiological bypass graft(s) of the extremities with rest pain, bilateral legs   A

I70.628   Atherosclerosis of nonbiological bypass graft(s) of the extremities with rest pain, other extremity   A

I70.629   Atherosclerosis of nonbiological bypass graft(s) of the extremities with rest pain, unspecified extremity   A ▽

√6th **I70.63**   **Atherosclerosis of nonbiological bypass graft(s) of the right leg with ulceration**
> INCLUDES   any condition classifiable to I70.611 and I70.621
> Use additional code to identify severity of ulcer (L97.-)

I70.631   Atherosclerosis of nonbiological bypass graft(s) of the right leg with ulceration of thigh   A

I70.632   Atherosclerosis of nonbiological bypass graft(s) of the right leg with ulceration of calf   A

I70.633   Atherosclerosis of nonbiological bypass graft(s) of the right leg with ulceration of ankle   A

I70.634   Atherosclerosis of nonbiological bypass graft(s) of the right leg with ulceration of heel and midfoot   A
> Atherosclerosis of nonbiological bypass graft(s) of right leg with ulceration of plantar surface of midfoot

I70.635   Atherosclerosis of nonbiological bypass graft(s) of the right leg with ulceration of other part of foot   A
> Atherosclerosis of nonbiological bypass graft(s) of the right leg with ulceration of toe

I70.638   Atherosclerosis of nonbiological bypass graft(s) of the right leg with ulceration of other part of lower leg   A

I70.639   Atherosclerosis of nonbiological bypass graft(s) of the right leg with ulceration of unspecified site   A ▽

√6th **I70.64**   **Atherosclerosis of nonbiological bypass graft(s) of the left leg with ulceration**
> INCLUDES   any condition classifiable to I70.612 and I70.622
> Use additional code to identify severity of ulcer (L97.-)

I70.641   Atherosclerosis of nonbiological bypass graft(s) of the left leg with ulceration of thigh   A

I70.642   Atherosclerosis of nonbiological bypass graft(s) of the left leg with ulceration of calf   A

I70.643   Atherosclerosis of nonbiological bypass graft(s) of the left leg with ulceration of ankle   A

I70.644   Atherosclerosis of nonbiological bypass graft(s) of the left leg with ulceration of heel and midfoot   A
> Atherosclerosis of nonbiological bypass graft(s) of left leg with ulceration of plantar surface of midfoot

I70.645   Atherosclerosis of nonbiological bypass graft(s) of the left leg with ulceration of other part of foot   A
> Atherosclerosis of nonbiological bypass graft(s) of the left leg with ulceration of toe

I70.648   Atherosclerosis of nonbiological bypass graft(s) of the left leg with ulceration of other part of lower leg   A

I70.649   Atherosclerosis of nonbiological bypass graft(s) of the left leg with ulceration of unspecified site   A ▽

I70.65   **Atherosclerosis of nonbiological bypass graft(s) of other extremity with ulceration**   A
> INCLUDES   any condition classifiable to I70.618 and I70.628
> Use additional code to identify severity of ulcer (L98.49)

√6th **I70.66**   **Atherosclerosis of nonbiological bypass graft(s) of the extremities with gangrene**
> INCLUDES   any condition classifiable to I70.61-, I70.62-, I70.63-, I70.64-, I70.65
> Use additional code to identify the severity of any ulcer (L97.-, L98.49-), if applicable

I70.661   Atherosclerosis of nonbiological bypass graft(s) of the extremities with gangrene, right leg   A

I70.662   Atherosclerosis of nonbiological bypass graft(s) of the extremities with gangrene, left leg   A

I70.663   Atherosclerosis of nonbiological bypass graft(s) of the extremities with gangrene, bilateral legs   A

EXCLUDES1 Not coded here   EXCLUDES2 Not included here   N Newborn Age : 0   P Pediatric Age : 0-17   M Maternity Age : 12-55   A Adult Age : 15-124

I70.668   **Atherosclerosis of nonbiological bypass graft(s) of the extremities with gangrene, other extremity**   [A]

I70.669   **Atherosclerosis of nonbiological bypass graft(s) of the extremities with gangrene, unspecified extremity**   [A] [▽]

✓6ᵗʰ   **I70.69**   **Other atherosclerosis of nonbiological bypass graft(s) of the extremities**

    I70.691   **Other atherosclerosis of nonbiological bypass graft(s) of the extremities, right leg**   [A]

    I70.692   **Other atherosclerosis of nonbiological bypass graft(s) of the extremities, left leg**   [A]

    I70.693   **Other atherosclerosis of nonbiological bypass graft(s) of the extremities, bilateral legs**   [A]

    I70.698   **Other atherosclerosis of nonbiological bypass graft(s) of the extremities, other extremity**   [A]

    I70.699   **Other atherosclerosis of nonbiological bypass graft(s) of the extremities, unspecified extremity**   [A] [▽]

✓5ᵗʰ   **I70.7**   **Atherosclerosis of other type of bypass graft(s) of the extremities**

> Use additional code, if applicable, to identify chronic total occlusion of artery of extremity (I70.92)

✓6ᵗʰ   **I70.70**   **Unspecified atherosclerosis of other type of bypass graft(s) of the extremities**

    I70.701   **Unspecified atherosclerosis of other type of bypass graft(s) of the extremities, right leg**   [A] [▽]

    I70.702   **Unspecified atherosclerosis of other type of bypass graft(s) of the extremities, left leg**   [A] [▽]

    I70.703   **Unspecified atherosclerosis of other type of bypass graft(s) of the extremities, bilateral legs**   [A] [▽]

    I70.708   **Unspecified atherosclerosis of other type of bypass graft(s) of the extremities, other extremity**   [A] [▽]

    I70.709   **Unspecified atherosclerosis of other type of bypass graft(s) of the extremities, unspecified extremity**   [A] [▽]

✓6ᵗʰ   **I70.71**   **Atherosclerosis of other type of bypass graft(s) of the extremities with intermittent claudication**

    I70.711   **Atherosclerosis of other type of bypass graft(s) of the extremities with intermittent claudication, right leg**   [A]

    I70.712   **Atherosclerosis of other type of bypass graft(s) of the extremities with intermittent claudication, left leg**   [A]

    I70.713   **Atherosclerosis of other type of bypass graft(s) of the extremities with intermittent claudication, bilateral legs**   [A]

    I70.718   **Atherosclerosis of other type of bypass graft(s) of the extremities with intermittent claudication, other extremity**   [A]

    I70.719   **Atherosclerosis of other type of bypass graft(s) of the extremities with intermittent claudication, unspecified extremity**   [A] [▽]

✓6ᵗʰ   **I70.72**   **Atherosclerosis of other type of bypass graft(s) of the extremities with rest pain**

> INCLUDES   any condition classifiable to I70.71-

    I70.721   **Atherosclerosis of other type of bypass graft(s) of the extremities with rest pain, right leg**   [A]

    I70.722   **Atherosclerosis of other type of bypass graft(s) of the extremities with rest pain, left leg**   [A]

    I70.723   **Atherosclerosis of other type of bypass graft(s) of the extremities with rest pain, bilateral legs**   [A]

    I70.728   **Atherosclerosis of other type of bypass graft(s) of the extremities with rest pain, other extremity**   [A]

    I70.729   **Atherosclerosis of other type of bypass graft(s) of the extremities with rest pain, unspecified extremity**   [A] [▽]

✓6ᵗʰ   **I70.73**   **Atherosclerosis of other type of bypass graft(s) of the right leg with ulceration**

> INCLUDES   any condition classifiable to I70.711 and I70.721
>
> Use additional code to identify severity of ulcer (L97.-)

    I70.731   **Atherosclerosis of other type of bypass graft(s) of the right leg with ulceration of thigh**   [A]

    I70.732   **Atherosclerosis of other type of bypass graft(s) of the right leg with ulceration of calf**   [A]

    I70.733   **Atherosclerosis of other type of bypass graft(s) of the right leg with ulceration of ankle**   [A]

    I70.734   **Atherosclerosis of other type of bypass graft(s) of the right leg with ulceration of heel and midfoot**   [A]

> Atherosclerosis of other type of bypass graft(s) of right leg with ulceration of plantar surface of midfoot

    I70.735   **Atherosclerosis of other type of bypass graft(s) of the right leg with ulceration of other part of foot**   [A]

> Atherosclerosis of other type of bypass graft(s) of right leg with ulceration of toe

    I70.738   **Atherosclerosis of other type of bypass graft(s) of the right leg with ulceration of other part of lower leg**   [A]

    I70.739   **Atherosclerosis of other type of bypass graft(s) of the right leg with ulceration of unspecified site**   [A] [▽]

✓6ᵗʰ   **I70.74**   **Atherosclerosis of other type of bypass graft(s) of the left leg with ulceration**

> INCLUDES   any condition classifiable to I70.712 and I70.722
>
> Use additional code to identify severity of ulcer (L97.-)

    I70.741   **Atherosclerosis of other type of bypass graft(s) of the left leg with ulceration of thigh**   [A]

    I70.742   **Atherosclerosis of other type of bypass graft(s) of the left leg with ulceration of calf**   [A]

    I70.743   **Atherosclerosis of other type of bypass graft(s) of the left leg with ulceration of ankle**   [A]

    I70.744   **Atherosclerosis of other type of bypass graft(s) of the left leg with ulceration of heel and midfoot**   [A]

> Atherosclerosis of other type of bypass graft(s) of left leg with ulceration of plantar surface of midfoot

    I70.745   **Atherosclerosis of other type of bypass graft(s) of the left leg with ulceration of other part of foot**   [A]

> Atherosclerosis of other type of bypass graft(s) of left leg with ulceration of toe

    I70.748   **Atherosclerosis of other type of bypass graft(s) of the left leg with ulceration of other part of lower leg**   [A]

    I70.749   **Atherosclerosis of other type of bypass graft(s) of the left leg with ulceration of unspecified site**   [A] [▽]

    I70.75   **Atherosclerosis of other type of bypass graft(s) of other extremity with ulceration**   [A]

> INCLUDES   any condition classifiable to I70.718 and I70.728
>
> Use additional code to identify severity of ulcer (L98.49)

✓ Additional Character Required   ✓x7ᵗʰ Placeholder Alert   Manifestation Dx   ▽ Unspecified Dx   ►◄ Revised Text   ● New Code   ▲ Revised Code Title

ICD-10-CM 2017   **631**

☑6ᵗʰ **I70.76** **Atherosclerosis of other type of bypass graft(s) of the extremities with gangrene**

> INCLUDES   any condition classifiable to I70.71-, I70.72-, I70.73-, I70.74-, I70.75
> Use additional code to identify the severity of any ulcer (L97.-, L98.49-), if applicable

    I70.761 **Atherosclerosis of other type of bypass graft(s) of the extremities with gangrene, right leg** Ⓐ

    I70.762 **Atherosclerosis of other type of bypass graft(s) of the extremities with gangrene, left leg** Ⓐ

    I70.763 **Atherosclerosis of other type of bypass graft(s) of the extremities with gangrene, bilateral legs** Ⓐ

    I70.768 **Atherosclerosis of other type of bypass graft(s) of the extremities with gangrene, other extremity** Ⓐ

    I70.769 **Atherosclerosis of other type of bypass graft(s) of the extremities with gangrene, unspecified extremity** Ⓐ ▽

☑6ᵗʰ **I70.79** **Other atherosclerosis of other type of bypass graft(s) of the extremities**

    I70.791 **Other atherosclerosis of other type of bypass graft(s) of the extremities, right leg** Ⓐ

    I70.792 **Other atherosclerosis of other type of bypass graft(s) of the extremities, left leg** Ⓐ

    I70.793 **Other atherosclerosis of other type of bypass graft(s) of the extremities, bilateral legs** Ⓐ

    I70.798 **Other atherosclerosis of other type of bypass graft(s) of the extremities, other extremity** Ⓐ

    I70.799 **Other atherosclerosis of other type of bypass graft(s) of the extremities, unspecified extremity** Ⓐ ▽

I70.8 **Atherosclerosis of other arteries** Ⓐ

> **TIP:** Arteriosclerosis of the iliac arteries is coded here.

☑5ᵗʰ **I70.9** **Other and unspecified atherosclerosis**

    I70.90 **Unspecified atherosclerosis** Ⓐ ▽

    I70.91 **Generalized atherosclerosis** Ⓐ

    I70.92 **Chronic total occlusion of artery of the extremities** Ⓐ

> Complete occlusion of artery of the extremities
> Total occlusion of artery of the extremities
> Code first atherosclerosis of arteries of the extremities (I70.2-, I70.3-, I70.4-, I70.5-, I70.6-, I70.7-)

☑4ᵗʰ **I71** **Aortic aneurysm and dissection**

> EXCLUDES 1   aortic ectasia (I77.81-)
> syphilitic aortic aneurysm (A52.01)
> traumatic aortic aneurysm (S25.09, S35.09)

☑5ᵗʰ **I71.0** **Dissection of aorta**

    I71.00 **Dissection of unspecified site of aorta** ▽

    I71.01 **Dissection of thoracic aorta**

    I71.02 **Dissection of abdominal aorta**

    I71.03 **Dissection of thoracoabdominal aorta**

I71.1 **Thoracic aortic aneurysm, ruptured**

I71.2 **Thoracic aortic aneurysm, without rupture**

I71.3 **Abdominal aortic aneurysm, ruptured**

I71.4 **Abdominal aortic aneurysm, without rupture**

I71.5 **Thoracoabdominal aortic aneurysm, ruptured**

I71.6 **Thoracoabdominal aortic aneurysm, without rupture**

I71.8 **Aortic aneurysm of unspecified site, ruptured** ▽

> Rupture of aorta NOS

I71.9 **Aortic aneurysm of unspecified site, without rupture** ▽

> Aneurysm of aorta
> Dilatation of aorta
> Hyaline necrosis of aorta

☑4ᵗʰ **I72** **Other aneurysm**

> INCLUDES   aneurysm (cirsoid) (false) (ruptured)
> EXCLUDES 2   acquired aneurysm (I77.0)
> aneurysm (of) aorta (I71.-)
> aneurysm (of) arteriovenous NOS (Q27.3-)
> carotid artery dissection (I77.71)
> cerebral (nonruptured) aneurysm (I67.1)
> coronary aneurysm (I25.4)
> coronary artery dissection (I25.42)
> dissection of artery NEC (I77.79)
> ▶dissection of precerebral artery, congenital (nonruptured) (Q28.1)◀
> heart aneurysm (I25.3)
> iliac artery dissection (I77.72)
> pulmonary artery aneurysm (I28.1)
> renal artery dissection (I77.73)
> retinal aneurysm (H35.0)
> ruptured cerebral aneurysm (I60.7)
> varicose aneurysm (I77.0)
> vertebral artery dissection (I77.74)

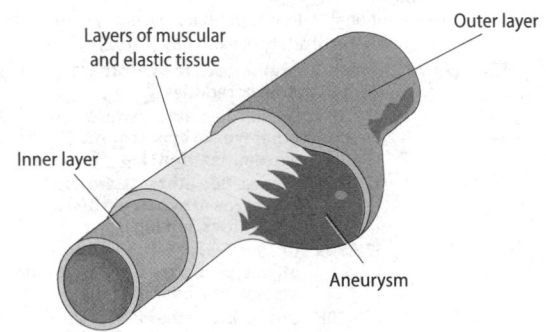

Aneurysm

Layers of muscular and elastic tissue

Outer layer

Inner layer

Aneurysm

I72.0 **Aneurysm of carotid artery**

> Aneurysm of common carotid artery
> Aneurysm of external carotid artery
> Aneurysm of internal carotid artery, extracranial portion
> EXCLUDES 1   aneurysm of internal carotid artery, intracranial portion (I67.1)
> aneurysm of internal carotid artery NOS (I67.1)

I72.1 **Aneurysm of artery of upper extremity**

I72.2 **Aneurysm of renal artery**

I72.3 **Aneurysm of iliac artery**

I72.4 **Aneurysm of artery of lower extremity**

● **I72.5** **Aneurysm of other precerebral arteries**

> Aneurysm of basilar artery (trunk)
> EXCLUDES 2   aneurysm of carotid artery (I72.0)
> aneurysm of vertebral artery (I72.6)
> dissection of carotid artery (I77.71)
> dissection of other precerebral arteries (I77.75)
> dissection of vertebral artery (I77.74)

● **I72.6** **Aneurysm of vertebral artery**

> EXCLUDES 2   dissection of vertebral artery (I77.74)

I72.8 **Aneurysm of other specified arteries**

I72.9 **Aneurysm of unspecified site** ▽

☑4ᵗʰ **I73** **Other peripheral vascular diseases**

> EXCLUDES 2   chilblains (T69.1)
> frostbite (T33-T34)
> immersion hand or foot (T69.0-)
> spasm of cerebral artery (G45.9)

☑5ᵗʰ **I73.0** **Raynaud's syndrome**

> Raynaud's disease
> Raynaud's phenomenon (secondary)

    I73.00 **Raynaud's syndrome without gangrene**

    I73.01 **Raynaud's syndrome with gangrene**

I73.1 **Thromboangiitis obliterans [Buerger's disease]**

EXCLUDES 1   Not coded here   EXCLUDES 2   Not included here   Ⓝ Newborn Age : 0   Ⓟ Pediatric Age : 0-17   Ⓜ Maternity Age : 12-55   Ⓐ Adult Age : 15-124

632   ICD-10-CM 2017

√5ᵗʰ **I73.8 Other specified peripheral vascular diseases**

     EXCLUDES 1 *diabetic (peripheral) angiopathy (E08-E13 with .51-.52)*

     I73.81 Erythromelalgia

     I73.89 Other specified peripheral vascular diseases
         Acrocyanosis
         Erythrocyanosis
         Simple acroparesthesia [Schultze's type]
         Vasomotor acroparesthesia [Nothnagel's type]

I73.9 Peripheral vascular disease, unspecified ▽
     Intermittent claudication
     Peripheral angiopathy NOS
     Spasm of artery
     EXCLUDES 1 *atherosclerosis of the extremities (I70.2-I70.7-)*

√4ᵗʰ **I74 Arterial embolism and thrombosis**

     INCLUDES   embolic infarction
             embolic occlusion
             thrombotic infarction
             thrombotic occlusion

Code first:
     embolism and thrombosis complicating abortion or ectopic or molar
         pregnancy (O00-O07, O08.2)
     embolism and thrombosis complicating pregnancy, childbirth and
         the puerperium (O88.-)
     EXCLUDES 2 *atheroembolism (I75.-)*
         basilar embolism and thrombosis (I63.0-I63.2, I65.1)
         carotid embolism and thrombosis (I63.0-I63.2, I65.2)
         cerebral embolism and thrombosis (I63.3-I63.5, I66.-)
         coronary embolism and thrombosis (I21-I25)
         mesenteric embolism and thrombosis ▶*(K55.0-)*◀
         ophthalmic embolism and thrombosis (H34.-)
         precerebral embolism and thrombosis NOS (I63.0 I63.2, I65.9)
         pulmonary embolism and thrombosis (I26.-)
         renal embolism and thrombosis (N28.0)
         retinal embolism and thrombosis (H34.-)
         septic embolism and thrombosis (I76)
         vertebral embolism and thrombosis (I63.0-I63.2, I65.0)

√5ᵗʰ **I74.0 Embolism and thrombosis of abdominal aorta**

     I74.01 Saddle embolus of abdominal aorta

     **I74.09 Other arterial embolism and thrombosis of
         abdominal aorta**
         Aortic bifurcation syndrome
         Aortoiliac obstruction
         Leriche's syndrome

√5ᵗʰ **I74.1 Embolism and thrombosis of other and unspecified parts of
aorta**

     I74.10 Embolism and thrombosis of unspecified ▽
         parts of aorta

     I74.11 Embolism and thrombosis of thoracic aorta

     I74.19 Embolism and thrombosis of other parts of aorta

I74.2 Embolism and thrombosis of arteries of the upper extremities

I74.3 Embolism and thrombosis of arteries of the lower extremities ●

I74.4 Embolism and thrombosis of arteries of extremities, ▽
unspecified
     Peripheral arterial embolism NOS

I74.5 Embolism and thrombosis of iliac artery

I74.8 Embolism and thrombosis of other arteries

I74.9 Embolism and thrombosis of unspecified artery ▽

√4ᵗʰ **I75 Atheroembolism**

     INCLUDES   atherothrombotic microembolism
             cholesterol embolism

√5ᵗʰ **I75.0 Atheroembolism of extremities**

     √6ᵗʰ **I75.01 Atheroembolism of upper extremity**

         I75.011 Atheroembolism of right upper extremity
         I75.012 Atheroembolism of left upper extremity
         **I75.013 Atheroembolism of bilateral upper
             extremities**
         I75.019 Atheroembolism of unspecified ▽
             upper extremity

     √6ᵗʰ **I75.02 Atheroembolism of lower extremity**

         I75.021 Atheroembolism of right lower extremity
         I75.022 Atheroembolism of left lower extremity
         **I75.023 Atheroembolism of bilateral lower
             extremities**
         I75.029 Atheroembolism of unspecified ▽
             lower extremity

√5ᵗʰ **I75.8 Atheroembolism of other sites**

     I75.81 Atheroembolism of kidney
         Use additional code for any associated acute kidney
             failure and chronic kidney disease (N17.-, N18.-)

     I75.89 Atheroembolism of other site

I76 Septic arterial embolism
     Code first underlying infection, such as:
         infective endocarditis (I33.0)
         lung abscess (J85.-)
     Use additional code to identify the site of the embolism (I74.-)
     EXCLUDES 2 *septic pulmonary embolism (I26.01, I26.90)*

√4ᵗʰ **I77 Other disorders of arteries and arterioles**

     EXCLUDES 2 *collagen (vascular) diseases (M30-M36)*
         hypersensitivity angiitis (M31.0)
         pulmonary artery (I28.-)

I77.0 Arteriovenous fistula, acquired
     Aneurysmal varix
     Arteriovenous aneurysm, acquired
     EXCLUDES 1 *arteriovenous aneurysm NOS (Q27.3-)*
         *presence of arteriovenous shunt (fistula) for dialysis
             (Z99.2)*
         traumatic - see injury of blood vessel by body region
     EXCLUDES 2 *cerebral (I67.1)*
         coronary (I25.4)

I77.1 Stricture of artery
     Narrowing of artery

I77.2 Rupture of artery
     Erosion of artery   Ulcer of artery
     Fistula of artery
     EXCLUDES 1 *traumatic rupture of artery - see injury of blood vessel
         by body region*

I77.3 Arterial fibromuscular dysplasia
     Fibromuscular hyperplasia (of) carotid artery
     Fibromuscular hyperplasia (of) renal artery

I77.4 Celiac artery compression syndrome

I77.5 Necrosis of artery

I77.6 Arteritis, unspecified ▽
     Aortitis NOS
     Endarteritis NOS
     EXCLUDES 1 *arteritis or endarteritis:*
         aortic arch (M31.4)
         cerebral NEC (I67.7)
         coronary (I25.89)
         deformans (I70.-)
         giant cell (M31.5., M31.6)
         obliterans (I70.-)
         senile (I70.-)

√5ᵗʰ **I77.7 Other arterial dissection**

     EXCLUDES 2 *dissection of aorta (I71.0-)*
         dissection of coronary artery (I25.42)

     I77.70 Dissection of unspecified artery ▽ ●

     I77.71 Dissection of carotid artery

     I77.72 Dissection of iliac artery

     I77.73 Dissection of renal artery

     I77.74 Dissection of vertebral artery
         EXCLUDES 2 ▶*aneurysm of vertebral artery (I72.6)*◀

     I77.75 Dissection of other precerebral arteries ●
         Dissection of basilar artery (trunk)
         EXCLUDES 2 *aneurysm of carotid artery (I72.0)*
         *aneurysm of other precerebral arteries
             (I72.5)*
         aneurysm of vertebral artery (I72.6)
         dissection of carotid artery (I77.71)
         dissection of vertebral artery (I77.74)

     I77.76 Dissection of artery of upper extremity ●

     I77.77 Dissection of artery of lower extremity ●

     I77.79 Dissection of other specified artery ▲

√5ᵗʰ **I77.8 Other specified disorders of arteries and arterioles**

     √6ᵗʰ **I77.81 Aortic ectasia**
         Ectasis aorta
         EXCLUDES 1 *aortic aneurysm and dissection (I71.0-)*
         I77.810 Thoracic aortic ectasia
         I77.811 Abdominal aortic ectasia
         I77.812 Thoracoabdominal aortic ectasia
         I77.819 Aortic ectasia, unspecified site ▽

☑ Additional Character Required   √x7ᵗʰ Placeholder Alert   Manifestation Dx   ▽Unspecified Dx   ▶◀ Revised Text   ● New Code   ▲ Revised Code Title

ICD-10-CM 2017   633

Chapter 9. Diseases of the Circulatory System

I77.89   Other specified disorders of arteries and arterioles

I77.9   Disorder of arteries and arterioles, unspecified ▽

√4ᵗʰ **I78**   **Diseases of capillaries**

    I78.0   **Hereditary hemorrhagic telangiectasia**
      Rendu-Osler-Weber disease

    I78.1   **Nevus, non-neoplastic**
      Araneus nevus
      Senile nevus
      Spider nevus
      Stellar nevus
      EXCLUDES 1   nevus NOS (D22.-)
            vascular NOS (Q82.5)
      EXCLUDES 2   blue nevus (D22.-)
            flammeus nevus (Q82.5)
            hairy nevus (D22.-)
            melanocytic nevus (D22.-)
            pigmented nevus (D22.-)
            portwine nevus (Q82.5)
            sanguineous nevus (Q82.5)
            strawberry nevus (Q82.5)
            verrucous nevus (Q82.5)

    I78.8   **Other diseases of capillaries**

    I78.9   **Disease of capillaries, unspecified** ▽

√4ᵗʰ **I79**   **Disorders of arteries, arterioles and capillaries in diseases classified elsewhere**

    I79.0   *Aneurysm of aorta in diseases classified elsewhere*
      Code first underlying disease
      EXCLUDES 1   syphilitic aneurysm (A52.01)

    I79.1   *Aortitis in diseases classified elsewhere*
      Code first underlying disease
      EXCLUDES 1   syphilitic aortitis (A52.02)

    I79.8   *Other disorders of arteries, arterioles and capillaries in diseases classified elsewhere*
      Code first underlying disease, such as:
       amyloidosis (E85.-)
      EXCLUDES 1   diabetic (peripheral) angiopathy (E08-E13 with .51-.52)
            syphilitic endarteritis (A52.09)
            tuberculous endarteritis (A18.89)

Diseases of veins, lymphatic vessels and lymph nodes, not elsewhere classified (I80-I89)

√4ᵗʰ **I80**   **Phlebitis and thrombophlebitis**

    [INCLUDES]   endophlebitis
          inflammation, vein
          periphlebitis
          suppurative phlebitis

    Code first:
      phlebitis and thrombophlebitis complicating abortion, ectopic or molar pregnancy (O00-O07, O08.7)
      phlebitis and thrombophlebitis complicating pregnancy, childbirth and the puerperium (O22.-, O87.-)
      EXCLUDES 1   venous embolism and thrombosis of lower extremities (I82.4-, I82.5-, I82.81-)

√5ᵗʰ   **I80.0**   **Phlebitis and thrombophlebitis of superficial vessels of lower extremities**
      Phlebitis and thrombophlebitis of femoropopliteal vein

      I80.00   **Phlebitis and thrombophlebitis of superficial vessels of unspecified lower extremity** ▽

      I80.01   **Phlebitis and thrombophlebitis of superficial vessels of right lower extremity**

      I80.02   **Phlebitis and thrombophlebitis of superficial vessels of left lower extremity**

      I80.03   **Phlebitis and thrombophlebitis of superficial vessels of lower extremities, bilateral**

√5ᵗʰ   **I80.1**   **Phlebitis and thrombophlebitis of femoral vein**

      I80.10   **Phlebitis and thrombophlebitis of unspecified femoral vein** ▽

      I80.11   **Phlebitis and thrombophlebitis of right femoral vein**

      I80.12   **Phlebitis and thrombophlebitis of left femoral vein**

      I80.13   **Phlebitis and thrombophlebitis of femoral vein, bilateral**

√5ᵗʰ   **I80.2**   **Phlebitis and thrombophlebitis of other and unspecified deep vessels of lower extremities**

      √6ᵗʰ   **I80.20**   **Phlebitis and thrombophlebitis of unspecified deep vessels of lower extremities**

        I80.201   **Phlebitis and thrombophlebitis of unspecified deep vessels of right lower extremity**

        I80.202   **Phlebitis and thrombophlebitis of unspecified deep vessels of left lower extremity**

        I80.203   **Phlebitis and thrombophlebitis of unspecified deep vessels of lower extremities, bilateral**

        I80.209   **Phlebitis and thrombophlebitis of unspecified deep vessels of unspecified lower extremity** ▽

      √6ᵗʰ   **I80.21**   **Phlebitis and thrombophlebitis of iliac vein**

        I80.211   **Phlebitis and thrombophlebitis of right iliac vein**

        I80.212   **Phlebitis and thrombophlebitis of left iliac vein**

        I80.213   **Phlebitis and thrombophlebitis of iliac vein, bilateral**

        I80.219   **Phlebitis and thrombophlebitis of unspecified iliac vein** ▽

      √6ᵗʰ   **I80.22**   **Phlebitis and thrombophlebitis of popliteal vein**

        I80.221   **Phlebitis and thrombophlebitis of right popliteal vein**

        I80.222   **Phlebitis and thrombophlebitis of left popliteal vein**

        I80.223   **Phlebitis and thrombophlebitis of popliteal vein, bilateral**

        I80.229   **Phlebitis and thrombophlebitis of unspecified popliteal vein** ▽

      √6ᵗʰ   **I80.23**   **Phlebitis and thrombophlebitis of tibial vein**

        I80.231   **Phlebitis and thrombophlebitis of right tibial vein**

        I80.232   **Phlebitis and thrombophlebitis of left tibial vein**

        I80.233   **Phlebitis and thrombophlebitis of tibial vein, bilateral**

        I80.239   **Phlebitis and thrombophlebitis of unspecified tibial vein** ▽

      √6ᵗʰ   **I80.29**   **Phlebitis and thrombophlebitis of other deep vessels of lower extremities**

        I80.291   **Phlebitis and thrombophlebitis of other deep vessels of right lower extremity**

        I80.292   **Phlebitis and thrombophlebitis of other deep vessels of left lower extremity**

        I80.293   **Phlebitis and thrombophlebitis of other deep vessels of lower extremity, bilateral**

        I80.299   **Phlebitis and thrombophlebitis of other deep vessels of unspecified lower extremity** ▽

    I80.3   **Phlebitis and thrombophlebitis of lower extremities, unspecified** ▽

    I80.8   **Phlebitis and thrombophlebitis of other sites**

    I80.9   **Phlebitis and thrombophlebitis of unspecified site** ▽

I81   **Portal vein thrombosis**
    Portal (vein) obstruction
    EXCLUDES 2   hepatic vein thrombosis (I82.0)
           phlebitis of portal vein (K75.1)

√4ᵗʰ **I82**   **Other venous embolism and thrombosis**
    Code first venous embolism and thrombosis complicating:
      abortion, ectopic or molar pregnancy (O00-O07, O08.7)
      pregnancy, childbirth and the puerperium (O22.-, O87.-)
    EXCLUDES 2   venous embolism and thrombosis (of):
           cerebral (I63.6, I67.6)
           coronary (I21-I25)
           intracranial and intraspinal, septic or NOS (G08)
           intracranial, nonpyogenic (I67.6)
           intraspinal, nonpyogenic (G95.1)
           mesenteric (K55.0-)
           portal (I81)
           pulmonary (I26.-)

    I82.0   **Budd-Chiari syndrome**
      Hepatic vein thrombosis

    I82.1   **Thrombophlebitis migrans**

√5ᵗʰ   **I82.2**   **Embolism and thrombosis of vena cava and other thoracic veins**

      √6ᵗʰ   **I82.21**   **Embolism and thrombosis of superior vena cava**

EXCLUDES 1   Not coded here   *EXCLUDES 2*   Not included here   N Newborn Age : 0   P Pediatric Age : 0-17   M Maternity Age : 12-55   A Adult Age : 15-124

634   ICD-10-CM 2017

I82.210 **Acute embolism and thrombosis of superior vena cava**
Embolism and thrombosis of superior vena cava NOS

I82.211 **Chronic embolism and thrombosis of superior vena cava**

√6ᵗʰ I82.22 **Embolism and thrombosis of inferior vena cava**

I82.220 **Acute embolism and thrombosis of inferior vena cava**
Embolism and thrombosis of inferior vena cava NOS

I82.221 **Chronic embolism and thrombosis of inferior vena cava**

√6ᵗʰ I82.29 **Embolism and thrombosis of other thoracic veins**
Embolism and thrombosis of brachiocephalic (innominate) vein

I82.290 **Acute embolism and thrombosis of other thoracic veins**

I82.291 **Chronic embolism and thrombosis of other thoracic veins**

I82.3 **Embolism and thrombosis of renal vein**

√5ᵗʰ I82.4 **Acute embolism and thrombosis of deep veins of lower extremity**

√6ᵗʰ I82.40 **Acute embolism and thrombosis of unspecified deep veins of lower extremity**
Deep vein thrombosis NOS
DVT NOS

EXCLUDES 1 *acute embolism and thrombosis of unspecified deep veins of distal lower extremity (I82.4Z-)*
acute embolism and thrombosis of unspecified deep veins of proximal lower extremity (I82.4Y-)

I82.401 **Acute embolism and thrombosis of unspecified deep veins of right lower extremity** ▽

I82.402 **Acute embolism and thrombosis of unspecified deep veins of left lower extremity** ▽

I82.403 **Acute embolism and thrombosis of unspecified deep veins of lower extremity, bilateral** ▽

I82.409 **Acute embolism and thrombosis of unspecified deep veins of unspecified lower extremity** ▽

√6ᵗʰ I82.41 **Acute embolism and thrombosis of femoral vein**

I82.411 **Acute embolism and thrombosis of right femoral vein**

I82.412 **Acute embolism and thrombosis of left femoral vein**

I82.413 **Acute embolism and thrombosis of femoral vein, bilateral**

I82.419 **Acute embolism and thrombosis of unspecified femoral vein** ▽

√6ᵗʰ I82.42 **Acute embolism and thrombosis of iliac vein**

I82.421 **Acute embolism and thrombosis of right iliac vein**

I82.422 **Acute embolism and thrombosis of left iliac vein**

I82.423 **Acute embolism and thrombosis of iliac vein, bilateral**

I82.429 **Acute embolism and thrombosis of unspecified iliac vein** ▽

√6ᵗʰ I82.43 **Acute embolism and thrombosis of popliteal vein**

I82.431 **Acute embolism and thrombosis of right popliteal vein**

I82.432 **Acute embolism and thrombosis of left popliteal vein**

I82.433 **Acute embolism and thrombosis of popliteal vein, bilateral**

I82.439 **Acute embolism and thrombosis of unspecified popliteal vein** ▽

√6ᵗʰ I82.44 **Acute embolism and thrombosis of tibial vein**

I82.441 **Acute embolism and thrombosis of right tibial vein**

I82.442 **Acute embolism and thrombosis of left tibial vein**

I82.443 **Acute embolism and thrombosis of tibial vein, bilateral**

I82.449 **Acute embolism and thrombosis of unspecified tibial vein** ▽

√6ᵗʰ I82.49 **Acute embolism and thrombosis of other specified deep vein of lower extremity**

I82.491 **Acute embolism and thrombosis of other specified deep vein of right lower extremity**

I82.492 **Acute embolism and thrombosis of other specified deep vein of left lower extremity**

I82.493 **Acute embolism and thrombosis of other specified deep vein of lower extremity, bilateral**

I82.499 **Acute embolism and thrombosis of other specified deep vein of unspecified lower extremity** ▽

√6ᵗʰ I82.4Y **Acute embolism and thrombosis of unspecified deep veins of proximal lower extremity**
Acute embolism and thrombosis of deep vein of thigh NOS
Acute embolism and thrombosis of deep vein of upper leg NOS

I82.4Y1 **Acute embolism and thrombosis of unspecified deep veins of right proximal lower extremity**

I82.4Y2 **Acute embolism and thrombosis of unspecified deep veins of left proximal lower extremity**

I82.4Y3 **Acute embolism and thrombosis of unspecified deep veins of proximal lower extremity, bilateral**

I82.4Y9 **Acute embolism and thrombosis of unspecified deep veins of unspecified proximal lower extremity** ▽

√6ᵗʰ I82.4Z **Acute embolism and thrombosis of unspecified deep veins of distal lower extremity**
Acute embolism and thrombosis of deep vein of calf NOS
Acute embolism and thrombosis of deep vein of lower leg NOS

I82.4Z1 **Acute embolism and thrombosis of unspecified deep veins of right distal lower extremity**

I82.4Z2 **Acute embolism and thrombosis of unspecified deep veins of left distal lower extremity**

I82.4Z3 **Acute embolism and thrombosis of unspecified deep veins of distal lower extremity, bilateral**

I82.4Z9 **Acute embolism and thrombosis of unspecified deep veins of unspecified distal lower extremity** ▽

√5ᵗʰ I82.5 **Chronic embolism and thrombosis of deep veins of lower extremity**
Use additional code, if applicable, for associated long-term (current) use of anticoagulants (Z79.01)

EXCLUDES 1 *personal history of venous embolism and thrombosis (Z86.718)*

√6ᵗʰ I82.50 **Chronic embolism and thrombosis of unspecified deep veins of lower extremity**

EXCLUDES 1 *chronic embolism and thrombosis of unspecified deep veins of distal lower extremity (I82.5Z-)*
chronic embolism and thrombosis of unspecified deep veins of proximal lower extremity (I82.5Y-)

I82.501 **Chronic embolism and thrombosis of unspecified deep veins of right lower extremity** ▽

I82.502 **Chronic embolism and thrombosis of unspecified deep veins of left lower extremity** ▽

I82.503 **Chronic embolism and thrombosis of unspecified deep veins of lower extremity, bilateral** ▽

I82.509 **Chronic embolism and thrombosis of unspecified deep veins of unspecified lower extremity** ▽

√6ᵗʰ I82.51 **Chronic embolism and thrombosis of femoral vein**

I82.511 **Chronic embolism and thrombosis of right femoral vein**

I82.512 **Chronic embolism and thrombosis of left femoral vein**

✔ Additional Character Required   √x7ᵗʰ Placeholder Alert   Manifestation Dx   ▽ Unspecified Dx   ▶◀ Revised Text   ● New Code   ▲ Revised Code Title

I82.513   Chronic embolism and thrombosis of femoral vein, bilateral

I82.519   Chronic embolism and thrombosis of unspecified femoral vein ▽

✓6ᵗʰ **I82.52**   Chronic embolism and thrombosis of iliac vein

I82.521   Chronic embolism and thrombosis of right iliac vein

I82.522   Chronic embolism and thrombosis of left iliac vein

I82.523   Chronic embolism and thrombosis of iliac vein, bilateral

I82.529   Chronic embolism and thrombosis of unspecified iliac vein ▽

✓6ᵗʰ **I82.53**   Chronic embolism and thrombosis of popliteal vein

I82.531   Chronic embolism and thrombosis of right popliteal vein

I82.532   Chronic embolism and thrombosis of left popliteal vein

I82.533   Chronic embolism and thrombosis of popliteal vein, bilateral

I82.539   Chronic embolism and thrombosis of unspecified popliteal vein ▽

✓6ᵗʰ **I82.54**   Chronic embolism and thrombosis of tibial vein

I82.541   Chronic embolism and thrombosis of right tibial vein

I82.542   Chronic embolism and thrombosis of left tibial vein

I82.543   Chronic embolism and thrombosis of tibial vein, bilateral

I82.549   Chronic embolism and thrombosis of unspecified tibial vein ▽

✓6ᵗʰ **I82.59**   Chronic embolism and thrombosis of other specified deep vein of lower extremity

I82.591   Chronic embolism and thrombosis of other specified deep vein of right lower extremity

I82.592   Chronic embolism and thrombosis of other specified deep vein of left lower extremity

I82.593   Chronic embolism and thrombosis of other specified deep vein of lower extremity, bilateral

I82.599   Chronic embolism and thrombosis of other specified deep vein of unspecified lower extremity ▽

✓6ᵗʰ **I82.5Y**   Chronic embolism and thrombosis of unspecified deep veins of proximal lower extremity

Chronic embolism and thrombosis of deep veins of thigh NOS

Chronic embolism and thrombosis of deep veins of upper leg NOS

I82.5Y1   Chronic embolism and thrombosis of unspecified deep veins of right proximal lower extremity

I82.5Y2   Chronic embolism and thrombosis of unspecified deep veins of left proximal lower extremity

I82.5Y3   Chronic embolism and thrombosis of unspecified deep veins of proximal lower extremity, bilateral

I82.5Y9   Chronic embolism and thrombosis of unspecified deep veins of unspecified proximal lower extremity ▽

✓6ᵗʰ **I82.5Z**   Chronic embolism and thrombosis of unspecified deep veins of distal lower extremity

Chronic embolism and thrombosis of deep veins of calf NOS

Chronic embolism and thrombosis of deep veins of lower leg NOS

I82.5Z1   Chronic embolism and thrombosis of unspecified deep veins of right distal lower extremity

I82.5Z2   Chronic embolism and thrombosis of unspecified deep veins of left distal lower extremity

I82.5Z3   Chronic embolism and thrombosis of unspecified deep veins of distal lower extremity, bilateral

I82.5Z9   Chronic embolism and thrombosis of unspecified deep veins of unspecified distal lower extremity ▽

✓5ᵗʰ **I82.6**   Acute embolism and thrombosis of veins of upper extremity

✓6ᵗʰ **I82.60**   Acute embolism and thrombosis of unspecified veins of upper extremity

I82.601   Acute embolism and thrombosis of unspecified veins of right upper extremity ▽

I82.602   Acute embolism and thrombosis of unspecified veins of left upper extremity ▽

I82.603   Acute embolism and thrombosis of unspecified veins of upper extremity, bilateral ▽

I82.609   Acute embolism and thrombosis of unspecified veins of unspecified upper extremity ▽

✓6ᵗʰ **I82.61**   Acute embolism and thrombosis of superficial veins of upper extremity

Acute embolism and thrombosis of antecubital vein

Acute embolism and thrombosis of basilic vein

Acute embolism and thrombosis of cephalic vein

I82.611   Acute embolism and thrombosis of superficial veins of right upper extremity

I82.612   Acute embolism and thrombosis of superficial veins of left upper extremity

I82.613   Acute embolism and thrombosis of superficial veins of upper extremity, bilateral

I82.619   Acute embolism and thrombosis of superficial veins of unspecified upper extremity ▽

✓6ᵗʰ **I82.62**   Acute embolism and thrombosis of deep veins of upper extremity

Acute embolism and thrombosis of brachial vein

Acute embolism and thrombosis of radial vein

Acute embolism and thrombosis of ulnar vein

I82.621   Acute embolism and thrombosis of deep veins of right upper extremity

I82.622   Acute embolism and thrombosis of deep veins of left upper extremity

I82.623   Acute embolism and thrombosis of deep veins of upper extremity, bilateral

I82.629   Acute embolism and thrombosis of deep veins of unspecified upper extremity ▽

✓5ᵗʰ **I82.7**   Chronic embolism and thrombosis of veins of upper extremity

Use additional code, if applicable, for associated long-term (current) use of anticoagulants (Z79.01)

EXCLUDES 1   *personal history of venous embolism and thrombosis (Z86.718)*

✓6ᵗʰ **I82.70**   Chronic embolism and thrombosis of unspecified veins of upper extremity

I82.701   Chronic embolism and thrombosis of unspecified veins of right upper extremity ▽

I82.702   Chronic embolism and thrombosis of unspecified veins of left upper extremity ▽

I82.703   Chronic embolism and thrombosis of unspecified veins of upper extremity, bilateral ▽

I82.709   Chronic embolism and thrombosis of unspecified veins of unspecified upper extremity ▽

✓6ᵗʰ **I82.71**   Chronic embolism and thrombosis of superficial veins of upper extremity

Chronic embolism and thrombosis of antecubital vein

Chronic embolism and thrombosis of basilic vein

Chronic embolism and thrombosis of cephalic vein

I82.711   Chronic embolism and thrombosis of superficial veins of right upper extremity

I82.712   Chronic embolism and thrombosis of superficial veins of left upper extremity

I82.713   Chronic embolism and thrombosis of superficial veins of upper extremity, bilateral

I82.719   Chronic embolism and thrombosis of superficial veins of unspecified upper extremity ▽

EXCLUDES 1 Not coded here   **EXCLUDES 2** Not included here   **N** Newborn Age : 0   **P** Pediatric Age : 0-17   **M** Maternity Age : 12-55   **A** Adult Age : 15-124

636   ICD-10-CM 2017

Chapter 9. Diseases of the Circulatory System

√6ᵗʰ **I82.72 Chronic embolism and thrombosis of deep veins of upper extremity**
Chronic embolism and thrombosis of brachial vein
Chronic embolism and thrombosis of radial vein
Chronic embolism and thrombosis of ulnar vein

I82.721 Chronic embolism and thrombosis of deep veins of right upper extremity

I82.722 Chronic embolism and thrombosis of deep veins of left upper extremity

I82.723 Chronic embolism and thrombosis of deep veins of upper extremity, bilateral

I82.729 Chronic embolism and thrombosis of deep veins of unspecified upper extremity ▽

√5ᵗʰ **I82.A Embolism and thrombosis of axillary vein**

√6ᵗʰ **I82.A1 Acute embolism and thrombosis of axillary vein**

I82.A11 Acute embolism and thrombosis of right axillary vein

I82.A12 Acute embolism and thrombosis of left axillary vein

I82.A13 Acute embolism and thrombosis of axillary vein, bilateral

I82.A19 Acute embolism and thrombosis of unspecified axillary vein ▽

√6ᵗʰ **I82.A2 Chronic embolism and thrombosis of axillary vein**

I82.A21 Chronic embolism and thrombosis of right axillary vein

I82.A22 Chronic embolism and thrombosis of left axillary vein

I82.A23 Chronic embolism and thrombosis of axillary vein, bilateral

I82.A29 Chronic embolism and thrombosis of unspecified axillary vein ▽

√5ᵗʰ **I82.B Embolism and thrombosis of subclavian vein**

√6ᵗʰ **I82.B1 Acute embolism and thrombosis of subclavian vein**

I82.B11 Acute embolism and thrombosis of right subclavian vein

I82.B12 Acute embolism and thrombosis of left subclavian vein

I82.B13 Acute embolism and thrombosis of subclavian vein, bilateral

I82.B19 Acute embolism and thrombosis of unspecified subclavian vein ▽

√6ᵗʰ **I82.B2 Chronic embolism and thrombosis of subclavian vein**

I82.B21 Chronic embolism and thrombosis of right subclavian vein

I82.B22 Chronic embolism and thrombosis of left subclavian vein

I82.B23 Chronic embolism and thrombosis of subclavian vein, bilateral

I82.B29 Chronic embolism and thrombosis of unspecified subclavian vein ▽

√5ᵗʰ **I82.C Embolism and thrombosis of internal jugular vein**

√6ᵗʰ **I82.C1 Acute embolism and thrombosis of internal jugular vein**

I82.C11 Acute embolism and thrombosis of right internal jugular vein

I82.C12 Acute embolism and thrombosis of left internal jugular vein

I82.C13 Acute embolism and thrombosis of internal jugular vein, bilateral

I82.C19 Acute embolism and thrombosis of unspecified internal jugular vein ▽

√6ᵗʰ **I82.C2 Chronic embolism and thrombosis of internal jugular vein**

I82.C21 Chronic embolism and thrombosis of right internal jugular vein

I82.C22 Chronic embolism and thrombosis of left internal jugular vein

I82.C23 Chronic embolism and thrombosis of internal jugular vein, bilateral

I82.C29 Chronic embolism and thrombosis of unspecified internal jugular vein ▽

√5ᵗʰ **I82.8 Embolism and thrombosis of other specified veins**
Use additional code, if applicable, for associated long-term (current) use of anticoagulants (Z79.01)

√6ᵗʰ **I82.81 Embolism and thrombosis of superficial veins of lower extremities**
Embolism and thrombosis of saphenous vein (greater) (lesser)

I82.811 Embolism and thrombosis of superficial veins of right lower extremities

I82.812 Embolism and thrombosis of superficial veins of left lower extremities

I82.813 Embolism and thrombosis of superficial veins of lower extremities, bilateral

I82.819 Embolism and thrombosis of superficial veins of unspecified lower extremities ▽

I82.89 Embolism and thrombosis of other specified veins

I82.890 Acute embolism and thrombosis of other specified veins

I82.891 Chronic embolism and thrombosis of other specified veins

√5ᵗʰ **I82.9 Embolism and thrombosis of unspecified vein**

I82.90 Acute embolism and thrombosis of unspecified vein ▽
Embolism of vein NOS
Thrombosis (vein) NOS

I82.91 Chronic embolism and thrombosis of unspecified vein ▽

√4ᵗʰ **I83 Varicose veins of lower extremities**
EXCLUDES 1 *varicose veins complicating pregnancy (O22.0-)*
varicose veins complicating the puerperium (O87.4)

√5ᵗʰ **I83.0 Varicose veins of lower extremities with ulcer**
Use additional code to identify severity of ulcer (L97.-)

√6ᵗʰ **I83.00 Varicose veins of unspecified lower extremity with ulcer**

I83.001 Varicose veins of unspecified lower extremity with ulcer of thigh A ▽

I83.002 Varicose veins of unspecified lower extremity with ulcer of calf A ▽

I83.003 Varicose veins of unspecified lower extremity with ulcer of ankle A ▽

I83.004 Varicose veins of unspecified lower extremity with ulcer of heel and midfoot A ▽
Varicose veins of unspecified lower extremity with ulcer of plantar surface of midfoot

I83.005 Varicose veins of unspecified lower extremity with ulcer other part of foot A ▽
Varicose veins of unspecified lower extremity with ulcer of toe

I83.008 Varicose veins of unspecified lower extremity with ulcer other part of lower leg A ▽

I83.009 Varicose veins of unspecified lower extremity with ulcer of unspecified site A ▽

√6ᵗʰ **I83.01 Varicose veins of right lower extremity with ulcer**

I83.011 Varicose veins of right lower extremity with ulcer of thigh A

I83.012 Varicose veins of right lower extremity with ulcer of calf A

I83.013 Varicose veins of right lower extremity with ulcer of ankle A

I83.014 Varicose veins of right lower extremity with ulcer of heel and midfoot A
Varicose veins of right lower extremity with ulcer of plantar surface of midfoot

I83.015 Varicose veins of right lower extremity with ulcer other part of foot A
Varicose veins of right lower extremity with ulcer of toe

I83.018 Varicose veins of right lower extremity with ulcer other part of lower leg A

I83.019 Varicose veins of right lower extremity with ulcer of unspecified site A ▽

√6ᵗʰ **I83.02 Varicose veins of left lower extremity with ulcer**

I83.021 Varicose veins of left lower extremity with ulcer of thigh A

I83.022   **Varicose veins of left lower extremity with ulcer of calf**   A

I83.023   **Varicose veins of left lower extremity with ulcer of ankle**   A

I83.024   **Varicose veins of left lower extremity with ulcer of heel and midfoot**   A
> Varicose veins of left lower extremity with ulcer of plantar surface of midfoot

I83.025   **Varicose veins of left lower extremity with ulcer other part of foot**   A
> Varicose veins of left lower extremity with ulcer of toe

I83.028   **Varicose veins of left lower extremity with ulcer other part of lower leg**   A

I83.029   **Varicose veins of left lower extremity with ulcer of unspecified site**   A ▽

√5ᵗʰ **I83.1**   **Varicose veins of lower extremities with inflammation**

I83.10   **Varicose veins of unspecified lower extremity with inflammation**   A ▽

I83.11   **Varicose veins of right lower extremity with inflammation**   A

I83.12   **Varicose veins of left lower extremity with inflammation**   A

√5ᵗʰ **I83.2**   **Varicose veins of lower extremities with both ulcer and inflammation**
> Use additional code to identify severity of ulcer (L97.-)

√6ᵗʰ **I83.20**   **Varicose veins of unspecified lower extremity with both ulcer and inflammation**

I83.201   **Varicose veins of unspecified lower extremity with both ulcer of thigh and inflammation**   A ▽

I83.202   **Varicose veins of unspecified lower extremity with both ulcer of calf and inflammation**   A ▽

I83.203   **Varicose veins of unspecified lower extremity with both ulcer of ankle and inflammation**   A ▽

I83.204   **Varicose veins of unspecified lower extremity with both ulcer of heel and midfoot and inflammation**   A ▽
> Varicose veins of unspecified lower extremity with both ulcer of plantar surface of midfoot and inflammation

I83.205   **Varicose veins of unspecified lower extremity with both ulcer of other part of foot and inflammation**   A ▽
> Varicose veins of unspecified lower extremity with both ulcer of toe and inflammation

I83.208   **Varicose veins of unspecified lower extremity with both ulcer of other part of lower extremity and inflammation**   A ▽

I83.209   **Varicose veins of unspecified lower extremity with both ulcer of unspecified site and inflammation**   A ▽

√6ᵗʰ **I83.21**   **Varicose veins of right lower extremity with both ulcer and inflammation**

I83.211   **Varicose veins of right lower extremity with both ulcer of thigh and inflammation**   A

I83.212   **Varicose veins of right lower extremity with both ulcer of calf and inflammation**   A

I83.213   **Varicose veins of right lower extremity with both ulcer of ankle and inflammation**   A

I83.214   **Varicose veins of right lower extremity with both ulcer of heel and midfoot and inflammation**   A
> Varicose veins of right lower extremity with both ulcer of plantar surface of midfoot and inflammation

I83.215   **Varicose veins of right lower extremity with both ulcer other part of foot and inflammation**   A
> Varicose veins of right lower extremity with both ulcer of toe and inflammation

I83.218   **Varicose veins of right lower extremity with both ulcer of other part of lower extremity and inflammation**   A

I83.219   **Varicose veins of right lower extremity with both ulcer of unspecified site and inflammation**   A ▽

√6ᵗʰ **I83.22**   **Varicose veins of left lower extremity with both ulcer and inflammation**

I83.221   **Varicose veins of left lower extremity with both ulcer of thigh and inflammation**   A

I83.222   **Varicose veins of left lower extremity with both ulcer of calf and inflammation**   A

I83.223   **Varicose veins of left lower extremity with both ulcer of ankle and inflammation**   A

I83.224   **Varicose veins of left lower extremity with both ulcer of heel and midfoot and inflammation**   A
> Varicose veins of left lower extremity with both ulcer of plantar surface of midfoot and inflammation

I83.225   **Varicose veins of left lower extremity with both ulcer other part of foot and inflammation**   A
> Varicose veins of left lower extremity with both ulcer of toe and inflammation

I83.228   **Varicose veins of left lower extremity with both ulcer of other part of lower extremity and inflammation**   A

I83.229   **Varicose veins of left lower extremity with both ulcer of unspecified site and inflammation**   A ▽

√5ᵗʰ **I83.8**   **Varicose veins of lower extremities with other complications**

√6ᵗʰ **I83.81**   **Varicose veins of lower extremities with pain**

I83.811   **Varicose veins of right lower extremities with pain**   A

I83.812   **Varicose veins of left lower extremities with pain**   A

I83.813   **Varicose veins of bilateral lower extremities with pain**   A

I83.819   **Varicose veins of unspecified lower extremities with pain**   A ▽

√6ᵗʰ **I83.89**   **Varicose veins of lower extremities with other complications**
> Varicose veins of lower extremities with edema
> Varicose veins of lower extremities with swelling

I83.891   **Varicose veins of right lower extremities with other complications**   A

I83.892   **Varicose veins of left lower extremities with other complications**   A

I83.893   **Varicose veins of bilateral lower extremities with other complications**   A

I83.899   **Varicose veins of unspecified lower extremities with other complications**   A ▽

√5ᵗʰ **I83.9**   **Asymptomatic varicose veins of lower extremities**
> Phlebectasia of lower extremities
> Varicose veins of lower extremities
> Varix of lower extremities

I83.90   **Asymptomatic varicose veins of unspecified lower extremity**   A ▽
> Varicose veins NOS

I83.91   **Asymptomatic varicose veins of right lower extremity**   A

I83.92   **Asymptomatic varicose veins of left lower extremity**   A

I83.93   **Asymptomatic varicose veins of bilateral lower extremities**   A

EXCLUDES 1 Not coded here   *EXCLUDES 2* Not included here   N Newborn Age : 0   P Pediatric Age : 0-17   M Maternity Age : 12-55   A Adult Age : 15-124

638

ICD-10-CM 2017

☑4ᵗʰ **I85 Esophageal varices**

Use additional code to identify:
alcohol abuse and dependence (F10.-)

☑5ᵗʰ **I85.0 Esophageal varices**

Idiopathic esophageal varices
Primary esophageal varices

I85.00 Esophageal varices without bleeding
Esophageal varices NOS

I85.01 Esophageal varices with bleeding

☑5ᵗʰ **I85.1 Secondary esophageal varices**

Esophageal varices secondary to alcoholic liver disease
Esophageal varices secondary to cirrhosis of liver
Esophageal varices secondary to schistosomiasis
Esophageal varices secondary to toxic liver disease
Code first underlying disease

I85.10 Secondary esophageal varices without bleeding

I85.11 Secondary esophageal varices with bleeding

☑4ᵗʰ **I86 Varicose veins of other sites**

EXCLUDES 1 *varicose veins of unspecified site (I83.9-)*
EXCLUDES 2 *retinal varices (H35.0-)*

I86.0 Sublingual varices

I86.1 Scrotal varices   ♂

Varicocele

I86.2 Pelvic varices

I86.3 Vulval varices   ♀

EXCLUDES 1 *vulval varices complicating childbirth and the*
puerperium (O87.8)
vulval varices complicating pregnancy (O22.1-)

I86.4 Gastric varices

I86.8 Varicose veins of other specified sites   Ⓐ

Varicose ulcer of nasal septum

☑4ᵗʰ **I87 Other disorders of veins**

☑5ᵗʰ **I87.0 Postthrombotic syndrome**

Chronic venous hypertension due to deep vein thrombosis
Postphlebitic syndrome

EXCLUDES 1 *chronic venous hypertension without deep vein*
thrombosis (I87.3-)

☑6ᵗʰ **I87.00 Postthrombotic syndrome without complications**

Asymptomatic postthrombotic syndrome

I87.001 Postthrombotic syndrome without complications of right lower extremity

I87.002 Postthrombotic syndrome without complications of left lower extremity

I87.003 Postthrombotic syndrome without complications of bilateral lower extremity

I87.009 Postthrombotic syndrome without ▽
complications of unspecified extremity
Postthrombotic syndrome NOS

☑6ᵗʰ **I87.01 Postthrombotic syndrome with ulcer**

Use additional code to specify site and severity of
ulcer (L97.-)

I87.011 Postthrombotic syndrome with ulcer of right lower extremity

I87.012 Postthrombotic syndrome with ulcer of left lower extremity

I87.013 Postthrombotic syndrome with ulcer of bilateral lower extremity

I87.019 Postthrombotic syndrome with ▽
ulcer of unspecified lower extremity

☑6ᵗʰ **I87.02 Postthrombotic syndrome with inflammation**

I87.021 Postthrombotic syndrome with inflammation of right lower extremity

I87.022 Postthrombotic syndrome with inflammation of left lower extremity

I87.023 Postthrombotic syndrome with inflammation of bilateral lower extremity

I87.029 Postthrombotic syndrome with ▽
inflammation of unspecified lower extremity

☑6ᵗʰ **I87.03 Postthrombotic syndrome with ulcer and inflammation**

Use additional code to specify site and severity of
ulcer (L97.-)

I87.031 Postthrombotic syndrome with ulcer and inflammation of right lower extremity

I87.032 Postthrombotic syndrome with ulcer and inflammation of left lower extremity

I87.033 Postthrombotic syndrome with ulcer and inflammation of bilateral lower extremity

I87.039 Postthrombotic syndrome with ▽
ulcer and inflammation of unspecified lower extremity

☑6ᵗʰ **I87.09 Postthrombotic syndrome with other complications**

I87.091 Postthrombotic syndrome with other complications of right lower extremity

I87.092 Postthrombotic syndrome with other complications of left lower extremity

I87.093 Postthrombotic syndrome with other complications of bilateral lower extremity

I87.099 Postthrombotic syndrome with ▽
other complications of unspecified lower extremity

I87.1 Compression of vein

Stricture of vein
Vena cava syndrome (inferior) (superior)

EXCLUDES 2 *compression of pulmonary vein (I28.8)*

I87.2 Venous insufficiency (chronic) (peripheral)

▶Stasis dermatitis◀
EXCLUDES 1 ▶*stasis dermatitis with varicose veins of lower*
extremities (I83.1-, I83.2-)◀

DEF: Insufficient drainage of venous blood in any part of body;
results in edema or dermatosis.

☑5ᵗʰ **I87.3 Chronic venous hypertension (idiopathic)**

Stasis edema
EXCLUDES 1 *chronic venous hypertension due to deep vein*
thrombosis (I87.0-)
varicose veins of lower extremities (I83.-)

☑6ᵗʰ **I87.30 Chronic venous hypertension (idiopathic) without complications**

Asymptomatic chronic venous hypertension
(idiopathic)

I87.301 Chronic venous hypertension (idiopathic) without complications of right lower extremity

I87.302 Chronic venous hypertension (idiopathic) without complications of left lower extremity

I87.303 Chronic venous hypertension (idiopathic) without complications of bilateral lower extremity

I87.309 Chronic venous hypertension ▽
(idiopathic) without complications of unspecified lower extremity
Chronic venous hypertension NOS

☑6ᵗʰ **I87.31 Chronic venous hypertension (idiopathic) with ulcer**

Use additional code to specify site and severity of
ulcer (L97.-)

I87.311 Chronic venous hypertension (idiopathic) with ulcer of right lower extremity

I87.312 Chronic venous hypertension (idiopathic) with ulcer of left lower extremity

I87.313 Chronic venous hypertension (idiopathic) with ulcer of bilateral lower extremity

I87.319 Chronic venous hypertension ▽
(idiopathic) with ulcer of unspecified lower extremity

☑6ᵗʰ **I87.32 Chronic venous hypertension (idiopathic) with inflammation**

I87.321 Chronic venous hypertension (idiopathic) with inflammation of right lower extremity

I87.322 Chronic venous hypertension (idiopathic) with inflammation of left lower extremity

I87.323 Chronic venous hypertension (idiopathic) with inflammation of bilateral lower extremity

I87.329 Chronic venous hypertension ▽
(idiopathic) with inflammation of unspecified lower extremity

☑6ᵗʰ **I87.33 Chronic venous hypertension (idiopathic) with ulcer and inflammation**

Use additional code to specify site and severity of
ulcer (L97.-)

I87.331 Chronic venous hypertension (idiopathic) with ulcer and inflammation of right lower extremity

---

☑ Additional Character Required   ☑x7ᵗʰ Placeholder Alert   Manifestation Dx   ▽ Unspecified Dx   ▶◀ Revised Text   ● New Code   ▲ Revised Code Title

I87.332 **Chronic venous hypertension (idiopathic) with ulcer and inflammation of** left lower **extremity**

I87.333 **Chronic venous hypertension (idiopathic) with ulcer and inflammation of** bilateral lower **extremity**

I87.339 **Chronic venous hypertension (idiopathic) with ulcer and inflammation of unspecified lower extremity** ▽

√6ᵗʰ I87.39 **Chronic venous hypertension (idiopathic) with other complications**

I87.391 **Chronic venous hypertension (idiopathic) with other complications of** right lower **extremity**

I87.392 **Chronic venous hypertension (idiopathic) with other complications of** left lower **extremity**

I87.393 **Chronic venous hypertension (idiopathic) with other complications of** bilateral lower **extremity**

I87.399 **Chronic venous hypertension (idiopathic) with other complications of unspecified lower extremity** ▽

I87.8 **Other specified disorders of veins**
Phlebosclerosis
Venofibrosis

I87.9 **Disorder of vein, unspecified** ▽

√4ᵗʰ **I88 Nonspecific lymphadenitis**
EXCLUDES 1   *acute lymphadenitis, except mesenteric (L04.-)*
enlarged lymph nodes NOS (R59.-)
human immunodeficiency virus [HIV] disease resulting in generalized lymphadenopathy (B20)

I88.0 **Nonspecific mesenteric lymphadenitis**
Mesenteric lymphadenitis (acute)(chronic)

I88.1 **Chronic lymphadenitis, except mesenteric**
Adenitis
Lymphadenitis

I88.8 **Other nonspecific lymphadenitis**

I88.9 **Nonspecific lymphadenitis, unspecified** ▽
Lymphadenitis NOS

√4ᵗʰ **I89 Other noninfective disorders of lymphatic vessels and lymph nodes**
EXCLUDES 1   *chylocele, tunica vaginalis (nonfilarial) NOS ▶(N50.89)◀*
enlarged lymph nodes NOS (R59.-)
filarial chylocele (B74.-)
hereditary lymphedema (Q82.0)

I89.0 **Lymphedema, not elsewhere classified**
Elephantiasis (nonfilarial) NOS
Lymphangiectasis
Obliteration, lymphatic vessel
Praecox lymphedema
Secondary lymphedema
EXCLUDES 1   *postmastectomy lymphedema (I97.2)*

I89.1 **Lymphangitis**
Chronic lymphangitis
Lymphangitis NOS
Subacute lymphangitis
EXCLUDES 1   *acute lymphangitis (L03.-)*

I89.8 **Other specified noninfective disorders of lymphatic vessels and lymph nodes**
Chylocele (nonfilarial)
Chylous ascites
Chylous cyst
Lipomelanotic reticulosis
Lymph node or vessel fistula
Lymph node or vessel infarction
Lymph node or vessel rupture

I89.9 **Noninfective disorder of lymphatic vessels and lymph nodes, unspecified** ▽
Disease of lymphatic vessels NOS

Other and unspecified disorders of the circulatory system (I95-I99)

√4ᵗʰ **I95 Hypotension**
EXCLUDES 1   *cardiovascular collapse (R57.9) (~R57.9)*
maternal hypotension syndrome (O26.5-)
nonspecific low blood pressure reading NOS (R03.1)

I95.0 **Idiopathic hypotension**

I95.1 **Orthostatic hypotension**
Hypotension, postural
EXCLUDES 1   *neurogenic orthostatic hypotension [Shy-Drager] (G90.3)*
orthostatic hypotension due to drugs (I95.2)

I95.2 **Hypotension due to drugs**
Orthostatic hypotension due to drugs
Use additional code for adverse effect, if applicable, to identify drug (T36-T50 with fifth or sixth character 5)

I95.3 **Hypotension of hemodialysis**
Intra-dialytic hypotension

√5ᵗʰ I95.8 **Other hypotension**

I95.81 **Postprocedural hypotension**

I95.89 **Other hypotension**
Chronic hypotension

I95.9 **Hypotension, unspecified** ▽

I96 **Gangrene, not elsewhere classified**
Gangrenous cellulitis
EXCLUDES 1   *gangrene in atherosclerosis of native arteries of the extremities (I70.26)*
gangrene in diabetes mellitus ▶(E08-E13 with .52)◀
gangrene in hernia (K40.1, K40.4, K41.1, K41.4, K42.1, K43.1-, K44.1, K45.1, K46.1)
gangrene in other peripheral vascular diseases (I73.-)
gangrene of certain specified sites - see Alphabetical Index
gas gangrene (A48.0)
pyoderma gangrenosum (L88)
AHA: 2013,2Q,34

√4ᵗʰ **I97 Intraoperative and postprocedural complications and disorders of circulatory system, not elsewhere classified**
EXCLUDES 2   *postprocedural shock (T81.1-)*

I97.0 **Postcardiotomy syndrome**

√5ᵗʰ I97.1 **Other postprocedural cardiac functional disturbances**
EXCLUDES 2   *acute pulmonary insufficiency following thoracic surgery (J95.1)*
intraoperative cardiac functional disturbances (I97.7-)

√6ᵗʰ I97.11 **Postprocedural cardiac insufficiency**

I97.110 **Postprocedural cardiac insufficiency following** cardiac surgery

I97.111 **Postprocedural cardiac insufficiency following** other surgery

√6ᵗʰ I97.12 **Postprocedural cardiac arrest**

I97.120 **Postprocedural cardiac arrest following** cardiac surgery

I97.121 **Postprocedural cardiac arrest following** other surgery

√6ᵗʰ I97.13 **Postprocedural heart failure**
Use additional code to identify the heart failure (I50.-)

I97.130 **Postprocedural heart failure following** cardiac surgery

I97.131 **Postprocedural heart failure following** other surgery

√6ᵗʰ I97.19 **Other postprocedural cardiac functional disturbances**
Use additional code, if applicable, to further specify disorder

I97.190 **Other postprocedural cardiac functional disturbances following** cardiac surgery

I97.191 **Other postprocedural cardiac functional disturbances following** other surgery

I97.2 **Postmastectomy lymphedema syndrome** Ⓐ
Elephantiasis due to mastectomy
Obliteration of lymphatic vessels

I97.3 **Postprocedural hypertension**

EXCLUDES 1   Not coded here   *EXCLUDES 2*   Not included here   Ⓝ Newborn Age : 0   Ⓟ Pediatric Age : 0-17   Ⓜ Maternity Age : 12-55   Ⓐ Adult Age : 15-124

640

ICD-10-CM 2017

✓5ᵗʰ **I97.4 Intraoperative hemorrhage and hematoma** of a circulatory system organ or structure complicating a procedure

> EXCLUDES 1   *intraoperative hemorrhage and hematoma of a circulatory system organ or structure due to accidental puncture and laceration during a procedure (I97.5-)*
>
> EXCLUDES 2   *intraoperative cerebrovascular hemorrhage complicating a procedure (G97.3-)*

✓6ᵗʰ **I97.41 Intraoperative hemorrhage and hematoma** of a circulatory system organ or structure complicating a circulatory system procedure

I97.410 Intraoperative hemorrhage and hematoma of a circulatory system organ or structure complicating a cardiac catheterization

I97.411 Intraoperative hemorrhage and hematoma of a circulatory system organ or structure complicating a cardiac bypass

I97.418 Intraoperative hemorrhage and hematoma of a circulatory system organ or structure complicating other circulatory system procedure

I97.42 Intraoperative hemorrhage and hematoma of a circulatory system organ or structure complicating other procedure

✓5ᵗʰ **I97.5 Accidental puncture and laceration** of a circulatory system organ or structure during a procedure

> EXCLUDES 2   *accidental puncture and laceration of brain during a procedure (G97.4-)*

I97.51 Accidental puncture and laceration of a circulatory system organ or structure during a circulatory system procedure

I97.52 Accidental puncture and laceration of a circulatory system organ or structure during other procedure

▲ ✓5ᵗʰ **I97.6 Postprocedural hemorrhage, hematoma and seroma** of a circulatory system organ or structure following a procedure

> EXCLUDES 2   *postprocedural cerebrovascular hemorrhage complicating a procedure (G97.5-)*

▲ ✓6ᵗʰ **I97.61 Postprocedural hemorrhage** of a circulatory system organ or structure following a circulatory system procedure

▲ **I97.610 Postprocedural hemorrhage** of a circulatory system organ or structure following a cardiac catheterization

▲ **I97.611 Postprocedural hemorrhage** of a circulatory system organ or structure following cardiac bypass

▲ **I97.618 Postprocedural hemorrhage** of a circulatory system organ or structure following other circulatory system procedure

▲ ✓6ᵗʰ **I97.62 Postprocedural hemorrhage, hematoma and seroma** of a circulatory system organ or structure following other procedure

● **I97.620 Postprocedural** hemorrhage **of a circulatory system organ or structure following other procedure**

● **I97.621 Postprocedural** hematoma **of a circulatory system organ or structure following other procedure**

● **I97.622 Postprocedural** seroma **of a circulatory system organ or structure following other procedure**

● **I97.63 Postprocedural** hematoma **of a circulatory system organ or structure following a** circulatory system procedure

● **I97.630 Postprocedural hematoma** of a circulatory system organ or structure following a cardiac catheterization

● **I97.631 Postprocedural hematoma** of a circulatory system organ or structure following cardiac bypass

● **I97.638 Postprocedural hematoma** of a circulatory system organ or structure following other circulatory system procedure

● **I97.64 Postprocedural** seroma **of a circulatory system organ or structure following a circulatory system procedure**

● **I97.640 Postprocedural seroma** of a circulatory system organ or structure following a cardiac catheterization

● **I97.641 Postprocedural seroma** of a circulatory system organ or structure following cardiac bypass

● **I97.648 Postprocedural seroma** of a circulatory system organ or structure following other circulatory system procedure

✓5ᵗʰ **I97.7 Intraoperative cardiac functional disturbances**

> EXCLUDES 2   *acute pulmonary insufficiency following thoracic surgery (J95.1)*
> *postprocedural cardiac functional disturbances (I97.1-)*

✓6ᵗʰ **I97.71 Intraoperative cardiac arrest**

I97.710 Intraoperative cardiac arrest during cardiac surgery

I97.711 Intraoperative cardiac arrest during other surgery

✓6ᵗʰ **I97.79 Other intraoperative cardiac functional disturbances**

> Use additional code, if applicable, to further specify disorder

I97.790 Other intraoperative cardiac functional disturbances during cardiac surgery

I97.791 Other intraoperative cardiac functional disturbances during other surgery

✓5ᵗʰ **I97.8 Other intraoperative and postprocedural complications and disorders of the circulatory system, not elsewhere classified**

> Use additional code, if applicable, to further specify disorder

✓6ᵗʰ **I97.81 Intraoperative cerebrovascular infarction**

I97.810 Intraoperative cerebrovascular infarction during cardiac surgery

I97.811 Intraoperative cerebrovascular infarction during other surgery

✓6ᵗʰ **I97.82 Postprocedural cerebrovascular infarction**

I97.820 Postprocedural cerebrovascular infarction following cardiac surgery

I97.821 Postprocedural cerebrovascular infarction following other surgery

I97.88 Other intraoperative complications of the circulatory system, not elsewhere classified

I97.89 Other postprocedural complications and disorders of the circulatory system, not elsewhere classified

✓4ᵗʰ **I99 Other and unspecified disorders of circulatory system**

I99.8 Other disorder of circulatory system

I99.9 Unspecified disorder of circulatory system   ▽

✓ Additional Character Required   ✓ₓ7ᵗʰ Placeholder Alert   Manifestation Dx   ▽ Unspecified Dx   ▶◀ Revised Text   ● New Code   ▲ Revised Code Title

Chapter 10. Diseases of the Respiratory System (J00–J99)

Chapter Specific Guidelines with Coding Examples

The chapter specific guidelines from the ICD-10-CM Official Guidelines for Coding and Reporting have been provided below. Along with these guidelines are coding examples, contained in the shaded boxes, that have been developed to help illustrate the coding and/or sequencing guidance found in these guidelines.

a. Chronic obstructive pulmonary disease [COPD] and asthma

1) Acute exacerbation of chronic obstructive bronchitis and asthma

The codes in categories J44 and J45 distinguish between uncomplicated cases and those in acute exacerbation. An acute exacerbation is a worsening or a decompensation of a chronic condition. An acute exacerbation is not equivalent to an infection superimposed on a chronic condition, though an exacerbation may be triggered by an infection.

Acute streptococcal bronchitis with acute exacerbation of COPD

J20.2   **Acute bronchitis due to streptococcus**

J44.0   **Chronic obstructive pulmonary disease with acute lower respiratory infection**

J44.1   **Chronic obstructive pulmonary disease with (acute) exacerbation**

Explanation: ICD-10-CM uses combination codes to create organism-specific classifications for acute bronchitis. Category J44 codes include combination codes with severity components, which differentiate between COPD with acute lower respiratory infection (acute bronchitis), COPD with acute exacerbation, and COPD without mention of a complication (unspecified).

An acute exacerbation is a worsening or a decompensation of a chronic condition. An acute exacerbation is not equivalent to an infection superimposed on a chronic condition, though an exacerbation may be triggered by an infection, as in this example.

Exacerbation of moderate persistent asthma with status asthmaticus

J45.42   **Moderate persistent asthma with status asthmaticus**

Explanation: Category J45 Asthma includes severity-specific subcategories and fifth-character codes to distinguish between uncomplicated cases, those in acute exacerbation, and those with status asthmaticus.

---

b. Acute respiratory failure

1) Acute respiratory failure as principal diagnosis

A code from subcategory J96.0, Acute respiratory failure, or subcategory J96.2, Acute and chronic respiratory failure, may be assigned as a principal diagnosis when it is the condition established after study to be chiefly responsible for occasioning the admission to the hospital, and the selection is supported by the Alphabetic Index and Tabular List. However, chapter-specific coding guidelines (such as obstetrics, poisoning, HIV, newborn) that provide sequencing direction take precedence.

Acute hypoxic respiratory failure due to COPD exacerbation

J96.01   **Acute respiratory failure with hypoxia**

J44.1   **Chronic obstructive pulmonary disease with (acute) exacerbation**

Explanation: Category J96 classifies respiratory failure with combination codes that designate the severity and the presence of hypoxia and hypercapnia. Code J96.01 is sequenced as the first-listed diagnosis, as the reason for the admission. Respiratory failure may be assigned as a principal diagnosis when it is the condition established after study to be chiefly responsible for occasioning the admission to the hospital and the selection is supported by the Alphabetic Index and Tabular List.

---

2) Acute respiratory failure as secondary diagnosis

Respiratory failure may be listed as a secondary diagnosis if it occurs after admission, or if it is present on admission, but does not meet the definition of principal diagnosis.

Acute respiratory failure due to accidental oxycodone overdose

T40.2X1A   **Poisoning by other opioids, accidental (unintentional), initial encounter**

J96.00   **Acute respiratory failure, unspecified whether with hypoxia or hypercapnia**

Explanation: Respiratory failure may be assigned as a principal diagnosis when it is the condition established after study to be chiefly responsible for occasioning the admission to the hospital, and the selection is supported by the Alphabetic Index and Tabular List. However, chapter-specific coding guidelines, such as poisoning, that provide sequencing direction take precedence. When coding a poisoning or reaction to the improper use of a medication (e.g. overdose, wrong substance given or taken in error, wrong route of administration), first assign the appropriate code from categories T36–T50. Use additional code(s) for all manifestations of the poisoning. In this instance, the respiratory failure is a manifestation of the poisoning and is sequenced as a secondary diagnosis.

Acute pneumococcal pneumonia with subsequent development of acute respiratory failure

J13   **Pneumonia due to Streptococcus pneumoniae**

J96.00   **Acute respiratory failure, unspecified whether with hypoxia or hypercapnia**

Explanation: Acute respiratory failure may be listed as a secondary diagnosis if it occurs after admission, or if it is present on admission but does not meet the definition of principal diagnosis.

---

3) Sequencing of acute respiratory failure and another acute condition

When a patient is admitted with respiratory failure and another acute condition, (e.g., myocardial infarction, cerebrovascular accident, aspiration pneumonia), the principal diagnosis will not be the same in every situation. This applies whether the other acute condition is a respiratory or nonrespiratory condition. Selection of the principal diagnosis will be dependent on the circumstances of admission. If both the respiratory failure and the other acute condition are equally responsible for occasioning the admission to the hospital, and there are no chapter-specific sequencing rules, the guideline regarding two or more diagnoses that equally meet the definition for principal diagnosis (Section II, C.) may be applied in these situations.

If the documentation is not clear as to whether acute respiratory failure and another condition are equally responsible for occasioning the admission, query the provider for clarification.

Acute pneumococcal pneumonia and acute respiratory failure, both present on admission

J96.00   **Acute respiratory failure, unspecified whether with hypoxia or hypercapnia**

J13   **Pneumonia due to Streptococcus pneumoniae**

Explanation: When a patient is admitted with respiratory failure and another acute condition, such as a bacterial pneumonia, the principal diagnosis is not the same in every situation. This applies whether the other acute condition is a respiratory or nonrespiratory condition. The principal diagnosis depends on the circumstances of admission.

---

c. Influenza due to certain identified influenza viruses

Code only confirmed cases of influenza due to certain identified influenza viruses (category J09), and due to other identified influenza virus (category J10). This is an exception to the hospital inpatient guideline Section II, H. (Uncertain Diagnosis).

In this context, "confirmation" does not require documentation of positive laboratory testing specific for avian or other novel influenza A or other identified influenza virus. However, coding should be based on the provider's diagnostic statement that the patient has avian influenza, or other novel influenza A, for category J09, or has another particular identified strain of influenza, such as H1N1 or H3N2, but not identified as novel or variant, for category J10.

If the provider records "suspected" or "possible" or "probable" avian influenza, or novel influenza, or other identified influenza, then the appropriate influenza code from category J11, Influenza due to unidentified influenza virus, should be assigned. A code from category J09, Influenza due to certain identified influenza viruses, should not be assigned nor should a code from category J10, Influenza due to other identified influenza virus.

Influenza due to avian influenza virus with pneumonia

J09.X1   **Influenza due to identified novel influenza A virus with pneumonia**

Explanation: Codes in category J09 Influenza due to certain identified influenza viruses should be assigned only for confirmed cases. "Confirmation" does not require positive laboratory testing of a specific influenza virus but does need to be based on the provider's diagnostic statement, which should not include terms such as "possible," "probable," or "suspected."

---

d. Ventilator associated pneumonia

1) Documentation of ventilator associated pneumonia

As with all procedural or postprocedural complications, code assignment is based on the provider's documentation of the relationship between the condition and the procedure.

Code J95.851, Ventilator associated pneumonia, should be assigned only when the provider has documented ventilator associated pneumonia (VAP). An additional code to identify the organism (e.g., Pseudomonas aeruginosa, code B96.5) should also be assigned. Do not assign an additional code from categories J12-J18 to identify the type of pneumonia.

Code J95.851 should not be assigned for cases where the patient has pneumonia and is on a mechanical ventilator and the provider has not specifically stated that the pneumonia is ventilator-associated pneumonia. If the documentation is unclear as to whether the patient has a pneumonia that is a complication attributable to the mechanical ventilator, query the provider.

2) Ventilator associated pneumonia develops after admission

A patient may be admitted with one type of pneumonia (e.g., code J13, Pneumonia due to Streptococcus pneumonia) and subsequently develop VAP. In this instance, the principal diagnosis would be the appropriate code from categories J12-J18 for the pneumonia diagnosed at the time of admission. Code J95.851, Ventilator associated pneumonia, would be assigned as an additional diagnosis when the provider has also documented the presence of ventilator associated pneumonia.

Patient with pneumonia due to *Klebsiella pneumoniae* develops superimposed MRSA ventilator-associated pneumonia

J15.0   **Pneumonia due to Klebsiella pneumoniae**

J95.851   **Ventilator associated pneumonia**

B95.62   **Methicillin resistant Staphylococcus aureus infection as the cause of diseases classified elsewhere**

Explanation: Code assignment for ventilator-associated pneumonia is based on the provider's documentation of the relationship between the condition and the procedure and is reported only when the provider has documented ventilator-associated pneumonia (VAP).

A patient may be admitted with one type of pneumonia and subsequently develop VAP. In this example, the principal diagnosis code describes the pneumonia diagnosed at the time of admission, with code J95.851 Ventilator associated pneumonia, assigned as secondary.

Chapter 10. Diseases of the Respiratory System (J00-J99)

NOTE When a respiratory condition is described as occurring in more than one site and is not specifically indexed, it should be classified to the lower anatomic site (e.g., tracheobronchitis to bronchitis in J40).

Use additional code, where applicable, to identify:
exposure to environmental tobacco smoke (Z77.22)
exposure to tobacco smoke in the perinatal period (P96.81)
►history of tobacco dependence (Z87.891)◄
occupational exposure to environmental tobacco smoke (Z57.31)
tobacco dependence (F17.-)
tobacco use (Z72.0)

EXCLUDES 2 certain conditions originating in the perinatal period (P04-P96)
certain infectious and parasitic diseases (A00-B99)
complications of pregnancy, childbirth and the puerperium (O00-O9A)
congenital malformations, deformations and chromosomal abnormalities (Q00-Q99)
endocrine, nutritional and metabolic diseases (E00-E88)
injury, poisoning and certain other consequences of external causes (S00-T88)
neoplasms (C00-D49)
smoke inhalation (T59.81-)
symptoms, signs and abnormal clinical and laboratory findings, not elsewhere classified (R00-R94)

This chapter contains the following blocks:
J00-J06   Acute upper respiratory infections
J09-J18   Influenza and pneumonia
J20-J22   Other acute lower respiratory infections
J30-J39   Other diseases of upper respiratory tract
J40-J47   Chronic lower respiratory diseases
J60-J70   Lung diseases due to external agents
J80-J84   Other respiratory diseases principally affecting the interstitium
J85-J86   Suppurative and necrotic conditions of the lower respiratory tract
J90-J94   Other diseases of the pleura
J95   Intraoperative and postprocedural complications and disorders of respiratory system, not elsewhere classified
J96-J99   Other diseases of the respiratory system

Acute upper respiratory infections (J00-J06)

EXCLUDES 1 chronic obstructive pulmonary disease with acute lower respiratory infection (J44.0)
influenza virus with other respiratory manifestations (J09.X2, J10.1, J11.1)

J00   Acute nasopharyngitis [common cold]
Acute rhinitis
Coryza (acute)
Infective nasopharyngitis NOS
Infective rhinitis
Nasal catarrh, acute
Nasopharyngitis NOS
EXCLUDES 1 acute pharyngitis (J02.-)
acute sore throat NOS (J02.9)
pharyngitis NOS (J02.9)
rhinitis NOS (J31.0)
sore throat NOS (J02.9)
EXCLUDES 2 allergic rhinitis (J30.1-J30.9)
chronic pharyngitis (J31.2)
chronic rhinitis (J31.0)
chronic sore throat (J31.2)
nasopharyngitis, chronic (J31.1)
vasomotor rhinitis (J30.0)

√4ᵗʰ J01   Acute sinusitis
INCLUDES acute abscess of sinus
acute empyema of sinus
acute infection of sinus
acute inflammation of sinus
acute suppuration of sinus
Use additional code (B95-B97) to identify infectious agent
EXCLUDES 1 sinusitis NOS (J32.9)
EXCLUDES 2 chronic sinusitis (J32.0-J32.8)

√5ᵗʰ J01.0   **Acute maxillary sinusitis**
Acute antritis
J01.00   **Acute maxillary sinusitis, unspecified** ▽
J01.01   **Acute recurrent maxillary sinusitis**

√5ᵗʰ J01.1   **Acute frontal sinusitis**
J01.10   **Acute frontal sinusitis, unspecified** ▽
J01.11   **Acute recurrent frontal sinusitis**

√5ᵗʰ J01.2   **Acute ethmoidal sinusitis**
J01.20   **Acute ethmoidal sinusitis, unspecified** ▽

J01.21   **Acute recurrent ethmoidal sinusitis**

√5ᵗʰ J01.3   **Acute sphenoidal sinusitis**
J01.30   **Acute sphenoidal sinusitis, unspecified** ▽
J01.31   **Acute recurrent sphenoidal sinusitis**

√5ᵗʰ J01.4   **Acute pansinusitis**
J01.40   **Acute pansinusitis, unspecified** ▽
J01.41   **Acute recurrent pansinusitis**

√5ᵗʰ J01.8   **Other acute sinusitis**
J01.80   **Other acute sinusitis**
Acute sinusitis involving more than one sinus but not pansinusitis
J01.81   **Other acute recurrent sinusitis**
Acute recurrent sinusitis involving more than one sinus but not pansinusitis

√5ᵗʰ J01.9   **Acute sinusitis, unspecified**
J01.90   **Acute sinusitis, unspecified** ▽
J01.91   **Acute recurrent sinusitis, unspecified** ▽

√4ᵗʰ J02   Acute pharyngitis
INCLUDES acute sore throat
EXCLUDES 1 acute laryngopharyngitis (J06.0)
peritonsillar abscess (J36)
pharyngeal abscess (J39.1)
retropharyngeal abscess (J39.0)
EXCLUDES 2 chronic pharyngitis (J31.2)

J02.0   **Streptococcal pharyngitis**
Septic pharyngitis
Streptococcal sore throat
EXCLUDES 2 scarlet fever (A38.-)

J02.8   **Acute pharyngitis due to other specified organisms**
Use additional code (B95-B97) to identify infectious agent
EXCLUDES 1 acute pharyngitis due to coxsackie virus (B08.5)
acute pharyngitis due to gonococcus (A54.5)
acute pharyngitis due to herpes [simplex] virus (B00.2)
acute pharyngitis due to infectious mononucleosis (B27.-)
enteroviral vesicular pharyngitis (B08.5)

J02.9   **Acute pharyngitis, unspecified** ▽
Gangrenous pharyngitis (acute)
Infective pharyngitis (acute) NOS
Pharyngitis (acute) NOS
Sore throat (acute) NOS
Suppurative pharyngitis (acute)
Ulcerative pharyngitis (acute)

√4ᵗʰ J03   Acute tonsillitis
EXCLUDES 1 acute sore throat (J02.-)
hypertrophy of tonsils (J35.1)
peritonsillar abscess (J36)
sore throat NOS (J02.9)
streptococcal sore throat (J02.0)
EXCLUDES 2 chronic tonsillitis (J35.0)

√5ᵗʰ J03.0   **Streptococcal tonsillitis**
J03.00   **Acute streptococcal tonsillitis, unspecified** ▽
J03.01   **Acute recurrent streptococcal tonsillitis**

√5ᵗʰ J03.8   **Acute tonsillitis due to other specified organisms**
Use additional code (B95-B97) to identify infectious agent
EXCLUDES 1 diphtheritic tonsillitis (A36.0)
herpesviral pharyngotonsillitis (B00.2)
streptococcal tonsillitis (J03.0)
tuberculous tonsillitis (A15.8)
Vincent's tonsillitis (A69.1)
J03.80   **Acute tonsillitis due to other specified organisms**
J03.81   **Acute recurrent tonsillitis due to other specified organisms**

√5ᵗʰ J03.9   **Acute tonsillitis, unspecified**
Follicular tonsillitis (acute)
Gangrenous tonsillitis (acute)
Infective tonsillitis (acute)
Tonsillitis (acute) NOS
Ulcerative tonsillitis (acute)
J03.90   **Acute tonsillitis, unspecified** ▽
J03.91   **Acute recurrent tonsillitis, unspecified** ▽

☑4ᵗʰ **J04 Acute laryngitis and tracheitis**
Use additional code (B95-B97) to identify infectious agent
EXCLUDES 1 *acute obstructive laryngitis [croup] and epiglottitis (J05.-)*
EXCLUDES 2 *laryngismus (stridulus) (J38.5)*

J04.0 Acute laryngitis
Edematous laryngitis (acute)
Laryngitis (acute) NOS
Subglottic laryngitis (acute)
Suppurative laryngitis (acute)
Ulcerative laryngitis (acute)
EXCLUDES 1 *acute obstructive laryngitis (J05.0)*
EXCLUDES 2 *chronic laryngitis (J37.0)*

☑5ᵗʰ **J04.1 Acute tracheitis**
Acute viral tracheitis
Catarrhal tracheitis (acute)
Tracheitis (acute) NOS
EXCLUDES 2 *chronic tracheitis (J42)*

   J04.10 Acute tracheitis without obstruction
   J04.11 Acute tracheitis with obstruction

J04.2 Acute laryngotracheitis
Laryngotracheitis NOS
Tracheitis (acute) with laryngitis (acute)
EXCLUDES 1 *acute obstructive laryngotracheitis (J05.0)*
EXCLUDES 2 *chronic laryngotracheitis (J37.1)*

☑5ᵗʰ **J04.3 Supraglottitis, unspecified**

   J04.30 Supraglottitis, unspecified, without obstruction ▽
   J04.31 Supraglottitis, unspecified, with obstruction ▽

☑4ᵗʰ **J05 Acute obstructive laryngitis [croup] and epiglottitis**
Use additional code (B95-B97) to identify infectious agent

J05.0 Acute obstructive laryngitis [croup]
Obstructive laryngitis (acute) NOS
Obstructive laryngotracheitis NOS
DEF: Acute laryngeal obstruction due to allergy, foreign body, or in the majority of cases a viral infection; symptoms include harsh, barking cough, hoarseness, and persistent high-pitched respiratory sound (stridor).

☑5ᵗʰ **J05.1 Acute epiglottitis**
EXCLUDES 2 *epiglottitis, chronic (J37.0)*

   J05.10 Acute epiglottitis without obstruction
Epiglottitis NOS
   J05.11 Acute epiglottitis with obstruction

☑4ᵗʰ **J06 Acute upper respiratory infections of multiple and unspecified sites**
EXCLUDES 1 *acute respiratory infection NOS (J22)*
streptococcal pharyngitis (J02.0)

J06.0 Acute laryngopharyngitis
J06.9 Acute upper respiratory infection, unspecified ▽
Upper respiratory disease, acute
Upper respiratory infection NOS

Influenza and pneumonia (J09-J18)

EXCLUDES 2 *allergic or eosinophilic pneumonia (J82)*
aspiration pneumonia NOS (J69.0)
meconium pneumonia (P24.01)
neonatal aspiration pneumonia (P24.-)
pneumonia due to solids and liquids (J69.-)
congenital pneumonia (P23.9)
lipid pneumonia (J69.1)
rheumatic pneumonia (I00)
ventilator associated pneumonia (J95.851)

☑4ᵗʰ **J09 Influenza due to certain identified influenza viruses**
EXCLUDES 1 *influenza due to other identified influenza virus (J10.-)*
influenza due to unidentified influenza virus (J11.-)
seasonal influenza due to other identified influenza virus (J10.-)
seasonal influenza due to unidentified influenza virus (J11.-)

☑5ᵗʰ **J09.X Influenza due to identified novel influenza A virus**
Avian influenza
Bird influenza
Influenza A/H5N1
Influenza of other animal origin, not bird or swine
Swine influenza virus (viruses that normally cause infections in pigs)

J09.X1 Influenza due to identified novel influenza A virus with pneumonia
Code also, if applicable, associated:
lung abscess (J85.1)
other specified type of pneumonia

J09.X2 Influenza due to identified novel influenza A virus with other respiratory manifestations
Influenza due to identified novel influenza A virus NOS
Influenza due to identified novel influenza A virus with laryngitis
Influenza due to identified novel influenza A virus with pharyngitis
Influenza due to identified novel influenza A virus with upper respiratory symptoms
Use additional code, if applicable, for associated:
pleural effusion (J91.8)
sinusitis (J01.-)

J09.X3 Influenza due to identified novel influenza A virus with gastrointestinal manifestations
Influenza due to identified novel influenza A virus gastroenteritis
EXCLUDES 1 *'intestinal flu' [viral gastroenteritis] (A08.-)*

J09.X9 Influenza due to identified novel influenza A virus with other manifestations
Influenza due to identified novel influenza A virus with encephalopathy
Influenza due to identified novel influenza A virus with myocarditis
Influenza due to identified novel influenza A virus with otitis media
Use additional code to identify manifestation

☑4ᵗʰ **J10 Influenza due to other identified influenza virus**
EXCLUDES 1 *influenza due to avian influenza virus (J09.X-)*
influenza due to swine flu (J09.X-)
influenza due to unidentifed influenza virus (J11.-)

☑5ᵗʰ **J10.0 Influenza due to other identified influenza virus with pneumonia**
Code also associated lung abscess, if applicable (J85.1)

   J10.00 Influenza due to other identified influenza virus with unspecified type of pneumonia ▽
   J10.01 Influenza due to other identified influenza virus with the same other identified influenza virus pneumonia
   J10.08 Influenza due to other identified influenza virus with other specified pneumonia
Code also other specified type of pneumonia

J10.1 Influenza due to other identified influenza virus with other respiratory manifestations
Influenza due to other identified influenza virus NOS
Influenza due to other identified influenza virus with laryngitis
Influenza due to other identified influenza virus with pharyngitis
Influenza due to other identified influenza virus with upper respiratory symptoms
Use additional code for associated pleural effusion, if applicable (J91.8)
Use additional code for associated sinusitis, if applicable (J01.-)

J10.2 Influenza due to other identified influenza virus with gastrointestinal manifestations
Influenza due to other identified influenza virus gastroenteritis
EXCLUDES 1 *"intestinal flu" [viral gastroenteritis] (A08.-)*

☑5ᵗʰ **J10.8 Influenza due to other identified influenza virus with other manifestations**
   J10.81 Influenza due to other identified influenza virus with encephalopathy
   J10.82 Influenza due to other identified influenza virus with myocarditis
   J10.83 Influenza due to other identified influenza virus with otitis media
Use additional code for any associated perforated tympanic membrane (H72.-)
   J10.89 Influenza due to other identified influenza virus with other manifestations
Use additional codes to identify the manifestations

☑4ᵗʰ **J11 Influenza due to unidentified influenza virus**

☑5ᵗʰ **J11.0 Influenza due to unidentified influenza virus with pneumonia**
Code also associated lung abscess, if applicable (J85.1)

Chapter 10. Diseases of the Respiratory System

J11.00   **Influenza due to unidentified influenza virus with unspecified type of pneumonia**
Influenza with pneumonia NOS

J11.08   **Influenza due to unidentified influenza virus with specified pneumonia**
Code also other specified type of pneumonia

J11.1   **Influenza due to unidentified influenza virus with other respiratory manifestations**
Influenza NOS
Influenzal laryngitis NOS
Influenzal pharyngitis NOS
Influenza with upper respiratory symptoms NOS
Use additional code for associated pleural effusion, if applicable (J91.8)
Use additional code for associated sinusitis, if applicable (J01.-)

J11.2   **Influenza due to unidentified influenza virus with gastrointestinal manifestations**
Influenza gastroenteritis NOS
EXCLUDES 1   *"intestinal flu" [viral gastroenteritis] (A08.-)*

✓5th **J11.8**   **Influenza due to unidentified influenza virus with other manifestations**

J11.81   **Influenza due to unidentified influenza virus with encephalopathy**
Influenzal encephalopathy NOS

J11.82   **Influenza due to unidentified influenza virus with myocarditis**
Influenzal myocarditis NOS

J11.83   **Influenza due to unidentified influenza virus with otitis media**
Influenzal otitis media NOS
Use additional code for any associated perforated tympanic membrane (H72.-)

J11.89   **Influenza due to unidentified influenza virus with other manifestations**
Use additional codes to identify the manifestations

✓4th **J12**   **Viral pneumonia, not elsewhere classified**
INCLUDES   bronchopneumonia due to viruses other than influenza viruses
Code first associated influenza, if applicable (J09.X1, J10.0-, J11.0-)
Code also associated abscess, if applicable (J85.1)
EXCLUDES 1   *aspiration pneumonia due to anesthesia during labor and delivery (O74.0)*
aspiration pneumonia due to anesthesia during pregnancy (O29)
aspiration pneumonia due to anesthesia during puerperium (O89.0)
aspiration pneumonia due to solids and liquids (J69.-)
aspiration pneumonia NOS (J69.0)
congenital pneumonia (P23.0)
congenital rubella pneumonitis (P35.0)
interstitial pneumonia NOS (J84.9)
lipid pneumonia (J69.1)
neonatal aspiration pneumonia (P24.-)
AHA: 2013,4Q,118

J12.0   **Adenoviral pneumonia**
J12.1   **Respiratory syncytial virus pneumonia**
J12.2   **Parainfluenza virus pneumonia**
J12.3   **Human metapneumovirus pneumonia**
✓5th **J12.8**   **Other viral pneumonia**

J12.81   **Pneumonia due to SARS-associated coronavirus**
Severe acute respiratory syndrome NOS

J12.89   **Other viral pneumonia**
J12.9   **Viral pneumonia, unspecified**   ▽

J13   **Pneumonia due to Streptococcus pneumoniae**
Bronchopneumonia due to S. pneumoniae
Code first associated influenza, if applicable (J09.X1, J10.0-, J11.0-)
Code also associated abscess, if applicable (J85.1)
EXCLUDES 1   *congenital pneumonia due to S. pneumoniae (P23.6)*
lobar pneumonia, unspecified organism (J18.1)
pneumonia due to other streptococci (J15.3-J15.4)
AHA: 2013,4Q,118

J14   **Pneumonia due to Hemophilus influenzae**
Bronchopneumonia due to H. influenzae
Code first associated influenza, if applicable (J09.X1, J10.0-, J11.0-)
Code also associated abscess, if applicable (J85.1)
EXCLUDES 1   *congenital pneumonia due to H. influenzae (P23.6)*
AHA: 2013,4Q,118

✓4th **J15**   **Bacterial pneumonia, not elsewhere classified**
INCLUDES   Bronchopneumonia due to bacteria other than S. pneumoniae and H. influenzae
Code first associated influenza, if applicable (J09.X1, J10.0-, -J11.0-)
Code also associated abscess, if applicable (J85.1)
EXCLUDES 1   *chlamydial pneumonia (J16.0)*
congenital pneumonia (P23.-)
Legionnaires' disease (A48.1)
spirochetal pneumonia (A69.8)
AHA: 2013,4Q,118

J15.0   **Pneumonia due to Klebsiella pneumoniae**
J15.1   **Pneumonia due to Pseudomonas**
✓5th **J15.2**   **Pneumonia due to staphylococcus**

J15.20   **Pneumonia due to staphylococcus, unspecified**   ▽

✓6th **J15.21**   **Pneumonia due to Staphylococcus aureus**

J15.211   **Pneumonia due to methicillin susceptible Staphylococcus aureus**
MSSA pneumonia
Pneumonia due to Staphylococcus aureus NOS

J15.212   **Pneumonia due to methicillin resistant Staphylococcus aureus**

J15.29   **Pneumonia due to other staphylococcus**

J15.3   **Pneumonia due to streptococcus, group B**
J15.4   **Pneumonia due to other streptococci**
EXCLUDES 1   *pneumonia due to streptococcus, group B (J15.3)*
pneumonia due to Streptococcus pneumoniae (J13)

J15.5   **Pneumonia due to Escherichia coli**
J15.6   **Pneumonia due to other aerobic Gram-negative bacteria**
Pneumonia due to Serratia marcescens
J15.7   **Pneumonia due to Mycoplasma pneumoniae**
J15.8   **Pneumonia due to other specified bacteria**
J15.9   **Unspecified bacterial pneumonia**   ▽
Pneumonia due to gram-positive bacteria

✓4th **J16**   **Pneumonia due to other infectious organisms, not elsewhere classified**
Code first associated influenza, if applicable (J09.X1, J10.0-, J11.0-)
Code also associated abscess, if applicable (J85.1)
EXCLUDES 1   *congenital pneumonia (P23.-)*
ornithosis (A70)
pneumocystosis (B59)
pneumonia NOS (J18.9)
AHA: 2013,4Q,118

J16.0   **Chlamydial pneumonia**
J16.8   **Pneumonia due to other specified infectious organisms**

J17   *Pneumonia in diseases classified elsewhere*
Code first underlying disease, such as:
Q fever (A78)
rheumatic fever (I00)
schistosomiasis (B65.0-B65.9)
EXCLUDES 1   *candidial pneumonia (B37.1)*
chlamydial pneumonia (J16.0)
gonorrheal pneumonia (A54.84)
histoplasmosis pneumonia (B39.0-B39.2)
measles pneumonia (B05.2)
nocardiosis pneumonia (A43.0)
pneumocystosis (B59)
pneumonia due to Pneumocystis carinii (B59)
pneumonia due to Pneumocystis jiroveci (B59)
pneumonia in actinomycosis (A42.0)
pneumonia in anthrax (A22.1)
pneumonia in ascariasis (B77.81)
pneumonia in aspergillosis (B44.0-B44.1)
pneumonia in coccidioidomycosis (B38.0-B38.2)
pneumonia in cytomegalovirus disease (B25.0)
pneumonia in toxoplasmosis (B58.3)
rubella pneumonia (B06.81)
salmonella pneumonia (A02.22)
spirochetal infection NEC with pneumonia (A69.8)
tularemia pneumonia (A21.2)
typhoid fever with pneumonia (A01.03)
varicella pneumonia (B01.2)
whooping cough with pneumonia (A37 with fifth character 1)
AHA: 2013,4Q,118

EXCLUDES 1 Not coded here   *EXCLUDES 2* Not included here   **N** Newborn Age : 0   **P** Pediatric Age : 0-17   **M** Maternity Age : 12-55   **A** Adult Age : 15-124

646   ICD-10-CM 2017

✓4th **J18 Pneumonia, unspecified organism**

Code first associated influenza, if applicable (J09.X1, J10.0-, J11.0-)

EXCLUDES 1 *abscess of lung with pneumonia (J85.1)*

aspiration pneumonia due to anesthesia during labor and delivery (O74.0)

aspiration pneumonia due to anesthesia during pregnancy (O29)

aspiration pneumonia due to anesthesia during puerperium (O89.0)

aspiration pneumonia due to solids and liquids (J69.-)

aspiration pneumonia NOS (J69.0)

congenital pneumonia (P23.0)

drug-induced interstitial lung disorder (J70.2-J70.4)

interstitial pneumonia NOS (J84.9)

lipid pneumonia (J69.1)

neonatal aspiration pneumonia (P24.-)

pneumonitis due to external agents (J67-J70)

pneumonitis due to fumes and vapors (J68.0)

usual interstitial pneumonia (J84.17)

AHA: 2013,4Q,118

J18.0 Bronchopneumonia, unspecified organism ▽

EXCLUDES 1 *hypostatic bronchopneumonia (J18.2)*

lipid pneumonia (J69.1)

EXCLUDES 2 *acute bronchiolitis (J21.-)*

chronic bronchiolitis (J44.9)

J18.1 Lobar pneumonia, unspecified organism ▽

J18.2 Hypostatic pneumonia, unspecified organism ▽

Hypostatic bronchopneumonia

Passive pneumonia

J18.8 Other pneumonia, unspecified organism ▽

J18.9 Pneumonia, unspecified organism ▽

AHA: 2014,3Q,4; 2013,4Q,119; 2012,4Q,94

Other acute lower respiratory infections (J20-J22)

EXCLUDES 2 *chronic obstructive pulmonary disease with acute lower respiratory infection (J44.0)*

✓4th **J20 Acute bronchitis**

INCLUDES acute and subacute bronchitis (with) bronchospasm

acute and subacute bronchitis (with) tracheitis

acute and subacute bronchitis (with) tracheobronchitis, acute

acute and subacute fibrinous bronchitis

acute and subacute membranous bronchitis

acute and subacute purulent bronchitis

acute and subacute septic bronchitis

EXCLUDES 1 *bronchitis NOS (J40)*

tracheobronchitis NOS (J40)

EXCLUDES 2 *acute bronchitis with bronchiectasis (J47.0)*

acute bronchitis with chronic obstructive asthma (J44.0)

acute bronchitis with chronic obstructive pulmonary disease (J44.0)

allergic bronchitis NOS (J45.909-)

bronchitis due to chemicals, fumes and vapors (J68.0)

chronic bronchitis NOS (J42)

chronic mucopurulent bronchitis (J41.1)

chronic obstructive bronchitis (J44.-)

chronic obstructive tracheobronchitis (J44.-)

chronic simple bronchitis (J41.0)

chronic tracheobronchitis (J42)

J20.0 Acute bronchitis due to Mycoplasma pneumoniae

J20.1 Acute bronchitis due to Hemophilus influenzae

J20.2 Acute bronchitis due to streptococcus

J20.3 Acute bronchitis due to coxsackievirus

J20.4 Acute bronchitis due to parainfluenza virus

J20.5 Acute bronchitis due to respiratory syncytial virus

J20.6 Acute bronchitis due to rhinovirus

J20.7 Acute bronchitis due to echovirus

J20.8 Acute bronchitis due to other specified organisms

J20.9 Acute bronchitis, unspecified ▽

✓4th **J21 Acute bronchiolitis**

INCLUDES acute bronchiolitis with bronchospasm

EXCLUDES 2 *respiratory bronchiolitis interstitial lung disease (J84.115)*

J21.0 Acute bronchiolitis due to respiratory syncytial virus

J21.1 Acute bronchiolitis due to human metapneumovirus

J21.8 Acute bronchiolitis due to other specified organisms

J21.9 Acute bronchiolitis, unspecified ▽

Bronchiolitis (acute)

EXCLUDES 1 *chronic bronchiolitis (J44.-)*

J22 Unspecified acute lower respiratory infection ▽

Acute (lower) respiratory (tract) infection NOS

EXCLUDES 1 *upper respiratory infection (acute) (J06.9)*

Other diseases of upper respiratory tract (J30-J39)

✓4th **J30 Vasomotor and allergic rhinitis**

INCLUDES spasmodic rhinorrhea

EXCLUDES 1 *allergic rhinitis with asthma (bronchial) (J45.909)*

rhinitis NOS (J31.0)

J30.0 Vasomotor rhinitis

J30.1 Allergic rhinitis due to pollen

Allergy NOS due to pollen

Hay fever

Pollinosis

J30.2 Other seasonal allergic rhinitis

J30.5 Allergic rhinitis due to food

✓5th **J30.8 Other allergic rhinitis**

J30.81 Allergic rhinitis due to animal (cat) (dog) hair and dander

J30.89 Other allergic rhinitis

Perennial allergic rhinitis

J30.9 Allergic rhinitis, unspecified ▽

✓4th **J31 Chronic rhinitis, nasopharyngitis and pharyngitis**

Use additional code to identify:

exposure to environmental tobacco smoke (Z77.22)

exposure to tobacco smoke in the perinatal period (P96.81)

►history of tobacco dependence (Z87.891)◄

occupational exposure to environmental tobacco smoke (Z57.31)

tobacco dependence (F17.-)

tobacco use (Z72.0)

J31.0 Chronic rhinitis

Atrophic rhinitis (chronic)

Granulomatous rhinitis (chronic)

Hypertrophic rhinitis (chronic)

Obstructive rhinitis (chronic)

Ozena

Purulent rhinitis (chronic)

Rhinitis (chronic) NOS

Ulcerative rhinitis (chronic)

EXCLUDES 1 *allergic rhinitis (J30.1-J30.9)*

vasomotor rhinitis (J30.0)

J31.1 Chronic nasopharyngitis

EXCLUDES 2 *acute nasopharyngitis (J00)*

J31.2 Chronic pharyngitis

Atrophic pharyngitis (chronic)

Chronic sore throat

Granular pharyngitis (chronic)

Hypertrophic pharyngitis (chronic)

EXCLUDES 2 *acute pharyngitis (J02.9)*

✓4th **J32 Chronic sinusitis**

INCLUDES sinus abscess

sinus empyema

sinus infection

sinus suppuration

Use additional code to identify:

exposure to environmental tobacco smoke (Z77.22)

exposure to tobacco smoke in the perinatal period (P96.81)

►history of tobacco dependence (Z87.891)◄

infectious agent (B95-B97)

occupational exposure to environmental tobacco smoke (Z57.31)

tobacco dependence (F17.-)

tobacco use (Z72.0)

EXCLUDES 2 *acute sinusitis (J01.-)*

J32.0 Chronic maxillary sinusitis

Antritis (chronic)

Maxillary sinusitis NOS

J32.1 Chronic frontal sinusitis

Frontal sinusitis NOS

J32.2 Chronic ethmoidal sinusitis

Ethmoidal sinusitis NOS

EXCLUDES 1 *Woakes' ethmoiditis (J33.1)*

☑ Additional Character Required ✗7th Placeholder Alert Manifestation Dx ▽ Unspecified Dx ►◄ Revised Text ● New Code ▲ Revised Code Title

ICD-10-CM 2017 **647**

Chapter 10. Diseases of the Respiratory System

J32.3   **Chronic sphenoidal sinusitis**
Sphenoidal sinusitis NOS

J32.4   **Chronic pansinusitis**
Pansinusitis NOS

J32.8   **Other chronic sinusitis**
Sinusitis (chronic) involving more than one sinus but not pansinusitis

J32.9   **Chronic sinusitis, unspecified**   ▽
Sinusitis (chronic) NOS

√4ᵗʰ **J33**   **Nasal polyp**
Use additional code to identify:
exposure to environmental tobacco smoke (Z77.22)
exposure to tobacco smoke in the perinatal period (P96.81)
▶history of tobacco dependence (Z87.891)◀
occupational exposure to environmental tobacco smoke (Z57.31)
tobacco dependence (F17.-)
tobacco use (Z72.0)
EXCLUDES 1 *adenomatous polyps (D14.0)*

J33.0   **Polyp of nasal cavity**
Choanal polyp
Nasopharyngeal polyp

J33.1   **Polypoid sinus degeneration**
Woakes' syndrome or ethmoiditis

J33.8   **Other polyp of sinus**
Accessory polyp of sinus
Ethmoidal polyp of sinus
Maxillary polyp of sinus
Sphenoidal polyp of sinus

J33.9   **Nasal polyp, unspecified**   ▽

√4ᵗʰ **J34**   **Other and unspecified disorders of nose and nasal sinuses**
EXCLUDES 2 *varicose ulcer of nasal septum (I86.8)*

J34.0   **Abscess, furuncle and carbuncle of nose**
Cellulitis of nose
Necrosis of nose
Ulceration of nose

J34.1   **Cyst and mucocele of nose and nasal sinus**

J34.2   **Deviated nasal septum**
Deflection or deviation of septum (nasal) (acquired)
EXCLUDES 1 *congenital deviated nasal septum (Q67.4)*

J34.3   **Hypertrophy of nasal turbinates**

√5ᵗʰ **J34.8**   **Other specified disorders of nose and nasal sinuses**

J34.81   **Nasal mucositis (ulcerative)**
Code also type of associated therapy, such as:
antineoplastic and immunosuppressive drugs (T45.1X-)
radiological procedure and radiotherapy (Y84.2)
EXCLUDES 2 *gastrointestinal mucositis (ulcerative) (K92.81)*
mucositis (ulcerative) of vagina and vulva (N76.81)
oral mucositis (ulcerative) (K12.3-)

J34.89   **Other specified disorders of nose and nasal sinuses**
Perforation of nasal septum NOS
Rhinolith

J34.9   **Unspecified disorder of nose and nasal sinuses**   ▽

√4ᵗʰ **J35**   **Chronic diseases of tonsils and adenoids**
Use additional code to identify:
exposure to environmental tobacco smoke (Z77.22)
exposure to tobacco smoke in the perinatal period (P96.81)
▶history of tobacco dependence (Z87.891)◀
occupational exposure to environmental tobacco smoke (Z57.31)
tobacco dependence (F17.-)
tobacco use (Z72.0)

√5ᵗʰ **J35.0**   **Chronic tonsillitis and adenoiditis**
EXCLUDES 2 *acute tonsillitis (J03.-)*

J35.01   **Chronic tonsillitis**
J35.02   **Chronic adenoiditis**
J35.03   **Chronic tonsillitis and adenoiditis**

J35.1   **Hypertrophy of tonsils**
Enlargement of tonsils
EXCLUDES 1 *hypertrophy of tonsils with tonsillitis (J35.0-)*

J35.2   **Hypertrophy of adenoids**
Enlargement of adenoids
EXCLUDES 1 *hypertrophy of adenoids with adenoiditis (J35.0-)*

J35.3   **Hypertrophy of tonsils with hypertrophy of adenoids**
EXCLUDES 1 *hypertrophy of tonsils and adenoids with tonsillitis and adenoiditis (J35.03)*

J35.8   **Other chronic diseases of tonsils and adenoids**
Adenoid vegetations
Amygdalolith
Calculus, tonsil
Cicatrix of tonsil (and adenoid)
Tonsillar tag
Ulcer of tonsil

J35.9   **Chronic disease of tonsils and adenoids, unspecified**   ▽
Disease (chronic) of tonsils and adenoids NOS

J36   **Peritonsillar abscess**
INCLUDES   abscess of tonsil
peritonsillar cellulitis
quinsy
Use additional code (B95-B97) to identify infectious agent
EXCLUDES 1 *acute tonsillitis (J03.-)*
chronic tonsillitis (J35.0)
retropharyngeal abscess (J39.0)
tonsillitis NOS (J03.9-)

√4ᵗʰ **J37**   **Chronic laryngitis and laryngotracheitis**
Use additional code to identify:
exposure to environmental tobacco smoke (Z77.22)
exposure to tobacco smoke in the perinatal period (P96.81)
▶history of tobacco dependence (Z87.891)◀
infectious agent (B95-B97)
occupational exposure to environmental tobacco smoke (Z57.31)
tobacco dependence (F17.-)
tobacco use (Z72.0)

J37.0   **Chronic laryngitis**
Catarrhal laryngitis
Hypertrophic laryngitis
Sicca laryngitis
EXCLUDES 2 *acute laryngitis (J04.0)*
obstructive (acute) laryngitis (J05.0)

J37.1   **Chronic laryngotracheitis**
Laryngitis, chronic, with tracheitis (chronic)
Tracheitis, chronic, with laryngitis
EXCLUDES 1 *chronic tracheitis (J42)*
EXCLUDES 2 *acute laryngotracheitis (J04.2)*
acute tracheitis (J04.1)

√4ᵗʰ **J38**   **Diseases of vocal cords and larynx, not elsewhere classified**
Use additional code to identify:
exposure to environmental tobacco smoke (Z77.22)
exposure to tobacco smoke in the perinatal period (P96.81)
▶history of tobacco dependence (Z87.891)◀
occupational exposure to environmental tobacco smoke (Z57.31)
tobacco dependence (F17.-)
tobacco use (Z72.0)
EXCLUDES 1 *congenital laryngeal stridor (P28.89)*
obstructive laryngitis (acute) (J05.0)
postprocedural subglottic stenosis (J95.5)
stridor (R06.1)
ulcerative laryngitis (J04.0)

√5ᵗʰ **J38.0**   **Paralysis of vocal cords and larynx**
Laryngoplegia
Paralysis of glottis

J38.00   **Paralysis of vocal cords and larynx, unspecified**   ▽
J38.01   **Paralysis of vocal cords and larynx, unilateral**
J38.02   **Paralysis of vocal cords and larynx, bilateral**

J38.1   **Polyp of vocal cord and larynx**
EXCLUDES 1 *adenomatous polyps (D14.1)*

J38.2   **Nodules of vocal cords**
Chorditis (fibrinous)(nodosa)(tuberosa)
Singer's nodes
Teacher's nodes

J38.3   **Other diseases of vocal cords**
Abscess of vocal cords
Cellulitis of vocal cords
Granuloma of vocal cords
Leukokeratosis of vocal cords
Leukoplakia of vocal cords

EXCLUDES 1 Not coded here   EXCLUDES 2 Not included here   N Newborn Age : 0   P Pediatric Age : 0-17   M Maternity Age : 12-55   A Adult Age : 15-124

J38.4 Edema of larynx
Edema (of) glottis
Subglottic edema
Supraglottic edema
EXCLUDES 1   *acute obstructive laryngitis [croup] (J05.0)*
         edematous laryngitis (J04.0)

J38.5 Laryngeal spasm
Laryngismus (stridulus)

J38.6 Stenosis of larynx

J38.7 Other diseases of larynx
Abscess of larynx
Cellulitis of larynx
Disease of larynx NOS
Necrosis of larynx
Pachyderma of larynx
Perichondritis of larynx
Ulcer of larynx

☑4ᵗʰ **J39 Other diseases of upper respiratory tract**
EXCLUDES 1   *acute respiratory infection NOS (J22)*
         acute upper respiratory infection (J06.9)
         upper respiratory inflammation due to chemicals, gases, fumes
         or vapors (J68.2)

J39.0 Retropharyngeal and parapharyngeal abscess
Peripharyngeal abscess
EXCLUDES 1   *peritonsillar abscess (J36)*

J39.1 Other abscess of pharynx
Cellulitis of pharynx
Nasopharyngeal abscess

J39.2 Other diseases of pharynx
Cyst of pharynx
Edema of pharynx
EXCLUDES 2   *chronic pharyngitis (J31.2)*
         ulcerative pharyngitis (J02.9)

J39.3 Upper respiratory tract hypersensitivity reaction, site ▽
unspecified
EXCLUDES 1   *hypersensitivity reaction of upper respiratory tract,*
         such as:
         extrinsic allergic alveolitis (J67.9)
         pneumoconiosis (J60-J67.9)

J39.8 Other specified diseases of upper respiratory tract

J39.9 Disease of upper respiratory tract, unspecified ▽

Chronic lower respiratory diseases (J40-J47)

EXCLUDES 1   *bronchitis due to chemicals, gases, fumes and vapors (J68.0)*
EXCLUDES 2   *cystic fibrosis (E84.-)*

J40 Bronchitis, not specified as acute or chronic ▽
Bronchitis NOS
Bronchitis with tracheitis NOS
Catarrhal bronchitis
Tracheobronchitis NOS
Use additional code to identify:
   exposure to environmental tobacco smoke (Z77.22)
   exposure to tobacco smoke in the perinatal period (P96.81)
   ►history of tobacco dependence (Z87.891)◄
   occupational exposure to environmental tobacco smoke (Z57.31)
   tobacco dependence (F17.-)
   tobacco use (Z72.0)
EXCLUDES 1   *acute bronchitis (J20.-)*
         allergic bronchitis NOS (J45.909-)
         asthmatic bronchitis NOS (J45.9-)
         bronchitis due to chemicals, fumes and vapors (J68.0)

☑4ᵗʰ **J41 Simple and mucopurulent chronic bronchitis**
Use additional code to identify:
   exposure to environmental tobacco smoke (Z77.22)
   exposure to tobacco smoke in the perinatal period (P96.81)
   ►history of tobacco dependence (Z87.891)◄
   occupational exposure to environmental tobacco smoke (Z57.31)
   tobacco dependence (F17.-)
   tobacco use (Z72.0)
EXCLUDES 1   *chronic bronchitis NOS (J42)*
         chronic obstructive bronchitis (J44.-)

J41.0 Simple chronic bronchitis

J41.1 Mucopurulent chronic bronchitis

J41.8 Mixed simple and mucopurulent chronic bronchitis

J42 Unspecified chronic bronchitis ▽
Chronic bronchitis NOS
Chronic tracheitis
Chronic tracheobronchitis
Use additional code to identify:
   exposure to environmental tobacco smoke (Z77.22)
   exposure to tobacco smoke in the perinatal period (P96.81)
   ►history of tobacco dependence (Z87.891)◄
   occupational exposure to environmental tobacco smoke (Z57.31)
   tobacco dependence (F17.-)
   tobacco use (Z72.0)
EXCLUDES 1   *chronic asthmatic bronchitis (J44.-)*
         chronic bronchitis with airways obstruction (J44.-)
         chronic emphysematous bronchitis (J44.-)
         chronic obstructive pulmonary disease NOS (J44.9)
         simple and mucopurulent chronic bronchitis (J41.-)

☑4ᵗʰ **J43 Emphysema**
Use additional code to identify:
   exposure to environmental tobacco smoke (Z77.22)
   ►history of tobacco dependence (Z87.891)◄
   occupational exposure to environmental tobacco smoke (Z57.31)
   tobacco dependence (F17.-)
   tobacco use (Z72.0)
EXCLUDES 1   *compensatory emphysema (J98.3)*
         emphysema due to inhalation of chemicals, gases, fumes or
         vapors (J68.4)
         emphysema with chronic (obstructive) bronchitis (J44.-)
         emphysematous (obstructive) bronchitis (J44.-)
         interstitial emphysema (J98.2)
         mediastinal emphysema (J98.2)
         neonatal interstitial emphysema (P25.0)
         surgical (subcutaneous) emphysema (T81.82)
         traumatic subcutaneous emphysema (T79.7)

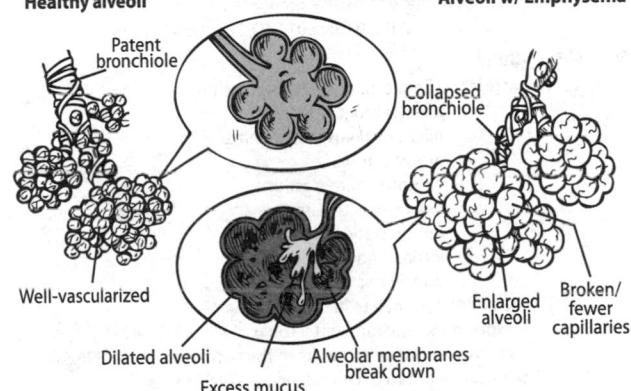

Emphysema

Healthy alveoli   Alveoli w/ Emphysema

Patent bronchiole   Collapsed bronchiole

Well-vascularized   Enlarged alveoli   Broken/ fewer capillaries

Dilated alveoli   Alveolar membranes break down

Excess mucus

J43.0 Unilateral pulmonary emphysema [MacLeod's syndrome]
Swyer-James syndrome
Unilateral emphysema
Unilateral hyperlucent lung
Unilateral pulmonary artery functional hypoplasia
Unilateral transparency of lung

J43.1 Panlobular emphysema
Panacinar emphysema

J43.2 Centrilobular emphysema

J43.8 Other emphysema

J43.9 Emphysema, unspecified ▽
Bullous emphysema (lung)(pulmonary)
Emphysema (lung)(pulmonary) NOS
Emphysematous bleb
Vesicular emphysema (lung)(pulmonary)

✓4th **J44 Other chronic obstructive pulmonary disease**

INCLUDES   asthma with chronic obstructive pulmonary disease
chronic asthmatic (obstructive) bronchitis
chronic bronchitis with airways obstruction
chronic bronchitis with emphysema
chronic emphysematous bronchitis
chronic obstructive asthma
chronic obstructive bronchitis
chronic obstructive tracheobronchitis

Code also type of asthma, if applicable (J45.-)
Use additional code to identify:
   exposure to environmental tobacco smoke (Z77.22)
   ▶history of tobacco dependence (Z87.891)◀
   occupational exposure to environmental tobacco smoke (Z57.31)
   tobacco dependence (F17.-)
   tobacco use (Z72.0)

EXCLUDES 1   bronchiectasis (J47.-)
chronic bronchitis NOS (J42)
chronic simple and mucopurulent bronchitis (J41.-)
chronic tracheitis (J42)
chronic tracheobronchitis (J42)
emphysema without chronic bronchitis (J43.-)

EXCLUDES 2   ▶lung diseases due to external agents (J60-J70)◀
AHA: 2013,4Q,109

J44.0 Chronic obstructive pulmonary disease with acute lower respiratory infection
   Use additional code to identify the infection

J44.1 Chronic obstructive pulmonary disease with (acute) exacerbation
   Decompensated COPD
   Decompensated COPD with (acute) exacerbation
   EXCLUDES 2   chronic obstructive pulmonary disease [COPD] with acute bronchitis (J44.0)
   AHA: 2016,1Q,35

J44.9 Chronic obstructive pulmonary disease, unspecified ▽
   Chronic obstructive airway disease NOS
   Chronic obstructive lung disease NOS
   AHA: 2016,1Q,36; 2014,4Q,21; 2013,4Q,109

✓4th **J45 Asthma**

INCLUDES   allergic (predominantly) asthma
allergic bronchitis NOS
allergic rhinitis with asthma
atopic asthma
extrinsic allergic asthma
hay fever with asthma
idiosyncratic asthma
intrinsic nonallergic asthma
nonallergic asthma

Use additional code to identify:
   exposure to environmental tobacco smoke (Z77.22)
   exposure to tobacco smoke in the perinatal period (P96.81)
   ▶history of tobacco dependence (Z87.891)◀
   occupational exposure to environmental tobacco smoke (Z57.31)
   tobacco dependence (F17.-)
   tobacco use (Z72.0)

EXCLUDES 1   detergent asthma (J69.8)
eosinophilic asthma (J82)
lung diseases due to external agents (J60-J70)
miner's asthma (J60)
wheezing NOS (R06.2)
wood asthma (J67.8)

EXCLUDES 2   asthma with chronic obstructive pulmonary disease (J44.9)
chronic asthmatic (obstructive) bronchitis (J44.9)
chronic obstructive asthma (J44.9)

AHA: 2012,4Q,99
DEF: Status asthmaticus: Severe, intractable episode of asthma that is unresponsive to normal therapeutic measures.

✓5th **J45.2 Mild intermittent asthma**

   J45.20 Mild intermittent asthma, uncomplicated
     Mild intermittent asthma NOS
   J45.21 Mild intermittent asthma with (acute) exacerbation
   J45.22 Mild intermittent asthma with status asthmaticus

✓5th **J45.3 Mild persistent asthma**

   J45.30 Mild persistent asthma, uncomplicated
     Mild persistent asthma NOS

   J45.31 Mild persistent asthma with (acute) exacerbation
     AHA: 2016,1Q,35
   J45.32 Mild persistent asthma with status asthmaticus

✓5th **J45.4 Moderate persistent asthma**

   J45.40 Moderate persistent asthma, uncomplicated
     Moderate persistent asthma NOS
   J45.41 Moderate persistent asthma with (acute) exacerbation
   J45.42 Moderate persistent asthma with status asthmaticus

✓5th **J45.5 Severe persistent asthma**

   J45.50 Severe persistent asthma, uncomplicated
     Severe persistent asthma NOS
   J45.51 Severe persistent asthma with (acute) exacerbation
   J45.52 Severe persistent asthma with status asthmaticus

✓5th **J45.9 Other and unspecified asthma**

   ✓6th **J45.90 Unspecified asthma**
     Asthmatic bronchitis NOS
     Childhood asthma NOS
     Late onset asthma

     J45.901 Unspecified asthma with (acute) exacerbation ▽
     J45.902 Unspecified asthma with status asthmaticus ▽
     J45.909 Unspecified asthma, uncomplicated ▽
       Asthma NOS

   ✓6th **J45.99 Other asthma**
     J45.990 Exercise induced bronchospasm
     J45.991 Cough variant asthma
     J45.998 Other asthma

✓4th **J47 Bronchiectasis**

INCLUDES   bronchiolectasis
Use additional code to identify:
   exposure to environmental tobacco smoke (Z77.22)
   exposure to tobacco smoke in the perinatal period (P96.81)
   ▶history of tobacco dependence (Z87.891)◀
   occupational exposure to environmental tobacco smoke (Z57.31)
   tobacco dependence (F17.-)
   tobacco use (Z72.0)

EXCLUDES 1   congenital bronchiectasis (Q33.4)
tuberculous bronchiectasis (current disease) (A15.0)

J47.0 Bronchiectasis with acute lower respiratory infection
   Bronchiectasis with acute bronchitis
   ▶Use additional code to identify the infection◀

J47.1 Bronchiectasis with (acute) exacerbation

J47.9 Bronchiectasis, uncomplicated ▽
   Bronchiectasis NOS

Lung diseases due to external agents (J60-J70)

EXCLUDES 2   asthma (J45.-)
malignant neoplasm of bronchus and lung (C34.-)

J60 Coalworker's pneumoconiosis 🅐
   Anthracosilicosis
   Anthracosis
   Black lung disease
   Coalworker's lung
   EXCLUDES 1   coalworker pneumoconiosis with tuberculosis, any type in A15 (J65)

J61 Pneumoconiosis due to asbestos and other mineral fibers 🅐
   Asbestosis
   EXCLUDES 1   pleural plaque with asbestosis (J92.0)
     pneumoconiosis with tuberculosis, any type in A15 (J65)

✓4th **J62 Pneumoconiosis due to dust containing silica**
   INCLUDES   silicotic fibrosis (massive) of lung
   EXCLUDES 1   pneumoconiosis with tuberculosis, any type in A15 (J65)
   J62.0 Pneumoconiosis due to talc dust
   J62.8 Pneumoconiosis due to other dust containing silica
     Silicosis NOS

✓4th **J63 Pneumoconiosis due to other inorganic dusts**
   EXCLUDES 1   pneumoconiosis with tuberculosis, any type in A15 (J65)
   J63.0 Aluminosis (of lung)
   J63.1 Bauxite fibrosis (of lung)
   J63.2 Berylliosis
   J63.3 Graphite fibrosis (of lung)

EXCLUDES 1 Not coded here   EXCLUDES 2 Not included here   N Newborn Age : 0   P Pediatric Age : 0-17   M Maternity Age : 12-55   🅐 Adult Age : 15-124

650   ICD-10-CM 2017

J63.4   **Siderosis**

J63.5   **Stannosis**

J63.6   **Pneumoconiosis due to other specified inorganic dusts**

J64 Unspecified pneumoconiosis   ▽

   EXCLUDES 1   *pneumonoconiosis with tuberculosis, any type in A15 (J65)*

J65 Pneumoconiosis associated with tuberculosis

   Any condition in J60-J64 with tuberculosis, any type in A15

   Silicotuberculosis

☑4ᵗʰ **J66 Airway disease due to specific organic dust**

   EXCLUDES 2   *allergic alveolitis (J67.-)*

         asbestosis (J61)

         bagassosis (J67.1)

         farmer's lung (J67.0)

         hypersensitivity pneumonitis due to organic dust (J67.-)

         reactive airways dysfunction syndrome (J68.3)

J66.0   **Byssinosis**

     Airway disease due to cotton dust

J66.1   **Flax-dressers' disease**

J66.2   **Cannabinosis**

J66.8   **Airway disease due to other specific organic dusts**

☑4ᵗʰ **J67 Hypersensitivity pneumonitis due to organic dust**

   INCLUDES   allergic alveolitis and pneumonitis due to inhaled organic dust and particles of fungal, actinomycetic or other origin

   EXCLUDES 1   *pneumonitis due to inhalation of chemicals, gases, fumes or vapors (J68.0)*

J67.0   **Farmer's lung**

     Harvester's lung

     Haymaker's lung

     Moldy hay disease

J67.1   **Bagassosis**

     Bagasse disease

     Bagasse pneumonitis

J67.2   **Bird fancier's lung**

     Budgerigar fancier's disease or lung

     Pigeon fancier's disease or lung

J67.3   **Suberosis**

     Corkhandler's disease or lung

     Corkworker's disease or lung

J67.4   **Maltworker's lung**

     Alveolitis due to Aspergillus clavatus

J67.5   **Mushroom-worker's lung**

J67.6   **Maple-bark-stripper's lung**

     Alveolitis due to Cryptostroma corticale

     Cryptostromosis

J67.7   **Air conditioner and humidifier lung**

     Allergic alveolitis due to fungal, thermophilic actinomycetes and other organisms growing in ventilation [air conditioning] systems

J67.8   **Hypersensitivity pneumonitis due to other organic dusts**

     Cheese-washer's lung

     Coffee-worker's lung

     Fish-meal worker's lung

     Furrier's lung

     Sequoiosis

J67.9   **Hypersensitivity pneumonitis due to unspecified organic dust**   ▽

     Allergic alveolitis (extrinsic) NOS

     Hypersensitivity pneumonitis NOS

☑4ᵗʰ **J68 Respiratory conditions due to inhalation of chemicals, gases, fumes and vapors**

     Code first (T51-T65) to identify cause

     Use additional code to identify associated respiratory conditions, such as:

     acute respiratory failure (J96.0-)

J68.0   **Bronchitis and pneumonitis due to chemicals, gases, fumes and vapors**

     Chemical bronchitis (acute)

J68.1   **Pulmonary edema due to chemicals, gases, fumes and vapors**

     Chemical pulmonary edema (acute) (chronic)

     EXCLUDES 1   *pulmonary edema (acute) (chronic) NOS (J81.-)*

J68.2   **Upper respiratory inflammation due to chemicals, gases, fumes and vapors, not elsewhere classified**

J68.3   **Other acute and subacute respiratory conditions due to chemicals, gases, fumes and vapors**

     Reactive airways dysfunction syndrome

J68.4   **Chronic respiratory conditions due to chemicals, gases, fumes and vapors**

     Emphysema (diffuse) (chronic) due to inhalation of chemicals, gases, fumes and vapors

     Obliterative bronchiolitis (chronic) (subacute) due to inhalation of chemicals, gases, fumes and vapors

     Pulmonary fibrosis (chronic) due to inhalation of chemicals, gases, fumes and vapors

     EXCLUDES 1   *chronic pulmonary edema due to chemicals, gases, fumes and vapors (J68.1)*

J68.8   **Other respiratory conditions due to chemicals, gases, fumes and vapors**

J68.9   **Unspecified respiratory condition due to chemicals, gases, fumes and vapors**   ▽

☑4ᵗʰ **J69 Pneumonitis due to solids and liquids**

   EXCLUDES 1   *neonatal aspiration syndromes (P24.-)*

         postprocedural pneumonitis (J95.4)

J69.0   **Pneumonitis due to inhalation of food and vomit**

     Aspiration pneumonia NOS

     Aspiration pneumonia (due to) food (regurgitated)

     Aspiration pneumonia (due to) gastric secretions

     Aspiration pneumonia (due to) milk

     Aspiration pneumonia (due to) vomit

     Code also any associated foreign body in respiratory tract (T17.-)

     EXCLUDES 1   *chemical pneumonitis due to anesthesia (J95.4)*

         obstetric aspiration pneumonia (O74.0)

J69.1   **Pneumonitis due to inhalation of oils and essences**

     Exogenous lipoid pneumonia

     Lipid pneumonia NOS

     Code first (T51-T65) to identify substance

     EXCLUDES 1   *endogenous lipoid pneumonia (J84.89)*

J69.8   **Pneumonitis due to inhalation of other solids and liquids**

     Pneumonitis due to aspiration of blood

     Pneumonitis due to aspiration of detergent

     Code first (T51-T65) to identify substance

☑4ᵗʰ **J70 Respiratory conditions due to other external agents**

J70.0   **Acute pulmonary manifestations due to radiation**

     Radiation pneumonitis

     Use additional code (W88-W90, X39.0-) to identify the external cause

J70.1   **Chronic and other pulmonary manifestations due to radiation**

     Fibrosis of lung following radiation

     Use additional code (W88-W90, X39.0-) to identify the external cause

J70.2   **Acute drug-induced interstitial lung disorders**

     Use additional code for adverse effect, if applicable, to identify drug (T36-T50 with fifth or sixth character 5)

     EXCLUDES 1   *interstitial pneumonia NOS (J84.9)*

         lymphoid interstitial pneumonia (J84.2)

J70.3   **Chronic drug-induced interstitial lung disorders**

     Use additional code for adverse effect, if applicable, to identify drug (T36-T50 with fifth or sixth character 5)

     EXCLUDES 1   *interstitial pneumonia NOS (J84.9)*

         lymphoid interstitial pneumonia (J84.2)

J70.4   **Drug-induced interstitial lung disorders, unspecified**   ▽

     Use additional code for adverse effect, if applicable, to identify drug (T36-T50 with fifth or sixth character 5)

     EXCLUDES 1   *interstitial pneumonia NOS (J84.9)*

         lymphoid interstitial pneumonia (J84.2)

J70.5   **Respiratory conditions due to smoke inhalation**

     Smoke inhalation NOS

     EXCLUDES 1   *smoke inhalation due to chemicals, gases, fumes and vapors (J68.9)*

     AHA: 2013,4Q,121

J70.8   **Respiratory conditions due to other specified external agents**

     Code first (T51-T65) to identify the external agent

J70.9   **Respiratory conditions due to unspecified external agent**   ▽

     Code first (T51-T65) to identify the external agent

☑ Additional Character Required   ☑x7ᵗʰ Placeholder Alert   Manifestation Dx   ▽ Unspecified Dx   ►◄ Revised Text   ● New Code   ▲ Revised Code Title

ICD-10-CM 2017

651

Other respiratory diseases principally affecting the interstitium (J80-J84)

J80 Acute respiratory distress syndrome
Acute respiratory distress syndrome in adult or child
Adult hyaline membrane disease
EXCLUDES 1 *respiratory distress syndrome in newborn (perinatal) (P22.0)*

√4th **J81 Pulmonary edema**
Use additional code to identify:
exposure to environmental tobacco smoke (Z77.22)
►history of tobacco dependence (Z87.891)◄
occupational exposure to environmental tobacco smoke (Z57.31)
tobacco dependence (F17.-)
tobacco use (Z72.0)
EXCLUDES 1 *chemical (acute) pulmonary edema (J68.1)*
hypostatic pneumonia (J18.2)
passive pneumonia (J18.2)
pulmonary edema due to external agents (J60-J70)
pulmonary edema with heart disease NOS (I50.1)
pulmonary edema with heart failure (I50.1)

J81.0 Acute pulmonary edema
Acute edema of lung

J81.1 Chronic pulmonary edema
Pulmonary congestion (chronic) (passive)
Pulmonary edema NOS

J82 Pulmonary eosinophilia, not elsewhere classified
Allergic pneumonia
Eosinophilic asthma
Eosinophilic pneumonia
Löffler's pneumonia
Tropical (pulmonary) eosinophilia NOS
EXCLUDES 1 *pulmonary eosinophilia due to aspergillosis (B44.-)*
pulmonary eosinophilia due to drugs (J70.2-J70.4)
pulmonary eosinophilia due to specified parasitic infection (B50-B83)
pulmonary eosinophilia due to systemic connective tissue disorders (M30-M36)
pulmonary infiltrate NOS (R91.8)

√4th **J84 Other interstitial pulmonary diseases**
EXCLUDES 1 *drug-induced interstitial lung disorders (J70.2-J70.4)*
interstitial emphysema (J98.2)
lung diseases due to external agents (J60-J70)

√5th **J84.0 Alveolar and parieto-alveolar conditions**
J84.01 Alveolar proteinosis
J84.02 Pulmonary alveolar microlithiasis
J84.03 *Idiopathic pulmonary hemosiderosis*
Essential brown induration of lung
Code first underlying disease, such as:
disorders of iron metabolism (E83.1-)
EXCLUDES 1 *acute idiopathic pulmonary hemorrhage in infants [AIPHI] (R04.81)*
J84.09 Other alveolar and parieto-alveolar conditions

√5th **J84.1 Other interstitial pulmonary diseases with fibrosis**
EXCLUDES 1 *pulmonary fibrosis (chronic) due to inhalation of chemicals, gases, fumes or vapors (J68.4)*
pulmonary fibrosis (chronic) following radiation (J70.1)

J84.10 Pulmonary fibrosis, unspecified ▽
Capillary fibrosis of lung
Cirrhosis of lung (chronic) NOS
Fibrosis of lung (atrophic) (chronic) (confluent) (massive) (perialveolar) (peribronchial) NOS
Induration of lung (chronic) NOS
Postinflammatory pulmonary fibrosis

√6th **J84.11 Idiopathic interstitial pneumonia**
EXCLUDES 1 *lymphoid interstitial pneumonia (J84.2)*
pneumocystis pneumonia (B59)
J84.111 Idiopathic interstitial pneumonia, not otherwise specified ▽
J84.112 Idiopathic pulmonary fibrosis
Cryptogenic fibrosing alveolitis
Idiopathic fibrosing alveolitis

J84.113 Idiopathic non-specific interstitial pneumonitis
EXCLUDES 1 *non-specific interstitial pneumonia NOS, or due to known underlying cause (J84.89)*
J84.114 Acute interstitial pneumonitis
Hamman-Rich syndrome
EXCLUDES 1 *pneumocystis pneumonia (B59)*
J84.115 Respiratory bronchiolitis interstitial lung disease
J84.116 Cryptogenic organizing pneumonia
EXCLUDES 1 *organizing pneumonia NOS, or due to known underlying cause (J84.89)*
J84.117 Desquamative interstitial pneumonia
J84.17 *Other interstitial pulmonary diseases with fibrosis in diseases classified elsewhere*
Interstitial pneumonia (nonspecific) (usual) due to collagen vascular disease
Interstitial pneumonia (nonspecific) (usual) in diseases classified elsewhere
Organizing pneumonia due to collagen vascular disease
Organizing pneumonia in diseases classified elsewhere
Code first underlying disease, such as:
progressive systemic sclerosis (M34.0)
rheumatoid arthritis (M05.00-M06.9)
systemic lupus erythematosis (M32.0-M32.9)

J84.2 Lymphoid interstitial pneumonia
Lymphoid interstitial pneumonitis

√5th **J84.8 Other specified interstitial pulmonary diseases**
EXCLUDES 1 *exogenous lipoid pneumonia (J69.1)*
unspecified lipoid pneumonia (J69.1)
J84.81 Lymphangioleiomyomatosis ♀
Lymphangiomyomatosis
J84.82 Adult pulmonary Langerhans cell histiocytosis 🅐
Adult PLCH
J84.83 Surfactant mutations of the lung
DEF: Genetic disorder resulting in insufficient secretion of a complex mixture of phospholipids and proteins that reduce surface tension in the alveoli following the onset of breathing to facilitate lung expansion in the newborn; leading indication for pediatric lung transplantation.
√6th **J84.84 Other interstitial lung diseases of childhood**
J84.841 Neuroendocrine cell hyperplasia of infancy
J84.842 Pulmonary interstitial glycogenosis
J84.843 Alveolar capillary dysplasia with vein misalignment
J84.848 Other interstitial lung diseases of childhood
J84.89 Other specified interstitial pulmonary diseases
Endogenous lipoid pneumonia
Interstitial pneumonitis
Non-specific interstitial pneumonitis NOS
Organizing pneumonia NOS
Code first, if applicable:
poisoning due to drug or toxin (T51-T65 with fifth or sixth character to indicate intent), for toxic pneumonopathy
underlying cause of pneumonopathy, if known
Use additional code, for adverse effect, to identify drug (T36-T50 with fifth or sixth character 5), if drug-induced
EXCLUDES 1 *cryptogenic organizing pneumonia (J84.116)*
idiopathic non-specific interstitial pneumonitis (J84.113)
lipoid pneumonia, exogenous or unspecified (J69.1)
lymphoid interstitial pneumonia (J84.2)

J84.9 Interstitial pulmonary disease, unspecified ▽
Interstitial pneumonia NOS

Suppurative and necrotic conditions of the lower respiratory tract (J85-J86)

✔4ᵗʰ **J85   Abscess of lung and mediastinum**
    Use additional code (B95-B97) to identify infectious agent
    J85.0   Gangrene and necrosis of lung
    J85.1   Abscess of lung with pneumonia
        Code also the type of pneumonia
    J85.2   Abscess of lung without pneumonia
        Abscess of lung NOS
    J85.3   Abscess of mediastinum

✔4ᵗʰ **J86   Pyothorax**
    Use additional code (B95-B97) to identify infectious agent
    EXCLUDES 1   *abscess of lung (J85.-)*
                 pyothorax due to tuberculosis (A15.6)
    J86.0   Pyothorax with fistula
        Bronchocutaneous fistula
        Bronchopleural fistula
        Hepatopleural fistula
        Mediastinal fistula
        Pleural fistula
        Thoracic fistula
        Any condition classifiable to J86.9 with fistula
        DEF: Purulent infection of respiratory cavity, with communication from cavity to another structure.
    J86.9   Pyothorax without fistula
        Abscess of pleura
        Abscess of thorax
        Empyema (chest) (lung) (pleura)
        Fibrinopurulent pleurisy
        Purulent pleurisy
        Pyopneumothorax
        Septic pleurisy
        Seropurulent pleurisy
        Suppurative pleurisy

Other diseases of the pleura (J90-J94)

J90   Pleural effusion, not elsewhere classified
    Encysted pleurisy
    Pleural effusion NOS
    Pleurisy with effusion (exudative) (serous)
    EXCLUDES 1   *chylous (pleural) effusion (J94.0)*
                 malignant pleural effusion (J91.0))
                 pleurisy NOS (R09.1)
                 tuberculous pleural effusion (A15.6)

Pleural Effusion

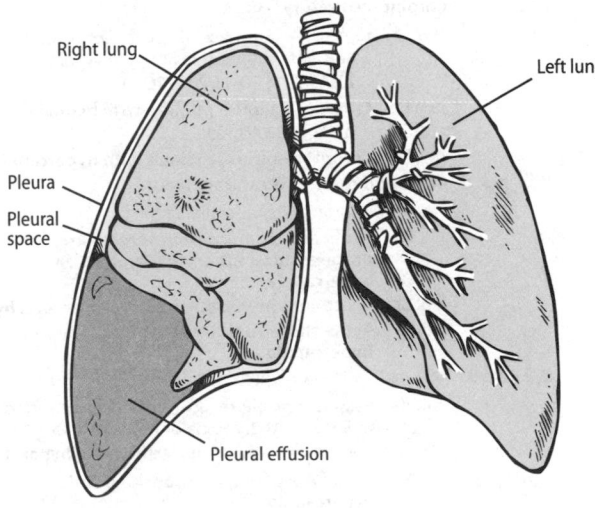

Right lung
Left lung
Pleura
Pleural space
Pleural effusion

✔4ᵗʰ **J91   Pleural effusion in conditions classified elsewhere**
    EXCLUDES 2   *pleural effusion in heart failure (I50.-)*
                 pleural effusion in systemic lupus erythematosus (M32.13)
    J91.0   *Malignant pleural effusion*
        Code first underlying neoplasm

J91.8   *Pleural effusion in other conditions classified elsewhere*
    Code first underlying disease, such as:
        filariasis (B74.0-B74.9)
        influenza (J09.X2, J10.1, J11.1)
    AHA: 2015,2Q,15

✔4ᵗʰ **J92   Pleural plaque**
    INCLUDES   pleural thickening
    J92.0   Pleural plaque with presence of asbestos
    J92.9   Pleural plaque without asbestos
        Pleural plaque NOS

✔4ᵗʰ **J93   Pneumothorax and air leak**
    EXCLUDES 1   *congenital or perinatal pneumothorax (P25.1)*
                 postprocedural air leak (J95.812)
                 postprocedural pneumothorax (J95.811)
                 pyopneumothorax (J86.-)
                 traumatic pneumothorax (S27.0)
                 tuberculous (current disease) pneumothorax (A15.-)
    J93.0   Spontaneous tension pneumothorax
✔5ᵗʰ **J93.1   Other spontaneous pneumothorax**
        J93.11   Primary spontaneous pneumothorax
        J93.12   Secondary spontaneous pneumothorax
            Code first underlying condition, such as:
                catamenial pneumothorax due to endometriosis (N80.8)
                cystic fibrosis (E84.-)
                eosinophilic pneumonia (J82)
                lymphangioleiomyomatosis (J84.81)
                malignant neoplasm of bronchus and lung (C34.-)
                Marfan's syndrome (Q87.4)
                pneumonia due to Pneumocystis carinii (B59)
                secondary malignant neoplasm of lung (C78.0-)
                spontaneous rupture of the esophagus (K22.3)
✔5ᵗʰ **J93.8   Other pneumothorax and air leak**
        J93.81   Chronic pneumothorax
        J93.82   Other air leak
            Persistent air leak
        J93.83   Other pneumothorax
            Acute pneumothorax
            Spontaneous pneumothorax NOS
    J93.9   Pneumothorax, unspecified   ▽
        Pneumothorax NOS

✔4ᵗʰ **J94   Other pleural conditions**
    EXCLUDES 1   *pleurisy NOS (R09.1)*
                 traumatic hemopneumothorax (S27.2)
                 traumatic hemothorax (S27.1)
                 tuberculous pleural conditions (current disease) (A15.-)
    J94.0   Chylous effusion
        Chyliform effusion
    J94.1   Fibrothorax
    J94.2   Hemothorax
        Hemopneumothorax
    J94.8   Other specified pleural conditions
        Hydropneumothorax
        Hydrothorax
    J94.9   Pleural condition, unspecified   ▽

Intraoperative and postprocedural complications and disorders of respiratory system, not elsewhere classified (J95)

✔4ᵗʰ **J95   Intraoperative and postprocedural complications and disorders of respiratory system, not elsewhere classified**
    EXCLUDES 2   *aspiration pneumonia (J69.-)*
                 emphysema (subcutaneous) resulting from a procedure (T81.82)
                 hypostatic pneumonia (J18.2)
                 pulmonary manifestations due to radiation (J70.0-J70.1)
✔5ᵗʰ **J95.0   Tracheostomy complications**
        J95.00   Unspecified tracheostomy complication   ▽
        J95.01   Hemorrhage from tracheostomy stoma
        J95.02   Infection of tracheostomy stoma
            Use additional code to identify type of infection, such as:
                cellulitis of neck (L03.8)
                sepsis (A40, A41.-)

Chapter 10. Diseases of the Respiratory System

J95.03   **Malfunction of tracheostomy stoma**
Mechanical complication of tracheostomy stoma
Obstruction of tracheostomy airway
Tracheal stenosis due to tracheostomy

J95.04   **Tracheo-esophageal fistula following tracheostomy**

J95.09   **Other tracheostomy complication**

J95.1   **Acute pulmonary insufficiency following thoracic surgery**
EXCLUDES 2   *functional disturbances following cardiac surgery (I97.0, I97.1-)*

J95.2   **Acute pulmonary insufficiency following nonthoracic surgery**
EXCLUDES 2   *functional disturbances following cardiac surgery (I97.0, I97.1-)*

J95.3   **Chronic pulmonary insufficiency following surgery**
EXCLUDES 2   *functional disturbances following cardiac surgery (I97.0, I97.1-)*

J95.4   **Chemical pneumonitis due to anesthesia**
Mendelson's syndrome
Postprocedural aspiration pneumonia
Use additional code for adverse effect, if applicable, to identify drug (T41.- with fifth or sixth character 5)
EXCLUDES 1   *aspiration pneumonitis due to anesthesia complicating labor and delivery (O74.0)*
aspiration pneumonitis due to anesthesia complicating pregnancy (O29)
aspiration pneumonitis due to anesthesia complicating the puerperium (O89.01)

J95.5   **Postprocedural subglottic stenosis**

✓5th **J95.6**   **Intraoperative hemorrhage and hematoma of a respiratory system organ or structure complicating a procedure**
EXCLUDES 1   *intraoperative hemorrhage and hematoma of a respiratory system organ or structure due to accidental puncture and laceration during procedure (J95.7-)*

J95.61   **Intraoperative hemorrhage and hematoma of a respiratory system organ or structure complicating a respiratory system procedure**

J95.62   **Intraoperative hemorrhage and hematoma of a respiratory system organ or structure complicating other procedure**

✓5th **J95.7**   **Accidental puncture and laceration of a respiratory system organ or structure during a procedure**
EXCLUDES 2   *postprocedural pneumothorax (J95.811)*

J95.71   **Accidental puncture and laceration of a respiratory system organ or structure during a respiratory system procedure**

J95.72   **Accidental puncture and laceration of a respiratory system organ or structure during other procedure**

✓5th **J95.8**   **Other intraoperative and postprocedural complications and disorders of respiratory system, not elsewhere classified**

✓6th **J95.81**   **Postprocedural pneumothorax and air leak**

J95.811   **Postprocedural pneumothorax**
J95.812   **Postprocedural air leak**

✓6th **J95.82**   **Postprocedural respiratory failure**
EXCLUDES 1   *Respiratory failure in other conditions (J96.-)*

J95.821   **Acute postprocedural respiratory failure**
Postprocedural respiratory failure NOS

J95.822   **Acute and chronic postprocedural respiratory failure**

▲ ✓6th **J95.83**   **Postprocedural hemorrhage of a respiratory system organ or structure following a procedure**

▲   **J95.830**   **Postprocedural hemorrhage of a respiratory system organ or structure following a respiratory system procedure**

▲   **J95.831**   **Postprocedural hemorrhage of a respiratory system organ or structure following other procedure**

J95.84   **Transfusion-related acute lung injury (TRALI)**
DEF: A relatively rare, but serious, pulmonary complication of blood transfusion, with acute respiratory distress, noncardiogenic pulmonary edema, cyanosis, hypoxemia, hypotension, fever, and chills.

✓6th **J95.85**   **Complication of respirator [ventilator]**

J95.850   **Mechanical complication of respirator**
EXCLUDES 1   *encounter for respirator [ventilator] dependence during power failure (Z99.12)*

J95.851   **Ventilator associated pneumonia**
Ventilator associated pneumonitis
Use additional code to identify the organism, if known (B95.-, B96.-, B97.-)
EXCLUDES 1   *ventilator lung in newborn (P27.8)*

J95.859   **Other complication of respirator [ventilator]**

✓6th **J95.86**   **Postprocedural hematoma and seroma of a respiratory system organ or structure following a procedure**

J95.860   **Postprocedural hematoma of a respiratory system organ or structure following a respiratory system procedure**

J95.861   **Postprocedural hematoma of a respiratory system organ or structure following other procedure**

J95.862   **Postprocedural seroma of a respiratory system organ or structure following a respiratory system procedure**

J95.863   **Postprocedural seroma of a respiratory system organ or structure following other procedure**

J95.88   **Other intraoperative complications of respiratory system, not elsewhere classified**

J95.89   **Other postprocedural complications and disorders of respiratory system, not elsewhere classified**
Use additional code to identify disorder, such as:
aspiration pneumonia (J69.-)
bacterial or viral pneumonia (J12-J18)
EXCLUDES 2   *acute pulmonary insufficiency following thoracic surgery (J95.1)*
postprocedural subglottic stenosis (J95.5)

Other diseases of the respiratory system (J96-J99)

✓4th **J96**   **Respiratory failure, not elsewhere classified**
EXCLUDES 1   *acute respiratory distress syndrome (J80)*
cardiorespiratory failure (R09.2)
newborn respiratory distress syndrome (P22.0)
postprocedural respiratory failure (J95.82-)
respiratory arrest (R09.2)
respiratory arrest of newborn (P28.81)
respiratory failure of newborn (P28.5)

✓5th **J96.0**   **Acute respiratory failure**

J96.00   **Acute respiratory failure, unspecified whether with hypoxia or hypercapnia** ▽
AHA: 2013,4Q,121

J96.01   **Acute respiratory failure with hypoxia**
J96.02   **Acute respiratory failure with hypercapnia**

✓5th **J96.1**   **Chronic respiratory failure**

J96.10   **Chronic respiratory failure, unspecified whether with hypoxia or hypercapnia** ▽
AHA: 2016,1Q,38; 2015,1Q,21

J96.11   **Chronic respiratory failure with hypoxia**
AHA: 2013,4Q,129

J96.12   **Chronic respiratory failure with hypercapnia**

✓5th **J96.2**   **Acute and chronic respiratory failure**
Acute on chronic respiratory failure

J96.20   **Acute and chronic respiratory failure, unspecified whether with hypoxia or hypercapnia** ▽

J96.21   **Acute and chronic respiratory failure with hypoxia**

J96.22   **Acute and chronic respiratory failure with hypercapnia**

✓5th **J96.9**   **Respiratory failure, unspecified**

J96.90   **Respiratory failure, unspecified, unspecified whether with hypoxia or hypercapnia** ▽

J96.91   **Respiratory failure, unspecified with hypoxia** ▽

J96.92   **Respiratory failure, unspecified with hypercapnia** ▽

EXCLUDES 1 Not coded here   EXCLUDES 2 Not included here   N Newborn Age : 0   P Pediatric Age : 0-17   M Maternity Age : 12-55   A Adult Age : 15-124

654   ICD-10-CM 2017

☑4ᵗʰ **J98 Other respiratory disorders**

Use additional code to identify:

exposure to environmental tobacco smoke (Z77.22)

exposure to tobacco smoke in the perinatal period (P96.81)

▶history of tobacco dependence (Z87.891)◀

occupational exposure to environmental tobacco smoke (Z57.31)

tobacco dependence (F17.-)

tobacco use (Z72.0)

EXCLUDES 1   *newborn apnea (P28.4)*

newborn sleep apnea (P28.3)

EXCLUDES 2   *apnea NOS (R06.81)*

sleep apnea (G47.3-)

☑5ᵗʰ **J98.0 Diseases of bronchus, not elsewhere classified**

J98.01 Acute bronchospasm

EXCLUDES 1   *acute bronchiolitis with bronchospasm (J21.-)*

acute bronchitis with bronchospasm (J20.-)

asthma (J45.-)

exercise induced bronchospasm (J45.990)

J98.09 Other diseases of bronchus, not elsewhere classified

Broncholithiasis

Calcification of bronchus

Stenosis of bronchus

Tracheobronchial collapse

Tracheobronchial dyskinesia

Ulcer of bronchus

☑5ᵗʰ **J98.1 Pulmonary collapse**

EXCLUDES 1   *therapeutic collapse of lung status (Z98.3)*

J98.11 Atelectasis

EXCLUDES 1   *newborn atelectasis*

tuberculous atelectasis (current disease) (A15)

J98.19 Other pulmonary collapse

J98.2 Interstitial emphysema

Mediastinal emphysema

EXCLUDES 1   *emphysema NOS (J43.9)*

emphysema in newborn (P25.0)

surgical emphysema (subcutaneous) (T81.82)

traumatic subcutaneous emphysema (T79.7)

J98.3 Compensatory emphysema

J98.4 Other disorders of lung

Calcification of lung

Cystic lung disease (acquired)

Lung disease NOS

Pulmolithiasis

EXCLUDES 1   *acute interstitial pneumonitis (J84.114)*

pulmonary insufficiency following surgery (J95.1-J95.2)

☑5ᵗʰ **J98.5 Diseases of mediastinum, not elsewhere classified**

EXCLUDES 2   *abscess of mediastinum (J85.3)*

● **J98.51 Mediastinitis**

Code first underlying condition, if applicable, such as postoperative mediastinitis (T81.-)

● **J98.59 Other diseases of mediastinum, not elsewhere classified**

Fibrosis of mediastinum

Hernia of mediastinum

Retraction of mediastinum

J98.6 Disorders of diaphragm

Diaphragmatitis

Paralysis of diaphragm

Relaxation of diaphragm

EXCLUDES 1   *congenital malformation of diaphragm NEC (Q79.1)*

congenital diaphragmatic hernia (Q79.0)

EXCLUDES 2   *diaphragmatic hernia (K44.-)*

J98.8 Other specified respiratory disorders

J98.9 Respiratory disorder, unspecified   ▽

Respiratory disease (chronic) NOS

J99 *Respiratory disorders in diseases classified elsewhere*

Code first underlying disease, such as:

amyloidosis (E85.-)

ankylosing spondylitis (M45)

congenital syphilis (A50.5)

cryoglobulinemia (D89.1)

early congenital syphilis (A50.0)

schistosomiasis (B65.0-B65.9)

EXCLUDES 1   *respiratory disorders in:*

amebiasis (A06.5)

blastomycosis (B40.0-B40.2)

candidiasis (B37.1)

coccidioidomycosis (B38.0-B38.2)

cystic fibrosis with pulmonary manifestations (E84.0)

dermatomyositis (M33.01, M33.11)

histoplasmosis (B39.0-B39.2)

late syphilis (A52.72, A52.73)

polymyositis (M33.21)

sicca syndrome (M35.02)

systemic lupus erythematosus (M32.13)

systemic sclerosis (M34.81)

Wegener's granulomatosis (M31.30-M31.31)

☑ Additional Character Required   ☑7ᵗʰ Placeholder Alert   Manifestation Dx   ▽ Unspecified Dx   ▶◀ Revised Text   ● New Code   ▲ Revised Code Title

Chapter 11. Diseases of the Digestive System (KØØ–K95)

Chapter Specific Coding Guidelines and Examples
Reserved for future guideline expansion.

Chapter 11. Diseases of the Digestive System (K00–K95)

EXCLUDES 2   certain conditions originating in the perinatal period (P04-P96)
certain infectious and parasitic diseases (A00-B99)
complications of pregnancy, childbirth and the puerperium (O00-O9A)
congenital malformations, deformations and chromosomal abnormalities (Q00-Q99)
endocrine, nutritional and metabolic diseases (E00-E88)
injury, poisoning and certain other consequences of external causes (S00-T88)
neoplasms (C00-D49)
symptoms, signs and abnormal clinical and laboratory findings, not elsewhere classified (R00-R94)

This chapter contains the following blocks:

K00-K14   Diseases of oral cavity and salivary glands
K20-K31   Diseases of esophagus, stomach and duodenum
K35-K38   Diseases of appendix
K40-K46   Hernia
K50-K52   Noninfective enteritis and colitis
K55-K64   Other diseases of intestines
K65-K68   Diseases of peritoneum and retroperitoneum
K70-K77   Diseases of liver
K80-K87   Disorders of gallbladder, biliary tract and pancreas
K90-K95   Other diseases of the digestive system

Diseases of oral cavity and salivary glands (K00-K14)

✓4ᵗʰ **K00   Disorders of tooth development and eruption**

   EXCLUDES 2   embedded and impacted teeth (K01.-)

K00.0   Anodontia
   Hypodontia
   Oligodontia
   EXCLUDES 1   acquired absence of teeth (K08.1-)

K00.1   Supernumerary teeth
   Distomolar
   Fourth molar
   Mesiodens
   Paramolar
   Supplementary teeth
   EXCLUDES 2   supernumerary roots (K00.2)

K00.2   Abnormalities of size and form of teeth
   Concrescence of teeth
   Dens evaginatus
   Dens in dente
   Dens invaginatus
   Enamel pearls
   Fusion of teeth
   Gemination of teeth
   Macrodontia
   Microdontia
   Peg-shaped [conical] teeth
   Supernumerary roots
   Taurodontism
   Tuberculum paramolare
   EXCLUDES 1   abnormalities of teeth due to congenital syphilis (A50.5)
       tuberculum Carabelli, which is regarded as a normal variation and should not be coded

K00.3   Mottled teeth
   Dental fluorosis
   Mottling of enamel
   Nonfluoride enamel opacities
   EXCLUDES 2   deposits [accretions] on teeth (K03.6)

K00.4   Disturbances in tooth formation
   Aplasia and hypoplasia of cementum
   Dilaceration of tooth
   Enamel hypoplasia (neonatal) (postnatal) (prenatal)
   Regional odontodysplasia
   Turner's tooth
   EXCLUDES 1   Hutchinson's teeth and mulberry molars in congenital syphilis (A50.5)
   EXCLUDES 2   mottled teeth (K00.3)

K00.5   Hereditary disturbances in tooth structure, not elsewhere classified
   Amelogenesis imperfecta
   Dentinogenesis imperfecta
   Odontogenesis imperfecta
   Dentinal dysplasia
   Shell teeth

K00.6   Disturbances in tooth eruption
   Dentia praecox
   Natal tooth
   Neonatal tooth
   Premature eruption of tooth
   Premature shedding of primary [deciduous] tooth
   Prenatal teeth
   Retained [persistent] primary tooth
   EXCLUDES 2   embedded and impacted teeth (K01.-)

K00.7   Teething syndrome

K00.8   Other disorders of tooth development
   Color changes during tooth formation
   Intrinsic staining of teeth NOS
   EXCLUDES 2   posteruptive color changes (K03.7)

K00.9   Disorder of tooth development, unspecified   ▽
   Disorder of odontogenesis NOS

✓4ᵗʰ **K01   Embedded and impacted teeth**
   EXCLUDES 1   abnormal position of fully erupted teeth (M26.3-)

K01.0   Embedded teeth

K01.1   Impacted teeth

✓4ᵗʰ **K02   Dental caries**
   INCLUDES   ►caries of dentine◄
     dental cavities
     ►early childhood caries◄
     ►pre-eruptive caries◄
     ►recurrent caries (dentino enamel junction) (enamel) (to the pulp)◄
     tooth decay

K02.3   Arrested dental caries
   Arrested coronal and root caries

✓5ᵗʰ **K02.5   Dental caries on pit and fissure surface**
   Dental caries on chewing surface of tooth

     K02.51   Dental caries on pit and fissure surface limited to enamel
       White spot lesions [initial caries] on pit and fissure surface of tooth

     K02.52   Dental caries on pit and fissure surface penetrating into dentin
       ►Primary dental caries, cervical origin◄

     K02.53   Dental caries on pit and fissure surface penetrating into pulp

✓5ᵗʰ **K02.6   Dental caries on smooth surface**

     K02.61   Dental caries on smooth surface limited to enamel
       White spot lesions [initial caries] on smooth surface of tooth

     K02.62   Dental caries on smooth surface penetrating into dentin

     K02.63   Dental caries on smooth surface penetrating into pulp

K02.7   Dental root caries

K02.9   Dental caries, unspecified   ▽

✓4ᵗʰ **K03   Other diseases of hard tissues of teeth**
   EXCLUDES 2   bruxism (F45.8)
     dental caries (K02.-)
     teeth-grinding NOS (F45.8)

K03.0   Excessive attrition of teeth
   Approximal wear of teeth
   Occlusal wear of teeth

K03.1   Abrasion of teeth
   Dentifrice abrasion of teeth
   Habitual abrasion of teeth
   Occupational abrasion of teeth
   Ritual abrasion of teeth
   Traditional abrasion of teeth
   Wedge defect NOS

K03.2   Erosion of teeth
   Erosion of teeth due to diet
   Erosion of teeth due to drugs and medicaments
   Erosion of teeth due to persistent vomiting
   Erosion of teeth NOS
   Idiopathic erosion of teeth
   Occupational erosion of teeth

K03.3   Pathological resorption of teeth
   Internal granuloma of pulp
   Resorption of teeth (external)

☑ Additional Character Required   ✓7ᵗʰ Placeholder Alert   Manifestation Dx   ▽ Unspecified Dx   ►◄ Revised Text   ● New Code   ▲ Revised Code Title

K03.4   **Hypercementosis**
Cementation hyperplasia

K03.5   **Ankylosis of teeth**

K03.6   **Deposits [accretions] on teeth**
Betel deposits [accretions] on teeth
Black deposits [accretions] on teeth
Extrinsic staining of teeth NOS
Green deposits [accretions] on teeth
Materia alba deposits [accretions] on teeth
Orange deposits [accretions] on teeth
Staining of teeth NOS
Subgingival dental calculus
Supragingival dental calculus
Tobacco deposits [accretions] on teeth

K03.7   **Posteruptive color changes of dental hard tissues**
EXCLUDES 2   *deposits [accretions] on teeth (K03.6)*

✓5ᵗʰ **K03.8**   **Other specified diseases of hard tissues of teeth**

    K03.81   **Cracked tooth**
        EXCLUDES 1   *asymptomatic craze lines in enamel - omit code*
        broken or fractured tooth due to trauma (S02.5)

    K03.89   **Other specified diseases of hard tissues of teeth**

K03.9   **Disease of hard tissues of teeth, unspecified**   ▽

✓4ᵗʰ **K04**   **Diseases of pulp and periapical tissues**

✓5ᵗʰ **K04.0**   **Pulpitis**
Acute pulpitis
Chronic (hyperplastic) (ulcerative) pulpitis

●   **K04.01**   **Reversible pulpitis**

●   **K04.02**   **Irreversible pulpitis**

K04.1   **Necrosis of pulp**
Pulpal gangrene

K04.2   **Pulp degeneration**
Denticles
Pulpal calcifications
Pulpal stones

K04.3   **Abnormal hard tissue formation in pulp**
Secondary or irregular dentine

K04.4   **Acute apical periodontitis of pulpal origin**
Acute apical periodontitis NOS
EXCLUDES 1   *acute periodontitis (K05.2-)*
DEF: Severe inflammation of the area surrounding the tip of a tooth's root; often secondary to infection or trauma.

K04.5   **Chronic apical periodontitis**
Apical or periapical granuloma
Apical periodontitis NOS
EXCLUDES 1   *chronic periodontitis (K05.3-)*

K04.6   **Periapical abscess with sinus**
Dental abscess with sinus
Dentoalveolar abscess with sinus

K04.7   **Periapical abscess without sinus**
Dental abscess without sinus
Dentoalveolar abscess without sinus
Periapical abscess without sinus

K04.8   **Radicular cyst**
Apical (periodontal) cyst
Periapical cyst
Residual radicular cyst
EXCLUDES 2   *lateral periodontal cyst (K09.0)*

✓5ᵗʰ **K04.9**   **Other and unspecified diseases of pulp and periapical tissues**

    K04.90   **Unspecified diseases of pulp and periapical tissues**   ▽

    K04.99   **Other diseases of pulp and periapical tissues**

✓4ᵗʰ **K05**   **Gingivitis and periodontal diseases**
Use additional code to identify:
alcohol abuse and dependence (F10.-)
exposure to environmental tobacco smoke (Z77.22)
exposure to tobacco smoke in the perinatal period (P96.81)
▶history of tobacco dependence (Z87.891)◀
occupational exposure to environmental tobacco smoke (Z57.31)
tobacco dependence (F17.-)
tobacco use (Z72.0)

✓5ᵗʰ **K05.0**   **Acute gingivitis**
    EXCLUDES 1   *acute necrotizing ulcerative gingivitis (A69.1)*
    herpesviral [herpes simplex] gingivostomatitis (B00.2)

    K05.00   **Acute gingivitis, plaque induced**
        Acute gingivitis NOS
        ▶Plaque induced gingival disease◀

    K05.01   **Acute gingivitis, non-plaque induced**

✓5ᵗʰ **K05.1**   **Chronic gingivitis**
Desquamative gingivitis (chronic)
Gingivitis (chronic) NOS
Hyperplastic gingivitis (chronic)
▶Pregnancy associated gingivitis◀
Simple marginal gingivitis (chronic)
Ulcerative gingivitis (chronic)
▶Code first, if applicable, diseases of the digestive system complicating pregnacy (O99.61-)◀

    K05.10   **Chronic gingivitis, plaque induced**
        Chronic gingivitis NOS
        Gingivitis NOS

    K05.11   **Chronic gingivitis, non-plaque induced**

✓5ᵗʰ **K05.2**   **Aggressive periodontitis**
Acute pericoronitis
EXCLUDES 1   *acute apical periodontitis (K04.4)*
    periapical abscess (K04.7)
    periapical abscess with sinus (K04.6)

    K05.20   **Aggressive periodontitis, unspecified**   ▽

   ✓6ᵗʰ **K05.21**   **Aggressive periodontitis, localized**
        Periodontal abscess

        K05.211   **Aggressive periodontitis, localized, slight**

        K05.212   **Aggressive periodontitis, localized, moderate**

        K05.213   **Aggressive periodontitis, localized, severe**

        K05.219   **Aggressive periodontitis, localized, unspecified severity**   ▽

   ✓6ᵗʰ **K05.22**   **Aggressive periodontitis, generalized**

        K05.221   **Aggressive periodontitis, generalized, slight**

        K05.222   **Aggressive periodontitis, generalized, moderate**

        K05.223   **Aggressive periodontitis, generalized, severe**

        K05.229   **Aggressive periodontitis, generalized, unspecified severity**   ▽

✓5ᵗʰ **K05.3**   **Chronic periodontitis**
Chronic pericoronitis
Complex periodontitis
Periodontitis NOS
Simplex periodontitis
EXCLUDES 1   *chronic apical periodontitis (K04.5)*

    K05.30   **Chronic periodontitis, unspecified**   ▽

   ✓6ᵗʰ **K05.31**   **Chronic periodontitis, localized**

        K05.311   **Chronic periodontitis, localized, slight**

        K05.312   **Chronic periodontitis, localized, moderate**

        K05.313   **Chronic periodontitis, localized, severe**

        K05.319   **Chronic periodontitis, localized, unspecified severity**   ▽

   ✓6ᵗʰ **K05.32**   **Chronic periodontitis, generalized**

        K05.321   **Chronic periodontitis, generalized, slight**

        K05.322   **Chronic periodontitis, generalized, moderate**

        K05.323   **Chronic periodontitis, generalized, severe**

        K05.329   **Chronic periodontitis, generalized, unspecified**   ▽

K05.4   **Periodontosis**
Juvenile periodontosis

K05.5   **Other periodontal diseases**
▶Combined periodontic-endodontic lesion◀
▶Narrow gingival width (of periodontal soft tissue)◀
EXCLUDES 2   *leukoplakia of gingiva (K13.21)*

K05.6   **Periodontal disease, unspecified**   ▽

EXCLUDES 1 Not coded here   *EXCLUDES 2* Not included here   **N** Newborn Age : 0   **P** Pediatric Age : 0-17   **M** Maternity Age : 12-55   **A** Adult Age : 15-124

658   ICD-10-CM 2017

✓4ᵗʰ **K06** **Other disorders of gingiva and edentulous alveolar ridge**

> EXCLUDES 2 *acute gingivitis (K05.0)*
> *atrophy of edentulous alveolar ridge (K08.2)*
> *chronic gingivitis (K05.1)*
> *gingivitis NOS (K05.1)*

K06.0 **Gingival recession**
> Gingival recession (generalized) (localized) (postinfective) (postprocedural)

K06.1 **Gingival enlargement**
> Gingival fibromatosis

K06.2 **Gingival and edentulous alveolar ridge lesions associated with trauma**
> Irritative hyperplasia of edentulous ridge [denture hyperplasia]
> Use additional code (Chapter 20) to identify external cause or denture status (Z97.2)

● **K06.3** **Horizontal alveolar bone loss**

K06.8 **Other specified disorders of gingiva and edentulous alveolar ridge**
> Fibrous epulis
> Flabby alveolar ridge
> Giant cell epulis
> Peripheral giant cell granuloma of gingiva
> Pyogenic granuloma of gingiva
> ▶Vertical ridge deficiency◀
> EXCLUDES 2 *gingival cyst (K09.0)*

K06.9 **Disorder of gingiva and edentulous alveolar ridge, unspecified** ▽

✓4ᵗʰ **K08** **Other disorders of teeth and supporting structures**

> EXCLUDES 2 *dentofacial anomalies [including malocclusion] (M26.-)*
> *disorders of jaw (M27.-)*

K08.0 **Exfoliation of teeth due to systemic causes**
> Code also underlying systemic condition

✓5ᵗʰ **K08.1** **Complete loss of teeth**
> Acquired loss of teeth, complete
> EXCLUDES 1 *congenital absence of teeth (K00.0)*
> *exfoliation of teeth due to systemic causes (K08.0)*
> *partial loss of teeth (K08.4-)*

   ✓6ᵗʰ **K08.10** **Complete loss of teeth, unspecified cause**

      K08.101 **Complete loss of teeth, unspecified cause, class I** ▽

      K08.102 **Complete loss of teeth, unspecified cause, class II** ▽

      K08.103 **Complete loss of teeth, unspecified cause, class III** ▽

      K08.104 **Complete loss of teeth, unspecified cause, class IV** ▽

      K08.109 **Complete loss of teeth, unspecified cause, unspecified class** ▽
> Edentulism NOS

   ✓6ᵗʰ **K08.11** **Complete loss of teeth due to trauma**

      K08.111 **Complete loss of teeth due to trauma, class I**

      K08.112 **Complete loss of teeth due to trauma, class II**

      K08.113 **Complete loss of teeth due to trauma, class III**

      K08.114 **Complete loss of teeth due to trauma, class IV**

      K08.119 **Complete loss of teeth due to trauma, unspecified class** ▽

   ✓6ᵗʰ **K08.12** **Complete loss of teeth due to periodontal diseases**

      K08.121 **Complete loss of teeth due to periodontal diseases, class I**

      K08.122 **Complete loss of teeth due to periodontal diseases, class II**

      K08.123 **Complete loss of teeth due to periodontal diseases, class III**

      K08.124 **Complete loss of teeth due to periodontal diseases, class IV**

      K08.129 **Complete loss of teeth due to periodontal diseases, unspecified class** ▽

   ✓6ᵗʰ **K08.13** **Complete loss of teeth due to caries**

      K08.131 **Complete loss of teeth due to caries, class I**

      K08.132 **Complete loss of teeth due to caries, class II**

      K08.133 **Complete loss of teeth due to caries, class III**

      K08.134 **Complete loss of teeth due to caries, class IV**

      K08.139 **Complete loss of teeth due to caries, unspecified class** ▽

   ✓6ᵗʰ **K08.19** **Complete loss of teeth due to other specified cause**

      K08.191 **Complete loss of teeth due to other specified cause, class I**

      K08.192 **Complete loss of teeth due to other specified cause, class II**

      K08.193 **Complete loss of teeth due to other specified cause, class III**

      K08.194 **Complete loss of teeth due to other specified cause, class IV**

      K08.199 **Complete loss of teeth due to other specified cause, unspecified class** ▽

✓5ᵗʰ **K08.2** **Atrophy of edentulous alveolar ridge**

   K08.20 **Unspecified atrophy of edentulous alveolar ridge** ▽
> Atrophy of the mandible NOS
> Atrophy of the maxilla NOS

   K08.21 **Minimal atrophy of the mandible**
> Minimal atrophy of the edentulous mandible

   K08.22 **Moderate atrophy of the mandible**
> Moderate atrophy of the edentulous mandible

   K08.23 **Severe atrophy of the mandible**
> Severe atrophy of the edentulous mandible

   K08.24 **Minimal atrophy of maxilla**
> Minimal atrophy of the edentulous maxilla

   K08.25 **Moderate atrophy of the maxilla**
> Moderate atrophy of the edentulous maxilla

   K08.26 **Severe atrophy of the maxilla**
> Severe atrophy of the edentulous maxilla

K08.3 **Retained dental root**

✓5ᵗʰ **K08.4** **Partial loss of teeth**
> Acquired loss of teeth, partial
> EXCLUDES 1 *complete loss of teeth (K08.1-)*
> *congenital absence of teeth (K00.0)*
> EXCLUDES 2 *exfoliation of teeth due to systemic causes (K08.0)*

   ✓6ᵗʰ **K08.40** **Partial loss of teeth, unspecified cause**

      K08.401 **Partial loss of teeth, unspecified cause, class I** ▽

      K08.402 **Partial loss of teeth, unspecified cause, class II** ▽

      K08.403 **Partial loss of teeth, unspecified cause, class III** ▽

      K08.404 **Partial loss of teeth, unspecified cause, class IV** ▽

      K08.409 **Partial loss of teeth, unspecified cause, unspecified class** ▽
> Tooth extraction status NOS

   ✓6ᵗʰ **K08.41** **Partial loss of teeth due to trauma**

      K08.411 **Partial loss of teeth due to trauma, class I**

      K08.412 **Partial loss of teeth due to trauma, class II**

      K08.413 **Partial loss of teeth due to trauma, class III**

      K08.414 **Partial loss of teeth due to trauma, class IV**

      K08.419 **Partial loss of teeth due to trauma, unspecified class** ▽

   ✓6ᵗʰ **K08.42** **Partial loss of teeth due to periodontal diseases**

      K08.421 **Partial loss of teeth due to periodontal diseases, class I**

      K08.422 **Partial loss of teeth due to periodontal diseases, class II**

      K08.423 **Partial loss of teeth due to periodontal diseases, class III**

      K08.424 **Partial loss of teeth due to periodontal diseases, class IV**

      K08.429 **Partial loss of teeth due to periodontal diseases, unspecified class** ▽

   ✓6ᵗʰ **K08.43** **Partial loss of teeth due to caries**

      K08.431 **Partial loss of teeth due to caries, class I**

      K08.432 **Partial loss of teeth due to caries, class II**

      K08.433 **Partial loss of teeth due to caries, class III**

✔ Additional Character Required   ✓7ᵗʰ Placeholder Alert   Manifestation Dx   ▽ Unspecified Dx   ▶◀ Revised Text   ● New Code   ▲ Revised Code Title

ICD-10-CM 2017   **659**

K06–K08.433

Chapter 11. Diseases of the Digestive System

K08.434   **Partial loss of teeth due to caries, class IV**

K08.439   **Partial loss of teeth due to caries, unspecified class** ▽

✓6ᵗʰ   **K08.49**   **Partial loss of teeth due to other specified cause**

K08.491   **Partial loss of teeth due to other specified cause, class I**

K08.492   **Partial loss of teeth due to other specified cause, class II**

K08.493   **Partial loss of teeth due to other specified cause, class III**

K08.494   **Partial loss of teeth due to other specified cause, class IV**

K08.499   **Partial loss of teeth due to other specified cause, unspecified class** ▽

✓5ᵗʰ   **K08.5**   **Unsatisfactory restoration of tooth**

Defective bridge, crown, filling

Defective dental restoration

EXCLUDES 1   *dental restoration status (Z98.811)*

EXCLUDES 2   *endosseous dental implant failure (M27.6-)*
     unsatisfactory endodontic treatment (M27.5-)

K08.50   **Unsatisfactory restoration of tooth, unspecified** ▽

Defective dental restoration NOS

K08.51   **Open restoration margins of tooth**

Dental restoration failure of marginal integrity

Open margin on tooth restoration

Poor gingival margin to tooth restoration

K08.52   **Unrepairable overhanging of dental restorative materials**

Overhanging of tooth restoration

✓6ᵗʰ   **K08.53**   **Fractured dental restorative material**

EXCLUDES 1   *cracked tooth (K03.81)*
     traumatic fracture of tooth (S02.5)

K08.530   **Fractured dental restorative material without loss of material**

K08.531   **Fractured dental restorative material with loss of material**

K08.539   **Fractured dental restorative material, unspecified** ▽

K08.54   **Contour of existing restoration of tooth biologically incompatible with oral health**

Dental restoration failure of periodontal anatomical integrity

Unacceptable contours of existing restoration of tooth

Unacceptable morphology of existing restoration of tooth

K08.55   **Allergy to existing dental restorative material**

Use additional code to identify the specific type of allergy

K08.56   **Poor aesthetic of existing restoration of tooth**

Dental restoration aesthetically inadequate or displeasing

K08.59   **Other unsatisfactory restoration of tooth**

Other defective dental restoration

✓5ᵗʰ   **K08.8**   **Other specified disorders of teeth and supporting structures**

●   **K08.81**   **Primary occlusal trauma**

●   **K08.82**   **Secondary occlusal trauma**

●   **K08.89**   **Other specified disorders of teeth and supporting structures**

Enlargement of alveolar ridge NOS

Insufficient anatomic crown height

Insufficient clinical crown length

Irregular alveolar process

Toothache NOS

K08.9   **Disorder of teeth and supporting structures, unspecified** ▽

✓4ᵗʰ   **K09**   **Cysts of oral region, not elsewhere classified**

INCLUDES   lesions showing histological features both of aneurysmal cyst and of another fibro-osseous lesion

EXCLUDES 2   *cysts of jaw (M27.0-, M27.4-)*
     radicular cyst (K04.8)

K09.0   **Developmental odontogenic cysts**

Dentigerous cyst

Eruption cyst

Follicular cyst

Gingival cyst

Lateral periodontal cyst

Primordial cyst

EXCLUDES 2   *keratocysts (D16.4, D16.5)*
     odontogenic keratocystic tumors (D16.4, D16.5)

K09.1   **Developmental (nonodontogenic) cysts of oral region**

Cyst (of) incisive canal

Cyst (of) palatine of papilla

Globulomaxillary cyst

Median palatal cyst

Nasoalveolar cyst

Nasolabial cyst

Nasopalatine duct cyst

K09.8   **Other cysts of oral region, not elsewhere classified**

Dermoid cyst

Epidermoid cyst

Lymphoepithelial cyst

Epstein's pearl

K09.9   **Cyst of oral region, unspecified** ▽

✓4ᵗʰ   **K11**   **Diseases of salivary glands**

Use additional code to identify:

alcohol abuse and dependence (F10.-)

exposure to environmental tobacco smoke (Z77.22)

exposure to tobacco smoke in the perinatal period (P96.81)

▶history of tobacco dependence (Z87.891)◀

occupational exposure to environmental tobacco smoke (Z57.31)

tobacco dependence (F17.-)

tobacco use (Z72.0)

K11.0   **Atrophy of salivary gland**

K11.1   **Hypertrophy of salivary gland**

✓5ᵗʰ   **K11.2**   **Sialoadenitis**

Parotitis

EXCLUDES 1   *epidemic parotitis (B26.-)*
     mumps (B26.-)
     uveoparotid fever [Heerfordt] (D86.89)

K11.20   **Sialoadenitis, unspecified** ▽

K11.21   **Acute sialoadenitis**

EXCLUDES 1   *acute recurrent sialoadenitis (K11.22)*

K11.22   **Acute recurrent sialoadenitis**

K11.23   **Chronic sialoadenitis**

K11.3   **Abscess of salivary gland**

K11.4   **Fistula of salivary gland**

EXCLUDES 1   *congenital fistula of salivary gland (Q38.4)*

K11.5   **Sialolithiasis**

Calculus of salivary gland or duct

Stone of salivary gland or duct

K11.6   **Mucocele of salivary gland**

Mucous extravasation cyst of salivary gland

Mucous retention cyst of salivary gland

Ranula

K11.7   **Disturbances of salivary secretion**

Hypoptyalism

Ptyalism

Xerostomia

EXCLUDES 2   *dry mouth NOS (R68.2)*

K11.8   **Other diseases of salivary glands**

Benign lymphoepithelial lesion of salivary gland

Mikulicz' disease

Necrotizing sialometaplasia

Sialectasia

Stenosis of salivary duct

Stricture of salivary duct

EXCLUDES 1   *sicca syndrome [Sjögren] (M35.0-)*

K11.9   **Disease of salivary gland, unspecified** ▽

Sialoadenopathy NOS

EXCLUDES 1 Not coded here   EXCLUDES 2 Not included here   N Newborn Age : 0   P Pediatric Age : 0-17   M Maternity Age : 12-55   A Adult Age : 15-124

660

ICD-10-CM 2017

☑4ᵗʰ **K12   Stomatitis and related lesions**

    Use additional code to identify:
      alcohol abuse and dependence (F10.-)
      exposure to environmental tobacco smoke (Z77.22)
      exposure to tobacco smoke in the perinatal period (P96.81)
      ►history of tobacco dependence (Z87.891)◄
      occupational exposure to environmental tobacco smoke (Z57.31)
      tobacco dependence (F17.-)
      tobacco use (Z72.0)

      EXCLUDES 1   cancrum oris (A69.0)
                   cheilitis (K13.0)
                   gangrenous stomatitis (A69.0)
                   herpesviral [herpes simplex] gingivostomatitis (B00.2)
                   noma (A69.0)

    K12.0   Recurrent oral aphthae
      Aphthous stomatitis (major) (minor)
      Bednar's aphthae
      Periadenitis mucosa necrotica recurrens
      Recurrent aphthous ulcer
      Stomatitis herpetiformis

    K12.1   Other forms of stomatitis
      Stomatitis NOS
      Denture stomatitis
      Ulcerative stomatitis
      Vesicular stomatitis
      EXCLUDES 1   acute necrotizing ulcerative stomatitis (A69.1)
                   Vincent's stomatitis (A69.1)

    K12.2   Cellulitis and abscess of mouth
      Cellulitis of mouth (floor)
      Submandibular abscess
      EXCLUDES 2   abscess of salivary gland (K11.3)
                   abscess of tongue (K14.0)
                   periapical abscess (K04.6-K04.7)
                   periodontal abscess (K05.21)
                   peritonsillar abscess (J36)

☑5ᵗʰ   **K12.3   Oral mucositis (ulcerative)**
      Mucositis (oral) (oropharyneal)
      EXCLUDES 2   gastrointestinal mucositis (ulcerative) (K92.81)
                   mucositis (ulcerative) of vagina and vulva (N76.81)
                   nasal mucositis (ulcerative) (J34.81)

      K12.30   Oral mucositis (ulcerative), unspecified   ▽

      K12.31   Oral mucositis (ulcerative) due to antineoplastic therapy
          Use additional code for adverse effect, if applicable, to identify antineoplastic and immunosuppressive drugs (T45.1X5)
         Use additional code for other antineoplastic therapy, such as:
           radiological procedure and radiotherapy (Y84.2)

      K12.32   Oral mucositis (ulcerative) due to other drugs
         Use additional code for adverse effect, if applicable, to identify drug (T36-T50 with fifth or sixth character 5)

      K12.33   Oral mucositis (ulcerative) due to radiation
         Use additional external cause code (W88-W90, X39.0-) to identify cause

      K12.39   Other oral mucositis (ulcerative)
         Viral oral mucositis (ulcerative)

☑4ᵗʰ **K13   Other diseases of lip and oral mucosa**
      INCLUDES   epithelial disturbances of tongue
    Use additional code to identify:
      alcohol abuse and dependence (F10.-)
      exposure to environmental tobacco smoke (Z77.22)
      exposure to tobacco smoke in the perinatal period (P96.81)
      ►history of tobacco dependence (Z87.891)◄
      occupational exposure to environmental tobacco smoke (Z57.31)
      tobacco dependence (F17.-)
      tobacco use (Z72.0)
      EXCLUDES 2   certain disorders of gingiva and edentulous alveolar ridge (K05-K06)
                   cysts of oral region (K09.-)
                   diseases of tongue (K14.-)
                   stomatitis and related lesions (K12.-)

    K13.0   Diseases of lips
      Abscess of lips
      Angular cheilitis
      Cellulitis of lips
      Cheilitis NOS
      Cheilodynia
      Cheilosis
      Exfoliative cheilitis
      Fistula of lips
      Glandular cheilitis
      Hypertrophy of lips
      Perlèche NEC
      EXCLUDES 1   ariboflavinosis (E53.0)
                   cheilitis due to radiation-related disorders (L55-L59)
                   congenital fistula of lips (Q38.0)
                   congenital hypertrophy of lips (Q18.6)
                   perlèche due to candidiasis (B37.83)
                   perlèche due to riboflavin deficiency (E53.0)

    K13.1   Cheek and lip biting

☑5ᵗʰ   **K13.2   Leukoplakia and other disturbances of oral epithelium, including tongue**
      EXCLUDES 1   carcinoma in situ of oral epithelium (D00.0-)
                   hairy leukoplakia (K13.3)

      K13.21   Leukoplakia of oral mucosa, including tongue
         Leukokeratosis of oral mucosa
         Leukoplakia of gingiva, lips, tongue
         EXCLUDES 1   hairy leukoplakia (K13.3)
                   leukokeratosis nicotina palati (K13.24)

      K13.22   Minimal keratinized residual ridge mucosa
         Minimal keratinization of alveolar ridge mucosa

      K13.23   Excessive keratinized residual ridge mucosa
         Excessive keratinization of alveolar ridge mucosa

      K13.24   Leukokeratosis nicotina palati
         Smoker's palate

      K13.29   Other disturbances of oral epithelium, including tongue
         Erythroplakia of mouth or tongue
         Focal epithelial hyperplasia of mouth or tongue
         Leukoedema of mouth or tongue
         Other oral epithelium disturbances

    K13.3   Hairy leukoplakia

    K13.4   Granuloma and granuloma-like lesions of oral mucosa
      Eosinophilic granuloma
      Granuloma pyogenicum
      Verrucous xanthoma

    K13.5   Oral submucous fibrosis
      Submucous fibrosis of tongue

    K13.6   Irritative hyperplasia of oral mucosa
      EXCLUDES 2   irritative hyperplasia of edentulous ridge [denture hyperplasia] (K06.2)

☑5ᵗʰ   **K13.7   Other and unspecified lesions of oral mucosa**

      K13.70   Unspecified lesions of oral mucosa   ▽

      K13.79   Other lesions of oral mucosa
         Focal oral mucinosis

☑4ᵗʰ **K14   Diseases of tongue**
    Use additional code to identify:
      alcohol abuse and dependence (F10.-)
      exposure to environmental tobacco smoke (Z77.22)
      ►history of tobacco dependence (Z87.891)◄
      occupational exposure to environmental tobacco smoke (Z57.31)
      tobacco dependence (F17.-)
      tobacco use (Z72.0)
      EXCLUDES 2   erythroplakia (K13.29)
                   focal epithelial hyperplasia (K13.29)
                   leukedema of tongue (K13.29)
                   leukoplakia of tongue (K13.21)
                   hairy leukoplakia (K13.3)
                   macroglossia (congenital) (Q38.2)
                   submucous fibrosis of tongue (K13.5)

    K14.0   Glossitis
      Abscess of tongue
      Ulceration (traumatic) of tongue
      EXCLUDES 1   atrophic glossitis (K14.4)

    K14.1   Geographic tongue
      Benign migratory glossitis
      Glossitis areata exfoliativa

    K14.2   Median rhomboid glossitis

☑ Additional Character Required   ☑x7ᵗʰ Placeholder Alert   Manifestation Dx   ▽ Unspecified Dx   ►◄ Revised Text   ● New Code   ▲ Revised Code Title

K14.3 Hypertrophy of tongue papillae
Black hairy tongue
Coated tongue
Hypertrophy of foliate papillae
Lingua villosa nigra

K14.4 Atrophy of tongue papillae
Atrophic glossitis

K14.5 Plicated tongue
Fissured tongue
Furrowed tongue
Scrotal tongue
EXCLUDES 1 *fissured tongue, congenital (Q38.3)*

K14.6 Glossodynia
Glossopyrosis
Painful tongue

K14.8 Other diseases of tongue
Atrophy of tongue
Crenated tongue
Enlargement of tongue
Glossocele
Glossoptosis
Hypertrophy of tongue

K14.9 Disease of tongue, unspecified   ▽
Glossopathy NOS

Diseases of esophagus, stomach and duodenum (K20-K31)

EXCLUDES 2 *hiatus hernia (K44.-)*

✓4ᵗʰ **K20 Esophagitis**
Use additional code to identify:
alcohol abuse and dependence (F10.-)
EXCLUDES 1 *erosion of esophagus (K22.1-)*
esophagitis with gastro-esophageal reflux disease (K21.0)
reflux esophagitis (K21.0)
ulcerative esophagitis (K22.1-)
EXCLUDES 2 *eosinophilic gastritis or gastroenteritis (K52.81)*

K20.0 Eosinophilic esophagitis

K20.8 Other esophagitis
Abscess of esophagus

K20.9 Esophagitis, unspecified   ▽
Esophagitis NOS

✓4ᵗʰ **K21 Gastro-esophageal reflux disease**
EXCLUDES 1 *newborn esophageal reflux (P78.83)*

K21.0 Gastro-esophageal reflux disease with esophagitis
Reflux esophagitis

K21.9 Gastro-esophageal reflux disease without esophagitis
Esophageal reflux NOS
AHA: 2016,1Q,18

✓4ᵗʰ **K22 Other diseases of esophagus**
EXCLUDES 2 *esophageal varices (I85.-)*

K22.0 Achalasia of cardia
Achalasia NOS
Cardiospasm
EXCLUDES 1 *congenital cardiospasm (Q39.5)*

✓5ᵗʰ **K22.1 Ulcer of esophagus**
Barrett's ulcer
Erosion of esophagus
Fungal ulcer of esophagus
Peptic ulcer of esophagus
Ulcer of esophagus due to ingestion of chemicals
Ulcer of esophagus due to ingestion of drugs and medicaments
Ulcerative esophagitis
Code first poisoning due to drug or toxin, if applicable (T36-T65 with fifth or sixth character 1-4 or 6)
Use additional code for adverse effect, if applicable, to identify drug (T36-T50 with fifth or sixth character 5)
EXCLUDES 1 *Barrett's esophagus (K22.7-)*

K22.10 Ulcer of esophagus without bleeding
Ulcer of esophagus NOS

K22.11 Ulcer of esophagus with bleeding
EXCLUDES 2 *bleeding esophageal varices (I85.01, I85.11)*

K22.2 Esophageal obstruction
Compression of esophagus
Constriction of esophagus
Stenosis of esophagus
Stricture of esophagus
EXCLUDES 1 *congenital stenosis or stricture of esophagus (Q39.3)*

K22.3 Perforation of esophagus
Rupture of esophagus
EXCLUDES 1 *traumatic perforation of (thoracic) esophagus (S27.8-)*

K22.4 Dyskinesia of esophagus
Corkscrew esophagus
Diffuse esophageal spasm
Spasm of esophagus
EXCLUDES 1 *cardiospasm (K22.0)*

K22.5 Diverticulum of esophagus, acquired
Esophageal pouch, acquired
EXCLUDES 1 *diverticulum of esophagus (congenital) (Q39.6)*

K22.6 Gastro-esophageal laceration-hemorrhage syndrome
Mallory-Weiss syndrome

✓5ᵗʰ **K22.7 Barrett's esophagus**
Barrett's disease
Barrett's syndrome
EXCLUDES 1 *Barrett's ulcer (K22.1)*
malignant neoplasm of esophagus (C15.-)
DEF: A metaplastic disorder in which specialized columnar epithelial cells replace the normal squamous epithelial cells; secondary to chronic gastroesophageal reflux damage to the mucosa; increases risk of developing adenocarcinoma.

K22.70 Barrett's esophagus without dysplasia
Barrett's esophagus NOS

✓6ᵗʰ **K22.71 Barrett's esophagus with dysplasia**

K22.710 Barrett's esophagus with low grade dysplasia

K22.711 Barrett's esophagus with high grade dysplasia

K22.719 Barrett's esophagus with dysplasia, unspecified   ▽

K22.8 Other specified diseases of esophagus
Hemorrhage of esophagus NOS
EXCLUDES 2 *esophageal varices (I85.-)*
Paterson-Kelly syndrome (D50.1)

K22.9 Disease of esophagus, unspecified   ▽

K23 *Disorders of esophagus in diseases classified elsewhere*
Code first underlying disease, such as:
congenital syphilis (A50.5)
EXCLUDES 1 *late syphilis (A52.79)*
megaesophagus due to Chagas' disease (B57.31)
tuberculosis (A18.83)

✓4ᵗʰ **K25 Gastric ulcer**
INCLUDES erosion (acute) of stomach
pylorus ulcer (peptic)
stomach ulcer (peptic)
Use additional code to identify:
alcohol abuse and dependence (F10.-)
EXCLUDES 1 *acute gastritis (K29.0-)*
peptic ulcer NOS (K27.-)

K25.0 Acute gastric ulcer with hemorrhage

K25.1 Acute gastric ulcer with perforation

K25.2 Acute gastric ulcer with both hemorrhage and perforation

K25.3 Acute gastric ulcer without hemorrhage or perforation

K25.4 Chronic or unspecified gastric ulcer with hemorrhage

K25.5 Chronic or unspecified gastric ulcer with perforation

K25.6 Chronic or unspecified gastric ulcer with both hemorrhage and perforation

K25.7 Chronic gastric ulcer without hemorrhage or perforation

K25.9 Gastric ulcer, unspecified as acute or chronic, without hemorrhage or perforation   ▽

✓4ᵗʰ **K26 Duodenal ulcer**
INCLUDES erosion (acute) of duodenum
duodenum ulcer (peptic)
postpyloric ulcer (peptic)
Use additional code to identify:
alcohol abuse and dependence (F10.-)
EXCLUDES 1 *peptic ulcer NOS (K27.-)*

K26.0 Acute duodenal ulcer with hemorrhage

K26.1 Acute duodenal ulcer with perforation

EXCLUDES 1 Not coded here   EXCLUDES 2 Not included here   N Newborn Age : 0   P Pediatric Age : 0-17   M Maternity Age : 12-55   A Adult Age : 15-124

662

ICD-10-CM 2017

K26.2 Acute **duodenal ulcer** with both hemorrhage and perforation

K26.3 Acute **duodenal ulcer** without hemorrhage or perforation

K26.4 Chronic or unspecified **duodenal ulcer** with hemorrhage
   AHA: 2016,1Q,14

K26.5 Chronic or unspecified **duodenal ulcer** with perforation

K26.6 Chronic or unspecified **duodenal ulcer** with both hemorrhage and perforation

K26.7 Chronic **duodenal ulcer** without hemorrhage or perforation

K26.9 Duodenal ulcer, unspecified as acute or chronic, ▽ without hemorrhage or perforation

✓4ᵗʰ **K27** Peptic **ulcer, site unspecified**

   INCLUDES gastroduodenal ulcer NOS
      peptic ulcer NOS
   Use additional code to identify:
      alcohol abuse and dependence (F10.-)
      EXCLUDES 1 peptic ulcer of newborn (P78.82)

K27.0 Acute **peptic ulcer, site unspecified,** with hemorrhage

K27.1 Acute **peptic ulcer, site unspecified,** with perforation

K27.2 Acute **peptic ulcer, site unspecified,** with both hemorrhage and perforation

K27.3 Acute **peptic ulcer, site unspecified,** without hemorrhage or perforation

K27.4 Chronic or unspecified **peptic ulcer, site unspecified,** with hemorrhage

K27.5 Chronic or unspecified **peptic ulcer, site unspecified,** with perforation

K27.6 Chronic or unspecified **peptic ulcer, site unspecified,** with both hemorrhage and perforation

K27.7 Chronic **peptic ulcer, site unspecified,** without hemorrhage or perforation

K27.9 Peptic ulcer, site unspecified, unspecified as acute or ▽ chronic, without hemorrhage or perforation

✓4ᵗʰ **K28** Gastrojejunal **ulcer**

   INCLUDES anastomotic ulcer (peptic) or erosion
      gastrocolic ulcer (peptic) or erosion
      gastrointestinal ulcer (peptic) or erosion
      gastrojejunal ulcer (peptic) or erosion
      jejunal ulcer (peptic) or erosion
      marginal ulcer (peptic) or erosion
      stomal ulcer (peptic) or erosion
   Use additional code to identify:
      alcohol abuse and dependence (F10.-)
      EXCLUDES 1 primary ulcer of small intestine (K63.3)

K28.0 Acute **gastrojejunal ulcer** with hemorrhage

K28.1 Acute **gastrojejunal ulcer** with perforation

K28.2 Acute **gastrojejunal ulcer** with both hemorrhage and perforation

K28.3 Acute **gastrojejunal ulcer** without hemorrhage or perforation

K28.4 Chronic or unspecified **gastrojejunal ulcer** with hemorrhage

K28.5 Chronic or unspecified **gastrojejunal ulcer** with perforation

K28.6 Chronic or unspecified **gastrojejunal ulcer** with both hemorrhage and perforation

K28.7 Chronic **gastrojejunal ulcer** without hemorrhage or perforation

K28.9 Gastrojejunal ulcer, unspecified as acute or chronic, ▽ without hemorrhage or perforation

✓4ᵗʰ **K29** Gastritis **and duodenitis**

   EXCLUDES 1 eosinophilic gastritis or gastroenteritis (K52.81)
      Zollinger-Ellison syndrome (E16.4)

✓5ᵗʰ **K29.0** Acute **gastritis**
   Use additional code to identify:
      alcohol abuse and dependence (F10.-)
      EXCLUDES 1 erosion (acute) of stomach (K25.-)

   K29.00 Acute **gastritis** without bleeding
   K29.01 Acute **gastritis** with bleeding

✓5ᵗʰ **K29.2** Alcoholic **gastritis**
   Use additional code to identify:
      alcohol abuse and dependence (F10.-)

   K29.20 Alcoholic **gastritis** without bleeding
   K29.21 Alcoholic **gastritis** with bleeding

✓5ᵗʰ **K29.3** Chronic superficial **gastritis**
   K29.30 Chronic superficial **gastritis** without bleeding
   K29.31 Chronic superficial **gastritis** with bleeding

✓5ᵗʰ **K29.4** Chronic atrophic **gastritis**
   Gastric atrophy
   K29.40 Chronic atrophic **gastritis** without bleeding

   K29.41 Chronic atrophic **gastritis** with bleeding

✓5ᵗʰ **K29.5** Unspecified chronic **gastritis**
   Chronic antral gastritis
   Chronic fundal gastritis

   K29.50 Unspecified chronic **gastritis** without ▽ bleeding
   K29.51 Unspecified chronic **gastritis** with bleeding ▽

✓6ᵗʰ **K29.6** Other **gastritis**
   Giant hypertrophic gastritis
   Granulomatous gastritis
   Ménétrier's disease
   K29.60 Other **gastritis** without bleeding
   K29.61 Other **gastritis** with bleeding

✓5ᵗʰ **K29.7** Gastritis, **unspecified**
   K29.70 Gastritis, unspecified, without bleeding ▽
   K29.71 Gastritis, unspecified, with bleeding ▽

✓5ᵗʰ **K29.8** Duodenitis
   K29.80 Duodenitis without bleeding
   K29.81 Duodenitis with bleeding

✓5ᵗʰ **K29.9** Gastroduodenitis, **unspecified**
   K29.90 Gastroduodenitis, unspecified, without ▽ bleeding
   K29.91 Gastroduodenitis, unspecified, with bleeding ▽

K30 Functional **dyspepsia**
   Indigestion
   EXCLUDES 1 dyspepsia NOS (R10.13)
      heartburn (R12)
      nervous dyspepsia (F45.8)
      neurotic dyspepsia (F45.8)
      psychogenic dyspepsia (F45.8)

✓4ᵗʰ **K31** Other **diseases of stomach and duodenum**
   INCLUDES functional disorders of stomach
   EXCLUDES 2 diabetic gastroparesis (E08.43, E09.43, E10.43, E11.43, E13.43)
      diverticulum of duodenum (K57.00-K57.13)

K31.0 Acute **dilatation of stomach**
   Acute distention of stomach

K31.1 Adult **hypertrophic pyloric stenosis** Ⓐ
   Pyloric stenosis NOS
   EXCLUDES 1 congenital or infantile pyloric stenosis (Q40.0)

K31.2 Hourglass **stricture and stenosis of stomach**
   EXCLUDES 1 congenital hourglass stomach (Q40.2)
      hourglass contraction of stomach (K31.89)

K31.3 Pylorospasm, **not elsewhere classified**
   EXCLUDES 1 congenital or infantile pylorospasm (Q40.0)
      neurotic pylorospasm (F45.8)
      psychogenic pylorospasm (F45.8)

K31.4 Gastric **diverticulum**
   EXCLUDES 1 congenital diverticulum of stomach (Q40.2)

K31.5 Obstruction **of duodenum**
   Constriction of duodenum
   Duodenal ileus (chronic)
   Stenosis of duodenum
   Stricture of duodenum
   Volvulus of duodenum
   EXCLUDES 1 congenital stenosis of duodenum (Q41.0)

K31.6 Fistula **of stomach and duodenum**
   Gastrocolic fistula
   Gastrojejunocolic fistula

K31.7 Polyp **of stomach and duodenum**
   EXCLUDES 1 adenomatous polyp of stomach (D13.1)

✓5ᵗʰ **K31.8** Other **specified diseases of stomach and duodenum**
   ✓6ᵗʰ **K31.81** Angiodysplasia **of stomach and duodenum**
      K31.811 Angiodysplasia **of stomach and duodenum** with bleeding
      K31.819 Angiodysplasia **of stomach and duodenum** without bleeding
         Angiodysplasia of stomach and duodenum NOS
   K31.82 Dieulafoy **lesion (hemorrhagic) of stomach and duodenum**
      EXCLUDES 2 Dieulafoy lesion of intestine (K63.81)
   K31.83 Achlorhydria

K31.84 Gastroparesis
Gastroparalysis
Code first underlying disease, if known, such as:
anorexia nervosa (F50.0-)
diabetes mellitus (E08.43, E09.43, E10.43, E11.43, E13.43)
scleroderma (M34.-)
AHA: 2013,4Q,114

K31.89 Other diseases of stomach and duodenum

K31.9 Disease of stomach and duodenum, unspecified ▽

Diseases of appendix (K35-K38)

✓4ᵗʰ **K35 Acute appendicitis**

K35.2 Acute appendicitis with generalized peritonitis
Appendicitis (acute) with generalized (diffuse) peritonitis following rupture or perforation of appendix
Perforated appendix NOS
Ruptured appendix NOS

K35.3 Acute appendicitis with localized peritonitis
▶Acute appendicitis with or without perforation or rupture with peritonitis NOS◀
Acute appendicitis with or without perforation or rupture with localized peritonitis
Acute appendicitis with peritoneal abscess

✓5ᵗʰ **K35.8 Other and unspecified acute appendicitis**

K35.80 Unspecified acute appendicitis ▽
Acute appendicitis NOS
Acute appendicitis without (localized) (generalized) peritonitis

K35.89 Other acute appendicitis

K36 Other appendicitis
Chronic appendicitis
Recurrent appendicitis

K37 Unspecified appendicitis ▽
EXCLUDES 1 unspecified appendicitis with peritonitis (K35.2-K35.3)

✓4ᵗʰ **K38 Other diseases of appendix**

K38.0 Hyperplasia of appendix

K38.1 Appendicular concretions
Fecalith of appendix
Stercolith of appendix

K38.2 Diverticulum of appendix

K38.3 Fistula of appendix

K38.8 Other specified diseases of appendix
Intussusception of appendix

K38.9 Disease of appendix, unspecified ▽

Hernia (K40-K46)

NOTE Hernia with both gangrene and obstruction is classified to hernia with gangrene.

INCLUDES acquired hernia
congenital [except diaphragmatic or hiatus] hernia
recurrent hernia

✓4ᵗʰ **K40 Inguinal hernia**
INCLUDES bubonocele
direct inguinal hernia
double inguinal hernia
indirect inguinal hernia
inguinal hernia NOS
oblique inguinal hernia
scrotal hernia

Hernia Sites

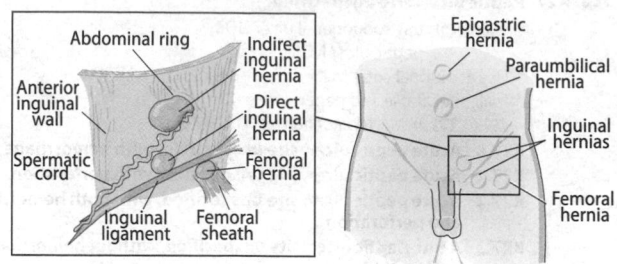

✓5ᵗʰ **K40.0 Bilateral inguinal hernia, with obstruction, without gangrene**
Inguinal hernia (bilateral) causing obstruction without gangrene
Incarcerated inguinal hernia (bilateral) without gangrene
Irreducible inguinal hernia (bilateral) without gangrene
Strangulated inguinal hernia (bilateral) without gangrene

K40.00 Bilateral inguinal hernia, with obstruction, without gangrene, not specified as recurrent
Bilateral inguinal hernia, with obstruction, without gangrene NOS

K40.01 Bilateral inguinal hernia, with obstruction, without gangrene, recurrent

✓5ᵗʰ **K40.1 Bilateral inguinal hernia, with gangrene**

K40.10 Bilateral inguinal hernia, with gangrene, not specified as recurrent
Bilateral inguinal hernia, with gangrene NOS

K40.11 Bilateral inguinal hernia, with gangrene, recurrent

✓5ᵗʰ **K40.2 Bilateral inguinal hernia, without obstruction or gangrene**

K40.20 Bilateral inguinal hernia, without obstruction or gangrene, not specified as recurrent
Bilateral inguinal hernia NOS

K40.21 Bilateral inguinal hernia, without obstruction or gangrene, recurrent

✓5ᵗʰ **K40.3 Unilateral inguinal hernia, with obstruction, without gangrene**
Inguinal hernia (unilateral) causing obstruction without gangrene
Incarcerated inguinal hernia (unilateral) without gangrene
Irreducible inguinal hernia (unilateral) without gangrene
Strangulated inguinal hernia (unilateral) without gangrene

K40.30 Unilateral inguinal hernia, with obstruction, without gangrene, not specified as recurrent
Inguinal hernia, with obstruction NOS
Unilateral inguinal hernia, with obstruction, without gangrene NOS

K40.31 Unilateral inguinal hernia, with obstruction, without gangrene, recurrent

✓5ᵗʰ **K40.4 Unilateral inguinal hernia, with gangrene**

K40.40 Unilateral inguinal hernia, with gangrene, not specified as recurrent
Inguinal hernia with gangrene NOS
Unilateral inguinal hernia with gangrene NOS

K40.41 Unilateral inguinal hernia, with gangrene, recurrent

✓5ᵗʰ **K40.9 Unilateral inguinal hernia, without obstruction or gangrene**

K40.90 Unilateral inguinal hernia, without obstruction or gangrene, not specified as recurrent
Inguinal hernia NOS
Unilateral inguinal hernia NOS

K40.91 Unilateral inguinal hernia, without obstruction or gangrene, recurrent

✓4ᵗʰ **K41 Femoral hernia**

  ✓5ᵗʰ **K41.0 Bilateral femoral hernia, with obstruction, without gangrene**
Femoral hernia (bilateral) causing obstruction, without gangrene
Incarcerated femoral hernia (bilateral), without gangrene
Irreducible femoral hernia (bilateral), without gangrene
Strangulated femoral hernia (bilateral), without gangrene

    K41.00 Bilateral femoral hernia, with obstruction, without gangrene, not specified as recurrent
Bilateral femoral hernia, with obstruction, without gangrene NOS

    K41.01 Bilateral femoral hernia, with obstruction, without gangrene, recurrent

  ✓5ᵗʰ **K41.1 Bilateral femoral hernia, with gangrene**

    K41.10 Bilateral femoral hernia, with gangrene, not specified as recurrent
Bilateral femoral hernia, with gangrene NOS

    K41.11 Bilateral femoral hernia, with gangrene, recurrent

  ✓5ᵗʰ **K41.2 Bilateral femoral hernia, without obstruction or gangrene**

    K41.20 Bilateral femoral hernia, without obstruction or gangrene, not specified as recurrent
Bilateral femoral hernia NOS

    K41.21 Bilateral femoral hernia, without obstruction or gangrene, recurrent

  ✓6ᵗʰ **K41.3 Unilateral femoral hernia, with obstruction, without gangrene**
Femoral hernia (unilateral) causing obstruction, without gangrene
Incarcerated femoral hernia (unilateral), without gangrene
Irreducible femoral hernia (unilateral), without gangrene
Strangulated femoral hernia (unilateral), without gangrene

    K41.30 Unilateral femoral hernia, with obstruction, without gangrene, not specified as recurrent
Femoral hernia, with obstruction NOS
Unilateral femoral hernia, with obstruction NOS

    K41.31 Unilateral femoral hernia, with obstruction, without gangrene, recurrent

  ✓5ᵗʰ **K41.4 Unilateral femoral hernia, with gangrene**

    K41.40 Unilateral femoral hernia, with gangrene, not specified as recurrent
Femoral hernia, with gangrene NOS
Unilateral femoral hernia, with gangrene NOS

    K41.41 Unilateral femoral hernia, with gangrene, recurrent

  ✓5ᵗʰ **K41.9 Unilateral femoral hernia, without obstruction or gangrene**

    K41.90 Unilateral femoral hernia, without obstruction or gangrene, not specified as recurrent
Femoral hernia NOS
Unilateral femoral hernia NOS

    K41.91 Unilateral femoral hernia, without obstruction or gangrene, recurrent

✓4ᵗʰ **K42 Umbilical hernia**
  INCLUDES paraumbilical hernia
  EXCLUDES 1 omphalocele (Q79.2)

  K42.0 Umbilical hernia with obstruction, without gangrene
Umbilical hernia causing obstruction, without gangrene
Incarcerated umbilical hernia, without gangrene
Irreducible umbilical hernia, without gangrene
Strangulated umbilical hernia, without gangrene

  K42.1 Umbilical hernia with gangrene
Gangrenous umbilical hernia

  K42.9 Umbilical hernia without obstruction or gangrene
Umbilical hernia NOS

✓4ᵗʰ **K43 Ventral hernia**

  K43.0 Incisional hernia with obstruction, without gangrene
Incisional hernia causing obstruction, without gangrene
Incarcerated incisional hernia, without gangrene
Irreducible incisional hernia, without gangrene
Strangulated incisional hernia, without gangrene

  K43.1 Incisional hernia with gangrene
Gangrenous incisional hernia

  K43.2 Incisional hernia without obstruction or gangrene
Incisional hernia NOS

  K43.3 Parastomal hernia with obstruction, without gangrene
Incarcerated parastomal hernia, without gangrene
Irreducible parastomal hernia, without gangrene
Parastomal hernia causing obstruction, without gangrene
Strangulated parastomal hernia, without gangrene

  K43.4 Parastomal hernia with gangrene
Gangrenous parastomal hernia

  K43.5 Parastomal hernia without obstruction or gangrene
Parastomal hernia NOS

  K43.6 Other and unspecified ventral hernia with obstruction, without gangrene ▽
Epigastric hernia causing obstruction, without gangrene
Hypogastric hernia causing obstruction, without gangrene
Incarcerated epigastric hernia without gangrene
Incarcerated hypogastric hernia without gangrene
Incarcerated midline hernia without gangrene
Incarcerated spigelian hernia without gangrene
Incarcerated subxiphoid hernia without gangrene
Irreducible epigastric hernia without gangrene
Irreducible hypogastric hernia without gangrene
Irreducible midline hernia without gangrene
Irreducible spigelian hernia without gangrene
Irreducible subxiphoid hernia without gangrene
Midline hernia causing obstruction, without gangrene
Spigelian hernia causing obstruction, without gangrene
Strangulated epigastric hernia without gangrene
Strangulated hypogastric hernia without gangrene
Strangulated midline hernia without gangrene
Strangulated spigelian hernia without gangrene
Strangulated subxiphoid hernia without gangrene
Subxiphoid hernia causing obstruction, without gangrene

  K43.7 Other and unspecified ventral hernia with gangrene ▽
Any condition listed under K43.6 specified as gangrenous

  K43.9 Ventral hernia without obstruction or gangrene ▽
Epigastric hernia
Ventral hernia NOS

✓4ᵗʰ **K44 Diaphragmatic hernia**
  INCLUDES hiatus hernia (esophageal) (sliding)
    paraesophageal hernia
  EXCLUDES 1 congenital diaphragmatic hernia (Q79.0)
    congenital hiatus hernia (Q40.1)

  K44.0 Diaphragmatic hernia with obstruction, without gangrene
Diaphragmatic hernia causing obstruction
Incarcerated diaphragmatic hernia
Irreducible diaphragmatic hernia
Strangulated diaphragmatic hernia

  K44.1 Diaphragmatic hernia with gangrene
Gangrenous diaphragmatic hernia

  K44.9 Diaphragmatic hernia without obstruction or gangrene
Diaphragmatic hernia NOS

✓4ᵗʰ **K45 Other abdominal hernia**
  INCLUDES abdominal hernia, specified site NEC
    lumbar hernia
    obturator hernia
    pudendal hernia
    retroperitoneal hernia
    sciatic hernia

  K45.0 Other specified abdominal hernia with obstruction, without gangrene
Other specified abdominal hernia causing obstruction
Other specified incarcerated abdominal hernia
Other specified irreducible abdominal hernia
Other specified strangulated abdominal hernia

  K45.1 Other specified abdominal hernia with gangrene
Any condition listed under K45 specified as gangrenous

  K45.8 Other specified abdominal hernia without obstruction or gangrene

✓4ᵗʰ **K46 Unspecified abdominal hernia**
  INCLUDES enterocele
    epiplocele
    hernia NOS
    interstitial hernia
    intestinal hernia
    intra-abdominal hernia
  EXCLUDES 1 vaginal enterocele (N81.5)

  K46.0 Unspecified abdominal hernia with obstruction, without gangrene ▽
Unspecified abdominal hernia causing obstruction
Unspecified incarcerated abdominal hernia
Unspecified irreducible abdominal hernia
Unspecified strangulated abdominal hernia

K46.1 **Unspecified abdominal hernia with gangrene** ▽
Any condition listed under K46 specified as gangrenous

K46.9 **Unspecified abdominal hernia without obstruction** ▽
or gangrene
Abdominal hernia NOS

Noninfective enteritis and colitis (K50-K52)

INCLUDES noninfective inflammatory bowel disease
EXCLUDES 1 irritable bowel syndrome (K58.-)
megacolon ▶(K59.3-)◀

✓4th **K50** **Crohn's disease [regional enteritis]**
INCLUDES granulomatous enteritis
Use additional code to identify manifestations, such as:
pyoderma gangrenosum (L88)
EXCLUDES 1 ulcerative colitis (K51.-)
AHA: 2012,4Q,104

✓5th **K50.0** **Crohn's disease of small intestine**
Crohn's disease [regional enteritis] of duodenum
Crohn's disease [regional enteritis] of ileum
Crohn's disease [regional enteritis] of jejunum
Regional ileitis
Terminal ileitis
EXCLUDES 1 Crohn's disease of both small and large intestine
(K50.8-)

K50.00 **Crohn's disease of small intestine without**
complications

✓6th **K50.01** **Crohn's disease of small intestine with**
complications

K50.011 **Crohn's disease of small intestine with**
rectal bleeding

K50.012 **Crohn's disease of small intestine with**
intestinal obstruction

K50.013 **Crohn's disease of small intestine with**
fistula

K50.014 **Crohn's disease of small intestine with**
abscess
AHA: 2012,4Q,104

K50.018 **Crohn's disease of small intestine with**
other complication

K50.019 **Crohn's disease of small intestine** ▽
with unspecified complications

✓5th **K50.1** **Crohn's disease of large intestine**
Crohn's disease [regional enteritis] of colon
Crohn's disease [regional enteritis] of large bowel
Crohn's disease [regional enteritis] of rectum
Granulomatous colitis
Regional colitis
EXCLUDES 1 Crohn's disease of both small and large intestine
(K50.8)

K50.10 **Crohn's disease of large intestine without**
complications

✓6th **K50.11** **Crohn's disease of large intestine with**
complications

K50.111 **Crohn's disease of large intestine with**
rectal bleeding

K50.112 **Crohn's disease of large intestine with**
intestinal obstruction

K50.113 **Crohn's disease of large intestine with**
fistula

K50.114 **Crohn's disease of large intestine with**
abscess

K50.118 **Crohn's disease of large intestine with**
other complication

K50.119 **Crohn's disease of large intestine** ▽
with unspecified complications

✓5th **K50.8** **Crohn's disease of both small and large intestine**

K50.80 **Crohn's disease of both small and large intestine**
without complications

✓6th **K50.81** **Crohn's disease of both small and large intestine**
with complications

K50.811 **Crohn's disease of both small and large**
intestine with rectal bleeding

K50.812 **Crohn's disease of both small and large**
intestine with intestinal obstruction

K50.813 **Crohn's disease of both small and large**
intestine with fistula

K50.814 **Crohn's disease of both small and large**
intestine with abscess

K50.818 **Crohn's disease of both small and large**
intestine with other complication

K50.819 **Crohn's disease of both small and** ▽
large intestine with unspecified
complications

✓5th **K50.9** **Crohn's disease, unspecified**

K50.90 **Crohn's disease, unspecified, without** ▽
complications
Crohn's disease NOS
Regional enteritis NOS

✓6th **K50.91** **Crohn's disease, unspecified, with complications**

K50.911 **Crohn's disease, unspecified, with** ▽
rectal bleeding

K50.912 **Crohn's disease, unspecified, with** ▽
intestinal obstruction

K50.913 **Crohn's disease, unspecified, with** ▽
fistula

K50.914 **Crohn's disease, unspecified, with** ▽
abscess

K50.918 **Crohn's disease, unspecified, with** ▽
other complication

K50.919 **Crohn's disease, unspecified, with** ▽
unspecified complications

✓4th **K51** **Ulcerative colitis**
Use additional code to identify manifestations, such as:
pyoderma gangrenosum (L88)
EXCLUDES 1 Crohn's disease [regional enteritis] (K50.-)

✓5th **K51.0** **Ulcerative (chronic) pancolitis**
Backwash ileitis

K51.00 **Ulcerative (chronic) pancolitis without**
complications
Ulcerative (chronic) pancolitis NOS

✓6th **K51.01** **Ulcerative (chronic) pancolitis with complications**

K51.011 **Ulcerative (chronic) pancolitis with rectal**
bleeding

K51.012 **Ulcerative (chronic) pancolitis with**
intestinal obstruction

K51.013 **Ulcerative (chronic) pancolitis with fistula**

K51.014 **Ulcerative (chronic) pancolitis with**
abscess

K51.018 **Ulcerative (chronic) pancolitis with other**
complication

K51.019 **Ulcerative (chronic) pancolitis with** ▽
unspecified complications

✓5th **K51.2** **Ulcerative (chronic) proctitis**

K51.20 **Ulcerative (chronic) proctitis without complications**
Ulcerative (chronic) proctitis NOS

✓6th **K51.21** **Ulcerative (chronic) proctitis with complications**

K51.211 **Ulcerative (chronic) proctitis with rectal**
bleeding

K51.212 **Ulcerative (chronic) proctitis with**
intestinal obstruction

K51.213 **Ulcerative (chronic) proctitis with fistula**

K51.214 **Ulcerative (chronic) proctitis with abscess**

K51.218 **Ulcerative (chronic) proctitis with other**
complication

K51.219 **Ulcerative (chronic) proctitis with** ▽
unspecified complications

✓5th **K51.3** **Ulcerative (chronic) rectosigmoiditis**

K51.30 **Ulcerative (chronic) rectosigmoiditis without**
complications
Ulcerative (chronic) rectosigmoiditis NOS

✓6th **K51.31** **Ulcerative (chronic) rectosigmoiditis with**
complications

K51.311 **Ulcerative (chronic) rectosigmoiditis with**
rectal bleeding

K51.312 **Ulcerative (chronic) rectosigmoiditis with**
intestinal obstruction

K51.313 **Ulcerative (chronic) rectosigmoiditis with**
fistula

K51.314 **Ulcerative (chronic) rectosigmoiditis with**
abscess

K51.318 **Ulcerative (chronic) rectosigmoiditis with**
other complication

K51.319 **Ulcerative (chronic)** ▽
rectosigmoiditis with unspecified
complications

EXCLUDES 1 Not coded here   EXCLUDES 2 Not included here   N Newborn Age : 0   P Pediatric Age : 0-17   M Maternity Age : 12-55   A Adult Age : 15-124

666   ICD-10-CM 2017

√5ᵗʰ **K51.4 Inflammatory polyps of colon**

> *EXCLUDES 1*   *adenomatous polyp of colon (D12.6)*
> *polyposis of colon (D12.6)*
> *polyps of colon NOS (K63.5)*

     K51.40 Inflammatory polyps of colon without **complications**
         Inflammatory polyps of colon NOS

     √6ᵗʰ **K51.41 Inflammatory polyps of colon** with **complications**

         K51.411 Inflammatory polyps of colon with rectal **bleeding**

         K51.412 Inflammatory polyps of colon with intestinal **obstruction**

         K51.413 Inflammatory polyps of colon with fistula

         K51.414 Inflammatory polyps of colon with abscess

         K51.418 Inflammatory polyps of colon with other complication

         K51.419 Inflammatory polyps of colon with unspecified **complications** ▽

√5ᵗʰ **K51.5 Left sided colitis**
     Left hemicolitis

     K51.50 Left sided colitis without **complications**
         Left sided colitis NOS

     √6ᵗʰ **K51.51 Left sided colitis** with **complications**

         K51.511 Left sided colitis with rectal **bleeding**

         K51.512 Left sided colitis with intestinal **obstruction**

         K51.513 Left sided colitis with fistula

         K51.514 Left sided colitis with abscess

         K51.518 Left sided colitis with other complication

         K51.519 Left sided colitis with unspecified complications ▽

√5ᵗʰ **K51.8 Other ulcerative colitis**

     K51.80 Other ulcerative colitis without **complications**

     √6ᵗʰ **K51.81 Other ulcerative colitis** with **complications**

         K51.811 Other ulcerative colitis with rectal **bleeding**

         K51.812 Other ulcerative colitis with intestinal **obstruction**

         K51.813 Other ulcerative colitis with fistula

         K51.814 Other ulcerative colitis with abscess

         K51.818 Other ulcerative colitis with other complication

         K51.819 Other ulcerative colitis with unspecified **complications** ▽

√5ᵗʰ **K51.9 Ulcerative colitis, unspecified**

     K51.90 Ulcerative colitis, unspecified, without **complications** ▽

     √6ᵗʰ **K51.91 Ulcerative colitis, unspecified,** with **complications**

         K51.911 Ulcerative colitis, unspecified with rectal **bleeding** ▽

         K51.912 Ulcerative colitis, unspecified with intestinal **obstruction** ▽

         K51.913 Ulcerative colitis, unspecified with fistula ▽

         K51.914 Ulcerative colitis, unspecified with abscess ▽

         K51.918 Ulcerative colitis, unspecified with other **complication** ▽

         K51.919 Ulcerative colitis, unspecified with unspecified **complications** ▽

√4ᵗʰ **K52 Other and unspecified noninfective gastroenteritis and colitis**

     K52.0 Gastroenteritis and colitis due to radiation

     K52.1 Toxic gastroenteritis and colitis
         Drug-induced gastroenteritis and colitis
         Code first (T51-T65) to identify toxic agent
         Use additional code for adverse effect, if applicable, to identify drug (T36-T50 with fifth or sixth character 5)

√5ᵗʰ **K52.2 Allergic and dietetic gastroenteritis and colitis**
     Food hypersensitivity gastroenteritis or colitis
     Use additional code to identify type of food allergy (Z91.01-, Z91.02-)

> *EXCLUDES 2*   ▶*allergic eosinophilic colitis (K52.82)*◀
> ▶*allergic eosinophilic esophagitis (K20.0)*◀
> ▶*allergic eosinophilic gastritis (K52.81)*◀
> ▶*allergic eosinophilic gastroenteritis (K52.81)*◀
> ▶*food protein-induced proctocolitis (K52.82)*◀

     DEF: True immunoglobulin E (IgE)-mediated allergic reaction of the lining of the stomach, intestines, or colon to food proteins; causes nausea, vomiting, diarrhea, and abdominal cramping.

     K52.21 Food protein-induced enterocolitis syndrome
         Use additional code for hypovolemic shock, if present (R57.1)

     K52.22 Food protein-induced enteropathy

     K52.29 Other allergic and dietetic gastroenteritis and colitis
         Food hypersensitivity gastroenteritis or colitis
         Immediate gastrointestinal hypersensitivity

     K52.3 Indeterminate colitis
     Colonic inflammatory bowel disease unclassified (IBDU)

> *EXCLUDES 1*   *unspecified colitis (K52.9)*

√5ᵗʰ **K52.8 Other specified noninfective gastroenteritis and colitis**

     K52.81 Eosinophilic gastritis or gastroenteritis
     Eosinophilic enteritis

> *EXCLUDES 2*   ▶*eosinophilic esophagitis (K20.0)*◀

     K52.82 Eosinophilic colitis
     ▶Allergic proctocolitis◀
     ▶Food-induced eosinophilic proctocolitis◀
     ▶Food protein-induced proctocolitis◀
     ▶Milk protein-induced proctocolitis◀

     K52.83 Microscopic colitis

         K52.831 Collagenous colitis

         K52.832 Lymphocytic colitis

         K52.838 Other microscopic colitis

         K52.839 Microscopic colitis, unspecified ▽

     K52.89 Other specified noninfective gastroenteritis and colitis

     K52.9 Noninfective gastroenteritis and colitis, unspecified ▽
     Colitis NOS
     Enteritis NOS
     Gastroenteritis NOS
     Ileitis NOS
     Jejunitis NOS
     Sigmoiditis NOS

> *EXCLUDES 1*   *diarrhea NOS (R19.7)*
> *functional diarrhea (K59.1)*
> *infectious gastroenteritis and colitis NOS (A09)*
> *neonatal diarrhea (noninfective) (P78.3)*
> *psychogenic diarrhea (F45.8)*

Other diseases of intestines (K55-K64)

√4ᵗʰ **K55 Vascular disorders of intestine**

> *EXCLUDES 1*   *necrotizing enterocolitis of newborn (P77.-)*

√5ᵗʰ **K55.0 Acute vascular disorders of intestine**
     Infarction of appendices epiploicae
     Mesenteric (artery) (vein) embolism
     Mesenteric (artery) (vein) infarction
     Mesenteric (artery) (vein) thrombosis

     K55.01 Acute (reversible) ischemia of small intestine

         K55.011 Focal (segmental) acute (reversible) ischemia of small intestine

         K55.012 Diffuse acute (reversible) ischemia of small intestine

         K55.019 Acute (reversible) ischemia of small intestine, extent unspecified ▽

     K55.02 Acute infarction of small intestine
         Gangrene of small intestine
         Necrosis of small intestine

         K55.021 Focal (segmental) acute infarction of small intestine

         K55.022 Diffuse acute infarction of small intestine

         K55.029 Acute infarction of small intestine, extent unspecified ▽

☑ Additional Character Required   √ₓ7ᵗʰ Placeholder Alert   Manifestation Dx   ▽ Unspecified Dx   ▶◀ Revised Text   ● New Code   ▲ Revised Code Title

ICD-10-CM 2017   667

K51.4–K55.029

Chapter 11. Diseases of the Digestive System

- **K55.03 Acute (reversible) ischemia of large intestine**
  - Acute fulminant ischemic colitis
  - Subacute ischemic colitis
  - **K55.031 Focal (segmental) acute (reversible) ischemia of large intestine**
  - **K55.032 Diffuse acute (reversible) ischemia of large intestine**
  - **K55.039 Acute (reversible) ischemia of large intestine, extent unspecified** ▽
- **K55.04 Acute infarction of large intestine**
  - Gangrene of large intestine
  - Necrosis of large intestine
  - **K55.041 Focal (segmental) acute infarction of large intestine**
  - **K55.042 Diffuse acute infarction of large intestine**
  - **K55.049 Acute infarction of large intestine, extent unspecified** ▽
- **K55.05 Acute (reversible) ischemia of intestine, part unspecified**
  - **K55.051 Focal (segmental) acute (reversible) ischemia of intestine, part unspecified**
  - **K55.052 Diffuse acute (reversible) ischemia of intestine, part unspecified**
  - **K55.059 Acute (reversible) ischemia of intestine, part and extent unspecified** ▽
- **K55.06 Acute infarction of intestine, part unspecified**
  - Acute intestinal infarction
  - Gangrene of intestine
  - Necrosis of intestine
  - **K55.061 Focal (segmental) acute infarction of intestine, part unspecified** ▽
  - **K55.062 Diffuse acute infarction of intestine, part unspecified** ▽
  - **K55.069 Acute infarction of intestine, part and extent unspecified** ▽
- **K55.1 Chronic vascular disorders of intestine**
  - Chronic ischemic colitis
  - Chronic ischemic enteritis
  - Chronic ischemic enterocolitis
  - Ischemic stricture of intestine
  - Mesenteric atherosclerosis
  - Mesenteric vascular insufficiency
- √5ᵗʰ **K55.2 Angiodysplasia of colon**
  - **K55.20 Angiodysplasia of colon without hemorrhage**
  - **K55.21 Angiodysplasia of colon with hemorrhage**
- **K55.3 Necrotizing enterocolitis**
  - EXCLUDES 1 *necrotizing enterocolitis of newborn (P77.-)*
  - EXCLUDES 2 *necrotizing enterocolitis due to Clostridium difficile (A04.7)*
  - **K55.30 Necrotizing enterocolitis, unspecified** ▽
    - Necrotizing enterocolitis, NOS
  - **K55.31 Stage 1 necrotizing enterocolitis**
    - Necrotizing enterocolitis without pneumatosis, without perforation
  - **K55.32 Stage 2 necrotizing enterocolitis**
    - Necrotizing enterocolitis with pneumatosis, without perforation
  - **K55.33 Stage 3 necrotizing enterocolitis**
    - Necrotizing enterocolitis with perforation
    - Necrotizing enterocolitis with pneumatosis and perforation
- **K55.8 Other vascular disorders of intestine**
- **K55.9 Vascular disorder of intestine, unspecified** ▽
  - Ischemic colitis
  - Ischemic enteritis
  - Ischemic enterocolitis

√4ᵗʰ **K56 Paralytic ileus and intestinal obstruction without hernia**
  - EXCLUDES 1 *congenital stricture or stenosis of intestine (Q41-Q42)*
    - *cystic fibrosis with meconium ileus (E84.11)*
    - *intestinal obstruction with hernia (K40-K46)*
    - *ischemic stricture of intestine (K55.1)*
    - *meconium ileus NOS (P76.0)*
    - *neonatal intestinal obstructions classifiable to P76.-*
    - *obstruction of duodenum (K31.5)*
    - *postprocedural intestinal obstruction (K91.3)*
    - *stenosis of anus or rectum (K62.4)*
  - **K56.0 Paralytic ileus**
    - Paralysis of bowel
    - Paralysis of colon
    - Paralysis of intestine
    - EXCLUDES 1 *gallstone ileus (K56.3)*
      - *ileus NOS (K56.7)*
      - *obstructive ileus NOS (K56.69)*
  - **K56.1 Intussusception**
    - Intussusception or invagination of bowel
    - Intussusception or invagination of colon
    - Intussusception or invagination of intestine
    - Intussusception or invagination of rectum
    - EXCLUDES 2 *intussusception of appendix (K38.8)*
  - **K56.2 Volvulus**
    - Strangulation of colon or intestine
    - Torsion of colon or intestine
    - Twist of colon or intestine
    - EXCLUDES 2 *volvulus of duodenum (K31.5)*
  - **K56.3 Gallstone ileus**
    - Obstruction of intestine by gallstone
  - √5ᵗʰ **K56.4 Other impaction of intestine**
    - **K56.41 Fecal impaction**
      - EXCLUDES 1 *constipation (K59.0-)*
        - *incomplete defecation (R15.0)*
    - **K56.49 Other impaction of intestine**
  - **K56.5 Intestinal adhesions [bands] with obstruction (postprocedural) (postinfection)**
    - Abdominal hernia due to adhesions with obstruction
    - Peritoneal adhesions [bands] with intestinal obstruction (postprocedural) (postinfection)
  - √5ᵗʰ **K56.6 Other and unspecified intestinal obstruction**
    - **K56.60 Unspecified intestinal obstruction** ▽
      - Intestinal obstruction NOS
      - EXCLUDES 1 *intestinal obstruction due to specified condition - code to condition*
    - **K56.69 Other intestinal obstruction**
      - Enterostenosis NOS
      - Obstructive ileus NOS
      - Occlusion of colon or intestine NOS
      - Stenosis of colon or intestine NOS
      - Stricture of colon or intestine NOS
      - EXCLUDES 1 *intestinal obstruction due to specified condition - code to condition*

EXCLUDES 1 Not coded here   EXCLUDES 2 Not included here   N Newborn Age : 0   P Pediatric Age : 0-17   M Maternity Age : 12-55   A Adult Age : 15-124

668   ICD-10-CM 2017

K56.7 **Ileus, unspecified** ▽
　　EXCLUDES 1 *obstructive ileus (K56.69)*

Volvulus

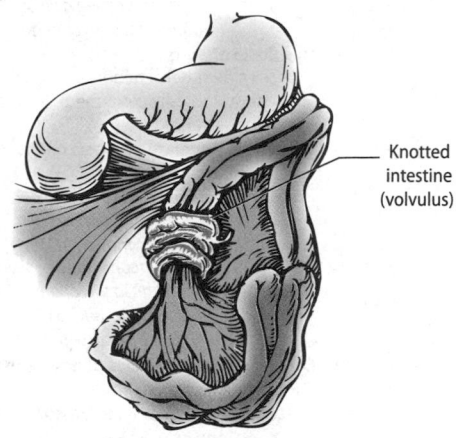

Knotted
intestine
(volvulus)

✓4ᵗʰ **K57** **Diverticular disease of intestine**
　　EXCLUDES 1 *congenital diverticulum of intestine (Q43.8)*
　　　　　　Meckel's diverticulum (Q43.0)
　　EXCLUDES 2 *diverticulum of appendix (K38.2)*

✓5ᵗʰ **K57.0** **Diverticulitis of** small intestine with perforation and abscess
　　Diverticulitis of small intestine with peritonitis
　　EXCLUDES 1 *diverticulitis of both small and large intestine with*
　　　　　　perforation and abscess (K57.4-)
　　K57.00 **Diverticulitis of small intestine with perforation and abscess** without bleeding
　　K57.01 **Diverticulitis of small intestine with perforation and abscess** with bleeding

✓5ᵗʰ **K57.1** **Diverticular disease of** small intestine without perforation or abscess
　　EXCLUDES 1 *diverticular disease of both small and large intestine*
　　　　　　without perforation or abscess (K57.5-)
　　K57.10 **Diverticulosis of small intestine without perforation or abscess** without bleeding
　　　　Diverticular disease of small intestine NOS
　　K57.11 **Diverticulosis of small intestine without perforation or abscess** with bleeding
　　K57.12 **Diverticulitis of small intestine without perforation or abscess** without bleeding
　　K57.13 **Diverticulitis of small intestine without perforation or abscess** with bleeding

✓5ᵗʰ **K57.2** **Diverticulitis of** large intestine with perforation and abscess
　　Diverticulitis of colon with peritonitis
　　EXCLUDES 1 *diverticulitis of both small and large intestine with*
　　　　　　perforation and abscess (K57.4-)
　　K57.20 **Diverticulitis of large intestine with perforation and abscess** without bleeding
　　K57.21 **Diverticulitis of large intestine with perforation and abscess** with bleeding

✓5ᵗʰ **K57.3** **Diverticular disease of** large intestine without perforation or abscess
　　EXCLUDES 1 *diverticular disease of both small and large intestine*
　　　　　　without perforation or abscess (K57.5-)
　　K57.30 **Diverticulosis of large intestine without perforation or abscess** without bleeding
　　　　Diverticular disease of colon NOS
　　K57.31 **Diverticulosis of large intestine without perforation or abscess** with bleeding
　　K57.32 **Diverticulitis of large intestine without perforation or abscess** without bleeding
　　K57.33 **Diverticulitis of large intestine without perforation or abscess** with bleeding

✓5ᵗʰ **K57.4** **Diverticulitis of both** small and large intestine with perforation and abscess
　　Diverticulitis of both small and large intestine with peritonitis
　　K57.40 **Diverticulitis of both small and large intestine with perforation and abscess** without bleeding
　　K57.41 **Diverticulitis of both small and large intestine with perforation and abscess** with bleeding

✓5ᵗʰ **K57.5** **Diverticular disease of** both small and large intestine without perforation or abscess
　　K57.50 **Diverticulosis of both small and large intestine without perforation or abscess** without bleeding
　　　　Diverticular disease of both small and large intestine NOS
　　K57.51 **Diverticulosis of both small and large intestine without perforation or abscess** with bleeding
　　K57.52 **Diverticulitis of both small and large intestine without perforation or abscess** without bleeding
　　K57.53 **Diverticulitis of both small and large intestine without perforation or abscess** with bleeding

✓5ᵗʰ **K57.8** **Diverticulitis of intestine, part unspecified, with perforation and abscess**
　　Diverticulitis of intestine NOS with peritonitis
　　K57.80 **Diverticulitis of intestine, part unspecified, with perforation and abscess** without bleeding ▽
　　K57.81 **Diverticulitis of intestine, part unspecified, with perforation and abscess** with bleeding ▽

✓5ᵗʰ **K57.9** **Diverticular disease of intestine, part unspecified, without perforation or abscess**
　　K57.90 **Diverticulosis of intestine, part unspecified, without perforation or abscess** without bleeding ▽
　　　　Diverticular disease of intestine NOS
　　K57.91 **Diverticulosis of intestine, part unspecified, without perforation or abscess** with bleeding ▽
　　K57.92 **Diverticulitis of intestine, part unspecified, without perforation or abscess** without bleeding ▽
　　K57.93 **Diverticulitis of intestine, part unspecified, without perforation or abscess** with bleeding ▽

✓4ᵗʰ **K58** **Irritable bowel syndrome**
　　INCLUDES irritable colon
　　　　spastic colon
　　K58.0 **Irritable bowel syndrome** with diarrhea
●　**K58.1** **Irritable bowel syndrome** with constipation
●　**K58.2** **Mixed** irritable bowel syndrome
●　**K58.8** **Other** irritable bowel syndrome
　　K58.9 **Irritable bowel syndrome** without diarrhea
　　　　Irritable bowel syndrome NOS

✓4ᵗʰ **K59** **Other functional intestinal disorders**
　　EXCLUDES 1 *change in bowel habit NOS (R19.4)*
　　　　　　intestinal malabsorption (K90.-)
　　　　　　psychogenic intestinal disorders (F45.8)
　　EXCLUDES 2 *functional disorders of stomach (K31.-)*

✓5ᵗʰ **K59.0** **Constipation**
　　▶Use additional code for adverse effect, if applicable, to identify drug (T36-T50 with fifth or sixth character 5) ◀
　　EXCLUDES 1 *fecal impaction (K56.41)*
　　　　　　incomplete defecation (R15.0)
　　K59.00 **Constipation, unspecified** ▽
　　K59.01 **Slow transit** constipation
　　K59.02 **Outlet dysfunction** constipation
●　**K59.03** **Drug induced** constipation
　　　　Use additional code for adverse effect, if applicable, to identify drug (T36-T50 with fifth or sixth character 5)
●　**K59.04** **Chronic idiopathic** constipation
　　　　Functional constipation
　　K59.09 **Other constipation**
　　　　▶Chronic constipation◀

　　K59.1 **Functional diarrhea**
　　EXCLUDES 1 *diarrhea NOS (R19.7)*
　　　　　　irritable bowel syndrome with diarrhea (K58.0)

　　K59.2 **Neurogenic bowel, not elsewhere classified**
　　　　DEF: Disorder of bowel due to spinal cord lesion due to injury or as a complication of conditions such as multiple sclerosis (MS) or spina bifida; loss of bowel control is the primary symptom, manifested as constipation or bowel incontinence.

✓5ᵗʰ **K59.3** **Megacolon, not elsewhere classified**
Dilatation of colon
▶Code first, if applicable (T51-T65) to identify toxic agent◀
EXCLUDES 1 *congenital megacolon (aganglionic) (Q43.1)*
megacolon (due to) (in) Chagas' disease (B57.32)
megacolon (due to) (in) Clostridium difficile (A04.7)
megacolon (due to) (in) Hirschsprung's disease (Q43.1)

● **K59.31** **Toxic megacolon**

● **K59.39** **Other megacolon**
Megacolon NOS

K59.4 **Anal spasm**
Proctalgia fugax

K59.8 **Other specified functional intestinal disorders**
Atony of colon
Pseudo-obstruction (acute) (chronic) of intestine

K59.9 **Functional intestinal disorder, unspecified** ▽

✓4ᵗʰ **K60** **Fissure and fistula of anal and rectal regions**
EXCLUDES 1 *fissure and fistula of anal and rectal regions with abscess or*
cellulitis (K61.-)
EXCLUDES 2 *anal sphincter tear (healed) (nontraumatic) (old) (K62.81)*

K60.0 **Acute anal fissure**
K60.1 **Chronic anal fissure**
K60.2 **Anal fissure, unspecified** ▽

K60.3 **Anal fistula**
K60.4 **Rectal fistula**
Fistula of rectum to skin
EXCLUDES 1 *rectovaginal fistula (N82.3)*
vesicorectal fistual (N32.1)

K60.5 **Anorectal fistula**

✓4ᵗʰ **K61** **Abscess of anal and rectal regions**
INCLUDES abscess of anal and rectal regions
cellulitis of anal and rectal regions

K61.0 **Anal abscess**
Perianal abscess
EXCLUDES 1 *intrasphincteric abscess (K61.4)*

K61.1 **Rectal abscess**
Perirectal abscess
EXCLUDES 1 *ischiorectal abscess (K61.3)*
AHA: 2012,4Q,104

K61.2 **Anorectal abscess**
K61.3 **Ischiorectal abscess**
Abscess of ischiorectal fossa

K61.4 **Intrasphincteric abscess**

✓4ᵗʰ **K62** **Other diseases of anus and rectum**
INCLUDES anal canal
EXCLUDES 2 *colostomy and enterostomy malfunction (K94.0-, K94.1-)*
fecal incontinence (R15.-)
hemorrhoids (K64.-)

K62.0 **Anal polyp**
K62.1 **Rectal polyp**
EXCLUDES 1 *adenomatous polyp (D12.8)*

K62.2 **Anal prolapse**
Prolapse of anal canal

K62.3 **Rectal prolapse**
Prolapse of rectal mucosa

K62.4 **Stenosis of anus and rectum**
Stricture of anus (sphincter)

K62.5 **Hemorrhage of anus and rectum**
EXCLUDES 1 *gastrointestinal bleeding NOS (K92.2)*
melena (K92.1)
neonatal rectal hemorrhage (P54.2)

K62.6 **Ulcer of anus and rectum**
Solitary ulcer of anus and rectum
Stercoral ulcer of anus and rectum
EXCLUDES 1 *fissure and fistula of anus and rectum (K60.-)*
ulcerative colitis (K51.-)

K62.7 **Radiation proctitis**
Use additional code to identify the type of radiation (W90.-)

✓5ᵗʰ **K62.8** **Other specified diseases of anus and rectum**
EXCLUDES 2 *ulcerative proctitis (K51.2)*

K62.81 **Anal sphincter tear (healed) (nontraumatic) (old)**
Tear of anus, nontraumatic
Use additional code for any associated fecal
incontinence (R15.-)
EXCLUDES 2 *anal fissure (K60.-)*
anal sphincter tear (healed) (old)
complicating delivery (O34.7-)
traumatic tear of anal sphincter (S31.831)

K62.82 **Dysplasia of anus**
Anal intraepithelial neoplasia I and II (AIN I and II)
(histologically confirmed)
Dysplasia of anus NOS
Mild and moderate dysplasia of anus (histologically
confirmed)
EXCLUDES 1 *abnormal results from anal cytologic*
examination without histologic
confirmation (R85.61-)
anal intraepithelial neoplasia III (D01.3)
carcinoma in situ of anus (D01.3)
HGSIL of anus (R85.613)
severe dysplasia of anus (D01.3)

K62.89 **Other specified diseases of anus and rectum**
Proctitis NOS
Use additional code for any associated fecal
incontinence (R15.-)

K62.9 **Disease of anus and rectum, unspecified** ▽

✓4ᵗʰ **K63** **Other diseases of intestine**

K63.0 **Abscess of intestine**
EXCLUDES 1 *abscess of intestine with Crohn's disease (K50.014,*
K50.114, K50.814, K50.914,)
abscess of intestine with diverticular disease (K57.0,
K57.2, K57.4, K57.8)
abscess of intestine with ulcerative colitis (K51.014,
K51.214, K51.314, K51.414, K51.514, K51.814,
K51.914)
EXCLUDES 2 *abscess of anal and rectal regions (K61.-)*
abscess of appendix (K35.3)

K63.1 **Perforation of intestine (nontraumatic)**
Perforation (nontraumatic) of rectum
EXCLUDES 1 *perforation (nontraumatic) of duodenum (K26.-)*
perforation (nontraumatic) of intestine with
diverticular disease (K57.0, K57.2, K57.4, K57.8)
EXCLUDES 2 *perforation (nontraumatic) of appendix (K35.2, K35.3)*

K63.2 **Fistula of intestine**
EXCLUDES 1 *fistula of duodenum (K31.6)*
fistula of intestine with Crohn's disease (K50.013,
K50.113, K50.813, K50.913)
fistula of intestine with ulcerative colitis (K51.013,
K51.213, K51.313, K51.413, K51.513, K51.813,
K51.913)
EXCLUDES 2 *fistula of anal and rectal regions (K60.-)*
fistula of appendix (K38.3)
intestinal-genital fistula, female (N82.2-N82.4)
vesicointestinal fistula (N32.1)

K63.3 **Ulcer of intestine**
Primary ulcer of small intestine
EXCLUDES 1 *duodenal ulcer (K26.-)*
gastrointestinal ulcer (K28.-)
gastrojejunal ulcer (K28.-)
jejunal ulcer (K28.-)
peptic ulcer, site unspecified (K27.-)
ulcer of intestine with perforation (K63.1)
ulcer of anus or rectum (K62.6)
ulcerative colitis (K51.-)

K63.4 **Enteroptosis**
K63.5 **Polyp of colon**
EXCLUDES 1 *adenomatous polyp of colon (D12.6)*
inflammatory polyp of colon (K51.4-)
polyposis of colon (D12.6)
AHA: 2015,2Q,14

✓5ᵗʰ **K63.8** **Other specified diseases of intestine**

K63.81 **Dieulafoy lesion of intestine**
EXCLUDES 2 *Dieulafoy lesion of stomach and duodenum*
(K31.82)

K63.89 **Other specified diseases of intestine**
AHA: 2013,2Q,31

K63.9 **Disease of intestine, unspecified** ▽

✓4ᵗʰ K64 Hemorrhoids and perianal venous thrombosis

INCLUDES piles

EXCLUDES 1 *hemorrhoids complicating childbirth and the puerperium (O87.2)*
hemorrhoids complicating pregnancy (O22.4)

Hemorrhoids

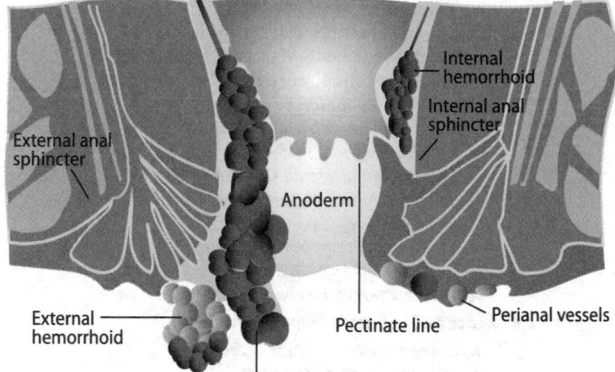

External anal sphincter
External hemorrhoid
Anoderm
Pectinate line
Prolapsing internal hemorrhoid
Internal hemorrhoid
Internal anal sphincter
Perianal vessels

K64.0 First degree hemorrhoids
Grade/stage I hemorrhoids
Hemorrhoids (bleeding) without prolapse outside of anal canal

K64.1 Second degree hemorrhoids
Grade/stage II hemorrhoids
Hemorrhoids (bleeding) that prolapse with straining, but retract spontaneously

K64.2 Third degree hemorrhoids
Grade/stage III hemorrhoids
Hemorrhoids (bleeding) that prolapse with straining and require manual replacement back inside anal canal

K64.3 Fourth degree hemorrhoids
Grade/stage IV hemorrhoids
Hemorrhoids (bleeding) with prolapsed tissue that cannot be manually replaced

K64.4 Residual hemorrhoidal skin tags
External hemorrhoids, NOS
Skin tags of anus

K64.5 Perianal venous thrombosis
External hemorrhoids with thrombosis
Perianal hematoma
Thrombosed hemorrhoids NOS

K64.8 Other hemorrhoids
Internal hemorrhoids, without mention of degree
Prolapsed hemorrhoids, degree not specified

K64.9 Unspecified hemorrhoids ▽
Hemorrhoids (bleeding) NOS
Hemorrhoids (bleeding) without mention of degree

Diseases of peritoneum and retroperitoneum (K65-K68)

✓4ᵗʰ K65 Peritonitis

Use additional code (B95-B97), to identify infectious agent

EXCLUDES 1 *acute appendicitis with generalized peritonitis (K35.2)*
aseptic peritonitis (T81.6)
benign paroxysmal peritonitis (E85.0)
chemical peritonitis (T81.6)
diverticulitis of both small and large intestine with peritonitis (K57.4-)
diverticulitis of colon with peritonitis (K57.2-)
diverticulitis of intestine, NOS, with peritonitis (K57.8-)
diverticulitis of small intestine with peritonitis (K57.0-)
gonococcal peritonitis (A54.85)
neonatal peritonitis (P78.0-P78.1)
pelvic peritonitis, female (N73.3-N73.5)
periodic familial peritonitis (E85.0)
peritonitis due to talc or other foreign substance (T81.6)
peritonitis in chlamydia (A74.81)
peritonitis in diphtheria (A36.89)
peritonitis in syphilis (late) (A52.74)
peritonitis in tuberculosis (A18.31)
peritonitis with or following abortion or ectopic or molar pregnancy (O00-O07, O08.0)
peritonitis with or following appendicitis (K35.-)
peritonitis with or following diverticular disease of intestine (K57.-)
puerperal peritonitis (O85)
retroperitoneal infections (K68.-)

K65.0 Generalized (acute) peritonitis
Pelvic peritonitis (acute), male
Subphrenic peritonitis (acute)
Suppurative peritonitis (acute)

K65.1 Peritoneal abscess
Abdominopelvic abscess
Abscess (of) omentum
Abscess (of) peritoneum
Mesenteric abscess
Retrocecal abscess
Subdiaphragmatic abscess
Subhepatic abscess
Subphrenic abscess

K65.2 Spontaneous bacterial peritonitis
EXCLUDES 1 *bacterial peritonitis NOS (K65.9)*

K65.3 Choleperitonitis
Peritonitis due to bile

K65.4 Sclerosing mesenteritis
Fat necrosis of peritoneum
(Idiopathic) sclerosing mesenteric fibrosis
Mesenteric lipodystrophy
Mesenteric panniculitis
Retractile mesenteritis

K65.8 Other peritonitis
Chronic proliferative peritonitis
Peritonitis due to urine

K65.9 Peritonitis, unspecified ▽
Bacterial peritonitis NOS
AHA: 2013,2Q,31

✓4ᵗʰ K66 Other disorders of peritoneum

EXCLUDES 2 *ascites (R18.-)*
peritoneal effusion (chronic) (R18.8)

K66.0 Peritoneal adhesions (postprocedural) (postinfection)
Adhesions (of) abdominal (wall)
Adhesions (of) diaphragm
Adhesions (of) intestine
Adhesions (of) male pelvis
Adhesions (of) omentum
Adhesions (of) stomach
Adhesive bands
Mesenteric adhesions
EXCLUDES 1 *female pelvic adhesions [bands] (N73.6)*
peritoneal adhesions with intestinal obstruction (K56.5)

K66.1 Hemoperitoneum
EXCLUDES 1 *traumatic hemoperitoneum (S36.8-)*

K66.8 Other specified disorders of peritoneum

K66.9 Disorder of peritoneum, unspecified ▽

✓ Additional Character Required   ✓7ᵗʰ Placeholder Alert   Manifestation Dx   ▽ Unspecified Dx   ►◄ Revised Text   ● New Code   ▲ Revised Code Title

Chapter 11. Diseases of the Digestive System

K67   *Disorders of peritoneum in infectious diseases classified elsewhere*

Code first underlying disease, such as :
congenital syphilis (A50.0)
helminthiasis (B65.0-B83.9)

> **EXCLUDES 1**   peritonitis in chlamydia (A74.81)
> peritonitis in diphtheria (A36.89)
> peritonitis in gonococcal (A54.85)
> peritonitis in syphilis (late) (A52.74)
> peritonitis in tuberculosis (A18.31)

✓4ᵗʰ **K68**   **Disorders of retroperitoneum**

✓5ᵗʰ   **K68.1**   **Retroperitoneal abscess**

     K68.11   **Postprocedural** retroperitoneal abscess

     K68.12   **Psoas muscle** abscess

     K68.19   **Other** retroperitoneal abscess

   K68.9   **Other disorders** of retroperitoneum

Diseases of liver (K70-K77)

> **EXCLUDES 1**   jaundice NOS (R17)
> **EXCLUDES 2**   hemochromatosis (E83.11-)
> Reye's syndrome (G93.7)
> viral hepatitis (B15-B19)
> Wilson's disease (E83.0)

✓4ᵗʰ **K70**   **Alcoholic liver disease**

Use additional code to identify:
alcohol abuse and dependence (F10.-)

   K70.0   **Alcoholic fatty liver**   A

✓5ᵗʰ   **K70.1**   **Alcoholic hepatitis**

     K70.10   **Alcoholic hepatitis** without ascites   A

     K70.11   **Alcoholic hepatitis** with ascites   A

   K70.2   **Alcoholic fibrosis and sclerosis** of liver   A

✓5ᵗʰ   **K70.3**   **Alcoholic cirrhosis** of liver

Alcoholic cirrhosis NOS

     K70.30   **Alcoholic cirrhosis of liver** without ascites   A

     K70.31   **Alcoholic cirrhosis of liver** with ascites   A

✓5ᵗʰ   **K70.4**   **Alcoholic hepatic failure**

Acute alcoholic hepatic failure
Alcoholic hepatic failure NOS
Chronic alcoholic hepatic failure
Subacute alcoholic hepatic failure

     K70.40   **Alcoholic hepatic failure** without coma   A

     K70.41   **Alcoholic hepatic failure** with coma   A

   K70.9   **Alcoholic liver disease, unspecified**   A ▽

✓4ᵗʰ **K71**   **Toxic liver disease**

> **INCLUDES**   drug-induced idiosyncratic (unpredictable) liver disease
> drug-induced toxic (predictable) liver disease

Code first poisoning due to drug or toxin, if applicable (T36-T65 with fifth or sixth character 1-4 or 6)
Use additional code for adverse effect, if applicable, to identify drug (T36-T50 with fifth or sixth character 5)

> **EXCLUDES 2**   alcoholic liver disease (K70.-)
> Budd-Chiari syndrome (I82.0)

   K71.0   **Toxic liver disease with cholestasis**

Cholestasis with hepatocyte injury
"Pure" cholestasis

✓5ᵗʰ   **K71.1**   **Toxic liver disease with hepatic necrosis**

Hepatic failure (acute) (chronic) due to drugs

     K71.10   **Toxic liver disease with hepatic necrosis,** without coma

     K71.11   **Toxic liver disease with hepatic necrosis,** with coma

   K71.2   **Toxic liver disease with acute hepatitis**

   K71.3   **Toxic liver disease with chronic persistent hepatitis**

   K71.4   **Toxic liver disease with chronic lobular hepatitis**

✓5ᵗʰ   **K71.5**   **Toxic liver disease with chronic active hepatitis**

Toxic liver disease with lupoid hepatitis

     K71.50   **Toxic liver disease with chronic active hepatitis** without ascites

     K71.51   **Toxic liver disease with chronic active hepatitis** with ascites

   K71.6   **Toxic liver disease with hepatitis, not elsewhere classified**

   K71.7   **Toxic liver disease with fibrosis and cirrhosis of liver**

   K71.8   **Toxic liver disease with other disorders of liver**

Toxic liver disease with focal nodular hyperplasia
Toxic liver disease with hepatic granulomas
Toxic liver disease with peliosis hepatis
Toxic liver disease with veno-occlusive disease of liver

   K71.9   **Toxic liver disease, unspecified**   ▽

✓4ᵗʰ **K72**   **Hepatic failure, not elsewhere classified**

> **INCLUDES**   fulminant hepatitis NEC, with hepatic failure
> hepatic encephalopathy NOS
> liver (cell) necrosis with hepatic failure
> malignant hepatitis NEC, with hepatic failure
> yellow liver atrophy or dystrophy

> **EXCLUDES 1**   alcoholic hepatic failure (K70.4)
> hepatic failure with toxic liver disease (K71.1-)
> icterus of newborn (P55-P59)
> postprocedural hepatic failure (K91.82)

> **EXCLUDES 2**   hepatic failure complicating abortion or ectopic or molar pregnancy (O00-O07, O08.8)
> hepatic failure complicating pregnancy, childbirth and the puerperium (O26.6-)
> ▶viral hepatitis with hepatic coma (B15-B19)◀

✓5ᵗʰ   **K72.0**   **Acute and subacute hepatic failure**

▶Acute non-viral hepatitis NOS◀

AHA: 2015,2Q,17; 2014,2Q,13

     K72.00   **Acute and subacute hepatic failure** without coma

     K72.01   **Acute and subacute hepatic failure** with coma

✓5ᵗʰ   **K72.1**   **Chronic hepatic failure**

     K72.10   **Chronic hepatic failure** without coma

     K72.11   **Chronic hepatic failure** with coma

✓5ᵗʰ   **K72.9**   **Hepatic failure, unspecified**

     K72.90   **Hepatic failure, unspecified** without coma   ▽

       AHA: 2016,2Q,35

     K72.91   **Hepatic failure, unspecified** with coma   ▽

Hepatic coma NOS

✓4ᵗʰ **K73**   **Chronic hepatitis, not elsewhere classified**

> **EXCLUDES 1**   alcoholic hepatitis (chronic) (K70.1-)
> drug-induced hepatitis (chronic) (K71.-)
> granulomatous hepatitis (chronic) NEC (K75.3)
> reactive, nonspecific hepatitis (chronic) (K75.2)
> viral hepatitis (chronic) (B15-B19)

   K73.0   **Chronic persistent hepatitis, not elsewhere classified**

   K73.1   **Chronic lobular hepatitis, not elsewhere classified**

   K73.2   **Chronic active hepatitis, not elsewhere classified**

   K73.8   **Other chronic hepatitis, not elsewhere classified**

   K73.9   **Chronic hepatitis, unspecified**   ▽

✓4ᵗʰ **K74**   **Fibrosis and cirrhosis of liver**

Code also, if applicable, viral hepatitis (acute) (chronic) (B15-B19)

> **EXCLUDES 1**   alcoholic cirrhosis (of liver) (K70.3)
> alcoholic fibrosis of liver (K70.2)
> cardiac sclerosis of liver (K76.1)
> cirrhosis (of liver) with toxic liver disease (K71.7)
> congenital cirrhosis (of liver) (P78.81)
> pigmentary cirrhosis (of liver) (E83.110)

   K74.0   **Hepatic fibrosis**

   K74.1   **Hepatic sclerosis**

   K74.2   **Hepatic fibrosis with hepatic sclerosis**

   K74.3   **Primary biliary cirrhosis**

Chronic nonsuppurative destructive cholangitis

   K74.4   **Secondary biliary cirrhosis**

   K74.5   **Biliary cirrhosis, unspecified**   ▽

✓5ᵗʰ   **K74.6**   **Other and unspecified cirrhosis of liver**

     K74.60   **Unspecified cirrhosis of liver**   ▽

Cirrhosis (of liver) NOS

     K74.69   **Other cirrhosis of liver**

Cryptogenic cirrhosis (of liver)
Macronodular cirrhosis (of liver)
Micronodular cirrhosis (of liver)
Mixed type cirrhosis (of liver)
Portal cirrhosis (of liver)
Postnecrotic cirrhosis (of liver)

EXCLUDES 1 Not coded here   **EXCLUDES 2** Not included here   N Newborn Age : 0   P Pediatric Age : 0-17   M Maternity Age : 12-55   A Adult Age : 15-124

672   ICD-10-CM 2017

✓4ᵗʰ **K75**   **Other inflammatory liver diseases**
> EXCLUDES 2   *toxic liver disease (K71.-)*

     K75.0   **Abscess of liver**
> Cholangitic hepatic abscess
> Hematogenic hepatic abscess
> Hepatic abscess NOS
> Lymphogenic hepatic abscess
> Pylephlebitic hepatic abscess
>> EXCLUDES 1   *amebic liver abscess (A06.4)*
>> *cholangitis without liver abscess (K83.0)*
>> *pylephlebitis without liver abscess (K75.1)*
>>> EXCLUDES 2   ►*acute or subacute hepatitis NOS (B17.9)*◄
>>> ►*acute or subacute non-viral hepatitis (K72.0)*◄
>>> ►*chronic hepatitis NEC (K73.8)*◄

     K75.1   **Phlebitis of portal vein**
> Pylephlebitis
>> EXCLUDES 1   *pylephlebitic liver abscess (K75.0)*

     K75.2   **Nonspecific reactive hepatitis**
>> EXCLUDES 1   *acute or subacute hepatitis (K72.0-)*
>> *chronic hepatitis NEC (K73.-)*
>> *viral hepatitis (B15-B19)*

     K75.3   **Granulomatous hepatitis, not elsewhere classified**
>> EXCLUDES 1   *acute or subacute hepatitis (K72.0-)*
>> *chronic hepatitis NEC (K73.-)*
>> *viral hepatitis (B15-B19)*

     K75.4   **Autoimmune hepatitis**
> Lupoid hepatitis NEC

✓5ᵗʰ   **K75.8**   **Other specified inflammatory liver diseases**
         K75.81   **Nonalcoholic steatohepatitis (NASH)**
         K75.89   **Other specified inflammatory liver diseases**

     K75.9   **Inflammatory liver disease, unspecified**   ▽
> Hepatitis NOS
>> EXCLUDES 1   *acute or subacute hepatitis (K72.0-)*
>> *chronic hepatitis NEC (K73.-)*
>> *viral hepatitis (B15-B19)*
> **AHA:** 2015,2Q,17

✓4ᵗʰ **K76**   **Other diseases of liver**
> EXCLUDES 2   *alcoholic liver disease (K70.-)*
> *amyloid degeneration of liver (E85.-)*
> *cystic disease of liver (congenital) (Q44.6)*
> *hepatic vein thrombosis (I82.0)*
> *hepatomegaly NOS (R16.0)*
> *pigmentary cirrhosis (of liver) (E83.110)*
> *portal vein thrombosis (I81)*
> *toxic liver disease (K71.-)*

     K76.0   **Fatty (change of) liver, not elsewhere classified**
> Nonalcoholic fatty liver disease (NAFLD)
>> EXCLUDES 1   *nonalcoholic steatohepatitis (NASH) (K75.81)*

     K76.1   **Chronic passive congestion of liver**
> Cardiac cirrhosis
> Cardiac sclerosis

     K76.2   **Central hemorrhagic necrosis of liver**
>> EXCLUDES 1   *liver necrosis with hepatic failure (K72.-)*

     K76.3   **Infarction of liver**
     K76.4   **Peliosis hepatis**
> Hepatic angiomatosis

     K76.5   **Hepatic veno-occlusive disease**
>> EXCLUDES 1   *Budd-Chiari syndrome (I82.0)*

     K76.6   **Portal hypertension**
> Use additional code for any associated complications, such as:
> portal hypertensive gastropathy (K31.89)

     K76.7   **Hepatorenal syndrome**
>> EXCLUDES 1   *hepatorenal syndrome following labor and delivery (O90.4)*
>> *postprocedural hepatorenal syndrome ►(K91.83)◄*

✓5ᵗʰ   **K76.8**   **Other specified diseases of liver**
         K76.81   **Hepatopulmonary syndrome**
> Code first underlying liver disease, such as:
> alcoholic cirrhosis of liver (K70.3-)
> cirrhosis of liver without mention of alcohol (K74.6-)
         K76.89   **Other specified diseases of liver**
> Cyst (simple) of liver
> Focal nodular hyperplasia of liver
> Hepatoptosis

     K76.9   **Liver disease, unspecified**   ▽

K77   *Liver disorders in diseases classified elsewhere*
> Code first underlying disease, such as:
> amyloidosis (E85.-)
> congenital syphilis (A50.0, A50.5)
> congenital toxoplasmosis (P37.1)
> schistosomiasis (B65.0-B65.9)
>> EXCLUDES 1   *alcoholic hepatitis (K70.1-)*
>> *alcoholic liver disease (K70.-)*
>> *cytomegaloviral hepatitis (B25.1)*
>> *herpesviral [herpes simplex] hepatitis (B00.81)*
>> *infectious mononucleosis with liver disease (B27.0-B27.9 with .9)*
>> *mumps hepatitis (B26.81)*
>> *sarcoidosis with liver disease (D86.89)*
>> *secondary syphilis with liver disease (A51.45)*
>> *syphilis (late) with liver disease (A52.74)*
>> *toxoplasmosis (acquired) hepatitis (B58.1)*
>> *tuberculosis with liver disease (A18.83)*

Disorders of gallbladder, biliary tract and pancreas (K80-K87)

✓4ᵗʰ **K80**   **Cholelithiasis**
> EXCLUDES 1   *retained cholelithiasis following cholecystectomy (K91.86)*

Cholelithiasis

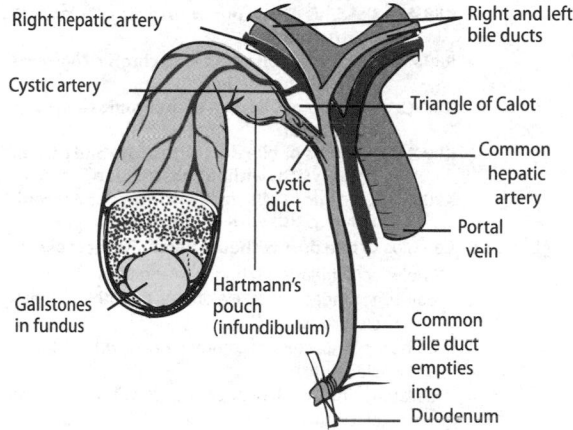

Right hepatic artery · Cystic artery · Cystic duct · Gallstones in fundus · Hartmann's pouch (infundibulum) · Right and left bile ducts · Triangle of Calot · Common hepatic artery · Portal vein · Common bile duct empties into Duodenum

✓5ᵗʰ   **K80.0**   **Calculus of gallbladder with acute cholecystitis**
> Any condition listed in K80.2 with acute cholecystitis
         K80.00   **Calculus of gallbladder with acute cholecystitis without obstruction**
         K80.01   **Calculus of gallbladder with acute cholecystitis with obstruction**

✓5ᵗʰ   **K80.1**   **Calculus of gallbladder with other cholecystitis**
         K80.10   **Calculus of gallbladder with chronic cholecystitis without obstruction**
> Cholelithiasis with cholecystitis NOS
         K80.11   **Calculus of gallbladder with chronic cholecystitis with obstruction**
         K80.12   **Calculus of gallbladder with acute and chronic cholecystitis without obstruction**
         K80.13   **Calculus of gallbladder with acute and chronic cholecystitis with obstruction**
         K80.18   **Calculus of gallbladder with other cholecystitis without obstruction**
         K80.19   **Calculus of gallbladder with other cholecystitis with obstruction**

✓5ᵗʰ   **K80.2**   **Calculus of gallbladder without cholecystitis**
> Cholecystolithiasis without cholecystitis
> Cholelithiasis (without cholecystitis)
> Colic (recurrent) of gallbladder (without cholecystitis)
> Gallstone (impacted) of cystic duct (without cholecystitis)
> Gallstone (impacted) of gallbladder (without cholecystitis)
         K80.20   **Calculus of gallbladder without cholecystitis without obstruction**
         K80.21   **Calculus of gallbladder without cholecystitis with obstruction**

✓ Additional Character Required   ✓x7ᵗʰ Placeholder Alert   Manifestation Dx   ▽ Unspecified Dx   ►◄ Revised Text   ● New Code   ▲ Revised Code Title

Chapter 11. Diseases of the Digestive System

✓5ᵗʰ K80.3 Calculus of bile duct with cholangitis

Any condition listed in K80.5 with cholangitis

K80.30 Calculus of bile duct with cholangitis, unspecified, without obstruction ▽

K80.31 Calculus of bile duct with cholangitis, unspecified, with obstruction ▽

K80.32 Calculus of bile duct with acute **cholangitis** without obstruction

K80.33 Calculus of bile duct with acute **cholangitis** with obstruction

K80.34 Calculus of bile duct with chronic **cholangitis** without obstruction

K80.35 Calculus of bile duct with chronic **cholangitis** with obstruction

K80.36 Calculus of bile duct with acute and chronic **cholangitis** without obstruction

K80.37 Calculus of bile duct with acute and chronic **cholangitis** with obstruction

✓5ᵗʰ K80.4 Calculus of bile duct with cholecystitis

Any condition listed in K80.5 with cholecystitis (with cholangitis)

K80.40 Calculus of bile duct with cholecystitis, unspecified, without obstruction ▽

K80.41 Calculus of bile duct with cholecystitis, unspecified, with obstruction ▽

K80.42 Calculus of bile duct with acute **cholecystitis** without obstruction

K80.43 Calculus of bile duct with acute **cholecystitis** with obstruction

K80.44 Calculus of bile duct with chronic **cholecystitis** without obstruction

K80.45 Calculus of bile duct with chronic **cholecystitis** with obstruction

K80.46 Calculus of bile duct with acute and chronic **cholecystitis** without obstruction

K80.47 Calculus of bile duct with acute and chronic **cholecystitis** with obstruction

✓5ᵗʰ K80.5 Calculus of bile duct without cholangitis or cholecystitis

Choledocholithiasis (without cholangitis or cholecystitis)

Gallstone (impacted) of bile duct NOS (without cholangitis or cholecystitis)

Gallstone (impacted) of common duct (without cholangitis or cholecystitis)

Gallstone (impacted) of hepatic duct (without cholangitis or cholecystitis)

Hepatic cholelithiasis (without cholangitis or cholecystitis)

Hepatic colic (recurrent) (without cholangitis or cholecystitis)

K80.50 Calculus of bile duct without cholangitis or cholecystitis without obstruction

K80.51 Calculus of bile duct without cholangitis or cholecystitis with obstruction

✓5ᵗʰ K80.6 Calculus of gallbladder and bile duct with cholecystitis

K80.60 Calculus of gallbladder and bile duct with cholecystitis, unspecified, without obstruction ▽

K80.61 Calculus of gallbladder and bile duct with cholecystitis, unspecified, with obstruction ▽

K80.62 Calculus of gallbladder and bile duct with acute **cholecystitis** without obstruction

K80.63 Calculus of gallbladder and bile duct with acute **cholecystitis** with obstruction

K80.64 Calculus of gallbladder and bile duct with chronic **cholecystitis** without obstruction

K80.65 Calculus of gallbladder and bile duct with chronic **cholecystitis** with obstruction

K80.66 Calculus of gallbladder and bile duct with acute and chronic **cholecystitis** without obstruction

K80.67 Calculus of gallbladder and bile duct with acute and chronic **cholecystitis** with obstruction

✓5ᵗʰ K80.7 Calculus of gallbladder and bile duct without cholecystitis

K80.70 Calculus of gallbladder and bile duct without cholecystitis without obstruction

K80.71 Calculus of gallbladder and bile duct without cholecystitis with obstruction

✓5ᵗʰ K80.8 Other cholelithiasis

K80.80 Other cholelithiasis without obstruction

K80.81 Other cholelithiasis with obstruction

✓4ᵗʰ K81 Cholecystitis

   EXCLUDES 1 *cholecystitis with cholelithiasis (K80.-)*

K81.0 Acute cholecystitis

Abscess of gallbladder

Angiocholecystitis

Emphysematous (acute) cholecystitis

Empyema of gallbladder

Gangrene of gallbladder

Gangrenous cholecystitis

Suppurative cholecystitis

K81.1 Chronic cholecystitis

K81.2 Acute cholecystitis with chronic cholecystitis

K81.9 Cholecystitis, unspecified ▽

✓4ᵗʰ K82 Other diseases of gallbladder

   EXCLUDES 1 *nonvisualization of gallbladder (R93.2)*
             postcholecystectomy syndrome (K91.5)

K82.0 Obstruction of gallbladder

Occlusion of cystic duct or gallbladder without cholelithiasis

Stenosis of cystic duct or gallbladder without cholelithiasis

Stricture of cystic duct or gallbladder without cholelithiasis

   EXCLUDES 1 *obstruction of gallbladder with cholelithiasis (K80.-)*

K82.1 Hydrops of gallbladder

Mucocele of gallbladder

K82.2 Perforation of gallbladder

Rupture of cystic duct or gallbladder

K82.3 Fistula of gallbladder

Cholecystocolic fistula

Cholecystoduodenal fistula

K82.4 Cholesterolosis of gallbladder

Strawberry gallbladder

   EXCLUDES 1 *cholesterolosis of gallbladder with cholecystitis (K81.-)*
             cholesterolosis of gallbladder with cholelithiasis (K80.-)

K82.8 Other specified diseases of gallbladder

Adhesions of cystic duct or gallbladder

Atrophy of cystic duct or gallbladder

Cyst of cystic duct or gallbladder

Dyskinesia of cystic duct or gallbladder

Hypertrophy of cystic duct or gallbladder

Nonfunctioning of cystic duct or gallbladder

Ulcer of cystic duct or gallbladder

K82.9 Disease of gallbladder, unspecified ▽

✓4ᵗʰ K83 Other diseases of biliary tract

   EXCLUDES 1 *postcholecystectomy syndrome (K91.5)*
   EXCLUDES 2 *conditions involving the gallbladder (K81-K82)*
             conditions involving the cystic duct (K81-K82)

K83.0 Cholangitis

Ascending cholangitis

Cholangitis NOS

Primary cholangitis

Recurrent cholangitis

Sclerosing cholangitis

Secondary cholangitis

Stenosing cholangitis

Suppurative cholangitis

   EXCLUDES 1 *cholangitic liver abscess (K75.0)*
             cholangitis with choledocholithiasis (K80.3-, K80.4-)
             chronic nonsuppurative destructive cholangitis (K74.3)

K83.1 Obstruction of bile duct

Occlusion of bile duct without cholelithiasis

Stenosis of bile duct without cholelithiasis

Stricture of bile duct without cholelithiasis

   EXCLUDES 1 *congenital obstruction of bile duct (Q44.3)*
             obstruction of bile duct with cholelithiasis (K80.-)

   AHA: 2016,1Q,18

K83.2 Perforation of bile duct

Rupture of bile duct

K83.3 Fistula of bile duct

Choledochoduodenal fistula

K83.4 Spasm of sphincter of Oddi

K83.5 Biliary cyst

K83.8 Other specified diseases of biliary tract

Adhesions of biliary tract

Atrophy of biliary tract

Hypertrophy of biliary tract

Ulcer of biliary tract

K83.9 Disease of biliary tract, unspecified ▽

EXCLUDES 1 Not coded here   **EXCLUDES 2** Not included here   **N** Newborn Age : 0   **P** Pediatric Age : 0-17   **M** Maternity Age : 12-55   **A** Adult Age : 15-124

674   ICD-10-CM 2017

☑4ᵗʰ **K85 Acute pancreatitis**

     INCLUDES   Acute (recurrent) pancreatitis

             Subacute pancreatitis

   ☑5ᵗʰ **K85.0 Idiopathic acute pancreatitis**

●   **K85.00 Idiopathic acute pancreatitis** without necrosis or infection

●   **K85.01 Idiopathic acute pancreatitis** with uninfected necrosis

●   **K85.02 Idiopathic acute pancreatitis** with infected necrosis

   ☑5ᵗʰ **K85.1 Biliary acute pancreatitis**

         Gallstone pancreatitis

●   **K85.10 Biliary acute pancreatitis** without necrosis or infection

●   **K85.11 Biliary acute pancreatitis** with uninfected necrosis

●   **K85.12 Biliary acute pancreatitis** with infected necrosis

   ☑5ᵗʰ **K85.2 Alcohol induced acute pancreatitis**

         EXCLUDES 2   *alcohol induced chronic pancreatitis (K86.0)*

●   **K85.20 Alcohol induced acute pancreatitis** without necrosis or infection

●   **K85.21 Alcohol induced acute pancreatitis** with uninfected necrosis

●   **K85.22 Alcohol induced acute pancreatitis** with infected necrosis

   ☑6ᵗʰ **K85.3 Drug induced acute pancreatitis**

         Use additional code for adverse effect, if applicable, to identify drug (T36-T50 with fifth or sixth character 5)

         Use additional code to identify drug abuse and dependence (F11.- F17.-)

●   **K85.30 Drug induced acute pancreatitis** without necrosis or infection

●   **K85.31 Drug induced acute pancreatitis** with uninfected necrosis

●   **K85.32 Drug induced acute pancreatitis** with infected necrosis

   ☑5ᵗʰ **K85.8 Other acute pancreatitis**

●   **K85.80 Other acute pancreatitis** without necrosis or infection

●   **K85.81 Other acute pancreatitis** with uninfected necrosis

●   **K85.82 Other acute pancreatitis** with infected necrosis

   ☑5ᵗʰ **K85.9 Acute pancreatitis, unspecified**   ▽

         Pancreatitis NOS

●   **K85.90 Acute pancreatitis** without necrosis or infection, **unspecified**   ▽

●   **K85.91 Acute pancreatitis** with uninfected necrosis, **unspecified**   ▽

●   **K85.92 Acute pancreatitis** with infected necrosis, **unspecified**   ▽

☑4ᵗʰ **K86 Other diseases of pancreas**

     EXCLUDES 2   *fibrocystic disease of pancreas (E84.-)*

                 islet cell tumor (of pancreas) (D13.7)

                 pancreatic steatorrhea (K90.3)

   K86.0 Alcohol-induced chronic pancreatitis

         Use additional code to identify:

            alcohol abuse and dependence (F10.-)

         ▶Code also exocrine pancreatic insufficiency (K86.81)◀

         EXCLUDES 2   *alcohol induced acute pancreatitis* ▶*(K85.2-)*◀

   K86.1 Other chronic pancreatitis

         Chronic pancreatitis NOS

         Infectious chronic pancreatitis

         Recurrent chronic pancreatitis

         Relapsing chronic pancreatitis

         ▶Code also exocrine pancreatic insufficiency (K86.81)◀

   K86.2 Cyst of pancreas

   K86.3 Pseudocyst of pancreas

   ☑5ᵗʰ **K86.8 Other specified diseases of pancreas**

●   **K86.81 Exocrine pancreatic insufficiency**

     K86.89 Other specified diseases of pancreas

         Aseptic pancreatic necrosis, unrelated to acute pancreatitis

         Atrophy of pancreas

         Calculus of pancreas

         Cirrhosis of pancreas

         Fibrosis of pancreas

         Pancreatic fat necrosis, unrelated to acute pancreatitis

         Pancreatic infantilism

         Pancreatic necrosis NOS, unrelated to acute pancreatitis

   K86.9 Disease of pancreas, unspecified   ▽

K87 *Disorders of gallbladder, biliary tract and pancreas in diseases classified elsewhere*

     Code first underlying disease

     EXCLUDES 1   *cytomegaloviral pancreatitis (B25.2)*

               mumps pancreatitis (B26.3)

               syphilitic gallbladder (A52.74)

               syphilitic pancreas (A52.74)

               tuberculosis of gallbladder (A18.83)

               tuberculosis of pancreas (A18.83)

Other diseases of the digestive system (K90-K95)

☑4ᵗʰ **K90 Intestinal malabsorption**

     EXCLUDES 1   *intestinal malabsorption following gastrointestinal surgery (K91.2)*

   K90.0 Celiac disease

         ▶Celiac disease with steatorrhea◀

         Gluten-sensitive enteropathy

         Nontropical sprue

         Use additional code for associated disorders including:

            dermatitis herpetiformis (L13.0)

            gluten ataxia (G32.81)

         ▶Code also exocrine pancreatic insufficiency (K86.81)◀

         DEF: Malabsorption syndrome due to gluten consumption; symptoms include fetid, bulky, frothy, oily stools, distended abdomen, gas, asthenia, electrolyte depletion, and vitamin B, D, and K deficiency.

   K90.1 Tropical sprue

         Sprue NOS

         Tropical steatorrhea

   K90.2 Blind loop syndrome, not elsewhere classified

         Blind loop syndrome NOS

         EXCLUDES 1   *congenital blind loop syndrome (Q43.8)*

                 postsurgical blind loop syndrome (K91.2)

   K90.3 Pancreatic steatorrhea

▲   ☑5ᵗʰ **K90.4 Other malabsorption due to intolerance**

         EXCLUDES 2   *gluten-sensitive enteropathy (K90.0)*

                 lactose intolerance (E73.-)

●   **K90.41 Non-celiac gluten sensitivity**

         Gluten sensitivity NOS

         Non-celiac gluten sensitive enteropathy

●   **K90.49 Malabsorption due to intolerance, not elsewhere classified**

         Malabsorption due to intolerance to carbohydrate

         Malabsorption due to intolerance to fat

         Malabsorption due to intolerance to protein

         Malabsorption due to intolerance to starch

   ☑5ᵗʰ **K90.8 Other intestinal malabsorption**

     K90.81 Whipple's disease

     K90.89 Other intestinal malabsorption

   K90.9 Intestinal malabsorption, unspecified   ▽

☑4ᵗʰ **K91 Intraoperative and postprocedural complications and disorders of digestive system, not elsewhere classified**

     EXCLUDES 2   *complications of artificial opening of digestive system (K94.-)*

                 complications of bariatric procedures (K95.-)

                 gastrojejunal ulcer (K28.-)

                 postprocedural (radiation) retroperitoneal abscess (K68.11)

                 radiation colitis (K52.0)

                 radiation gastroenteritis (K52.0)

                 radiation proctitis (K62.7)

   K91.0 Vomiting following gastrointestinal surgery

K91.1   **Postgastric surgery syndromes**
> Dumping syndrome
> Postgastrectomy syndrome
> Postvagotomy syndrome

K91.2   **Postsurgical malabsorption, not elsewhere classified**
> Postsurgical blind loop syndrome
> EXCLUDES 1   *malabsorption osteomalacia in adults (M83.2)*
> *malabsorption osteoporosis, postsurgical (M80.8-, M81.8)*

K91.3   **Postprocedural intestinal obstruction**

K91.5   **Postcholecystectomy syndrome**

√5ᵗʰ **K91.6**   **Intraoperative hemorrhage and hematoma of a digestive system organ or structure complicating a procedure**
> EXCLUDES 1   *intraoperative hemorrhage and hematoma of a digestive system organ or structure due to accidental puncture and laceration during a procedure (K91.7-)*

▲   **K91.61**   **Intraoperative hemorrhage and hematoma of a digestive system organ or structure complicating a digestive system procedure**

    K91.62   **Intraoperative hemorrhage and hematoma of a digestive system organ or structure complicating other procedure**

√5ᵗʰ **K91.7**   **Accidental puncture and laceration of a digestive system organ or structure during a procedure**

    K91.71   **Accidental puncture and laceration of a digestive system organ or structure during a digestive system procedure**

    K91.72   **Accidental puncture and laceration of a digestive system organ or structure during other procedure**

√5ᵗʰ **K91.8**   **Other intraoperative and postprocedural complications and disorders of digestive system**

    K91.81   **Other intraoperative complications of digestive system**

    K91.82   **Postprocedural hepatic failure**

    K91.83   **Postprocedural hepatorenal syndrome**

▲   √6ᵗʰ **K91.84**   **Postprocedural hemorrhage of a digestive system organ or structure following a procedure**

▲   **K91.840**   **Postprocedural hemorrhage of a digestive system organ or structure following a digestive system procedure**
>   **AHA:** 2016,1Q,15

▲   **K91.841**   **Postprocedural hemorrhage of a digestive system organ or structure following other procedure**

    √6ᵗʰ **K91.85**   **Complications of intestinal pouch**

      K91.850   **Pouchitis**
> Inflammation of internal ileoanal pouch
> **DEF:** Inflammatory complication of an existing surgically created ileoanal pouch, resulting in multiple GI complaints, including diarrhea, abdominal pain, rectal bleeding, fecal urgency, or incontinence.

      K91.858   **Other complications of intestinal pouch**

    K91.86   **Retained cholelithiasis following cholecystectomy**

●   **K91.87**   **Postprocedural hematoma and seroma of a digestive system organ or structure following a procedure**

●   **K91.870**   **Postprocedural hematoma of a digestive system organ or structure following a digestive system procedure**

●   **K91.871**   **Postprocedural hematoma of a digestive system organ or structure following other procedure**

●   **K91.872**   **Postprocedural seroma of a digestive system organ or structure following a digestive system procedure**

●   **K91.873**   **Postprocedural seroma of a digestive system organ or structure following other procedure**

    K91.89   **Other postprocedural complications and disorders of digestive system**
> Use additional code, if applicable, to further specify disorder
> EXCLUDES 2   *postprocedural retroperitoneal abscess (K68.11)*

√4ᵗʰ **K92**   **Other diseases of digestive system**
> EXCLUDES 1   *neonatal gastrointestinal hemorrhage (P54.0-P54.3)*

K92.0   **Hematemesis**

K92.1   **Melena**
> EXCLUDES 1   *occult blood in feces (R19.5)*

K92.2   **Gastrointestinal hemorrhage, unspecified**   ▽
> Gastric hemorrhage NOS
> Intestinal hemorrhage NOS
> EXCLUDES 1   *acute hemorrhagic gastritis (K29.01)*
> *hemorrhage of anus and rectum (K62.5)*
> *angiodysplasia of stomach with hemorrhage (K31.811)*
> *diverticular disease with hemorrhage (K57.-)*
> *gastritis and duodenitis with hemorrhage (K29.-)*
> *peptic ulcer with hemorrhage (K25-K28)*

√5ᵗʰ **K92.8**   **Other specified diseases of the digestive system**

    K92.81   **Gastrointestinal mucositis (ulcerative)**
> Code also type of associated therapy, such as:
> antineoplastic and immunosuppressive drugs (T45.1X-)
> radiological procedure and radiotherapy (Y84.2)
> EXCLUDES 2   *mucositis (ulcerative) of vagina and vulva (N76.81)*
> *nasal mucositis (ulcerative) (J34.81)*
> *oral mucositis (ulcerative) (K12.3-)*

    K92.89   **Other specified diseases of the digestive system**

K92.9   **Disease of digestive system, unspecified**   ▽

√4ᵗʰ **K94**   **Complications of artificial openings of the digestive system**

√5ᵗʰ **K94.0**   **Colostomy complications**

    K94.00   **Colostomy complication, unspecified**   ▽

    K94.01   **Colostomy hemorrhage**

    K94.02   **Colostomy infection**
> Use additional code to specify type of infection, such as:
> cellulitis of abdominal wall (L03.311)
> sepsis (A40.-, A41.-)

    K94.03   **Colostomy malfunction**
> Mechanical complication of colostomy

    K94.09   **Other complications of colostomy**

√5ᵗʰ **K94.1**   **Enterostomy complications**

    K94.10   **Enterostomy complication, unspecified**   ▽

    K94.11   **Enterostomy hemorrhage**

    K94.12   **Enterostomy infection**
> Use additional code to specify type of infection, such as:
> cellulitis of abdominal wall (L03.311)
> sepsis (A40.-, A41.-)

    K94.13   **Enterostomy malfunction**
> Mechanical complication of enterostomy

    K94.19   **Other complications of enterostomy**

√5ᵗʰ **K94.2**   **Gastrostomy complications**

    K94.20   **Gastrostomy complication, unspecified**   ▽

    K94.21   **Gastrostomy hemorrhage**

    K94.22   **Gastrostomy infection**
> Use additional code to specify type of infection, such as:
> cellulitis of abdominal wall (L03.311)
> sepsis (A40.-, A41.-)

    K94.23   **Gastrostomy malfunction**
> Mechanical complication of gastrostomy

    K94.29   **Other complications of gastrostomy**

√5ᵗʰ **K94.3**   **Esophagostomy complications**

    K94.30   **Esophagostomy complications, unspecified**   ▽

    K94.31   **Esophagostomy hemorrhage**

    K94.32   **Esophagostomy infection**
> Use additional code to identify the infection

    K94.33   **Esophagostomy malfunction**
> Mechanical complication of esophagostomy

    K94.39   **Other complications of esophagostomy**

√4ᵗʰ **K95**   **Complications of bariatric procedures**

√5ᵗʰ **K95.0**   **Complications of gastric band procedure**

    K95.01   **Infection due to gastric band procedure**
> Use additional code to specify type of infection or organism, such as:
> bacterial and viral infectious agents (B95.-, B96.-)
> cellulitis of abdominal wall (L03.311)
> sepsis (A40.-, A41.-)

EXCLUDES 1   Not coded here   EXCLUDES 2   Not included here   N Newborn Age : 0   P Pediatric Age : 0-17   M Maternity Age : 12-55   A Adult Age : 15-124

676   ICD-10-CM 2017

K95.09   **Other complications of gastric band procedure**
Use additional code, if applicable, to further specify complication

☑5ᵗʰ **K95.8**   **Complications of other bariatric procedure**

　　EXCLUDES 1   *complications of gastric band surgery (K95.0-)*

K95.81   **Infection due to other bariatric procedure**
Use additional code to specify type of infection or organism, such as:
bacterial and viral infectious agents (B95.-, B96.-)
cellulitis of abdominal wall (L03.311)
sepsis (A40.-, A41.-)

K95.89   **Other complications of other bariatric procedure**
Use additional code, if applicable, to further specify complication

☑ Additional Character Required　　☑7ᵗʰ Placeholder Alert　　Manifestation Dx　　▽ Unspecified Dx　　▶◀ Revised Text　　● New Code　　▲ Revised Code Title

ICD-10-CM 2017　　**677**

Chapter 12. Diseases of the Skin and Subcutaneous Tissue (L00–L99)

Chapter Specific Guidelines with Coding Examples

The chapter specific guidelines from the ICD-10-CM Official Guidelines for Coding and Reporting have been provided below. Along with these guidelines are coding examples, contained in the shaded boxes, that have been developed to help illustrate the coding and/or sequencing guidance found in these guidelines.

a. Pressure ulcer stage codes

1) Pressure ulcer stages

Codes from category L89, Pressure ulcer, identify the site of the pressure ulcer as well as the stage of the ulcer.

The ICD-10-CM classifies pressure ulcer stages based on severity, which is designated by stages 1-4, unspecified stage and unstageable.

Assign as many codes from category L89 as needed to identify all the pressure ulcers the patient has, if applicable.

> Stage 4 pressure ulcer right heel, 9 x 10 cm that invades the muscle and fascia; stage 2 pressure ulcer of left elbow
>
> **L89.614**   **Pressure ulcer of right heel, stage 4**
>
> **L89.022**   **Pressure ulcer of left elbow, stage 2**
>
> *Explanation:* Patient has a right heel pressure ulcer documented as stage 4 and a left elbow pressure ulcer documented as stage 2. Combination codes from category L89 Pressure ulcer, identify the site of the pressure ulcer as well as the stage. Assign as many codes from category L89 as needed to identify all the pressure ulcers the patient has.

2) Unstageable pressure ulcers

Assignment of the code for unstageable pressure ulcer (L89.--0) should be based on the clinical documentation. These codes are used for pressure ulcers whose stage cannot be clinically determined (e.g., the ulcer is covered by eschar or has been treated with a skin or muscle graft) and pressure ulcers that are documented as deep tissue injury but not documented as due to trauma. This code should not be confused with the codes for unspecified stage (L89.--9). When there is no documentation regarding the stage of the pressure ulcer, assign the appropriate code for unspecified stage (L89.--9).

> Pressure ulcer of the right lower back documented as unstageable due to the presence of thick eschar covering the ulcer
>
> **L89.130**   **Pressure ulcer of right lower back, unstageable**
>
> *Explanation:* Codes for unstageable pressure ulcers are assigned when the stage cannot be clinically determined (e.g., the ulcer is covered by eschar or has been treated with a skin or muscle graft).

3) Documented pressure ulcer stage

Assignment of the pressure ulcer stage code should be guided by clinical documentation of the stage or documentation of the terms found in the Alphabetic Index. For clinical terms describing the stage that are not found in the Alphabetic Index, and there is no documentation of the stage, the provider should be queried.

> Left heel pressure ulcer with partial thickness skin loss involving the dermis
>
> **L89.622**   **Pressure ulcer of left heel, stage 2**
>
> *Explanation:* Code assignment for the pressure ulcer stage should be guided by either the clinical documentation of the stage or the documentation of terms found in the Alphabetic Index. The clinical documentation describing the left heel pressure ulcer "partial thickness skin loss involving the dermis" matches the ICD-10-CM index parenthetical description for stage 2 "(abrasion, blister, partial thickness skin loss involving epidermis and/or dermis)."

4) Patients admitted with pressure ulcers documented as healed

No code is assigned if the documentation states that the pressure ulcer is completely healed.

> Patient receiving follow-up examination of a completely healed pressure ulcer of the foot
>
> **Z09**   **Encounter for follow-up examination after completed treatment for conditions other than malignant neoplasm**
>
> **Z87.2**   **Personal history of diseases of the skin and subcutaneous tissue**
>
> *Explanation:* Assign only codes for the reason for the encounter and the personal history of the pressure ulcer. Personal history code Z87.2 includes conditions classifiable to L00–L99 such as pressure ulcer. No code is assigned for a pressure ulcer documented as completely healed.

5) Patients admitted with pressure ulcers documented as healing

Pressure ulcers described as healing should be assigned the appropriate pressure ulcer stage code based on the documentation in the medical record. If the documentation does not provide information about the stage of the healing pressure ulcer, assign the appropriate code for unspecified stage.

If the documentation is unclear as to whether the patient has a current (new) pressure ulcer or if the patient is being treated for a healing pressure ulcer, query the provider.

For ulcers that were present on admission but healed at the time of discharge, assign the code for the site and stage of the pressure ulcer at the time of admission.

> Healing stage 2 sacral pressure ulcer, resolved at time of discharge
>
> **L89.152**   **Pressure ulcer of sacral region, stage 2**
>
> *Explanation:* Although completely healed upon discharge, the pressure ulcer required observation and/or treatment and should be coded based on the site and stage upon admission.

6) Patient admitted with pressure ulcer evolving into another stage during the admission

If a patient is admitted with a pressure ulcer at one stage and it progresses to a higher stage, **two separate codes should be assigned: one code for the site and stage of the ulcer on admission and a second code for the same ulcer site and the highest stage reported during the stay.**

> Stage 3 right hip pressure ulcer worsened during admission to a stage 4
>
> **L89.213**   **Pressure ulcer of right hip, stage 3**
>
> **L89.214**   **Pressure ulcer of right hip, stage 4**
>
> *Explanation:* A pressure ulcer that progresses from a lower stage to a higher stage is assigned two codes, one for the documented stage upon admission and one for the documented stage at discharge.

Chapter 12. Diseases of the Skin and Subcutaneous Tissue (L00-L99)

EXCLUDES 2   *certain conditions originating in the perinatal period (P04-P96)*
certain infectious and parasitic diseases (A00-B99)
complications of pregnancy, childbirth and the puerperium (O00-O9A)
congenital malformations, deformations, and chromosomal abnormalities (Q00-Q99)
endocrine, nutritional and metabolic diseases (E00-E88)
lipomelanotic reticulosis (I89.8)
neoplasms (C00-D49)
symptoms, signs and abnormal clinical and laboratory findings, not elsewhere classified (R00-R94)
systemic connective tissue disorders (M30-M36)
viral warts (B07.-)

This chapter contains the following blocks:

L00-L08   Infections of the skin and subcutaneous tissue
L10-L14   Bullous disorders
L20-L30   Dermatitis and eczema
L40-L45   Papulosquamous disorders
L49-L54   Urticaria and erythema
L55-L59   Radiation-related disorders of the skin and subcutaneous tissue
L60-L75   Disorders of skin appendages
L76   Intraoperative and postprocedural complications of skin and subcutaneous tissue
L80-L99   Other disorders of the skin and subcutaneous tissue

Infections of the skin and subcutaneous tissue (L00-L08)

Use additional code (B95-B97) to identify infectious agent
EXCLUDES 2   *hordeolum (H00.0)*
infective dermatitis (L30.3)
local infections of skin classified in Chapter 1
lupus panniculitis (L93.2)
panniculitis NOS (M79.3)
panniculitis of neck and back (M54.0-)
perlèche NOS (K13.0)
perlèche due to candidiasis (B37.0)
perlèche due to riboflavin deficiency (E53.0)
pyogenic granuloma (L98.0)
relapsing panniculitis [Weber-Christian] (M35.6)
viral warts (B07.-)
zoster (B02.-)

L00   **Staphylococcal scalded skin syndrome**
Ritter's disease
Use additional code to identify percentage of skin exfoliation (L49.-)
EXCLUDES 1   *bullous impetigo (L01.03)*
pemphigus neonatorum (L01.03)
toxic epidermal necrolysis [Lyell] (L51.2)

☑4th **L01**   **Impetigo**
EXCLUDES 1   *impetigo herpetiformis (L40.1)*

   ☑5th **L01.0**   **Impetigo**
Impetigo contagiosa
Impetigo vulgaris
    L01.00   **Impetigo, unspecified**   ▽
Impetigo NOS
    L01.01   **Non-bullous impetigo**
    L01.02   **Bockhart's impetigo**
Impetigo follicularis
Perifolliculitis NOS
Superficial pustular perifolliculitis
    L01.03   **Bullous impetigo**
Impetigo neonatorum
Pemphigus neonatorum
    L01.09   **Other impetigo**
Ulcerative impetigo
   L01.1   **Impetiginization of other dermatoses**

☑4th **L02**   **Cutaneous abscess, furuncle and carbuncle**
Use additional code to identify organism (B95-B96)
EXCLUDES 2   *abscess of anus and rectal regions (K61.-)*
abscess of female genital organs (external) (N76.4)
abscess of male genital organs (external) (N48.2, N49.-)

   ☑5th **L02.0**   **Cutaneous abscess, furuncle and carbuncle of face**
EXCLUDES 2   *abscess of ear, external (H60.0)*
abscess of eyelid (H00.0)
abscess of head [any part, except face] (L02.8)
abscess of lacrimal gland (H04.0)
abscess of lacrimal passages (H04.3)
abscess of mouth (K12.2)
abscess of nose (J34.0)
abscess of orbit (H05.0)
submandibular abscess (K12.2)
    L02.01   **Cutaneous abscess of face**
    L02.02   **Furuncle of face**
Boil of face
Folliculitis of face
    L02.03   **Carbuncle of face**

   ☑5th **L02.1**   **Cutaneous abscess, furuncle and carbuncle of neck**
    L02.11   **Cutaneous abscess of neck**
    L02.12   **Furuncle of neck**
Boil of neck
Folliculitis of neck
    L02.13   **Carbuncle of neck**

   ☑5th **L02.2**   **Cutaneous abscess, furuncle and carbuncle of trunk**
EXCLUDES 1   *non-newborn omphalitis (L08.82)*
omphalitis of newborn (P38.-)
EXCLUDES 2   *abscess of breast ►(N61.1)◄*
abscess of buttocks (L02.3)
abscess of female external genital organs (N76.4)
abscess of hip (L02.4)
abscess of male external genital organs (N48.2, N49.-)

    ☑6th **L02.21**   **Cutaneous abscess of trunk**
     L02.211   **Cutaneous abscess of abdominal wall**
     L02.212   **Cutaneous abscess of back [any part, except buttock]**
     L02.213   **Cutaneous abscess of chest wall**
     L02.214   **Cutaneous abscess of groin**
     L02.215   **Cutaneous abscess of perineum**
     L02.216   **Cutaneous abscess of umbilicus**
     L02.219   **Cutaneous abscess of trunk, unspecified**   ▽

    ☑6th **L02.22**   **Furuncle of trunk**
Boil of trunk
Folliculitis of trunk
     L02.221   **Furuncle of abdominal wall**
     L02.222   **Furuncle of back [any part, except buttock]**
     L02.223   **Furuncle of chest wall**
     L02.224   **Furuncle of groin**
     L02.225   **Furuncle of perineum**
     L02.226   **Furuncle of umbilicus**
     L02.229   **Furuncle of trunk, unspecified**   ▽

    ☑6th **L02.23**   **Carbuncle of trunk**
     L02.231   **Carbuncle of abdominal wall**
     L02.232   **Carbuncle of back [any part, except buttock]**
     L02.233   **Carbuncle of chest wall**
     L02.234   **Carbuncle of groin**
     L02.235   **Carbuncle of perineum**
     L02.236   **Carbuncle of umbilicus**
     L02.239   **Carbuncle of trunk, unspecified**   ▽

   ☑5th **L02.3**   **Cutaneous abscess, furuncle and carbuncle of buttock**
EXCLUDES 1   *pilonidal cyst with abscess (L05.01)*
    L02.31   **Cutaneous abscess of buttock**
Cutaneous abscess of gluteal region
    L02.32   **Furuncle of buttock**
Boil of buttock
Folliculitis of buttock
Furuncle of gluteal region
    L02.33   **Carbuncle of buttock**
Carbuncle of gluteal region

   ☑5th **L02.4**   **Cutaneous abscess, furuncle and carbuncle of limb**
EXCLUDES 2   *cutaneous abscess, furuncle and carbuncle of groin (L02.214, L02.224, L02.234)*
cutaneous abscess, furuncle and carbuncle of hand (L02.5-)
cutaneous abscess, furuncle and carbuncle of foot (L02.6-)

☑ Additional Character Required   ☑x7th Placeholder Alert   Manifestation Dx   ▽ Unspecified Dx   ►◄ Revised Text   ● New Code   ▲ Revised Code Title

√6th **L02.41** Cutaneous abscess **of limb**
  L02.411 Cutaneous abscess of **right axilla**
  L02.412 Cutaneous abscess of **left axilla**
  L02.413 Cutaneous abscess of **right upper limb**
  L02.414 Cutaneous abscess of **left upper limb**
  L02.415 Cutaneous abscess of **right lower limb**
  L02.416 Cutaneous abscess of **left lower limb**
  L02.419 Cutaneous abscess **of limb, unspecified**   ▽

√6th **L02.42** Furuncle **of limb**
  Boil of limb
  Folliculitis of limb
  L02.421 Furuncle of **right axilla**
  L02.422 Furuncle of **left axilla**
  L02.423 Furuncle of **right upper limb**
  L02.424 Furuncle of **left upper limb**
  L02.425 Furuncle of **right lower limb**
  L02.426 Furuncle of **left lower limb**
  L02.429 Furuncle of limb, unspecified   ▽

√6th **L02.43** Carbuncle **of limb**
  L02.431 Carbuncle of **right axilla**
  L02.432 Carbuncle of **left axilla**
  L02.433 Carbuncle of **right upper limb**
  L02.434 Carbuncle of **left upper limb**
  L02.435 Carbuncle of **right lower limb**
  L02.436 Carbuncle of **left lower limb**
  L02.439 Carbuncle of limb, unspecified   ▽

√5th **L02.5** Cutaneous abscess, furuncle and carbuncle of **hand**

√6th **L02.51** Cutaneous abscess **of hand**
  L02.511 Cutaneous abscess of **right hand**
  L02.512 Cutaneous abscess of **left hand**
  L02.519 Cutaneous abscess of unspecified hand   ▽

√6th **L02.52** Furuncle **hand**
  Boil of hand
  Folliculitis of hand
  L02.521 Furuncle **right hand**
  L02.522 Furuncle **left hand**
  L02.529 Furuncle unspecified hand   ▽

√6th **L02.53** Carbuncle **of hand**
  L02.531 Carbuncle of **right hand**
  L02.532 Carbuncle of **left hand**
  L02.539 Carbuncle of unspecified hand   ▽

√5th **L02.6** Cutaneous abscess, furuncle and carbuncle of **foot**

√6th **L02.61** Cutaneous abscess **of foot**
  L02.611 Cutaneous abscess of **right foot**
  L02.612 Cutaneous abscess of **left foot**
  L02.619 Cutaneous abscess of unspecified foot   ▽

√6th **L02.62** Furuncle **of foot**
  Boil of foot
  Folliculitis of foot
  L02.621 Furuncle of **right foot**
  L02.622 Furuncle of **left foot**
  L02.629 Furuncle of unspecified foot   ▽

√6th **L02.63** Carbuncle **of foot**
  L02.631 Carbuncle of **right foot**
  L02.632 Carbuncle of **left foot**
  L02.639 Carbuncle of unspecified foot   ▽

√5th **L02.8** Cutaneous abscess, furuncle and carbuncle of other sites

√6th **L02.81** Cutaneous abscess **of other sites**
  L02.811 Cutaneous abscess of **head [any part, except face]**
  L02.818 Cutaneous abscess of **other sites**

√6th **L02.82** Furuncle **of other sites**
  Boil of other sites
  Folliculitis of other sites
  L02.821 Furuncle of **head [any part, except face]**
  L02.828 Furuncle of **other sites**

√6th **L02.83** Carbuncle **of other sites**
  L02.831 Carbuncle of **head [any part, except face]**
  L02.838 Carbuncle of **other sites**

√5th **L02.9** Cutaneous abscess, furuncle and carbuncle, unspecified
  L02.91 Cutaneous abscess, **unspecified**   ▽
  L02.92 Furuncle, **unspecified**   ▽
    Boil NOS
    Furunculosis NOS
  L02.93 Carbuncle, **unspecified**   ▽

√4th **L03** Cellulitis and acute lymphangitis
  EXCLUDES 2 cellulitis of anal and rectal region (K61.-)
    cellulitis of external auditory canal (H60.1)
    cellulitis of eyelid (H00.0)
    cellulitis of female external genital organs (N76.4)
    cellulitis of lacrimal apparatus (H04.3)
    cellulitis of male external genital organs (N48.2, N49.-)
    cellulitis of mouth (K12.2)
    cellulitis of nose (J34.0)
    eosinophilic cellulitis [Wells] (L98.3)
    febrile neutrophilic dermatosis [Sweet] (L98.2)
    lymphangitis (chronic) (subacute) (I89.1)

√5th **L03.0** Cellulitis and acute lymphangitis of **finger and toe**
  Infection of nail   Paronychia
  Onychia   Perionychia

√6th **L03.01** Cellulitis **of finger**
  Felon
  Whitlow
  EXCLUDES 1 herpetic whitlow (B00.89)
  DEF: Felon: Superficial bacterial skin infection at the tip of the finger.
  L03.011 Cellulitis of **right finger**
  L03.012 Cellulitis of **left finger**
  L03.019 Cellulitis of **unspecified finger**   ▽

√6th **L03.02** Acute lymphangitis **of finger**
  Hangnail with lymphangitis of finger
  L03.021 Acute lymphangitis of **right finger**
  L03.022 Acute lymphangitis of **left finger**
  L03.029 Acute lymphangitis of unspecified finger   ▽

√6th **L03.03** Cellulitis **of toe**
  L03.031 Cellulitis of **right toe**
  L03.032 Cellulitis of **left toe**
  L03.039 Cellulitis of **unspecified toe**   ▽

√6th **L03.04** Acute lymphangitis **of toe**
  Hangnail with lymphangitis of toe
  L03.041 Acute lymphangitis of **right toe**
  L03.042 Acute lymphangitis of **left toe**
  L03.049 Acute lymphangitis of unspecified toe   ▽

√5th **L03.1** Cellulitis and acute lymphangitis of other parts of limb

√6th **L03.11** Cellulitis **of other parts of limb**
  EXCLUDES 2 cellulitis of fingers (L03.01-)
    cellulitis of toes (L03.03-)
    groin (L03.314)
  L03.111 Cellulitis of **right axilla**
  L03.112 Cellulitis of **left axilla**
  L03.113 Cellulitis of **right upper limb**
  L03.114 Cellulitis of **left upper limb**
  L03.115 Cellulitis of **right lower limb**
  L03.116 Cellulitis of **left lower limb**
  L03.119 Cellulitis of **unspecified part of limb**   ▽

√6th **L03.12** Acute lymphangitis **of other parts of limb**
  EXCLUDES 2 acute lymphangitis of fingers (L03.2-)
    acute lymphangitis of groin (L03.324)
    acute lymphangitis of toes (L03.04-)
  L03.121 Acute lymphangitis of **right axilla**
  L03.122 Acute lymphangitis of **left axilla**
  L03.123 Acute lymphangitis of **right upper limb**
  L03.124 Acute lymphangitis of **left upper limb**
  L03.125 Acute lymphangitis of **right lower limb**
  L03.126 Acute lymphangitis of **left lower limb**
  L03.129 Acute lymphangitis of unspecified part of limb   ▽

√6th **L03.2** Cellulitis and acute lymphangitis of **face and neck**

√6th **L03.21** Cellulitis and acute lymphangitis of **face**

L03.211 Cellulitis of face
> EXCLUDES 2 ▶abscess of orbit (H05.01-)◀
> cellulitis of ear (H60.1-)
> cellulitis of eyelid (H00.0-)
> cellulitis of head (L03.81)
> cellulitis of lacrimal apparatus (H04.3)
> cellulitis of lip (K13.0)
> cellulitis of mouth (K12.2)
> cellulitis of nose (internal) (J34.0)
> cellulitis of orbit ▶(H05.01-)◀
> cellulitis of scalp (L03.81)

AHA: 2013,4Q,123

L03.212 Acute lymphangitis of face
L03.213 Periorbital cellulitis
     Preseptal cellulitis

✓6th **L03.22 Cellulitis and acute lymphangitis of neck**
L03.221 Cellulitis of neck
L03.222 Acute lymphangitis of neck

✓5th **L03.3 Cellulitis and acute lymphangitis of trunk**

✓6th **L03.31 Cellulitis of trunk**
> EXCLUDES 2 cellulitis of anal and rectal regions (K61.-)
> cellulitis of breast NOS ▶(N61.0)◀
> cellulitis of female external genital organs (N76.4)
> cellulitis of male external genital organs (N48.2, N49.-)
> omphalitis of newborn (P38.-)
> puerperal cellulitis of breast (O91.2)

L03.311 Cellulitis of abdominal wall
> EXCLUDES 2 cellulitis of umbilicus (L03.316)
> cellulitis of groin (L03.314)

L03.312 Cellulitis of back [any part except buttock]
L03.313 Cellulitis of chest wall
L03.314 Cellulitis of groin
L03.315 Cellulitis of perineum
L03.316 Cellulitis of umbilicus
L03.317 Cellulitis of buttock
L03.319 Cellulitis of trunk, unspecified ▽

✓6th **L03.32 Acute lymphangitis of trunk**
L03.321 Acute lymphangitis of abdominal wall
L03.322 Acute lymphangitis of back [any part except buttock]
L03.323 Acute lymphangitis of chest wall
L03.324 Acute lymphangitis of groin
L03.325 Acute lymphangitis of perineum
L03.326 Acute lymphangitis of umbilicus
L03.327 Acute lymphangitis of buttock
L03.329 Acute lymphangitis of trunk, unspecified ▽

✓5th **L03.8 Cellulitis and acute lymphangitis of other sites**

✓6th **L03.81 Cellulitis of other sites**
L03.811 Cellulitis of head [any part, except face]
     Cellulitis of scalp
> EXCLUDES 2 cellulitis of face (L03.211)

L03.818 Cellulitis of other sites

✓6th **L03.89 Acute lymphangitis of other sites**
L03.891 Acute lymphangitis of head [any part, except face]
L03.898 Acute lymphangitis of other sites

✓5th **L03.9 Cellulitis and acute lymphangitis, unspecified**
L03.90 Cellulitis, unspecified ▽
L03.91 Acute lymphangitis, unspecified ▽
> EXCLUDES 1 lymphangitis NOS (I89.1)

✓4th **L04 Acute lymphadenitis**
> INCLUDES abscess (acute) of lymph nodes, except mesenteric
> acute lymphadenitis, except mesenteric
> EXCLUDES 1 chronic or subacute lymphadenitis, except mesenteric (I88.1)
> enlarged lymph nodes (R59.-)
> human immunodeficiency virus [HIV] disease resulting in generalized lymphadenopathy (B20)
> lymphadenitis NOS (I88.9)
> nonspecific mesenteric lymphadenitis (I88.0)

L04.0 Acute lymphadenitis of face, head and neck
L04.1 Acute lymphadenitis of trunk

L04.2 Acute lymphadenitis of upper limb
     Acute lymphadenitis of axilla
     Acute lymphadenitis of shoulder

L04.3 Acute lymphadenitis of lower limb
     Acute lymphadenitis of hip
> EXCLUDES 2 acute lymphadenitis of groin (L04.1)

L04.8 Acute lymphadenitis of other sites
L04.9 Acute lymphadenitis, unspecified ▽

✓4th **L05 Pilonidal cyst and sinus**

✓5th **L05.0 Pilonidal cyst and sinus with abscess**
L05.01 Pilonidal cyst with abscess
     Pilonidal abscess
     Pilonidal dimple with abscess
     Postanal dimple with abscess
> EXCLUDES 2 ▶congenital sacral dimple (Q82.6)◀
> ▶parasacral dimple (Q82.6)◀

L05.02 Pilonidal sinus with abscess
     Coccygeal fistula with abscess
     Coccygeal sinus with abscess
     Pilonidal fistula with abscess

✓5th **L05.9 Pilonidal cyst and sinus without abscess**
L05.91 Pilonidal cyst without abscess
     Pilonidal dimple
     Postanal dimple
     Pilonidal cyst NOS
> EXCLUDES 2 ▶congenital sacral dimple (Q82.6)◀
> ▶parasacral dimple (Q82.6)◀

L05.92 Pilonidal sinus without abscess
     Coccygeal fistula
     Coccygeal sinus without abscess
     Pilonidal fistula

✓4th **L08 Other local infections of skin and subcutaneous tissue**
L08.0 Pyoderma
     Dermatitis gangrenosa
     Purulent dermatitis
     Septic dermatitis
     Suppurative dermatitis
> EXCLUDES 1 pyoderma gangrenosum (L88)
> pyoderma vegetans (L08.81)

L08.1 Erythrasma
✓5th **L08.8 Other specified local infections of the skin and subcutaneous tissue**
L08.81 Pyoderma vegetans
> EXCLUDES 1 pyoderma gangrenosum (L88)
> pyoderma NOS (L08.0)

L08.82 Omphalitis not of newborn
> EXCLUDES 1 omphalitis of newborn (P38.-)

L08.89 Other specified local infections of the skin and subcutaneous tissue

L08.9 Local infection of the skin and subcutaneous tissue, unspecified ▽

Bullous disorders (L10-L14)

> EXCLUDES 1 benign familial pemphigus [Hailey-Hailey] (Q82.8)
> staphylococcal scalded skin syndrome (L00)
> toxic epidermal necrolysis [Lyell] (L51.2)

✓4th **L10 Pemphigus**
> EXCLUDES 1 pemphigus neonatorum (L01.03)

L10.0 Pemphigus vulgaris
L10.1 Pemphigus vegetans
L10.2 Pemphigus foliaceous
L10.3 Brazilian pemphigus [fogo selvagem]
L10.4 Pemphigus erythematosus
     Senear-Usher syndrome
L10.5 Drug-induced pemphigus
     Use additional code for adverse effect, if applicable, to identify drug (T36-T50 with fifth or sixth character 5)

✓5th **L10.8 Other pemphigus**
L10.81 Paraneoplastic pemphigus
L10.89 Other pemphigus
L10.9 Pemphigus, unspecified ▽

✓4th **L11 Other acantholytic disorders**
L11.0 Acquired keratosis follicularis
> EXCLUDES 1 keratosis follicularis (congenital) [Darier-White] (Q82.8)

L11.1 Transient acantholytic dermatosis [Grover]

☑ Additional Character Required   ✓7th Placeholder Alert   Manifestation Dx   ▽ Unspecified Dx   ▶◀ Revised Text   ● New Code   ▲ Revised Code Title

L11.8   Other specified acantholytic disorders

L11.9   Acantholytic disorder, unspecified   ▽

√4ᵗʰ **L12   Pemphigoid**

> *EXCLUDES 1*   herpes gestationis (O26.4-)
> impetigo herpetiformis (L40.1)

L12.0   Bullous pemphigoid

L12.1   Cicatricial pemphigoid
> Benign mucous membrane pemphigoid

L12.2   Chronic bullous disease of childhood   Ⓟ
> Juvenile dermatitis herpetiformis

√5ᵗʰ **L12.3   Acquired epidermolysis bullosa**
> *EXCLUDES 1*   epidermolysis bullosa (congenital) (Q81.-)

    L12.30   Acquired epidermolysis bullosa, unspecified   ▽

    L12.31   Epidermolysis bullosa due to drug
> Use additional code for adverse effect, if applicable, to identify drug (T36-T50 with fifth or sixth character 5)

    L12.35   Other acquired epidermolysis bullosa

L12.8   Other pemphigoid

L12.9   Pemphigoid, unspecified   ▽

√4ᵗʰ **L13   Other bullous disorders**

L13.0   Dermatitis herpetiformis
> Duhring's disease
> Hydroa herpetiformis
> *EXCLUDES 1*   juvenile dermatitis herpetiformis (L12.2)
>   senile dermatitis herpetiformis (L12.0)
> **DEF:** Skin disease to which people are genetically predisposed resulting from an immunological response to gluten; seen as an extremely pruritic eruption of various lesions that frequently heal, leaving hyperpigmentation or hypopigmentation and occasionally scarring; usually associated with an asymptomatic gluten-sensitive enteropathy.

L13.1   Subcorneal pustular dermatitis
> Sneddon-Wilkinson disease

L13.8   Other specified bullous disorders

L13.9   Bullous disorder, unspecified   ▽

L14   *Bullous disorders in diseases classified elsewhere*
> Code first underlying disease

Dermatitis and eczema (L20-L30)

> **NOTE**   In this block the terms dermatitis and eczema are used synonymously and interchangeably.
>
> *EXCLUDES 2*   chronic (childhood) granulomatous disease (D71)
>   dermatitis gangrenosa (L08.0)
>   dermatitis herpetiformis (L13.0)
>   dry skin dermatitis (L85.3)
>   factitial dermatitis (L98.1)
>   perioral dermatitis (L71.0)
>   radiation-related disorders of the skin and subcutaneous tissue (L55-L59)
>   stasis dermatitis ▶(I87.2)◀

√4ᵗʰ **L20   Atopic dermatitis**

L20.0   Besnier's prurigo

√5ᵗʰ **L20.8   Other atopic dermatitis**
> *EXCLUDES 2*   circumscribed neurodermatitis (L28.0)

    L20.81   Atopic neurodermatitis
> Diffuse neurodermatitis

    L20.82   Flexural eczema

    L20.83   Infantile (acute) (chronic) eczema   Ⓟ

    L20.84   Intrinsic (allergic) eczema

    L20.89   Other atopic dermatitis

L20.9   Atopic dermatitis, unspecified   ▽

√4ᵗʰ **L21   Seborrheic dermatitis**
> *EXCLUDES 2*   infective dermatitis (L30.3)
>   seborrheic keratosis (L82.-)

L21.0   Seborrhea capitis   Ⓟ
> Cradle cap

L21.1   Seborrheic infantile dermatitis   Ⓟ

L21.8   Other seborrheic dermatitis

L21.9   Seborrheic dermatitis, unspecified   ▽
> Seborrhea NOS

L22   Diaper dermatitis
> Diaper erythema
> Diaper rash
> Psoriasiform diaper rash

√4ᵗʰ **L23   Allergic contact dermatitis**
> *EXCLUDES 1*   allergy NOS (T78.40)
>   contact dermatitis NOS (L25.9)
>   dermatitis NOS (L30.9)
> *EXCLUDES 2*   dermatitis due to substances taken internally (L27.-)
>   dermatitis of eyelid (H01.1-)
>   diaper dermatitis (L22)
>   eczema of external ear (H60.5-)
>   irritant contact dermatitis (L24.-)
>   perioral dermatitis (L71.0)
>   radiation-related disorders of the skin and subcutaneous tissue (L55-L59)

L23.0   Allergic contact dermatitis due to metals
> Allergic contact dermatitis due to chromium
> Allergic contact dermatitis due to nickel

L23.1   Allergic contact dermatitis due to adhesives

L23.2   Allergic contact dermatitis due to cosmetics

L23.3   Allergic contact dermatitis due to drugs in contact with skin
> Use additional code for adverse effect, if applicable, to identify drug (T36-T50 with fifth or sixth character 5)
> *EXCLUDES 2*   dermatitis due to ingested drugs and medicaments (L27.0-L27.1)

L23.4   Allergic contact dermatitis due to dyes

L23.5   Allergic contact dermatitis due to other chemical products
> Allergic contact dermatitis due to cement
> Allergic contact dermatitis due to insecticide
> Allergic contact dermatitis due to plastic
> Allergic contact dermatitis due to rubber

L23.6   Allergic contact dermatitis due to food in contact with the skin
> *EXCLUDES 2*   dermatitis due to ingested food (L27.2)

L23.7   Allergic contact dermatitis due to plants, except food
> *EXCLUDES 2*   allergy NOS due to pollen (J30.1)

√5ᵗʰ **L23.8   Allergic contact dermatitis due to other agents**

    L23.81   Allergic contact dermatitis due to animal (cat) (dog) dander
> Allergic contact dermatitis due to animal (cat) (dog) hair

    L23.89   Allergic contact dermatitis due to other agents

L23.9   Allergic contact dermatitis, unspecified cause   ▽
> Allergic contact eczema NOS

√4ᵗʰ **L24   Irritant contact dermatitis**
> *EXCLUDES 1*   allergy NOS (T78.40)
>   contact dermatitis NOS (L25.9)
>   dermatitis NOS (L30.9)
> *EXCLUDES 2*   allergic contact dermatitis (L23.-)
>   dermatitis due to substances taken internally (L27.-)
>   dermatitis of eyelid (H01.1-)
>   diaper dermatitis (L22)
>   eczema of external ear (H60.5-)
>   perioral dermatitis (L71.0)
>   radiation-related disorders of the skin and subcutaneous tissue (L55-L59)

L24.0   Irritant contact dermatitis due to detergents

L24.1   Irritant contact dermatitis due to oils and greases

L24.2   Irritant contact dermatitis due to solvents
> Irritant contact dermatitis due to chlorocompound
> Irritant contact dermatitis due to cyclohexane
> Irritant contact dermatitis due to ester
> Irritant contact dermatitis due to glycol
> Irritant contact dermatitis due to hydrocarbon
> Irritant contact dermatitis due to ketone

L24.3   Irritant contact dermatitis due to cosmetics

L24.4   Irritant contact dermatitis due to drugs in contact with skin
> Use additional code for adverse effect, if applicable, to identify drug (T36-T50 with fifth or sixth character 5)

L24.5   Irritant contact dermatitis due to other chemical products
> Irritant contact dermatitis due to cement
> Irritant contact dermatitis due to insecticide
> Irritant contact dermatitis due to plastic
> Irritant contact dermatitis due to rubber

EXCLUDES 1 Not coded here   *EXCLUDES 2* Not included here   Ⓝ Newborn Age : 0   Ⓟ Pediatric Age : 0-17   Ⓜ Maternity Age : 12-55   Ⓐ Adult Age : 15-124

682   ICD-10-CM 2017

L24.6   **Irritant contact dermatitis due to** food in contact with skin
    EXCLUDES 2   *dermatitis due to ingested food (L27.2)*

L24.7   **Irritant contact dermatitis due to** plants, except food
    EXCLUDES 2   *allergy NOS to pollen (J30.1)*

√5ᵗʰ **L24.8**   **Irritant contact dermatitis due to other agents**

    L24.81   **Irritant contact dermatitis due to** metals
       Irritant contact dermatitis due to chromium
       Irritant contact dermatitis due to nickel

    L24.89   **Irritant contact dermatitis due to other agents**
       Irritant contact dermatitis due to dyes

L24.9   **Irritant contact dermatitis, unspecified cause** ▽
    Irritant contact eczema NOS

√4ᵗʰ **L25**   **Unspecified contact dermatitis**
    EXCLUDES 1   *allergic contact dermatitis (L23.-)*
       allergy NOS (T78.40)
       dermatitis NOS (L30.9)
       irritant contact dermatitis (L24.-)
    EXCLUDES 2   *dermatitis due to ingested substances (L27.-)*
       dermatitis of eyelid (H01.1-)
       eczema of external ear (H60.5-)
       perioral dermatitis (L71.0)
       radiation-related disorders of the skin and subcutaneous tissue (L55-L59)

L25.0   **Unspecified contact dermatitis due to** cosmetics ▽

L25.1   **Unspecified contact dermatitis due to** drugs in contact with skin ▽
    Use additional code for adverse effect, if applicable, to identify drug (T36-T50 with fifth or sixth character 5)
    EXCLUDES 2   *dermatitis due to ingested drugs and medicaments (L27.0-L27.1)*

L25.2   **Unspecified contact dermatitis due to** dyes ▽

L25.3   **Unspecified contact dermatitis due to** other chemical products ▽
    Unspecified contact dermatitis due to cement
    Unspecified contact dermatitis due to insecticide

L25.4   **Unspecified contact dermatitis due to** food in contact with skin ▽
    EXCLUDES 2   *dermatitis due to ingested food (L27.2)*

L25.5   **Unspecified contact dermatitis due to** plants, except food ▽
    EXCLUDES 1   *nettle rash (L50.9)*
    EXCLUDES 2   *allergy NOS due to pollen (J30.1)*

L25.8   **Unspecified contact dermatitis due to other agents** ▽

L25.9   **Unspecified contact dermatitis, unspecified cause** ▽
    Contact dermatitis (occupational) NOS
    Contact eczema (occupational) NOS

L26   **Exfoliative** dermatitis
    Hebra's pityriasis
    EXCLUDES 1   *Ritter's disease (L00)*

√4ᵗʰ **L27**   **Dermatitis** due to substances taken internally
    EXCLUDES 1   *allergy NOS (T78.40)*
    EXCLUDES 2   *adverse food reaction, except dermatitis (T78.0-T78.1)*
       contact dermatitis (L23-L25)
       drug photoallergic response (L56.1)
       drug phototoxic response (L56.0)
       urticaria (L50.-)

L27.0   **Generalized** skin eruption due to drugs and medicaments taken internally
    Use additional code for adverse effect, if applicable, to identify drug (T36-T50 with fifth or sixth character 5)

L27.1   **Localized** skin eruption due to drugs and medicaments taken internally
    Use additional code for adverse effect, if applicable, to identify drug (T36-T50 with fifth or sixth character 5)

L27.2   **Dermatitis** due to ingested food
    EXCLUDES 2   *dermatitis due to food in contact with skin (L23.6, L24.6, L25.4)*

L27.8   **Dermatitis due to other substances taken internally**

L27.9   **Dermatitis due to unspecified substance taken internally** ▽

√4ᵗʰ **L28**   **Lichen simplex chronicus and prurigo**

L28.0   **Lichen simplex chronicus**
    Circumscribed neurodermatitis
    Lichen NOS

L28.1   **Prurigo nodularis**

L28.2   **Other prurigo**
    Prurigo NOS
    Prurigo Hebra
    Prurigo mitis
    Urticaria papulosa

√4ᵗʰ **L29**   **Pruritus**
    EXCLUDES 1   *neurotic excoriation (L98.1)*
       psychogenic pruritus (F45.8)

L29.0   **Pruritus** ani

L29.1   **Pruritus** scroti   ♂

L29.2   **Pruritus** vulvae   ♀

L29.3   **Anogenital** pruritus, unspecified ▽

L29.8   **Other pruritus**

L29.9   **Pruritus, unspecified** ▽
    Itch NOS

√4ᵗʰ **L30**   **Other and unspecified dermatitis**
    EXCLUDES 2   *contact dermatitis (L23-L25)*
       dry skin dermatitis (L85.3)
       small plaque parapsoriasis (L41.3)
       stasis dermatitis ▶(I87.2)◀

L30.0   **Nummular dermatitis**

L30.1   **Dyshidrosis [pompholyx]**

L30.2   **Cutaneous autosensitization**
    Candidid [levurid]
    Dermatophytid
    Eczematid

L30.3   **Infective dermatitis**
    Infectious eczematoid dermatitis

L30.4   **Erythema intertrigo**

L30.5   **Pityriasis alba**

L30.8   **Other specified dermatitis**

L30.9   **Dermatitis, unspecified** ▽
    Eczema NOS

Papulosquamous disorders (L40-L45)

√4ᵗʰ **L40**   **Psoriasis**

L40.0   **Psoriasis** vulgaris
    Nummular psoriasis
    Plaque psoriasis

L40.1   **Generalized pustular** psoriasis
    Impetigo herpetiformis
    Von Zumbusch's disease

L40.2   **Acrodermatitis continua**

L40.3   **Pustulosis palmaris et plantaris**

L40.4   **Guttate** psoriasis

√5ᵗʰ **L40.5**   **Arthropathic** psoriasis

    L40.50   **Arthropathic psoriasis, unspecified** ▽

    L40.51   **Distal interphalangeal** psoriatic arthropathy

    L40.52   **Psoriatic arthritis** mutilans

    L40.53   **Psoriatic** spondylitis

    L40.54   **Psoriatic** juvenile arthropathy

    L40.59   **Other psoriatic arthropathy**

L40.8   **Other psoriasis**
    Flexural psoriasis

L40.9   **Psoriasis, unspecified** ▽

√4ᵗʰ **L41**   **Parapsoriasis**
    EXCLUDES 1   *poikiloderma vasculare atrophicans (L94.5)*

L41.0   **Pityriasis lichenoides et varioliformis acuta**
    Mucha-Habermann disease

L41.1   **Pityriasis lichenoides chronica**

L41.3   **Small plaque** parapsoriasis

L41.4   **Large plaque** parapsoriasis

L41.5   **Retiform** parapsoriasis

L41.8   **Other parapsoriasis**

L41.9   **Parapsoriasis, unspecified** ▽

L42   **Pityriasis rosea**

√4ᵗʰ **L43**   **Lichen planus**
    EXCLUDES 1   *lichen planopilaris (L66.1)*

L43.0   **Hypertrophic** lichen planus

L43.1   **Bullous** lichen planus

☑ Additional Character Required   √x7ᵗʰ Placeholder Alert   Manifestation Dx   ▽ Unspecified Dx   ▶◀ Revised Text   ● New Code   ▲ Revised Code Title

ICD-10-CM 2017   683

L43.2   **Lichenoid** drug reaction
     Use additional code for adverse effect, if applicable, to identify drug (T36-T50 with fifth or sixth character 5)

L43.3   Subacute (active) lichen planus
     Lichen planus tropicus

L43.8   **Other lichen planus**

L43.9   **Lichen planus, unspecified** ▽

✓4ᵗʰ **L44**   **Other papulosquamous disorders**

L44.0   **Pityriasis rubra pilaris**

L44.1   **Lichen nitidus**
     DEF: Chronic, inflammatory, asymptomatic skin disorder, characterized by numerous glistening, flat-topped, discrete, skin-colored micropapules, most often on the penis, lower abdomen, inner thighs, wrists, forearms, breasts and buttocks.

L44.2   **Lichen striatus**

L44.3   **Lichen ruber moniliformis**

L44.4   **Infantile papular acrodermatitis [Gianotti-Crosti]**   ℙ

L44.8   **Other specified papulosquamous disorders**

L44.9   **Papulosquamous disorder, unspecified** ▽

L45   *Papulosquamous disorders in diseases classified elsewhere*
     Code first underlying disease

Urticaria and erythema (L49-L54)

EXCLUDES 1   *Lyme disease (A69.2-) (~A69.2-A69.29)*
         rosacea (L71.-)

✓4ᵗʰ **L49**   **Exfoliation due to erythematous conditions according to extent of body surface involved**
     Code first erythematous condition causing exfoliation, such as:
     Ritter's disease (L00)
     (Staphylococcal) scalded skin syndrom (L00)
     Stevens-Johnson syndrome (L51.1)
     Stevens-Johnson syndrome-toxic epidermal necrolysis overlap syndrome (L51.3)
     Toxic epidermal necrolysis (L51.2)

L49.0   **Exfoliation due to erythematous condition involving less than 10 percent of body surface**
     Exfoliation due to erythematous condition NOS

L49.1   **Exfoliation due to erythematous condition involving 10-19 percent of body surface**

L49.2   **Exfoliation due to erythematous condition involving 20-29 percent of body surface**

L49.3   **Exfoliation due to erythematous condition involving 30-39 percent of body surface**

L49.4   **Exfoliation due to erythematous condition involving 40-49 percent of body surface**

L49.5   **Exfoliation due to erythematous condition involving 50-59 percent of body surface**

L49.6   **Exfoliation due to erythematous condition involving 60-69 percent of body surface**

L49.7   **Exfoliation due to erythematous condition involving 70-79 percent of body surface**

L49.8   **Exfoliation due to erythematous condition involving 80-89 percent of body surface**

L49.9   **Exfoliation due to erythematous condition involving 90 or more percent of body surface**

✓4ᵗʰ **L50**   **Urticaria**

EXCLUDES 1   *allergic contact dermatitis (L23.-)*
         angioneurotic edema (T78.3)
         giant urticaria (T78.3)
         hereditary angio-edema (D84.1)
         Quincke's edema (T78.3)
         serum urticaria (T80.6-)
         solar urticaria (L56.3)
         urticaria neonatorum (P83.8)
         urticaria papulosa (L28.2)
         urticaria pigmentosa (Q82.2)

L50.0   **Allergic urticaria**

L50.1   **Idiopathic urticaria**

L50.2   **Urticaria due to cold and heat**
     EXCLUDES 2   ▶*familial cold urticaria (M04.2)*◀

L50.3   **Dermatographic urticaria**

L50.4   **Vibratory urticaria**

L50.5   **Cholinergic urticaria**

L50.6   **Contact urticaria**

L50.8   **Other urticaria**
     Chronic urticaria
     Recurrent periodic urticaria

L50.9   **Urticaria, unspecified** ▽

✓4ᵗʰ **L51**   **Erythema multiforme**
     Use additional code for adverse effect, if applicable, to identify drug (T36-T50 with fifth or sixth character 5)
     Use additional code to identify associated manifestations, such as:
     arthropathy associated with dermatological disorders (M14.8-)
     conjunctival edema (H11.42)
     conjunctivitis (H10.22-)
     corneal scars and opacities (H17.-)
     corneal ulcer (H16.0-)
     edema of eyelid (H02.84)
     inflammation of eyelid (H01.8)
     keratoconjunctivitis sicca (H16.22-)
     mechanical lagophthalmos (H02.22-)
     stomatitis (K12.-)
     symblepharon (H11.23-)
     Use additional code to identify percentage of skin exfoliation (L49.-)
     EXCLUDES 1   *Ritter's disease (L00)*
              staphylococcal scalded skin syndrome (L00)

L51.0   **Nonbullous erythema multiforme**

L51.1   **Stevens-Johnson syndrome**

L51.2   **Toxic epidermal necrolysis [Lyell]**

L51.3   **Stevens-Johnson syndrome-toxic epidermal necrolysis overlap syndrome**
     SJS-TEN overlap syndrome

L51.8   **Other erythema multiforme**

L51.9   **Erythema multiforme, unspecified** ▽
     Erythema iris
     Erythema multiforme major NOS
     Erythema multiforme minor NOS
     Herpes iris

L52   **Erythema nodosum**
     EXCLUDES 1   *tuberculous erythema nodosum (A18.4)*

✓4ᵗʰ **L53**   **Other erythematous conditions**
     EXCLUDES 1   *erythema ab igne (L59.0)*
              erythema due to external agents in contact with skin (L23-L25)
              erythema intertrigo (L30.4)

L53.0   **Toxic erythema**
     Code first poisoning due to drug or toxin, if applicable (T36-T65 with fifth or sixth character 1-4 or 6)
     Use additional code for adverse effect, if applicable, to identify drug (T36-T50 with fifth or sixth character 5)
     EXCLUDES 1   *neonatal erythema toxicum (P83.1)*

L53.1   **Erythema annulare centrifugum**

L53.2   **Erythema marginatum**

L53.3   **Other chronic figurate erythema**

L53.8   **Other specified erythematous conditions**

L53.9   **Erythematous condition, unspecified** ▽
     Erythema NOS
     Erythroderma NOS

L54   *Erythema in diseases classified elsewhere*
     Code first underlying disease

Radiation-related disorders of the skin and subcutaneous tissue (L55-L59)

✓4ᵗʰ **L55**   **Sunburn**

L55.0   **Sunburn of first degree**

L55.1   **Sunburn of second degree**

L55.2   **Sunburn of third degree**

L55.9   **Sunburn, unspecified** ▽

✓4ᵗʰ **L56**   **Other acute skin changes due to ultraviolet radiation**
     Use additional code to identify the source of the ultraviolet radiation (W89, X32)

L56.0   **Drug phototoxic response**
     Use additional code for adverse effect, if applicable, to identify drug (T36-T50 with fifth or sixth character 5)

L56.1   **Drug photoallergic response**
     Use additional code for adverse effect, if applicable, to identify drug (T36-T50 with fifth or sixth character 5)

L56.2   **Photocontact dermatitis [berloque dermatitis]**

L56.3   **Solar urticaria**

EXCLUDES 1   Not coded here   EXCLUDES 2   Not included here   N   Newborn Age : 0   ℙ   Pediatric Age : 0-17   M   Maternity Age : 12-55   A   Adult Age : 15-124

684   ICD-10-CM 2017

L56.4 Polymorphous light eruption

L56.5 Disseminated superficial actinic porokeratosis (DSAP)

L56.8 Other specified acute skin changes due to ultraviolet radiation

L56.9 Acute skin change due to ultraviolet radiation, unspecified ▽

✓4ᵗʰ **L57 Skin changes due to chronic exposure to nonionizing radiation**

Use additional code to identify the source of the ultraviolet radiation (W89, X32)

L57.0 Actinic keratosis

Keratosis NOS

Senile keratosis

Solar keratosis

L57.1 Actinic reticuloid

L57.2 Cutis rhomboidalis nuchae

L57.3 Poikiloderma of Civatte

L57.4 Cutis laxa senilis

Elastosis senilis

L57.5 Actinic granuloma

L57.8 Other skin changes due to chronic exposure to nonionizing radiation

Farmer's skin

Sailor's skin

Solar dermatitis

L57.9 Skin changes due to chronic exposure to nonionizing radiation, unspecified ▽

✓4ᵗʰ **L58 Radiodermatitis**

Use additional code to identify the source of the radiation (W88, W90)

L58.0 Acute radiodermatitis

L58.1 Chronic radiodermatitis

L58.9 Radiodermatitis, unspecified ▽

✓4ᵗʰ **L59 Other disorders of skin and subcutaneous tissue related to radiation**

L59.0 Erythema ab igne [dermatitis ab igne]

L59.8 Other specified disorders of the skin and subcutaneous tissue related to radiation

L59.9 Disorder of the skin and subcutaneous tissue related to radiation, unspecified ▽

Disorders of skin appendages (L60-L75)

EXCLUDES 1 *congenital malformations of integument (Q84.-)*

✓4ᵗʰ **L60 Nail disorders**

EXCLUDES 2 *clubbing of nails (R68.3)*

onychia and paronychia (L03.0-)

L60.0 Ingrowing nail

L60.1 Onycholysis

L60.2 Onychogryphosis

L60.3 Nail dystrophy

L60.4 Beau's lines

L60.5 Yellow nail syndrome

L60.8 Other nail disorders

L60.9 Nail disorder, unspecified ▽

L62 *Nail disorders in diseases classified elsewhere*

Code first underlying disease, such as:

pachydermoperiostosis (M89.4-)

✓4ᵗʰ **L63 Alopecia areata**

L63.0 Alopecia (capitis) totalis

L63.1 Alopecia universalis

L63.2 Ophiasis

L63.8 Other alopecia areata

L63.9 Alopecia areata, unspecified ▽

✓4ᵗʰ **L64 Androgenic alopecia**

INCLUDES male-pattern baldness

L64.0 Drug-induced androgenic alopecia

Use additional code for adverse effect, if applicable, to identify drug (T36-T50 with fifth or sixth character 5)

L64.8 Other androgenic alopecia

L64.9 Androgenic alopecia, unspecified ▽

✓4ᵗʰ **L65 Other nonscarring hair loss**

Use additional code for adverse effect, if applicable, to identify drug (T36-T50 with fifth or sixth character 5)

EXCLUDES 1 *trichotillomania (F63.3)*

L65.0 Telogen effluvium

L65.1 Anagen effluvium

L65.2 Alopecia mucinosa

L65.8 Other specified nonscarring hair loss

L65.9 Nonscarring hair loss, unspecified ▽

Alopecia NOS

✓4ᵗʰ **L66 Cicatricial alopecia [scarring hair loss]**

L66.0 Pseudopelade

L66.1 Lichen planopilaris

Follicular lichen planus

L66.2 Folliculitis decalvans

L66.3 Perifolliculitis capitis abscedens

L66.4 Folliculitis ulerythematosa reticulata

L66.8 Other cicatricial alopecia

AHA: 2015,1Q,19

L66.9 Cicatricial alopecia, unspecified ▽

✓4ᵗʰ **L67 Hair color and hair shaft abnormalities**

EXCLUDES 1 *monilethrix (Q84.1)*

pili annulati (Q84.1)

telogen effluvium (L65.0)

L67.0 Trichorrhexis nodosa

L67.1 Variations in hair color

Canities

Greyness, hair (premature)

Heterochromia of hair

Poliosis circumscripta, acquired

Poliosis NOS

L67.8 Other hair color and hair shaft abnormalities

Fragilitas crinium

L67.9 Hair color and hair shaft abnormality, unspecified ▽

✓4ᵗʰ **L68 Hypertrichosis**

INCLUDES excess hair

EXCLUDES 1 *congenital hypertrichosis (Q84.2)*

persistent lanugo (Q84.2)

L68.0 Hirsutism

L68.1 Acquired hypertrichosis lanuginosa

L68.2 Localized hypertrichosis

L68.3 Polytrichia

L68.8 Other hypertrichosis

L68.9 Hypertrichosis, unspecified ▽

✓4ᵗʰ **L70 Acne**

EXCLUDES 2 *acne keloid (L73.0)*

L70.0 Acne vulgaris

L70.1 Acne conglobata

L70.2 Acne varioliformis

Acne necrotica miliaris

L70.3 Acne tropica

L70.4 Infantile acne P

▲ **L70.5 Acné excoriée**

▶Acné excoriée des jeunes filles◀

Picker's acne

L70.8 Other acne

L70.9 Acne, unspecified ▽

✓4ᵗʰ **L71 Rosacea**

Use additional code for adverse effect, if applicable, to identify drug (T36-T50 with fifth or sixth character 5)

L71.0 Perioral dermatitis

L71.1 Rhinophyma

L71.8 Other rosacea

L71.9 Rosacea, unspecified ▽

✓4ᵗʰ **L72 Follicular cysts of skin and subcutaneous tissue**

L72.0 Epidermal cyst

✓5ᵗʰ **L72.1 Pilar and trichodermal cyst**

L72.11 Pilar cyst

L72.12 Trichodermal cyst

Trichilemmal (proliferating) cyst

L72.2 Steatocystoma multiplex

L72.3 Sebaceous cyst

EXCLUDES 2 *pilar cyst (L72.11)*

trichilemmal (proliferating) cyst (L72.12)

L72.8 Other follicular cysts of the skin and subcutaneous tissue

L72.9 Follicular cyst of the skin and subcutaneous tissue, unspecified ▽

☑ Additional Character Required   ✓x7ᵗʰ Placeholder Alert   Manifestation Dx   ▽ Unspecified Dx   ▶◀ Revised Text   ● New Code   ▲ Revised Code Title

✓4ᵗʰ **L73 Other follicular disorders**

L73.0 **Acne keloid**

L73.1 **Pseudofolliculitis barbae**

L73.2 **Hidradenitis suppurativa**

L73.8 **Other specified follicular disorders**
Sycosis barbae

L73.9 **Follicular disorder, unspecified**   ▽

✓4ᵗʰ **L74 Eccrine sweat disorders**

EXCLUDES 2 *generalized hyperhidrosis (R61)*

L74.0 **Miliaria** rubra

L74.1 **Miliaria** crystallina

L74.2 **Miliaria** profunda
Miliaria tropicalis

L74.3 **Miliaria, unspecified**   ▽

L74.4 **Anhidrosis**
Hypohidrosis

✓5ᵗʰ L74.5 **Focal hyperhidrosis**

✓6ᵗʰ L74.51 **Primary** **focal hyperhidrosis**

L74.510 **Primary focal hyperhidrosis,** axilla
L74.511 **Primary focal hyperhidrosis,** face
L74.512 **Primary focal hyperhidrosis,** palms
L74.513 **Primary focal hyperhidrosis,** soles
L74.519 **Primary focal hyperhidrosis, unspecified**   ▽

L74.52 **Secondary** **focal hyperhidrosis**
Frey's syndrome

L74.8 **Other eccrine sweat disorders**

L74.9 **Eccrine sweat disorder, unspecified**   ▽
Sweat gland disorder NOS

✓4ᵗʰ **L75 Apocrine sweat disorders**

EXCLUDES 1 *dyshidrosis (L30.1)*
hidradenitis suppurativa (L73.2)

L75.0 **Bromhidrosis**

L75.1 **Chromhidrosis**

L75.2 **Apocrine miliaria**
Fox-Fordyce disease

L75.8 **Other apocrine sweat disorders**

L75.9 **Apocrine sweat disorder, unspecified**   ▽

Intraoperative and postprocedural complications of skin and subcutaneous tissue (L76)

✓4ᵗʰ **L76 Intraoperative and postprocedural complications of skin and subcutaneous tissue**

✓5ᵗʰ L76.0 **Intraoperative hemorrhage and hematoma of skin and subcutaneous tissue complicating a procedure**

EXCLUDES 1 *intraoperative hemorrhage and hematoma of skin and subcutaneous tissue due to accidental puncture and laceration during a procedure (L76.1-)*

L76.01 **Intraoperative hemorrhage and hematoma of skin and subcutaneous tissue complicating a dermatologic procedure**

L76.02 **Intraoperative hemorrhage and hematoma of skin and subcutaneous tissue complicating other procedure**

✓5ᵗʰ L76.1 **Accidental puncture and laceration of skin and subcutaneous tissue during a procedure**

L76.11 **Accidental puncture and laceration of skin and subcutaneous tissue during a dermatologic procedure**

L76.12 **Accidental puncture and laceration of skin and subcutaneous tissue during other procedure**

▲ ✓5ᵗʰ L76.2 **Postprocedural hemorrhage of skin and subcutaneous tissue following a procedure**

▲ L76.21 **Postprocedural hemorrhage of skin and subcutaneous tissue following a dermatologic procedure**

▲ L76.22 **Postprocedural hemorrhage of skin and subcutaneous tissue following other procedure**

● ✓5ᵗʰ L76.3 **Postprocedural hematoma and seroma of skin and subcutaneous tissue following a procedure**

● L76.31 **Postprocedural hematoma of skin and subcutaneous tissue following a dermatologic procedure**

● L76.32 **Postprocedural hematoma of skin and subcutaneous tissue following other procedure**

● L76.33 **Postprocedural seroma of skin and subcutaneous tissue following a dermatologic procedure**

● L76.34 **Postprocedural seroma of skin and subcutaneous tissue following other procedure**

✓5ᵗʰ L76.8 **Other intraoperative and postprocedural complications of skin and subcutaneous tissue**
Use additional code, if applicable, to further specify disorder

L76.81 **Other intraoperative complications of skin and subcutaneous tissue**

L76.82 **Other postprocedural complications of skin and subcutaneous tissue**

Other disorders of the skin and subcutaneous tissue (L80-L99)

L80 Vitiligo

EXCLUDES 2 *vitiligo of eyelids (H02.73-)*
vitiligo of vulva (N90.89)

DEF: Persistent, progressive development of nonpigmented white patches on otherwise normal skin.

✓4ᵗʰ **L81 Other disorders of pigmentation**

EXCLUDES 1 *birthmark NOS (Q82.5)*
Peutz-Jeghers syndrome (Q85.8)
EXCLUDES 2 *nevus - see Alphabetical Index*

L81.0 **Postinflammatory hyperpigmentation**

L81.1 **Chloasma**

L81.2 **Freckles**

L81.3 **Café au lait spots**

L81.4 **Other melanin hyperpigmentation**
Lentigo

L81.5 **Leukoderma, not elsewhere classified**

L81.6 **Other disorders of diminished melanin formation**

L81.7 **Pigmented purpuric dermatosis**
Angioma serpiginosum

L81.8 **Other specified disorders of pigmentation**
Iron pigmentation
Tattoo pigmentation

L81.9 **Disorder of pigmentation, unspecified**   ▽

✓4ᵗʰ **L82 Seborrheic keratosis**

INCLUDES ▶basal cell papilloma◀
dermatosis papulosa nigra
Leser-Trélat disease
EXCLUDES 2 *seborrheic dermatitis (L21.-)*

L82.0 **Inflamed** **seborrheic keratosis**

L82.1 **Other seborrheic keratosis**
Seborrheic keratosis NOS

L83 Acanthosis nigricans
Confluent and reticulated papillomatosis

L84 Corns and callosities
Callus
Clavus

✓4ᵗʰ **L85 Other epidermal thickening**

EXCLUDES 2 *hypertrophic disorders of the skin (L91.-)*

L85.0 **Acquired ichthyosis**
EXCLUDES 1 *congenital ichthyosis (Q80.-)*

L85.1 **Acquired keratosis [keratoderma] palmaris et plantaris**
EXCLUDES 1 *inherited keratosis palmaris et plantaris (Q82.8)*

L85.2 **Keratosis punctata (palmaris et plantaris)**

L85.3 **Xerosis cutis**
Dry skin dermatitis

L85.8 **Other specified epidermal thickening**
Cutaneous horn

L85.9 **Epidermal thickening, unspecified**   ▽

L86 *Keratoderma in diseases classified elsewhere*
Code first underlying disease, such as:
Reiter's disease (M02.3-)
EXCLUDES 1 *gonococcal keratoderma (A54.89)*
gonococcal keratosis (A54.89)
keratoderma due to vitamin A deficiency (E50.8)
keratosis due to vitamin A deficiency (E50.8)
xeroderma due to vitamin A deficiency (E50.8)

✓4ᵗʰ **L87 Transepidermal elimination disorders**

EXCLUDES 1 *granuloma annulare (perforating) (L92.0)*

L87.0 **Keratosis follicularis et parafollicularis in cutem penetrans**
Hyperkeratosis follicularis penetrans
Kyrle disease

L87.1 **Reactive perforating collagenosis**

L87.2 **Elastosis perforans serpiginosa**

EXCLUDES 1 Not coded here   EXCLUDES 2 Not included here   N Newborn Age : 0   P Pediatric Age : 0-17   M Maternity Age : 12-55   A Adult Age : 15-124

L87.8 **Other transepidermal elimination disorders**

L87.9 **Transepidermal elimination disorder, unspecified** ▽

L88 **Pyoderma gangrenosum**
Phagedenic pyoderma
EXCLUDES 1 *dermatitis gangrenosa (L08.0)*
DEF: Persistent debilitating skin disease characterized by irregular, boggy, blue-red ulcerations, with central healing and undermined edges.

☑4ᵗʰ L89 **Pressure ulcer**
INCLUDES bed sore
decubitus ulcer
plaster ulcer
pressure area
pressure sore
Code first any associated gangrene (I96)
EXCLUDES 2 *decubitus (trophic) ulcer of cervix (uteri) (N86)*
diabetic ulcers (E08.621, E08.622, E09.621, E09.622, E10.621, E10.622, E11.621, E11.622, E13.621, E13.622)
non-pressure chronic ulcer of skin (L97.-)
skin infections (L00-L08)
varicose ulcer (I83.0, I83.2)

Four Stages of Pressure Ulcer

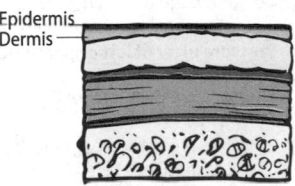

Stage 1
Persistent focal erythema

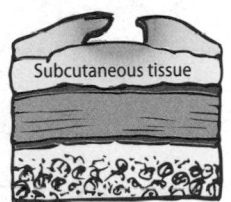

Stage 2
Abrasion, blister, partial thickness skin loss involving epidermis and/or dermis

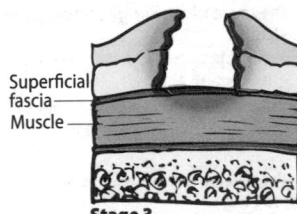

Stage 3
Full thickness skin loss involving damage or necrosis of subcutaneous tissue

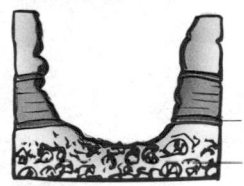

Stage 4
Necrosis of soft tissues through to underlying muscle, tendon, or bone

☑5ᵗʰ L89.0 **Pressure ulcer of** elbow

☑6ᵗʰ L89.00 **Pressure ulcer of unspecified elbow**

L89.000 **Pressure ulcer of unspecified elbow, unstageable** ▽

L89.001 **Pressure ulcer of unspecified elbow, stage 1** ▽
Healing pressure ulcer of unspecified elbow, stage 1
Pressure pre-ulcer skin changes limited to persistent focal edema, unspecified elbow

L89.002 **Pressure ulcer of unspecified elbow, stage 2** ▽
Healing pressure ulcer of unspecified elbow, stage 2
Pressure ulcer with abrasion, blister, partial thickness skin loss involving epidermis and/or dermis, unspecified elbow

L89.003 **Pressure ulcer of unspecified elbow, stage 3** ▽
Healing pressure ulcer of unspecified elbow, stage 3
Pressure ulcer with full thickness skin loss involving damage or necrosis of subcutaneous tissue, unspecified elbow

L89.004 **Pressure ulcer of unspecified elbow, stage 4** ▽
Healing pressure ulcer of unspecified elbow, stage 4
Pressure ulcer with necrosis of soft tissues through to underlying muscle, tendon, or bone, unspecified elbow

L89.009 **Pressure ulcer of unspecified elbow, unspecified stage** ▽
Healing pressure ulcer of elbow NOS
Healing pressure ulcer of unspecified elbow, unspecified stage

☑6ᵗʰ L89.01 **Pressure ulcer of** right **elbow**

L89.010 **Pressure ulcer of right elbow, unstageable**

L89.011 **Pressure ulcer of right elbow, stage 1**
Healing pressure ulcer of right elbow, stage 1
Pressure pre-ulcer skin changes limited to persistent focal edema, right elbow

L89.012 **Pressure ulcer of right elbow, stage 2**
Healing pressure ulcer of right elbow, stage 2
Pressure ulcer with abrasion, blister, partial thickness skin loss involving epidermis and/or dermis, right elbow

L89.013 **Pressure ulcer of right elbow, stage 3**
Healing pressure ulcer of right elbow, stage 3
Pressure ulcer with full thickness skin loss involving damage or necrosis of subcutaneous tissue, right elbow

L89.014 **Pressure ulcer of right elbow, stage 4**
Healing pressure ulcer of right elbow, stage 4
Pressure ulcer with necrosis of soft tissues through to underlying muscle, tendon, or bone, right elbow

L89.019 **Pressure ulcer of right elbow, unspecified stage** ▽
Healing pressure right of elbow NOS
Healing pressure ulcer of unspecified elbow, unspecified stage

☑6ᵗʰ L89.02 **Pressure ulcer of** left **elbow**

L89.020 **Pressure ulcer of left elbow, unstageable**

L89.021 **Pressure ulcer of left elbow, stage 1**
Healing pressure ulcer of left elbow, stage 1
Pressure pre-ulcer skin changes limited to persistent focal edema, left elbow

L89.022 **Pressure ulcer of left elbow, stage 2**
Healing pressure ulcer of left elbow, stage 2
Pressure ulcer with abrasion, blister, partial thickness skin loss involving epidermis and/or dermis, left elbow

L89.023 **Pressure ulcer of left elbow, stage 3**
Healing pressure ulcer of left elbow, stage 3
Pressure ulcer with full thickness skin loss involving damage or necrosis of subcutaneous tissue, left elbow

L89.024 **Pressure ulcer of left elbow, stage 4**
Healing pressure ulcer of left elbow, stage 4
Pressure ulcer with necrosis of soft tissues through to underlying muscle, tendon, or bone, left elbow

L89.029 **Pressure ulcer of left elbow, unspecified stage** ▽
Healing pressure ulcer of left of elbow NOS
Healing pressure ulcer of unspecified elbow, unspecified stage

☑5ᵗʰ L89.1 **Pressure ulcer of** back

☑6ᵗʰ L89.10 **Pressure ulcer of unspecified part of back**

L89.100 **Pressure ulcer of unspecified part of back, unstageable** ▽

L89.101   **Pressure ulcer of unspecified part of back,** stage 1   ▽

Healing pressure ulcer of unspecified part of back, stage 1

Pressure pre-ulcer skin changes limited to persistent focal edema, unspecified part of back

L89.102   **Pressure ulcer of unspecified part of back,** stage 2   ▽

Healing pressure ulcer of unspecified part of back, stage 2

Pressure ulcer with abrasion, blister, partial thickness skin loss involving epidermis and/or dermis, unspecified part of back

L89.103   **Pressure ulcer of unspecified part of back,** stage 3   ▽

Healing pressure ulcer of unspecified part of back, stage 3

Pressure ulcer with full thickness skin loss involving damage or necrosis of subcutaneous tissue, unspecified part of back

L89.104   **Pressure ulcer of unspecified part of back,** stage 4   ▽

Healing pressure ulcer of unspecified part of back, stage 4

Pressure ulcer with necrosis of soft tissues through to underlying muscle, tendon, or bone, unspecified part of back

L89.109   **Pressure ulcer of unspecified part of back, unspecified stage**   ▽

Healing pressure ulcer of unspecified part of back NOS

Healing pressure ulcer of unspecified part of back, unspecified stage

√6ᵗʰ   **L89.11**   **Pressure ulcer of** right upper **back**

Pressure ulcer of right shoulder blade

L89.110   **Pressure ulcer of right upper back, unstageable**

L89.111   **Pressure ulcer of right upper back, stage 1**

Healing pressure ulcer of right upper back, stage 1

Pressure pre-ulcer skin changes limited to persistent focal edema, right upper back

L89.112   **Pressure ulcer of right upper back, stage 2**

Healing pressure ulcer of right upper back, stage 2

Pressure ulcer with abrasion, blister, partial thickness skin loss involving epidermis and/or dermis, right upper back

L89.113   **Pressure ulcer of right upper back, stage 3**

Healing pressure ulcer of right upper back, stage 3

Pressure ulcer with full thickness skin loss involving damage or necrosis of subcutaneous tissue, right upper back

L89.114   **Pressure ulcer of right upper back, stage 4**

Healing pressure ulcer of right upper back, stage 4

Pressure ulcer with necrosis of soft tissues through to underlying muscle, tendon, or bone, right upper back

L89.119   **Pressure ulcer of right upper back, unspecified stage**   ▽

Healing pressure ulcer of right upper back NOS

Healing pressure ulcer of right upper back, unspecified stage

√6ᵗʰ   **L89.12**   **Pressure ulcer of** left upper **back**

Pressure ulcer of left shoulder blade

L89.120   **Pressure ulcer of left upper back, unstageable**

L89.121   **Pressure ulcer of left upper back,** stage 1

Healing pressure ulcer of left upper back, stage 1

Pressure pre-ulcer skin changes limited to persistent focal edema, left upper back

L89.122   **Pressure ulcer of left upper back,** stage 2

Healing pressure ulcer of left upper back, stage 2

Pressure ulcer with abrasion, blister, partial thickness skin loss involving epidermis and/or dermis, left upper back

L89.123   **Pressure ulcer of left upper back,** stage 3

Healing pressure ulcer of left upper back, stage 3

Pressure ulcer with full thickness skin loss involving damage or necrosis of subcutaneous tissue, left upper back

L89.124   **Pressure ulcer of left upper back,** stage 4

Healing pressure ulcer of left upper back, stage 4

Pressure ulcer with necrosis of soft tissues through to underlying muscle, tendon, or bone, left upper back

L89.129   **Pressure ulcer of left upper back, unspecified stage**   ▽

Healing pressure ulcer of left upper back NOS

Healing pressure ulcer of left upper back, unspecified stage

√6ᵗʰ   **L89.13**   **Pressure ulcer of** right lower **back**

L89.130   **Pressure ulcer of right lower back, unstageable**

L89.131   **Pressure ulcer of right lower back, stage 1**

Healing pressure ulcer of right lower back, stage 1

Pressure pre-ulcer skin changes limited to persistent focal edema, right lower back

L89.132   **Pressure ulcer of right lower back, stage 2**

Healing pressure ulcer of right lower back, stage 2

Pressure ulcer with abrasion, blister, partial thickness skin loss involving epidermis and/or dermis, right lower back

L89.133   **Pressure ulcer of right lower back, stage 3**

Healing pressure ulcer of right lower back, stage 3

Pressure ulcer with full thickness skin loss involving damage or necrosis of subcutaneous tissue, right lower back

L89.134   **Pressure ulcer of right lower back, stage 4**

Healing pressure ulcer of right lower back, stage 4

Pressure ulcer with necrosis of soft tissues through to underlying muscle, tendon, or bone, right lower back

L89.139   **Pressure ulcer of right lower back, unspecified stage**   ▽

Healing pressure ulcer of right lower back NOS

Healing pressure ulcer of right lower back, unspecified stage

√6ᵗʰ   **L89.14**   **Pressure ulcer of** left lower **back**

L89.140   **Pressure ulcer of left lower back, unstageable**

L89.141   **Pressure ulcer of left lower back,** stage 1

Healing pressure ulcer of left lower back, stage 1

Pressure pre-ulcer skin changes limited to persistent focal edema, left lower back

EXCLUDES 1 Not coded here   EXCLUDES 2 Not included here   Ⓝ Newborn Age : 0   Ⓟ Pediatric Age : 0-17   Ⓜ Maternity Age : 12-55   Ⓐ Adult Age : 15-124

688

ICD-10-CM 2017

L89.142 Pressure ulcer of left lower back, stage 2
Healing pressure ulcer of left lower back, stage 2
Pressure ulcer with abrasion, blister, partial thickness skin loss involving epidermis and/or dermis, left lower back

L89.143 Pressure ulcer of left lower back, stage 3
Healing pressure ulcer of left lower back, stage 3
Pressure ulcer with full thickness skin loss involving damage or necrosis of subcutaneous tissue, left lower back

L89.144 Pressure ulcer of left lower back, stage 4
Healing pressure ulcer of left lower back, stage 4
Pressure ulcer with necrosis of soft tissues through to underlying muscle, tendon, or bone, left lower back

L89.149 Pressure ulcer of left lower back, unspecified stage ▽
Healing pressure ulcer of left lower back NOS
Healing pressure ulcer of left lower back, unspecified stage

✓6ᵗʰ L89.15 Pressure ulcer of sacral region
Pressure ulcer of coccyx
Pressure ulcer of tailbone

L89.150 Pressure ulcer of sacral region, unstageable

L89.151 Pressure ulcer of sacral region, stage 1
Healing pressure ulcer of sacral region, stage 1
Pressure pre-ulcer skin changes limited to persistent focal edema, sacral region

L89.152 Pressure ulcer of sacral region, stage 2
Healing pressure ulcer of sacral region, stage 2
Pressure ulcer with abrasion, blister, partial thickness skin loss involving epidermis and/or dermis, sacral region

L89.153 Pressure ulcer of sacral region, stage 3
Healing pressure ulcer of sacral region, stage 3
Pressure ulcer with full thickness skin loss involving damage or necrosis of subcutaneous tissue, sacral region

L89.154 Pressure ulcer of sacral region, stage 4
Healing pressure ulcer of sacral region, stage 4
Pressure ulcer with necrosis of soft tissues through to underlying muscle, tendon, or bone, sacral region

L89.159 Pressure ulcer of sacral region, unspecified stage ▽
Healing pressure ulcer of sacral region NOS
Healing pressure ulcer of sacral region, unspecified stage

✓5ᵗʰ L89.2 Pressure ulcer of hip

✓6ᵗʰ L89.20 Pressure ulcer of unspecified hip

L89.200 Pressure ulcer of unspecified hip, unstageable ▽

L89.201 Pressure ulcer of unspecified hip, stage 1 ▽
Healing pressure ulcer of unspecified hip back, stage 1
Pressure pre-ulcer skin changes limited to persistent focal edema, unspecified hip

L89.202 Pressure ulcer of unspecified hip, stage 2 ▽
Healing pressure ulcer of unspecified hip, stage 2
Pressure ulcer with abrasion, blister, partial thickness skin loss involving epidermis and/or dermis, unspecified hip

L89.203 Pressure ulcer of unspecified hip, stage 3 ▽
Healing pressure ulcer of unspecified hip, stage 3
Pressure ulcer with full thickness skin loss involving damage or necrosis of subcutaneous tissue, unspecified hip

L89.204 Pressure ulcer of unspecified hip, stage 4 ▽
Healing pressure ulcer of unspecified hip, stage 4
Pressure ulcer with necrosis of soft tissues through to underlying muscle, tendon, or bone, unspecified hip

L89.209 Pressure ulcer of unspecified hip, unspecified stage ▽
Healing pressure ulcer of unspecified hip NOS
Healing pressure ulcer of unspecified hip, unspecified stage

✓6ᵗʰ L89.21 Pressure ulcer of right hip

L89.210 Pressure ulcer of right hip, unstageable

L89.211 Pressure ulcer of right hip, stage 1
Healing pressure ulcer of right hip back, stage 1
Pressure pre-ulcer skin changes limited to persistent focal edema, right hip

L89.212 Pressure ulcer of right hip, stage 2
Healing pressure ulcer of right hip, stage 2
Pressure ulcer with abrasion, blister, partial thickness skin loss involving epidermis and/or dermis, right hip

L89.213 Pressure ulcer of right hip, stage 3
Healing pressure ulcer of right hip, stage 3
Pressure ulcer with full thickness skin loss involving damage or necrosis of subcutaneous tissue, right hip

L89.214 Pressure ulcer of right hip, stage 4
Healing pressure ulcer of right hip, stage 4
Pressure ulcer with necrosis of soft tissues through to underlying muscle, tendon, or bone, right hip

L89.219 Pressure ulcer of right hip, unspecified stage ▽
Healing pressure ulcer of right hip NOS
Healing pressure ulcer of right hip, unspecified stage

✓6ᵗʰ L89.22 Pressure ulcer of left hip

L89.220 Pressure ulcer of left hip, unstageable

L89.221 Pressure ulcer of left hip, stage 1
Healing pressure ulcer of left hip back, stage 1
Pressure pre-ulcer skin changes limited to persistent focal edema, left hip

L89.222 Pressure ulcer of left hip, stage 2
Healing pressure ulcer of left hip, stage 2
Pressure ulcer with abrasion, blister, partial thickness skin loss involving epidermis and/or dermis, left hip

L89.223 Pressure ulcer of left hip, stage 3
Healing pressure ulcer of left hip, stage 3
Pressure ulcer with full thickness skin loss involving damage or necrosis of subcutaneous tissue, left hip

L89.224 Pressure ulcer of left hip, stage 4
Healing pressure ulcer of left hip, stage 4
Pressure ulcer with necrosis of soft tissues through to underlying muscle, tendon, or bone, left hip

L89.229 Pressure ulcer of left hip, unspecified stage ▽
Healing pressure ulcer of left hip NOS
Healing pressure ulcer of left hip, unspecified stage

Chapter 12. Diseases of the Skin and Subcutaneous Tissue

L89.3–L89.501

√5ᵗʰ **L89.3**   **Pressure ulcer of** buttock

    √6ᵗʰ **L89.30**   **Pressure ulcer of unspecified buttock**

       L89.300   **Pressure ulcer of unspecified buttock,** unstageable ▽

       L89.301   **Pressure ulcer of unspecified buttock,** stage 1 ▽
          Healing pressure ulcer of unspecified buttock, stage 1
          Pressure pre-ulcer skin changes limited to persistent focal edema, unspecified buttock

       L89.302   **Pressure ulcer of unspecified buttock,** stage 2 ▽
          Healing pressure ulcer of unspecified buttock, stage 2
          Pressure ulcer with abrasion, blister, partial thickness skin loss involving epidermis and/or dermis, unspecified buttock

       L89.303   **Pressure ulcer of unspecified buttock,** stage 3 ▽
          Healing pressure ulcer of unspecified buttock, stage 3
          Pressure ulcer with full thickness skin loss involving damage or necrosis of subcutaneous tissue, unspecified buttock

       L89.304   **Pressure ulcer of unspecified buttock,** stage 4 ▽
          Healing pressure ulcer of unspecified buttock, stage 4
          Pressure ulcer with necrosis of soft tissues through to underlying muscle, tendon, or bone, unspecified buttock

       L89.309   **Pressure ulcer of unspecified buttock, unspecified stage** ▽
          Healing pressure ulcer of unspecified buttock NOS
          Healing pressure ulcer of unspecified buttock, unspecified stage

    √6ᵗʰ **L89.31**   **Pressure ulcer of** right **buttock**

       L89.310   **Pressure ulcer of right buttock,** unstageable

       L89.311   **Pressure ulcer of right buttock,** stage 1
          Healing pressure ulcer of right buttock, stage 1
          Pressure pre-ulcer skin changes limited to persistent focal edema, right buttock

       L89.312   **Pressure ulcer of right buttock,** stage 2
          Healing pressure ulcer of right buttock, stage 2
          Pressure ulcer with abrasion, blister, partial thickness skin loss involving epidermis and/or dermis, right buttock

       L89.313   **Pressure ulcer of right buttock,** stage 3
          Healing pressure ulcer of right buttock, stage 3
          Pressure ulcer with full thickness skin loss involving damage or necrosis of subcutaneous tissue, right buttock

       L89.314   **Pressure ulcer of right buttock,** stage 4
          Healing pressure ulcer of right buttock, stage 4
          Pressure ulcer with necrosis of soft tissues through to underlying muscle, tendon, or bone, right buttock

       L89.319   **Pressure ulcer of right buttock, unspecified stage** ▽
          Healing pressure ulcer of right buttock NOS
          Healing pressure ulcer of right buttock, unspecified stage

    √6ᵗʰ **L89.32**   **Pressure ulcer of** left **buttock**

       L89.320   **Pressure ulcer of left buttock,** unstageable

       L89.321   **Pressure ulcer of left buttock,** stage 1
          Healing pressure ulcer of left buttock, stage 1
          Pressure pre-ulcer skin changes limited to persistent focal edema, left buttock

       L89.322   **Pressure ulcer of left buttock,** stage 2
          Healing pressure ulcer of left buttock, stage 2
          Pressure ulcer with abrasion, blister, partial thickness skin loss involving epidermis and/or dermis, left buttock

       L89.323   **Pressure ulcer of left buttock,** stage 3
          Healing pressure ulcer of left buttock, stage 3
          Pressure ulcer with full thickness skin loss involving damage or necrosis of subcutaneous tissue, left buttock

       L89.324   **Pressure ulcer of left buttock,** stage 4
          Healing pressure ulcer of left buttock, stage 4
          Pressure ulcer with necrosis of soft tissues through to underlying muscle, tendon, or bone, left buttock

       L89.329   **Pressure ulcer of left buttock, unspecified stage** ▽
          Healing pressure ulcer of left buttock NOS
          Healing pressure ulcer of left buttock, unspecified stage

√5ᵗʰ **L89.4**   **Pressure ulcer of contiguous site of** back, buttock and hip

       L89.40   **Pressure ulcer of contiguous site of back, buttock and hip, unspecified stage** ▽
          Healing pressure ulcer of contiguous site of back, buttock and hip NOS
          Healing pressure ulcer of contiguous site of back, buttock and hip, unspecified stage

       L89.41   **Pressure ulcer of contiguous site of back, buttock and hip,** stage 1
          Healing pressure ulcer of contiguous site of back, buttock and hip, stage 1
          Pressure pre-ulcer skin changes limited to persistent focal edema, contiguous site of back, buttock and hip

       L89.42   **Pressure ulcer of contiguous site of back, buttock and hip,** stage 2
          Healing pressure ulcer of contiguous site of back, buttock and hip, stage 2
          Pressure ulcer with abrasion, blister, partial thickness skin loss involving epidermis and/or dermis, contiguous site of back, buttock and hip

       L89.43   **Pressure ulcer of contiguous site of back, buttock and hip,** stage 3
          Healing pressure ulcer of contiguous site of back, buttock and hip, stage 3
          Pressure ulcer with full thickness skin loss involving damage or necrosis of subcutaneous tissue, contiguous site of back, buttock and hip

       L89.44   **Pressure ulcer of contiguous site of back, buttock and hip,** stage 4
          Healing pressure ulcer of contiguous site of back, buttock and hip, stage 4
          Pressure ulcer with necrosis of soft tissues through to underlying muscle, tendon, or bone, contiguous site of back, buttock and hip

       L89.45   **Pressure ulcer of contiguous site of back, buttock and hip,** unstageable

√5ᵗʰ **L89.5**   **Pressure ulcer of** ankle

    √6ᵗʰ **L89.50**   **Pressure ulcer of unspecified ankle**

       L89.500   **Pressure ulcer of unspecified ankle,** unstageable ▽

       L89.501   **Pressure ulcer of unspecified ankle,** stage 1 ▽
          Healing pressure ulcer of unspecified ankle, stage 1
          Pressure pre-ulcer skin changes limited to persistent focal edema, unspecified ankle

EXCLUDES 1 Not coded here   EXCLUDES 2 Not included here   N Newborn Age : 0   P Pediatric Age : 0-17   M Maternity Age : 12-55   A Adult Age : 15-124

690   ICD-10-CM 2017

  L89.502 **Pressure ulcer of unspecified** ▽
        ankle, stage 2
        Healing pressure ulcer of unspecified ankle, stage 2
        Pressure ulcer with abrasion, blister, partial thickness skin loss involving epidermis and/or dermis, unspecified ankle

  L89.503 **Pressure ulcer of unspecified** ▽
        ankle, stage 3
        Healing pressure ulcer of unspecified ankle, stage 3
        Pressure ulcer with full thickness skin loss involving damage or necrosis of subcutaneous tissue, unspecified ankle

  L89.504 **Pressure ulcer of unspecified** ▽
        ankle, stage 4
        Healing pressure ulcer of unspecified ankle, stage 4
        Pressure ulcer with necrosis of soft tissues through to underlying muscle, tendon, or bone, unspecified ankle

  L89.509 **Pressure ulcer of unspecified** ▽
        ankle, unspecified stage
        Healing pressure ulcer of unspecified ankle NOS
        Healing pressure ulcer of unspecified ankle, unspecified stage

✓6ᵗʰ **L89.51 Pressure ulcer of right ankle**

  L89.510 **Pressure ulcer of right ankle, unstageable**
  L89.511 **Pressure ulcer of right ankle, stage 1**
        Healing pressure ulcer of right ankle, stage 1
        Pressure pre-ulcer skin changes limited to persistent focal edema, right ankle

  L89.512 **Pressure ulcer of right ankle, stage 2**
        Healing pressure ulcer of right ankle, stage 2
        Pressure ulcer with abrasion, blister, partial thickness skin loss involving epidermis and/or dermis, right ankle

  L89.513 **Pressure ulcer of right ankle, stage 3**
        Healing pressure ulcer of right ankle, stage 3
        Pressure ulcer with full thickness skin loss involving damage or necrosis of subcutaneous tissue, right ankle

  L89.514 **Pressure ulcer of right ankle, stage 4**
        Healing pressure ulcer of right ankle, stage 4
        Pressure ulcer with necrosis of soft tissues through to underlying muscle, tendon, or bone, right ankle

  L89.519 **Pressure ulcer of right ankle,** ▽
        unspecified stage
        Healing pressure ulcer of right ankle NOS
        Healing pressure ulcer of right ankle, unspecified stage

✓6ᵗʰ **L89.52 Pressure ulcer of left ankle**

  L89.520 **Pressure ulcer of left ankle, unstageable**
  L89.521 **Pressure ulcer of left ankle, stage 1**
        Healing pressure ulcer of left ankle, stage 1
        ▶Pressure pre-ulcer skin changes limited to persistent focal edema, left ankle◀

  L89.522 **Pressure ulcer of left ankle, stage 2**
        Healing pressure ulcer of left ankle, stage 2
        Pressure ulcer with abrasion, blister, partial thickness skin loss involving epidermis and/or dermis, left ankle

  L89.523 **Pressure ulcer of left ankle, stage 3**
        Healing pressure ulcer of left ankle, stage 3
        Pressure ulcer with full thickness skin loss involving damage or necrosis of subcutaneous tissue, left ankle

  L89.524 **Pressure ulcer of left ankle, stage 4**
        Healing pressure ulcer of left ankle, stage 4
        Pressure ulcer with necrosis of soft tissues through to underlying muscle, tendon, or bone, left ankle

  L89.529 **Pressure ulcer of left ankle,** ▽
        unspecified stage
        Healing pressure ulcer of left ankle NOS
        Healing pressure ulcer of left ankle, unspecified stage

✓5ᵗʰ **L89.6 Pressure ulcer of heel**

  ✓6ᵗʰ **L89.60 Pressure ulcer of unspecified heel**

  L89.600 **Pressure ulcer of unspecified heel,** ▽
        unstageable
  L89.601 **Pressure ulcer of unspecified heel,** ▽
        stage 1
        Healing pressure ulcer of unspecified heel, stage 1
        Pressure pre-ulcer skin changes limited to persistent focal edema, unspecified heel

  L89.602 **Pressure ulcer of unspecified heel,** ▽
        stage 2
        Healing pressure ulcer of unspecified heel, stage 2
        Pressure ulcer with abrasion, blister, partial thickness skin loss involving epidermis and/or dermis, unspecified heel

  L89.603 **Pressure ulcer of unspecified heel,** ▽
        stage 3
        Healing pressure ulcer of unspecified heel, stage 3
        Pressure ulcer with full thickness skin loss involving damage or necrosis of subcutaneous tissue, unspecified heel

  L89.604 **Pressure ulcer of unspecified heel,** ▽
        stage 4
        Healing pressure ulcer of unspecified heel, stage 4
        Pressure ulcer with necrosis of soft tissues through to underlying muscle, tendon, or bone, unspecified heel

  L89.609 **Pressure ulcer of unspecified heel,** ▽
        unspecified stage
        Healing pressure ulcer of unspecified heel NOS
        Healing pressure ulcer of unspecified heel, unspecified stage

✓6ᵗʰ **L89.61 Pressure ulcer of right heel**

  L89.610 **Pressure ulcer of right heel, unstageable**
  L89.611 **Pressure ulcer of right heel, stage 1**
        Healing pressure ulcer of right heel, stage 1
        Pressure pre-ulcer skin changes limited to persistent focal edema, right heel

  L89.612 **Pressure ulcer of right heel, stage 2**
        Healing pressure ulcer of right heel, stage 2
        Pressure ulcer with abrasion, blister, partial thickness skin loss involving epidermis and/or dermis, right heel

  L89.613 **Pressure ulcer of right heel, stage 3**
        Healing pressure ulcer of right heel, stage 3
        Pressure ulcer with full thickness skin loss involving damage or necrosis of subcutaneous tissue, right heel

  L89.614 **Pressure ulcer of right heel, stage 4**
        Healing pressure ulcer of right heel, stage 4
        Pressure ulcer with necrosis of soft tissues through to underlying muscle, tendon, or bone, right heel

---

✔ Additional Character Required   ✔x7ᵗʰ Placeholder Alert   Manifestation Dx   ▽ Unspecified Dx   ▶◀ Revised Text   ● New Code   ▲ Revised Code Title

L89.619 Pressure ulcer of right heel, unspecified stage ▽
Healing pressure ulcer of right heel NOS
Healing pressure ulcer of unspecified heel, right stage

√6ᵗʰ **L89.62 Pressure ulcer of left heel**

L89.620 Pressure ulcer of left heel, unstageable

L89.621 Pressure ulcer of left heel, stage 1
Healing pressure ulcer of left heel, stage 1
Pressure pre-ulcer skin changes limited to persistent focal edema, left heel

L89.622 Pressure ulcer of left heel, stage 2
Healing pressure ulcer of left heel, stage 2
Pressure ulcer with abrasion, blister, partial thickness skin loss involving epidermis and/or dermis, left heel

L89.623 Pressure ulcer of left heel, stage 3
Healing pressure ulcer of left heel, stage 3
Pressure ulcer with full thickness skin loss involving damage or necrosis of subcutaneous tissue, left heel

L89.624 Pressure ulcer of left heel, stage 4
Healing pressure ulcer of left heel, stage 4
Pressure ulcer with necrosis of soft tissues through to underlying muscle, tendon, or bone, left heel

L89.629 Pressure ulcer of left heel, unspecified stage ▽
Healing pressure ulcer of left heel NOS
Healing pressure ulcer of left heel, unspecified stage

√5ᵗʰ **L89.8 Pressure ulcer of other site**

√6ᵗʰ **L89.81 Pressure ulcer of head**
Pressure ulcer of face

L89.810 Pressure ulcer of head, unstageable

L89.811 Pressure ulcer of head, stage 1
Healing pressure ulcer of head, stage 1
Pressure pre-ulcer skin changes limited to persistent focal edema, head

L89.812 Pressure ulcer of head, stage 2
Healing pressure ulcer of head, stage 2
Pressure ulcer with abrasion, blister, partial thickness skin loss involving epidermis and/or dermis, head

L89.813 Pressure ulcer of head, stage 3
Healing pressure ulcer of head, stage 3
Pressure ulcer with full thickness skin loss involving damage or necrosis of subcutaneous tissue, head

L89.814 Pressure ulcer of head, stage 4
Healing pressure ulcer of head, stage 4
Pressure ulcer with necrosis of soft tissues through to underlying muscle, tendon, or bone, head

L89.819 Pressure ulcer of head, unspecified stage ▽
Healing pressure ulcer of head NOS
Healing pressure ulcer of head, unspecified stage

√6ᵗʰ **L89.89 Pressure ulcer of other site**

L89.890 Pressure ulcer of other site, unstageable

L89.891 Pressure ulcer of other site, stage 1
Healing pressure ulcer of other site, stage 1
Pressure pre-ulcer skin changes limited to persistent focal edema, other site

L89.892 Pressure ulcer of other site, stage 2
Healing pressure ulcer of other site, stage 2
Pressure ulcer with abrasion, blister, partial thickness skin loss involving epidermis and/or dermis, other site

L89.893 Pressure ulcer of other site, stage 3
Healing pressure ulcer of other site, stage 3
Pressure ulcer with full thickness skin loss involving damage or necrosis of subcutaneous tissue, other site

L89.894 Pressure ulcer of other site, stage 4
Healing pressure ulcer of other site, stage 4
Pressure ulcer with necrosis of soft tissues through to underlying muscle, tendon, or bone, other site

L89.899 Pressure ulcer of other site, unspecified stage ▽
Healing pressure ulcer of other site NOS
Healing pressure ulcer of other site, unspecified stage

√5ᵗʰ **L89.9 Pressure ulcer of unspecified site**

L89.90 Pressure ulcer of unspecified site, unspecified stage ▽
Healing pressure ulcer of unspecified site NOS
Healing pressure ulcer of unspecified site, unspecified stage

L89.91 Pressure ulcer of unspecified site, stage 1 ▽
Healing pressure ulcer of unspecified site, stage 1
Pressure pre-ulcer skin changes limited to persistent focal edema, unspecified site

L89.92 Pressure ulcer of unspecified site, stage 2 ▽
Healing pressure ulcer of unspecified site, stage 2
Pressure ulcer with abrasion, blister, partial thickness skin loss involving epidermis and/or dermis, unspecified site

L89.93 Pressure ulcer of unspecified site, stage 3 ▽
Healing pressure ulcer of unspecified site, stage 3
Pressure ulcer with full thickness skin loss involving damage or necrosis of subcutaneous tissue, unspecified site

L89.94 Pressure ulcer of unspecified site, stage 4 ▽
Healing pressure ulcer of unspecified site, stage 4
Pressure ulcer with necrosis of soft tissues through to underlying muscle, tendon, or bone, unspecified site

L89.95 Pressure ulcer of unspecified site, unstageable ▽

√4ᵗʰ **L90 Atrophic disorders of skin**

L90.0 Lichen sclerosus et atrophicus
EXCLUDES 2 *lichen sclerosus of external female genital organs (N90.4)*
lichen sclerosus of external male genital organs (N48.0)

L90.1 Anetoderma of Schweninger-Buzzi

L90.2 Anetoderma of Jadassohn-Pellizzari

L90.3 Atrophoderma of Pasini and Pierini

L90.4 Acrodermatitis chronica atrophicans

L90.5 Scar conditions and fibrosis of skin
Adherent scar (skin)
Cicatrix
Disfigurement of skin due to scar
Fibrosis of skin NOS
Scar NOS
EXCLUDES 2 *hypertrophic scar (L91.0)*
keloid scar (L91.0)
AHA: 2016,2Q,5; 2015,1Q,19

L90.6 Striae atrophicae

L90.8 Other atrophic disorders of skin

L90.9 Atrophic disorder of skin, unspecified ▽

√4ᵗʰ **L91 Hypertrophic disorders of skin**

L91.0 Hypertrophic scar
Keloid
Keloid scar
EXCLUDES 2 *acne keloid (L73.0)*
scar NOS (L90.5)

DEF: Overgrowth of scar tissue due to excess amounts of collagen during connective tissue repair; occurs mainly on upper trunk, and face.

L91.8 Other hypertrophic disorders of the skin

L91.9 Hypertrophic disorder of the skin, unspecified ▽

EXCLUDES 1 Not coded here   *EXCLUDES 2* Not included here   N Newborn Age : 0   P Pediatric Age : 0-17   M Maternity Age : 12-55   A Adult Age : 15-124

692   ICD-10-CM 2017

✓4ᵗʰ **L92 Granulomatous disorders of skin and subcutaneous tissue**

    EXCLUDES 2 *actinic granuloma (L57.5)*

    L92.0 Granuloma annulare
       Perforating granuloma annulare

    L92.1 Necrobiosis lipoidica, not elsewhere classified
       EXCLUDES 1 *necrobiosis lipoidica associated with diabetes mellitus (E08-E13 with .620)*

    L92.2 Granuloma faciale [eosinophilic granuloma of skin]

    L92.3 Foreign body granuloma of the skin and subcutaneous tissue
       Use additional code to identify the type of retained foreign body (Z18.-)

    L92.8 Other granulomatous disorders of the skin and subcutaneous tissue

    L92.9 Granulomatous disorder of the skin and subcutaneous ▽
       tissue, unspecified

✓4ᵗʰ **L93 Lupus erythematosus**

    Use additional code for adverse effect, if applicable, to identify drug (T36-T50 with fifth or sixth character 5)

    EXCLUDES 1 *lupus exedens (A18.4)*
          lupus vulgaris (A18.4)
          scleroderma (M34.-)
          systemic lupus erythematosus (M32.-)

    L93.0 Discoid lupus erythematosus
       Lupus erythematosus NOS

    L93.1 Subacute cutaneous lupus erythematosus

    L93.2 Other local lupus erythematosus
       Lupus erythematosus profundus
       Lupus panniculitis

✓4ᵗʰ **L94 Other localized connective tissue disorders**

    EXCLUDES 1 *systemic connective tissue disorders (M30-M36)*

    L94.0 Localized scleroderma [morphea]
       Circumscribed scleroderma

    L94.1 Linear scleroderma
       En coup de sabre lesion

    L94.2 Calcinosis cutis

    L94.3 Sclerodactyly

    L94.4 Gottron's papules

    L94.5 Poikiloderma vasculare atrophicans

    L94.6 Ainhum

    L94.8 Other specified locallzed connective tissue disorders

    L94.9 Localized connective tissue disorder, unspecified ▽

✓4ᵗʰ **L95 Vasculitis limited to skin, not elsewhere classified**

    EXCLUDES 1 *angioma serpiginosum (L81.7)*
          Henoch(-Schönlein) purpura (D69.0)
          hypersensitivity angiitis (M31.0)
          lupus panniculitis (L93.2)
          panniculitis NOS (M79.3)
          panniculitis of neck and back (M54.0-)
          polyarteritis nodosa (M30.0)
          relapsing panniculitis (M35.6)
          rheumatoid vasculitis (M05.2)
          serum sickness (T80.6-)
          urticaria (L50.-)
          Wegener's granulomatosis (M31.3-)

    L95.0 Livedoid vasculitis
       Atrophie blanche (en plaque)

    L95.1 Erythema elevatum diutinum

    L95.8 Other vasculitis limited to the skin

    L95.9 Vasculitis limited to the skin, unspecified ▽

✓4ᵗʰ **L97 Non-pressure chronic ulcer of lower limb, not elsewhere classified**

    INCLUDES chronic ulcer of skin of lower limb NOS
          non-healing ulcer of skin
          non-infected sinus of skin
          trophic ulcer NOS
          tropical ulcer NOS
          ulcer of skin of lower limb NOS

    Code first any associated underlying condition, such as:
       any associated gangrene (I96)
       atherosclerosis of the lower extremities (I70.23-, I70.24-, I70.33-, I70.34-, I70.43-, I70.44-, I70.53-, I70.54-, I70.63-, I70.64-, I70.73-, I70.74-)
       chronic venous hypertension (I87.31-, I87.33-)
       diabetic ulcers (E08.621, E08.622, E09.621, E09.622, E10.621, E10.622, E11.621, E11.622, E13.621, E13.622)
       postphlebitic syndrome (I87.01-, I87.03-)
       postthrombotic syndrome (I87.01-, I87.03-)
       varicose ulcer (I83.0-, I83.2-)

    EXCLUDES 2 *pressure ulcer (pressure area) (L89.-)*
          skin infections (L00-L08)
          specific infections classified to A00-B99

    ✓5ᵗʰ **L97.1 Non-pressure chronic ulcer of thigh**

       ✓6ᵗʰ **L97.10 Non-pressure chronic ulcer of unspecified thigh**

          L97.101 Non-pressure chronic ulcer of ▽
             unspecified thigh limited to breakdown of skin

          L97.102 Non-pressure chronic ulcer of ▽
             unspecified thigh with fat layer exposed

          L97.103 Non-pressure chronic ulcer of ▽
             unspecified thigh with necrosis of muscle

          L97.104 Non-pressure chronic ulcer of ▽
             unspecified thigh with necrosis of bone

          L97.109 Non-pressure chronic ulcer of ▽
             unspecified thigh with unspecified severity

       ✓6ᵗʰ **L97.11 Non-pressure chronic ulcer of right thigh**

          L97.111 Non-pressure chronic ulcer of right thigh limited to breakdown of skin

          L97.112 Non-pressure chronic ulcer of right thigh with fat layer exposed

          L97.113 Non-pressure chronic ulcer of right thigh with necrosis of muscle

          L97.114 Non-pressure chronic ulcer of right thigh with necrosis of bone

          L97.119 Non-pressure chronic ulcer of right ▽
             thigh with unspecified severity

       ✓6ᵗʰ **L97.12 Non-pressure chronic ulcer of left thigh**

          L97.121 Non-pressure chronic ulcer of left thigh limited to breakdown of skin

          L97.122 Non-pressure chronic ulcer of left thigh with fat layer exposed

          L97.123 Non-pressure chronic ulcer of left thigh with necrosis of muscle

          L97.124 Non-pressure chronic ulcer of left thigh with necrosis of bone

          L97.129 Non-pressure chronic ulcer of left ▽
             thigh with unspecified severity

    ✓5ᵗʰ **L97.2 Non-pressure chronic ulcer of calf**

       ✓6ᵗʰ **L97.20 Non-pressure chronic ulcer of unspecified calf**

          L97.201 Non-pressure chronic ulcer of ▽
             unspecified calf limited to breakdown of skin

          L97.202 Non-pressure chronic ulcer of ▽
             unspecified calf with fat layer exposed

          L97.203 Non-pressure chronic ulcer of ▽
             unspecified calf with necrosis of muscle

          L97.204 Non-pressure chronic ulcer of ▽
             unspecified calf with necrosis of bone

          L97.209 Non-pressure chronic ulcer of ▽
             unspecified calf with unspecified severity

       ✓6ᵗʰ **L97.21 Non-pressure chronic ulcer of right calf**

          L97.211 Non-pressure chronic ulcer of right calf limited to breakdown of skin

---

✔ Additional Character Required   ✓x7ᵗʰ Placeholder Alert   Manifestation Dx   ▽ Unspecified Dx   ▶◀ Revised Text   ● New Code   ▲ Revised Code Title

    L97.212 Non-pressure chronic ulcer of right calf with fat layer exposed

    L97.213 Non-pressure chronic ulcer of right calf with necrosis of muscle

    L97.214 Non-pressure chronic ulcer of right calf with necrosis of bone

    L97.219 Non-pressure chronic ulcer of right calf with unspecified severity ▽

✓6th **L97.22** Non-pressure chronic ulcer of left calf

    L97.221 Non-pressure chronic ulcer of left calf limited to breakdown of skin

    L97.222 Non-pressure chronic ulcer of left calf with fat layer exposed

    L97.223 Non-pressure chronic ulcer of left calf with necrosis of muscle

    L97.224 Non-pressure chronic ulcer of left calf with necrosis of bone

    L97.229 Non-pressure chronic ulcer of left calf with unspecified severity ▽

✓5th **L97.3** Non-pressure chronic ulcer of ankle

  ✓6th **L97.30** Non-pressure chronic ulcer of unspecified ankle

    L97.301 Non-pressure chronic ulcer of unspecified ankle limited to breakdown of skin ▽

    L97.302 Non-pressure chronic ulcer of unspecified ankle with fat layer exposed ▽

    L97.303 Non-pressure chronic ulcer of unspecified ankle with necrosis of muscle ▽

    L97.304 Non-pressure chronic ulcer of unspecified ankle with necrosis of bone ▽

    L97.309 Non-pressure chronic ulcer of unspecified ankle with unspecified severity ▽

  ✓6th **L97.31** Non-pressure chronic ulcer of right ankle

    L97.311 Non-pressure chronic ulcer of right ankle limited to breakdown of skin

    L97.312 Non-pressure chronic ulcer of right ankle with fat layer exposed

    L97.313 Non-pressure chronic ulcer of right ankle with necrosis of muscle

    L97.314 Non-pressure chronic ulcer of right ankle with necrosis of bone

    L97.319 Non-pressure chronic ulcer of right ankle with unspecified severity ▽

  ✓6th **L97.32** Non-pressure chronic ulcer of left ankle

    L97.321 Non-pressure chronic ulcer of left ankle limited to breakdown of skin

    L97.322 Non-pressure chronic ulcer of left ankle with fat layer exposed

    L97.323 Non-pressure chronic ulcer of left ankle with necrosis of muscle

    L97.324 Non-pressure chronic ulcer of left ankle with necrosis of bone

    L97.329 Non-pressure chronic ulcer of left ankle with unspecified severity ▽

✓5th **L97.4** Non-pressure chronic ulcer of heel and midfoot

  Non-pressure chronic ulcer of plantar surface of midfoot

  ✓6th **L97.40** Non-pressure chronic ulcer of unspecified heel and midfoot

    L97.401 Non-pressure chronic ulcer of unspecified heel and midfoot limited to breakdown of skin ▽

    L97.402 Non-pressure chronic ulcer of unspecified heel and midfoot with fat layer exposed ▽

    L97.403 Non-pressure chronic ulcer of unspecified heel and midfoot with necrosis of muscle ▽

    L97.404 Non-pressure chronic ulcer of unspecified heel and midfoot with necrosis of bone ▽

    L97.409 Non-pressure chronic ulcer of unspecified heel and midfoot with unspecified severity ▽

  ✓6th **L97.41** Non-pressure chronic ulcer of right heel and midfoot

    L97.411 Non-pressure chronic ulcer of right heel and midfoot limited to breakdown of skin

    L97.412 Non-pressure chronic ulcer of right heel and midfoot with fat layer exposed

    L97.413 Non-pressure chronic ulcer of right heel and midfoot with necrosis of muscle

    L97.414 Non-pressure chronic ulcer of right heel and midfoot with necrosis of bone

    L97.419 Non-pressure chronic ulcer of right heel and midfoot with unspecified severity ▽

  ✓6th **L97.42** Non-pressure chronic ulcer of left heel and midfoot

    L97.421 Non-pressure chronic ulcer of left heel and midfoot limited to breakdown of skin

        AHA: 2016,1Q,12

    L97.422 Non-pressure chronic ulcer of left heel and midfoot with fat layer exposed

    L97.423 Non-pressure chronic ulcer of left heel and midfoot with necrosis of muscle

    L97.424 Non-pressure chronic ulcer of left heel and midfoot with necrosis of bone

    L97.429 Non-pressure chronic ulcer of left heel and midfoot with unspecified severity ▽

✓5th **L97.5** Non-pressure chronic ulcer of other part of foot

  Non-pressure chronic ulcer of toe

  ✓6th **L97.50** Non-pressure chronic ulcer of other part of unspecified foot

    L97.501 Non-pressure chronic ulcer of other part of unspecified foot limited to breakdown of skin ▽

    L97.502 Non-pressure chronic ulcer of other part of unspecified foot with fat layer exposed ▽

    L97.503 Non-pressure chronic ulcer of other part of unspecified foot with necrosis of muscle ▽

    L97.504 Non-pressure chronic ulcer of other part of unspecified foot with necrosis of bone ▽

    L97.509 Non-pressure chronic ulcer of other part of unspecified foot with unspecified severity ▽

  ✓6th **L97.51** Non-pressure chronic ulcer of other part of right foot

    L97.511 Non-pressure chronic ulcer of other part of right foot limited to breakdown of skin

    L97.512 Non-pressure chronic ulcer of other part of right foot with fat layer exposed

    L97.513 Non-pressure chronic ulcer of other part of right foot with necrosis of muscle

    L97.514 Non-pressure chronic ulcer of other part of right foot with necrosis of bone

    L97.519 Non-pressure chronic ulcer of other part of right foot with unspecified severity ▽

  ✓6th **L97.52** Non-pressure chronic ulcer of other part of left foot

    L97.521 Non-pressure chronic ulcer of other part of left foot limited to breakdown of skin

    L97.522 Non-pressure chronic ulcer of other part of left foot with fat layer exposed

    L97.523 Non-pressure chronic ulcer of other part of left foot with necrosis of muscle

    L97.524 Non-pressure chronic ulcer of other part of left foot with necrosis of bone

    L97.529 Non-pressure chronic ulcer of other part of left foot with unspecified severity ▽

✓5th **L97.8** Non-pressure chronic ulcer of other part of lower leg

  ✓6th **L97.80** Non-pressure chronic ulcer of other part of unspecified lower leg

    L97.801 Non-pressure chronic ulcer of other part of unspecified lower leg limited to breakdown of skin ▽

    L97.802 Non-pressure chronic ulcer of other part of unspecified lower leg with fat layer exposed ▽

    L97.803 Non-pressure chronic ulcer of other part of unspecified lower leg with necrosis of muscle ▽

    L97.804 Non-pressure chronic ulcer of other part of unspecified lower leg with necrosis of bone ▽

EXCLUDES 1 Not coded here   EXCLUDES 2 Not included here   N Newborn Age : 0   P Pediatric Age : 0-17   M Maternity Age : 12-55   A Adult Age : 15-124

694   ICD-10-CM 2017

L97.809 Non-pressure chronic ulcer of other part of unspecified lower leg with unspecified severity ▽

✓6ᵗʰ **L97.81** Non-pressure chronic ulcer of other part of right lower leg

L97.811 Non-pressure chronic ulcer of other part of right lower leg limited to breakdown of skin

L97.812 Non-pressure chronic ulcer of other part of right lower leg with fat layer exposed

L97.813 Non-pressure chronic ulcer of other part of right lower leg with necrosis of muscle

L97.814 Non-pressure chronic ulcer of other part of right lower leg with necrosis of bone

L97.819 Non-pressure chronic ulcer of other part of right lower leg with unspecified severity ▽

✓6ᵗʰ **L97.82** Non-pressure chronic ulcer of other part of left lower leg

L97.821 Non-pressure chronic ulcer of other part of left lower leg limited to breakdown of skin

L97.822 Non-pressure chronic ulcer of other part of left lower leg with fat layer exposed

L97.823 Non-pressure chronic ulcer of other part of left lower leg with necrosis of muscle

L97.824 Non-pressure chronic ulcer of other part of left lower leg with necrosis of bone

L97.829 Non-pressure chronic ulcer of other part of left lower leg with unspecified severity ▽

✓5ᵗʰ **L97.9** Non-pressure chronic ulcer of unspecified part of lower leg

✓6ᵗʰ **L97.90** Non-pressure chronic ulcer of unspecified part of unspecified lower leg

L97.901 Non-pressure chronic ulcer of unspecified part of unspecified lower leg limited to breakdown of skin ▽

L97.902 Non-pressure chronic ulcer of unspecified part of unspecified lower leg with fat layer exposed ▽

L97.903 Non-pressure chronic ulcer of unspecified part of unspecified lower leg with necrosis of muscle ▽

L97.904 Non-pressure chronic ulcer of unspecified part of unspecified lower leg with necrosis of bone ▽

L97.909 Non-pressure chronic ulcer of unspecified part of unspecified lower leg with unspecified severity ▽

✓6ᵗʰ **L97.91** Non-pressure chronic ulcer of unspecified part of right lower leg

L97.911 Non-pressure chronic ulcer of unspecified part of right lower leg limited to breakdown of skin ▽

L97.912 Non-pressure chronic ulcer of unspecified part of right lower leg with fat layer exposed ▽

L97.913 Non-pressure chronic ulcer of unspecified part of right lower leg with necrosis of muscle ▽

L97.914 Non-pressure chronic ulcer of unspecified part of right lower leg with necrosis of bone ▽

L97.919 Non-pressure chronic ulcer of unspecified part of right lower leg with unspecified severity ▽

✓6ᵗʰ **L97.92** Non-pressure chronic ulcer of unspecified part of left lower leg

L97.921 Non-pressure chronic ulcer of unspecified part of left lower leg limited to breakdown of skin ▽

L97.922 Non-pressure chronic ulcer of unspecified part of left lower leg with fat layer exposed ▽

L97.923 Non-pressure chronic ulcer of unspecified part of left lower leg with necrosis of muscle ▽

L97.924 Non-pressure chronic ulcer of unspecified part of left lower leg with necrosis of bone ▽

L97.929 Non-pressure chronic ulcer of unspecified part of left lower leg with unspecified severity ▽

✓4ᵗʰ **L98** Other disorders of skin and subcutaneous tissue, not elsewhere classified

L98.0 Pyogenic granuloma

EXCLUDES 2 *pyogenic granuloma of gingiva (K06.8)*
pyogenic granuloma of maxillary alveolar ridge (K04.5)
pyogenic granuloma of oral mucosa (K13.4)

L98.1 Factitial dermatitis
Neurotic excoriation
EXCLUDES 1 ►*excoriation (skin-picking) disorder (F42.4)*◄

L98.2 Febrile neutrophilic dermatosis [Sweet]

L98.3 Eosinophilic cellulitis [Wells]

✓5ᵗʰ **L98.4** Non-pressure chronic ulcer of skin, not elsewhere classified
Chronic ulcer of skin NOS
Tropical ulcer NOS
Ulcer of skin NOS
EXCLUDES 2 *gangrene (I96)*
pressure ulcer (pressure area) (L89.-)
skin infections (L00-L08)
specific infections classified to A00-B99
ulcer of lower limb NEC (L97.-)
varicose ulcer (I83.0-I82.2)

✓6ᵗʰ **L98.41** Non-pressure chronic ulcer of buttock

L98.411 Non-pressure chronic ulcer of buttock limited to breakdown of skin

L98.412 Non-pressure chronic ulcer of buttock with fat layer exposed

L98.413 Non-pressure chronic ulcer of buttock with necrosis of muscle

L98.414 Non-pressure chronic ulcer of buttock with necrosis of bone

L98.419 Non-pressure chronic ulcer of buttock with unspecified severity ▽

✓6ᵗʰ **L98.42** Non-pressure chronic ulcer of back

L98.421 Non-pressure chronic ulcer of back limited to breakdown of skin

L98.422 Non-pressure chronic ulcer of back with fat layer exposed

L98.423 Non-pressure chronic ulcer of back with necrosis of muscle

L98.424 Non-pressure chronic ulcer of back with necrosis of bone

L98.429 Non-pressure chronic ulcer of back with unspecified severity ▽

✓6ᵗʰ **L98.49** Non-pressure chronic ulcer of skin of other sites
Non-pressure chronic ulcer of skin NOS

L98.491 Non-pressure chronic ulcer of skin of other sites limited to breakdown of skin

L98.492 Non-pressure chronic ulcer of skin of other sites with fat layer exposed

L98.493 Non-pressure chronic ulcer of skin of other sites with necrosis of muscle

L98.494 Non-pressure chronic ulcer of skin of other sites with necrosis of bone

L98.499 Non-pressure chronic ulcer of skin of other sites with unspecified severity ▽

L98.5 Mucinosis of the skin
Focal mucinosis
Lichen myxedematosus
Reticular erythematous mucinosis
EXCLUDES 1 *focal oral mucinosis (K13.79)*
myxedema (E03.9)

L98.6 Other infiltrative disorders of the skin and subcutaneous tissue
EXCLUDES 1 *hyalinosis cutis et mucosae (E78.89)*

● **L98.7** Excessive and redundant skin and subcutaneous tissue
Loose or sagging skin, following bariatric surgery weight loss
Loose or sagging skin following dietary weight loss
Loose or sagging skin, NOS
EXCLUDES 2 *acquired excess or redundant skin of eyelid (H02.3-)*
congenital excess or redundant skin of eyelid (Q10.3)
skin changes due to chronic exposure to nonionizing radiation (L57.-)

L98.8 Other specified disorders of the skin and subcutaneous tissue
AHA: 2013,2Q,32

L98.9 Disorder of the skin and subcutaneous tissue, unspecified ▽

✓ Additional Character Required   ✓x7ᵗʰ Placeholder Alert   Manifestation Dx   ▽ Unspecified Dx   ►◄ Revised Text   ● New Code   ▲ Revised Code Title

L99 *Other disorders of skin and subcutaneous tissue in diseases classified elsewhere*

Code first underlying disease, such as:

amyloidosis (E85.-)

EXCLUDES 1   skin disorders in diabetes (E08-E13 with .62)
skin disorders in gonorrhea (A54.89)
skin disorders in syphilis (A51.31, A52.79)

EXCLUDES 1 Not coded here   EXCLUDES 2 Not included here   N Newborn Age : 0   P Pediatric Age : 0-17   M Maternity Age : 12-55   A Adult Age : 15-124

Chapter 13. Diseases of the Musculoskeletal System and Connective Tissue (M00–M99)

Chapter Specific Guidelines with Coding Examples

The chapter specific guidelines from the ICD-10-CM Official Guidelines for Coding and Reporting have been provided below. Along with these guidelines are coding examples, contained in the shaded boxes, that have been developed to help illustrate the coding and/or sequencing guidance found in these guidelines.

a. Site and laterality

Most of the codes within Chapter 13 have site and laterality designations. The site represents the bone, joint or the muscle involved. For some conditions where more than one bone, joint or muscle is usually involved, such as osteoarthritis, there is a "multiple sites" code available. For categories where no multiple site code is provided and more than one bone, joint or muscle is involved, multiple codes should be used to indicate the different sites involved.

> Right elbow infective bursitis
>
> **M71.121   Other infective bursitis, right elbow**
>
> *Explanation:* Most of the codes within chapter 13 have site and laterality designations. The site represents the bone, joint, or the muscle involved.

> Rheumatoid arthritis of multiple sites without rheumatoid factor
>
> **M06.09   Rheumatoid arthritis without rheumatoid factor, multiple sites**
>
> *Explanation:* For some conditions where more than one bone, joint or muscle is usually involved, such as osteoarthritis, there is a "multiple sites" code available.

> Osteomyelitis of the fourth thoracic and second lumbar vertebrae
>
> **M46.24   Osteomyelitis of vertebra, thoracic region**
>
> **M46.26   Osteomyelitis of vertebra, lumbar region**
>
> *Explanation:* For categories without a multiple site code and more than one bone, joint, or muscle is involved, multiple codes should be used to indicate the different sites involved.

1) Bone versus joint

For certain conditions, the bone may be affected at the upper or lower end, (e.g., avascular necrosis of bone, M87, Osteoporosis, M80, M81). Though the portion of the bone affected may be at the joint, the site designation will be the bone, not the joint.

> Idiopathic avascular necrosis of the femoral head of the left hip joint
>
> **M87.052   Idiopathic aseptic necrosis of left femur**
>
> *Explanation:* For certain conditions such as avascular necrosis, the bone may be affected at the joint, but the site designation is the bone, not the joint.

b. Acute traumatic versus chronic or recurrent musculoskeletal conditions

Many musculoskeletal conditions are a result of previous injury or trauma to a site, or are recurrent conditions. Bone, joint or muscle conditions that are the result of a healed injury are usually found in chapter 13. Recurrent bone, joint or muscle conditions are also usually found in chapter 13. Any current, acute injury should be coded to the appropriate injury code from chapter 19. Chronic or recurrent conditions should generally be coded with a code from chapter 13. If it is difficult to determine from the documentation in the record which code is best to describe a condition, query the provider.

> Acute traumatic bucket handle tear of right medial meniscus
>
> **S83.211A   Bucket-handle tear of medial meniscus, current injury, right knee, initial encounter**
>
> *Explanation:* Any current, acute injury is not coded in chapter 13. It should instead be coded to the appropriate injury code from chapter 19.

> Old bucket handle tear of right medial meniscus
>
> **M23.203   Derangement of unspecified medial meniscus due to old tear or injury, right knee**
>
> *Explanation:* Chronic or recurrent conditions should generally be coded with a code from chapter 13.

c. Coding of pathologic fractures

7th character A is for use as long as the patient is receiving active treatment for the fracture. While the patient may be seen by a new or different provider over the course of treatment for a pathological fracture, assignment of the 7th character is based on whether the patient is undergoing active treatment and not whether the provider is seeing the patient for the first time.

> Pathologic fracture of left foot, unknown cause, currently under active treatment by a follow-up provider
>
> **M84.475A   Pathological fracture, left foot, initial encounter for fracture**
>
> *Explanation:* Seventh character A is for use as long as the patient is receiving active treatment for a pathologic fracture. Examples of active treatment are surgical treatment, emergency department encounter, evaluation, and continuing treatment by the same or a different physician.
>
> The seventh character is based on whether the patient is undergoing active treatment and not whether the provider is seeing the patient for the first time.

7th character D is to be used for encounters after the patient has completed active treatment. The other 7th characters, listed under each subcategory in the Tabular List, are to be used for subsequent encounters for **routine care of fractures during the healing and recovery phase as well as** treatment of problems associated with the healing, such as malunions, nonunions, and sequelae.

Care for complications of surgical treatment for fracture repairs during the healing or recovery phase should be coded with the appropriate complication codes.

See Section I.C.19. Coding of traumatic fractures.

d. Osteoporosis

Osteoporosis is a systemic condition, meaning that all bones of the musculoskeletal system are affected. Therefore, site is not a component of the codes under category M81, Osteoporosis without current pathological fracture. The site codes under category M80, Osteoporosis with current pathological fracture, identify the site of the fracture, not the osteoporosis.

1) Osteoporosis without pathological fracture

Category M81, Osteoporosis without current pathological fracture, is for use for patients with osteoporosis who do not currently have a pathologic fracture due to the osteoporosis, even if they have had a fracture in the past. For patients with a history of osteoporosis fractures, status code Z87.310, Personal history of (healed) osteoporosis fracture, should follow the code from M81.

> Age-related osteoporosis with healed osteoporotic fracture of the lumbar vertebra
>
> **M81.0   Age-related osteoporosis without current pathological fracture**
>
> **Z87.310   Personal history of (healed) osteoporosis fracture**
>
> *Explanation:* Category M81 is used for patients with osteoporosis who do not currently have a pathologic fracture due to the osteoporosis. To report a previous (healed) fracture, status code Z87.310 Personal history of (healed) osteoporosis fracture, should follow the code from M81.

2) Osteoporosis with current pathological fracture

Category M80, Osteoporosis with current pathological fracture, is for patients who have a current pathologic fracture at the time of an encounter. The codes under M80 identify the site of the fracture. A code from category M80, not a traumatic fracture code, should be used for any patient with known osteoporosis who suffers a fracture, even if the patient had a minor fall or trauma, if that fall or trauma would not usually break a normal, healthy bone.

> Disuse osteoporosis with current fracture of right shoulder sustained lifting a grocery bag, initial encounter
>
> **M80.811A   Other osteoporosis with current pathological fracture, right shoulder, initial encounter for fracture**
>
> *Explanation:* A code from category M80, not a traumatic fracture code, should be used for any patient with known osteoporosis who suffers a fracture, even if the patient had a minor fall or trauma, if that fall or trauma would not usually break a normal, healthy bone.

Muscle/Tendon Table

ICD-10-CM categorizes certain muscles and tendons in the upper and lower extremities by their action (e.g., extension, flexion), their anatomical location (e.g., posterior, anterior), and/or whether they are intrinsic or extrinsic to a certain anatomical area. The Muscle/Tendon Table is provided at the beginning of chapters 13 and 19 as a resource to help users when code selection depends on one or more of these characteristics. Please note that this table is not all-inclusive, and proper code assignment should be based on the provider's documentation.

Body Region	Muscle	Extensor Tendon	Flexor Tendon	Other Tendon
Shoulder				
	Deltoid	Posterior deltoid	Anterior deltoid	
	Rotator cuff			
	Infraspinatus			Infraspinatus
	Subscapularis			Subscapularis
	Supraspinatus			Supraspinatus
	Teres minor			Teres minor
	Teres major	Teres major		
Upper arm				
	Anterior muscles			
	Biceps brachii — long head		Biceps brachii — long head	
	Biceps brachii — short head		Biceps brachii — short head	
	Brachialis		Brachialis	
	Coracobrachialis		Coracobrachialis	
	Posterior muscles			
	Triceps brachii	Triceps brachii		
Forearm				
	Anterior muscles			
	Flexors			
	Deep			
	Flexor digitorum profundus		Flexor digitorum profundus	
	Flexor pollicis longus		Flexor pollicis longus	
	Intermediate			
	Flexor digitorum superficialis		Flexor digitorum superficialis	
	Superficial			
	Flexor carpi radialis		Flexor carpi radialis	
	Flexor carpi ulnaris		Flexor carpi ulnaris	
	Palmaris longus		Palmaris longus	
	Pronators			
	Pronator quadratus			Pronator quadratus
	Pronator teres			Pronator teres
	Posterior muscles			
	Extensors			
	Deep			
	Abductor pollicis longus			Abductor pollicis longus
	Extensor indicis	Extensor indicis		
	Extensor pollicis brevis	Extensor pollicis brevis		
	Extensor pollicis longus	Extensor pollicis longus		
	Superficial			
	Brachioradialis			Brachioradialis
	Extensor carpi radialis brevis	Extensor carpi radialis brevis		
	Extensor carpi radialis longus	Extensor carpi radialis longus		
	Extensor carpi ulnaris	Extensor carpi ulnaris		
	Extensor digiti minimi	Extensor digiti minimi		
	Extensor digitorum	Extensor digitorum		
	Anconeus	Anconeus		
	Supinator			Supinator

Body Region	Muscle	Extensor Tendon	Flexor Tendon	Other Tendon
Hand				
Extrinsic — attach to a site in the forearm as well as a site in the hand with action related to hand movement at the wrist				
	Extensor carpi radialis brevis	Extensor carpi radialis brevis		
	Extensor carpi radialis longus	Extensor carpie radialis longus		
	Extensor carpi ulnaris	Extensor carpi ulnaris		
	Flexor carpi radialis		Flexor carpi radialis	
	Flexor carpi ulnaris		Flexor carpi ulnaris	
	Flexor digitorum superficialis		Flexor digitorum superficialis	
	Palmaris longus		Palmaris longus	
Extrinsic — attach to a site in the forearm as well as a site in the hand with action in the hand related to finger movement				
	Adductor pollicis longus			Adductor pollicis longus
	Extensor digiti minimi	Extensor digiti minimi		
	Extensor digitorum	Extensor digitorum		
	Extensor indicis	Extensor indicis		
	Flexor digitorum profundus		Flexor digitorum profundus	
	Flexor digitorum superficialis		Flexor digitorum superficialis	
Extrinsic — attach to a site in the forearm as well as a site in the hand with action in the hand related to thumb movement				
	Extensor pollicis brevis	Extensor pollicis brevis		
	Extensor pollicis longus	Extensor pollicis longus		
	Flexor pollicis longus		Flexor pollicis longus	
Intrinsic — found within the hand only				
	Adductor pollicis			Adductor pollicis
	Dorsal Interossei	Dorsal interossei	Dorsal interossei	
	Lumbricals	Lumbricals	Lumbricals	
	Palmaris brevis			Palmaris brevis
	Palmar interossei	Palmar interossei	Palmar interossei	
	Hypothenar muscles			
	Abductor digiti minimi			Abductor digiti minimi
	Flexor digiti minimi brevis		Flexor digiti minimi brevis	
	Oppenens digiti minimi		Oppenens digiti minimi	
	Thenar muscles			
	Abductor pollicis brevis			Abductor pollicis brevis
	Flexor pollicis brevis		Flexor pollicis brevis	
	Oppenens pollicis		Oppenens pollicis	
Thigh				
	Anterior muscles			
	Iliopsoas		Iliopsoas	
	Pectineus		Pectineus	
	Quadriceps	Quadriceps		
	Rectus femoris	Rectus femoris — Extends knee	Rectus femoris — Flexes hip	
	Vastus intermedius	Vastus intermedius		
	Vastus lateralis	Vastus lateralis		
	Vastus medialis	Vastus medialis		
	Sartorius		Sartorius	
	Medial muscles			
	Adductor brevis			Adductor brevis
	Adductor longus			Adductor longus
	Adductor magnus			Adductor magnus
	Gracilis			Gracilis
	Obturator externus			Obturator externus
	Posterior muscles			
	Hamstring	Hamstring — Extends hip	Hamstring — Flexes knee	
	Biceps femoris	Biceps femoris	Biceps femoris	
	Semimembranosus	Semimembranosus	Semimembranosus	
	Semitendinosus	Semitendinosus	Semitendinosus	

Body Region	Muscle	Extensor Tendon	Flexor Tendon	Other Tendon
Lower leg				
	Anterior muscles			
	Extensor digitorum longus	Extensor digitorum longus		
	Extensor hallucis longus	Extensor hallucis longus		
	Fibularis (peroneus) tertius	Fibularis (peroneus) tertius		
	Tibialis anterior	Tibialis anterior		Tibialis anterior
	Lateral muscles			
	Fibularis (peroneus) brevis		Fibularis (peroneus) brevis	
	Fibularis (peroneus) longus		Fibularis (peroneus) longus	
	Posterior muscles			
	Deep			
	Flexor digitorum longus		Flexor digitorum longus	
	Flexor hallucis longus		Flexor hallucis longus	
	Popliteus		Popliteus	
	Tibialis posterior		Tibialis posterior	
	Superficial			
	Gastrocnemius		Gastrocnemius	
	Plantaris		Plantaris	
	Soleus		Soleus	
				Calcaneal (Achilles)
Ankle/Foot				
Extrinsic — attach to a site in the lower leg as well as a site in the foot with action related to foot movement at the ankle				
	Plantaris		Plantaris	
	Soleus		Soleus	
	Tibialis anterior	Tibialis anterior		
	Tibialis posterior		Tibialis posterior	
Extrinsic — attach to a site in the lower leg as well as a site in the foot with action in the foot related to toe movement				
	Extensor digitorum longus	Extensor digitorum longus		
	Extensor hallicus longus	Extensor hallicus longus		
	Flexor digitorum longus		Flexor digitorum longus	
	Flexor hallucis longus		Flexor hallucis longus	
Intrinsic — found within the ankle/foot only				
	Dorsal muscles			
	Extensor digitorum brevis	Extensor digitorum brevis		
	Extensor hallucis brevis	Extensor hallucis brevis		
	Plantar muscles			
	Abductor digiti minimi		Abductor digiti minimi	
	Abductor hallucis		Abductor hallucis	
	Dorsal interossei	Dorsal interossei	Dorsal interossei	
	Flexor digiti minimi brevis		Flexor digiti minimi brevis	
	Flexor digitorum brevis		Flexor digitorum brevis	
	Flexor hallucis brevis		Flexor hallucis brevis	
	Lumbricals	Lumbricals	Lumbricals	
	Quadratus plantae		Quadratus plantae	
	Plantar interossei	Plantar interossei	Plantar interossei	

Chapter 13. Diseases of the Musculoskeletal System and Connective Tissue (M00-M99)

NOTE Use an external cause code following the code for the musculoskeletal condition, if applicable, to identify the cause of the musculoskeletal condition

EXCLUDES 2 *arthropathic psoriasis (L40.5-)*
certain conditions originating in the perinatal period (P04-P96)
certain infectious and parasitic diseases (A00-B99)
compartment syndrome (traumatic) (T79.A-)
complications of pregnancy, childbirth and the puerperium (O00-O9A)
congenital malformations, deformations, and chromosomal abnormalities (Q00-Q99)
endocrine, nutritional and metabolic diseases (E00-E88)
injury, poisoning and certain other consequences of external causes (S00-T88)
neoplasms (C00-D49)
symptoms, signs and abnormal clinical and laboratory findings, not elsewhere classified (R00-R94)

This chapter contains the following blocks:

M00-M02 Infectious arthropathies
▶M04 Autoinflammatory syndromes◀
M05-M14 Inflammatory polyarthropathies
M15-M19 Osteoarthritis
M20-M25 Other joint disorders
M26-M27 Dentofacial anomalies [including malocclusion] and other disorders of jaw
M30-M36 Systemic connective tissue disorders
M40-M43 Deforming dorsopathies
M45-M49 Spondylopathies
M50-M54 Other dorsopathies
M60-M63 Disorders of muscles
M65-M67 Disorders of synovium and tendon
M70-M79 Other soft tissue disorders
M80-M85 Disorders of bone density and structure
M86-M90 Other osteopathies
M91-M94 Chondropathies
M95 Other disorders of the musculoskeletal system and connective tissue
M96 Intraoperative and postprocedural complications and disorders of musculoskeletal system, not elsewhere classified
▶M97 Periprosthetic fracture around internal prosthetic joint◀
M99 Biomechanical lesions, not elsewhere classified

Arthropathies (M00-M25)

INCLUDES disorders affecting predominantly peripheral (limb) joints

Infectious arthropathies (M00-M02)

NOTE This block comprises arthropathies due to microbiological agents. Distinction is made between the following types of etiological relationship:
  a) direct infection of joint, where organisms invade synovial tissue and microbial antigen is present in the joint;
  b) indirect infection, which may be of two types: a reactive arthropathy, where microbial infection of the body is established but neither organisms nor antigens can be identified in the joint, and a postinfective arthropathy, where microbial antigen is present but recovery of an organism is inconstant and evidence of local multiplication is lacking.

✓4ᵗʰ **M00 Pyogenic arthritis**

  ✓5ᵗʰ **M00.0 Staphylococcal arthritis and polyarthritis**

    Use additional code (B95.61-B95.8) to identify bacterial agent
    EXCLUDES 2 *infection and inflammatory reaction due to internal joint prosthesis (T84.5-)*

    M00.00 Staphylococcal arthritis, unspecified joint ▽

    ✓6ᵗʰ **M00.01 Staphylococcal arthritis, shoulder**

      M00.011 Staphylococcal arthritis, right shoulder
      M00.012 Staphylococcal arthritis, left shoulder
      M00.019 Staphylococcal arthritis, unspecified shoulder ▽

    ✓6ᵗʰ **M00.02 Staphylococcal arthritis, elbow**

      M00.021 Staphylococcal arthritis, right elbow
      M00.022 Staphylococcal arthritis, left elbow
      M00.029 Staphylococcal arthritis, unspecified elbow ▽

    ✓6ᵗʰ **M00.03 Staphylococcal arthritis, wrist**
      Staphylococcal arthritis of carpal bones
      M00.031 Staphylococcal arthritis, right wrist
      M00.032 Staphylococcal arthritis, left wrist
      M00.039 Staphylococcal arthritis, unspecified wrist ▽

    ✓6ᵗʰ **M00.04 Staphylococcal arthritis, hand**
      Staphylococcal arthritis of metacarpus and phalanges
      M00.041 Staphylococcal arthritis, right hand

      M00.042 Staphylococcal arthritis, left hand
      M00.049 Staphylococcal arthritis, unspecified hand ▽

  ✓6ᵗʰ **M00.05 Staphylococcal arthritis, hip**

    M00.051 Staphylococcal arthritis, right hip
    M00.052 Staphylococcal arthritis, left hip
    M00.059 Staphylococcal arthritis, unspecified hip

  ✓6ᵗʰ **M00.06 Staphylococcal arthritis, knee**

    M00.061 Staphylococcal arthritis, right knee
    M00.062 Staphylococcal arthritis, left knee
    M00.069 Staphylococcal arthritis, unspecified knee ▽

  ✓6ᵗʰ **M00.07 Staphylococcal arthritis, ankle and foot**
    Staphylococcal arthritis, tarsus, metatarsus and phalanges
    M00.071 Staphylococcal arthritis, right ankle and foot
    M00.072 Staphylococcal arthritis, left ankle and foot
    M00.079 Staphylococcal arthritis, unspecified ankle and foot ▽

  M00.08 Staphylococcal arthritis, vertebrae
  M00.09 Staphylococcal polyarthritis

  ✓5ᵗʰ **M00.1 Pneumococcal arthritis and polyarthritis**

    M00.10 Pneumococcal arthritis, unspecified joint ▽

    ✓6ᵗʰ **M00.11 Pneumococcal arthritis, shoulder**

      M00.111 Pneumococcal arthritis, right shoulder
      M00.112 Pneumococcal arthritis, left shoulder
      M00.119 Pneumococcal arthritis, unspecified shoulder ▽

    ✓6ᵗʰ **M00.12 Pneumococcal arthritis, elbow**

      M00.121 Pneumococcal arthritis, right elbow
      M00.122 Pneumococcal arthritis, left elbow
      M00.129 Pneumococcal arthritis, unspecified elbow ▽

    ✓6ᵗʰ **M00.13 Pneumococcal arthritis, wrist**
      Pneumococcal arthritis of carpal bones
      M00.131 Pneumococcal arthritis, right wrist
      M00.132 Pneumococcal arthritis, left wrist
      M00.139 Pneumococcal arthritis, unspecified wrist ▽

    ✓6ᵗʰ **M00.14 Pneumococcal arthritis, hand**
      Pneumococcal arthritis of metacarpus and phalanges
      M00.141 Pneumococcal arthritis, right hand
      M00.142 Pneumococcal arthritis, left hand
      M00.149 Pneumococcal arthritis, unspecified hand ▽

    ✓6ᵗʰ **M00.15 Pneumococcal arthritis, hip**

      M00.151 Pneumococcal arthritis, right hip
      M00.152 Pneumococcal arthritis, left hip
      M00.159 Pneumococcal arthritis, unspecified hip ▽

    ✓6ᵗʰ **M00.16 Pneumococcal arthritis, knee**

      M00.161 Pneumococcal arthritis, right knee
      M00.162 Pneumococcal arthritis, left knee
      M00.169 Pneumococcal arthritis, unspecified knee ▽

    ✓6ᵗʰ **M00.17 Pneumococcal arthritis, ankle and foot**
      Pneumococcal arthritis, tarsus, metatarsus and phalanges
      M00.171 Pneumococcal arthritis, right ankle and foot
      M00.172 Pneumococcal arthritis, left ankle and foot
      M00.179 Pneumococcal arthritis, unspecified ankle and foot ▽

    M00.18 Pneumococcal arthritis, vertebrae
    M00.19 Pneumococcal polyarthritis

  ✓5ᵗʰ **M00.2 Other streptococcal arthritis and polyarthritis**
    Use additional code (B95.0-B95.2, B95.4-B95.5) to identify bacterial agent

    M00.20 Other streptococcal arthritis, unspecified joint ▽

    ✓6ᵗʰ **M00.21 Other streptococcal arthritis, shoulder**

      M00.211 Other streptococcal arthritis, right shoulder
      M00.212 Other streptococcal arthritis, left shoulder

✓ Additional Character Required   ✓x7ᵗʰ Placeholder Alert   Manifestation Dx   ▽ Unspecified Dx   ▶◀ Revised Text   ● New Code   ▲ Revised Code Title

ICD-10-CM 2017   701

M00.219 **Other streptococcal arthritis, unspecified shoulder** ▽

✓6ᵗʰ M00.22 **Other streptococcal arthritis, elbow**

M00.221 **Other streptococcal arthritis, right elbow**

M00.222 **Other streptococcal arthritis, left elbow**

M00.229 **Other streptococcal arthritis, unspecified elbow** ▽

✓6ᵗʰ M00.23 **Other streptococcal arthritis, wrist**

Other streptococcal arthritis of carpal bones

M00.231 **Other streptococcal arthritis, right wrist**

M00.232 **Other streptococcal arthritis, left wrist**

M00.239 **Other streptococcal arthritis, unspecified wrist** ▽

✓6ᵗʰ M00.24 **Other streptococcal arthritis, hand**

Other streptococcal arthritis metacarpus and phalanges

M00.241 **Other streptococcal arthritis, right hand**

M00.242 **Other streptococcal arthritis, left hand**

M00.249 **Other streptococcal arthritis, unspecified hand** ▽

✓6ᵗʰ M00.25 **Other streptococcal arthritis, hip**

M00.251 **Other streptococcal arthritis, right hip**

M00.252 **Other streptococcal arthritis, left hip**

M00.259 **Other streptococcal arthritis, unspecified hip** ▽

✓6ᵗʰ M00.26 **Other streptococcal arthritis, knee**

M00.261 **Other streptococcal arthritis, right knee**

M00.262 **Other streptococcal arthritis, left knee**

M00.269 **Other streptococcal arthritis, unspecified knee** ▽

✓6ᵗʰ M00.27 **Other streptococcal arthritis, ankle and foot**

Other streptococcal arthritis, tarsus, metatarsus and phalanges

M00.271 **Other streptococcal arthritis, right ankle and foot**

M00.272 **Other streptococcal arthritis, left ankle and foot**

M00.279 **Other streptococcal arthritis, unspecified ankle and foot** ▽

M00.28 **Other streptococcal arthritis, vertebrae**

M00.29 **Other streptococcal polyarthritis**

✓5ᵗʰ M00.8 **Arthritis and polyarthritis due to other bacteria**

Use additional code (B96) to identify bacteria

M00.80 **Arthritis due to other bacteria, unspecified joint** ▽

✓6ᵗʰ M00.81 **Arthritis due to other bacteria, shoulder**

M00.811 **Arthritis due to other bacteria, right shoulder**

M00.812 **Arthritis due to other bacteria, left shoulder**

M00.819 **Arthritis due to other bacteria, unspecified shoulder** ▽

✓6ᵗʰ M00.82 **Arthritis due to other bacteria, elbow**

M00.821 **Arthritis due to other bacteria, right elbow**

M00.822 **Arthritis due to other bacteria, left elbow**

M00.829 **Arthritis due to other bacteria, unspecified elbow** ▽

✓6ᵗʰ M00.83 **Arthritis due to other bacteria, wrist**

Arthritis due to other bacteria, carpal bones

M00.831 **Arthritis due to other bacteria, right wrist**

M00.832 **Arthritis due to other bacteria, left wrist**

M00.839 **Arthritis due to other bacteria, unspecified wrist** ▽

✓6ᵗʰ M00.84 **Arthritis due to other bacteria, hand**

Arthritis due to other bacteria, metacarpus and phalanges

M00.841 **Arthritis due to other bacteria, right hand**

M00.842 **Arthritis due to other bacteria, left hand**

M00.849 **Arthritis due to other bacteria, unspecified hand** ▽

✓6ᵗʰ M00.85 **Arthritis due to other bacteria, hip**

M00.851 **Arthritis due to other bacteria, right hip**

M00.852 **Arthritis due to other bacteria, left hip**

M00.859 **Arthritis due to other bacteria, unspecified hip** ▽

✓6ᵗʰ M00.86 **Arthritis due to other bacteria, knee**

M00.861 **Arthritis due to other bacteria, right knee**

M00.862 **Arthritis due to other bacteria, left knee**

M00.869 **Arthritis due to other bacteria, unspecified knee** ▽

✓6ᵗʰ M00.87 **Arthritis due to other bacteria, ankle and foot**

Arthritis due to other bacteria, tarsus, metatarsus, and phalanges

M00.871 **Arthritis due to other bacteria, right ankle and foot**

M00.872 **Arthritis due to other bacteria, left ankle and foot**

M00.879 **Arthritis due to other bacteria, unspecified ankle and foot** ▽

M00.88 **Arthritis due to other bacteria, vertebrae**

M00.89 **Polyarthritis due to other bacteria**

M00.9 **Pyogenic arthritis, unspecified** ▽

Infective arthritis NOS

✓4ᵗʰ **M01** **Direct infections of joint in infectious and parasitic diseases classified elsewhere**

Code first underlying disease, such as:

leprosy [Hansen's disease] (A30.-)

mycoses (B35-B49)

O'nyong-nyong fever (A92.1)

paratyphoid fever (A01.1-A01.4)

> **EXCLUDES 1** arthropathy in Lyme disease (A69.23)
> gonococcal arthritis (A54.42)
> meningococcal arthritis (A39.83)
> mumps arthritis (B26.85)
> postinfective arthropathy (M02.-)
> postmeningococcal arthritis (A39.84)
> reactive arthritis (M02.3)
> rubella arthritis (B06.82)
> sarcoidosis arthritis (D86.86)
> typhoid fever arthritis (A01.04)
> tuberculosis arthritis (A18.01-A18.02)

✓5ᵗʰ **M01.X** **Direct infection of joint in infectious and parasitic diseases classified elsewhere**

M01.X0 *Direct infection of unspecified joint in infectious and parasitic diseases classified elsewhere* ▽

✓6ᵗʰ M01.X1 *Direct infection of shoulder joint in infectious and parasitic diseases classified elsewhere*

M01.X11 *Direct infection of right shoulder in infectious and parasitic diseases classified elsewhere*

M01.X12 *Direct infection of left shoulder in infectious and parasitic diseases classified elsewhere*

M01.X19 *Direct infection of unspecified shoulder in infectious and parasitic diseases classified elsewhere* ▽

✓6ᵗʰ M01.X2 *Direct infection of elbow in infectious and parasitic diseases classified elsewhere*

M01.X21 *Direct infection of right elbow in infectious and parasitic diseases classified elsewhere*

M01.X22 *Direct infection of left elbow in infectious and parasitic diseases classified elsewhere*

M01.X29 *Direct infection of unspecified elbow in infectious and parasitic diseases classified elsewhere* ▽

✓6ᵗʰ M01.X3 *Direct infection of wrist in infectious and parasitic diseases classified elsewhere*

Direct infection of carpal bones in infectious and parasitic diseases classified elsewhere

M01.X31 *Direct infection of right wrist in infectious and parasitic diseases classified elsewhere*

M01.X32 *Direct infection of left wrist in infectious and parasitic diseases classified elsewhere*

M01.X39 *Direct infection of unspecified wrist in infectious and parasitic diseases classified elsewhere* ▽

✓6ᵗʰ M01.X4 *Direct infection of hand in infectious and parasitic diseases classified elsewhere*

Direct infection of metacarpus and phalanges in infectious and parasitic diseases classified elsewhere

M01.X41 *Direct infection of right hand in infectious and parasitic diseases classified elsewhere*

M01.X42 *Direct infection of left hand in infectious and parasitic diseases classified elsewhere*

M01.X49 *Direct infection of unspecified hand in infectious and parasitic diseases classified elsewhere* ▽

EXCLUDES 1 Not coded here   **EXCLUDES 2** Not included here   Ⓝ Newborn Age : 0   Ⓟ Pediatric Age : 0-17   Ⓜ Maternity Age : 12-55   Ⓐ Adult Age : 15-124

702

ICD-10-CM 2017

√6ᵗʰ **M01.X5** **Direct infection of** hip **in infectious and parasitic diseases classified elsewhere**

    M01.X51 *Direct infection of* right *hip in infectious and parasitic diseases classified elsewhere*

    M01.X52 *Direct infection of* left *hip in infectious and parasitic diseases classified elsewhere*

    M01.X59 *Direct infection of unspecified hip in infectious and parasitic diseases classified elsewhere* ▽

√6ᵗʰ **M01.X6** **Direct infection of** knee **in infectious and parasitic diseases classified elsewhere**

    M01.X61 *Direct infection of* right *knee in infectious and parasitic diseases classified elsewhere*

    M01.X62 *Direct infection of* left *knee in infectious and parasitic diseases classified elsewhere*

    M01.X69 *Direct infection of unspecified knee in infectious and parasitic diseases classified elsewhere* ▽

√6ᵗʰ **M01.X7** **Direct infection of** ankle and foot **in infectious and parasitic diseases classified elsewhere**

    Direct infection of tarsus, metatarsus and phalanges in infectious and parasitic diseases classified elsewhere

    M01.X71 *Direct infection of* right *ankle and foot in infectious and parasitic diseases classified elsewhere*

    M01.X72 *Direct infection of* left *ankle and foot in infectious and parasitic diseases classified elsewhere*

    M01.X79 *Direct infection of unspecified ankle and foot in infectious and parasitic diseases classified elsewhere* ▽

  M01.X8 *Direct Infection of* vertebrae *in infectious and parasitic diseases classified elsewhere*

  M01.X9 *Direct infection of* multiple joints *in infectious and parasitic diseases classified elsewhere*

√4ᵗʰ **M02** **Postinfective and reactive arthropathies**

  Code first underlying disease, such as:
    congenital syphilis [Clutton's joints] (A50.5)
    enteritis due to Yersinia enterocolitica (A04.6)
    infective endocarditis (I33.0)
    viral hepatitis (B15-B19)

    EXCLUDES 1 *Behçet's disease (M35.2)*
        direct infections of joint in infectious and parasitic diseases classified elsewhere (M01.-)
        mumps arthritis (B26.85)
        postmeningococcal arthritis (A39.84)
        rheumatic fever (I00)
        rubella arthritis (B06.82)
        syphilis arthritis (late) (A52.77)
        tabetic arthropathy [Charcôt's] (A52.16)

√5ᵗʰ **M02.0** **Arthropathy** following intestinal bypass

  M02.00 **Arthropathy following intestinal bypass, unspecified site** ▽

√6ᵗʰ **M02.01** **Arthropathy following intestinal bypass,** shoulder

    M02.011 **Arthropathy following intestinal bypass,** right **shoulder**

    M02.012 **Arthropathy following intestinal bypass,** left **shoulder**

    M02.019 **Arthropathy following intestinal bypass, unspecified shoulder** ▽

√6ᵗʰ **M02.02** **Arthropathy following intestinal bypass,** elbow

    M02.021 **Arthropathy following intestinal bypass,** right **elbow**

    M02.022 **Arthropathy following intestinal bypass,** left **elbow**

    M02.029 **Arthropathy following intestinal bypass, unspecified elbow** ▽

√6ᵗʰ **M02.03** **Arthropathy following intestinal bypass,** wrist

    Arthropathy following intestinal bypass, carpal bones

    M02.031 **Arthropathy following intestinal bypass,** right **wrist**

    M02.032 **Arthropathy following intestinal bypass,** left **wrist**

    M02.039 **Arthropathy following intestinal bypass, unspecified wrist** ▽

√6ᵗʰ **M02.04** **Arthropathy following intestinal bypass,** hand

    Arthropathy following intestinal bypass, metacarpals and phalanges

    M02.041 **Arthropathy following intestinal bypass,** right **hand**

    M02.042 **Arthropathy following intestinal bypass,** left **hand**

    M02.049 **Arthropathy following intestinal bypass, unspecified hand** ▽

√6ᵗʰ **M02.05** **Arthropathy following intestinal bypass,** hip

    M02.051 **Arthropathy following intestinal bypass,** right **hip**

    M02.052 **Arthropathy following intestinal bypass,** left **hip**

    M02.059 **Arthropathy following intestinal bypass, unspecified hip** ▽

√6ᵗʰ **M02.06** **Arthropathy following intestinal bypass,** knee

    M02.061 **Arthropathy following intestinal bypass,** right **knee**

    M02.062 **Arthropathy following intestinal bypass,** left **knee**

    M02.069 **Arthropathy following intestinal bypass, unspecified knee** ▽

√6ᵗʰ **M02.07** **Arthropathy following intestinal bypass,** ankle and foot

    Arthropathy following intestinal bypass, tarsus, metatarsus and phalanges

    M02.071 **Arthropathy following intestinal bypass,** right **ankle and foot**

    M02.072 **Arthropathy following intestinal bypass,** left **ankle and foot**

    M02.079 **Arthropathy following intestinal bypass, unspecified ankle and foot** ▽

  M02.08 **Arthropathy following intestinal bypass,** vertebrae

  M02.09 **Arthropathy following intestinal bypass,** multiple sites

√5ᵗʰ **M02.1** Postdysenteric **arthropathy**

  M02.10 **Postdysenteric arthropathy, unspecified site** ▽

√6ᵗʰ **M02.11** **Postdysenteric arthropathy,** shoulder

    M02.111 **Postdysenteric arthropathy,** right **shoulder**

    M02.112 **Postdysenteric arthropathy,** left **shoulder**

    M02.119 **Postdysenteric arthropathy, unspecified shoulder** ▽

√6ᵗʰ **M02.12** **Postdysenteric arthropathy,** elbow

    M02.121 **Postdysenteric arthropathy,** right **elbow**

    M02.122 **Postdysenteric arthropathy,** left **elbow**

    M02.129 **Postdysenteric arthropathy, unspecified elbow** ▽

√6ᵗʰ **M02.13** **Postdysenteric arthropathy,** wrist

    Postdysenteric arthropathy, carpal bones

    M02.131 **Postdysenteric arthropathy,** right **wrist**

    M02.132 **Postdysenteric arthropathy,** left **wrist**

    M02.139 **Postdysenteric arthropathy, unspecified wrist** ▽

√6ᵗʰ **M02.14** **Postdysenteric arthropathy,** hand

    Postdysenteric arthropathy, metacarpus and phalanges

    M02.141 **Postdysenteric arthropathy,** right **hand**

    M02.142 **Postdysenteric arthropathy,** left **hand**

    M02.149 **Postdysenteric arthropathy, unspecified hand** ▽

√6ᵗʰ **M02.15** **Postdysenteric arthropathy,** hip

    M02.151 **Postdysenteric arthropathy,** right **hip**

    M02.152 **Postdysenteric arthropathy,** left **hip**

    M02.159 **Postdysenteric arthropathy, unspecified hip** ▽

√6ᵗʰ **M02.16** **Postdysenteric arthropathy,** knee

    M02.161 **Postdysenteric arthropathy,** right **knee**

    M02.162 **Postdysenteric arthropathy,** left **knee**

    M02.169 **Postdysenteric arthropathy, unspecified knee** ▽

√6ᵗʰ **M02.17** **Postdysenteric arthropathy,** ankle and foot

    Postdysenteric arthropathy, tarsus, metatarsus and phalanges

    M02.171 **Postdysenteric arthropathy,** right **ankle and foot**

    M02.172 **Postdysenteric arthropathy,** left **ankle and foot**

    M02.179 **Postdysenteric arthropathy, unspecified ankle and foot** ▽

  M02.18 **Postdysenteric arthropathy,** vertebrae

  M02.19 **Postdysenteric arthropathy,** multiple sites

☑ Additional Character Required   ✗7ᵗʰ Placeholder Alert   Manifestation Dx   ▽ Unspecified Dx   ►◄ Revised Text   ● New Code   ▲ Revised Code Title

Chapter 13. Diseases of the Musculoskeletal System and Connective Tissue

✓5th **M02.2** Postimmunization arthropathy

    M02.20 Postimmunization arthropathy, unspecified site ▽

    ✓6th **M02.21** Postimmunization arthropathy, shoulder

        M02.211 Postimmunization arthropathy, right shoulder

        M02.212 Postimmunization arthropathy, left shoulder

        M02.219 Postimmunization arthropathy, unspecified shoulder ▽

    ✓6th **M02.22** Postimmunization arthropathy, elbow

        M02.221 Postimmunization arthropathy, right elbow

        M02.222 Postimmunization arthropathy, left elbow

        M02.229 Postimmunization arthropathy, unspecified elbow ▽

    ✓6th **M02.23** Postimmunization arthropathy, wrist

        Postimmunization arthropathy, carpal bones

        M02.231 Postimmunization arthropathy, right wrist

        M02.232 Postimmunization arthropathy, left wrist

        M02.239 Postimmunization arthropathy, unspecified wrist ▽

    ✓6th **M02.24** Postimmunization arthropathy, hand

        Postimmunization arthropathy, metacarpus and phalanges

        M02.241 Postimmunization arthropathy, right hand

        M02.242 Postimmunization arthropathy, left hand

        M02.249 Postimmunization arthropathy, unspecified hand ▽

    ✓6th **M02.25** Postimmunization arthropathy, hip

        M02.251 Postimmunization arthropathy, right hip

        M02.252 Postimmunization arthropathy, left hip

        M02.259 Postimmunization arthropathy, unspecified hip ▽

    ✓6th **M02.26** Postimmunization arthropathy, knee

        M02.261 Postimmunization arthropathy, right knee

        M02.262 Postimmunization arthropathy, left knee

        M02.269 Postimmunization arthropathy, unspecified knee ▽

    ✓6th **M02.27** Postimmunization arthropathy, ankle and foot

        Postimmunization arthropathy, tarsus, metatarsus and phalanges

        M02.271 Postimmunization arthropathy, right ankle and foot

        M02.272 Postimmunization arthropathy, left ankle and foot

        M02.279 Postimmunization arthropathy, unspecified ankle and foot ▽

    M02.28 Postimmunization arthropathy, vertebrae

    M02.29 Postimmunization arthropathy, multiple sites

✓5th **M02.3** Reiter's disease

    Reactive arthritis

    M02.30 Reiter's disease, unspecified site ▽

    ✓6th **M02.31** Reiter's disease, shoulder

        M02.311 Reiter's disease, right shoulder

        M02.312 Reiter's disease, left shoulder

        M02.319 Reiter's disease, unspecified shoulder ▽

    ✓6th **M02.32** Reiter's disease, elbow

        M02.321 Reiter's disease, right elbow

        M02.322 Reiter's disease, left elbow

        M02.329 Reiter's disease, unspecified elbow ▽

    ✓6th **M02.33** Reiter's disease, wrist

        Reiter's disease, carpal bones

        M02.331 Reiter's disease, right wrist

        M02.332 Reiter's disease, left wrist

        M02.339 Reiter's disease, unspecified wrist ▽

    ✓6th **M02.34** Reiter's disease, hand

        Reiter's disease, metacarpus and phalanges

        M02.341 Reiter's disease, right hand

        M02.342 Reiter's disease, left hand

        M02.349 Reiter's disease, unspecified hand

    ✓6th **M02.35** Reiter's disease, hip

        M02.351 Reiter's disease, right hip

        M02.352 Reiter's disease, left hip

        M02.359 Reiter's disease, unspecified hip ▽

    ✓6th **M02.36** Reiter's disease, knee

        M02.361 Reiter's disease, right knee

        M02.362 Reiter's disease, left knee

        M02.369 Reiter's disease, unspecified knee ▽

    ✓6th **M02.37** Reiter's disease, ankle and foot

        Reiter's disease, tarsus, metatarsus and phalanges

        M02.371 Reiter's disease, right ankle and foot

        M02.372 Reiter's disease, left ankle and foot

        M02.379 Reiter's disease, unspecified ankle and foot ▽

    M02.38 Reiter's disease, vertebrae

    M02.39 Reiter's disease, multiple sites

✓5th **M02.8** Other reactive arthropathies

    M02.80 *Other reactive arthropathies, unspecified site* ▽

    ✓6th **M02.81** Other reactive arthropathies, shoulder

        M02.811 *Other reactive arthropathies, right shoulder*

        M02.812 *Other reactive arthropathies, left shoulder*

        M02.819 *Other reactive arthropathies, unspecified shoulder* ▽

    ✓6th **M02.82** Other reactive arthropathies, elbow

        M02.821 *Other reactive arthropathies, right elbow*

        M02.822 *Other reactive arthropathies, left elbow*

        M02.829 *Other reactive arthropathies, unspecified elbow* ▽

    ✓6th **M02.83** Other reactive arthropathies, wrist

        Other reactive arthropathies, carpal bones

        M02.831 *Other reactive arthropathies, right wrist*

        M02.832 *Other reactive arthropathies, left wrist*

        M02.839 *Other reactive arthropathies, unspecified wrist* ▽

    ✓6th **M02.84** Other reactive arthropathies, hand

        Other reactive arthropathies, metacarpus and phalanges

        M02.841 *Other reactive arthropathies, right hand*

        M02.842 *Other reactive arthropathies, left hand*

        M02.849 *Other reactive arthropathies, unspecified hand* ▽

    ✓6th **M02.85** Other reactive arthropathies, hip

        M02.851 *Other reactive arthropathies, right hip*

        M02.852 *Other reactive arthropathies, left hip*

        M02.859 *Other reactive arthropathies, unspecified hip* ▽

    ✓6th **M02.86** Other reactive arthropathies, knee

        M02.861 *Other reactive arthropathies, right knee*

        M02.862 *Other reactive arthropathies, left knee*

        M02.869 *Other reactive arthropathies, unspecified knee* ▽

    ✓6th **M02.87** Other reactive arthropathies, ankle and foot

        Other reactive arthropathies, tarsus, metatarsus and phalanges

        M02.871 *Other reactive arthropathies, right ankle and foot*

        M02.872 *Other reactive arthropathies, left ankle and foot*

        M02.879 *Other reactive arthropathies, unspecified ankle and foot* ▽

    M02.88 *Other reactive arthropathies, vertebrae*

    M02.89 *Other reactive arthropathies, multiple sites*

M02.9 *Reactive arthropathy, unspecified* ▽

▶Autoinflammatory syndromes (M04)◀

● **M04** Autoinflammatory syndromes

    EXCLUDES 2 Crohn's disease (K50.-)

● **M04.1** Periodic fever syndromes

    Familial Mediterranean fever

    Hyperimmunoglobin D syndrome

    Mevalonate kinase deficiency

    Tumor necrosis factor receptor associated periodic syndrome [TRAPS]

EXCLUDES 1 Not coded here   EXCLUDES 2 Not included here   N Newborn Age : 0   P Pediatric Age : 0-17   M Maternity Age : 12-55   A Adult Age : 15-124

704   ICD-10-CM 2017

●   **M04.2 Cryopyrin-associated periodic syndromes**

     Chronic infantile neurological, cutaneous and articular syndrome [CINCA]

     Familial cold autoinflammatory syndrome

     Familial cold urticaria

     Muckle-Wells syndrome

     Neonatal onset multisystemic inflammatory disorder [NOMID]

●   **M04.8 Other autoinflammatory syndromes**

     Blau syndrome

     Deficiency of interleukin 1 receptor antagonist [DIRA]

     Majeed syndrome

     Periodic fever, aphthous stomatitis, pharyngitis, and adenopathy syndrome [PFAPA]

     Pyogenic arthritis, pyoderma gangrenosum, and acne syndrome [PAPA]

●   **M04.9 Autoinflammatory syndrome, unspecified** ▽

Inflammatory polyarthropathies (M05-M14)

✓4ᵗʰ **M05 Rheumatoid arthritis with rheumatoid factor**

     EXCLUDES 1   *rheumatic fever (I00)*

                  juvenile rheumatoid arthritis (M08.-)

                  rheumatoid arthritis of spine (M45.-)

✓5ᵗʰ   **M05.0 Felty's syndrome**

     Rheumatoid arthritis with splenoadenomegaly and leukopenia

     M05.00 Felty's syndrome, unspecified site ▽

✓6ᵗʰ   **M05.01 Felty's syndrome, shoulder**

       M05.011 Felty's syndrome, right shoulder

       M05.012 Felty's syndrome, left shoulder

       M05.019 Felty's syndrome, unspecified shoulder ▽

✓6ᵗʰ   **M05.02 Felty's syndrome, elbow**

       M05.021 Felty's syndrome, right elbow

       M05.022 Felty's syndrome, left elbow

       M05.029 Felty's syndrome, unspecified elbow ▽

✓6ᵗʰ   **M05.03 Felty's syndrome, wrist**

       Felty's syndrome, carpal bones

       M05.031 Felty's syndrome, right wrist

       M05.032 Felty's syndrome, left wrist

       M05.039 Felty's syndrome, unspecified wrist ▽

✓6ᵗʰ   **M05.04 Felty's syndrome, hand**

       Felty's syndrome, metacarpus and phalanges

       M05.041 Felty's syndrome, right hand

       M05.042 Felty's syndrome, left hand

       M05.049 Felty's syndrome, unspecified hand ▽

✓6ᵗʰ   **M05.05 Felty's syndrome, hip**

       M05.051 Felty's syndrome, right hip

       M05.052 Felty's syndrome, left hip

       M05.059 Felty's syndrome, unspecified hip ▽

✓6ᵗʰ   **M05.06 Felty's syndrome, knee**

       M05.061 Felty's syndrome, right knee

       M05.062 Felty's syndrome, left knee

       M05.069 Felty's syndrome, unspecified knee ▽

✓6ᵗʰ   **M05.07 Felty's syndrome, ankle and foot**

       Felty's syndrome, tarsus, metatarsus and phalanges

       M05.071 Felty's syndrome, right ankle and foot

       M05.072 Felty's syndrome, left ankle and foot

       M05.079 Felty's syndrome, unspecified ankle and foot ▽

     M05.09 Felty's syndrome, multiple sites

✓5ᵗʰ   **M05.1 Rheumatoid lung disease with rheumatoid arthritis**

     DEF: Lung disorders associated with rheumatoid arthritis.

     M05.10 Rheumatoid lung disease with rheumatoid arthritis of unspecified site ▽

✓6ᵗʰ   **M05.11 Rheumatoid lung disease with rheumatoid arthritis of shoulder**

       M05.111 Rheumatoid lung disease with rheumatoid arthritis of right shoulder

       M05.112 Rheumatoid lung disease with rheumatoid arthritis of left shoulder

       M05.119 Rheumatoid lung disease with rheumatoid arthritis of unspecified shoulder ▽

✓6ᵗʰ   **M05.12 Rheumatoid lung disease with rheumatoid arthritis of elbow**

       M05.121 Rheumatoid lung disease with rheumatoid arthritis of right elbow

       M05.122 Rheumatoid lung disease with rheumatoid arthritis of left elbow

       M05.129 Rheumatoid lung disease with rheumatoid arthritis of unspecified elbow ▽

✓6ᵗʰ   **M05.13 Rheumatoid lung disease with rheumatoid arthritis of wrist**

       Rheumatoid lung disease with rheumatoid arthritis, carpal bones

       M05.131 Rheumatoid lung disease with rheumatoid arthritis of right wrist

       M05.132 Rheumatoid lung disease with rheumatoid arthritis of left wrist

       M05.139 Rheumatoid lung disease with rheumatoid arthritis of unspecified wrist ▽

✓6ᵗʰ   **M05.14 Rheumatoid lung disease with rheumatoid arthritis of hand**

       Rheumatoid lung disease with rheumatoid arthritis, metacarpus and phalanges

       M05.141 Rheumatoid lung disease with rheumatoid arthritis of right hand

       M05.142 Rheumatoid lung disease with rheumatoid arthritis of left hand

       M05.149 Rheumatoid lung disease with rheumatoid arthritis of unspecified hand ▽

✓6ᵗʰ   **M05.15 Rheumatoid lung disease with rheumatoid arthritis of hip**

       M05.151 Rheumatoid lung disease with rheumatoid arthritis of right hip

       M05.152 Rheumatoid lung disease with rheumatoid arthritis of left hip

       M05.159 Rheumatoid lung disease with rheumatoid arthritis of unspecified hip ▽

✓6ᵗʰ   **M05.16 Rheumatoid lung disease with rheumatoid arthritis of knee**

       M05.161 Rheumatoid lung disease with rheumatoid arthritis of right knee

       M05.162 Rheumatoid lung disease with rheumatoid arthritis of left knee

       M05.169 Rheumatoid lung disease with rheumatoid arthritis of unspecified knee ▽

✓6ᵗʰ   **M05.17 Rheumatoid lung disease with rheumatoid arthritis of ankle and foot**

       Rheumatoid lung disease with rheumatoid arthritis, tarsus, metatarsus and phalanges

       M05.171 Rheumatoid lung disease with rheumatoid arthritis of right ankle and foot

       M05.172 Rheumatoid lung disease with rheumatoid arthritis of left ankle and foot

       M05.179 Rheumatoid lung disease with rheumatoid arthritis of unspecified ankle and foot ▽

     M05.19 Rheumatoid lung disease with rheumatoid arthritis of multiple sites

✓5ᵗʰ   **M05.2 Rheumatoid vasculitis with rheumatoid arthritis**

     M05.20 Rheumatoid vasculitis with rheumatoid arthritis of unspecified site ▽

✓6ᵗʰ   **M05.21 Rheumatoid vasculitis with rheumatoid arthritis of shoulder**

       M05.211 Rheumatoid vasculitis with rheumatoid arthritis of right shoulder

       M05.212 Rheumatoid vasculitis with rheumatoid arthritis of left shoulder

       M05.219 Rheumatoid vasculitis with rheumatoid arthritis of unspecified shoulder ▽

✓6ᵗʰ   **M05.22 Rheumatoid vasculitis with rheumatoid arthritis of elbow**

       M05.221 Rheumatoid vasculitis with rheumatoid arthritis of right elbow

       M05.222 Rheumatoid vasculitis with rheumatoid arthritis of left elbow

---

✓ Additional Character Required   ✓x7ᵗʰ Placeholder Alert   Manifestation Dx   ▽ Unspecified Dx   ►◄ Revised Text   ● New Code   ▲ Revised Code Title

M05.229 Rheumatoid vasculitis with rheumatoid arthritis of unspecified elbow ▽

✓6ᵗʰ **M05.23** Rheumatoid vasculitis with rheumatoid arthritis of wrist
     Rheumatoid vasculitis with rheumatoid arthritis, carpal bones

M05.231 Rheumatoid vasculitis with rheumatoid arthritis of right wrist

M05.232 Rheumatoid vasculitis with rheumatoid arthritis of left wrist

M05.239 Rheumatoid vasculitis with rheumatoid arthritis of unspecified wrist ▽

✓6ᵗʰ **M05.24** Rheumatoid vasculitis with rheumatoid arthritis of hand
     Rheumatoid vasculitis with rheumatoid arthritis, metacarpus and phalanges

M05.241 Rheumatoid vasculitis with rheumatoid arthritis of right hand

M05.242 Rheumatoid vasculitis with rheumatoid arthritis of left hand

M05.249 Rheumatoid vasculitis with rheumatoid arthritis of unspecified hand ▽

✓6ᵗʰ **M05.25** Rheumatoid vasculitis with rheumatoid arthritis of hip

M05.251 Rheumatoid vasculitis with rheumatoid arthritis of right hip

M05.252 Rheumatoid vasculitis with rheumatoid arthritis of left hip

M05.259 Rheumatoid vasculitis with rheumatoid arthritis of unspecified hip ▽

✓6ᵗʰ **M05.26** Rheumatoid vasculitis with rheumatoid arthritis of knee

M05.261 Rheumatoid vasculitis with rheumatoid arthritis of right knee

M05.262 Rheumatoid vasculitis with rheumatoid arthritis of left knee

M05.269 Rheumatoid vasculitis with rheumatoid arthritis of unspecified knee ▽

✓6ᵗʰ **M05.27** Rheumatoid vasculitis with rheumatoid arthritis of ankle and foot
     Rheumatoid vasculitis with rheumatoid arthritis, tarsus, metatarsus and phalanges

M05.271 Rheumatoid vasculitis with rheumatoid arthritis of right ankle and foot

M05.272 Rheumatoid vasculitis with rheumatoid arthritis of left ankle and foot

M05.279 Rheumatoid vasculitis with rheumatoid arthritis of unspecified ankle and foot ▽

M05.29 Rheumatoid vasculitis with rheumatoid arthritis of multiple sites

✓5ᵗʰ **M05.3** Rheumatoid heart disease with rheumatoid arthritis
     Rheumatoid carditis
     Rheumatoid endocarditis
     Rheumatoid myocarditis
     Rheumatoid pericarditis

M05.30 Rheumatoid heart disease with rheumatoid arthritis of unspecified site ▽

✓6ᵗʰ **M05.31** Rheumatoid heart disease with rheumatoid arthritis of shoulder

M05.311 Rheumatoid heart disease with rheumatoid arthritis of right shoulder

M05.312 Rheumatoid heart disease with rheumatoid arthritis of left shoulder

M05.319 Rheumatoid heart disease with rheumatoid arthritis of unspecified shoulder ▽

✓6ᵗʰ **M05.32** Rheumatoid heart disease with rheumatoid arthritis of elbow

M05.321 Rheumatoid heart disease with rheumatoid arthritis of right elbow

M05.322 Rheumatoid heart disease with rheumatoid arthritis of left elbow

M05.329 Rheumatoid heart disease with rheumatoid arthritis of unspecified elbow ▽

✓6ᵗʰ **M05.33** Rheumatoid heart disease with rheumatoid arthritis of wrist
     Rheumatoid heart disease with rheumatoid arthritis, carpal bones

M05.331 Rheumatoid heart disease with rheumatoid arthritis of right wrist

M05.332 Rheumatoid heart disease with rheumatoid arthritis of left wrist

M05.339 Rheumatoid heart disease with rheumatoid arthritis of unspecified wrist ▽

✓6ᵗʰ **M05.34** Rheumatoid heart disease with rheumatoid arthritis of hand
     Rheumatoid heart disease with rheumatoid arthritis, metacarpus and phalanges

M05.341 Rheumatoid heart disease with rheumatoid arthritis of right hand

M05.342 Rheumatoid heart disease with rheumatoid arthritis of left hand

M05.349 Rheumatoid heart disease with rheumatoid arthritis of unspecified hand ▽

✓6ᵗʰ **M05.35** Rheumatoid heart disease with rheumatoid arthritis of hip

M05.351 Rheumatoid heart disease with rheumatoid arthritis of right hip

M05.352 Rheumatoid heart disease with rheumatoid arthritis of left hip

M05.359 Rheumatoid heart disease with rheumatoid arthritis of unspecified hip ▽

✓6ᵗʰ **M05.36** Rheumatoid heart disease with rheumatoid arthritis of knee

M05.361 Rheumatoid heart disease with rheumatoid arthritis of right knee

M05.362 Rheumatoid heart disease with rheumatoid arthritis of left knee

M05.369 Rheumatoid heart disease with rheumatoid arthritis of unspecified knee ▽

✓6ᵗʰ **M05.37** Rheumatoid heart disease with rheumatoid arthritis of ankle and foot
     Rheumatoid heart disease with rheumatoid arthritis, tarsus, metatarsus and phalanges

M05.371 Rheumatoid heart disease with rheumatoid arthritis of right ankle and foot

M05.372 Rheumatoid heart disease with rheumatoid arthritis of left ankle and foot

M05.379 Rheumatoid heart disease with rheumatoid arthritis of unspecified ankle and foot ▽

M05.39 Rheumatoid heart disease with rheumatoid arthritis of multiple sites

✓5ᵗʰ **M05.4** Rheumatoid myopathy with rheumatoid arthritis

M05.40 Rheumatoid myopathy with rheumatoid arthritis of unspecified site ▽

✓6ᵗʰ **M05.41** Rheumatoid myopathy with rheumatoid arthritis of shoulder

M05.411 Rheumatoid myopathy with rheumatoid arthritis of right shoulder

M05.412 Rheumatoid myopathy with rheumatoid arthritis of left shoulder

M05.419 Rheumatoid myopathy with rheumatoid arthritis of unspecified shoulder ▽

✓6ᵗʰ **M05.42** Rheumatoid myopathy with rheumatoid arthritis of elbow

M05.421 Rheumatoid myopathy with rheumatoid arthritis of right elbow

M05.422 Rheumatoid myopathy with rheumatoid arthritis of left elbow

M05.429 Rheumatoid myopathy with rheumatoid arthritis of unspecified elbow ▽

✓6ᵗʰ **M05.43** Rheumatoid myopathy with rheumatoid arthritis of wrist
     Rheumatoid myopathy with rheumatoid arthritis, carpal bones

M05.431 Rheumatoid myopathy with rheumatoid arthritis of right wrist

M05.432 Rheumatoid myopathy with rheumatoid arthritis of left wrist

EXCLUDES 1 Not coded here   **EXCLUDES 2** Not included here   **N** Newborn Age : 0   **P** Pediatric Age : 0-17   **M** Maternity Age : 12-55   **A** Adult Age : 15-124

706   ICD-10-CM 2017

      M05.439 **Rheumatoid myopathy with** ▽
           rheumatoid arthritis of
           unspecified wrist

✓6ᵗʰ **M05.44** **Rheumatoid myopathy with rheumatoid arthritis of hand**
    Rheumatoid myopathy with rheumatoid arthritis, metacarpus and phalanges

      M05.441 **Rheumatoid myopathy with rheumatoid arthritis of right hand**

      M05.442 **Rheumatoid myopathy with rheumatoid arthritis of left hand**

      M05.449 **Rheumatoid myopathy with rheumatoid arthritis of unspecified hand** ▽

✓6ᵗʰ **M05.45** **Rheumatoid myopathy with rheumatoid arthritis of hip**

      M05.451 **Rheumatoid myopathy with rheumatoid arthritis of right hip**

      M05.452 **Rheumatoid myopathy with rheumatoid arthritis of left hip**

      M05.459 **Rheumatoid myopathy with rheumatoid arthritis of unspecified hip** ▽

✓6ᵗʰ **M05.46** **Rheumatoid myopathy with rheumatoid arthritis of knee**

      M05.461 **Rheumatoid myopathy with rheumatoid arthritis of right knee**

      M05.462 **Rheumatoid myopathy with rheumatoid arthritis of left knee**

      M05.469 **Rheumatoid myopathy with rheumatoid arthritis of unspecified knee** ▽

✓6ᵗʰ **M05.47** **Rheumatoid myopathy with rheumatoid arthritis of ankle and foot**
    Rheumatoid myopathy with rheumatoid arthritis, tarsus, metatarsus and phalanges

      M05.471 **Rheumatoid myopathy with rheumatoid arthritis of right ankle and foot**

      M05.472 **Rheumatoid myopathy with rheumatoid arthritis of left ankle and foot**

      M05.479 **Rheumatoid myopathy with rheumatoid arthritis of unspecified ankle and foot** ▽

    M05.49 **Rheumatoid myopathy with rheumatoid arthritis of multiple sites**

✓5ᵗʰ **M05.5** **Rheumatoid polyneuropathy with rheumatoid arthritis**

    M05.50 **Rheumatoid polyneuropathy with rheumatoid arthritis of unspecified site** ▽

✓6ᵗʰ **M05.51** **Rheumatoid polyneuropathy with rheumatoid arthritis of shoulder**

      M05.511 **Rheumatoid polyneuropathy with rheumatoid arthritis of right shoulder**

      M05.512 **Rheumatoid polyneuropathy with rheumatoid arthritis of left shoulder**

      M05.519 **Rheumatoid polyneuropathy with rheumatoid arthritis of unspecified shoulder** ▽

✓6ᵗʰ **M05.52** **Rheumatoid polyneuropathy with rheumatoid arthritis of elbow**

      M05.521 **Rheumatoid polyneuropathy with rheumatoid arthritis of right elbow**

      M05.522 **Rheumatoid polyneuropathy with rheumatoid arthritis of left elbow**

      M05.529 **Rheumatoid polyneuropathy with rheumatoid arthritis of unspecified elbow** ▽

✓6ᵗʰ **M05.53** **Rheumatoid polyneuropathy with rheumatoid arthritis of wrist**
    Rheumatoid polyneuropathy with rheumatoid arthritis, carpal bones

      M05.531 **Rheumatoid polyneuropathy with rheumatoid arthritis of right wrist**

      M05.532 **Rheumatoid polyneuropathy with rheumatoid arthritis of left wrist**

      M05.539 **Rheumatoid polyneuropathy with rheumatoid arthritis of unspecified wrist** ▽

✓6ᵗʰ **M05.54** **Rheumatoid polyneuropathy with rheumatoid arthritis of hand**
    Rheumatoid polyneuropathy with rheumatoid arthritis, metacarpus and phalanges

      M05.541 **Rheumatoid polyneuropathy with rheumatoid arthritis of right hand**

      M05.542 **Rheumatoid polyneuropathy with rheumatoid arthritis of left hand**

      M05.549 **Rheumatoid polyneuropathy with rheumatoid arthritis of unspecified hand** ▽

✓6ᵗʰ **M05.55** **Rheumatoid polyneuropathy with rheumatoid arthritis of hip**

      M05.551 **Rheumatoid polyneuropathy with rheumatoid arthritis of right hip**

      M05.552 **Rheumatoid polyneuropathy with rheumatoid arthritis of left hip**

      M05.559 **Rheumatoid polyneuropathy with rheumatoid arthritis of unspecified hip** ▽

✓6ᵗʰ **M05.56** **Rheumatoid polyneuropathy with rheumatoid arthritis of knee**

      M05.561 **Rheumatoid polyneuropathy with rheumatoid arthritis of right knee**

      M05.562 **Rheumatoid polyneuropathy with rheumatoid arthritis of left knee**

      M05.569 **Rheumatoid polyneuropathy with rheumatoid arthritis of unspecified knee** ▽

✓6ᵗʰ **M05.57** **Rheumatoid polyneuropathy with rheumatoid arthritis of ankle and foot**
    Rheumatoid polyneuropathy with rheumatoid arthritis, tarsus, metatarsus and phalanges

      M05.571 **Rheumatoid polyneuropathy with rheumatoid arthritis of right ankle and foot**

      M05.572 **Rheumatoid polyneuropathy with rheumatoid arthritis of left ankle and foot**

      M05.579 **Rheumatoid polyneuropathy with rheumatoid arthritis of unspecified ankle and foot** ▽

    M05.59 **Rheumatoid polyneuropathy with rheumatoid arthritis of multiple sites**

✓5ᵗʰ **M05.6** **Rheumatoid arthritis with involvement of other organs and systems**

    M05.60 **Rheumatoid arthritis of unspecified site with involvement of other organs and systems** ▽

✓6ᵗʰ **M05.61** **Rheumatoid arthritis of shoulder with involvement of other organs and systems**

      M05.611 **Rheumatoid arthritis of right shoulder with involvement of other organs and systems**

      M05.612 **Rheumatoid arthritis of left shoulder with involvement of other organs and systems**

      M05.619 **Rheumatoid arthritis of unspecified shoulder with involvement of other organs and systems** ▽

✓6ᵗʰ **M05.62** **Rheumatoid arthritis of elbow with involvement of other organs and systems**

      M05.621 **Rheumatoid arthritis of right elbow with involvement of other organs and systems**

      M05.622 **Rheumatoid arthritis of left elbow with involvement of other organs and systems**

      M05.629 **Rheumatoid arthritis of unspecified elbow with involvement of other organs and systems** ▽

✓6ᵗʰ **M05.63** **Rheumatoid arthritis of wrist with involvement of other organs and systems**
    Rheumatoid arthritis of carpal bones with involvement of other organs and systems

      M05.631 **Rheumatoid arthritis of right wrist with involvement of other organs and systems**

      M05.632 **Rheumatoid arthritis of left wrist with involvement of other organs and systems**

      M05.639 **Rheumatoid arthritis of unspecified wrist with involvement of other organs and systems** ▽

✓6ᵗʰ **M05.64** **Rheumatoid arthritis of hand with involvement of other organs and systems**
    Rheumatoid arthritis of metacarpus and phalanges with involvement of other organs and systems

      M05.641 **Rheumatoid arthritis of right hand with involvement of other organs and systems**

      M05.642 **Rheumatoid arthritis of left hand with involvement of other organs and systems**

☑ Additional Character Required   ✓x7ᵗʰ Placeholder Alert   Manifestation Dx   ▽ Unspecified Dx   ►◄ Revised Text   ● New Code   ▲ Revised Code Title

ICD-10-CM 2017   707

M05.649 Rheumatoid arthritis of unspecified hand with involvement of other organs and systems ▽

✓6ᵗʰ M05.65 **Rheumatoid arthritis of hip with involvement of other organs and systems**

M05.651 Rheumatoid arthritis of right hip with involvement of other organs and systems

M05.652 Rheumatoid arthritis of left hip with involvement of other organs and systems

M05.659 Rheumatoid arthritis of unspecified hip with involvement of other organs and systems ▽

✓6ᵗʰ M05.66 **Rheumatoid arthritis of knee with involvement of other organs and systems**

M05.661 Rheumatoid arthritis of right knee with involvement of other organs and systems

M05.662 Rheumatoid arthritis of left knee with involvement of other organs and systems

M05.669 Rheumatoid arthritis of unspecified knee with involvement of other organs and systems ▽

✓6ᵗʰ M05.67 **Rheumatoid arthritis of ankle and foot with involvement of other organs and systems**

Rheumatoid arthritis of tarsus, metatarsus and phalanges with involvement of other organs and systems

M05.671 Rheumatoid arthritis of right ankle and foot with involvement of other organs and systems

M05.672 Rheumatoid arthritis of left ankle and foot with involvement of other organs and systems

M05.679 Rheumatoid arthritis of unspecified ankle and foot with involvement of other organs and systems ▽

M05.69 **Rheumatoid arthritis of multiple sites with involvement of other organs and systems**

✓5ᵗʰ M05.7 **Rheumatoid arthritis with rheumatoid factor without organ or systems involvement**

M05.70 Rheumatoid arthritis with rheumatoid factor of unspecified site without organ or systems involvement ▽

✓6ᵗʰ M05.71 **Rheumatoid arthritis with rheumatoid factor of shoulder without organ or systems involvement**

M05.711 Rheumatoid arthritis with rheumatoid factor of right shoulder without organ or systems involvement

M05.712 Rheumatoid arthritis with rheumatoid factor of left shoulder without organ or systems involvement

M05.719 Rheumatoid arthritis with rheumatoid factor of unspecified shoulder without organ or systems involvement ▽

✓6ᵗʰ M05.72 **Rheumatoid arthritis with rheumatoid factor of elbow without organ or systems involvement**

M05.721 Rheumatoid arthritis with rheumatoid factor of right elbow without organ or systems involvement

M05.722 Rheumatoid arthritis with rheumatoid factor of left elbow without organ or systems involvement

M05.729 Rheumatoid arthritis with rheumatoid factor of unspecified elbow without organ or systems involvement ▽

✓6ᵗʰ M05.73 **Rheumatoid arthritis with rheumatoid factor of wrist without organ or systems involvement**

M05.731 Rheumatoid arthritis with rheumatoid factor of right wrist without organ or systems involvement

M05.732 Rheumatoid arthritis with rheumatoid factor of left wrist without organ or systems involvement

M05.739 Rheumatoid arthritis with rheumatoid factor of unspecified wrist without organ or systems involvement ▽

✓6ᵗʰ M05.74 **Rheumatoid arthritis with rheumatoid factor of hand without organ or systems involvement**

M05.741 Rheumatoid arthritis with rheumatoid factor of right hand without organ or systems involvement

M05.742 Rheumatoid arthritis with rheumatoid factor of left hand without organ or systems involvement

M05.749 Rheumatoid arthritis with rheumatoid factor of unspecified hand without organ or systems involvement ▽

✓6ᵗʰ M05.75 **Rheumatoid arthritis with rheumatoid factor of hip without organ or systems involvement**

M05.751 Rheumatoid arthritis with rheumatoid factor of right hip without organ or systems involvement

M05.752 Rheumatoid arthritis with rheumatoid factor of left hip without organ or systems involvement

M05.759 Rheumatoid arthritis with rheumatoid factor of unspecified hip without organ or systems involvement ▽

✓6ᵗʰ M05.76 **Rheumatoid arthritis with rheumatoid factor of knee without organ or systems involvement**

M05.761 Rheumatoid arthritis with rheumatoid factor of right knee without organ or systems involvement

M05.762 Rheumatoid arthritis with rheumatoid factor of left knee without organ or systems involvement

M05.769 Rheumatoid arthritis with rheumatoid factor of unspecified knee without organ or systems involvement ▽

✓6ᵗʰ M05.77 **Rheumatoid arthritis with rheumatoid factor of ankle and foot without organ or systems involvement**

M05.771 Rheumatoid arthritis with rheumatoid factor of right ankle and foot without organ or systems involvement

M05.772 Rheumatoid arthritis with rheumatoid factor of left ankle and foot without organ or systems involvement

M05.779 Rheumatoid arthritis with rheumatoid factor of unspecified ankle and foot without organ or systems involvement ▽

M05.79 **Rheumatoid arthritis with rheumatoid factor of multiple sites without organ or systems involvement**

✓5ᵗʰ M05.8 **Other rheumatoid arthritis with rheumatoid factor**

M05.80 Other rheumatoid arthritis with rheumatoid factor of unspecified site ▽

✓6ᵗʰ M05.81 **Other rheumatoid arthritis with rheumatoid factor of shoulder**

M05.811 Other rheumatoid arthritis with rheumatoid factor of right shoulder

M05.812 Other rheumatoid arthritis with rheumatoid factor of left shoulder

M05.819 Other rheumatoid arthritis with rheumatoid factor of unspecified shoulder ▽

✓6ᵗʰ M05.82 **Other rheumatoid arthritis with rheumatoid factor of elbow**

M05.821 Other rheumatoid arthritis with rheumatoid factor of right elbow

M05.822 Other rheumatoid arthritis with rheumatoid factor of left elbow

M05.829 Other rheumatoid arthritis with rheumatoid factor of unspecified elbow ▽

✓6ᵗʰ M05.83 **Other rheumatoid arthritis with rheumatoid factor of wrist**

M05.831 Other rheumatoid arthritis with rheumatoid factor of right wrist

M05.832 Other rheumatoid arthritis with rheumatoid factor of left wrist

M05.839 Other rheumatoid arthritis with rheumatoid factor of unspecified wrist ▽

✓6ᵗʰ M05.84 **Other rheumatoid arthritis with rheumatoid factor of hand**

M05.841 Other rheumatoid arthritis with rheumatoid factor of right hand

EXCLUDES 1 Not coded here   EXCLUDES 2 Not included here   N Newborn Age : 0   P Pediatric Age : 0-17   M Maternity Age : 12-55   A Adult Age : 15-124

708
ICD-10-CM 2017

M05.842 Other rheumatoid arthritis with rheumatoid factor of left hand

M05.849 Other rheumatoid arthritis with rheumatoid factor of unspecified hand ▽

✓6ᵗʰ **M05.85** Other rheumatoid arthritis with rheumatoid factor of hip

   M05.851 Other rheumatoid arthritis with rheumatoid factor of right hip

   M05.852 Other rheumatoid arthritis with rheumatoid factor of left hip

   M05.859 Other rheumatoid arthritis with rheumatoid factor of unspecified hip ▽

✓6ᵗʰ **M05.86** Other rheumatoid arthritis with rheumatoid factor of knee

   M05.861 Other rheumatoid arthritis with rheumatoid factor of right knee

   M05.862 Other rheumatoid arthritis with rheumatoid factor of left knee

   M05.869 Other rheumatoid arthritis with rheumatoid factor of unspecified knee ▽

✓6ᵗʰ **M05.87** Other rheumatoid arthritis with rheumatoid factor of ankle and foot

   M05.871 Other rheumatoid arthritis with rheumatoid factor of right ankle and foot

   M05.872 Other rheumatoid arthritis with rheumatoid factor of left ankle and foot

   M05.879 Other rheumatoid arthritis with rheumatoid factor of unspecified ankle and foot ▽

M05.89 Other rheumatoid arthritis with rheumatoid factor of multiple sites

M05.9 Rheumatoid arthritis with rheumatoid factor, unspecified ▽

✓4ᵗʰ **M06** Other rheumatoid arthritis

✓5ᵗʰ **M06.0** Rheumatoid arthritis without rheumatoid factor

M06.00 Rheumatoid arthritis without rheumatoid factor, unspecified site ▽

✓6ᵗʰ **M06.01** Rheumatoid arthritis without rheumatoid factor, shoulder

   M06.011 Rheumatoid arthritis without rheumatoid factor, right shoulder

   M06.012 Rheumatoid arthritis without rheumatoid factor, left shoulder

   M06.019 Rheumatoid arthritis without rheumatoid factor, unspecified shoulder ▽

✓6ᵗʰ **M06.02** Rheumatoid arthritis without rheumatoid factor, elbow

   M06.021 Rheumatoid arthritis without rheumatoid factor, right elbow

   M06.022 Rheumatoid arthritis without rheumatoid factor, left elbow

   M06.029 Rheumatoid arthritis without rheumatoid factor, unspecified elbow ▽

✓6ᵗʰ **M06.03** Rheumatoid arthritis without rheumatoid factor, wrist

   M06.031 Rheumatoid arthritis without rheumatoid factor, right wrist

   M06.032 Rheumatoid arthritis without rheumatoid factor, left wrist

   M06.039 Rheumatoid arthritis without rheumatoid factor, unspecified wrist ▽

✓6ᵗʰ **M06.04** Rheumatoid arthritis without rheumatoid factor, hand

   M06.041 Rheumatoid arthritis without rheumatoid factor, right hand

   M06.042 Rheumatoid arthritis without rheumatoid factor, left hand

   M06.049 Rheumatoid arthritis without rheumatoid factor, unspecified hand ▽

✓6ᵗʰ **M06.05** Rheumatoid arthritis without rheumatoid factor, hip

   M06.051 Rheumatoid arthritis without rheumatoid factor, right hip

   M06.052 Rheumatoid arthritis without rheumatoid factor, left hip

   M06.059 Rheumatoid arthritis without rheumatoid factor, unspecified hip ▽

✓6ᵗʰ **M06.06** Rheumatoid arthritis without rheumatoid factor, knee

   M06.061 Rheumatoid arthritis without rheumatoid factor, right knee

   M06.062 Rheumatoid arthritis without rheumatoid factor, left knee

   M06.069 Rheumatoid arthritis without rheumatoid factor, unspecified knee ▽

✓6ᵗʰ **M06.07** Rheumatoid arthritis without rheumatoid factor, ankle and foot

   M06.071 Rheumatoid arthritis without rheumatoid factor, right ankle and foot

   M06.072 Rheumatoid arthritis without rheumatoid factor, left ankle and foot

   M06.079 Rheumatoid arthritis without rheumatoid factor, unspecified ankle and foot ▽

M06.08 Rheumatoid arthritis without rheumatoid factor, vertebrae

M06.09 Rheumatoid arthritis without rheumatoid factor, multiple sites

M06.1 Adult-onset Still's disease ▲

   EXCLUDES 1 Still's disease NOS (M08.2-)

✓5ᵗʰ **M06.2** Rheumatoid bursitis

M06.20 Rheumatoid bursitis, unspecified site ▽

✓6ᵗʰ **M06.21** Rheumatoid bursitis, shoulder

   M06.211 Rheumatoid bursitis, right shoulder

   M06.212 Rheumatoid bursitis, left shoulder

   M06.219 Rheumatoid bursitis, unspecified shoulder ▽

✓6ᵗʰ **M06.22** Rheumatoid bursitis, elbow

   M06.221 Rheumatoid bursitis, right elbow

   M06.222 Rheumatoid bursitis, left elbow

   M06.229 Rheumatoid bursitis, unspecified elbow ▽

✓6ᵗʰ **M06.23** Rheumatoid bursitis, wrist

   M06.231 Rheumatoid bursitis, right wrist

   M06.232 Rheumatoid bursitis, left wrist

   M06.239 Rheumatoid bursitis, unspecified wrist ▽

✓6ᵗʰ **M06.24** Rheumatoid bursitis, hand

   M06.241 Rheumatoid bursitis, right hand

   M06.242 Rheumatoid bursitis, left hand

   M06.249 Rheumatoid bursitis, unspecified hand ▽

✓6ᵗʰ **M06.25** Rheumatoid bursitis, hip

   M06.251 Rheumatoid bursitis, right hip

   M06.252 Rheumatoid bursitis, left hip

   M06.259 Rheumatoid bursitis, unspecified hip ▽

✓6ᵗʰ **M06.26** Rheumatoid bursitis, knee

   M06.261 Rheumatoid bursitis, right knee

   M06.262 Rheumatoid bursitis, left knee

   M06.269 Rheumatoid bursitis, unspecified knee ▽

✓6ᵗʰ **M06.27** Rheumatoid bursitis, ankle and foot

   M06.271 Rheumatoid bursitis, right ankle and foot

   M06.272 Rheumatoid bursitis, left ankle and foot

   M06.279 Rheumatoid bursitis, unspecified ankle and foot ▽

M06.28 Rheumatoid bursitis, vertebrae

M06.29 Rheumatoid bursitis, multiple sites

✓5ᵗʰ **M06.3** Rheumatoid nodule

M06.30 Rheumatoid nodule, unspecified site ▽

✓6ᵗʰ **M06.31** Rheumatoid nodule, shoulder

   M06.311 Rheumatoid nodule, right shoulder

   M06.312 Rheumatoid nodule, left shoulder

   M06.319 Rheumatoid nodule, unspecified shoulder ▽

✓6ᵗʰ **M06.32** Rheumatoid nodule, elbow

   M06.321 Rheumatoid nodule, right elbow

   M06.322 Rheumatoid nodule, left elbow

   M06.329 Rheumatoid nodule, unspecified elbow ▽

☑ Additional Character Required   ✓x7ᵗʰ Placeholder Alert   Manifestation Dx   ▽ Unspecified Dx   ►◄ Revised Text   ● New Code   ▲ Revised Code Title

Chapter 13. Diseases of the Musculoskeletal System and Connective Tissue

✓6th **M06.33 Rheumatoid nodule,** wrist
- **M06.331 Rheumatoid nodule,** right **wrist**
- **M06.332 Rheumatoid nodule,** left **wrist**
- **M06.339 Rheumatoid nodule,** unspecified **wrist** ▽

✓6th **M06.34 Rheumatoid nodule,** hand
- **M06.341 Rheumatoid nodule,** right **hand**
- **M06.342 Rheumatoid nodule,** left **hand**
- **M06.349 Rheumatoid nodule,** unspecified **hand** ▽

✓6th **M06.35 Rheumatoid nodule,** hip
- **M06.351 Rheumatoid nodule,** right **hip**
- **M06.352 Rheumatoid nodule,** left **hip**
- **M06.359 Rheumatoid nodule,** unspecified **hip** ▽

✓6th **M06.36 Rheumatoid nodule,** knee
- **M06.361 Rheumatoid nodule,** right **knee**
- **M06.362 Rheumatoid nodule,** left **knee**
- **M06.369 Rheumatoid nodule,** unspecified **knee** ▽

✓6th **M06.37 Rheumatoid nodule,** ankle and foot
- **M06.371 Rheumatoid nodule,** right **ankle and foot**
- **M06.372 Rheumatoid nodule,** left **ankle and foot**
- **M06.379 Rheumatoid nodule,** unspecified **ankle and foot** ▽

M06.38 Rheumatoid nodule, vertebrae
M06.39 Rheumatoid nodule, multiple sites

M06.4 Inflammatory polyarthropathy
> EXCLUDES 1 *polyarthritis NOS (M13.0)*

✓5th **M06.8 Other specified rheumatoid arthritis**
- **M06.80 Other specified rheumatoid arthritis,** unspecified site ▽

✓6th **M06.81 Other specified rheumatoid arthritis,** shoulder
- **M06.811 Other specified rheumatoid arthritis,** right **shoulder**
- **M06.812 Other specified rheumatoid arthritis,** left **shoulder**
- **M06.819 Other specified rheumatoid arthritis,** unspecified **shoulder** ▽

✓6th **M06.82 Other specified rheumatoid arthritis,** elbow
- **M06.821 Other specified rheumatoid arthritis,** right **elbow**
- **M06.822 Other specified rheumatoid arthritis,** left **elbow**
- **M06.829 Other specified rheumatoid arthritis,** unspecified **elbow** ▽

✓6th **M06.83 Other specified rheumatoid arthritis,** wrist
- **M06.831 Other specified rheumatoid arthritis,** right **wrist**
- **M06.832 Other specified rheumatoid arthritis,** left **wrist**
- **M06.839 Other specified rheumatoid arthritis,** unspecified **wrist** ▽

✓6th **M06.84 Other specified rheumatoid arthritis,** hand
- **M06.841 Other specified rheumatoid arthritis,** right **hand**
- **M06.842 Other specified rheumatoid arthritis,** left **hand**
- **M06.849 Other specified rheumatoid arthritis,** unspecified **hand** ▽

✓6th **M06.85 Other specified rheumatoid arthritis,** hip
- **M06.851 Other specified rheumatoid arthritis,** right **hip**
- **M06.852 Other specified rheumatoid arthritis,** left **hip**
- **M06.859 Other specified rheumatoid arthritis,** unspecified **hip** ▽

✓6th **M06.86 Other specified rheumatoid arthritis,** knee
- **M06.861 Other specified rheumatoid arthritis,** right **knee**
- **M06.862 Other specified rheumatoid arthritis,** left **knee**
- **M06.869 Other specified rheumatoid arthritis,** unspecified **knee** ▽

✓6th **M06.87 Other specified rheumatoid arthritis,** ankle and foot
- **M06.871 Other specified rheumatoid arthritis,** right **ankle and foot**
- **M06.872 Other specified rheumatoid arthritis,** left **ankle and foot**
- **M06.879 Other specified rheumatoid arthritis,** unspecified **ankle and foot** ▽

M06.88 Other specified rheumatoid arthritis, vertebrae
M06.89 Other specified rheumatoid arthritis, multiple sites

M06.9 Rheumatoid arthritis, unspecified ▽

✓4th **M07 Enteropathic arthropathies**

Code also associated enteropathy, such as:
   regional enteritis [Crohn's disease] (K50.-)
   ulcerative colitis (K51.-)
> EXCLUDES 1 *psoriatic arthropathies (L40.5-)*

✓5th **M07.6 Enteropathic arthropathies**
- **M07.60 Enteropathic arthropathies, unspecified site** ▽

✓6th **M07.61 Enteropathic arthropathies,** shoulder
- **M07.611 Enteropathic arthropathies,** right **shoulder**
- **M07.612 Enteropathic arthropathies,** left **shoulder**
- **M07.619 Enteropathic arthropathies,** unspecified **shoulder** ▽

✓6th **M07.62 Enteropathic arthropathies,** elbow
- **M07.621 Enteropathic arthropathies,** right **elbow**
- **M07.622 Enteropathic arthropathies,** left **elbow**
- **M07.629 Enteropathic arthropathies,** unspecified **elbow** ▽

✓6th **M07.63 Enteropathic arthropathies,** wrist
- **M07.631 Enteropathic arthropathies,** right **wrist**
- **M07.632 Enteropathic arthropathies,** left **wrist**
- **M07.639 Enteropathic arthropathies,** unspecified **wrist** ▽

✓6th **M07.64 Enteropathic arthropathies,** hand
- **M07.641 Enteropathic arthropathies,** right **hand**
- **M07.642 Enteropathic arthropathies,** left **hand**
- **M07.649 Enteropathic arthropathies,** unspecified **hand** ▽

✓6th **M07.65 Enteropathic arthropathies,** hip
- **M07.651 Enteropathic arthropathies,** right **hip**
- **M07.652 Enteropathic arthropathies,** left **hip**
- **M07.659 Enteropathic arthropathies,** unspecified **hip** ▽

✓6th **M07.66 Enteropathic arthropathies,** knee
- **M07.661 Enteropathic arthropathies,** right **knee**
- **M07.662 Enteropathic arthropathies,** left **knee**
- **M07.669 Enteropathic arthropathies,** unspecified **knee** ▽

✓6th **M07.67 Enteropathic arthropathies,** ankle and foot
- **M07.671 Enteropathic arthropathies,** right **ankle and foot**
- **M07.672 Enteropathic arthropathies,** left **ankle and foot**
- **M07.679 Enteropathic arthropathies,** unspecified **ankle and foot** ▽

M07.68 Enteropathic arthropathies, vertebrae
M07.69 Enteropathic arthropathies, multiple sites

✓4th **M08 Juvenile arthritis**

Code also any associated underlying condition, such as:
   regional enteritis [Crohn's disease] (K50.-)
   ulcerative colitis (K51.-)
> EXCLUDES 1 *arthropathy in Whipple's disease (M14.8)*
> *Felty's syndrome (M05.0)*
> *juvenile dermatomyositis (M33.0-)*
> *psoriatic juvenile arthropathy (L40.54)*

✓5th **M08.0 Unspecified juvenile rheumatoid arthritis**

Juvenile rheumatoid arthritis with or without rheumatoid factor
- **M08.00 Unspecified juvenile rheumatoid arthritis of unspecified site** ▽

✓6th **M08.01 Unspecified juvenile rheumatoid arthritis,** shoulder
- **M08.011 Unspecified juvenile rheumatoid arthritis,** right **shoulder** ▽
- **M08.012 Unspecified juvenile rheumatoid arthritis,** left **shoulder** ▽
- **M08.019 Unspecified juvenile rheumatoid arthritis,** unspecified **shoulder** ▽

✓6th **M08.02 Unspecified juvenile rheumatoid arthritis of** elbow
- **M08.021 Unspecified juvenile rheumatoid arthritis,** right **elbow** ▽
- **M08.022 Unspecified juvenile rheumatoid arthritis,** left **elbow** ▽

EXCLUDES 1 Not coded here   EXCLUDES 2 Not included here   Ⓝ Newborn Age : 0   Ⓟ Pediatric Age : 0-17   Ⓜ Maternity Age : 12-55   Ⓐ Adult Age : 15-124

M08.029   Unspecified juvenile rheumatoid arthritis, unspecified elbow ▽

√6ᵗʰ M08.03   Unspecified juvenile rheumatoid arthritis, wrist

M08.031   Unspecified juvenile rheumatoid arthritis, right wrist ▽

M08.032   Unspecified juvenile rheumatoid arthritis, left wrist ▽

M08.039   Unspecified juvenile rheumatoid arthritis, unspecified wrist ▽

√6ᵗʰ M08.04   Unspecified juvenile rheumatoid arthritis, hand

M08.041   Unspecified juvenile rheumatoid arthritis, right hand ▽

M08.042   Unspecified juvenile rheumatoid arthritis, left hand ▽

M08.049   Unspecified juvenile rheumatoid arthritis, unspecified hand ▽

√6ᵗʰ M08.05   Unspecified juvenile rheumatoid arthritis, hip

M08.051   Unspecified juvenile rheumatoid arthritis, right hip ▽

M08.052   Unspecified juvenile rheumatoid arthritis, left hip ▽

M08.059   Unspecified juvenile rheumatoid arthritis, unspecified hip ▽

√6ᵗʰ M08.06   Unspecified juvenile rheumatoid arthritis, knee

M08.061   Unspecified juvenile rheumatoid arthritis, right knee ▽

M08.062   Unspecified juvenile rheumatoid arthritis, left knee ▽

M08.069   Unspecified juvenile rheumatoid arthritis, unspecified knee ▽

√6ᵗʰ M08.07   Unspecified juvenile rheumatoid arthritis, ankle and foot

M08.071   Unspecified juvenile rheumatoid arthritis, right ankle and foot ▽

M08.072   Unspecified juvenile rheumatoid arthritis, left ankle and foot ▽

M08.079   Unspecified juvenile rheumatoid arthritis, unspecified ankle and foot ▽

M08.08   Unspecified juvenile rheumatoid arthritis, vertebrae ▽

M08.09   Unspecified juvenile rheumatoid arthritis, multiple sites ▽

M08.1   Juvenile ankylosing spondylitis
    EXCLUDES 1   ankylosing spondylitis in adults (M45.0-)

√5ᵗʰ M08.2   Juvenile rheumatoid arthritis with systemic onset
    Still's disease NOS
    EXCLUDES 1   adult-onset Still's disease (M06.1-)

M08.20   Juvenile rheumatoid arthritis with systemic onset, unspecified site ▽

√6ᵗʰ M08.21   Juvenile rheumatoid arthritis with systemic onset, shoulder

M08.211   Juvenile rheumatoid arthritis with systemic onset, right shoulder

M08.212   Juvenile rheumatoid arthritis with systemic onset, left shoulder

M08.219   Juvenile rheumatoid arthritis with systemic onset, unspecified shoulder ▽

√6ᵗʰ M08.22   Juvenile rheumatoid arthritis with systemic onset, elbow

M08.221   Juvenile rheumatoid arthritis with systemic onset, right elbow

M08.222   Juvenile rheumatoid arthritis with systemic onset, left elbow

M08.229   Juvenile rheumatoid arthritis with systemic onset, unspecified elbow

√6ᵗʰ M08.23   Juvenile rheumatoid arthritis with systemic onset, wrist

M08.231   Juvenile rheumatoid arthritis with systemic onset, right wrist

M08.232   Juvenile rheumatoid arthritis with systemic onset, left wrist

M08.239   Juvenile rheumatoid arthritis with systemic onset, unspecified wrist ▽

√6ᵗʰ M08.24   Juvenile rheumatoid arthritis with systemic onset, hand

M08.241   Juvenile rheumatoid arthritis with systemic onset, right hand

M08.242   Juvenile rheumatoid arthritis with systemic onset, left hand

M08.249   Juvenile rheumatoid arthritis with systemic onset, unspecified hand ▽

√6ᵗʰ M08.25   Juvenile rheumatoid arthritis with systemic onset, hip

M08.251   Juvenile rheumatoid arthritis with systemic onset, right hip

M08.252   Juvenile rheumatoid arthritis with systemic onset, left hip

M08.259   Juvenile rheumatoid arthritis with systemic onset, unspecified hip

√6ᵗʰ M08.26   Juvenile rheumatoid arthritis with systemic onset, knee

M08.261   Juvenile rheumatoid arthritis with systemic onset, right knee

M08.262   Juvenile rheumatoid arthritis with systemic onset, left knee

M08.269   Juvenile rheumatoid arthritis with systemic onset, unspecified knee ▽

√6ᵗʰ M08.27   Juvenile rheumatoid arthritis with systemic onset, ankle and foot

M08.271   Juvenile rheumatoid arthritis with systemic onset, right ankle and foot

M08.272   Juvenile rheumatoid arthritis with systemic onset, left ankle and foot

M08.279   Juvenile rheumatoid arthritis with systemic onset, unspecified ankle and foot ▽

M08.28   Juvenile rheumatoid arthritis with systemic onset, vertebrae

M08.29   Juvenile rheumatoid arthritis with systemic onset, multiple sites

M08.3   Juvenile rheumatoid polyarthritis (seronegative)

√6ᵗʰ M08.4   Pauciarticular juvenile rheumatoid arthritis

M08.40   Pauciarticular juvenile rheumatoid arthritis, unspecified site ▽

√6ᵗʰ M08.41   Pauciarticular juvenile rheumatoid arthritis, shoulder

M08.411   Pauciarticular juvenile rheumatoid arthritis, right shoulder

M08.412   Pauciarticular juvenile rheumatoid arthritis, left shoulder

M08.419   Pauciarticular juvenile rheumatoid arthritis, unspecified shoulder ▽

√6ᵗʰ M08.42   Pauciarticular juvenile rheumatoid arthritis, elbow

M08.421   Pauciarticular juvenile rheumatoid arthritis, right elbow

M08.422   Pauciarticular juvenile rheumatoid arthritis, left elbow

M08.429   Pauciarticular juvenile rheumatoid arthritis, unspecified elbow ▽

√6ᵗʰ M08.43   Pauciarticular juvenile rheumatoid arthritis, wrist

M08.431   Pauciarticular juvenile rheumatoid arthritis, right wrist

M08.432   Pauciarticular juvenile rheumatoid arthritis, left wrist

M08.439   Pauciarticular juvenile rheumatoid arthritis, unspecified wrist ▽

√6ᵗʰ M08.44   Pauciarticular juvenile rheumatoid arthritis, hand

M08.441   Pauciarticular juvenile rheumatoid arthritis, right hand

M08.442   Pauciarticular juvenile rheumatoid arthritis, left hand

M08.449   Pauciarticular juvenile rheumatoid arthritis, unspecified hand ▽

√6ᵗʰ M08.45   Pauciarticular juvenile rheumatoid arthritis, hip

M08.451   Pauciarticular juvenile rheumatoid arthritis, right hip

M08.452   Pauciarticular juvenile rheumatoid arthritis, left hip

M08.459   Pauciarticular juvenile rheumatoid arthritis, unspecified hip ▽

√6ᵗʰ M08.46   Pauciarticular juvenile rheumatoid arthritis, knee

M08.461   Pauciarticular juvenile rheumatoid arthritis, right knee

M08.462   Pauciarticular juvenile rheumatoid arthritis, left knee

M08.469   Pauciarticular juvenile rheumatoid arthritis, unspecified knee ▽

√6ᵗʰ M08.47   Pauciarticular juvenile rheumatoid arthritis, ankle and foot

M08.471   Pauciarticular juvenile rheumatoid arthritis, right ankle and foot

☑ Additional Character Required   P-T Placeholder Alert   Manifestation Dx   ▽ Unspecified Dx   ►◄ Revised Text   ● New Code   ▲ Revised Code Title

ICD-10-CM 2017   711

M08.472 **Pauciarticular juvenile rheumatoid arthritis,** left **ankle and foot**

M08.479 **Pauciarticular juvenile rheumatoid arthritis, unspecified ankle and foot** ▽

M08.48 **Pauciarticular juvenile rheumatoid arthritis,** vertebrae

✓5ᵗʰ **M08.8** **Other juvenile arthritis**

M08.80 **Other juvenile arthritis, unspecified site** ▽

✓6ᵗʰ M08.81 **Other juvenile arthritis,** shoulder

M08.811 **Other juvenile arthritis,** right **shoulder**

M08.812 **Other juvenile arthritis,** left **shoulder**

M08.819 **Other juvenile arthritis, unspecified shoulder** ▽

✓6ᵗʰ M08.82 **Other juvenile arthritis,** elbow

M08.821 **Other juvenile arthritis,** right **elbow**

M08.822 **Other juvenile arthritis,** left **elbow**

M08.829 **Other juvenile arthritis, unspecified elbow** ▽

✓6ᵗʰ M08.83 **Other juvenile arthritis,** wrist

M08.831 **Other juvenile arthritis,** right **wrist**

M08.832 **Other juvenile arthritis,** left **wrist**

M08.839 **Other juvenile arthritis, unspecified wrist** ▽

✓6ᵗʰ M08.84 **Other juvenile arthritis,** hand

M08.841 **Other juvenile arthritis,** right **hand**

M08.842 **Other juvenile arthritis,** left **hand**

M08.849 **Other juvenile arthritis, unspecified hand** ▽

✓6ᵗʰ M08.85 **Other juvenile arthritis,** hip

M08.851 **Other juvenile arthritis,** right **hip**

M08.852 **Other juvenile arthritis,** left **hip**

M08.859 **Other juvenile arthritis, unspecified hip** ▽

✓6ᵗʰ M08.86 **Other juvenile arthritis,** knee

M08.861 **Other juvenile arthritis,** right **knee**

M08.862 **Other juvenile arthritis,** left **knee**

M08.869 **Other juvenile arthritis, unspecified knee** ▽

✓6ᵗʰ M08.87 **Other juvenile arthritis,** ankle and foot

M08.871 **Other juvenile arthritis,** right **ankle and foot**

M08.872 **Other juvenile arthritis,** left **ankle and foot**

M08.879 **Other juvenile arthritis, unspecified ankle and foot** ▽

M08.88 **Other juvenile arthritis, other specified site**
Other juvenile arthritis, vertebrae

M08.89 **Other juvenile arthritis,** multiple sites

✓5ᵗʰ **M08.9** **Juvenile arthritis, unspecified**

EXCLUDES 1 *juvenile rheumatoid arthritis, unspecified (M08.0-)*

M08.90 **Juvenile arthritis, unspecified, unspecified site** ▽

✓6ᵗʰ M08.91 **Juvenile arthritis, unspecified,** shoulder

M08.911 **Juvenile arthritis, unspecified,** right **shoulder** ▽

M08.912 **Juvenile arthritis, unspecified,** left **shoulder** ▽

M08.919 **Juvenile arthritis, unspecified, unspecified shoulder** ▽

✓6ᵗʰ M08.92 **Juvenile arthritis, unspecified,** elbow

M08.921 **Juvenile arthritis, unspecified,** right **elbow** ▽

M08.922 **Juvenile arthritis, unspecified,** left **elbow** ▽

M08.929 **Juvenile arthritis, unspecified, unspecified elbow** ▽

✓6ᵗʰ M08.93 **Juvenile arthritis, unspecified,** wrist

M08.931 **Juvenile arthritis, unspecified,** right **wrist** ▽

M08.932 **Juvenile arthritis, unspecified,** left **wrist** ▽

M08.939 **Juvenile arthritis, unspecified, unspecified wrist** ▽

✓6ᵗʰ M08.94 **Juvenile arthritis, unspecified,** hand

M08.941 **Juvenile arthritis, unspecified,** right **hand** ▽

M08.942 **Juvenile arthritis, unspecified,** left **hand** ▽

M08.949 **Juvenile arthritis, unspecified, unspecified hand** ▽

✓6ᵗʰ M08.95 **Juvenile arthritis, unspecified,** hip

M08.951 **Juvenile arthritis, unspecified,** right **hip** ▽

M08.952 **Juvenile arthritis, unspecified,** left **hip** ▽

M08.959 **Juvenile arthritis, unspecified, unspecified hip** ▽

✓6ᵗʰ M08.96 **Juvenile arthritis, unspecified,** knee

M08.961 **Juvenile arthritis, unspecified,** right **knee** ▽

M08.962 **Juvenile arthritis, unspecified,** left **knee** ▽

M08.969 **Juvenile arthritis, unspecified, unspecified knee** ▽

✓6ᵗʰ M08.97 **Juvenile arthritis, unspecified,** ankle and foot

M08.971 **Juvenile arthritis, unspecified,** right **ankle and foot** ▽

M08.972 **Juvenile arthritis, unspecified,** left **ankle and foot** ▽

M08.979 **Juvenile arthritis, unspecified, unspecified ankle and foot** ▽

M08.98 **Juvenile arthritis, unspecified,** vertebrae ▽

M08.99 **Juvenile arthritis, unspecified,** multiple sites ▽

✓4ᵗʰ **M1A** **Chronic gout**

Use additional code to identify:
autonomic neuropathy in diseases classified elsewhere (G99.0)
calculus of urinary tract in diseases classified elsewhere (N22)
cardiomyopathy in diseases classified elsewhere (I43)
disorders of external ear in diseases classified elsewhere (H61.1-, H62.8-)
disorders of iris and ciliary body in diseases classified elsewhere (H22)
glomerular disorders in diseases classified elsewhere (N08)

EXCLUDES 1 *gout NOS (M10.-)*

EXCLUDES 2 ▶*acute gout (M10.-)*◀

The appropriate 7th character is to be added to each code from category M1A.
0   without tophus (tophi)
1   with tophus (tophi)

✓5ᵗʰ **M1A.0** **Idiopathic chronic gout**

Chronic gouty bursitis
Primary chronic gout

✓x7ᵗʰ M1A.00 **Idiopathic chronic gout, unspecified site** ▽

✓6ᵗʰ M1A.01 **Idiopathic chronic gout,** shoulder

✓7ᵗʰ M1A.011 **Idiopathic chronic gout,** right **shoulder**

✓7ᵗʰ M1A.012 **Idiopathic chronic gout,** left **shoulder**

✓7ᵗʰ M1A.019 **Idiopathic chronic gout, unspecified shoulder** ▽

✓6ᵗʰ M1A.02 **Idiopathic chronic gout,** elbow

✓7ᵗʰ M1A.021 **Idiopathic chronic gout,** right **elbow**

✓7ᵗʰ M1A.022 **Idiopathic chronic gout,** left **elbow**

✓7ᵗʰ M1A.029 **Idiopathic chronic gout, unspecified elbow** ▽

✓6ᵗʰ M1A.03 **Idiopathic chronic gout,** wrist

✓7ᵗʰ M1A.031 **Idiopathic chronic gout,** right **wrist**

✓7ᵗʰ M1A.032 **Idiopathic chronic gout,** left **wrist**

✓7ᵗʰ M1A.039 **Idiopathic chronic gout, unspecified wrist** ▽

✓6ᵗʰ M1A.04 **Idiopathic chronic gout,** hand

✓7ᵗʰ M1A.041 **Idiopathic chronic gout,** right **hand**

✓7ᵗʰ M1A.042 **Idiopathic chronic gout,** left **hand**

✓7ᵗʰ M1A.049 **Idiopathic chronic gout, unspecified hand** ▽

✓6ᵗʰ M1A.05 **Idiopathic chronic gout,** hip

✓7ᵗʰ M1A.051 **Idiopathic chronic gout,** right **hip**

✓7ᵗʰ M1A.052 **Idiopathic chronic gout,** left **hip**

✓7ᵗʰ M1A.059 **Idiopathic chronic gout, unspecified hip** ▽

✓6ᵗʰ M1A.06 **Idiopathic chronic gout,** knee

✓7ᵗʰ M1A.061 **Idiopathic chronic gout,** right **knee**

EXCLUDES 1 Not coded here   **EXCLUDES 2** Not included here   Ⓝ Newborn Age : 0   Ⓟ Pediatric Age : 0-17   Ⓜ Maternity Age : 12-55   Ⓐ Adult Age : 15-124

712   ICD-10-CM 2017

√7ᵗʰ **M1A.062** Idiopathic chronic gout, left knee

√7ᵗʰ **M1A.069** Idiopathic chronic gout, unspecified knee ▽

√6ᵗʰ **M1A.07** Idiopathic chronic gout, ankle and foot

     √7ᵗʰ **M1A.071** Idiopathic chronic gout, right ankle and foot

     √7ᵗʰ **M1A.072** Idiopathic chronic gout, left ankle and foot

     √7ᵗʰ **M1A.079** Idiopathic chronic gout, unspecified ankle and foot ▽

√x7ᵗʰ **M1A.08** Idiopathic chronic gout, vertebrae

√x7ᵗʰ **M1A.09** Idiopathic chronic gout, multiple sites

√5ᵗʰ **M1A.1** Lead-induced chronic gout

     Code first toxic effects of lead and its compounds (T56.0-)

√x7ᵗʰ **M1A.10** Lead-induced chronic gout, unspecified site ▽

√6ᵗʰ **M1A.11** Lead-induced chronic gout, shoulder

     √7ᵗʰ **M1A.111** Lead-induced chronic gout, right shoulder

     √7ᵗʰ **M1A.112** Lead-induced chronic gout, left shoulder

     √7ᵗʰ **M1A.119** Lead-induced chronic gout, unspecified shoulder ▽

√6ᵗʰ **M1A.12** Lead-induced chronic gout, elbow

     √7ᵗʰ **M1A.121** Lead-induced chronic gout, right elbow

     √7ᵗʰ **M1A.122** Lead-induced chronic gout, left elbow

     √7ᵗʰ **M1A.129** Lead-induced chronic gout, unspecified elbow ▽

√6ᵗʰ **M1A.13** Lead-induced chronic gout, wrist

     √7ᵗʰ **M1A.131** Lead-induced chronic gout, right wrist

     √7ᵗʰ **M1A.132** Lead-induced chronic gout, left wrist

     √7ᵗʰ **M1A.139** Lead-induced chronic gout, unspecified wrist ▽

√6ᵗʰ **M1A.14** Lead-induced chronic gout, hand

     √7ᵗʰ **M1A.141** Lead-induced chronic gout, right hand

     √7ᵗʰ **M1A.142** Lead-induced chronic gout, left hand

     √7ᵗʰ **M1A.149** Lead-induced chronic gout, unspecified hand ▽

√6ᵗʰ **M1A.15** Lead-induced chronic gout, hip

     √7ᵗʰ **M1A.151** Lead-induced chronic gout, right hip

     √7ᵗʰ **M1A.152** Lead-induced chronic gout, left hip

     √7ᵗʰ **M1A.159** Lead-induced chronic gout, unspecified hip ▽

√6ᵗʰ **M1A.16** Lead-induced chronic gout, knee

     √7ᵗʰ **M1A.161** Lead-induced chronic gout, right knee

     √7ᵗʰ **M1A.162** Lead-induced chronic gout, left knee

     √7ᵗʰ **M1A.169** Lead-induced chronic gout, unspecified knee ▽

√6ᵗʰ **M1A.17** Lead-induced chronic gout, ankle and foot

     √7ᵗʰ **M1A.171** Lead-induced chronic gout, right ankle and foot

     √7ᵗʰ **M1A.172** Lead-induced chronic gout, left ankle and foot

     √7ᵗʰ **M1A.179** Lead-induced chronic gout, unspecified ankle and foot ▽

√x7ᵗʰ **M1A.18** Lead-induced chronic gout, vertebrae

√x7ᵗʰ **M1A.19** Lead-induced chronic gout, multiple sites

√5ᵗʰ **M1A.2** Drug-induced chronic gout

     Use additional code for adverse effect, if applicable, to identify drug (T36-T50 with fifth or sixth character 5)

√x7ᵗʰ **M1A.20** Drug-induced chronic gout, unspecified site ▽

√6ᵗʰ **M1A.21** Drug-induced chronic gout, shoulder

     √7ᵗʰ **M1A.211** Drug-induced chronic gout, right shoulder

     √7ᵗʰ **M1A.212** Drug-induced chronic gout, left shoulder

     √7ᵗʰ **M1A.219** Drug-induced chronic gout, unspecified shoulder ▽

√6ᵗʰ **M1A.22** Drug-induced chronic gout, elbow

     √7ᵗʰ **M1A.221** Drug-induced chronic gout, right elbow

     √7ᵗʰ **M1A.222** Drug-induced chronic gout, left elbow

     √7ᵗʰ **M1A.229** Drug-induced chronic gout, unspecified elbow ▽

√6ᵗʰ **M1A.23** Drug-induced chronic gout, wrist

     √7ᵗʰ **M1A.231** Drug-induced chronic gout, right wrist

     √7ᵗʰ **M1A.232** Drug-induced chronic gout, left wrist

√7ᵗʰ **M1A.239** Drug-induced chronic gout, unspecified wrist ▽

√6ᵗʰ **M1A.24** Drug-induced chronic gout, hand

     √7ᵗʰ **M1A.241** Drug-induced chronic gout, right hand

     √7ᵗʰ **M1A.242** Drug-induced chronic gout, left hand

     √7ᵗʰ **M1A.249** Drug-induced chronic gout, unspecified hand

√6ᵗʰ **M1A.25** Drug-induced chronic gout, hip

     √7ᵗʰ **M1A.251** Drug-induced chronic gout, right hip

     √7ᵗʰ **M1A.252** Drug-induced chronic gout, left hip

     √7ᵗʰ **M1A.259** Drug-induced chronic gout, unspecified hip ▽

√6ᵗʰ **M1A.26** Drug-induced chronic gout, knee

     √7ᵗʰ **M1A.261** Drug-induced chronic gout, right knee

     √7ᵗʰ **M1A.262** Drug-induced chronic gout, left knee

     √7ᵗʰ **M1A.269** Drug-induced chronic gout, unspecified knee ▽

√6ᵗʰ **M1A.27** Drug-induced chronic gout, ankle and foot

     √7ᵗʰ **M1A.271** Drug-induced chronic gout, right ankle and foot

     √7ᵗʰ **M1A.272** Drug-induced chronic gout, left ankle and foot

     √7ᵗʰ **M1A.279** Drug-induced chronic gout, unspecified ankle and foot ▽

√x7ᵗʰ **M1A.28** Drug-induced chronic gout, vertebrae

√x7ᵗʰ **M1A.29** Drug-induced chronic gout, multiple sites

√5ᵗʰ **M1A.3** Chronic gout due to renal impairment

     Code first associated renal disease

√x7ᵗʰ **M1A.30** Chronic gout due to renal impairment, unspecified site ▽

√6ᵗʰ **M1A.31** Chronic gout due to renal impairment, shoulder

     √7ᵗʰ **M1A.311** Chronic gout due to renal impairment, right shoulder

     √7ᵗʰ **M1A.312** Chronic gout due to renal impairment, left shoulder

     √7ᵗʰ **M1A.319** Chronic gout due to renal impairment, unspecified shoulder ▽

√6ᵗʰ **M1A.32** Chronic gout due to renal impairment, elbow

     √7ᵗʰ **M1A.321** Chronic gout due to renal impairment, right elbow

     √7ᵗʰ **M1A.322** Chronic gout due to renal impairment, left elbow

     √7ᵗʰ **M1A.329** Chronic gout due to renal impairment, unspecified elbow ▽

√6ᵗʰ **M1A.33** Chronic gout due to renal impairment, wrist

     √7ᵗʰ **M1A.331** Chronic gout due to renal impairment, right wrist

     √7ᵗʰ **M1A.332** Chronic gout due to renal impairment, left wrist

     √7ᵗʰ **M1A.339** Chronic gout due to renal impairment, unspecified wrist ▽

√6ᵗʰ **M1A.34** Chronic gout due to renal impairment, hand

     √7ᵗʰ **M1A.341** Chronic gout due to renal impairment, right hand

     √7ᵗʰ **M1A.342** Chronic gout due to renal impairment, left hand

     √7ᵗʰ **M1A.349** Chronic gout due to renal impairment, unspecified hand ▽

√6ᵗʰ **M1A.35** Chronic gout due to renal impairment, hip

     √7ᵗʰ **M1A.351** Chronic gout due to renal impairment, right hip

     √7ᵗʰ **M1A.352** Chronic gout due to renal impairment, left hip

     √7ᵗʰ **M1A.359** Chronic gout due to renal impairment, unspecified hip ▽

√6ᵗʰ **M1A.36** Chronic gout due to renal impairment, knee

     √7ᵗʰ **M1A.361** Chronic gout due to renal impairment, right knee

     √7ᵗʰ **M1A.362** Chronic gout due to renal impairment, left knee

     √7ᵗʰ **M1A.369** Chronic gout due to renal impairment, unspecified knee ▽

√6ᵗʰ **M1A.37** Chronic gout due to renal impairment, ankle and foot

     √7ᵗʰ **M1A.371** Chronic gout due to renal impairment, right ankle and foot

     √7ᵗʰ **M1A.372** Chronic gout due to renal impairment, left ankle and foot

---

✔ Additional Character Required   √x7ᵗʰ Placeholder Alert   Manifestation Dx   ▽ Unspecified Dx   ▶◀ Revised Text   ● New Code   ▲ Revised Code Title

√7ᵗʰ **M1A.379** Chronic gout due to renal impairment, unspecified ankle and foot ▽

√x7ᵗʰ **M1A.38** Chronic gout due to renal impairment, vertebrae

√x7ᵗʰ **M1A.39** Chronic gout due to renal impairment, multiple sites

√5ᵗʰ **M1A.4** Other secondary chronic gout

Code first associated condition

√x7ᵗʰ **M1A.40** Other secondary chronic gout, unspecified site ▽

√6ᵗʰ **M1A.41** Other secondary chronic gout, shoulder

√7ᵗʰ **M1A.411** Other secondary chronic gout, right shoulder

√7ᵗʰ **M1A.412** Other secondary chronic gout, left shoulder

√7ᵗʰ **M1A.419** Other secondary chronic gout, unspecified shoulder ▽

√6ᵗʰ **M1A.42** Other secondary chronic gout, elbow

√7ᵗʰ **M1A.421** Other secondary chronic gout, right elbow

√7ᵗʰ **M1A.422** Other secondary chronic gout, left elbow

√7ᵗʰ **M1A.429** Other secondary chronic gout, unspecified elbow ▽

√6ᵗʰ **M1A.43** Other secondary chronic gout, wrist

√7ᵗʰ **M1A.431** Other secondary chronic gout, right wrist

√7ᵗʰ **M1A.432** Other secondary chronic gout, left wrist

√7ᵗʰ **M1A.439** Other secondary chronic gout, unspecified wrist ▽

√6ᵗʰ **M1A.44** Other secondary chronic gout, hand

√7ᵗʰ **M1A.441** Other secondary chronic gout, right hand

√7ᵗʰ **M1A.442** Other secondary chronic gout, left hand

√7ᵗʰ **M1A.449** Other secondary chronic gout, unspecified hand ▽

√6ᵗʰ **M1A.45** Other secondary chronic gout, hip

√7ᵗʰ **M1A.451** Other secondary chronic gout, right hip

√7ᵗʰ **M1A.452** Other secondary chronic gout, left hip

√7ᵗʰ **M1A.459** Other secondary chronic gout, unspecified hip ▽

√6ᵗʰ **M1A.46** Other secondary chronic gout, knee

√7ᵗʰ **M1A.461** Other secondary chronic gout, right knee

√7ᵗʰ **M1A.462** Other secondary chronic gout, left knee

√7ᵗʰ **M1A.469** Other secondary chronic gout, unspecified knee ▽

√6ᵗʰ **M1A.47** Other secondary chronic gout, ankle and foot

√7ᵗʰ **M1A.471** Other secondary chronic gout, right ankle and foot

√7ᵗʰ **M1A.472** Other secondary chronic gout, left ankle and foot

√7ᵗʰ **M1A.479** Other secondary chronic gout, unspecified ankle and foot ▽

√x7ᵗʰ **M1A.48** Other secondary chronic gout, vertebrae

√x7ᵗʰ **M1A.49** Other secondary chronic gout, multiple sites

√x7ᵗʰ **M1A.9** Chronic gout, unspecified ▽

√4ᵗʰ **M10** Gout

Acute gout
Gout attack
Gout flare
Podagra
Use additional code to identify:
autonomic neuropathy in diseases classified elsewhere (G99.0)
calculus of urinary tract in diseases classified elsewhere (N22)
cardiomyopathy in diseases classified elsewhere (I43)
disorders of external ear in diseases classified elsewhere (H61.1-, H62.8-)
disorders of iris and ciliary body in diseases classified elsewhere (H22)
glomerular disorders in diseases classified elsewhere (N08)
EXCLUDES 2 ▶chronic gout (M1A.-)◀
DEF: Purine and pyrimidine metabolic disorders; manifested by hyperuricemia and recurrent acute inflammatory arthritis; monosodium urate or monohydrate crystals may be deposited in and around the joints, leading to joint destruction and severe crippling.

√5ᵗʰ **M10.0** Idiopathic gout

Gouty bursitis
Primary gout

M10.00 Idiopathic gout, unspecified site ▽

√6ᵗʰ **M10.01** Idiopathic gout, shoulder

M10.011 Idiopathic gout, right shoulder

M10.012 Idiopathic gout, left shoulder

M10.019 Idiopathic gout, unspecified shoulder ▽

√6ᵗʰ **M10.02** Idiopathic gout, elbow

M10.021 Idiopathic gout, right elbow

M10.022 Idiopathic gout, left elbow

M10.029 Idiopathic gout, unspecified elbow ▽

√6ᵗʰ **M10.03** Idiopathic gout, wrist

M10.031 Idiopathic gout, right wrist

M10.032 Idiopathic gout, left wrist

M10.039 Idiopathic gout, unspecified wrist ▽

√6ᵗʰ **M10.04** Idiopathic gout, hand

M10.041 Idiopathic gout, right hand

M10.042 Idiopathic gout, left hand

M10.049 Idiopathic gout, unspecified hand ▽

√6ᵗʰ **M10.05** Idiopathic gout, hip

M10.051 Idiopathic gout, right hip

M10.052 Idiopathic gout, left hip

M10.059 Idiopathic gout, unspecified hip ▽

√6ᵗʰ **M10.06** Idiopathic gout, knee

M10.061 Idiopathic gout, right knee

M10.062 Idiopathic gout, left knee

M10.069 Idiopathic gout, unspecified knee ▽

√6ᵗʰ **M10.07** Idiopathic gout, ankle and foot

M10.071 Idiopathic gout, right ankle and foot

M10.072 Idiopathic gout, left ankle and foot

M10.079 Idiopathic gout, unspecified ankle and foot ▽

M10.08 Idiopathic gout, vertebrae

M10.09 Idiopathic gout, multiple sites

√5ᵗʰ **M10.1** Lead-induced gout

Code first toxic effects of lead and its compounds (T56.0-)

M10.10 Lead-induced gout, unspecified site ▽

√6ᵗʰ **M10.11** Lead-induced gout, shoulder

M10.111 Lead-induced gout, right shoulder

M10.112 Lead-induced gout, left shoulder

M10.119 Lead-induced gout, unspecified shoulder ▽

√6ᵗʰ **M10.12** Lead-induced gout, elbow

M10.121 Lead-induced gout, right elbow

M10.122 Lead-induced gout, left elbow

M10.129 Lead-induced gout, unspecified elbow ▽

√6ᵗʰ **M10.13** Lead-induced gout, wrist

M10.131 Lead-induced gout, right wrist

M10.132 Lead-induced gout, left wrist

M10.139 Lead-induced gout, unspecified wrist ▽

√6ᵗʰ **M10.14** Lead-induced gout, hand

M10.141 Lead-induced gout, right hand

M10.142 Lead-induced gout, left hand

M10.149 Lead-induced gout, unspecified hand ▽

√6ᵗʰ **M10.15** Lead-induced gout, hip

M10.151 Lead-induced gout, right hip

M10.152 Lead-induced gout, left hip

M10.159 Lead-induced gout, unspecified hip ▽

√6ᵗʰ **M10.16** Lead-induced gout, knee

M10.161 Lead-induced gout, right knee

M10.162 Lead-induced gout, left knee

M10.169 Lead-induced gout, unspecified knee ▽

√6ᵗʰ **M10.17** Lead-induced gout, ankle and foot

M10.171 Lead-induced gout, right ankle and foot

M10.172 Lead-induced gout, left ankle and foot

M10.179 Lead-induced gout, unspecified ankle and foot ▽

M10.18 Lead-induced gout, vertebrae

M10.19 Lead-induced gout, multiple sites

EXCLUDES 1 Not coded here   **EXCLUDES 2** Not included here   N Newborn Age : 0   P Pediatric Age : 0-17   M Maternity Age : 12-55   A Adult Age : 15-124

714
ICD-10-CM 2017

✓5ᵗʰ **M10.2** Drug-induced **gout**

Use additional code for adverse effect, if applicable, to identify drug (T36-T50 with fifth or sixth character 5)

M10.20 Drug-induced gout, unspecified site ▽

✓6ᵗʰ **M10.21** Drug-induced gout, shoulder
- **M10.211** Drug-induced gout, right shoulder
- **M10.212** Drug-induced gout, left shoulder
- **M10.219** Drug-induced gout, unspecified shoulder ▽

✓6ᵗʰ **M10.22** Drug-induced gout, elbow
- **M10.221** Drug-induced gout, right elbow
- **M10.222** Drug-induced gout, left elbow
- **M10.229** Drug-induced gout, unspecified elbow ▽

✓6ᵗʰ **M10.23** Drug-induced gout, wrist
- **M10.231** Drug-induced gout, right wrist
- **M10.232** Drug-induced gout, left wrist
- **M10.239** Drug-induced gout, unspecified wrist ▽

✓6ᵗʰ **M10.24** Drug-induced gout, hand
- **M10.241** Drug-induced gout, right hand
- **M10.242** Drug-induced gout, left hand
- **M10.249** Drug-induced gout, unspecified hand ▽

✓6ᵗʰ **M10.25** Drug-induced gout, hip
- **M10.251** Drug-induced gout, right hip
- **M10.252** Drug-induced gout, left hip
- **M10.259** Drug-induced gout, unspecified hip ▽

✓6ᵗʰ **M10.26** Drug-induced gout, knee
- **M10.261** Drug-induced gout, right knee
- **M10.262** Drug-induced gout, left knee
- **M10.269** Drug-induced gout, unspecified knee ▽

✓6ᵗʰ **M10.27** Drug-induced gout, ankle and foot
- **M10.271** Drug-induced gout, right ankle and foot
- **M10.272** Drug-induced gout, left ankle and foot
- **M10.279** Drug-induced gout, unspecified ankle and foot ▽

M10.28 Drug-induced gout, vertebrae

M10.29 Drug-induced gout, multiple sites

✓5ᵗʰ **M10.3** Gout due to renal impairment

Code first associated renal disease

M10.30 Gout due to renal impairment, unspecified site ▽

✓6ᵗʰ **M10.31** Gout due to renal impairment, shoulder
- **M10.311** Gout due to renal impairment, right shoulder
- **M10.312** Gout due to renal impairment, left shoulder
- **M10.319** Gout due to renal impairment, unspecified shoulder ▽

✓6ᵗʰ **M10.32** Gout due to renal impairment, elbow
- **M10.321** Gout due to renal impairment, right elbow
- **M10.322** Gout due to renal impairment, left elbow
- **M10.329** Gout due to renal impairment, unspecified elbow ▽

✓6ᵗʰ **M10.33** Gout due to renal impairment, wrist
- **M10.331** Gout due to renal impairment, right wrist
- **M10.332** Gout due to renal impairment, left wrist
- **M10.339** Gout due to renal impairment, unspecified wrist ▽

✓6ᵗʰ **M10.34** Gout due to renal impairment, hand
- **M10.341** Gout due to renal impairment, right hand
- **M10.342** Gout due to renal impairment, left hand
- **M10.349** Gout due to renal impairment, unspecified hand ▽

✓6ᵗʰ **M10.35** Gout due to renal impairment, hip
- **M10.351** Gout due to renal impairment, right hip
- **M10.352** Gout due to renal impairment, left hip
- **M10.359** Gout due to renal impairment, unspecified hip ▽

✓6ᵗʰ **M10.36** Gout due to renal impairment, knee
- **M10.361** Gout due to renal impairment, right knee
- **M10.362** Gout due to renal impairment, left knee

M10.369 Gout due to renal impairment, unspecified knee ▽

✓6ᵗʰ **M10.37** Gout due to renal impairment, ankle and foot
- **M10.371** Gout due to renal impairment, right ankle and foot
- **M10.372** Gout due to renal impairment, left ankle and foot
- **M10.379** Gout due to renal impairment, unspecified ankle and foot ▽

M10.38 Gout due to renal impairment, vertebrae

M10.39 Gout due to renal impairment, multiple sites

✓5ᵗʰ **M10.4** Other secondary gout

Code first associated condition

M10.40 Other secondary gout, unspecified site ▽

✓6ᵗʰ **M10.41** Other secondary gout, shoulder
- **M10.411** Other secondary gout, right shoulder
- **M10.412** Other secondary gout, left shoulder
- **M10.419** Other secondary gout, unspecified shoulder ▽

✓6ᵗʰ **M10.42** Other secondary gout, elbow
- **M10.421** Other secondary gout, right elbow
- **M10.422** Other secondary gout, left elbow
- **M10.429** Other secondary gout, unspecified elbow ▽

✓6ᵗʰ **M10.43** Other secondary gout, wrist
- **M10.431** Other secondary gout, right wrist
- **M10.432** Other secondary gout, left wrist
- **M10.439** Other secondary gout, unspecified wrist ▽

✓6ᵗʰ **M10.44** Other secondary gout, hand
- **M10.441** Other secondary gout, right hand
- **M10.442** Other secondary gout, left hand
- **M10.449** Other secondary gout, unspecified hand ▽

✓6ᵗʰ **M10.45** Other secondary gout, hip
- **M10.451** Other secondary gout, right hip
- **M10.452** Other secondary gout, left hip
- **M10.459** Other secondary gout, unspecified hip ▽

✓6ᵗʰ **M10.46** Other secondary gout, knee
- **M10.461** Other secondary gout, right knee
- **M10.462** Other secondary gout, left knee
- **M10.469** Other secondary gout, unspecified knee ▽

✓6ᵗʰ **M10.47** Other secondary gout, ankle and foot
- **M10.471** Other secondary gout, right ankle and foot
- **M10.472** Other secondary gout, left ankle and foot
- **M10.479** Other secondary gout, unspecified ankle and foot ▽

M10.48 Other secondary gout, vertebrae

M10.49 Other secondary gout, multiple sites

M10.9 Gout, unspecified ▽

Gout NOS

✓4ᵗʰ **M11** Other crystal arthropathies

✓5ᵗʰ **M11.0** Hydroxyapatite deposition disease

M11.00 Hydroxyapatite deposition disease, unspecified site ▽

✓6ᵗʰ **M11.01** Hydroxyapatite deposition disease, shoulder
- **M11.011** Hydroxyapatite deposition disease, right shoulder
- **M11.012** Hydroxyapatite deposition disease, left shoulder
- **M11.019** Hydroxyapatite deposition disease, unspecified shoulder ▽

✓6ᵗʰ **M11.02** Hydroxyapatite deposition disease, elbow
- **M11.021** Hydroxyapatite deposition disease, right elbow
- **M11.022** Hydroxyapatite deposition disease, left elbow
- **M11.029** Hydroxyapatite deposition disease, unspecified elbow ▽

✓6ᵗʰ **M11.03** Hydroxyapatite deposition disease, wrist
- **M11.031** Hydroxyapatite deposition disease, right wrist
- **M11.032** Hydroxyapatite deposition disease, left wrist

☑ Additional Character Required   ✓x7ᵗʰ Placeholder Alert   Manifestation Dx   ▽ Unspecified Dx   ►◄ Revised Text   ● New Code   ▲ Revised Code Title

ICD-10-CM 2017   715

M11.039 Hydroxyapatite deposition disease, unspecified wrist ▽

✓6ᵗʰ M11.04 Hydroxyapatite deposition disease, hand

M11.041 Hydroxyapatite deposition disease, right hand

M11.042 Hydroxyapatite deposition disease, left hand

M11.049 Hydroxyapatite deposition disease, unspecified hand ▽

✓6ᵗʰ M11.05 Hydroxyapatite deposition disease, hip

M11.051 Hydroxyapatite deposition disease, right hip

M11.052 Hydroxyapatite deposition disease, left hip

M11.059 Hydroxyapatite deposition disease, unspecified hip ▽

✓6ᵗʰ M11.06 Hydroxyapatite deposition disease, knee

M11.061 Hydroxyapatite deposition disease, right knee

M11.062 Hydroxyapatite deposition disease, left knee

M11.069 Hydroxyapatite deposition disease, unspecified knee ▽

✓6ᵗʰ M11.07 Hydroxyapatite deposition disease, ankle and foot

M11.071 Hydroxyapatite deposition disease, right ankle and foot

M11.072 Hydroxyapatite deposition disease, left ankle and foot

M11.079 Hydroxyapatite deposition disease, unspecified ankle and foot ▽

M11.08 Hydroxyapatite deposition disease, vertebrae

M11.09 Hydroxyapatite deposition disease, multiple sites

✓5ᵗʰ M11.1 Familial chondrocalcinosis

M11.10 Familial chondrocalcinosis, unspecified site ▽

✓6ᵗʰ M11.11 Familial chondrocalcinosis, shoulder

M11.111 Familial chondrocalcinosis, right shoulder

M11.112 Familial chondrocalcinosis, left shoulder

M11.119 Familial chondrocalcinosis, unspecified shoulder ▽

✓6ᵗʰ M11.12 Familial chondrocalcinosis, elbow

M11.121 Familial chondrocalcinosis, right elbow

M11.122 Familial chondrocalcinosis, left elbow

M11.129 Familial chondrocalcinosis, unspecified elbow ▽

✓6ᵗʰ M11.13 Familial chondrocalcinosis, wrist

M11.131 Familial chondrocalcinosis, right wrist

M11.132 Familial chondrocalcinosis, left wrist

M11.139 Familial chondrocalcinosis, unspecified wrist ▽

✓6ᵗʰ M11.14 Familial chondrocalcinosis, hand

M11.141 Familial chondrocalcinosis, right hand

M11.142 Familial chondrocalcinosis, left hand

M11.149 Familial chondrocalcinosis, unspecified hand ▽

✓6ᵗʰ M11.15 Familial chondrocalcinosis, hip

M11.151 Familial chondrocalcinosis, right hip

M11.152 Familial chondrocalcinosis, left hip

M11.159 Familial chondrocalcinosis, unspecified hip ▽

✓6ᵗʰ M11.16 Familial chondrocalcinosis, knee

M11.161 Familial chondrocalcinosis, right knee

M11.162 Familial chondrocalcinosis, left knee

M11.169 Familial chondrocalcinosis, unspecified knee ▽

✓6ᵗʰ M11.17 Familial chondrocalcinosis, ankle and foot

M11.171 Familial chondrocalcinosis, right ankle and foot

M11.172 Familial chondrocalcinosis, left ankle and foot

M11.179 Familial chondrocalcinosis, unspecified ankle and foot ▽

M11.18 Familial chondrocalcinosis, vertebrae

M11.19 Familial chondrocalcinosis, multiple sites

✓5ᵗʰ M11.2 Other chondrocalcinosis

Chondrocalcinosis NOS

M11.20 Other chondrocalcinosis, unspecified site ▽

✓6ᵗʰ M11.21 Other chondrocalcinosis, shoulder

M11.211 Other chondrocalcinosis, right shoulder

M11.212 Other chondrocalcinosis, left shoulder

M11.219 Other chondrocalcinosis, unspecified shoulder ▽

✓6ᵗʰ M11.22 Other chondrocalcinosis, elbow

M11.221 Other chondrocalcinosis, right elbow

M11.222 Other chondrocalcinosis, left elbow

M11.229 Other chondrocalcinosis, unspecified elbow ▽

✓6ᵗʰ M11.23 Other chondrocalcinosis, wrist

M11.231 Other chondrocalcinosis, right wrist

M11.232 Other chondrocalcinosis, left wrist

M11.239 Other chondrocalcinosis, unspecified wrist ▽

✓6ᵗʰ M11.24 Other chondrocalcinosis, hand

M11.241 Other chondrocalcinosis, right hand

M11.242 Other chondrocalcinosis, left hand

M11.249 Other chondrocalcinosis, unspecified hand ▽

✓6ᵗʰ M11.25 Other chondrocalcinosis, hip

M11.251 Other chondrocalcinosis, right hip

M11.252 Other chondrocalcinosis, left hip

M11.259 Other chondrocalcinosis, unspecified hip ▽

✓6ᵗʰ M11.26 Other chondrocalcinosis, knee

M11.261 Other chondrocalcinosis, right knee

M11.262 Other chondrocalcinosis, left knee

M11.269 Other chondrocalcinosis, unspecified knee ▽

✓6ᵗʰ M11.27 Other chondrocalcinosis, ankle and foot

M11.271 Other chondrocalcinosis, right ankle and foot

M11.272 Other chondrocalcinosis, left ankle and foot

M11.279 Other chondrocalcinosis, unspecified ankle and foot ▽

M11.28 Other chondrocalcinosis, vertebrae

M11.29 Other chondrocalcinosis, multiple sites

✓5ᵗʰ M11.8 Other specified crystal arthropathies

M11.80 Other specified crystal arthropathies, unspecified site ▽

✓6ᵗʰ M11.81 Other specified crystal arthropathies, shoulder

M11.811 Other specified crystal arthropathies, right shoulder

M11.812 Other specified crystal arthropathies, left shoulder

M11.819 Other specified crystal arthropathies, unspecified shoulder ▽

✓6ᵗʰ M11.82 Other specified crystal arthropathies, elbow

M11.821 Other specified crystal arthropathies, right elbow

M11.822 Other specified crystal arthropathies, left elbow

M11.829 Other specified crystal arthropathies, unspecified elbow ▽

✓6ᵗʰ M11.83 Other specified crystal arthropathies, wrist

M11.831 Other specified crystal arthropathies, right wrist

M11.832 Other specified crystal arthropathies, left wrist

M11.839 Other specified crystal arthropathies, unspecified wrist ▽

✓6ᵗʰ M11.84 Other specified crystal arthropathies, hand

M11.841 Other specified crystal arthropathies, right hand

M11.842 Other specified crystal arthropathies, left hand

M11.849 Other specified crystal arthropathies, unspecified hand ▽

✓6ᵗʰ M11.85 Other specified crystal arthropathies, hip

M11.851 Other specified crystal arthropathies, right hip

M11.852 Other specified crystal arthropathies, left hip

M11.859 Other specified crystal arthropathies, unspecified hip ▽

EXCLUDES 1   Not coded here   EXCLUDES 2   Not included here   N Newborn Age : 0   P Pediatric Age : 0-17   M Maternity Age : 12-55   A Adult Age : 15-124

716   ICD-10-CM 2017

✓6ᵗʰ **M11.86 Other specified crystal arthropathies,** knee

     M11.861 Other specified crystal arthropathies, right knee

     M11.862 Other specified crystal arthropathies, left knee

     M11.869 Other specified crystal arthropathies, unspecified knee ▽

✓6ᵗʰ **M11.87 Other specified crystal arthropathies,** ankle and foot

     M11.871 Other specified crystal arthropathies, right ankle and foot

     M11.872 Other specified crystal arthropathies, left ankle and foot

     M11.879 Other specified crystal arthropathies, unspecified ankle and foot ▽

M11.88 Other specified crystal arthropathies, vertebrae

M11.89 Other specified crystal arthropathies, multiple sites

M11.9 Crystal arthropathy, unspecified ▽

✓4ᵗʰ **M12 Other and unspecified arthropathy**

     EXCLUDES 1   *arthrosis (M15-M19)*

                cricoarytenoid arthropathy (J38.7)

✓5ᵗʰ **M12.0 Chronic postrheumatic arthropathy [Jaccoud]**

     M12.00 Chronic postrheumatic arthropathy [Jaccoud], unspecified site ▽

     ✓6ᵗʰ **M12.01 Chronic postrheumatic arthropathy [Jaccoud],** shoulder

         M12.011 Chronic postrheumatic arthropathy [Jaccoud], right shoulder

         M12.012 Chronic postrheumatic arthropathy [Jaccoud], left shoulder

         M12.019 Chronic postrheumatic arthropathy [Jaccoud], unspecified shoulder ▽

     ✓6ᵗʰ **M12.02 Chronic postrheumatic arthropathy [Jaccoud],** elbow

         M12.021 Chronic postrheumatic arthropathy [Jaccoud], right elbow

         M12.022 Chronic postrheumatic arthropathy [Jaccoud], left elbow

         M12.029 Chronic postrheumatic arthropathy [Jaccoud], unspecified elbow ▽

     ✓6ᵗʰ **M12.03 Chronic postrheumatic arthropathy [Jaccoud],** wrist

         M12.031 Chronic postrheumatic arthropathy [Jaccoud], right wrist

         M12.032 Chronic postrheumatic arthropathy [Jaccoud], left wrist

         M12.039 Chronic postrheumatic arthropathy [Jaccoud], unspecified wrist ▽

     ✓6ᵗʰ **M12.04 Chronic postrheumatic arthropathy [Jaccoud],** hand

         M12.041 Chronic postrheumatic arthropathy [Jaccoud], right hand

         M12.042 Chronic postrheumatic arthropathy [Jaccoud], left hand

         M12.049 Chronic postrheumatic arthropathy [Jaccoud], unspecified hand ▽

     ✓6ᵗʰ **M12.05 Chronic postrheumatic arthropathy [Jaccoud],** hip

         M12.051 Chronic postrheumatic arthropathy [Jaccoud], right hip

         M12.052 Chronic postrheumatic arthropathy [Jaccoud], left hip

         M12.059 Chronic postrheumatic arthropathy [Jaccoud], unspecified hip ▽

     ✓6ᵗʰ **M12.06 Chronic postrheumatic arthropathy [Jaccoud],** knee

         M12.061 Chronic postrheumatic arthropathy [Jaccoud], right knee

         M12.062 Chronic postrheumatic arthropathy [Jaccoud], left knee

         M12.069 Chronic postrheumatic arthropathy [Jaccoud], unspecified knee ▽

     ✓6ᵗʰ **M12.07 Chronic postrheumatic arthropathy [Jaccoud],** ankle and foot

         M12.071 Chronic postrheumatic arthropathy [Jaccoud], right ankle and foot

         M12.072 Chronic postrheumatic arthropathy [Jaccoud], left ankle and foot

         M12.079 Chronic postrheumatic arthropathy [Jaccoud], unspecified ankle and foot ▽

     M12.08 Chronic postrheumatic arthropathy [Jaccoud], other specified site

         Chronic postrheumatic arthropathy [Jaccoud], vertebrae

     M12.09 Chronic postrheumatic arthropathy [Jaccoud], multiple sites

✓5ᵗʰ **M12.1 Kaschin-Beck disease**

     Osteochondroarthrosis deformans endemica

     M12.10 Kaschin-Beck disease, unspecified site ▽

     ✓6ᵗʰ **M12.11 Kaschin-Beck disease,** shoulder

         M12.111 Kaschin-Beck disease, right shoulder

         M12.112 Kaschin-Beck disease, left shoulder

         M12.119 Kaschin-Beck disease, unspecified shoulder ▽

     ✓6ᵗʰ **M12.12 Kaschin-Beck disease,** elbow

         M12.121 Kaschin-Beck disease, right elbow

         M12.122 Kaschin-Beck disease, left elbow

         M12.129 Kaschin-Beck disease, unspecified elbow ▽

     ✓6ᵗʰ **M12.13 Kaschin-Beck disease,** wrist

         M12.131 Kaschin-Beck disease, right wrist

         M12.132 Kaschin-Beck disease, left wrist

         M12.139 Kaschin-Beck disease, unspecified wrist ▽

     ✓6ᵗʰ **M12.14 Kaschin-Beck disease,** hand

         M12.141 Kaschin-Beck disease, right hand

         M12.142 Kaschin-Beck disease, left hand

         M12.149 Kaschin-Beck disease, unspecified hand ▽

     ✓6ᵗʰ **M12.15 Kaschin-Beck disease,** hip

         M12.151 Kaschin-Beck disease, right hip

         M12.152 Kaschin-Beck disease, left hip

         M12.159 Kaschin-Beck disease, unspecified hip ▽

     ✓6ᵗʰ **M12.16 Kaschin-Beck disease,** knee

         M12.161 Kaschin-Beck disease, right knee

         M12.162 Kaschin-Beck disease, left knee

         M12.169 Kaschin-Beck disease, unspecified knee ▽

     ✓6ᵗʰ **M12.17 Kaschin-Beck disease,** ankle and foot

         M12.171 Kaschin-Beck disease, right ankle and foot

         M12.172 Kaschin-Beck disease, left ankle and foot

         M12.179 Kaschin-Beck disease, unspecified ankle and foot ▽

     M12.18 Kaschin-Beck disease, vertebrae

     M12.19 Kaschin-Beck disease, multiple sites

✓5ᵗʰ **M12.2 Villonodular synovitis (pigmented)**

     M12.20 Villonodular synovitis (pigmented), unspecified site ▽

     ✓6ᵗʰ **M12.21 Villonodular synovitis (pigmented),** shoulder

         M12.211 Villonodular synovitis (pigmented), right shoulder

         M12.212 Villonodular synovitis (pigmented), left shoulder

         M12.219 Villonodular synovitis (pigmented), unspecified shoulder ▽

     ✓6ᵗʰ **M12.22 Villonodular synovitis (pigmented),** elbow

         M12.221 Villonodular synovitis (pigmented), right elbow

         M12.222 Villonodular synovitis (pigmented), left elbow

         M12.229 Villonodular synovitis (pigmented), unspecified elbow ▽

     ✓6ᵗʰ **M12.23 Villonodular synovitis (pigmented),** wrist

         M12.231 Villonodular synovitis (pigmented), right wrist

         M12.232 Villonodular synovitis (pigmented), left wrist

         M12.239 Villonodular synovitis (pigmented), unspecified wrist ▽

     ✓6ᵗʰ **M12.24 Villonodular synovitis (pigmented),** hand

         M12.241 Villonodular synovitis (pigmented), right hand

---

☑ Additional Character Required   ✓7ᵗʰ Placeholder Alert   Manifestation Dx   ▽ Unspecified Dx   ▶◄ Revised Text   ● New Code   ▲ Revised Code Title

ICD-10-CM 2017   717

Chapter 13. Diseases of the Musculoskeletal System and Connective Tissue

M12.242–M12.569

           M12.242 Villonodular synovitis (pigmented), left hand
           M12.249 Villonodular synovitis (pigmented), unspecified hand ▽
- ✓6ᵗʰ M12.25 Villonodular synovitis (pigmented), hip
           M12.251 Villonodular synovitis (pigmented), right hip
           M12.252 Villonodular synovitis (pigmented), left hip
           M12.259 Villonodular synovitis (pigmented), unspecified hip ▽
- ✓6ᵗʰ M12.26 Villonodular synovitis (pigmented), knee
           M12.261 Villonodular synovitis (pigmented), right knee
           M12.262 Villonodular synovitis (pigmented), left knee
           M12.269 Villonodular synovitis (pigmented), unspecified knee ▽
- ✓6ᵗʰ M12.27 Villonodular synovitis (pigmented), ankle and foot
           M12.271 Villonodular synovitis (pigmented), right ankle and foot
           M12.272 Villonodular synovitis (pigmented), left ankle and foot
           M12.279 Villonodular synovitis (pigmented), unspecified ankle and foot ▽
     M12.28 Villonodular synovitis (pigmented), other specified site
         Villonodular synovitis (pigmented), vertebrae
     M12.29 Villonodular synovitis (pigmented), multiple sites
- ✓5ᵗʰ **M12.3 Palindromic rheumatism**
     M12.30 Palindromic rheumatism, unspecified site ▽
- ✓6ᵗʰ M12.31 Palindromic rheumatism, shoulder
           M12.311 Palindromic rheumatism, right shoulder
           M12.312 Palindromic rheumatism, left shoulder
           M12.319 Palindromic rheumatism, unspecified shoulder ▽
- ✓6ᵗʰ M12.32 Palindromic rheumatism, elbow
           M12.321 Palindromic rheumatism, right elbow
           M12.322 Palindromic rheumatism, left elbow
           M12.329 Palindromic rheumatism, unspecified elbow ▽
- ✓6ᵗʰ M12.33 Palindromic rheumatism, wrist
           M12.331 Palindromic rheumatism, right wrist
           M12.332 Palindromic rheumatism, left wrist
           M12.339 Palindromic rheumatism, unspecified wrist ▽
- ✓6ᵗʰ M12.34 Palindromic rheumatism, hand
           M12.341 Palindromic rheumatism, right hand
           M12.342 Palindromic rheumatism, left hand
           M12.349 Palindromic rheumatism, unspecified hand ▽
- ✓6ᵗʰ M12.35 Palindromic rheumatism, hip
           M12.351 Palindromic rheumatism, right hip
           M12.352 Palindromic rheumatism, left hip
           M12.359 Palindromic rheumatism, unspecified hip ▽
- ✓6ᵗʰ M12.36 Palindromic rheumatism, knee
           M12.361 Palindromic rheumatism, right knee
           M12.362 Palindromic rheumatism, left knee
           M12.369 Palindromic rheumatism, unspecified knee ▽
- ✓6ᵗʰ M12.37 Palindromic rheumatism, ankle and foot
           M12.371 Palindromic rheumatism, right ankle and foot
           M12.372 Palindromic rheumatism, left ankle and foot
           M12.379 Palindromic rheumatism, unspecified ankle and foot ▽
     M12.38 Palindromic rheumatism, other specified site
         Palindromic rheumatism, vertebrae
     M12.39 Palindromic rheumatism, multiple sites
- ✓5ᵗʰ **M12.4 Intermittent hydrarthrosis**
     M12.40 Intermittent hydrarthrosis, unspecified site ▽
- ✓6ᵗʰ M12.41 Intermittent hydrarthrosis, shoulder
           M12.411 Intermittent hydrarthrosis, right shoulder
           M12.412 Intermittent hydrarthrosis, left shoulder

           M12.419 Intermittent hydrarthrosis, unspecified shoulder ▽
- ✓6ᵗʰ M12.42 Intermittent hydrarthrosis, elbow
           M12.421 Intermittent hydrarthrosis, right elbow
           M12.422 Intermittent hydrarthrosis, left elbow
           M12.429 Intermittent hydrarthrosis, unspecified elbow ▽
- ✓6ᵗʰ M12.43 Intermittent hydrarthrosis, wrist
           M12.431 Intermittent hydrarthrosis, right wrist
           M12.432 Intermittent hydrarthrosis, left wrist
           M12.439 Intermittent hydrarthrosis, unspecified wrist ▽
- ✓6ᵗʰ M12.44 Intermittent hydrarthrosis, hand
           M12.441 Intermittent hydrarthrosis, right hand
           M12.442 Intermittent hydrarthrosis, left hand
           M12.449 Intermittent hydrarthrosis, unspecified hand ▽
- ✓6ᵗʰ M12.45 Intermittent hydrarthrosis, hip
           M12.451 Intermittent hydrarthrosis, right hip
           M12.452 Intermittent hydrarthrosis, left hip
           M12.459 Intermittent hydrarthrosis, unspecified hip ▽
- ✓6ᵗʰ M12.46 Intermittent hydrarthrosis, knee
           M12.461 Intermittent hydrarthrosis, right knee
           M12.462 Intermittent hydrarthrosis, left knee
           M12.469 Intermittent hydrarthrosis, unspecified knee ▽
- ✓6ᵗʰ M12.47 Intermittent hydrarthrosis, ankle and foot
           M12.471 Intermittent hydrarthrosis, right ankle and foot
           M12.472 Intermittent hydrarthrosis, left ankle and foot
           M12.479 Intermittent hydrarthrosis, unspecified ankle and foot ▽
     M12.48 Intermittent hydrarthrosis, other site
     M12.49 Intermittent hydrarthrosis, multiple sites
- ✓5ᵗʰ **M12.5 Traumatic arthropathy**
        EXCLUDES 1   *current injury–see Alphabetic Index*
          post-traumatic osteoarthritis of first carpometacarpal joint (M18.2-M18.3)
          post-traumatic osteoarthritis of hip (M16.4-M16.5)
          post-traumatic osteoarthritis of knee (M17.2-M17.3)
          post-traumatic osteoarthritis NOS (M19.1-)
          post-traumatic osteoarthritis of other single joints (M19.1-)
        AHA: 2015,1Q,17
     M12.50 Traumatic arthropathy, unspecified site ▽
- ✓6ᵗʰ M12.51 Traumatic arthropathy, shoulder
           M12.511 Traumatic arthropathy, right shoulder
           M12.512 Traumatic arthropathy, left shoulder
           M12.519 Traumatic arthropathy, unspecified shoulder ▽
- ✓6ᵗʰ M12.52 Traumatic arthropathy, elbow
           M12.521 Traumatic arthropathy, right elbow
           M12.522 Traumatic arthropathy, left elbow
           M12.529 Traumatic arthropathy, unspecified elbow ▽
- ✓6ᵗʰ M12.53 Traumatic arthropathy, wrist
           M12.531 Traumatic arthropathy, right wrist
           M12.532 Traumatic arthropathy, left wrist
           M12.539 Traumatic arthropathy, unspecified wrist ▽
- ✓6ᵗʰ M12.54 Traumatic arthropathy, hand
           M12.541 Traumatic arthropathy, right hand
           M12.542 Traumatic arthropathy, left hand
           M12.549 Traumatic arthropathy, unspecified hand ▽
- ✓6ᵗʰ M12.55 Traumatic arthropathy, hip
           M12.551 Traumatic arthropathy, right hip
           M12.552 Traumatic arthropathy, left hip
           M12.559 Traumatic arthropathy, unspecified hip ▽
- ✓6ᵗʰ M12.56 Traumatic arthropathy, knee
           M12.561 Traumatic arthropathy, right knee
           M12.562 Traumatic arthropathy, left knee
           M12.569 Traumatic arthropathy, unspecified knee ▽

EXCLUDES 1 Not coded here   **EXCLUDES 2** Not included here   **N** Newborn Age : 0   **P** Pediatric Age : 0-17   **M** Maternity Age : 12-55   **A** Adult Age : 15-124

718   ICD-10-CM 2017

√6ᵗʰ **M12.57 Traumatic arthropathy, ankle and foot**

    M12.571 Traumatic arthropathy, right ankle and foot

    M12.572 Traumatic arthropathy, left ankle and foot

    M12.579 Traumatic arthropathy, unspecified ankle and foot ▽

M12.58 Traumatic arthropathy, other specified site

    Traumatic arthropathy, vertebrae

M12.59 Traumatic arthropathy, multiple sites

√5ᵗʰ **M12.8 Other specific arthropathies, not elsewhere classified**

    Transient arthropathy

M12.80 Other specific arthropathies, not elsewhere classified, unspecified site ▽

√6ᵗʰ **M12.81 Other specific arthropathies, not elsewhere classified, shoulder**

    M12.811 Other specific arthropathies, not elsewhere classified, right shoulder

    M12.812 Other specific arthropathies, not elsewhere classified, left shoulder

    M12.819 Other specific arthropathies, not elsewhere classified, unspecified shoulder ▽

√6ᵗʰ **M12.82 Other specific arthropathies, not elsewhere classified, elbow**

    M12.821 Other specific arthropathies, not elsewhere classified, right elbow

    M12.822 Other specific arthropathies, not elsewhere classified, left elbow

    M12.829 Other specific arthropathies, not elsewhere classified, unspecified elbow ▽

√6ᵗʰ **M12.83 Other specific arthropathies, not elsewhere classified, wrist**

    M12.831 Other specific arthropathies, not elsewhere classified, right wrist

    M12.832 Other specific arthropathies, not elsewhere classified, left wrist

    M12.839 Other specific arthropathies, not elsewhere classified, unspecified wrist ▽

√6ᵗʰ **M12.84 Other specific arthropathies, not elsewhere classified, hand**

    M12.841 Other specific arthropathies, not elsewhere classified, right hand

    M12.842 Other specific arthropathies, not elsewhere classified, left hand

    M12.849 Other specific arthropathies, not elsewhere classified, unspecified hand ▽

√6ᵗʰ **M12.85 Other specific arthropathies, not elsewhere classified, hip**

    M12.851 Other specific arthropathies, not elsewhere classified, right hip

    M12.852 Other specific arthropathies, not elsewhere classified, left hip

    M12.859 Other specific arthropathies, not elsewhere classified, unspecified hip ▽

√6ᵗʰ **M12.86 Other specific arthropathies, not elsewhere classified, knee**

    M12.861 Other specific arthropathies, not elsewhere classified, right knee

    M12.862 Other specific arthropathies, not elsewhere classified, left knee

    M12.869 Other specific arthropathies, not elsewhere classified, unspecified knee ▽

√6ᵗʰ **M12.87 Other specific arthropathies, not elsewhere classified, ankle and foot**

    M12.871 Other specific arthropathies, not elsewhere classified, right ankle and foot

    M12.872 Other specific arthropathies, not elsewhere classified, left ankle and foot

    M12.879 Other specific arthropathies, not elsewhere classified, unspecified ankle and foot ▽

M12.88 Other specific arthropathies, not elsewhere classified, other specified site

    Other specific arthropathies, not elsewhere classified, vertebrae

M12.89 Other specific arthropathies, not elsewhere classified, multiple sites

M12.9 Arthropathy, unspecified ▽

√4ᵗʰ **M13 Other arthritis**

    EXCLUDES 1 arthrosis (M15-M19)
              osteoarthritis (M15-M19)

M13.0 Polyarthritis, unspecified ▽

√5ᵗʰ **M13.1 Monoarthritis, not elsewhere classified**

M13.10 Monoarthritis, not elsewhere classified, unspecified site ▽

√6ᵗʰ **M13.11 Monoarthritis, not elsewhere classified, shoulder**

    M13.111 Monoarthritis, not elsewhere classified, right shoulder

    M13.112 Monoarthritis, not elsewhere classified, left shoulder

    M13.119 Monoarthritis, not elsewhere classified, unspecified shoulder ▽

√6ᵗʰ **M13.12 Monoarthritis, not elsewhere classified, elbow**

    M13.121 Monoarthritis, not elsewhere classified, right elbow

    M13.122 Monoarthritis, not elsewhere classified, left elbow

    M13.129 Monoarthritis, not elsewhere classified, unspecified elbow ▽

√6ᵗʰ **M13.13 Monoarthritis, not elsewhere classified, wrist**

    M13.131 Monoarthritis, not elsewhere classified, right wrist

    M13.132 Monoarthritis, not elsewhere classified, left wrist

    M13.139 Monoarthritis, not elsewhere classified, unspecified wrist ▽

√6ᵗʰ **M13.14 Monoarthritis, not elsewhere classified, hand**

    M13.141 Monoarthritis, not elsewhere classified, right hand

    M13.142 Monoarthritis, not elsewhere classified, left hand

    M13.149 Monoarthritis, not elsewhere classified, unspecified hand ▽

√6ᵗʰ **M13.15 Monoarthritis, not elsewhere classified, hip**

    M13.151 Monoarthritis, not elsewhere classified, right hip

    M13.152 Monoarthritis, not elsewhere classified, left hip

    M13.159 Monoarthritis, not elsewhere classified, unspecified hip ▽

√6ᵗʰ **M13.16 Monoarthritis, not elsewhere classified, knee**

    M13.161 Monoarthritis, not elsewhere classified, right knee

    M13.162 Monoarthritis, not elsewhere classified, left knee

    M13.169 Monoarthritis, not elsewhere classified, unspecified knee ▽

√6ᵗʰ **M13.17 Monoarthritis, not elsewhere classified, ankle and foot**

    M13.171 Monoarthritis, not elsewhere classified, right ankle and foot

    M13.172 Monoarthritis, not elsewhere classified, left ankle and foot

    M13.179 Monoarthritis, not elsewhere classified, unspecified ankle and foot ▽

√5ᵗʰ **M13.8 Other specified arthritis**

    Allergic arthritis

    EXCLUDES 1 osteoarthritis (M15-M19)

M13.80 Other specified arthritis, unspecified site ▽

√6ᵗʰ **M13.81 Other specified arthritis, shoulder**

    M13.811 Other specified arthritis, right shoulder
    M13.812 Other specified arthritis, left shoulder
    M13.819 Other specified arthritis, unspecified shoulder ▽

√6ᵗʰ **M13.82 Other specified arthritis, elbow**

    M13.821 Other specified arthritis, right elbow
    M13.822 Other specified arthritis, left elbow
    M13.829 Other specified arthritis, unspecified elbow ▽

√6ᵗʰ **M13.83 Other specified arthritis, wrist**

    M13.831 Other specified arthritis, right wrist
    M13.832 Other specified arthritis, left wrist
    M13.839 Other specified arthritis, unspecified wrist ▽

☑ Additional Character Required   √xᵀ Placeholder Alert   Manifestation Dx   ▽ Unspecified Dx   ▶◀ Revised Text   ● New Code   ▲ Revised Code Title

ICD-10-CM 2017   719

√6th **M13.84** **Other specified arthritis, hand**

M13.841 Other specified arthritis, right hand

M13.842 Other specified arthritis, left hand

M13.849 Other specified arthritis, unspecified hand ▽

√6th **M13.85** **Other specified arthritis, hip**

M13.851 Other specified arthritis, right hip

M13.852 Other specified arthritis, left hip

M13.859 Other specified arthritis, unspecified hip ▽

√6th **M13.86** **Other specified arthritis, knee**

M13.861 Other specified arthritis, right knee

M13.862 Other specified arthritis, left knee

M13.869 Other specified arthritis, unspecified knee ▽

√6th **M13.87** **Other specified arthritis, ankle and foot**

M13.871 Other specified arthritis, right ankle and foot

M13.872 Other specified arthritis, left ankle and foot

M13.879 Other specified arthritis, unspecified ankle and foot ▽

M13.88 Other specified arthritis, other site

M13.89 Other specified arthritis, multiple sites

√4th **M14** **Arthropathies in other diseases classified elsewhere**

EXCLUDES 1 arthropathy in:
diabetes mellitus (E08-E13 with .61-)
hematological disorders (M36.2-M36.3)
hypersensitivity reactions (M36.4)
neoplastic disease (M36.1)
neurosyphillis (A52.16)
sarcoidosis (D86.86)
enteropathic arthropathies (M07.-)
juvenile psoriatic arthropathy (L40.54)
lipoid dermatoarthritis (E78.81)

√5th **M14.6** **Charcôt's joint**

Neuropathic arthropathy

EXCLUDES 1 Charcôt's joint in diabetes mellitus (E08-E13 with .610)
Charcôt's joint in tabes dorsalis (A52.16)

M14.60 Charcôt's joint, unspecified site ▽

√6th **M14.61** **Charcôt's joint, shoulder**

M14.611 Charcôt's joint, right shoulder

M14.612 Charcôt's joint, left shoulder

M14.619 Charcôt's joint, unspecified shoulder ▽

√6th **M14.62** **Charcôt's joint, elbow**

M14.621 Charcôt's joint, right elbow

M14.622 Charcôt's joint, left elbow

M14.629 Charcôt's joint, unspecified elbow ▽

√6th **M14.63** **Charcôt's joint, wrist**

M14.631 Charcôt's joint, right wrist

M14.632 Charcôt's joint, left wrist

M14.639 Charcôt's joint, unspecified wrist ▽

√6th **M14.64** **Charcôt's joint, hand**

M14.641 Charcôt's joint, right hand

M14.642 Charcôt's joint, left hand

M14.649 Charcôt's joint, unspecified hand ▽

√6th **M14.65** **Charcôt's joint, hip**

M14.651 Charcôt's joint, right hip

M14.652 Charcôt's joint, left hip

M14.659 Charcôt's joint, unspecified hip ▽

√6th **M14.66** **Charcôt's joint, knee**

M14.661 Charcôt's joint, right knee

M14.662 Charcôt's joint, left knee

M14.669 Charcôt's joint, unspecified knee ▽

√6th **M14.67** **Charcôt's joint, ankle and foot**

M14.671 Charcôt's joint, right ankle and foot

M14.672 Charcôt's joint, left ankle and foot

M14.679 Charcôt's joint, unspecified ankle and foot ▽

M14.68 Charcôt's joint, vertebrae

M14.69 Charcôt's joint, multiple sites

√5th **M14.8** **Arthropathies in other specified diseases classified elsewhere**

Code first underlying disease, such as:
amyloidosis (E85.-)
erythema multiforme (L51.-)
erythema nodosum (L52)
hemochromatosis (E83.11-)
hyperparathyroidism (E21.-)
hypothyroidism (E00-E03)
sickle-cell disorders (D57.-)
thyrotoxicosis [hyperthyroidism] (E05.-)
Whipple's disease (K90.81)

M14.80 *Arthropathies in other specified diseases classified elsewhere, unspecified site* ▽

√6th **M14.81** **Arthropathies in other specified diseases classified elsewhere, shoulder**

M14.811 *Arthropathies in other specified diseases classified elsewhere, right shoulder*

M14.812 *Arthropathies in other specified diseases classified elsewhere, left shoulder*

M14.819 *Arthropathies in other specified diseases classified elsewhere, unspecified shoulder* ▽

√6th **M14.82** **Arthropathies in other specified diseases classified elsewhere, elbow**

M14.821 *Arthropathies in other specified diseases classified elsewhere, right elbow*

M14.822 *Arthropathies in other specified diseases classified elsewhere, left elbow*

M14.829 *Arthropathies in other specified diseases classified elsewhere, unspecified elbow* ▽

√6th **M14.83** **Arthropathies in other specified diseases classified elsewhere, wrist**

M14.831 *Arthropathies in other specified diseases classified elsewhere, right wrist*

M14.832 *Arthropathies in other specified diseases classified elsewhere, left wrist*

M14.839 *Arthropathies in other specified diseases classified elsewhere, unspecified wrist* ▽

√6th **M14.84** **Arthropathies in other specified diseases classified elsewhere, hand**

M14.841 *Arthropathies in other specified diseases classified elsewhere, right hand*

M14.842 *Arthropathies in other specified diseases classified elsewhere, left hand*

M14.849 *Arthropathies in other specified diseases classified elsewhere, unspecified hand* ▽

√6th **M14.85** **Arthropathies in other specified diseases classified elsewhere, hip**

M14.851 *Arthropathies in other specified diseases classified elsewhere, right hip*

M14.852 *Arthropathies in other specified diseases classified elsewhere, left hip*

M14.859 *Arthropathies in other specified diseases classified elsewhere, unspecified hip* ▽

√6th **M14.86** **Arthropathies in other specified diseases classified elsewhere, knee**

M14.861 *Arthropathies in other specified diseases classified elsewhere, right knee*

M14.862 *Arthropathies in other specified diseases classified elsewhere, left knee*

M14.869 *Arthropathies in other specified diseases classified elsewhere, unspecified knee* ▽

√6th **M14.87** **Arthropathies in other specified diseases classified elsewhere, ankle and foot**

M14.871 *Arthropathies in other specified diseases classified elsewhere, right ankle and foot*

M14.872 *Arthropathies in other specified diseases classified elsewhere, left ankle and foot*

M14.879 *Arthropathies in other specified diseases classified elsewhere, unspecified ankle and foot* ▽

M14.88 *Arthropathies in other specified diseases classified elsewhere, vertebrae*

M14.89 *Arthropathies in other specified diseases classified elsewhere, multiple sites*

EXCLUDES 1 Not coded here　　　EXCLUDES 2 Not included here　　　N Newborn Age : 0　　　P Pediatric Age : 0-17　　　M Maternity Age : 12-55　　　A Adult Age : 15-124

Osteoarthritis (M15-M19)

EXCLUDES 2 *osteoarthritis of spine (M47.-)*

☑4ᵗʰ M15 Polyosteoarthritis

INCLUDES arthritis of multiple sites
EXCLUDES 1 *bilateral involvement of single joint (M16-M19)*

M15.0 Primary generalized (osteo)arthritis

M15.1 Heberden's nodes (with arthropathy)
Interphalangeal distal osteoarthritis

M15.2 Bouchard's nodes (with arthropathy)
Juxtaphalangeal distal osteoarthritis

M15.3 Secondary multiple arthritis
Post-traumatic polyosteoarthritis

M15.4 Erosive (osteo)arthritis

M15.8 Other polyosteoarthritis

M15.9 Polyosteoarthritis, unspecified ▽
Generalized osteoarthritis NOS

☑4ᵗʰ M16 Osteoarthritis of hip

M16.0 Bilateral primary osteoarthritis of hip

☑5ᵗʰ **M16.1 Unilateral primary osteoarthritis of hip**
Primary osteoarthritis of hip NOS

    M16.10 Unilateral primary osteoarthritis, unspecified hip ▽

    M16.11 Unilateral primary osteoarthritis, right hip

    M16.12 Unilateral primary osteoarthritis, left hip

M16.2 Bilateral osteoarthritis resulting from hip dysplasia

☑5ᵗʰ **M16.3 Unilateral osteoarthritis resulting from hip dysplasia**
Dysplastic osteoarthritis of hip NOS

    M16.30 Unilateral osteoarthritis resulting from hip dysplasia, unspecified hip ▽

    M16.31 Unilateral osteoarthritis resulting from hip dysplasia, right hip

    M16.32 Unilateral osteoarthritis resulting from hip dysplasia, left hip

M16.4 Bilateral post-traumatic osteoarthritis of hip

☑5ᵗʰ **M16.5 Unilateral post-traumatic osteoarthritis of hip**
Post-traumatic osteoarthritis of hip NOS

    M16.50 Unilateral post-traumatic osteoarthritis, unspecified hip ▽

    M16.51 Unilateral post-traumatic osteoarthritis, right hip

    M16.52 Unilateral post-traumatic osteoarthritis, left hip

M16.6 Other bilateral secondary osteoarthritis of hip

M16.7 Other unilateral secondary osteoarthritis of hip
Secondary osteoarthritis of hip NOS

M16.9 Osteoarthritis of hip, unspecified ▽

☑4ᵗʰ M17 Osteoarthritis of knee

M17.0 Bilateral primary osteoarthritis of knee

☑5ᵗʰ **M17.1 Unilateral primary osteoarthritis of knee**
Primary osteoarthritis of knee NOS

    M17.10 Unilateral primary osteoarthritis, unspecified knee ▽

    M17.11 Unilateral primary osteoarthritis, right knee

    M17.12 Unilateral primary osteoarthritis, left knee

M17.2 Bilateral post-traumatic osteoarthritis of knee

☑5ᵗʰ **M17.3 Unilateral post-traumatic osteoarthritis of knee**
Post-traumatic osteoarthritis of knee NOS

    M17.30 Unilateral post-traumatic osteoarthritis, unspecified knee ▽

    M17.31 Unilateral post-traumatic osteoarthritis, right knee

    M17.32 Unilateral post-traumatic osteoarthritis, left knee

M17.4 Other bilateral secondary osteoarthritis of knee

M17.5 Other unilateral secondary osteoarthritis of knee
Secondary osteoarthritis of knee NOS

M17.9 Osteoarthritis of knee, unspecified ▽

☑4ᵗʰ M18 Osteoarthritis of first carpometacarpal joint

M18.0 Bilateral primary osteoarthritis of first carpometacarpal joints

☑5ᵗʰ **M18.1 Unilateral primary osteoarthritis of first carpometacarpal joint**
Primary osteoarthritis of first carpometacarpal joint NOS

    M18.10 Unilateral primary osteoarthritis of first carpometacarpal joint, unspecified hand ▽

    M18.11 Unilateral primary osteoarthritis of first carpometacarpal joint, right hand

    M18.12 Unilateral primary osteoarthritis of first carpometacarpal joint, left hand

M18.2 Bilateral post-traumatic osteoarthritis of first carpometacarpal joints

☑5ᵗʰ **M18.3 Unilateral post-traumatic osteoarthritis of first carpometacarpal joint**
Post-traumatic osteoarthritis of first carpometacarpal joint NOS

    M18.30 Unilateral post-traumatic osteoarthritis of first carpometacarpal joint, unspecified hand ▽

    M18.31 Unilateral post-traumatic osteoarthritis of first carpometacarpal joint, right hand

    M18.32 Unilateral post-traumatic osteoarthritis of first carpometacarpal joint, left hand

M18.4 Other bilateral secondary osteoarthritis of first carpometacarpal joints

☑5ᵗʰ **M18.5 Other unilateral secondary osteoarthritis of first carpometacarpal joint**
Secondary osteoarthritis of first carpometacarpal joint NOS

    M18.50 Other unilateral secondary osteoarthritis of first carpometacarpal joint, unspecified hand ▽

    M18.51 Other unilateral secondary osteoarthritis of first carpometacarpal joint, right hand

    M18.52 Other unilateral secondary osteoarthritis of first carpometacarpal joint, left hand

M18.9 Osteoarthritis of first carpometacarpal joint, unspecified ▽

☑4ᵗʰ M19 Other and unspecified osteoarthritis

EXCLUDES 1 *polyarthritis (M15.-)*
EXCLUDES 2 *arthrosis of spine (M47.-)*
hallux rigidus (M20.2)
osteoarthritis of spine (M47.-)

☑5ᵗʰ **M19.0 Primary osteoarthritis of other joints**

☑6ᵗʰ **M19.01 Primary osteoarthritis, shoulder**

    M19.011 Primary osteoarthritis, right shoulder

    M19.012 Primary osteoarthritis, left shoulder

    M19.019 Primary osteoarthritis, unspecified shoulder ▽

☑6ᵗʰ **M19.02 Primary osteoarthritis, elbow**

    M19.021 Primary osteoarthritis, right elbow

    M19.022 Primary osteoarthritis, left elbow

    M19.029 Primary osteoarthritis, unspecified elbow ▽

☑6ᵗʰ **M19.03 Primary osteoarthritis, wrist**

    M19.031 Primary osteoarthritis, right wrist

    M19.032 Primary osteoarthritis, left wrist

    M19.039 Primary osteoarthritis, unspecified wrist ▽

☑6ᵗʰ **M19.04 Primary osteoarthritis, hand**

    EXCLUDES 2 *primary osteoarthritis of first carpometacarpal joint (M18.0-, M18.1-)*

    M19.041 Primary osteoarthritis, right hand

    M19.042 Primary osteoarthritis, left hand

    M19.049 Primary osteoarthritis, unspecified hand ▽

☑6ᵗʰ **M19.07 Primary osteoarthritis ankle and foot**

    M19.071 Primary osteoarthritis, right ankle and foot

    M19.072 Primary osteoarthritis, left ankle and foot

    M19.079 Primary osteoarthritis, unspecified ankle and foot ▽

☑5ᵗʰ **M19.1 Post-traumatic osteoarthritis of other joints**

☑6ᵗʰ **M19.11 Post-traumatic osteoarthritis, shoulder**

    M19.111 Post-traumatic osteoarthritis, right shoulder

    M19.112 Post-traumatic osteoarthritis, left shoulder

    M19.119 Post-traumatic osteoarthritis, unspecified shoulder ▽

☑6ᵗʰ **M19.12 Post-traumatic osteoarthritis, elbow**

    M19.121 Post-traumatic osteoarthritis, right elbow

    M19.122 Post-traumatic osteoarthritis, left elbow

    M19.129 Post-traumatic osteoarthritis, unspecified elbow ▽

☑6ᵗʰ **M19.13 Post-traumatic osteoarthritis, wrist**

    M19.131 Post-traumatic osteoarthritis, right wrist

    M19.132 Post-traumatic osteoarthritis, left wrist

    M19.139 Post-traumatic osteoarthritis, unspecified wrist ▽

☑ Additional Character Required   ☑7ᵗʰ Placeholder Alert   Manifestation Dx   ▽ Unspecified Dx   ►◄ Revised Text   ● New Code   ▲ Revised Code Title

√6ᵗʰ M19.14 Post-traumatic osteoarthritis, hand

> EXCLUDES 2   *post-traumatic osteoarthritis of first carpometacarpal joint (M18.2-, M18.3-)*

     M19.141 Post-traumatic osteoarthritis, right hand
     M19.142 Post-traumatic osteoarthritis, left hand
     M19.149 Post-traumatic osteoarthritis, unspecified hand ▽

√6ᵗʰ M19.17 Post-traumatic osteoarthritis, ankle and foot

     M19.171 Post-traumatic osteoarthritis, right ankle and foot
     M19.172 Post-traumatic osteoarthritis, left ankle and foot
     M19.179 Post-traumatic osteoarthritis, unspecified ankle and foot ▽

√5ᵗʰ M19.2 Secondary osteoarthritis of other joints

√6ᵗʰ M19.21 Secondary osteoarthritis, shoulder

     M19.211 Secondary osteoarthritis, right shoulder
     M19.212 Secondary osteoarthritis, left shoulder
     M19.219 Secondary osteoarthritis, unspecified shoulder ▽

√6ᵗʰ M19.22 Secondary osteoarthritis, elbow

     M19.221 Secondary osteoarthritis, right elbow
     M19.222 Secondary osteoarthritis, left elbow
     M19.229 Secondary osteoarthritis, unspecified elbow ▽

√6ᵗʰ M19.23 Secondary osteoarthritis, wrist

     M19.231 Secondary osteoarthritis, right wrist
     M19.232 Secondary osteoarthritis, left wrist
     M19.239 Secondary osteoarthritis, unspecified wrist ▽

√6ᵗʰ M19.24 Secondary osteoarthritis, hand

     M19.241 Secondary osteoarthritis, right hand
     M19.242 Secondary osteoarthritis, left hand
     M19.249 Secondary osteoarthritis, unspecified hand ▽

√6ᵗʰ M19.27 Secondary osteoarthritis, ankle and foot

     M19.271 Secondary osteoarthritis, right ankle and foot
     M19.272 Secondary osteoarthritis, left ankle and foot
     M19.279 Secondary osteoarthritis, unspecified ankle and foot ▽

√5ᵗʰ M19.9 Osteoarthritis, unspecified site

     M19.90 Unspecified osteoarthritis, unspecified site ▽
         Arthrosis NOS
         Arthritis NOS
         Osteoarthritis NOS

     M19.91 Primary osteoarthritis, unspecified site ▽
         Primary osteoarthritis NOS

     M19.92 Post-traumatic osteoarthritis, unspecified site ▽
         Post-traumatic osteoarthritis NOS

     M19.93 Secondary osteoarthritis, unspecified site ▽
         Secondary osteoarthritis NOS

Other joint disorders (M20-M25)

> EXCLUDES 2   *joints of the spine (M40-M54)*

√4ᵗʰ M20 Acquired deformities of fingers and toes

> EXCLUDES 1   *acquired absence of fingers and toes (Z89.-)*
> *congenital absence of fingers and toes (Q71.3-, Q72.3-)*
> *congenital deformities and malformations of fingers and toes (Q66.-, Q68-Q70, Q74.-)*

√5ᵗʰ M20.0 Deformity of finger(s)

> EXCLUDES 1   *clubbing of fingers (R68.3)*
> *palmar fascial fibromatosis [Dupuytren] (M72.0)*
> *trigger finger (M65.3)*

√6ᵗʰ M20.00 Unspecified deformity of finger(s)

     M20.001 Unspecified deformity of right finger(s) ▽
     M20.002 Unspecified deformity of left finger(s) ▽
     M20.009 Unspecified deformity of unspecified finger(s) ▽

√6ᵗʰ M20.01 Mallet finger

     M20.011 Mallet finger of right finger(s)
     M20.012 Mallet finger of left finger(s)

     M20.019 Mallet finger of unspecified finger(s)

√6ᵗʰ M20.02 Boutonnière deformity

     M20.021 Boutonnière deformity of right finger(s)
     M20.022 Boutonnière deformity of left finger(s)
     M20.029 Boutonnière deformity of unspecified finger(s)

√6ᵗʰ M20.03 Swan-neck deformity

     M20.031 Swan-neck deformity of right finger(s)
     M20.032 Swan-neck deformity of left finger(s)
     M20.039 Swan-neck deformity of unspecified finger(s) ▽

√6ᵗʰ M20.09 Other deformity of finger(s)

     M20.091 Other deformity of right finger(s)
     M20.092 Other deformity of left finger(s)
     M20.099 Other deformity of finger(s), unspecified finger(s) ▽

√5ᵗʰ M20.1 Hallux valgus (acquired)

> EXCLUDES 2   ▶*bunion (M21.6-)*◀

Hallux Valgus (Bunion)

Hallux valgus bunion

Medial eminence of metatarsal bone

Right foot

     M20.10 Hallux valgus (acquired), unspecified foot ▽
     M20.11 Hallux valgus (acquired), right foot
     M20.12 Hallux valgus (acquired), left foot

√5ᵗʰ M20.2 Hallux rigidus

     M20.20 Hallux rigidus, unspecified foot ▽
     M20.21 Hallux rigidus, right foot
     M20.22 Hallux rigidus, left foot

√5ᵗʰ M20.3 Hallux varus (acquired)

     M20.30 Hallux varus (acquired), unspecified foot ▽
     M20.31 Hallux varus (acquired), right foot
     M20.32 Hallux varus (acquired), left foot

√5ᵗʰ M20.4 Other hammer toe(s) (acquired)

     M20.40 Other hammer toe(s) (acquired), unspecified foot ▽
     M20.41 Other hammer toe(s) (acquired), right foot
     M20.42 Other hammer toe(s) (acquired), left foot

√5ᵗʰ M20.5 Other deformities of toe(s) (acquired)

√6ᵗʰ M20.5X Other deformities of toe(s) (acquired)

     M20.5X1 Other deformities of toe(s) (acquired), right foot
     M20.5X2 Other deformities of toe(s) (acquired), left foot
     M20.5X9 Other deformities of toe(s) (acquired), unspecified foot ▽

√5ᵗʰ M20.6 Acquired deformities of toe(s), unspecified

     M20.60 Acquired deformities of toe(s), unspecified, unspecified foot ▽
     M20.61 Acquired deformities of toe(s), unspecified, right foot ▽
     M20.62 Acquired deformities of toe(s), unspecified, left foot ▽

EXCLUDES 1 Not coded here   EXCLUDES 2 Not included here   N Newborn Age : 0   P Pediatric Age : 0-17   M Maternity Age : 12-55   A Adult Age : 15-124

722   ICD-10-CM 2017

✓4ᵗʰ M21 Other acquired deformities of limbs

EXCLUDES 1   acquired absence of limb (Z89.-)
congenital absence of limbs (Q71-Q73)
congenital deformities and malformations of limbs (Q65-Q66, Q68-Q74)

EXCLUDES 2   acquired deformities of fingers or toes (M20.-)
coxa plana (M91.2)

✓5ᵗʰ M21.0 Valgus deformity, not elsewhere classified

EXCLUDES 1   metatarsus valgus (Q66.6)
talipes calcaneovalgus (Q66.4)

    M21.00 Valgus deformity, not elsewhere classified, unspecified site ▽

✓6ᵗʰ M21.02 Valgus deformity, not elsewhere classified, elbow
Cubitus valgus
    M21.021 Valgus deformity, not elsewhere classified, right elbow
    M21.022 Valgus deformity, not elsewhere classified, left elbow
    M21.029 Valgus deformity, not elsewhere classified, unspecified elbow ▽

✓6ᵗʰ M21.05 Valgus deformity, not elsewhere classified, hip
    M21.051 Valgus deformity, not elsewhere classified, right hip
    M21.052 Valgus deformity, not elsewhere classified, left hip
    M21.059 Valgus deformity, not elsewhere classified, unspecified hip ▽

✓6ᵗʰ M21.06 Valgus deformity, not elsewhere classified, knee
Genu valgum
Knock knee
    M21.061 Valgus deformity, not elsewhere classified, right knee
    M21.062 Valgus deformity, not elsewhere classified, left knee
    M21.069 Valgus deformity, not elsewhere classified, unspecified knee ▽

✓6ᵗʰ M21.07 Valgus deformity, not elsewhere classified, ankle
    M21.071 Valgus deformity, not elsewhere classified, right ankle
    M21.072 Valgus deformity, not elsewhere classified, left ankle
    M21.079 Valgus deformity, not elsewhere classified, unspecified ankle ▽

✓5ᵗʰ M21.1 Varus deformity, not elsewhere classified

EXCLUDES 1   metatarsus varus ►(Q66.22)◄
tibia vara (M92.5)

    M21.10 Varus deformity, not elsewhere classified, unspecified site ▽

✓6ᵗʰ M21.12 Varus deformity, not elsewhere classified, elbow
Cubitus varus, elbow
    M21.121 Varus deformity, not elsewhere classified, right elbow
    M21.122 Varus deformity, not elsewhere classified, left elbow
    M21.129 Varus deformity, not elsewhere classified, unspecified elbow ▽

✓6ᵗʰ M21.15 Varus deformity, not elsewhere classified, hip
    M21.151 Varus deformity, not elsewhere classified, right hip
    M21.152 Varus deformity, not elsewhere classified, left hip
    M21.159 Varus deformity, not elsewhere classified, unspecified ▽

✓6ᵗʰ M21.16 Varus deformity, not elsewhere classified, knee
Bow leg
Genu varum
    M21.161 Varus deformity, not elsewhere classified, right knee
    M21.162 Varus deformity, not elsewhere classified, left knee
    M21.169 Varus deformity, not elsewhere classified, unspecified knee ▽

✓6ᵗʰ M21.17 Varus deformity, not elsewhere classified, ankle
    M21.171 Varus deformity, not elsewhere classified, right ankle
    M21.172 Varus deformity, not elsewhere classified, left ankle
    M21.179 Varus deformity, not elsewhere classified, unspecified ankle ▽

✓5ᵗʰ M21.2 Flexion deformity

    M21.20 Flexion deformity, unspecified site

✓6ᵗʰ M21.21 Flexion deformity, shoulder
    M21.211 Flexion deformity, right shoulder
    M21.212 Flexion deformity, left shoulder
    M21.219 Flexion deformity, unspecified shoulder

✓6ᵗʰ M21.22 Flexion deformity, elbow
    M21.221 Flexion deformity, right elbow
    M21.222 Flexion deformity, left elbow
    M21.229 Flexion deformity, unspecified elbow ▽

✓6ᵗʰ M21.23 Flexion deformity, wrist
    M21.231 Flexion deformity, right wrist
    M21.232 Flexion deformity, left wrist
    M21.239 Flexion deformity, unspecified wrist ▽

✓6ᵗʰ M21.24 Flexion deformity, finger joints
    M21.241 Flexion deformity, right finger joints
    M21.242 Flexion deformity, left finger joints
    M21.249 Flexion deformity, unspecified finger joints ▽

✓6ᵗʰ M21.25 Flexion deformity, hip
    M21.251 Flexion deformity, right hip
    M21.252 Flexion deformity, left hip
    M21.259 Flexion deformity, unspecified hip ▽

✓6ᵗʰ M21.26 Flexion deformity, knee
    M21.261 Flexion deformity, right knee
    M21.262 Flexion deformity, left knee
    M21.269 Flexion deformity, unspecified knee ▽

✓6ᵗʰ M21.27 Flexion deformity, ankle and toes
    M21.271 Flexion deformity, right ankle and toes
    M21.272 Flexion deformity, left ankle and toes
    M21.279 Flexion deformity, unspecified ankle and toes ▽

✓5ᵗʰ M21.3 Wrist or foot drop (acquired)

✓6ᵗʰ M21.33 Wrist drop (acquired)
    M21.331 Wrist drop, right wrist
    M21.332 Wrist drop, left wrist
    M21.339 Wrist drop, unspecified wrist ▽

✓6ᵗʰ M21.37 Foot drop (acquired)
    M21.371 Foot drop, right foot
    M21.372 Foot drop, left foot
    M21.379 Foot drop, unspecified foot ▽

✓5ᵗʰ M21.4 Flat foot [pes planus] (acquired)

EXCLUDES 1   congenital pes planus (Q66.5-)

    M21.40 Flat foot [pes planus] (acquired), unspecified foot ▽
    M21.41 Flat foot [pes planus] (acquired), right foot
    M21.42 Flat foot [pes planus] (acquired), left foot

✓5ᵗʰ M21.5 Acquired clawhand, clubhand, clawfoot and clubfoot

EXCLUDES 1   clubfoot, not specified as acquired (Q66.89)

✓6ᵗʰ M21.51 Acquired clawhand
    M21.511 Acquired clawhand, right hand
    M21.512 Acquired clawhand, left hand
    M21.519 Acquired clawhand, unspecified hand ▽

✓6ᵗʰ M21.52 Acquired clubhand
    M21.521 Acquired clubhand, right hand
    M21.522 Acquired clubhand, left hand
    M21.529 Acquired clubhand, unspecified hand ▽

✓6ᵗʰ M21.53 Acquired clawfoot
DEF: High foot arch with hyperextended toes at metatarsophalangeal joint and flexed toes at distal joints.
    M21.531 Acquired clawfoot, right foot
    M21.532 Acquired clawfoot, left foot
    M21.539 Acquired clawfoot, unspecified foot ▽

✓6ᵗʰ M21.54 Acquired clubfoot
    M21.541 Acquired clubfoot, right foot
    M21.542 Acquired clubfoot, left foot

☑ Additional Character Required   ✓x7ᵗʰ Placeholder Alert   Manifestation Dx   ▽ Unspecified Dx   ►◄ Revised Text   ● New Code   ▲ Revised Code Title

ICD-10-CM 2017   723

M21.549   **Acquired clubfoot, unspecified foot** ▽

✓5ᵗʰ **M21.6   Other acquired deformities of foot**

> EXCLUDES 2   *deformities of toe (acquired) ▶(M20.1-M20.6-)◀*

● ✓6ᵗʰ **M21.61   Bunion**
●   M21.611   **Bunion of** right **foot**
●   M21.612   **Bunion of** left **foot**
●   M21.619   **Bunion of unspecified foot** ▽

● ✓6ᵗʰ **M21.62   Bunionette**
●   M21.621   **Bunionette of** right **foot**
●   M21.622   **Bunionette of** left **foot**
●   M21.629   **Bunionette of unspecified foot** ▽

✓6ᵗʰ **M21.6X   Other acquired deformities of foot**
    M21.6X1   **Other acquired deformities of** right **foot**
    M21.6X2   **Other acquired deformities of** left **foot**
    M21.6X9   **Other acquired deformities of unspecified foot** ▽

✓5ᵗʰ **M21.7   Unequal limb length (acquired)**

> **NOTE**   The site used should correspond to the shorter limb

    M21.70   **Unequal limb length (acquired), unspecified site** ▽

✓6ᵗʰ **M21.72   Unequal limb length (acquired),** humerus
    M21.721   **Unequal limb length (acquired),** right **humerus**
    M21.722   **Unequal limb length (acquired),** left **humerus**
    M21.729   **Unequal limb length (acquired), unspecified humerus** ▽

✓6ᵗʰ **M21.73   Unequal limb length (acquired),** ulna and radius
    M21.731   **Unequal limb length (acquired),** right **ulna**
    M21.732   **Unequal limb length (acquired),** left ulna
    M21.733   **Unequal limb length (acquired),** right **radius**
    M21.734   **Unequal limb length (acquired),** left **radius**
    M21.739   **Unequal limb length (acquired), unspecified ulna and radius** ▽

✓6ᵗʰ **M21.75   Unequal limb length (acquired),** femur
    M21.751   **Unequal limb length (acquired),** right **femur**
    M21.752   **Unequal limb length (acquired),** left **femur**
    M21.759   **Unequal limb length (acquired), unspecified femur** ▽

✓6ᵗʰ **M21.76   Unequal limb length (acquired),** tibia and fibula
    M21.761   **Unequal limb length (acquired),** right **tibia**
    M21.762   **Unequal limb length (acquired),** left tibia
    M21.763   **Unequal limb length (acquired),** right **fibula**
    M21.764   **Unequal limb length (acquired),** left **fibula**
    M21.769   **Unequal limb length (acquired), unspecified tibia and fibula** ▽

✓5ᵗʰ **M21.8   Other specified acquired deformities of limbs**

> EXCLUDES 2   *coxa plana (M91.2)*

    M21.80   **Other specified acquired deformities of unspecified limb** ▽

✓6ᵗʰ **M21.82   Other specified acquired deformities of** upper arm
    M21.821   **Other specified acquired deformities of right upper arm**
    M21.822   **Other specified acquired deformities of left upper arm**
    M21.829   **Other specified acquired deformities of unspecified upper arm** ▽

✓6ᵗʰ **M21.83   Other specified acquired deformities of** forearm
    M21.831   **Other specified acquired deformities of right forearm**
    M21.832   **Other specified acquired deformities of left forearm**
    M21.839   **Other specified acquired deformities of unspecified forearm** ▽

✓6ᵗʰ **M21.85   Other specified acquired deformities of** thigh
    M21.851   **Other specified acquired deformities of right thigh**

    M21.852   **Other specified acquired deformities of** left **thigh**
    M21.859   **Other specified acquired deformities of unspecified thigh** ▽

✓6ᵗʰ **M21.86   Other specified acquired deformities of** lower leg
    M21.861   **Other specified acquired deformities of** right **lower leg**
    M21.862   **Other specified acquired deformities of** left **lower leg**
    M21.869   **Other specified acquired deformities of unspecified lower leg** ▽

✓5ᵗʰ **M21.9   Unspecified acquired deformity of** limb and hand
    M21.90   **Unspecified acquired deformity of unspecified limb** ▽

✓6ᵗʰ **M21.92   Unspecified acquired deformity of** upper arm
    M21.921   **Unspecified acquired deformity of** right **upper arm** ▽
    M21.922   **Unspecified acquired deformity of** left **upper arm** ▽
    M21.929   **Unspecified acquired deformity of unspecified upper arm** ▽

✓6ᵗʰ **M21.93   Unspecified acquired deformity of** forearm
    M21.931   **Unspecified acquired deformity of** right **forearm** ▽
    M21.932   **Unspecified acquired deformity of** left **forearm** ▽
    M21.939   **Unspecified acquired deformity of unspecified forearm** ▽

✓6ᵗʰ **M21.94   Unspecified acquired deformity of** hand
    M21.941   **Unspecified acquired deformity of hand,** right **hand** ▽
    M21.942   **Unspecified acquired deformity of hand,** left **hand** ▽
    M21.949   **Unspecified acquired deformity of hand, unspecified hand** ▽

✓6ᵗʰ **M21.95   Unspecified acquired deformity of** thigh
    M21.951   **Unspecified acquired deformity of** right **thigh** ▽
    M21.952   **Unspecified acquired deformity of** left **thigh** ▽
    M21.959   **Unspecified acquired deformity of unspecified thigh** ▽

✓6ᵗʰ **M21.96   Unspecified acquired deformity of** lower leg
    M21.961   **Unspecified acquired deformity of** right **lower leg** ▽
    M21.962   **Unspecified acquired deformity of** left **lower leg** ▽
    M21.969   **Unspecified acquired deformity of unspecified lower leg** ▽

✓4ᵗʰ **M22   Disorder of patella**

> EXCLUDES 1   *traumatic dislocation of patella (S83.0-)*

✓5ᵗʰ **M22.0   Recurrent dislocation of patella**
    M22.00   **Recurrent dislocation of patella, unspecified knee** ▽
    M22.01   **Recurrent dislocation of patella,** right **knee**
    M22.02   **Recurrent dislocation of patella,** left **knee**

✓5ᵗʰ **M22.1   Recurrent subluxation of patella**
    Incomplete dislocation of patella
    M22.10   **Recurrent subluxation of patella, unspecified knee** ▽
    M22.11   **Recurrent subluxation of patella,** right **knee**
    M22.12   **Recurrent subluxation of patella,** left **knee**

✓5ᵗʰ **M22.2   Patellofemoral disorders**
✓6ᵗʰ **M22.2X   Patellofemoral disorders**
    M22.2X1   **Patellofemoral disorders,** right **knee**
    M22.2X2   **Patellofemoral disorders,** left **knee**
    M22.2X9   **Patellofemoral disorders, unspecified knee** ▽

✓5ᵗʰ **M22.3   Other derangements of patella**
✓6ᵗʰ **M22.3X   Other derangements of patella**
    M22.3X1   **Other derangements of patella,** right **knee**
    M22.3X2   **Other derangements of patella,** left **knee**
    M22.3X9   **Other derangements of patella, unspecified knee** ▽

✓5ᵗʰ **M22.4   Chondromalacia patellae**
    M22.40   **Chondromalacia patellae, unspecified knee** ▽

EXCLUDES 1 Not coded here   **EXCLUDES 2** Not included here   Ⓝ Newborn Age : 0   Ⓟ Pediatric Age : 0-17   Ⓜ Maternity Age : 12-55   Ⓐ Adult Age : 15-124

724   ICD-10-CM 2017

M22.41   Chondromalacia patellae, right knee

M22.42   Chondromalacia patellae, left knee

√5th M22.8   **Other disorders of patella**

    √6th M22.8X   Other disorders of patella

       M22.8X1   Other disorders of patella, right knee

       M22.8X2   Other disorders of patella, left knee

       M22.8X9   Other disorders of patella, unspecified knee   ▽

√5th M22.9   **Unspecified disorder of patella**

    M22.90   Unspecified disorder of patella, unspecified knee   ▽

    M22.91   Unspecified disorder of patella, right knee   ▽

    M22.92   Unspecified disorder of patella, left knee   ▽

√4th **M23**   **Internal derangement of knee**

    EXCLUDES 1   *ankylosis (M24.66)*

         current injury - see injury of knee and lower leg (S80-S89)

         deformity of knee (M21.-)

         osteochondritis dissecans (M93.2)

         recurrent dislocation or subluxation of joints (M24.4)

         recurrent dislocation or subluxation of patella (M22.0-M22.1)

√5th M23.0   **Cystic meniscus**

    √6th M23.00   **Cystic meniscus, unspecified meniscus**

        Cystic meniscus, unspecified lateral meniscus

        Cystic meniscus, unspecified medial meniscus

       M23.000   Cystic meniscus, unspecified lateral meniscus, right knee

       M23.001   Cystic meniscus, unspecified lateral meniscus, left knee

       M23.002   Cystic meniscus, unspecified lateral meniscus, unspecified knee   ▽

       M23.003   Cystic meniscus, unspecified medial meniscus, right knee

       M23.004   Cystic meniscus, unspecified medial meniscus, left knee

       M23.005   Cystic meniscus, unspecified medial meniscus, unspecified knee   ▽

       M23.006   Cystic meniscus, unspecified meniscus, right knee

       M23.007   Cystic meniscus, unspecified meniscus, left knee

       M23.009   Cystic meniscus, unspecified meniscus, unspecified knee   ▽

    √6th M23.01   **Cystic meniscus, anterior horn of medial meniscus**

       M23.011   Cystic meniscus, anterior horn of medial meniscus, right knee

       M23.012   Cystic meniscus, anterior horn of medial meniscus, left knee

       M23.019   Cystic meniscus, anterior horn of medial meniscus, unspecified knee   ▽

    √6th M23.02   **Cystic meniscus, posterior horn of medial meniscus**

       M23.021   Cystic meniscus, posterior horn of medial meniscus, right knee

       M23.022   Cystic meniscus, posterior horn of medial meniscus, left knee

       M23.029   Cystic meniscus, posterior horn of medial meniscus, unspecified knee   ▽

    √6th M23.03   **Cystic meniscus, other medial meniscus**

       M23.031   Cystic meniscus, other medial meniscus, right knee

       M23.032   Cystic meniscus, other medial meniscus, left knee

       M23.039   Cystic meniscus, other medial meniscus, unspecified knee   ▽

    √6th M23.04   **Cystic meniscus, anterior horn of lateral meniscus**

       M23.041   Cystic meniscus, anterior horn of lateral meniscus, right knee

       M23.042   Cystic meniscus, anterior horn of lateral meniscus, left knee

       M23.049   Cystic meniscus, anterior horn of lateral meniscus, unspecified knee   ▽

    √6th M23.05   **Cystic meniscus, posterior horn of lateral meniscus**

       M23.051   Cystic meniscus, posterior horn of lateral meniscus, right knee

       M23.052   Cystic meniscus, posterior horn of lateral meniscus, left knee

       M23.059   Cystic meniscus, posterior horn of lateral meniscus, unspecified knee   ▽

    √6th M23.06   **Cystic meniscus, other lateral meniscus**

       M23.061   Cystic meniscus, other lateral meniscus, right knee

       M23.062   Cystic meniscus, other lateral meniscus, left knee

       M23.069   Cystic meniscus, other lateral meniscus, unspecified knee   ▽

√5th M23.2   **Derangement of meniscus due to old tear or injury**

        Old bucket-handle tear

Derangement of Meniscus

Overhead view of right knee

Bucket handle tear

Radial tear

Meniscus

    √6th M23.20   **Derangement of unspecified meniscus due to old tear or injury**

        Derangement of unspecified lateral meniscus due to old tear or injury

        Derangement of unspecified medial meniscus due to old tear or injury

       M23.200   Derangement of unspecified lateral meniscus due to old tear or injury, right knee

       M23.201   Derangement of unspecified lateral meniscus due to old tear or injury, left knee

       M23.202   Derangement of unspecified lateral meniscus due to old tear or injury, unspecified knee   ▽

       M23.203   Derangement of unspecified medial meniscus due to old tear or injury, right knee

       M23.204   Derangement of unspecified medial meniscus due to old tear or injury, left knee

       M23.205   Derangement of unspecified medial meniscus due to old tear or injury, unspecified knee   ▽

       M23.206   Derangement of unspecified meniscus due to old tear or injury, right knee

       M23.207   Derangement of unspecified meniscus due to old tear or injury, left knee

       M23.209   Derangement of unspecified meniscus due to old tear or injury, unspecified knee   ▽

    √6th M23.21   **Derangement of anterior horn of medial meniscus due to old tear or injury**

       M23.211   Derangement of anterior horn of medial meniscus due to old tear or injury, right knee

       M23.212   Derangement of anterior horn of medial meniscus due to old tear or injury, left knee

       M23.219   Derangement of anterior horn of medial meniscus due to old tear or injury, unspecified knee   ▽

    √6th M23.22   **Derangement of posterior horn of medial meniscus due to old tear or injury**

       M23.221   Derangement of posterior horn of medial meniscus due to old tear or injury, right knee

✔ Additional Character Required   √x7th Placeholder Alert   Manifestation Dx   ▽ Unspecified Dx   ►◄ Revised Text   ● New Code   ▲ Revised Code Title

ICD-10-CM 2017   725

M23.222 Derangement of posterior horn of medial meniscus due to old tear or injury, left knee

M23.229 Derangement of posterior horn of medial meniscus due to old tear or injury, unspecified knee ▽

✓6ᵗʰ **M23.23** Derangement of other medial meniscus due to old tear or injury

M23.231 Derangement of other medial meniscus due to old tear or injury, right knee

M23.232 Derangement of other medial meniscus due to old tear or injury, left knee

M23.239 Derangement of other medial meniscus due to old tear or injury, unspecified knee ▽

✓6ᵗʰ **M23.24** Derangement of anterior horn of lateral meniscus due to old tear or injury

M23.241 Derangement of anterior horn of lateral meniscus due to old tear or injury, right knee

M23.242 Derangement of anterior horn of lateral meniscus due to old tear or injury, left knee

M23.249 Derangement of anterior horn of lateral meniscus due to old tear or injury, unspecified knee ▽

✓6ᵗʰ **M23.25** Derangement of posterior horn of lateral meniscus due to old tear or injury

M23.251 Derangement of posterior horn of lateral meniscus due to old tear or injury, right knee

M23.252 Derangement of posterior horn of lateral meniscus due to old tear or injury, left knee

M23.259 Derangement of posterior horn of lateral meniscus due to old tear or injury, unspecified knee ▽

✓6ᵗʰ **M23.26** Derangement of other lateral meniscus due to old tear or injury

M23.261 Derangement of other lateral meniscus due to old tear or injury, right knee

M23.262 Derangement of other lateral meniscus due to old tear or injury, left knee

M23.269 Derangement of other lateral meniscus due to old tear or injury, unspecified knee ▽

✓5ᵗʰ **M23.3** Other meniscus derangements

Degenerate meniscus
Detached meniscus
Retained meniscus

✓6ᵗʰ **M23.30** Other meniscus derangements, unspecified meniscus

Other meniscus derangements, unspecified lateral meniscus

Other meniscus derangements, unspecified medial meniscus

M23.300 Other meniscus derangements, unspecified lateral meniscus, right knee ▽

M23.301 Other meniscus derangements, unspecified lateral meniscus, left knee ▽

M23.302 Other meniscus derangements, unspecified lateral meniscus, unspecified knee ▽

M23.303 Other meniscus derangements, unspecified medial meniscus, right knee ▽

M23.304 Other meniscus derangements, unspecified medial meniscus, left knee ▽

M23.305 Other meniscus derangements, unspecified medial meniscus, unspecified knee ▽

M23.306 Other meniscus derangements, unspecified meniscus, right knee ▽

M23.307 Other meniscus derangements, unspecified meniscus, left knee ▽

M23.309 Other meniscus derangements, unspecified meniscus, unspecified knee ▽

✓6ᵗʰ **M23.31** Other meniscus derangements, anterior horn of medial meniscus

M23.311 Other meniscus derangements, anterior horn of medial meniscus, right knee

M23.312 Other meniscus derangements, anterior horn of medial meniscus, left knee

M23.319 Other meniscus derangements, anterior horn of medial meniscus, unspecified knee ▽

✓6ᵗʰ **M23.32** Other meniscus derangements, posterior horn of medial meniscus

M23.321 Other meniscus derangements, posterior horn of medial meniscus, right knee

M23.322 Other meniscus derangements, posterior horn of medial meniscus, left knee

M23.329 Other meniscus derangements, posterior horn of medial meniscus, unspecified knee ▽

✓6ᵗʰ **M23.33** Other meniscus derangements, other medial meniscus

M23.331 Other meniscus derangements, other medial meniscus, right knee

M23.332 Other meniscus derangements, other medial meniscus, left knee

M23.339 Other meniscus derangements, other medial meniscus, unspecified knee ▽

✓6ᵗʰ **M23.34** Other meniscus derangements, anterior horn of lateral meniscus

M23.341 Other meniscus derangements, anterior horn of lateral meniscus, right knee

M23.342 Other meniscus derangements, anterior horn of lateral meniscus, left knee

M23.349 Other meniscus derangements, anterior horn of lateral meniscus, unspecified knee ▽

✓6ᵗʰ **M23.35** Other meniscus derangements, posterior horn of lateral meniscus

M23.351 Other meniscus derangements, posterior horn of lateral meniscus, right knee

M23.352 Other meniscus derangements, posterior horn of lateral meniscus, left knee

M23.359 Other meniscus derangements, posterior horn of lateral meniscus, unspecified knee ▽

✓6ᵗʰ **M23.36** Other meniscus derangements, other lateral meniscus

M23.361 Other meniscus derangements, other lateral meniscus, right knee

M23.362 Other meniscus derangements, other lateral meniscus, left knee

M23.369 Other meniscus derangements, other lateral meniscus, unspecified knee ▽

✓5ᵗʰ **M23.4** Loose body in knee

M23.40 Loose body in knee, unspecified knee ▽

M23.41 Loose body in knee, right knee

M23.42 Loose body in knee, left knee

✓5ᵗʰ **M23.5** Chronic instability of knee

M23.50 Chronic instability of knee, unspecified knee ▽

M23.51 Chronic instability of knee, right knee

M23.52 Chronic instability of knee, left knee

✓5ᵗʰ **M23.6** Other spontaneous disruption of ligament(s) of knee

✓6ᵗʰ **M23.60** Other spontaneous disruption of unspecified ligament of knee

M23.601 Other spontaneous disruption of unspecified ligament of right knee ▽

M23.602 Other spontaneous disruption of unspecified ligament of left knee ▽

M23.609 Other spontaneous disruption of unspecified ligament of unspecified knee ▽

✓6ᵗʰ **M23.61** Other spontaneous disruption of anterior cruciate ligament of knee

M23.611 Other spontaneous disruption of anterior cruciate ligament of right knee

M23.612 Other spontaneous disruption of anterior cruciate ligament of left knee

M23.619 Other spontaneous disruption of anterior cruciate ligament of unspecified knee ▽

EXCLUDES 1 Not coded here   *EXCLUDES 2* Not included here   Ⓝ Newborn Age : 0   Ⓟ Pediatric Age : 0-17   Ⓜ Maternity Age : 12-55   Ⓐ Adult Age : 15-124

726   ICD-10-CM 2017

√6ᵗʰ **M23.62** **Other spontaneous disruption of** posterior cruciate **ligament of knee**

     M23.621 Other spontaneous disruption of posterior cruciate ligament of right knee

     M23.622 Other spontaneous disruption of posterior cruciate ligament of left knee

     M23.629 Other spontaneous disruption of posterior cruciate ligament of unspecified knee ▽

√6ᵗʰ **M23.63** **Other spontaneous disruption of** medial collateral **ligament of knee**

     M23.631 Other spontaneous disruption of medial collateral ligament of right knee

     M23.632 Other spontaneous disruption of medial collateral ligament of left knee

     M23.639 Other spontaneous disruption of medial collateral ligament of unspecified knee ▽

√6ᵗʰ **M23.64** **Other spontaneous disruption of** lateral collateral **ligament of knee**

     M23.641 Other spontaneous disruption of lateral collateral ligament of right knee

     M23.642 Other spontaneous disruption of lateral collateral ligament of left knee

     M23.649 Other spontaneous disruption of lateral collateral ligament of unspecified knee ▽

√6ᵗʰ **M23.67** **Other spontaneous disruption of** capsular **ligament of knee**

     M23.671 Other spontaneous disruption of capsular ligament of right knee

     M23.672 Other spontaneous disruption of capsular ligament of left knee

     M23.679 Other spontaneous disruption of capsular ligament of unspecified knee ▽

√5ᵗʰ **M23.8** **Other internal derangements of knee**

   Laxity of ligament of knee
   Snapping knee

√6ᵗʰ **M23.8X** **Other internal derangements of knee**

     M23.8X1 Other internal derangements of right knee

     M23.8X2 Other internal derangements of left knee

     M23.8X9 Other internal derangements of unspecified knee ▽

√5ᵗʰ **M23.9** **Unspecified internal derangement of knee**

     M23.90 Unspecified internal derangement of unspecified knee ▽

     M23.91 Unspecified internal derangement of right knee ▽

     M23.92 Unspecified internal derangement of left knee ▽

√4ᵗʰ **M24** **Other specific joint derangements**

   EXCLUDES 1   current injury - see injury of joint by body region
   EXCLUDES 2   ganglion (M67.4)
           snapping knee (M23.8-)
           temporomandibular joint disorders (M26.6-)

√5ᵗʰ **M24.0** **Loose body in joint**

   EXCLUDES 2   loose body in knee (M23.4)

     M24.00 Loose body in unspecified joint ▽

√6ᵗʰ **M24.01** **Loose body in** shoulder

     M24.011 Loose body in right shoulder
     M24.012 Loose body in left shoulder
     M24.019 Loose body in unspecified shoulder ▽

√6ᵗʰ **M24.02** **Loose body in** elbow

     M24.021 Loose body in right elbow
     M24.022 Loose body in left elbow
     M24.029 Loose body in unspecified elbow ▽

√6ᵗʰ **M24.03** **Loose body in** wrist

     M24.031 Loose body in right wrist
     M24.032 Loose body in left wrist
     M24.039 Loose body in unspecified wrist ▽

√6ᵗʰ **M24.04** **Loose body in** finger joints

     M24.041 Loose body in right finger joint(s)
     M24.042 Loose body in left finger joint(s)
     M24.049 Loose body in unspecified finger joint(s) ▽

√6ᵗʰ **M24.05** **Loose body in** hip

     M24.051 Loose body in right hip

     M24.052 Loose body in left hip
     M24.059 Loose body in unspecified hip ▽

√6ᵗʰ **M24.07** **Loose body in** ankle and toe joints

     M24.071 Loose body in right ankle
     M24.072 Loose body in left ankle
     M24.073 Loose body in unspecified ankle ▽
     M24.074 Loose body in right toe joint(s)
     M24.075 Loose body in left toe joint(s)
     M24.076 Loose body in unspecified toe joints ▽

     M24.08 Loose body, other site

√5ᵗʰ **M24.1** **Other articular cartilage disorders**

   EXCLUDES 2   chondrocalcinosis (M11.1, M11.2-)
           internal derangement of knee (M23.-)
           metastatic calcification (E83.5)
           ochronosis (E70.2)

     M24.10 Other articular cartilage disorders, unspecified site ▽

√6ᵗʰ **M24.11** **Other articular cartilage disorders,** shoulder

     M24.111 Other articular cartilage disorders, right shoulder

     M24.112 Other articular cartilage disorders, left shoulder

     M24.119 Other articular cartilage disorders, unspecified shoulder ▽

√6ᵗʰ **M24.12** **Other articular cartilage disorders,** elbow

     M24.121 Other articular cartilage disorders, right elbow

     M24.122 Other articular cartilage disorders, left elbow

     M24.129 Other articular cartilage disorders, unspecified elbow ▽

√6ᵗʰ **M24.13** **Other articular cartilage disorders,** wrist

     M24.131 Other articular cartilage disorders, right wrist

     M24.132 Other articular cartilage disorders, left wrist

     M24.139 Other articular cartilage disorders, unspecified wrist ▽

√6ᵗʰ **M24.14** **Other articular cartilage disorders,** hand

     M24.141 Other articular cartilage disorders, right hand

     M24.142 Other articular cartilage disorders, left hand

     M24.149 Other articular cartilage disorders, unspecified hand ▽

√6ᵗʰ **M24.15** **Other articular cartilage disorders,** hip

     M24.151 Other articular cartilage disorders, right hip

     M24.152 Other articular cartilage disorders, left hip

     M24.159 Other articular cartilage disorders, unspecified hip ▽

√6ᵗʰ **M24.17** **Other articular cartilage disorders,** ankle and foot

     M24.171 Other articular cartilage disorders, right ankle

     M24.172 Other articular cartilage disorders, left ankle

     M24.173 Other articular cartilage disorders, unspecified ankle ▽

     M24.174 Other articular cartilage disorders, right foot

     M24.175 Other articular cartilage disorders, left foot

     M24.176 Other articular cartilage disorders, unspecified foot ▽

√5ᵗʰ **M24.2** **Disorder of ligament**

   Instability secondary to old ligament injury
   Ligamentous laxity NOS
   EXCLUDES 1   familial ligamentous laxity (M35.7)
   EXCLUDES 2   internal derangement of knee (M23.5-M23.89)

     M24.20 Disorder of ligament, unspecified site ▽

√6ᵗʰ **M24.21** **Disorder of ligament,** shoulder

     M24.211 Disorder of ligament, right shoulder
     M24.212 Disorder of ligament, left shoulder
     M24.219 Disorder of ligament, unspecified shoulder ▽

√6ᵗʰ **M24.22** **Disorder of ligament,** elbow

     M24.221 Disorder of ligament, right elbow

☑ Additional Character Required   √x7ᵗʰ Placeholder Alert   Manifestation Dx   ▽ Unspecified Dx   ▶◀ Revised Text   ● New Code   ▲ Revised Code Title

M24.222 Disorder of ligament, left elbow
M24.229 Disorder of ligament, unspecified elbow ▽

√6ᵗʰ **M24.23** **Disorder of ligament, wrist**
M24.231 Disorder of ligament, right wrist
M24.232 Disorder of ligament, left wrist
M24.239 Disorder of ligament, unspecified wrist ▽

√6ᵗʰ **M24.24** **Disorder of ligament, hand**
M24.241 Disorder of ligament, right hand
M24.242 Disorder of ligament, left hand
M24.249 Disorder of ligament, unspecified hand ▽

√6ᵗʰ **M24.25** **Disorder of ligament, hip**
M24.251 Disorder of ligament, right hip
M24.252 Disorder of ligament, left hip
M24.259 Disorder of ligament, unspecified hip ▽

√6ᵗʰ **M24.27** **Disorder of ligament, ankle and foot**
M24.271 Disorder of ligament, right ankle
M24.272 Disorder of ligament, left ankle
M24.273 Disorder of ligament, unspecified ankle ▽
M24.274 Disorder of ligament, right foot
M24.275 Disorder of ligament, left foot
M24.276 Disorder of ligament, unspecified foot ▽

M24.28 **Disorder of ligament, vertebrae**

√5ᵗʰ **M24.3** **Pathological dislocation of joint, not elsewhere classified**
EXCLUDES 1 congenital dislocation or displacement of joint - see congenital malformations and deformations of the musculoskeletal system (Q65-Q79)
current injury - see injury of joints and ligaments by body region
recurrent dislocation of joint (M24.4-)

M24.30 **Pathological dislocation of unspecified joint, not elsewhere classified** ▽

√6ᵗʰ **M24.31** **Pathological dislocation of shoulder, not elsewhere classified**
M24.311 Pathological dislocation of right shoulder, not elsewhere classified
M24.312 Pathological dislocation of left shoulder, not elsewhere classified
M24.319 Pathological dislocation of unspecified shoulder, not elsewhere classified ▽

√6ᵗʰ **M24.32** **Pathological dislocation of elbow, not elsewhere classified**
M24.321 Pathological dislocation of right elbow, not elsewhere classified
M24.322 Pathological dislocation of left elbow, not elsewhere classified
M24.329 Pathological dislocation of unspecified elbow, not elsewhere classified ▽

√6ᵗʰ **M24.33** **Pathological dislocation of wrist, not elsewhere classified**
M24.331 Pathological dislocation of right wrist, not elsewhere classified
M24.332 Pathological dislocation of left wrist, not elsewhere classified
M24.339 Pathological dislocation of unspecified wrist, not elsewhere classified ▽

√6ᵗʰ **M24.34** **Pathological dislocation of hand, not elsewhere classified**
M24.341 Pathological dislocation of right hand, not elsewhere classified
M24.342 Pathological dislocation of left hand, not elsewhere classified
M24.349 Pathological dislocation of unspecified hand, not elsewhere classified ▽

√6ᵗʰ **M24.35** **Pathological dislocation of hip, not elsewhere classified**
M24.351 Pathological dislocation of right hip, not elsewhere classified
M24.352 Pathological dislocation of left hip, not elsewhere classified

M24.359 Pathological dislocation of unspecified hip, not elsewhere classified ▽

√6ᵗʰ **M24.36** **Pathological dislocation of knee, not elsewhere classified**
M24.361 Pathological dislocation of right knee, not elsewhere classified
M24.362 Pathological dislocation of left knee, not elsewhere classified
M24.369 Pathological dislocation of unspecified knee, not elsewhere classified ▽

√6ᵗʰ **M24.37** **Pathological dislocation of ankle and foot, not elsewhere classified**
M24.371 Pathological dislocation of right ankle, not elsewhere classified
M24.372 Pathological dislocation of left ankle, not elsewhere classified
M24.373 Pathological dislocation of unspecified ankle, not elsewhere classified ▽
M24.374 Pathological dislocation of right foot, not elsewhere classified
M24.375 Pathological dislocation of left foot, not elsewhere classified
M24.376 Pathological dislocation of unspecified foot, not elsewhere classified ▽

√5ᵗʰ **M24.4** **Recurrent dislocation of joint**
Recurrent subluxation of joint
EXCLUDES 2 recurrent dislocation of patella (M22.0-M22.1)
recurrent vertebral dislocation (M43.3-, M43.4, M43.5-)

M24.40 **Recurrent dislocation, unspecified joint** ▽

√6ᵗʰ **M24.41** **Recurrent dislocation, shoulder**
M24.411 Recurrent dislocation, right shoulder
M24.412 Recurrent dislocation, left shoulder
M24.419 Recurrent dislocation, unspecified shoulder ▽

√6ᵗʰ **M24.42** **Recurrent dislocation, elbow**
M24.421 Recurrent dislocation, right elbow
M24.422 Recurrent dislocation, left elbow
M24.429 Recurrent dislocation, unspecified elbow ▽

√6ᵗʰ **M24.43** **Recurrent dislocation, wrist**
M24.431 Recurrent dislocation, right wrist
M24.432 Recurrent dislocation, left wrist
M24.439 Recurrent dislocation, unspecified wrist ▽

√6ᵗʰ **M24.44** **Recurrent dislocation, hand and finger(s)**
M24.441 Recurrent dislocation, right hand
M24.442 Recurrent dislocation, left hand
M24.443 Recurrent dislocation, unspecified hand ▽
M24.444 Recurrent dislocation, right finger
M24.445 Recurrent dislocation, left finger
M24.446 Recurrent dislocation, unspecified finger ▽

√6ᵗʰ **M24.45** **Recurrent dislocation, hip**
M24.451 Recurrent dislocation, right hip
M24.452 Recurrent dislocation, left hip
M24.459 Recurrent dislocation, unspecified hip ▽

√6ᵗʰ **M24.46** **Recurrent dislocation, knee**
M24.461 Recurrent dislocation, right knee
M24.462 Recurrent dislocation, left knee
M24.469 Recurrent dislocation, unspecified knee ▽

√6ᵗʰ **M24.47** **Recurrent dislocation, ankle, foot and toes**
M24.471 Recurrent dislocation, right ankle
M24.472 Recurrent dislocation, left ankle
M24.473 Recurrent dislocation, unspecified ankle ▽
M24.474 Recurrent dislocation, right foot
M24.475 Recurrent dislocation, left foot
M24.476 Recurrent dislocation, unspecified foot ▽
M24.477 Recurrent dislocation, right toe(s)
M24.478 Recurrent dislocation, left toe(s)
M24.479 Recurrent dislocation, unspecified toe(s) ▽

✓5ᵗʰ **M24.5** **Contracture of joint**

　　EXCLUDES 1 *contracture of muscle without contracture of joint (M62.4-)*
　　　　contracture of tendon (sheath) without contracture of joint (M62.4-)
　　　　Dupuytren's contracture (M72.0)
　　EXCLUDES 2 *acquired deformities of limbs (M20-M21)*
　　AHA: 2016,2Q,6

　　M24.50 Contracture, unspecified joint　　　▽

✓6ᵗʰ **M24.51** Contracture, shoulder
　　M24.511 Contracture, right shoulder
　　M24.512 Contracture, left shoulder
　　M24.519 Contracture, unspecified shoulder　▽

✓6ᵗʰ **M24.52** Contracture, elbow
　　M24.521 Contracture, right elbow
　　M24.522 Contracture, left elbow
　　M24.529 Contracture, unspecified elbow　▽

✓6ᵗʰ **M24.53** Contracture, wrist
　　M24.531 Contracture, right wrist
　　M24.532 Contracture, left wrist
　　M24.539 Contracture, unspecified wrist　▽

✓6ᵗʰ **M24.54** Contracture, hand
　　M24.541 Contracture, right hand
　　M24.542 Contracture, left hand
　　M24.549 Contracture, unspecified hand　▽

✓6ᵗʰ **M24.55** Contracture, hip
　　M24.551 Contracture, right hip
　　M24.552 Contracture, left hip
　　M24.559 Contracture, unspecified hip　▽

✓6ᵗʰ **M24.56** Contracture, knee
　　M24.561 Contracture, right knee
　　M24.562 Contracture, left knee
　　M24.569 Contracture, unspecified knee　▽

✓6ᵗʰ **M24.57** Contracture, ankle and foot
　　M24.571 Contracture, right ankle
　　M24.572 Contracture, left ankle
　　M24.573 Contracture, unspecified ankle　▽
　　M24.574 Contracture, right foot
　　M24.575 Contracture, left foot
　　M24.576 Contracture, unspecified foot　▽

✓5ᵗʰ **M24.6** **Ankylosis of joint**

　　EXCLUDES 1 *stiffness of joint without ankylosis (M25.6-)*
　　EXCLUDES 2 *spine (M43.2-)*

　　M24.60 Ankylosis, unspecified joint　　　▽

✓6ᵗʰ **M24.61** Ankylosis, shoulder
　　M24.611 Ankylosis, right shoulder
　　M24.612 Ankylosis, left shoulder
　　M24.619 Ankylosis, unspecified shoulder　▽

✓6ᵗʰ **M24.62** Ankylosis, elbow
　　M24.621 Ankylosis, right elbow
　　M24.622 Ankylosis, left elbow
　　M24.629 Ankylosis, unspecified elbow　▽

✓6ᵗʰ **M24.63** Ankylosis, wrist
　　M24.631 Ankylosis, right wrist
　　M24.632 Ankylosis, left wrist
　　M24.639 Ankylosis, unspecified wrist　▽

✓6ᵗʰ **M24.64** Ankylosis, hand
　　M24.641 Ankylosis, right hand
　　M24.642 Ankylosis, left hand
　　M24.649 Ankylosis, unspecified hand　▽

✓6ᵗʰ **M24.65** Ankylosis, hip
　　M24.651 Ankylosis, right hip
　　M24.652 Ankylosis, left hip
　　M24.659 Ankylosis, unspecified hip　▽

✓6ᵗʰ **M24.66** Ankylosis, knee
　　M24.661 Ankylosis, right knee
　　M24.662 Ankylosis, left knee
　　M24.669 Ankylosis, unspecified knee　▽

✓6ᵗʰ **M24.67** Ankylosis, ankle and foot
　　M24.671 Ankylosis, right ankle
　　M24.672 Ankylosis, left ankle
　　M24.673 Ankylosis, unspecified ankle　▽

　　M24.674 Ankylosis, right foot
　　M24.675 Ankylosis, left foot
　　M24.676 Ankylosis, unspecified foot　▽

　M24.7 **Protrusio acetabuli**

✓5ᵗʰ **M24.8** **Other specific joint derangements, not elsewhere classified**

　　EXCLUDES 2 *iliotibial band syndrome (M76.3)*

　　M24.80 Other specific joint derangements of unspecified joint, not elsewhere classified　▽

✓6ᵗʰ **M24.81** Other specific joint derangements of shoulder, not elsewhere classified
　　M24.811 Other specific joint derangements of right shoulder, not elsewhere classified
　　M24.812 Other specific joint derangements of left shoulder, not elsewhere classified
　　M24.819 Other specific joint derangements of unspecified shoulder, not elsewhere classified　▽

✓6ᵗʰ **M24.82** Other specific joint derangements of elbow, not elsewhere classified
　　M24.821 Other specific joint derangements of right elbow, not elsewhere classified
　　M24.822 Other specific joint derangements of left elbow, not elsewhere classified
　　M24.829 Other specific joint derangements of unspecified elbow, not elsewhere classified　▽

✓6ᵗʰ **M24.83** Other specific joint derangements of wrist, not elsewhere classified
　　M24.831 Other specific joint derangements of right wrist, not elsewhere classified
　　M24.832 Other specific joint derangements of left wrist, not elsewhere classified
　　M24.839 Other specific joint derangements of unspecified wrist, not elsewhere classified　▽

✓6ᵗʰ **M24.84** Other specific joint derangements of hand, not elsewhere classified
　　M24.841 Other specific joint derangements of right hand, not elsewhere classified
　　M24.842 Other specific joint derangements of left hand, not elsewhere classified
　　M24.849 Other specific joint derangements of unspecified hand, not elsewhere classified　▽

✓6ᵗʰ **M24.85** Other specific joint derangements of hip, not elsewhere classified
　　Irritable hip
　　M24.851 Other specific joint derangements of right hip, not elsewhere classified
　　M24.852 Other specific joint derangements of left hip, not elsewhere classified
　　M24.859 Other specific joint derangements of unspecified hip, not elsewhere classified　▽

✓6ᵗʰ **M24.87** Other specific joint derangements of ankle and foot, not elsewhere classified
　　M24.871 Other specific joint derangements of right ankle, not elsewhere classified
　　M24.872 Other specific joint derangements of left ankle, not elsewhere classified
　　M24.873 Other specific joint derangements of unspecified ankle, not elsewhere classified　▽
　　M24.874 Other specific joint derangements of right foot, not elsewhere classified
　　M24.875 Other specific joint derangements left foot, not elsewhere classified
　　M24.876 Other specific joint derangements of unspecified foot, not elsewhere classified　▽

　M24.9 **Joint derangement, unspecified**　▽

✓4ᵗʰ **M25** **Other joint disorder, not elsewhere classified**

　　EXCLUDES 2 *abnormality of gait and mobility (R26.-)*
　　　　acquired deformities of limb (M20-M21)
　　　　calcification of bursa (M71.4-)
　　　　calcification of shoulder (joint) (M75.3)
　　　　calcification of tendon (M65.2-)
　　　　difficulty in walking (R26.2)
　　　　temporomandibular joint disorder (M26.6-)

☑ Additional Character Required　　✓7ᵗʰ Placeholder Alert　　Manifestation Dx　　▽ Unspecified Dx　　▶◀ Revised Text　　● New Code　　▲ Revised Code Title

ICD-10-CM 2017　　　　　　　　　　　　　　　　　　　　　　　　　　　　　　　　**729**

Chapter 13. Diseases of the Musculoskeletal System and Connective Tissue

✓5th **M25.0 Hemarthrosis**

> EXCLUDES 1   *current injury - see injury of joint by body region*
> *hemophilic arthropathy (M36.2)*

     M25.00   Hemarthrosis, unspecified joint ▽

     ✓6th   M25.01   Hemarthrosis, shoulder

         M25.011   Hemarthrosis, right shoulder
         M25.012   Hemarthrosis, left shoulder
         M25.019   Hemarthrosis, unspecified shoulder ▽

     ✓6th   M25.02   Hemarthrosis, elbow

         M25.021   Hemarthrosis, right elbow
         M25.022   Hemarthrosis, left elbow
         M25.029   Hemarthrosis, unspecified elbow ▽

     ✓6th   M25.03   Hemarthrosis, wrist

         M25.031   Hemarthrosis, right wrist
         M25.032   Hemarthrosis, left wrist
         M25.039   Hemarthrosis, unspecified wrist ▽

     ✓6th   M25.04   Hemarthrosis, hand

         M25.041   Hemarthrosis, right hand
         M25.042   Hemarthrosis, left hand
         M25.049   Hemarthrosis, unspecified hand ▽

     ✓6th   M25.05   Hemarthrosis, hip

         M25.051   Hemarthrosis, right hip
         M25.052   Hemarthrosis, left hip
         M25.059   Hemarthrosis, unspecified hip ▽

     ✓6th   M25.06   Hemarthrosis, knee

         M25.061   Hemarthrosis, right knee
         M25.062   Hemarthrosis, left knee
         M25.069   Hemarthrosis, unspecified knee ▽

     ✓6th   M25.07   Hemarthrosis, ankle and foot

         M25.071   Hemarthrosis, right ankle
         M25.072   Hemarthrosis, left ankle
         M25.073   Hemarthrosis, unspecified ankle ▽
         M25.074   Hemarthrosis, right foot
         M25.075   Hemarthrosis, left foot
         M25.076   Hemarthrosis, unspecified foot ▽

     M25.08   Hemarthrosis, other specified site
         Hemarthrosis, vertebrae

✓5th **M25.1 Fistula of joint**

     M25.10   Fistula, unspecified joint ▽

     ✓6th   M25.11   Fistula, shoulder

         M25.111   Fistula, right shoulder
         M25.112   Fistula, left shoulder
         M25.119   Fistula, unspecified shoulder ▽

     ✓6th   M25.12   Fistula, elbow

         M25.121   Fistula, right elbow
         M25.122   Fistula, left elbow
         M25.129   Fistula, unspecified elbow ▽

     ✓6th   M25.13   Fistula, wrist

         M25.131   Fistula, right wrist
         M25.132   Fistula, left wrist
         M25.139   Fistula, unspecified wrist ▽

     ✓6th   M25.14   Fistula, hand

         M25.141   Fistula, right hand
         M25.142   Fistula, left hand
         M25.149   Fistula, unspecified hand ▽

     ✓6th   M25.15   Fistula, hip

         M25.151   Fistula, right hip
         M25.152   Fistula, left hip
         M25.159   Fistula, unspecified hip ▽

     ✓6th   M25.16   Fistula, knee

         M25.161   Fistula, right knee
         M25.162   Fistula, left knee
         M25.169   Fistula, unspecified knee ▽

     ✓6th   M25.17   Fistula, ankle and foot

         M25.171   Fistula, right ankle
         M25.172   Fistula, left ankle
         M25.173   Fistula, unspecified ankle ▽
         M25.174   Fistula, right foot
         M25.175   Fistula, left foot
         M25.176   Fistula, unspecified foot

     M25.18   Fistula, other specified site
         Fistula, vertebrae

✓5th **M25.2 Flail joint**

     M25.20   Flail joint, unspecified joint ▽

     ✓6th   M25.21   Flail joint, shoulder

         M25.211   Flail joint, right shoulder
         M25.212   Flail joint, left shoulder
         M25.219   Flail joint, unspecified shoulder ▽

     ✓6th   M25.22   Flail joint, elbow

         M25.221   Flail joint, right elbow
         M25.222   Flail joint, left elbow
         M25.229   Flail joint, unspecified elbow ▽

     ✓6th   M25.23   Flail joint, wrist

         M25.231   Flail joint, right wrist
         M25.232   Flail joint, left wrist
         M25.239   Flail joint, unspecified wrist ▽

     ✓6th   M25.24   Flail joint, hand

         M25.241   Flail joint, right hand
         M25.242   Flail joint, left hand
         M25.249   Flail joint, unspecified hand ▽

     ✓6th   M25.25   Flail joint, hip

         M25.251   Flail joint, right hip
         M25.252   Flail joint, left hip
         M25.259   Flail joint, unspecified hip ▽

     ✓6th   M25.26   Flail joint, knee

         M25.261   Flail joint, right knee
         M25.262   Flail joint, left knee
         M25.269   Flail joint, unspecified knee ▽

     ✓6th   M25.27   Flail joint, ankle and foot

         M25.271   Flail joint, right ankle and foot
         M25.272   Flail joint, left ankle and foot
         M25.279   Flail joint, unspecified ankle and foot ▽

     M25.28   Flail joint, other site

✓5th **M25.3 Other instability of joint**

> EXCLUDES 1   *instability of joint secondary to old ligament injury*
> *(M24.2-)*
> *instability of joint secondary to removal of joint*
> *prosthesis (M96.8-)*
> EXCLUDES 2   *spinal instabilities (M53.2-)*

     M25.30   Other instability, unspecified joint ▽

     ✓6th   M25.31   Other instability, shoulder

         M25.311   Other instability, right shoulder
         M25.312   Other instability, left shoulder
         M25.319   Other instability, unspecified shoulder ▽

     ✓6th   M25.32   Other instability, elbow

         M25.321   Other instability, right elbow
         M25.322   Other instability, left elbow
         M25.329   Other instability, unspecified elbow ▽

     ✓6th   M25.33   Other instability, wrist

         M25.331   Other instability, right wrist
         M25.332   Other instability, left wrist
         M25.339   Other instability, unspecified wrist ▽

     ✓6th   M25.34   Other instability, hand

         M25.341   Other instability, right hand
         M25.342   Other instability, left hand
         M25.349   Other instability, unspecified hand ▽

     ✓6th   M25.35   Other instability, hip

         M25.351   Other instability, right hip
         M25.352   Other instability, left hip
         M25.359   Other instability, unspecified hip ▽

     ✓6th   M25.36   Other instability, knee

         M25.361   Other instability, right knee
         M25.362   Other instability, left knee
         M25.369   Other instability, unspecified knee ▽

     ✓6th   M25.37   Other instability, ankle and foot

         M25.371   Other instability, right ankle
         M25.372   Other instability, left ankle
         M25.373   Other instability, unspecified ankle ▽
         M25.374   Other instability, right foot

EXCLUDES 1   Not coded here   EXCLUDES 2   Not included here   N Newborn Age : 0   P Pediatric Age : 0-17   M Maternity Age : 12-55   A Adult Age : 15-124

730   ICD-10-CM 2017

M25.375   Other instability, left foot
M25.376   Other instability, unspecified foot ▽

√5ᵗʰ **M25.4   Effusion of joint**

EXCLUDES 1   hydrarthrosis in yaws (A66.6)
intermittent hydrarthrosis (M12.4-)
other infective (teno)synovitis (M65.1-)

M25.40   **Effusion, unspecified joint** ▽

√6ᵗʰ   M25.41   **Effusion, shoulder**
M25.411   Effusion, right shoulder
M25.412   Effusion, left shoulder
M25.419   Effusion, unspecified shoulder ▽

√6ᵗʰ   M25.42   **Effusion, elbow**
M25.421   Effusion, right elbow
M25.422   Effusion, left elbow
M25.429   Effusion, unspecified elbow ▽

√6ᵗʰ   M25.43   **Effusion, wrist**
M25.431   Effusion, right wrist
M25.432   Effusion, left wrist
M25.439   Effusion, unspecified wrist ▽

√6ᵗʰ   M25.44   **Effusion, hand**
M25.441   Effusion, right hand
M25.442   Effusion, left hand
M25.449   Effusion, unspecified hand ▽

√6ᵗʰ   M25.45   **Effusion, hip**
M25.451   Effusion, right hip
M25.452   Effusion, left hip
M25.459   Effusion, unspecified hip ▽

√6ᵗʰ   M25.46   **Effusion, knee**
M25.461   Effusion, right knee
M25.462   Effusion, left knee
M25.469   Effusion, unspecified knee ▽

√6ᵗʰ   M25.47   **Effusion, ankle and foot**
M25.471   Effusion, right ankle
M25.472   Effusion, left ankle
M25.473   Effusion, unspecified ankle ▽
M25.474   Effusion, right foot
M25.475   Effusion, left foot
M25.476   Effusion, unspecified foot ▽

M25.48   **Effusion, other site**

√5ᵗʰ **M25.5   Pain in joint**

EXCLUDES 2   pain in hand (M79.64-)
pain in fingers (M79.64-)
pain in foot (M79.67-)
pain in limb (M79.6-)
pain in toes (M79.67-)

M25.50   **Pain in unspecified joint** ▽

√6ᵗʰ   M25.51   **Pain in shoulder**
M25.511   Pain in right shoulder
M25.512   Pain in left shoulder
M25.519   Pain in unspecified shoulder ▽

√6ᵗʰ   M25.52   **Pain in elbow**
M25.521   Pain in right elbow
M25.522   Pain in left elbow
M25.529   Pain in unspecified elbow ▽

√6ᵗʰ   M25.53   **Pain in wrist**
M25.531   Pain in right wrist
M25.532   Pain in left wrist
M25.539   Pain in unspecified wrist ▽

● √6ᵗʰ   M25.54   **Pain in joints of hand**
●   M25.541   Pain in joints of right hand
●   M25.542   Pain in joints of left hand
●   M25.549   Pain in joints of unspecified hand ▽
     Pain in joints of hand NOS

√6ᵗʰ   M25.55   **Pain in hip**
M25.551   Pain in right hip
M25.552   Pain in left hip
M25.559   Pain in unspecified hip ▽

√6ᵗʰ   M25.56   **Pain in knee**
M25.561   Pain in right knee
M25.562   Pain in left knee
M25.569   Pain in unspecified knee ▽

√6ᵗʰ   M25.57   **Pain in ankle and joints of foot**
M25.571   Pain in right ankle and joints of right foot
M25.572   Pain in left ankle and joints of left foot
M25.579   Pain in unspecified ankle and joints of unspecified foot ▽

√5ᵗʰ **M25.6   Stiffness of joint, not elsewhere classified**

EXCLUDES 1   ankylosis of joint (M24.6-)
contracture of joint (M24.5-)

M25.60   **Stiffness of unspecified joint, not elsewhere classified** ▽

√6ᵗʰ   M25.61   **Stiffness of shoulder, not elsewhere classified**
M25.611   Stiffness of right shoulder, not elsewhere classified
M25.612   Stiffness of left shoulder, not elsewhere classified
M25.619   Stiffness of unspecified shoulder, not elsewhere classified ▽

√6ᵗʰ   M25.62   **Stiffness of elbow, not elsewhere classified**
M25.621   Stiffness of right elbow, not elsewhere classified
M25.622   Stiffness of left elbow, not elsewhere classified
M25.629   Stiffness of unspecified elbow, not elsewhere classified ▽

√6ᵗʰ   M25.63   **Stiffness of wrist, not elsewhere classified**
M25.631   Stiffness of right wrist, not elsewhere classified
M25.632   Stiffness of left wrist, not elsewhere classified
M25.639   Stiffness of unspecified wrist, not elsewhere classified ▽

√6ᵗʰ   M25.64   **Stiffness of hand, not elsewhere classified**
M25.641   Stiffness of right hand, not elsewhere classified
M25.642   Stiffness of left hand, not elsewhere classified
M25.649   Stiffness of unspecified hand, not elsewhere classified ▽

√6ᵗʰ   M25.65   **Stiffness of hip, not elsewhere classified**
M25.651   Stiffness of right hip, not elsewhere classified
M25.652   Stiffness of left hip, not elsewhere classified
M25.659   Stiffness of unspecified hip, not elsewhere classified ▽

√6ᵗʰ   M25.66   **Stiffness of knee, not elsewhere classified**
M25.661   Stiffness of right knee, not elsewhere classified
M25.662   Stiffness of left knee, not elsewhere classified
M25.669   Stiffness of unspecified knee, not elsewhere classified ▽

√6ᵗʰ   M25.67   **Stiffness of ankle and foot, not elsewhere classified**
M25.671   Stiffness of right ankle, not elsewhere classified
M25.672   Stiffness of left ankle, not elsewhere classified
M25.673   Stiffness of unspecified ankle, not elsewhere classified ▽
M25.674   Stiffness of right foot, not elsewhere classified
M25.675   Stiffness of left foot, not elsewhere classified
M25.676   Stiffness of unspecified foot, not elsewhere classified ▽

√5ᵗʰ **M25.7   Osteophyte**

M25.70   **Osteophyte, unspecified joint** ▽

√6ᵗʰ   M25.71   **Osteophyte, shoulder**
M25.711   Osteophyte, right shoulder
M25.712   Osteophyte, left shoulder
M25.719   Osteophyte, unspecified shoulder ▽

√6ᵗʰ   M25.72   **Osteophyte, elbow**
M25.721   Osteophyte, right elbow
M25.722   Osteophyte, left elbow
M25.729   Osteophyte, unspecified elbow ▽

√6ᵗʰ   M25.73   **Osteophyte, wrist**
M25.731   Osteophyte, right wrist
M25.732   Osteophyte, left wrist
M25.739   Osteophyte, unspecified wrist ▽

☑ Additional Character Required   √7ᵗʰ Placeholder Alert   Manifestation Dx   ▽ Unspecified Dx   ►◄ Revised Text   ● New Code   ▲ Revised Code Title

ICD-10-CM 2017   731

✓6ᵗʰ **M25.74 Osteophyte,** hand
     M25.741 Osteophyte, right **hand**
     M25.742 Osteophyte, left **hand**
     M25.749 Osteophyte, unspecified **hand** ▽

✓6ᵗʰ **M25.75 Osteophyte,** hip
     M25.751 Osteophyte, right **hip**
     M25.752 Osteophyte, left **hip**
     M25.759 Osteophyte, unspecified **hip** ▽

✓6ᵗʰ **M25.76 Osteophyte,** knee
     M25.761 Osteophyte, right **knee**
     M25.762 Osteophyte, left **knee**
     M25.769 Osteophyte, unspecified **knee** ▽

✓6ᵗʰ **M25.77 Osteophyte,** ankle and foot
     M25.771 Osteophyte, right **ankle**
     M25.772 Osteophyte, left **ankle**
     M25.773 Osteophyte, unspecified **ankle** ▽
     M25.774 Osteophyte, right **foot**
     M25.775 Osteophyte, left **foot**
     M25.776 Osteophyte, unspecified **foot** ▽

     M25.78 Osteophyte, vertebrae

✓5ᵗʰ **M25.8 Other specified joint disorders**
     M25.80 Other specified joint disorders, unspecified joint ▽

✓6ᵗʰ **M25.81 Other specified joint disorders,** shoulder
     M25.811 Other specified joint disorders, right **shoulder**
     M25.812 Other specified joint disorders, left **shoulder**
     M25.819 Other specified joint disorders, unspecified shoulder ▽

✓6ᵗʰ **M25.82 Other specified joint disorders,** elbow
     M25.821 Other specified joint disorders, right **elbow**
     M25.822 Other specified joint disorders, left **elbow**
     M25.829 Other specified joint disorders, unspecified elbow ▽

✓6ᵗʰ **M25.83 Other specified joint disorders,** wrist
     M25.831 Other specified joint disorders, right **wrist**
     M25.832 Other specified joint disorders, left **wrist**
     M25.839 Other specified joint disorders, unspecified wrist ▽

✓6ᵗʰ **M25.84 Other specified joint disorders,** hand
     M25.841 Other specified joint disorders, right **hand**
     M25.842 Other specified joint disorders, left **hand**
     M25.849 Other specified joint disorders, unspecified hand ▽

✓6ᵗʰ **M25.85 Other specified joint disorders,** hip

     AHA: 2014,4Q,25
     M25.851 Other specified joint disorders, right **hip**
     M25.852 Other specified joint disorders, left **hip**
     M25.859 Other specified joint disorders, unspecified hip ▽

✓6ᵗʰ **M25.86 Other specified joint disorders,** knee
     M25.861 Other specified joint disorders, right **knee**
     M25.862 Other specified joint disorders, left **knee**
     M25.869 Other specified joint disorders, unspecified knee ▽

✓6ᵗʰ **M25.87 Other specified joint disorders,** ankle and foot
     M25.871 Other specified joint disorders, right **ankle and foot**
     M25.872 Other specified joint disorders, left **ankle and foot**
     M25.879 Other specified joint disorders, unspecified ankle and foot ▽

     M25.9 Joint disorder, unspecified ▽

Dentofacial anomalies [including malocclusion] and other disorders of jaw (M26-M27)

EXCLUDES 1   hemifacial atrophy or hypertrophy (Q67.4)
           unilateral condylar hyperplasia or hypoplasia (M27.8)

✓4ᵗʰ **M26 Dentofacial anomalies [including malocclusion]**

✓5ᵗʰ **M26.0 Major anomalies of jaw size**
     EXCLUDES 1   acromegaly (E22.0)
              Robin's syndrome (Q87.0)
     M26.00 Unspecified anomaly of jaw size ▽

     M26.01 Maxillary hyperplasia
     M26.02 Maxillary hypoplasia
         AHA: 2014,3Q,23
     M26.03 Mandibular hyperplasia
     M26.04 Mandibular hypoplasia
     M26.05 Macrogenia
     M26.06 Microgenia
     M26.07 Excessive tuberosity of jaw
         Entire maxillary tuberosity
     M26.09 Other specified anomalies of jaw size

✓5ᵗʰ **M26.1 Anomalies of jaw-cranial base relationship**
     M26.10 Unspecified anomaly of jaw-cranial base relationship ▽
     M26.11 Maxillary asymmetry
     M26.12 Other jaw asymmetry
     M26.19 Other specified anomalies of jaw-cranial base relationship

✓5ᵗʰ **M26.2 Anomalies of dental arch relationship**
     M26.20 Unspecified anomaly of dental arch relationship ▽

✓6ᵗʰ **M26.21 Malocclusion, Angle's class**
     M26.211 Malocclusion, Angle's class I
         Neutro-occlusion
     M26.212 Malocclusion, Angle's class II
         Disto-occlusion Division I
         Disto-occlusion Division II
     M26.213 Malocclusion, Angle's class III
         Mesio-occlusion
     M26.219 Malocclusion, Angle's class, unspecified ▽

✓6ᵗʰ **M26.22 Open occlusal relationship**
     M26.220 Open anterior **occlusal relationship**
         Anterior openbite
     M26.221 Open posterior **occlusal relationship**
         Posterior openbite
     M26.23 Excessive horizontal overlap
         Excessive horizontal overjet
     M26.24 Reverse articulation
         Crossbite (anterior) (posterior)
     M26.25 Anomalies of interarch distance
     M26.29 Other anomalies of dental arch relationship
         Midline deviation of dental arch
         Overbite (excessive) deep
         Overbite (excessive) horizontal
         Overbite (excessive) vertical
         Posterior lingual occlusion of mandibular teeth

✓5ᵗʰ **M26.3 Anomalies of tooth position of fully erupted tooth or teeth**
     EXCLUDES 2   embedded and impacted teeth (K01.-)
     M26.30 Unspecified anomaly of tooth position of fully erupted tooth or teeth ▽
         Abnormal spacing of fully erupted tooth or teeth NOS
         Displacement of fully erupted tooth or teeth NOS
         Transposition of fully erupted tooth or teeth NOS
     M26.31 Crowding of fully erupted teeth
     M26.32 Excessive spacing of fully erupted teeth
         Diastema of fully erupted tooth or teeth NOS
     M26.33 Horizontal displacement of fully erupted tooth or teeth
         Tipped tooth or teeth
         Tipping of fully erupted tooth
     M26.34 Vertical displacement of fully erupted tooth or teeth
         Extruded tooth
         Infraeruption of tooth or teeth
         Supraeruption of tooth or teeth
     M26.35 Rotation of fully erupted tooth or teeth
     M26.36 Insufficient interocclusal distance of fully erupted teeth (ridge)
         Lack of adequate intermaxillary vertical dimension of fully erupted teeth
     M26.37 Excessive interocclusal distance of fully erupted teeth
         Excessive intermaxillary vertical dimension of fully erupted teeth
         Loss of occlusal vertical dimension of fully erupted teeth
     M26.39 Other anomalies of tooth position of fully erupted tooth or teeth

EXCLUDES 1   Not coded here   EXCLUDES 2   Not included here   N Newborn Age : 0   P Pediatric Age : 0-17   M Maternity Age : 12-55   A Adult Age : 15-124

732   ICD-10-CM 2017

M26.4 Malocclusion, unspecified ▽

✓5ᵗʰ **M26.5 Dentofacial functional abnormalities**

> EXCLUDES 1   *bruxism (F45.8)*
> *teeth-grinding NOS (F45.8)*

  M26.50 Dentofacial functional abnormalities, unspecified ▽

  M26.51 Abnormal jaw closure

  M26.52 Limited mandibular range of motion

  M26.53 Deviation in opening and closing of the mandible

  M26.54 Insufficient anterior guidance
     Insufficient anterior occlusal guidance

  M26.55 Centric occlusion maximum intercuspation discrepancy
> EXCLUDES 1   *centric occlusion NOS (M26.59)*

  M26.56 Non-working side interference
     Balancing side interference

  M26.57 Lack of posterior occlusal support

  M26.59 Other dentofacial functional abnormalities
     Centric occlusion (of teeth) NOS
     Malocclusion due to abnormal swallowing
     Malocclusion due to mouth breathing
     Malocclusion due to tongue, lip or finger habits

✓5ᵗʰ **M26.6 Temporomandibular joint disorders**

> EXCLUDES 2   *current temporomandibular joint dislocation (S03.0)*
> *current temporomandibular joint sprain (S03.4)*

  ✓6ᵗʰ **M26.60 Temporomandibular joint disorder, unspecified**

●   **M26.601 Right temporomandibular joint disorder, unspecified** ▽

●   **M26.602 Left temporomandibular joint disorder, unspecified** ▽

●   **M26.603 Bilateral temporomandibular joint disorder, unspecified** ▽

●   **M26.609 Unspecified temporomandibular joint disorder, unspecified side** ▽
       Temporomandibular joint disorder NOS

  ✓6ᵗʰ **M26.61 Adhesions and ankylosis of temporomandibular joint**

●   **M26.611 Adhesions and ankylosis of right temporomandibular joint**

●   **M26.612 Adhesions and ankylosis of left temporomandibular joint**

●   **M26.613 Adhesions and ankylosis of bilateral temporomandibular joint**

●   **M26.619 Adhesions and ankylosis of temporomandibular joint, unspecified side** ▽

  ✓6ᵗʰ **M26.62 Arthralgia of temporomandibular joint**

●   **M26.621 Arthralgia of right temporomandibular joint**

●   **M26.622 Arthralgia of left temporomandibular joint**

●   **M26.623 Arthralgia of bilateral temporomandibular joint**

●   **M26.629 Arthralgia of temporomandibular joint, unspecified side** ▽

  ✓6ᵗʰ **M26.63 Articular disc disorder of temporomandibular joint**

●   **M26.631 Articular disc disorder of right temporomandibular joint**

●   **M26.632 Articular disc disorder of left temporomandibular joint**

●   **M26.633 Articular disc disorder of bilateral temporomandibular joint**

●   **M26.639 Articular disc disorder of temporomandibular joint, unspecified side** ▽

  M26.69 Other specified disorders of temporomandibular joint

✓5ᵗʰ **M26.7 Dental alveolar anomalies**

  M26.70 Unspecified alveolar anomaly ▽

  M26.71 Alveolar maxillary hyperplasia

  M26.72 Alveolar mandibular hyperplasia

  M26.73 Alveolar maxillary hypoplasia

  M26.74 Alveolar mandibular hypoplasia

  M26.79 Other specified alveolar anomalies

✓5ᵗʰ **M26.8 Other dentofacial anomalies**

  M26.81 Anterior soft tissue impingement
     Anterior soft tissue impingement on teeth

  M26.82 Posterior soft tissue impingement
     Posterior soft tissue impingement on teeth

  M26.89 Other dentofacial anomalies

M26.9 Dentofacial anomaly, unspecified ▽

✓4ᵗʰ **M27 Other diseases of jaws**

M27.0 Developmental disorders of jaws
   Latent bone cyst of jaw
   Stafne's cyst
   Torus mandibularis
   Torus palatinus

M27.1 Giant cell granuloma, central
   Giant cell granuloma NOS
> EXCLUDES 1   *peripheral giant cell granuloma (K06.8)*

M27.2 Inflammatory conditions of jaws
   Osteitis of jaw(s)
   Osteomyelitis (neonatal) jaw(s)
   Osteoradionecrosis jaw(s)
   Periostitis jaw(s)
   Sequestrum of jaw bone
   Use additional code (W88-W90, X39.0) to identify radiation, if radiation-induced
> EXCLUDES 2   *osteonecrosis of jaw due to drug (M87.180)*

M27.3 Alveolitis of jaws
   Alveolar osteitis
   Dry socket

✓5ᵗʰ **M27.4 Other and unspecified cysts of jaw**
> EXCLUDES 1   *cysts of oral region (K09.-)*
> *latent bone cyst of jaw (M27.0)*
> *Stafne's cyst (M27.0)*

  M27.40 Unspecified cyst of jaw ▽
     Cyst of jaw NOS

  M27.49 Other cysts of jaw
     Aneurysmal cyst of jaw
     Hemorrhagic cyst of jaw
     Traumatic cyst of jaw

✓5ᵗʰ **M27.5 Periradicular pathology associated with previous endodontic treatment**

  M27.51 Perforation of root canal space due to endodontic treatment

  M27.52 Endodontic overfill

  M27.53 Endodontic underfill

  M27.59 Other periradicular pathology associated with previous endodontic treatment

✓5ᵗʰ **M27.6 Endosseous dental implant failure**

  M27.61 Osseointegration failure of dental implant
     Hemorrhagic complications of dental implant placement
     Iatrogenic osseointegration failure of dental implant
     Osseointegration failure of dental implant due to complications of systemic disease
     Osseointegration failure of dental implant due to poor bone quality
     Pre-integration failure of dental implant NOS
     Pre-osseointegration failure of dental implant

  M27.62 Post-osseointegration biological failure of dental implant
     Failure of dental implant due to lack of attached gingiva
     Failure of dental implant due to occlusal trauma (caused by poor prosthetic design)
     Failure of dental implant due to parafunctional habits
     Failure of dental implant due to periodontal infection (peri-implantitis)
     Failure of dental implant due to poor oral hygiene
     Iatrogenic post-osseointegration failure of dental implant
     Post-osseointegration failure of dental implant due to complications of systemic disease

☑ Additional Character Required   ✓7ᵗʰ Placeholder Alert   Manifestation Dx   ▽ Unspecified Dx   ►◄ Revised Text   ● New Code   ▲ Revised Code Title

ICD-10-CM 2017   733

M27.63   **Post-osseointegration mechanical failure of dental implant**
    Failure of dental prosthesis causing loss of dental implant
    Fracture of dental implant
    EXCLUDES 2   *cracked tooth (K03.81)*
       fractured dental restorative material with loss of material (K08.531)
       fractured dental restorative material without loss of material (K08.530)
       fractured tooth (S02.5)

M27.69   **Other endosseous dental implant failure**
    Dental implant failure NOS

M27.8   **Other specified diseases of jaws**
    Cherubism
    Exostosis
    Fibrous dysplasia
    Unilateral condylar hyperplasia
    Unilateral condylar hypoplasia
    EXCLUDES 1   *jaw pain (R68.84)*

M27.9   **Disease of jaws, unspecified** ▽

Systemic connective tissue disorders (M30-M36)

INCLUDES   autoimmune disease NOS
    collagen (vascular) disease NOS
    systemic autoimmune disease
    systemic collagen (vascular) disease
EXCLUDES 1   *autoimmune disease, single organ or single cell-type-code to relevant condition category*

✓4ᵗʰ **M30**   **Polyarteritis nodosa and related conditions**
    EXCLUDES 1   *microscopic polyarteritis (M31.7)*

M30.0   **Polyarteritis nodosa**

M30.1   **Polyarteritis with lung involvement [Churg-Strauss]**
    Allergic granulomatous angiitis

M30.2   **Juvenile polyarteritis**

M30.3   **Mucocutaneous lymph node syndrome [Kawasaki]**

M30.8   **Other conditions related to polyarteritis nodosa**
    Polyangiitis overlap syndrome

✓4ᵗʰ **M31**   **Other necrotizing vasculopathies**

M31.0   **Hypersensitivity angiitis**
    Goodpasture's syndrome

M31.1   **Thrombotic microangiopathy**
    Thrombotic thrombocytopenic purpura

M31.2   **Lethal midline granuloma**

✓5ᵗʰ **M31.3**   **Wegener's granulomatosis**
    Necrotizing respiratory granulomatosis

    M31.30   **Wegener's granulomatosis without renal involvement**
       Wegener's granulomatosis NOS

    M31.31   **Wegener's granulomatosis with renal involvement**

M31.4   **Aortic arch syndrome [Takayasu]**

M31.5   **Giant cell arteritis with polymyalgia rheumatica**

M31.6   **Other giant cell arteritis**

M31.7   **Microscopic polyangiitis**
    Microscopic polyarteritis
    EXCLUDES 1   *polyarteritis nodosa (M30.0)*

M31.8   **Other specified necrotizing vasculopathies**
    Hypocomplementemic vasculitis
    Septic vasculitis

M31.9   **Necrotizing vasculopathy, unspecified** ▽

✓4ᵗʰ **M32**   **Systemic lupus erythematosus (SLE)**
    EXCLUDES 1   *lupus erythematosus (discoid) (NOS) (L93.0)*

M32.0   **Drug-induced systemic lupus erythematosus**
    Use additional code for adverse effect, if applicable, to identify drug (T36-T50 with fifth or sixth character 5)

✓5ᵗʰ **M32.1**   **Systemic lupus erythematosus with organ or system involvement**

    M32.10   **Systemic lupus erythematosus, organ or system involvement unspecified** ▽

    M32.11   **Endocarditis in systemic lupus erythematosus**
       Libman-Sacks disease

    M32.12   **Pericarditis in systemic lupus erythematosus**
       Lupus pericarditis

    M32.13   **Lung involvement in systemic lupus erythematosus**
       Pleural effusion due to systemic lupus erythematosus

    M32.14   **Glomerular disease in systemic lupus erythematosus**
       Lupus renal disease NOS
       AHA: 2013,4Q,125

    M32.15   **Tubulo-interstitial nephropathy in systemic lupus erythematosus**

    M32.19   **Other organ or system involvement in systemic lupus erythematosus**

M32.8   **Other forms of systemic lupus erythematosus**

M32.9   **Systemic lupus erythematosus, unspecified** ▽
    SLE NOS
    Systemic lupus erythematosus NOS
    Systemic lupus erythematosus without organ involvement

✓4ᵗʰ **M33**   **Dermatopolymyositis**

✓5ᵗʰ **M33.0**   **Juvenile dermatopolymyositis**

    M33.00   **Juvenile dermatopolymyositis, organ involvement unspecified** ▽

    M33.01   **Juvenile dermatopolymyositis with respiratory involvement**

    M33.02   **Juvenile dermatopolymyositis with myopathy**

    M33.09   **Juvenile dermatopolymyositis with other organ involvement**

✓5ᵗʰ **M33.1**   **Other dermatopolymyositis**

    M33.10   **Other dermatopolymyositis, organ involvement unspecified** ▽

    M33.11   **Other dermatopolymyositis with respiratory involvement**

    M33.12   **Other dermatopolymyositis with myopathy**

    M33.19   **Other dermatopolymyositis with other organ involvement**

✓5ᵗʰ **M33.2**   **Polymyositis**

    M33.20   **Polymyositis, organ involvement unspecified** ▽

    M33.21   **Polymyositis with respiratory involvement**

    M33.22   **Polymyositis with myopathy**

    M33.29   **Polymyositis with other organ involvement**

✓5ᵗʰ **M33.9**   **Dermatopolymyositis, unspecified**

    M33.90   **Dermatopolymyositis, unspecified, organ involvement unspecified** ▽

    M33.91   **Dermatopolymyositis, unspecified with respiratory involvement** ▽

    M33.92   **Dermatopolymyositis, unspecified with myopathy** ▽

    M33.99   **Dermatopolymyositis, unspecified with other organ involvement** ▽

✓4ᵗʰ **M34**   **Systemic sclerosis [scleroderma]**
    EXCLUDES 1   *circumscribed scleroderma (L94.0)*
       neonatal scleroderma (P83.8)

M34.0   **Progressive systemic sclerosis**

M34.1   **CR(E)ST syndrome**
    Combination of calcinosis, Raynaud's phenomenon, esophageal dysfunction, sclerodactyly, telangiectasia

M34.2   **Systemic sclerosis induced by drug and chemical**
    Code first poisoning due to drug or toxin, if applicable (T36-T65 with fifth or sixth character 1-4 or 6)
    Use additional code for adverse effect, if applicable, to identify drug (T36-T50 with fifth or sixth character 5)

✓5ᵗʰ **M34.8**   **Other forms of systemic sclerosis**

    M34.81   **Systemic sclerosis with lung involvement**
    M34.82   **Systemic sclerosis with myopathy**
    M34.83   **Systemic sclerosis with polyneuropathy**
    M34.89   **Other systemic sclerosis**

M34.9   **Systemic sclerosis, unspecified** ▽

✓4ᵗʰ **M35**   **Other systemic involvement of connective tissue**
    EXCLUDES 1   *reactive perforating collagenosis (L87.1)*

✓5ᵗʰ **M35.0**   **Sicca syndrome [Sjögren]**
    DEF: Autoimmune disease; associated with keratoconjunctivitis, laryngopharyngitis, rhinitis, dry mouth, enlarged parotid gland, and chronic polyarthritis.

    M35.00   **Sicca syndrome, unspecified** ▽

    M35.01   **Sicca syndrome with keratoconjunctivitis**

    M35.02   **Sicca syndrome with lung involvement**

    M35.03   **Sicca syndrome with myopathy**

EXCLUDES 1   Not coded here   EXCLUDES 2   Not included here   N Newborn Age : 0   P Pediatric Age : 0-17   M Maternity Age : 12-55   A Adult Age : 15-124

734   ICD-10-CM 2017

M35.04 **Sicca syndrome with tubulo-interstitial nephropathy**
Renal tubular acidosis in sicca syndrome

M35.09 **Sicca syndrome with other organ involvement**

M35.1 **Other overlap syndromes**
Mixed connective tissue disease
EXCLUDES 1 *polyangiitis overlap syndrome (M30.8)*

M35.2 **Behçet's disease**

M35.3 **Polymyalgia rheumatica**
EXCLUDES 1 *polymyalgia rheumatica with giant cell arteritis (M31.5)*

M35.4 **Diffuse (eosinophilic) fasciitis**

M35.5 **Multifocal fibrosclerosis**

M35.6 **Relapsing panniculitis [Weber-Christian]**
EXCLUDES 1 *lupus panniculitis (L93.2)*
panniculitis NOS (M79.3-)

M35.7 **Hypermobility syndrome**
Familial ligamentous laxity
EXCLUDES 1 *Ehlers-Danlos syndrome (Q79.6)*
ligamentous laxity, NOS (M24.2-)

M35.8 **Other specified systemic involvement of connective tissue**

M35.9 **Systemic involvement of connective tissue, unspecified** ▽
Autoimmune disease (systemic) NOS
Collagen (vascular) disease NOS

☑4ᵗʰ **M36 Systemic disorders of connective tissue in diseases classified elsewhere**
EXCLUDES 2 *arthropathies in diseases classified elsewhere (M14.-)*

M36.0 *Dermato(poly)myositis in neoplastic disease*
Code first underlying neoplasm (C00-D49)

M36.1 *Arthropathy in neoplastic disease*
Code first underlying neoplasm, such as:
leukemia (C91-C95)
malignant histiocytosis (C96.A)
multiple myeloma (C90.0)

M36.2 *Hemophilic arthropathy*
Hemarthrosis in hemophilic arthropathy
Code first underlying disease, such as:
factor VIII deficiency (D66)
with vascular defect (D68.0)
factor IX deficiency (D67)
hemophilia (classical) (D66)
hemophilia B (D67)
hemophilia C (D68.1)

M36.3 *Arthropathy in other blood disorders*

M36.4 *Arthropathy in hypersensitivity reactions classified elsewhere*
Code first underlying disease, such as:
Henoch (-Schönlein) purpura (D69.0)
serum sickness (T80.6-)

M36.8 *Systemic disorders of connective tissue in other diseases classified elsewhere*
Code first underlying disease, such as:
alkaptonuria (E70.2)
hypogammaglobulinemia (D80.-)
ochronosis (E70.2)

Dorsopathies (M40-M54)

Deforming dorsopathies (M40-M43)

☑4ᵗʰ **M40 Kyphosis and lordosis**
EXCLUDES 1 *congenital kyphosis and lordosis (Q76.4)*
kyphoscoliosis (M41.-)
postprocedural kyphosis and lordosis (M96.-)

Kyphosis and Lordosis

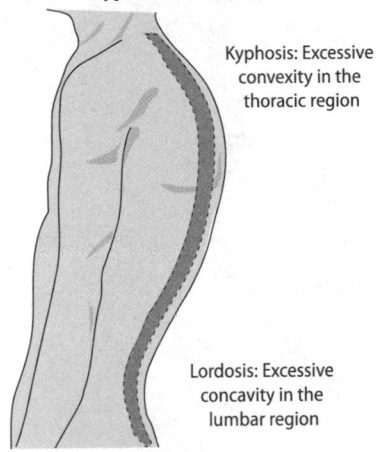

Kyphosis: Excessive convexity in the thoracic region

Lordosis: Excessive concavity in the lumbar region

☑5ᵗʰ **M40.0 Postural kyphosis**
EXCLUDES 1 *osteochondrosis of spine (M42.-)*
M40.00 **Postural kyphosis, site unspecified** ▽
M40.03 **Postural kyphosis, cervicothoracic region**
M40.04 **Postural kyphosis, thoracic region**
M40.05 **Postural kyphosis, thoracolumbar region**

☑5ᵗʰ **M40.1 Other secondary kyphosis**
M40.10 **Other secondary kyphosis, site unspecified** ▽
M40.12 **Other secondary kyphosis, cervical region**
M40.13 **Other secondary kyphosis, cervicothoracic region**
M40.14 **Other secondary kyphosis, thoracic region**
M40.15 **Other secondary kyphosis, thoracolumbar region**

☑5ᵗʰ **M40.2 Other and unspecified kyphosis**
☑6ᵗʰ **M40.20 Unspecified kyphosis**
M40.202 **Unspecified kyphosis, cervical region** ▽
M40.203 **Unspecified kyphosis, cervicothoracic region** ▽
M40.204 **Unspecified kyphosis, thoracic region** ▽
M40.205 **Unspecified kyphosis, thoracolumbar region** ▽
M40.209 **Unspecified kyphosis, site unspecified** ▽

☑6ᵗʰ **M40.29 Other kyphosis**
M40.292 **Other kyphosis, cervical region**
M40.293 **Other kyphosis, cervicothoracic region**
M40.294 **Other kyphosis, thoracic region**
M40.295 **Other kyphosis, thoracolumbar region**
M40.299 **Other kyphosis, site unspecified** ▽

☑5ᵗʰ **M40.3 Flatback syndrome**
M40.30 **Flatback syndrome, site unspecified** ▽
M40.35 **Flatback syndrome, thoracolumbar region**
M40.36 **Flatback syndrome, lumbar region**
M40.37 **Flatback syndrome, lumbosacral region**

☑5ᵗʰ **M40.4 Postural lordosis**
Acquired lordosis
M40.40 **Postural lordosis, site unspecified** ▽
M40.45 **Postural lordosis, thoracolumbar region**
M40.46 **Postural lordosis, lumbar region**
M40.47 **Postural lordosis, lumbosacral region**

☑5ᵗʰ **M40.5 Lordosis, unspecified**
M40.50 **Lordosis, unspecified, site unspecified** ▽
M40.55 **Lordosis, unspecified, thoracolumbar region**

☑ Additional Character Required   ✓x7ᵗʰ Placeholder Alert   Manifestation Dx   ▽ Unspecified Dx   ►◄ Revised Text   ● New Code   ▲ Revised Code Title

ICD-10-CM 2017   **735**

M40.56 Lordosis, unspecified, **lumbar region**
M40.57 Lordosis, unspecified, **lumbosacral region**

✓4ᵗʰ **M41 Scoliosis**

> **INCLUDES** kyphoscoliosis
> **EXCLUDES 1** congenital scoliosis due to bony malformation (Q76.3)
> congenital scoliosis NOS (Q67.5)
> kyphoscoliotic heart disease (I27.1)
> postprocedural scoliosis (M96.-)
> postural congenital scoliosis (Q67.5)

Scoliosis

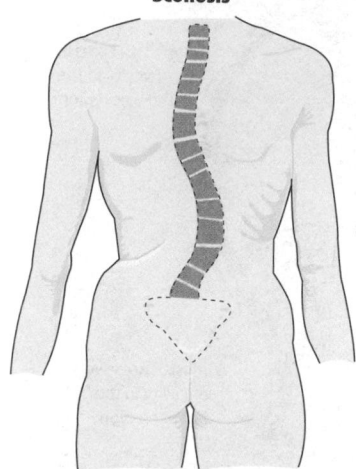

Lateral curvature of spine

✓6ᵗʰ **M41.0 Infantile idiopathic scoliosis**

> **AHA:** 2014,4Q,26

M41.00 **Infantile idiopathic scoliosis, site unspecified** ▽
M41.02 **Infantile idiopathic scoliosis, cervical region**
M41.03 **Infantile idiopathic scoliosis, cervicothoracic region**
M41.04 **Infantile idiopathic scoliosis, thoracic region**
M41.05 **Infantile idiopathic scoliosis, thoracolumbar region**
M41.06 **Infantile idiopathic scoliosis, lumbar region**
M41.07 **Infantile idiopathic scoliosis, lumbosacral region**
M41.08 **Infantile idiopathic scoliosis, sacral and sacrococcygeal region**

✓5ᵗʰ **M41.1 Juvenile and adolescent idiopathic scoliosis**

✓6ᵗʰ **M41.11 Juvenile idiopathic scoliosis**

> **AHA:** 2014,4Q,28

M41.112 **Juvenile idiopathic scoliosis, cervical region**
M41.113 **Juvenile idiopathic scoliosis, cervicothoracic region**
M41.114 **Juvenile idiopathic scoliosis, thoracic region**
M41.115 **Juvenile idiopathic scoliosis, thoracolumbar region**
M41.116 **Juvenile idiopathic scoliosis, lumbar region**
M41.117 **Juvenile idiopathic scoliosis, lumbosacral region**
M41.119 **Juvenile idiopathic scoliosis, site unspecified** ▽

✓6ᵗʰ **M41.12 Adolescent scoliosis**

M41.122 **Adolescent idiopathic scoliosis, cervical region**
M41.123 **Adolescent idiopathic scoliosis, cervicothoracic region**
M41.124 **Adolescent idiopathic scoliosis, thoracic region**
M41.125 **Adolescent idiopathic scoliosis, thoracolumbar region**
M41.126 **Adolescent idiopathic scoliosis, lumbar region**
M41.127 **Adolescent idiopathic scoliosis, lumbosacral region**
M41.129 **Adolescent idiopathic scoliosis, site unspecified** ▽

✓5ᵗʰ **M41.2 Other idiopathic scoliosis**

M41.20 **Other idiopathic scoliosis, site unspecified** ▽

M41.22 **Other idiopathic scoliosis, cervical region**
M41.23 **Other idiopathic scoliosis, cervicothoracic region**
M41.24 **Other idiopathic scoliosis, thoracic region**
M41.25 **Other idiopathic scoliosis, thoracolumbar region**
M41.26 **Other idiopathic scoliosis, lumbar region**
M41.27 **Other idiopathic scoliosis, lumbosacral region**

✓5ᵗʰ **M41.3 Thoracogenic scoliosis**

M41.30 **Thoracogenic scoliosis, site unspecified** ▽
M41.34 **Thoracogenic scoliosis, thoracic region**
M41.35 **Thoracogenic scoliosis, thoracolumbar region**

✓5ᵗʰ **M41.4 Neuromuscular scoliosis**

> Scoliosis secondary to cerebral palsy, Friedreich's ataxia, poliomyelitis and other neuromuscular disorders
> Code also underlying condition
> **AHA:** 2014,4Q,27

M41.40 **Neuromuscular scoliosis, site unspecified** ▽
M41.41 **Neuromuscular scoliosis, occipito-atlanto-axial region**
M41.42 **Neuromuscular scoliosis, cervical region**
M41.43 **Neuromuscular scoliosis, cervicothoracic region**
M41.44 **Neuromuscular scoliosis, thoracic region**
M41.45 **Neuromuscular scoliosis, thoracolumbar region**
M41.46 **Neuromuscular scoliosis, lumbar region**
M41.47 **Neuromuscular scoliosis, lumbosacral region**

✓5ᵗʰ **M41.5 Other secondary scoliosis**

M41.50 **Other secondary scoliosis, site unspecified** ▽
M41.52 **Other secondary scoliosis, cervical region**
M41.53 **Other secondary scoliosis, cervicothoracic region**
M41.54 **Other secondary scoliosis, thoracic region**
M41.55 **Other secondary scoliosis, thoracolumbar region**
M41.56 **Other secondary scoliosis, lumbar region**
M41.57 **Other secondary scoliosis, lumbosacral region**

✓5ᵗʰ **M41.8 Other forms of scoliosis**

M41.80 **Other forms of scoliosis, site unspecified** ▽
M41.82 **Other forms of scoliosis, cervical region**
M41.83 **Other forms of scoliosis, cervicothoracic region**
M41.84 **Other forms of scoliosis, thoracic region**
M41.85 **Other forms of scoliosis, thoracolumbar region**
M41.86 **Other forms of scoliosis, lumbar region**
M41.87 **Other forms of scoliosis, lumbosacral region**

M41.9 **Scoliosis, unspecified** ▽

✓4ᵗʰ **M42 Spinal osteochondrosis**

✓5ᵗʰ **M42.0 Juvenile osteochondrosis of spine**

> Calvé's disease
> Scheuermann's disease
> **EXCLUDES 1** postural kyphosis (M40.0)

M42.00 **Juvenile osteochondrosis of spine, site unspecified** ▽
M42.01 **Juvenile osteochondrosis of spine, occipito-atlanto-axial region**
M42.02 **Juvenile osteochondrosis of spine, cervical region**
M42.03 **Juvenile osteochondrosis of spine, cervicothoracic region**
M42.04 **Juvenile osteochondrosis of spine, thoracic region**
M42.05 **Juvenile osteochondrosis of spine, thoracolumbar region**
M42.06 **Juvenile osteochondrosis of spine, lumbar region**
M42.07 **Juvenile osteochondrosis of spine, lumbosacral region**
M42.08 **Juvenile osteochondrosis of spine, sacral and sacrococcygeal region**
M42.09 **Juvenile osteochondrosis of spine, multiple sites in spine**

✓5ᵗʰ **M42.1 Adult osteochondrosis of spine**

M42.10 **Adult osteochondrosis of spine, site unspecified** Ⓐ ▽
M42.11 **Adult osteochondrosis of spine, occipito-atlanto-axial region** Ⓐ
M42.12 **Adult osteochondrosis of spine, cervical region** Ⓐ
M42.13 **Adult osteochondrosis of spine, cervicothoracic region** Ⓐ
M42.14 **Adult osteochondrosis of spine, thoracic region** Ⓐ
M42.15 **Adult osteochondrosis of spine, thoracolumbar region** Ⓐ

M42.16   Adult osteochondrosis of spine, lumbar region   🅰

M42.17   Adult osteochondrosis of spine, lumbosacral region   🅰

M42.18   Adult osteochondrosis of spine, sacral and sacrococcygeal region   🅰

M42.19   Adult osteochondrosis of spine, multiple sites in spine   🅰

M42.9   Spinal osteochondrosis, unspecified   ▽

✓4th M43   Other deforming dorsopathies

EXCLUDES 1   *congenital spondylolysis and spondylolisthesis (Q76.2)*
hemivertebra (Q76.3-Q76.4)
Klippel-Feil syndrome (Q76.1)
lumbarization and sacralization (Q76.4)
platyspondylisis (Q76.4)
spina bifida occulta (Q76.0)
spinal curvature in osteoporosis (M80.-)
spinal curvature in Paget's disease of bone [osteitis deformans] (M88.-)

✓5th M43.0   Spondylolysis

EXCLUDES 1   *congenital spondylolysis (Q76.2)*
spondylolisthesis (M43.1)

M43.00   Spondylolysis, site unspecified   ▽

M43.01   Spondylolysis, occipito-atlanto-axial region

M43.02   Spondylolysis, cervical region

M43.03   Spondylolysis, cervicothoracic region

M43.04   Spondylolysis, thoracic region

M43.05   Spondylolysis, thoracolumbar region

M43.06   Spondylolysis, lumbar region

M43.07   Spondylolysis, lumbosacral region

M43.08   Spondylolysis, sacral and sacrococcygeal region

M43.09   Spondylolysis, multiple sites in spine

✓5th M43.1   Spondylolisthesis

EXCLUDES 1   *acute traumatic of lumbosacral region (S33.1)*
acute traumatic of sites other than lumbosacral- code to Fracture, vertebra, by region
congenital spondylolisthesis (Q76.2)

M43.10   Spondylolisthesis, site unspecified   ▽

M43.11   Spondylolisthesis, occipito-atlanto-axial region

M43.12   Spondylolisthesis, cervical region

M43.13   Spondylolisthesis, cervicothoracic region

M43.14   Spondylolisthesis, thoracic region

M43.15   Spondylolisthesis, thoracolumbar region

M43.16   Spondylolisthesis, lumbar region

M43.17   Spondylolisthesis, lumbosacral region

M43.18   Spondylolisthesis, sacral and sacrococcygeal region

M43.19   Spondylolisthesis, multiple sites in spine

✓5th M43.2   Fusion of spine

Ankylosis of spinal joint

EXCLUDES 1   *ankylosing spondylitis (M45.0-)*
congenital fusion of spine (Q76.4)

EXCLUDES 2   *arthrodesis status (Z98.1)*
pseudoarthrosis after fusion or arthrodesis (M96.0)

M43.20   Fusion of spine, site unspecified   ▽

M43.21   Fusion of spine, occipito-atlanto-axial region

M43.22   Fusion of spine, cervical region

M43.23   Fusion of spine, cervicothoracic region

M43.24   Fusion of spine, thoracic region

M43.25   Fusion of spine, thoracolumbar region

M43.26   Fusion of spine, lumbar region

M43.27   Fusion of spine, lumbosacral region

M43.28   Fusion of spine, sacral and sacrococcygeal region

M43.3   Recurrent atlantoaxial dislocation with myelopathy

M43.4   Other recurrent atlantoaxial dislocation

✓5th M43.5   Other recurrent vertebral dislocation

EXCLUDES 1   *biomechanical lesions NEC (M99.-)*

✓6th M43.5X   Other recurrent vertebral dislocation

M43.5X2   Other recurrent vertebral dislocation, cervical region

M43.5X3   Other recurrent vertebral dislocation, cervicothoracic region

M43.5X4   Other recurrent vertebral dislocation, thoracic region

M43.5X5   Other recurrent vertebral dislocation, thoracolumbar region

M43.5X6   Other recurrent vertebral dislocation, lumbar region

M43.5X7   Other recurrent vertebral dislocation, lumbosacral region

M43.5X8   Other recurrent vertebral dislocation, sacral and sacrococcygeal region

M43.5X9   Other recurrent vertebral dislocation, site unspecified   ▽

M43.6   Torticollis

EXCLUDES 1   *congenital (sternomastoid) torticollis (Q68.0)*
current injury - see Injury, of spine, by body region
ocular torticollis (R29.891)
psychogenic torticollis (F45.8)
spasmodic torticollis (G24.3)
torticollis due to birth injury (P15.2)

✓5th M43.8   Other specified deforming dorsopathies

EXCLUDES 2   *kyphosis and lordosis (M40.-)*
scoliosis (M41.-)

✓6th M43.8X   Other specified deforming dorsopathies

M43.8X1   Other specified deforming dorsopathies, occipito-atlanto-axial region

M43.8X2   Other specified deforming dorsopathies, cervical region

M43.8X3   Other specified deforming dorsopathies, cervicothoracic region

M43.8X4   Other specified deforming dorsopathies, thoracic region

M43.8X5   Other specified deforming dorsopathies, thoracolumbar region

M43.8X6   Other specified deforming dorsopathies, lumbar region

M43.8X7   Other specified deforming dorsopathies, lumbosacral region

M43.8X8   Other specified deforming dorsopathies, sacral and sacrococcygeal region

M43.8X9   Other specified deforming dorsopathies, site unspecified   ▽

M43.9   Deforming dorsopathy, unspecified   ▽

Curvature of spine NOS

Spondylopathies (M45-M49)

✓4th M45   Ankylosing spondylitis

Rheumatoid arthritis of spine

EXCLUDES 1   *arthropathy in Reiter's disease (M02.3-)*
juvenile (ankylosing) spondylitis (M08.1)

EXCLUDES 2   *Behçet's disease (M35.2)*

M45.0   Ankylosing spondylitis of multiple sites in spine

M45.1   Ankylosing spondylitis of occipito-atlanto-axial region

M45.2   Ankylosing spondylitis of cervical region

M45.3   Ankylosing spondylitis of cervicothoracic region

M45.4   Ankylosing spondylitis of thoracic region

M45.5   Ankylosing spondylitis of thoracolumbar region

M45.6   Ankylosing spondylitis lumbar region

M45.7   Ankylosing spondylitis of lumbosacral region

M45.8   Ankylosing spondylitis sacral and sacrococcygeal region

M45.9   Ankylosing spondylitis of unspecified sites in spine   ▽

✓4th M46   Other inflammatory spondylopathies

✓5th M46.0   Spinal enthesopathy

Disorder of ligamentous or muscular attachments of spine

M46.00   Spinal enthesopathy, site unspecified   ▽

M46.01   Spinal enthesopathy, occipito-atlanto-axial region

M46.02   Spinal enthesopathy, cervical region

M46.03   Spinal enthesopathy, cervicothoracic region

M46.04   Spinal enthesopathy, thoracic region

M46.05   Spinal enthesopathy, thoracolumbar region

M46.06   Spinal enthesopathy, lumbar region

M46.07   Spinal enthesopathy, lumbosacral region

M46.08   Spinal enthesopathy, sacral and sacrococcygeal region

M46.09   Spinal enthesopathy, multiple sites in spine

M46.1   Sacroiliitis, not elsewhere classified

✓5th M46.2   Osteomyelitis of vertebra

M46.20   Osteomyelitis of vertebra, site unspecified   ▽

M46.21   Osteomyelitis of vertebra, occipito-atlanto-axial region

M46.22   Osteomyelitis of vertebra, cervical region

☑ Additional Character Required   ✓x7th Placeholder Alert   Manifestation Dx   ▽ Unspecified Dx   ►◄ Revised Text   ● New Code   ▲ Revised Code Title

ICD-10-CM 2017   **737**

M46.23 **Osteomyelitis of vertebra,** cervicothoracic **region**

M46.24 **Osteomyelitis of vertebra,** thoracic **region**

M46.25 **Osteomyelitis of vertebra,** thoracolumbar **region**

M46.26 **Osteomyelitis of vertebra,** lumbar **region**

M46.27 **Osteomyelitis of vertebra,** lumbosacral **region**

M46.28 **Osteomyelitis of vertebra,** sacral and sacrococcygeal **region**

√5ᵗʰ M46.3 **Infection of intervertebral disc (pyogenic)**

Use additional code (B95-B97) to identify infectious agent

M46.30 **Infection of intervertebral disc (pyogenic), site unspecified**

M46.31 **Infection of intervertebral disc (pyogenic),** occipito-atlanto-axial **region**

M46.32 **Infection of intervertebral disc (pyogenic),** cervical **region**

M46.33 **Infection of intervertebral disc (pyogenic),** cervicothoracic **region**

M46.34 **Infection of intervertebral disc (pyogenic),** thoracic **region**

M46.35 **Infection of intervertebral disc (pyogenic),** thoracolumbar **region**

M46.36 **Infection of intervertebral disc (pyogenic),** lumbar **region**

M46.37 **Infection of intervertebral disc (pyogenic),** lumbosacral **region**

M46.38 **Infection of intervertebral disc (pyogenic),** sacral and sacrococcygeal **region**

M46.39 **Infection of intervertebral disc (pyogenic),** multiple sites **in spine**

√5ᵗʰ M46.4 **Discitis, unspecified**

M46.40 **Discitis, unspecified, site unspecified** ▽

M46.41 **Discitis, unspecified,** occipito-atlanto-axial **region** ▽

M46.42 **Discitis, unspecified,** cervical **region** ▽

M46.43 **Discitis, unspecified,** cervicothoracic **region** ▽

M46.44 **Discitis, unspecified,** thoracic **region** ▽

M46.45 **Discitis, unspecified,** thoracolumbar **region** ▽

M46.46 **Discitis, unspecified,** lumbar **region** ▽

M46.47 **Discitis, unspecified,** lumbosacral **region** ▽

M46.48 **Discitis, unspecified,** sacral and sacrococcygeal **region** ▽

M46.49 **Discitis, unspecified,** multiple sites **in spine** ▽

√5ᵗʰ M46.5 **Other infective spondylopathies**

M46.50 **Other infective spondylopathies, site unspecified** ▽

M46.51 **Other infective spondylopathies,** occipito-atlanto-axial **region**

M46.52 **Other infective spondylopathies,** cervical **region**

M46.53 **Other infective spondylopathies,** cervicothoracic **region**

M46.54 **Other infective spondylopathies,** thoracic **region**

M46.55 **Other infective spondylopathies,** thoracolumbar **region**

M46.56 **Other infective spondylopathies,** lumbar **region**

M46.57 **Other infective spondylopathies,** lumbosacral **region**

M46.58 **Other infective spondylopathies,** sacral and sacrococcygeal **region**

M46.59 **Other infective spondylopathies,** multiple sites **in spine**

√5ᵗʰ M46.8 **Other specified inflammatory spondylopathies**

M46.80 **Other specified inflammatory spondylopathies, site unspecified** ▽

M46.81 **Other specified inflammatory spondylopathies,** occipito-atlanto-axial **region**

M46.82 **Other specified inflammatory spondylopathies,** cervical **region**

M46.83 **Other specified inflammatory spondylopathies,** cervicothoracic **region**

M46.84 **Other specified inflammatory spondylopathies,** thoracic **region**

M46.85 **Other specified inflammatory spondylopathies,** thoracolumbar **region**

M46.86 **Other specified inflammatory spondylopathies,** lumbar **region**

M46.87 **Other specified inflammatory spondylopathies,** lumbosacral **region**

M46.88 **Other specified inflammatory spondylopathies,** sacral and sacrococcygeal **region**

M46.89 **Other specified inflammatory spondylopathies,** multiple sites **in spine**

√5ᵗʰ M46.9 **Unspecified inflammatory spondylopathy**

M46.90 **Unspecified inflammatory spondylopathy, site unspecified** ▽

M46.91 **Unspecified inflammatory spondylopathy,** occipito-atlanto-axial **region** ▽

M46.92 **Unspecified inflammatory spondylopathy,** cervical **region** ▽

M46.93 **Unspecified inflammatory spondylopathy,** cervicothoracic **region** ▽

M46.94 **Unspecified inflammatory spondylopathy,** thoracic **region** ▽

M46.95 **Unspecified inflammatory spondylopathy,** thoracolumbar **region** ▽

M46.96 **Unspecified inflammatory spondylopathy,** lumbar **region** ▽

M46.97 **Unspecified inflammatory spondylopathy,** lumbosacral **region** ▽

M46.98 **Unspecified inflammatory spondylopathy,** sacral and sacrococcygeal **region** ▽

M46.99 **Unspecified inflammatory spondylopathy,** multiple sites **in spine** ▽

√4ᵗʰ **M47 Spondylosis**

INCLUDES arthrosis or osteoarthritis of spine
degeneration of facet joints

√5ᵗʰ M47.0 **Anterior spinal and vertebral artery** compression syndromes

√6ᵗʰ M47.01 Anterior spinal artery compression syndromes

M47.011 **Anterior spinal artery compression syndromes,** occipito-atlanto-axial **region**

M47.012 **Anterior spinal artery compression syndromes,** cervical **region**

M47.013 **Anterior spinal artery compression syndromes,** cervicothoracic **region**

M47.014 **Anterior spinal artery compression syndromes,** thoracic **region**

M47.015 **Anterior spinal artery compression syndromes,** thoracolumbar **region**

M47.016 **Anterior spinal artery compression syndromes,** lumbar **region**

M47.019 **Anterior spinal artery compression syndromes, site unspecified** ▽

√6ᵗʰ M47.02 Vertebral artery compression syndromes

M47.021 **Vertebral artery compression syndromes,** occipito-atlanto-axial **region**

M47.022 **Vertebral artery compression syndromes,** cervical **region**

M47.029 **Vertebral artery compression syndromes, site unspecified** ▽

√5ᵗʰ M47.1 **Other spondylosis** with myelopathy

Spondylogenic compression of spinal cord
EXCLUDES 1 vertebral subluxation (M43.3-M43.59)

M47.10 **Other spondylosis with myelopathy, site unspecified** ▽

M47.11 **Other spondylosis with myelopathy,** occipito-atlanto-axial **region**

M47.12 **Other spondylosis with myelopathy,** cervical **region**

M47.13 **Other spondylosis with myelopathy,** cervicothoracic **region**

M47.14 **Other spondylosis with myelopathy,** thoracic **region**

M47.15 **Other spondylosis with myelopathy,** thoracolumbar **region**

M47.16 **Other spondylosis with myelopathy,** lumbar **region**

√5ᵗʰ M47.2 **Other spondylosis** with radiculopathy

M47.20 **Other spondylosis with radiculopathy, site unspecified** ▽

M47.21 **Other spondylosis with radiculopathy,** occipito-atlanto-axial **region**

M47.22 **Other spondylosis with radiculopathy,** cervical **region**

M47.23 **Other spondylosis with radiculopathy,** cervicothoracic **region**

M47.24 **Other spondylosis with radiculopathy,** thoracic **region**

M47.25 **Other spondylosis with radiculopathy,** thoracolumbar **region**

M47.26 **Other spondylosis with radiculopathy,** lumbar **region**

EXCLUDES 1 Not coded here   EXCLUDES 2 Not included here   N Newborn Age : 0   P Pediatric Age : 0-17   M Maternity Age : 12-55   A Adult Age : 15-124

738   ICD-10-CM 2017

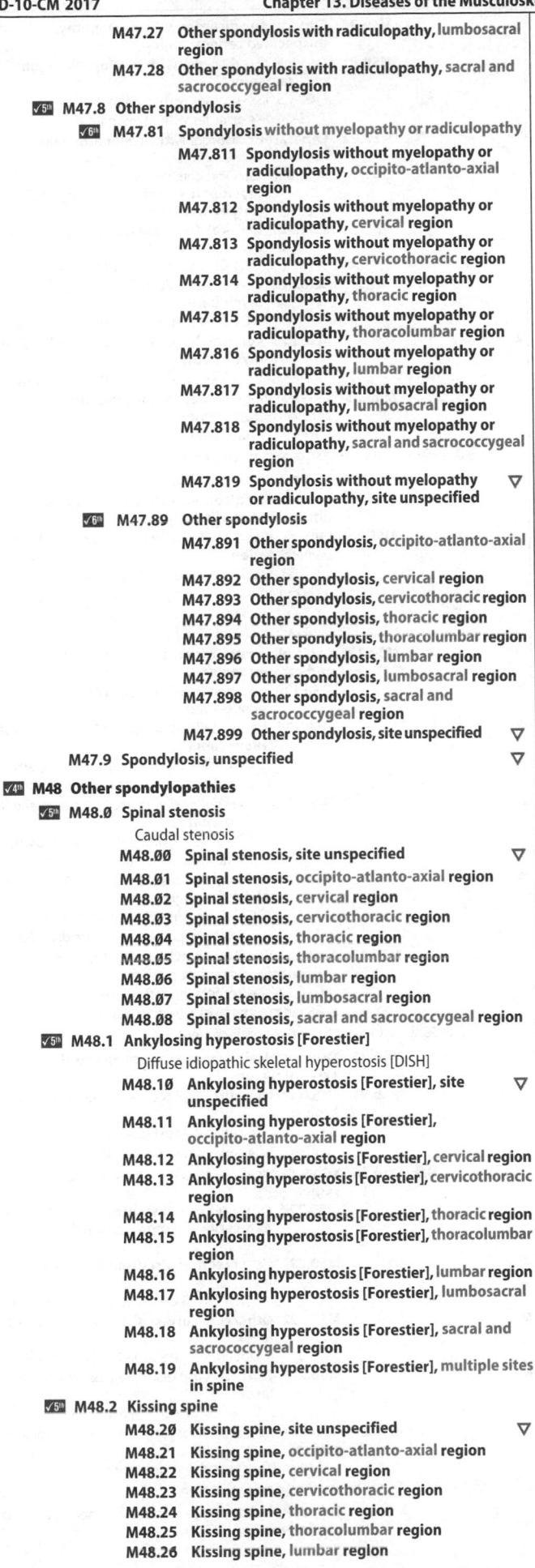

M47.27   **Other spondylosis with radiculopathy, lumbosacral region**

M47.28   **Other spondylosis with radiculopathy, sacral and sacrococcygeal region**

√5ᵗʰ **M47.8**   **Other spondylosis**

√6ᵗʰ **M47.81**   **Spondylosis without myelopathy or radiculopathy**

M47.811   **Spondylosis without myelopathy or radiculopathy, occipito-atlanto-axial region**

M47.812   **Spondylosis without myelopathy or radiculopathy, cervical region**

M47.813   **Spondylosis without myelopathy or radiculopathy, cervicothoracic region**

M47.814   **Spondylosis without myelopathy or radiculopathy, thoracic region**

M47.815   **Spondylosis without myelopathy or radiculopathy, thoracolumbar region**

M47.816   **Spondylosis without myelopathy or radiculopathy, lumbar region**

M47.817   **Spondylosis without myelopathy or radiculopathy, lumbosacral region**

M47.818   **Spondylosis without myelopathy or radiculopathy, sacral and sacrococcygeal region**

M47.819   **Spondylosis without myelopathy or radiculopathy, site unspecified** ▽

√6ᵗʰ **M47.89**   **Other spondylosis**

M47.891   **Other spondylosis, occipito-atlanto-axial region**

M47.892   **Other spondylosis, cervical region**

M47.893   **Other spondylosis, cervicothoracic region**

M47.894   **Other spondylosis, thoracic region**

M47.895   **Other spondylosis, thoracolumbar region**

M47.896   **Other spondylosis, lumbar region**

M47.897   **Other spondylosis, lumbosacral region**

M47.898   **Other spondylosis, sacral and sacrococcygeal region**

M47.899   **Other spondylosis, site unspecified** ▽

M47.9   **Spondylosis, unspecified** ▽

√4ᵗʰ **M48**   **Other spondylopathies**

√5ᵗʰ **M48.0**   **Spinal stenosis**

Caudal stenosis

M48.00   **Spinal stenosis, site unspecified** ▽

M48.01   **Spinal stenosis, occipito-atlanto-axial region**

M48.02   **Spinal stenosis, cervical region**

M48.03   **Spinal stenosis, cervicothoracic region**

M48.04   **Spinal stenosis, thoracic region**

M48.05   **Spinal stenosis, thoracolumbar region**

M48.06   **Spinal stenosis, lumbar region**

M48.07   **Spinal stenosis, lumbosacral region**

M48.08   **Spinal stenosis, sacral and sacrococcygeal region**

√5ᵗʰ **M48.1**   **Ankylosing hyperostosis [Forestier]**

Diffuse idiopathic skeletal hyperostosis [DISH]

M48.10   **Ankylosing hyperostosis [Forestier], site unspecified** ▽

M48.11   **Ankylosing hyperostosis [Forestier], occipito-atlanto-axial region**

M48.12   **Ankylosing hyperostosis [Forestier], cervical region**

M48.13   **Ankylosing hyperostosis [Forestier], cervicothoracic region**

M48.14   **Ankylosing hyperostosis [Forestier], thoracic region**

M48.15   **Ankylosing hyperostosis [Forestier], thoracolumbar region**

M48.16   **Ankylosing hyperostosis [Forestier], lumbar region**

M48.17   **Ankylosing hyperostosis [Forestier], lumbosacral region**

M48.18   **Ankylosing hyperostosis [Forestier], sacral and sacrococcygeal region**

M48.19   **Ankylosing hyperostosis [Forestier], multiple sites in spine**

√5ᵗʰ **M48.2**   **Kissing spine**

M48.20   **Kissing spine, site unspecified** ▽

M48.21   **Kissing spine, occipito-atlanto-axial region**

M48.22   **Kissing spine, cervical region**

M48.23   **Kissing spine, cervicothoracic region**

M48.24   **Kissing spine, thoracic region**

M48.25   **Kissing spine, thoracolumbar region**

M48.26   **Kissing spine, lumbar region**

M48.27   **Kissing spine, lumbosacral region**

√5ᵗʰ **M48.3**   **Traumatic spondylopathy**

M48.30   **Traumatic spondylopathy, site unspecified** ▽

M48.31   **Traumatic spondylopathy, occipito-atlanto-axial region**

M48.32   **Traumatic spondylopathy, cervical region**

M48.33   **Traumatic spondylopathy, cervicothoracic region**

M48.34   **Traumatic spondylopathy, thoracic region**

M48.35   **Traumatic spondylopathy, thoracolumbar region**

M48.36   **Traumatic spondylopathy, lumbar region**

M48.37   **Traumatic spondylopathy, lumbosacral region**

M48.38   **Traumatic spondylopathy, sacral and sacrococcygeal region**

√5ᵗʰ **M48.4**   **Fatigue fracture of vertebra**

Stress fracture of vertebra

EXCLUDES 1   *pathological fracture NOS (M84.4-)*
pathological fracture of vertebra due to neoplasm (M84.58)
pathological fracture of vertebra due to osteoporosis (M80.-)
pathological fracture of vertebra due to other diagnosis (M84.68)
traumatic fracture of vertebrae (S12.0-S12.3-, S22.0-, S32.0-)

The appropriate 7th character is to be added to each code from subcategory M48.4.
A   initial encounter for fracture
D   subsequent encounter for fracture with routine healing
G   subsequent encounter for fracture with delayed healing
S   sequela of fracture

√x7ᵗʰ **M48.40**   **Fatigue fracture of vertebra, site unspecified** ▽

√x7ᵗʰ **M48.41**   **Fatigue fracture of vertebra, occipito-atlanto-axial region**

√x7ᵗʰ **M48.42**   **Fatigue fracture of vertebra, cervical region**

√x7ᵗʰ **M48.43**   **Fatigue fracture of vertebra, cervicothoracic region**

√x7ᵗʰ **M48.44**   **Fatigue fracture of vertebra, thoracic region**

√x7ᵗʰ **M48.45**   **Fatigue fracture of vertebra, thoracolumbar region**

√x7ᵗʰ **M48.46**   **Fatigue fracture of vertebra, lumbar region**

√x7ᵗʰ **M48.47**   **Fatigue fracture of vertebra, lumbosacral region**

√x7ᵗʰ **M48.48**   **Fatigue fracture of vertebra, sacral and sacrococcygeal region**

√5ᵗʰ **M48.5**   **Collapsed vertebra, not elsewhere classified**

Collapsed vertebra NOS
►Compression fracture of vertebra NOS◄
Wedging of vertebra NOS

EXCLUDES 1   *current injury - see Injury of spine, by body region*
fatigue fracture of vertebra (M48.4)
pathological fracture NOS (M84.4-)
pathological fracture of vertebra due to neoplasm (M84.58)
pathological fracture of vertebra due to osteoporosis (M80.-)
pathological fracture of vertebra due to other diagnosis (M84.68)
stress fracture of vertebra (M48.4-)
traumatic fracture of vertebra (S12.-, S22.-, S32.-)

The appropriate 7th character is to be added to each code from subcategory M48.5.
A   initial encounter for fracture
D   subsequent encounter for fracture with routine healing
G   subsequent encounter for fracture with delayed healing
S   sequela of fracture

√x7ᵗʰ **M48.50**   **Collapsed vertebra, not elsewhere classified, site unspecified** ▽

√x7ᵗʰ **M48.51**   **Collapsed vertebra, not elsewhere classified, occipito-atlanto-axial region**

√x7ᵗʰ **M48.52**   **Collapsed vertebra, not elsewhere classified, cervical region**

√x7ᵗʰ **M48.53**   **Collapsed vertebra, not elsewhere classified, cervicothoracic region**

√x7ᵗʰ **M48.54**   **Collapsed vertebra, not elsewhere classified, thoracic region**

√x7ᵗʰ **M48.55**   **Collapsed vertebra, not elsewhere classified, thoracolumbar region**

√x7ᵗʰ **M48.56**   **Collapsed vertebra, not elsewhere classified, lumbar region**

☑ Additional Character Required   √x7ᵗʰ Placeholder Alert   Manifestation Dx   ▽ Unspecified Dx   ►◄ Revised Text   ● New Code   ▲ Revised Code Title

ICD-10-CM 2017   739

√x7ᵗʰ M48.57   **Collapsed vertebra, not elsewhere classified, lumbosacral region**

√x7ᵗʰ M48.58   **Collapsed vertebra, not elsewhere classified,** sacral and sacrococcygeal **region**

√5ᵗʰ M48.8   **Other specified spondylopathies**

Ossification of posterior longitudinal ligament

√6ᵗʰ M48.8X   **Other specified spondylopathies**

M48.8X1   **Other specified spondylopathies, occipito-atlanto-axial region**

M48.8X2   **Other specified spondylopathies,** cervical **region**

M48.8X3   **Other specified spondylopathies, cervicothoracic region**

M48.8X4   **Other specified spondylopathies,** thoracic **region**

M48.8X5   **Other specified spondylopathies, thoracolumbar region**

M48.8X6   **Other specified spondylopathies,** lumbar **region**

M48.8X7   **Other specified spondylopathies, lumbosacral region**

M48.8X8   **Other specified spondylopathies,** sacral and sacrococcygeal **region**

M48.8X9   **Other specified spondylopathies, site unspecified**

M48.9   **Spondylopathy, unspecified**

√4ᵗʰ M49   **Spondylopathies in diseases classified elsewhere**

INCLUDES   curvature of spine in diseases classified elsewhere
deformity of spine in diseases classified elsewhere
kyphosis in diseases classified elsewhere
scoliosis in diseases classified elsewhere
spondylopathy in diseases classified elsewhere

Code first underlying disease, such as:
brucellosis (A23.-)
Charcôt-Marie-Tooth disease (G60.0)
enterobacterial infections (A01-A04)
osteitis fibrosa cystica (E21.0)

EXCLUDES 1   curvature of spine in tuberculosis [Pott's] (A18.01)
enteropathic arthropathies (M07.-)
gonococcal spondylitis (A54.41)
neuropathic spondylopathy in syringomyelia (G95.0)
neuropathic spondylopathy in tabes dorsalis (A52.11)
neuropathic [tabes dorsalis] spondylitis (A52.11)
nonsyphilitic neuropathic spondylopathy NEC (G98.0)
spondylitis in syphilis (acquired) (A52.77)
tuberculous spondylitis (A18.01)
typhoid fever spondylitis (A01.05)

√5ᵗʰ M49.8   **Spondylopathy in diseases classified elsewhere**

M49.80   *Spondylopathy in diseases classified elsewhere, site unspecified*

M49.81   *Spondylopathy in diseases classified elsewhere, occipito-atlanto-axial region*

M49.82   *Spondylopathy in diseases classified elsewhere, cervical region*

M49.83   *Spondylopathy in diseases classified elsewhere, cervicothoracic region*

M49.84   *Spondylopathy in diseases classified elsewhere, thoracic region*

M49.85   *Spondylopathy in diseases classified elsewhere, thoracolumbar region*

M49.86   *Spondylopathy in diseases classified elsewhere, lumbar region*

M49.87   *Spondylopathy in diseases classified elsewhere, lumbosacral region*

M49.88   *Spondylopathy in diseases classified elsewhere,* sacral and sacrococcygeal *region*

M49.89   *Spondylopathy in diseases classified elsewhere, multiple sites in spine*

Other dorsopathies (M50-M54)

EXCLUDES 1   current injury - see injury of spine by body region
discitis NOS (M46.4-)

√4ᵗʰ M50   **Cervical disc disorders**

NOTE   Code to the most superior level of disorder

INCLUDES   cervicothoracic disc disorders
cervicothoracic disc disorders with cervicalgia

AHA: 2016,1Q,17

√5ᵗʰ M50.0   **Cervical disc disorder** with myelopathy

M50.00   **Cervical disc disorder with myelopathy, unspecified cervical region**

M50.01   **Cervical disc disorder with myelopathy,** high cervical **region**

C2-C3 disc disorder with myelopathy
C3-C4 disc disorder with myelopathy

√6ᵗʰ M50.02   **Cervical disc disorder with myelopathy,** mid-cervical **region**

M50.020   **Cervical disc disorder with myelopathy, mid-cervical region, unspecified level**

M50.021   **Cervical disc disorder at** C4-C5 **level with myelopathy**

C4-C5 disc disorder with myelopathy

M50.022   **Cervical disc disorder at** C5-C6 **level with myelopathy**

C5-C6 disc disorder with myelopathy

M50.023   **Cervical disc disorder at** C6-C7 **level with myelopathy**

C6-C7 disc disorder with myelopathy

M50.03   **Cervical disc disorder with myelopathy, cervicothoracic region**

C7-T1 disc disorder with myelopathy

√5ᵗʰ M50.1   **Cervical disc disorder** with radiculopathy

EXCLUDES 2   brachial radiculitis NOS (M54.13)

M50.10   **Cervical disc disorder with radiculopathy, unspecified cervical region**

M50.11   **Cervical disc disorder with radiculopathy,** high cervical **region**

C2-C3 disc disorder with radiculopathy
C3 radiculopathy due to disc disorder
C3-C4 disc disorder with radiculopathy
C4 radiculopathy due to disc disorder

√6ᵗʰ M50.12   **Cervical disc disorder with radiculopathy, mid-cervical region**

M50.120   **Mid-cervical disc disorder, unspecified**

M50.121   **Cervical disc disorder at** C4-C5 **level with radiculopathy**

C4-C5 disc disorder with radiculopathy
C5 radiculopathy due to disc disorder

M50.122   **Cervical disc disorder at** C5-C6 **level with radiculopathy**

C5-C6 disc disorder with radiculopathy
C6 radiculopathy due to disc disorder

M50.123   **Cervical disc disorder at** C6-C7 **level with radiculopathy**

C6-C7 disc disorder with radiculopathy
C7 radiculopathy due to disc disorder

M50.13   **Cervical disc disorder with radiculopathy, cervicothoracic region**

C7-T1 disc disorder with radiculopathy
C8 radiculopathy due to disc disorder

√5ᵗʰ M50.2   **Other cervical disc** displacement

M50.20   **Other cervical disc displacement, unspecified cervical region**

M50.21   **Other cervical disc displacement,** high cervical **region**

Other C2-C3 cervical disc displacement
Other C3-C4 cervical disc displacement

√6ᵗʰ M50.22   **Other cervical disc displacement,** mid-cervical **region**

M50.220   **Other cervical disc displacement, mid-cervical region, unspecified level**

M50.221   **Other cervical disc displacement at** C4-C5 **level**

Other C4-C5 cervical disc displacement

M50.222   **Other cervical disc displacement at** C5-C6 **level**

Other C5-C6 cervical disc displacement

M50.223   **Other cervical disc displacement at** C6-C7 **level**

Other C6-C7 cervical disc displacement

M50.23   **Other cervical disc displacement,** cervicothoracic **region**

Other C7-T1 cervical disc displacement

√6ᵗʰ M50.3   **Other cervical disc** degeneration

M50.30   **Other cervical disc degeneration, unspecified cervical region**

EXCLUDES 1 Not coded here   **EXCLUDES 2** Not included here   **N** Newborn Age : 0   **P** Pediatric Age : 0-17   **M** Maternity Age : 12-55   **A** Adult Age : 15-124

740   ICD-10-CM 2017

M50.31 Other cervical disc degeneration, high cervical region
  Other C2-C3 cervical disc degeneration
  Other C3-C4 cervical disc degeneration

✓6th **M50.32** Other cervical disc degeneration, mid-cervical region

● **M50.320** Other cervical disc degeneration, mid-cervical region, unspecified level ▽

● **M50.321** Other cervical disc degeneration at C4-C5 level
  Other C4-C5 cervical disc degeneration

● **M50.322** Other cervical disc degeneration at C5-C6 level
  Other C5-C6 cervical disc degeneration

● **M50.323** Other cervical disc degeneration at C6-C7 level
  Other C6-C7 cervical disc degeneration

M50.33 Other cervical disc degeneration, cervicothoracic region
  Other C7-T1 cervical disc degeneration

✓5th **M50.8** Other cervical disc disorders

M50.80 Other cervical disc disorders, unspecified cervical region ▽

M50.81 Other cervical disc disorders, high cervical region
  Other C2-C3 cervical disc disorders
  Other C3-C4 cervical disc disorders

✓6th **M50.82** Other cervical disc disorders, mid-cervical region

● **M50.820** Other cervical disc disorders, mid-cervical region, unspecified level ▽

● **M50.821** Other cervical disc disorders at C4-C5 level
  Other C4-C5 cervical disc disorders

● **M50.822** Other cervical disc disorders at C5-C6 level
  Other C5-C6 cervical disc disorders

● **M50.823** Other cervical disc disorders at C6-C7 level
  Other C6-C7 cervical disc disorders

M50.83 Other cervical disc disorders, cervicothoracic region
  Other C7-T1 cervical disc disorders

✓5th **M50.9** Cervical disc disorder, unspecified

M50.90 Cervical disc disorder, unspecified, unspecified cervical region ▽

M50.91 Cervical disc disorder, unspecified, high cervical region ▽
  C2-C3 cervical disc disorder, unspecified
  C3-C4 cervical disc disorder, unspecified

✓6th **M50.92** Cervical disc disorder, unspecified, mid-cervical region

● **M50.920** Unspecified cervical disc disorder, mid-cervical region, unspecified level ▽

● **M50.921** Unspecified cervical disc disorder at C4-C5 level ▽
  Unspecified C4-C5 cervical disc disorder

● **M50.922** Unspecified cervical disc disorder at C5-C6 level ▽
  Unspecified C5-C6 cervical disc disorder

● **M50.923** Unspecified cervical disc disorder at C6-C7 level ▽
  Unspecified C6-C7 cervical disc disorder

M50.93 Cervical disc disorder, unspecified, cervicothoracic region ▽
  C7-T1 cervical disc disorder, unspecified

✓4th **M51** Thoracic, thoracolumbar, and lumbosacral intervertebral disc disorders

  EXCLUDES 2 cervical and cervicothoracic disc disorders (M50.-)
    sacral and sacrococcygeal disorders (M53.3)

✓5th **M51.0** Thoracic, thoracolumbar and lumbosacral intervertebral disc disorders with myelopathy

M51.04 Intervertebral disc disorders with myelopathy, thoracic region

M51.05 Intervertebral disc disorders with myelopathy, thoracolumbar region

M51.06 Intervertebral disc disorders with myelopathy, lumbar region

✓5th **M51.1** Thoracic, thoracolumbar and lumbosacral intervertebral disc disorders with radiculopathy
  Sciatica due to intervertebral disc disorder
  EXCLUDES 1 lumbar radiculitis NOS (M54.16)
    sciatica NOS (M54.3)

M51.14 Intervertebral disc disorders with radiculopathy, thoracic region

M51.15 Intervertebral disc disorders with radiculopathy, thoracolumbar region

M51.16 Intervertebral disc disorders with radiculopathy, lumbar region

M51.17 Intervertebral disc disorders with radiculopathy, lumbosacral region

✓5th **M51.2** Other thoracic, thoracolumbar and lumbosacral intervertebral disc displacement
  Lumbago due to displacement of intervertebral disc

Displacement Intervertebral Disc

Normal Top View   Herniated Top View

M51.24 Other intervertebral disc displacement, thoracic region

M51.25 Other intervertebral disc displacement, thoracolumbar region

M51.26 Other intervertebral disc displacement, lumbar region

M51.27 Other intervertebral disc displacement, lumbosacral region

✓5th **M51.3** Other thoracic, thoracolumbar and lumbosacral intervertebral disc degeneration
  AHA: 2013,3Q,22

M51.34 Other intervertebral disc degeneration, thoracic region

M51.35 Other intervertebral disc degeneration, thoracolumbar region

M51.36 Other intervertebral disc degeneration, lumbar region

M51.37 Other intervertebral disc degeneration, lumbosacral region

✓5th **M51.4** Schmorl's nodes
  DEF: Irregular bone defect in the margin of the vertebral body; causes herniation into end plate of vertebral body.

M51.44 Schmorl's nodes, thoracic region

M51.45 Schmorl's nodes, thoracolumbar region

M51.46 Schmorl's nodes, lumbar region

M51.47 Schmorl's nodes, lumbosacral region

✓5th **M51.8** Other thoracic, thoracolumbar and lumbosacral intervertebral disc disorders

M51.84 Other intervertebral disc disorders, thoracic region

M51.85 Other intervertebral disc disorders, thoracolumbar region

M51.86 Other intervertebral disc disorders, lumbar region

M51.87 Other intervertebral disc disorders, lumbosacral region

M51.9 Unspecified thoracic, thoracolumbar and lumbosacral intervertebral disc disorder ▽

✓4th **M53** Other and unspecified dorsopathies, not elsewhere classified

M53.0 Cervicocranial syndrome
  Posterior cervical sympathetic syndrome

M53.1 Cervicobrachial syndrome
  EXCLUDES 2 cervical disc disorder (M50.-)
    thoracic outlet syndrome (G54.0)

Chapter 13. Diseases of the Musculoskeletal System and Connective Tissue

✓5ᵗʰ **M53.2 Spinal instabilities**
  ✓6ᵗʰ **M53.2X Spinal instabilities**
    M53.2X1 Spinal instabilities, occipito-atlanto-axial region
    M53.2X2 Spinal instabilities, cervical region
    M53.2X3 Spinal instabilities, cervicothoracic region
    M53.2X4 Spinal instabilities, thoracic region
    M53.2X5 Spinal instabilities, thoracolumbar region
    M53.2X6 Spinal instabilities, lumbar region
    M53.2X7 Spinal instabilities, lumbosacral region
    M53.2X8 Spinal instabilities, sacral and sacrococcygeal region
    M53.2X9 Spinal instabilities, site unspecified ▽

  M53.3 Sacrococcygeal disorders, not elsewhere classified
    Coccygodynia

✓5ᵗʰ **M53.8 Other specified dorsopathies**
    M53.80 Other specified dorsopathies, site unspecified ▽
    M53.81 Other specified dorsopathies, occipito-atlanto-axial region
    M53.82 Other specified dorsopathies, cervical region
    M53.83 Other specified dorsopathies, cervicothoracic region
    M53.84 Other specified dorsopathies, thoracic region
    M53.85 Other specified dorsopathies, thoracolumbar region
    M53.86 Other specified dorsopathies, lumbar region
    M53.87 Other specified dorsopathies, lumbosacral region
    M53.88 Other specified dorsopathies, sacral and sacrococcygeal region

  M53.9 Dorsopathy, unspecified ▽

✓4ᵗʰ **M54 Dorsalgia**
    EXCLUDES 1   psychogenic dorsalgia (F45.41)

✓5ᵗʰ **M54.0 Panniculitis affecting regions of neck and back**
    EXCLUDES 1   lupus panniculitis (L93.2)
         panniculitis NOS (M79.3)
         relapsing [Weber-Christian] panniculitis (M35.6)
    M54.00 Panniculitis affecting regions of neck and back, site unspecified ▽
    M54.01 Panniculitis affecting regions of neck and back, occipito-atlanto-axial region
    M54.02 Panniculitis affecting regions of neck and back, cervical region
    M54.03 Panniculitis affecting regions of neck and back, cervicothoracic region
    M54.04 Panniculitis affecting regions of neck and back, thoracic region
    M54.05 Panniculitis affecting regions of neck and back, thoracolumbar region
    M54.06 Panniculitis affecting regions of neck and back, lumbar region
    M54.07 Panniculitis affecting regions of neck and back, lumbosacral region
    M54.08 Panniculitis affecting regions of neck and back, sacral and sacrococcygeal region
    M54.09 Panniculitis affecting regions, neck and back, multiple sites in spine

✓5ᵗʰ **M54.1 Radiculopathy**
    Brachial neuritis or radiculitis NOS
    Lumbar neuritis or radiculitis NOS
    Lumbosacral neuritis or radiculitis NOS
    Thoracic neuritis or radiculitis NOS
    Radiculitis NOS
    EXCLUDES 1   neuralgia and neuritis NOS (M79.2)
         radiculopathy with cervical disc disorder (M50.1)
         radiculopathy with lumbar and other intervertebral disc disorder (M51.1-)
         radiculopathy with spondylosis (M47.2-)
    M54.10 Radiculopathy, site unspecified ▽
    M54.11 Radiculopathy, occipito-atlanto-axial region
    M54.12 Radiculopathy, cervical region
    M54.13 Radiculopathy, cervicothoracic region
    M54.14 Radiculopathy, thoracic region
    M54.15 Radiculopathy, thoracolumbar region
    M54.16 Radiculopathy, lumbar region
    M54.17 Radiculopathy, lumbosacral region
    M54.18 Radiculopathy, sacral and sacrococcygeal region

M54.2 Cervicalgia
    EXCLUDES 1   cervicalgia due to intervertebral cervical disc disorder (M50.-)

✓5ᵗʰ **M54.3 Sciatica**
    EXCLUDES 1   lesion of sciatic nerve (G57.0)
         sciatica due to intervertebral disc disorder (M51.1-)
         sciatica with lumbago (M54.4-)
    M54.30 Sciatica, unspecified side ▽
    M54.31 Sciatica, right side
    M54.32 Sciatica, left side

✓5ᵗʰ **M54.4 Lumbago with sciatica**
    EXCLUDES 1   lumbago with sciatica due to intervertebral disc disorder (M51.1-)
    AHA: 2016,2Q,7
    M54.40 Lumbago with sciatica, unspecified side ▽
    M54.41 Lumbago with sciatica, right side
    M54.42 Lumbago with sciatica, left side

M54.5 Low back pain
    Loin pain
    Lumbago NOS
    EXCLUDES 1   low back strain (S39.012)
         lumbago due to intervertebral disc displacement (M51.2-)
         lumbago with sciatica (M54.4-)

M54.6 Pain in thoracic spine
    EXCLUDES 1   pain in thoracic spine due to intervertebral disc disorder (M51.-)

✓5ᵗʰ **M54.8 Other dorsalgia**
    EXCLUDES 1   dorsalgia in thoracic region (M54.6)
         low back pain (M54.5)
    M54.81 Occipital neuralgia
    M54.89 Other dorsalgia

M54.9 Dorsalgia, unspecified ▽
    Backache NOS
    Back pain NOS

Soft tissue disorders (M60-M79)

Disorders of muscles (M60-M63)

EXCLUDES 1   dermatopolymyositis (M33.-)
     muscular dystrophies and myopathies (G71-G72)
     myopathy in amyloidosis (E85.-)
     myopathy in polyarteritis nodosa (M30.0)
     myopathy in rheumatoid arthritis (M05.32)
     myopathy in scleroderma (M34.-)
     myopathy in Sjögren's syndrome (M35.03)
     myopathy in systemic lupus erythematosus (M32.-)

✓4ᵗʰ **M60 Myositis**
    EXCLUDES 2   inclusion body myositis [IBM] (G72.41)

✓5ᵗʰ **M60.0 Infective myositis**
    Tropical pyomyositis
    Use additional code (B95-B97) to identify infectious agent
    ✓6ᵗʰ **M60.00 Infective myositis, unspecified site**
        M60.000 Infective myositis, unspecified right arm
             Infective myositis, right upper limb NOS
        M60.001 Infective myositis, unspecified left arm
             Infective myositis, left upper limb NOS
        M60.002 Infective myositis, unspecified arm ▽
             Infective myositis, upper limb NOS
        M60.003 Infective myositis, unspecified right leg
             Infective myositis, right lower limb NOS
        M60.004 Infective myositis, unspecified left leg
             Infective myositis, left lower limb NOS
        M60.005 Infective myositis, unspecified leg ▽
             Infective myositis, lower limb NOS
        M60.009 Infective myositis, unspecified site ▽
    ✓6ᵗʰ **M60.01 Infective myositis, shoulder**
        M60.011 Infective myositis, right shoulder
        M60.012 Infective myositis, left shoulder
        M60.019 Infective myositis, unspecified shoulder ▽
    ✓6ᵗʰ **M60.02 Infective myositis, upper arm**
        M60.021 Infective myositis, right upper arm
        M60.022 Infective myositis, left upper arm
        M60.029 Infective myositis, unspecified upper arm ▽

EXCLUDES 1 Not coded here   EXCLUDES 2 Not included here   N Newborn Age : 0   P Pediatric Age : 0-17   M Maternity Age : 12-55   A Adult Age : 15-124

742   ICD-10-CM 2017

M53.2–M60.029

✓6ᵗʰ **M60.03** Infective myositis, forearm
     M60.031 Infective myositis, right forearm
     M60.032 Infective myositis, left forearm
     M60.039 Infective myositis, unspecified forearm ▽

✓6ᵗʰ **M60.04** Infective myositis, hand and fingers
     M60.041 Infective myositis, right hand
     M60.042 Infective myositis, left hand
     M60.043 Infective myositis, unspecified hand ▽
     M60.044 Infective myositis, right finger(s)
     M60.045 Infective myositis, left finger(s)
     M60.046 Infective myositis, unspecified finger(s) ▽

✓6ᵗʰ **M60.05** Infective myositis, thigh
     M60.051 Infective myositis, right thigh
     M60.052 Infective myositis, left thigh
     M60.059 Infective myositis, unspecified thigh ▽

✓6ᵗʰ **M60.06** Infective myositis, lower leg
     M60.061 Infective myositis, right lower leg
     M60.062 Infective myositis, left lower leg
     M60.069 Infective myositis, unspecified lower leg ▽

✓6ᵗʰ **M60.07** Infective myositis, ankle, foot and toes
     M60.070 Infective myositis, right ankle
     M60.071 Infective myositis, left ankle
     M60.072 Infective myositis, unspecified ankle ▽
     M60.073 Infective myositis, right foot
     M60.074 Infective myositis, left foot
     M60.075 Infective myositis, unspecified foot ▽
     M60.076 Infective myositis, right toe(s)
     M60.077 Infective myositis, left toe(s)
     M60.078 Infective myositis, unspecified toe(s) ▽

     M60.08 Infective myositis, other site
     M60.09 Infective myositis, multiple sites

✓5ᵗʰ **M60.1** Interstitial myositis
     M60.10 Interstitial myositis of unspecified site ▽

✓6ᵗʰ **M60.11** Interstitial myositis, shoulder
     M60.111 Interstitial myositis, right shoulder
     M60.112 Interstitial myositis, left shoulder
     M60.119 Interstitial myositis, unspecified shoulder ▽

✓6ᵗʰ **M60.12** Interstitial myositis, upper arm
     M60.121 Interstitial myositis, right upper arm
     M60.122 Interstitial myositis, left upper arm
     M60.129 Interstitial myositis, unspecified upper arm ▽

✓6ᵗʰ **M60.13** Interstitial myositis, forearm
     M60.131 Interstitial myositis, right forearm
     M60.132 Interstitial myositis, left forearm
     M60.139 Interstitial myositis, unspecified forearm ▽

✓6ᵗʰ **M60.14** Interstitial myositis, hand
     M60.141 Interstitial myositis, right hand
     M60.142 Interstitial myositis, left hand
     M60.149 Interstitial myositis, unspecified hand ▽

✓6ᵗʰ **M60.15** Interstitial myositis, thigh
     M60.151 Interstitial myositis, right thigh
     M60.152 Interstitial myositis, left thigh
     M60.159 Interstitial myositis, unspecified thigh ▽

✓6ᵗʰ **M60.16** Interstitial myositis, lower leg
     M60.161 Interstitial myositis, right lower leg
     M60.162 Interstitial myositis, left lower leg
     M60.169 Interstitial myositis, unspecified lower leg ▽

✓6ᵗʰ **M60.17** Interstitial myositis, ankle and foot
     M60.171 Interstitial myositis, right ankle and foot
     M60.172 Interstitial myositis, left ankle and foot
     M60.179 Interstitial myositis, unspecified ankle and foot ▽

     M60.18 Interstitial myositis, other site

     M60.19 Interstitial myositis, multiple sites

✓5ᵗʰ **M60.2** Foreign body granuloma of soft tissue, not elsewhere classified
     Use additional code to identify the type of retained foreign body (Z18.-)
     EXCLUDES 1 foreign body granuloma of skin and subcutaneous tissue (L92.3)

     M60.20 Foreign body granuloma of soft tissue, not elsewhere classified, unspecified site ▽

✓6ᵗʰ **M60.21** Foreign body granuloma of soft tissue, not elsewhere classified, shoulder
     M60.211 Foreign body granuloma of soft tissue, not elsewhere classified, right shoulder
     M60.212 Foreign body granuloma of soft tissue, not elsewhere classified, left shoulder
     M60.219 Foreign body granuloma of soft tissue, not elsewhere classified, unspecified shoulder ▽

✓6ᵗʰ **M60.22** Foreign body granuloma of soft tissue, not elsewhere classified, upper arm
     M60.221 Foreign body granuloma of soft tissue, not elsewhere classified, right upper arm
     M60.222 Foreign body granuloma of soft tissue, not elsewhere classified, left upper arm
     M60.229 Foreign body granuloma of soft tissue, not elsewhere classified, unspecified upper arm ▽

✓6ᵗʰ **M60.23** Foreign body granuloma of soft tissue, not elsewhere classified, forearm
     M60.231 Foreign body granuloma of soft tissue, not elsewhere classified, right forearm
     M60.232 Foreign body granuloma of soft tissue, not elsewhere classified, left forearm
     M60.239 Foreign body granuloma of soft tissue, not elsewhere classified, unspecified forearm ▽

✓6ᵗʰ **M60.24** Foreign body granuloma of soft tissue, not elsewhere classified, hand
     M60.241 Foreign body granuloma of soft tissue, not elsewhere classified, right hand
     M60.242 Foreign body granuloma of soft tissue, not elsewhere classified, left hand
     M60.249 Foreign body granuloma of soft tissue, not elsewhere classified, unspecified hand ▽

✓6ᵗʰ **M60.25** Foreign body granuloma of soft tissue, not elsewhere classified, thigh
     M60.251 Foreign body granuloma of soft tissue, not elsewhere classified, right thigh
     M60.252 Foreign body granuloma of soft tissue, not elsewhere classified, left thigh
     M60.259 Foreign body granuloma of soft tissue, not elsewhere classified, unspecified thigh ▽

✓6ᵗʰ **M60.26** Foreign body granuloma of soft tissue, not elsewhere classified, lower leg
     M60.261 Foreign body granuloma of soft tissue, not elsewhere classified, right lower leg
     M60.262 Foreign body granuloma of soft tissue, not elsewhere classified, left lower leg
     M60.269 Foreign body granuloma of soft tissue, not elsewhere classified, unspecified lower leg ▽

✓6ᵗʰ **M60.27** Foreign body granuloma of soft tissue, not elsewhere classified, ankle and foot
     M60.271 Foreign body granuloma of soft tissue, not elsewhere classified, right ankle and foot
     M60.272 Foreign body granuloma of soft tissue, not elsewhere classified, left ankle and foot
     M60.279 Foreign body granuloma of soft tissue, not elsewhere classified, unspecified ankle and foot ▽

     M60.28 Foreign body granuloma of soft tissue, not elsewhere classified, other site

✓5ᵗʰ **M60.8** Other myositis
     M60.80 Other myositis, unspecified site ▽

✓6ᵗʰ **M60.81** Other myositis shoulder
     M60.811 Other myositis, right shoulder
     M60.812 Other myositis, left shoulder
     M60.819 Other myositis, unspecified shoulder ▽

✓ Additional Character Required   ✕✗7ᵗʰ Placeholder Alert   Manifestation Dx   ▽ Unspecified Dx   ▶◀ Revised Text   ● New Code   ▲ Revised Code Title

ICD-10-CM 2017   **743**

✓6ᵗʰ **M60.82** **Other myositis,** upper arm

 M60.821 **Other myositis,** right **upper arm**
 M60.822 **Other myositis,** left **upper arm**
 M60.829 **Other myositis,** unspecified upper arm ▽

✓6ᵗʰ **M60.83** **Other myositis,** forearm

 M60.831 **Other myositis,** right **forearm**
 M60.832 **Other myositis,** left **forearm**
 M60.839 **Other myositis,** unspecified forearm ▽

✓6ᵗʰ **M60.84** **Other myositis,** hand

 M60.841 **Other myositis,** right **hand**
 M60.842 **Other myositis,** left **hand**
 M60.849 **Other myositis,** unspecified hand ▽

✓6ᵗʰ **M60.85** **Other myositis,** thigh

 M60.851 **Other myositis,** right **thigh**
 M60.852 **Other myositis,** left **thigh**
 M60.859 **Other myositis,** unspecified thigh ▽

✓6ᵗʰ **M60.86** **Other myositis,** lower leg

 M60.861 **Other myositis,** right **lower leg**
 M60.862 **Other myositis,** left **lower leg**
 M60.869 **Other myositis,** unspecified lower leg ▽

✓6ᵗʰ **M60.87** **Other myositis,** ankle and foot

 M60.871 **Other myositis,** right **ankle and foot**
 M60.872 **Other myositis,** left **ankle and foot**
 M60.879 **Other myositis,** unspecified ankle and foot ▽

 M60.88 **Other myositis, other site**
 M60.89 **Other myositis,** multiple sites

 M60.9 **Myositis, unspecified** ▽

✓4ᵗʰ **M61** **Calcification and ossification of muscle**

✓5ᵗʰ **M61.0** **Myositis ossificans** traumatica

 M61.00 **Myositis ossificans traumatica, unspecified site** ▽

✓6ᵗʰ **M61.01** **Myositis ossificans traumatica,** shoulder

 M61.011 **Myositis ossificans traumatica, right shoulder**
 M61.012 **Myositis ossificans traumatica, left shoulder**
 M61.019 **Myositis ossificans traumatica, unspecified shoulder** ▽

✓6ᵗʰ **M61.02** **Myositis ossificans traumatica,** upper arm

 M61.021 **Myositis ossificans traumatica, right upper arm**
 M61.022 **Myositis ossificans traumatica,** left **upper arm**
 M61.029 **Myositis ossificans traumatica, unspecified upper arm** ▽

✓6ᵗʰ **M61.03** **Myositis ossificans traumatica,** forearm

 M61.031 **Myositis ossificans traumatica, right forearm**
 M61.032 **Myositis ossificans traumatica,** left **forearm**
 M61.039 **Myositis ossificans traumatica, unspecified forearm** ▽

✓6ᵗʰ **M61.04** **Myositis ossificans traumatica,** hand

 M61.041 **Myositis ossificans traumatica,** right **hand**
 M61.042 **Myositis ossificans traumatica,** left **hand**
 M61.049 **Myositis ossificans traumatica, unspecified hand** ▽

✓6ᵗʰ **M61.05** **Myositis ossificans traumatica,** thigh

 M61.051 **Myositis ossificans traumatica,** right **thigh**
 M61.052 **Myositis ossificans traumatica,** left **thigh**
 M61.059 **Myositis ossificans traumatica, unspecified thigh** ▽

✓6ᵗʰ **M61.06** **Myositis ossificans traumatica,** lower leg

 M61.061 **Myositis ossificans traumatica, right lower leg**
 M61.062 **Myositis ossificans traumatica,** left **lower leg**
 M61.069 **Myositis ossificans traumatica, unspecified lower leg** ▽

✓6ᵗʰ **M61.07** **Myositis ossificans traumatica,** ankle and foot

 M61.071 **Myositis ossificans traumatica,** right **ankle and foot**

 M61.072 **Myositis ossificans traumatica,** left **ankle and foot**
 M61.079 **Myositis ossificans traumatica, unspecified ankle and foot** ▽

 M61.08 **Myositis ossificans traumatica, other site**
 M61.09 **Myositis ossificans traumatica,** multiple sites

✓5ᵗʰ **M61.1** **Myositis ossificans** progressiva

 Fibrodysplasia ossificans progressiva

 M61.10 **Myositis ossificans progressiva, unspecified site** ▽

✓6ᵗʰ **M61.11** **Myositis ossificans progressiva,** shoulder

 M61.111 **Myositis ossificans progressiva,** right **shoulder**
 M61.112 **Myositis ossificans progressiva,** left **shoulder**
 M61.119 **Myositis ossificans progressiva, unspecified shoulder** ▽

✓6ᵗʰ **M61.12** **Myositis ossificans progressiva,** upper arm

 M61.121 **Myositis ossificans progressiva,** right **upper arm**
 M61.122 **Myositis ossificans progressiva,** left **upper arm**
 M61.129 **Myositis ossificans progressiva, unspecified arm** ▽

✓6ᵗʰ **M61.13** **Myositis ossificans progressiva,** forearm

 M61.131 **Myositis ossificans progressiva,** right **forearm**
 M61.132 **Myositis ossificans progressiva,** left **forearm**
 M61.139 **Myositis ossificans progressiva, unspecified forearm** ▽

✓6ᵗʰ **M61.14** **Myositis ossificans progressiva,** hand and finger(s)

 M61.141 **Myositis ossificans progressiva,** right **hand**
 M61.142 **Myositis ossificans progressiva,** left **hand**
 M61.143 **Myositis ossificans progressiva, unspecified hand** ▽
 M61.144 **Myositis ossificans progressiva,** right **finger(s)**
 M61.145 **Myositis ossificans progressiva,** left **finger(s)**
 M61.146 **Myositis ossificans progressiva, unspecified finger(s)** ▽

✓6ᵗʰ **M61.15** **Myositis ossificans progressiva,** thigh

 M61.151 **Myositis ossificans progressiva,** right **thigh**
 M61.152 **Myositis ossificans progressiva,** left **thigh**
 M61.159 **Myositis ossificans progressiva, unspecified thigh** ▽

✓6ᵗʰ **M61.16** **Myositis ossificans progressiva,** lower leg

 M61.161 **Myositis ossificans progressiva,** right **lower leg**
 M61.162 **Myositis ossificans progressiva,** left **lower leg**
 M61.169 **Myositis ossificans progressiva, unspecified lower leg** ▽

✓6ᵗʰ **M61.17** **Myositis ossificans progressiva,** ankle, foot and toe(s)

 M61.171 **Myositis ossificans progressiva,** right **ankle**
 M61.172 **Myositis ossificans progressiva,** left **ankle**
 M61.173 **Myositis ossificans progressiva, unspecified ankle** ▽
 M61.174 **Myositis ossificans progressiva,** right **foot**
 M61.175 **Myositis ossificans progressiva,** left **foot**
 M61.176 **Myositis ossificans progressiva, unspecified foot**
 M61.177 **Myositis ossificans progressiva,** right **toe(s)**
 M61.178 **Myositis ossificans progressiva,** left **toe(s)**
 M61.179 **Myositis ossificans progressiva, unspecified toe(s)** ▽

 M61.18 **Myositis ossificans progressiva, other site**
 M61.19 **Myositis ossificans progressiva,** multiple sites

✓5ᵗʰ **M61.2** **Paralytic calcification and ossification of muscle**

 Myositis ossificans associated with quadriplegia or paraplegia

 M61.20 **Paralytic calcification and ossification of muscle, unspecified site** ▽

EXCLUDES 1 Not coded here   **EXCLUDES 2** Not included here   **N** Newborn Age : 0   **P** Pediatric Age : 0-17   **M** Maternity Age : 12-55   **A** Adult Age : 15-124

744   ICD-10-CM 2017

✓6ᵗʰ **M61.21** Paralytic calcification and ossification of muscle, shoulder

     M61.211 Paralytic calcification and ossification of muscle, right shoulder

     M61.212 Paralytic calcification and ossification of muscle, left shoulder

     M61.219 Paralytic calcification and ossification of muscle, unspecified shoulder ▽

✓6ᵗʰ **M61.22** Paralytic calcification and ossification of muscle, upper arm

     M61.221 Paralytic calcification and ossification of muscle, right upper arm

     M61.222 Paralytic calcification and ossification of muscle, left upper arm

     M61.229 Paralytic calcification and ossification of muscle, unspecified upper arm ▽

✓6ᵗʰ **M61.23** Paralytic calcification and ossification of muscle, forearm

     M61.231 Paralytic calcification and ossification of muscle, right forearm

     M61.232 Paralytic calcification and ossification of muscle, left forearm

     M61.239 Paralytic calcification and ossification of muscle, unspecified forearm ▽

✓6ᵗʰ **M61.24** Paralytic calcification and ossification of muscle, hand

     M61.241 Paralytic calcification and ossification of muscle, right hand

     M61.242 Paralytic calcification and ossification of muscle, left hand

     M61.249 Paralytic calcification and ossification of muscle, unspecified hand ▽

✓6ᵗʰ **M61.25** Paralytic calcification and ossification of muscle, thigh

     M61.251 Paralytic calcification and ossification of muscle, right thigh

     M61.252 Paralytic calcification and ossification of muscle, left thigh

     M61.259 Paralytic calcification and ossification of muscle, unspecified thigh ▽

✓6ᵗʰ **M61.26** Paralytic calcification and ossification of muscle, lower leg

     M61.261 Paralytic calcification and ossification of muscle, right lower leg

     M61.262 Paralytic calcification and ossification of muscle, left lower leg

     M61.269 Paralytic calcification and ossification of muscle, unspecified lower leg ▽

✓6ᵗʰ **M61.27** Paralytic calcification and ossification of muscle, ankle and foot

     M61.271 Paralytic calcification and ossification of muscle, right ankle and foot

     M61.272 Paralytic calcification and ossification of muscle, left ankle and foot

     M61.279 Paralytic calcification and ossification of muscle, unspecified ankle and foot ▽

     M61.28 Paralytic calcification and ossification of muscle, other site

     M61.29 Paralytic calcification and ossification of muscle, multiple sites

✓5ᵗʰ **M61.3** Calcification and ossification of muscles associated with burns

     Myositis ossificans associated with burns

     M61.30 Calcification and ossification of muscles associated with burns, unspecified site ▽

✓6ᵗʰ **M61.31** Calcification and ossification of muscles associated with burns, shoulder

     M61.311 Calcification and ossification of muscles associated with burns, right shoulder

     M61.312 Calcification and ossification of muscles associated with burns, left shoulder

     M61.319 Calcification and ossification of muscles associated with burns, unspecified shoulder ▽

✓6ᵗʰ **M61.32** Calcification and ossification of muscles associated with burns, upper arm

     M61.321 Calcification and ossification of muscles associated with burns, right upper arm

     M61.322 Calcification and ossification of muscles associated with burns, left upper arm

     M61.329 Calcification and ossification of muscles associated with burns, unspecified upper arm ▽

✓6ᵗʰ **M61.33** Calcification and ossification of muscles associated with burns, forearm

     M61.331 Calcification and ossification of muscles associated with burns, right forearm

     M61.332 Calcification and ossification of muscles associated with burns, left forearm

     M61.339 Calcification and ossification of muscles associated with burns, unspecified forearm ▽

✓6ᵗʰ **M61.34** Calcification and ossification of muscles associated with burns, hand

     M61.341 Calcification and ossification of muscles associated with burns, right hand

     M61.342 Calcification and ossification of muscles associated with burns, left hand

     M61.349 Calcification and ossification of muscles associated with burns, unspecified hand ▽

✓6ᵗʰ **M61.35** Calcification and ossification of muscles associated with burns, thigh

     M61.351 Calcification and ossification of muscles associated with burns, right thigh

     M61.352 Calcification and ossification of muscles associated with burns, left thigh

     M61.359 Calcification and ossification of muscles associated with burns, unspecified thigh ▽

✓6ᵗʰ **M61.36** Calcification and ossification of muscles associated with burns, lower leg

     M61.361 Calcification and ossification of muscles associated with burns, right lower leg

     M61.362 Calcification and ossification of muscles associated with burns, left lower leg

     M61.369 Calcification and ossification of muscles associated with burns, unspecified lower leg ▽

✓6ᵗʰ **M61.37** Calcification and ossification of muscles associated with burns, ankle and foot

     M61.371 Calcification and ossification of muscles associated with burns, right ankle and foot

     M61.372 Calcification and ossification of muscles associated with burns, left ankle and foot

     M61.379 Calcification and ossification of muscles associated with burns, unspecified ankle and foot ▽

     M61.38 Calcification and ossification of muscles associated with burns, other site

     M61.39 Calcification and ossification of muscles associated with burns, multiple sites

✓5ᵗʰ **M61.4** Other calcification of muscle

     EXCLUDES 1   *calcific tendinitis NOS (M65.2-)*
                          calcific tendinitis of shoulder (M75.3)

     M61.40 Other calcification of muscle, unspecified site ▽

✓6ᵗʰ **M61.41** Other calcification of muscle, shoulder

     M61.411 Other calcification of muscle, right shoulder

     M61.412 Other calcification of muscle, left shoulder

     M61.419 Other calcification of muscle, unspecified shoulder ▽

✓6ᵗʰ **M61.42** Other calcification of muscle, upper arm

     M61.421 Other calcification of muscle, right upper arm

     M61.422 Other calcification of muscle, left upper arm

     M61.429 Other calcification of muscle, unspecified upper arm ▽

✓6ᵗʰ **M61.43** Other calcification of muscle, forearm

     M61.431 Other calcification of muscle, right forearm

     M61.432 Other calcification of muscle, left forearm

     M61.439 Other calcification of muscle, unspecified forearm ▽

✓6ᵗʰ **M61.44** Other calcification of muscle, hand

     M61.441 Other calcification of muscle, right hand

☑ Additional Character Required   ✓x7ᵗʰ Placeholder Alert   Manifestation Dx   ▽ Unspecified Dx   ►◄ Revised Text   ● New Code   ▲ Revised Code Title

ICD-10-CM 2017   745

M61.442 **Other calcification of muscle**, left hand
M61.449 **Other calcification of muscle**, unspecified hand   ▽

√6ᵗʰ **M61.45** **Other calcification of muscle**, thigh

M61.451 **Other calcification of muscle**, right thigh
M61.452 **Other calcification of muscle**, left thigh
M61.459 **Other calcification of muscle**, unspecified thigh

√6ᵗʰ **M61.46** **Other calcification of muscle**, lower leg

M61.461 **Other calcification of muscle**, right lower leg
M61.462 **Other calcification of muscle**, left lower leg
M61.469 **Other calcification of muscle**, unspecified lower leg   ▽

√6ᵗʰ **M61.47** **Other calcification of muscle**, ankle and foot

M61.471 **Other calcification of muscle**, right ankle and foot
M61.472 **Other calcification of muscle**, left ankle and foot
M61.479 **Other calcification of muscle**, unspecified ankle and foot   ▽

M61.48 **Other calcification of muscle**, other site
M61.49 **Other calcification of muscle**, multiple sites

√5ᵗʰ **M61.5** **Other** ossification of muscle

M61.50 **Other ossification of muscle**, unspecified site   ▽

√6ᵗʰ **M61.51** **Other ossification of muscle**, shoulder

M61.511 **Other ossification of muscle**, right shoulder
M61.512 **Other ossification of muscle**, left shoulder
M61.519 **Other ossification of muscle**, unspecified shoulder   ▽

√6ᵗʰ **M61.52** **Other ossification of muscle**, upper arm

M61.521 **Other ossification of muscle**, right upper arm
M61.522 **Other ossification of muscle**, left upper arm
M61.529 **Other ossification of muscle**, unspecified upper arm   ▽

√6ᵗʰ **M61.53** **Other ossification of muscle**, forearm

M61.531 **Other ossification of muscle**, right forearm
M61.532 **Other ossification of muscle**, left forearm
M61.539 **Other ossification of muscle**, unspecified forearm   ▽

√6ᵗʰ **M61.54** **Other ossification of muscle**, hand

M61.541 **Other ossification of muscle**, right hand
M61.542 **Other ossification of muscle**, left hand
M61.549 **Other ossification of muscle**, unspecified hand   ▽

√6ᵗʰ **M61.55** **Other ossification of muscle**, thigh

M61.551 **Other ossification of muscle**, right thigh
M61.552 **Other ossification of muscle**, left thigh
M61.559 **Other ossification of muscle**, unspecified thigh   ▽

√6ᵗʰ **M61.56** **Other ossification of muscle**, lower leg

M61.561 **Other ossification of muscle**, right lower leg
M61.562 **Other ossification of muscle**, left lower leg
M61.569 **Other ossification of muscle**, unspecified lower leg   ▽

√6ᵗʰ **M61.57** **Other ossification of muscle**, ankle and foot

M61.571 **Other ossification of muscle**, right ankle and foot
M61.572 **Other ossification of muscle**, left ankle and foot
M61.579 **Other ossification of muscle**, unspecified ankle and foot   ▽

M61.58 **Other ossification of muscle**, other site
M61.59 **Other ossification of muscle**, multiple sites

M61.9 **Calcification and ossification of muscle, unspecified**   ▽

√4ᵗʰ **M62** **Other disorders of muscle**

EXCLUDES 1   *alcoholic myopathy (G72.1)*
cramp and spasm (R25.2)
drug-induced myopathy (G72.0)
myalgia (M79.1)
stiff-man syndrome (G25.82)
EXCLUDES 2   *nontraumatic hematoma of muscle (M79.81)*

√5ᵗʰ **M62.0** **Separation of muscle (nontraumatic)**

Diastasis of muscle
EXCLUDES 1   *diastasis recti complicating pregnancy, labor and delivery (O71.8)*
traumatic separation of muscle - see strain of muscle by body region

M62.00 **Separation of muscle (nontraumatic), unspecified site**   ▽

√6ᵗʰ **M62.01** **Separation of muscle (nontraumatic)**, shoulder

M62.011 **Separation of muscle (nontraumatic)**, right shoulder
M62.012 **Separation of muscle (nontraumatic)**, left shoulder
M62.019 **Separation of muscle (nontraumatic), unspecified shoulder**   ▽

√6ᵗʰ **M62.02** **Separation of muscle (nontraumatic)**, upper arm

M62.021 **Separation of muscle (nontraumatic)**, right upper arm
M62.022 **Separation of muscle (nontraumatic)**, left upper arm
M62.029 **Separation of muscle (nontraumatic), unspecified upper arm**   ▽

√6ᵗʰ **M62.03** **Separation of muscle (nontraumatic)**, forearm

M62.031 **Separation of muscle (nontraumatic)**, right forearm
M62.032 **Separation of muscle (nontraumatic)**, left forearm
M62.039 **Separation of muscle (nontraumatic), unspecified forearm**   ▽

√6ᵗʰ **M62.04** **Separation of muscle (nontraumatic)**, hand

M62.041 **Separation of muscle (nontraumatic)**, right hand
M62.042 **Separation of muscle (nontraumatic)**, left hand
M62.049 **Separation of muscle (nontraumatic), unspecified hand**   ▽

√6ᵗʰ **M62.05** **Separation of muscle (nontraumatic)**, thigh

M62.051 **Separation of muscle (nontraumatic)**, right thigh
M62.052 **Separation of muscle (nontraumatic)**, left thigh
M62.059 **Separation of muscle (nontraumatic), unspecified thigh**   ▽

√6ᵗʰ **M62.06** **Separation of muscle (nontraumatic)**, lower leg

M62.061 **Separation of muscle (nontraumatic)**, right lower leg
M62.062 **Separation of muscle (nontraumatic)**, left lower leg
M62.069 **Separation of muscle (nontraumatic), unspecified lower leg**   ▽

√6ᵗʰ **M62.07** **Separation of muscle (nontraumatic)**, ankle and foot

M62.071 **Separation of muscle (nontraumatic)**, right ankle and foot
M62.072 **Separation of muscle (nontraumatic)**, left ankle and foot
M62.079 **Separation of muscle (nontraumatic), unspecified ankle and foot**   ▽

M62.08 **Separation of muscle (nontraumatic)**, other site

√5ᵗʰ **M62.1** **Other rupture of muscle (nontraumatic)**

EXCLUDES 1   *traumatic rupture of muscle - see strain of muscle by body region*
EXCLUDES 2   *rupture of tendon (M66.-)*

M62.10 **Other rupture of muscle (nontraumatic), unspecified site**   ▽

√6ᵗʰ **M62.11** **Other rupture of muscle (nontraumatic)**, shoulder

M62.111 **Other rupture of muscle (nontraumatic)**, right shoulder

M62.112   Other rupture of muscle (nontraumatic), **left** shoulder

M62.119   Other rupture of muscle (nontraumatic), unspecified shoulder ▽

✓6ᵗʰ   **M62.12**   Other rupture of muscle (nontraumatic), upper arm

M62.121   Other rupture of muscle (nontraumatic), **right** upper arm

M62.122   Other rupture of muscle (nontraumatic), **left** upper arm

M62.129   Other rupture of muscle (nontraumatic), unspecified upper arm ▽

✓6ᵗʰ   **M62.13**   Other rupture of muscle (nontraumatic), forearm

M62.131   Other rupture of muscle (nontraumatic), **right** forearm

M62.132   Other rupture of muscle (nontraumatic), **left** forearm

M62.139   Other rupture of muscle (nontraumatic), unspecified forearm ▽

✓6ᵗʰ   **M62.14**   Other rupture of muscle (nontraumatic), hand

M62.141   Other rupture of muscle (nontraumatic), **right** hand

M62.142   Other rupture of muscle (nontraumatic), **left** hand

M62.149   Other rupture of muscle (nontraumatic), unspecified hand ▽

✓6ᵗʰ   **M62.15**   Other rupture of muscle (nontraumatic), thigh

M62.151   Other rupture of muscle (nontraumatic), **right** thigh

M62.152   Other rupture of muscle (nontraumatic), **left** thigh

M62.159   Other rupture of muscle (nontraumatic), unspecified thigh ▽

✓6ᵗʰ   **M62.16**   Other rupture of muscle (nontraumatic), lower leg

M62.161   Other rupture of muscle (nontraumatic), **right** lower leg

M62.162   Other rupture of muscle (nontraumatic), **left** lower leg

M62.169   Other rupture of muscle (nontraumatic), unspecified lower leg ▽

✓6ᵗʰ   **M62.17**   Other rupture of muscle (nontraumatic), ankle and foot

M62.171   Other rupture of muscle (nontraumatic), **right** ankle and foot

M62.172   Other rupture of muscle (nontraumatic), **left** ankle and foot

M62.179   Other rupture of muscle (nontraumatic), unspecified ankle and foot ▽

M62.18   Other rupture of muscle (nontraumatic), other site

✓5ᵗʰ   **M62.2**   **Nontraumatic ischemic infarction of muscle**

EXCLUDES 1   *compartment syndrome (traumatic) (T79.A-)*
nontraumatic compartment syndrome (M79.A-)
rhabdomyolysis (M62.82)
traumatic ischemia of muscle (T79.6)
Volkmann's ischemic contracture (T79.6)

M62.20   Nontraumatic ischemic infarction of muscle, unspecified site ▽

✓6ᵗʰ   **M62.21**   Nontraumatic ischemic infarction of muscle, shoulder

M62.211   Nontraumatic ischemic infarction of muscle, **right** shoulder

M62.212   Nontraumatic ischemic infarction of muscle, **left** shoulder

M62.219   Nontraumatic ischemic infarction of muscle, unspecified shoulder ▽

✓6ᵗʰ   **M62.22**   Nontraumatic ischemic infarction of muscle, upper arm

M62.221   Nontraumatic ischemic infarction of muscle, **right** upper arm

M62.222   Nontraumatic ischemic infarction of muscle, **left** upper arm

M62.229   Nontraumatic ischemic infarction of muscle, unspecified upper arm ▽

✓6ᵗʰ   **M62.23**   Nontraumatic ischemic infarction of muscle, forearm

M62.231   Nontraumatic ischemic infarction of muscle, **right** forearm

M62.232   Nontraumatic ischemic infarction of muscle, **left** forearm

M62.239   Nontraumatic ischemic infarction of muscle, unspecified forearm ▽

✓6ᵗʰ   **M62.24**   Nontraumatic ischemic infarction of muscle, hand

M62.241   Nontraumatic ischemic infarction of muscle, **right** hand

M62.242   Nontraumatic ischemic infarction of muscle, **left** hand

M62.249   Nontraumatic ischemic infarction of muscle, unspecified hand ▽

✓6ᵗʰ   **M62.25**   Nontraumatic ischemic infarction of muscle, thigh

M62.251   Nontraumatic ischemic infarction of muscle, **right** thigh

M62.252   Nontraumatic ischemic infarction of muscle, **left** thigh

M62.259   Nontraumatic ischemic infarction of muscle, unspecified thigh ▽

✓6ᵗʰ   **M62.26**   Nontraumatic ischemic infarction of muscle, lower leg

M62.261   Nontraumatic ischemic infarction of muscle, **right** lower leg

M62.262   Nontraumatic ischemic infarction of muscle, **left** lower leg

M62.269   Nontraumatic ischemic infarction of muscle, unspecified lower leg ▽

✓6ᵗʰ   **M62.27**   Nontraumatic ischemic infarction of muscle, ankle and foot

M62.271   Nontraumatic ischemic infarction of muscle, **right** ankle and foot

M62.272   Nontraumatic ischemic infarction of muscle, **left** ankle and foot

M62.279   Nontraumatic ischemic infarction of muscle, unspecified ankle and foot ▽

M62.28   Nontraumatic ischemic infarction of muscle, other site

M62.3   **Immobility syndrome (paraplegic)**

✓5ᵗʰ   **M62.4**   **Contracture of muscle**

Contracture of tendon (sheath)

EXCLUDES 1   *contracture of joint (M24.5-)*

M62.40   Contracture of muscle, unspecified site ▽

✓6ᵗʰ   **M62.41**   Contracture of muscle, shoulder

M62.411   Contracture of muscle, **right** shoulder

M62.412   Contracture of muscle, **left** shoulder

M62.419   Contracture of muscle, unspecified shoulder ▽

✓6ᵗʰ   **M62.42**   Contracture of muscle, upper arm

M62.421   Contracture of muscle, **right** upper arm

M62.422   Contracture of muscle, **left** upper arm

M62.429   Contracture of muscle, unspecified upper arm ▽

✓6ᵗʰ   **M62.43**   Contracture of muscle, forearm

M62.431   Contracture of muscle, **right** forearm

M62.432   Contracture of muscle, **left** forearm

M62.439   Contracture of muscle, unspecified forearm ▽

✓6ᵗʰ   **M62.44**   Contracture of muscle, hand

M62.441   Contracture of muscle, **right** hand

M62.442   Contracture of muscle, **left** hand

M62.449   Contracture of muscle, unspecified hand ▽

✓6ᵗʰ   **M62.45**   Contracture of muscle, thigh

M62.451   Contracture of muscle, **right** thigh

M62.452   Contracture of muscle, **left** thigh

M62.459   Contracture of muscle, unspecified thigh ▽

✓6ᵗʰ   **M62.46**   Contracture of muscle, lower leg

M62.461   Contracture of muscle, **right** lower leg

M62.462   Contracture of muscle, **left** lower leg

M62.469   Contracture of muscle, unspecified lower leg ▽

✓6ᵗʰ   **M62.47**   Contracture of muscle, ankle and foot

M62.471   Contracture of muscle, **right** ankle and foot

M62.472   Contracture of muscle, **left** ankle and foot

M62.479   Contracture of muscle, unspecified ankle and foot ▽

M62.48   Contracture of muscle, other site

M62.49   **Contracture of muscle,** multiple sites

√5ᵗʰ M62.5   **Muscle wasting and atrophy, not elsewhere classified**

Disuse atrophy NEC

EXCLUDES 1   *neuralgic amyotrophy (G54.5)*
progressive muscular atrophy (G12.29)
▶*sarcopenia (M62.84)*◀

EXCLUDES 2   *pelvic muscle wasting (N81.84)*

M62.50   **Muscle wasting and atrophy, not elsewhere classified, unspecified site**

√6ᵗʰ M62.51   **Muscle wasting and atrophy, not elsewhere classified, shoulder**

M62.511   **Muscle wasting and atrophy, not elsewhere classified, right shoulder**

M62.512   **Muscle wasting and atrophy, not elsewhere classified, left shoulder**

M62.519   **Muscle wasting and atrophy, not elsewhere classified, unspecified shoulder**

√6ᵗʰ M62.52   **Muscle wasting and atrophy, not elsewhere classified, upper arm**

M62.521   **Muscle wasting and atrophy, not elsewhere classified, right upper arm**

M62.522   **Muscle wasting and atrophy, not elsewhere classified, left upper arm**

M62.529   **Muscle wasting and atrophy, not elsewhere classified, unspecified upper arm**

√6ᵗʰ M62.53   **Muscle wasting and atrophy, not elsewhere classified, forearm**

M62.531   **Muscle wasting and atrophy, not elsewhere classified, right forearm**

M62.532   **Muscle wasting and atrophy, not elsewhere classified, left forearm**

M62.539   **Muscle wasting and atrophy, not elsewhere classified, unspecified forearm**

√6ᵗʰ M62.54   **Muscle wasting and atrophy, not elsewhere classified, hand**

M62.541   **Muscle wasting and atrophy, not elsewhere classified, right hand**

M62.542   **Muscle wasting and atrophy, not elsewhere classified, left hand**

M62.549   **Muscle wasting and atrophy, not elsewhere classified, unspecified hand**

√6ᵗʰ M62.55   **Muscle wasting and atrophy, not elsewhere classified, thigh**

M62.551   **Muscle wasting and atrophy, not elsewhere classified, right thigh**

M62.552   **Muscle wasting and atrophy, not elsewhere classified, left thigh**

M62.559   **Muscle wasting and atrophy, not elsewhere classified, unspecified thigh**

√6ᵗʰ M62.56   **Muscle wasting and atrophy, not elsewhere classified, lower leg**

M62.561   **Muscle wasting and atrophy, not elsewhere classified, right lower leg**

M62.562   **Muscle wasting and atrophy, not elsewhere classified, left lower leg**

M62.569   **Muscle wasting and atrophy, not elsewhere classified, unspecified lower leg**

√6ᵗʰ M62.57   **Muscle wasting and atrophy, not elsewhere classified, ankle and foot**

M62.571   **Muscle wasting and atrophy, not elsewhere classified, right ankle and foot**

M62.572   **Muscle wasting and atrophy, not elsewhere classified, left ankle and foot**

M62.579   **Muscle wasting and atrophy, not elsewhere classified, unspecified ankle and foot**

M62.58   **Muscle wasting and atrophy, not elsewhere classified, other site**

M62.59   **Muscle wasting and atrophy, not elsewhere classified, multiple sites**

√5ᵗʰ M62.8   **Other specified disorders of muscle**

EXCLUDES 2   *nontraumatic hematoma of muscle (M79.81)*

M62.81   **Muscle weakness (generalized)**

EXCLUDES 1   ▶*muscle weakness in sarcopenia (M62.84)*◀

M62.82   **Rhabdomyolysis**

EXCLUDES 1   *traumatic rhabdomyolysis (T79.6)*

√6ᵗʰ M62.83   **Muscle spasm**

M62.830   **Muscle spasm of back**

M62.831   **Muscle spasm of calf**

Charley-horse

M62.838   **Other muscle spasm**

M62.84   **Sarcopenia**

Age-related sarcopenia

Code first underlying disease, if applicable, such as:
disorders of myoneural junction and muscle disease in diseases classified elsewhere (G73.-)
other and unspecified myopathies (G72.-)
primary disorders of muscles (G71.-)

M62.89   **Other specified disorders of muscle**

Muscle (sheath) hernia

M62.9   **Disorder of muscle, unspecified**

√4ᵗʰ M63   **Disorders of muscle in diseases classified elsewhere**

Code first underlying disease, such as:
leprosy (A30.-)
neoplasm (C49.-, C79.89, D21.-, D48.1)
schistosomiasis (B65.-)
trichinellosis (B75)

EXCLUDES 1   *myopathy in cysticercosis (B69.81)*
myopathy in endocrine diseases (G73.7)
myopathy in metabolic diseases (G73.7)
myopathy in sarcoidosis (D86.87)
myopathy in secondary syphilis (A51.49)
myopathy in syphilis (late) (A52.78)
myopathy in toxoplasmosis (B58.82)
myopathy in tuberculosis (A18.09)

√5ᵗʰ M63.8   **Disorders of muscle in diseases classified elsewhere**

M63.80   *Disorders of muscle in diseases classified elsewhere, unspecified site*

√6ᵗʰ M63.81   **Disorders of muscle in diseases classified elsewhere, shoulder**

M63.811   *Disorders of muscle in diseases classified elsewhere, right shoulder*

M63.812   *Disorders of muscle in diseases classified elsewhere, left shoulder*

M63.819   *Disorders of muscle in diseases classified elsewhere, unspecified shoulder*

√6ᵗʰ M63.82   **Disorders of muscle in diseases classified elsewhere, upper arm**

M63.821   *Disorders of muscle in diseases classified elsewhere, right upper arm*

M63.822   *Disorders of muscle in diseases classified elsewhere, left upper arm*

M63.829   *Disorders of muscle in diseases classified elsewhere, unspecified upper arm*

√6ᵗʰ M63.83   **Disorders of muscle in diseases classified elsewhere, forearm**

M63.831   *Disorders of muscle in diseases classified elsewhere, right forearm*

M63.832   *Disorders of muscle in diseases classified elsewhere, left forearm*

M63.839   *Disorders of muscle in diseases classified elsewhere, unspecified forearm*

√6ᵗʰ M63.84   **Disorders of muscle in diseases classified elsewhere, hand**

M63.841   *Disorders of muscle in diseases classified elsewhere, right hand*

M63.842   *Disorders of muscle in diseases classified elsewhere, left hand*

M63.849   *Disorders of muscle in diseases classified elsewhere, unspecified hand*

√6ᵗʰ M63.85   **Disorders of muscle in diseases classified elsewhere, thigh**

M63.851   *Disorders of muscle in diseases classified elsewhere, right thigh*

M63.852   *Disorders of muscle in diseases classified elsewhere, left thigh*

M63.859   *Disorders of muscle in diseases classified elsewhere, unspecified thigh*

EXCLUDES 1 Not coded here   *EXCLUDES 2* Not included here   N Newborn Age : 0   P Pediatric Age : 0-17   M Maternity Age : 12-55   A Adult Age : 15-124

748   ICD-10-CM 2017

✓6ᵗʰ **M63.86** Disorders of muscle in diseases classified elsewhere, lower leg

    M63.861 *Disorders of muscle in diseases classified elsewhere, right lower leg*

    M63.862 *Disorders of muscle in diseases classified elsewhere, left lower leg*

    M63.869 *Disorders of muscle in diseases classified elsewhere, unspecified lower leg* ▽

✓6ᵗʰ **M63.87** Disorders of muscle in diseases classified elsewhere, ankle and foot

    M63.871 *Disorders of muscle in diseases classified elsewhere, right ankle and foot*

    M63.872 *Disorders of muscle in diseases classified elsewhere, left ankle and foot*

    M63.879 *Disorders of muscle in diseases classified elsewhere, unspecified ankle and foot* ▽

  M63.88 *Disorders of muscle in diseases classified elsewhere, other site*

  M63.89 *Disorders of muscle in diseases classified elsewhere, multiple sites*

Disorders of synovium and tendon (M65-M67)

✓4ᵗʰ **M65 Synovitis and tenosynovitis**

  EXCLUDES 1 *chronic crepitant synovitis of hand and wrist (M70.0-)*
        current injury - see injury of ligament or tendon by body region
        soft tissue disorders related to use, overuse and pressure (M70.-)

✓5ᵗʰ **M65.0 Abscess of tendon sheath**

    Use additional code (B95-B96) to identify bacterial agent.

  M65.00 Abscess of tendon sheath, unspecified site ▽

✓6ᵗʰ **M65.01** Abscess of tendon sheath, shoulder

    M65.011 Abscess of tendon sheath, right shoulder
    M65.012 Abscess of tendon sheath, left shoulder
    M65.019 Abscess of tendon sheath, unspecified shoulder ▽

✓6ᵗʰ **M65.02** Abscess of tendon sheath, upper arm

    M65.021 Abscess of tendon sheath, right upper arm
    M65.022 Abscess of tendon sheath, left upper arm
    M65.029 Abscess of tendon sheath, unspecified upper arm ▽

✓6ᵗʰ **M65.03** Abscess of tendon sheath, forearm

    M65.031 Abscess of tendon sheath, right forearm
    M65.032 Abscess of tendon sheath, left forearm
    M65.039 Abscess of tendon sheath, unspecified forearm ▽

✓6ᵗʰ **M65.04** Abscess of tendon sheath, hand

    M65.041 Abscess of tendon sheath, right hand
    M65.042 Abscess of tendon sheath, left hand
    M65.049 Abscess of tendon sheath, unspecified hand ▽

✓6ᵗʰ **M65.05** Abscess of tendon sheath, thigh

    M65.051 Abscess of tendon sheath, right thigh
    M65.052 Abscess of tendon sheath, left thigh
    M65.059 Abscess of tendon sheath, unspecified thigh ▽

✓6ᵗʰ **M65.06** Abscess of tendon sheath, lower leg

    M65.061 Abscess of tendon sheath, right lower leg
    M65.062 Abscess of tendon sheath, left lower leg
    M65.069 Abscess of tendon sheath, unspecified lower leg ▽

✓6ᵗʰ **M65.07** Abscess of tendon sheath, ankle and foot

    M65.071 Abscess of tendon sheath, right ankle and foot
    M65.072 Abscess of tendon sheath, left ankle and foot
    M65.079 Abscess of tendon sheath, unspecified ankle and foot ▽

  M65.08 Abscess of tendon sheath, other site

✓5ᵗʰ **M65.1 Other infective (teno)synovitis**

  M65.10 Other infective (teno)synovitis, unspecified site ▽

✓6ᵗʰ **M65.11** Other infective (teno)synovitis, shoulder

    M65.111 Other infective (teno)synovitis, right shoulder
    M65.112 Other infective (teno)synovitis, left shoulder

    M65.119 Other infective (teno)synovitis, unspecified shoulder ▽

✓6ᵗʰ **M65.12** Other infective (teno)synovitis, elbow

    M65.121 Other infective (teno)synovitis, right elbow
    M65.122 Other infective (teno)synovitis, left elbow
    M65.129 Other infective (teno)synovitis, unspecified elbow ▽

✓6ᵗʰ **M65.13** Other infective (teno)synovitis, wrist

    M65.131 Other infective (teno)synovitis, right wrist
    M65.132 Other infective (teno)synovitis, left wrist
    M65.139 Other infective (teno)synovitis, unspecified wrist ▽

✓6ᵗʰ **M65.14** Other infective (teno)synovitis, hand

    M65.141 Other infective (teno)synovitis, right hand
    M65.142 Other infective (teno)synovitis, left hand
    M65.149 Other infective (teno)synovitis, unspecified hand ▽

✓6ᵗʰ **M65.15** Other infective (teno)synovitis, hip

    M65.151 Other infective (teno)synovitis, right hip
    M65.152 Other infective (teno)synovitis, left hip
    M65.159 Other infective (teno)synovitis, unspecified hip ▽

✓6ᵗʰ **M65.16** Other infective (teno)synovitis, knee

    M65.161 Other infective (teno)synovitis, right knee
    M65.162 Other infective (teno)synovitis, left knee
    M65.169 Other infective (teno)synovitis, unspecified knee ▽

✓6ᵗʰ **M65.17** Other infective (teno)synovitis, ankle and foot

    M65.171 Other infective (teno)synovitis, right ankle and foot
    M65.172 Other infective (teno)synovitis, left ankle and foot
    M65.179 Other infective (teno)synovitis, unspecified ankle and foot ▽

  M65.18 Other infective (teno)synovitis, other site
  M65.19 Other infective (teno)synovitis, multiple sites

✓5ᵗʰ **M65.2 Calcific tendinitis**

  EXCLUDES 1 *tendinitis as classified in M75-M77*
        calcified tendinitis of shoulder (M75.3)

  M65.20 Calcific tendinitis, unspecified site ▽

✓6ᵗʰ **M65.22** Calcific tendinitis, upper arm

    M65.221 Calcific tendinitis, right upper arm
    M65.222 Calcific tendinitis, left upper arm
    M65.229 Calcific tendinitis, unspecified upper arm ▽

✓6ᵗʰ **M65.23** Calcific tendinitis, forearm

    M65.231 Calcific tendinitis, right forearm
    M65.232 Calcific tendinitis, left forearm
    M65.239 Calcific tendinitis, unspecified forearm ▽

✓6ᵗʰ **M65.24** Calcific tendinitis, hand

    M65.241 Calcific tendinitis, right hand
    M65.242 Calcific tendinitis, left hand
    M65.249 Calcific tendinitis, unspecified hand ▽

✓6ᵗʰ **M65.25** Calcific tendinitis, thigh

    M65.251 Calcific tendinitis, right thigh
    M65.252 Calcific tendinitis, left thigh
    M65.259 Calcific tendinitis, unspecified thigh ▽

✓6ᵗʰ **M65.26** Calcific tendinitis, lower leg

    M65.261 Calcific tendinitis, right lower leg
    M65.262 Calcific tendinitis, left lower leg
    M65.269 Calcific tendinitis, unspecified lower leg ▽

✓6ᵗʰ **M65.27** Calcific tendinitis, ankle and foot

    M65.271 Calcific tendinitis, right ankle and foot
    M65.272 Calcific tendinitis, left ankle and foot
    M65.279 Calcific tendinitis, unspecified ankle and foot ▽

  M65.28 Calcific tendinitis, other site
  M65.29 Calcific tendinitis, multiple sites

✓5ᵗʰ **M65.3 Trigger finger**

    Nodular tendinous disease

  M65.30 Trigger finger, unspecified finger ▽

☑ Additional Character Required   ✓x7ᵗʰ Placeholder Alert   Manifestation Dx   ▽ Unspecified Dx   ►◄ Revised Text   ● New Code   ▲ Revised Code Title

ICD-10-CM 2017   **749**

✓6ᵗʰ **M65.31** **Trigger** thumb
- M65.311 **Trigger thumb, right** thumb
- M65.312 **Trigger thumb, left** thumb
- M65.319 **Trigger thumb, unspecified** thumb ▽

✓6ᵗʰ **M65.32** **Trigger finger,** index finger
- M65.321 **Trigger finger, right** index finger
- M65.322 **Trigger finger, left** index finger
- M65.329 **Trigger finger, unspecified** index finger ▽

✓6ᵗʰ **M65.33** **Trigger finger,** middle finger
- M65.331 **Trigger finger, right** middle finger
- M65.332 **Trigger finger, left** middle finger
- M65.339 **Trigger finger, unspecified** middle finger ▽

✓6ᵗʰ **M65.34** **Trigger finger,** ring finger
- M65.341 **Trigger finger, right** ring finger
- M65.342 **Trigger finger, left** ring finger
- M65.349 **Trigger finger, unspecified** ring finger ▽

✓6ᵗʰ **M65.35** **Trigger finger,** little finger
- M65.351 **Trigger finger, right** little finger
- M65.352 **Trigger finger, left** little finger
- M65.359 **Trigger finger, unspecified** little finger ▽

M65.4 **Radial styloid tenosynovitis [de Quervain]**

✓5ᵗʰ **M65.8** **Other synovitis and tenosynovitis**
- **M65.80** **Other synovitis and tenosynovitis, unspecified site** ▽
- ✓6ᵗʰ **M65.81** **Other synovitis and tenosynovitis,** shoulder
  - M65.811 **Other synovitis and tenosynovitis, right** shoulder
  - M65.812 **Other synovitis and tenosynovitis, left** shoulder
  - M65.819 **Other synovitis and tenosynovitis, unspecified** shoulder ▽
- ✓6ᵗʰ **M65.82** **Other synovitis and tenosynovitis,** upper arm
  - M65.821 **Other synovitis and tenosynovitis, right** upper arm
  - M65.822 **Other synovitis and tenosynovitis, left** upper arm
  - M65.829 **Other synovitis and tenosynovitis, unspecified** upper arm ▽
- ✓6ᵗʰ **M65.83** **Other synovitis and tenosynovitis,** forearm
  - M65.831 **Other synovitis and tenosynovitis, right** forearm
  - M65.832 **Other synovitis and tenosynovitis, left** forearm
  - M65.839 **Other synovitis and tenosynovitis, unspecified** forearm ▽
- ✓6ᵗʰ **M65.84** **Other synovitis and tenosynovitis,** hand
  - M65.841 **Other synovitis and tenosynovitis, right** hand
  - M65.842 **Other synovitis and tenosynovitis, left** hand
  - M65.849 **Other synovitis and tenosynovitis, unspecified** hand ▽
- ✓6ᵗʰ **M65.85** **Other synovitis and tenosynovitis,** thigh
  - M65.851 **Other synovitis and tenosynovitis, right** thigh
  - M65.852 **Other synovitis and tenosynovitis, left** thigh
  - M65.859 **Other synovitis and tenosynovitis, unspecified** thigh ▽
- ✓6ᵗʰ **M65.86** **Other synovitis and tenosynovitis,** lower leg
  - M65.861 **Other synovitis and tenosynovitis, right** lower leg
  - M65.862 **Other synovitis and tenosynovitis, left** lower leg
  - M65.869 **Other synovitis and tenosynovitis, unspecified** lower leg ▽
- ✓6ᵗʰ **M65.87** **Other synovitis and tenosynovitis,** ankle and foot
  - M65.871 **Other synovitis and tenosynovitis, right** ankle and foot
  - M65.872 **Other synovitis and tenosynovitis, left** ankle and foot
  - M65.879 **Other synovitis and tenosynovitis, unspecified** ankle and foot ▽
- **M65.88** **Other synovitis and tenosynovitis, other site**
- **M65.89** **Other synovitis and tenosynovitis,** multiple sites

M65.9 **Synovitis and tenosynovitis, unspecified** ▽

✓4ᵗʰ **M66** **Spontaneous rupture of synovium and tendon**

> INCLUDES rupture that occurs when a normal force is applied to tissues that are inferred to have less than normal strength
>
> EXCLUDES 2 *rotator cuff syndrome (M75.1-)*
>
> *rupture where an abnormal force is applied to normal tissue - see injury of tendon by body region*

M66.0 **Rupture of** popliteal cyst

✓5ᵗʰ **M66.1** **Rupture of** synovium
> Rupture of synovial cyst
>
> EXCLUDES 2 *rupture of popliteal cyst (M66.0)*
- **M66.10** **Rupture of synovium, unspecified joint** ▽
- ✓6ᵗʰ **M66.11** **Rupture of synovium,** shoulder
  - M66.111 **Rupture of synovium, right** shoulder
  - M66.112 **Rupture of synovium, left** shoulder
  - M66.119 **Rupture of synovium, unspecified** shoulder ▽
- ✓6ᵗʰ **M66.12** **Rupture of synovium,** elbow
  - M66.121 **Rupture of synovium, right** elbow
  - M66.122 **Rupture of synovium, left** elbow
  - M66.129 **Rupture of synovium, unspecified** elbow ▽
- ✓6ᵗʰ **M66.13** **Rupture of synovium,** wrist
  - M66.131 **Rupture of synovium, right** wrist
  - M66.132 **Rupture of synovium, left** wrist
  - M66.139 **Rupture of synovium, unspecified** wrist ▽
- ✓6ᵗʰ **M66.14** **Rupture of synovium,** hand and fingers
  - M66.141 **Rupture of synovium, right** hand
  - M66.142 **Rupture of synovium, left** hand
  - M66.143 **Rupture of synovium, unspecified** hand ▽
  - M66.144 **Rupture of synovium, right** finger(s)
  - M66.145 **Rupture of synovium, left** finger(s)
  - M66.146 **Rupture of synovium, unspecified** finger(s) ▽
- ✓6ᵗʰ **M66.15** **Rupture of synovium,** hip
  - M66.151 **Rupture of synovium, right** hip
  - M66.152 **Rupture of synovium, left** hip
  - M66.159 **Rupture of synovium, unspecified** hip ▽
- ✓6ᵗʰ **M66.17** **Rupture of synovium,** ankle, foot and toes
  - M66.171 **Rupture of synovium, right** ankle
  - M66.172 **Rupture of synovium, left** ankle
  - M66.173 **Rupture of synovium, unspecified** ankle ▽
  - M66.174 **Rupture of synovium, right** foot
  - M66.175 **Rupture of synovium, left** foot
  - M66.176 **Rupture of synovium, unspecified** foot ▽
  - M66.177 **Rupture of synovium, right** toe(s)
  - M66.178 **Rupture of synovium, left** toe(s)
  - M66.179 **Rupture of synovium, unspecified** toe(s) ▽
- **M66.18** **Rupture of synovium, other site**

✓5ᵗʰ **M66.2** **Spontaneous rupture of** extensor tendons
> **TIP:** Refer to the Muscle/Tendon table at the beginning of the chapter
- **M66.20** **Spontaneous rupture of extensor tendons, unspecified site** ▽
- ✓6ᵗʰ **M66.21** **Spontaneous rupture of extensor tendons,** shoulder
  - M66.211 **Spontaneous rupture of extensor tendons, right** shoulder
  - M66.212 **Spontaneous rupture of extensor tendons, left** shoulder
  - M66.219 **Spontaneous rupture of extensor tendons, unspecified** shoulder ▽
- ✓6ᵗʰ **M66.22** **Spontaneous rupture of extensor tendons,** upper arm
  - M66.221 **Spontaneous rupture of extensor tendons, right** upper arm
  - M66.222 **Spontaneous rupture of extensor tendons, left** upper arm
  - M66.229 **Spontaneous rupture of extensor tendons, unspecified** upper arm ▽
- ✓6ᵗʰ **M66.23** **Spontaneous rupture of extensor tendons,** forearm
  - M66.231 **Spontaneous rupture of extensor tendons, right** forearm

EXCLUDES 1 Not coded here   EXCLUDES 2 Not included here   N Newborn Age : 0   P Pediatric Age : 0-17   M Maternity Age : 12-55   A Adult Age : 15-124

750
ICD-10-CM 2017

M66.232   Spontaneous rupture of extensor tendons, left forearm

M66.239   Spontaneous rupture of extensor tendons, unspecified forearm ▽

☑6ᵗʰ   **M66.24**   Spontaneous rupture of extensor tendons, hand

M66.241   Spontaneous rupture of extensor tendons, right hand

M66.242   Spontaneous rupture of extensor tendons, left hand

M66.249   Spontaneous rupture of extensor tendons, unspecified hand ▽

☑6ᵗʰ   **M66.25**   Spontaneous rupture of extensor tendons, thigh

M66.251   Spontaneous rupture of extensor tendons, right thigh

M66.252   Spontaneous rupture of extensor tendons, left thigh

M66.259   Spontaneous rupture of extensor tendons, unspecified thigh ▽

☑6ᵗʰ   **M66.26**   Spontaneous rupture of extensor tendons, lower leg

M66.261   Spontaneous rupture of extensor tendons, right lower leg

M66.262   Spontaneous rupture of extensor tendons, left lower leg

M66.269   Spontaneous rupture of extensor tendons, unspecified lower leg ▽

☑6ᵗʰ   **M66.27**   Spontaneous rupture of extensor tendons, ankle and foot

M66.271   Spontaneous rupture of extensor tendons, right ankle and foot

M66.272   Spontaneous rupture of extensor tendons, left ankle and foot

M66.279   Spontaneous rupture of extensor tendons, unspecified ankle and foot ▽

M66.28   Spontaneous rupture of extensor tendons, other site

M66.29   Spontaneous rupture of extensor tendons, multiple sites

☑5ᵗʰ   **M66.3**   **Spontaneous rupture of** flexor tendons

> **TIP:** Refer to the Muscle/Tendon table at the beginning of this chapter

M66.30   Spontaneous rupture of flexor tendons, unspecified site ▽

☑6ᵗʰ   **M66.31**   Spontaneous rupture of flexor tendons, shoulder

M66.311   Spontaneous rupture of flexor tendons, right shoulder

M66.312   Spontaneous rupture of flexor tendons, left shoulder

M66.319   Spontaneous rupture of flexor tendons, unspecified shoulder ▽

☑6ᵗʰ   **M66.32**   Spontaneous rupture of flexor tendons, upper arm

M66.321   Spontaneous rupture of flexor tendons, right upper arm

M66.322   Spontaneous rupture of flexor tendons, left upper arm

M66.329   Spontaneous rupture of flexor tendons, unspecified upper arm ▽

☑6ᵗʰ   **M66.33**   Spontaneous rupture of flexor tendons, forearm

M66.331   Spontaneous rupture of flexor tendons, right forearm

M66.332   Spontaneous rupture of flexor tendons, left forearm

M66.339   Spontaneous rupture of flexor tendons, unspecified forearm ▽

☑6ᵗʰ   **M66.34**   Spontaneous rupture of flexor tendons, hand

M66.341   Spontaneous rupture of flexor tendons, right hand

M66.342   Spontaneous rupture of flexor tendons, left hand

M66.349   Spontaneous rupture of flexor tendons, unspecified hand ▽

☑6ᵗʰ   **M66.35**   Spontaneous rupture of flexor tendons, thigh

M66.351   Spontaneous rupture of flexor tendons, right thigh

M66.352   Spontaneous rupture of flexor tendons, left thigh

M66.359   Spontaneous rupture of flexor tendons, unspecified thigh ▽

☑6ᵗʰ   **M66.36**   Spontaneous rupture of flexor tendons, lower leg

M66.361   Spontaneous rupture of flexor tendons, right lower leg

M66.362   Spontaneous rupture of flexor tendons, left lower leg

M66.369   Spontaneous rupture of flexor tendons, unspecified lower leg ▽

☑6ᵗʰ   **M66.37**   Spontaneous rupture of flexor tendons, ankle and foot

M66.371   Spontaneous rupture of flexor tendons, right ankle and foot

M66.372   Spontaneous rupture of flexor tendons, left ankle and foot

M66.379   Spontaneous rupture of flexor tendons, unspecified ankle and foot ▽

M66.38   Spontaneous rupture of flexor tendons, other site

M66.39   Spontaneous rupture of flexor tendons, multiple sites

☑5ᵗʰ   **M66.8**   **Spontaneous rupture of** other tendons

> **TIP:** Refer to the Muscle/Tendon table at the beginning of this chapter

M66.80   Spontaneous rupture of other tendons, unspecified site ▽

☑6ᵗʰ   **M66.81**   Spontaneous rupture of other tendons, shoulder

M66.811   Spontaneous rupture of other tendons, right shoulder

M66.812   Spontaneous rupture of other tendons, left shoulder

M66.819   Spontaneous rupture of other tendons, unspecified shoulder ▽

☑6ᵗʰ   **M66.82**   Spontaneous rupture of other tendons, upper arm

M66.821   Spontaneous rupture of other tendons, right upper arm

M66.822   Spontaneous rupture of other tendons, left upper arm

M66.829   Spontaneous rupture of other tendons, unspecified upper arm ▽

☑6ᵗʰ   **M66.83**   Spontaneous rupture of other tendons, forearm

M66.831   Spontaneous rupture of other tendons, right forearm

M66.832   Spontaneous rupture of other tendons, left forearm

M66.839   Spontaneous rupture of other tendons, unspecified forearm ▽

☑6ᵗʰ   **M66.84**   Spontaneous rupture of other tendons, hand

M66.841   Spontaneous rupture of other tendons, right hand

M66.842   Spontaneous rupture of other tendons, left hand

M66.849   Spontaneous rupture of other tendons, unspecified hand ▽

☑6ᵗʰ   **M66.85**   Spontaneous rupture of other tendons, thigh

M66.851   Spontaneous rupture of other tendons, right thigh

M66.852   Spontaneous rupture of other tendons, left thigh

M66.859   Spontaneous rupture of other tendons, unspecified thigh ▽

☑6ᵗʰ   **M66.86**   Spontaneous rupture of other tendons, lower leg

M66.861   Spontaneous rupture of other tendons, right lower leg

M66.862   Spontaneous rupture of other tendons, left lower leg

M66.869   Spontaneous rupture of other tendons, unspecified lower leg ▽

☑6ᵗʰ   **M66.87**   Spontaneous rupture of other tendons, ankle and foot

M66.871   Spontaneous rupture of other tendons, right ankle and foot

M66.872   Spontaneous rupture of other tendons, left ankle and foot

M66.879   Spontaneous rupture of other tendons, unspecified ankle and foot ▽

M66.88   Spontaneous rupture of other tendons, other

M66.89   Spontaneous rupture of other tendons, multiple sites

M66.9   **Spontaneous rupture of unspecified tendon** ▽

Rupture at musculotendinous junction, nontraumatic

☑ Additional Character Required   ✓x7ᵗʰ Placeholder Alert   Manifestation Dx   ▽ Unspecified Dx   ▶◀ Revised Text   ● New Code   ▲ Revised Code Title

ICD-10-CM 2017   **751**

√4ᵗʰ **M67** **Other disorders of synovium and tendon**

> **EXCLUDES 1**   *palmar fascial fibromatosis [Dupuytren] (M72.0)*
> *tendinitis NOS (M77.9-)*
> *xanthomatosis localized to tendons (E78.2)*

√5ᵗʰ **M67.0** **Short Achilles tendon (acquired)**

    M67.00 **Short Achilles tendon (acquired), unspecified ankle** ▽

    M67.01 **Short Achilles tendon (acquired), right ankle**

    M67.02 **Short Achilles tendon (acquired), left ankle**

√5ᵗʰ **M67.2** **Synovial hypertrophy, not elsewhere classified**

> **EXCLUDES 1**   *villonodular synovitis (pigmented) (M12.2-)*

    M67.20 **Synovial hypertrophy, not elsewhere classified, unspecified site** ▽

√6ᵗʰ **M67.21** **Synovial hypertrophy, not elsewhere classified, shoulder**

    M67.211 **Synovial hypertrophy, not elsewhere classified, right shoulder**

    M67.212 **Synovial hypertrophy, not elsewhere classified, left shoulder**

    M67.219 **Synovial hypertrophy, not elsewhere classified, unspecified shoulder** ▽

√6ᵗʰ **M67.22** **Synovial hypertrophy, not elsewhere classified, upper arm**

    M67.221 **Synovial hypertrophy, not elsewhere classified, right upper arm**

    M67.222 **Synovial hypertrophy, not elsewhere classified, left upper arm**

    M67.229 **Synovial hypertrophy, not elsewhere classified, unspecified upper arm** ▽

√6ᵗʰ **M67.23** **Synovial hypertrophy, not elsewhere classified, forearm**

    M67.231 **Synovial hypertrophy, not elsewhere classified, right forearm**

    M67.232 **Synovial hypertrophy, not elsewhere classified, left forearm**

    M67.239 **Synovial hypertrophy, not elsewhere classified, unspecified forearm** ▽

√6ᵗʰ **M67.24** **Synovial hypertrophy, not elsewhere classified, hand**

    M67.241 **Synovial hypertrophy, not elsewhere classified, right hand**

    M67.242 **Synovial hypertrophy, not elsewhere classified, left hand**

    M67.249 **Synovial hypertrophy, not elsewhere classified, unspecified hand** ▽

√6ᵗʰ **M67.25** **Synovial hypertrophy, not elsewhere classified, thigh**

    M67.251 **Synovial hypertrophy, not elsewhere classified, right thigh**

    M67.252 **Synovial hypertrophy, not elsewhere classified, left thigh**

    M67.259 **Synovial hypertrophy, not elsewhere classified, unspecified thigh** ▽

√6ᵗʰ **M67.26** **Synovial hypertrophy, not elsewhere classified, lower leg**

    M67.261 **Synovial hypertrophy, not elsewhere classified, right lower leg**

    M67.262 **Synovial hypertrophy, not elsewhere classified, left lower leg**

    M67.269 **Synovial hypertrophy, not elsewhere classified, unspecified lower leg** ▽

√6ᵗʰ **M67.27** **Synovial hypertrophy, not elsewhere classified, ankle and foot**

    M67.271 **Synovial hypertrophy, not elsewhere classified, right ankle and foot**

    M67.272 **Synovial hypertrophy, not elsewhere classified, left ankle and foot**

    M67.279 **Synovial hypertrophy, not elsewhere classified, unspecified ankle and foot** ▽

    M67.28 **Synovial hypertrophy, not elsewhere classified, other site**

    M67.29 **Synovial hypertrophy, not elsewhere classified, multiple sites**

√5ᵗʰ **M67.3** **Transient synovitis**

    Toxic synovitis

> **EXCLUDES 1**   *palindromic rheumatism (M12.3-)*

    M67.30 **Transient synovitis, unspecified site** ▽

√6ᵗʰ **M67.31** **Transient synovitis, shoulder**

    M67.311 **Transient synovitis, right shoulder**

    M67.312 **Transient synovitis, left shoulder**

    M67.319 **Transient synovitis, unspecified shoulder** ▽

√6ᵗʰ **M67.32** **Transient synovitis, elbow**

    M67.321 **Transient synovitis, right elbow**

    M67.322 **Transient synovitis, left elbow**

    M67.329 **Transient synovitis, unspecified elbow** ▽

√6ᵗʰ **M67.33** **Transient synovitis, wrist**

    M67.331 **Transient synovitis, right wrist**

    M67.332 **Transient synovitis, left wrist**

    M67.339 **Transient synovitis, unspecified wrist** ▽

√6ᵗʰ **M67.34** **Transient synovitis, hand**

    M67.341 **Transient synovitis, right hand**

    M67.342 **Transient synovitis, left hand**

    M67.349 **Transient synovitis, unspecified hand** ▽

√6ᵗʰ **M67.35** **Transient synovitis, hip**

    M67.351 **Transient synovitis, right hip**

    M67.352 **Transient synovitis, left hip**

    M67.359 **Transient synovitis, unspecified hip** ▽

√6ᵗʰ **M67.36** **Transient synovitis, knee**

    M67.361 **Transient synovitis, right knee**

    M67.362 **Transient synovitis, left knee**

    M67.369 **Transient synovitis, unspecified knee** ▽

√6ᵗʰ **M67.37** **Transient synovitis, ankle and foot**

    M67.371 **Transient synovitis, right ankle and foot**

    M67.372 **Transient synovitis, left ankle and foot**

    M67.379 **Transient synovitis, unspecified ankle and foot** ▽

    M67.38 **Transient synovitis, other site**

    M67.39 **Transient synovitis, multiple sites**

√5ᵗʰ **M67.4** **Ganglion**

    Ganglion of joint or tendon (sheath)

> **EXCLUDES 1**   *ganglion in yaws (A66.6)*
> **EXCLUDES 2**   *cyst of bursa (M71.2-M71.3)*
> *cyst of synovium (M71.2-M71.3)*

    M67.40 **Ganglion, unspecified site** ▽

√6ᵗʰ **M67.41** **Ganglion, shoulder**

    M67.411 **Ganglion, right shoulder**

    M67.412 **Ganglion, left shoulder**

    M67.419 **Ganglion, unspecified shoulder** ▽

√6ᵗʰ **M67.42** **Ganglion, elbow**

    M67.421 **Ganglion, right elbow**

    M67.422 **Ganglion, left elbow**

    M67.429 **Ganglion, unspecified elbow** ▽

√6ᵗʰ **M67.43** **Ganglion, wrist**

    M67.431 **Ganglion, right wrist**

    M67.432 **Ganglion, left wrist**

    M67.439 **Ganglion, unspecified wrist** ▽

√6ᵗʰ **M67.44** **Ganglion, hand**

    M67.441 **Ganglion, right hand**

    M67.442 **Ganglion, left hand**

    M67.449 **Ganglion, unspecified hand** ▽

√6ᵗʰ **M67.45** **Ganglion, hip**

    M67.451 **Ganglion, right hip**

    M67.452 **Ganglion, left hip**

    M67.459 **Ganglion, unspecified hip** ▽

√6ᵗʰ **M67.46** **Ganglion, knee**

    M67.461 **Ganglion, right knee**

    M67.462 **Ganglion, left knee**

    M67.469 **Ganglion, unspecified knee** ▽

√6ᵗʰ **M67.47** **Ganglion, ankle and foot**

    M67.471 **Ganglion, right ankle and foot**

    M67.472 **Ganglion, left ankle and foot**

EXCLUDES 1 Not coded here   **EXCLUDES 2** Not included here   **N** Newborn Age : 0   **P** Pediatric Age : 0-17   **M** Maternity Age : 12-55   **A** Adult Age : 15-124

752   ICD-10-CM 2017

M67.479   **Ganglion, unspecified ankle and foot** ▽

M67.48   **Ganglion, other site**

M67.49   **Ganglion, multiple sites**

✓5ᵗʰ **M67.5   Plica syndrome**

     Plica knee

M67.5Ø   **Plica syndrome, unspecified knee** ▽

M67.51   **Plica syndrome, right knee**

M67.52   **Plica syndrome, left knee**

✓5ᵗʰ **M67.8   Other specified disorders of synovium and tendon**

M67.8Ø   **Other specified disorders of synovium and tendon, unspecified site** ▽

✓6ᵗʰ M67.81   **Other specified disorders of synovium and tendon, shoulder**

M67.811   **Other specified disorders of synovium, right shoulder**

M67.812   **Other specified disorders of synovium, left shoulder**

M67.813   **Other specified disorders of tendon, right shoulder**

M67.814   **Other specified disorders of tendon, left shoulder**

M67.819   **Other specified disorders of synovium and tendon, unspecified shoulder** ▽

✓6ᵗʰ M67.82   **Other specified disorders of synovium and tendon, elbow**

M67.821   **Other specified disorders of synovium, right elbow**

M67.822   **Other specified disorders of synovium, left elbow**

M67.823   **Other specified disorders of tendon, right elbow**

M67.824   **Other specified disorders of tendon, left elbow**

M67.829   **Other specified disorders of synovium and tendon, unspecified elbow** ▽

✓6ᵗʰ M67.83   **Other specified disorders of synovium and tendon, wrist**

M67.831   **Other specified disorders of synovium, right wrist**

M67.832   **Other specified disorders of synovium, left wrist**

M67.833   **Other specified disorders of tendon, right wrist**

M67.834   **Other specified disorders of tendon, left wrist**

M67.839   **Other specified disorders of synovium and tendon, unspecified forearm** ▽

✓6ᵗʰ M67.84   **Other specified disorders of synovium and tendon, hand**

M67.841   **Other specified disorders of synovium, right hand**

M67.842   **Other specified disorders of synovium, left hand**

M67.843   **Other specified disorders of tendon, right hand**

M67.844   **Other specified disorders of tendon, left hand**

M67.849   **Other specified disorders of synovium and tendon, unspecified hand** ▽

✓6ᵗʰ M67.85   **Other specified disorders of synovium and tendon, hip**

M67.851   **Other specified disorders of synovium, right hip**

M67.852   **Other specified disorders of synovium, left hip**

M67.853   **Other specified disorders of tendon, right hip**

M67.854   **Other specified disorders of tendon, left hip**

M67.859   **Other specified disorders of synovium and tendon, unspecified hip** ▽

✓6ᵗʰ M67.86   **Other specified disorders of synovium and tendon, knee**

M67.861   **Other specified disorders of synovium, right knee**

M67.862   **Other specified disorders of synovium, left knee**

M67.863   **Other specified disorders of tendon, right knee**

M67.864   **Other specified disorders of tendon, left knee**

M67.869   **Other specified disorders of synovium and tendon, unspecified knee** ▽

✓6ᵗʰ M67.87   **Other specified disorders of synovium and tendon, ankle and foot**

M67.871   **Other specified disorders of synovium, right ankle and foot**

M67.872   **Other specified disorders of synovium, left ankle and foot**

M67.873   **Other specified disorders of tendon, right ankle and foot**

M67.874   **Other specified disorders of tendon, left ankle and foot**

M67.879   **Other specified disorders of synovium and tendon, unspecified ankle and foot** ▽

M67.88   **Other specified disorders of synovium and tendon, other site**

M67.89   **Other specified disorders of synovium and tendon, multiple sites**

✓5ᵗʰ **M67.9   Unspecified disorder of synovium and tendon**

M67.9Ø   **Unspecified disorder of synovium and tendon, unspecified site** ▽

✓6ᵗʰ M67.91   **Unspecified disorder of synovium and tendon, shoulder**

M67.911   **Unspecified disorder of synovium and tendon, right shoulder** ▽

M67.912   **Unspecified disorder of synovium and tendon, left shoulder** ▽

M67.919   **Unspecified disorder of synovium and tendon, unspecified shoulder** ▽

✓6ᵗʰ M67.92   **Unspecified disorder of synovium and tendon, upper arm**

M67.921   **Unspecified disorder of synovium and tendon, right upper arm** ▽

M67.922   **Unspecified disorder of synovium and tendon, left upper arm** ▽

M67.929   **Unspecified disorder of synovium and tendon, unspecified upper arm** ▽

✓6ᵗʰ M67.93   **Unspecified disorder of synovium and tendon, forearm**

M67.931   **Unspecified disorder of synovium and tendon, right forearm** ▽

M67.932   **Unspecified disorder of synovium and tendon, left forearm** ▽

M67.939   **Unspecified disorder of synovium and tendon, unspecified forearm** ▽

✓6ᵗʰ M67.94   **Unspecified disorder of synovium and tendon, hand**

M67.941   **Unspecified disorder of synovium and tendon, right hand** ▽

M67.942   **Unspecified disorder of synovium and tendon, left hand** ▽

M67.949   **Unspecified disorder of synovium and tendon, unspecified hand** ▽

✓6ᵗʰ M67.95   **Unspecified disorder of synovium and tendon, thigh**

M67.951   **Unspecified disorder of synovium and tendon, right thigh** ▽

M67.952   **Unspecified disorder of synovium and tendon, left thigh** ▽

M67.959   **Unspecified disorder of synovium and tendon, unspecified thigh** ▽

✓6ᵗʰ M67.96   **Unspecified disorder of synovium and tendon, lower leg**

M67.961   **Unspecified disorder of synovium and tendon, right lower leg** ▽

M67.962   **Unspecified disorder of synovium and tendon, left lower leg** ▽

M67.969   **Unspecified disorder of synovium and tendon, unspecified lower leg** ▽

✓6ᵗʰ M67.97   **Unspecified disorder of synovium and tendon, ankle and foot**

M67.971   **Unspecified disorder of synovium and tendon, right ankle and foot** ▽

M67.972   **Unspecified disorder of synovium and tendon, left ankle and foot** ▽

☑ Additional Character Required   ✓x7ᵗʰ Placeholder Alert   Manifestation Dx   ▽ Unspecified Dx   ▶◀ Revised Text   ● New Code   ▲ Revised Code Title

ICD-10-CM 2017   753

M67.979 Unspecified disorder of synovium and tendon, unspecified ankle and foot ▽

M67.98 Unspecified disorder of synovium and tendon, other site ▽

M67.99 Unspecified disorder of synovium and tendon, multiple sites ▽

Other soft tissue disorders (M70-M79)

✓4th **M70** Soft tissue disorders related to use, overuse and pressure

INCLUDES soft tissue disorders of occupational origin

Use additional external cause code to identify activity causing disorder (Y93.-)

EXCLUDES 1 bursitis NOS (M71.9-)

EXCLUDES 2 bursitis of shoulder (M75.5)
enthesopathies (M76-M77)
pressure ulcer (pressure area) (L89.-)

✓5th **M70.0** Crepitant synovitis (acute) (chronic) of hand and wrist

✓6th **M70.03** Crepitant synovitis (acute) (chronic), wrist

M70.031 Crepitant synovitis (acute) (chronic), right wrist

M70.032 Crepitant synovitis (acute) (chronic), left wrist

M70.039 Crepitant synovitis (acute) (chronic), unspecified wrist ▽

✓6th **M70.04** Crepitant synovitis (acute) (chronic), hand

M70.041 Crepitant synovitis (acute) (chronic), right hand

M70.042 Crepitant synovitis (acute) (chronic), left hand

M70.049 Crepitant synovitis (acute) (chronic), unspecified hand ▽

✓5th **M70.1** Bursitis of hand

M70.10 Bursitis, unspecified hand ▽

M70.11 Bursitis, right hand

M70.12 Bursitis, left hand

✓5th **M70.2** Olecranon bursitis

M70.20 Olecranon bursitis, unspecified elbow ▽

M70.21 Olecranon bursitis, right elbow

M70.22 Olecranon bursitis, left elbow

✓5th **M70.3** Other bursitis of elbow

M70.30 Other bursitis of elbow, unspecified elbow ▽

M70.31 Other bursitis of elbow, right elbow

M70.32 Other bursitis of elbow, left elbow

✓5th **M70.4** Prepatellar bursitis

M70.40 Prepatellar bursitis, unspecified knee ▽

M70.41 Prepatellar bursitis, right knee

M70.42 Prepatellar bursitis, left knee

Knee Bursae

✓5th **M70.5** Other bursitis of knee

M70.50 Other bursitis of knee, unspecified knee ▽

M70.51 Other bursitis of knee, right knee

M70.52 Other bursitis of knee, left knee

✓5th **M70.6** Trochanteric bursitis

Trochanteric tendinitis

M70.60 Trochanteric bursitis, unspecified hip ▽

M70.61 Trochanteric bursitis, right hip

M70.62 Trochanteric bursitis, left hip

✓5th **M70.7** Other bursitis of hip

Ischial bursitis

M70.70 Other bursitis of hip, unspecified hip ▽

M70.71 Other bursitis of hip, right hip

M70.72 Other bursitis of hip, left hip

✓5th **M70.8** Other soft tissue disorders related to use, overuse and pressure

M70.80 Other soft tissue disorders related to use, overuse and pressure of unspecified site ▽

✓6th **M70.81** Other soft tissue disorders related to use, overuse and pressure of shoulder

M70.811 Other soft tissue disorders related to use, overuse and pressure, right shoulder

M70.812 Other soft tissue disorders related to use, overuse and pressure, left shoulder

M70.819 Other soft tissue disorders related to use, overuse and pressure, unspecified shoulder ▽

✓6th **M70.82** Other soft tissue disorders related to use, overuse and pressure of upper arm

M70.821 Other soft tissue disorders related to use, overuse and pressure, right upper arm

M70.822 Other soft tissue disorders related to use, overuse and pressure, left upper arm

M70.829 Other soft tissue disorders related to use, overuse and pressure, unspecified upper arms ▽

✓6th **M70.83** Other soft tissue disorders related to use, overuse and pressure of forearm

M70.831 Other soft tissue disorders related to use, overuse and pressure, right forearm

M70.832 Other soft tissue disorders related to use, overuse and pressure, left forearm

M70.839 Other soft tissue disorders related to use, overuse and pressure, unspecified forearm ▽

✓6th **M70.84** Other soft tissue disorders related to use, overuse and pressure of hand

M70.841 Other soft tissue disorders related to use, overuse and pressure, right hand

M70.842 Other soft tissue disorders related to use, overuse and pressure, left hand

M70.849 Other soft tissue disorders related to use, overuse and pressure, unspecified hand ▽

✓6th **M70.85** Other soft tissue disorders related to use, overuse and pressure of thigh

M70.851 Other soft tissue disorders related to use, overuse and pressure, right thigh

M70.852 Other soft tissue disorders related to use, overuse and pressure, left thigh

M70.859 Other soft tissue disorders related to use, overuse and pressure, unspecified thigh ▽

✓6th **M70.86** Other soft tissue disorders related to use, overuse and pressure lower leg

M70.861 Other soft tissue disorders related to use, overuse and pressure, right lower leg

M70.862 Other soft tissue disorders related to use, overuse and pressure, left lower leg

M70.869 Other soft tissue disorders related to use, overuse and pressure, unspecified leg ▽

✓6th **M70.87** Other soft tissue disorders related to use, overuse and pressure of ankle and foot

M70.871 Other soft tissue disorders related to use, overuse and pressure, right ankle and foot

M70.872 Other soft tissue disorders related to use, overuse and pressure, left ankle and foot

M70.879 Other soft tissue disorders related to use, overuse and pressure, unspecified ankle and foot ▽

M70.88 Other soft tissue disorders related to use, overuse and pressure other site

EXCLUDES 1 Not coded here   EXCLUDES 2 Not included here   N Newborn Age : 0   P Pediatric Age : 0-17   M Maternity Age : 12-55   A Adult Age : 15-124

754   ICD-10-CM 2017

M70.89 Other soft tissue disorders related to use, overuse and pressure multiple sites

✓5ᵗʰ **M70.9** Unspecified soft tissue disorder related to use, overuse and pressure

    M70.90 Unspecified soft tissue disorder related to use, overuse and pressure of unspecified site ▽

✓6ᵗʰ **M70.91** Unspecified soft tissue disorder related to use, overuse and pressure of shoulder

    M70.911 Unspecified soft tissue disorder related to use, overuse and pressure, right shoulder ▽

    M70.912 Unspecified soft tissue disorder related to use, overuse and pressure, left shoulder ▽

    M70.919 Unspecified soft tissue disorder related to use, overuse and pressure, unspecified shoulder ▽

✓6ᵗʰ **M70.92** Unspecified soft tissue disorder related to use, overuse and pressure of upper arm

    M70.921 Unspecified soft tissue disorder related to use, overuse and pressure, right upper arm ▽

    M70.922 Unspecified soft tissue disorder related to use, overuse and pressure, left upper arm ▽

    M70.929 Unspecified soft tissue disorder related to use, overuse and pressure, unspecified upper arm ▽

✓6ᵗʰ **M70.93** Unspecified soft tissue disorder related to use, overuse and pressure of forearm

    M70.931 Unspecified soft tissue disorder related to use, overuse and pressure, right forearm ▽

    M70.932 Unspecified soft tissue disorder related to use, overuse and pressure, left forearm ▽

    M70.939 Unspecified soft tissue disorder related to use, overuse and pressure, unspecified forearm ▽

✓6ᵗʰ **M70.94** Unspecified soft tissue disorder related to use, overuse and pressure of hand

    M70.941 Unspecified soft tissue disorder related to use, overuse and pressure, right hand ▽

    M70.942 Unspecified soft tissue disorder related to use, overuse and pressure, left hand ▽

    M70.949 Unspecified soft tissue disorder related to use, overuse and pressure, unspecified hand ▽

✓6ᵗʰ **M70.95** Unspecified soft tissue disorder related to use, overuse and pressure of thigh

    M70.951 Unspecified soft tissue disorder related to use, overuse and pressure, right thigh ▽

    M70.952 Unspecified soft tissue disorder related to use, overuse and pressure, left thigh ▽

    M70.959 Unspecified soft tissue disorder related to use, overuse and pressure, unspecified thigh ▽

✓6ᵗʰ **M70.96** Unspecified soft tissue disorder related to use, overuse and pressure lower leg

    M70.961 Unspecified soft tissue disorder related to use, overuse and pressure, right lower leg ▽

    M70.962 Unspecified soft tissue disorder related to use, overuse and pressure, left lower leg ▽

    M70.969 Unspecified soft tissue disorder related to use, overuse and pressure, unspecified lower leg ▽

✓6ᵗʰ **M70.97** Unspecified soft tissue disorder related to use, overuse and pressure of ankle and foot

    M70.971 Unspecified soft tissue disorder related to use, overuse and pressure, right ankle and foot ▽

    M70.972 Unspecified soft tissue disorder related to use, overuse and pressure, left ankle and foot ▽

    M70.979 Unspecified soft tissue disorder related to use, overuse and pressure, unspecified ankle and foot ▽

M70.98 Unspecified soft tissue disorder related to use, overuse and pressure other ▽

M70.99 Unspecified soft tissue disorder related to use, overuse and pressure multiple sites ▽

✓4ᵗʰ **M71** Other bursopathies

    EXCLUDES 1   bunion (M20.1)

         bursitis related to use, overuse or pressure (M70.-)

         enthesopathies (M76-M77)

✓5ᵗʰ **M71.0** Abscess of bursa

    Use additional code (B95.-, B96.-) to identify causative organism

    M71.00 Abscess of bursa, unspecified site ▽

✓6ᵗʰ **M71.01** Abscess of bursa, shoulder

    M71.011 Abscess of bursa, right shoulder

    M71.012 Abscess of bursa, left shoulder

    M71.019 Abscess of bursa, unspecified shoulder ▽

✓6ᵗʰ **M71.02** Abscess of bursa, elbow

    M71.021 Abscess of bursa, right elbow

    M71.022 Abscess of bursa, left elbow

    M71.029 Abscess of bursa, unspecified elbow ▽

✓6ᵗʰ **M71.03** Abscess of bursa, wrist

    M71.031 Abscess of bursa, right wrist

    M71.032 Abscess of bursa, left wrist

    M71.039 Abscess of bursa, unspecified wrist ▽

✓6ᵗʰ **M71.04** Abscess of bursa, hand

    M71.041 Abscess of bursa, right hand

    M71.042 Abscess of bursa, left hand

    M71.049 Abscess of bursa, unspecified hand ▽

✓6ᵗʰ **M71.05** Abscess of bursa, hip

    M71.051 Abscess of bursa, right hip

    M71.052 Abscess of bursa, left hip

    M71.059 Abscess of bursa, unspecified hip ▽

✓6ᵗʰ **M71.06** Abscess of bursa, knee

    M71.061 Abscess of bursa, right knee

    M71.062 Abscess of bursa, left knee

    M71.069 Abscess of bursa, unspecified knee ▽

✓6ᵗʰ **M71.07** Abscess of bursa, ankle and foot

    M71.071 Abscess of bursa, right ankle and foot

    M71.072 Abscess of bursa, left ankle and foot

    M71.079 Abscess of bursa, unspecified ankle and foot ▽

    M71.08 Abscess of bursa, other site

    M71.09 Abscess of bursa, multiple sites

✓5ᵗʰ **M71.1** Other infective bursitis

    Use additional code (B95.-, B96.-) to identify causative organism

    M71.10 Other infective bursitis, unspecified site ▽

✓6ᵗʰ **M71.11** Other infective bursitis, shoulder

    M71.111 Other infective bursitis, right shoulder

    M71.112 Other infective bursitis, left shoulder

    M71.119 Other infective bursitis, unspecified shoulder ▽

✓6ᵗʰ **M71.12** Other infective bursitis, elbow

    M71.121 Other infective bursitis, right elbow

    M71.122 Other infective bursitis, left elbow

    M71.129 Other infective bursitis, unspecified elbow ▽

✓6ᵗʰ **M71.13** Other infective bursitis, wrist

    M71.131 Other infective bursitis, right wrist

    M71.132 Other infective bursitis, left wrist

    M71.139 Other infective bursitis, unspecified wrist ▽

✓6ᵗʰ **M71.14** Other infective bursitis, hand

    M71.141 Other infective bursitis, right hand

    M71.142 Other infective bursitis, left hand

    M71.149 Other infective bursitis, unspecified hand ▽

✓6ᵗʰ **M71.15** Other infective bursitis, hip

    M71.151 Other infective bursitis, right hip

    M71.152 Other infective bursitis, left hip

    M71.159 Other infective bursitis, unspecified hip ▽

✓6ᵗʰ **M71.16** Other infective bursitis, knee

    M71.161 Other infective bursitis, right knee

    M71.162 Other infective bursitis, left knee

☑ Additional Character Required   ✓x7ᵗʰ Placeholder Alert   Manifestation Dx   ▽ Unspecified Dx   ►◄ Revised Text   ● New Code   ▲ Revised Code Title

M71.169   Other infective bursitis, unspecified knee ▽

✓6ᵗʰ   M71.17   Other infective bursitis, ankle and foot

    M71.171   Other infective bursitis, right ankle and foot

    M71.172   Other infective bursitis, left ankle and foot

    M71.179   Other infective bursitis, unspecified ankle and foot ▽

M71.18   Other infective bursitis, other site

M71.19   Other infective bursitis, multiple sites

✓5ᵗʰ   M71.2   Synovial cyst of popliteal space [Baker]

    EXCLUDES 1   synovial cyst of popliteal space with rupture (M66.0)

M71.20   Synovial cyst of popliteal space [Baker], unspecified knee ▽

M71.21   Synovial cyst of popliteal space [Baker], right knee

M71.22   Synovial cyst of popliteal space [Baker], left knee

✓5ᵗʰ   M71.3   Other bursal cyst

    Synovial cyst NOS

    EXCLUDES 1   synovial cyst with rupture (M66.1-)

M71.30   Other bursal cyst, unspecified site ▽

✓6ᵗʰ   M71.31   Other bursal cyst, shoulder

    M71.311   Other bursal cyst, right shoulder

    M71.312   Other bursal cyst, left shoulder

    M71.319   Other bursal cyst, unspecified shoulder ▽

✓6ᵗʰ   M71.32   Other bursal cyst, elbow

    M71.321   Other bursal cyst, right elbow

    M71.322   Other bursal cyst, left elbow

    M71.329   Other bursal cyst, unspecified elbow ▽

✓6ᵗʰ   M71.33   Other bursal cyst, wrist

    M71.331   Other bursal cyst, right wrist

    M71.332   Other bursal cyst, left wrist

    M71.339   Other bursal cyst, unspecified wrist ▽

✓6ᵗʰ   M71.34   Other bursal cyst, hand

    M71.341   Other bursal cyst, right hand

    M71.342   Other bursal cyst, left hand

    M71.349   Other bursal cyst, unspecified hand ▽

✓6ᵗʰ   M71.35   Other bursal cyst, hip

    M71.351   Other bursal cyst, right hip

    M71.352   Other bursal cyst, left hip

    M71.359   Other bursal cyst, unspecified hip ▽

✓6ᵗʰ   M71.37   Other bursal cyst, ankle and foot

    M71.371   Other bursal cyst, right ankle and foot

    M71.372   Other bursal cyst, left ankle and foot

    M71.379   Other bursal cyst, unspecified ankle and foot ▽

M71.38   Other bursal cyst, other site

M71.39   Other bursal cyst, multiple sites

✓5ᵗʰ   M71.4   Calcium deposit in bursa

    EXCLUDES 2   calcium deposit in bursa of shoulder (M75.3)

M71.40   Calcium deposit in bursa, unspecified site ▽

✓6ᵗʰ   M71.42   Calcium deposit in bursa, elbow

    M71.421   Calcium deposit in bursa, right elbow

    M71.422   Calcium deposit in bursa, left elbow

    M71.429   Calcium deposit in bursa, unspecified elbow ▽

✓6ᵗʰ   M71.43   Calcium deposit in bursa, wrist

    M71.431   Calcium deposit in bursa, right wrist

    M71.432   Calcium deposit in bursa, left wrist

    M71.439   Calcium deposit in bursa, unspecified wrist ▽

✓6ᵗʰ   M71.44   Calcium deposit in bursa, hand

    M71.441   Calcium deposit in bursa, right hand

    M71.442   Calcium deposit in bursa, left hand

    M71.449   Calcium deposit in bursa, unspecified hand ▽

✓6ᵗʰ   M71.45   Calcium deposit in bursa, hip

    M71.451   Calcium deposit in bursa, right hip

    M71.452   Calcium deposit in bursa, left hip

    M71.459   Calcium deposit in bursa, unspecified hip ▽

✓6ᵗʰ   M71.46   Calcium deposit in bursa, knee

    M71.461   Calcium deposit in bursa, right knee

M71.462   Calcium deposit in bursa, left knee

M71.469   Calcium deposit in bursa, unspecified knee ▽

✓6ᵗʰ   M71.47   Calcium deposit in bursa, ankle and foot

    M71.471   Calcium deposit in bursa, right ankle and foot

    M71.472   Calcium deposit in bursa, left ankle and foot

    M71.479   Calcium deposit in bursa, unspecified ankle and foot ▽

M71.48   Calcium deposit in bursa, other site

M71.49   Calcium deposit in bursa, multiple sites

✓5ᵗʰ   M71.5   Other bursitis, not elsewhere classified

    EXCLUDES 1   bursitis NOS (M71.9-)

    EXCLUDES 2   bursitis of shoulder (M75.5)

        bursitis of tibial collateral [Pellegrini-Stieda] ▶(M76.4-)◀

M71.50   Other bursitis, not elsewhere classified, unspecified site ▽

✓6ᵗʰ   M71.52   Other bursitis, not elsewhere classified, elbow

    M71.521   Other bursitis, not elsewhere classified, right elbow

    M71.522   Other bursitis, not elsewhere classified, left elbow

    M71.529   Other bursitis, not elsewhere classified, unspecified elbow ▽

✓6ᵗʰ   M71.53   Other bursitis, not elsewhere classified, wrist

    M71.531   Other bursitis, not elsewhere classified, right wrist

    M71.532   Other bursitis, not elsewhere classified, left wrist

    M71.539   Other bursitis, not elsewhere classified, unspecified wrist ▽

✓6ᵗʰ   M71.54   Other bursitis, not elsewhere classified, hand

    M71.541   Other bursitis, not elsewhere classified, right hand

    M71.542   Other bursitis, not elsewhere classified, left hand

    M71.549   Other bursitis, not elsewhere classified, unspecified hand ▽

✓6ᵗʰ   M71.55   Other bursitis, not elsewhere classified, hip

    M71.551   Other bursitis, not elsewhere classified, right hip

    M71.552   Other bursitis, not elsewhere classified, left hip

    M71.559   Other bursitis, not elsewhere classified, unspecified hip ▽

✓6ᵗʰ   M71.56   Other bursitis, not elsewhere classified, knee

    M71.561   Other bursitis, not elsewhere classified, right knee

    M71.562   Other bursitis, not elsewhere classified, left knee

    M71.569   Other bursitis, not elsewhere classified, unspecified knee ▽

✓6ᵗʰ   M71.57   Other bursitis, not elsewhere classified, ankle and foot

    M71.571   Other bursitis, not elsewhere classified, right ankle and foot

    M71.572   Other bursitis, not elsewhere classified, left ankle and foot

    M71.579   Other bursitis, not elsewhere classified, unspecified ankle and foot ▽

M71.58   Other bursitis, not elsewhere classified, other site

✓5ᵗʰ   M71.8   Other specified bursopathies

M71.80   Other specified bursopathies, unspecified site ▽

✓6ᵗʰ   M71.81   Other specified bursopathies, shoulder

    M71.811   Other specified bursopathies, right shoulder

    M71.812   Other specified bursopathies, left shoulder

    M71.819   Other specified bursopathies, unspecified shoulder ▽

✓6ᵗʰ   M71.82   Other specified bursopathies, elbow

    M71.821   Other specified bursopathies, right elbow

    M71.822   Other specified bursopathies, left elbow

    M71.829   Other specified bursopathies, unspecified elbow ▽

EXCLUDES 1 Not coded here   EXCLUDES 2 Not included here   N Newborn Age : 0   P Pediatric Age : 0-17   M Maternity Age : 12-55   A Adult Age : 15-124

756   ICD-10-CM 2017

✓6ᵗʰ **M71.83** **Other specified bursopathies,** wrist

M71.831 Other specified bursopathies, right **wrist**
M71.832 Other specified bursopathies, left **wrist**
M71.839 Other specified bursopathies, unspecified **wrist** ▽

✓6ᵗʰ **M71.84** **Other specified bursopathies,** hand

M71.841 Other specified bursopathies, right **hand**
M71.842 Other specified bursopathies, left **hand**
M71.849 Other specified bursopathies, unspecified **hand** ▽

✓6ᵗʰ **M71.85** **Other specified bursopathies,** hip

M71.851 Other specified bursopathies, right **hip**
M71.852 Other specified bursopathies, left **hip**
M71.859 Other specified bursopathies, unspecified **hip** ▽

✓6ᵗʰ **M71.86** **Other specified bursopathies,** knee

M71.861 Other specified bursopathies, right **knee**
M71.862 Other specified bursopathies, left **knee**
M71.869 Other specified bursopathies, unspecified **knee** ▽

✓6ᵗʰ **M71.87** **Other specified bursopathies,** ankle and foot

M71.871 Other specified bursopathies, right **ankle and foot**
M71.872 Other specified bursopathies, left **ankle and foot**
M71.879 Other specified bursopathies, unspecified **ankle and foot** ▽

M71.88 **Other specified bursopathies, other site**
M71.89 **Other specified bursopathies,** multiple sites

M71.9 **Bursopathy, unspecified** ▽
Bursitis NOS

✓4ᵗʰ **M72** **Fibroblastic disorders**

EXCLUDES 2 retroperitoneal fibromatosis (D48.3)

M72.0 **Palmar fascial fibromatosis [Dupuytren]** Ⓐ

DEF: Dupuytren's contracture: Flexion deformity of finger, due to shortened, thickened fibrosing of palmar fascia; cause unknown; associated with long-standing epilepsy.

M72.1 **Knuckle pads**
M72.2 **Plantar fascial fibromatosis**
Plantar fasciitis
M72.4 **Pseudosarcomatous fibromatosis**
Nodular fasciitis
M72.6 **Necrotizing fasciitis**
Use additional code (B95.-, B96.-) to identify causative organism
M72.8 **Other fibroblastic disorders**
Abscess of fascia
Fasciitis NEC
Other infective fasciitis
Use additional code to (B95.-, B96.-) identify causative organism
EXCLUDES 1 diffuse (eosinophilic) fasciitis (M35.4)
necrotizing fasciitis (M72.6)
nodular fasciitis (M72.4)
perirenal fasciitis NOS (N13.5)
perirenal fasciitis with infection (N13.6)
plantar fasciitis (M72.2)
M72.9 **Fibroblastic disorder, unspecified** ▽
Fasciitis NOS
Fibromatosis NOS

✓4ᵗʰ **M75** **Shoulder lesions**

EXCLUDES 2 shoulder-hand syndrome (M89.0-)

✓5ᵗʰ **M75.0** **Adhesive capsulitis of shoulder**
Frozen shoulder
Periarthritis of shoulder
AHA: 2015,2Q,23
M75.00 **Adhesive capsulitis of unspecified shoulder** ▽
M75.01 **Adhesive capsulitis of** right **shoulder**
M75.02 **Adhesive capsulitis of** left **shoulder**

✓5ᵗʰ **M75.1** **Rotator cuff tear or rupture, not specified as traumatic**
Rotator cuff syndrome
Supraspinatus syndrome
Supraspinatus tear or rupture, not specified as traumatic
EXCLUDES 1 tear of rotator cuff, traumatic (S46.01-)
✓6ᵗʰ **M75.10** **Unspecified rotator cuff tear or rupture, not specified as traumatic**

M75.100 Unspecified rotator cuff tear or rupture of unspecified shoulder, not specified as traumatic ▽
M75.101 Unspecified rotator cuff tear or rupture of right shoulder, not specified as traumatic ▽
M75.102 Unspecified rotator cuff tear or rupture of left shoulder, not specified as traumatic ▽

✓6ᵗʰ **M75.11** Incomplete rotator cuff tear or rupture not specified as traumatic

M75.110 Incomplete rotator cuff tear or rupture of unspecified shoulder, not specified as traumatic ▽
M75.111 Incomplete rotator cuff tear or rupture of right shoulder, not specified as traumatic
M75.112 Incomplete rotator cuff tear or rupture of left shoulder, not specified as traumatic

✓6ᵗʰ **M75.12** Complete rotator cuff tear or rupture not specified as traumatic

M75.120 Complete rotator cuff tear or rupture of unspecified shoulder, not specified as traumatic ▽
M75.121 Complete rotator cuff tear or rupture of right shoulder, not specified as traumatic
M75.122 Complete rotator cuff tear or rupture of left shoulder, not specified as traumatic

✓5ᵗʰ **M75.2** **Bicipital** tendinitis

M75.20 **Bicipital tendinitis, unspecified shoulder** ▽
M75.21 **Bicipital tendinitis,** right **shoulder**
M75.22 **Bicipital tendinitis,** left **shoulder**

✓5ᵗʰ **M75.3** **Calcific** tendinitis of shoulder
Calcified bursa of shoulder
M75.30 **Calcific tendinitis of unspecified shoulder** ▽
M75.31 **Calcific tendinitis of** right **shoulder**
M75.32 **Calcific tendinitis of** left **shoulder**

✓5ᵗʰ **M75.4** **Impingement** syndrome **of shoulder**
M75.40 **Impingement syndrome of unspecified shoulder** ▽
M75.41 **Impingement syndrome of** right **shoulder**
M75.42 **Impingement syndrome of** left **shoulder**

✓5ᵗʰ **M75.5** **Bursitis** of shoulder
M75.50 **Bursitis of unspecified shoulder** ▽
M75.51 **Bursitis of** right **shoulder**
M75.52 **Bursitis of** left **shoulder**

✓5ᵗʰ **M75.8** **Other shoulder lesions**
M75.80 **Other shoulder lesions, unspecified shoulder** ▽
M75.81 **Other shoulder lesions,** right **shoulder**
M75.82 **Other shoulder lesions,** left **shoulder**

✓5ᵗʰ **M75.9** **Shoulder lesion, unspecified**
M75.90 **Shoulder lesion, unspecified, unspecified shoulder** ▽
M75.91 **Shoulder lesion, unspecified,** right **shoulder** ▽
M75.92 **Shoulder lesion, unspecified,** left **shoulder** ▽

✓4ᵗʰ **M76** **Enthesopathies, lower limb, excluding foot**

EXCLUDES 2 bursitis due to use, overuse and pressure (M70.-)
enthesopathies of ankle and foot (M77.5-)

✓5ᵗʰ **M76.0** **Gluteal** tendinitis
M76.00 **Gluteal tendinitis, unspecified hip** ▽
M76.01 **Gluteal tendinitis,** right **hip**
M76.02 **Gluteal tendinitis,** left **hip**

✓5ᵗʰ **M76.1** **Psoas** tendinitis
M76.10 **Psoas tendinitis, unspecified hip** ▽
M76.11 **Psoas tendinitis,** right **hip**
M76.12 **Psoas tendinitis,** left **hip**

✓5ᵗʰ **M76.2** **Iliac crest** spur
M76.20 **Iliac crest spur, unspecified hip** ▽
M76.21 **Iliac crest spur,** right **hip**
M76.22 **Iliac crest spur,** left **hip**

✓5ᵗʰ **M76.3** **Iliotibial band** syndrome
M76.30 **Iliotibial band syndrome, unspecified leg** ▽
M76.31 **Iliotibial band syndrome,** right **leg**
M76.32 **Iliotibial band syndrome,** left **leg**

Chapter 13. Diseases of the Musculoskeletal System and Connective Tissue

M71.83–M76.32

√5th M76.4 Tibial collateral bursitis [Pellegrini-Stieda]

   M76.40 Tibial collateral bursitis [Pellegrini-Stieda], unspecified leg ▽

   M76.41 Tibial collateral bursitis [Pellegrini-Stieda], right leg

   M76.42 Tibial collateral bursitis [Pellegrini-Stieda], left leg

√5th M76.5 Patellar tendinitis

   M76.50 Patellar tendinitis, unspecified knee ▽

   M76.51 Patellar tendinitis, right knee

   M76.52 Patellar tendinitis, left knee

√5th M76.6 Achilles tendinitis

   Achilles bursitis

   M76.60 Achilles tendinitis, unspecified leg ▽

   M76.61 Achilles tendinitis, right leg

   M76.62 Achilles tendinitis, left leg

√5th M76.7 Peroneal tendinitis

   M76.70 Peroneal tendinitis, unspecified leg ▽

   M76.71 Peroneal tendinitis, right leg

   M76.72 Peroneal tendinitis, left leg

√5th M76.8 Other specified enthesopathies of lower limb, excluding foot

   √6th M76.81 Anterior tibial syndrome

      M76.811 Anterior tibial syndrome, right leg

      M76.812 Anterior tibial syndrome, left leg

      M76.819 Anterior tibial syndrome, unspecified leg ▽

   √6th M76.82 Posterior tibial tendinitis

      M76.821 Posterior tibial tendinitis, right leg

      M76.822 Posterior tibial tendinitis, left leg

      M76.829 Posterior tibial tendinitis, unspecified leg ▽

   √6th M76.89 Other specified enthesopathies of lower limb, excluding foot

      M76.891 Other specified enthesopathies of right lower limb, excluding foot

      M76.892 Other specified enthesopathies of left lower limb, excluding foot

      M76.899 Other specified enthesopathies of unspecified lower limb, excluding foot ▽

   M76.9 Unspecified enthesopathy, lower limb, excluding foot ▽

√4th M77 Other enthesopathies

   EXCLUDES 1 bursitis NOS (M71.9-)

   EXCLUDES 2 bursitis due to use, overuse and pressure (M70.-)

      osteophyte (M25.7)

      spinal enthesopathy (M46.0-)

√5th M77.0 Medial epicondylitis

   M77.00 Medial epicondylitis, unspecified elbow ▽

   M77.01 Medial epicondylitis, right elbow

   M77.02 Medial epicondylitis, left elbow

√5th M77.1 Lateral epicondylitis

   Tennis elbow

   M77.10 Lateral epicondylitis, unspecified elbow ▽

   M77.11 Lateral epicondylitis, right elbow

   M77.12 Lateral epicondylitis, left elbow

√5th M77.2 Periarthritis of wrist

   M77.20 Periarthritis, unspecified wrist ▽

   M77.21 Periarthritis, right wrist

   M77.22 Periarthritis, left wrist

√5th M77.3 Calcaneal spur

   M77.30 Calcaneal spur, unspecified foot ▽

   M77.31 Calcaneal spur, right foot

   M77.32 Calcaneal spur, left foot

√5th M77.4 Metatarsalgia

   EXCLUDES 1 Morton's metatarsalgia (G57.6)

   M77.40 Metatarsalgia, unspecified foot ▽

   M77.41 Metatarsalgia, right foot

   M77.42 Metatarsalgia, left foot

√5th M77.5 Other enthesopathy of foot

   M77.50 Other enthesopathy of unspecified foot ▽

   M77.51 Other enthesopathy of right foot

   M77.52 Other enthesopathy of left foot

   M77.8 Other enthesopathies, not elsewhere classified

M77.9 Enthesopathy, unspecified ▽

   Bone spur NOS

   Capsulitis NOS

   Periarthritis NOS

   Tendinitis NOS

√4th M79 Other and unspecified soft tissue disorders, not elsewhere classified

   EXCLUDES 1 psychogenic rheumatism (F45.8)

      soft tissue pain, psychogenic (F45.41)

M79.0 Rheumatism, unspecified ▽

   EXCLUDES 1 fibromyalgia (M79.7)

      palindromic rheumatism (M12.3-)

M79.1 Myalgia

   Myofascial pain syndrome

   EXCLUDES 1 fibromyalgia (M79.7)

      myositis (M60.-)

M79.2 Neuralgia and neuritis, unspecified ▽

   EXCLUDES 1 brachial radiculitis NOS (M54.1)

      lumbosacral radiculitis NOS (M54.1)

      mononeuropathies (G56-G58)

      radiculitis NOS (M54.1)

      sciatica (M54.3-M54.4)

M79.3 Panniculitis, unspecified ▽

   EXCLUDES 1 lupus panniculitis (L93.2)

      neck and back panniculitis (M54.0-)

      relapsing [Weber-Christian] panniculitis (M35.6)

M79.4 Hypertrophy of (infrapatellar) fat pad

M79.5 Residual foreign body in soft tissue

   EXCLUDES 1 foreign body granuloma of skin and subcutaneous tissue (L92.3)

      foreign body granuloma of soft tissue (M60.2-)

√5th M79.6 Pain in limb, hand, foot, fingers and toes

   EXCLUDES 2 pain in joint (M25.5-)

   √6th M79.60 Pain in limb, unspecified

      M79.601 Pain in right arm

         Pain in right upper limb NOS

      M79.602 Pain in left arm

         Pain in left upper limb NOS

      M79.603 Pain in arm, unspecified ▽

         Pain in upper limb NOS

      M79.604 Pain in right leg

         Pain in right lower limb NOS

      M79.605 Pain in left leg

         Pain in left lower limb NOS

      M79.606 Pain in leg, unspecified ▽

         Pain in lower limb NOS

      M79.609 Pain in unspecified limb ▽

         Pain in limb NOS

   √6th M79.62 Pain in upper arm

      Pain in axillary region

      M79.621 Pain in right upper arm

      M79.622 Pain in left upper arm

      M79.629 Pain in unspecified upper arm ▽

   √6th M79.63 Pain in forearm

      M79.631 Pain in right forearm

      M79.632 Pain in left forearm

      M79.639 Pain in unspecified forearm ▽

   √6th M79.64 Pain in hand and fingers

      M79.641 Pain in right hand

      M79.642 Pain in left hand

      M79.643 Pain in unspecified hand ▽

      M79.644 Pain in right finger(s)

      M79.645 Pain in left finger(s)

      M79.646 Pain in unspecified finger(s) ▽

   √6th M79.65 Pain in thigh

      M79.651 Pain in right thigh

      M79.652 Pain in left thigh

      M79.659 Pain in unspecified thigh ▽

   √6th M79.66 Pain in lower leg

      M79.661 Pain in right lower leg

      M79.662 Pain in left lower leg

      M79.669 Pain in unspecified lower leg ▽

   √6th M79.67 Pain in foot and toes

      M79.671 Pain in right foot

EXCLUDES 1 Not coded here   *EXCLUDES 2* Not included here   N Newborn Age : 0   P Pediatric Age : 0-17   M Maternity Age : 12-55   A Adult Age : 15-124

758   ICD-10-CM 2017

M79.672 **Pain in** left foot
M79.673 **Pain in** unspecified foot   ▽
M79.674 **Pain in** right toe(s)
M79.675 **Pain in** left toe(s)
M79.676 **Pain in** unspecified toe(s)   ▽

M79.7 **Fibromyalgia**
Fibromyositis
Fibrositis
Myofibrositis

✓5ᵗʰ M79.A **Nontraumatic compartment syndrome**
Code first, if applicable, associated postprocedural complication
EXCLUDES 1 *compartment syndrome NOS (T79.A-)*
fibromyalgia (M79.7)
nontraumatic ischemic infarction of muscle (M62.2-)
traumatic compartment syndrome (T79.A-)

✓6ᵗʰ M79.A1 **Nontraumatic compartment syndrome of** upper extremity
Nontraumatic compartment syndrome of shoulder, arm, forearm, wrist, hand, and fingers
M79.A11 **Nontraumatic compartment syndrome of** right **upper extremity**
M79.A12 **Nontraumatic compartment syndrome of** left **upper extremity**
M79.A19 **Nontraumatic compartment syndrome of unspecified upper extremity**   ▽

✓6ᵗʰ M79.A2 **Nontraumatic compartment syndrome of** lower extremity
Nontraumatic compartment syndrome of hip, buttock, thigh, leg, foot, and toes
M79.A21 **Nontraumatic compartment syndrome of** right **lower extremity**
M79.A22 **Nontraumatic compartment syndrome of** left **lower extremity**
M79.A29 **Nontraumatic compartment syndrome of unspecified lower extremity**   ▽

M79.A3 **Nontraumatic compartment syndrome of** abdomen
M79.A9 **Nontraumatic compartment syndrome of other sites**

✓6ᵗʰ M79.8 **Other specified soft tissue disorders**
M79.81 **Nontraumatic hematoma of soft tissue**
Nontraumatic hematoma of muscle
Nontraumatic seroma of muscle and soft tissue
M79.89 **Other specified soft tissue disorders**
Polyalgia

M79.9 **Soft tissue disorder, unspecified**   ▽

Osteopathies and chondropathies (M80-M94)

Disorders of bone density and structure (M80-M85)

✓4ᵗʰ **M80 Osteoporosis** with current pathological fracture
INCLUDES osteoporosis with current fragility fracture
Use additional code to identify major osseous defect, if applicable (M89.7-)
EXCLUDES 1 *collapsed vertebra NOS (M48.5)*
pathological fracture NOS (M84.4)
wedging of vertebra NOS (M48.5)
EXCLUDES 2 *personal history of (healed) osteoporosis fracture (Z87.310)*

The appropriate 7th character is to be added to each code from category M80:
A   initial encounter for fracture
D   subsequent encounter for fracture with routine healing
G   subsequent encounter for fracture with delayed healing
K   subsequent encounter for fracture with nonunion
P   subsequent encounter for fracture with malunion
S   sequela

✓5ᵗʰ M80.0 Age-related **osteoporosis with current pathological fracture**
Involutional osteoporosis with current pathological fracture
Osteoporosis NOS with current pathological fracture
Postmenopausal osteoporosis with current pathological fracture
Senile osteoporosis with current pathological fracture
✓x7ᵗʰ M80.00 **Age-related osteoporosis with current pathological fracture, unspecified site**   Ⓐ ▽
✓6ᵗʰ M80.01 **Age-related osteoporosis with current pathological fracture,** shoulder

✓7ᵗʰ M80.011 **Age-related osteoporosis with current pathological fracture,** right **shoulder**   Ⓐ
✓7ᵗʰ M80.012 **Age-related osteoporosis with current pathological fracture,** left **shoulder**   Ⓐ
✓7ᵗʰ M80.019 **Age-related osteoporosis with current pathological fracture, unspecified shoulder**   Ⓐ ▽

✓6ᵗʰ M80.02 **Age-related osteoporosis with current pathological fracture,** humerus
✓7ᵗʰ M80.021 **Age-related osteoporosis with current pathological fracture,** right **humerus**   Ⓐ
✓7ᵗʰ M80.022 **Age-related osteoporosis with current pathological fracture,** left **humerus**   Ⓐ
✓7ᵗʰ M80.029 **Age-related osteoporosis with current pathological fracture, unspecified humerus**   Ⓐ ▽

✓6ᵗʰ M80.03 **Age-related osteoporosis with current pathological fracture,** forearm
Age-related osteoporosis with current pathological fracture of wrist
✓7ᵗʰ M80.031 **Age-related osteoporosis with current pathological fracture,** right **forearm**   Ⓐ
✓7ᵗʰ M80.032 **Age-related osteoporosis with current pathological fracture,** left **forearm**   Ⓐ
✓7ᵗʰ M80.039 **Age-related osteoporosis with current pathological fracture, unspecified forearm**   Ⓐ ▽

✓6ᵗʰ M80.04 **Age-related osteoporosis with current pathological fracture,** hand
✓7ᵗʰ M80.041 **Age-related osteoporosis with current pathological fracture,** right **hand**   Ⓐ
✓7ᵗʰ M80.042 **Age-related osteoporosis with current pathological fracture,** left **hand**   Ⓐ
✓7ᵗʰ M80.049 **Age-related osteoporosis with current pathological fracture, unspecified hand**   Ⓐ ▽

✓6ᵗʰ M80.05 **Age-related osteoporosis with current pathological fracture,** femur
Age-related osteoporosis with current pathological fracture of hip
✓7ᵗʰ M80.051 **Age-related osteoporosis with current pathological fracture,** right **femur**   Ⓐ
✓7ᵗʰ M80.052 **Age-related osteoporosis with current pathological fracture,** left **femur**   Ⓐ
✓7ᵗʰ M80.059 **Age-related osteoporosis with current pathological fracture, unspecified femur**   Ⓐ ▽

✓6ᵗʰ M80.06 **Age-related osteoporosis with current pathological fracture,** lower leg
✓7ᵗʰ M80.061 **Age-related osteoporosis with current pathological fracture,** right **lower leg**   Ⓐ
✓7ᵗʰ M80.062 **Age-related osteoporosis with current pathological fracture,** left **lower leg**   Ⓐ
✓7ᵗʰ M80.069 **Age-related osteoporosis with current pathological fracture, unspecified lower leg**   Ⓐ ▽

✓6ᵗʰ M80.07 **Age-related osteoporosis with current pathological fracture,** ankle and foot
✓7ᵗʰ M80.071 **Age-related osteoporosis with current pathological fracture,** right **ankle and foot**   Ⓐ
✓7ᵗʰ M80.072 **Age-related osteoporosis with current pathological fracture,** left **ankle and foot**   Ⓐ
✓7ᵗʰ M80.079 **Age-related osteoporosis with current pathological fracture, unspecified ankle and foot**   Ⓐ ▽

✓x7ᵗʰ M80.08 **Age-related osteoporosis with current pathological fracture,** vertebra(e)   Ⓐ

√5ᵗʰ **M80.8** **Other osteoporosis with current pathological fracture**

Drug-induced osteoporosis with current pathological fracture

Idiopathic osteoporosis with current pathological fracture

Osteoporosis of disuse with current pathological fracture

Postoophorectomy osteoporosis with current pathological fracture

Postsurgical malabsorption osteoporosis with current pathological fracture

Post-traumatic osteoporosis with current pathological fracture

Use additional code for adverse effect, if applicable, to identify drug (T36-T50 with fifth or sixth character 5)

√×7ᵗʰ **M80.80** **Other osteoporosis with current pathological fracture, unspecified site** ▽

√6ᵗʰ **M80.81** **Other osteoporosis with current pathological fracture, shoulder**

√7ᵗʰ **M80.811** Other osteoporosis with current pathological fracture, **right shoulder**

√7ᵗʰ **M80.812** Other osteoporosis with current pathological fracture, **left shoulder**

√7ᵗʰ **M80.819** Other osteoporosis with current pathological fracture, unspecified **shoulder** ▽

√6ᵗʰ **M80.82** **Other osteoporosis with current pathological fracture, humerus**

√7ᵗʰ **M80.821** Other osteoporosis with current pathological fracture, **right humerus**

√7ᵗʰ **M80.822** Other osteoporosis with current pathological fracture, **left humerus**

√7ᵗʰ **M80.829** Other osteoporosis with current pathological fracture, unspecified **humerus** ▽

√6ᵗʰ **M80.83** **Other osteoporosis with current pathological fracture, forearm**

Other osteoporosis with current pathological fracture of wrist

√7ᵗʰ **M80.831** Other osteoporosis with current pathological fracture, **right forearm**

√7ᵗʰ **M80.832** Other osteoporosis with current pathological fracture, **left forearm**

√7ᵗʰ **M80.839** Other osteoporosis with current pathological fracture, unspecified **forearm** ▽

√6ᵗʰ **M80.84** **Other osteoporosis with current pathological fracture, hand**

√7ᵗʰ **M80.841** Other osteoporosis with current pathological fracture, **right hand**

√7ᵗʰ **M80.842** Other osteoporosis with current pathological fracture, **left hand**

√7ᵗʰ **M80.849** Other osteoporosis with current pathological fracture, unspecified **hand** ▽

√6ᵗʰ **M80.85** **Other osteoporosis with current pathological fracture, femur**

Other osteoporosis with current pathological fracture of hip

√7ᵗʰ **M80.851** Other osteoporosis with current pathological fracture, **right femur**

√7ᵗʰ **M80.852** Other osteoporosis with current pathological fracture, **left femur**

√7ᵗʰ **M80.859** Other osteoporosis with current pathological fracture, unspecified **femur** ▽

√6ᵗʰ **M80.86** **Other osteoporosis with current pathological fracture, lower leg**

√7ᵗʰ **M80.861** Other osteoporosis with current pathological fracture, **right lower leg**

√7ᵗʰ **M80.862** Other osteoporosis with current pathological fracture, **left lower leg**

√7ᵗʰ **M80.869** Other osteoporosis with current pathological fracture, unspecified **lower leg** ▽

√6ᵗʰ **M80.87** **Other osteoporosis with current pathological fracture, ankle and foot**

√7ᵗʰ **M80.871** Other osteoporosis with current pathological fracture, **right ankle and foot**

√7ᵗʰ **M80.872** Other osteoporosis with current pathological fracture, **left ankle and foot**

√7ᵗʰ **M80.879** Other osteoporosis with current pathological fracture, unspecified **ankle and foot** ▽

√×7ᵗʰ **M80.88** **Other osteoporosis with current pathological fracture, vertebra(e)**

√4ᵗʰ **M81** **Osteoporosis** **without current pathological fracture**

Use additional code to identify:

major osseous defect, if applicable (M89.7-)

personal history of (healed) osteoporosis fracture, if applicable (Z87.310)

EXCLUDES 1 *osteoporosis with current pathological fracture (M80.-)*

Sudeck's atrophy (M89.0)

M81.0 **Age-related osteoporosis without current pathological fracture** Ⓐ

Involutional osteoporosis without current pathological fracture

Osteoporosis NOS

Postmenopausal osteoporosis without current pathological fracture

Senile osteoporosis without current pathological fracture

M81.6 **Localized osteoporosis [Lequesne]**

EXCLUDES 1 *Sudeck's atrophy (M89.0)*

M81.8 **Other osteoporosis without current pathological fracture**

Drug-induced osteoporosis without current pathological fracture

Idiopathic osteoporosis without current pathological fracture

Osteoporosis of disuse without current pathological fracture

Postoophorectomy osteoporosis without current pathological fracture

Postsurgical malabsorption osteoporosis without current pathological fracture

Post-traumatic osteoporosis without current pathological fracture

Use additional code for adverse effect, if applicable, to identify drug (T36-T50 with fifth or sixth character 5)

√4ᵗʰ **M83** **Adult osteomalacia**

EXCLUDES 1 *infantile and juvenile osteomalacia (E55.0)*

renal osteodystrophy (N25.0)

rickets (active) (E55.0)

rickets (active) sequelae (E64.3)

vitamin D-resistant osteomalacia (E83.3)

vitamin D-resistant rickets (active) (E83.3)

M83.0 **Puerperal osteomalacia** Ⓜ ♀

M83.1 **Senile osteomalacia** Ⓐ

M83.2 **Adult osteomalacia due to malabsorption** Ⓐ

Postsurgical malabsorption osteomalacia in adults

M83.3 **Adult osteomalacia due to malnutrition** Ⓐ

M83.4 **Aluminum bone disease**

M83.5 **Other drug-induced osteomalacia in adults** Ⓐ

Use additional code for adverse effect, if applicable, to identify drug (T36-T50 with fifth or sixth character 5)

M83.8 **Other adult osteomalacia** Ⓐ

M83.9 **Adult osteomalacia, unspecified** Ⓐ ▽

√4ᵗʰ **M84** **Disorder of continuity of bone**

EXCLUDES 2 *traumatic fracture of bone-see fracture, by site*

√5ᵗʰ **M84.3** **Stress fracture**

Fatigue fracture

March fracture

Stress fracture NOS

Stress reaction

Use additional external cause code(s) to identify the cause of the stress fracture

EXCLUDES 1 *pathological fracture due to osteoporosis (M80.-)*

pathological fracture NOS (M84.4.-)

traumatic fracture (S12.-, S22.-, S32.-, S42.-, S52.-, S62.-, S72.-, S82.-, S92.-)

EXCLUDES 2 *personal history of (healed) stress (fatigue) fracture (Z87.312)*

stress fracture of vertebra (M48.4-)

> The appropriate 7th character is to be added to each code from subcategory M84.3.
>
> A   initial encounter for fracture
> D   subsequent encounter for fracture with routine healing
> G   subsequent encounter for fracture with delayed healing
> K   subsequent encounter for fracture with nonunion
> P   subsequent encounter for fracture with malunion
> S   sequela

√×7ᵗʰ **M84.30** **Stress fracture, unspecified site** ▽

√6ᵗʰ **M84.31** **Stress fracture, shoulder**

√7ᵗʰ **M84.311** **Stress fracture, right shoulder**

EXCLUDES 1 Not coded here   **EXCLUDES 2** Not included here   Ⓝ Newborn Age : 0   Ⓟ Pediatric Age : 0-17   Ⓜ Maternity Age : 12-55   Ⓐ Adult Age : 15-124

760

ICD-10-CM 2017

√7ᵗʰ M84.312   Stress fracture, left shoulder

√7ᵗʰ M84.319   Stress fracture, unspecified shoulder ▽

√6ᵗʰ M84.32   Stress fracture, humerus

√7ᵗʰ M84.321   Stress fracture, right humerus

√7ᵗʰ M84.322   Stress fracture, left humerus

√7ᵗʰ M84.329   Stress fracture, unspecified humerus ▽

√6ᵗʰ M84.33   Stress fracture, ulna and radius

√7ᵗʰ M84.331   Stress fracture, right ulna

√7ᵗʰ M84.332   Stress fracture, left ulna

√7ᵗʰ M84.333   Stress fracture, right radius

√7ᵗʰ M84.334   Stress fracture, left radius

√7ᵗʰ M84.339   Stress fracture, unspecified ulna and radius ▽

√6ᵗʰ M84.34   Stress fracture, hand and fingers

√7ᵗʰ M84.341   Stress fracture, right hand

√7ᵗʰ M84.342   Stress fracture, left hand

√7ᵗʰ M84.343   Stress fracture, unspecified hand ▽

√7ᵗʰ M84.344   Stress fracture, right finger(s)

√7ᵗʰ M84.345   Stress fracture, left finger(s)

√7ᵗʰ M84.346   Stress fracture, unspecified finger(s) ▽

√6ᵗʰ M84.35   Stress fracture, pelvis and femur

Stress fracture, hip

√7ᵗʰ M84.350   Stress fracture, pelvis

√7ᵗʰ M84.351   Stress fracture, right femur

√7ᵗʰ M84.352   Stress fracture, left femur

√7ᵗʰ M84.353   Stress fracture, unspecified femur ▽

√7ᵗʰ M84.359   Stress fracture, hip, unspecified ▽

√6ᵗʰ M84.36   Stress fracture, tibia and fibula

√7ᵗʰ M84.361   Stress fracture, right tibia

√7ᵗʰ M84.362   Stress fracture, left tibia

√7ᵗʰ M84.363   Stress fracture, right fibula

√7ᵗʰ M84.364   Stress fracture, left fibula

√7ᵗʰ M84.369   Stress fracture, unspecified tibia and fibula ▽

√6ᵗʰ M84.37   Stress fracture, ankle, foot and toes

√7ᵗʰ M84.371   Stress fracture, right ankle

√7ᵗʰ M84.372   Stress fracture, left ankle

√7ᵗʰ M84.373   Stress fracture, unspecified ankle ▽

√7ᵗʰ M84.374   Stress fracture, right foot

√7ᵗʰ M84.375   Stress fracture, left foot

√7ᵗʰ M84.376   Stress fracture, unspecified foot ▽

√7ᵗʰ M84.377   Stress fracture, right toe(s)

√7ᵗʰ M84.378   Stress fracture, left toe(s)

√7ᵗʰ M84.379   Stress fracture, unspecified toe(s) ▽

√x7ᵗʰ M84.38   Stress fracture, other site

EXCLUDES 2   stress fracture of vertebra (M48.4-)

√5ᵗʰ M84.4   Pathological fracture, not elsewhere classified

Chronic fracture

Pathological fracture NOS

EXCLUDES 1   collapsed vertebra NEC (M48.5)

pathological fracture in neoplastic disease (M84.5-)

pathological fracture in osteoporosis (M80.-)

pathological fracture in other disease (M84.6-)

stress fracture (M84.3-)

traumatic fracture (S12.-, S22.-, S32.-, S42.-, S52.-, S62.-, S72.-, S82.-, S92.-)

EXCLUDES 2   personal history of (healed) pathological fracture (Z87.311)

The appropriate 7th character is to be added to each code from subcategory M84.4.

A   initial encounter for fracture

D   subsequent encounter for fracture with routine healing

G   subsequent encounter for fracture with delayed healing

K   subsequent encounter for fracture with nonunion

P   subsequent encounter for fracture with malunion

S   sequela

√x7ᵗʰ M84.40   Pathological fracture, unspecified site ▽

√6ᵗʰ M84.41   Pathological fracture, shoulder

√7ᵗʰ M84.411   Pathological fracture, right shoulder

√7ᵗʰ M84.412   Pathological fracture, left shoulder

√7ᵗʰ M84.419   Pathological fracture, unspecified shoulder ▽

√6ᵗʰ M84.42   Pathological fracture, humerus

√7ᵗʰ M84.421   Pathological fracture, right humerus

√7ᵗʰ M84.422   Pathological fracture, left humerus

√7ᵗʰ M84.429   Pathological fracture, unspecified humerus ▽

√6ᵗʰ M84.43   Pathological fracture, ulna and radius

√7ᵗʰ M84.431   Pathological fracture, right ulna

√7ᵗʰ M84.432   Pathological fracture, left ulna

√7ᵗʰ M84.433   Pathological fracture, right radius

√7ᵗʰ M84.434   Pathological fracture, left radius

√7ᵗʰ M84.439   Pathological fracture, unspecified ulna and radius ▽

√6ᵗʰ M84.44   Pathological fracture, hand and fingers

√7ᵗʰ M84.441   Pathological fracture, right hand

√7ᵗʰ M84.442   Pathological fracture, left hand

√7ᵗʰ M84.443   Pathological fracture, unspecified hand ▽

√7ᵗʰ M84.444   Pathological fracture, right finger(s)

√7ᵗʰ M84.445   Pathological fracture, left finger(s)

√7ᵗʰ M84.446   Pathological fracture, unspecified finger(s) ▽

√6ᵗʰ M84.45   Pathological fracture, femur and pelvis

√7ᵗʰ M84.451   Pathological fracture, right femur

√7ᵗʰ M84.452   Pathological fracture, left femur

√7ᵗʰ M84.453   Pathological fracture, unspecified femur ▽

√7ᵗʰ M84.454   Pathological fracture, pelvis

√7ᵗʰ M84.459   Pathological fracture, hip, unspecified ▽

√6ᵗʰ M84.46   Pathological fracture, tibia and fibula

√7ᵗʰ M84.461   Pathological fracture, right tibia

√7ᵗʰ M84.462   Pathological fracture, left tibia

√7ᵗʰ M84.463   Pathological fracture, right fibula

√7ᵗʰ M84.464   Pathological fracture, left fibula

√7ᵗʰ M84.469   Pathological fracture, unspecified tibia and fibula ▽

√6ᵗʰ M84.47   Pathological fracture, ankle, foot and toes

√7ᵗʰ M84.471   Pathological fracture, right ankle

√7ᵗʰ M84.472   Pathological fracture, left ankle

√7ᵗʰ M84.473   Pathological fracture, unspecified ankle ▽

√7ᵗʰ M84.474   Pathological fracture, right foot

√7ᵗʰ M84.475   Pathological fracture, left foot

√7ᵗʰ M84.476   Pathological fracture, unspecified foot ▽

√7ᵗʰ M84.477   Pathological fracture, right toe(s)

√7ᵗʰ M84.478   Pathological fracture, left toe(s)

√7ᵗʰ M84.479   Pathological fracture, unspecified toe(s) ▽

√x7ᵗʰ M84.48   Pathological fracture, other site

√5ᵗʰ M84.5   Pathological fracture in neoplastic disease

Code also underlying neoplasm

The appropriate 7th character is to be added to each code from subcategory M84.5.

A   initial encounter for fracture

D   subsequent encounter for fracture with routine healing

G   subsequent encounter for fracture with delayed healing

K   subsequent encounter for fracture with nonunion

P   subsequent encounter for fracture with malunion

S   sequela

√x7ᵗʰ M84.50   Pathological fracture in neoplastic disease, unspecified site ▽

√6ᵗʰ M84.51   Pathological fracture in neoplastic disease, shoulder

√7ᵗʰ M84.511   Pathological fracture in neoplastic disease, right shoulder

√7ᵗʰ M84.512   Pathological fracture in neoplastic disease, left shoulder

√7ᵗʰ M84.519   Pathological fracture in neoplastic disease, unspecified shoulder ▽

☑ Additional Character Required   √x7ᵗʰ Placeholder Alert   Manifestation Dx   ▽ Unspecified Dx   ►◄ Revised Text   ● New Code   ▲ Revised Code Title

M84.52 Pathological fracture in neoplastic disease, humerus
> **M84.521** Pathological fracture in neoplastic disease, right **humerus**
> **M84.522** Pathological fracture in neoplastic disease, left **humerus**
> **M84.529** Pathological fracture in neoplastic disease, unspecified humerus ▽

M84.53 Pathological fracture in neoplastic disease, ulna and radius
> **M84.531** Pathological fracture in neoplastic disease, right ulna
> **M84.532** Pathological fracture in neoplastic disease, left ulna
> **M84.533** Pathological fracture in neoplastic disease, right radius
> **M84.534** Pathological fracture in neoplastic disease, left radius
> **M84.539** Pathological fracture in neoplastic disease, unspecified ulna and radius ▽

M84.54 Pathological fracture in neoplastic disease, hand
> **M84.541** Pathological fracture in neoplastic disease, right **hand**
> **M84.542** Pathological fracture in neoplastic disease, left **hand**
> **M84.549** Pathological fracture in neoplastic disease, unspecified hand ▽

M84.55 Pathological fracture in neoplastic disease, pelvis and femur
> **M84.550** Pathological fracture in neoplastic disease, pelvis
> **M84.551** Pathological fracture in neoplastic disease, right femur
> **M84.552** Pathological fracture in neoplastic disease, left femur
> **M84.553** Pathological fracture in neoplastic disease, unspecified femur ▽
> **M84.559** Pathological fracture in neoplastic disease, hip, unspecified ▽

M84.56 Pathological fracture in neoplastic disease, tibia and fibula
> **M84.561** Pathological fracture in neoplastic disease, right tibia
> **M84.562** Pathological fracture in neoplastic disease, left tibia
> **M84.563** Pathological fracture in neoplastic disease, right fibula
> **M84.564** Pathological fracture in neoplastic disease, left fibula
> **M84.569** Pathological fracture in neoplastic disease, unspecified tibia and fibula ▽

M84.57 Pathological fracture in neoplastic disease, ankle and foot
> **M84.571** Pathological fracture in neoplastic disease, right ankle
> **M84.572** Pathological fracture in neoplastic disease, left ankle
> **M84.573** Pathological fracture in neoplastic disease, unspecified ankle ▽
> **M84.574** Pathological fracture in neoplastic disease, right foot
> **M84.575** Pathological fracture in neoplastic disease, left foot
> **M84.576** Pathological fracture in neoplastic disease, unspecified foot ▽

M84.58 Pathological fracture in neoplastic disease, other specified site
> Pathological fracture in neoplastic disease, vertebrae

M84.6 Pathological fracture in other disease
> Code also underlying condition
> _EXCLUDES 1_ _pathological fracture in osteoporosis (M80.-)_
>
> The appropriate 7th character is to be added to each code from subcategory M84.6.
> A   initial encounter for fracture
> D   subsequent encounter for fracture with routine healing
> G   subsequent encounter for fracture with delayed healing
> K   subsequent encounter for fracture with nonunion
> P   subsequent encounter for fracture with malunion
> S   sequela

M84.60 Pathological fracture in other disease, unspecified site ▽

M84.61 Pathological fracture in other disease, shoulder
> **M84.611** Pathological fracture in other disease, right **shoulder**
> **M84.612** Pathological fracture in other disease, left **shoulder**
> **M84.619** Pathological fracture in other disease, unspecified shoulder ▽

M84.62 Pathological fracture in other disease, humerus
> **M84.621** Pathological fracture in other disease, right **humerus**
> **M84.622** Pathological fracture in other disease, left **humerus**
> **M84.629** Pathological fracture in other disease, unspecified humerus ▽

M84.63 Pathological fracture in other disease, ulna and radius
> **M84.631** Pathological fracture in other disease, right ulna
> **M84.632** Pathological fracture in other disease, left ulna
> **M84.633** Pathological fracture in other disease, right radius
> **M84.634** Pathological fracture in other disease, left radius
> **M84.639** Pathological fracture in other disease, unspecified ulna and radius ▽

M84.64 Pathological fracture in other disease, hand
> **M84.641** Pathological fracture in other disease, right **hand**
> **M84.642** Pathological fracture in other disease, left **hand**
> **M84.649** Pathological fracture in other disease, unspecified hand ▽

M84.65 Pathological fracture in other disease, pelvis and femur
> **M84.650** Pathological fracture in other disease, pelvis
> **M84.651** Pathological fracture in other disease, right femur
> **M84.652** Pathological fracture in other disease, left femur
> **M84.653** Pathological fracture in other disease, unspecified femur ▽
> **M84.659** Pathological fracture in other disease, hip, unspecified ▽

M84.66 Pathological fracture in other disease, tibia and fibula
> **M84.661** Pathological fracture in other disease, right tibia
> **M84.662** Pathological fracture in other disease, left tibia
> **M84.663** Pathological fracture in other disease, right fibula
> **M84.664** Pathological fracture in other disease, left fibula
> **M84.669** Pathological fracture in other disease, unspecified tibia and fibula ▽

M84.67 Pathological fracture in other disease, ankle and foot
> **M84.671** Pathological fracture in other disease, right ankle
> **M84.672** Pathological fracture in other disease, left ankle
> **M84.673** Pathological fracture in other disease, unspecified ankle ▽
> **M84.674** Pathological fracture in other disease, right foot
> **M84.675** Pathological fracture in other disease, left foot
> **M84.676** Pathological fracture in other disease, unspecified foot ▽

M84.68 Pathological fracture in other disease, other site

EXCLUDES 1 Not coded here   _EXCLUDES 2_ Not included here   N Newborn Age : 0   P Pediatric Age : 0-17   M Maternity Age : 12-55   A Adult Age : 15-124

762   ICD-10-CM 2017

●   ✓5ᵗʰ **M84.7**   Nontraumatic fracture, not elsewhere classified

●   ✓6ᵗʰ **M84.75**   Atypical femoral fracture

> The appropriate 7th character is to be added to each code from M84.75:
> A   initial encounter for fracture
> D   subsequent encounter for fracture with routine healing
> G   subsequent encounter for fracture with delayed healing
> K   subsequent encounter for fracture with nonunion
> P   subsequent encounter for fracture with malunion
> S   sequela

●   ✓7ᵗʰ **M84.750**   Atypical femoral fracture, unspecified   ▽

●   ✓7ᵗʰ **M84.751**   Incomplete atypical femoral fracture, right leg

●   ✓7ᵗʰ **M84.752**   Incomplete atypical femoral fracture, left leg

●   ✓7ᵗʰ **M84.753**   Incomplete atypical femoral fracture, unspecified leg   ▽

●   ✓7ᵗʰ **M84.754**   Complete transverse atypical femoral fracture, right leg

●   ✓7ᵗʰ **M84.755**   Complete transverse atypical femoral fracture, left leg

●   ✓7ᵗʰ **M84.756**   Complete transverse atypical femoral fracture, unspecified leg   ▽

●   ✓7ᵗʰ **M84.757**   Complete oblique atypical femoral fracture, right leg

●   ✓7ᵗʰ **M84.758**   Complete oblique atypical femoral fracture, left leg

●   ✓7ᵗʰ **M84.759**   Complete oblique atypical femoral fracture, unspecified leg   ▽

   ✓5ᵗʰ **M84.8**   Other disorders of continuity of bone

     M84.80   Other disorders of continuity of bone, unspecified site   ▽

     ✓6ᵗʰ **M84.81**   Other disorders of continuity of bone, shoulder

      M84.811   Other disorders of continuity of bone, right shoulder

      M84.812   Other disorders of continuity of bone, left shoulder

      M84.819   Other disorders of continuity of bone, unspecified shoulder   ▽

     ✓6ᵗʰ **M84.82**   Other disorders of continuity of bone, humerus

      M84.821   Other disorders of continuity of bone, right humerus

      M84.822   Other disorders of continuity of bone, left humerus

      M84.829   Other disorders of continuity of bone, unspecified humerus   ▽

     ✓6ᵗʰ **M84.83**   Other disorders of continuity of bone, ulna and radius

      M84.831   Other disorders of continuity of bone, right ulna

      M84.832   Other disorders of continuity of bone, left ulna

      M84.833   Other disorders of continuity of bone, right radius

      M84.834   Other disorders of continuity of bone, left radius

      M84.839   Other disorders of continuity of bone, unspecified ulna and radius   ▽

     ✓6ᵗʰ **M84.84**   Other disorders of continuity of bone, hand

      M84.841   Other disorders of continuity of bone, right hand

      M84.842   Other disorders of continuity of bone, left hand

      M84.849   Other disorders of continuity of bone, unspecified hand   ▽

     ✓6ᵗʰ **M84.85**   Other disorders of continuity of bone, pelvic region and thigh

      M84.851   Other disorders of continuity of bone, right pelvic region and thigh

      M84.852   Other disorders of continuity of bone, left pelvic region and thigh

      M84.859   Other disorders of continuity of bone, unspecified pelvic region and thigh   ▽

     ✓6ᵗʰ **M84.86**   Other disorders of continuity of bone, tibia and fibula

      M84.861   Other disorders of continuity of bone, right tibia

      M84.862   Other disorders of continuity of bone, left tibia

      M84.863   Other disorders of continuity of bone, right fibula

      M84.864   Other disorders of continuity of bone, left fibula

      M84.869   Other disorders of continuity of bone, unspecified tibia and fibula   ▽

     ✓6ᵗʰ **M84.87**   Other disorders of continuity of bone, ankle and foot

      M84.871   Other disorders of continuity of bone, right ankle and foot

      M84.872   Other disorders of continuity of bone, left ankle and foot

      M84.879   Other disorders of continuity of bone, unspecified ankle and foot   ▽

     M84.88   Other disorders of continuity of bone, other site

   M84.9   Disorder of continuity of bone, unspecified   ▽

✓4ᵗʰ **M85**   **Other disorders of bone density and structure**

> EXCLUDES 1   osteogenesis imperfecta (Q78.0)
> osteopetrosis (Q78.2)
> osteopoikilosis (Q78.8)
> polyostotic fibrous dysplasia (Q78.1)

   ✓5ᵗʰ **M85.0**   Fibrous dysplasia (monostotic)

> EXCLUDES 2   fibrous dysplasia of jaw (M27.8)

     M85.00   Fibrous dysplasia (monostotic), unspecified site   ▽

     ✓6ᵗʰ **M85.01**   Fibrous dysplasia (monostotic), shoulder

      M85.011   Fibrous dysplasia (monostotic), right shoulder

      M85.012   Fibrous dysplasia (monostotic), left shoulder

      M85.019   Fibrous dysplasia (monostotic), unspecified shoulder   ▽

     ✓6ᵗʰ **M85.02**   Fibrous dysplasia (monostotic), upper arm

      M85.021   Fibrous dysplasia (monostotic), right upper arm

      M85.022   Fibrous dysplasia (monostotic), left upper arm

      M85.029   Fibrous dysplasia (monostotic), unspecified upper arm   ▽

     ✓6ᵗʰ **M85.03**   Fibrous dysplasia (monostotic), forearm

      M85.031   Fibrous dysplasia (monostotic), right forearm

      M85.032   Fibrous dysplasia (monostotic), left forearm

      M85.039   Fibrous dysplasia (monostotic), unspecified forearm   ▽

     ✓6ᵗʰ **M85.04**   Fibrous dysplasia (monostotic), hand

      M85.041   Fibrous dysplasia (monostotic), right hand

      M85.042   Fibrous dysplasia (monostotic), left hand

      M85.049   Fibrous dysplasia (monostotic), unspecified hand   ▽

     ✓6ᵗʰ **M85.05**   Fibrous dysplasia (monostotic), thigh

      M85.051   Fibrous dysplasia (monostotic), right thigh

      M85.052   Fibrous dysplasia (monostotic), left thigh

      M85.059   Fibrous dysplasia (monostotic), unspecified thigh   ▽

     ✓6ᵗʰ **M85.06**   Fibrous dysplasia (monostotic), lower leg

      M85.061   Fibrous dysplasia (monostotic), right lower leg

      M85.062   Fibrous dysplasia (monostotic), left lower leg

      M85.069   Fibrous dysplasia (monostotic), unspecified lower leg   ▽

     ✓6ᵗʰ **M85.07**   Fibrous dysplasia (monostotic), ankle and foot

      M85.071   Fibrous dysplasia (monostotic), right ankle and foot

      M85.072   Fibrous dysplasia (monostotic), left ankle and foot

      M85.079   Fibrous dysplasia (monostotic), unspecified ankle and foot   ▽

     M85.08   Fibrous dysplasia (monostotic), other site

     M85.09   Fibrous dysplasia (monostotic), multiple sites

✓ Additional Character Required   ✓x7ᵗʰ Placeholder Alert   Manifestation Dx   ▽Unspecified Dx   ►◄ Revised Text   ● New Code   ▲ Revised Code Title

ICD-10-CM 2017   763

√5ᵗʰ **M85.1** **Skeletal fluorosis**
    M85.10 Skeletal fluorosis, unspecified site ▽
    √6ᵗʰ **M85.11** Skeletal fluorosis, shoulder
        M85.111 Skeletal fluorosis, right shoulder
        M85.112 Skeletal fluorosis, left shoulder
        M85.119 Skeletal fluorosis, unspecified shoulder ▽
    √6ᵗʰ **M85.12** Skeletal fluorosis, upper arm
        M85.121 Skeletal fluorosis, right upper arm
        M85.122 Skeletal fluorosis, left upper arm
        M85.129 Skeletal fluorosis, unspecified upper arm ▽
    √6ᵗʰ **M85.13** Skeletal fluorosis, forearm
        M85.131 Skeletal fluorosis, right forearm
        M85.132 Skeletal fluorosis, left forearm
        M85.139 Skeletal fluorosis, unspecified forearm ▽
    √6ᵗʰ **M85.14** Skeletal fluorosis, hand
        M85.141 Skeletal fluorosis, right hand
        M85.142 Skeletal fluorosis, left hand
        M85.149 Skeletal fluorosis, unspecified hand ▽
    √6ᵗʰ **M85.15** Skeletal fluorosis, thigh
        M85.151 Skeletal fluorosis, right thigh
        M85.152 Skeletal fluorosis, left thigh
        M85.159 Skeletal fluorosis, unspecified thigh ▽
    √6ᵗʰ **M85.16** Skeletal fluorosis, lower leg
        M85.161 Skeletal fluorosis, right lower leg
        M85.162 Skeletal fluorosis, left lower leg
        M85.169 Skeletal fluorosis, unspecified lower leg ▽
    √6ᵗʰ **M85.17** Skeletal fluorosis, ankle and foot
        M85.171 Skeletal fluorosis, right ankle and foot
        M85.172 Skeletal fluorosis, left ankle and foot
        M85.179 Skeletal fluorosis, unspecified ankle and foot ▽
    M85.18 Skeletal fluorosis, other site
    M85.19 Skeletal fluorosis, multiple sites
M85.2 **Hyperostosis of skull**
√5ᵗʰ **M85.3** **Osteitis condensans**
    M85.30 Osteitis condensans, unspecified site ▽
    √6ᵗʰ **M85.31** Osteitis condensans, shoulder
        M85.311 Osteitis condensans, right shoulder
        M85.312 Osteitis condensans, left shoulder
        M85.319 Osteitis condensans, unspecified shoulder ▽
    √6ᵗʰ **M85.32** Osteitis condensans, upper arm
        M85.321 Osteitis condensans, right upper arm
        M85.322 Osteitis condensans, left upper arm
        M85.329 Osteitis condensans, unspecified upper arm ▽
    √6ᵗʰ **M85.33** Osteitis condensans, forearm
        M85.331 Osteitis condensans, right forearm
        M85.332 Osteitis condensans, left forearm
        M85.339 Osteitis condensans, unspecified forearm ▽
    √6ᵗʰ **M85.34** Osteitis condensans, hand
        M85.341 Osteitis condensans, right hand
        M85.342 Osteitis condensans, left hand
        M85.349 Osteitis condensans, unspecified hand ▽
    √6ᵗʰ **M85.35** Osteitis condensans, thigh
        M85.351 Osteitis condensans, right thigh
        M85.352 Osteitis condensans, left thigh
        M85.359 Osteitis condensans, unspecified thigh ▽
    √6ᵗʰ **M85.36** Osteitis condensans, lower leg
        M85.361 Osteitis condensans, right lower leg
        M85.362 Osteitis condensans, left lower leg
        M85.369 Osteitis condensans, unspecified lower leg ▽
    √6ᵗʰ **M85.37** Osteitis condensans, ankle and foot
        M85.371 Osteitis condensans, right ankle and foot
        M85.372 Osteitis condensans, left ankle and foot
        M85.379 Osteitis condensans, unspecified ankle and foot ▽

    M85.38 Osteitis condensans, other site
    M85.39 Osteitis condensans, multiple sites
√5ᵗʰ **M85.4** **Solitary bone cyst**
    EXCLUDES 2 solitary cyst of jaw (M27.4)
    M85.40 Solitary bone cyst, unspecified site ▽
    √6ᵗʰ **M85.41** Solitary bone cyst, shoulder
        M85.411 Solitary bone cyst, right shoulder
        M85.412 Solitary bone cyst, left shoulder
        M85.419 Solitary bone cyst, unspecified shoulder ▽
    √6ᵗʰ **M85.42** Solitary bone cyst, humerus
        M85.421 Solitary bone cyst, right humerus
        M85.422 Solitary bone cyst, left humerus
        M85.429 Solitary bone cyst, unspecified humerus ▽
    √6ᵗʰ **M85.43** Solitary bone cyst, ulna and radius
        M85.431 Solitary bone cyst, right ulna and radius
        M85.432 Solitary bone cyst, left ulna and radius
        M85.439 Solitary bone cyst, unspecified ulna and radius ▽
    √6ᵗʰ **M85.44** Solitary bone cyst, hand
        M85.441 Solitary bone cyst, right hand
        M85.442 Solitary bone cyst, left hand
        M85.449 Solitary bone cyst, unspecified hand ▽
    √6ᵗʰ **M85.45** Solitary bone cyst, pelvis
        M85.451 Solitary bone cyst, right pelvis
        M85.452 Solitary bone cyst, left pelvis
        M85.459 Solitary bone cyst, unspecified pelvis ▽
    √6ᵗʰ **M85.46** Solitary bone cyst, tibia and fibula
        M85.461 Solitary bone cyst, right tibia and fibula
        M85.462 Solitary bone cyst, left tibia and fibula
        M85.469 Solitary bone cyst, unspecified tibia and fibula ▽
    √6ᵗʰ **M85.47** Solitary bone cyst, ankle and foot
        M85.471 Solitary bone cyst, right ankle and foot
        M85.472 Solitary bone cyst, left ankle and foot
        M85.479 Solitary bone cyst, unspecified ankle and foot ▽
    M85.48 Solitary bone cyst, other site
√5ᵗʰ **M85.5** **Aneurysmal bone cyst**
    EXCLUDES 2 aneurysmal cyst of jaw (M27.4)
    DEF: Solitary bone lesion, bulges into periosteum; marked by calcified rim.
    M85.50 Aneurysmal bone cyst, unspecified site ▽
    √6ᵗʰ **M85.51** Aneurysmal bone cyst, shoulder
        M85.511 Aneurysmal bone cyst, right shoulder
        M85.512 Aneurysmal bone cyst, left shoulder
        M85.519 Aneurysmal bone cyst, unspecified shoulder ▽
    √6ᵗʰ **M85.52** Aneurysmal bone cyst, upper arm
        M85.521 Aneurysmal bone cyst, right upper arm
        M85.522 Aneurysmal bone cyst, left upper arm
        M85.529 Aneurysmal bone cyst, unspecified upper arm ▽
    √6ᵗʰ **M85.53** Aneurysmal bone cyst, forearm
        M85.531 Aneurysmal bone cyst, right forearm
        M85.532 Aneurysmal bone cyst, left forearm
        M85.539 Aneurysmal bone cyst, unspecified forearm ▽
    √6ᵗʰ **M85.54** Aneurysmal bone cyst, hand
        M85.541 Aneurysmal bone cyst, right hand
        M85.542 Aneurysmal bone cyst, left hand
        M85.549 Aneurysmal bone cyst, unspecified hand ▽
    √6ᵗʰ **M85.55** Aneurysmal bone cyst, thigh
        M85.551 Aneurysmal bone cyst, right thigh
        M85.552 Aneurysmal bone cyst, left thigh
        M85.559 Aneurysmal bone cyst, unspecified thigh ▽
    √6ᵗʰ **M85.56** Aneurysmal bone cyst, lower leg
        M85.561 Aneurysmal bone cyst, right lower leg
        M85.562 Aneurysmal bone cyst, left lower leg
        M85.569 Aneurysmal bone cyst, unspecified lower leg ▽

EXCLUDES 1 Not coded here   *EXCLUDES 2* Not included here   N Newborn Age : 0   P Pediatric Age : 0-17   M Maternity Age : 12-55   A Adult Age : 15-124

764   ICD-10-CM 2017

✓6ᵗʰ **M85.57** **Aneurysmal bone cyst,** ankle and foot

     M85.571 **Aneurysmal bone cyst,** right ankle and foot

     M85.572 **Aneurysmal bone cyst,** left ankle and foot

     M85.579 **Aneurysmal bone cyst,** unspecified ankle and foot ▽

     M85.58 **Aneurysmal bone cyst, other site**

     M85.59 **Aneurysmal bone cyst,** multiple sites

✓5ᵗʰ **M85.6** **Other cyst of bone**

     EXCLUDES 1   *cyst of jaw NEC (M27.4)*
         osteitis fibrosa cystica generalisata [von Recklinghausen's disease of bone] (E21.0)

     M85.60 **Other cyst of bone, unspecified site** ▽

✓6ᵗʰ **M85.61** **Other cyst of bone,** shoulder

     M85.611 **Other cyst of bone,** right shoulder

     M85.612 **Other cyst of bone,** left shoulder

     M85.619 **Other cyst of bone, unspecified shoulder** ▽

✓6ᵗʰ **M85.62** **Other cyst of bone,** upper arm

     M85.621 **Other cyst of bone,** right upper arm

     M85.622 **Other cyst of bone,** left upper arm

     M85.629 **Other cyst of bone, unspecified upper arm** ▽

✓6ᵗʰ **M85.63** **Other cyst of bone,** forearm

     M85.631 **Other cyst of bone,** right forearm

     M85.632 **Other cyst of bone,** left forearm

     M85.639 **Other cyst of bone, unspecified forearm** ▽

✓6ᵗʰ **M85.64** **Other cyst of bone,** hand

     M85.641 **Other cyst of bone,** right hand

     M85.642 **Other cyst of bone,** left hand

     M85.649 **Other cyst of bone, unspecified hand** ▽

✓6ᵗʰ **M85.65** **Other cyst of bone,** thigh

     M85.651 **Other cyst of bone,** right thigh

     M85.652 **Other cyst of bone,** left thigh

     M85.659 **Other cyst of bone, unspecified thigh** ▽

✓6ᵗʰ **M85.66** **Other cyst of bone,** lower leg

     M85.661 **Other cyst of bone,** right lower leg

     M85.662 **Other cyst of bone,** left lower leg

     M85.669 **Other cyst of bone, unspecified lower leg** ▽

✓6ᵗʰ **M85.67** **Other cyst of bone,** ankle and foot

     M85.671 **Other cyst of bone,** right ankle and foot

     M85.672 **Other cyst of bone,** left ankle and foot

     M85.679 **Other cyst of bone, unspecified ankle and foot** ▽

     M85.68 **Other cyst of bone, other site**

     M85.69 **Other cyst of bone,** multiple sites

✓5ᵗʰ **M85.8** **Other specified disorders of bone density and structure**

     Hyperostosis of bones, except skull
     Osteosclerosis, acquired

     EXCLUDES 1   *diffuse idiopathic skeletal hyperostosis [DISH] (M48.1)*
         osteosclerosis congenita (Q77.4)
         osteosclerosis fragilitas (generalista) (Q78.2)
         osteosclerosis myelofibrosis (D75.81)

     M85.80 **Other specified disorders of bone density and structure, unspecified site** ▽

✓6ᵗʰ **M85.81** **Other specified disorders of bone density and structure,** shoulder

     M85.811 **Other specified disorders of bone density and structure,** right shoulder

     M85.812 **Other specified disorders of bone density and structure,** left shoulder

     M85.819 **Other specified disorders of bone density and structure, unspecified shoulder** ▽

✓6ᵗʰ **M85.82** **Other specified disorders of bone density and structure,** upper arm

     M85.821 **Other specified disorders of bone density and structure,** right upper arm

     M85.822 **Other specified disorders of bone density and structure,** left upper arm

     M85.829 **Other specified disorders of bone density and structure, unspecified upper arm** ▽

✓6ᵗʰ **M85.83** **Other specified disorders of bone density and structure,** forearm

     M85.831 **Other specified disorders of bone density and structure,** right forearm

     M85.832 **Other specified disorders of bone density and structure,** left forearm

     M85.839 **Other specified disorders of bone density and structure, unspecified forearm** ▽

✓6ᵗʰ **M85.84** **Other specified disorders of bone density and structure,** hand

     M85.841 **Other specified disorders of bone density and structure,** right hand

     M85.842 **Other specified disorders of bone density and structure,** left hand

     M85.849 **Other specified disorders of bone density and structure, unspecified hand** ▽

✓6ᵗʰ **M85.85** **Other specified disorders of bone density and structure,** thigh

     M85.851 **Other specified disorders of bone density and structure,** right thigh

     M85.852 **Other specified disorders of bone density and structure,** left thigh

     M85.859 **Other specified disorders of bone density and structure, unspecified thigh** ▽

✓6ᵗʰ **M85.86** **Other specified disorders of bone density and structure,** lower leg

     M85.861 **Other specified disorders of bone density and structure,** right lower leg

     M85.862 **Other specified disorders of bone density and structure,** left lower leg

     M85.869 **Other specified disorders of bone density and structure, unspecified lower leg** ▽

✓6ᵗʰ **M85.87** **Other specified disorders of bone density and structure,** ankle and foot

     M85.871 **Other specified disorders of bone density and structure,** right ankle and foot

     M85.872 **Other specified disorders of bone density and structure,** left ankle and foot

     M85.879 **Other specified disorders of bone density and structure, unspecified ankle and foot** ▽

     M85.88 **Other specified disorders of bone density and structure, other site**

     M85.89 **Other specified disorders of bone density and structure,** multiple sites

     M85.9 **Disorder of bone density and structure, unspecified** ▽

Other osteopathies (M86-M90)

     EXCLUDES 1   *postprocedural osteopathies (M96.-)*

✓4ᵗʰ **M86** **Osteomyelitis**

     Use additional code (B95-B97) to identify infectious agent
     Use additional code to identify major osseous defect, if applicable (M89.7-)

     EXCLUDES 1   *osteomyelitis due to:*
         echinococcus (B67.2)
         gonococcus (A54.43)
         salmonella (A02.24)

     EXCLUDES 2   *osteomyelitis of:*
         orbit (H05.0-)
         petrous bone (H70.2-)
         vertebra (M46.2-)

✓5ᵗʰ **M86.0** **Acute hematogenous osteomyelitis**

     M86.00 **Acute hematogenous osteomyelitis, unspecified site** ▽

✓6ᵗʰ **M86.01** **Acute hematogenous osteomyelitis,** shoulder

     M86.011 **Acute hematogenous osteomyelitis,** right shoulder

     M86.012 **Acute hematogenous osteomyelitis,** left shoulder

     M86.019 **Acute hematogenous osteomyelitis, unspecified shoulder** ▽

✓6ᵗʰ **M86.02** **Acute hematogenous osteomyelitis,** humerus

     M86.021 **Acute hematogenous osteomyelitis,** right humerus

     M86.022 **Acute hematogenous osteomyelitis,** left humerus

✓ Additional Character Required   ✓x7ᵗʰ Placeholder Alert   Manifestation Dx   ▽ Unspecified Dx   ►◄ Revised Text   ● New Code   ▲ Revised Code Title

ICD-10-CM 2017   765

M86.029   Acute hematogenous osteomyelitis, unspecified humerus   ▽

✓6ᵗʰ M86.03   Acute hematogenous osteomyelitis, radius and ulna

M86.031   Acute hematogenous osteomyelitis, right radius and ulna

M86.032   Acute hematogenous osteomyelitis, left radius and ulna

M86.039   Acute hematogenous osteomyelitis, unspecified radius and ulna   ▽

✓6ᵗʰ M86.04   Acute hematogenous osteomyelitis, hand

M86.041   Acute hematogenous osteomyelitis, right hand

M86.042   Acute hematogenous osteomyelitis, left hand

M86.049   Acute hematogenous osteomyelitis, unspecified hand   ▽

✓6ᵗʰ M86.05   Acute hematogenous osteomyelitis, femur

M86.051   Acute hematogenous osteomyelitis, right femur

M86.052   Acute hematogenous osteomyelitis, left femur

M86.059   Acute hematogenous osteomyelitis, unspecified femur   ▽

✓6ᵗʰ M86.06   Acute hematogenous osteomyelitis, tibia and fibula

M86.061   Acute hematogenous osteomyelitis, right tibia and fibula

M86.062   Acute hematogenous osteomyelitis, left tibia and fibula

M86.069   Acute hematogenous osteomyelitis, unspecified tibia and fibula   ▽

✓6ᵗʰ M86.07   Acute hematogenous osteomyelitis, ankle and foot

M86.071   Acute hematogenous osteomyelitis, right ankle and foot

M86.072   Acute hematogenous osteomyelitis, left ankle and foot

M86.079   Acute hematogenous osteomyelitis, unspecified ankle and foot   ▽

M86.08   Acute hematogenous osteomyelitis, other sites

M86.09   Acute hematogenous osteomyelitis, multiple sites

✓5ᵗʰ M86.1   Other acute osteomyelitis

M86.10   Other acute osteomyelitis, unspecified site   ▽

✓6ᵗʰ M86.11   Other acute osteomyelitis, shoulder

M86.111   Other acute osteomyelitis, right shoulder

M86.112   Other acute osteomyelitis, left shoulder

M86.119   Other acute osteomyelitis, unspecified shoulder   ▽

✓6ᵗʰ M86.12   Other acute osteomyelitis, humerus

M86.121   Other acute osteomyelitis, right humerus

M86.122   Other acute osteomyelitis, left humerus

M86.129   Other acute osteomyelitis, unspecified humerus   ▽

✓6ᵗʰ M86.13   Other acute osteomyelitis, radius and ulna

M86.131   Other acute osteomyelitis, right radius and ulna

M86.132   Other acute osteomyelitis, left radius and ulna

M86.139   Other acute osteomyelitis, unspecified radius and ulna   ▽

✓6ᵗʰ M86.14   Other acute osteomyelitis, hand

M86.141   Other acute osteomyelitis, right hand

M86.142   Other acute osteomyelitis, left hand

M86.149   Other acute osteomyelitis, unspecified hand   ▽

✓6ᵗʰ M86.15   Other acute osteomyelitis, femur

M86.151   Other acute osteomyelitis, right femur

M86.152   Other acute osteomyelitis, left femur

M86.159   Other acute osteomyelitis, unspecified femur   ▽

✓6ᵗʰ M86.16   Other acute osteomyelitis, tibia and fibula

M86.161   Other acute osteomyelitis, right tibia and fibula

M86.162   Other acute osteomyelitis, left tibia and fibula

M86.169   Other acute osteomyelitis, unspecified tibia and fibula   ▽

✓6ᵗʰ M86.17   Other acute osteomyelitis, ankle and foot

M86.171   Other acute osteomyelitis, right ankle and foot

M86.172   Other acute osteomyelitis, left ankle and foot

M86.179   Other acute osteomyelitis, unspecified ankle and foot   ▽

M86.18   Other acute osteomyelitis, other site

M86.19   Other acute osteomyelitis, multiple sites

✓5ᵗʰ M86.2   Subacute osteomyelitis

M86.20   Subacute osteomyelitis, unspecified site   ▽

✓6ᵗʰ M86.21   Subacute osteomyelitis, shoulder

M86.211   Subacute osteomyelitis, right shoulder

M86.212   Subacute osteomyelitis, left shoulder

M86.219   Subacute osteomyelitis, unspecified shoulder

✓6ᵗʰ M86.22   Subacute osteomyelitis, humerus

M86.221   Subacute osteomyelitis, right humerus

M86.222   Subacute osteomyelitis, left humerus

M86.229   Subacute osteomyelitis, unspecified humerus   ▽

✓6ᵗʰ M86.23   Subacute osteomyelitis, radius and ulna

M86.231   Subacute osteomyelitis, right radius and ulna

M86.232   Subacute osteomyelitis, left radius and ulna

M86.239   Subacute osteomyelitis, unspecified radius and ulna   ▽

✓6ᵗʰ M86.24   Subacute osteomyelitis, hand

M86.241   Subacute osteomyelitis, right hand

M86.242   Subacute osteomyelitis, left hand

M86.249   Subacute osteomyelitis, unspecified hand   ▽

✓6ᵗʰ M86.25   Subacute osteomyelitis, femur

M86.251   Subacute osteomyelitis, right femur

M86.252   Subacute osteomyelitis, left femur

M86.259   Subacute osteomyelitis, unspecified femur   ▽

✓6ᵗʰ M86.26   Subacute osteomyelitis, tibia and fibula

M86.261   Subacute osteomyelitis, right tibia and fibula

M86.262   Subacute osteomyelitis, left tibia and fibula

M86.269   Subacute osteomyelitis, unspecified tibia and fibula   ▽

✓6ᵗʰ M86.27   Subacute osteomyelitis, ankle and foot

M86.271   Subacute osteomyelitis, right ankle and foot

M86.272   Subacute osteomyelitis, left ankle and foot

M86.279   Subacute osteomyelitis, unspecified ankle and foot   ▽

M86.28   Subacute osteomyelitis, other site

M86.29   Subacute osteomyelitis, multiple sites

✓5ᵗʰ M86.3   Chronic multifocal osteomyelitis

M86.30   Chronic multifocal osteomyelitis, unspecified site   ▽

✓6ᵗʰ M86.31   Chronic multifocal osteomyelitis, shoulder

M86.311   Chronic multifocal osteomyelitis, right shoulder

M86.312   Chronic multifocal osteomyelitis, left shoulder

M86.319   Chronic multifocal osteomyelitis, unspecified shoulder   ▽

✓6ᵗʰ M86.32   Chronic multifocal osteomyelitis, humerus

M86.321   Chronic multifocal osteomyelitis, right humerus

M86.322   Chronic multifocal osteomyelitis, left humerus

M86.329   Chronic multifocal osteomyelitis, unspecified humerus   ▽

✓6ᵗʰ M86.33   Chronic multifocal osteomyelitis, radius and ulna

M86.331   Chronic multifocal osteomyelitis, right radius and ulna

M86.332   Chronic multifocal osteomyelitis, left radius and ulna

M86.339   Chronic multifocal osteomyelitis, unspecified radius and ulna   ▽

EXCLUDES 1   Not coded here   EXCLUDES 2   Not included here   N   Newborn Age : 0   P   Pediatric Age : 0-17   M   Maternity Age : 12-55   A   Adult Age : 15-124

766   ICD-10-CM 2017

✓6ᵗʰ **M86.34 Chronic multifocal osteomyelitis, hand**

     M86.341 Chronic multifocal osteomyelitis, right hand

     M86.342 Chronic multifocal osteomyelitis, left hand

     M86.349 Chronic multifocal osteomyelitis, unspecified hand ▽

✓6ᵗʰ **M86.35 Chronic multifocal osteomyelitis, femur**

     M86.351 Chronic multifocal osteomyelitis, right femur

     M86.352 Chronic multifocal osteomyelitis, left femur

     M86.359 Chronic multifocal osteomyelitis, unspecified femur ▽

✓6ᵗʰ **M86.36 Chronic multifocal osteomyelitis, tibia and fibula**

     M86.361 Chronic multifocal osteomyelitis, right tibia and fibula

     M86.362 Chronic multifocal osteomyelitis, left tibia and fibula

     M86.369 Chronic multifocal osteomyelitis, unspecified tibia and fibula ▽

✓6ᵗʰ **M86.37 Chronic multifocal osteomyelitis, ankle and foot**

     M86.371 Chronic multifocal osteomyelitis, right ankle and foot

     M86.372 Chronic multifocal osteomyelitis, left ankle and foot

     M86.379 Chronic multifocal osteomyelitis, unspecified ankle and foot ▽

     M86.38 Chronic multifocal osteomyelitis, other site

     M86.39 Chronic multifocal osteomyelitis, multiple sites

✓5ᵗʰ **M86.4 Chronic osteomyelitis with draining sinus**

     M86.40 Chronic osteomyelitis with draining sinus, unspecified site ▽

✓6ᵗʰ **M86.41 Chronic osteomyelitis with draining sinus, shoulder**

     M86.411 Chronic osteomyelitis with draining sinus, right shoulder

     M86.412 Chronic osteomyelitis with draining sinus, left shoulder

     M86.419 Chronic osteomyelitis with draining sinus, unspecified shoulder ▽

✓6ᵗʰ **M86.42 Chronic osteomyelitis with draining sinus, humerus**

     M86.421 Chronic osteomyelitis with draining sinus, right humerus

     M86.422 Chronic osteomyelitis with draining sinus, left humerus

     M86.429 Chronic osteomyelitis with draining sinus, unspecified humerus ▽

✓6ᵗʰ **M86.43 Chronic osteomyelitis with draining sinus, radius and ulna**

     M86.431 Chronic osteomyelitis with draining sinus, right radius and ulna

     M86.432 Chronic osteomyelitis with draining sinus, left radius and ulna

     M86.439 Chronic osteomyelitis with draining sinus, unspecified radius and ulna ▽

✓6ᵗʰ **M86.44 Chronic osteomyelitis with draining sinus, hand**

     M86.441 Chronic osteomyelitis with draining sinus, right hand

     M86.442 Chronic osteomyelitis with draining sinus, left hand

     M86.449 Chronic osteomyelitis with draining sinus, unspecified hand ▽

✓6ᵗʰ **M86.45 Chronic osteomyelitis with draining sinus, femur**

     M86.451 Chronic osteomyelitis with draining sinus, right femur

     M86.452 Chronic osteomyelitis with draining sinus, left femur

     M86.459 Chronic osteomyelitis with draining sinus, unspecified femur ▽

✓6ᵗʰ **M86.46 Chronic osteomyelitis with draining sinus, tibia and fibula**

     M86.461 Chronic osteomyelitis with draining sinus, right tibia and fibula

     M86.462 Chronic osteomyelitis with draining sinus, left tibia and fibula

     M86.469 Chronic osteomyelitis with draining sinus, unspecified tibia and fibula ▽

✓6ᵗʰ **M86.47 Chronic osteomyelitis with draining sinus, ankle and foot**

     M86.471 Chronic osteomyelitis with draining sinus, right ankle and foot

     M86.472 Chronic osteomyelitis with draining sinus, left ankle and foot

     M86.479 Chronic osteomyelitis with draining sinus, unspecified ankle and foot ▽

     M86.48 Chronic osteomyelitis with draining sinus, other site

     M86.49 Chronic osteomyelitis with draining sinus, multiple sites

✓5ᵗʰ **M86.5 Other chronic hematogenous osteomyelitis**

     M86.50 Other chronic hematogenous osteomyelitis, unspecified site ▽

✓6ᵗʰ **M86.51 Other chronic hematogenous osteomyelitis, shoulder**

     M86.511 Other chronic hematogenous osteomyelitis, right shoulder

     M86.512 Other chronic hematogenous osteomyelitis, left shoulder

     M86.519 Other chronic hematogenous osteomyelitis, unspecified shoulder ▽

✓6ᵗʰ **M86.52 Other chronic hematogenous osteomyelitis, humerus**

     M86.521 Other chronic hematogenous osteomyelitis, right humerus

     M86.522 Other chronic hematogenous osteomyelitis, left humerus

     M86.529 Other chronic hematogenous osteomyelitis, unspecified humerus ▽

✓6ᵗʰ **M86.53 Other chronic hematogenous osteomyelitis, radius and ulna**

     M86.531 Other chronic hematogenous osteomyelitis, right radius and ulna

     M86.532 Other chronic hematogenous osteomyelitis, left radius and ulna

     M86.539 Other chronic hematogenous osteomyelitis, unspecified radius and ulna ▽

✓6ᵗʰ **M86.54 Other chronic hematogenous osteomyelitis, hand**

     M86.541 Other chronic hematogenous osteomyelitis, right hand

     M86.542 Other chronic hematogenous osteomyelitis, left hand

     M86.549 Other chronic hematogenous osteomyelitis, unspecified hand ▽

✓6ᵗʰ **M86.55 Other chronic hematogenous osteomyelitis, femur**

     M86.551 Other chronic hematogenous osteomyelitis, right femur

     M86.552 Other chronic hematogenous osteomyelitis, left femur

     M86.559 Other chronic hematogenous osteomyelitis, unspecified femur ▽

✓6ᵗʰ **M86.56 Other chronic hematogenous osteomyelitis, tibia and fibula**

     M86.561 Other chronic hematogenous osteomyelitis, right tibia and fibula

     M86.562 Other chronic hematogenous osteomyelitis, left tibia and fibula

     M86.569 Other chronic hematogenous osteomyelitis, unspecified tibia and fibula ▽

✓6ᵗʰ **M86.57 Other chronic hematogenous osteomyelitis, ankle and foot**

     M86.571 Other chronic hematogenous osteomyelitis, right ankle and foot

     M86.572 Other chronic hematogenous osteomyelitis, left ankle and foot

     M86.579 Other chronic hematogenous osteomyelitis, unspecified ankle and foot ▽

     M86.58 Other chronic hematogenous osteomyelitis, other site

     M86.59 Other chronic hematogenous osteomyelitis, multiple sites

✓5ᵗʰ **M86.6 Other chronic osteomyelitis**

     M86.60 Other chronic osteomyelitis, unspecified site ▽

✓ Additional Character Required   ✓ᴛ⁷ᵗʰ Placeholder Alert   Manifestation Dx   ▽ Unspecified Dx   ▶◀ Revised Text   ● New Code   ▲ Revised Code Title

√6ᵗʰ **M86.61** **Other chronic osteomyelitis,** shoulder

     M86.611 **Other chronic osteomyelitis,** right shoulder

     M86.612 **Other chronic osteomyelitis,** left shoulder

     M86.619 **Other chronic osteomyelitis,** unspecified shoulder ▽

√6ᵗʰ **M86.62** **Other chronic osteomyelitis,** humerus

     M86.621 **Other chronic osteomyelitis,** right humerus

     M86.622 **Other chronic osteomyelitis,** left humerus

     M86.629 **Other chronic osteomyelitis,** unspecified humerus ▽

√6ᵗʰ **M86.63** **Other chronic osteomyelitis,** radius and ulna

     M86.631 **Other chronic osteomyelitis,** right radius and ulna

     M86.632 **Other chronic osteomyelitis,** left radius and ulna

     M86.639 **Other chronic osteomyelitis,** unspecified radius and ulna ▽

√6ᵗʰ **M86.64** **Other chronic osteomyelitis,** hand

     M86.641 **Other chronic osteomyelitis,** right hand

     M86.642 **Other chronic osteomyelitis,** left hand

     M86.649 **Other chronic osteomyelitis,** unspecified hand ▽

√6ᵗʰ **M86.65** **Other chronic osteomyelitis,** thigh

     M86.651 **Other chronic osteomyelitis,** right thigh

     M86.652 **Other chronic osteomyelitis,** left thigh

     M86.659 **Other chronic osteomyelitis,** unspecified thigh ▽

√6ᵗʰ **M86.66** **Other chronic osteomyelitis,** tibia and fibula

     M86.661 **Other chronic osteomyelitis,** right tibia and fibula

     M86.662 **Other chronic osteomyelitis,** left tibia and fibula

     M86.669 **Other chronic osteomyelitis,** unspecified tibia and fibula ▽

√6ᵗʰ **M86.67** **Other chronic osteomyelitis,** ankle and foot

     M86.671 **Other chronic osteomyelitis,** right ankle and foot

         AHA: 2016,1Q,13

     M86.672 **Other chronic osteomyelitis,** left ankle and foot

     M86.679 **Other chronic osteomyelitis,** unspecified ankle and foot ▽

   M86.68 **Other chronic osteomyelitis, other site**

   M86.69 **Other chronic osteomyelitis,** multiple sites

√5ᵗʰ **M86.8** **Other osteomyelitis**

   Brodie's abscess

√6ᵗʰ **M86.8X** **Other osteomyelitis**

     M86.8X0 **Other osteomyelitis,** multiple sites

     M86.8X1 **Other osteomyelitis,** shoulder

     M86.8X2 **Other osteomyelitis,** upper arm

     M86.8X3 **Other osteomyelitis,** forearm

     M86.8X4 **Other osteomyelitis,** hand

     M86.8X5 **Other osteomyelitis,** thigh

     M86.8X6 **Other osteomyelitis,** lower leg

     M86.8X7 **Other osteomyelitis,** ankle and foot

     M86.8X8 **Other osteomyelitis,** other site

     M86.8X9 **Other osteomyelitis,** unspecified sites ▽

   M86.9 **Osteomyelitis, unspecified** ▽

     Infection of bone NOS

     Periostitis without osteomyelitis

√4ᵗʰ **M87** **Osteonecrosis**

   INCLUDES   avascular necrosis of bone

   Use additional code to identify major osseous defect, if applicable (M89.7-)

   EXCLUDES 1   *juvenile osteonecrosis (M91-M92)*

          osteochondropathies (M90-M93)

√5ᵗʰ **M87.0** **Idiopathic aseptic necrosis of bone**

   M87.00 **Idiopathic aseptic necrosis of unspecified bone** ▽

√6ᵗʰ **M87.01** **Idiopathic aseptic necrosis of** shoulder

     Idiopathic aseptic necrosis of clavicle and scapula

     M87.011 **Idiopathic aseptic necrosis of** right shoulder

     M87.012 **Idiopathic aseptic necrosis of** left shoulder

     M87.019 **Idiopathic aseptic necrosis of** unspecified shoulder ▽

√6ᵗʰ **M87.02** **Idiopathic aseptic necrosis of** humerus

     M87.021 **Idiopathic aseptic necrosis of** right humerus

     M87.022 **Idiopathic aseptic necrosis of** left humerus

     M87.029 **Idiopathic aseptic necrosis of** unspecified humerus ▽

√6ᵗʰ **M87.03** **Idiopathic aseptic necrosis of** radius, ulna and carpus

     M87.031 **Idiopathic aseptic necrosis of** right radius

     M87.032 **Idiopathic aseptic necrosis of** left radius

     M87.033 **Idiopathic aseptic necrosis of** unspecified radius ▽

     M87.034 **Idiopathic aseptic necrosis of** right ulna

     M87.035 **Idiopathic aseptic necrosis of** left ulna

     M87.036 **Idiopathic aseptic necrosis of** unspecified ulna ▽

     M87.037 **Idiopathic aseptic necrosis of** right carpus

     M87.038 **Idiopathic aseptic necrosis of** left carpus

     M87.039 **Idiopathic aseptic necrosis of** unspecified carpus ▽

√6ᵗʰ **M87.04** **Idiopathic aseptic necrosis of** hand and fingers

     Idiopathic aseptic necrosis of metacarpals and phalanges of hands

     M87.041 **Idiopathic aseptic necrosis of** right hand

     M87.042 **Idiopathic aseptic necrosis of** left hand

     M87.043 **Idiopathic aseptic necrosis of** unspecified hand ▽

     M87.044 **Idiopathic aseptic necrosis of** right finger(s)

     M87.045 **Idiopathic aseptic necrosis of** left finger(s)

     M87.046 **Idiopathic aseptic necrosis of** unspecified finger(s) ▽

√6ᵗʰ **M87.05** **Idiopathic aseptic necrosis of** pelvis and femur

     M87.050 **Idiopathic aseptic necrosis of** pelvis

     M87.051 **Idiopathic aseptic necrosis of** right femur

     M87.052 **Idiopathic aseptic necrosis of** left femur

     M87.059 **Idiopathic aseptic necrosis of** unspecified femur ▽

     Idiopathic aseptic necrosis of hip NOS

√6ᵗʰ **M87.06** **Idiopathic aseptic necrosis of** tibia and fibula

     M87.061 **Idiopathic aseptic necrosis of** right tibia

     M87.062 **Idiopathic aseptic necrosis of** left tibia

     M87.063 **Idiopathic aseptic necrosis of** unspecified tibia ▽

     M87.064 **Idiopathic aseptic necrosis of** right fibula

     M87.065 **Idiopathic aseptic necrosis of** left fibula

     M87.066 **Idiopathic aseptic necrosis of** unspecified fibula ▽

√6ᵗʰ **M87.07** **Idiopathic aseptic necrosis of** ankle, foot and toes

     Idiopathic aseptic necrosis of metatarsus, tarsus, and phalanges of toes

     M87.071 **Idiopathic aseptic necrosis of** right ankle

     M87.072 **Idiopathic aseptic necrosis of** left ankle

     M87.073 **Idiopathic aseptic necrosis of** unspecified ankle ▽

     M87.074 **Idiopathic aseptic necrosis of** right foot

     M87.075 **Idiopathic aseptic necrosis of** left foot

     M87.076 **Idiopathic aseptic necrosis of** unspecified foot ▽

     M87.077 **Idiopathic aseptic necrosis of** right toe(s)

     M87.078 **Idiopathic aseptic necrosis of** left toe(s)

     M87.079 **Idiopathic aseptic necrosis of** unspecified toe(s) ▽

   M87.08 **Idiopathic aseptic necrosis of bone, other site**

   M87.09 **Idiopathic aseptic necrosis of bone,** multiple sites

√5ᵗʰ **M87.1** **Osteonecrosis** due to drugs

   Use additional code for adverse effect, if applicable, to identify drug (T36-T50 with fifth or sixth character 5)

   M87.10 **Osteonecrosis due to drugs, unspecified bone** ▽

√6ᵗʰ **M87.11** **Osteonecrosis due to drugs,** shoulder

     M87.111 **Osteonecrosis due to drugs,** right shoulder

     M87.112 **Osteonecrosis due to drugs,** left shoulder

     M87.119 **Osteonecrosis due to drugs,** unspecified shoulder ▽

EXCLUDES 1 Not coded here   EXCLUDES 2 Not included here   N Newborn Age : 0   P Pediatric Age : 0-17   M Maternity Age : 12-55   A Adult Age : 15-124

768   ICD-10-CM 2017

✓6th **M87.12 Osteonecrosis due to drugs, humerus**

     M87.121 Osteonecrosis due to drugs, right humerus

     M87.122 Osteonecrosis due to drugs, left humerus

     M87.129 Osteonecrosis due to drugs, unspecified humerus ▽

✓6th **M87.13 Osteonecrosis due to drugs of radius, ulna and carpus**

     M87.131 Osteonecrosis due to drugs of right radius

     M87.132 Osteonecrosis due to drugs of left radius

     M87.133 Osteonecrosis due to drugs of unspecified radius ▽

     M87.134 Osteonecrosis due to drugs of right ulna

     M87.135 Osteonecrosis due to drugs of left ulna

     M87.136 Osteonecrosis due to drugs of unspecified ulna ▽

     M87.137 Osteonecrosis due to drugs of right carpus

     M87.138 Osteonecrosis due to drugs of left carpus

     M87.139 Osteonecrosis due to drugs of unspecified carpus ▽

✓6th **M87.14 Osteonecrosis due to drugs, hand and fingers**

     M87.141 Osteonecrosis due to drugs, right hand

     M87.142 Osteonecrosis due to drugs, left hand

     M87.143 Osteonecrosis due to drugs, unspecified hand

     M87.144 Osteonecrosis due to drugs, right finger(s)

     M87.145 Osteonecrosis due to drugs, left finger(s)

     M87.146 Osteonecrosis due to drugs, unspecified finger(s) ▽

✓6th **M87.15 Osteonecrosis due to drugs, pelvis and femur**

     M87.150 Osteonecrosis due to drugs, pelvis

     M87.151 Osteonecrosis due to drugs, right femur

     M87.152 Osteonecrosis due to drugs, left femur

     M87.159 Osteonecrosis due to drugs, unspecified femur ▽

✓6th **M87.16 Osteonecrosis due to drugs, tibia and fibula**

     M87.161 Osteonecrosis due to drugs, right tibia

     M87.162 Osteonecrosis due to drugs, left tibia

     M87.163 Osteonecrosis due to drugs, unspecified tibia ▽

     M87.164 Osteonecrosis due to drugs, right fibula

     M87.165 Osteonecrosis due to drugs, left fibula

     M87.166 Osteonecrosis due to drugs, unspecified fibula ▽

✓6th **M87.17 Osteonecrosis due to drugs, ankle, foot and toes**

     M87.171 Osteonecrosis due to drugs, right ankle

     M87.172 Osteonecrosis due to drugs, left ankle

     M87.173 Osteonecrosis due to drugs, unspecified ankle ▽

     M87.174 Osteonecrosis due to drugs, right foot

     M87.175 Osteonecrosis due to drugs, left foot

     M87.176 Osteonecrosis due to drugs, unspecified foot

     M87.177 Osteonecrosis due to drugs, right toe(s)

     M87.178 Osteonecrosis due to drugs, left toe(s)

     M87.179 Osteonecrosis due to drugs, unspecified toe(s) ▽

✓6th **M87.18 Osteonecrosis due to drugs, other site**

     M87.180 Osteonecrosis due to drugs, jaw

     M87.188 Osteonecrosis due to drugs, other site

     M87.19 Osteonecrosis due to drugs, multiple sites

✓5th **M87.2 Osteonecrosis due to previous trauma**

     M87.20 Osteonecrosis due to previous trauma, unspecified bone ▽

✓6th **M87.21 Osteonecrosis due to previous trauma, shoulder**

     M87.211 Osteonecrosis due to previous trauma, right shoulder

     M87.212 Osteonecrosis due to previous trauma, left shoulder

     M87.219 Osteonecrosis due to previous trauma, unspecified shoulder ▽

✓6th **M87.22 Osteonecrosis due to previous trauma, humerus**

     M87.221 Osteonecrosis due to previous trauma, right humerus

     M87.222 Osteonecrosis due to previous trauma, left humerus

     M87.229 Osteonecrosis due to previous trauma, unspecified humerus ▽

✓6th **M87.23 Osteonecrosis due to previous trauma of radius, ulna and carpus**

     M87.231 Osteonecrosis due to previous trauma of right radius

     M87.232 Osteonecrosis due to previous trauma of left radius

     M87.233 Osteonecrosis due to previous trauma of unspecified radius ▽

     M87.234 Osteonecrosis due to previous trauma of right ulna

     M87.235 Osteonecrosis due to previous trauma of left ulna

     M87.236 Osteonecrosis due to previous trauma of unspecified ulna ▽

     M87.237 Osteonecrosis due to previous trauma of right carpus

     M87.238 Osteonecrosis due to previous trauma of left carpus

     M87.239 Osteonecrosis due to previous trauma of unspecified carpus ▽

✓6th **M87.24 Osteonecrosis due to previous trauma, hand and fingers**

     M87.241 Osteonecrosis due to previous trauma, right hand

     M87.242 Osteonecrosis due to previous trauma, left hand

     M87.243 Osteonecrosis due to previous trauma, unspecified hand ▽

     M87.244 Osteonecrosis due to previous trauma, right finger(s)

     M87.245 Osteonecrosis due to previous trauma, left finger(s)

     M87.246 Osteonecrosis due to previous trauma, unspecified finger(s) ▽

✓6th **M87.25 Osteonecrosis due to previous trauma, pelvis and femur**

     M87.250 Osteonecrosis due to previous trauma, pelvis

     M87.251 Osteonecrosis due to previous trauma, right femur

     M87.252 Osteonecrosis due to previous trauma, left femur

     M87.256 Osteonecrosis due to previous trauma, unspecified femur ▽

✓6th **M87.26 Osteonecrosis due to previous trauma, tibia and fibula**

     M87.261 Osteonecrosis due to previous trauma, right tibia

     M87.262 Osteonecrosis due to previous trauma, left tibia

     M87.263 Osteonecrosis due to previous trauma, unspecified tibia ▽

     M87.264 Osteonecrosis due to previous trauma, right fibula

     M87.265 Osteonecrosis due to previous trauma, left fibula

     M87.266 Osteonecrosis due to previous trauma, unspecified fibula ▽

✓6th **M87.27 Osteonecrosis due to previous trauma, ankle, foot and toes**

     M87.271 Osteonecrosis due to previous trauma, right ankle

     M87.272 Osteonecrosis due to previous trauma, left ankle

     M87.273 Osteonecrosis due to previous trauma, unspecified ankle ▽

     M87.274 Osteonecrosis due to previous trauma, right foot

     M87.275 Osteonecrosis due to previous trauma, left foot

     M87.276 Osteonecrosis due to previous trauma, unspecified foot ▽

     M87.277 Osteonecrosis due to previous trauma, right toe(s)

     M87.278 Osteonecrosis due to previous trauma, left toe(s)

     M87.279 Osteonecrosis due to previous trauma, unspecified toe(s) ▽

     M87.28 Osteonecrosis due to previous trauma, other site

     M87.29 Osteonecrosis due to previous trauma, multiple sites

☑ Additional Character Required   ✓x7th Placeholder Alert   Manifestation Dx   ▽ Unspecified Dx   ►◄ Revised Text   ● New Code   ▲ Revised Code Title

ICD-10-CM 2017

769

√5th **M87.3** Other secondary osteonecrosis

M87.30 Other secondary osteonecrosis, unspecified bone ▽

√6th **M87.31** Other secondary osteonecrosis, shoulder

M87.311 Other secondary osteonecrosis, right shoulder

M87.312 Other secondary osteonecrosis, left shoulder

M87.319 Other secondary osteonecrosis, unspecified shoulder ▽

√6th **M87.32** Other secondary osteonecrosis, humerus

M87.321 Other secondary osteonecrosis, right humerus

M87.322 Other secondary osteonecrosis, left humerus

M87.329 Other secondary osteonecrosis, unspecified humerus ▽

√6th **M87.33** Other secondary osteonecrosis of radius, ulna and carpus

M87.331 Other secondary osteonecrosis of right radius

M87.332 Other secondary osteonecrosis of left radius

M87.333 Other secondary osteonecrosis of unspecified radius ▽

M87.334 Other secondary osteonecrosis of right ulna

M87.335 Other secondary osteonecrosis of left ulna

M87.336 Other secondary osteonecrosis of unspecified ulna ▽

M87.337 Other secondary osteonecrosis of right carpus

M87.338 Other secondary osteonecrosis of left carpus

M87.339 Other secondary osteonecrosis of unspecified carpus ▽

√6th **M87.34** Other secondary osteonecrosis, hand and fingers

M87.341 Other secondary osteonecrosis, right hand

M87.342 Other secondary osteonecrosis, left hand

M87.343 Other secondary osteonecrosis, unspecified hand ▽

M87.344 Other secondary osteonecrosis, right finger(s)

M87.345 Other secondary osteonecrosis, left finger(s)

M87.346 Other secondary osteonecrosis, unspecified finger(s) ▽

√6th **M87.35** Other secondary osteonecrosis, pelvis and femur

M87.350 Other secondary osteonecrosis, pelvis

M87.351 Other secondary osteonecrosis, right femur

M87.352 Other secondary osteonecrosis, left femur

M87.353 Other secondary osteonecrosis, unspecified femur ▽

√6th **M87.36** Other secondary osteonecrosis, tibia and fibula

M87.361 Other secondary osteonecrosis, right tibia

M87.362 Other secondary osteonecrosis, left tibia

M87.363 Other secondary osteonecrosis, unspecified tibia ▽

M87.364 Other secondary osteonecrosis, right fibula

M87.365 Other secondary osteonecrosis, left fibula

M87.366 Other secondary osteonecrosis, unspecified fibula ▽

√6th **M87.37** Other secondary osteonecrosis, ankle and foot

M87.371 Other secondary osteonecrosis, right ankle

M87.372 Other secondary osteonecrosis, left ankle

M87.373 Other secondary osteonecrosis, unspecified ankle ▽

M87.374 Other secondary osteonecrosis, right foot

M87.375 Other secondary osteonecrosis, left foot

M87.376 Other secondary osteonecrosis, unspecified foot ▽

M87.377 Other secondary osteonecrosis, right toe(s)

M87.378 Other secondary osteonecrosis, left toe(s)

M87.379 Other secondary osteonecrosis, unspecified toe(s) ▽

M87.38 Other secondary osteonecrosis, other site

M87.39 Other secondary osteonecrosis, multiple sites

√5th **M87.8** Other osteonecrosis

M87.80 Other osteonecrosis, unspecified bone ▽

√6th **M87.81** Other osteonecrosis, shoulder

M87.811 Other osteonecrosis, right shoulder

M87.812 Other osteonecrosis, left shoulder

M87.819 Other osteonecrosis, unspecified shoulder ▽

√6th **M87.82** Other osteonecrosis, humerus

M87.821 Other osteonecrosis, right humerus

M87.822 Other osteonecrosis, left humerus

M87.829 Other osteonecrosis, unspecified humerus ▽

√6th **M87.83** Other osteonecrosis of radius, ulna and carpus

M87.831 Other osteonecrosis of right radius

M87.832 Other osteonecrosis of left radius

M87.833 Other osteonecrosis of unspecified radius ▽

M87.834 Other osteonecrosis of right ulna

M87.835 Other osteonecrosis of left ulna

M87.836 Other osteonecrosis of unspecified ulna ▽

M87.837 Other osteonecrosis of right carpus

M87.838 Other osteonecrosis of left carpus

M87.839 Other osteonecrosis of unspecified carpus ▽

√6th **M87.84** Other osteonecrosis, hand and fingers

M87.841 Other osteonecrosis, right hand

M87.842 Other osteonecrosis, left hand

M87.843 Other osteonecrosis, unspecified hand ▽

M87.844 Other osteonecrosis, right finger(s)

M87.845 Other osteonecrosis, left finger(s)

M87.849 Other osteonecrosis, unspecified finger(s) ▽

√6th **M87.85** Other osteonecrosis, pelvis and femur

M87.850 Other osteonecrosis, pelvis

M87.851 Other osteonecrosis, right femur

M87.852 Other osteonecrosis, left femur

M87.859 Other osteonecrosis, unspecified femur ▽

√6th **M87.86** Other osteonecrosis, tibia and fibula

M87.861 Other osteonecrosis, right tibia

M87.862 Other osteonecrosis, left tibia

M87.863 Other osteonecrosis, unspecified tibia ▽

M87.864 Other osteonecrosis, right fibula

M87.865 Other osteonecrosis, left fibula

M87.869 Other osteonecrosis, unspecified fibula ▽

√6th **M87.87** Other osteonecrosis, ankle, foot and toes

M87.871 Other osteonecrosis, right ankle

M87.872 Other osteonecrosis, left ankle

M87.873 Other osteonecrosis, unspecified ankle ▽

M87.874 Other osteonecrosis, right foot

M87.875 Other osteonecrosis, left foot

M87.876 Other osteonecrosis, unspecified foot ▽

M87.877 Other osteonecrosis, right toe(s)

M87.878 Other osteonecrosis, left toe(s)

M87.879 Other osteonecrosis, unspecified toe(s) ▽

M87.88 Other osteonecrosis, other site

M87.89 Other osteonecrosis, multiple sites

M87.9 Osteonecrosis, unspecified ▽

Necrosis of bone NOS

√4th **M88** **Osteitis deformans [Paget's disease of bone]**

EXCLUDES 1 osteitis deformans in neoplastic disease (M90.6)

M88.0 Osteitis deformans of skull

M88.1 Osteitis deformans of vertebrae

√5th **M88.8** Osteitis deformans of other bones

√6th **M88.81** Osteitis deformans of shoulder

M88.811 Osteitis deformans of right shoulder

M88.812 Osteitis deformans of left shoulder

EXCLUDES 1 Not coded here · *EXCLUDES 2* Not included here · N Newborn Age : 0 · P Pediatric Age : 0-17 · M Maternity Age : 12-55 · A Adult Age : 15-124

770

ICD-10-CM 2017

             M88.819   **Osteitis deformans of** unspecified shoulder ▽

✓6ᵗʰ **M88.82**   **Osteitis deformans of** upper arm

             M88.821   **Osteitis deformans of** right **upper arm**
             M88.822   **Osteitis deformans of** left **upper arm**
             M88.829   **Osteitis deformans of** unspecified upper arm ▽

✓6ᵗʰ **M88.83**   **Osteitis deformans of** forearm

             M88.831   **Osteitis deformans of** right **forearm**
             M88.832   **Osteitis deformans of** left **forearm**
             M88.839   **Osteitis deformans of** unspecified forearm ▽

✓6ᵗʰ **M88.84**   **Osteitis deformans of** hand

             M88.841   **Osteitis deformans of** right **hand**
             M88.842   **Osteitis deformans of** left **hand**
             M88.849   **Osteitis deformans of** unspecified hand ▽

✓6ᵗʰ **M88.85**   **Osteitis deformans of** thigh

             M88.851   **Osteitis deformans of** right **thigh**
             M88.852   **Osteitis deformans of** left **thigh**
             M88.859   **Osteitis deformans of** unspecified thigh ▽

✓6ᵗʰ **M88.86**   **Osteitis deformans of** lower leg

             M88.861   **Osteitis deformans of** right **lower leg**
             M88.862   **Osteitis deformans of** left **lower leg**
             M88.869   **Osteitis deformans of** unspecified lower leg ▽

✓6ᵗʰ **M88.87**   **Osteitis deformans of** ankle and foot

             M88.871   **Osteitis deformans of** right **ankle and foot**
             M88.872   **Osteitis deformans of** left **ankle and foot**
             M88.879   **Osteitis deformans of** unspecified ankle and foot ▽

        M88.88   **Osteitis deformans of other bones**
             EXCLUDES 2   *osteitis deformans of skull (M88.0)*
                     osteitis deformans of vertebrae (M88.1)

        M88.89   **Osteitis deformans of** multiple sites
     M88.9   **Osteitis deformans of unspecified bone** ▽

✓4ᵗʰ **M89**   **Other disorders of bone**

    ✓5ᵗʰ **M89.0**   **Algoneurodystrophy**

       Shoulder-hand syndrome
       Sudeck's atrophy
       EXCLUDES 1   *causalgia, lower limb (G57.7-)*
                 causalgia, upper limb (G56.4-)
                 complex regional pain syndrome II, lower limb (G57.7-)
                 complex regional pain syndrome II, upper limb (G56.4-)
                 reflex sympathetic dystrophy (G90.5-)

        M89.00   **Algoneurodystrophy, unspecified site** ▽

    ✓6ᵗʰ **M89.01**   **Algoneurodystrophy,** shoulder

             M89.011   **Algoneurodystrophy,** right **shoulder**
             M89.012   **Algoneurodystrophy,** left **shoulder**
             M89.019   **Algoneurodystrophy,** unspecified shoulder ▽

    ✓6ᵗʰ **M89.02**   **Algoneurodystrophy,** upper arm

             M89.021   **Algoneurodystrophy,** right **upper arm**
             M89.022   **Algoneurodystrophy,** left **upper arm**
             M89.029   **Algoneurodystrophy,** unspecified upper arm ▽

    ✓6ᵗʰ **M89.03**   **Algoneurodystrophy,** forearm

             M89.031   **Algoneurodystrophy,** right **forearm**
             M89.032   **Algoneurodystrophy,** left **forearm**
             M89.039   **Algoneurodystrophy,** unspecified forearm ▽

    ✓6ᵗʰ **M89.04**   **Algoneurodystrophy,** hand

             M89.041   **Algoneurodystrophy,** right **hand**
             M89.042   **Algoneurodystrophy,** left **hand**
             M89.049   **Algoneurodystrophy,** unspecified hand ▽

    ✓6ᵗʰ **M89.05**   **Algoneurodystrophy,** thigh

             M89.051   **Algoneurodystrophy,** right **thigh**
             M89.052   **Algoneurodystrophy,** left **thigh**
             M89.059   **Algoneurodystrophy,** unspecified thigh ▽

    ✓6ᵗʰ **M89.06**   **Algoneurodystrophy,** lower leg

             M89.061   **Algoneurodystrophy,** right **lower leg**
             M89.062   **Algoneurodystrophy,** left **lower leg**

             M89.069   **Algoneurodystrophy, unspecified lower leg** ▽

    ✓6ᵗʰ **M89.07**   **Algoneurodystrophy,** ankle and foot

             M89.071   **Algoneurodystrophy,** right **ankle and foot**
             M89.072   **Algoneurodystrophy,** left **ankle and foot**
             M89.079   **Algoneurodystrophy,** unspecified ankle and foot

        M89.08   **Algoneurodystrophy, other site**
        M89.09   **Algoneurodystrophy,** multiple sites

    ✓5ᵗʰ **M89.1**   **Physeal arrest**

       Arrest of growth plate
       Epiphyseal arrest
       Growth plate arrest

    ✓6ᵗʰ **M89.12**   **Physeal arrest, humerus**

             M89.121   **Complete physeal arrest,** right proximal humerus
             M89.122   **Complete physeal arrest,** left proximal humerus
             M89.123   **Partial physeal arrest,** right proximal humerus
             M89.124   **Partial physeal arrest,** left proximal humerus
             M89.125   **Complete physeal arrest,** right distal humerus
             M89.126   **Complete physeal arrest,** left distal humerus
             M89.127   **Partial physeal arrest,** right distal humerus
             M89.128   **Partial physeal arrest,** left distal **humerus**
             M89.129   **Physeal arrest, humerus, unspecified** ▽

    ✓6ᵗʰ **M89.13**   **Physeal arrest,** forearm

             M89.131   **Complete physeal arrest,** right distal radius
             M89.132   **Complete physeal arrest,** left distal radius
             M89.133   **Partial physeal arrest,** right distal radius
             M89.134   **Partial physeal arrest,** left distal radius
             M89.138   **Other physeal arrest of forearm**
             M89.139   **Physeal arrest, forearm, unspecified** ▽

    ✓6ᵗʰ **M89.15**   **Physeal arrest,** femur

             M89.151   **Complete physeal arrest,** right proximal femur
             M89.152   **Complete physeal arrest,** left proximal femur
             M89.153   **Partial physeal arrest,** right proximal femur
             M89.154   **Partial physeal arrest,** left proximal **femur**
             M89.155   **Complete physeal arrest,** right distal femur
             M89.156   **Complete physeal arrest,** left distal **femur**
             M89.157   **Partial physeal arrest,** right distal **femur**
             M89.158   **Partial physeal arrest,** left distal **femur**
             M89.159   **Physeal arrest, femur, unspecified** ▽

    ✓6ᵗʰ **M89.16**   **Physeal arrest,** lower leg

             M89.160   **Complete physeal arrest,** right proximal tibia
             M89.161   **Complete physeal arrest,** left proximal tibia
             M89.162   **Partial physeal arrest,** right proximal **tibia**
             M89.163   **Partial physeal arrest,** left proximal **tibia**
             M89.164   **Complete physeal arrest,** right distal **tibia**
             M89.165   **Complete physeal arrest,** left distal **tibia**
             M89.166   **Partial physeal arrest,** right distal **tibia**
             M89.167   **Partial physeal arrest,** left distal **tibia**
             M89.168   **Other physeal arrest of lower leg**
             M89.169   **Physeal arrest, lower leg, unspecified** ▽

        M89.18   **Physeal arrest, other site**

    ✓5ᵗʰ **M89.2**   **Other disorders of bone development and growth**

        M89.20   **Other disorders of bone development and growth, unspecified site** ▽

    ✓6ᵗʰ **M89.21**   **Other disorders of bone development and growth, shoulder**

             M89.211   **Other disorders of bone development and growth,** right **shoulder**
             M89.212   **Other disorders of bone development and growth,** left **shoulder**

✓ Additional Character Required   x7ᵗʰ Placeholder Alert   Manifestation Dx   ▽ Unspecified Dx   ►◄ Revised Text   ● New Code   ▲ Revised Code Title

ICD-10-CM 2017   **771**

M89.219   Other disorders of bone development and growth, unspecified shoulder ▽

√6ᵗʰ M89.22   Other disorders of bone development and growth, humerus

    M89.221   Other disorders of bone development and growth, right humerus

    M89.222   Other disorders of bone development and growth, left humerus

    M89.229   Other disorders of bone development and growth, unspecified humerus ▽

√6ᵗʰ M89.23   Other disorders of bone development and growth, ulna and radius

    M89.231   Other disorders of bone development and growth, right ulna

    M89.232   Other disorders of bone development and growth, left ulna

    M89.233   Other disorders of bone development and growth, right radius

    M89.234   Other disorders of bone development and growth, left radius

    M89.239   Other disorders of bone development and growth, unspecified ulna and radius ▽

√6ᵗʰ M89.24   Other disorders of bone development and growth, hand

    M89.241   Other disorders of bone development and growth, right hand

    M89.242   Other disorders of bone development and growth, left hand

    M89.249   Other disorders of bone development and growth, unspecified hand ▽

√6ᵗʰ M89.25   Other disorders of bone development and growth, femur

    M89.251   Other disorders of bone development and growth, right femur

    M89.252   Other disorders of bone development and growth, left femur

    M89.259   Other disorders of bone development and growth, unspecified femur ▽

√6ᵗʰ M89.26   Other disorders of bone development and growth, tibia and fibula

    M89.261   Other disorders of bone development and growth, right tibia

    M89.262   Other disorders of bone development and growth, left tibia

    M89.263   Other disorders of bone development and growth, right fibula

    M89.264   Other disorders of bone development and growth, left fibula

    M89.269   Other disorders of bone development and growth, unspecified lower leg ▽

√6ᵗʰ M89.27   Other disorders of bone development and growth, ankle and foot

    M89.271   Other disorders of bone development and growth, right ankle and foot

    M89.272   Other disorders of bone development and growth, left ankle and foot

    M89.279   Other disorders of bone development and growth, unspecified ankle and foot ▽

M89.28   Other disorders of bone development and growth, other site

M89.29   Other disorders of bone development and growth, multiple sites

√5ᵗʰ M89.3   Hypertrophy of bone

    M89.30   Hypertrophy of bone, unspecified site ▽

√6ᵗʰ M89.31   Hypertrophy of bone, shoulder

    M89.311   Hypertrophy of bone, right shoulder

    M89.312   Hypertrophy of bone, left shoulder

    M89.319   Hypertrophy of bone, unspecified shoulder ▽

√6ᵗʰ M89.32   Hypertrophy of bone, humerus

    M89.321   Hypertrophy of bone, right humerus

    M89.322   Hypertrophy of bone, left humerus

    M89.329   Hypertrophy of bone, unspecified humerus ▽

√6ᵗʰ M89.33   Hypertrophy of bone, ulna and radius

    M89.331   Hypertrophy of bone, right ulna

    M89.332   Hypertrophy of bone, left ulna

    M89.333   Hypertrophy of bone, right radius

    M89.334   Hypertrophy of bone, left radius

    M89.339   Hypertrophy of bone, unspecified ulna and radius ▽

√6ᵗʰ M89.34   Hypertrophy of bone, hand

    M89.341   Hypertrophy of bone, right hand

    M89.342   Hypertrophy of bone, left hand

    M89.349   Hypertrophy of bone, unspecified hand ▽

√6ᵗʰ M89.35   Hypertrophy of bone, femur

    M89.351   Hypertrophy of bone, right femur

    M89.352   Hypertrophy of bone, left femur

    M89.359   Hypertrophy of bone, unspecified femur ▽

√6ᵗʰ M89.36   Hypertrophy of bone, tibia and fibula

    M89.361   Hypertrophy of bone, right tibia

    M89.362   Hypertrophy of bone, left tibia

    M89.363   Hypertrophy of bone, right fibula

    M89.364   Hypertrophy of bone, left fibula

    M89.369   Hypertrophy of bone, unspecified tibia and fibula ▽

√6ᵗʰ M89.37   Hypertrophy of bone, ankle and foot

    M89.371   Hypertrophy of bone, right ankle and foot

    M89.372   Hypertrophy of bone, left ankle and foot

    M89.379   Hypertrophy of bone, unspecified ankle and foot ▽

M89.38   Hypertrophy of bone, other site

M89.39   Hypertrophy of bone, multiple sites

√5ᵗʰ M89.4   Other hypertrophic osteoarthropathy

    Marie-Bamberger disease
    Pachydermoperiostosis

    M89.40   Other hypertrophic osteoarthropathy, unspecified site ▽

√6ᵗʰ M89.41   Other hypertrophic osteoarthropathy, shoulder

    M89.411   Other hypertrophic osteoarthropathy, right shoulder

    M89.412   Other hypertrophic osteoarthropathy, left shoulder

    M89.419   Other hypertrophic osteoarthropathy, unspecified shoulder ▽

√6ᵗʰ M89.42   Other hypertrophic osteoarthropathy, upper arm

    M89.421   Other hypertrophic osteoarthropathy, right upper arm

    M89.422   Other hypertrophic osteoarthropathy, left upper arm

    M89.429   Other hypertrophic osteoarthropathy, unspecified upper arm ▽

√6ᵗʰ M89.43   Other hypertrophic osteoarthropathy, forearm

    M89.431   Other hypertrophic osteoarthropathy, right forearm

    M89.432   Other hypertrophic osteoarthropathy, left forearm

    M89.439   Other hypertrophic osteoarthropathy, unspecified forearm ▽

√6ᵗʰ M89.44   Other hypertrophic osteoarthropathy, hand

    M89.441   Other hypertrophic osteoarthropathy, right hand

    M89.442   Other hypertrophic osteoarthropathy, left hand

    M89.449   Other hypertrophic osteoarthropathy, unspecified hand ▽

√6ᵗʰ M89.45   Other hypertrophic osteoarthropathy, thigh

    M89.451   Other hypertrophic osteoarthropathy, right thigh

    M89.452   Other hypertrophic osteoarthropathy, left thigh

    M89.459   Other hypertrophic osteoarthropathy, unspecified thigh ▽

√6ᵗʰ M89.46   Other hypertrophic osteoarthropathy, lower leg

    M89.461   Other hypertrophic osteoarthropathy, right lower leg

EXCLUDES 1   Not coded here   EXCLUDES 2   Not included here   N Newborn Age : 0   P Pediatric Age : 0-17   M Maternity Age : 12-55   A Adult Age : 15-124

772   ICD-10-CM 2017

M89.462　**Other hypertrophic osteoarthropathy, left lower leg**

M89.469　**Other hypertrophic osteoarthropathy, unspecified lower leg** ▽

✓6ᵗʰ　M89.47　**Other hypertrophic osteoarthropathy, ankle and foot**

M89.471　**Other hypertrophic osteoarthropathy, right ankle and foot**

M89.472　**Other hypertrophic osteoarthropathy, left ankle and foot**

M89.479　**Other hypertrophic osteoarthropathy, unspecified ankle and foot** ▽

M89.48　**Other hypertrophic osteoarthropathy, other site**

M89.49　**Other hypertrophic osteoarthropathy, multiple sites**

✓5ᵗʰ　**M89.5　Osteolysis**

Use additional code to identify major osseous defect, if applicable (M89.7-)

EXCLUDES 2　*periprosthetic osteolysis of internal prosthetic joint (T84.05-)*

M89.50　**Osteolysis, unspecified site** ▽

✓6ᵗʰ　M89.51　**Osteolysis, shoulder**

M89.511　**Osteolysis, right shoulder**

M89.512　**Osteolysis, left shoulder**

M89.519　**Osteolysis, unspecified shoulder** ▽

✓6ᵗʰ　M89.52　**Osteolysis, upper arm**

M89.521　**Osteolysis, right upper arm**

M89.522　**Osteolysis, left upper arm**

M89.529　**Osteolysis, unspecified upper arm** ▽

✓6ᵗʰ　M89.53　**Osteolysis, forearm**

M89.531　**Osteolysis, right forearm**

M89.532　**Osteolysis, left forearm**

M89.539　**Osteolysis, unspecified forearm** ▽

✓6ᵗʰ　M89.54　**Osteolysis, hand**

M89.541　**Osteolysis, right hand**

M89.542　**Osteolysis, left hand**

M89.549　**Osteolysis, unspecified hand** ▽

✓6ᵗʰ　M89.55　**Osteolysis, thigh**

M89.551　**Osteolysis, right thigh**

M89.552　**Osteolysis, left thigh**

M89.559　**Osteolysis, unspecified thigh** ▽

✓6ᵗʰ　M89.56　**Osteolysis, lower leg**

M89.561　**Osteolysis, right lower leg**

M89.562　**Osteolysis, left lower leg**

M89.569　**Osteolysis, unspecified lower leg** ▽

✓6ᵗʰ　M89.57　**Osteolysis, ankle and foot**

M89.571　**Osteolysis, right ankle and foot**

M89.572　**Osteolysis, left ankle and foot**

M89.579　**Osteolysis, unspecified ankle and foot** ▽

M89.58　**Osteolysis, other site**

M89.59　**Osteolysis, multiple sites**

✓5ᵗʰ　**M89.6　Osteopathy after poliomyelitis**

Use additional code (B91) to identify previous poliomyelitis

EXCLUDES 1　*postpolio syndrome (G14)*

M89.60　**Osteopathy after poliomyelitis, unspecified site** ▽

✓6ᵗʰ　M89.61　**Osteopathy after poliomyelitis, shoulder**

M89.611　**Osteopathy after poliomyelitis, right shoulder**

M89.612　**Osteopathy after poliomyelitis, left shoulder**

M89.619　**Osteopathy after poliomyelitis, unspecified shoulder** ▽

✓6ᵗʰ　M89.62　**Osteopathy after poliomyelitis, upper arm**

M89.621　**Osteopathy after poliomyelitis, right upper arm**

M89.622　**Osteopathy after poliomyelitis, left upper arm**

M89.629　**Osteopathy after poliomyelitis, unspecified upper arm** ▽

✓6ᵗʰ　M89.63　**Osteopathy after poliomyelitis, forearm**

M89.631　**Osteopathy after poliomyelitis, right forearm**

M89.632　**Osteopathy after poliomyelitis, left forearm**

M89.639　**Osteopathy after poliomyelitis, unspecified forearm** ▽

✓6ᵗʰ　M89.64　**Osteopathy after poliomyelitis, hand**

M89.641　**Osteopathy after poliomyelitis, right hand**

M89.642　**Osteopathy after poliomyelitis, left hand**

M89.649　**Osteopathy after poliomyelitis, unspecified hand** ▽

✓6ᵗʰ　M89.65　**Osteopathy after poliomyelitis, thigh**

M89.651　**Osteopathy after poliomyelitis, right thigh**

M89.652　**Osteopathy after poliomyelitis, left thigh**

M89.659　**Osteopathy after poliomyelitis, unspecified thigh** ▽

✓6ᵗʰ　M89.66　**Osteopathy after poliomyelitis, lower leg**

M89.661　**Osteopathy after poliomyelitis, right lower leg**

M89.662　**Osteopathy after poliomyelitis, left lower leg**

M89.669　**Osteopathy after poliomyelitis, unspecified lower leg** ▽

✓6ᵗʰ　M89.67　**Osteopathy after poliomyelitis, ankle and foot**

M89.671　**Osteopathy after poliomyelitis, right ankle and foot**

M89.672　**Osteopathy after poliomyelitis, left ankle and foot**

M89.679　**Osteopathy after poliomyelitis, unspecified ankle and foot** ▽

M89.68　**Osteopathy after poliomyelitis, other site**

M89.69　**Osteopathy after poliomyelitis, multiple sites**

✓5ᵗʰ　**M89.7　Major osseous defect**

Code first underlying disease, if known, such as:

aseptic necrosis of bone (M87.-)

malignant neoplasm of bone (C40.-)

osteolysis (M89.5)

osteomyelitis (M86.-)

osteonecrosis (M87.-)

osteoporosis (M80.-, M81.-)

periprosthetic osteolysis (T84.05-)

M89.70　**Major osseous defect, unspecified site** ▽

✓6ᵗʰ　M89.71　**Major osseous defect, shoulder region**

Major osseous defect clavicle or scapula

M89.711　**Major osseous defect, right shoulder region**

M89.712　**Major osseous defect, left shoulder region**

M89.719　**Major osseous defect, unspecified shoulder region** ▽

✓6ᵗʰ　M89.72　**Major osseous defect, humerus**

M89.721　**Major osseous defect, right humerus**

M89.722　**Major osseous defect, left humerus**

M89.729　**Major osseous defect, unspecified humerus** ▽

✓6ᵗʰ　M89.73　**Major osseous defect, forearm**

Major osseous defect of radius and ulna

M89.731　**Major osseous defect, right forearm**

M89.732　**Major osseous defect, left forearm**

M89.739　**Major osseous defect, unspecified forearm** ▽

✓6ᵗʰ　M89.74　**Major osseous defect, hand**

Major osseous defect of carpus, fingers, metacarpus

M89.741　**Major osseous defect, right hand**

M89.742　**Major osseous defect, left hand**

M89.749　**Major osseous defect, unspecified hand** ▽

✓6ᵗʰ　M89.75　**Major osseous defect, pelvic region and thigh**

Major osseous defect of femur and pelvis

M89.751　**Major osseous defect, right pelvic region and thigh**

M89.752　**Major osseous defect, left pelvic region and thigh**

M89.759　**Major osseous defect, unspecified pelvic region and thigh** ▽

✓6ᵗʰ　M89.76　**Major osseous defect, lower leg**

Major osseous defect of fibula and tibia

M89.761　**Major osseous defect, right lower leg**

M89.762　**Major osseous defect, left lower leg**

☑ **Additional Character Required**　　ᵛˣ⁷ᵗʰ **Placeholder Alert**　　**Manifestation Dx**　　▽ Unspecified Dx　　▶◀ Revised Text　　● New Code　　▲ Revised Code Title

    M89.769 **Major osseous defect, unspecified lower leg** ▽

✓6ᵗʰ M89.77 **Major osseous defect, ankle and foot**

    Major osseous defect of metatarsus, tarsus, toes

    M89.771 **Major osseous defect, right ankle and foot**

    M89.772 **Major osseous defect, left ankle and foot**

    M89.779 **Major osseous defect, unspecified ankle and foot**

M89.78 **Major osseous defect, other site**

M89.79 **Major osseous defect, multiple sites**

✓5ᵗʰ M89.8 **Other specified disorders of bone**

    Infantile cortical hyperostoses

    Post-traumatic subperiosteal ossification

✓6ᵗʰ M89.8X **Other specified disorders of bone**

    M89.8X0 **Other specified disorders of bone, multiple sites**

    M89.8X1 **Other specified disorders of bone, shoulder**

    M89.8X2 **Other specified disorders of bone, upper arm**

    M89.8X3 **Other specified disorders of bone, forearm**

    M89.8X4 **Other specified disorders of bone, hand**

    M89.8X5 **Other specified disorders of bone, thigh**

    M89.8X6 **Other specified disorders of bone, lower leg**

    M89.8X7 **Other specified disorders of bone, ankle and foot**

    M89.8X8 **Other specified disorders of bone, other site**

    M89.8X9 **Other specified disorders of bone, unspecified site** ▽

M89.9 **Disorder of bone, unspecified** ▽

✓4ᵗʰ **M90** **Osteopathies in diseases classified elsewhere**

    EXCLUDES 1 osteochondritis, osteomyelitis, and osteopathy (in):
      cryptococcosis (B45.3)
      diabetes mellitus ▶(E08-E13 with .69-)◀
      gonococcal (A54.43)
      neurogenic syphilis (A52.11)
      renal osteodystrophy (N25.0)
      salmonellosis (A02.24)
      secondary syphilis (A51.46)
      syphilis (late) (A52.77)

✓5ᵗʰ **M90.5** **Osteonecrosis in diseases classified elsewhere**

    Code first underlying disease, such as:
      caisson disease (T70.3)
      hemoglobinopathy (D50-D64)

    M90.50 *Osteonecrosis in diseases classified elsewhere, unspecified site* ▽

✓6ᵗʰ M90.51 **Osteonecrosis in diseases classified elsewhere, shoulder**

    M90.511 *Osteonecrosis in diseases classified elsewhere, right shoulder*

    M90.512 *Osteonecrosis in diseases classified elsewhere, left shoulder*

    M90.519 *Osteonecrosis in diseases classified elsewhere, unspecified shoulder* ▽

✓6ᵗʰ M90.52 **Osteonecrosis in diseases classified elsewhere, upper arm**

    M90.521 *Osteonecrosis in diseases classified elsewhere, right upper arm*

    M90.522 *Osteonecrosis in diseases classified elsewhere, left upper arm*

    M90.529 *Osteonecrosis in diseases classified elsewhere, unspecified upper arm* ▽

✓6ᵗʰ M90.53 **Osteonecrosis in diseases classified elsewhere, forearm**

    M90.531 *Osteonecrosis in diseases classified elsewhere, right forearm*

    M90.532 *Osteonecrosis in diseases classified elsewhere, left forearm*

    M90.539 *Osteonecrosis in diseases classified elsewhere, unspecified forearm* ▽

✓6ᵗʰ M90.54 **Osteonecrosis in diseases classified elsewhere, hand**

    M90.541 *Osteonecrosis in diseases classified elsewhere, right hand*

    M90.542 *Osteonecrosis in diseases classified elsewhere, left hand*

    M90.549 *Osteonecrosis in diseases classified elsewhere, unspecified hand* ▽

✓6ᵗʰ M90.55 **Osteonecrosis in diseases classified elsewhere, thigh**

    M90.551 *Osteonecrosis in diseases classified elsewhere, right thigh*

    M90.552 *Osteonecrosis in diseases classified elsewhere, left thigh*

    M90.559 *Osteonecrosis in diseases classified elsewhere, unspecified thigh* ▽

✓6ᵗʰ M90.56 **Osteonecrosis in diseases classified elsewhere, lower leg**

    M90.561 *Osteonecrosis in diseases classified elsewhere, right lower leg*

    M90.562 *Osteonecrosis in diseases classified elsewhere, left lower leg*

    M90.569 *Osteonecrosis in diseases classified elsewhere, unspecified lower leg*

✓6ᵗʰ M90.57 **Osteonecrosis in diseases classified elsewhere, ankle and foot**

    M90.571 *Osteonecrosis in diseases classified elsewhere, right ankle and foot*

    M90.572 *Osteonecrosis in diseases classified elsewhere, left ankle and foot*

    M90.579 *Osteonecrosis in diseases classified elsewhere, unspecified ankle and foot* ▽

M90.58 *Osteonecrosis in diseases classified elsewhere, other site*

M90.59 *Osteonecrosis in diseases classified elsewhere, multiple sites*

✓5ᵗʰ **M90.6** **Osteitis deformans in neoplastic diseases**

    Osteitis deformans in malignant neoplasm of bone
    Code first the neoplasm (C40.-, C41.-)

    EXCLUDES 1 *osteitis deformans [Paget's disease of bone] (M88.-)*

    M90.60 *Osteitis deformans in neoplastic diseases, unspecified site* ▽

✓6ᵗʰ M90.61 **Osteitis deformans in neoplastic diseases, shoulder**

    M90.611 *Osteitis deformans in neoplastic diseases, right shoulder*

    M90.612 *Osteitis deformans in neoplastic diseases, left shoulder*

    M90.619 *Osteitis deformans in neoplastic diseases, unspecified shoulder* ▽

✓6ᵗʰ M90.62 **Osteitis deformans in neoplastic diseases, upper arm**

    M90.621 *Osteitis deformans in neoplastic diseases, right upper arm*

    M90.622 *Osteitis deformans in neoplastic diseases, left upper arm*

    M90.629 *Osteitis deformans in neoplastic diseases, unspecified upper arm* ▽

✓6ᵗʰ M90.63 **Osteitis deformans in neoplastic diseases, forearm**

    M90.631 *Osteitis deformans in neoplastic diseases, right forearm*

    M90.632 *Osteitis deformans in neoplastic diseases, left forearm*

    M90.639 *Osteitis deformans in neoplastic diseases, unspecified forearm* ▽

✓6ᵗʰ M90.64 **Osteitis deformans in neoplastic diseases, hand**

    M90.641 *Osteitis deformans in neoplastic diseases, right hand*

    M90.642 *Osteitis deformans in neoplastic diseases, left hand*

    M90.649 *Osteitis deformans in neoplastic diseases, unspecified hand* ▽

✓6ᵗʰ M90.65 **Osteitis deformans in neoplastic diseases, thigh**

    M90.651 *Osteitis deformans in neoplastic diseases, right thigh*

    M90.652 *Osteitis deformans in neoplastic diseases, left thigh*

    M90.659 *Osteitis deformans in neoplastic diseases, unspecified thigh* ▽

✓6ᵗʰ M90.66 **Osteitis deformans in neoplastic diseases, lower leg**

    M90.661 *Osteitis deformans in neoplastic diseases, right lower leg*

    M90.662 *Osteitis deformans in neoplastic diseases, left lower leg*

    M90.669 *Osteitis deformans in neoplastic diseases, unspecified lower leg* ▽

EXCLUDES 1 Not coded here   **EXCLUDES 2** Not included here   **N** Newborn Age : 0   **P** Pediatric Age : 0-17   **M** Maternity Age : 12-55   **A** Adult Age : 15-124

774   ICD-10-CM 2017

✓6ᵗʰ **M90.67 Osteitis deformans in neoplastic diseases, ankle and foot**

     M90.671 *Osteitis deformans in neoplastic diseases, right ankle and foot*

     M90.672 *Osteitis deformans in neoplastic diseases, left ankle and foot*

     M90.679 *Osteitis deformans in neoplastic diseases, unspecified ankle and foot* ▽

M90.68 *Osteitis deformans in neoplastic diseases, other site*

M90.69 *Osteitis deformans in neoplastic diseases, multiple sites*

✓5ᵗʰ **M90.8 Osteopathy in diseases classified elsewhere**

     Code first underlying disease, such as:
       rickets (E55.0)
       vitamin-D-resistant rickets (E83.3)

     M90.80 *Osteopathy in diseases classified elsewhere, unspecified site* ▽

✓6ᵗʰ **M90.81 Osteopathy in diseases classified elsewhere, shoulder**

     M90.811 *Osteopathy in diseases classified elsewhere, right shoulder*

     M90.812 *Osteopathy in diseases classified elsewhere, left shoulder*

     M90.819 *Osteopathy in diseases classified elsewhere, unspecified shoulder* ▽

✓6ᵗʰ **M90.82 Osteopathy in diseases classified elsewhere, upper arm**

     M90.821 *Osteopathy in diseases classified elsewhere, right upper arm*

     M90.822 *Osteopathy in diseases classified elsewhere, left upper arm*

     M90.829 *Osteopathy in diseases classified elsewhere, unspecified upper arm* ▽

✓6ᵗʰ **M90.83 Osteopathy in diseases classified elsewhere, forearm**

     M90.831 *Osteopathy in diseases classified elsewhere, right forearm*

     M90.832 *Osteopathy in diseases classified elsewhere, left forearm*

     M90.839 *Osteopathy in diseases classified elsewhere, unspecified forearm* ▽

✓6ᵗʰ **M90.84 Osteopathy in diseases classified elsewhere, hand**

     M90.841 *Osteopathy in diseases classified elsewhere, right hand*

     M90.842 *Osteopathy in diseases classified elsewhere, left hand*

     M90.849 *Osteopathy in diseases classified elsewhere, unspecified hand* ▽

✓6ᵗʰ **M90.85 Osteopathy in diseases classified elsewhere, thigh**

     M90.851 *Osteopathy in diseases classified elsewhere, right thigh*

     M90.852 *Osteopathy in diseases classified elsewhere, left thigh*

     M90.859 *Osteopathy in diseases classified elsewhere, unspecified thigh* ▽

✓6ᵗʰ **M90.86 Osteopathy in diseases classified elsewhere, lower leg**

     M90.861 *Osteopathy in diseases classified elsewhere, right lower leg*

     M90.862 *Osteopathy in diseases classified elsewhere, left lower leg*

     M90.869 *Osteopathy in diseases classified elsewhere, unspecified lower leg* ▽

✓6ᵗʰ **M90.87 Osteopathy in diseases classified elsewhere, ankle and foot**

     M90.871 *Osteopathy in diseases classified elsewhere, right ankle and foot*

     M90.872 *Osteopathy in diseases classified elsewhere, left ankle and foot*

     M90.879 *Osteopathy in diseases classified elsewhere, unspecified ankle and foot* ▽

M90.88 *Osteopathy in diseases classified elsewhere, other site*

M90.89 *Osteopathy in diseases classified elsewhere, multiple sites*

Chondropathies (M91-M94)

EXCLUDES 1 *postprocedural chondropathies (M96.-)*

✓4ᵗʰ **M91 Juvenile osteochondrosis of hip and pelvis**

     EXCLUDES 1 *slipped upper femoral epiphysis (nontraumatic) (M93.0)*

     M91.0 Juvenile osteochondrosis of pelvis

       Osteochondrosis (juvenile) of acetabulum
       Osteochondrosis (juvenile) of iliac crest [Buchanan]
       Osteochondrosis (juvenile) of ischiopubic synchondrosis [van Neck]
       Osteochondrosis (juvenile) of symphysis pubis [Pierson]

✓5ᵗʰ **M91.1 Juvenile osteochondrosis of head of femur [Legg-Calvé-Perthes]**

     M91.10 **Juvenile osteochondrosis of head of femur [Legg-Calvé-Perthes], unspecified leg** ▽

     M91.11 **Juvenile osteochondrosis of head of femur [Legg-Calvé-Perthes], right leg**

     M91.12 **Juvenile osteochondrosis of head of femur [Legg-Calvé-Perthes], left leg**

✓5ᵗʰ **M91.2 Coxa plana**

     Hip deformity due to previous juvenile osteochondrosis

     M91.20 **Coxa plana, unspecified hip** ▽

     M91.21 **Coxa plana, right hip**

     M91.22 **Coxa plana, left hip**

✓5ᵗʰ **M91.3 Pseudocoxalgia**

     M91.30 **Pseudocoxalgia, unspecified hip** ▽

     M91.31 **Pseudocoxalgia, right hip**

     M91.32 **Pseudocoxalgia, left hip**

✓5ᵗʰ **M91.4 Coxa magna**

     M91.40 **Coxa magna, unspecified hip** ▽

     M91.41 **Coxa magna, right hip**

     M91.42 **Coxa magna, left hip**

✓5ᵗʰ **M91.8 Other juvenile osteochondrosis of hip and pelvis**

     Juvenile osteochondrosis after reduction of congenital dislocation of hip

     M91.80 **Other juvenile osteochondrosis of hip and pelvis, unspecified leg** ▽

     M91.81 **Other juvenile osteochondrosis of hip and pelvis, right leg**

     M91.82 **Other Juvenile osteochondrosis of hip and pelvis, left leg**

✓5ᵗʰ **M91.9 Juvenile osteochondrosis of hip and pelvis, unspecified**

     M91.90 **Juvenile osteochondrosis of hip and pelvis, unspecified, unspecified leg** ▽

     M91.91 **Juvenile osteochondrosis of hip and pelvis, unspecified, right leg** ▽

     M91.92 **Juvenile osteochondrosis of hip and pelvis, unspecified, left leg** ▽

✓4ᵗʰ **M92 Other juvenile osteochondrosis**

✓5ᵗʰ **M92.0 Juvenile osteochondrosis of humerus**

     Osteochondrosis (juvenile) of capitulum of humerus [Panner]
     Osteochondrosis (juvenile) of head of humerus [Haas]

     M92.00 **Juvenile osteochondrosis of humerus, unspecified arm** ▽

     M92.01 **Juvenile osteochondrosis of humerus, right arm**

     M92.02 **Juvenile osteochondrosis of humerus, left arm**

✓5ᵗʰ **M92.1 Juvenile osteochondrosis of radius and ulna**

     Osteochondrosis (juvenile) of lower ulna [Burns]
     Osteochondrosis (juvenile) of radial head [Brailsford]

     M92.10 **Juvenile osteochondrosis of radius and ulna, unspecified arm** ▽

     M92.11 **Juvenile osteochondrosis of radius and ulna, right arm**

     M92.12 **Juvenile osteochondrosis of radius and ulna, left arm**

✓5ᵗʰ **M92.2 Juvenile osteochondrosis, hand**

     ✓6ᵗʰ **M92.20 Unspecified juvenile osteochondrosis, hand**

       M92.201 **Unspecified juvenile osteochondrosis, right hand** ▽

       M92.202 **Unspecified juvenile osteochondrosis, left hand** ▽

       M92.209 **Unspecified juvenile osteochondrosis, unspecified hand** ▽

     ✓6ᵗʰ **M92.21 Osteochondrosis (juvenile) of carpal lunate [Kienböck]**

       M92.211 **Osteochondrosis (juvenile) of carpal lunate [Kienböck], right hand**

☑ Additional Character Required   ᵛˣ⁷ᵗʰ Placeholder Alert   Manifestation Dx   ▽ Unspecified Dx   ►◄ Revised Text   ● New Code   ▲ Revised Code Title

ICD-10-CM 2017   775

Chapter 13. Diseases of the Musculoskeletal System and Connective Tissue

M92.212 Osteochondrosis (juvenile) of carpal lunate [Kienböck], left hand

M92.219 Osteochondrosis (juvenile) of carpal lunate [Kienböck], unspecified hand ▽

✓6ᵗʰ **M92.22** Osteochondrosis (juvenile) of metacarpal heads [Mauclaire]

M92.221 Osteochondrosis (juvenile) of metacarpal heads [Mauclaire], right hand

M92.222 Osteochondrosis (juvenile) of metacarpal heads [Mauclaire], left hand

M92.229 Osteochondrosis (juvenile) of metacarpal heads [Mauclaire], unspecified hand ▽

✓6ᵗʰ **M92.29** Other juvenile osteochondrosis, hand

M92.291 Other juvenile osteochondrosis, right hand

M92.292 Other juvenile osteochondrosis, left hand

M92.299 Other juvenile osteochondrosis, unspecified hand ▽

✓5ᵗʰ **M92.3** Other juvenile osteochondrosis, upper limb

M92.30 Other juvenile osteochondrosis, unspecified upper limb ▽

M92.31 Other juvenile osteochondrosis, right upper limb

M92.32 Other juvenile osteochondrosis, left upper limb

✓5ᵗʰ **M92.4** Juvenile osteochondrosis of patella

Osteochondrosis (juvenile) of primary patellar center [Köhler]

Osteochondrosis (juvenile) of secondary patellar centre [Sinding Larsen]

M92.40 Juvenile osteochondrosis of patella, unspecified knee ▽

M92.41 Juvenile osteochondrosis of patella, right knee

M92.42 Juvenile osteochondrosis of patella, left knee

✓5ᵗʰ **M92.5** Juvenile osteochondrosis of tibia and fibula

Osteochondrosis (juvenile) of proximal tibia [Blount]

Osteochondrosis (juvenile) of tibial tubercle [Osgood-Schlatter]

Tibia vara

M92.50 Juvenile osteochondrosis of tibia and fibula, unspecified leg ▽

M92.51 Juvenile osteochondrosis of tibia and fibula, right leg

M92.52 Juvenile osteochondrosis of tibia and fibula, left leg

✓5ᵗʰ **M92.6** Juvenile osteochondrosis of tarsus

Osteochondrosis (juvenile) of calcaneum [Sever]

Osteochondrosis (juvenile) of os tibiale externum [Haglund]

Osteochondrosis (juvenile) of talus [Diaz]

Osteochondrosis (juvenile) of tarsal navicular [Köhler]

M92.60 Juvenile osteochondrosis of tarsus, unspecified ankle ▽

M92.61 Juvenile osteochondrosis of tarsus, right ankle

M92.62 Juvenile osteochondrosis of tarsus, left ankle

✓5ᵗʰ **M92.7** Juvenile osteochondrosis of metatarsus

Osteochondrosis (juvenile) of fifth metatarsus [Iselin]

Osteochondrosis (juvenile) of second metatarsus [Freiberg]

M92.70 Juvenile osteochondrosis of metatarsus, unspecified foot ▽

M92.71 Juvenile osteochondrosis of metatarsus, right foot

M92.72 Juvenile osteochondrosis of metatarsus, left foot

M92.8 Other specified juvenile osteochondrosis

Calcaneal apophysitis

M92.9 Juvenile osteochondrosis, unspecified ▽

Juvenile apophysitis NOS

Juvenile epiphysitis NOS

Juvenile osteochondritis NOS

Juvenile osteochondrosis NOS

✓4ᵗʰ **M93** Other osteochondropathies

EXCLUDES 2   *osteochondrosis of spine (M42.-)*

✓5ᵗʰ **M93.0** Slipped upper femoral epiphysis (nontraumatic)

Use additional code for associated chondrolysis (M94.3)

✓6ᵗʰ **M93.00** Unspecified slipped upper femoral epiphysis (nontraumatic)

M93.001 Unspecified slipped upper femoral epiphysis (nontraumatic), right hip ▽

M93.002 Unspecified slipped upper femoral epiphysis (nontraumatic), left hip ▽

M93.003 Unspecified slipped upper femoral epiphysis (nontraumatic), unspecified hip ▽

✓6ᵗʰ **M93.01** Acute slipped upper femoral epiphysis (nontraumatic)

M93.011 Acute slipped upper femoral epiphysis (nontraumatic), right hip

M93.012 Acute slipped upper femoral epiphysis (nontraumatic), left hip

M93.013 Acute slipped upper femoral epiphysis (nontraumatic), unspecified hip ▽

✓6ᵗʰ **M93.02** Chronic slipped upper femoral epiphysis (nontraumatic)

M93.021 Chronic slipped upper femoral epiphysis (nontraumatic), right hip

M93.022 Chronic slipped upper femoral epiphysis (nontraumatic), left hip

M93.023 Chronic slipped upper femoral epiphysis (nontraumatic), unspecified hip ▽

✓6ᵗʰ **M93.03** Acute on chronic slipped upper femoral epiphysis (nontraumatic)

M93.031 Acute on chronic slipped upper femoral epiphysis (nontraumatic), right hip

M93.032 Acute on chronic slipped upper femoral epiphysis (nontraumatic), left hip

M93.033 Acute on chronic slipped upper femoral epiphysis (nontraumatic), unspecified hip ▽

M93.1 Kienböck's disease of adults   A

Adult osteochondrosis of carpal lunates

✓5ᵗʰ **M93.2** Osteochondritis dissecans

M93.20 Osteochondritis dissecans of unspecified site ▽

✓6ᵗʰ **M93.21** Osteochondritis dissecans of shoulder

M93.211 Osteochondritis dissecans, right shoulder

M93.212 Osteochondritis dissecans, left shoulder

M93.219 Osteochondritis dissecans, unspecified shoulder ▽

✓6ᵗʰ **M93.22** Osteochondritis dissecans of elbow

M93.221 Osteochondritis dissecans, right elbow

M93.222 Osteochondritis dissecans, left elbow

M93.229 Osteochondritis dissecans, unspecified elbow ▽

✓6ᵗʰ **M93.23** Osteochondritis dissecans of wrist

M93.231 Osteochondritis dissecans, right wrist

M93.232 Osteochondritis dissecans, left wrist

M93.239 Osteochondritis dissecans, unspecified wrist ▽

✓6ᵗʰ **M93.24** Osteochondritis dissecans of joints of hand

M93.241 Osteochondritis dissecans, joints of right hand

M93.242 Osteochondritis dissecans, joints of left hand

M93.249 Osteochondritis dissecans, joints of unspecified hand ▽

✓6ᵗʰ **M93.25** Osteochondritis dissecans of hip

M93.251 Osteochondritis dissecans, right hip

M93.252 Osteochondritis dissecans, left hip

M93.259 Osteochondritis dissecans, unspecified hip ▽

✓6ᵗʰ **M93.26** Osteochondritis dissecans knee

M93.261 Osteochondritis dissecans, right knee

M93.262 Osteochondritis dissecans, left knee

M93.269 Osteochondritis dissecans, unspecified knee ▽

✓6ᵗʰ **M93.27** Osteochondritis dissecans of ankle and joints of foot

M93.271 Osteochondritis dissecans, right ankle and joints of right foot

M93.272 Osteochondritis dissecans, left ankle and joints of left foot

M93.279 Osteochondritis dissecans, unspecified ankle and joints of foot ▽

M93.28 Osteochondritis dissecans other site

M93.29 Osteochondritis dissecans multiple sites

✓5ᵗʰ **M93.8** Other specified osteochondropathies

M93.80 Other specified osteochondropathies of unspecified site ▽

✓6ᵗʰ **M93.81** Other specified osteochondropathies of shoulder

M93.811 Other specified osteochondropathies, right shoulder

EXCLUDES 1 Not coded here   EXCLUDES 2 Not included here   N Newborn Age : 0   P Pediatric Age : 0-17   M Maternity Age : 12-55   A Adult Age : 15-124

776   ICD-10-CM 2017

M93.812 Other specified osteochondropathies, left shoulder

M93.819 Other specified osteochondropathies, unspecified shoulder ▽

✓6th M93.82 Other specified osteochondropathies of upper arm

M93.821 Other specified osteochondropathies, right upper arm

M93.822 Other specified osteochondropathies, left upper arm

M93.829 Other specified osteochondropathies, unspecified upper arm ▽

✓6th M93.83 Other specified osteochondropathies of forearm

M93.831 Other specified osteochondropathies, right forearm

M93.832 Other specified osteochondropathies, left forearm

M93.839 Other specified osteochondropathies, unspecified forearm ▽

✓6th M93.84 Other specified osteochondropathies of hand

M93.841 Other specified osteochondropathies, right hand

M93.842 Other specified osteochondropathies, left hand

M93.849 Other specified osteochondropathies, unspecified hand ▽

✓6th M93.85 Other specified osteochondropathies of thigh

M93.851 Other specified osteochondropathies, right thigh

M93.852 Other specified osteochondropathies, left thigh

M93.859 Other specified osteochondropathies, unspecified thigh ▽

✓6th M93.86 Other specified osteochondropathies lower leg

M93.861 Other specified osteochondropathies, right lower leg

M93.862 Other specified osteochondropathies, left lower leg

M93.869 Other specified osteochondropathies, unspecified lower leg ▽

✓6th M93.87 Other specified osteochondropathies of ankle and foot

M93.871 Other specified osteochondropathies, right ankle and foot

M93.872 Other specified osteochondropathies, left ankle and foot

M93.879 Other specified osteochondropathies, unspecified ankle and foot ▽

M93.88 Other specified osteochondropathies other site

M93.89 Other specified osteochondropathies multiple sites

✓5th M93.9 Osteochondropathy, unspecified

Apophysitis NOS
Epiphysitis NOS
Osteochondritis NOS
Osteochondrosis NOS

M93.90 Osteochondropathy, unspecified of unspecified site ▽

✓6th M93.91 Osteochondropathy, unspecified of shoulder

M93.911 Osteochondropathy, unspecified, right shoulder ▽

M93.912 Osteochondropathy, unspecified, left shoulder ▽

M93.919 Osteochondropathy, unspecified, unspecified shoulder ▽

✓6th M93.92 Osteochondropathy, unspecified of upper arm

M93.921 Osteochondropathy, unspecified, right upper arm ▽

M93.922 Osteochondropathy, unspecified, left upper arm ▽

M93.929 Osteochondropathy, unspecified, unspecified upper arm ▽

✓6th M93.93 Osteochondropathy, unspecified of forearm

M93.931 Osteochondropathy, unspecified, right forearm ▽

M93.932 Osteochondropathy, unspecified, left forearm ▽

M93.939 Osteochondropathy, unspecified, unspecified forearm ▽

✓6th M93.94 Osteochondropathy, unspecified of hand

M93.941 Osteochondropathy, unspecified, right hand ▽

M93.942 Osteochondropathy, unspecified, left hand ▽

M93.949 Osteochondropathy, unspecified, unspecified hand ▽

✓6th M93.95 Osteochondropathy, unspecified of thigh

M93.951 Osteochondropathy, unspecified, right thigh ▽

M93.952 Osteochondropathy, unspecified, left thigh ▽

M93.959 Osteochondropathy, unspecified, unspecified thigh ▽

✓6th M93.96 Osteochondropathy, unspecified lower leg

M93.961 Osteochondropathy, unspecified, right lower leg ▽

M93.962 Osteochondropathy, unspecified, left lower leg ▽

M93.969 Osteochondropathy, unspecified, unspecified lower leg ▽

✓6th M93.97 Osteochondropathy, unspecified of ankle and foot

M93.971 Osteochondropathy, unspecified, right ankle and foot ▽

M93.972 Osteochondropathy, unspecified, left ankle and foot ▽

M93.979 Osteochondropathy, unspecified, unspecified ankle and foot ▽

M93.98 Osteochondropathy, unspecified other site ▽

M93.99 Osteochondropathy, unspecified multiple sites ▽

✓4th M94 Other disorders of cartilage

M94.0 Chondrocostal junction syndrome [Tietze]
Costochondritis

M94.1 Relapsing polychondritis

✓5th M94.2 Chondromalacia

EXCLUDES 1 chondromalacia patellae (M22.4)

M94.20 Chondromalacia, unspecified site ▽

✓6th M94.21 Chondromalacia, shoulder

M94.211 Chondromalacia, right shoulder
M94.212 Chondromalacia, left shoulder
M94.219 Chondromalacia, unspecified shoulder ▽

✓6th M94.22 Chondromalacia, elbow

M94.221 Chondromalacia, right elbow
M94.222 Chondromalacia, left elbow
M94.229 Chondromalacia, unspecified elbow ▽

✓6th M94.23 Chondromalacia, wrist

M94.231 Chondromalacia, right wrist
M94.232 Chondromalacia, left wrist
M94.239 Chondromalacia, unspecified wrist ▽

✓6th M94.24 Chondromalacia, joints of hand

M94.241 Chondromalacia, joints of right hand
M94.242 Chondromalacia, joints of left hand
M94.249 Chondromalacia, joints of unspecified hand ▽

✓6th M94.25 Chondromalacia, hip

M94.251 Chondromalacia, right hip
M94.252 Chondromalacia, left hip
M94.259 Chondromalacia, unspecified hip ▽

✓6th M94.26 Chondromalacia, knee

M94.261 Chondromalacia, right knee
M94.262 Chondromalacia, left knee
M94.269 Chondromalacia, unspecified knee ▽

✓6th M94.27 Chondromalacia, ankle and joints of foot

M94.271 Chondromalacia, right ankle and joints of right foot

M94.272 Chondromalacia, left ankle and joints of left foot

M94.279 Chondromalacia, unspecified ankle and joints of foot ▽

M94.28 Chondromalacia, other site

☑ Additional Character Required   ✓x7th Placeholder Alert   Manifestation Dx   ▽ Unspecified Dx   ►◄ Revised Text   ● New Code   ▲ Revised Code Title

ICD-10-CM 2017   777

M94.29 Chondromalacia, **multiple sites**

✓5ᵗʰ **M94.3** **Chondrolysis**

Code first any associated slipped upper femoral epiphysis (nontraumatic) (M93.0-)

✓6ᵗʰ **M94.35** **Chondrolysis, hip**

M94.351 Chondrolysis, **right** hip

M94.352 Chondrolysis, **left** hip

M94.359 Chondrolysis, **unspecified** hip ▽

✓5ᵗʰ **M94.8** **Other specified disorders of cartilage**

✓6ᵗʰ **M94.8X** **Other specified disorders of cartilage**

M94.8X0 Other specified disorders of cartilage, **multiple sites**

M94.8X1 Other specified disorders of cartilage, **shoulder**

M94.8X2 Other specified disorders of cartilage, **upper arm**

M94.8X3 Other specified disorders of cartilage, **forearm**

M94.8X4 Other specified disorders of cartilage, **hand**

M94.8X5 Other specified disorders of cartilage, **thigh**

M94.8X6 Other specified disorders of cartilage, **lower leg**

M94.8X7 Other specified disorders of cartilage, **ankle and foot**

M94.8X8 Other specified disorders of cartilage, **other site**

M94.8X9 Other specified disorders of cartilage, **unspecified sites** ▽

M94.9 Disorder of cartilage, unspecified ▽

Other disorders of the musculoskeletal system and connective tissue (M95)

✓4ᵗʰ **M95** **Other acquired deformities of musculoskeletal system and connective tissue**

EXCLUDES 2　*acquired absence of limbs and organs (Z89-Z90)*
acquired deformities of limbs (M20-M21)
congenital malformations and deformations of the musculoskeletal system (Q65-Q79)
deforming dorsopathies (M40-M43)
dentofacial anomalies [including malocclusion] (M26.-)
postprocedural musculoskeletal disorders (M96.-)

M95.0 **Acquired deformity of nose**

EXCLUDES 2　*deviated nasal septum (J34.2)*

✓5ᵗʰ **M95.1** **Cauliflower ear**

EXCLUDES 2　*other acquired deformities of ear (H61.1)*

M95.10 Cauliflower ear, unspecified ear ▽

M95.11 Cauliflower ear, **right** ear

M95.12 Cauliflower ear, **left** ear

M95.2 Other acquired **deformity of head**

M95.3 Acquired **deformity of neck**

M95.4 Acquired **deformity of chest and rib**

　AHA: 2014,4Q,26-27

M95.5 Acquired **deformity of pelvis**

EXCLUDES 1　*maternal care for known or suspected disproportion (O33.-)*

M95.8 Other specified acquired deformities of musculoskeletal system

M95.9 Acquired deformity of musculoskeletal system, unspecified ▽

Intraoperative and postprocedural complications and disorders of musculoskeletal system, not elsewhere classified (M96)

✓4ᵗʰ **M96** **Intraoperative and postprocedural complications and disorders of musculoskeletal system, not elsewhere classified**

EXCLUDES 2　*arthropathy following intestinal bypass (M02.0-)*
complications of internal orthopedic prosthetic devices, implants and grafts (T84.-)
disorders associated with osteoporosis (M80)
▶*periprosthetic fracture around internal prosthetic joint (M97.-)*◀
presence of functional implants and other devices (Z96-Z97)

M96.0 **Pseudarthrosis after fusion or arthrodesis**

M96.1 **Postlaminectomy syndrome, not elsewhere classified**

M96.2 **Postradiation kyphosis**

M96.3 **Postlaminectomy kyphosis**

M96.4 **Postsurgical lordosis**

M96.5 **Postradiation scoliosis**

✓5ᵗʰ **M96.6** **Fracture of bone following insertion of orthopedic implant, joint prosthesis, or bone plate**

Intraoperative fracture of bone during insertion of orthopedic implant, joint prosthesis, or bone plate

EXCLUDES 2　*complication of internal orthopedic devices, implants or grafts (T84.-)*

✓6ᵗʰ **M96.62** **Fracture of humerus following insertion of orthopedic implant, joint prosthesis, or bone plate**

M96.621 **Fracture of humerus following insertion of orthopedic implant, joint prosthesis, or bone plate, right arm**

M96.622 **Fracture of humerus following insertion of orthopedic implant, joint prosthesis, or bone plate, left arm**

M96.629 **Fracture of humerus following insertion of orthopedic implant, joint prosthesis, or bone plate, unspecified arm** ▽

✓6ᵗʰ **M96.63** **Fracture of radius or ulna following insertion of orthopedic implant, joint prosthesis, or bone plate**

M96.631 **Fracture of radius or ulna following insertion of orthopedic implant, joint prosthesis, or bone plate, right arm**

M96.632 **Fracture of radius or ulna following insertion of orthopedic implant, joint prosthesis, or bone plate, left arm**

M96.639 **Fracture of radius or ulna following insertion of orthopedic implant, joint prosthesis, or bone plate, unspecified arm** ▽

M96.65 **Fracture of pelvis following insertion of orthopedic implant, joint prosthesis, or bone plate**

✓6ᵗʰ **M96.66** **Fracture of femur following insertion of orthopedic implant, joint prosthesis, or bone plate**

M96.661 **Fracture of femur following insertion of orthopedic implant, joint prosthesis, or bone plate, right leg**

M96.662 **Fracture of femur following insertion of orthopedic implant, joint prosthesis, or bone plate, left leg**

M96.669 **Fracture of femur following insertion of orthopedic implant, joint prosthesis, or bone plate, unspecified leg** ▽

✓6ᵗʰ **M96.67** **Fracture of tibia or fibula following insertion of orthopedic implant, joint prosthesis, or bone plate**

M96.671 **Fracture of tibia or fibula following insertion of orthopedic implant, joint prosthesis, or bone plate, right leg**

M96.672 **Fracture of tibia or fibula following insertion of orthopedic implant, joint prosthesis, or bone plate, left leg**

M96.679 **Fracture of tibia or fibula following insertion of orthopedic implant, joint prosthesis, or bone plate, unspecified leg** ▽

M96.69 **Fracture of other bone following insertion of orthopedic implant, joint prosthesis, or bone plate**

✓5ᵗʰ **M96.8** **Other intraoperative and postprocedural complications and disorders of musculoskeletal system, not elsewhere classified**

✓6ᵗʰ **M96.81** Intraoperative hemorrhage and hematoma of a musculoskeletal structure complicating a procedure

EXCLUDES 1　*intraoperative hemorrhage and hematoma of a musculoskeletal structure due to accidental puncture and laceration during a procedure (M96.82-)*

M96.810 **Intraoperative hemorrhage and hematoma of a musculoskeletal structure complicating a musculoskeletal system procedure**

M96.811 **Intraoperative hemorrhage and hematoma of a musculoskeletal structure complicating other procedure**

✓6ᵗʰ **M96.82** Accidental puncture and laceration of a musculoskeletal structure during a procedure

M96.820 **Accidental puncture and laceration of a musculoskeletal structure during a musculoskeletal system procedure**

M96.821 **Accidental puncture and laceration of a musculoskeletal structure during other procedure**

EXCLUDES 1　Not coded here　　　　EXCLUDES 2　Not included here　　　N Newborn Age : 0　　　P Pediatric Age : 0-17　　　M Maternity Age : 12-55　　　A Adult Age : 15-124

778　　　ICD-10-CM 2017

▲ ☑6ᵗʰ **M96.83** Postprocedural hemorrhage **of a musculoskeletal structure following a procedure**

▲ **M96.830** Postprocedural hemorrhage **of a musculoskeletal structure following a** musculoskeletal system procedure

▲ **M96.831** Postprocedural hemorrhage **of a musculoskeletal structure following** other procedure

● ☑6ᵗʰ **M96.84** Postprocedural hematoma and seroma **of a musculoskeletal structure following a procedure**

● **M96.840** Postprocedural hematoma **of a musculoskeletal structure following a** musculoskeletal system procedure

● **M96.841** Postprocedural hematoma **of a musculoskeletal structure following** other procedure

● **M96.842** Postprocedural seroma **of a musculoskeletal structure following a** musculoskeletal system procedure

● **M96.843** Postprocedural seroma **of a musculoskeletal structure following** other procedure

M96.89 **Other intraoperative and postprocedural complications and disorders of the musculoskeletal system**
Instability of joint secondary to removal of joint prosthesis
Use additional code, if applicable, to further specify disorder

▶Periprosthetic fractures around internal prosthetic joint (M97)◀

●☑4ᵗʰ **M97** **Periprosthetic fracture around internal prosthetic joint**
EXCLUDES 2 *breakage (fracture) of prosthetic joint (T84.01-)*
fracture of bone following insertion of orthopedic implant, joint prosthesis or bone plate (M96.6-)

The appropriate 7th character is to be added to each code from category M97
A initial encounter
D subsequent encounter
S sequela

● ☑5ᵗʰ **M97.0** **Periprosthetic fracture around internal prosthetic hip joint**

● ☑x7ᵗʰ **M97.01** **Periprosthetic fracture around internal prosthetic right hip joint**

● ☑x7ᵗʰ **M97.02** **Periprosthetic fracture around internal prosthetic left hip joint**

● ☑5ᵗʰ **M97.1** **Periprosthetic fracture around internal prosthetic knee joint**

● ☑x7ᵗʰ **M97.11** **Periprosthetic fracture around internal prosthetic right knee joint**

● ☑x7ᵗʰ **M97.12** **Periprosthetic fracture around internal prosthetic left knee joint**

● ☑5ᵗʰ **M97.2** **Periprosthetic fracture around internal prosthetic ankle joint**

● ☑x7ᵗʰ **M97.21** **Periprosthetic fracture around internal prosthetic right ankle joint**

● ☑x7ᵗʰ **M97.22** **Periprosthetic fracture around internal prosthetic left ankle joint**

● ☑5ᵗʰ **M97.3** **Periprosthetic fracture around internal prosthetic shoulder joint**

● ☑x7ᵗʰ **M97.31** **Periprosthetic fracture around internal prosthetic right shoulder joint**

● ☑x7ᵗʰ **M97.32** **Periprosthetic fracture around internal prosthetic left shoulder joint**

● ☑5ᵗʰ **M97.4** **Periprosthetic fracture around internal prosthetic elbow joint**

● ☑x7ᵗʰ **M97.41** **Periprosthetic fracture around internal prosthetic right elbow joint**

● ☑x7ᵗʰ **M97.42** **Periprosthetic fracture around internal prosthetic left elbow joint**

● ☑x7ᵗʰ **M97.8** **Periprosthetic fracture around** other **internal prosthetic joint**
Periprosthetic fracture around internal prosthetic finger joint
Periprosthetic fracture around internal prosthetic spinal joint
Periprosthetic fracture around internal prosthetic toe joint
Periprosthetic fracture around internal prosthetic wrist joint
Use additional code to identify the joint (Z96.6-)

● ☑x7ᵗʰ **M97.9** **Periprosthetic fracture around unspecified internal prosthetic joint** ▽

Biomechanical lesions, not elsewhere classified (M99)

☑4ᵗʰ **M99** **Biomechanical lesions, not elsewhere classified**
NOTE This category should not be used if the condition can be classified elsewhere.

☑5ᵗʰ **M99.0** **Segmental and somatic dysfunction**

M99.00 **Segmental and somatic dysfunction of** head **region**
M99.01 **Segmental and somatic dysfunction of** cervical **region**
M99.02 **Segmental and somatic dysfunction of** thoracic **region**
M99.03 **Segmental and somatic dysfunction of** lumbar **region**
M99.04 **Segmental and somatic dysfunction of** sacral **region**
M99.05 **Segmental and somatic dysfunction of** pelvic **region**
M99.06 **Segmental and somatic dysfunction of** lower **extremity**
M99.07 **Segmental and somatic dysfunction of** upper **extremity**
M99.08 **Segmental and somatic dysfunction of** rib cage
M99.09 **Segmental and somatic dysfunction of** abdomen and other **regions**

☑5ᵗʰ **M99.1** **Subluxation complex (vertebral)**

M99.10 **Subluxation complex (vertebral) of** head **region**
M99.11 **Subluxation complex (vertebral) of** cervical **region**
M99.12 **Subluxation complex (vertebral) of** thoracic **region**
M99.13 **Subluxation complex (vertebral) of** lumbar **region**
M99.14 **Subluxation complex (vertebral) of** sacral **region**
M99.15 **Subluxation complex (vertebral) of** pelvic **region**
M99.16 **Subluxation complex (vertebral) of** lower extremity
M99.17 **Subluxation complex (vertebral) of** upper extremity
M99.18 **Subluxation complex (vertebral) of** rib cage
M99.19 **Subluxation complex (vertebral) of** abdomen and other **regions**

☑5ᵗʰ **M99.2** **Subluxation stenosis of neural canal**

M99.20 **Subluxation stenosis of neural canal of** head **region**
M99.21 **Subluxation stenosis of neural canal of** cervical **region**
M99.22 **Subluxation stenosis of neural canal of** thoracic **region**
M99.23 **Subluxation stenosis of neural canal of** lumbar **region**
M99.24 **Subluxation stenosis of neural canal of** sacral **region**
M99.25 **Subluxation stenosis of neural canal of** pelvic **region**
M99.26 **Subluxation stenosis of neural canal of** lower **extremity**
M99.27 **Subluxation stenosis of neural canal of** upper **extremity**
M99.28 **Subluxation stenosis of neural canal of** rib cage
M99.29 **Subluxation stenosis of neural canal of** abdomen and other **regions**

☑5ᵗʰ **M99.3** **Osseous stenosis of neural canal**

M99.30 **Osseous stenosis of neural canal of** head **region**
M99.31 **Osseous stenosis of neural canal of** cervical **region**
M99.32 **Osseous stenosis of neural canal of** thoracic **region**
M99.33 **Osseous stenosis of neural canal of** lumbar **region**
M99.34 **Osseous stenosis of neural canal of** sacral **region**
M99.35 **Osseous stenosis of neural canal of** pelvic **region**
M99.36 **Osseous stenosis of neural canal of** lower extremity
M99.37 **Osseous stenosis of neural canal of** upper extremity
M99.38 **Osseous stenosis of neural canal of** rib cage
M99.39 **Osseous stenosis of neural canal of** abdomen and other **regions**

☑5ᵗʰ **M99.4** **Connective tissue stenosis of neural canal**

M99.40 **Connective tissue stenosis of neural canal of** head **region**
M99.41 **Connective tissue stenosis of neural canal of** cervical **region**
M99.42 **Connective tissue stenosis of neural canal of** thoracic **region**
M99.43 **Connective tissue stenosis of neural canal of** lumbar **region**
M99.44 **Connective tissue stenosis of neural canal of** sacral **region**
M99.45 **Connective tissue stenosis of neural canal of** pelvic **region**

M99.46   **Connective tissue stenosis of neural canal of** lower **extremity**

M99.47   **Connective tissue stenosis of neural canal of** upper **extremity**

M99.48   **Connective tissue stenosis of neural canal of** rib **cage**

M99.49   **Connective tissue stenosis of neural canal of** abdomen and other **regions**

√5ᵗʰ   **M99.5**   **Intervertebral disc stenosis of neural canal**

M99.50   **Intervertebral disc stenosis of neural canal of** head **region**

M99.51   **Intervertebral disc stenosis of neural canal of** cervical **region**

M99.52   **Intervertebral disc stenosis of neural canal of** thoracic **region**

M99.53   **Intervertebral disc stenosis of neural canal of** lumbar **region**

M99.54   **Intervertebral disc stenosis of neural canal of** sacral **region**

M99.55   **Intervertebral disc stenosis of neural canal of** pelvic **region**

M99.56   **Intervertebral disc stenosis of neural canal of** lower **extremity**

M99.57   **Intervertebral disc stenosis of neural canal of** upper **extremity**

M99.58   **Intervertebral disc stenosis of neural canal of** rib **cage**

M99.59   **Intervertebral disc stenosis of neural canal of** abdomen and other **regions**

√5ᵗʰ   **M99.6**   **Osseous and subluxation stenosis of intervertebral foramina**

M99.60   **Osseous and subluxation stenosis of intervertebral foramina of** head **region**

M99.61   **Osseous and subluxation stenosis of intervertebral foramina of** cervical **region**

M99.62   **Osseous and subluxation stenosis of intervertebral foramina of** thoracic **region**

M99.63   **Osseous and subluxation stenosis of intervertebral foramina of** lumbar **region**

M99.64   **Osseous and subluxation stenosis of intervertebral foramina of** sacral **region**

M99.65   **Osseous and subluxation stenosis of intervertebral foramina of** pelvic **region**

M99.66   **Osseous and subluxation stenosis of intervertebral foramina of** lower extremity

M99.67   **Osseous and subluxation stenosis of intervertebral foramina of** upper extremity

M99.68   **Osseous and subluxation stenosis of intervertebral foramina of** rib cage

M99.69   **Osseous and subluxation stenosis of intervertebral foramina of** abdomen and other **regions**

√5ᵗʰ   **M99.7**   **Connective tissue and disc stenosis of intervertebral foramina**

M99.70   **Connective tissue and disc stenosis of intervertebral foramina of** head **region**

M99.71   **Connective tissue and disc stenosis of intervertebral foramina of** cervical **region**

M99.72   **Connective tissue and disc stenosis of intervertebral foramina of** thoracic **region**

M99.73   **Connective tissue and disc stenosis of intervertebral foramina of** lumbar **region**

M99.74   **Connective tissue and disc stenosis of intervertebral foramina of** sacral **region**

M99.75   **Connective tissue and disc stenosis of intervertebral foramina of** pelvic **region**

M99.76   **Connective tissue and disc stenosis of intervertebral foramina of** lower **extremity**

M99.77   **Connective tissue and disc stenosis of intervertebral foramina of** upper **extremity**

M99.78   **Connective tissue and disc stenosis of intervertebral foramina of** rib **cage**

M99.79   **Connective tissue and disc stenosis of intervertebral foramina of** abdomen and other **regions**

√5ᵗʰ   **M99.8**   **Other biomechanical lesions**

M99.80   **Other biomechanical lesions of** head **region**

M99.81   **Other biomechanical lesions of** cervical **region**

M99.82   **Other biomechanical lesions of** thoracic **region**

M99.83   **Other biomechanical lesions of** lumbar **region**

M99.84   **Other biomechanical lesions of** sacral **region**

M99.85   **Other biomechanical lesions of** pelvic **region**

M99.86   **Other biomechanical lesions of** lower extremity

M99.87   **Other biomechanical lesions of** upper extremity

M99.88   **Other biomechanical lesions of** rib cage

M99.89   **Other biomechanical lesions of** abdomen and other **regions**

M99.9   **Biomechanical lesion, unspecified**   ▽

EXCLUDES 1   Not coded here   EXCLUDES 2   Not included here   N   Newborn Age : 0   P   Pediatric Age : 0-17   M   Maternity Age : 12-55   A   Adult Age : 15-124

780   ICD-10-CM 2017

Chapter 14. Diseases of Genitourinary System (NØØ–N99)

Chapter Specific Guidelines with Coding Examples

The chapter specific guidelines from the ICD-10-CM Official Guidelines for Coding and Reporting have been provided below. Along with these guidelines are coding examples, contained in the shaded boxes, that have been developed to help illustrate the coding and/or sequencing guidance found in these guidelines.

a. Chronic kidney disease

1) Stages of chronic kidney disease (CKD)

The ICD-10-CM classifies CKD based on severity. The severity of CKD is designated by stages 1-5. Stage 2, code N18.2, equates to mild CKD; stage 3, code N18.3, equates to moderate CKD; and stage 4, code N18.4, equates to severe CKD. Code N18.6, End stage renal disease (ESRD), is assigned when the provider has documented end-stage-renal disease (ESRD).

If both a stage of CKD and ESRD are documented, assign code N18.6 only.

> **Stage 5 chronic kidney disease with ESRD requiring chronic dialysis**
>
> **N18.6**   **End stage renal disease**
>
> **Z99.2**   **Dependence on renal dialysis**
>
> *Explanation:* The diagnostic statement indicates the patient has chronic kidney disease, documented both as stage 5 and as ESRD requiring chronic dialysis. Code N18.6 End stage renal disease (ESRD), is assigned when the provider has documented end-stage-renal disease (ESRD). If both a stage of CKD and ESRD are documented, assign code N18.6 only.

2) Chronic kidney disease and kidney transplant status

Patients who have undergone kidney transplant may still have some form of chronic kidney disease (CKD) because the kidney transplant may not fully restore kidney function. Therefore, the presence of CKD alone does not constitute a transplant complication. Assign the appropriate N18 code for the patient's stage of CKD and code Z94.Ø, Kidney transplant status. If a transplant complication such as failure or rejection or other transplant complication is documented, see section I.C.19.g for information on coding complications of a kidney transplant. If the documentation is unclear as to whether the patient has a complication of the transplant, query the provider.

> **Patient with residual chronic kidney disease stage 1 after kidney transplant**
>
> **N18.1**   **Chronic kidney disease, stage 1**
>
> **Z94.Ø**   **Kidney transplant status**
>
> *Explanation:* Patients who have undergone kidney transplant may still have some form of chronic kidney disease (CKD) because the kidney transplant may not fully restore kidney function. The presence of CKD alone does not constitute a transplant complication. Assign the appropriate N18 code for the patient's stage of CKD and code Z94.Ø Kidney transplant status.

3) Chronic kidney disease with other conditions

Patients with CKD may also suffer from other serious conditions, most commonly diabetes mellitus and hypertension. The sequencing of the CKD code in relationship to codes for other contributing conditions is based on the conventions in the Tabular List.

See I.C.9. Hypertensive chronic kidney disease.

See I.C.19. Chronic kidney disease and kidney transplant complications.

> **Type 1 diabetic chronic kidney disease, stage 2**
>
> **E10.22**   **Type 1 diabetes mellitus with diabetic chronic kidney disease**
>
> **N18.2**   **Chronic kidney disease, stage 2 (mild)**
>
> *Explanation:* Patients with CKD may also suffer from other serious conditions such as diabetes mellitus. The sequencing of the CKD code in relationship to codes for other contributing conditions is based on the conventions in the Tabular List. Diabetic CKD code E10.22 includes an instructional note to "Use additional code to identify stage of chronic kidney disease (N18.1–N18.6)," thus providing sequencing direction.

Chapter 14. Diseases of the Genitourinary System (N00-N99)

> **EXCLUDES 2** *certain conditions originating in the perinatal period (P04-P96)*
> *certain infectious and parasitic diseases (A00-B99)*
> *complications of pregnancy, childbirth and the puerperium (O00-O9A)*
> *congenital malformations, deformations and chromosomal abnormalities (Q00-Q99)*
> *endocrine, nutritional and metabolic diseases (E00-E88)*
> *injury, poisoning and certain other consequences of external causes (S00-T88)*
> *neoplasms (C00-D49)*
> *symptoms, signs and abnormal clinical and laboratory findings, not elsewhere classified (R00-R94)*

This chapter contains the following blocks:

N00-N08   Glomerular diseases
N10-N16   Renal tubulo-interstitial diseases
N17-N19   Acute kidney failure and chronic kidney disease
N20-N23   Urolithiasis
N25-N29   Other disorders of kidney and ureter
N30-N39   Other diseases of the urinary system
N40-N53   Diseases of male genital organs
N60-N65   Disorders of breast
N70-N77   Inflammatory diseases of female pelvic organs
N80-N98   Noninflammatory disorders of female genital tract
N99   Intraoperative and postprocedural complications and disorders of genitourinary system, not elsewhere classified

Glomerular diseases (N00-N08)

Code also any associated kidney failure (N17-N19).
> **EXCLUDES 1** *hypertensive chronic kidney disease (I12.-)*

√4ᵗʰ **N00   Acute nephritic syndrome**

> **INCLUDES**   acute glomerular disease
> acute glomerulonephritis
> acute nephritis
> **EXCLUDES 1** *acute tubulo-interstitial nephritis (N10)*
> *nephritic syndrome NOS (N05.-)*

N00.0   Acute nephritic syndrome with minor glomerular abnormality
Acute nephritic syndrome with minimal change lesion

N00.1   Acute nephritic syndrome with focal and segmental glomerular lesions
Acute nephritic syndrome with focal and segmental hyalinosis
Acute nephritic syndrome with focal and segmental sclerosis
Acute nephritic syndrome with focal glomerulonephritis

N00.2   Acute nephritic syndrome with diffuse membranous glomerulonephritis

N00.3   Acute nephritic syndrome with diffuse mesangial proliferative glomerulonephritis

N00.4   Acute nephritic syndrome with diffuse endocapillary proliferative glomerulonephritis

N00.5   Acute nephritic syndrome with diffuse mesangiocapillary glomerulonephritis
Acute nephritic syndrome with membranoproliferative glomerulonephritis, types 1 and 3, or NOS

N00.6   Acute nephritic syndrome with dense deposit disease
Acute nephritic syndrome with membranoproliferative glomerulonephritis, type 2

N00.7   Acute nephritic syndrome with diffuse crescentic glomerulonephritis
Acute nephritic syndrome with extracapillary glomerulonephritis

N00.8   Acute nephritic syndrome with other morphologic changes
Acute nephritic syndrome with proliferative glomerulonephritis NOS

N00.9   Acute nephritic syndrome with unspecified morphologic changes ▽

√4ᵗʰ **N01   Rapidly progressive nephritic syndrome**

> **INCLUDES**   rapidly progressive glomerular disease
> rapidly progressive glomerulonephritis
> rapidly progressive nephritis
> **EXCLUDES 1** *nephritic syndrome NOS (N05.-)*

N01.0   Rapidly progressive nephritic syndrome with minor glomerular abnormality
Rapidly progressive nephritic syndrome with minimal change lesion

N01.1   Rapidly progressive nephritic syndrome with focal and segmental glomerular lesions
Rapidly progressive nephritic syndrome with focal and segmental hyalinosis
Rapidly progressive nephritic syndrome with focal and segmental sclerosis
Rapidly progressive nephritic syndrome with focal glomerulonephritis

N01.2   Rapidly progressive nephritic syndrome with diffuse membranous glomerulonephritis

N01.3   Rapidly progressive nephritic syndrome with diffuse mesangial proliferative glomerulonephritis

N01.4   Rapidly progressive nephritic syndrome with diffuse endocapillary proliferative glomerulonephritis

N01.5   Rapidly progressive nephritic syndrome with diffuse mesangiocapillary glomerulonephritis
Rapidly progressive nephritic syndrome with membranoproliferative glomerulonephritis, types 1 and 3, or NOS

N01.6   Rapidly progressive nephritic syndrome with dense deposit disease
Rapidly progressive nephritic syndrome with membranoproliferative glomerulonephritis, type 2

N01.7   Rapidly progressive nephritic syndrome with diffuse crescentic glomerulonephritis
Rapidly progressive nephritic syndrome with extracapillary glomerulonephritis

N01.8   Rapidly progressive nephritic syndrome with other morphologic changes
Rapidly progressive nephritic syndrome with proliferative glomerulonephritis NOS

N01.9   Rapidly progressive nephritic syndrome with unspecified morphologic changes ▽

√4ᵗʰ **N02   Recurrent and persistent hematuria**

> **EXCLUDES 1** *acute cystitis with hematuria (N30.01)*
> *hematuria NOS (R31.9)*
> *hematuria not associated with specified morphologic lesions (R31.-)*

N02.0   Recurrent and persistent hematuria with minor glomerular abnormality
Recurrent and persistent hematuria with minimal change lesion

N02.1   Recurrent and persistent hematuria with focal and segmental glomerular lesions
Recurrent and persistent hematuria with focal and segmental hyalinosis
Recurrent and persistent hematuria with focal and segmental sclerosis
Recurrent and persistent hematuria with focal glomerulonephritis

N02.2   Recurrent and persistent hematuria with diffuse membranous glomerulonephritis

N02.3   Recurrent and persistent hematuria with diffuse mesangial proliferative glomerulonephritis

N02.4   Recurrent and persistent hematuria with diffuse endocapillary proliferative glomerulonephritis

N02.5   Recurrent and persistent hematuria with diffuse mesangiocapillary glomerulonephritis
Recurrent and persistent hematuria with membranoproliferative glomerulonephritis, types 1 and 3, or NOS

N02.6   Recurrent and persistent hematuria with dense deposit disease
Recurrent and persistent hematuria with membranoproliferative glomerulonephritis, type 2

N02.7   Recurrent and persistent hematuria with diffuse crescentic glomerulonephritis
Recurrent and persistent hematuria with extracapillary glomerulonephritis

N02.8   Recurrent and persistent hematuria with other morphologic changes
Recurrent and persistent hematuria with proliferative glomerulonephritis NOS

N02.9   Recurrent and persistent hematuria with unspecified morphologic changes ▽

EXCLUDES 1 Not coded here   **EXCLUDES 2** Not included here   N Newborn Age : 0   P Pediatric Age : 0-17   M Maternity Age : 12-55   A Adult Age : 15-124

782   ICD-10-CM 2017

✓4ᵗʰ **N03 Chronic nephritic syndrome**

    INCLUDES chronic glomerular disease
             chronic glomerulonephritis
             chronic nephritis

    EXCLUDES 1 *chronic tubulo-interstitial nephritis (N11.-)*
             diffuse sclerosing glomerulonephritis (N05.8-)
             nephritic syndrome NOS (N05.-)

DEF: Slow, progressive type of nephritis characterized by inflammation of the capillary loops in the glomeruli of the kidney, which leads to renal failure.

N03.0 Chronic nephritic syndrome with minor glomerular abnormality
    Chronic nephritic syndrome with minimal change lesion

N03.1 Chronic nephritic syndrome with focal and segmental glomerular lesions
    Chronic nephritic syndrome with focal and segmental hyalinosis
    Chronic nephritic syndrome with focal and segmental sclerosis
    Chronic nephritic syndrome with focal glomerulonephritis

N03.2 Chronic nephritic syndrome with diffuse membranous glomerulonephritis

N03.3 Chronic nephritic syndrome with diffuse mesangial proliferative glomerulonephritis

N03.4 Chronic nephritic syndrome with diffuse endocapillary proliferative glomerulonephritis

N03.5 Chronic nephritic syndrome with diffuse mesangiocapillary glomerulonephritis
    Chronic nephritic syndrome with membranoproliferative glomerulonephritis, types 1 and 3, or NOS

N03.6 Chronic nephritic syndrome with dense deposit disease
    Chronic nephritic syndrome with membranoproliferative glomerulonephritis, type 2

N03.7 Chronic nephritic syndrome with diffuse crescentic glomerulonephritis
    Chronic nephritic syndrome with extracapillary glomerulonephritis

N03.8 Chronic nephritic syndrome with other morphologic changes
    Chronic nephritic syndrome with proliferative glomerulonephritis NOS

N03.9 Chronic nephritic syndrome with unspecified morphologic changes ▽

✓4ᵗʰ **N04 Nephrotic syndrome**

    INCLUDES congenital nephrotic syndrome
             lipoid nephrosis

N04.0 Nephrotic syndrome with minor glomerular abnormality
    Nephrotic syndrome with minimal change lesion

N04.1 Nephrotic syndrome with focal and segmental glomerular lesions
    Nephrotic syndrome with focal and segmental hyalinosis
    Nephrotic syndrome with focal and segmental sclerosis
    Nephrotic syndrome with focal glomerulonephritis

N04.2 Nephrotic syndrome with diffuse membranous glomerulonephritis

N04.3 Nephrotic syndrome with diffuse mesangial proliferative glomerulonephritis

N04.4 Nephrotic syndrome with diffuse endocapillary proliferative glomerulonephritis

N04.5 Nephrotic syndrome with diffuse mesangiocapillary glomerulonephritis
    Nephrotic syndrome with membranoproliferative glomerulonephritis, types 1 and 3, or NOS

N04.6 Nephrotic syndrome with dense deposit disease
    Nephrotic syndrome with membranoproliferative glomerulonephritis, type 2

N04.7 Nephrotic syndrome with diffuse crescentic glomerulonephritis
    Nephrotic syndrome with extracapillary glomerulonephritis

N04.8 Nephrotic syndrome with other morphologic changes
    Nephrotic syndrome with proliferative glomerulonephritis NOS

N04.9 Nephrotic syndrome with unspecified morphologic changes ▽

✓4ᵗʰ **N05 Unspecified nephritic syndrome**

    INCLUDES glomerular disease NOS
             glomerulonephritis NOS
             nephritis NOS
             nephropathy NOS and renal disease NOS with morphological lesion specified in .0-.8

    EXCLUDES 1 *nephropathy NOS with no stated morphological lesion (N28.9)*
             renal disease NOS with no stated morphological lesion (N28.9)
             tubulo-interstitial nephritis NOS (N12)

N05.0 Unspecified nephritic syndrome with minor glomerular abnormality ▽
    Unspecified nephritic syndrome with minimal change lesion

N05.1 Unspecified nephritic syndrome with focal and segmental glomerular lesions ▽
    Unspecified nephritic syndrome with focal and segmental hyalinosis
    Unspecified nephritic syndrome with focal and segmental sclerosis
    Unspecified nephritic syndrome with focal glomerulonephritis

N05.2 Unspecified nephritic syndrome with diffuse membranous glomerulonephritis ▽

N05.3 Unspecified nephritic syndrome with diffuse mesangial proliferative glomerulonephritis ▽

N05.4 Unspecified nephritic syndrome with diffuse endocapillary proliferative glomerulonephritis ▽

N05.5 Unspecified nephritic syndrome with diffuse mesangiocapillary glomerulonephritis ▽
    Unspecified nephritic syndrome with membranoproliferative glomerulonephritis, types 1 and 3, or NOS

N05.6 Unspecified nephritic syndrome with dense deposit disease ▽
    Unspecified nephritic syndrome with membranoproliferative glomerulonephritis, type 2

N05.7 Unspecified nephritic syndrome with diffuse crescentic glomerulonephritis ▽
    Unspecified nephritic syndrome with extracapillary glomerulonephritis

N05.8 Unspecified nephritic syndrome with other morphologic changes ▽
    Unspecified nephritic syndrome with proliferative glomerulonephritis NOS

N05.9 Unspecified nephritic syndrome with unspecified morphologic changes ▽

✓4ᵗʰ **N06 Isolated proteinuria with specified morphological lesion**

    EXCLUDES 1 *proteinuria not associated with specific morphologic lesions (R80.0)*

N06.0 Isolated proteinuria with minor glomerular abnormality
    Isolated proteinuria with minimal change lesion

N06.1 Isolated proteinuria with focal and segmental glomerular lesions
    Isolated proteinuria with focal and segmental hyalinosis
    Isolated proteinuria with focal and segmental sclerosis
    Isolated proteinuria with focal glomerulonephritis

N06.2 Isolated proteinuria with diffuse membranous glomerulonephritis

N06.3 Isolated proteinuria with diffuse mesangial proliferative glomerulonephritis

N06.4 Isolated proteinuria with diffuse endocapillary proliferative glomerulonephritis

N06.5 Isolated proteinuria with diffuse mesangiocapillary glomerulonephritis
    Isolated proteinuria with membranoproliferative glomerulonephritis, types 1 and 3, or NOS

N06.6 Isolated proteinuria with dense deposit disease
    Isolated proteinuria with membranoproliferative glomerulonephritis, type 2

N06.7 Isolated proteinuria with diffuse crescentic glomerulonephritis
    Isolated proteinuria with extracapillary glomerulonephritis

N06.8 Isolated proteinuria with other morphologic lesion
    Isolated proteinuria with proliferative glomerulonephritis NOS

N06.9 Isolated proteinuria with unspecified morphologic lesion ▽

✓ Additional Character Required   ✓x7ᵗʰ Placeholder Alert   Manifestation Dx   ▽ Unspecified Dx   ►◄ Revised Text   ● New Code   ▲ Revised Code Title

Chapter 14. Diseases of the Genitourinary System

☑4ᵗʰ **N07** **Hereditary nephropathy, not elsewhere classified**

EXCLUDES 2   *Alport's syndrome (Q87.81-)*
hereditary amyloid nephropathy (E85.-)
nail patella syndrome (Q87.2)
non-neuropathic heredofamilial amyloidosis (E85.-)

N07.0 **Hereditary nephropathy, not elsewhere classified with** minor glomerular abnormality
Hereditary nephropathy, not elsewhere classified with minimal change lesion

N07.1 **Hereditary nephropathy, not elsewhere classified with** focal and segmental glomerular lesions
Hereditary nephropathy, not elsewhere classified with focal and segmental hyalinosis
Hereditary nephropathy, not elsewhere classified with focal and segmental sclerosis
Hereditary nephropathy, not elsewhere classified with focal glomerulonephritis

N07.2 **Hereditary nephropathy, not elsewhere classified with diffuse membranous glomerulonephritis**

N07.3 **Hereditary nephropathy, not elsewhere classified with diffuse mesangial proliferative glomerulonephritis**

N07.4 **Hereditary nephropathy, not elsewhere classified with diffuse endocapillary proliferative glomerulonephritis**

N07.5 **Hereditary nephropathy, not elsewhere classified with diffuse mesangiocapillary glomerulonephritis**
Hereditary nephropathy, not elsewhere classified with membranoproliferative glomerulonephritis, types 1 and 3, or NOS

N07.6 **Hereditary nephropathy, not elsewhere classified with** dense deposit disease
Hereditary nephropathy, not elsewhere classified with membranoproliferative glomerulonephritis, type 2

N07.7 **Hereditary nephropathy, not elsewhere classified with diffuse crescentic glomerulonephritis**
Hereditary nephropathy, not elsewhere classified with extracapillary glomerulonephritis

N07.8 **Hereditary nephropathy, not elsewhere classified with other morphologic lesions**
Hereditary nephropathy, not elsewhere classified with proliferative glomerulonephritis NOS

N07.9 **Hereditary nephropathy, not elsewhere classified with unspecified morphologic lesions** ▽

N08 *Glomerular disorders in diseases classified elsewhere*
Glomerulonephritis
Nephritis
Nephropathy
Code first underlying disease, such as:
amyloidosis (E85.-)
congenital syphilis (A50.5)
cryoglobulinemia (D89.1)
disseminated intravascular coagulation (D65)
gout (M1A.-, M10.-)
microscopic polyangiitis (M31.7)
multiple myeloma (C90.0-)
sepsis (A40.0-A41.9)
sickle-cell disease (D57.0-D57.8)

EXCLUDES 1   *glomerulonephritis, nephritis and nephropathy (in):*
antiglomerular basement membrane disease (M31.0)
diabetes (E08-E13 with .21)
gonococcal (A54.21)
Goodpasture's syndrome (M31.0)
hemolytic-uremic syndrome (D59.3)
lupus (M32.14)
mumps (B26.83)
syphilis (A52.75)
systemic lupus erythematosus (M32.14)
Wegener's granulomatosis (M31.31)
pyelonephritis in diseases classified elsewhere (N16)
renal tubulo-interstitial disorders classified elsewhere (N16)

Renal tubulo-interstitial diseases (N10-N16)

INCLUDES   pyelonephritis
EXCLUDES 1   *pyeloureteritis cystica (N28.85)*

▲ **N10** **Acute pyelonephritis**
Acute infectious interstitial nephritis
Acute pyelitis
►Acute tubulo-interstitial nephritis◄
Hemoglobin nephrosis
Myoglobin nephrosis
Use additional code (B95-B97), to identify infectious agent

☑4ᵗʰ **N11** **Chronic tubulo-interstitial nephritis**

INCLUDES   chronic infectious interstitial nephritis
chronic pyelitis
chronic pyelonephritis
Use additional code (B95-B97), to identify infectious agent

N11.0 **Nonobstructive reflux-associated** chronic pyelonephritis
Pyelonephritis (chronic) associated with (vesicoureteral) reflux
EXCLUDES 1   *vesicoureteral reflux NOS (N13.70)*

N11.1 **Chronic** obstructive **pyelonephritis**
Pyelonephritis (chronic) associated with anomaly of pelviureteric junction
Pyelonephritis (chronic) associated with anomaly of pyeloureteric junction
Pyelonephritis (chronic) associated with crossing of vessel
Pyelonephritis (chronic) associated with kinking of ureter
Pyelonephritis (chronic) associated with obstruction of ureter
Pyelonephritis (chronic) associated with stricture of pelviureteric junction
Pyelonephritis (chronic) associated with stricture of ureter
EXCLUDES 1   *calculous pyelonephritis (N20.9)*
obstructive uropathy (N13.-)

N11.8 **Other chronic tubulo-interstitial nephritis**
Nonobstructive chronic pyelonephritis NOS

N11.9 **Chronic tubulo-interstitial nephritis, unspecified** ▽
Chronic interstitial nephritis NOS
Chronic pyelitis NOS
Chronic pyelonephritis NOS

N12 **Tubulo-interstitial nephritis, not specified as acute or chronic**
Interstitial nephritis NOS
Pyelitis NOS
Pyelonephritis NOS
EXCLUDES 1   *calculous pyelonephritis (N20.9)*

☑4ᵗʰ **N13** **Obstructive and reflux uropathy**

EXCLUDES 2   *calculus of kidney and ureter without hydronephrosis (N20.-)*
congenital obstructive defects of renal pelvis and ureter (Q62.0-Q62.3)
hydronephrosis with ureteropelvic junction obstruction (Q62.1)
obstructive pyelonephritis (N11.1)

● **N13.0** **Hydronephrosis with ureteropelvic junction obstruction**
Hydronephrosis due to acquired occlusion of ureteropelvic junction
EXCLUDES 2   *hydronephrosis with ureteropelvic junction obstruction due to calculus (N13.2)*

N13.1 **Hydronephrosis with ureteral stricture, not elsewhere classified**
EXCLUDES 1   *hydronephrosis with ureteral stricture with infection (N13.6)*

N13.2 **Hydronephrosis with renal and ureteral calculous obstruction**
EXCLUDES 1   *hydronephrosis with renal and ureteral calculous obstruction with infection (N13.6)*

☑5ᵗʰ **N13.3** **Other and unspecified hydronephrosis**
EXCLUDES 1   *hydronephrosis with infection (N13.6)*
N13.30 **Unspecified hydronephrosis** ▽
N13.39 **Other hydronephrosis**

N13.4 **Hydroureter**
EXCLUDES 1   *congenital hydroureter (Q62.3-)*
hydroureter with infection (N13.6)
vesicoureteral-reflux with hydroureter (N13.73-)

N13.5 **Crossing vessel and stricture of ureter without hydronephrosis**
Kinking and stricture of ureter without hydronephrosis
EXCLUDES 1   *crossing vessel and stricture of ureter without hydronephrosis with infection (N13.6)*

N13.6 **Pyonephrosis**
►Conditions in N13.0-N13.5 with infection◄
Obstructive uropathy with infection
Use additional code (B95-B97), to identify infectious agent

EXCLUDES 1   Not coded here   EXCLUDES 2   Not included here   N Newborn Age : 0   P Pediatric Age : 0-17   M Maternity Age : 12-55   A Adult Age : 15-124

784   ICD-10-CM 2017

☑5ᵗʰ **N13.7** **Vesicoureteral-reflux**
> *EXCLUDES 1*   reflux-associated pyelonephritis (N11.0)

N13.70   **Vesicoureteral-reflux, unspecified**   ▽
> Vesicoureteral-reflux NOS

N13.71   **Vesicoureteral-reflux** without reflux nephropathy

☑6ᵗʰ **N13.72**   **Vesicoureteral-reflux** with reflux nephropathy without hydroureter

     N13.721   **Vesicoureteral-reflux with reflux nephropathy without hydroureter, unilateral**

     N13.722   **Vesicoureteral-reflux with reflux nephropathy without hydroureter, bilateral**

     N13.729   **Vesicoureteral-reflux with reflux**   ▽
            nephropathy without hydroureter, unspecified

☑6ᵗʰ **N13.73**   **Vesicoureteral-reflux** with reflux nephropathy with hydroureter

     N13.731   **Vesicoureteral-reflux with reflux nephropathy with hydroureter,** unilateral

     N13.732   **Vesicoureteral-reflux with reflux nephropathy with hydroureter,** bilateral

     N13.739   **Vesicoureteral-reflux with reflux**   ▽
            nephropathy with hydroureter, unspecified

N13.8   **Other obstructive and reflux uropathy**
> Urinary tract obstruction due to specified cause
> Code first, if applicable, any causal condition, such as:
>   enlarged prostate (N40.1)

N13.9   **Obstructive and reflux uropathy, unspecified**   ▽
> Urinary tract obstruction NOS

☑4ᵗʰ **N14**   **Drug- and heavy-metal-induced tubulo-interstitial and tubular conditions**
> Code first poisoning due to drug or toxin, if applicable (T36-T65 with fifth or sixth character 1-4 or 6)
> Use additional code for adverse effect, if applicable, to identify drug (T36-T50 with fifth or sixth character 5)

N14.0   **Analgesic nephropathy**

N14.1   **Nephropathy induced by other drugs, medicaments and biological substances**

N14.2   **Nephropathy induced by unspecified drug, medicament or biological substance**   ▽

N14.3   **Nephropathy induced by heavy metals**

N14.4   **Toxic nephropathy, not elsewhere classified**

☑4ᵗʰ **N15**   **Other renal tubulo-interstitial diseases**

N15.0   **Balkan nephropathy**
> Balkan endemic nephropathy

N15.1   **Renal and perinephric abscess**

N15.8   **Other specified renal tubulo-interstitial diseases**

N15.9   **Renal tubulo-interstitial disease, unspecified**   ▽
> Infection of kidney NOS
> *EXCLUDES 1*   urinary tract infection NOS (N39.0)

N16   *Renal tubulo-interstitial disorders in diseases classified elsewhere*
> Pyelonephritis
> Tubulo-interstitial nephritis
> Code first underlying disease, such as:
>   brucellosis (A23.0-A23.9)
>   cryoglobulinemia (D89.1)
>   glycogen storage disease (E74.0)
>   leukemia (C91-C95)
>   lymphoma (C81.0-C85.9, C96.0-C96.9)
>   multiple myeloma (C90.0-)
>   sepsis (A40.0-A41.9)
>   Wilson's disease (E83.0)
> *EXCLUDES 1*   diphtheritic pyelonephritis and tubulo-interstitial nephritis (A36.84)
>   pyelonephritis and tubulo-interstitial nephritis in candidiasis (B37.49)
>   pyelonephritis and tubulo-interstitial nephritis in cystinosis (E72.04)
>   pyelonephritis and tubulo-interstitial nephritis in salmonella infection (A02.25)
>   pyelonephritis and tubulo-interstitial nephritis in sarcoidosis (D86.84)
>   pyelonephritis and tubulo-interstitial nephritis in sicca syndrome [Sjogren's] (M35.04)
>   pyelonephritis and tubulo-interstitial nephritis in systemic lupus erythematosus (M32.15)
>   pyelonephritis and tubulo-interstitial nephritis in toxoplasmosis (B58.83)
>   renal tubular degeneration in diabetes (E08-E13 with .29)
>   syphilitic pyelonephritis and tubulo-interstitial nephritis (A52.75)

Acute kidney failure and chronic kidney disease (N17-N19)

> *EXCLUDES 2*   congenital renal failure (P96.0)
>   drug- and heavy-metal-induced tubulo-interstitial and tubular conditions (N14.-)
>   extrarenal uremia (R39.2)
>   hemolytic-uremic syndrome (D59.3)
>   hepatorenal syndrome (K76.7)
>   postpartum hepatorenal syndrome (O90.4)
>   posttraumatic renal failure (T79.5)
>   prerenal uremia (R39.2)
>   renal failure complicating abortion or ectopic or molar pregnancy (O00-O07, O08.4)
>   renal failure following labor and delivery (O90.4)
>   renal failure postprocedural (N99.0)

☑4ᵗʰ **N17**   **Acute kidney failure**
> Code also associated underlying condition
> *EXCLUDES 1*   posttraumatic renal failure (T79.5)
> **AHA:** 2013,4Q,124

N17.0   **Acute kidney failure with tubular necrosis**
> Acute tubular necrosis
> Renal tubular necrosis
> Tubular necrosis NOS

N17.1   **Acute kidney failure with acute cortical necrosis**
> Acute cortical necrosis
> Cortical necrosis NOS
> Renal cortical necrosis

N17.2   **Acute kidney failure with medullary necrosis**
> Medullary [papillary] necrosis NOS
> Acute medullary [papillary] necrosis
> Renal medullary [papillary] necrosis

N17.8   **Other acute kidney failure**

N17.9   **Acute kidney failure, unspecified**   ▽
> Acute kidney injury (nontraumatic)
> *EXCLUDES 2*   traumatic kidney injury (S37.0-)

☑4ᵗʰ **N18**   **Chronic kidney disease (CKD)**
> Code first any associated:
>   diabetic chronic kidney disease (E08.22, E09.22, E10.22, E11.22, E13.22)
>   hypertensive chronic kidney disease (I12.-, I13.-)
> Use additional code to identify kidney transplant status, if applicable, (Z94.0)
> **AHA:** 2013,1Q,24

N18.1   **Chronic kidney disease, stage 1**

N18.2   **Chronic kidney disease, stage 2 (mild)**

N18.3   **Chronic kidney disease, stage 3 (moderate)**

N18.4   **Chronic kidney disease, stage 4 (severe)**

☑ Additional Character Required   ☑7ᵗʰ Placeholder Alert   Manifestation Dx   ▽ Unspecified Dx   ►◄ Revised Text   ● New Code   ▲ Revised Code Title

ICD-10-CM 2017   **785**

N18.5 Chronic kidney disease, stage 5
     EXCLUDES 1   *chronic kidney disease, stage 5 requiring chronic dialysis (N18.6)*

N18.6 End stage renal disease
     Chronic kidney disease requiring chronic dialysis
     Use additional code to identify dialysis status (Z99.2)
     AHA: 2016,1Q,12; 2013,4Q,124-125

N18.9 Chronic kidney disease, unspecified   ▽
     Chronic renal disease
     Chronic renal failure NOS
     Chronic renal insufficiency
     Chronic uremia

N19 Unspecified kidney failure   ▽
     Uremia NOS
     EXCLUDES 1   *acute kidney failure (N17.-)*
         chronic kidney disease (N18.-)
         chronic uremia (N18.9)
         extrarenal uremia (R39.2)
         prerenal uremia (R39.2)
         renal insufficiency (acute) (N28.9)
         uremia of newborn (P96.0)

Urolithiasis (N20-N23)

AHA: 2015,2Q,8

√4ᵗʰ N20 Calculus of kidney and ureter
     Calculous pyelonephritis
     EXCLUDES 1   *nephrocalcinosis (E83.5)*
         that with hydronephrosis (N13.2)

N20.0 Calculus of kidney
     Nephrolithiasis NOS
     Renal calculus
     Renal stone
     Staghorn calculus
     Stone in kidney

N20.1 Calculus of ureter
     Ureteric stone

N20.2 Calculus of kidney with calculus of ureter

N20.9 Urinary calculus, unspecified   ▽

√4ᵗʰ N21 Calculus of lower urinary tract
     INCLUDES   calculus of lower urinary tract with cystitis and urethritis

N21.0 Calculus in bladder
     Calculus in diverticulum of bladder
     Urinary bladder stone
     EXCLUDES 2   *staghorn calculus (N20.0)*

N21.1 Calculus in urethra
     EXCLUDES 2   *calculus of prostate (N42.0)*

N21.8 Other lower urinary tract calculus

N21.9 Calculus of lower urinary tract, unspecified   ▽
     EXCLUDES 1   *calculus of urinary tract NOS (N20.9)*

N22 *Calculus of urinary tract in diseases classified elsewhere*
     Code first underlying disease, such as:
     gout (M1A.-, M10.-)
     schistosomiasis (B65.0-B65.9)

N23 Unspecified renal colic   ▽

Other disorders of kidney and ureter (N25-N29)

     EXCLUDES 2   *disorders of kidney and ureter with urolithiasis (N20-N23)*

√4ᵗʰ N25 Disorders resulting from impaired renal tubular function
     EXCLUDES 1   *metabolic disorders classifiable to E70-E88*

N25.0 Renal osteodystrophy
     Azotemic osteodystrophy
     Phosphate-losing tubular disorders
     Renal rickets
     Renal short stature

N25.1 Nephrogenic diabetes insipidus
     EXCLUDES 1   *diabetes insipidus NOS (E23.2)*

√5ᵗʰ N25.8 Other disorders resulting from impaired renal tubular function

N25.81 Secondary hyperparathyroidism of renal origin
     EXCLUDES 1   *secondary hyperparathyroidism, non-renal (E21.1)*
     DEF: Parathyroid dysfunction caused by chronic renal failure; phosphate clearance is impaired, phosphate is released from bone, vitamin D is not produced, intestinal calcium absorption is low, and blood levels of calcium are lowered, causing excessive production of parathyroid hormone.

N25.89 Other disorders resulting from impaired renal tubular function
     Hypokalemic nephropathy
     Lightwood-Albright syndrome
     Renal tubular acidosis NOS

N25.9 Disorder resulting from impaired renal tubular function, unspecified   ▽

√4ᵗʰ N26 Unspecified contracted kidney
     EXCLUDES 1   *contracted kidney due to hypertension (I12.-)*
         diffuse sclerosing glomerulonephritis (N05.8.-)
         hypertensive nephrosclerosis (arteriolar) (arteriosclerotic) (I12.-)
         small kidney of unknown cause (N27.-)

N26.1 Atrophy of kidney (terminal)

N26.2 Page kidney

N26.9 Renal sclerosis, unspecified   ▽

√4ᵗʰ N27 Small kidney of unknown cause
     INCLUDES   oligonephronia

N27.0 Small kidney, unilateral

N27.1 Small kidney, bilateral

N27.9 Small kidney, unspecified   ▽

√4ᵗʰ N28 Other disorders of kidney and ureter, not elsewhere classified

N28.0 Ischemia and infarction of kidney
     Renal artery embolism
     Renal artery obstruction
     Renal artery occlusion
     Renal artery thrombosis
     Renal infarct
     EXCLUDES 1   *atherosclerosis of renal artery (extrarenal part) (I70.1)*
         congenital stenosis of renal artery (Q27.1)
         Goldblatt's kidney (I70.1)

N28.1 Cyst of kidney, acquired
     Cyst (multiple)(solitary) of kidney, acquired
     EXCLUDES 1   *cystic kidney disease (congenital) (Q61.-)*

√5ᵗʰ N28.8 Other specified disorders of kidney and ureter
     EXCLUDES 1   *hydroureter (N13.4)*
         ureteric stricture with hydronephrosis (N13.1)
         ureteric stricture without hydronephrosis (N13.5)

N28.81 Hypertrophy of kidney
N28.82 Megaloureter
N28.83 Nephroptosis
N28.84 Pyelitis cystica
N28.85 Pyeloureteritis cystica
N28.86 Ureteritis cystica
N28.89 Other specified disorders of kidney and ureter

N28.9 Disorder of kidney and ureter, unspecified   ▽
     Nephropathy NOS
     Renal disease (acute) NOS
     Renal insufficiency (acute)
     EXCLUDES 1   *chronic renal insufficiency (N18.9)*
         unspecified nephritic syndrome (N05.-)
     AHA: 2016,1Q,13

N29 *Other disorders of kidney and ureter in diseases classified elsewhere*
     Code first underlying disease, such as:
     amyloidosis (E85.-)
     nephrocalcinosis (E83.5)
     schistosomiasis (B65.0-B65.9)
     EXCLUDES 1   *disorders of kidney and ureter in:*
         cystinosis (E72.0)
         gonorrhea (A54.21)
         syphilis (A52.75)
         tuberculosis (A18.11)

EXCLUDES 1 Not coded here   EXCLUDES 2 Not included here   N Newborn Age : 0   P Pediatric Age : 0-17   M Maternity Age : 12-55   A Adult Age : 15-124

786   ICD-10-CM 2017

Other diseases of the urinary system (N30-N39)

EXCLUDES 1 *urinary infection (complicating):*
abortion or ectopic or molar pregnancy (O00-O07, O08.8)
pregnancy, childbirth and the puerperium (O23.-, O75.3, O86.2-)

✓4th **N30 Cystitis**
Use additional code to identify infectious agent (B95 B97)
EXCLUDES 1 *prostatocystitis (N41.3)*

✓5th **N30.0 Acute cystitis**
EXCLUDES 1 *irradiation cystitis (N30.4-)*
trigonitis (N30.3-)

N30.00 Acute cystitis without hematuria
N30.01 Acute cystitis with hematuria

✓5th **N30.1 Interstitial cystitis (chronic)**
N30.10 Interstitial cystitis (chronic) without hematuria
N30.11 Interstitial cystitis (chronic) with hematuria

✓5th **N30.2 Other chronic cystitis**
N30.20 Other chronic cystitis without hematuria
N30.21 Other chronic cystitis with hematuria

✓5th **N30.3 Trigonitis**
Urethrotrigonitis
N30.30 Trigonitis without hematuria
N30.31 Trigonitis with hematuria

✓5th **N30.4 Irradiation cystitis**
N30.40 Irradiation cystitis without hematuria
N30.41 Irradiation cystitis with hematuria

✓5th **N30.8 Other cystitis**
Abscess of bladder
N30.80 Other cystitis without hematuria
N30.81 Other cystitis with hematuria

✓5th **N30.9 Cystitis, unspecified**
N30.90 Cystitis, unspecified without hematuria ▽
N30.91 Cystitis, unspecified with hematuria ▽

✓4th **N31 Neuromuscular dysfunction of bladder, not elsewhere classified**
Use additional code to identify any associated urinary incontinence (N39.3-N39.4-)
EXCLUDES 1 *cord bladder NOS (G95.89)*
neurogenic bladder due to cauda equina syndrome (G83.4)
neuromuscular dysfunction due to spinal cord lesion (G95.89)

N31.0 Uninhibited neuropathic bladder, not elsewhere classified
N31.1 Reflex neuropathic bladder, not elsewhere classified
N31.2 Flaccid neuropathic bladder, not elsewhere classified
Atonic (motor) (sensory) neuropathic bladder
Autonomous neuropathic bladder
Nonreflex neuropathic bladder

N31.8 Other neuromuscular dysfunction of bladder
N31.9 Neuromuscular dysfunction of bladder, unspecified ▽
Neurogenic bladder dysfunction NOS

✓4th **N32 Other disorders of bladder**
EXCLUDES 2 *calculus of bladder (N21.0)*
cystocele (N81.1-)
hernia or prolapse of bladder, female (N81.1-)

N32.0 Bladder-neck obstruction
Bladder-neck stenosis (acquired)
EXCLUDES 1 *congenital bladder-neck obstruction (Q64.3-)*
DEF: Bladder outlet and vesicourethral obstruction; occurs as a consequence of benign prostatic hypertrophy or prostatic cancer; may also occur in either sex due to strictures, radiation, cystoscopy, catheterization, injury, infection, blood clots, bladder cancer, impaction, or other disease that compresses the bladder neck.

N32.1 Vesicointestinal fistula
Vesicorectal fistula
N32.2 Vesical fistula, not elsewhere classified
EXCLUDES 1 *fistula between bladder and female genital tract (N82.0-N82.1)*
N32.3 Diverticulum of bladder
EXCLUDES 1 *congenital diverticulum of bladder (Q64.6)*
diverticulitis of bladder (N30.8-)

✓5th **N32.8 Other specified disorders of bladder**
N32.81 Overactive bladder
Detrusor muscle hyperactivity
EXCLUDES 1 *frequent urination due to specified bladder condition - code to condition*

N32.89 Other specified disorders of bladder
Bladder hemorrhage
Bladder hypertrophy
Calcified bladder
Contracted bladder
N32.9 Bladder disorder, unspecified ▽

N33 *Bladder disorders in diseases classified elsewhere*
Code first underlying disease, such as:
schistosomiasis (B65.0-B65.9)
EXCLUDES 1 *bladder disorder in syphilis (A52.76)*
bladder disorder in tuberculosis (A18.12)
candidal cystitis (B37.41)
chlamydial cystitis (A56.01)
cystitis in gonorrhea (A54.01)
cystitis in neurogenic bladder (N31.-)
diphtheritic cystitis (A36.85)
syphilitic cystitis (A52.76)
trichomonal cystitis (A59.03)

✓4th **N34 Urethritis and urethral syndrome**
Use additional code (B95-B97), to identify infectious agent
EXCLUDES 2 *Reiter's disease (M02.3-)*
urethritis in diseases with a predominantly sexual mode of transmission (A50-A64)
urethrotrigonitis (N30.3-)

N34.0 Urethral abscess
Abscess (of) Cowper's gland
Abscess (of) Littré's gland
Abscess (of) urethral (gland)
Periurethral abscess
EXCLUDES 1 *urethral caruncle (N36.2)*

N34.1 Nonspecific urethritis
Nongonococcal urethritis
Nonvenereal urethritis

N34.2 Other urethritis
Meatitis, urethral
Postmenopausal urethritis
Ulcer of urethra (meatus)
Urethritis NOS

N34.3 Urethral syndrome, unspecified ▽

✓4th **N35 Urethral stricture**
EXCLUDES 1 *congenital urethral stricture (Q64.3-)*
postprocedural urethral stricture (N99.1-)

✓5th **N35.0 Post-traumatic urethral stricture**
Urethral stricture due to injury
EXCLUDES 1 *postprocedural urethral stricture (N99.1-)*

✓6th **N35.01 Post-traumatic urethral stricture, male**
N35.010 Post-traumatic urethral stricture, male, meatal ♂
N35.011 Post-traumatic bulbous urethral stricture
N35.012 Post-traumatic membranous urethral stricture
N35.013 Post-traumatic anterior urethral stricture
N35.014 Post-traumatic urethral stricture, male, unspecified ♂ ▽

✓6th **N35.02 Post-traumatic urethral stricture, female**
N35.021 Urethral stricture due to childbirth ♀
N35.028 Other post-traumatic urethral stricture, female ♀

✓5th **N35.1 Postinfective urethral stricture, not elsewhere classified**
EXCLUDES 1 *gonococcal urethral stricture (A54.01)*
syphilitic urethral stricture (A52.76)
urethral stricture associated with schistosomiasis (B65.-, N29)

✓6th **N35.11 Postinfective urethral stricture, not elsewhere classified, male**
N35.111 Postinfective urethral stricture, not elsewhere classified, male, meatal ♂
N35.112 Postinfective bulbous urethral stricture, not elsewhere classified
N35.113 Postinfective membranous urethral stricture, not elsewhere classified
N35.114 Postinfective anterior urethral stricture, not elsewhere classified
N35.119 Postinfective urethral stricture, not elsewhere classified, male, unspecified ♂ ▽

✓ Additional Character Required   ✓7th Placeholder Alert   Manifestation Dx   ▽ Unspecified Dx   ▶◀ Revised Text   ● New Code   ▲ Revised Code Title

    N35.12 Postinfective urethral stricture, not elsewhere classified, female ♀

N35.8 Other urethral stricture
> EXCLUDES 1 *postprocedural urethral stricture (N99.1-)*

N35.9 Urethral stricture, unspecified ▽

✓4ᵗʰ **N36 Other disorders of urethra**

N36.0 Urethral fistula
Urethroperineal fistula
Urethrorectal fistula
Urinary fistula NOS
> EXCLUDES 1 *urethroscrotal fistula ▶(N50.89)◀*
> *urethrovaginal fistula (N82.1)*
> *urethrovesicovaginal fistula (N82.1)*

N36.1 Urethral diverticulum

N36.2 Urethral caruncle

✓5ᵗʰ **N36.4 Urethral functional and muscular disorders**
Use additional code to identify associated urinary stress incontinence (N39.3)

    N36.41 Hypermobility of urethra

    N36.42 Intrinsic sphincter deficiency (ISD)

    N36.43 Combined hypermobility of urethra and intrinsic sphincter deficiency

    N36.44 Muscular disorders of urethra
Bladder sphincter dyssynergy

N36.5 Urethral false passage

N36.8 Other specified disorders of urethra
> EXCLUDES 1 *▶congenital urethrocele (Q64.7)◀*
> *▶female urethrocele (N81.0)◀*

N36.9 Urethral disorder, unspecified ▽

N37 *Urethral disorders in diseases classified elsewhere*
Code first underlying disease
> EXCLUDES 1 *urethritis (in):*
> *candidal infection (B37.41)*
> *chlamydial (A56.01)*
> *gonorrhea (A54.01)*
> *syphilis (A52.76)*
> *trichomonal infection (A59.03)*
> *tuberculosis (A18.13)*

✓4ᵗʰ **N39 Other disorders of urinary system**
> EXCLUDES 2 *hematuria NOS (R31.-)*
> *recurrent or persistent hematuria (N02.-)*
> *recurrent or persistent hematuria with specified morphological lesion (N02.-)*
> *proteinuria NOS (R80.-)*

N39.0 Urinary tract infection, site not specified ▽
Use additional code (B95-B97), to identify infectious agent
> EXCLUDES 1 *candidiasis of urinary tract (B37.4-)*
> *neonatal urinary tract infection (P39.3)*
> *urinary tract infection of specified site, such as:*
> *cystitis (N30.-)*
> *urethritis (N34.-)*

    AHA: 2012,4Q,94

N39.3 Stress incontinence (female) (male)
Code also any associated overactive bladder (N32.81)
> EXCLUDES 1 *mixed incontinence (N39.46)*

✓5ᵗʰ **N39.4 Other specified urinary incontinence**
Code also any associated overactive bladder (N32.81)
> EXCLUDES 1 *enuresis NOS (R32)*
> *functional urinary incontinence (R39.81)*
> *urinary incontinence associated with cognitive impairment (R39.81)*
> *urinary incontinence NOS (R32)*
> *urinary incontinence of nonorganic origin (F98.0)*

    N39.41 Urge incontinence
> EXCLUDES 1 *mixed incontinence (N39.46)*

    N39.42 Incontinence without sensory awareness
▶Insensible (urinary) incontinence◀

    N39.43 Post-void dribbling

    N39.44 Nocturnal enuresis

    N39.45 Continuous leakage

    N39.46 Mixed incontinence
Urge and stress incontinence

✓6ᵗʰ   **N39.49 Other specified urinary incontinence**

      N39.490 Overflow incontinence

      N39.491 Coital incontinence

      N39.492 Postural (urinary) incontinence

      N39.498 Other specified urinary incontinence
Reflex incontinence
Total incontinence

N39.8 Other specified disorders of urinary system

N39.9 Disorder of urinary system, unspecified ▽

Diseases of male genital organs (N40-N53)

▲ ✓4ᵗʰ **N40 Benign prostatic hyperplasia**
> INCLUDES adenofibromatous hypertrophy of prostate
> benign hypertrophy of the prostate
> benign prostatic hypertrophy
> BPH
> ▶enlarged prostate◀
> nodular prostate
> polyp of prostate
> EXCLUDES 1 *benign neoplasms of prostate (adenoma, benign) (fibroadenoma) (fibroma) (myoma) (D29.1)*
> EXCLUDES 2 *malignant neoplasm of prostate (C61)*

▲ **N40.0 Benign prostatic hyperplasia without lower urinary tract symptoms** A ♂
Enlarged prostate NOS
Enlarged prostate without LUTS

▲ **N40.1 Benign prostatic hyperplasia with lower urinary tract symptoms** A ♂
Enlarged prostate with LUTS
Use additional code for associated symptoms, when specified:
incomplete bladder emptying (R39.14)
nocturia (R35.1)
straining on urination (R39.16)
urinary frequency (R35.0)
urinary hesitancy (R39.11)
urinary incontinence (N39.4-)
urinary obstruction (N13.8)
urinary retention (R33.8)
urinary urgency (R39.15)
weak urinary stream (R39.12)

N40.2 Nodular prostate without lower urinary tract symptoms A ♂
Nodular prostate without LUTS

N40.3 Nodular prostate with lower urinary tract symptoms A ♂
Use additional code for associated symptoms, when specified:
incomplete bladder emptying (R39.14)
nocturia (R35.1)
straining on urination (R39.16)
urinary frequency (R35.0)
urinary hesitancy (R39.11)
urinary incontinence (N39.4-)
urinary obstruction (N13.8)
urinary retention (R33.8)
urinary urgency (R39.15)
weak urinary stream (R39.12)

✓4ᵗʰ **N41 Inflammatory diseases of prostate**
Use additional code (B95-B97), to identify infectious agent

N41.0 Acute prostatitis A ♂

N41.1 Chronic prostatitis A ♂

N41.2 Abscess of prostate A ♂

N41.3 Prostatocystitis A ♂

N41.4 Granulomatous prostatitis A ♂

N41.8 Other inflammatory diseases of prostate A ♂

N41.9 Inflammatory disease of prostate, unspecified A ♂ ▽
Prostatitis NOS

✓4ᵗʰ **N42 Other and unspecified disorders of prostate**

N42.0 Calculus of prostate A ♂
Prostatic stone

N42.1 Congestion and hemorrhage of prostate A ♂
> EXCLUDES 1 *enlarged prostate (N40.-)*
> *hematuria (R31.-)*
> *hyperplasia of prostate (N40.-)*
> *inflammatory diseases of prostate (N41.-)*

EXCLUDES 1 Not coded here   EXCLUDES 2 Not included here   N Newborn Age : 0   P Pediatric Age : 0-17   M Maternity Age : 12-55   A Adult Age : 15-124

788   ICD-10-CM 2017

Chapter 14. Diseases of the Genitourinary System

✓5ᵗʰ **N42.3**   **Dysplasia of prostate**

●   **N42.30**   **Unspecified dysplasia of prostate**   ▽

●   **N42.31**   **Prostatic intraepithelial neoplasia**

PIN

Prostatic intraepithelial neoplasia I (PIN I)

Prostatic intraepithelial neoplasia II (PIN II)

EXCLUDES 1   *prostatic intraepithelial neoplasia III (PIN III) (DØ7.5)*

DEF: Abnormality of shape and size of the intraepithelial tissues of the prostate; premalignant condition characterized by stalks and absence of a basilar cell layer; synonyms are intraductal dysplasia, large acinar atypical hyperplasia, atypical primary hyperplasia, hyperplasia with malignant changes, marked atypia, or duct-acinar dysplasia.

●   **N42.32**   **Atypical small acinar proliferation of prostate**

●   **N42.39**   **Other dysplasia of prostate**

✓5ᵗʰ **N42.8**   **Other specified disorders of prostate**

     N42.81   **Prostatodynia syndrome**   A ♂

       Painful prostate syndrome

     N42.82   **Prostatosis syndrome**   A ♂

     N42.83   **Cyst of prostate**   A ♂

     N42.89   **Other specified disorders of prostate**   A ♂

   N42.9   **Disorder of prostate, unspecified**   A ♂ ▽

✓4ᵗʰ **N43**   **Hydrocele and spermatocele**

INCLUDES   hydrocele of spermatic cord, testis or tunica vaginalis

EXCLUDES 1   *congenital hydrocele (P83.5)*

   N43.Ø   **Encysted hydrocele**   ♂

   N43.1   **Infected hydrocele**   ♂

       Use additional code (B95-B97), to identify infectious agent

   N43.2   **Other hydrocele**   ♂

Hydrocele

Normal   Noncommunicating hydrocele   Communicating hydrocele   Hydrocele of the cord

Testicle

Scrotum

   N43.3   **Hydrocele, unspecified**   ♂ ▽

✓5ᵗʰ **N43.4**   **Spermatocele of epididymis**

       Spermatic cyst

     N43.40   **Spermatocele of epididymis, unspecified**   ♂ ▽

     N43.41   **Spermatocele of epididymis, single**   ♂

     N43.42   **Spermatocele of epididymis, multiple**   ♂

✓4ᵗʰ **N44**   **Noninflammatory disorders of testis**

✓5ᵗʰ **N44.Ø**   **Torsion of testis**

     N44.00   **Torsion of testis, unspecified**   ♂ ▽

     N44.01   **Extravaginal torsion of spermatic cord**   ♂

     N44.02   **Intravaginal torsion of spermatic cord**   ♂

       Torsion of spermatic cord NOS

     N44.03   **Torsion of appendix testis**   ♂

     N44.04   **Torsion of appendix epididymis**   ♂

   N44.1   **Cyst of tunica albuginea testis**   ♂

   N44.2   **Benign cyst of testis**   ♂

   N44.8   **Other noninflammatory disorders of the testis**   ♂

✓4ᵗʰ **N45**   **Orchitis and epididymitis**

       Use additional code (B95-B97), to identify infectious agent

   N45.1   **Epididymitis**   ♂

   N45.2   **Orchitis**   ♂

   N45.3   **Epididymo-orchitis**   ♂

   N45.4   **Abscess of epididymis or testis**   ♂

✓4ᵗʰ **N46**   **Male infertility**

EXCLUDES 1   *vasectomy status (Z98.52)*

✓5ᵗʰ **N46.Ø**   **Azoospermia**

       Absolute male infertility

       Male infertility due to germinal (cell) aplasia

       Male infertility due to spermatogenic arrest (complete)

     N46.Ø1   **Organic azoospermia**   A ♂

       Azoospermia NOS

✓6ᵗʰ   **N46.Ø2**   **Azoospermia due to extratesticular causes**

       Code also associated cause

       N46.Ø21   **Azoospermia due to drug therapy**   A ♂

       N46.Ø22   **Azoospermia due to infection**   A ♂

       N46.Ø23   **Azoospermia due to obstruction of efferent ducts**   A ♂

       N46.Ø24   **Azoospermia due to radiation**   A ♂

       N46.Ø25   **Azoospermia due to systemic disease**   A ♂

       N46.Ø29   **Azoospermia due to other extratesticular causes**   A ♂

✓5ᵗʰ **N46.1**   **Oligospermia**

       Male Infertility due to germinal cell desquamation

       Male infertility due to hypospermatogenesis

       Male infertility due to incomplete spermatogenic arrest

     N46.11   **Organic oligospermia**   A ♂

       Oligospermia NOS

✓6ᵗʰ   **N46.12**   **Oligospermia due to extratesticular causes**

       Code also associated cause

       N46.121   **Oligospermia due to drug therapy**   A ♂

       N46.122   **Oligospermia due to infection**   A ♂

       N46.123   **Oligospermia due to obstruction of efferent ducts**   A ♂

       N46.124   **Oligospermia due to radiation**   A ♂

       N46.125   **Oligospermia due to systemic disease**   A ♂

       N46.129   **Oligospermia due to other extratesticular causes**   A ♂

   N46.8   **Other male infertility**   A ♂

   N46.9   **Male infertility, unspecified**   A ♂ ▽

✓4ᵗʰ **N47**   **Disorders of prepuce**

   N47.Ø   **Adherent prepuce, newborn**   N ♂

   N47.1   **Phimosis**   ♂

   N47.2   **Paraphimosis**   ♂

   N47.3   **Deficient foreskin**   ♂

   N47.4   **Benign cyst of prepuce**   ♂

   N47.5   **Adhesions of prepuce and glans penis**   ♂

   N47.6   **Balanoposthitis**   ♂

       Use additional code (B95-B97), to identify infectious agent

       EXCLUDES 1   *balanitis (N48.1)*

   N47.7   **Other inflammatory diseases of prepuce**   ♂

       Use additional code (B95-B97), to identify infectious agent

   N47.8   **Other disorders of prepuce**   ♂

✓4ᵗʰ **N48**   **Other disorders of penis**

   N48.Ø   **Leukoplakia of penis**   ♂

       Balanitis xerotica obliterans

       Kraurosis of penis

       Lichen sclerosus of external male genital organs

       EXCLUDES 1   *carcinoma in situ of penis (DØ7.4)*

✓ Additional Character Required   ✓x7ᵗʰ Placeholder Alert   Manifestation Dx   ▽ Unspecified Dx   ►◄ Revised Text   ● New Code   ▲ Revised Code Title

ICD-10-CM 2017   **789**

Chapter 14. Diseases of the Genitourinary System

N48.1   Balanitis ♂

     Use additional code (B95-B97), to identify infectious agent

     EXCLUDES 1   *amebic balanitis (A06.8)*
           balanitis xerotica obliterans (N48.0)
           candidal balanitis (B37.42)
           gonococcal balanitis (A54.23)
           herpesviral [herpes simplex] balanitis (A60.01)

✓5ᵗʰ **N48.2   Other inflammatory disorders of penis**

     Use additional code (B95-B97), to identify infectious agent

     EXCLUDES 1   *balanitis (N48.1)*
           balanitis xerotica obliterans (N48.0)
           balanoposthitis (N47.6)

     N48.21   Abscess of corpus cavernosum and penis ♂

     N48.22   Cellulitis of corpus cavernosum and penis ♂

     N48.29   Other inflammatory disorders of penis ♂

✓5ᵗʰ **N48.3   Priapism**

     Painful erection

     Code first underlying cause

     N48.30   Priapism, unspecified ♂ ▽

     N48.31   Priapism due to trauma ♂

     N48.32   *Priapism due to disease classified elsewhere* ♂

     N48.33   Priapism, drug-induced ♂

     N48.39   Other priapism ♂

N48.5   Ulcer of penis ♂

N48.6   Induration penis plastica ♂

     Peyronie's disease

     Plastic induration of penis

✓5ᵗʰ **N48.8   Other specified disorders of penis**

     N48.81   Thrombosis of superficial vein of penis ♂

     N48.82   Acquired torsion of penis ♂

         Acquired torsion of penis NOS

         EXCLUDES 1   *congenital torsion of penis (Q55.63)*

     N48.83   Acquired buried penis ♂

         EXCLUDES 1   *congenital hidden penis (Q55.64)*

     N48.89   Other specified disorders of penis ♂

N48.9   Disorder of penis, unspecified ♂ ▽

✓4ᵗʰ **N49   Inflammatory disorders of male genital organs, not elsewhere classified**

     Use additional code (B95-B97), to identify infectious agent

     EXCLUDES 1   *inflammation of penis (N48.1, N48.2-)*
           orchitis and epididymitis (N45.-)

N49.0   Inflammatory disorders of seminal vesicle ♂

     Vesiculitis NOS

N49.1   Inflammatory disorders of spermatic cord, tunica vaginalis and vas deferens ♂

     Vasitis

N49.2   Inflammatory disorders of scrotum ♂

N49.3   Fournier gangrene ♂

N49.8   Inflammatory disorders of other specified male genital organs ♂

     Inflammation of multiple sites in male genital organs

N49.9   Inflammatory disorder of unspecified male genital organ ♂ ▽

     Abscess of unspecified male genital organ

     Boil of unspecified male genital organ

     Carbuncle of unspecified male genital organ

     Cellulitis of unspecified male genital organ

✓4ᵗʰ **N50   Other and unspecified disorders of male genital organs**

     EXCLUDES 2   *torsion of testis (N44.0-)*

N50.0   Atrophy of testis ♂

N50.1   Vascular disorders of male genital organs ♂

     Hematocele, NOS, of male genital organs

     Hemorrhage of male genital organs

     Thrombosis of male genital organs

N50.3   Cyst of epididymis ♂

✓5ᵗʰ **N50.8   Other specified disorders of male genital organs**

     ● **N50.81   Testicular pain**

         ● **N50.811   Right testicular pain**

         ● **N50.812   Left testicular pain**

         ● **N50.819   Testicular pain, unspecified** ▽

     N50.82   Scrotal pain

● **N50.89   Other specified disorders of the male genital organs**

     Atrophy of scrotum, seminal vesicle, spermatic cord, tunica vaginalis and vas deferens

     Chylocele, tunica vaginalis (nonfilarial) NOS

     Edema of scrotum, seminal vesicle, spermatic cord, tunica vaginalis and vas deferens

     Hypertrophy of scrotum, seminal vesicle, spermatic cord, tunica vaginalis and vas deferens

     Stricture of spermatic cord, tunica vaginalis, and vas deferens

     Ulcer of scrotum, seminal vesicle, spermatic cord, testis, tunica vaginalis and vas deferens

     Urethroscrotal fistula

N50.9   Disorder of male genital organs, unspecified ♂ ▽

N51   *Disorders of male genital organs in diseases classified elsewhere* ♂

     Code first underlying disease, such as:

     filariasis (B74.0-B74.9)

     EXCLUDES 1   *amebic balanitis (A06.8)*
           candidal balanitis (B37.42)
           gonococcal balanitis (A54.23)
           gonococcal prostatitis (A54.22)
           herpesviral [herpes simplex] balanitis (A60.01)
           trichomonal prostatitis (A59.02)
           tuberculous prostatitis (A18.14)

✓4ᵗʰ **N52   Male erectile dysfunction**

     EXCLUDES 1   *psychogenic impotence (F52.21)*

✓5ᵗʰ **N52.0   Vasculogenic erectile dysfunction**

     N52.01   Erectile dysfunction due to arterial insufficiency Ⓐ ♂

     N52.02   Corporo-venous occlusive erectile dysfunction Ⓐ ♂

     N52.03   Combined arterial insufficiency and corporo-venous occlusive erectile dysfunction Ⓐ ♂

N52.1   *Erectile dysfunction due to diseases classified elsewhere* Ⓐ ♂

     Code first underlying disease

N52.2   Drug-induced erectile dysfunction Ⓐ ♂

▲ ✓5ᵗʰ **N52.3   Postprocedural erectile dysfunction**

     N52.31   Erectile dysfunction following radical prostatectomy Ⓐ ♂

     N52.32   Erectile dysfunction following radical cystectomy Ⓐ ♂

     N52.33   Erectile dysfunction following urethral surgery Ⓐ ♂

     N52.34   Erectile dysfunction following simple prostatectomy Ⓐ ♂

     ● **N52.35   Erectile dysfunction following radiation therapy**

     ● **N52.36   Erectile dysfunction following interstitial seed therapy**

     ● **N52.37   Erectile dysfunction following prostate ablative therapy**

         Erectile dysfunction following cryotherapy

         Erectile dysfunction following other prostate ablative therapies

         Erectile dysfunction following ultrasound ablative therapies

▲   **N52.39   Other and unspecified postprocedural erectile dysfunction** Ⓐ ♂ ▽

N52.8   Other male erectile dysfunction Ⓐ ♂

N52.9   Male erectile dysfunction, unspecified Ⓐ ♂ ▽

     Impotence NOS

✓4ᵗʰ **N53   Other male sexual dysfunction**

     EXCLUDES 1   *psychogenic sexual dysfunction (F52.-)*

✓5ᵗʰ **N53.1   Ejaculatory dysfunction**

     EXCLUDES 1   *premature ejaculation (F52.4)*

     N53.11   Retarded ejaculation ♂

     N53.12   Painful ejaculation ♂

     N53.13   Anejaculatory orgasm ♂

     N53.14   Retrograde ejaculation ♂

     N53.19   Other ejaculatory dysfunction ♂

         Ejaculatory dysfunction NOS

N53.8   Other male sexual dysfunction ♂

N53.9   Unspecified male sexual dysfunction ♂ ▽

EXCLUDES 1   Not coded here   EXCLUDES 2   Not included here   Ⓝ Newborn Age : 0   Ⓟ Pediatric Age : 0-17   Ⓜ Maternity Age : 12-55   Ⓐ Adult Age : 15-124

790   ICD-10-CM 2017

Disorders of breast (N60-N65)

EXCLUDES 1 *disorders of breast associated with childbirth (O91-O92)*

☑4ᵗʰ **N60 Benign mammary dysplasia**
> INCLUDES fibrocystic mastopathy

☑5ᵗʰ **N60.0 Solitary cyst of breast**
> Cyst of breast
>
> **N60.01 Solitary cyst of right breast**
> **N60.02 Solitary cyst of left breast**
> **N60.09 Solitary cyst of unspecified breast** ▽

☑5ᵗʰ **N60.1 Diffuse cystic mastopathy**
> Cystic breast
> Fibrocystic disease of breast
> EXCLUDES 1 *diffuse cystic mastopathy with epithelial proliferation (N60.3-)*
>
> **N60.11 Diffuse cystic mastopathy of right breast** Ⓐ
> **N60.12 Diffuse cystic mastopathy of left breast** Ⓐ
> **N60.19 Diffuse cystic mastopathy of unspecified breast** Ⓐ ▽

☑5ᵗʰ **N60.2 Fibroadenosis of breast**
> Adenofibrosis of breast
> EXCLUDES 2 *fibroadenoma of breast (D24.-)*
>
> **N60.21 Fibroadenosis of right breast**
> **N60.22 Fibroadenosis of left breast**
> **N60.29 Fibroadenosis of unspecified breast** ▽

☑5ᵗʰ **N60.3 Fibrosclerosis of breast**
> Cystic mastopathy with epithelial proliferation
>
> **N60.31 Fibrosclerosis of right breast**
> **N60.32 Fibrosclerosis of left breast**
> **N60.39 Fibrosclerosis of unspecified breast** ▽

☑5ᵗʰ **N60.4 Mammary duct ectasia**
> **N60.41 Mammary duct ectasia of right breast**
> **N60.42 Mammary duct ectasia of left breast**
> **N60.49 Mammary duct ectasia of unspecified breast** ▽

☑5ᵗʰ **N60.8 Other benign mammary dysplasias**
> **N60.81 Other benign mammary dysplasias of right breast**
> **N60.82 Other benign mammary dysplasias of left breast**
> **N60.89 Other benign mammary dysplasias of unspecified breast** ▽

☑5ᵗʰ **N60.9 Unspecified benign mammary dysplasia**
> **N60.91 Unspecified benign mammary dysplasia of right breast** ▽
> **N60.92 Unspecified benign mammary dysplasia of left breast** ▽
> **N60.99 Unspecified benign mammary dysplasia of unspecified breast** ▽

☑4ᵗʰ **N61 Inflammatory disorders of breast**
> EXCLUDES 1 *inflammatory carcinoma of breast (C50.9)*
> *inflammatory disorder of breast associated with childbirth (O91.-)*
> *neonatal infective mastitis (P39.0)*
> *thrombophlebitis of breast [Mondor's disease] (I80.8)*

● **N61.0 Mastitis without abscess**
> Infective mastitis (acute) (nonpuerperal) (subacute)
> Mastitis (acute) (nonpuerperal) (subacute) NOS
> Cellulitis (acute) (nonpuerperal) (subacute) of breast NOS
> Cellulitis (acute) (nonpuerperal) (subacute) of nipple NOS

● **N61.1 Abscess of the breast and nipple**
> Abscess (acute) (chronic) (nonpuerperal) of areola
> Abscess (acute) (chronic) (nonpuerperal) of breast
> Carbuncle of breast
> Mastitis with abscess

N62 Hypertrophy of breast
> Gynecomastia
> Hypertrophy of breast NOS
> Massive pubertal hypertrophy of breast
> EXCLUDES 1 *breast engorgement of newborn (P83.4)*
> *disproportion of reconstructed breast (N65.1)*

N63 Unspecified lump in breast ▽
> Nodule(s) NOS in breast

☑4ᵗʰ **N64 Other disorders of breast**
> EXCLUDES 2 *mechanical complication of breast prosthesis and implant (T85.4-)*

N64.0 Fissure and fistula of nipple

N64.1 Fat necrosis of breast
> Fat necrosis (segmental) of breast
> Code first breast necrosis due to breast graft ▶(T85.898)◀

N64.2 Atrophy of breast

N64.3 Galactorrhea not associated with childbirth

N64.4 Mastodynia

☑5ᵗʰ **N64.5 Other signs and symptoms in breast**
> EXCLUDES 2 *abnormal findings on diagnostic imaging of breast (R92.-)*
>
> **N64.51 Induration of breast**
> **N64.52 Nipple discharge**
> > EXCLUDES 1 *abnormal findings in nipple discharge (R89.-)*
> **N64.53 Retraction of nipple**
> **N64.59 Other signs and symptoms in breast**

☑5ᵗʰ **N64.8 Other specified disorders of breast**
> **N64.81 Ptosis of breast** Ⓐ
> > EXCLUDES 1 *ptosis of native breast in relation to reconstructed breast (N65.1)*
> **N64.82 Hypoplasia of breast** Ⓐ
> > Micromastia
> > EXCLUDES 1 *congenital absence of breast (Q83.0)*
> > *hypoplasia of native breast in relation to reconstructed breast (N65.1)*
> **N64.89 Other specified disorders of breast**
> > Galactocele
> > Subinvolution of breast (postlactational)

N64.9 Disorder of breast, unspecified ▽

☑4ᵗʰ **N65 Deformity and disproportion of reconstructed breast**
> **N65.0 Deformity of reconstructed breast** Ⓐ
> > Contour irregularity in reconstructed breast
> > Excess tissue in reconstructed breast
> > Misshapen reconstructed breast
> **N65.1 Disproportion of reconstructed breast** Ⓐ
> > Breast asymmetry between native breast and reconstructed breast
> > Disproportion between native breast and reconstructed breast

Inflammatory diseases of female pelvic organs (N70-N77)

EXCLUDES 1 *inflammatory diseases of female pelvic organs complicating:*
abortion or ectopic or molar pregnancy (O00-O07, O08.0)
pregnancy, childbirth and the puerperium (O23.-, O75.3, O85, O86.-)

☑4ᵗʰ **N70 Salpingitis and oophoritis**
> INCLUDES abscess (of) fallopian tube
> abscess (of) ovary
> pyosalpinx
> salpingo-oophoritis
> tubo-ovarian abscess
> tubo-ovarian inflammatory disease
> Use additional code (B95-B97), to identify infectious agent
> EXCLUDES 1 *gonococcal infection (A54.24)*
> *tuberculous infection (A18.17)*

☑5ᵗʰ **N70.0 Acute salpingitis and oophoritis**
> **N70.01 Acute salpingitis** ♀
> **N70.02 Acute oophoritis** ♀
> **N70.03 Acute salpingitis and oophoritis** ♀

☑5ᵗʰ **N70.1 Chronic salpingitis and oophoritis**
> Hydrosalpinx
> **N70.11 Chronic salpingitis** ♀
> **N70.12 Chronic oophoritis** ♀
> **N70.13 Chronic salpingitis and oophoritis** ♀

☑5ᵗʰ **N70.9 Salpingitis and oophoritis, unspecified**
> **N70.91 Salpingitis, unspecified** ♀ ▽
> **N70.92 Oophoritis, unspecified** ♀ ▽
> **N70.93 Salpingitis and oophoritis, unspecified** ♀ ▽

☑ Additional Character Required   ᵥₓ₇ᵗʰ Placeholder Alert   Manifestation Dx   ▽ Unspecified Dx   ▶◀ Revised Text   ● New Code   ▲ Revised Code Title

ICD-10-CM 2017

791

✓4ᵗʰ **N71** **Inflammatory disease of uterus, except cervix**

     INCLUDES   endo (myo) metritis
                     metritis
                     myometritis
                     pyometra
                     uterine abscess

     Use additional code (B95-B97), to identify infectious agent
        EXCLUDES 1   *hyperplastic endometritis (N85.0-)*
                     infection of uterus following delivery (O85, O86.-)

     N71.0 **Acute inflammatory disease of uterus**   ♀

     N71.1 **Chronic inflammatory disease of uterus**   ♀

     N71.9 **Inflammatory disease of uterus, unspecified**   ♀ ▽

N72 **Inflammatory disease of cervix uteri**   ♀

     INCLUDES   cervicitis (with or without erosion or ectropion)
                     endocervicitis (with or without erosion or ectropion)
                     exocervicitis (with or without erosion or ectropion)

     Use additional code (B95-B97), to identify infectious agent
        EXCLUDES 1   *erosion and ectropion of cervix without cervicitis (N86)*

✓4ᵗʰ **N73** **Other female pelvic inflammatory diseases**

     Use additional code (B95-B97), to identify infectious agent

     N73.0 **Acute parametritis and pelvic cellulitis**   ♀

         Abscess of broad ligament
         Abscess of parametrium
         Pelvic cellulitis, female
         DEF: Parametritis: Inflammation of the parametrium; pelvic
         cellulitis is a synonym for parametritis.

     N73.1 **Chronic parametritis and pelvic cellulitis**   ♀

         Any condition in N73.0 specified as chronic
           EXCLUDES 1   *tuberculous parametritis and pelvic cellultis (A18.17)*

     N73.2 **Unspecified parametritis and pelvic cellulitis**   ♀ ▽

         Any condition in N73.0 unspecified whether acute or chronic

     N73.3 **Female acute pelvic peritonitis**   ♀

     N73.4 **Female chronic pelvic peritonitis**   ♀

           EXCLUDES 1   *tuberculous pelvic (female) peritonitis (A18.17)*

     N73.5 **Female pelvic peritonitis, unspecified**   ♀ ▽

     N73.6 **Female pelvic peritoneal adhesions (postinfective)**   ♀

           EXCLUDES 2   *postprocedural pelvic peritoneal adhesions (N99.4)*
         AHA: 2014,1Q,6

     N73.8 **Other specified female pelvic inflammatory diseases**   ♀

     N73.9 **Female pelvic inflammatory disease, unspecified**   ♀ ▽

         Female pelvic infection or inflammation NOS

N74 *Female pelvic inflammatory disorders in diseases classified*   ♀
     elsewhere

     Code first underlying disease
        EXCLUDES 1   *chlamydial cervicitis (A56.02)*
                     chlamydial pelvic inflammatory disease (A56.11)
                     gonococcal cervicitis (A54.03)
                     gonococcal pelvic inflammatory disease (A54.24)
                     herpesviral [herpes simplex] cervicitis (A60.03)
                     herpesviral [herpes simplex] pelvic inflammatory disease
                         (A60.09)
                     syphilitic cervicitis (A52.76)
                     syphilitic pelvic inflammatory disease (A52.76)
                     trichomonal cervicitis (A59.09)
                     tuberculous cervicitis (A18.16)
                     tuberculous pelvic inflammatory disease (A18.17)

✓4ᵗʰ **N75** **Diseases of Bartholin's gland**

     N75.0 **Cyst of Bartholin's gland**   ♀

     N75.1 **Abscess of Bartholin's gland**   ♀

     N75.8 **Other diseases of Bartholin's gland**   ♀

         Bartholinitis

     N75.9 **Disease of Bartholin's gland, unspecified**   ♀ ▽

✓4ᵗʰ **N76** **Other inflammation of vagina and vulva**

     Use additional code (B95-B97), to identify infectious agent
        EXCLUDES 2   *senile (atrophic) vaginitis (N95.2)*
                     vulvar vestibulitis (N94.810)

     N76.0 **Acute vaginitis**   ♀

         Acute vulvovaginitis
         Vaginitis NOS
         Vulvovaginitis NOS

     N76.1 **Subacute and chronic vaginitis**   ♀

         Chronic vulvovaginitis
         Subacute vulvovaginitis

     N76.2 **Acute vulvitis**   ♀

         Vulvitis NOS

     N76.3 **Subacute and chronic vulvitis**   ♀

     N76.4 **Abscess of vulva**   ♀

         Furuncle of vulva

     N76.5 **Ulceration of vagina**   ♀

     N76.6 **Ulceration of vulva**   ♀

✓5ᵗʰ **N76.8** **Other specified inflammation of vagina and vulva**

         N76.81 **Mucositis (ulcerative) of vagina and vulva**   ♀

              Code also type of associated therapy, such as:
                antineoplastic and immunosuppressive drugs
                   (T45.1X-)
                radiological procedure and radiotherapy (Y84.2)
                EXCLUDES 2   *gastrointestinal mucositis (ulcerative)*
                         (K92.81)
                        nasal mucositis (ulcerative) (J34.81)
                        oral mucositis (ulcerative) (K12.3-)

         N76.89 **Other specified inflammation of vagina and**   ♀
                   vulva

✓4ᵗʰ **N77** **Vulvovaginal ulceration and inflammation in diseases classified**
     elsewhere

     N77.0 *Ulceration of vulva in diseases classified elsewhere*   ♀

         Code first underlying disease, such as:
           Behçet's disease (M35.2)
           EXCLUDES 1   *ulceration of vulva in gonococcal infection (A54.02)*
                     ulceration of vulva in herpesviral [herpes simplex]
                       infection (A60.04)
                     ulceration of vulva in syphilis (A51.0)
                     ulceration of vulva in tuberculosis (A18.18)

     N77.1 *Vaginitis, vulvitis and vulvovaginitis in diseases*   ♀
              classified elsewhere

         Code first underlying disease, such as:
           pinworm (B80)
           EXCLUDES 1   *candidal vulvovaginitis (B37.3)*
                     chlamydial vulvovaginitis (A56.02)
                     gonococcal vulvovaginitis (A54.02)
                     herpesviral [herpes simplex] vulvovaginitis (A60.04)
                     trichomonal vulvovaginitis (A59.01)
                     tuberculous vulvovaginitis (A18.18)
                     vulvovaginitis in early syphilis (A51.0)
                     vulvovaginitis in late syphilis (A52.76)

Noninflammatory disorders of female genital tract (N80-N98)

✓4ᵗʰ **N80** **Endometriosis**

     N80.0 **Endometriosis of uterus**   ♀

         Adenomyosis
           EXCLUDES 1   *stromal endometriosis (D39.0)*

     N80.1 **Endometriosis of ovary**   ♀

     N80.2 **Endometriosis of fallopian tube**   ♀

     N80.3 **Endometriosis of pelvic peritoneum**   ♀

     N80.4 **Endometriosis of rectovaginal septum and vagina**   ♀

     N80.5 **Endometriosis of intestine**   ♀

     N80.6 **Endometriosis in cutaneous scar**   ♀

     N80.8 **Other endometriosis**   ♀

     N80.9 **Endometriosis, unspecified**   ♀ ▽

☑️4ᵗʰ **N81 Female genital prolapse**

> EXCLUDES 1   *genital prolapse complicating pregnancy, labor or delivery (O34.5-)*
> *prolapse and hernia of ovary and fallopian tube ▶(N83.4-)◀*
> *prolapse of vaginal vault after hysterectomy (N99.3)*

Types of Pelvic Organ Prolapse

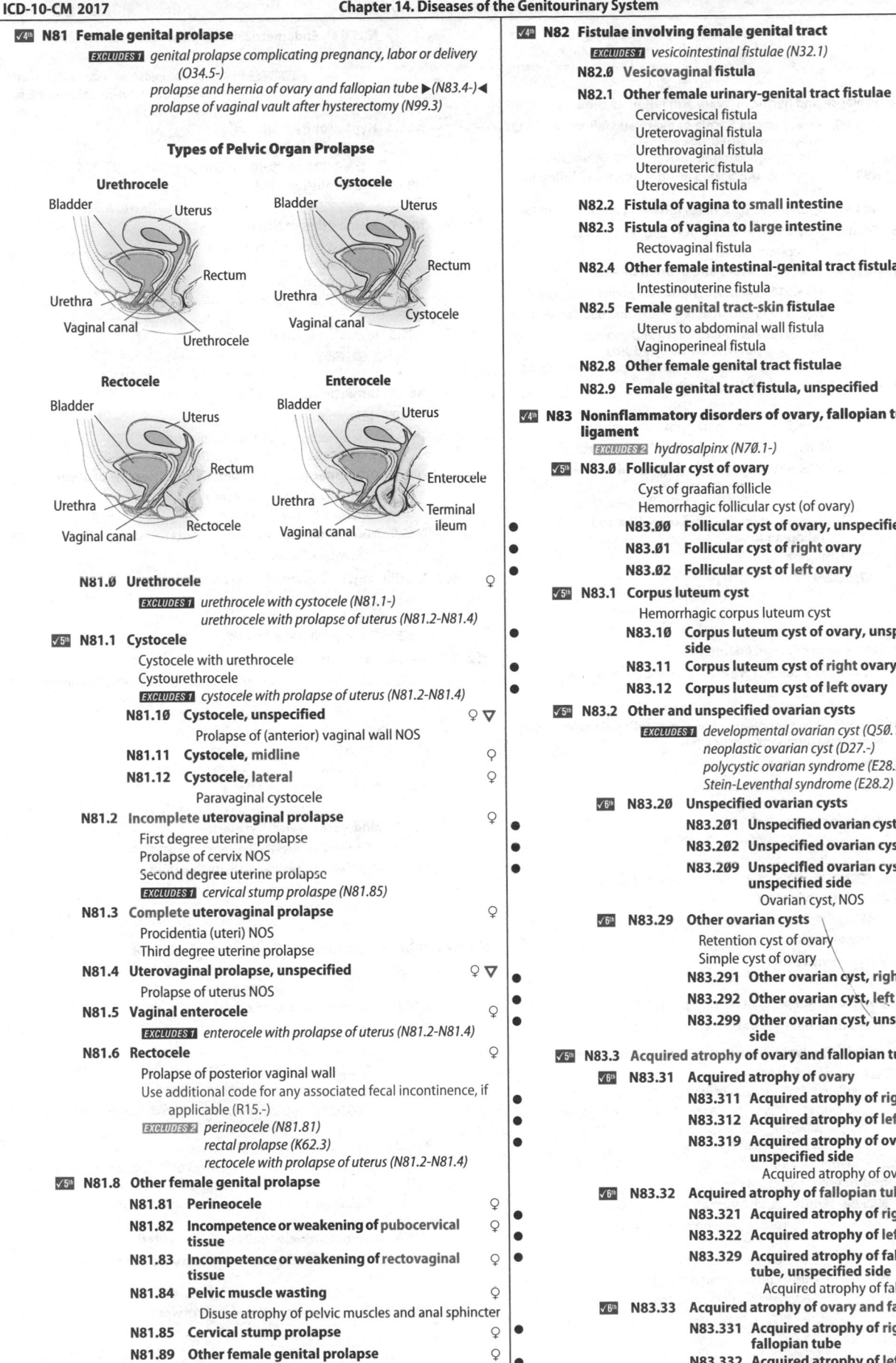

N81.0 Urethrocele   ♀

> EXCLUDES 1   *urethrocele with cystocele (N81.1-)*
> *urethrocele with prolapse of uterus (N81.2-N81.4)*

☑️5ᵗʰ **N81.1 Cystocele**

Cystocele with urethrocele
Cystourethrocele

> EXCLUDES 1   *cystocele with prolapse of uterus (N81.2-N81.4)*

N81.10 Cystocele, unspecified   ♀ ▽

Prolapse of (anterior) vaginal wall NOS

N81.11 Cystocele, midline   ♀

N81.12 Cystocele, lateral   ♀

Paravaginal cystocele

N81.2 Incomplete uterovaginal prolapse   ♀

First degree uterine prolapse
Prolapse of cervix NOS
Second degree uterine prolapse

> EXCLUDES 1   *cervical stump prolaspe (N81.85)*

N81.3 Complete uterovaginal prolapse   ♀

Procidentia (uteri) NOS
Third degree uterine prolapse

N81.4 Uterovaginal prolapse, unspecified   ♀ ▽

Prolapse of uterus NOS

N81.5 Vaginal enterocele   ♀

> EXCLUDES 1   *enterocele with prolapse of uterus (N81.2-N81.4)*

N81.6 Rectocele   ♀

Prolapse of posterior vaginal wall
Use additional code for any associated fecal incontinence, if applicable (R15.-)

> EXCLUDES 2   *perineocele (N81.81)*
> *rectal prolapse (K62.3)*
> *rectocele with prolapse of uterus (N81.2-N81.4)*

☑️5ᵗʰ **N81.8 Other female genital prolapse**

N81.81 Perineocele   ♀

N81.82 Incompetence or weakening of pubocervical tissue   ♀

N81.83 Incompetence or weakening of rectovaginal tissue   ♀

N81.84 Pelvic muscle wasting   ♀

Disuse atrophy of pelvic muscles and anal sphincter

N81.85 Cervical stump prolapse   ♀

N81.89 Other female genital prolapse   ♀

Deficient perineum
Old laceration of muscles of pelvic floor

N81.9 Female genital prolapse, unspecified   ♀ ▽

☑️4ᵗʰ **N82 Fistulae involving female genital tract**

> EXCLUDES 1   *vesicointestinal fistulae (N32.1)*

N82.0 Vesicovaginal fistula   ♀

N82.1 Other female urinary-genital tract fistulae   ♀

Cervicovesical fistula
Ureterovaginal fistula
Urethrovaginal fistula
Uteroureteric fistula
Uterovesical fistula

N82.2 Fistula of vagina to small intestine   ♀

N82.3 Fistula of vagina to large intestine   ♀

Rectovaginal fistula

N82.4 Other female intestinal-genital tract fistulae   ♀

Intestinouterine fistula

N82.5 Female genital tract-skin fistulae   ♀

Uterus to abdominal wall fistula
Vaginoperineal fistula

N82.8 Other female genital tract fistulae   ♀

N82.9 Female genital tract fistula, unspecified   ♀ ▽

☑️4ᵗʰ **N83 Noninflammatory disorders of ovary, fallopian tube and broad ligament**

> EXCLUDES 2   *hydrosalpinx (N70.1-)*

☑️5ᵗʰ **N83.0 Follicular cyst of ovary**

Cyst of graafian follicle
Hemorrhagic follicular cyst (of ovary)

● **N83.00 Follicular cyst of ovary, unspecified side**   ▽

● **N83.01 Follicular cyst of right ovary**

● **N83.02 Follicular cyst of left ovary**

☑️5ᵗʰ **N83.1 Corpus luteum cyst**

Hemorrhagic corpus luteum cyst

● **N83.10 Corpus luteum cyst of ovary, unspecified side**   ▽

N83.11 Corpus luteum cyst of right ovary

N83.12 Corpus luteum cyst of left ovary

☑️5ᵗʰ **N83.2 Other and unspecified ovarian cysts**

> EXCLUDES 1   *developmental ovarian cyst (Q50.1)*
> *neoplastic ovarian cyst (D27.-)*
> *polycystic ovarian syndrome (E28.2)*
> *Stein-Leventhal syndrome (E28.2)*

☑️6ᵗʰ **N83.20 Unspecified ovarian cysts**

● **N83.201 Unspecified ovarian cyst, right side**   ▽

● **N83.202 Unspecified ovarian cyst, left side**   ▽

● **N83.209 Unspecified ovarian cyst, unspecified side**   ▽

Ovarian cyst, NOS

☑️6ᵗʰ **N83.29 Other ovarian cysts**

Retention cyst of ovary
Simple cyst of ovary

● **N83.291 Other ovarian cyst, right side**

● **N83.292 Other ovarian cyst, left side**

● **N83.299 Other ovarian cyst, unspecified side**   ▽

☑️5ᵗʰ **N83.3 Acquired atrophy of ovary and fallopian tube**

☑️6ᵗʰ **N83.31 Acquired atrophy of ovary**

● **N83.311 Acquired atrophy of right ovary**

● **N83.312 Acquired atrophy of left ovary**

● **N83.319 Acquired atrophy of ovary, unspecified side**   ▽

Acquired atrophy of ovary, NOS

☑️6ᵗʰ **N83.32 Acquired atrophy of fallopian tube**

● **N83.321 Acquired atrophy of right fallopian tube**

● **N83.322 Acquired atrophy of left fallopian tube**

● **N83.329 Acquired atrophy of fallopian tube, unspecified side**   ▽

Acquired atrophy of fallopian tube, NOS

☑️6ᵗʰ **N83.33 Acquired atrophy of ovary and fallopian tube**

● **N83.331 Acquired atrophy of right ovary and fallopian tube**

N83.332 Acquired atrophy of left ovary and fallopian tube

☑️ Additional Character Required   ☑️x7ᵗʰ Placeholder Alert   Manifestation Dx   ▽ Unspecified Dx   ▶◀ Revised Text   ● New Code   ▲ Revised Code Title

N83.339 **Acquired atrophy of ovary and fallopian tube, unspecified side** ▽
Acquired atrophy of ovary and fallopian tube, NOS

✓5ᵗʰ **N83.4** **Prolapse and hernia** of ovary and fallopian tube

N83.40 **Prolapse and hernia of ovary and fallopian tube, unspecified side** ▽
Prolapse and hernia of ovary and fallopian tube, NOS

N83.41 **Prolapse and hernia of right ovary and fallopian tube**

N83.42 **Prolapse and hernia of left ovary and fallopian tube**

✓5ᵗʰ **N83.5** **Torsion** of ovary, ovarian pedicle and fallopian tube
Torsion of accessory tube

✓6ᵗʰ **N83.51** **Torsion of ovary and ovarian pedicle**

N83.511 **Torsion of right ovary and ovarian pedicle**

N83.512 **Torsion of left ovary and ovarian pedicle**

N83.519 **Torsion of ovary and ovarian pedicle, unspecified side** ▽
Torsion of ovary and ovarian pedicle, NOS

✓6ᵗʰ **N83.52** **Torsion of fallopian tube**
Torsion of hydatid of Morgagni

N83.521 **Torsion of right fallopian tube**

N83.522 **Torsion of left fallopian tube**

N83.529 **Torsion of fallopian tube, unspecified side** ▽
Torsion of fallopian tube, NOS

N83.53 **Torsion of ovary, ovarian pedicle and fallopian tube** ♀

N83.6 **Hematosalpinx** ♀
EXCLUDES 1 hematosalpinx (with) (in):
hematocolpos (N89.7)
hematometra (N85.7)
tubal pregnancy ▶(O00.1-)◀

N83.7 **Hematoma of broad ligament** ♀

N83.8 **Other noninflammatory disorders of ovary, fallopian tube and broad ligament** ♀
Broad ligament laceration syndrome [Allen-Masters]

N83.9 **Noninflammatory disorder of ovary, fallopian tube and broad ligament, unspecified** ♀ ▽

✓4ᵗʰ **N84** **Polyp of female genital tract**
EXCLUDES 1 adenomatous polyp (D28.-)
placental polyp (O90.89)

N84.0 **Polyp of corpus uteri** ♀
Polyp of endometrium
Polyp of uterus NOS
EXCLUDES 1 polypoid endometrial hyperplasia (N85.0-)

N84.1 **Polyp of cervix uteri** ♀
Mucous polyp of cervix

N84.2 **Polyp of vagina** ♀

N84.3 **Polyp of vulva** ♀
Polyp of labia

N84.8 **Polyp of other parts of female genital tract** ♀

N84.9 **Polyp of female genital tract, unspecified** ♀ ▽

✓4ᵗʰ **N85** **Other noninflammatory disorders of uterus, except cervix**
EXCLUDES 1 endometriosis (N80.-)
inflammatory diseases of uterus (N71.-)
noninflammatory disorders of cervix, except malposition (N86-N88)
polyp of corpus uteri (N84.0)
uterine prolapse (N81.-)

✓5ᵗʰ **N85.0** **Endometrial hyperplasia**

N85.00 **Endometrial hyperplasia, unspecified** ♀ ▽
Hyperplasia (adenomatous) (cystic) (glandular) of endometrium
Hyperplastic endometritis

N85.01 **Benign endometrial hyperplasia** ♀
Endometrial hyperplasia (complex) (simple) without atypia

N85.02 **Endometrial intraepithelial neoplasia [EIN]** ♀
Endometrial hyperplasia with atypia
EXCLUDES 1 malignant neoplasm of endometrium (with endometrial intraepithelial neoplasia [EIN]) (C54.1)

N85.2 **Hypertrophy of uterus** ♀
Bulky or enlarged uterus
EXCLUDES 1 puerperal hypertrophy of uterus (O90.89)

N85.3 **Subinvolution of uterus** ♀
EXCLUDES 1 puerperal subinvolution of uterus (O90.89)

N85.4 **Malposition of uterus** ♀
Anteversion of uterus
Retroflexion of uterus
Retroversion of uterus
EXCLUDES 1 malposition of uterus complicating pregnancy, labor or delivery (O34.5-, O65.5)

N85.5 **Inversion of uterus** ♀
EXCLUDES 1 current obstetric trauma (O71.2)
postpartum inversion of uterus (O71.2)

N85.6 **Intrauterine synechiae** ♀

N85.7 **Hematometra** ♀
Hematosalpinx with hematometra
EXCLUDES 1 hematometra with hematocolpos (N89.7)

N85.8 **Other specified noninflammatory disorders of uterus** ♀
Atrophy of uterus, acquired
Fibrosis of uterus NOS

N85.9 **Noninflammatory disorder of uterus, unspecified** ♀ ▽
Disorder of uterus NOS

N86 **Erosion and ectropion of cervix uteri** ♀
Decubitus (trophic) ulcer of cervix
Eversion of cervix
EXCLUDES 1 erosion and ectropion of cervix with cervicitis (N72)

✓4ᵗʰ **N87** **Dysplasia of cervix uteri**
EXCLUDES 1 abnormal results from cervical cytologic examination without histologic confirmation (R87.61-)
carcinoma in situ of cervix uteri (D06.-)
cervical intraepithelial neoplasia III [CIN III] (D06.-)
HGSIL of cervix (R87.613)
severe dysplasia of cervix uteri (D06.-)

N87.0 **Mild cervical dysplasia** ♀
Cervical intraepithelial neoplasia I [CIN I]

N87.1 **Moderate cervical dysplasia** ♀
Cervical intraepithelial neoplasia II [CIN II]

N87.9 **Dysplasia of cervix uteri, unspecified** ♀ ▽
Anaplasia of cervix
Cervical atypism
Cervical dysplasia NOS

✓4ᵗʰ **N88** **Other noninflammatory disorders of cervix uteri**
EXCLUDES 2 inflammatory disease of cervix (N72)
polyp of cervix (N84.1)

N88.0 **Leukoplakia of cervix uteri** ♀

N88.1 **Old laceration of cervix uteri** ♀
Adhesions of cervix
EXCLUDES 1 current obstetric trauma (O71.3)

N88.2 **Stricture and stenosis of cervix uteri** ♀
EXCLUDES 1 stricture and stenosis of cervix uteri complicating labor (O65.5)

N88.3 **Incompetence of cervix uteri** ♀
Investigation and management of (suspected) cervical incompetence in a nonpregnant woman
EXCLUDES 1 cervical incompetence complicating pregnancy (O34.3-)

N88.4 **Hypertrophic elongation of cervix uteri** ♀

N88.8 **Other specified noninflammatory disorders of cervix uteri** ♀
EXCLUDES 1 current obstetric trauma (O71.3)

N88.9 **Noninflammatory disorder of cervix uteri, unspecified** ♀ ▽

EXCLUDES 1 Not coded here   EXCLUDES 2 Not included here   N Newborn Age : 0   P Pediatric Age : 0-17   M Maternity Age : 12-55   A Adult Age : 15-124

794

ICD-10-CM 2017

☑4ᵗʰ **N89 Other noninflammatory disorders of vagina**

> EXCLUDES 1   *abnormal results from vaginal cytologic examination without histologic confirmation (R87.62-)*
> *carcinoma in situ of vagina (D07.2)*
> *HGSIL of vagina (R87.623)*
> *inflammation of vagina (N76.-)*
> *senile (atrophic) vaginitis (N95.2)*
> *severe dysplasia of vagina (D07.2)*
> *trichomonal leukorrhea (A59.00)*
> *vaginal intraepithelial neoplasia [VAIN], grade III (D07.2)*

N89.0 Mild vaginal dysplasia   ♀

     Vaginal intraepithelial neoplasia [VAIN], grade I

N89.1 Moderate vaginal dysplasia   ♀

     Vaginal intraepithelial neoplasia [VAIN], grade II

N89.3 Dysplasia of vagina, unspecified   ♀ ▽

N89.4 Leukoplakia of vagina   ♀

N89.5 Stricture and atresia of vagina   ♀

     Vaginal adhesions
     Vaginal stenosis

> EXCLUDES 1   *congenital atresia or stricture (Q52.4)*
> *postprocedural adhesions of vagina (N99.2)*

N89.6 Tight hymenal ring   ♀

     Rigid hymen
     Tight introitus

> EXCLUDES 1   *imperforate hymen (Q52.3)*

N89.7 Hematocolpos   ♀

     Hematocolpos with hematometra or hematosalpinx

N89.8 Other specified noninflammatory disorders of vagina   ♀

     Leukorrhea NOS
     Old vaginal laceration
     Pessary ulcer of vagina

> EXCLUDES 1   *current obstetric trauma (O70.-, O71.4, O71.7-O71.8)*
> *old laceration involving muscles of pelvic floor (N81.8)*

N89.9 Noninflammatory disorder of vagina, unspecified   ♀ ▽

☑4ᵗʰ **N90 Other noninflammatory disorders of vulva and perineum**

> EXCLUDES 1   *anogenital (venereal) warts (A63.0)*
> *carcinoma in situ of vulva (D07.1)*
> *condyloma acuminatum (A63.0)*
> *current obstetric trauma (O70.-, O71.7-O71.8)*
> *inflammation of vulva (N76.)*
> *severe dysplasia of vulva (D07.1)*
> *vulvar intraepithelial neoplasm III [VIN III] (D07.1)*

N90.0 Mild vulvar dysplasia   ♀

     Vulvar intraepithelial neoplasia [VIN], grade I

N90.1 Moderate vulvar dysplasia   ♀

     Vulvar intraepithelial neoplasia [VIN], grade II

N90.3 Dysplasia of vulva, unspecified   ♀ ▽

N90.4 Leukoplakia of vulva   ♀

     Dystrophy of vulva
     Kraurosis of vulva
     Lichen sclerosus of external female genital organs

N90.5 Atrophy of vulva   ♀

     Stenosis of vulva

☑5ᵗʰ **N90.6 Hypertrophy of vulva**

•   **N90.60 Unspecified hypertrophy of vulva**   ▽

       Unspecified hypertrophy of labia

•   **N90.61 Childhood asymmetric labium majus enlargement**

       CALME

•   **N90.69 Other specified hypertrophy of vulva**

       Other specified hypertrophy of labia

N90.7 Vulvar cyst   ♀

☑5ᵗʰ **N90.8 Other specified noninflammatory disorders of vulva and perineum**

☑6ᵗʰ   **N90.81 Female genital mutilation status**

       Female genital cutting status

     N90.810 Female genital mutilation status, unspecified   ♀ ▽

         Female genital cutting status, unspecified
         Female genital mutilation status NOS

     N90.811 Female genital mutilation Type I status   ♀

         Clitorectomy status
         Female genital cutting Type I status

     N90.812 Female genital mutilation Type II status   ♀

         Clitorectomy with excision of labia minora status
         Female genital cutting Type II status

     N90.813 Female genital mutilation Type III status   ♀

         Female genital cutting Type III status
         Infibulation status

     N90.818 Other female genital mutilation status   ♀

         Female genital cutting Type IV status
         Female genital mutilation Type IV status
         Other female genital cutting status

   N90.89 Other specified noninflammatory disorders of vulva and perineum   ♀

       Adhesions of vulva
       Hypertrophy of clitoris

N90.9 Noninflammatory disorder of vulva and perineum, unspecified   ♀ ▽

☑4ᵗʰ **N91 Absent, scanty and rare menstruation**

> EXCLUDES 1   *ovarian dysfunction (E28.-)*

N91.0 Primary amenorrhea   ♀

N91.1 Secondary amenorrhea   ♀

N91.2 Amenorrhea, unspecified   ♀ ▽

N91.3 Primary oligomenorrhea   ♀

N91.4 Secondary oligomenorrhea   ♀

N91.5 Oligomenorrhea, unspecified   ♀ ▽

     Hypomenorrhea NOS

☑4ᵗʰ **N92 Excessive, frequent and irregular menstruation**

> EXCLUDES 1   *postmenopausal bleeding (N95.0)*
> *precocious puberty (menstruation) (E30.1)*

N92.0 Excessive and frequent menstruation with regular cycle   ♀

     Heavy periods NOS
     Menorrhagia NOS
     Polymenorrhea

N92.1 Excessive and frequent menstruation with irregular cycle   ♀

     Irregular intermenstrual bleeding
     Irregular, shortened intervals between menstrual bleeding
     Menometrorrhagia
     Metrorrhagia

N92.2 Excessive menstruation at puberty   P ♀

     Excessive bleeding associated with onset of menstrual periods
     Pubertal menorrhagia
     Puberty bleeding

N92.3 Ovulation bleeding   ♀

     Regular intermenstrual bleeding

N92.4 Excessive bleeding in the premenopausal period   ♀

     Climacteric menorrhagia or metrorrhagia
     Menopausal menorrhagia or metrorrhagia
     Preclimacteric menorrhagia or metrorrhagia
     Premenopausal menorrhagia or metrorrhagia

N92.5 Other specified irregular menstruation   ♀

N92.6 Irregular menstruation, unspecified   ♀ ▽

     Irregular bleeding NOS
     Irregular periods NOS

> EXCLUDES 1   *irregular menstruation with:*
> *lengthened intervals or scanty bleeding (N91.3-N91.5)*
> *shortened intervals or excessive bleeding (N92.1)*

☑4ᵗʰ **N93 Other abnormal uterine and vaginal bleeding**

> EXCLUDES 1   *neonatal vaginal hemorrhage (P54.6)*
> *precocious puberty (menstruation) (E30.1)*
> *pseudomenses (P54.6)*

N93.0 Postcoital and contact bleeding   ♀

•   **N93.1 Pre-pubertal vaginal bleeding**

☑ Additional Character Required   ☑x7ᵗʰ Placeholder Alert   Manifestation Dx   ▽ Unspecified Dx   ►◄ Revised Text   ● New Code   ▲ Revised Code Title

ICD-10-CM 2017   795

Chapter 14. Diseases of the Genitourinary System

N93.8   **Other specified abnormal uterine and vaginal bleeding** ♀

Dysfunctional or functional uterine or vaginal bleeding NOS

N93.9   **Abnormal uterine and vaginal bleeding, unspecified** ♀ ▽

✓4ᵗʰ **N94**   **Pain and other conditions associated with female genital organs and menstrual cycle**

N94.0   **Mittelschmerz** ♀

✓5ᵗʰ **N94.1**   **Dyspareunia**

     EXCLUDES 1   *psychogenic dyspareunia (F52.6)*

●   **N94.10**   **Unspecified dyspareunia** ▽

●   **N94.11**   **Superficial (introital) dyspareunia**

●   **N94.12**   **Deep dyspareunia**

●   **N94.19**   **Other specified dyspareunia**

N94.2   **Vaginismus** ♀

     EXCLUDES 1   *psychogenic vaginismus (F52.5)*

N94.3   **Premenstrual tension syndrome** ♀

     Code also associated menstrual migraine (G43.82-, G43.83-)

     EXCLUDES 1   ▶*premenstrual dysphoric disorder (F32.81)*◀

N94.4   **Primary dysmenorrhea**

N94.5   **Secondary dysmenorrhea** ♀

N94.6   **Dysmenorrhea, unspecified** ♀ ▽

     EXCLUDES 1   *psychogenic dysmenorrhea (F45.8)*

✓5ᵗʰ **N94.8**   **Other specified conditions associated with female genital organs and menstrual cycle**

✓6ᵗʰ   **N94.81**   **Vulvodynia**

        N94.810   **Vulvar vestibulitis** ♀

        N94.818   **Other vulvodynia** ♀

        N94.819   **Vulvodynia, unspecified** ♀ ▽

          Vulvodynia NOS

    N94.89   **Other specified conditions associated with female genital organs and menstrual cycle** ♀

N94.9   **Unspecified condition associated with female genital organs and menstrual cycle** ♀ ▽

✓4ᵗʰ **N95**   **Menopausal and other perimenopausal disorders**

     Menopausal and other perimenopausal disorders due to naturally occurring (age-related) menopause and perimenopause

     EXCLUDES 1   *excessive bleeding in the premenopausal period (N92.4)*
         menopausal and perimenopausal disorders due to artificial or premature menopause (E89.4-, E28.31-)
         premature menopause (E28.31-)

     EXCLUDES 2   *postmenopausal osteoporosis (M81.0-)*
         postmenopausal osteoporosis with current pathological fracture (M80.0-)
         postmenopausal urethritis (N34.2)

N95.0   **Postmenopausal bleeding** ♀

N95.1   **Menopausal and female climacteric states** ♀

     Symptoms such as flushing, sleeplessness, headache, lack of concentration, associated with natural (age-related) menopause

     Use additional code for associated symptoms

     EXCLUDES 1   *asymptomatic menopausal state (Z78.0)*
         symptoms associated with artificial menopause (E89.41)
         symptoms associated with premature menopause (E28.310)

N95.2   **Postmenopausal atrophic vaginitis** ♀

     Senile (atrophic) vaginitis

N95.8   **Other specified menopausal and perimenopausal disorders** ♀

N95.9   **Unspecified menopausal and perimenopausal disorder** ♀ ▽

N96   **Recurrent pregnancy loss** ♀

     Investigation or care in a nonpregnant woman with history of recurrent pregnancy loss

     EXCLUDES 1   *recurrent pregnancy loss with current pregnancy (O26.2-)*

✓4ᵗʰ **N97**   **Female infertility**

     INCLUDES   inability to achieve a pregnancy
         sterility, female NOS

     EXCLUDES 1   *female infertility associated with:*
         hypopituitarism (E23.0)
         Stein-Leventhal syndrome (E28.2)

     EXCLUDES 2   *incompetence of cervix uteri (N88.3)*

     DEF: Infertility: Inability to conceive for at least one year with regular intercourse.

     DEF: Primary infertility: Infertility occurring in patients who have never conceived.

     DEF: Secondary infertility: Infertility occurring in patients who have previously conceived.

N97.0   **Female infertility associated with anovulation** ♀

N97.1   **Female infertility of tubal origin** ♀

     Female infertility associated with congenital anomaly of tube
     Female infertility due to tubal block
     Female infertility due to tubal occlusion
     Female infertility due to tubal stenosis

N97.2   **Female infertility of uterine origin** ♀

     Female infertility associated with congenital anomaly of uterus
     Female infertility due to nonimplantation of ovum

N97.8   **Female infertility of other origin** ♀

N97.9   **Female infertility, unspecified** ♀ ▽

✓4ᵗʰ **N98**   **Complications associated with artificial fertilization**

N98.0   **Infection associated with artificial insemination** ♀

N98.1   **Hyperstimulation of ovaries** ♀

     Hyperstimulation of ovaries NOS
     Hyperstimulation of ovaries associated with induced ovulation

N98.2   **Complications of attempted introduction of fertilized ovum following in vitro fertilization** ♀

N98.3   **Complications of attempted introduction of embryo in embryo transfer** ♀

N98.8   **Other complications associated with artificial fertilization** ♀

N98.9   **Complication associated with artificial fertilization, unspecified** ♀ ▽

Intraoperative and postprocedural complications and disorders of genitourinary system, not elsewhere classified (N99)

✓4ᵗʰ **N99**   **Intraoperative and postprocedural complications and disorders of genitourinary system, not elsewhere classified**

     EXCLUDES 2   *irradiation cystitis (N30.4-)*
         postoophorectomy osteoporosis with current pathological fracture (M80.8-)
         postoophorectomy osteoporosis without current pathological fracture (M81.8)

N99.0   **Postprocedural (acute) (chronic) kidney failure**

     Use additional code to type of kidney disease

✓5ᵗʰ **N99.1**   **Postprocedural urethral stricture**

     Postcatheterization urethral stricture

✓6ᵗʰ   **N99.11**   **Postprocedural urethral stricture, male**

        N99.110   **Postprocedural urethral stricture, male, meatal** ♂

        N99.111   **Postprocedural bulbous urethral stricture**

        N99.112   **Postprocedural membranous urethral stricture**

        N99.113   **Postprocedural anterior bulbous urethral stricture**

        N99.114   **Postprocedural urethral stricture, male, unspecified** ♂ ▽

●   **N99.115**   **Postprocedural fossa navicularis urethral stricture**

    N99.12   **Postprocedural urethral stricture, female** ♀

N99.2   **Postprocedural adhesions of vagina** ♀

N99.3   **Prolapse of vaginal vault after hysterectomy** ♀

N99.4   **Postprocedural pelvic peritoneal adhesions**

     EXCLUDES 2   *pelvic peritoneal adhesions NOS (N73.6)*
         postinfective pelvic peritoneal adhesions (N73.6)

✓5ᵗʰ **N99.5**   **Complications of stoma of urinary tract**

     EXCLUDES 2   ▶*mechanical complication of urinary catheter (T83.0-)*◀

✓6ᵗʰ   **N99.51**   **Complication of cystostomy**

        N99.510   **Cystostomy hemorrhage**

EXCLUDES 1   Not coded here   EXCLUDES 2   Not included here   N Newborn Age : 0   P Pediatric Age : 0-17   M Maternity Age : 12-55   A Adult Age : 15-124

796   ICD-10-CM 2017

        N99.511   Cystostomy infection
        N99.512   Cystostomy malfunction
        N99.518   Other cystostomy complication

▲   √6ᵗʰ   **N99.52**   Complication of incontinent external stoma of urinary tract

▲   **N99.520**   Hemorrhage of incontinent external stoma of urinary tract

▲   **N99.521**   Infection of incontinent external stoma of urinary tract

▲   **N99.522**   Malfunction of incontinent external stoma of urinary tract

●   **N99.523**   Herniation of incontinent stoma of urinary tract

●   **N99.524**   Stenosis of incontinent stoma of urinary tract

▲   **N99.528**   Other complication of incontinent external stoma of urinary tract

▲   √6ᵗʰ   **N99.53**   Complication of continent stoma of urinary tract

▲   **N99.530**   Hemorrhage of continent stoma of urinary tract

▲   **N99.531**   Infection of continent stoma of urinary tract

▲   **N99.532**   Malfunction of continent stoma of urinary tract

●   **N99.533**   Herniation of continent stoma of urinary tract

●   **N99.534**   Stenosis of continent stoma of urinary tract

▲   **N99.538**   Other complication of continent stoma of urinary tract

√5ᵗʰ   **N99.6**   Intraoperative hemorrhage and hematoma of a genitourinary system organ or structure complicating a procedure

       EXCLUDES 1   intraoperative hemorrhage and hematoma of a genitourinary system organ or structure due to accidental puncture or laceration during a procedure (N99.7-)

      N99.61   Intraoperative hemorrhage and hematoma of a genitourinary system organ or structure complicating a genitourinary system procedure

      N99.62   Intraoperative hemorrhage and hematoma of a genitourinary system organ or structure complicating other procedure

√5ᵗʰ   **N99.7**   Accidental puncture and laceration of a genitourinary system organ or structure during a procedure

      N99.71   Accidental puncture and laceration of a genitourinary system organ or structure during a genitourinary system procedure

      N99.72   Accidental puncture and laceration of a genitourinary system organ or structure during other procedure

√5ᵗʰ   **N99.8**   Other intraoperative and postprocedural complications and disorders of genitourinary system

      N99.81   Other intraoperative complications of genitourinary system

▲   √6ᵗʰ   **N99.82**   Postprocedural hemorrhage of a genitourinary system organ or structure following a procedure

▲   **N99.820**   Postprocedural hemorrhage of a genitourinary system organ or structure following a genitourinary system procedure

▲   **N99.821**   Postprocedural hemorrhage of a genitourinary system organ or structure following other procedure

      N99.83   Residual ovary syndrome   ♀

●   **N99.84**   Postprocedural hematoma and seroma of a genitourinary system organ or structure following a procedure

●   **N99.840**   Postprocedural hematoma of a genitourinary system organ or structure following a genitourinary system procedure

●   **N99.841**   Postprocedural hematoma of a genitourinary system organ or structure following other procedure

●   **N99.842**   Postprocedural seroma of a genitourinary system organ or structure following a genitourinary system procedure

●   **N99.843**   Postprocedural seroma of a genitourinary system organ or structure following other procedure

      N99.89   Other postprocedural complications and disorders of genitourinary system

---

☑ Additional Character Required   √7ᵗʰ Placeholder Alert   Manifestation Dx   ▽ Unspecified Dx   ►◄ Revised Text   ● New Code   ▲ Revised Code Title

Chapter 15. Pregnancy, Childbirth and the Puerperium (O00–O9A)

Chapter Specific Guidelines with Coding Examples

The chapter specific guidelines from the ICD-10-CM Official Guidelines for Coding and Reporting have been provided below. Along with these guidelines are coding examples, contained in the shaded boxes, that have been developed to help illustrate the coding and/or sequencing guidance found in these guidelines.

a. General rules for obstetric cases

1) Codes from Chapter 15 and sequencing priority

Obstetric cases require codes from chapter 15, codes in the range O00–O9A, Pregnancy, Childbirth, and the Puerperium. Chapter 15 codes have sequencing priority over codes from other chapters. Additional codes from other chapters may be used in conjunction with chapter 15 codes to further specify conditions. Should the provider document that the pregnancy is incidental to the encounter, then code Z33.1, Pregnant state, incidental, should be used in place of any chapter 15 codes. It is the provider's responsibility to state that the condition being treated is not affecting the pregnancy.

Bladder abscess in pregnant patient at 25 weeks' gestation	
O23.12	**Infections of bladder in pregnancy, second trimester**
N30.80	**Other cystitis without hematuria**
Z3A.25	**25 weeks gestation of pregnancy**

Explanation: The documentation does not indicate that the pregnancy is incidental or in any way unaffected by the bladder abscess; therefore, an obstetrics code should be sequenced first. An additional code was provided to identify the specific bladder condition as this information is not called out specifically in the obstetrics code.

2) Chapter 15 codes used only on the maternal record

Chapter 15 codes are to be used only on the maternal record, never on the record of the newborn.

3) Final character for trimester

The majority of codes in Chapter 15 have a final character indicating the trimester of pregnancy. The timeframes for the trimesters are indicated at the beginning of the chapter. If trimester is not a component of a code, it is because the condition always occurs in a specific trimester, or the concept of trimester of pregnancy is not applicable. Certain codes have characters for only certain trimesters because the condition does not occur in all trimesters, but it may occur in more than just one. Assignment of the final character for trimester should be based on the provider's documentation of the trimester (or number of weeks) for the current admission/encounter. This applies to the assignment of trimester for pre-existing conditions as well as those that develop during or are due to the pregnancy. The provider's documentation of the number of weeks may be used to assign the appropriate code identifying the trimester.

Whenever delivery occurs during the current admission, and there is an "in childbirth" option for the obstetric complication being coded, the "in childbirth" code should be assigned.

Pregnant patient at 21 weeks' gestation admitted with excessive vomiting	
O21.2	**Late vomiting of pregnancy**
Z3A.21	**21 weeks gestation of pregnancy**

Explanation: Category O21 classifies vomiting in pregnancy. Although code selection is based on whether the vomiting is before or after 20 completed weeks, these codes are not further classified by trimester. If vomiting only in the second trimester was documented, the provider should be queried for the specific week of gestation, as this will affect code selection.

4) Selection of trimester for inpatient admissions that encompass more than one trimester

In instances when a patient is admitted to a hospital for complications of pregnancy during one trimester and remains in the hospital into a subsequent trimester, the trimester character for the antepartum complication code should be assigned on the basis of the trimester when the complication developed, not the trimester of the discharge. If the condition developed prior to the current admission/encounter or represents a pre-existing condition, the trimester character for the trimester at the time of the admission/encounter should be assigned.

Patient admitted at 27 6/7 weeks' gestation for hemorrhaging from partial placenta previa; three days after admission at 28 1/7 weeks' gestation, she developed gestational hypertension	
O44.32	**Partial placenta previa with hemorrhage, second trimester**
O13.3	**Gestational [pregnancy-induced] hypertension without significant proteinuria, third trimester**
Z3A.27	**27 weeks gestation of pregnancy**

Explanation: The patient presented with hemorrhaging from partial placenta previa while still in her 27th week, which falls within the second trimester. The gestational hypertension did not occur until three days after admission, putting the patient in her 28th week of pregnancy or what is considered to be the third trimester. The weeks of gestation captured by a code from category Z3A should represent only the gestational weeks upon admission.

5) Unspecified trimester

Each category that includes codes for trimester has a code for "unspecified trimester." The "unspecified trimester" code should rarely be used, such as when the documentation in the record is insufficient to determine the trimester and it is not possible to obtain clarification.

6) 7th character for fetus identification

Where applicable, a 7th character is to be assigned for certain categories (O31, O32, O33.3 - O33.6, O35, O36, O40, O41, O60.1, O60.2, O64, and O69) to identify the fetus for which the complication code applies.

Assign 7th character "0":

- For single gestations
- When the documentation in the record is insufficient to determine the fetus affected and it is not possible to obtain clarification.
- When it is not possible to clinically determine which fetus is affected.

Maternal patient with twin gestations is seen after ultrasound identifies fetus B to be in breech presentation	
O32.1XX2	**Maternal care for breech presentation, fetus 2**

Explanation: The documentation indicates that although there are two fetuses, only one fetus is determined to be in breech presentation. Whether fetus 2 or fetus B is used, the coder can assign the seventh character of 2 to identify the second fetus as the one in breech.

b. Selection of OB principal or first-listed diagnosis

1) Routine outpatient prenatal visits

For routine outpatient prenatal visits when no complications are present, a code from category Z34, Encounter for supervision of normal pregnancy, should be used as the first-listed diagnosis. These codes should not be used in conjunction with chapter 15 codes.

2) *Supervision of high-risk pregnancy*

Codes from category O09, Supervision of high-risk pregnancy, are intended for use only during the prenatal period. For complications during the labor or delivery episode as a result of a high-risk pregnancy, assign the applicable complication codes from Chapter 15. If there are no complications during the labor or delivery episode, assign code O80, Encounter for full-term uncomplicated delivery.

For routine prenatal outpatient visits for patients with high-risk pregnancies, a code from category O09, Supervision of high-risk pregnancy, should be used as the first-listed diagnosis. Secondary chapter 15 codes may be used in conjunction with these codes if appropriate.

36-year-old admitted in labor with second child at 39 weeks' gestation, delivered a healthy baby, delivery complicated by tear of fourchette that was repaired	
O70.0	**First degree perineal laceration during delivery**
Z3A.39	**39 weeks gestation of pregnancy**
Z37.0	**Single live birth**

Explanation: Although this patient is over 35 and having her second child (elderly multigravida), do not append a code from subcategory O09.52-. A code describing the tear of the fourchette, which complicated the delivery, should be used in addition to the applicable Z codes.

3) Episodes when no delivery occurs

In episodes when no delivery occurs, the principal diagnosis should correspond to the principal complication of the pregnancy which necessitated the encounter. Should more than one complication exist, all of which are treated or monitored, any of the complications codes may be sequenced first.

4) When a delivery occurs

When an obstetric patient is admitted and delivers during that admission, the condition that prompted the admission should be sequenced as the principal diagnosis. If multiple conditions prompted the admission, sequence the one most related to the delivery as the principal diagnosis. A code for any complication of the delivery should be assigned as an additional diagnosis. In cases of cesarean delivery, if the patient was admitted with a condition that resulted in the performance of a cesarean procedure, that condition should be selected as the principal diagnosis. If the reason for the admission was unrelated to the condition resulting in the cesarean delivery, the condition related to the reason for the admission should be selected as the principal diagnosis.

Maternal patient with diet-controlled gestational diabetes was admitted at 38 weeks' gestation in obstructed labor due to footling presentation; cesarean performed for the malpresentation

O64.8XX0	Obstructed labor due to other malposition and malpresentation, not applicable or unspecified
O24.420	Gestational diabetes mellitus in childbirth, diet controlled
Z3A.38	38 weeks gestation of pregnancy
Z37.0	Single live birth

Explanation: The obstructed labor necessitated the cesarean procedure.

At 39 weeks' gestation, a maternal patient presents with hemorrhage with coagulation defect; the next day the patient goes into labor and eventually delivers via cesarean section due to arrested active phase of labor

O46.003	Antepartum hemorrhage with coagulation defect, unspecified, third trimester
O62.1	Secondary uterine inertia
Z3A.39	39 weeks gestation of pregnancy
Z37.0	Single live birth

Explanation: The patient was admitted because of the antepartum hemorrhage with coagulation defect. The arrested active phase, although the reason for the cesarean delivery, did not develop until later into the stay.

5) Outcome of delivery

A code from category Z37, Outcome of delivery, should be included on every maternal record when a delivery has occurred. These codes are not to be used on subsequent records or on the newborn record.

c. Pre-existing conditions versus conditions due to the pregnancy

Certain categories in Chapter 15 distinguish between conditions of the mother that existed prior to pregnancy (pre-existing) and those that are a direct result of pregnancy. When assigning codes from Chapter 15, it is important to assess if a condition was pre-existing prior to pregnancy or developed during or due to the pregnancy in order to assign the correct code.

Categories that do not distinguish between pre-existing and pregnancy-related conditions may be used for either. It is acceptable to use codes specifically for the puerperium with codes complicating pregnancy and childbirth if a condition arises postpartum during the delivery encounter.

d. Pre-existing hypertension in pregnancy

Category O10, Pre-existing hypertension complicating pregnancy, childbirth and the puerperium, includes codes for hypertensive heart and hypertensive chronic kidney disease. When assigning one of the O10 codes that includes hypertensive heart disease or hypertensive chronic kidney disease, it is necessary to add a secondary code from the appropriate hypertension category to specify the type of heart failure or chronic kidney disease.

See Section I.C.9. Hypertension.

e. Fetal conditions affecting the management of the mother

1) Codes from categories O35 and O36

Codes from categories O35, Maternal care for known or suspected fetal abnormality and damage, and O36, Maternal care for other fetal problems, are assigned only when the fetal condition is actually responsible for modifying the management of the mother, i.e., by requiring diagnostic studies, additional observation, special care, or termination of pregnancy. The fact that the fetal condition exists does not justify assigning a code from this series to the mother's record.

A patient is seen for spotting 15 weeks into her pregnancy; the doctors also suspect fetal hydrocephalus

O26.852	Spotting complicating pregnancy, second trimester
Z3A.15	15 weeks gestation of pregnancy

Explanation: Whether the fetal hydrocephalus was suspected or confirmed, an additional code is not warranted for this condition as the documentation does not indicate that this fetal condition is in any way altering the management of the mother or complicating her pregnancy.

2) In utero surgery

In cases when surgery is performed on the fetus, a diagnosis code from category O35, Maternal care for known or suspected fetal abnormality and damage, should be assigned identifying the fetal condition. Assign the appropriate procedure code for the procedure performed.

No code from Chapter 16, the perinatal codes, should be used on the mother's record to identify fetal conditions. Surgery performed in utero on a fetus is still to be coded as an obstetric encounter.

f. HIV infection in pregnancy, childbirth and the puerperium

During pregnancy, childbirth or the puerperium, a patient admitted because of an HIV-related illness should receive a principal diagnosis from subcategory O98.7-, Human immunodeficiency [HIV] disease complicating pregnancy, childbirth and the puerperium, followed by the code(s) for the HIV-related illness(es).

Patients with asymptomatic HIV infection status admitted during pregnancy, childbirth, or the puerperium should receive codes of O98.7- and Z21, Asymptomatic human immunodeficiency virus [HIV] infection status.

A previously asymptomatic HIV patient who is 13 weeks pregnant is admitted with oral thrush

O98.711	Human immunodeficiency virus [HIV] disease complicating pregnancy, first trimester
B20	Human immunodeficiency virus [HIV] disease
B37.0	Candidal stomatitis
Z3A.13	13 weeks gestation of pregnancy

Explanation: Because oral thrush is an HIV-related condition, this patient is now considered to have HIV disease. An obstetrics code indicating that HIV is complicating the pregnancy is coded first, followed by B20 for HIV disease as well as a code for the oral thrush.

g. Diabetes mellitus in pregnancy

Diabetes mellitus is a significant complicating factor in pregnancy. Pregnant women who are diabetic should be assigned a code from category O24, Diabetes mellitus in pregnancy, childbirth, and the puerperium, first, followed by the appropriate diabetes code(s) (E08-E13) from Chapter 4.

h. Long term use of insulin and oral hypoglycemics

Code Z79.4, Long-term (current) use of insulin, or **code Z79.84, Long-term (current) use of oral hypoglycemic drugs,** should also be assigned if the diabetes mellitus is being treated with insulin **or oral medications. If the patient is treated with both oral medications and insulin, only the code for insulin-controlled should be assigned.**

i. Gestational (pregnancy induced) diabetes

Gestational (pregnancy induced) diabetes can occur during the second and third trimester of pregnancy in women who were not diabetic prior to pregnancy. Gestational diabetes can cause complications in the pregnancy similar to those of pre-existing diabetes mellitus. It also puts the woman at greater risk of developing diabetes after the pregnancy. Codes for gestational diabetes are in subcategory O24.4, Gestational diabetes mellitus. No other code from category O24, Diabetes mellitus in pregnancy, childbirth, and the puerperium, should be used with a code from O24.4.

The codes under subcategory O24.4 include diet controlled, insulin controlled, **and controlled by oral hypoglycemic drugs.** If a patient with gestational diabetes is treated with both diet and insulin, only the code for insulin-controlled is required. **If a patient with gestational diabetes is treated with both diet and oral hypoglycemic medications, only the code for "controlled by oral hypoglycemic drugs" is required.** Code Z79.4, Long-term (current) use of insulin **or code Z79.84, Long-term (current) use of oral hypoglycemic drugs,** should not be assigned with codes from subcategory O24.4.

An abnormal glucose tolerance in pregnancy is assigned a code from subcategory O99.81, Abnormal glucose complicating pregnancy, childbirth, and the puerperium.

j. Sepsis and septic shock complicating abortion, pregnancy, childbirth and the puerperium

When assigning a chapter 15 code for sepsis complicating abortion, pregnancy, childbirth, and the puerperium, a code for the specific type of infection should be assigned as an additional diagnosis. If severe sepsis is present, a code from subcategory R65.2, Severe sepsis, and code(s) for associated organ dysfunction(s) should also be assigned as additional diagnoses.

> Patient is seen several days after a miscarriage with sepsis; cultures return MSSA
>
> **O03.87**   **Sepsis following complete or unspecified spontaneous abortion**
>
> **B95.61**   **Methicillin susceptible Staphylococcus aureus infection as the cause of diseases classified elsewhere**
>
> *Explanation:* The type of infection that caused this patient to become septic was methicillin susceptible *Staphylococcus aureus* (MSSA), which as a secondary code helps capture all aspects related to this patient's septic condition.

k. Puerperal sepsis

Code O85, Puerperal sepsis, should be assigned with a secondary code to identify the causal organism (e.g., for a bacterial infection, assign a code from category B95-B96, Bacterial infections in conditions classified elsewhere). A code from category A40, Streptococcal sepsis, or A41, Other sepsis, should not be used for puerperal sepsis. If applicable, use additional codes to identify severe sepsis (R65.2-) and any associated acute organ dysfunction.

l. Alcohol and tobacco use during pregnancy, childbirth and the puerperium

1) Alcohol use during pregnancy, childbirth and the puerperium

Codes under subcategory O99.31, Alcohol use complicating pregnancy, childbirth, and the puerperium, should be assigned for any pregnancy case when a mother uses alcohol during the pregnancy or postpartum. A secondary code from category F10, Alcohol related disorders, should also be assigned to identify manifestations of the alcohol use.

2) Tobacco use during pregnancy, childbirth and the puerperium

Codes under subcategory O99.33, Smoking (tobacco) complicating pregnancy, childbirth, and the puerperium, should be assigned for any pregnancy case when a mother uses any type of tobacco product during the pregnancy or postpartum. A secondary code from category F17, Nicotine dependence, should also be assigned to identify the type of nicotine dependence.

m. Poisoning, toxic effects, adverse effects and underdosing in a pregnant patient

A code from subcategory O9A.2, Injury, poisoning and certain other consequences of external causes complicating pregnancy, childbirth, and the puerperium, should be sequenced first, followed by the appropriate injury, poisoning, toxic effect, adverse effect or underdosing code, and then the additional code(s) that specifies the condition caused by the poisoning, toxic effect, adverse effect or underdosing.

See Section I.C.19. Adverse effects, poisoning, underdosing and toxic effects.

> Patient admitted with accidental carbon monoxide poisoning from a gas heating implement; the patient is 18 weeks' pregnant
>
> **O9A.212**   **Injury, poisoning and certain other consequences of external causes complicating pregnancy, second trimester**
>
> **T58.11XA**   **Toxic effect of carbon monoxide from utility gas, accidental (unintentional), initial encounter**
>
> **Z3A.18**   **18 weeks gestation of pregnancy**
>
> *Explanation:* Although the carbon monoxide poisoning is the reason the patient was admitted, a code from the obstetrics chapter must be sequenced first. Chapter 15 codes have sequencing priority over codes from other chapters.

n. Normal delivery, code O80

1) Encounter for full term uncomplicated delivery

Code O80 should be assigned when a woman is admitted for a full-term normal delivery and delivers a single, healthy infant without any complications antepartum, during the delivery, or postpartum during the delivery episode. Code O80 is always a principal diagnosis. It is not to be used if any other code from chapter 15 is needed to describe a current complication of the antenatal, delivery, or perinatal period. Additional codes from other chapters may be used with code O80 if they are not related to or are in any way complicating the pregnancy.

2) Uncomplicated delivery with resolved antepartum complication

Code O80 may be used if the patient had a complication at some point during the pregnancy, but the complication is not present at the time of the admission for delivery.

> Patient presents in labor at 39 weeks' gestation and delivers a healthy newborn; patient had abnormal glucose levels in her first trimester, which have since resolved
>
> **O80**   **Encounter for full-term uncomplicated delivery**
>
> **Z37.0**   **Single live birth**
>
> *Explanation:* The abnormal glucose levels during the first trimester cannot be coded if they are not affecting the patient's current trimester. Without additional complications associated with the pregnancy, fetus, or mother, code O80 is appropriate.

3) Outcome of delivery for O80

Z37.0, Single live birth, is the only outcome of delivery code appropriate for use with O80.

o. The peripartum and postpartum periods

1) Peripartum and postpartum periods

The postpartum period begins immediately after delivery and continues for six weeks following delivery. The peripartum period is defined as the last month of pregnancy to five months postpartum.

2) Peripartum and postpartum complication

A postpartum complication is any complication occurring within the six-week period.

3) Pregnancy-related complications after 6 week period

Chapter 15 codes may also be used to describe pregnancy-related complications after the peripartum or postpartum period if the provider documents that a condition is pregnancy related.

> Patient admitted for varicose veins. She had a baby boy three months ago; the varicose veins started to appear one month ago. The doctor attributes the patient's pregnancy as the cause of the varicose veins, which continue to be painful and bother the patient. She is seeking surgical relief.
>
> **O87.4**   **Varicose veins of the lower extremity in the puerperium**
>
> *Explanation:* Although the varicose veins occurred several months after the delivery of the newborn, the doctor attributed the varicose veins to pregnancy and therefore a code from chapter 15 is appropriate.

4) Admission for routine postpartum care following delivery outside hospital

When the mother delivers outside the hospital prior to admission and is admitted for routine postpartum care and no complications are noted, code Z39.0, Encounter for care and examination of mother immediately after delivery, should be assigned as the principal diagnosis.

5) Pregnancy associated cardiomyopathy

Pregnancy associated cardiomyopathy, code O90.3, is unique in that it may be diagnosed in the third trimester of pregnancy but may continue to progress months after delivery. For this reason, it is referred to as peripartum cardiomyopathy. Code O90.3 is only for use when the cardiomyopathy develops as a result of pregnancy in a woman who did not have pre-existing heart disease.

p. Code O94, Sequelae of complication of pregnancy, childbirth, and the puerperium

1) Code O94

Code O94, Sequelae of complication of pregnancy, childbirth, and the puerperium, is for use in those cases when an initial complication of a pregnancy develops a sequelae requiring care or treatment at a future date.

2) After the initial postpartum period

This code may be used at any time after the initial postpartum period.

3) Sequencing of code O94

This code, like all sequela codes, is to be sequenced following the code describing the sequelae of the complication.

q. *Termination of pregnancy and spontaneous abortions*

1) Abortion with liveborn fetus

When an attempted termination of pregnancy results in a liveborn fetus, assign code Z33.2, Encounter for elective termination of pregnancy and a code from category Z37, Outcome of Delivery.

2) Retained products of conception following an abortion

Subsequent encounters for retained products of conception following a spontaneous abortion or elective termination of pregnancy are assigned the appropriate code from category O03, Spontaneous abortion, or codes O07.4, Failed attempted termination of pregnancy without complication and Z33.2, Encounter for elective termination of pregnancy. This advice is appropriate even when the patient was discharged previously with a discharge diagnosis of complete abortion.

Patient was seen two days ago for complete spontaneous abortion but returns today for urinary tract infection (UTI) with ultrasound showing retained products of conception

O03.38   Urinary tract infection following incomplete spontaneous abortion

Explanation: Although the diagnosis from the patient's previous stay indicated that the patient had a complete abortion, it is now determined that there were actually retained products of conception (POC). An abortion with retained POC is considered incomplete and in this case resulted in the patient developing a UTI.

---

3) Complications leading to abortion

Codes from Chapter 15 may be used as additional codes to identify any documented complications of the pregnancy in conjunction with codes in categories in O07 and O08.

r. Abuse in a pregnant patient

For suspected or confirmed cases of abuse of a pregnant patient, a code(s) from subcategories O9A.3, Physical abuse complicating pregnancy, childbirth, and the puerperium, O9A.4, Sexual abuse complicating pregnancy, childbirth, and the puerperium, and O9A.5, Psychological abuse complicating pregnancy, childbirth, and the puerperium, should be sequenced first, followed by the appropriate codes (if applicable) to identify any associated current injury due to physical abuse, sexual abuse, and the perpetrator of abuse.

See Section I.C.19. Adult and child abuse, neglect and other maltreatment.

Chapter 15. Pregnancy, Childbirth and the Puerperium
(O00–O9A)

> **NOTE**   CODES FROM THIS CHAPTER ARE FOR USE ONLY ON MATERNAL RECORDS, NEVER ON NEWBORN RECORDS
>
> Codes from this chapter are for use for conditions related to or aggravated by the pregnancy, childbirth, or by the puerperium (maternal causes or obstetric causes)
> Trimesters are counted from the first day of the last menstrual period. They are defined as follows:
> 1st trimester- less than 14 weeks 0 days
> 2nd trimester- 14 weeks 0 days to less than 28 weeks 0 days
> 3rd trimester- 28 weeks 0 days until delivery
> ▶Use additional code from category Z3A, Weeks of gestation, to identify the specific week of the pregnancy, if known.◀
> *EXCLUDES 1*   *supervision of normal pregnancy (Z34.-)*
> *EXCLUDES 2*   *mental and behavioral disorders associated with the puerperium (F53)*
> *obstetrical tetanus (A34)*
> *postpartum necrosis of pituitary gland (E23.0)*
> *puerperal osteomalacia (M83.0)*
> **AHA:** 2016,1Q,3-5; 2014,3Q,17

This chapter contains the following blocks:

O00-O08   Pregnancy with abortive outcome
O09   Supervision of high risk pregnancy
O10-O16   Edema, proteinuria and hypertensive disorders in pregnancy, childbirth and the puerperium
O20-O29   Other maternal disorders predominantly related to pregnancy
O30-O48   Maternal care related to the fetus and amniotic cavity and possible delivery problems
O60-O77   Complications of labor and delivery
O80-O82   Encounter for delivery
O85-O92   Complications predominantly related to the puerperium
O94-O9A   Other obstetric conditions, not elsewhere classified

Pregnancy with abortive outcome (O00–O08)

EXCLUDES 1   *continuing pregnancy in multiple gestation after abortion of one fetus or more (O31.1-, O31.3-)*

✓4ᵗʰ O00 Ectopic pregnancy
> *INCLUDES*   ruptured ectopic pregnancy
> Use additional code from category O08 to identify any associated complication
> **AHA:** 2014,3Q,17

✓5ᵗʰ O00.0 Abdominal pregnancy
> *EXCLUDES 1*   *maternal care for viable fetus in abdominal pregnancy (O36.7-)*

- **O00.00 Abdominal pregnancy without intrauterine pregnancy**
  Abdominal pregnancy NOS
- **O00.01 Abdominal pregnancy with intrauterine pregnancy**

✓5ᵗʰ O00.1 Tubal pregnancy
Fallopian pregnancy
Rupture of (fallopian) tube due to pregnancy
Tubal abortion

- **O00.10 Tubal pregnancy without intrauterine pregnancy**
  Tubal pregnancy NOS
- **O00.11 Tubal pregnancy with intrauterine pregnancy**

✓5ᵗʰ O00.2 Ovarian pregnancy

- **O00.20 Ovarian pregnancy without intrauterine pregnancy**
  Ovarian pregnancy NOS
- **O00.21 Ovarian pregnancy with intrauterine pregnancy**

✓6ᵗʰ O00.8 Other ectopic pregnancy
Cervical pregnancy
Cornual pregnancy
Intraligamentous pregnancy
Mural pregnancy

- **O00.80 Other ectopic pregnancy without intrauterine pregnancy**
  Other ectopic pregnancy NOS
- **O00.81 Other ectopic pregnancy with intrauterine pregnancy**

✓5ᵗʰ O00.9 Ectopic pregnancy, unspecified

- **O00.90 Unspecified ectopic pregnancy without intrauterine pregnancy**   ▽
  Ectopic pregnancy NOS
- **O00.91 Unspecified ectopic pregnancy with intrauterine pregnancy**   ▽

✓4ᵗʰ O01 Hydatidiform mole
> Use additional code from category O08 to identify any associated complication
> *EXCLUDES 1*   *chorioadenoma (destruens) (D39.2)*
> *malignant hydatidiform mole (D39.2)*
> **AHA:** 2014,3Q,17
> **DEF:** Abnormal product of pregnancy; marked by mass of cysts resembling bunch of grapes due to chorionic villi proliferation and dissolution; must be surgically removed.

O01.0 Classical hydatidiform mole   Ⓜ ♀
Complete hydatidiform mole

O01.1 Incomplete and partial hydatidiform mole   Ⓜ ♀

O01.9 Hydatidiform mole, unspecified   Ⓜ ♀ ▽
Trophoblastic disease NOS
Vesicular mole NOS

✓4ᵗʰ O02 Other abnormal products of conception
> Use additional code from category O08 to identify any associated complication
> *EXCLUDES 1*   *papyraceous fetus (O31.0-)*
> **AHA:** 2014,3Q,17

O02.0 Blighted ovum and nonhydatidiform mole   Ⓜ ♀
Carneous mole
Fleshy mole
Intrauterine mole NOS
Molar pregnancy NEC
Pathological ovum

O02.1 Missed abortion   Ⓜ ♀
Early fetal death, before completion of 20 weeks of gestation, with retention of dead fetus
> *EXCLUDES 1*   *failed induced abortion (O07.-)*
> *fetal death (intrauterine) (late) (O36.4)*
> *missed abortion with blighted ovum (O02.0)*
> *missed abortion with hydatidiform mole (O01.-)*
> *missed abortion with nonhydatidiform (O02.0)*
> *missed abortion with other abnormal products of conception (O02.8-)*
> *missed delivery (O36.4)*
> *stillbirth (P95)*

✓5ᵗʰ O02.8 Other specified abnormal products of conception
> *EXCLUDES 1*   *abnormal products of conception with blighted ovum (O02.0)*
> *abnormal products of conception with hydatidiform mole (O01.-)*
> *abnormal products of conception with nonhydatidiform mole (O02.0)*

- **O02.81 Inappropriate change in quantitative human chorionic gonadotropin (hCG) in early pregnancy**   Ⓜ ♀
  Biochemical pregnancy
  Chemical pregnancy
  Inappropriate level of quantitative human chorionic gonadotropin (hCG) for gestational age in early pregnancy
- **O02.89 Other abnormal products of conception**   Ⓜ ♀

O02.9 Abnormal product of conception, unspecified   Ⓜ ♀ ▽

✓4ᵗʰ O03 Spontaneous abortion
> **NOTE**   Incomplete abortion includes retained products of conception following spontaneous abortion
> *INCLUDES*   miscarriage

O03.0 Genital tract and pelvic infection following incomplete spontaneous abortion   Ⓜ ♀
Endometritis following incomplete spontaneous abortion
Oophoritis following incomplete spontaneous abortion
Parametritis following incomplete spontaneous abortion
Pelvic peritonitis following incomplete spontaneous abortion
Salpingitis following incomplete spontaneous abortion
Salpingo-oophoritis following incomplete spontaneous abortion
> *EXCLUDES 1*   *sepsis following incomplete spontaneous abortion (O03.37)*
> *urinary tract infection following incomplete spontaneous abortion (O03.38)*

O03.1   **Delayed or excessive hemorrhage following** M ♀
incomplete **spontaneous abortion**

Afibrinogenemia following incomplete spontaneous abortion
Defibrination syndrome following incomplete spontaneous abortion
Hemolysis following incomplete spontaneous abortion
Intravascular coagulation following incomplete spontaneous abortion

O03.2   **Embolism following incomplete spontaneous abortion** M ♀

Air embolism following incomplete spontaneous abortion
Amniotic fluid embolism following incomplete spontaneous abortion
Blood-clot embolism following incomplete spontaneous abortion
Embolism NOS following incomplete spontaneous abortion
Fat embolism following incomplete spontaneous abortion
Pulmonary embolism following incomplete spontaneous abortion
Pyemic embolism following incomplete spontaneous abortion
Septic or septicopyemic embolism following incomplete spontaneous abortion
Soap embolism following incomplete spontaneous abortion

✓5ᵗʰ **O03.3**   **Other and unspecified complications following incomplete spontaneous abortion**

O03.30   **Unspecified complication following** M ♀ ▽
incomplete **spontaneous abortion**

O03.31   **Shock following incomplete spontaneous** M ♀
abortion

Circulatory collapse following incomplete spontaneous abortion
Shock (postprocedural) following incomplete spontaneous abortion
EXCLUDES 1   *shock due to infection following incomplete spontaneous abortion (O03.37)*

O03.32   **Renal failure following incomplete** M ♀
spontaneous abortion

Kidney failure (acute) following incomplete spontaneous abortion
Oliguria following incomplete spontaneous abortion
Renal shutdown following incomplete spontaneous abortion
Renal tubular necrosis following incomplete spontaneous abortion
Uremia following incomplete spontaneous abortion

O03.33   **Metabolic disorder following incomplete** M ♀
spontaneous abortion

O03.34   **Damage to pelvic organs following** M ♀
incomplete **spontaneous abortion**

Laceration, perforation, tear or chemical damage of bladder following incomplete spontaneous abortion
Laceration, perforation, tear or chemical damage of bowel following incomplete spontaneous abortion
Laceration, perforation, tear or chemical damage of broad ligament following incomplete spontaneous abortion
Laceration, perforation, tear or chemical damage of cervix following incomplete spontaneous abortion
Laceration, perforation, tear or chemical damage of periurethral tissue following incomplete spontaneous abortion
Laceration, perforation, tear or chemical damage of uterus following incomplete spontaneous abortion
Laceration, perforation, tear or chemical damage of vagina following incomplete spontaneous abortion

O03.35   **Other venous complications following** M ♀
incomplete **spontaneous abortion**

O03.36   **Cardiac arrest following incomplete** M ♀
spontaneous abortion

O03.37   **Sepsis following incomplete spontaneous** M ♀
abortion

Use additional code to identify infectious agent (B95-B97)
Use additional code to identify severe sepsis, if applicable (R65.2-)
EXCLUDES 1   *septic or septicopyemic embolism following incomplete spontaneous abortion (O03.2)*

O03.38   **Urinary tract infection following incomplete** M ♀
spontaneous abortion

Cystitis following incomplete spontaneous abortion

O03.39   **Incomplete spontaneous abortion with other** M ♀
complications

O03.4   **Incomplete spontaneous abortion without** M ♀
complication

O03.5   **Genital tract and pelvic infection following complete** M ♀
or unspecified spontaneous abortion

Endometritis following complete or unspecified spontaneous abortion
Oophoritis following complete or unspecified spontaneous abortion
Parametritis following complete or unspecified spontaneous abortion
Pelvic peritonitis following complete or unspecified spontaneous abortion
Salpingitis following complete or unspecified spontaneous abortion
Salpingo-oophoritis following complete or unspecified spontaneous abortion
EXCLUDES 1   *sepsis following complete or unspecified spontaneous abortion (O03.87)*
urinary tract infection following complete or unspecified spontaneous abortion (O03.88)

O03.6   **Delayed or excessive hemorrhage following complete** M ♀
or unspecified spontaneous abortion

Afibrinogenemia following complete or unspecified spontaneous abortion
Defibrination syndrome following complete or unspecified spontaneous abortion
Hemolysis following complete or unspecified spontaneous abortion
Intravascular coagulation following complete or unspecified spontaneous abortion

O03.7   **Embolism following complete or unspecified** M ♀
spontaneous abortion

Air embolism following complete or unspecified spontaneous abortion
Amniotic fluid embolism following complete or unspecified spontaneous abortion
Blood-clot embolism following complete or unspecified spontaneous abortion
Embolism NOS following complete or unspecified spontaneous abortion
Fat embolism following complete or unspecified spontaneous abortion
Pulmonary embolism following complete or unspecified spontaneous abortion
Pyemic embolism following complete or unspecified spontaneous abortion
Septic or septicopyemic embolism following complete or unspecified spontaneous abortion
Soap embolism following complete or unspecified spontaneous abortion

✓5ᵗʰ **O03.8**   **Other and unspecified complications following complete or unspecified spontaneous abortion**

O03.80   **Unspecified complication following** M ♀ ▽
complete or unspecified spontaneous abortion

O03.81   **Shock following complete or unspecified** M ♀
spontaneous abortion

Circulatory collapse following complete or unspecified spontaneous abortion
Shock (postprocedural) following complete or unspecified spontaneous abortion
EXCLUDES 1   *shock due to infection following complete or unspecified spontaneous abortion (O03.87)*

✔ Additional Character Required   ✓7ᵗʰ Placeholder Alert   Manifestation Dx   ▽ Unspecified Dx   ►◄ Revised Text   ● New Code   ▲ Revised Code Title

ICD-10-CM 2017   803

O03.82   **Renal failure following complete or unspecified spontaneous abortion**   Ⓜ ♀

Kidney failure (acute) following complete or unspecified spontaneous abortion

Oliguria following complete or unspecified spontaneous abortion

Renal shutdown following complete or unspecified spontaneous abortion

Renal tubular necrosis following complete or unspecified spontaneous abortion

Uremia following complete or unspecified spontaneous abortion

O03.83   **Metabolic disorder following complete or unspecified spontaneous abortion**   Ⓜ ♀

O03.84   **Damage to pelvic organs following complete or unspecified spontaneous abortion**   Ⓜ ♀

Laceration, perforation, tear or chemical damage of bladder following complete or unspecified spontaneous abortion

Laceration, perforation, tear or chemical damage of bowel following complete or unspecified spontaneous abortion

Laceration, perforation, tear or chemical damage of broad ligament following complete or unspecified spontaneous abortion

Laceration, perforation, tear or chemical damage of cervix following complete or unspecified spontaneous abortion

Laceration, perforation, tear or chemical damage of periurethral tissue following complete or unspecified spontaneous abortion

Laceration, perforation, tear or chemical damage of uterus following complete or unspecified spontaneous abortion

Laceration, perforation, tear or chemical damage of vagina following complete or unspecified spontaneous abortion

O03.85   **Other venous complications following complete or unspecified spontaneous abortion**   Ⓜ ♀

O03.86   **Cardiac arrest following complete or unspecified spontaneous abortion**   Ⓜ ♀

O03.87   **Sepsis following complete or unspecified spontaneous abortion**   Ⓜ ♀

Use additional code to identify infectious agent (B95-B97)

Use additional code to identify severe sepsis, if applicable (R65.2-)

EXCLUDES 1   *septic or septicopyemic embolism following complete or unspecified spontaneous abortion (O03.7)*

O03.88   **Urinary tract infection following complete or unspecified spontaneous abortion**   Ⓜ ♀

Cystitis following complete or unspecified spontaneous abortion

O03.89   **Complete or unspecified spontaneous abortion with other complications**   Ⓜ ♀

O03.9   **Complete or unspecified spontaneous abortion without complication**   Ⓜ ♀ ▽

Miscarriage NOS

Spontaneous abortion NOS

✓4ᵗʰ **O04**   **Complications following (induced) termination of pregnancy**

INCLUDES   complications following (induced) termination of pregnancy

EXCLUDES 1   *encounter for elective termination of pregnancy, uncomplicated (Z33.2)*

failed attempted termination of pregnancy (O07.-)

O04.5   **Genital tract and pelvic infection following (induced) termination of pregnancy**   Ⓜ ♀

Endometritis following (induced) termination of pregnancy

Oophoritis following (induced) termination of pregnancy

Parametritis following (induced) termination of pregnancy

Pelvic peritonitis following (induced) termination of pregnancy

Salpingitis following (induced) termination of pregnancy

Salpingo-oophoritis following (induced) termination of pregnancy

EXCLUDES 1   *sepsis following (induced) termination of pregnancy (O04.87)*

urinary tract infection following (induced) termination of pregnancy (O04.88)

O04.6   **Delayed or excessive hemorrhage following (induced) termination of pregnancy**   Ⓜ ♀

Afibrinogenemia following (induced) termination of pregnancy

Defibrination syndrome following (induced) termination of pregnancy

Hemolysis following (induced) termination of pregnancy

Intravascular coagulation following (induced) termination of pregnancy

O04.7   **Embolism following (induced) termination of pregnancy**   Ⓜ ♀

Air embolism following (induced) termination of pregnancy

Amniotic fluid embolism following (induced) termination of pregnancy

Blood-clot embolism following (induced) termination of pregnancy

Embolism NOS following (induced) termination of pregnancy

Fat embolism following (induced) termination of pregnancy

Pulmonary embolism following (induced) termination of pregnancy

Pyemic embolism following (induced) termination of pregnancy

Septic or septicopyemic embolism following (induced) termination of pregnancy

Soap embolism following (induced) termination of pregnancy

✓5ᵗʰ **O04.8**   **(Induced) termination of pregnancy with other and unspecified complications**

O04.80   **(Induced) termination of pregnancy with unspecified complications**   Ⓜ ♀ ▽

O04.81   **Shock following (induced) termination of pregnancy**   Ⓜ ♀

Circulatory collapse following (induced) termination of pregnancy

Shock (postprocedural) following (induced) termination of pregnancy

EXCLUDES 1   *shock due to infection following (induced) termination of pregnancy (O04.87)*

O04.82   **Renal failure following (induced) termination of pregnancy**   Ⓜ ♀

Kidney failure (acute) following (induced) termination of pregnancy

Oliguria following (induced) termination of pregnancy

Renal shutdown following (induced) termination of pregnancy

Renal tubular necrosis following (induced) termination of pregnancy

Uremia following (induced) termination of pregnancy

O04.83   **Metabolic disorder following (induced) termination of pregnancy**   Ⓜ ♀

EXCLUDES 1 Not coded here   **EXCLUDES 2** Not included here   Ⓝ Newborn Age : 0   Ⓟ Pediatric Age : 0-17   Ⓜ Maternity Age : 12-55   Ⓐ Adult Age : 15-124

804

O03.82–O04.83

ICD-10-CM 2017

O04.84 **Damage to pelvic organs following (induced)** Ⓜ ♀
termination of pregnancy
Laceration, perforation, tear or chemical damage of
bladder following (induced) termination of
pregnancy
Laceration, perforation, tear or chemical damage of
bowel following (induced) termination of
pregnancy
Laceration, perforation, tear or chemical damage of
broad ligament following (induced) termination
of pregnancy
Laceration, perforation, tear or chemical damage of
cervix following (induced) termination of
pregnancy
Laceration, perforation, tear or chemical damage of
periurethral tissue following (induced)
termination of pregnancy
Laceration, perforation, tear or chemical damage of
uterus following (induced) termination of
pregnancy
Laceration, perforation, tear or chemical damage of
vagina following (induced) termination of
pregnancy

O04.85 **Other venous complications following** Ⓜ ♀
(induced) termination of pregnancy

O04.86 **Cardiac arrest following (induced)** Ⓜ ♀
termination of pregnancy

O04.87 **Sepsis following (induced) termination of** Ⓜ ♀
pregnancy
Use additional code to identify infectious agent
(B95-B97)
Use additional code to identify severe sepsis, if
applicable (R65.2-)
EXCLUDES 1 *septic or septicopyemic embolism following*
(induced) termination of pregnancy
(O04.7)

O04.88 **Urinary tract infection following (induced)** Ⓜ ♀
termination of pregnancy
Cystitis following (induced) termination of pregnancy

O04.89 **(Induced) termination of pregnancy with** ♀
other complications

☑4ᵗʰ **O07** **Failed attempted termination of pregnancy**
INCLUDES failure of attempted induction of termination of pregnancy
incomplete elective abortion
EXCLUDES 1 *incomplete spontaneous abortion (O03.0-)*

O07.0 **Genital tract and pelvic infection following failed** Ⓜ ♀
attempted termination of pregnancy
Endometritis following failed attempted termination of
pregnancy
Oophoritis following failed attempted termination of pregnancy
Parametritis following failed attempted termination of
pregnancy
Pelvic peritonitis following failed attempted termination of
pregnancy
Salpingitis following failed attempted termination of pregnancy
Salpingo-oophoritis following failed attempted termination of
pregnancy
EXCLUDES 1 *sepsis following failed attempted termination of*
pregnancy (O07.37)
urinary tract infection following failed attempted
termination of pregnancy (O07.38)

O07.1 **Delayed or excessive hemorrhage following failed** Ⓜ ♀
attempted termination of pregnancy
Afibrinogenemia following failed attempted termination of
pregnancy
Defibrination syndrome following failed attempted termination
of pregnancy
Hemolysis following failed attempted termination of pregnancy
Intravascular coagulation following failed attempted
termination of pregnancy

O07.2 **Embolism following failed attempted termination of** Ⓜ ♀
pregnancy
Air embolism following failed attempted termination of
pregnancy
Amniotic fluid embolism following failed attempted termination
of pregnancy
Blood-clot embolism following failed attempted termination
of pregnancy
Embolism NOS following failed attempted termination of
pregnancy
Fat embolism following failed attempted termination of
pregnancy
Pulmonary embolism following failed attempted termination
of pregnancy
Pyemic embolism following failed attempted termination of
pregnancy
Septic or septicopyemic embolism following failed attempted
termination of pregnancy
Soap embolism following failed attempted termination of
pregnancy

☑5ᵗʰ **O07.3** **Failed attempted termination of pregnancy with other and**
unspecified complications

O07.30 **Failed attempted termination of pregnancy** Ⓜ ♀ ▽
with unspecified complications

O07.31 **Shock following failed attempted** Ⓜ ♀
termination of pregnancy
Circulatory collapse following failed attempted
termination of pregnancy
Shock (postprocedural) following failed attempted
termination of pregnancy
EXCLUDES 1 *shock due to infection following failed*
attempted termination of pregnancy
(O07.37)

O07.32 **Renal failure following failed attempted** Ⓜ ♀
termination of pregnancy
Kidney failure (acute) following failed attempted
termination of pregnancy
Oliguria following failed attempted termination of
pregnancy
Renal shutdown following failed attempted
termination of pregnancy
Renal tubular necrosis following failed attempted
termination of pregnancy
Uremia following failed attempted termination of
pregnancy

O07.33 **Metabolic disorder following failed** Ⓜ ♀
attempted termination of pregnancy

O07.34 **Damage to pelvic organs following failed** Ⓜ ♀
attempted termination of pregnancy
Laceration, perforation, tear or chemical damage of
bladder following failed attempted termination
of pregnancy
Laceration, perforation, tear or chemical damage of
bowel following failed attempted termination
of pregnancy
Laceration, perforation, tear or chemical damage of
broad ligament following failed attempted
termination of pregnancy
Laceration, perforation, tear or chemical damage of
cervix following failed attempted termination
of pregnancy
Laceration, perforation, tear or chemical damage of
periurethral tissue following failed attempted
termination of pregnancy
Laceration, perforation, tear or chemical damage of
uterus following failed attempted termination
of pregnancy
Laceration, perforation, tear or chemical damage of
vagina following failed attempted termination
of pregnancy

O07.35 **Other venous complications following failed** Ⓜ ♀
attempted termination of pregnancy

O07.36 **Cardiac arrest following failed attempted** Ⓜ ♀
termination of pregnancy

O07.37 **Sepsis following failed attempted termination of pregnancy** Ⓜ ♀
Use additional code (B95-B97), to identify infectious agent
Use additional code (R65.2-) to identify severe sepsis, if applicable
> **EXCLUDES 1** *septic or septicopyemic embolism following failed attempted termination of pregnancy (O07.2)*

O07.38 **Urinary tract infection following failed attempted termination of pregnancy** Ⓜ ♀
Cystitis following failed attempted termination of pregnancy

O07.39 **Failed attempted termination of pregnancy with other complications** Ⓜ ♀

O07.4 **Failed attempted termination of pregnancy** without complication Ⓜ ♀

✓4ᵗʰ **O08** **Complications following ectopic and molar pregnancy**
This category is for use with categories O00-O02 to identify any associated complications

O08.0 **Genital tract and pelvic infection following ectopic and molar pregnancy** Ⓜ ♀
Endometritis following ectopic and molar pregnancy
Oophoritis following ectopic and molar pregnancy
Parametritis following ectopic and molar pregnancy
Pelvic peritonitis following ectopic and molar pregnancy
Salpingitis following ectopic and molar pregnancy
Salpingo-oophoritis following ectopic and molar pregnancy
> **EXCLUDES 1** *sepsis following ectopic and molar pregnancy (O08.82)*
> *urinary tract infection (O08.83)*

O08.1 **Delayed or excessive hemorrhage following ectopic and molar pregnancy** Ⓜ ♀
Afibrinogenemia following ectopic and molar pregnancy
Defibrination syndrome following ectopic and molar pregnancy
Hemolysis following ectopic and molar pregnancy
Intravascular coagulation following ectopic and molar pregnancy
> **EXCLUDES 1** *delayed or excessive hemorrhage due to incomplete abortion (O03.1)*

O08.2 **Embolism following ectopic and molar pregnancy** Ⓜ ♀
Air embolism following ectopic and molar pregnancy
Amniotic fluid embolism following ectopic and molar pregnancy
Blood-clot embolism following ectopic and molar pregnancy
Embolism NOS following ectopic and molar pregnancy
Fat embolism following ectopic and molar pregnancy
Pulmonary embolism following ectopic and molar pregnancy
Pyemic embolism following ectopic and molar pregnancy
Septic or septicopyemic embolism following ectopic and molar pregnancy
Soap embolism following ectopic and molar pregnancy

O08.3 **Shock following ectopic and molar pregnancy** Ⓜ ♀
Circulatory collapse following ectopic and molar pregnancy
Shock (postprocedural) following ectopic and molar pregnancy
> **EXCLUDES 1** *shock due to infection following ectopic and molar pregnancy (O08.82)*

O08.4 **Renal failure following ectopic and molar pregnancy** Ⓜ ♀
Kidney failure (acute) following ectopic and molar pregnancy
Oliguria following ectopic and molar pregnancy
Renal shutdown following ectopic and molar pregnancy
Renal tubular necrosis following ectopic and molar pregnancy
Uremia following ectopic and molar pregnancy

O08.5 **Metabolic disorders following an ectopic and molar pregnancy** Ⓜ ♀

O08.6 **Damage to pelvic organs and tissues following an ectopic and molar pregnancy** Ⓜ ♀
Laceration, perforation, tear or chemical damage of bladder following an ectopic and molar pregnancy
Laceration, perforation, tear or chemical damage of bowel following an ectopic and molar pregnancy
Laceration, perforation, tear or chemical damage of broad ligament following an ectopic and molar pregnancy
Laceration, perforation, tear or chemical damage of cervix following an ectopic and molar pregnancy
Laceration, perforation, tear or chemical damage of periurethral tissue following an ectopic and molar pregnancy
Laceration, perforation, tear or chemical damage of uterus following an ectopic and molar pregnancy
Laceration, perforation, tear or chemical damage of vagina following an ectopic and molar pregnancy

O08.7 **Other venous complications following an ectopic and molar pregnancy** Ⓜ ♀

✓5ᵗʰ **O08.8** **Other complications following an ectopic and molar pregnancy**

O08.81 **Cardiac arrest following an ectopic and molar pregnancy** Ⓜ ♀

O08.82 **Sepsis following ectopic and molar pregnancy** Ⓜ ♀
Use additional code (B95-B97), to identify infectious agent
Use additional code (R65.2-) to identify severe sepsis, if applicable
> **EXCLUDES 1** *septic or septicopyemic embolism following ectopic and molar pregnancy (O08.2)*

O08.83 **Urinary tract infection following an ectopic and molar pregnancy** Ⓜ ♀
Cystitis following an ectopic and molar pregnancy

O08.89 **Other complications following an ectopic and molar pregnancy** Ⓜ ♀

O08.9 **Unspecified complication following an ectopic and molar pregnancy** Ⓜ ♀ ▽

Supervision of high risk pregnancy (O09)

✓4ᵗʰ **O09** **Supervision of** high risk **pregnancy**

✓5ᵗʰ **O09.0** **Supervision of pregnancy with** history of infertility

O09.00 **Supervision of pregnancy with history of infertility, unspecified trimester** Ⓜ ♀ ▽

O09.01 **Supervision of pregnancy with history of infertility, first trimester** Ⓜ ♀

O09.02 **Supervision of pregnancy with history of infertility, second trimester** Ⓜ ♀

O09.03 **Supervision of pregnancy with history of infertility, third trimester** Ⓜ ♀

▲ ✓5ᵗʰ **O09.1** **Supervision of pregnancy with** history of ectopic **pregnancy**

▲ **O09.10** **Supervision of pregnancy with history of ectopic pregnancy, unspecified trimester** Ⓜ ♀ ▽

▲ **O09.11** **Supervision of pregnancy with history of ectopic pregnancy, first trimester** Ⓜ ♀

▲ **O09.12** **Supervision of pregnancy with history of ectopic pregnancy, second trimester** Ⓜ ♀

▲ **O09.13** **Supervision of pregnancy with history of ectopic pregnancy, third trimester** Ⓜ ♀

● **O09.A** **Supervision of pregnancy with** history of molar **pregnancy**

● **O09.A0** **Supervision of pregnancy with history of molar pregnancy, unspecified trimester** ▽

● **O09.A1** **Supervision of pregnancy with history of molar pregnancy, first trimester**

● **O09.A2** **Supervision of pregnancy with history of molar pregnancy, second trimester**

● **O09.A3** **Supervision of pregnancy with history of molar pregnancy, third trimester**

✓5ᵗʰ **O09.2** **Supervision of pregnancy with other poor reproductive or obstetric history**
> **EXCLUDES 2** *pregnancy care for patient with history of recurrent pregnancy loss (O26.2-)*

✓6ᵗʰ **O09.21** **Supervision of pregnancy with history of** pre-term labor

O09.211 **Supervision of pregnancy with history of pre-term labor, first trimester** Ⓜ ♀

O09.212 **Supervision of pregnancy with history of pre-term labor, second trimester** Ⓜ ♀

O09.213 Supervision of pregnancy with history of pre-term labor, third trimester Ⓜ♀

O09.219 Supervision of pregnancy with history of pre-term labor, unspecified trimester Ⓜ♀▽

✓6ᵗʰ **O09.29** Supervision of pregnancy with other poor reproductive or obstetric history
> Supervision of pregnancy with history of neonatal death
> Supervision of pregnancy with history of stillbirth

O09.291 Supervision of pregnancy with other poor reproductive or obstetric history, first trimester Ⓜ♀

O09.292 Supervision of pregnancy with other poor reproductive or obstetric history, second trimester Ⓜ♀

O09.293 Supervision of pregnancy with other poor reproductive or obstetric history, third trimester Ⓜ♀

O09.299 Supervision of pregnancy with other poor reproductive or obstetric history, unspecified trimester Ⓜ♀▽

✓5ᵗʰ **O09.3** Supervision of pregnancy with insufficient antenatal care
> Supervision of concealed pregnancy
> Supervision of hidden pregnancy

O09.30 Supervision of pregnancy with insufficient antenatal care, unspecified trimester Ⓜ♀▽

O09.31 Supervision of pregnancy with insufficient antenatal care, first trimester Ⓜ♀

O09.32 Supervision of pregnancy with insufficient antenatal care, second trimester Ⓜ♀

O09.33 Supervision of pregnancy with insufficient antenatal care, third trimester Ⓜ♀

✓5ᵗʰ **O09.4** Supervision of pregnancy with grand multiparity

O09.40 Supervision of pregnancy with grand multiparity, unspecified trimester Ⓜ♀▽

O09.41 Supervision of pregnancy with grand multiparity, first trimester Ⓜ♀

O09.42 Supervision of pregnancy with grand multiparity, second trimester Ⓜ♀

O09.43 Supervision of pregnancy with grand multiparity, third trimester Ⓜ♀

✓6ᵗʰ **O09.5** Supervision of elderly primigravida and multigravida
> Pregnancy for a female 35 years and older at expected date of delivery

✓6ᵗʰ **O09.51** Supervision of elderly primigravida

O09.511 Supervision of elderly primigravida, first trimester Ⓜ♀

O09.512 Supervision of elderly primigravida, second trimester Ⓜ♀

O09.513 Supervision of elderly primigravida, third trimester Ⓜ♀

O09.519 Supervision of elderly primigravida, unspecified trimester Ⓜ♀▽

✓6ᵗʰ **O09.52** Supervision of elderly multigravida

O09.521 Supervision of elderly multigravida, first trimester Ⓜ♀

O09.522 Supervision of elderly multigravida, second trimester Ⓜ♀

O09.523 Supervision of elderly multigravida, third trimester Ⓜ♀

O09.529 Supervision of elderly multigravida, unspecified trimester Ⓜ♀▽

✓5ᵗʰ **O09.6** Supervision of young primigravida and multigravida
> Supervision of pregnancy for a female less than 16 years old at expected date of delivery

✓6ᵗʰ **O09.61** Supervision of young primigravida

O09.611 Supervision of young primigravida, first trimester Ⓜ♀

O09.612 Supervision of young primigravida, second trimester Ⓜ♀

O09.613 Supervision of young primigravida, third trimester Ⓜ♀

O09.619 Supervision of young primigravida, unspecified trimester Ⓜ♀▽

✓6ᵗʰ **O09.62** Supervision of young multigravida

O09.621 Supervision of young multigravida, first trimester Ⓜ♀

O09.622 Supervision of young multigravida, second trimester Ⓜ♀

O09.623 Supervision of young multigravida, third trimester Ⓜ♀

O09.629 Supervision of young multigravida, unspecified trimester Ⓜ♀▽

✓5ᵗʰ **O09.7** Supervision of high risk pregnancy due to social problems

O09.70 Supervision of high risk pregnancy due to social problems, unspecified trimester Ⓜ♀▽

O09.71 Supervision of high risk pregnancy due to social problems, first trimester Ⓜ♀

O09.72 Supervision of high risk pregnancy due to social problems, second trimester Ⓜ♀

O09.73 Supervision of high risk pregnancy due to social problems, third trimester Ⓜ♀

✓5ᵗʰ **O09.8** Supervision of other high risk pregnancies

✓6ᵗʰ **O09.81** Supervision of pregnancy resulting from assisted reproductive technology
> Supervision of pregnancy resulting from in-vitro fertilization
>
> *EXCLUDES 2* ▶*gestational carrier status (Z33.3)*◀

O09.811 Supervision of pregnancy resulting from assisted reproductive technology, first trimester Ⓜ♀

O09.812 Supervision of pregnancy resulting from assisted reproductive technology, second trimester Ⓜ♀

O09.813 Supervision of pregnancy resulting from assisted reproductive technology, third trimester Ⓜ♀

O09.819 Supervision of pregnancy resulting from assisted reproductive technology, unspecified trimester Ⓜ♀▽

✓6ᵗʰ **O09.82** Supervision of pregnancy with history of in utero procedure during previous pregnancy

O09.821 Supervision of pregnancy with history of in utero procedure during previous pregnancy, first trimester Ⓜ♀

O09.822 Supervision of pregnancy with history of in utero procedure during previous pregnancy, second trimester Ⓜ♀

O09.823 Supervision of pregnancy with history of in utero procedure during previous pregnancy, third trimester Ⓜ♀

O09.829 Supervision of pregnancy with history of in utero procedure during previous pregnancy, unspecified trimester Ⓜ♀▽
> *EXCLUDES 1* *supervision of pregnancy affected by in utero procedure during current pregnancy (O35.7)*

✓6ᵗʰ **O09.89** Supervision of other high risk pregnancies

O09.891 Supervision of other high risk pregnancies, first trimester Ⓜ♀

O09.892 Supervision of other high risk pregnancies, second trimester Ⓜ♀

O09.893 Supervision of other high risk pregnancies, third trimester Ⓜ♀

O09.899 Supervision of other high risk pregnancies, unspecified trimester Ⓜ♀▽

✓5ᵗʰ **O09.9** Supervision of high risk pregnancy, unspecified

O09.90 Supervision of high risk pregnancy, unspecified, unspecified trimester Ⓜ♀▽

O09.91 Supervision of high risk pregnancy, unspecified, first trimester Ⓜ♀▽

O09.92 Supervision of high risk pregnancy, unspecified, second trimester Ⓜ♀▽

O09.93 Supervision of high risk pregnancy, unspecified, third trimester Ⓜ♀▽

☑ Additional Character Required   ✓7ᵗʰ Placeholder Alert   Manifestation Dx   ▽ Unspecified Dx   ▶◀ Revised Text   ● New Code   ▲ Revised Code Title

ICD-10-CM 2017   807

Edema, proteinuria and hypertensive disorders in pregnancy, childbirth and the puerperium (O10-O16)

✓4ᵗʰ **O10 Pre-existing hypertension complicating pregnancy, childbirth and the puerperium**

> INCLUDES   pre-existing hypertension with pre-existing proteinuria complicating pregnancy, childbirth and the puerperium
>
> EXCLUDES 2   *pre-existing hypertension with superimposed pre-eclampsia complicating pregnancy, childbirth and the puerperium (O11.-)*

✓5ᵗʰ **O10.0 Pre-existing essential hypertension complicating pregnancy, childbirth and the puerperium**

> Any condition in I10 specified as a reason for obstetric care during pregnancy, childbirth or the puerperium

   ✓6ᵗʰ **O10.01 Pre-existing essential hypertension complicating pregnancy**

     O10.011 Pre-existing essential hypertension complicating pregnancy, first trimester   Ⓜ ♀

     O10.012 Pre-existing essential hypertension complicating pregnancy, second trimester   Ⓜ ♀

     O10.013 Pre-existing essential hypertension complicating pregnancy, third trimester   Ⓜ ♀

     O10.019 Pre-existing essential hypertension complicating pregnancy, unspecified trimester   Ⓜ ♀ ▽

   O10.02 Pre-existing essential hypertension complicating childbirth   Ⓜ ♀

   O10.03 Pre-existing essential hypertension complicating the puerperium   Ⓜ ♀

✓5ᵗʰ **O10.1 Pre-existing hypertensive heart disease complicating pregnancy, childbirth and the puerperium**

> Any condition in I11 specified as a reason for obstetric care during pregnancy, childbirth or the puerperium
>
> Use additional code from I11 to identify the type of hypertensive heart disease

   ✓6ᵗʰ **O10.11 Pre-existing hypertensive heart disease complicating pregnancy**

     O10.111 Pre-existing hypertensive heart disease complicating pregnancy, first trimester   Ⓜ ♀

     O10.112 Pre-existing hypertensive heart disease complicating pregnancy, second trimester   Ⓜ ♀

     O10.113 Pre-existing hypertensive heart disease complicating pregnancy, third trimester   Ⓜ ♀

     O10.119 Pre-existing hypertensive heart disease complicating pregnancy, unspecified trimester   Ⓜ ♀ ▽

   O10.12 Pre-existing hypertensive heart disease complicating childbirth   Ⓜ ♀

   O10.13 Pre-existing hypertensive heart disease complicating the puerperium   Ⓜ ♀

✓5ᵗʰ **O10.2 Pre-existing hypertensive chronic kidney disease complicating pregnancy, childbirth and the puerperium**

> Any condition in I12 specified as a reason for obstetric care during pregnancy, childbirth or the puerperium
>
> Use additional code from I12 to identify the type of hypertensive chronic kidney disease

   ✓6ᵗʰ **O10.21 Pre-existing hypertensive chronic kidney disease complicating pregnancy**

     O10.211 Pre-existing hypertensive chronic kidney disease complicating pregnancy, first trimester   Ⓜ ♀

     O10.212 Pre-existing hypertensive chronic kidney disease complicating pregnancy, second trimester   Ⓜ ♀

     O10.213 Pre-existing hypertensive chronic kidney disease complicating pregnancy, third trimester   Ⓜ ♀

     O10.219 Pre-existing hypertensive chronic kidney disease complicating pregnancy, unspecified trimester   Ⓜ ♀ ▽

   O10.22 Pre-existing hypertensive chronic kidney disease complicating childbirth   Ⓜ ♀

   O10.23 Pre-existing hypertensive chronic kidney disease complicating the puerperium   Ⓜ ♀

✓5ᵗʰ **O10.3 Pre-existing hypertensive heart and chronic kidney disease complicating pregnancy, childbirth and the puerperium**

> Any condition in I13 specified as a reason for obstetric care during pregnancy, childbirth or the puerperium
>
> Use additional code from I13 to identify the type of hypertensive heart and chronic kidney disease

   ✓6ᵗʰ **O10.31 Pre-existing hypertensive heart and chronic kidney disease complicating pregnancy**

     O10.311 Pre-existing hypertensive heart and chronic kidney disease complicating pregnancy, first trimester   Ⓜ ♀

     O10.312 Pre-existing hypertensive heart and chronic kidney disease complicating pregnancy, second trimester   Ⓜ ♀

     O10.313 Pre-existing hypertensive heart and chronic kidney disease complicating pregnancy, third trimester   Ⓜ ♀

     O10.319 Pre-existing hypertensive heart and chronic kidney disease complicating pregnancy, unspecified trimester   Ⓜ ♀ ▽

   O10.32 Pre-existing hypertensive heart and chronic kidney disease complicating childbirth   Ⓜ ♀

   O10.33 Pre-existing hypertensive heart and chronic kidney disease complicating the puerperium   Ⓜ ♀

✓5ᵗʰ **O10.4 Pre-existing secondary hypertension complicating pregnancy, childbirth and the puerperium**

> Any condition in I15 specified as a reason for obstetric care during pregnancy, childbirth or the puerperium
>
> Use additional code from I15 to identify the type of secondary hypertension

   ✓6ᵗʰ **O10.41 Pre-existing secondary hypertension complicating pregnancy**

     O10.411 Pre-existing secondary hypertension complicating pregnancy, first trimester   Ⓜ ♀

     O10.412 Pre-existing secondary hypertension complicating pregnancy, second trimester   Ⓜ ♀

     O10.413 Pre-existing secondary hypertension complicating pregnancy, third trimester   Ⓜ ♀

     O10.419 Pre-existing secondary hypertension complicating pregnancy, unspecified trimester   Ⓜ ♀ ▽

   O10.42 Pre-existing secondary hypertension complicating childbirth   Ⓜ ♀

   O10.43 Pre-existing secondary hypertension complicating the puerperium   Ⓜ ♀

✓5ᵗʰ **O10.9 Unspecified pre-existing hypertension complicating pregnancy, childbirth and the puerperium**

   ✓6ᵗʰ **O10.91 Unspecified pre-existing hypertension complicating pregnancy**

     O10.911 Unspecified pre-existing hypertension complicating pregnancy, first trimester   Ⓜ ♀ ▽

     O10.912 Unspecified pre-existing hypertension complicating pregnancy, second trimester   Ⓜ ♀ ▽

     O10.913 Unspecified pre-existing hypertension complicating pregnancy, third trimester   Ⓜ ♀ ▽

     O10.919 Unspecified pre-existing hypertension complicating pregnancy, unspecified trimester   Ⓜ ♀ ▽

   O10.92 Unspecified pre-existing hypertension complicating childbirth   Ⓜ ♀ ▽

   O10.93 Unspecified pre-existing hypertension complicating the puerperium   Ⓜ ♀ ▽

✓4ᵗʰ **O11 Pre-existing hypertension with pre-eclampsia**

> INCLUDES   conditions in O10 complicated by pre-eclampsia
> pre-eclampsia superimposed pre-existing in hypertension
>
> Use additional code from O10 to identify the type of hypertension

   O11.1 Pre-existing hypertension with pre-eclampsia, first trimester   Ⓜ ♀

   O11.2 Pre-existing hypertension with pre-eclampsia, second trimester   Ⓜ ♀

   O11.3 Pre-existing hypertension with pre-eclampsia, third trimester   Ⓜ ♀

EXCLUDES 1 Not coded here   EXCLUDES 2 Not included here   Ⓝ Newborn Age : 0   Ⓟ Pediatric Age : 0-17   Ⓜ Maternity Age : 12-55   Ⓐ Adult Age : 15-124

- **O11.4** **Pre-existing hypertension with pre-eclampsia, complicating childbirth**
- **O11.5** **Pre-existing hypertension with pre-eclampsia, complicating the puerperium**
- **O11.9** **Pre-existing hypertension with pre-eclampsia, unspecified trimester**   M ♀ ▽

✓4ᵗʰ **O12** **Gestational [pregnancy-induced] edema and proteinuria** without hypertension

   ✓5ᵗʰ **O12.0** **Gestational** edema
- **O12.00** **Gestational edema, unspecified trimester**   M ♀ ▽
- **O12.01** **Gestational edema, first trimester**   M ♀
- **O12.02** **Gestational edema, second trimester**   M ♀
- **O12.03** **Gestational edema, third trimester**   M ♀
- **O12.04** **Gestational edema, complicating childbirth**
- **O12.05** **Gestational edema, complicating the puerperium**

   ✓5ᵗʰ **O12.1** **Gestational** proteinuria
- **O12.10** **Gestational proteinuria, unspecified trimester**   M ♀ ▽
- **O12.11** **Gestational proteinuria, first trimester**   M ♀
- **O12.12** **Gestational proteinuria, second trimester**   M ♀
- **O12.13** **Gestational proteinuria, third trimester**   M ♀
- **O12.14** **Gestational proteinuria, complicating childbirth**
- **O12.15** **Gestational proteinuria, complicating the puerperium**

   ✓5ᵗʰ **O12.2** **Gestational** edema with proteinuria
- **O12.20** **Gestational edema with proteinuria, unspecified trimester**   M ♀ ▽
- **O12.21** **Gestational edema with proteinuria, first trimester**   M ♀
- **O12.22** **Gestational edema with proteinuria, second trimester**   M ♀
- **O12.23** **Gestational edema with proteinuria, third trimester**   M ♀
- **O12.24** **Gestational edema with proteinuria, complicating childbirth**
- **O12.25** **Gestational edema with proteinuria, complicating the puerperium**

✓4ᵗʰ **O13** **Gestational [pregnancy-induced] hypertension without significant proteinuria**

   INCLUDES   gestational hypertension NOS
     ►transient hypertension of pregnancy◄
   AHA: 2016,1Q,5

- **O13.1** **Gestational [pregnancy-induced] hypertension without significant proteinuria, first trimester**   M ♀
- **O13.2** **Gestational [pregnancy-induced] hypertension without significant proteinuria, second trimester**   M ♀
- **O13.3** **Gestational [pregnancy-induced] hypertension without significant proteinuria, third trimester**   M ♀
- **O13.4** **Gestational [pregnancy-induced] hypertension without significant proteinuria, complicating childbirth**
- **O13.5** **Gestational [pregnancy-induced] hypertension without significant proteinuria, complicating the puerperium**
- **O13.9** **Gestational [pregnancy-induced] hypertension without significant proteinuria, unspecified trimester**   M ♀ ▽

✓4ᵗʰ **O14** **Pre-eclampsia**

   EXCLUDES 1   pre-existing hypertension with pre-eclampsia (O11)

   ✓5ᵗʰ **O14.0** **Mild to moderate** pre-eclampsia
- **O14.00** **Mild to moderate pre-eclampsia, unspecified trimester**   M ♀ ▽
- **O14.02** **Mild to moderate pre-eclampsia, second trimester**   M ♀
- **O14.03** **Mild to moderate pre-eclampsia, third trimester**   M ♀
- **O14.04** **Mild to moderate pre-eclampsia, complicating childbirth**
- **O14.05** **Mild to moderate pre-eclampsia, complicating the puerperium**

   ✓5ᵗʰ **O14.1** **Severe** pre-eclampsia

     EXCLUDES 1   HELLP syndrome (O14.2-)

- **O14.10** **Severe pre-eclampsia, unspecified trimester**   M ♀ ▽
- **O14.12** **Severe pre-eclampsia, second trimester**   M ♀
- **O14.13** **Severe pre-eclampsia, third trimester**   M ♀
- **O14.14** **Severe pre-eclampsia complicating childbirth**
- **O14.15** **Severe pre-eclampsia, complicating the puerperium**

   ✓5ᵗʰ **O14.2** **HELLP syndrome**

     Severe pre-eclampsia with hemolysis, elevated liver enzymes and low platelet count (HELLP)

- **O14.20** **HELLP syndrome (HELLP), unspecified trimester**   M ♀ ▽
- **O14.22** **HELLP syndrome (HELLP), second trimester**   M ♀
- **O14.23** **HELLP syndrome (HELLP), third trimester**   M ♀
- **O14.24** **HELLP syndrome, complicating childbirth**
- **O14.25** **HELLP syndrome, complicating the puerperium**

   ✓5ᵗʰ **O14.9** **Unspecified pre-eclampsia**
- **O14.90** **Unspecified pre-eclampsia, unspecified trimester**   M ♀ ▽
- **O14.92** **Unspecified pre-eclampsia, second trimester**   M ♀ ▽
- **O14.93** **Unspecified pre-eclampsia, third trimester**   M ♀ ▽
- **O14.94** **Unspecified pre-eclampsia, complicating childbirth**   ▽
- **O14.95** **Unspecified pre-eclampsia, complicating the puerperium**   ▽

✓4ᵗʰ **O15** **Eclampsia**

   INCLUDES   convulsions following conditions in O10-O14 and O16

   ▲   ✓5ᵗʰ **O15.0** **Eclampsia** complicating pregnancy
- ▲ **O15.00** **Eclampsia complicating pregnancy, unspecified trimester**   M ♀ ▽
- ▲ **O15.02** **Eclampsia complicating pregnancy, second trimester**   ♀
- ▲ **O15.03** **Eclampsia complicating pregnancy, third trimester**   M ♀

- ▲ **O15.1** **Eclampsia complicating labor**   M ♀
- ▲ **O15.2** **Eclampsia complicating the puerperium**   M ♀
- **O15.9** **Eclampsia, unspecified as to time period**   M ♀ ▽
     Eclampsia NOS

✓4ᵗʰ **O16** **Unspecified maternal hypertension**
- **O16.1** **Unspecified maternal hypertension, first trimester**   M ♀ ▽
- **O16.2** **Unspecified maternal hypertension, second trimester**   M ♀ ▽
- **O16.3** **Unspecified maternal hypertension, third trimester**   M ♀ ▽
- **O16.4** **Unspecified maternal hypertension, complicating childbirth**   ▽
- **O16.5** **Unspecified maternal hypertension, complicating the puerperium**   ▽
- **O16.9** **Unspecified maternal hypertension, unspecified trimester**   M ♀ ▽

Other maternal disorders predominantly related to pregnancy (O20–O29)

   EXCLUDES 2   maternal care related to the fetus and amniotic cavity and possible delivery problems (O30–O48)
     maternal diseases classifiable elsewhere but complicating pregnancy, labor and delivery, and the puerperium (O98–O99)

✓4ᵗʰ **O20** **Hemorrhage in early pregnancy**

   INCLUDES   hemorrhage before completion of 20 weeks gestation
   EXCLUDES 1   pregnancy with abortive outcome (O00–O08)

- **O20.0** **Threatened abortion**   M ♀
     Hemorrhage specified as due to threatened abortion
     DEF: Bloody discharge during pregnancy; cervix may be dilated and pregnancy threatened, but the pregnancy is not terminated.
- **O20.8** **Other hemorrhage in early pregnancy**   M ♀
- **O20.9** **Hemorrhage in early pregnancy, unspecified**   M ♀ ▽

✓4ᵗʰ **O21** **Excessive vomiting in pregnancy**
- **O21.0** **Mild hyperemesis gravidarum**   M ♀
     Hyperemesis gravidarum, mild or unspecified, starting before the end of the 20th week of gestation
- **O21.1** **Hyperemesis gravidarum with metabolic disturbance**   M ♀
     Hyperemesis gravidarum, starting before the end of the 20th week of gestation, with metabolic disturbance such as carbohydrate depletion
     Hyperemesis gravidarum, starting before the end of the 20th week of gestation, with metabolic disturbance such as dehydration
     Hyperemesis gravidarum, starting before the end of the 20th week of gestation, with metabolic disturbance such as electrolyte imbalance

☑ Additional Character Required   ✓x7ᵗʰ Placeholder Alert   Manifestation Dx   ▽ Unspecified Dx   ►◄ Revised Text   ● New Code   ▲ Revised Code Title

ICD-10-CM 2017   809

Chapter 15. Pregnancy, Childbirth and the Puerperium

O21.2   **Late vomiting of pregnancy**   Ⓜ ♀

Excessive vomiting starting after 20 completed weeks of gestation

O21.8   **Other vomiting complicating pregnancy**   Ⓜ ♀

Vomiting due to diseases classified elsewhere, complicating pregnancy

Use additional code, to identify cause

O21.9   **Vomiting of pregnancy, unspecified**   Ⓜ ♀ ▽

✓4th **O22**   **Venous complications and hemorrhoids in pregnancy**

EXCLUDES 1   venous complications of:
     abortion NOS (O03.9)
     ectopic or molar pregnancy (O08.7)
     failed attempted abortion (O07.35)
     induced abortion (O04.85)
     spontaneous abortion (O03.89)

EXCLUDES 2   obstetric pulmonary embolism (O88.-)
     venous complications and hemorrhoids of childbirth and the puerperium (O87.-)

✓5th **O22.0**   **Varicose veins of lower extremity in pregnancy**

Varicose veins NOS in pregnancy

O22.00   **Varicose veins of lower extremity in pregnancy, unspecified trimester**   Ⓜ ♀ ▽

O22.01   **Varicose veins of lower extremity in pregnancy, first trimester**   Ⓜ ♀

O22.02   **Varicose veins of lower extremity in pregnancy, second trimester**   Ⓜ ♀

O22.03   **Varicose veins of lower extremity in pregnancy, third trimester**   Ⓜ ♀

✓5th **O22.1**   **Genital varices in pregnancy**

Perineal varices in pregnancy
Vaginal varices in pregnancy
Vulval varices in pregnancy

O22.10   **Genital varices in pregnancy, unspecified trimester**   Ⓜ ♀ ▽

O22.11   **Genital varices in pregnancy, first trimester**   Ⓜ ♀

O22.12   **Genital varices in pregnancy, second trimester**   Ⓜ ♀

O22.13   **Genital varices in pregnancy, third trimester**   Ⓜ ♀

✓5th **O22.2**   **Superficial thrombophlebitis in pregnancy**

Phlebitis in pregnancy NOS
Thrombophlebitis of legs in pregnancy
Thrombosis in pregnancy NOS
Use additional code to identify the superficial thrombophlebitis (I80.0-)

O22.20   **Superficial thrombophlebitis in pregnancy, unspecified trimester**   Ⓜ ♀ ▽

O22.21   **Superficial thrombophlebitis in pregnancy, first trimester**   Ⓜ ♀

O22.22   **Superficial thrombophlebitis in pregnancy, second trimester**   Ⓜ ♀

O22.23   **Superficial thrombophlebitis in pregnancy, third trimester**   Ⓜ ♀

✓5th **O22.3**   **Deep phlebothrombosis in pregnancy**

Deep vein thrombosis, antepartum
Use additional code to identify the deep vein thrombosis (I82.4-, I82.5-, I82.62-. I82.72-)
Use additional code, if applicable, for associated long-term (current) use of anticoagulants (Z79.01)

O22.30   **Deep phlebothrombosis in pregnancy, unspecified trimester**   Ⓜ ♀ ▽

O22.31   **Deep phlebothrombosis in pregnancy, first trimester**   Ⓜ ♀

O22.32   **Deep phlebothrombosis in pregnancy, second trimester**   Ⓜ ♀

O22.33   **Deep phlebothrombosis in pregnancy, third trimester**   Ⓜ ♀

✓5th **O22.4**   **Hemorrhoids in pregnancy**

O22.40   **Hemorrhoids in pregnancy, unspecified trimester**   Ⓜ ♀ ▽

O22.41   **Hemorrhoids in pregnancy, first trimester**   Ⓜ ♀

O22.42   **Hemorrhoids in pregnancy, second trimester**   Ⓜ ♀

O22.43   **Hemorrhoids in pregnancy, third trimester**   Ⓜ ♀

✓5th **O22.5**   **Cerebral venous thrombosis in pregnancy**

Cerebrovenous sinus thrombosis in pregnancy

O22.50   **Cerebral venous thrombosis in pregnancy, unspecified trimester**   Ⓜ ♀ ▽

O22.51   **Cerebral venous thrombosis in pregnancy, first trimester**   Ⓜ ♀

O22.52   **Cerebral venous thrombosis in pregnancy, second trimester**   Ⓜ ♀

O22.53   **Cerebral venous thrombosis in pregnancy, third trimester**   Ⓜ ♀

✓5th **O22.8**   **Other venous complications in pregnancy**

✓6th **O22.8X**   **Other venous complications in pregnancy**

O22.8X1   **Other venous complications in pregnancy, first trimester**   Ⓜ ♀

O22.8X2   **Other venous complications in pregnancy, second trimester**   Ⓜ ♀

O22.8X3   **Other venous complications in pregnancy, third trimester**   Ⓜ ♀

O22.8X9   **Other venous complications in pregnancy, unspecified trimester**   Ⓜ ♀ ▽

✓5th **O22.9**   **Venous complication in pregnancy, unspecified**

Gestational phlebitis NOS
Gestational phlebopathy NOS
Gestational thrombosis NOS

O22.90   **Venous complication in pregnancy, unspecified, unspecified trimester**   Ⓜ ♀ ▽

O22.91   **Venous complication in pregnancy, unspecified, first trimester**   Ⓜ ♀ ▽

O22.92   **Venous complication in pregnancy, unspecified, second trimester**   Ⓜ ♀ ▽

O22.93   **Venous complication in pregnancy, unspecified, third trimester**   Ⓜ ♀ ▽

✓4th **O23**   **Infections of genitourinary tract in pregnancy**

Use additional code to identify organism (B95.-, B96.-)

EXCLUDES 2   gonococcal infections complicating pregnancy, childbirth and the puerperium (O98.2)
     infections with a predominantly sexual mode of transmission NOS complicating pregnancy, childbirth and the puerperium (O98.3)
     syphilis complicating pregnancy, childbirth and the puerperium (O98.1)
     tuberculosis of genitourinary system complicating pregnancy, childbirth and the puerperium (O98.0)
     venereal disease NOS complicating pregnancy, childbirth and the puerperium (O98.3)

✓5th **O23.0**   **Infections of kidney in pregnancy**

Pyelonephritis in pregnancy

O23.00   **Infections of kidney in pregnancy, unspecified trimester**   Ⓜ ♀ ▽

O23.01   **Infections of kidney in pregnancy, first trimester**   Ⓜ ♀

O23.02   **Infections of kidney in pregnancy, second trimester**   Ⓜ ♀

O23.03   **Infections of kidney in pregnancy, third trimester**   Ⓜ ♀

✓5th **O23.1**   **Infections of bladder in pregnancy**

O23.10   **Infections of bladder in pregnancy, unspecified trimester**   Ⓜ ♀ ▽

O23.11   **Infections of bladder in pregnancy, first trimester**   Ⓜ ♀

O23.12   **Infections of bladder in pregnancy, second trimester**   Ⓜ ♀

O23.13   **Infections of bladder in pregnancy, third trimester**   Ⓜ ♀

✓5th **O23.2**   **Infections of urethra in pregnancy**

O23.20   **Infections of urethra in pregnancy, unspecified trimester**   Ⓜ ♀ ▽

O23.21   **Infections of urethra in pregnancy, first trimester**   Ⓜ ♀

O23.22   **Infections of urethra in pregnancy, second trimester**   Ⓜ ♀

O23.23   **Infections of urethra in pregnancy, third trimester**   Ⓜ ♀

✓5th **O23.3**   **Infections of other parts of urinary tract in pregnancy**

O23.30   **Infections of other parts of urinary tract in pregnancy, unspecified trimester**   Ⓜ ♀ ▽

O23.31   **Infections of other parts of urinary tract in pregnancy, first trimester**   Ⓜ ♀

O23.32   **Infections of other parts of urinary tract in pregnancy, second trimester**   Ⓜ ♀

O23.33   **Infections of other parts of urinary tract in pregnancy, third trimester**   Ⓜ ♀

EXCLUDES 1 Not coded here   EXCLUDES 2 Not included here   Ⓝ Newborn Age : 0   Ⓟ Pediatric Age : 0-17   Ⓜ Maternity Age : 12-55   Ⓐ Adult Age : 15-124

810   ICD-10-CM 2017

Chapter 15. Pregnancy, Childbirth and the Puerperium

✓5th **O23.4** **Unspecified infection of urinary tract in pregnancy**

    O23.40 Unspecified infection of urinary tract in pregnancy, unspecified trimester   Ⓜ♀▽

    O23.41 Unspecified infection of urinary tract in pregnancy, first trimester   Ⓜ♀▽

    O23.42 Unspecified infection of urinary tract in pregnancy, second trimester   Ⓜ♀▽

    O23.43 Unspecified infection of urinary tract in pregnancy, third trimester   Ⓜ♀▽

✓5th **O23.5** **Infections of the genital tract in pregnancy**

  ✓6th **O23.51** **Infection of cervix in pregnancy**

      O23.511 Infections of cervix in pregnancy, first trimester   Ⓜ♀

      O23.512 Infections of cervix in pregnancy, second trimester   Ⓜ♀

      O23.513 Infections of cervix in pregnancy, third trimester   Ⓜ♀

      O23.519 Infections of cervix in pregnancy, unspecified trimester   Ⓜ♀▽

  ✓6th **O23.52** **Salpingo-oophoritis in pregnancy**

    Oophoritis in pregnancy

    Salpingitis in pregnancy

      O23.521 Salpingo-oophoritis in pregnancy, first trimester   Ⓜ♀

      O23.522 Salpingo-oophoritis in pregnancy, second trimester   Ⓜ♀

      O23.523 Salpingo-oophoritis in pregnancy, third trimester   Ⓜ♀

      O23.529 Salpingo-oophoritis in pregnancy, unspecified trimester   Ⓜ♀▽

  ✓6th **O23.59** **Infection of other part of genital tract in pregnancy**

      O23.591 Infection of other part of genital tract in pregnancy, first trimester   Ⓜ♀

      O23.592 Infection of other part of genital tract in pregnancy, second trimester   Ⓜ♀

      O23.593 Infection of other part of genital tract in pregnancy, third trimester   Ⓜ♀

      O23.599 Infection of other part of genital tract in pregnancy, unspecified trimester   Ⓜ♀▽

  ✓6th **O23.9** **Unspecified genitourinary tract infection in pregnancy**

    Genitourinary tract infection in pregnancy NOS

    O23.90 Unspecified genitourinary tract infection in pregnancy, unspecified trimester   Ⓜ♀▽

    O23.91 Unspecified genitourinary tract infection in pregnancy, first trimester   Ⓜ♀▽

    O23.92 Unspecified genitourinary tract infection in pregnancy, second trimester   Ⓜ♀▽

    O23.93 Unspecified genitourinary tract infection in pregnancy, third trimester   Ⓜ♀▽

✓4th **O24** **Diabetes mellitus in pregnancy, childbirth and the puerperium**

▲ ✓5th **O24.0** **Pre-existing type 1 diabetes mellitus, in pregnancy, childbirth and the puerperium**

    Juvenile onset diabetes mellitus, in pregnancy, childbirth and the puerperium

    Ketosis-prone diabetes mellitus in pregnancy, childbirth and the puerperium

    Use additional code from category E10 to further identify any manifestations

▲ ✓6th **O24.01** **Pre-existing type 1 diabetes mellitus, in pregnancy**

▲   **O24.011** Pre-existing type 1 diabetes mellitus, in pregnancy, first trimester   Ⓜ♀

▲   **O24.012** Pre-existing type 1 diabetes mellitus, in pregnancy, second trimester   Ⓜ♀

▲   **O24.013** Pre-existing type 1 diabetes mellitus, in pregnancy, third trimester   Ⓜ♀

▲   **O24.019** Pre-existing type 1 diabetes mellitus, in pregnancy, unspecified trimester   Ⓜ♀▽

▲   **O24.02** Pre-existing type 1 diabetes mellitus, in childbirth   Ⓜ♀

▲   **O24.03** Pre-existing type 1 diabetes mellitus, in the puerperium   Ⓜ♀

▲ ✓5th **O24.1** **Pre-existing type 2 diabetes mellitus, in pregnancy, childbirth and the puerperium**

    Insulin-resistant diabetes mellitus in pregnancy, childbirth and the puerperium

    Use additional code (for):

      from category E11 to further identify any manifestations

      long-term (current) use of insulin (Z79.4)

▲ ✓6th **O24.11** **Pre-existing type 2 diabetes mellitus, in pregnancy**

▲   **O24.111** Pre-existing type 2 diabetes mellitus, in pregnancy, first trimester   Ⓜ♀

    O24.112 Pre-existing type 2 diabetes mellitus, in pregnancy, second trimester   Ⓜ♀

    O24.113 Pre-existing type 2 diabetes mellitus, in pregnancy, third trimester   Ⓜ♀

▲   **O24.119** Pre-existing type 2 diabetes mellitus, in pregnancy, unspecified trimester   Ⓜ♀▽

▲   **O24.12** Pre-existing type 2 diabetes mellitus, in childbirth   Ⓜ♀

▲   **O24.13** Pre-existing type 2 diabetes mellitus, in the puerperium   Ⓜ♀

✓5th **O24.3** **Unspecified pre-existing diabetes mellitus in pregnancy, childbirth and the puerperium**

    Use additional code (for):

      from category E11 to further identify any manifestation

      long-term (current) use of insulin (Z79.4)

  ✓6th **O24.31** **Unspecified pre-existing diabetes mellitus in pregnancy**

      O24.311 Unspecified pre-existing diabetes mellitus in pregnancy, first trimester   Ⓜ♀▽

      O24.312 Unspecified pre-existing diabetes mellitus in pregnancy, second trimester   Ⓜ♀▽

      O24.313 Unspecified pre-existing diabetes mellitus in pregnancy, third trimester   Ⓜ♀▽

      O24.319 Unspecified pre-existing diabetes mellitus in pregnancy, unspecified trimester   Ⓜ♀▽

    O24.32 Unspecified pre-existing diabetes mellitus in childbirth   Ⓜ♀▽

    O24.33 Unspecified pre-existing diabetes mellitus in the puerperium   Ⓜ♀▽

✓5th **O24.4** **Gestational diabetes mellitus**

    Diabetes mellitus arising in pregnancy

    Gestational diabetes mellitus NOS

  ✓6th **O24.41** **Gestational diabetes mellitus in pregnancy**

      O24.410 Gestational diabetes mellitus in pregnancy, diet controlled   Ⓜ♀

      O24.414 Gestational diabetes mellitus in pregnancy, insulin controlled   Ⓜ♀

●   **O24.415** Gestational diabetes mellitus in pregnancy, controlled by oral hypoglycemic drugs

        Gestational diabetes mellitus in pregnancy, controlled by oral antidiabetic drugs

      O24.419 Gestational diabetes mellitus in pregnancy, unspecified control   Ⓜ♀▽

        AHA: 2015,4Q,34

  ✓6th **O24.42** **Gestational diabetes mellitus in childbirth**

    AHA: 2016,1Q,5

      O24.420 Gestational diabetes mellitus in childbirth, diet controlled   Ⓜ♀

      O24.424 Gestational diabetes mellitus in childbirth, insulin controlled   Ⓜ♀

●   **O24.425** Gestational diabetes mellitus in childbirth, controlled by oral hypoglycemic drugs

        Gestational diabetes mellitus in childbirth, controlled by oral antidiabetic drugs

      O24.429 Gestational diabetes mellitus in childbirth, unspecified control   Ⓜ♀▽

        AHA: 2015,4Q,34

  ✓6th **O24.43** **Gestational diabetes mellitus in the puerperium**

      O24.430 Gestational diabetes mellitus in the puerperium, diet controlled   Ⓜ♀

✓ Additional Character Required   ✓x7th Placeholder Alert   Manifestation Dx   ▽ Unspecified Dx   ►◄ Revised Text   ● New Code   ▲ Revised Code Title

ICD-10-CM 2017   811

Chapter 15. Pregnancy, Childbirth and the Puerperium

O24.434   **Gestational diabetes mellitus in the puerperium, insulin controlled**   Ⓜ ♀

O24.435   **Gestational diabetes mellitus in puerperium, controlled by oral hypoglycemic drugs**
Gestational diabetes mellitus in puerperium, controlled by oral antidiabetic drugs

O24.439   **Gestational diabetes mellitus in the puerperium, unspecified control**   Ⓜ ♀ ▽
    AHA: 2015,4Q,34

✓5ᵗʰ **O24.8**   **Other pre-existing diabetes mellitus in pregnancy, childbirth, and the puerperium**
Use additional code (for):
,   from categories E08, E09 and E13 to further identify any manifestation
long-term (current) use of insulin (Z79.4)

✓6ᵗʰ **O24.81**   **Other pre-existing diabetes mellitus in pregnancy**

O24.811   **Other pre-existing diabetes mellitus in pregnancy, first trimester**   Ⓜ ♀

O24.812   **Other pre-existing diabetes mellitus in pregnancy, second trimester**   Ⓜ ♀

O24.813   **Other pre-existing diabetes mellitus in pregnancy, third trimester**   Ⓜ ♀

O24.819   **Other pre-existing diabetes mellitus in pregnancy, unspecified trimester**   Ⓜ ♀ ▽

O24.82   **Other pre-existing diabetes mellitus in childbirth**   Ⓜ ♀

O24.83   **Other pre-existing diabetes mellitus in the puerperium**   Ⓜ ♀

✓5ᵗʰ **O24.9**   **Unspecified diabetes mellitus in pregnancy, childbirth and the puerperium**
Use additional code for long-term (current) use of insulin (Z79.4)

✓6ᵗʰ **O24.91**   **Unspecified diabetes mellitus in pregnancy**

O24.911   **Unspecified diabetes mellitus in pregnancy, first trimester**   Ⓜ ♀ ▽

O24.912   **Unspecified diabetes mellitus in pregnancy, second trimester**   Ⓜ ♀ ▽

O24.913   **Unspecified diabetes mellitus in pregnancy, third trimester**   Ⓜ ♀ ▽

O24.919   **Unspecified diabetes mellitus in pregnancy, unspecified trimester**   Ⓜ ♀ ▽

O24.92   **Unspecified diabetes mellitus in childbirth**   Ⓜ ♀ ▽

O24.93   **Unspecified diabetes mellitus in the puerperium**   Ⓜ ♀ ▽

✓4ᵗʰ **O25**   **Malnutrition in pregnancy, childbirth and the puerperium**

✓5ᵗʰ **O25.1**   **Malnutrition in pregnancy**

O25.10   **Malnutrition in pregnancy, unspecified trimester**   Ⓜ ♀ ▽

O25.11   **Malnutrition in pregnancy, first trimester**   Ⓜ ♀

O25.12   **Malnutrition in pregnancy, second trimester**   Ⓜ ♀

O25.13   **Malnutrition in pregnancy, third trimester**   Ⓜ ♀

O25.2   **Malnutrition in childbirth**   Ⓜ ♀

O25.3   **Malnutrition in the puerperium**   Ⓜ ♀

✓4ᵗʰ **O26**   **Maternal care for other conditions predominantly related to pregnancy**

✓5ᵗʰ **O26.0**   **Excessive weight gain in pregnancy**
    EXCLUDES 2   gestational edema (O12.0, O12.2)

O26.00   **Excessive weight gain in pregnancy, unspecified trimester**   Ⓜ ♀ ▽

O26.01   **Excessive weight gain in pregnancy, first trimester**   Ⓜ ♀

O26.02   **Excessive weight gain in pregnancy, second trimester**   Ⓜ ♀

O26.03   **Excessive weight gain in pregnancy, third trimester**   Ⓜ ♀

✓5ᵗʰ **O26.1**   **Low weight gain in pregnancy**

O26.10   **Low weight gain in pregnancy, unspecified trimester**   Ⓜ ♀ ▽

O26.11   **Low weight gain in pregnancy, first trimester**   Ⓜ ♀

O26.12   **Low weight gain in pregnancy, second trimester**   Ⓜ ♀

O26.13   **Low weight gain in pregnancy, third trimester**   Ⓜ ♀

✓5ᵗʰ **O26.2**   **Pregnancy care for patient with recurrent pregnancy loss**

O26.20   **Pregnancy care for patient with recurrent pregnancy loss, unspecified trimester**   Ⓜ ♀ ▽

O26.21   **Pregnancy care for patient with recurrent pregnancy loss, first trimester**   Ⓜ ♀

O26.22   **Pregnancy care for patient with recurrent pregnancy loss, second trimester**   Ⓜ ♀

O26.23   **Pregnancy care for patient with recurrent pregnancy loss, third trimester**   Ⓜ ♀

✓5ᵗʰ **O26.3**   **Retained intrauterine contraceptive device in pregnancy**

O26.30   **Retained intrauterine contraceptive device in pregnancy, unspecified trimester**   Ⓜ ♀ ▽

O26.31   **Retained intrauterine contraceptive device in pregnancy, first trimester**   Ⓜ ♀

O26.32   **Retained intrauterine contraceptive device in pregnancy, second trimester**   Ⓜ ♀

O26.33   **Retained intrauterine contraceptive device in pregnancy, third trimester**   Ⓜ ♀

✓5ᵗʰ **O26.4**   **Herpes gestationis**

O26.40   **Herpes gestationis, unspecified trimester**   Ⓜ ♀ ▽

O26.41   **Herpes gestationis, first trimester**   Ⓜ ♀

O26.42   **Herpes gestationis, second trimester**   Ⓜ ♀

O26.43   **Herpes gestationis, third trimester**   Ⓜ ♀

✓5ᵗʰ **O26.5**   **Maternal hypotension syndrome**
Supine hypotensive syndrome

O26.50   **Maternal hypotension syndrome, unspecified trimester**   Ⓜ ♀ ▽

O26.51   **Maternal hypotension syndrome, first trimester**   Ⓜ ♀

O26.52   **Maternal hypotension syndrome, second trimester**   Ⓜ ♀

O26.53   **Maternal hypotension syndrome, third trimester**   Ⓜ ♀

✓5ᵗʰ **O26.6**   **Liver and biliary tract disorders in pregnancy, childbirth and the puerperium**
Use additional code to identify the specific disorder
    EXCLUDES 2   hepatorenal syndrome following labor and delivery (O90.4)

✓6ᵗʰ **O26.61**   **Liver and biliary tract disorders in pregnancy**

O26.611   **Liver and biliary tract disorders in pregnancy, first trimester**   Ⓜ ♀

O26.612   **Liver and biliary tract disorders in pregnancy, second trimester**   Ⓜ ♀

O26.613   **Liver and biliary tract disorders in pregnancy, third trimester**   Ⓜ ♀

O26.619   **Liver and biliary tract disorders in pregnancy, unspecified trimester**   Ⓜ ♀ ▽

O26.62   **Liver and biliary tract disorders in childbirth**   Ⓜ ♀

O26.63   **Liver and biliary tract disorders in the puerperium**   Ⓜ ♀

✓5ᵗʰ **O26.7**   **Subluxation of symphysis (pubis) in pregnancy, childbirth and the puerperium**
    EXCLUDES 1   traumatic separation of symphysis (pubis) during childbirth (O71.6)

✓6ᵗʰ **O26.71**   **Subluxation of symphysis (pubis) in pregnancy**

O26.711   **Subluxation of symphysis (pubis) in pregnancy, first trimester**   Ⓜ ♀

O26.712   **Subluxation of symphysis (pubis) in pregnancy, second trimester**   Ⓜ ♀

O26.713   **Subluxation of symphysis (pubis) in pregnancy, third trimester**   Ⓜ ♀

O26.719   **Subluxation of symphysis (pubis) in pregnancy, unspecified trimester**   Ⓜ ♀ ▽

O26.72   **Subluxation of symphysis (pubis) in childbirth**   Ⓜ ♀

O26.73   **Subluxation of symphysis (pubis) in the puerperium**   Ⓜ ♀

✓5ᵗʰ **O26.8**   **Other specified pregnancy related conditions**

✓6ᵗʰ **O26.81**   **Pregnancy related exhaustion and fatigue**

O26.811   **Pregnancy related exhaustion and fatigue, first trimester**   Ⓜ ♀

O26.812   **Pregnancy related exhaustion and fatigue, second trimester**   Ⓜ ♀

O26.813   **Pregnancy related exhaustion and fatigue, third trimester**   Ⓜ ♀

O26.819   **Pregnancy related exhaustion and fatigue, unspecified trimester**   Ⓜ ♀ ▽

EXCLUDES 1 Not coded here   *EXCLUDES 2* Not included here   Ⓝ Newborn Age : 0   Ⓟ Pediatric Age : 0-17   Ⓜ Maternity Age : 12-55   Ⓐ Adult Age : 15-124

812   **ICD-10-CM 2017**

√6ᵗʰ **O26.82 Pregnancy related peripheral neuritis**

     O26.821 Pregnancy related peripheral neuritis, first trimester Ⓜ ♀

     O26.822 Pregnancy related peripheral neuritis, second trimester Ⓜ ♀

     O26.823 Pregnancy related peripheral neuritis, third trimester Ⓜ ♀

     O26.829 Pregnancy related peripheral neuritis, unspecified trimester Ⓜ ♀ ▽

√6ᵗʰ **O26.83 Pregnancy related renal disease**

     Use additional code to identify the specific disorder

     O26.831 Pregnancy related renal disease, first trimester Ⓜ ♀

     O26.832 Pregnancy related renal disease, second trimester Ⓜ ♀

     O26.833 Pregnancy related renal disease, third trimester Ⓜ ♀

     O26.839 Pregnancy related renal disease, unspecified trimester Ⓜ ♀ ▽

√6ᵗʰ **O26.84 Uterine size-date discrepancy complicating pregnancy**

     EXCLUDES 1 encounter for suspected problem with fetal growth ruled out (Z03.74)

     O26.841 Uterine size-date discrepancy, first trimester Ⓜ ♀

     O26.842 Uterine size-date discrepancy, second trimester Ⓜ ♀

     O26.843 Uterine size-date discrepancy, third trimester Ⓜ ♀

     O26.849 Uterine size-date discrepancy, unspecified trimester Ⓜ ♀ ▽

√6ᵗʰ **O26.85 Spotting complicating pregnancy**

     O26.851 Spotting complicating pregnancy, first trimester Ⓜ ♀

     O26.852 Spotting complicating pregnancy, second trimester Ⓜ ♀

     O26.853 Spotting complicating pregnancy, third trimester Ⓜ ♀

     O26.859 Spotting complicating pregnancy, unspecified trimester Ⓜ ♀ ▽

O26.86 Pruritic urticarial papules and plaques of pregnancy (PUPPP) Ⓜ ♀

     Polymorphic eruption of pregnancy

√6ᵗʰ **O26.87 Cervical shortening**

     EXCLUDES 1 encounter for suspected cervical shortening ruled out (Z03.75)

     DEF: A cervix that has shortened to < 25 mm before the 24th week of pregnancy; warning sign for impending premature delivery; treated by cervical cerclage placement or progesterone.

     O26.872 Cervical shortening, second trimester Ⓜ ♀

     O26.873 Cervical shortening, third trimester Ⓜ ♀

     O26.879 Cervical shortening, unspecified trimester Ⓜ ♀ ▽

√6ᵗʰ **O26.89 Other specified pregnancy related conditions**

     AHA: 2015,3Q,40

     O26.891 Other specified pregnancy related conditions, first trimester Ⓜ ♀

     O26.892 Other specified pregnancy related conditions, second trimester Ⓜ ♀

     O26.893 Other specified pregnancy related conditions, third trimester Ⓜ ♀

     O26.899 Other specified pregnancy related conditions, unspecified trimester Ⓜ ♀ ▽

√5ᵗʰ **O26.9 Pregnancy related conditions, unspecified**

     O26.90 Pregnancy related conditions, unspecified, unspecified trimester Ⓜ ♀ ▽

     O26.91 Pregnancy related conditions, unspecified, first trimester Ⓜ ♀ ▽

     O26.92 Pregnancy related conditions, unspecified, second trimester Ⓜ ♀ ▽

     O26.93 Pregnancy related conditions, unspecified, third trimester Ⓜ ♀ ▽

√4ᵗʰ **O28 Abnormal findings on antenatal screening of mother**

     EXCLUDES 1 diagnostic findings classified elsewhere - see Alphabetical Index

O28.0 Abnormal hematological finding on antenatal screening of mother Ⓜ ♀

O28.1 Abnormal biochemical finding on antenatal screening of mother Ⓜ ♀

O28.2 Abnormal cytological finding on antenatal screening of mother Ⓜ ♀

O28.3 Abnormal ultrasonic finding on antenatal screening of mother Ⓜ ♀

O28.4 Abnormal radiological finding on antenatal screening of mother Ⓜ ♀

O28.5 Abnormal chromosomal and genetic finding on antenatal screening of mother Ⓜ ♀

O28.8 Other abnormal findings on antenatal screening of mother Ⓜ ♀

O28.9 Unspecified abnormal findings on antenatal screening of mother Ⓜ ♀ ▽

√4ᵗʰ **O29 Complications of anesthesia during pregnancy**

     INCLUDES maternal complications arising from the administration of a general, regional or local anesthetic, analgesic or other sedation during pregnancy

     Use additional code, if necessary, to identify the complication

     EXCLUDES 2 complications of anesthesia during labor and delivery (O74.-)
     complications of anesthesia during the puerperium (O89.-)

√5ᵗʰ **O29.0 Pulmonary complications of anesthesia during pregnancy**

     √6ᵗʰ **O29.01 Aspiration pneumonitis due to anesthesia during pregnancy**

       Inhalation of stomach contents or secretions NOS due to anesthesia during pregnancy

       Mendelson's syndrome due to anesthesia during pregnancy

       O29.011 Aspiration pneumonitis due to anesthesia during pregnancy, first trimester Ⓜ ♀

       O29.012 Aspiration pneumonitis due to anesthesia during pregnancy, second trimester Ⓜ ♀

       O29.013 Aspiration pneumonitis due to anesthesia during pregnancy, third trimester Ⓜ ♀

       O29.019 Aspiration pneumonitis due to anesthesia during pregnancy, unspecified trimester Ⓜ ♀ ▽

     √6ᵗʰ **O29.02 Pressure collapse of lung due to anesthesia during pregnancy**

       O29.021 Pressure collapse of lung due to anesthesia during pregnancy, first trimester Ⓜ ♀

       O29.022 Pressure collapse of lung due to anesthesia during pregnancy, second trimester Ⓜ ♀

       O29.023 Pressure collapse of lung due to anesthesia during pregnancy, third trimester Ⓜ ♀

       O29.029 Pressure collapse of lung due to anesthesia during pregnancy, unspecified trimester Ⓜ ♀ ▽

     √6ᵗʰ **O29.09 Other pulmonary complications of anesthesia during pregnancy**

       O29.091 Other pulmonary complications of anesthesia during pregnancy, first trimester Ⓜ ♀

       O29.092 Other pulmonary complications of anesthesia during pregnancy, second trimester Ⓜ ♀

       O29.093 Other pulmonary complications of anesthesia during pregnancy, third trimester Ⓜ ♀

       O29.099 Other pulmonary complications of anesthesia during pregnancy, unspecified trimester Ⓜ ♀ ▽

√5ᵗʰ **O29.1 Cardiac complications of anesthesia during pregnancy**

     √6ᵗʰ **O29.11 Cardiac arrest due to anesthesia during pregnancy**

       O29.111 Cardiac arrest due to anesthesia during pregnancy, first trimester Ⓜ ♀

       O29.112 Cardiac arrest due to anesthesia during pregnancy, second trimester Ⓜ ♀

       O29.113 Cardiac arrest due to anesthesia during pregnancy, third trimester Ⓜ ♀

       O29.119 Cardiac arrest due to anesthesia during pregnancy, unspecified trimester Ⓜ ♀ ▽

✔ Additional Character Required   √x7ᵗʰ Placeholder Alert   Manifestation Dx   ▽ Unspecified Dx   ▶◀ Revised Text   ● New Code   ▲ Revised Code Title

✓6ᵗʰ **O29.12   Cardiac failure due to anesthesia during pregnancy**

O29.121   Cardiac failure due to anesthesia Ⓜ ♀
during pregnancy, first trimester

O29.122   Cardiac failure due to anesthesia Ⓜ ♀
**during pregnancy, second
trimester**

O29.123   Cardiac failure due to anesthesia Ⓜ ♀
during pregnancy, third trimester

O29.129   Cardiac failure due to anesthesia Ⓜ ♀ ▽
**during pregnancy, unspecified
trimester**

✓6ᵗʰ **O29.19   Other cardiac complications of anesthesia during
pregnancy**

O29.191   Other cardiac complications of Ⓜ ♀
**anesthesia during pregnancy, first
trimester**

O29.192   Other cardiac complications of Ⓜ ♀
**anesthesia during pregnancy,
second trimester**

O29.193   Other cardiac complications of Ⓜ ♀
**anesthesia during pregnancy,
third trimester**

O29.199   Other cardiac complications of Ⓜ ♀ ▽
**anesthesia during pregnancy,
unspecified trimester**

✓5ᵗʰ **O29.2   Central nervous system complications of anesthesia during
pregnancy**

✓6ᵗʰ **O29.21   Cerebral anoxia due to anesthesia during
pregnancy**

O29.211   Cerebral anoxia due to anesthesia Ⓜ ♀
during pregnancy, first trimester

O29.212   Cerebral anoxia due to anesthesia Ⓜ ♀
**during pregnancy, second
trimester**

O29.213   Cerebral anoxia due to anesthesia Ⓜ ♀
during pregnancy, third trimester

O29.219   Cerebral anoxia due to anesthesia Ⓜ ♀ ▽
**during pregnancy, unspecified
trimester**

✓6ᵗʰ **O29.29   Other central nervous system complications of
anesthesia during pregnancy**

O29.291   Other central nervous system Ⓜ ♀
**complications of anesthesia
during pregnancy, first trimester**

O29.292   Other central nervous system Ⓜ ♀
**complications of anesthesia
during pregnancy, second
trimester**

O29.293   Other central nervous system Ⓜ ♀
**complications of anesthesia
during pregnancy, third trimester**

O29.299   Other central nervous system Ⓜ ♀ ▽
**complications of anesthesia
during pregnancy, unspecified
trimester**

✓5ᵗʰ **O29.3   Toxic reaction to local anesthesia during pregnancy**

✓6ᵗʰ **O29.3X   Toxic reaction to local anesthesia during pregnancy**

O29.3X1   Toxic reaction to local anesthesia Ⓜ ♀
during pregnancy, first trimester

O29.3X2   Toxic reaction to local anesthesia Ⓜ ♀
**during pregnancy, second
trimester**

O29.3X3   Toxic reaction to local anesthesia Ⓜ ♀
during pregnancy, third trimester

O29.3X9   Toxic reaction to local anesthesia Ⓜ ♀ ▽
**during pregnancy, unspecified
trimester**

✓5ᵗʰ **O29.4   Spinal and epidural anesthesia induced headache during
pregnancy**

O29.40   Spinal and epidural anesthesia induced Ⓜ ♀ ▽
**headache during pregnancy, unspecified
trimester**

O29.41   Spinal and epidural anesthesia induced Ⓜ ♀
headache during pregnancy, first trimester

O29.42   Spinal and epidural anesthesia induced Ⓜ ♀
**headache during pregnancy, second
trimester**

O29.43   Spinal and epidural anesthesia induced Ⓜ ♀
headache during pregnancy, third trimester

✓5ᵗʰ **O29.5   Other complications of spinal and epidural anesthesia during
pregnancy**

✓6ᵗʰ **O29.5X   Other complications of spinal and epidural
anesthesia during pregnancy**

O29.5X1   Other complications of spinal and Ⓜ ♀
**epidural anesthesia during
pregnancy, first trimester**

O29.5X2   Other complications of spinal and Ⓜ ♀
**epidural anesthesia during
pregnancy, second trimester**

O29.5X3   Other complications of spinal and Ⓜ ♀
**epidural anesthesia during
pregnancy, third trimester**

O29.5X9   Other complications of spinal and Ⓜ ♀ ▽
**epidural anesthesia during
pregnancy, unspecified trimester**

✓5ᵗʰ **O29.6   Failed or difficult intubation for anesthesia during pregnancy**

O29.60   Failed or difficult intubation for anesthesia Ⓜ ♀ ▽
during pregnancy, unspecified trimester

O29.61   Failed or difficult intubation for anesthesia Ⓜ ♀
during pregnancy, first trimester

O29.62   Failed or difficult intubation for anesthesia Ⓜ ♀
during pregnancy, second trimester

O29.63   Failed or difficult intubation for anesthesia Ⓜ ♀
during pregnancy, third trimester

✓5ᵗʰ **O29.8   Other complications of anesthesia during pregnancy**

✓6ᵗʰ **O29.8X   Other complications of anesthesia during
pregnancy**

O29.8X1   Other complications of anesthesia Ⓜ ♀
during pregnancy, first trimester

O29.8X2   Other complications of anesthesia Ⓜ ♀
**during pregnancy, second
trimester**

O29.8X3   Other complications of anesthesia Ⓜ ♀
during pregnancy, third trimester

O29.8X9   Other complications of anesthesia Ⓜ ♀ ▽
**during pregnancy, unspecified
trimester**

✓5ᵗʰ **O29.9   Unspecified complication of anesthesia during pregnancy**

O29.90   Unspecified complication of anesthesia Ⓜ ♀ ▽
during pregnancy, unspecified trimester

O29.91   Unspecified complication of anesthesia Ⓜ ♀ ▽
during pregnancy, first trimester

O29.92   Unspecified complication of anesthesia Ⓜ ♀ ▽
during pregnancy, second trimester

O29.93   Unspecified complication of anesthesia Ⓜ ♀ ▽
during pregnancy, third trimester

Maternal care related to the fetus and amniotic cavity and possible delivery problems (O30-O48)

✓4ᵗʰ **O30   Multiple gestation**

Code also any complications specific to multiple gestation

✓5ᵗʰ **O30.0   Twin pregnancy**

✓6ᵗʰ **O30.00   Twin pregnancy, unspecified number of placenta
and unspecified number of amniotic sacs**

O30.001   Twin pregnancy, unspecified Ⓜ ♀ ▽
**number of placenta and
unspecified number of amniotic
sacs, first trimester**

O30.002   Twin pregnancy, unspecified Ⓜ ♀ ▽
**number of placenta and
unspecified number of amniotic
sacs, second trimester**

O30.003   Twin pregnancy, unspecified Ⓜ ♀ ▽
**number of placenta and
unspecified number of amniotic
sacs, third trimester**

O30.009   Twin pregnancy, unspecified Ⓜ ♀ ▽
**number of placenta and
unspecified number of amniotic
sacs, unspecified trimester**

✓6ᵗʰ **O30.01   Twin pregnancy, monochorionic/monoamniotic**

Twin pregnancy, one placenta, one amniotic sac

EXCLUDES 1 conjoined twins (O30.02-)

O30.011   Twin pregnancy, Ⓜ ♀
**monochorionic/monoamniotic,
first trimester**

O30.012   Twin pregnancy, Ⓜ ♀
**monochorionic/monoamniotic,
second trimester**

O30.013   Twin pregnancy, Ⓜ ♀
**monochorionic/monoamniotic,
third trimester**

EXCLUDES 1 Not coded here   *EXCLUDES 2* Not included here   Ⓝ Newborn Age : 0   Ⓟ Pediatric Age : 0-17   Ⓜ Maternity Age : 12-55   Ⓐ Adult Age : 15-124

814   ICD-10-CM 2017

O30.019   Twin pregnancy, monochorionic/monoamniotic, unspecified trimester   M ♀ ▽

✓6ᵗʰ   **O30.02**   **Conjoined** twin pregnancy

O30.021   Conjoined twin pregnancy, first trimester   M ♀

O30.022   Conjoined twin pregnancy, second trimester   M ♀

O30.023   Conjoined twin pregnancy, third trimester   M ♀

O30.029   Conjoined twin pregnancy, unspecified trimester   M ♀ ▽

✓6ᵗʰ   **O30.03**   Twin pregnancy, **monochorionic/diamniotic**

Twin pregnancy, one placenta, two amniotic sacs

O30.031   Twin pregnancy, monochorionic/diamniotic, first trimester   M ♀

O30.032   Twin pregnancy, monochorionic/diamniotic, second trimester   M ♀

O30.033   Twin pregnancy, monochorionic/diamniotic, third trimester   M ♀

O30.039   Twin pregnancy, monochorionic/diamniotic, unspecified trimester   M ♀ ▽

✓6ᵗʰ   **O30.04**   Twin pregnancy, **dichorionic/diamniotic**

Twin pregnancy, two placentae, two amniotic sacs

O30.041   Twin pregnancy, dichorionic/diamniotic, first trimester   M ♀

O30.042   Twin pregnancy, dichorionic/diamniotic, second trimester   M ♀

O30.043   Twin pregnancy, dichorionic/diamniotic, third trimester   M ♀

O30.049   Twin pregnancy, dichorionic/diamniotic, unspecified trimester   M ♀ ▽

✓6ᵗʰ   **O30.09**   Twin pregnancy, unable to determine number of placenta and number of amniotic sacs

O30.091   Twin pregnancy, unable to determine number of placenta and number of amniotic sacs, first trimester   M ♀

O30.092   Twin pregnancy, unable to determine number of placenta and number of amniotic sacs, second trimester   M ♀

O30.093   Twin pregnancy, unable to determine number of placenta and number of amniotic sacs, third trimester   M ♀

O30.099   Twin pregnancy, unable to determine number of placenta and number of amniotic sacs, unspecified trimester   M ♀ ▽

✓5ᵗʰ   **O30.1**   **Triplet pregnancy**

✓6ᵗʰ   **O30.10**   Triplet pregnancy, unspecified number of placenta and unspecified number of amniotic sacs

     AHA: 2016,2Q,8

O30.101   Triplet pregnancy, unspecified number of placenta and unspecified number of amniotic sacs, first trimester   M ♀ ▽

O30.102   Triplet pregnancy, unspecified number of placenta and unspecified number of amniotic sacs, second trimester   M ♀ ▽

O30.103   Triplet pregnancy, unspecified number of placenta and unspecified number of amniotic sacs, third trimester   M ♀ ▽

O30.109   Triplet pregnancy, unspecified number of placenta and unspecified number of amniotic sacs, unspecified trimester   M ♀ ▽

✓6ᵗʰ   **O30.11**   Triplet pregnancy with two or more monochorionic fetuses

O30.111   Triplet pregnancy with two or more monochorionic fetuses, first trimester   M ♀

O30.112   Triplet pregnancy with two or more monochorionic fetuses, second trimester   M ♀

O30.113   Triplet pregnancy with two or more monochorionic fetuses, third trimester   M ♀

O30.119   Triplet pregnancy with two or more monochorionic fetuses, unspecified trimester   M ♀ ▽

✓6ᵗʰ   **O30.12**   Triplet pregnancy with two or more monoamniotic fetuses

O30.121   Triplet pregnancy with two or more monoamniotic fetuses, first trimester   M ♀

O30.122   Triplet pregnancy with two or more monoamniotic fetuses, second trimester   M ♀

O30.123   Triplet pregnancy with two or more monoamniotic fetuses, third trimester   M ♀

O30.129   Triplet pregnancy with two or more monoamniotic fetuses, unspecified trimester   M ♀ ▽

✓6ᵗʰ   **O30.19**   Triplet pregnancy, unable to determine number of placenta and number of amniotic sacs

O30.191   Triplet pregnancy, unable to determine number of placenta and number of amniotic sacs, first trimester   M ♀

O30.192   Triplet pregnancy, unable to determine number of placenta and number of amniotic sacs, second trimester   M ♀

O30.193   Triplet pregnancy, unable to determine number of placenta and number of amniotic sacs, third trimester   M ♀

O30.199   Triplet pregnancy, unable to determine number of placenta and number of amniotic sacs, unspecified trimester   M ♀ ▽

✓5ᵗʰ   **O30.2**   **Quadruplet pregnancy**

✓6ᵗʰ   **O30.20**   Quadruplet pregnancy, unspecified number of placenta and unspecified number of amniotic sacs

O30.201   Quadruplet pregnancy, unspecified number of placenta and unspecified number of amniotic sacs, first trimester   M ♀ ▽

O30.202   Quadruplet pregnancy, unspecified number of placenta and unspecified number of amniotic sacs, second trimester   M ♀ ▽

O30.203   Quadruplet pregnancy, unspecified number of placenta and unspecified number of amniotic sacs, third trimester   M ♀ ▽

O30.209   Quadruplet pregnancy, unspecified number of placenta and unspecified number of amniotic sacs, unspecified trimester   M ♀ ▽

✓6ᵗʰ   **O30.21**   Quadruplet pregnancy with two or more monochorionic fetuses

O30.211   Quadruplet pregnancy with two or more monochorionic fetuses, first trimester   M ♀

O30.212   Quadruplet pregnancy with two or more monochorionic fetuses, second trimester   M ♀

O30.213   Quadruplet pregnancy with two or more monochorionic fetuses, third trimester   M ♀

O30.219   Quadruplet pregnancy with two or more monochorionic fetuses, unspecified trimester   M ♀ ▽

✓6ᵗʰ   **O30.22**   Quadruplet pregnancy with two or more monoamniotic fetuses

O30.221   Quadruplet pregnancy with two or more monoamniotic fetuses, first trimester   M ♀

O30.222   Quadruplet pregnancy with two or more monoamniotic fetuses, second trimester   M ♀

☑ Additional Character Required   ✓x7ᵗʰ Placeholder Alert   Manifestation Dx   ▽ Unspecified Dx   ►◄ Revised Text   ● New Code   ▲ Revised Code Title

O30.223 **Quadruplet pregnancy with two** Ⓜ ♀
or more monoamniotic fetuses,
third trimester

O30.229 **Quadruplet pregnancy with two** Ⓜ ♀ ▽
or more monoamniotic fetuses,
unspecified trimester

√6ᵗʰ **O30.29** **Quadruplet pregnancy, unable to determine**
number of placenta and number of amniotic sacs

O30.291 **Quadruplet pregnancy, unable to** Ⓜ ♀
determine number of placenta and
number of amniotic sacs, first
trimester

O30.292 **Quadruplet pregnancy, unable to** Ⓜ ♀
determine number of placenta and
number of amniotic sacs, second
trimester

O30.293 **Quadruplet pregnancy, unable to** Ⓜ ♀
determine number of placenta and
number of amniotic sacs, third
trimester

O30.299 **Quadruplet pregnancy, unable to** Ⓜ ♀ ▽
determine number of placenta and
number of amniotic sacs,
unspecified trimester

√5ᵗʰ **O30.8** **Other specified multiple gestation**

Multiple gestation pregnancy greater then quadruplets

√6ᵗʰ **O30.80** **Other specified multiple gestation, unspecified**
number of placenta and unspecified number of
amniotic sacs

O30.801 **Other specified multiple gestation,** Ⓜ ♀ ▽
unspecified number of placenta
and unspecified number of
amniotic sacs, first trimester

O30.802 **Other specified multiple gestation,** Ⓜ ♀ ▽
unspecified number of placenta
and unspecified number of
amniotic sacs, second trimester

O30.803 **Other specified multiple gestation,** Ⓜ ♀ ▽
unspecified number of placenta
and unspecified number of
amniotic sacs, third trimester

O30.809 **Other specified multiple gestation,** Ⓜ ♀ ▽
unspecified number of placenta
and unspecified number of
amniotic sacs, unspecified
trimester

√6ᵗʰ **O30.81** **Other specified multiple gestation with two or more**
monochorionic fetuses

O30.811 **Other specified multiple gestation** Ⓜ ♀
with two or more monochorionic
fetuses, first trimester

O30.812 **Other specified multiple gestation** Ⓜ ♀
with two or more monochorionic
fetuses, second trimester

O30.813 **Other specified multiple gestation** Ⓜ ♀
with two or more monochorionic
fetuses, third trimester

O30.819 **Other specified multiple gestation** Ⓜ ♀ ▽
with two or more monochorionic
fetuses, unspecified trimester

√6ᵗʰ **O30.82** **Other specified multiple gestation with two or more**
monoamniotic fetuses

O30.821 **Other specified multiple gestation** Ⓜ ♀
with two or more monoamniotic
fetuses, first trimester

O30.822 **Other specified multiple gestation** Ⓜ ♀
with two or more monoamniotic
fetuses, second trimester

O30.823 **Other specified multiple gestation** Ⓜ ♀
with two or more monoamniotic
fetuses, third trimester

O30.829 **Other specified multiple gestation** Ⓜ ♀ ▽
with two or more monoamniotic
fetuses, unspecified trimester

√6ᵗʰ **O30.89** **Other specified multiple gestation, unable to**
determine number of placenta and number of
amniotic sacs

O30.891 **Other specified multiple gestation,** Ⓜ ♀
unable to determine number of
placenta and number of amniotic
sacs, first trimester

O30.892 **Other specified multiple gestation,** Ⓜ ♀
unable to determine number of
placenta and number of amniotic
sacs, second trimester

O30.893 **Other specified multiple gestation,** Ⓜ ♀
unable to determine number of
placenta and number of amniotic
sacs, third trimester

O30.899 **Other specified multiple gestation,** Ⓜ ♀ ▽
unable to determine number of
placenta and number of amniotic
sacs, unspecified trimester

√5ᵗʰ **O30.9** **Multiple gestation, unspecified**

Multiple pregnancy NOS

O30.90 **Multiple gestation, unspecified, unspecified** Ⓜ ♀ ▽
trimester

O30.91 **Multiple gestation, unspecified, first** Ⓜ ♀ ▽
trimester

O30.92 **Multiple gestation, unspecified, second** Ⓜ ♀ ▽
trimester

O30.93 **Multiple gestation, unspecified, third** Ⓜ ♀ ▽
trimester

√4ᵗʰ **O31** **Complications specific to multiple gestation**

EXCLUDES 2   *delayed delivery of second twin, triplet, etc. (O63.2)*
malpresentation of one fetus or more (O32.9)
placental transfusion syndromes (O43.0-)

AHA: 2012,4Q,107

One of the following 7th characters is to be assigned to each code
under category O31. 7th character 0 is for single gestations and
multiple gestations where the fetus is unspecified. 7th characters 1
through 9 are for cases of multiple gestations to identify the fetus for
which the code applies. The appropriate code from category O30,
Multiple gestation, must also be assigned when assigning a code
from category O31 that has a 7th character of 1 through 9.

0   not applicable or unspecified
1   fetus 1
2   fetus 2
3   fetus 3
4   fetus 4
5   fetus 5
9   fetus 9

√5ᵗʰ **O31.0** **Papyraceous fetus**

Fetus compressus

√7ᵗʰ **O31.00** **Papyraceous fetus, unspecified trimester** Ⓜ ♀ ▽

√7ᵗʰ **O31.01** **Papyraceous fetus, first trimester** Ⓜ ♀

√7ᵗʰ **O31.02** **Papyraceous fetus, second trimester** Ⓜ ♀

√7ᵗʰ **O31.03** **Papyraceous fetus, third trimester** Ⓜ ♀

√5ᵗʰ **O31.1** **Continuing pregnancy after spontaneous abortion of one**
fetus or more

√7ᵗʰ **O31.10** **Continuing pregnancy after spontaneous** Ⓜ ♀ ▽
abortion of one fetus or more, unspecified
trimester

√7ᵗʰ **O31.11** **Continuing pregnancy after spontaneous** Ⓜ ♀
abortion of one fetus or more, first trimester

√7ᵗʰ **O31.12** **Continuing pregnancy after spontaneous** Ⓜ ♀
abortion of one fetus or more, second
trimester

√7ᵗʰ **O31.13** **Continuing pregnancy after spontaneous** Ⓜ ♀
abortion of one fetus or more, third
trimester

√5ᵗʰ **O31.2** **Continuing pregnancy after intrauterine death of one fetus**
or more

√7ᵗʰ **O31.20** **Continuing pregnancy after intrauterine** Ⓜ ♀ ▽
death of one fetus or more, unspecified
trimester

√7ᵗʰ **O31.21** **Continuing pregnancy after intrauterine** Ⓜ ♀
death of one fetus or more, first trimester

√7ᵗʰ **O31.22** **Continuing pregnancy after intrauterine** Ⓜ ♀
death of one fetus or more, second trimester

√7ᵗʰ **O31.23** **Continuing pregnancy after intrauterine** Ⓜ ♀
death of one fetus or more, third trimester

√5ᵗʰ **O31.3** **Continuing pregnancy after elective fetal reduction of one**
fetus or more

Continuing pregnancy after selective termination of one fetus
or more

√7ᵗʰ **O31.30** **Continuing pregnancy after elective fetal** Ⓜ ♀ ▽
reduction of one fetus or more, unspecified
trimester

√7ᵗʰ **O31.31** **Continuing pregnancy after elective fetal** Ⓜ ♀
reduction of one fetus or more, first
trimester

EXCLUDES 1   Not coded here   EXCLUDES 2   Not included here   Ⓝ Newborn Age : 0   Ⓟ Pediatric Age : 0-17   Ⓜ Maternity Age : 12-55   Ⓐ Adult Age : 15-124

816

ICD-10-CM 2017

√x7ᵗʰ **O31.32**　**Continuing pregnancy after elective fetal reduction of one fetus or more, second trimester**　Ⓜ ♀

√x7ᵗʰ **O31.33**　**Continuing pregnancy after elective fetal reduction of one fetus or more, third trimester**　Ⓜ ♀

√5ᵗʰ **O31.8**　**Other complications specific to multiple gestation**

　√6ᵗʰ **O31.8X**　**Other complications specific to multiple gestation**

　　√7ᵗʰ **O31.8X1**　**Other complications specific to multiple gestation, first trimester**　Ⓜ ♀

　　√7ᵗʰ **O31.8X2**　**Other complications specific to multiple gestation, second trimester**　Ⓜ ♀

　　√7ᵗʰ **O31.8X3**　**Other complications specific to multiple gestation, third trimester**　Ⓜ ♀

　　√7ᵗʰ **O31.8X9**　**Other complications specific to multiple gestation, unspecified trimester**　Ⓜ ♀ ▽

√4ᵗʰ **O32**　**Maternal care for malpresentation of fetus**

　INCLUDES　the listed conditions as a reason for observation, hospitalization or other obstetric care of the mother, or for cesarean delivery before onset of labor

　EXCLUDES 1　*malpresentation of fetus with obstructed labor (O64.-)*

　AHA: 2012,4Q,107

One of the following 7th characters is to be assigned to each code under category O32. 7th character Ø is for single gestations and multiple gestations where the fetus is unspecified. 7th characters 1 through 9 are for cases of multiple gestations to identify the fetus for which the code applies. The appropriate code from category O3Ø, Multiple gestation, must also be assigned when assigning a code from category O32 that has a 7th character of 1 through 9.

　Ø　not applicable or unspecified
　1　fetus 1
　2　fetus 2
　3　fetus 3
　4　fetus 4
　5　fetus 5
　9　other fetus

√x7ᵗʰ **O32.Ø**　**Maternal care for** unstable lie　Ⓜ ♀

√x7ᵗʰ **O32.1**　**Maternal care for** breech presentation　Ⓜ ♀

　Maternal care for buttocks presentation
　Maternal care for complete breech
　Maternal care for frank breech
　　EXCLUDES 1　*footling presentation (O32.8)*
　　　　　　　incomplete breech (O32.8)

√x7ᵗʰ **O32.2**　**Maternal care for** transverse and oblique lie　Ⓜ ♀

　Maternal care for oblique presentation
　Maternal care for transverse presentation

√x7ᵗʰ **O32.3**　**Maternal care for** face, brow and chin presentation　Ⓜ ♀

√x7ᵗʰ **O32.4**　**Maternal care for** high head at term　Ⓜ ♀

　Maternal care for failure of head to enter pelvic brim

√x7ᵗʰ **O32.6**　**Maternal care for** compound presentation　Ⓜ ♀

√x7ᵗʰ **O32.8**　**Maternal care for** other malpresentation of fetus　Ⓜ ♀

　Maternal care for footling presentation
　Maternal care for incomplete breech

√x7ᵗʰ **O32.9**　**Maternal care for** malpresentation of fetus, unspecified　Ⓜ ♀ ▽

√4ᵗʰ **O33**　**Maternal care for disproportion**

　INCLUDES　the listed conditions as a reason for observation, hospitalization or other obstetric care of the mother, or for cesarean delivery before onset of labor

　EXCLUDES 1　*disproportion with obstructed labor (O65-O66)*

O33.Ø　**Maternal care for disproportion due to** deformity of maternal pelvic bones　Ⓜ ♀

　Maternal care for disproportion due to pelvic deformity causing disproportion NOS

O33.1　**Maternal care for disproportion due to** generally contracted pelvis　Ⓜ ♀

　Maternal care for disproportion due to contracted pelvis NOS causing disproportion

O33.2　**Maternal care for disproportion due to** inlet contraction of pelvis　Ⓜ ♀

　Maternal care for disproportion due to inlet contraction (pelvis) causing disproportion

---

√x7ᵗʰ **O33.3**　**Maternal care for disproportion due to** outlet contraction of pelvis　Ⓜ ♀

　Maternal care for disproportion due to mid-cavity contraction (pelvis)
　Maternal care for disproportion due to outlet contraction (pelvis)

One of the following 7th characters is to be assigned to code O33.3. 7th character Ø is for single gestations and multiple gestations where the fetus is unspecified. 7th characters 1 through 9 are for cases of multiple gestations to identify the fetus for which the code applies. The appropriate code from category O3Ø, Multiple gestation, must also be assigned when assigning code O33.3 with a 7th character of 1 through 9.

　Ø　not applicable or unspecified
　1　fetus 1
　2　fetus 2
　3　fetus 3
　4　fetus 4
　5　fetus 5
　9　other fetus

√x7ᵗʰ **O33.4**　**Maternal care for disproportion of mixed maternal and fetal origin**　Ⓜ ♀

One of the following 7th characters is to be assigned to code O33.4. 7th character Ø is for single gestations and multiple gestations where the fetus is unspecified. 7th characters 1 through 9 are for cases of multiple gestations to identify the fetus for which the code applies. The appropriate code from category O3Ø, Multiple gestation, must also be assigned when assigning code O33.4 with a 7th character of 1 through 9.

　Ø　not applicable or unspecified
　1　fetus 1
　2　fetus 2
　3　fetus 3
　4　fetus 4
　5　fetus 5
　9　other fetus

√x7ᵗʰ **O33.5**　**Maternal care for disproportion due to unusually large fetus**　Ⓜ ♀

　Maternal care for disproportion due to disproportion of fetal origin with normally formed fetus
　Maternal care for disproportion due to fetal disproportion NOS

One of the following 7th characters is to be assigned to code O33.5. 7th character Ø is for single gestations and multiple gestations where the fetus is unspecified. 7th characters 1 through 9 are for cases of multiple gestations to identify the fetus for which the code applies. The appropriate code from category O3Ø, Multiple gestation, must also be assigned when assigning code O33.5 with a 7th character of 1 through 9.

　Ø　not applicable or unspecified
　1　fetus 1
　2　fetus 2
　3　fetus 3
　4　fetus 4
　5　fetus 5
　9　other fetus

√x7ᵗʰ **O33.6**　**Maternal care for disproportion due to hydrocephalic fetus**　Ⓜ ♀

One of the following 7th characters is to be assigned to code O33.6. 7th character Ø is for single gestations and multiple gestations where the fetus is unspecified. 7th characters 1 through 9 are for cases of multiple gestations to identify the fetus for which the code applies. The appropriate code from category O3Ø, Multiple gestation, must also be assigned when assigning code O33.6 with a 7th character of 1 through 9.

　Ø　not applicable or unspecified
　1　fetus 1
　2　fetus 2
　3　fetus 3
　4　fetus 4
　5　fetus 5
　9　other fetus

☑ Additional Character Required　　√x7ᵗʰ Placeholder Alert　　Manifestation Dx　　▽ Unspecified Dx　　►◄ Revised Text　　● New Code　　▲ Revised Code Title

ICD-10-CM 2017　　　　　　817

✓x7ᵗʰ O33.7 **Maternal care for disproportion due to other fetal deformities**

Maternal care for disproportion due to fetal ascites

Maternal care for disproportion due to fetal hydrops

Maternal care for disproportion due to fetal meningomyelocele

Maternal care for disproportion due to fetal sacral teratoma

Maternal care for disproportion due to fetal tumor

EXCLUDES 1 *obstructed labor due to other fetal deformities (O66.3)*

One of the following 7th characters is to be assigned to code O33.7. 7th character Ø is for single gestations and multiple gestations where the fetus is unspecified. 7th characters 1 through 9 are for cases of multiple gestations to identify the fetus for which the code applies. The appropriate code from category O30, Multiple gestation, must also be assigned when assigning code O33.7 with a 7th character of 1 through 9.

Ø   not applicable or unspecified

1   fetus 1

2   fetus 2

3   fetus 3

4   fetus 4

5   fetus 5

9   other fetus

O33.8 **Maternal care for disproportion of other origin**   Ⓜ ♀

O33.9 **Maternal care for disproportion, unspecified**   Ⓜ ♀ ▽

Maternal care for disproportion due to cephalopelvic disproportion NOS

Maternal care for disproportion due to fetopelvic disproportion NOS

✓4ᵗʰ O34 Maternal care for abnormality of pelvic organs

INCLUDES   the listed conditions as a reason for hospitalization or other obstetric care of the mother, or for cesarean delivery before onset of labor

Code first any associated obstructed labor (O65.5)

Use additional code for specific condition

✓5ᵗʰ O34.0 **Maternal care for congenital malformation of uterus**

▶Maternal care for double uterus◀

▶Maternal care for uterus bicornis◀

O34.00 **Maternal care for unspecified congenital malformation of uterus, unspecified trimester**   Ⓜ ♀ ▽

O34.01 **Maternal care for unspecified congenital malformation of uterus, first trimester**   Ⓜ ♀ ▽

O34.02 **Maternal care for unspecified congenital malformation of uterus, second trimester**   Ⓜ ♀ ▽

O34.03 **Maternal care for unspecified congenital malformation of uterus, third trimester**   Ⓜ ♀ ▽

✓5ᵗʰ O34.1 **Maternal care for benign tumor of corpus uteri**

EXCLUDES 2 *maternal care for benign tumor of cervix (O34.4-)*
maternal care for malignant neoplasm of uterus (O9A.1-)

O34.10 **Maternal care for benign tumor of corpus uteri, unspecified trimester**   Ⓜ ♀ ▽

O34.11 **Maternal care for benign tumor of corpus uteri, first trimester**   Ⓜ ♀

O34.12 **Maternal care for benign tumor of corpus uteri, second trimester**   Ⓜ ♀

O34.13 **Maternal care for benign tumor of corpus uteri, third trimester**   Ⓜ ♀

✓5ᵗʰ O34.2 **Maternal care due to uterine scar from previous surgery**

✓6ᵗʰ O34.21 **Maternal care for scar from previous cesarean delivery**

● **O34.211** **Maternal care for low transverse scar from previous cesarean delivery**

● **O34.212** **Maternal care for vertical scar from previous cesarean delivery**

Maternal care for classical scar from previous cesarean delivery

● **O34.219** **Maternal care for unspecified type scar from previous cesarean delivery**   ▽

O34.29 **Maternal care due to uterine scar from other previous surgery**   Ⓜ ♀

▶Maternal care due to uterine scar from other transmural uterine incision◀

✓5ᵗʰ O34.3 **Maternal care for** cervical incompetence

Maternal care for cerclage with or without cervical incompetence

Maternal care for Shirodkar suture with or without cervical incompetence

O34.30 **Maternal care for cervical incompetence, unspecified trimester**   Ⓜ ♀ ▽

O34.31 **Maternal care for cervical incompetence, first trimester**   Ⓜ ♀

O34.32 **Maternal care for cervical incompetence, second trimester**   Ⓜ ♀

O34.33 **Maternal care for cervical incompetence, third trimester**   Ⓜ ♀

✓5ᵗʰ O34.4 **Maternal care for** other abnormalities of cervix

O34.40 **Maternal care for other abnormalities of cervix, unspecified trimester**   Ⓜ ♀ ▽

O34.41 **Maternal care for other abnormalities of cervix, first trimester**   Ⓜ ♀

O34.42 **Maternal care for other abnormalities of cervix, second trimester**   Ⓜ ♀

O34.43 **Maternal care for other abnormalities of cervix, third trimester**   Ⓜ ♀

✓5ᵗʰ O34.5 **Maternal care for** other abnormalities of gravid uterus

✓6ᵗʰ O34.51 **Maternal care for** incarceration of gravid uterus

O34.511 **Maternal care for incarceration of gravid uterus, first trimester**   Ⓜ ♀

O34.512 **Maternal care for incarceration of gravid uterus, second trimester**   Ⓜ ♀

O34.513 **Maternal care for incarceration of gravid uterus, third trimester**   Ⓜ ♀

O34.519 **Maternal care for incarceration of gravid uterus, unspecified trimester**   Ⓜ ♀ ▽

✓6ᵗʰ O34.52 **Maternal care for** prolapse of gravid uterus

O34.521 **Maternal care for prolapse of gravid uterus, first trimester**   Ⓜ ♀

O34.522 **Maternal care for prolapse of gravid uterus, second trimester**   Ⓜ ♀

O34.523 **Maternal care for prolapse of gravid uterus, third trimester**   Ⓜ ♀

O34.529 **Maternal care for prolapse of gravid uterus, unspecified trimester**   Ⓜ ♀ ▽

✓6ᵗʰ O34.53 **Maternal care for** retroversion of gravid uterus

O34.531 **Maternal care for retroversion of gravid uterus, first trimester**   Ⓜ ♀

O34.532 **Maternal care for retroversion of gravid uterus, second trimester**   Ⓜ ♀

O34.533 **Maternal care for retroversion of gravid uterus, third trimester**   Ⓜ ♀

O34.539 **Maternal care for retroversion of gravid uterus, unspecified trimester**   Ⓜ ♀ ▽

✓6ᵗʰ O34.59 **Maternal care for other abnormalities of gravid uterus**

O34.591 **Maternal care for other abnormalities of gravid uterus, first trimester**   Ⓜ ♀

O34.592 **Maternal care for other abnormalities of gravid uterus, second trimester**   Ⓜ ♀

O34.593 **Maternal care for other abnormalities of gravid uterus, third trimester**   Ⓜ ♀

O34.599 **Maternal care for other abnormalities of gravid uterus, unspecified trimester**   Ⓜ ♀ ▽

✓5ᵗʰ O34.6 **Maternal care for** abnormality of vagina

EXCLUDES 2 *maternal care for vaginal varices in pregnancy (O22.1-)*

O34.60 **Maternal care for abnormality of vagina, unspecified trimester**   Ⓜ ♀ ▽

O34.61 **Maternal care for abnormality of vagina, first trimester**   Ⓜ ♀

O34.62 **Maternal care for abnormality of vagina, second trimester**   Ⓜ ♀

O34.63 **Maternal care for abnormality of vagina, third trimester**   Ⓜ ♀

EXCLUDES 1 Not coded here   EXCLUDES 2 Not included here   Ⓝ Newborn Age : 0   Ⓟ Pediatric Age : 0-17   Ⓜ Maternity Age : 12-55   Ⓐ Adult Age : 15-124

818   ICD-10-CM 2017

√5ᵗʰ **O34.7 Maternal care for** abnormality of vulva and perineum

    EXCLUDES 2 *maternal care for perineal and vulval varices in pregnancy (O22.1-)*

    O34.70 Maternal care for abnormality of vulva and Ⓜ ♀ ▽ **perineum, unspecified trimester**

    O34.71 Maternal care for abnormality of vulva and Ⓜ ♀ **perineum, first trimester**

    O34.72 Maternal care for abnormality of vulva and ♀ **perineum, second trimester**

    O34.73 Maternal care for abnormality of vulva and Ⓜ ♀ **perineum, third trimester**

√5ᵗʰ **O34.8 Maternal care for** other abnormalities of pelvic organs

    O34.80 Maternal care for other abnormalities of Ⓜ ♀ ▽ **pelvic organs, unspecified trimester**

    O34.81 Maternal care for other abnormalities of Ⓜ ♀ **pelvic organs, first trimester**

    O34.82 Maternal care for other abnormalities of Ⓜ ♀ **pelvic organs, second trimester**

    O34.83 Maternal care for other abnormalities of Ⓜ ♀ **pelvic organs, third trimester**

√5ᵗʰ **O34.9 Maternal care for** abnormality of pelvic organ, unspecified

    O34.90 Maternal care for abnormality of pelvic Ⓜ ♀ ▽ **organ, unspecified, unspecified trimester**

    O34.91 Maternal care for abnormality of pelvic Ⓜ ♀ ▽ **organ, unspecified, first trimester**

    O34.92 Maternal care for abnormality of pelvic Ⓜ ♀ ▽ **organ, unspecified, second trimester**

    O34.93 Maternal care for abnormality of pelvic Ⓜ ♀ ▽ **organ, unspecified, third trimester**

√4ᵗʰ **O35 Maternal care for known or suspected fetal abnormality and damage**

    INCLUDES the listed conditions in the fetus as a reason for hospitalization or other obstetric care to the mother, or for termination of pregnancy

    Code also any associated maternal condition

    EXCLUDES 1 *encounter for suspected maternal and fetal conditions ruled out (Z03.7-)*

> One of the following 7th characters is to be assigned to each code under category O35. 7th character Ø is for single gestations and multiple gestations where the fetus is unspecified. 7th characters 1 through 9 are for cases of multiple gestations to identify the fetus for which the code applies. The appropriate code from category O30, Multiple gestation, must also be assigned when assigning a code from category O35 that has a 7th character of 1 through 9.
>
> Ø   not applicable or unspecified
> 1   fetus 1
> 2   fetus 2
> 3   fetus 3
> 4   fetus 4
> 5   fetus 5
> 9   other fetus

√x7ᵗʰ **O35.0 Maternal care for (suspected)** central nervous system Ⓜ ♀ **malformation in fetus**

    Maternal care for fetal anencephaly

    Maternal care for fetal hydrocephalus

    Maternal care for fetal spina bifida

    EXCLUDES 2 *chromosomal abnormality in fetus (O35.1)*

√x7ᵗʰ **O35.1 Maternal care for (suspected)** chromosomal Ⓜ ♀ **abnormality in fetus**

√x7ᵗʰ **O35.2 Maternal care for (suspected)** hereditary disease in Ⓜ ♀ **fetus**

    EXCLUDES 2 *chromosomal abnormality in fetus (O35.1)*

√x7ᵗʰ **O35.3 Maternal care for (suspected)** damage to fetus from Ⓜ ♀ **viral disease in mother**

    Maternal care for damage to fetus from maternal cytomegalovirus infection

    Maternal care for damage to fetus from maternal rubella

√x7ᵗʰ **O35.4 Maternal care for (suspected)** damage to fetus from Ⓜ ♀ **alcohol**

√x7ᵗʰ **O35.5 Maternal care for (suspected)** damage to fetus by Ⓜ ♀ **drugs**

    Maternal care for damage to fetus from drug addiction

√x7ᵗʰ **O35.6 Maternal care for (suspected)** damage to fetus by Ⓜ ♀ **radiation**

√x7ᵗʰ **O35.7 Maternal care for (suspected)** damage to fetus by Ⓜ ♀ **other medical procedures**

    Maternal care for damage to fetus by amniocentesis

    Maternal care for damage to fetus by biopsy procedures

    Maternal care for damage to fetus by hematological investigation

    Maternal care for damage to fetus by intrauterine contraceptive device

    Maternal care for damage to fetus by intrauterine surgery

√x7ᵗʰ **O35.8 Maternal care for other (suspected)** fetal abnormality Ⓜ ♀ **and damage**

    Maternal care for damage to fetus from maternal listeriosis

    Maternal care for damage to fetus from maternal toxoplasmosis

√x7ᵗʰ **O35.9 Maternal care for (suspected)** fetal abnormality and Ⓜ ♀ ▽ **damage, unspecified**

√4ᵗʰ **O36 Maternal care for other fetal problems**

    INCLUDES the listed conditions in the fetus as a reason for hospitalization or other obstetric care of the mother, or for termination of pregnancy

    EXCLUDES 1 *encounter for suspected maternal and fetal conditions ruled out (Z03.7-)*

       placental transfusion syndromes (O43.0-)

    EXCLUDES 2 *labor and delivery complicated by fetal stress (O77.-)*

    AHA: 2015,3Q,40

> One of the following 7th characters is to be assigned to each code under category O36. 7th character Ø is for single gestations and multiple gestations where the fetus is unspecified. 7th characters 1 through 9 are for cases of multiple gestations to identify the fetus for which the code applies. The appropriate code from category O30, Multiple gestation, must also be assigned when assigning a code from category O36 that has a 7th character of 1 through 9.
>
> Ø   not applicable or unspecified
> 1   fetus 1
> 2   fetus 2
> 3   fetus 3
> 4   fetus 4
> 5   fetus 5
> 9   other fetus

√5ᵗʰ **O36.0 Maternal care for rhesus isoimmunization**

    Maternal care for Rh incompatibility (with hydrops fetalis)

    √6ᵗʰ **O36.01 Maternal care for** anti-D [Rh] antibodies

       AHA: 2014,4Q,17

       √7ᵗʰ **O36.011 Maternal care for anti-D [Rh]** Ⓜ ♀ **antibodies, first trimester**

       √7ᵗʰ **O36.012 Maternal care for anti-D [Rh]** Ⓜ ♀ **antibodies, second trimester**

       √7ᵗʰ **O36.013 Maternal care for anti-D [Rh]** Ⓜ ♀ **antibodies, third trimester**

       √7ᵗʰ **O36.019 Maternal care for anti-D [Rh]** Ⓜ ♀ ▽ **antibodies, unspecified trimester**

    √6ᵗʰ **O36.09 Maternal care for other rhesus isoimmunization**

       √7ᵗʰ **O36.091 Maternal care for other rhesus** Ⓜ ♀ **isoimmunization, first trimester**

       √7ᵗʰ **O36.092 Maternal care for other rhesus** Ⓜ ♀ **isoimmunization, second trimester**

       √7ᵗʰ **O36.093 Maternal care for other rhesus** Ⓜ ♀ **isoimmunization, third trimester**

       √7ᵗʰ **O36.099 Maternal care for other rhesus** Ⓜ ♀ ▽ **isoimmunization, unspecified trimester**

√5ᵗʰ **O36.1 Maternal care for other isoimmunization**

    Maternal care for ABO isoimmunization

    √6ᵗʰ **O36.11 Maternal care for** Anti-A sensitization

       Maternal care for isoimmunization NOS (with hydrops fetalis)

       √7ᵗʰ **O36.111 Maternal care for Anti-A** Ⓜ ♀ **sensitization, first trimester**

       √7ᵗʰ **O36.112 Maternal care for Anti-A** Ⓜ ♀ **sensitization, second trimester**

       √7ᵗʰ **O36.113 Maternal care for Anti-A** Ⓜ ♀ **sensitization, third trimester**

       √7ᵗʰ **O36.119 Maternal care for Anti-A** Ⓜ ♀ ▽ **sensitization, unspecified trimester**

    √6ᵗʰ **O36.19 Maternal care for other isoimmunization**

       Maternal care for Anti-B sensitization

       √7ᵗʰ **O36.191 Maternal care for other** Ⓜ ♀ **isoimmunization, first trimester**

☑ Additional Character Required   √x7ᵗʰ Placeholder Alert   Manifestation Dx   ▽ Unspecified Dx   ►◄ Revised Text   ● New Code   ▲ Revised Code Title

ICD-10-CM 2017   819

√7ᵗʰ **O36.192 Maternal care for other isoimmunization, second trimester** Ⓜ ♀

√7ᵗʰ **O36.193 Maternal care for other isoimmunization, third trimester** Ⓜ ♀

√7ᵗʰ **O36.199 Maternal care for other isoimmunization, unspecified trimester** Ⓜ ♀ ▽

√5ᵗʰ **O36.2 Maternal care for hydrops fetalis**

Maternal care for hydrops fetalis NOS

Maternal care for hydrops fetalis not associated with isoimmunization

> **EXCLUDES 1** *hydrops fetalis associated with ABO isoimmunization (O36.1-)*
>
> *hydrops fetalis associated with rhesus isoimmunization (O36.0-)*

√x7ᵗʰ **O36.20 Maternal care for hydrops fetalis, unspecified trimester** Ⓜ ♀ ▽

√x7ᵗʰ **O36.21 Maternal care for hydrops fetalis, first trimester** Ⓜ ♀

√x7ᵗʰ **O36.22 Maternal care for hydrops fetalis, second trimester** Ⓜ ♀

√x7ᵗʰ **O36.23 Maternal care for hydrops fetalis, third trimester** Ⓜ ♀

√x7ᵗʰ **O36.4 Maternal care for intrauterine death** Ⓜ ♀

Maternal care for intrauterine fetal death NOS

Maternal care for intrauterine fetal death after completion of 20 weeks of gestation

Maternal care for late fetal death

Maternal care for missed delivery

> **EXCLUDES 1** *missed abortion (O02.1)*
>
> *stillbirth (P95)*

√5ᵗʰ **O36.5 Maternal care for known or suspected poor fetal growth**

√6ᵗʰ **O36.51 Maternal care for known or suspected placental insufficiency**

√7ᵗʰ **O36.511 Maternal care for known or suspected placental insufficiency, first trimester** Ⓜ ♀

√7ᵗʰ **O36.512 Maternal care for known or suspected placental insufficiency, second trimester** Ⓜ ♀

√7ᵗʰ **O36.513 Maternal care for known or suspected placental insufficiency, third trimester** Ⓜ ♀

√7ᵗʰ **O36.519 Maternal care for known or suspected placental insufficiency, unspecified trimester** Ⓜ ♀ ▽

√6ᵗʰ **O36.59 Maternal care for other known or suspected poor fetal growth**

Maternal care for known or suspected light-for-dates NOS

Maternal care for known or suspected small-for-dates NOS

√7ᵗʰ **O36.591 Maternal care for other known or suspected poor fetal growth, first trimester** Ⓜ ♀

√7ᵗʰ **O36.592 Maternal care for other known or suspected poor fetal growth, second trimester** Ⓜ ♀

√7ᵗʰ **O36.593 Maternal care for other known or suspected poor fetal growth, third trimester** Ⓜ ♀

√7ᵗʰ **O36.599 Maternal care for other known or suspected poor fetal growth, unspecified trimester** Ⓜ ♀ ▽

√5ᵗʰ **O36.6 Maternal care for excessive fetal growth**

Maternal care for known or suspected large-for-dates

√x7ᵗʰ **O36.60 Maternal care for excessive fetal growth, unspecified trimester** Ⓜ ♀ ▽

√x7ᵗʰ **O36.61 Maternal care for excessive fetal growth, first trimester** Ⓜ ♀

√x7ᵗʰ **O36.62 Maternal care for excessive fetal growth, second trimester** Ⓜ ♀

√x7ᵗʰ **O36.63 Maternal care for excessive fetal growth, third trimester** Ⓜ ♀

√5ᵗʰ **O36.7 Maternal care for viable fetus in abdominal pregnancy**

√x7ᵗʰ **O36.70 Maternal care for viable fetus in abdominal pregnancy, unspecified trimester** Ⓜ ♀ ▽

√x7ᵗʰ **O36.71 Maternal care for viable fetus in abdominal pregnancy, first trimester** Ⓜ ♀

√x7ᵗʰ **O36.72 Maternal care for viable fetus in abdominal pregnancy, second trimester** Ⓜ ♀

√7ᵗʰ **O36.73 Maternal care for viable fetus in abdominal pregnancy, third trimester** Ⓜ ♀

√5ᵗʰ **O36.8 Maternal care for other specified fetal problems**

√x7ᵗʰ **O36.80 Pregnancy with inconclusive fetal viability**

Encounter to determine fetal viability of pregnancy

√6ᵗʰ **O36.81 Decreased fetal movements**

√7ᵗʰ **O36.812 Decreased fetal movements, second trimester** Ⓜ ♀

√7ᵗʰ **O36.813 Decreased fetal movements, third trimester** Ⓜ ♀

√7ᵗʰ **O36.819 Decreased fetal movements, unspecified trimester** Ⓜ ♀ ▽

√6ᵗʰ **O36.82 Fetal anemia and thrombocytopenia**

√7ᵗʰ **O36.821 Fetal anemia and thrombocytopenia, first trimester** Ⓜ ♀

√7ᵗʰ **O36.822 Fetal anemia and thrombocytopenia, second trimester** Ⓜ ♀

√7ᵗʰ **O36.823 Fetal anemia and thrombocytopenia, third trimester** Ⓜ ♀

√7ᵗʰ **O36.829 Fetal anemia and thrombocytopenia, unspecified trimester** Ⓜ ♀ ▽

√6ᵗʰ **O36.89 Maternal care for other specified fetal problems**

√7ᵗʰ **O36.891 Maternal care for other specified fetal problems, first trimester** Ⓜ ♀

√7ᵗʰ **O36.892 Maternal care for other specified fetal problems, second trimester** Ⓜ ♀

√7ᵗʰ **O36.893 Maternal care for other specified fetal problems, third trimester** Ⓜ ♀

√7ᵗʰ **O36.899 Maternal care for other specified fetal problems, unspecified trimester** Ⓜ ♀ ▽

√5ᵗʰ **O36.9 Maternal care for fetal problem, unspecified**

√x7ᵗʰ **O36.90 Maternal care for fetal problem, unspecified, unspecified trimester** Ⓜ ♀ ▽

√x7ᵗʰ **O36.91 Maternal care for fetal problem, unspecified, first trimester** Ⓜ ♀ ▽

√x7ᵗʰ **O36.92 Maternal care for fetal problem, unspecified, second trimester** Ⓜ ♀ ▽

√x7ᵗʰ **O36.93 Maternal care for fetal problem, unspecified, third trimester** Ⓜ ♀ ▽

√4ᵗʰ **O40 Polyhydramnios**

> **INCLUDES** hydramnios
>
> **EXCLUDES 1** *encounter for suspected maternal and fetal conditions ruled out (Z03.7-)*

AHA: 2016,1Q,4

One of the following 7th characters is to be assigned to each code under category O40. 7th character 0 is for single gestations and multiple gestations where the fetus is unspecified. 7th characters 1 through 9 are for cases of multiple gestations to identify the fetus for which the code applies. The appropriate code from category O30, Multiple gestation, must also be assigned when assigning a code from category O40 that has a 7th character of 1 through 9.

0   not applicable or unspecified

1   fetus 1

2   fetus 2

3   fetus 3

4   fetus 4

5   fetus 5

9   other fetus

√x7ᵗʰ **O40.1 Polyhydramnios, first trimester** Ⓜ ♀

√x7ᵗʰ **O40.2 Polyhydramnios, second trimester** Ⓜ ♀

√x7ᵗʰ **O40.3 Polyhydramnios, third trimester** Ⓜ ♀

√x7ᵗʰ **O40.9 Polyhydramnios, unspecified trimester** Ⓜ ♀ ▽

EXCLUDES 1 Not coded here   **EXCLUDES 2** Not included here   Ⓝ Newborn Age : 0   Ⓟ Pediatric Age : 0-17   Ⓜ Maternity Age : 12-55   Ⓐ Adult Age : 15-124

820

ICD-10-CM 2017

✓4ᵗʰ **O41 Other disorders of amniotic fluid and membranes**

> **EXCLUDES 1** *encounter for suspected maternal and fetal conditions ruled out (Z03.7-)*

> One of the following 7th characters is to be assigned to each code under category O41. 7th character Ø is for single gestations and multiple gestations where the fetus is unspecified. 7th characters 1 through 9 are for cases of multiple gestations to identify the fetus for which the code applies. The appropriate code from category O30, Multiple gestation, must also be assigned when assigning a code from category O41 that has a 7th character of 1 through 9.
>
> Ø   not applicable or unspecified
> 1   fetus 1
> 2   fetus 2
> 3   fetus 3
> 4   fetus 4
> 5   fetus 5
> 9   other fetus

✓5ᵗʰ **O41.Ø Oligohydramnios**

   Oligohydramnios without rupture of membranes

✓x7ᵗʰ **O41.00 Oligohydramnios, unspecified trimester** Ⓜ♀▽

✓x7ᵗʰ **O41.01 Oligohydramnios, first trimester** Ⓜ♀

✓x7ᵗʰ **O41.02 Oligohydramnios, second trimester** Ⓜ♀

✓x7ᵗʰ **O41.03 Oligohydramnios, third trimester** Ⓜ♀

✓6ᵗʰ **O41.1 Infection of amniotic sac and membranes**

✓6ᵗʰ **O41.10 Infection of amniotic sac and membranes, unspecified**

✓7ᵗʰ **O41.101 Infection of amniotic sac and membranes, unspecified, first trimester** Ⓜ♀▽

✓7ᵗʰ **O41.102 Infection of amniotic sac and membranes, unspecified, second trimester** Ⓜ♀▽

✓7ᵗʰ **O41.103 Infection of amniotic sac and membranes, unspecified, third trimester** Ⓜ♀▽

✓7ᵗʰ **O41.109 Infection of amniotic sac and membranes, unspecified, unspecified trimester** Ⓜ♀▽

✓6ᵗʰ **O41.12 Chorioamnionitis**

✓7ᵗʰ **O41.121 Chorioamnionitis, first trimester** Ⓜ♀

✓7ᵗʰ **O41.122 Chorioamnionitis, second trimester** Ⓜ♀

✓7ᵗʰ **O41.123 Chorioamnionitis, third trimester** Ⓜ♀

✓7ᵗʰ **O41.129 Chorioamnionitis, unspecified trimester** Ⓜ♀▽

✓6ᵗʰ **O41.14 Placentitis**

✓7ᵗʰ **O41.141 Placentitis, first trimester** Ⓜ♀

✓7ᵗʰ **O41.142 Placentitis, second trimester** Ⓜ♀

✓7ᵗʰ **O41.143 Placentitis, third trimester** Ⓜ♀

✓7ᵗʰ **O41.149 Placentitis, unspecified trimester** Ⓜ♀▽

✓5ᵗʰ **O41.8 Other specified disorders of amniotic fluid and membranes**

✓6ᵗʰ **O41.8X Other specified disorders of amniotic fluid and membranes**

✓7ᵗʰ **O41.8X1 Other specified disorders of amniotic fluid and membranes, first trimester** Ⓜ♀

✓7ᵗʰ **O41.8X2 Other specified disorders of amniotic fluid and membranes, second trimester** Ⓜ♀

✓7ᵗʰ **O41.8X3 Other specified disorders of amniotic fluid and membranes, third trimester** Ⓜ♀

✓7ᵗʰ **O41.8X9 Other specified disorders of amniotic fluid and membranes, unspecified trimester** Ⓜ♀▽

✓5ᵗʰ **O41.9 Disorder of amniotic fluid and membranes, unspecified**

✓x7ᵗʰ **O41.90 Disorder of amniotic fluid and membranes, unspecified, unspecified trimester** Ⓜ♀▽

✓x7ᵗʰ **O41.91 Disorder of amniotic fluid and membranes, unspecified, first trimester** Ⓜ♀▽

✓x7ᵗʰ **O41.92 Disorder of amniotic fluid and membranes, unspecified, second trimester** Ⓜ♀▽

✓x7ᵗʰ **O41.93 Disorder of amniotic fluid and membranes, unspecified, third trimester** Ⓜ♀▽

✓4ᵗʰ **O42 Premature rupture of membranes**

   AHA: 2016,1Q,3

✓5ᵗʰ **O42.0 Premature rupture of membranes, onset of labor within 24 hours of rupture**

O42.00 Premature rupture of membranes, onset of labor within 24 hours of rupture, unspecified weeks of gestation Ⓜ♀▽

✓6ᵗʰ **O42.01 Preterm premature rupture of membranes, onset of labor within 24 hours of rupture**

   Premature rupture of membranes before 37 completed weeks of gestation

O42.011 Preterm premature rupture of membranes, onset of labor within 24 hours of rupture, first trimester Ⓜ♀

O42.012 Preterm premature rupture of membranes, onset of labor within 24 hours of rupture, second trimester Ⓜ♀

O42.013 Preterm premature rupture of membranes, onset of labor within 24 hours of rupture, third trimester Ⓜ♀

O42.019 Preterm premature rupture of membranes, onset of labor within 24 hours of rupture, unspecified trimester Ⓜ♀▽

O42.02 Full-term premature rupture of membranes, onset of labor within 24 hours of rupture Ⓜ♀

   ►Premature rupture of membranes at or after 37 completed weeks of gestation, onset of labor within 24 hours of rupture◄

✓5ᵗʰ **O42.1 Premature rupture of membranes, onset of labor more than 24 hours following rupture**

   AHA: 2016,1Q,5

O42.10 Premature rupture of membranes, onset of labor more than 24 hours following rupture, unspecified weeks of gestation Ⓜ♀▽

✓6ᵗʰ **O42.11 Preterm premature rupture of membranes, onset of labor more than 24 hours following rupture**

   Premature rupture of membranes before 37 completed weeks of gestation

O42.111 Preterm premature rupture of membranes, onset of labor more than 24 hours following rupture, first trimester Ⓜ♀

O42.112 Preterm premature rupture of membranes, onset of labor more than 24 hours following rupture, second trimester Ⓜ♀

O42.113 Preterm premature rupture of membranes, onset of labor more than 24 hours following rupture, third trimester Ⓜ♀

O42.119 Preterm premature rupture of membranes, onset of labor more than 24 hours following rupture, unspecified trimester Ⓜ♀▽

O42.12 Full-term premature rupture of membranes, onset of labor more than 24 hours following rupture Ⓜ♀

   ►Premature rupture of membranes at or after 37 completed weeks of gestation, onset of labor within 24 hours of rupture◄

✓5ᵗʰ **O42.9 Premature rupture of membranes, unspecified as to length of time between rupture and onset of labor**

O42.90 Premature rupture of membranes, unspecified as to length of time between rupture and onset of labor, unspecified weeks of gestation Ⓜ♀▽

✓6ᵗʰ **O42.91 Preterm premature rupture of membranes, unspecified as to length of time between rupture and onset of labor**

   Premature rupture of membranes before 37 completed weeks of gestation

O42.911 Preterm premature rupture of membranes, unspecified as to length of time between rupture and onset of labor, first trimester Ⓜ♀▽

O42.912 Preterm premature rupture of membranes, unspecified as to length of time between rupture and onset of labor, second trimester Ⓜ♀▽

☑ Additional Character Required   ✓x7ᵗʰ Placeholder Alert   Manifestation Dx   ▽ Unspecified Dx   ►◄ Revised Text   ● New Code   ▲ Revised Code Title

O42.913 **Preterm premature rupture of membranes, unspecified as to length of time between rupture and onset of labor, third trimester** Ⓜ ♀ ▽

O42.919 **Preterm premature rupture of membranes, unspecified as to length of time between rupture and onset of labor, unspecified trimester** Ⓜ ♀ ▽

O42.92 **Full-term premature rupture of membranes, unspecified as to length of time between rupture and onset of labor** Ⓜ ♀ ▽
  ▶ Premature rupture of membranes at or after 37 completed weeks of gestation, unspecified as to length of time between rupture and onset of labor ◀

✓4ᵗʰ **O43 Placental disorders**
  EXCLUDES 2 *maternal care for poor fetal growth due to placental insufficiency (O36.5-)*
  placenta previa (O44.-)
  placental polyp (O90.89)
  placentitis (O41.14-)
  premature separation of placenta [abruptio placentae] (O45.-)

✓5ᵗʰ **O43.0 Placental transfusion syndromes**

  ✓6ᵗʰ **O43.01 Fetomaternal placental transfusion syndrome**
    Maternofetal placental transfusion syndrome

    O43.011 **Fetomaternal placental transfusion syndrome, first trimester** Ⓜ ♀

    O43.012 **Fetomaternal placental transfusion syndrome, second trimester** Ⓜ ♀

    O43.013 **Fetomaternal placental transfusion syndrome, third trimester** Ⓜ ♀

    O43.019 **Fetomaternal placental transfusion syndrome, unspecified trimester** Ⓜ ♀ ▽

  ✓6ᵗʰ **O43.02 Fetus-to-fetus placental transfusion syndrome**

    O43.021 **Fetus-to-fetus placental transfusion syndrome, first trimester** Ⓜ ♀

    O43.022 **Fetus-to-fetus placental transfusion syndrome, second trimester** Ⓜ ♀

    O43.023 **Fetus-to-fetus placental transfusion syndrome, third trimester** Ⓜ ♀

    O43.029 **Fetus-to-fetus placental transfusion syndrome, unspecified trimester** Ⓜ ♀ ▽

✓5ᵗʰ **O43.1 Malformation of placenta**

  ✓6ᵗʰ **O43.10 Malformation of placenta, unspecified**
    Abnormal placenta NOS

    O43.101 **Malformation of placenta, unspecified, first trimester** Ⓜ ♀ ▽

    O43.102 **Malformation of placenta, unspecified, second trimester** Ⓜ ♀ ▽

    O43.103 **Malformation of placenta, unspecified, third trimester** Ⓜ ♀ ▽

    O43.109 **Malformation of placenta, unspecified, unspecified trimester** Ⓜ ♀ ▽

  ✓6ᵗʰ **O43.11 Circumvallate placenta**

    O43.111 **Circumvallate placenta, first trimester** Ⓜ ♀

    O43.112 **Circumvallate placenta, second trimester** Ⓜ ♀

    O43.113 **Circumvallate placenta, third trimester** Ⓜ ♀

    O43.119 **Circumvallate placenta, unspecified trimester** Ⓜ ♀ ▽

  ✓6ᵗʰ **O43.12 Velamentous insertion of umbilical cord**

    O43.121 **Velamentous insertion of umbilical cord, first trimester** Ⓜ ♀

    O43.122 **Velamentous insertion of umbilical cord, second trimester** Ⓜ ♀

    O43.123 **Velamentous insertion of umbilical cord, third trimester** Ⓜ ♀

    O43.129 **Velamentous insertion of umbilical cord, unspecified trimester** Ⓜ ♀ ▽

  ✓6ᵗʰ O43.19 **Other malformation of placenta**

    O43.191 **Other malformation of placenta, first trimester** Ⓜ ♀

    O43.192 **Other malformation of placenta, second trimester** Ⓜ ♀

    O43.193 **Other malformation of placenta, third trimester** Ⓜ ♀

    O43.199 **Other malformation of placenta, unspecified trimester** Ⓜ ♀ ▽

✓5ᵗʰ **O43.2 Morbidly adherent placenta**
    Code also associated third stage postpartum hemorrhage, if applicable (O72.0)
    EXCLUDES 1 *retained placenta (O73.-)*

  ✓6ᵗʰ **O43.21 Placenta accreta**

    O43.211 **Placenta accreta, first trimester** Ⓜ ♀

    O43.212 **Placenta accreta, second trimester** Ⓜ ♀

    O43.213 **Placenta accreta, third trimester** Ⓜ ♀

    O43.219 **Placenta accreta, unspecified trimester** Ⓜ ♀ ▽

  ✓6ᵗʰ **O43.22 Placenta increta**

    O43.221 **Placenta increta, first trimester** Ⓜ ♀

    O43.222 **Placenta increta, second trimester** Ⓜ ♀

    O43.223 **Placenta increta, third trimester** Ⓜ ♀

    O43.229 **Placenta increta, unspecified trimester** Ⓜ ♀ ▽

  ✓6ᵗʰ **O43.23 Placenta percreta**

    O43.231 **Placenta percreta, first trimester** Ⓜ ♀

    O43.232 **Placenta percreta, second trimester** Ⓜ ♀

    O43.233 **Placenta percreta, third trimester** Ⓜ ♀

    O43.239 **Placenta percreta, unspecified trimester** Ⓜ ♀ ▽

✓5ᵗʰ **O43.8 Other placental disorders**

  ✓6ᵗʰ **O43.81 Placental infarction**

    O43.811 **Placental infarction, first trimester** Ⓜ ♀

    O43.812 **Placental infarction, second trimester** Ⓜ ♀

    O43.813 **Placental infarction, third trimester** Ⓜ ♀

    O43.819 **Placental infarction, unspecified trimester** Ⓜ ♀ ▽

  ✓6ᵗʰ **O43.89 Other placental disorders**
    Placental dysfunction

    O43.891 **Other placental disorders, first trimester** Ⓜ ♀

    O43.892 **Other placental disorders, second trimester** Ⓜ ♀

    O43.893 **Other placental disorders, third trimester** Ⓜ ♀

    O43.899 **Other placental disorders, unspecified trimester** Ⓜ ♀ ▽

✓5ᵗʰ **O43.9 Unspecified placental disorder**

    O43.90 **Unspecified placental disorder, unspecified trimester** Ⓜ ♀ ▽

    O43.91 **Unspecified placental disorder, first trimester** Ⓜ ♀ ▽

    O43.92 **Unspecified placental disorder, second trimester** Ⓜ ♀ ▽

    O43.93 **Unspecified placental disorder, third trimester** Ⓜ ♀ ▽

✓4ᵗʰ **O44 Placenta previa**

▲ ✓5ᵗʰ **O44.0 Complete placenta previa NOS or without hemorrhage**
    ▶ Placenta previa NOS ◀

▲   O44.00 **Complete placenta previa NOS or without hemorrhage, unspecified trimester** Ⓜ ♀ ▽

▲   O44.01 **Complete placenta previa NOS or without hemorrhage, first trimester** Ⓜ ♀

▲   O44.02 **Complete placenta previa NOS or without hemorrhage, second trimester** Ⓜ ♀

▲   O44.03 **Complete placenta previa NOS or without hemorrhage, third trimester** Ⓜ ♀

▲ ✓5ᵗʰ **O44.1 Complete placenta previa with hemorrhage**
    EXCLUDES 1 *labor and delivery complicated by hemorrhage from vasa previa (O69.4)*

▲   O44.10 **Complete placenta previa with hemorrhage, unspecified trimester** Ⓜ ♀ ▽

EXCLUDES 1 Not coded here   EXCLUDES 2 Not included here   Ⓝ Newborn Age : 0   Ⓟ Pediatric Age : 0-17   Ⓜ Maternity Age : 12-55   Ⓐ Adult Age : 15-124

822   ICD-10-CM 2017

▲ **O44.11** **Complete placenta previa with hemorrhage,** Ⓜ ♀
first trimester

▲ **O44.12** **Complete placenta previa with hemorrhage,** Ⓜ ♀
second trimester

▲ **O44.13** **Complete placenta previa with hemorrhage,** Ⓜ ♀
third trimester

● ✓5ᵗʰ **O44.2** **Partial placenta previa without hemorrhage**
Marginal placenta previa, NOS or without hemorrhage

● **O44.20** **Partial placenta previa NOS or without** ▽
hemorrhage, unspecified trimester

O44.21 **Partial placenta previa NOS or without hemorrhage,**
first trimester

O44.22 **Partial placenta previa NOS or without hemorrhage,**
second trimester

O44.23 **Partial placenta previa NOS or without hemorrhage,**
third trimester

● ✓5ᵗʰ **O44.3** **Partial placenta previa with hemorrhage**
Marginal placenta previa with hemorrhage

● **O44.30** **Partial placenta previa with hemorrhage,** ▽
unspecified trimester

● **O44.31** **Partial placenta previa with hemorrhage, first**
trimester

● **O44.32** **Partial placenta previa with hemorrhage, second**
trimester

● **O44.33** **Partial placenta previa with hemorrhage, third**
trimester

● ✓5ᵗʰ **O44.4** **Low lying placenta NOS or without hemorrhage**
Low implantation of placenta NOS or without hemorrhage

● **O44.40** **Low lying placenta NOS or without** ▽
hemorrhage, unspecified trimester

● **O44.41** **Low lying placenta NOS or without hemorrhage,**
first trimester

● **O44.42** **Low lying placenta NOS or without hemorrhage,**
second trimester

● **O44.43** **Low lying placenta NOS or without hemorrhage,**
third trimester

● ✓5ᵗʰ **O44.5** **Low lying placenta with hemorrhage**
Low implantation of placenta with hemorrhage

● **O44.50** **Low lying placenta with hemorrhage,** ▽
unspecified trimester

● **O44.51** **Low lying placenta with hemorrhage, first trimester**

● **O44.52** **Low lying placenta with hemorrhage, second**
trimester

● **O44.53** **Low lying placenta with hemorrhage, third**
trimester

✓4ᵗʰ **O45** **Premature separation of placenta [abruptio placentae]**

✓5ᵗʰ **O45.0** **Premature separation of placenta with coagulation defect**

✓6ᵗʰ **O45.00** **Premature separation of placenta with coagulation**
defect, unspecified

O45.001 **Premature separation of placenta** Ⓜ ♀ ▽
with coagulation defect,
unspecified, first trimester

O45.002 **Premature separation of placenta** Ⓜ ♀ ▽
with coagulation defect,
unspecified, second trimester

O45.003 **Premature separation of placenta** Ⓜ ♀ ▽
with coagulation defect,
unspecified, third trimester

O45.009 **Premature separation of placenta** Ⓜ ♀ ▽
with coagulation defect,
unspecified, unspecified trimester

✓6ᵗʰ **O45.01** **Premature separation of placenta with**
afibrinogenemia
Premature separation of placenta with
hypofibrinogenemia

O45.011 **Premature separation of placenta** Ⓜ ♀
with afibrinogenemia, first
trimester

O45.012 **Premature separation of placenta** Ⓜ ♀
with afibrinogenemia, second
trimester

O45.013 **Premature separation of placenta** Ⓜ ♀
with afibrinogenemia, third
trimester

O45.019 **Premature separation of placenta** Ⓜ ♀ ▽
with afibrinogenemia, unspecified
trimester

✓6ᵗʰ **O45.02** **Premature separation of placenta with**
disseminated intravascular coagulation

O45.021 **Premature separation of placenta** Ⓜ ♀
with disseminated intravascular
coagulation, first trimester

O45.022 **Premature separation of placenta** Ⓜ ♀
with disseminated intravascular
coagulation, second trimester

O45.023 **Premature separation of placenta** Ⓜ ♀
with disseminated intravascular
coagulation, third trimester

O45.029 **Premature separation of placenta** Ⓜ♀▽
with disseminated intravascular
coagulation, unspecified trimester

✓6ᵗʰ **O45.09** **Premature separation of placenta with other**
coagulation defect

O45.091 **Premature separation of placenta** Ⓜ ♀
with other coagulation defect, first
trimester

O45.092 **Premature separation of placenta** Ⓜ ♀
with other coagulation defect,
second trimester

O45.093 **Premature separation of placenta** Ⓜ ♀
with other coagulation defect,
third trimester

O45.099 **Premature separation of placenta** Ⓜ♀▽
with other coagulation defect,
unspecified trimester

✓5ᵗʰ **O45.8** **Other premature separation of placenta**

✓6ᵗʰ **O45.8X** **Other premature separation of placenta**

O45.8X1 **Other premature separation of** Ⓜ ♀
placenta, first trimester

O45.8X2 **Other premature separation of** Ⓜ ♀
placenta, second trimester

O45.8X3 **Other premature separation of** Ⓜ ♀
placenta, third trimester

O45.8X9 **Other premature separation of** Ⓜ♀▽
placenta, unspecified trimester

✓5ᵗʰ **O45.9** **Premature separation of placenta, unspecified**
Abruptio placentae NOS

O45.90 **Premature separation of placenta,** Ⓜ♀▽
unspecified, unspecified trimester

O45.91 **Premature separation of placenta,** Ⓜ♀▽
unspecified, first trimester

O45.92 **Premature separation of placenta,** Ⓜ♀▽
unspecified, second trimester

O45.93 **Premature separation of placenta,** Ⓜ♀▽
unspecified, third trimester

✓4ᵗʰ **O46** **Antepartum hemorrhage, not elsewhere classified**

EXCLUDES 1 *hemorrhage in early pregnancy (O20.-)*
intrapartum hemorrhage NEC (O67.-)
placenta previa (O44.-)
premature separation of placenta [abruptio placentae] (O45.-)

✓5ᵗʰ **O46.0** **Antepartum hemorrhage with coagulation defect**

✓6ᵗʰ **O46.00** **Antepartum hemorrhage with coagulation defect,**
unspecified

O46.001 **Antepartum hemorrhage with** Ⓜ♀▽
coagulation defect, unspecified,
first trimester

O46.002 **Antepartum hemorrhage with** Ⓜ♀▽
coagulation defect, unspecified,
second trimester

O46.003 **Antepartum hemorrhage with** Ⓜ♀▽
coagulation defect, unspecified,
third trimester

O46.009 **Antepartum hemorrhage with** Ⓜ♀▽
coagulation defect, unspecified,
unspecified trimester

✓6ᵗʰ **O46.01** **Antepartum hemorrhage with afibrinogenemia**
Antepartum hemorrhage with hypofibrinogenemia

O46.011 **Antepartum hemorrhage with** Ⓜ ♀
afibrinogenemia, first trimester

O46.012 **Antepartum hemorrhage with** Ⓜ ♀
afibrinogenemia, second trimester

O46.013 **Antepartum hemorrhage with** Ⓜ ♀
afibrinogenemia, third trimester

O46.019 **Antepartum hemorrhage with** Ⓜ♀▽
afibrinogenemia, unspecified
trimester

✓6ᵗʰ **O46.02** **Antepartum hemorrhage with disseminated**
intravascular coagulation

O46.021 **Antepartum hemorrhage with** Ⓜ ♀
disseminated intravascular
coagulation, first trimester

✓ Additional Character Required   ✓x7ᵗʰ Placeholder Alert   Manifestation Dx   ▽ Unspecified Dx   ►◄ Revised Text   ● New Code   ▲ Revised Code Title

ICD-10-CM 2017   823

Chapter 15. Pregnancy, Childbirth and the Puerperium

O46.022-O62.1

        O46.022 Antepartum hemorrhage with disseminated intravascular coagulation, second trimester Ⓜ ♀

        O46.023 Antepartum hemorrhage with disseminated intravascular coagulation, third trimester Ⓜ ♀

        O46.029 Antepartum hemorrhage with disseminated intravascular coagulation, unspecified trimester Ⓜ ♀ ▽

✓6ᵗʰ **O46.09 Antepartum hemorrhage with other coagulation defect**

        O46.091 Antepartum hemorrhage with other coagulation defect, first trimester Ⓜ ♀

        O46.092 Antepartum hemorrhage with other coagulation defect, second trimester Ⓜ ♀

        O46.093 Antepartum hemorrhage with other coagulation defect, third trimester Ⓜ ♀

        O46.099 Antepartum hemorrhage with other coagulation defect, unspecified trimester Ⓜ ♀ ▽

✓5ᵗʰ **O46.8 Other antepartum hemorrhage**

  ✓6ᵗʰ **O46.8X Other antepartum hemorrhage**

        O46.8X1 Other antepartum hemorrhage, first trimester Ⓜ ♀

        O46.8X2 Other antepartum hemorrhage, second trimester Ⓜ ♀

        O46.8X3 Other antepartum hemorrhage, third trimester Ⓜ ♀

        O46.8X9 Other antepartum hemorrhage, unspecified trimester Ⓜ ♀ ▽

✓5ᵗʰ **O46.9 Antepartum hemorrhage, unspecified**

    O46.90 Antepartum hemorrhage, unspecified, unspecified trimester Ⓜ ♀ ▽

    O46.91 Antepartum hemorrhage, unspecified, first trimester Ⓜ ♀ ▽

    O46.92 Antepartum hemorrhage, unspecified, second trimester Ⓜ ♀ ▽

    O46.93 Antepartum hemorrhage, unspecified, third trimester Ⓜ ♀ ▽

✓4ᵗʰ **O47 False labor**

  INCLUDES Braxton Hicks contractions
         threatened labor
  EXCLUDES 1 *preterm labor (O60.-)*

  ✓5ᵗʰ **O47.0 False labor before 37 completed weeks of gestation**

    O47.00 False labor before 37 completed weeks of gestation, unspecified trimester Ⓜ ♀ ▽

    O47.02 False labor before 37 completed weeks of gestation, second trimester Ⓜ ♀

    O47.03 False labor before 37 completed weeks of gestation, third trimester Ⓜ ♀

  O47.1 False labor at or after 37 completed weeks of gestation Ⓜ ♀

  O47.9 False labor, unspecified Ⓜ ♀ ▽

✓4ᵗʰ **O48 Late pregnancy**

  O48.0 Post-term pregnancy Ⓜ ♀

     Pregnancy over 40 completed weeks to 42 completed weeks gestation

  O48.1 Prolonged pregnancy Ⓜ ♀

     Pregnancy which has advanced beyond 42 completed weeks gestation
    AHA: 2016,1Q,5

Complications of labor and delivery (O60-O77)

✓4ᵗʰ **O60 Preterm labor**

  INCLUDES onset (spontaneous) of labor before 37 completed weeks of gestation
  EXCLUDES 1 *false labor (O47.0-)*
         threatened labor NOS (O47.0-)

  ✓5ᵗʰ **O60.0 Preterm labor without delivery**

    O60.00 Preterm labor without delivery, unspecified trimester Ⓜ ♀ ▽

    O60.02 Preterm labor without delivery, second trimester Ⓜ ♀

    O60.03 Preterm labor without delivery, third trimester Ⓜ ♀

✓5ᵗʰ **O60.1 Preterm labor with preterm delivery**
  AHA: 2016,2Q,10

One of the following 7th characters is to be assigned to each code under subcategory O60.1. 7th character 0 is for single gestations and multiple gestations where the fetus is unspecified. 7th characters 1 through 9 are for cases of multiple gestations to identify the fetus for which the code applies. The appropriate code from category O30, Multiple gestation, must also be assigned when assigning a code from subcategory O60.1 that has a 7th character of 1 through 9.
  0   not applicable or unspecified
  1   fetus 1
  2   fetus 2
  3   fetus 3
  4   fetus 4
  5   fetus 5
  9   other fetus

  ✓x7ᵗʰ **O60.10 Preterm labor with preterm delivery, unspecified trimester** Ⓜ ♀ ▽
       Preterm labor with delivery NOS

  ✓x7ᵗʰ **O60.12 Preterm labor second trimester with preterm delivery second trimester** Ⓜ ♀

  ✓x7ᵗʰ **O60.13 Preterm labor second trimester with preterm delivery third trimester** Ⓜ ♀

  ✓x7ᵗʰ **O60.14 Preterm labor third trimester with preterm delivery third trimester** Ⓜ ♀

✓5ᵗʰ **O60.2 Term delivery with preterm labor**

One of the following 7th characters is to be assigned to each code under subcategory O60.2. 7th character 0 is for single gestations and multiple gestations where the fetus is unspecified. 7th characters 1 through 9 are for cases of multiple gestations to identify the fetus for which the code applies. The appropriate code from category O30, Multiple gestation, must also be assigned when assigning a code from subcategory O60.2 that has a 7th character of 1 through 9.
  0   not applicable or unspecified
  1   fetus 1
  2   fetus 2
  3   fetus 3
  4   fetus 4
  5   fetus 5
  9   other fetus

  ✓x7ᵗʰ **O60.20 Term delivery with preterm labor, unspecified trimester** Ⓜ ♀ ▽

  ✓x7ᵗʰ **O60.22 Term delivery with preterm labor, second trimester** Ⓜ ♀

  ✓x7ᵗʰ **O60.23 Term delivery with preterm labor, third trimester** Ⓜ ♀

✓4ᵗʰ **O61 Failed induction of labor**

  O61.0 Failed medical induction of labor Ⓜ ♀
     Failed induction (of labor) by oxytocin
     Failed induction (of labor) by prostaglandins

  O61.1 Failed instrumental induction of labor Ⓜ ♀
     Failed mechanical induction (of labor)
     Failed surgical induction (of labor)

  O61.8 Other failed induction of labor Ⓜ ♀

  O61.9 Failed induction of labor, unspecified Ⓜ ♀ ▽

✓4ᵗʰ **O62 Abnormalities of forces of labor**

  O62.0 Primary inadequate contractions Ⓜ ♀
     Failure of cervical dilatation
     Primary hypotonic uterine dysfunction
     Uterine inertia during latent phase of labor

  O62.1 Secondary uterine inertia Ⓜ ♀
     Arrested active phase of labor
     Secondary hypotonic uterine dysfunction

EXCLUDES 1 Not coded here   **EXCLUDES 2** Not included here   Ⓝ Newborn Age : 0   Ⓟ Pediatric Age : 0-17   Ⓜ Maternity Age : 12-55   Ⓐ Adult Age : 15-124

824   ICD-10-CM 2017

O62.2 Other uterine inertia M ♀
Atony of uterus without hemorrhage
Atony of uterus NOS
Desultory labor
Hypotonic uterine dysfunction NOS
Irregular labor
Poor contractions
Slow slope active phase of labor
Uterine inertia NOS
> EXCLUDES 1 atony of uterus with hemorrhage (postpartum) (O72.1)
> postpartum atony of uterus without hemorrhage (O75.89)

O62.3 Precipitate labor M ♀

O62.4 Hypertonic, incoordinate, and prolonged uterine contractions M ♀
Cervical spasm
Contraction ring dystocia
Dyscoordinate labor
Hour-glass contraction of uterus
Hypertonic uterine dysfunction
Incoordinate uterine action
Tetanic contractions
Uterine dystocia NOS
Uterine spasm
> EXCLUDES 1 dystocia (fetal) (maternal) NOS (O66.9)

O62.8 Other abnormalities of forces of labor M ♀

O62.9 Abnormality of forces of labor, unspecified M ♀ ▽

✓4ᵗʰ **O63 Long labor**

O63.0 Prolonged first stage (of labor) M ♀

O63.1 Prolonged second stage (of labor) M ♀

O63.2 Delayed delivery of second twin, triplet, etc. M ♀

O63.9 Long labor, unspecified M ♀ ▽
Prolonged labor NOS

✓4ᵗʰ **O64 Obstructed labor due to malposition and malpresentation of fetus**

One of the following 7th characters is to be assigned to each code under category O64. 7th character Ø is for single gestations and multiple gestations where the fetus is unspecified. 7th characters 1 through 9 are for cases of multiple gestations to identify the fetus for which the code applies. The appropriate code from category O30, Multiple gestation, must also be assigned when assigning a code from category O64 that has a 7th character of 1 through 9.
Ø not applicable or unspecified
1 fetus 1
2 fetus 2
3 fetus 3
4 fetus 4
5 fetus 5
9 other fetus

Fetal Malposition

Breech
Mother's pelvis
Shoulder (arm prolapse)
Compound (extremity together with head)
Face (mentum)
Oblique

✓x7ᵗʰ **O64.0 Obstructed labor due to incomplete rotation of fetal head** M ♀
Deep transverse arrest
Obstructed labor due to persistent occipitoiliac (position)
Obstructed labor due to persistent occipitoposterior (position)
Obstructed labor due to persistent occipitosacral (position)
Obstructed labor due to persistent occipitotransverse (position)

✓x7ᵗʰ **O64.1 Obstructed labor due to breech presentation** M ♀
Obstructed labor due to buttocks presentation
Obstructed labor due to complete breech presentation
Obstructed labor due to frank breech presentation

✓x7ᵗʰ **O64.2 Obstructed labor due to face presentation** M ♀
Obstructed labor due to chin presentation

✓x7ᵗʰ **O64.3 Obstructed labor due to brow presentation** M ♀

✓x7ᵗʰ **O64.4 Obstructed labor due to shoulder presentation** M ♀
Prolapsed arm
> EXCLUDES 1 impacted shoulders (O66.0)
> shoulder dystocia (O66.0)

✓x7ᵗʰ **O64.5 Obstructed labor due to compound presentation** M ♀

✓x7ᵗʰ **O64.8 Obstructed labor due to other malposition and malpresentation** M ♀
Obstructed labor due to footling presentation
Obstructed labor due to incomplete breech presentation

✓x7ᵗʰ **O64.9 Obstructed labor due to malposition and malpresentation, unspecified** M ♀ ▽

✓4ᵗʰ **O65 Obstructed labor due to maternal pelvic abnormality**

O65.0 Obstructed labor due to deformed pelvis M ♀

O65.1 Obstructed labor due to generally contracted pelvis M ♀

O65.2 Obstructed labor due to pelvic inlet contraction M ♀

O65.3 Obstructed labor due to pelvic outlet and mid-cavity contraction M ♀

O65.4 Obstructed labor due to fetopelvic disproportion, unspecified M ♀ ▽
> EXCLUDES 1 dystocia due to abnormality of fetus (O66.2-O66.3)

O65.5 Obstructed labor due to abnormality of maternal pelvic organs M ♀
Obstructed labor due to conditions listed in O34.-
Use additional code to identify abnormality of pelvic organs O34.-

O65.8 Obstructed labor due to other maternal pelvic abnormalities M ♀

O65.9 Obstructed labor due to maternal pelvic abnormality, unspecified M ♀ ▽

✓4ᵗʰ **O66 Other obstructed labor**

O66.0 Obstructed labor due to shoulder dystocia M ♀
Impacted shoulders

O66.1 Obstructed labor due to locked twins M ♀

O66.2 Obstructed labor due to unusually large fetus M ♀

O66.3 Obstructed labor due to other abnormalities of fetus M ♀
Dystocia due to fetal ascites
Dystocia due to fetal hydrops
Dystocia due to fetal meningomyelocele
Dystocia due to fetal sacral teratoma
Dystocia due to fetal tumor
Dystocia due to hydrocephalic fetus
Use additional code to identify cause of obstruction

✓5ᵗʰ **O66.4 Failed trial of labor**

O66.40 Failed trial of labor, unspecified M ♀ ▽

O66.41 Failed attempted vaginal birth after previous cesarean delivery M ♀
Code first rupture of uterus, if applicable (O71.0-, O71.1)

O66.5 Attempted application of vacuum extractor and forceps M ♀
Attempted application of vacuum or forceps, with subsequent delivery by forceps or cesarean delivery

O66.6 Obstructed labor due to other multiple fetuses M ♀

O66.8 Other specified obstructed labor M ♀
Use additional code to identify cause of obstruction

O66.9 Obstructed labor, unspecified M ♀ ▽
Dystocia NOS
Fetal dystocia NOS
Maternal dystocia NOS

✓ Additional Character Required   ✓x7ᵗʰ Placeholder Alert   Manifestation Dx   ▽ Unspecified Dx   ►◄ Revised Text   ● New Code   ▲ Revised Code Title
ICD-10-CM 2017   825

Chapter 15. Pregnancy, Childbirth and the Puerperium   O62.2–O66.9

✓4th **O67　Labor and delivery complicated by intrapartum hemorrhage, not elsewhere classified**

> EXCLUDES 1 *antepartum hemorrhage NEC (O46.-)*
> *placenta previa (O44.-)*
> *premature separation of placenta [abruptio placentae] (O45.-)*
> EXCLUDES 2 *postpartum hemorrhage (O72.-)*

O67.0　Intrapartum hemorrhage with coagulation defect Ⓜ ♀

> Intrapartum hemorrhage (excessive) associated with afibrinogenemia
> Intrapartum hemorrhage (excessive) associated with disseminated intravascular coagulation
> Intrapartum hemorrhage (excessive) associated with hyperfibrinolysis
> Intrapartum hemorrhage (excessive) associated with hypofibrinogenemia

O67.8　Other intrapartum hemorrhage Ⓜ ♀

> Excessive intrapartum hemorrhage

O67.9　Intrapartum hemorrhage, unspecified Ⓜ ♀ ▽

O68　Labor and delivery complicated by abnormality of fetal Ⓜ ♀
acid-base balance

> Fetal acidemia complicating labor and delivery
> Fetal acidosis complicating labor and delivery
> Fetal alkalosis complicating labor and delivery
> Fetal metabolic acidemia complicating labor and delivery
> EXCLUDES 1 *fetal stress NOS (O77.9)*
> *labor and delivery complicated by electrocardiographic evidence of fetal stress (O77.8)*
> *labor and delivery complicated by ultrasonic evidence of fetal stress (O77.8)*
> EXCLUDES 2 *abnormality in fetal heart rate or rhythm (O76)*
> *labor and delivery complicated by meconium in amniotic fluid (O77.0)*

✓4th **O69　Labor and delivery complicated by umbilical cord complications**

> AHA: 2016,1Q,5

> One of the following 7th characters is to be assigned to each code under category O69. 7th character 0 is for single gestations and multiple gestations where the fetus is unspecified. 7th characters 1 through 9 are for cases of multiple gestations to identify the fetus for which the code applies. The appropriate code from category O30, Multiple gestation, must also be assigned when assigning a code from category O69 that has a 7th character of 1 through 9.
> 0　not applicable or unspecified
> 1　fetus 1
> 2　fetus 2
> 3　fetus 3
> 4　fetus 4
> 5　fetus 5
> 9　other fetus

✓x7th **O69.0　Labor and delivery complicated by prolapse of cord** Ⓜ ♀

> DEF: Abnormal presentation of fetus; marked by protruding umbilical cord during labor; can cause fetal death.

✓x7th **O69.1　Labor and delivery complicated by cord around neck,** Ⓜ ♀
with compression

> EXCLUDES 1 *labor and delivery complicated by cord around neck, without compression (O69.81)*

✓x7th **O69.2　Labor and delivery complicated by other cord** Ⓜ ♀
entanglement, with compression

> Labor and delivery complicated by compression of cord NOS
> Labor and delivery complicated by entanglement of cords of twins in monoamniotic sac
> Labor and delivery complicated by knot in cord
> EXCLUDES 1 *labor and delivery complicated by other cord entanglement, without compression (O69.82)*

✓x7th **O69.3　Labor and delivery complicated by short cord** Ⓜ ♀

✓x7th **O69.4　Labor and delivery complicated by vasa previa** Ⓜ ♀

> Labor and delivery complicated by hemorrhage from vasa previa

✓x7th **O69.5　Labor and delivery complicated by vascular lesion of** Ⓜ ♀
cord

> Labor and delivery complicated by cord bruising
> Labor and delivery complicated by cord hematoma
> Labor and delivery complicated by thrombosis of umbilical vessels

✓5th **O69.8　Labor and delivery complicated by other cord complications**

> ✓x7th **O69.81　Labor and delivery complicated by cord** Ⓜ ♀
> **around neck, without compression**
> AHA: 2016,1Q,5

✓x7th **O69.82　Labor and delivery complicated by other** Ⓜ ♀
cord entanglement, without compression

✓x7th **O69.89　Labor and delivery complicated by other** Ⓜ ♀
cord complications

✓x7th **O69.9　Labor and delivery complicated by cord complication,** Ⓜ ♀ ▽
unspecified

✓4th **O70　Perineal laceration during delivery**

> INCLUDES episiotomy extended by laceration
> EXCLUDES 1 *obstetric high vaginal laceration alone (O71.4)*
> AHA: 2016,2Q,34; 2016,1Q,3-4,5

O70.0　First degree perineal laceration during delivery Ⓜ ♀

> Perineal laceration, rupture or tear involving fourchette during delivery
> Perineal laceration, rupture or tear involving labia during delivery
> Perineal laceration, rupture or tear involving skin during delivery
> Perineal laceration, rupture or tear involving vagina during delivery
> Perineal laceration, rupture or tear involving vulva during delivery
> Slight perineal laceration, rupture or tear during delivery

O70.1　Second degree perineal laceration during delivery Ⓜ ♀

> Perineal laceration, rupture or tear during delivery as in O70.0, also involving pelvic floor
> Perineal laceration, rupture or tear during delivery as in O70.0, also involving perineal muscles
> Perineal laceration, rupture or tear during delivery as in O70.0, also involving vaginal muscles
> EXCLUDES 1 *perineal laceration involving anal sphincter (O70.2)*

✓5th **O70.2　Third degree perineal laceration during delivery**

> Perineal laceration, rupture or tear during delivery as in O70.1, also involving anal sphincter
> Perineal laceration, rupture or tear during delivery as in O70.1, also involving rectovaginal septum
> Perineal laceration, rupture or tear during delivery as in O70.1, also involving sphincter NOS
> EXCLUDES 1 *anal sphincter tear during delivery without third degree perineal laceration (O70.4)*
> *perineal laceration involving anal or rectal mucosa (O70.3)*

● **O70.20　Third degree perineal laceration during** ▽
delivery, unspecified

● **O70.21　Third degree perineal laceration during delivery,**
IIIa

> Third degree perineal laceration during delivery with less than 50% of external anal sphincter (EAS) thickness torn

● **O70.22　Third degree perineal laceration during delivery,**
IIIb

> Third degree perineal laceration during delivery with more than 50% external anal sphincter (EAS) thickness torn

● **O70.23　Third degree perineal laceration during delivery,**
IIIc

> Third degree perineal laceration during delivery with both external anal sphincter (EAS) and internal anal sphincter (IAS) torn

O70.3　Fourth degree perineal laceration during delivery Ⓜ ♀

> Perineal laceration, rupture or tear during delivery as in O70.2, also involving anal mucosa
> Perineal laceration, rupture or tear during delivery as in O70.2, also involving rectal mucosa

O70.4　Anal sphincter tear complicating delivery, not Ⓜ ♀
associated with third degree laceration

> EXCLUDES 1 *anal sphincter tear with third degree perineal laceration (O70.2)*

O70.9　Perineal laceration during delivery, unspecified Ⓜ ♀ ▽

✓4th **O71　Other obstetric trauma**

> INCLUDES obstetric damage from instruments

✓5th **O71.0　Rupture of uterus (spontaneous) before onset of labor**

> EXCLUDES 1 *disruption of (current) cesarean delivery wound (O90.0)*
> *laceration of uterus, NEC (O71.1)*

O71.00　Rupture of uterus before onset of labor, Ⓜ ♀ ▽
unspecified trimester

EXCLUDES 1 Not coded here　　EXCLUDES 2 Not included here　　Ⓝ Newborn Age : 0　　Ⓟ Pediatric Age : 0-17　　Ⓜ Maternity Age : 12-55　　Ⓐ Adult Age : 15-124

826

ICD-10-CM 2017

O71.02 **Rupture of uterus before onset of labor, second trimester** Ⓜ ♀

O71.03 **Rupture of uterus before onset of labor, third trimester** Ⓜ ♀

O71.1 **Rupture of uterus during labor** Ⓜ ♀

Rupture of uterus not stated as occurring before onset of labor

EXCLUDES 1 *disruption of cesarean delivery wound (O90.0)*
laceration of uterus, NEC (O71.81)

O71.2 **Postpartum inversion of uterus** Ⓜ ♀

O71.3 **Obstetric laceration of cervix** Ⓜ ♀

Annular detachment of cervix

O71.4 **Obstetric high vaginal laceration alone** Ⓜ ♀

Laceration of vaginal wall without perineal laceration

EXCLUDES 1 *obstetric high vaginal laceration with perineal laceration (O70.-)*

AHA: 2016,1Q,5

O71.5 **Other obstetric injury to pelvic organs** Ⓜ ♀

Obstetric injury to bladder
Obstetric injury to urethra

EXCLUDES 2 *obstetric periurethral trauma (O71.82)*

AHA: 2014,4Q,18

O71.6 **Obstetric damage to pelvic joints and ligaments** Ⓜ ♀

Obstetric avulsion of inner symphyseal cartilage
Obstetric damage to coccyx
Obstetric traumatic separation of symphysis (pubis)

O71.7 **Obstetric hematoma of pelvis** Ⓜ ♀

Obstetric hematoma of perineum
Obstetric hematoma of vagina
Obstetric hematoma of vulva

✓5ᵗʰ **O71.8** **Other specified obstetric trauma**

O71.81 **Laceration of uterus, not elsewhere classified** Ⓜ ♀

O71.82 **Other specified trauma to perineum and vulva** Ⓜ ♀

Obstetric periurethral trauma

AHA: 2016,1Q,4; 2014,4Q,18

O71.89 **Other specified obstetric trauma** Ⓜ ♀

O71.9 **Obstetric trauma, unspecified** Ⓜ ♀ ▽

✓4ᵗʰ **O72** **Postpartum hemorrhage**

INCLUDES hemorrhage after delivery of fetus or infant

O72.0 **Third-stage hemorrhage** Ⓜ ♀

Hemorrhage associated with retained, trapped or adherent placenta
Retained placenta NOS
Code also type of adherent placenta (O43.2-)

O72.1 **Other immediate postpartum hemorrhage** Ⓜ ♀

Hemorrhage following delivery of placenta
Postpartum hemorrhage (atonic) NOS
Uterine atony with hemorrhage

EXCLUDES 1 *uterine atony NOS (O62.2)*
uterine atony without hemorrhage (O62.2)
postpartum atony of uterus without hemorrhage (O75.89)

AHA: 2016,1Q,4

O72.2 **Delayed and secondary postpartum hemorrhage** Ⓜ ♀

Hemorrhage associated with retained portions of placenta or membranes after the first 24 hours following delivery of placenta
Retained products of conception NOS, following delivery

O72.3 **Postpartum coagulation defects** Ⓜ ♀

Postpartum afibrinogenemia
Postpartum fibrinolysis

✓4ᵗʰ **O73** **Retained placenta and membranes, without hemorrhage**

EXCLUDES 1 *placenta accreta (O43.21-)*
placenta increta (O43.22-)
placenta percreta (O43.23-)

O73.0 **Retained placenta without hemorrhage** Ⓜ ♀

Adherent placenta, without hemorrhage
Trapped placenta without hemorrhage

O73.1 **Retained portions of placenta and membranes, without hemorrhage** Ⓜ ♀

Retained products of conception following delivery, without hemorrhage

✓4ᵗʰ **O74** **Complications of anesthesia during labor and delivery**

INCLUDES maternal complications arising from the administration of a general, regional or local anesthetic, analgesic or other sedation during labor and delivery

Use additional code, if applicable, to identify specific complication

O74.0 **Aspiration pneumonitis due to anesthesia during labor and delivery** Ⓜ ♀

Inhalation of stomach contents or secretions NOS due to anesthesia during labor and delivery
Mendelson's syndrome due to anesthesia during labor and delivery

O74.1 **Other pulmonary complications of anesthesia during labor and delivery** Ⓜ ♀

O74.2 **Cardiac complications of anesthesia during labor and delivery** Ⓜ ♀

O74.3 **Central nervous system complications of anesthesia during labor and delivery** Ⓜ ♀

O74.4 **Toxic reaction to local anesthesia during labor and delivery** Ⓜ ♀

O74.5 **Spinal and epidural anesthesia-induced headache during labor and delivery** Ⓜ ♀

O74.6 **Other complications of spinal and epidural anesthesia during labor and delivery** Ⓜ ♀

O74.7 **Failed or difficult intubation for anesthesia during labor and delivery** Ⓜ ♀

O74.8 **Other complications of anesthesia during labor and delivery** Ⓜ ♀

O74.9 **Complication of anesthesia during labor and delivery, unspecified** Ⓜ ♀ ▽

✓4ᵗʰ **O75** **Other complications of labor and delivery, not elsewhere classified**

EXCLUDES 2 *puerperal (postpartum) infection (O86.)*
puerperal (postpartum) sepsis (O85)

O75.0 **Maternal distress during labor and delivery** Ⓜ ♀

O75.1 **Shock during or following labor and delivery** Ⓜ ♀

Obstetric shock following labor and delivery

O75.2 **Pyrexia during labor, not elsewhere classified** Ⓜ ♀

O75.3 **Other infection during labor** Ⓜ ♀

Sepsis during labor
Use additional code (B95-B97), to identify infectious agent

O75.4 **Other complications of obstetric surgery and procedures** Ⓜ ♀

Cardiac arrest following obstetric surgery or procedures
Cardiac failure following obstetric surgery or procedures
Cerebral anoxia following obstetric surgery or procedures
Pulmonary edema following obstetric surgery or procedures
Use additional code to identify specific complication

EXCLUDES 2 *complications of anesthesia during labor and delivery (O74.-)*
disruption of obstetrical (surgical) wound (O90.0-O90.1)
hematoma of obstetrical (surgical) wound (O90.2)
infection of obstetrical (surgical) wound (O86.0)

O75.5 **Delayed delivery after artificial rupture of membranes** Ⓜ ♀

✓5ᵗʰ **O75.8** **Other specified complications of labor and delivery**

O75.81 **Maternal exhaustion complicating labor and delivery** Ⓜ ♀

O75.82 **Onset (spontaneous) of labor after 37 completed weeks of gestation but before 39 completed weeks gestation, with delivery by (planned) cesarean section** Ⓜ ♀

Delivery by (planned) cesarean section occurring after 37 completed weeks of gestation but before 39 completed weeks gestation due to (spontaneous) onset of labor
Code first to specify reason for planned cesarean section such as:
cephalopelvic disproportion (normally formed fetus) (O33.9)
previous cesarean delivery (O34.21)

O75.89 **Other specified complications of labor and delivery** Ⓜ ♀

O75.9 **Complication of labor and delivery, unspecified** Ⓜ ♀ ▽

☑ Additional Character Required   ✓x7ᵗʰ Placeholder Alert   Manifestation Dx   ▽ Unspecified Dx   ►◄ Revised Text   ● New Code   ▲ Revised Code Title

ICD-10-CM 2017   827

Chapter 15. Pregnancy, Childbirth and the Puerperium *(side tab)*

O76 Abnormality in fetal heart rate and rhythm complicating labor and delivery Ⓜ♀

    Depressed fetal heart rate tones complicating labor and delivery

    Fetal bradycardia complicating labor and delivery

    Fetal heart rate decelerations complicating labor and delivery

    Fetal heart rate irregularity complicating labor and delivery

    Fetal heart rate abnormal variability complicating labor and delivery

    Fetal tachycardia complicating labor and delivery

    Non-reassuring fetal heart rate or rhythm complicating labor and delivery

    EXCLUDES 1 *fetal stress NOS (O77.9)*

        labor and delivery complicated by electrocardiographic evidence of fetal stress (O77.8)

        labor and delivery complicated by ultrasonic evidence of fetal stress (O77.8)

    EXCLUDES 2 *fetal metabolic acidemia (O68)*

        other fetal stress (O77.0-O77.1)

    AHA: 2013,4Q,118

✓4ᵗʰ **O77 Other fetal stress complicating labor and delivery**

  O77.0 Labor and delivery complicated by meconium in amniotic fluid Ⓜ♀

    AHA: 2013,4Q,117-118

  O77.1 Fetal stress in labor or delivery due to drug administration Ⓜ♀

  O77.8 Labor and delivery complicated by other evidence of fetal stress Ⓜ♀

    Labor and delivery complicated by electrocardiographic evidence of fetal stress

    Labor and delivery complicated by ultrasonic evidence of fetal stress

    EXCLUDES 1 *abnormality of fetal acid-base balance (O68)*

        abnormality in fetal heart rate or rhythm (O76)

        fetal metabolic acidemia (O68)

  O77.9 Labor and delivery complicated by fetal stress, unspecified Ⓜ♀▽

    EXCLUDES 1 *abnormality of fetal acid-base balance (O68)*

        abnormality in fetal heart rate or rhythm (O76)

        fetal metabolic acidemia (O68)

Encounter for delivery (O80-O82)

O80 Encounter for full-term uncomplicated delivery Ⓜ♀

  NOTE   Delivery requiring minimal or no assistance, with or without episiotomy, without fetal manipulation [e.g., rotation version] or instrumentation [forceps] of a spontaneous, cephalic, vaginal, full-term, single, live-born infant. This code is for use as a single diagnosis code and is not to be used with any other code from chapter 15.

    Use additional code to indicate outcome of delivery (Z37.0)

    AHA: 2014,2Q,9

O82 Encounter for cesarean delivery without indication Ⓜ♀

    Use additional code to indicate outcome of delivery (Z37.0)

Complications predominantly related to the puerperium (O85-O92)

EXCLUDES 2 *mental and behavioral disorders associated with the puerperium (F53)*

    obstetrical tetanus (A34)

    puerperal osteomalacia (M83.0)

O85 Puerperal sepsis Ⓜ♀

    Postpartum sepsis

    Puerperal peritonitis

    Puerperal pyemia

    Use additional code (B95-B97), to identify infectious agent

    Use additional code (R65.2-) to identify severe sepsis, if applicable

    EXCLUDES 1 *fever of unknown origin following delivery (O86.4)*

        genital tract infection following delivery (O86.1-)

        obstetric pyemic and septic embolism (O88.3-)

        puerperal septic thrombophlebitis (O86.81)

        urinary tract infection following delivery (O86.2-)

    EXCLUDES 2 *sepsis during labor (O75.3)*

✓4ᵗʰ **O86 Other puerperal infections**

    Use additional code (B95-B97), to identify infectious agent

    EXCLUDES 2 *infection during labor (O75.3)*

        obstetrical tetanus (A34)

  O86.0 Infection of obstetric surgical wound Ⓜ♀

    Infected cesarean delivery wound following delivery

    Infected perineal repair following delivery

✓5ᵗʰ **O86.1 Other infection of genital tract following delivery**

  O86.11 Cervicitis following delivery Ⓜ♀

  O86.12 Endometritis following delivery Ⓜ♀

  O86.13 Vaginitis following delivery Ⓜ♀

  O86.19 Other infection of genital tract following delivery Ⓜ♀

✓5ᵗʰ **O86.2 Urinary tract infection following delivery**

  O86.20 Urinary tract infection following delivery, unspecified Ⓜ♀▽

    Puerperal urinary tract infection NOS

  O86.21 Infection of kidney following delivery Ⓜ♀

  O86.22 Infection of bladder following delivery Ⓜ♀

    Infection of urethra following delivery

  O86.29 Other urinary tract infection following delivery Ⓜ♀

  O86.4 Pyrexia of unknown origin following delivery Ⓜ♀

    Puerperal infection NOS following delivery

    Puerperal pyrexia NOS following delivery

    EXCLUDES 2 *pyrexia during labor (O75.2)*

✓5ᵗʰ **O86.8 Other specified puerperal infections**

  O86.81 Puerperal septic thrombophlebitis Ⓜ♀

  O86.89 Other specified puerperal infections Ⓜ♀

✓4ᵗʰ **O87 Venous complications and hemorrhoids in the puerperium**

    INCLUDES venous complications in labor, delivery and the puerperium

    EXCLUDES 2 *obstetric embolism (O88.-)*

        puerperal septic thrombophlebitis (O86.81)

        venous complications in pregnancy (O22.-)

  O87.0 Superficial thrombophlebitis in the puerperium Ⓜ♀

    Puerperal phlebitis NOS

    Puerperal thrombosis NOS

  O87.1 Deep phlebothrombosis in the puerperium Ⓜ♀

    Deep vein thrombosis, postpartum

    Pelvic thrombophlebitis, postpartum

    Use additional code to identify the deep vein thrombosis (I82.4-, I82.5-, I82.62-. I82.72-)

    Use additional code, if applicable, for associated long-term (current) use of anticoagulants (Z79.01)

  O87.2 Hemorrhoids in the puerperium Ⓜ♀

  O87.3 Cerebral venous thrombosis in the puerperium Ⓜ♀

    Cerebrovenous sinus thrombosis in the puerperium

  O87.4 Varicose veins of lower extremity in the puerperium Ⓜ♀

  O87.8 Other venous complications in the puerperium Ⓜ♀

    Genital varices in the puerperium

  O87.9 Venous complication in the puerperium, unspecified Ⓜ♀▽

    Puerperal phlebopathy NOS

✓4ᵗʰ **O88 Obstetric embolism**

    EXCLUDES 1 *embolism complicating abortion NOS (O03.2)*

        embolism complicating ectopic or molar pregnancy (O08.2)

        embolism complicating failed attempted abortion (O07.2)

        embolism complicating induced abortion (O04.7)

        embolism complicating spontaneous abortion (O03.2, O03.7)

✓5ᵗʰ **O88.0 Obstetric air embolism**

    DEF: Sudden blocking of pulmonary artery or right ventricle with air or nitrogen bubbles.

  ✓6ᵗʰ **O88.01 Obstetric air embolism in pregnancy**

    O88.011 Air embolism in pregnancy, first trimester Ⓜ♀

    O88.012 Air embolism in pregnancy, second trimester Ⓜ♀

    O88.013 Air embolism in pregnancy, third trimester Ⓜ♀

    O88.019 Air embolism in pregnancy, unspecified trimester Ⓜ♀▽

  O88.02 Air embolism in childbirth Ⓜ♀

  O88.03 Air embolism in the puerperium Ⓜ♀

✓5ᵗʰ **O88.1 Amniotic fluid embolism**

    Anaphylactoid syndrome in pregnancy

  ✓6ᵗʰ **O88.11 Amniotic fluid embolism in pregnancy**

    O88.111 Amniotic fluid embolism in pregnancy, first trimester Ⓜ♀

EXCLUDES 1 Not coded here   EXCLUDES 2 Not included here   Ⓝ Newborn Age : 0   Ⓟ Pediatric Age : 0-17   Ⓜ Maternity Age : 12-55   Ⓐ Adult Age : 15-124

828   ICD-10-CM 2017

           O88.112   **Amniotic fluid embolism in** Ⓜ♀
                     pregnancy, second trimester

           O88.113   **Amniotic fluid embolism in** Ⓜ♀
                     pregnancy, third trimester

           O88.119   **Amniotic fluid embolism in** Ⓜ♀▽
                     pregnancy, unspecified trimester

       O88.12   **Amniotic fluid embolism in** childbirth   Ⓜ♀

       O88.13   **Amniotic fluid embolism in the** puerperium   Ⓜ♀

✓5ᵗʰ **O88.2**   **Obstetric** thromboembolism

   ✓6ᵗʰ **O88.21**   **Thromboembolism in** pregnancy

          Obstetric (pulmonary) embolism NOS

          O88.211   **Thromboembolism in pregnancy,** Ⓜ♀
                  first trimester

          O88.212   **Thromboembolism in pregnancy,** Ⓜ♀
                  second trimester

          O88.213   **Thromboembolism in pregnancy,** Ⓜ♀
                  third trimester

          O88.219   **Thromboembolism in pregnancy,** Ⓜ♀▽
                  unspecified trimester

       O88.22   **Thromboembolism in** childbirth   Ⓜ♀

       O88.23   **Thromboembolism in the** puerperium   Ⓜ♀

          Puerperal (pulmonary) embolism NOS

✓5ᵗʰ **O88.3**   **Obstetric** pyemic and septic embolism

   ✓6ᵗʰ **O88.31**   **Pyemic and septic embolism in** pregnancy

          O88.311   **Pyemic and septic embolism in** Ⓜ♀
                  pregnancy, first trimester

          O88.312   **Pyemic and septic embolism in** Ⓜ♀
                  pregnancy, second trimester

          O88.313   **Pyemic and septic embolism in** Ⓜ♀
                  pregnancy, third trimester

          O88.319   **Pyemic and septic embolism in** Ⓜ♀▽
                  pregnancy, unspecified trimester

       O88.32   **Pyemic and septic embolism in** childbirth   Ⓜ♀

       O88.33   **Pyemic and septic embolism in the** Ⓜ♀
          puerperium

✓5ᵗʰ **O88.8**   **Other obstetric embolism**

       Obstetric fat embolism

   ✓6ᵗʰ **O88.81**   **Other embolism in** pregnancy

          O88.811   **Other embolism in pregnancy, first** Ⓜ♀
                  trimester

          O88.812   **Other embolism in pregnancy,** Ⓜ♀
                  second trimester

          O88.813   **Other embolism in pregnancy,** Ⓜ♀
                  third trimester

          O88.819   **Other embolism in pregnancy,** Ⓜ♀▽
                  unspecified trimester

       O88.82   **Other embolism in** childbirth   Ⓜ♀

       O88.83   **Other embolism in the** puerperium   Ⓜ♀

✓4ᵗʰ **O89**   **Complications of anesthesia during the puerperium**

     INCLUDES   maternal complications arising from the administration of a general, regional or local anesthetic, analgesic or other sedation during the puerperium

     Use additional code, if applicable, to identify specific complication

   ✓5ᵗʰ **O89.0**   **Pulmonary complications of anesthesia during the puerperium**

       O89.01   **Aspiration pneumonitis due to anesthesia** Ⓜ♀
          during the puerperium

          Inhalation of stomach contents or secretions NOS due to anesthesia during the puerperium

          Mendelson's syndrome due to anesthesia during the puerperium

       O89.09   **Other pulmonary complications of** Ⓜ♀
          anesthesia during the puerperium

   O89.1   **Cardiac complications of anesthesia during the** Ⓜ♀
       puerperium

   O89.2   **Central nervous system complications of anesthesia** Ⓜ♀
       during the puerperium

   O89.3   **Toxic reaction to local anesthesia during the** Ⓜ♀
       puerperium

   O89.4   **Spinal and epidural anesthesia-induced headache** Ⓜ♀
       during the puerperium

   O89.5   **Other complications of spinal and epidural anesthesia** Ⓜ♀
       during the puerperium

   O89.6   **Failed or difficult intubation for anesthesia during** Ⓜ♀
       the puerperium

   O89.8   **Other complications of anesthesia during the** Ⓜ♀
       puerperium

   O89.9   **Complication of anesthesia during the puerperium,** Ⓜ♀▽
       unspecified

✓4ᵗʰ **O90**   **Complications of the puerperium, not elsewhere classified**

   O90.0   **Disruption of cesarean delivery wound**   Ⓜ♀

       Dehiscence of cesarean delivery wound

       EXCLUDES 1   *rupture of uterus (spontaneous) before onset of labor (O71.0-)*

                rupture of uterus during labor (O71.1)

   O90.1   **Disruption of perineal obstetric wound**   Ⓜ♀

       Disruption of wound of episiotomy

       Disruption of wound of perineal laceration

       Secondary perineal tear

   O90.2   **Hematoma of obstetric wound**   Ⓜ♀

   O90.3   **Peripartum cardiomyopathy**   Ⓜ♀

       Conditions in I42.- arising during pregnancy and the puerperium

       EXCLUDES 1   *pre-existing heart disease complicating pregnancy and the puerperium (O99.4-)*

       DEF: Any structural or functional abnormality of the ventricular myocardium, noninflammatory disease of obscure or unknown etiology with onset during the postpartum period.

   O90.4   **Postpartum acute kidney failure**   Ⓜ♀

       Hepatorenal syndrome following labor and delivery

   O90.5   **Postpartum thyroiditis**   Ⓜ♀

   O90.6   **Postpartum mood disturbance**   Ⓜ♀

       Postpartum blues

       Postpartum dysphoria

       Postpartum sadness

       EXCLUDES 1   *postpartum depression (F53)*

                puerperal psychosis (F53)

   ✓5ᵗʰ **O90.8**   **Other complications of the puerperium, not elsewhere classified**

       O90.81   **Anemia of the puerperium**   Ⓜ♀

          Postpartum anemia NOS

          EXCLUDES 1   *pre-existing anemia complicating the puerperium (O99.03)*

       O90.89   **Other complications of the puerperium, not** Ⓜ♀
          elsewhere classified

          Placental polyp

   O90.9   **Complication of the puerperium, unspecified**   Ⓜ♀▽

✓4ᵗʰ **O91**   **Infections of breast associated with pregnancy, the puerperium and lactation**

     Use additional code to identify infection

   ✓5ᵗʰ **O91.0**   **Infection of nipple associated with pregnancy, the puerperium and lactation**

     ✓6ᵗʰ **O91.01**   **Infection of nipple associated with pregnancy**

       Gestational abscess of nipple

          O91.011   **Infection of nipple associated with** Ⓜ♀
                  pregnancy, first trimester

          O91.012   **Infection of nipple associated with** Ⓜ♀
                  pregnancy, second trimester

          O91.013   **Infection of nipple associated with** Ⓜ♀
                  pregnancy, third trimester

          O91.019   **Infection of nipple associated with** Ⓜ♀▽
                  pregnancy, unspecified trimester

       O91.02   **Infection of nipple associated with the** Ⓜ♀
          puerperium

          Puerperal abscess of nipple

       O91.03   **Infection of nipple associated with lactation**   Ⓜ♀

          Abscess of nipple associated with lactation

   ✓5ᵗʰ **O91.1**   **Abscess of breast associated with pregnancy, the puerperium and lactation**

     ✓6ᵗʰ **O91.11**   **Abscess of breast associated with pregnancy**

       Gestational mammary abscess

       Gestational purulent mastitis

       Gestational subareolar abscess

          O91.111   **Abscess of breast associated with** Ⓜ♀
                  pregnancy, first trimester

          O91.112   **Abscess of breast associated with** Ⓜ♀
                  pregnancy, second trimester

          O91.113   **Abscess of breast associated with** Ⓜ♀
                  pregnancy, third trimester

          O91.119   **Abscess of breast associated with** Ⓜ♀▽
                  pregnancy, unspecified trimester

O91.12 **Abscess of breast associated with the puerperium**　Ⓜ♀
Puerperal mammary abscess
Puerperal purulent mastitis
Puerperal subareolar abscess

O91.13 **Abscess of breast associated with lactation**　Ⓜ♀
Mammary abscess associated with lactation
Purulent mastitis associated with lactation
Subareolar abscess associated with lactation

✓5ᵗʰ **O91.2** **Nonpurulent mastitis associated with pregnancy, the puerperium and lactation**

✓6ᵗʰ **O91.21** **Nonpurulent mastitis associated with pregnancy**
Gestational interstitial mastitis
Gestational lymphangitis of breast
Gestational mastitis NOS
Gestational parenchymatous mastitis

O91.211 **Nonpurulent mastitis associated with pregnancy, first trimester**　Ⓜ♀

O91.212 **Nonpurulent mastitis associated with pregnancy, second trimester**　Ⓜ♀

O91.213 **Nonpurulent mastitis associated with pregnancy, third trimester**　Ⓜ♀

O91.219 **Nonpurulent mastitis associated with pregnancy, unspecified trimester**　Ⓜ♀▽

O91.22 **Nonpurulent mastitis associated with the puerperium**　Ⓜ♀
Puerperal interstitial mastitis
Puerperal lymphangitis of breast
Puerperal mastitis NOS
Puerperal parenchymatous mastitis

O91.23 **Nonpurulent mastitis associated with lactation**　Ⓜ♀
Interstitial mastitis associated with lactation
Lymphangitis of breast associated with lactation
Mastitis NOS associated with lactation
Parenchymatous mastitis associated with lactation

✓4ᵗʰ **O92** **Other disorders of breast and disorders of lactation associated with pregnancy and the puerperium**

✓5ᵗʰ **O92.0** **Retracted nipple associated with pregnancy, the puerperium, and lactation**

✓6ᵗʰ **O92.01** **Retracted nipple associated with pregnancy**

O92.011 **Retracted nipple associated with pregnancy, first trimester**　Ⓜ♀

O92.012 **Retracted nipple associated with pregnancy, second trimester**　Ⓜ♀

O92.013 **Retracted nipple associated with pregnancy, third trimester**　Ⓜ♀

O92.019 **Retracted nipple associated with pregnancy, unspecified trimester**　Ⓜ♀▽

O92.02 **Retracted nipple associated with the puerperium**　Ⓜ♀

O92.03 **Retracted nipple associated with lactation**　Ⓜ♀

✓5ᵗʰ **O92.1** **Cracked nipple associated with pregnancy, the puerperium, and lactation**
Fissure of nipple, gestational or puerperal

✓6ᵗʰ **O92.11** **Cracked nipple associated with pregnancy**

O92.111 **Cracked nipple associated with pregnancy, first trimester**　Ⓜ♀

O92.112 **Cracked nipple associated with pregnancy, second trimester**　Ⓜ♀

O92.113 **Cracked nipple associated with pregnancy, third trimester**　Ⓜ♀

O92.119 **Cracked nipple associated with pregnancy, unspecified trimester**　Ⓜ♀▽

O92.12 **Cracked nipple associated with the puerperium**　Ⓜ♀

O92.13 **Cracked nipple associated with lactation**　Ⓜ♀

✓5ᵗʰ **O92.2** **Other and unspecified disorders of breast associated with pregnancy and the puerperium**

O92.20 **Unspecified disorder of breast associated with pregnancy and the puerperium**　Ⓜ♀▽

O92.29 **Other disorders of breast associated with pregnancy and the puerperium**　Ⓜ♀

O92.3 **Agalactia**　Ⓜ♀
Primary agalactia
EXCLUDES 1　*elective agalactia (O92.5)*
　　secondary agalactia (O92.5)
　　therapeutic agalactia (O92.5)

O92.4 **Hypogalactia**　Ⓜ♀

O92.5 **Suppressed lactation**　Ⓜ♀
Elective agalactia
Secondary agalactia
Therapeutic agalactia
EXCLUDES 1　*primary agalactia (O92.3)*

O92.6 **Galactorrhea**　Ⓜ♀

✓5ᵗʰ **O92.7** **Other and unspecified disorders of lactation**

O92.70 **Unspecified disorders of lactation**　Ⓜ♀▽

O92.79 **Other disorders of lactation**　Ⓜ♀
Puerperal galactocele

Other obstetric conditions, not elsewhere classified (O94-O9A)

O94 **Sequelae of complication of pregnancy, childbirth, and the puerperium**　Ⓜ♀

> **NOTE**　This category is to be used to indicate conditions in O00-O77.-, O85-O94 and O98-O9A.- as the cause of late effects. The sequelae include conditions specified as such, or as late effects, which may occur at any time after the puerperium

Code first condition resulting from (sequela) of complication of pregnancy, childbirth, and the puerperium

✓4ᵗʰ **O98** **Maternal infectious and parasitic diseases classifiable elsewhere but complicating pregnancy, childbirth and the puerperium**
INCLUDES　the listed conditions when complicating the pregnant state, when aggravated by the pregnancy, or as a reason for obstetric care
Use additional code (Chapter 1), to identify specific infectious or parasitic disease
EXCLUDES 2　*herpes gestationis (O26.4-)*
　　infectious carrier state (O99.82-, O99.83-)
　　obstetrical tetanus (A34)
　　puerperal infection (O86.-)
　　puerperal sepsis (O85)
　　when the reason for maternal care is that the disease is known or suspected to have affected the fetus (O35-O36)

✓5ᵗʰ **O98.0** **Tuberculosis complicating pregnancy, childbirth and the puerperium**
Conditions in A15-A19

✓6ᵗʰ **O98.01** **Tuberculosis complicating pregnancy**

O98.011 **Tuberculosis complicating pregnancy, first trimester**　Ⓜ♀

O98.012 **Tuberculosis complicating pregnancy, second trimester**　Ⓜ♀

O98.013 **Tuberculosis complicating pregnancy, third trimester**　Ⓜ♀

O98.019 **Tuberculosis complicating pregnancy, unspecified trimester**　Ⓜ♀▽

O98.02 **Tuberculosis complicating childbirth**　Ⓜ♀

O98.03 **Tuberculosis complicating the puerperium**　Ⓜ♀

✓5ᵗʰ **O98.1** **Syphilis complicating pregnancy, childbirth and the puerperium**
Conditions in A50-A53

✓6ᵗʰ **O98.11** **Syphilis complicating pregnancy**

O98.111 **Syphilis complicating pregnancy, first trimester**　Ⓜ♀

O98.112 **Syphilis complicating pregnancy, second trimester**　Ⓜ♀

O98.113 **Syphilis complicating pregnancy, third trimester**　Ⓜ♀

O98.119 **Syphilis complicating pregnancy, unspecified trimester**　Ⓜ♀▽

O98.12 **Syphilis complicating childbirth**　Ⓜ♀

O98.13 **Syphilis complicating the puerperium**　Ⓜ♀

✓5ᵗʰ **O98.2** **Gonorrhea complicating pregnancy, childbirth and the puerperium**
Conditions in A54.-

✓6ᵗʰ **O98.21** **Gonorrhea complicating pregnancy**

O98.211 **Gonorrhea complicating pregnancy, first trimester**　Ⓜ♀

EXCLUDES 1　Not coded here　　EXCLUDES 2　Not included here　　Ⓝ Newborn Age : 0　　Ⓟ Pediatric Age : 0-17　　Ⓜ Maternity Age : 12-55　　Ⓐ Adult Age : 15-124

O98.212 **Gonorrhea complicating** M ♀
pregnancy, second trimester

O98.213 **Gonorrhea complicating** M ♀
pregnancy, third trimester

O98.219 **Gonorrhea complicating** M ♀ ▽
pregnancy, unspecified trimester

O98.22 **Gonorrhea complicating** childbirth M ♀

O98.23 **Gonorrhea complicating the** puerperium M ♀

✓5th O98.3 **Other infections with a predominantly sexual mode of transmission complicating pregnancy, childbirth and the puerperium**
Conditions in A55-A64

✓6th O98.31 **Other infections with a predominantly sexual mode of transmission complicating** pregnancy

O98.311 **Other infections with a** M ♀
predominantly sexual mode of
transmission complicating
pregnancy, first trimester

O98.312 **Other infections with a** M ♀
predominantly sexual mode of
transmission complicating
pregnancy, second trimester

O98.313 **Other infections with a** M ♀
predominantly sexual mode of
transmission complicating
pregnancy, third trimester

O98.319 **Other infections with a** M ♀ ▽
predominantly sexual mode of
transmission complicating
pregnancy, unspecified trimester

O98.32 **Other infections with a predominantly** M ♀
sexual mode of transmission complicating
childbirth

O98.33 **Other infections with a predominantly** M ♀
sexual mode of transmission complicating
the puerperium

✓5th O98.4 **Viral hepatitis complicating pregnancy, childbirth and the puerperium**
Conditions in B15-B19

✓6th O98.41 **Viral hepatitis complicating** pregnancy

O98.411 **Viral hepatitis complicating** M ♀
pregnancy, first trimester

O98.412 **Viral hepatitis complicating** M ♀
pregnancy, second trimester

O98.413 **Viral hepatitis complicating** M ♀
pregnancy, third trimester

O98.419 **Viral hepatitis complicating** M ♀ ▽
pregnancy, unspecified trimester

O98.42 **Viral hepatitis complicating** childbirth M ♀

O98.43 **Viral hepatitis complicating the** puerperium M ♀

✓5th O98.5 **Other viral diseases complicating pregnancy, childbirth and the puerperium**
Conditions in A80-B09, B25-B34, R87.81-, R87.82-
EXCLUDES 1 *human immunodeficiency virus [HIV] disease complicating pregnancy, childbirth and the puerperium (O98.7-)*

✓6th O98.51 **Other viral diseases complicating** pregnancy

O98.511 **Other viral diseases complicating** M ♀
pregnancy, first trimester

O98.512 **Other viral diseases complicating** M ♀
pregnancy, second trimester

O98.513 **Other viral diseases complicating** M ♀
pregnancy, third trimester

O98.519 **Other viral diseases complicating** M ♀ ▽
pregnancy, unspecified trimester

O98.52 **Other viral diseases complicating** childbirth M ♀

O98.53 **Other viral diseases complicating the** M ♀
puerperium

✓5th O98.6 **Protozoal diseases complicating pregnancy, childbirth and the puerperium**
Conditions in B50-B64

✓6th O98.61 **Protozoal diseases complicating** pregnancy

O98.611 **Protozoal diseases complicating** M ♀
pregnancy, first trimester

O98.612 **Protozoal diseases complicating** M ♀
pregnancy, second trimester

O98.613 **Protozoal diseases complicating** M ♀
pregnancy, third trimester

O98.619 **Protozoal diseases complicating** M ♀ ▽
pregnancy, unspecified trimester

O98.62 **Protozoal diseases complicating** childbirth M ♀

O98.63 **Protozoal diseases complicating the** M ♀
puerperium

✓5th O98.7 **Human immunodeficiency virus [HIV] disease complicating pregnancy, childbirth and the puerperium**
Use additional code to identify the type of HIV disease:
acquired immune deficiency syndrome (AIDS) (B20)
asymptomatic HIV status (Z21)
HIV positive NOS (Z21)
symptomatic HIV disease (B20)

✓6th O98.71 **Human immunodeficiency virus [HIV] disease complicating** pregnancy

O98.711 **Human immunodeficiency virus** M ♀
[HIV] disease complicating
pregnancy, first trimester

O98.712 **Human immunodeficiency virus** M ♀
[HIV] disease complicating
pregnancy, second trimester

O98.713 **Human immunodeficiency virus** M ♀
[HIV] disease complicating
pregnancy, third trimester

O98.719 **Human immunodeficiency virus** M ♀ ▽
[HIV] disease complicating
pregnancy, unspecified trimester

O98.72 **Human immunodeficiency virus [HIV]** M ♀
disease complicating childbirth

O98.73 **Human immunodeficiency virus [HIV]** M ♀
disease complicating the puerperium

✓5th O98.8 **Other maternal infectious and parasitic diseases complicating pregnancy, childbirth and the puerperium**

✓6th O98.81 **Other maternal infectious and parasitic diseases complicating** pregnancy

O98.811 **Other maternal infectious and** M ♀
parasitic diseases complicating
pregnancy, first trimester

O98.812 **Other maternal infectious and** M ♀
parasitic diseases complicating
pregnancy, second trimester

O98.813 **Other maternal infectious and** M ♀
parasitic diseases complicating
pregnancy, third trimester

O98.819 **Other maternal infectious and** M ♀ ▽
parasitic diseases complicating
pregnancy, unspecified trimester

O98.82 **Other maternal infectious and parasitic** M ♀
diseases complicating childbirth

O98.83 **Other maternal infectious and parasitic** M ♀
diseases complicating the puerperium

✓5th O98.9 **Unspecified maternal infectious and parasitic disease complicating pregnancy, childbirth and the puerperium**

✓6th O98.91 **Unspecified maternal infectious and parasitic disease complicating** pregnancy

O98.911 **Unspecified maternal infectious** M ♀ ▽
and parasitic disease complicating
pregnancy, first trimester

O98.912 **Unspecified maternal infectious** M ♀ ▽
and parasitic disease complicating
pregnancy, second trimester

O98.913 **Unspecified maternal infectious** M ♀ ▽
and parasitic disease complicating
pregnancy, third trimester

O98.919 **Unspecified maternal infectious** M ♀ ▽
and parasitic disease complicating
pregnancy, unspecified trimester

O98.92 **Unspecified maternal infectious and** M ♀ ▽
parasitic disease complicating childbirth

O98.93 **Unspecified maternal infectious and** M ♀ ▽
parasitic disease complicating the
puerperium

✓4th O99 **Other maternal diseases classifiable elsewhere but complicating pregnancy, childbirth and the puerperium**
INCLUDES conditions which complicate the pregnant state, are aggravated by the pregnancy or are a main reason for obstetric care
Use additional code to identify specific condition
EXCLUDES 2 *when the reason for maternal care is that the condition is known or suspected to have affected the fetus (O35-O36)*

✓6th O99.0 **Anemia complicating pregnancy, childbirth and the puerperium**
Conditions in D50-D64
EXCLUDES 1 *anemia arising in the puerperium (O90.81)*
postpartum anemia NOS (O90.81)

☑ Additional Character Required   vx7th Placeholder Alert   Manifestation Dx   ▽ Unspecified Dx   ►◄ Revised Text   ● New Code   ▲ Revised Code Title

ICD-10-CM 2017   831

✓6ᵗʰ **O99.01 Anemia complicating pregnancy**

AHA: 2016,1Q,4

O99.011 Anemia complicating pregnancy, first trimester Ⓜ♀

O99.012 Anemia complicating pregnancy, second trimester Ⓜ♀

O99.013 Anemia complicating pregnancy, third trimester Ⓜ♀

O99.019 Anemia complicating pregnancy, unspecified trimester Ⓜ♀▽

O99.02 Anemia complicating childbirth Ⓜ♀

O99.03 Anemia complicating the puerperium Ⓜ♀

> EXCLUDES 1 *postpartum anemia not pre-existing prior to delivery (O90.81)*

✓5ᵗʰ **O99.1 Other diseases of the blood and blood-forming organs and certain disorders involving the immune mechanism complicating pregnancy, childbirth and the puerperium**

Conditions in D65-D89

> EXCLUDES 2 *hemorrhage with coagulation defects (O45.-, O46.0-, O67.0, O72.3)*

✓6ᵗʰ **O99.11 Other diseases of the blood and blood-forming organs and certain disorders involving the immune mechanism complicating pregnancy**

O99.111 Other diseases of the blood and blood-forming organs and certain disorders involving the immune mechanism complicating pregnancy, first trimester Ⓜ♀

O99.112 Other diseases of the blood and blood-forming organs and certain disorders involving the immune mechanism complicating pregnancy, second trimester Ⓜ♀

O99.113 Other diseases of the blood and blood-forming organs and certain disorders involving the immune mechanism complicating pregnancy, third trimester Ⓜ♀

O99.119 Other diseases of the blood and blood-forming organs and certain disorders involving the immune mechanism complicating pregnancy, unspecified trimester Ⓜ♀▽

O99.12 Other diseases of the blood and blood-forming organs and certain disorders involving the immune mechanism complicating childbirth Ⓜ♀

O99.13 Other diseases of the blood and blood-forming organs and certain disorders involving the immune mechanism complicating the puerperium Ⓜ♀

✓5ᵗʰ **O99.2 Endocrine, nutritional and metabolic diseases complicating pregnancy, childbirth and the puerperium**

Conditions in E00-E88

> EXCLUDES 2 *diabetes mellitus (O24.-)*
> *malnutrition (O25.-)*
> *postpartum thyroiditis (O90.5)*

✓6ᵗʰ **O99.21 Obesity complicating pregnancy, childbirth, and the puerperium**

Use additional code to identify the type of obesity (E66.-)

O99.210 Obesity complicating pregnancy, unspecified trimester Ⓜ♀▽

O99.211 Obesity complicating pregnancy, first trimester Ⓜ♀

O99.212 Obesity complicating pregnancy, second trimester Ⓜ♀

O99.213 Obesity complicating pregnancy, third trimester Ⓜ♀

O99.214 Obesity complicating childbirth Ⓜ♀

O99.215 Obesity complicating the puerperium Ⓜ♀

✓6ᵗʰ **O99.28 Other endocrine, nutritional and metabolic diseases complicating pregnancy, childbirth and the puerperium**

O99.280 Endocrine, nutritional and metabolic diseases complicating pregnancy, unspecified trimester ♀▽

O99.281 Endocrine, nutritional and metabolic diseases complicating pregnancy, first trimester Ⓜ♀

O99.282 Endocrine, nutritional and metabolic diseases complicating pregnancy, second trimester Ⓜ♀

O99.283 Endocrine, nutritional and metabolic diseases complicating pregnancy, third trimester Ⓜ♀

O99.284 Endocrine, nutritional and metabolic diseases complicating childbirth Ⓜ♀

O99.285 Endocrine, nutritional and metabolic diseases complicating the puerperium Ⓜ♀

✓5ᵗʰ **O99.3 Mental disorders and diseases of the nervous system complicating pregnancy, childbirth and the puerperium**

✓6ᵗʰ **O99.31 Alcohol use complicating pregnancy, childbirth, and the puerperium**

Use additional code(s) from F10 to identify manifestations of the alcohol use

O99.310 Alcohol use complicating pregnancy, unspecified trimester Ⓜ♀▽

O99.311 Alcohol use complicating pregnancy, first trimester Ⓜ♀

O99.312 Alcohol use complicating pregnancy, second trimester Ⓜ♀

O99.313 Alcohol use complicating pregnancy, third trimester Ⓜ♀

O99.314 Alcohol use complicating childbirth Ⓜ♀

O99.315 Alcohol use complicating the puerperium Ⓜ♀

✓6ᵗʰ **O99.32 Drug use complicating pregnancy, childbirth, and the puerperium**

Use additional code(s) from F11-F16 and F18-F19 to identify manifestations of the drug use

O99.320 Drug use complicating pregnancy, unspecified trimester Ⓜ♀▽

O99.321 Drug use complicating pregnancy, first trimester Ⓜ♀

O99.322 Drug use complicating pregnancy, second trimester Ⓜ♀

O99.323 Drug use complicating pregnancy, third trimester Ⓜ♀

O99.324 Drug use complicating childbirth Ⓜ♀

O99.325 Drug use complicating the puerperium Ⓜ♀

✓6ᵗʰ **O99.33 Tobacco use disorder complicating pregnancy, childbirth, and the puerperium**

▶Smoking complicating pregnancy, childbirth, and the puerperium◀

▶Use additional code from category F17 to identify type of tobacco nicotine dependence◀

O99.330 Smoking (tobacco) complicating pregnancy, unspecified trimester Ⓜ♀▽

O99.331 Smoking (tobacco) complicating pregnancy, first trimester Ⓜ♀

O99.332 Smoking (tobacco) complicating pregnancy, second trimester Ⓜ♀

O99.333 Smoking (tobacco) complicating pregnancy, third trimester Ⓜ♀

O99.334 Smoking (tobacco) complicating childbirth Ⓜ♀

O99.335 Smoking (tobacco) complicating the puerperium Ⓜ♀

✓6ᵗʰ **O99.34 Other mental disorders complicating pregnancy, childbirth, and the puerperium**

Conditions in F01-F09 and F20-F99

> EXCLUDES 2 *postpartum mood disturbance (O90.6)*
> *postnatal psychosis (F53)*
> *puerperal psychosis (F53)*

O99.340 Other mental disorders complicating pregnancy, unspecified trimester Ⓜ♀▽

O99.341 Other mental disorders complicating pregnancy, first trimester Ⓜ♀

O99.342 Other mental disorders complicating pregnancy, second trimester Ⓜ♀

O99.343 Other mental disorders complicating pregnancy, third trimester Ⓜ♀

O99.344 Other mental disorders complicating childbirth Ⓜ♀

EXCLUDES 1 Not coded here   EXCLUDES 2 Not included here   Ⓝ Newborn Age : 0   Ⓟ Pediatric Age : 0-17   Ⓜ Maternity Age : 12-55   Ⓐ Adult Age : 15-124

O99.345 **Other mental disorders complicating the** puerperium   M ♀

√6ᵗʰ O99.35 **Diseases of the** nervous system **complicating pregnancy, childbirth, and the puerperium**
Conditions in G00-G99
EXCLUDES 2 *pregnancy related peripheral neuritis (O26.8-)*

O99.350 **Diseases of the nervous system complicating pregnancy, unspecified trimester**   M ♀ ▽

O99.351 **Diseases of the nervous system complicating pregnancy,** first **trimester**   M ♀

O99.352 **Diseases of the nervous system complicating pregnancy,** second **trimester**   M ♀

O99.353 **Diseases of the nervous system complicating pregnancy,** third **trimester**   M ♀

O99.354 **Diseases of the nervous system complicating** childbirth   M ♀

O99.355 **Diseases of the nervous system complicating the** puerperium   M ♀

√5ᵗʰ O99.4 **Diseases of the** circulatory system **complicating pregnancy, childbirth and the puerperium**
Conditions in I00-I99
EXCLUDES 1 *peripartum cardiomyopathy (O90.3)*
EXCLUDES 2 *hypertensive disorders (O10-O16)*
obstetric embolism (O88.-)
venous complications and cerebrovenous sinus thrombosis in labor, childbirth and the puerperium (O87.-)
venous complications and cerebrovenous sinus thrombosis in pregnancy (O22.-)
AHA: 2016,2Q,8

√6ᵗʰ O99.41 **Diseases of the circulatory system complicating pregnancy**

O99.411 **Diseases of the circulatory system complicating pregnancy,** first **trimester**   M ♀

O99.412 **Diseases of the circulatory system complicating pregnancy,** second **trimester**   M ♀

O99.413 **Diseases of the circulatory system complicating pregnancy,** third **trimester**   M ♀

O99.419 **Diseases of the circulatory system complicating pregnancy, unspecified trimester**   M ♀ ▽

O99.42 **Diseases of the circulatory system complicating** childbirth   M ♀

O99.43 **Diseases of the circulatory system complicating the** puerperium   M ♀

√5ᵗʰ O99.5 **Diseases of the** respiratory system **complicating pregnancy, childbirth and the puerperium**
Conditions in J00-J99

√6ᵗʰ O99.51 **Diseases of the respiratory system complicating pregnancy**

O99.511 **Diseases of the respiratory system complicating pregnancy,** first **trimester**   M ♀

O99.512 **Diseases of the respiratory system complicating pregnancy,** second **trimester**   M ♀

O99.513 **Diseases of the respiratory system complicating pregnancy,** third **trimester**   M ♀

O99.519 **Diseases of the respiratory system complicating pregnancy, unspecified trimester**   M ♀ ▽

O99.52 **Diseases of the respiratory system complicating** childbirth   M ♀

O99.53 **Diseases of the respiratory system complicating the** puerperium   M ♀

√5ᵗʰ O99.6 **Diseases of the** digestive system **complicating pregnancy, childbirth and the puerperium**
Conditions in K00-K93
EXCLUDES 2 ▶*hemorrhoids in pregnancy (O22.4-)*◀
liver and biliary tract disorders in pregnancy, childbirth and the puerperium (O26.6-)

√6ᵗʰ O99.61 **Diseases of the digestive system complicating pregnancy**
AHA: 2016,1Q,4

O99.611 **Diseases of the digestive system complicating pregnancy,** first **trimester**   M ♀

O99.612 **Diseases of the digestive system complicating pregnancy,** second **trimester**   M ♀

O99.613 **Diseases of the digestive system complicating pregnancy,** third **trimester**   M ♀

O99.619 **Diseases of the digestive system complicating pregnancy, unspecified trimester**   M ♀ ▽

O99.62 **Diseases of the digestive system complicating** childbirth   M ♀

O99.63 **Diseases of the digestive system complicating the** puerperium   M ♀

√5ᵗʰ O99.7 **Diseases of the** skin and subcutaneous tissue **complicating pregnancy, childbirth and the puerperium**
Conditions in L00-L99
EXCLUDES 2 *herpes gestationis (O26.4)*
pruritic urticarial papules and plaques of pregnancy (PUPPP) (O26.86)

√6ᵗʰ O99.71 **Diseases of the skin and subcutaneous tissue complicating pregnancy**

O99.711 **Diseases of the skin and subcutaneous tissue complicating pregnancy, first trimester**   M ♀

O99.712 **Diseases of the skin and subcutaneous tissue complicating pregnancy,** second trimester   M ♀

O99.713 **Diseases of the skin and subcutaneous tissue complicating pregnancy, third trimester**   M ♀

O99.719 **Diseases of the skin and subcutaneous tissue complicating pregnancy, unspecified trimester**   M ♀ ▽

O99.72 **Diseases of the skin and subcutaneous tissue complicating** childbirth   M ♀

O99.73 **Diseases of the skin and subcutaneous tissue complicating the** puerperium   M ♀

√5ᵗʰ O99.8 **Other specified diseases and conditions complicating pregnancy, childbirth and the puerperium**
Conditions in D00-D48, H00-H95, M00-N99, and Q00-Q99
Use additional code to identify condition
EXCLUDES 2 *genitourinary infections in pregnancy (O23.-)*
infection of genitourinary tract following delivery (O86.1-O86.3)
malignant neoplasm complicating pregnancy, childbirth and the puerperium (O9A.1-)
maternal care for known or suspected abnormality of maternal pelvic organs (O34.-)
postpartum acute kidney failure (O90.4)
traumatic injuries in pregnancy (O9A.2-)

√6ᵗʰ O99.81 **Abnormal glucose complicating pregnancy, childbirth and the puerperium**
EXCLUDES 1 *gestational diabetes (O24.4-)*

O99.810 **Abnormal glucose complicating pregnancy**   M ♀

O99.814 **Abnormal glucose complicating childbirth**   M ♀

O99.815 **Abnormal glucose complicating the puerperium**   M ♀

√6ᵗʰ O99.82 **Streptococcus B carrier state complicating pregnancy, childbirth and the puerperium**
EXCLUDES 1 ▶*carrier of streptococcus group B (GBS) in a nonpregnant woman (Z22.330)*◀

O99.820 **Streptococcus B carrier state complicating pregnancy**   M ♀

O99.824 **Streptococcus B carrier state complicating childbirth**   M ♀

O99.825 **Streptococcus B carrier state complicating the puerperium**   M ♀

√6ᵗʰ O99.83 **Other infection carrier state complicating pregnancy, childbirth and the puerperium**
Use additional code to identify the carrier state (Z22.-)

O99.830 **Other infection carrier state complicating pregnancy**   M ♀

O99.834 **Other infection carrier state complicating childbirth**   M ♀

Chapter 15. Pregnancy, Childbirth and the Puerperium

O99.835   **Other infection carrier state complicating the puerperium**   Ⓜ ♀

✓6ᵗʰ **O99.84**   **Bariatric surgery status complicating pregnancy, childbirth and the puerperium**

Gastric banding status complicating pregnancy, childbirth and the puerperium

Gastric bypass status for obesity complicating pregnancy, childbirth and the puerperium

Obesity surgery status complicating pregnancy, childbirth and the puerperium

O99.840   **Bariatric surgery status complicating pregnancy, unspecified trimester**   Ⓜ ♀ ▽

O99.841   **Bariatric surgery status complicating pregnancy, first trimester**   Ⓜ ♀

O99.842   **Bariatric surgery status complicating pregnancy, second trimester**   Ⓜ ♀

O99.843   **Bariatric surgery status complicating pregnancy, third trimester**   Ⓜ ♀

O99.844   **Bariatric surgery status complicating childbirth**   Ⓜ ♀

O99.845   **Bariatric surgery status complicating the puerperium**   Ⓜ ♀

O99.89   **Other specified diseases and conditions complicating pregnancy, childbirth and the puerperium**   Ⓜ ♀

✓4ᵗʰ **O9A**   **Maternal malignant neoplasms, traumatic injuries and abuse classifiable elsewhere but complicating pregnancy, childbirth and the puerperium**

✓5ᵗʰ **O9A.1**   **Malignant neoplasm complicating pregnancy, childbirth and the puerperium**

Conditions in C00-C96

Use additional code to identify neoplasm

> EXCLUDES 2 *maternal care for benign tumor of corpus uteri (O34.1-)*
> *maternal care for benign tumor of cervix (O34.4-)*

AHA: 2015,3Q,19

✓6ᵗʰ **O9A.11**   **Malignant neoplasm complicating pregnancy**

O9A.111   **Malignant neoplasm complicating pregnancy, first trimester**   Ⓜ ♀

O9A.112   **Malignant neoplasm complicating pregnancy, second trimester**   Ⓜ ♀

O9A.113   **Malignant neoplasm complicating pregnancy, third trimester**   Ⓜ ♀

O9A.119   **Malignant neoplasm complicating pregnancy, unspecified trimester**   Ⓜ ♀ ▽

O9A.12   **Malignant neoplasm complicating childbirth**   Ⓜ ♀

O9A.13   **Malignant neoplasm complicating the puerperium**   Ⓜ ♀

✓5ᵗʰ **O9A.2**   **Injury, poisoning and certain other consequences of external causes complicating pregnancy, childbirth and the puerperium**

Conditions in S00-T88, except T74 and T76

Use additional code(s) to identify the injury or poisoning

> EXCLUDES 2 *physical, sexual and psychological abuse complicating pregnancy, childbirth and the puerperium (O9A.3-, O9A.4-, O9A.5-)*

✓6ᵗʰ **O9A.21**   **Injury, poisoning and certain other consequences of external causes complicating pregnancy**

O9A.211   **Injury, poisoning and certain other consequences of external causes complicating pregnancy, first trimester**   Ⓜ ♀

O9A.212   **Injury, poisoning and certain other consequences of external causes complicating pregnancy, second trimester**   Ⓜ ♀

O9A.213   **Injury, poisoning and certain other consequences of external causes complicating pregnancy, third trimester**   Ⓜ ♀

O9A.219   **Injury, poisoning and certain other consequences of external causes complicating pregnancy, unspecified trimester**   Ⓜ ♀ ▽

O9A.22   **Injury, poisoning and certain other consequences of external causes complicating childbirth**   Ⓜ ♀

O9A.23   **Injury, poisoning and certain other consequences of external causes complicating the puerperium**   Ⓜ ♀

✓5ᵗʰ **O9A.3**   **Physical abuse complicating pregnancy, childbirth and the puerperium**

Conditions in T74.11 or T76.11

Use additional code (if applicable):

> to identify any associated current injury due to physical abuse
> to identify the perpetrator of abuse (Y07.-)

> EXCLUDES 2 *sexual abuse complicating pregnancy, childbirth and the puerperium (O9A.4)*

✓6ᵗʰ **O9A.31**   **Physical abuse complicating pregnancy**

O9A.311   **Physical abuse complicating pregnancy, first trimester**   Ⓜ ♀

O9A.312   **Physical abuse complicating pregnancy, second trimester**   Ⓜ ♀

O9A.313   **Physical abuse complicating pregnancy, third trimester**   Ⓜ ♀

O9A.319   **Physical abuse complicating pregnancy, unspecified trimester**   Ⓜ ♀ ▽

O9A.32   **Physical abuse complicating childbirth**   Ⓜ ♀

O9A.33   **Physical abuse complicating the puerperium**   Ⓜ ♀

✓5ᵗʰ **O9A.4**   **Sexual abuse complicating pregnancy, childbirth and the puerperium**

Conditions in T74.21 or T76.21

Use additional code (if applicable):

> to identify any associated current injury due to sexual abuse
> to identify the perpetrator of abuse (Y07.-)

✓6ᵗʰ **O9A.41**   **Sexual abuse complicating pregnancy**

O9A.411   **Sexual abuse complicating pregnancy, first trimester**   Ⓜ ♀

O9A.412   **Sexual abuse complicating pregnancy, second trimester**   Ⓜ ♀

O9A.413   **Sexual abuse complicating pregnancy, third trimester**   Ⓜ ♀

O9A.419   **Sexual abuse complicating pregnancy, unspecified trimester**   Ⓜ ♀ ▽

O9A.42   **Sexual abuse complicating childbirth**   Ⓜ ♀

O9A.43   **Sexual abuse complicating the puerperium**   Ⓜ ♀

✓5ᵗʰ **O9A.5**   **Psychological abuse complicating pregnancy, childbirth and the puerperium**

Conditions in T74.31 or T76.31

Use additional code to identify the perpetrator of abuse (Y07.-)

✓6ᵗʰ **O9A.51**   **Psychological abuse complicating pregnancy**

O9A.511   **Psychological abuse complicating pregnancy, first trimester**   Ⓜ ♀

O9A.512   **Psychological abuse complicating pregnancy, second trimester**   Ⓜ ♀

O9A.513   **Psychological abuse complicating pregnancy, third trimester**   Ⓜ ♀

O9A.519   **Psychological abuse complicating pregnancy, unspecified trimester**   Ⓜ ♀ ▽

O9A.52   **Psychological abuse complicating childbirth**   Ⓜ ♀

O9A.53   **Psychological abuse complicating the puerperium**   Ⓜ ♀

EXCLUDES 1 Not coded here   EXCLUDES 2 Not included here   Ⓝ Newborn Age : 0   Ⓟ Pediatric Age : 0-17   Ⓜ Maternity Age : 12-55   Ⓐ Adult Age : 15-124

834   ICD-10-CM 2017

Chapter 16. Certain Conditions Originating in the Perinatal Period (P00–P96)

Chapter Specific Guidelines with Coding Examples

The chapter specific guidelines from the ICD-10-CM Official Guidelines for Coding and Reporting have been provided below. Along with these guidelines are coding examples, contained in the shaded boxes, that have been developed to help illustrate the coding and/or sequencing guidance found in these guidelines.

For coding and reporting purposes the perinatal period is defined as before birth through the 28th day following birth. The following guidelines are provided for reporting purposes

a. General perinatal rules

1) Use of Chapter 16 codes

Codes in this chapter are <u>never</u> for use on the maternal record. Codes from Chapter 15, the obstetric chapter, are never permitted on the newborn record. Chapter 16 codes may be used throughout the life of the patient if the condition is still present.

2) Principal diagnosis for birth record

When coding the birth episode in a newborn record, assign a code from category Z38, Liveborn infants according to place of birth and type of delivery, as the principal diagnosis. A code from category Z38 is assigned only once, to a newborn at the time of birth. If a newborn is transferred to another institution, a code from category Z38 should not be used at the receiving hospital.

A code from category Z38 is used only on the newborn record, not on the mother's record.

> Newborn delivered via vaginal delivery in Rural Hospital A, experienced meconium aspiration resulting in pneumonia. Rural Hospital A is not equipped to handle the extensive respiratory therapy this baby needs and transfers the patient to Metropolis Hospital B, where the pneumonia resolves and the newborn is eventually discharged.
>
> *Rural Hospital A*
>
> **Z38.00**   **Single liveborn infant, delivered vaginally**
>
> **P24.01**   **Meconium aspiration with respiratory symptoms**
>
> *Metropolis Hospital B*
>
> **P24.01**   **Meconium aspiration with respiratory symptoms**
>
> *Explanation:* A code from category Z38 is a one-time use only code. The hospital that actually delivered the newborn, in this case Rural Hospital A, can append a code from category Z38 but for the delivery admission only. Once the patient is transferred or discharged, the Z38 category no longer applies for that patient.
>
> The reason for the transfer to Metropolis Hospital B was for the respiratory symptoms (pneumonia) the newborn was exhibiting secondary to aspirating meconium.

3) Use of codes from other chapters with codes from Chapter 16

Codes from other chapters may be used with codes from chapter 16 if the codes from the other chapters provide more specific detail. Codes for signs and symptoms may be assigned when a definitive diagnosis has not been established. If the reason for the encounter is a perinatal condition, the code from chapter 16 should be sequenced first.

4) Use of Chapter 16 codes after the perinatal period

Should a condition originate in the perinatal period, and continue throughout the life of the patient, the perinatal code should continue to be used regardless of the patient's age.

> A 7-year-old patient with history of birth injury that resulted in Erb's palsy is seen for subscapularis release
>
> **P14.0**   **Erb's paralysis due to birth injury**
>
> *Explanation:* Although in this instance Erb's palsy is specifically related to a birth injury, it has not resolved and continues to be a health concern. A perinatal code is appropriate even though this patient is beyond the perinatal period.

5) Birth process or community acquired conditions

If a newborn has a condition that may be either due to the birth process or community acquired and the documentation does not indicate which it is, the default is due to the birth process and the code from Chapter 16 should be used. If the condition is community-acquired, a code from Chapter 16 should not be assigned.

6) Code all clinically significant conditions

All clinically significant conditions noted on routine newborn examination should be coded. A condition is clinically significant if it requires:

clinical evaluation; or

therapeutic treatment; or

diagnostic procedures; or

extended length of hospital stay; or

increased nursing care and/or monitoring; or

has implications for future health care needs

Note: The perinatal guidelines listed above are the same as the general coding guidelines for "additional diagnoses", except for the final point regarding implications for future health care needs. Codes should be assigned for conditions that have been specified by the provider as having implications for future health care needs.

b. Observation and evaluation of newborns for suspected conditions not found

1)
Assign a code from category Z05, Observation and evaluation of newborns and infants for suspected conditions ruled out, to identify those instances when a healthy newborn is evaluated for a suspected condition that is determined after study not to be present. Do not use a code from category Z05 when the patient has identified signs or symptoms of a suspected problem; in such cases code the sign or symptom.

2)
A code from category Z05 may also be assigned as a principal or first-listed code for readmissions or encounters when the code from category Z38 code no longer applies. Codes from category Z05 are for use only for healthy newborns and infants for which no condition after study is found to be present.

3) Z05 on a birth record

A code from category Z05 is to be used as a secondary code after the code from category Z38, Liveborn infants according to place of birth and type of delivery.

> Newborn delivered via vaginal delivery; previous ultrasounds showed what appeared to be an abnormality of the right kidney. Kidney function tests were performed and ultrasounds taken and any genitourinary conditions ruled out.
>
> **Z38.00**   **Single liveborn infant, delivered vaginally**
>
> **Z05.6**   **Observation and evaluation of newborn for suspected genitourinary condition ruled out**
>
> *Explanation:* The newborn had no signs or symptoms of kidney or other genitourinary condition but was evaluated after delivery due to the abnormal prenatal ultrasound findings. A Z code describing the type and place of birth should be coded first, followed by a Z05 category code for the work performed to rule out a suspected genitourinary condition.

c. Coding additional perinatal diagnoses

1) Assigning codes for conditions that require treatment

Assign codes for conditions that require treatment or further investigation, prolong the length of stay, or require resource utilization.

2) Codes for conditions specified as having implications for future health care needs

Assign codes for conditions that have been specified by the provider as having implications for future health care needs.

Note: This guideline should not be used for adult patients.

> An abnormal noise was heard in the left hip of a post-term newborn during a physical examination. The pediatrician would like to follow the patient after discharge as a hip click can be an early sign of hip dysplasia. The newborn was delivered via cesarean at 41 weeks.
>
> **Z38.01   Single liveborn infant, delivered by cesarean**
>
> **P08.21   Post-term newborn**
>
> **R29.4   Clicking hip**
>
> *Explanation:* The abnormal hip noise or click is appended as a secondary diagnosis not only because it is an abnormal finding upon examination, but also due to its potential to be part of a bigger health issue. The hip dysplasia has not yet been diagnosed and does not warrant a code at this time.

d. Prematurity and fetal growth retardation

Providers utilize different criteria in determining prematurity. A code for prematurity should not be assigned unless it is documented. Assignment of codes in categories P05, Disorders of newborn related to slow fetal growth and fetal malnutrition, and P07, Disorders of newborn related to short gestation and low birth weight, not elsewhere classified, should be based on the recorded birth weight and estimated gestational age. Codes from category P05 should not be assigned with codes from category P07.

When both birth weight and gestational age are available, two codes from category P07 should be assigned, with the code for birth weight sequenced before the code for gestational age.

e. Low birth weight and immaturity status

Codes from category P07, Disorders of newborn related to short gestation and low birth weight, not elsewhere classified, are for use for a child or adult who was premature or had a low birth weight as a newborn and this is affecting the patient's current health status.

See Section I.C.21. Factors influencing health status and contact with health services, Status.

> A 35-year-old patient, who weighed 659 grams at birth, is seen for heart disease documented as being a consequence of the low birth weight
>
> **I51.9   Heart disease, unspecified**
>
> **P07.02   Extremely low birth weight newborn, 500–749 grams**
>
> *Explanation:* A code from subcategories P07.0- and P07.1- is appropriate, regardless of the age of the patient, as long as the documentation provides a clear link between the patient's current illness and the low birth weight.

f. Bacterial sepsis of newborn

Category P36, Bacterial sepsis of newborn, includes congenital sepsis. If a perinate is documented as having sepsis without documentation of congenital or community acquired, the default is congenital and a code from category P36 should be assigned. If the P36 code includes the causal organism, an additional code from category B95, Streptococcus, Staphylococcus, and Enterococcus as the cause of diseases classified elsewhere, or B96, Other bacterial agents as the cause of diseases classified elsewhere, should not be assigned. If the P36 code does not include the causal organism, assign an additional code from category B96. If applicable, use additional codes to identify severe sepsis (R65.2-) and any associated acute organ dysfunction.

> A full-term infant develops severe sepsis 24 hours after discharge from the hospital and is readmitted; cultures identified *E. coli* as the infective agent
>
> **P36.4   Sepsis of newborn due to Escherichia coli**
>
> **R65.20   Severe sepsis without septic shock**
>
> *Explanation:* Even though this newborn was discharged and could have acquired *E. coli* from his/her external environment, due to the lack of documentation specifying specifically how this pathogen was acquired, the default is to code the *E. coli* sepsis as congenital. A code from chapter 1, "Certain Infectious and Parasitic Diseases," is not required because the perinatal sepsis code identifies both the sepsis and the bacteria causing the sepsis.

g. Stillbirth

Code P95, Stillbirth, is only for use in institutions that maintain separate records for stillbirths. No other code should be used with P95. Code P95 should not be used on the mother's record.

Chapter 16. Certain Conditions Originating in the Perinatal Period (P00-P96)

NOTE Codes from this chapter are for use on newborn records only, never on maternal records.

INCLUDES conditions that have their origin in the fetal or perinatal period (before birth through the first 28 days after birth) even if morbidity occurs later

EXCLUDES 2 *congenital malformations, deformations and chromosomal abnormalities (Q00-Q99)*
endocrine, nutritional and metabolic diseases (E00-E88)
injury, poisoning and certain other consequences of external causes (S00-T88)
neoplasms (C00-D49)
tetanus neonatorum (A33)

This chapter contains the following blocks:

P00-P04   Newborn affected by maternal factors and by complications of pregnancy, labor, and delivery
P05-P08   Disorders of newborn related to length of gestation and fetal growth
P09   Abnormal findings on neonatal screening
P10-P15   Birth trauma
P19-P29   Respiratory and cardiovascular disorders specific to the perinatal period
P35-P39   Infections specific to the perinatal period
P50-P61   Hemorrhagic and hematological disorders of newborn
P70-P74   Transitory endocrine and metabolic disorders specific to newborn
P76-P78   Digestive system disorders of newborn
P80-P83   Conditions involving the integument and temperature regulation of newborn
P84   Other problems with newborn
P90-P96   Other disorders originating in the perinatal period

Newborn affected by maternal factors and by complications of pregnancy, labor, and delivery (P00-P04)

NOTE ▶These codes are for use when the listed maternal conditions are specified as the cause of confirmed morbidity or potential morbidity which have their origin in the perinatal period (before birth through the first 28 days after birth).◀

▲ ✔4ᵗʰ **P00** **Newborn affected by maternal conditions that may be unrelated to present pregnancy**
Code first any current condition in newborn
EXCLUDES 2 ▶*encounter for observation of newborn for suspected diseases and conditions ruled out (Z05.-)*◀
▶*newborn affected by maternal complications of pregnancy (P01.-)*◀
newborn affected by maternal endocrine and metabolic disorders (P70-P74)
newborn affected by noxious substances transmitted via placenta or breast milk (P04.-)

▲   **P00.0** **Newborn affected by maternal hypertensive disorders**
▶Newborn affected by maternal conditions classifiable to O10-O11, O13-O16◀

▲   **P00.1** **Newborn affected by maternal renal and urinary tract diseases**
▶Newborn affected by maternal conditions classifiable to N00-N39◀

▲   **P00.2** **Newborn affected by maternal infectious and parasitic diseases**
▶Newborn affected by maternal infectious disease classifiable to A00-B99, J09 and J10◀
EXCLUDES 1 *infections specific to the perinatal period (P35-P39)*
maternal genital tract or other localized infections (P00.8)
AHA: 2015,3Q,20

▲   **P00.3** **Newborn affected by other maternal circulatory and respiratory diseases**
▶Newborn affected by maternal conditions classifiable to I00-I99, J00-J99, Q20-Q34 and not included in P00.0, P00.2◀

▲   **P00.4** **Newborn affected by maternal nutritional disorders**
▶Newborn affected by maternal disorders classifiable to E40-E64◀
Maternal malnutrition NOS

▲   **P00.5** **Newborn affected by maternal injury**
▶Newborn affected by maternal conditions classifiable to O9A.2-◀

▲   **P00.6** **Newborn affected by surgical procedure on mother**
▶Newborn affected by amniocentesis◀
EXCLUDES 1 *Cesarean delivery for present delivery (P03.4)*
damage to placenta from amniocentesis, Cesarean delivery or surgical induction (P02.1)
previous surgery to uterus or pelvic organs (P03.89)
EXCLUDES 2 *newborn affected by complication of (fetal) intrauterine procedure (P96.5)*

▲   **P00.7** **Newborn affected by other medical procedures on mother, not elsewhere classified**
▶Newborn affected by radiation to mother◀
EXCLUDES 1 *damage to placenta from amniocentesis, cesarean delivery or surgical induction (P02.1)*
newborn affected by other complications of labor and delivery (P03.-)

▲ ✔5ᵗʰ **P00.8** **Newborn affected by other maternal conditions**
▲   **P00.81** **Newborn affected by periodontal disease in mother**
▲   **P00.89** **Newborn affected by other maternal conditions**
▶Newborn affected by conditions classifiable to T80-T88◀
▶Newborn affected by maternal genital tract or other localized infections◀
▶Newborn affected by maternal systemic lupus erythematosus◀

▲   **P00.9** **Newborn affected by unspecified maternal condition** ▽

▲ ✔4ᵗʰ **P01** **Newborn affected by maternal complications of pregnancy**
Code first any current condition in newborn
EXCLUDES 2 ▶*encounter for observation of newborn for suspected diseases and conditions ruled out (Z05.-)*◀

▲   **P01.0** **Newborn affected by incompetent cervix**

▲   **P01.1** **Newborn affected by premature rupture of membranes**

▲   **P01.2** **Newborn affected by oligohydramnios**
EXCLUDES 1 *oligohydramnios due to premature rupture of membranes (P01.1)*

▲   **P01.3** **Newborn affected by polyhydramnios**
▶Newborn affected by hydramnios◀

▲   **P01.4** **Newborn affected by ectopic pregnancy**
▶Newborn affected by abdominal pregnancy◀

▲   **P01.5** **Newborn affected by multiple pregnancy**
▶Newborn affected by triplet (pregnancy)◀
▶Newborn affected by twin (pregnancy)◀

▲   **P01.6** **Newborn affected by maternal death**

▲   **P01.7** **Newborn affected by malpresentation before labor**
▶Newborn affected by breech presentation before labor◀
▶Newborn affected by external version before labor◀
▶Newborn affected by face presentation before labor◀
▶Newborn affected by transverse lie before labor◀
▶Newborn affected by unstable lie before labor◀

▲   **P01.8** **Newborn affected by other maternal complications of pregnancy**

▲   **P01.9** **Newborn affected by maternal complication of pregnancy, unspecified** ▽

▲ ✔4ᵗʰ **P02** **Newborn affected by complications of placenta, cord and membranes**
Code first any current condition in newborn
EXCLUDES 2 ▶*encounter for observation of newborn for suspected diseases and conditions ruled out (Z05.-)*◀

▲   **P02.0** **Newborn affected by placenta previa**
DEF: Placenta developed in lower segment of uterus; can cause hemorrhaging leading to preterm delivery.

▲   **P02.1** **Newborn affected by other forms of placental separation and hemorrhage**
▶Newborn affected by abruptio placenta◀
▶Newborn affected by accidental hemorrhage◀
▶Newborn affected by antepartum hemorrhage◀
▶Newborn affected by damage to placenta from amniocentesis, cesarean delivery or surgical induction◀
▶Newborn affected by maternal blood loss◀
▶Newborn affected by premature separation of placenta◀

▲ ✔5ᵗʰ **P02.2** **Newborn affected by other and unspecified morphological and functional abnormalities of placenta**
▲   **P02.20** **Newborn affected by unspecified morphological and functional abnormalities of placenta** ▽

☑ Additional Character Required   ✔x7ᵗʰ Placeholder Alert   Manifestation Dx   ▽ Unspecified Dx   ▶◀ Revised Text   ● New Code   ▲ Revised Code Title

Chapter 16. Certain Conditions Originating in the Perinatal Period

▲   **P02.29**   **Newborn affected by** other **morphological and functional abnormalities of placenta**
- ▶Newborn affected by placental dysfunction◀
- ▶Newborn affected by placental infarction◀
- ▶Newborn affected by placental insufficiency◀

▲   **P02.3**   **Newborn affected by placental transfusion syndromes**
- ▶Newborn affected by placental and cord abnormalities resulting in twin-to-twin or other transplacental transfusion◀

▲   **P02.4**   **Newborn affected by prolapsed cord**

▲   **P02.5**   **Newborn affected by** other **compression of umbilical cord**
- ▶Newborn affected by umbilical cord (tightly) around neck◀
- ▶Newborn affected by entanglement of umbilical cord◀
- ▶Newborn affected by knot in umbilical cord◀

▲ ✓5ᵗʰ   **P02.6**   **Newborn affected by other and unspecified** conditions of umbilical cord

▲   **P02.60**   **Newborn affected by unspecified conditions of umbilical cord** ▽

▲   **P02.69**   **Newborn affected by other conditions of umbilical cord**
- ▶Newborn affected by short umbilical cord◀
- ▶Newborn affected by vasa previa◀
- EXCLUDES 1 *newborn affected by single umbilical artery (Q27.0)*

▲   **P02.7**   **Newborn affected by chorioamnionitis**
- ▶Newborn affected by amnionitis◀
- ▶Newborn affected by membranitis◀
- ▶Newborn affected by placentitis◀

▲   **P02.8**   **Newborn affected by** other **abnormalities of membranes**

▲   **P02.9**   **Newborn affected by abnormality of membranes, unspecified** ▽

▲ ✓4ᵗʰ   **P03**   **Newborn affected by other complications of labor and delivery**

Code first any current condition in newborn

EXCLUDES 2 ▶*encounter for observation of newborn for suspected diseases and conditions ruled out (Z05.-)* ◀

▲   **P03.0**   **Newborn affected by breech delivery and extraction**

▲   **P03.1**   **Newborn affected by** other **malpresentation, malposition and disproportion during labor and delivery**
- ▶Newborn affected by contracted pelvis◀
- ▶Newborn affected by conditions classifiable to O64-O66◀
- ▶Newborn affected by persistent occipitoposterior◀
- ▶Newborn affected by transverse lie◀

▲   **P03.2**   **Newborn affected by forceps delivery**

▲   **P03.3**   **Newborn affected by delivery by vacuum extractor [ventouse]**

▲   **P03.4**   **Newborn affected by Cesarean delivery**

▲   **P03.5**   **Newborn affected by precipitate delivery**
- ▶Newborn affected by rapid second stage◀

▲   **P03.6**   **Newborn affected by abnormal uterine contractions**
- ▶Newborn affected by conditions classifiable to O62.-, except O62.3◀
- ▶Newborn affected by hypertonic labor◀
- ▶Newborn affected by uterine inertia◀

▲ ✓5ᵗʰ   **P03.8**   **Newborn affected by** other **specified complications of labor and delivery**

▲ ✓6ᵗʰ   **P03.81**   **Newborn affected by abnormality in fetal (intrauterine) heart rate or rhythm**
- EXCLUDES 1 *neonatal cardiac dysrhythmia (P29.1-)*

▲   **P03.810**   **Newborn affected by abnormality in fetal (intrauterine) heart rate or rhythm before the onset of labor**

▲   **P03.811**   **Newborn affected by abnormality in fetal (intrauterine) heart rate or rhythm during labor**

▲   **P03.819**   **Newborn affected by abnormality in fetal (intrauterine) heart rate or rhythm, unspecified as to time of onset** ▽

    P03.82   **Meconium passage during delivery**
- EXCLUDES 1 *meconium aspiration (P24.00, P24.01)*
- *meconium staining (P96.83)*

▲   **P03.89**   **Newborn affected by** other **specified complications of labor and delivery**
- ▶Newborn affected by abnormality of maternal soft tissues◀
- ▶Newborn affected by conditions classifiable to O60-O75 and by procedures used in labor and delivery not included in P02.- and P03.0-P03.6◀
- ▶Newborn affected by induction of labor◀

▲   **P03.9**   **Newborn affected by complication of labor and delivery, unspecified** ▽

▲ ✓4ᵗʰ   **P04**   **Newborn affected by noxious substances transmitted via placenta or breast milk**

   INCLUDES   nonteratogenic effects of substances transmitted via placenta

   EXCLUDES 2   *congenital malformations (Q00-Q99)*
- ▶ *encounter for observation of newborn for suspected diseases and conditions ruled out (Z05.-)* ◀
- *neonatal jaundice from excessive hemolysis due to drugs or toxins transmitted from mother (P58.4)*
- *newborn in contact with and (suspected) exposures hazardous to health not transmitted via placenta or breast milk (Z77.-)*

▲   **P04.0**   **Newborn affected by maternal anesthesia and analgesia in pregnancy, labor and delivery**
- ▶Newborn affected by reactions and intoxications from maternal opiates and tranquilizers administered during labor and delivery◀

▲   **P04.1**   **Newborn affected by** other **maternal medication**
- ▶Newborn affected by cancer chemotherapy◀
- ▶Newborn affected by cytotoxic drugs◀
- EXCLUDES 1 *dysmorphism due to warfarin (Q86.2)*
- *fetal hydantoin syndrome (Q86.1)*
- *maternal use of drugs of addiction (P04.4-)*

▲   **P04.2**   **Newborn affected by maternal** use of tobacco
- ▶Newborn affected by exposure in utero to tobacco smoke◀
- EXCLUDES 2 *newborn exposure to environmental tobacco smoke (P96.81)*

▲   **P04.3**   **Newborn affected by maternal** use of alcohol
- EXCLUDES 1 *fetal alcohol syndrome (Q86.0)*

▲ ✓5ᵗʰ   **P04.4**   **Newborn affected by maternal use of drugs of addiction**

▲   **P04.41**   **Newborn affected by maternal** use of cocaine
- "Crack baby"

▲   **P04.49**   **Newborn affected by maternal use of** other drugs of addiction
- EXCLUDES 2 ▶*newborn affected by maternal anesthesia and analgesia (P04.0)*◀
- *withdrawal symptoms from maternal use of drugs of addiction (P96.1)*

▲   **P04.5**   **Newborn affected by maternal use of** nutritional chemical substances

▲   **P04.6**   **Newborn affected by maternal** exposure to environmental chemical substances

▲   **P04.8**   **Newborn affected by other maternal** noxious substances

▲   **P04.9**   **Newborn affected by maternal noxious substance, unspecified** ▽

Disorders of newborn related to length of gestation and fetal growth (P05-P08)

✓4ᵗʰ   **P05**   **Disorders of newborn related to slow fetal growth and fetal malnutrition**

✓5ᵗʰ   **P05.0**   **Newborn light for gestational age**

Newborn light-for-dates
- ▶Weight below but length above 10th percentile for gestational age◀

   P05.00   **Newborn light for gestational age, unspecified weight** ▽

   P05.01   **Newborn light for gestational age, less than 500 grams**

   P05.02   **Newborn light for gestational age, 500-749 grams**

   P05.03   **Newborn light for gestational age, 750-999 grams**

   P05.04   **Newborn light for gestational age, 1000-1249 grams**

   P05.05   **Newborn light for gestational age, 1250-1499 grams**

   P05.06   **Newborn light for gestational age, 1500-1749 grams**

   P05.07   **Newborn light for gestational age, 1750-1999 grams**

EXCLUDES 1 Not coded here   EXCLUDES 2 Not included here   N Newborn Age : 0   P Pediatric Age : 0-17   M Maternity Age : 12-55   A Adult Age : 15-124

●   **P05.08**   Newborn light for gestational age, 2000-2499 grams

●   **P05.09**   Newborn light for gestational age, 2500 grams and over

Newborn light for gestational age, other

✓5ᵗʰ   **P05.1**   Newborn small for gestational age

Newborn small-and-light-for-dates

Newborn small-for-dates

►Weight and length below 10th percentile for gestational age◄

P05.10   Newborn small for gestational age, unspecified weight   ▽

P05.11   Newborn small for gestational age, less than 500 grams

P05.12   Newborn small for gestational age, 500-749 grams

P05.13   Newborn small for gestational age, 750-999 grams

P05.14   Newborn small for gestational age, 1000-1249 grams

P05.15   Newborn small for gestational age, 1250-1499 grams

P05.16   Newborn small for gestational age, 1500-1749 grams

P05.17   Newborn small for gestational age, 1750-1999 grams

P05.18   Newborn small for gestational age, 2000-2499 grams

P05.19   Newborn small for gestational age, other

Newborn small for gestational age, 2500 grams and over

P05.2   Newborn affected by fetal (intrauterine) malnutrition not light or small for gestational age

Infant, not light or small for gestational age, showing signs of fetal malnutrition, such as dry, peeling skin and loss of subcutaneous tissue

EXCLUDES 1   newborn affected by fetal malnutrition with light for gestational age (P05.0-)

newborn affected by fetal malnutrition with small for gestational age (P05.1-)

P05.9   Newborn affected by slow intrauterine growth, unspecified   ▽

Newborn affected by fetal growth retardation NOS

✓4ᵗʰ   **P07**   Disorders of newborn related to short gestation and low birth weight, not elsewhere classified

NOTE   When both birth weight and gestational age of the newborn are available, both should be coded with birth weight sequenced before gestational age

INCLUDES   the listed conditions, without further specification, as the cause of morbidity or additional care, in newborn

✓5ᵗʰ   **P07.0**   Extremely low birth weight newborn

Newborn birth weight 999 g. or less

EXCLUDES 1   ►low birth weight due to slow fetal growth and fetal malnutrition (P05.-)◄

P07.00   Extremely low birth weight newborn, unspecified weight   ▽

P07.01   Extremely low birth weight newborn, less than 500 grams

P07.02   Extremely low birth weight newborn, 500-749 grams

P07.03   Extremely low birth weight newborn, 750-999 grams

✓5ᵗʰ   **P07.1**   Other low birth weight newborn

Newborn birth weight 1000-2499 g.

EXCLUDES 1   ►low birth weight due to slow fetal growth and fetal malnutrition (P05.-)◄

P07.10   Other low birth weight newborn, unspecified weight   ▽

P07.14   Other low birth weight newborn, 1000-1249 grams

P07.15   Other low birth weight newborn, 1250-1499 grams

P07.16   Other low birth weight newborn, 1500-1749 grams

P07.17   Other low birth weight newborn, 1750-1999 grams

P07.18   Other low birth weight newborn, 2000-2499 grams

✓5ᵗʰ   **P07.2**   Extreme immaturity of newborn

Less than 28 completed weeks (less than 196 completed days) of gestation.

P07.20   Extreme immaturity of newborn, unspecified weeks of gestation   ▽

Gestational age less than 28 completed weeks NOS

P07.21   Extreme immaturity of newborn, gestational age less than 23 completed weeks

Extreme immaturity of newborn, gestational age less than 23 weeks, 0 days

P07.22   Extreme immaturity of newborn, gestational age 23 completed weeks

Extreme immaturity of newborn, gestational age 23 weeks, 0 days through 23 weeks, 6 days

P07.23   Extreme immaturity of newborn, gestational age 24 completed weeks

Extreme immaturity of newborn, gestational age 24 weeks, 0 days through 24 weeks, 6 days

P07.24   Extreme immaturity of newborn, gestational age 25 completed weeks

Extreme immaturity of newborn, gestational age 25 weeks, 0 days through 25 weeks, 6 days

P07.25   Extreme immaturity of newborn, gestational age 26 completed weeks

Extreme immaturity of newborn, gestational age 26 weeks, 0 days through 26 weeks, 6 days

P07.26   Extreme immaturity of newborn, gestational age 27 completed weeks

Extreme immaturity of newborn, gestational age 27 weeks, 0 days through 27 weeks, 6 days

✓5ᵗʰ   **P07.3**   Preterm [premature] newborn [other]

28 completed weeks or more but less than 37 completed weeks (196 completed days but less than 259 completed days) of gestation

Prematurity NOS

P07.30   Preterm newborn, unspecified weeks of gestation   ▽

P07.31   Preterm newborn, gestational age 28 completed weeks

Preterm newborn, gestational age 28 weeks, 0 days through 28 weeks, 6 days

P07.32   Preterm newborn, gestational age 29 completed weeks

Preterm newborn, gestational age 29 weeks, 0 days through 29 weeks, 6 days

P07.33   Preterm newborn, gestational age 30 completed weeks

Preterm newborn, gestational age 30 weeks, 0 days through 30 weeks, 6 days

P07.34   Preterm newborn, gestational age 31 completed weeks

Preterm newborn, gestational age 31 weeks, 0 days through 31 weeks, 6 days

P07.35   Preterm newborn, gestational age 32 completed weeks

Preterm newborn, gestational age 32 weeks, 0 days through 32 weeks, 6 days

P07.36   Preterm newborn, gestational age 33 completed weeks

Preterm newborn, gestational age 33 weeks, 0 days through 33 weeks, 6 days

P07.37   Preterm newborn, gestational age 34 completed weeks

Preterm newborn, gestational age 34 weeks, 0 days through 34 weeks, 6 days

P07.38   Preterm newborn, gestational age 35 completed weeks

Preterm newborn, gestational age 35 weeks, 0 days through 35 weeks, 6 days

P07.39   Preterm newborn, gestational age 36 completed weeks

Preterm newborn, gestational age 36 weeks, 0 days through 36 weeks, 6 days

✓4ᵗʰ   **P08**   Disorders of newborn related to long gestation and high birth weight

NOTE   When both birth weight and gestational age of the newborn are available, priority of assignment should be given to birth weight

INCLUDES   the listed conditions, without further specification, as causes of morbidity or additional care, in newborn

P08.0   Exceptionally large newborn baby

Usually implies a birth weight of 4500 g. or more

EXCLUDES 1   syndrome of infant of diabetic mother (P70.1)

syndrome of infant of mother with gestational diabetes (P70.0)

☑ Additional Character Required   ✓x7ᵗʰ Placeholder Alert   Manifestation Dx   ▽ Unspecified Dx   ►◄ Revised Text   ● New Code   ▲ Revised Code Title

ICD-10-CM 2017   839

P05.08–P08.0

Chapter 16. Certain Conditions Originating in the Perinatal Period

P08.1   Other heavy for gestational age newborn
Other newborn heavy- or large-for-dates regardless of period of gestation
Usually implies a birth weight of 4000 g. to 4499 g.
> EXCLUDES 1   *newborn with a birth weight of 4500 or more (P08.0)*
> *syndrome of infant of diabetic mother (P70.1)*
> *syndrome of infant of mother with gestational diabetes (P70.0).*

✓5ᵗʰ **P08.2   Late newborn, not heavy for gestational age**
AHA: 2014,1Q,14
P08.21   Post-term newborn
Newborn with gestation period over 40 completed weeks to 42 completed weeks
P08.22   Prolonged gestation of newborn
Newborn with gestation period over 42 completed weeks (294 days or more), not heavy- or large-for-dates.
Postmaturity NOS

Abnormal findings on neonatal screening (P09)

P09   Abnormal findings on neonatal screening
Use additional code to identify signs, symptoms and conditions associated with the screening
> EXCLUDES 2   *nonspecific serologic evidence of human immunodeficiency virus [HIV] (R75)*

Birth trauma (P10-P15)

✓4ᵗʰ **P10   Intracranial laceration and hemorrhage due to birth injury**
> EXCLUDES 1   *intracranial hemorrhage of newborn NOS (P52.9)*
> *intracranial hemorrhage of newborn due to anoxia or hypoxia (P52.-)*
> *nontraumatic intracranial hemorrhage of newborn (P52.-)*

P10.0   Subdural hemorrhage due to birth injury
Subdural hematoma (localized) due to birth injury
> EXCLUDES 1   *subdural hemorrhage accompanying tentorial tear (P10.4)*

P10.1   Cerebral hemorrhage due to birth injury
P10.2   Intraventricular hemorrhage due to birth injury
P10.3   Subarachnoid hemorrhage due to birth injury
P10.4   Tentorial tear due to birth injury
P10.8   Other intracranial lacerations and hemorrhages due to birth injury
P10.9   Unspecified intracranial laceration and hemorrhage due to birth injury ▽

✓4ᵗʰ **P11   Other birth injuries to central nervous system**
P11.0   Cerebral edema due to birth injury
P11.1   Other specified brain damage due to birth injury
P11.2   Unspecified brain damage due to birth injury ▽
P11.3   Birth injury to facial nerve
Facial palsy due to birth injury
P11.4   Birth injury to other cranial nerves
P11.5   Birth injury to spine and spinal cord
Fracture of spine due to birth injury
P11.9   Birth injury to central nervous system, unspecified ▽

✓4ᵗʰ **P12   Birth injury to scalp**
P12.0   Cephalhematoma due to birth injury
P12.1   Chignon (from vacuum extraction) due to birth injury
P12.2   Epicranial subaponeurotic hemorrhage due to birth injury
Subgaleal hemorrhage
P12.3   Bruising of scalp due to birth injury
P12.4   Injury of scalp of newborn due to monitoring equipment
Sampling incision of scalp of newborn
Scalp clip (electrode) injury of newborn
✓5ᵗʰ **P12.8   Other birth injuries to scalp**
P12.81   Caput succedaneum
P12.89   Other birth injuries to scalp
P12.9   Birth injury to scalp, unspecified ▽

✓4ᵗʰ **P13   Birth injury to skeleton**
> EXCLUDES 2   *birth injury to spine (P11.5)*

P13.0   Fracture of skull due to birth injury
P13.1   Other birth injuries to skull
> EXCLUDES 1   *cephalhematoma (P12.0)*

P13.2   Birth injury to femur
P13.3   Birth injury to other long bones
P13.4   Fracture of clavicle due to birth injury
P13.8   Birth injuries to other parts of skeleton
P13.9   Birth injury to skeleton, unspecified ▽

✓4ᵗʰ **P14   Birth injury to peripheral nervous system**
P14.0   Erb's paralysis due to birth injury
P14.1   Klumpke's paralysis due to birth injury
P14.2   Phrenic nerve paralysis due to birth injury
P14.3   Other brachial plexus birth injuries
P14.8   Birth injuries to other parts of peripheral nervous system
P14.9   Birth injury to peripheral nervous system, unspecified ▽

✓4ᵗʰ **P15   Other birth injuries**
P15.0   Birth injury to liver
Rupture of liver due to birth injury
P15.1   Birth injury to spleen
Rupture of spleen due to birth injury
P15.2   Sternomastoid injury due to birth injury
P15.3   Birth injury to eye
Subconjunctival hemorrhage due to birth injury
Traumatic glaucoma due to birth injury
P15.4   Birth injury to face
Facial congestion due to birth injury
P15.5   Birth injury to external genitalia
P15.6   Subcutaneous fat necrosis due to birth injury
P15.8   Other specified birth injuries
TIP: Use for any injury of newborn from scalpel.
P15.9   Birth injury, unspecified ▽

Respiratory and cardiovascular disorders specific to the perinatal period (P19-P29)

✓4ᵗʰ **P19   Metabolic acidemia in newborn**
> INCLUDES   metabolic acidemia in newborn

P19.0   Metabolic acidemia in newborn first noted before onset of labor
P19.1   Metabolic acidemia in newborn first noted during labor
P19.2   Metabolic acidemia noted at birth
P19.9   Metabolic acidemia, unspecified ▽

✓4ᵗʰ **P22   Respiratory distress of newborn**
> EXCLUDES 1   *respiratory arrest of newborn (P28.81)*
> *respiratory failure of newborn NOS (P28.5)*

P22.0   Respiratory distress syndrome of newborn
Cardiorespiratory distress syndrome of newborn
Hyaline membrane disease
Idiopathic respiratory distress syndrome [IRDS or RDS] of newborn
Pulmonary hypoperfusion syndrome
Respiratory distress syndrome, type I
DEF: Severe chest contractions upon air intake and expiratory grunting; infant appears blue due to oxygen deficiency and has rapid respiratory rate; formerly called hyaline membrane disease.

P22.1   Transient tachypnea of newborn
Idiopathic tachypnea of newborn
Respiratory distress syndrome, type II
Wet lung syndrome
P22.8   Other respiratory distress of newborn
P22.9   Respiratory distress of newborn, unspecified ▽

✓4ᵗʰ **P23   Congenital pneumonia**
> INCLUDES   infective pneumonia acquired in utero or during birth
> EXCLUDES 1   *neonatal pneumonia resulting from aspiration (P24.-)*

P23.0   Congenital pneumonia due to viral agent
Use additional code (B97) to identify organism
> EXCLUDES 1   *congenital rubella pneumonitis (P35.0)*

P23.1   Congenital pneumonia due to Chlamydia
P23.2   Congenital pneumonia due to staphylococcus
P23.3   Congenital pneumonia due to streptococcus, group B
P23.4   Congenital pneumonia due to Escherichia coli
P23.5   Congenital pneumonia due to Pseudomonas

| EXCLUDES 1 Not coded here | EXCLUDES 2 Not included here | Ⓝ Newborn Age : 0 | Ⓟ Pediatric Age : 0-17 | Ⓜ Maternity Age : 12-55 | Ⓐ Adult Age : 15-124 |

P23.6 Congenital pneumonia due to other bacterial agents
Congenital pneumonia due to Hemophilus influenzae
Congenital pneumonia due to Klebsiella pneumoniae
Congenital pneumonia due to Mycoplasma
Congenital pneumonia due to Streptococcus, except group B
Use additional code (B95-B96) to identify organism

P23.8 Congenital pneumonia due to other organisms

P23.9 Congenital pneumonia, unspecified   ▽

√4ᵗʰ **P24 Neonatal aspiration**
INCLUDES aspiration in utero and during delivery

√5ᵗʰ **P24.0 Meconium aspiration**
EXCLUDES 1 meconium passage (without aspiration) during delivery (P03.82)
meconium staining (P96.83)

P24.00 Meconium aspiration without respiratory symptoms
Meconium aspiration NOS

P24.01 Meconium aspiration with respiratory symptoms
Meconium aspiration pneumonia
Meconium aspiration pneumonitis
Meconium aspiration syndrome NOS
Use additional code to identify any secondary pulmonary hypertension, if applicable (I27.2)

√5ᵗʰ **P24.1 Neonatal aspiration of (clear) amniotic fluid and mucus**
Neonatal aspiration of liquor (amnii)

P24.10 Neonatal aspiration of (clear) amniotic fluid and mucus without respiratory symptoms
Neonatal aspiration of amniotic fluid and mucus NOS

P24.11 Neonatal aspiration of (clear) amniotic fluid and mucus with respiratory symptoms
Neonatal aspiration of amniotic fluid and mucus with pneumonia
Neonatal aspiration of amniotic fluid and mucus with pneumonitis
Use additional code to identify any secondary pulmonary hypertension, if applicable (I27.2)

√5ᵗʰ **P24.2 Neonatal aspiration of blood**

P24.20 Neonatal aspiration of blood without respiratory symptoms
Neonatal aspiration of blood NOS

P24.21 Neonatal aspiration of blood with respiratory symptoms
Neonatal aspiration of blood with pneumonia
Neonatal aspiration of blood with pneumonitis
Use additional code to identify any secondary pulmonary hypertension, if applicable (I27.2)

√5ᵗʰ **P24.3 Neonatal aspiration of milk and regurgitated food**
Neonatal aspiration of stomach contents

P24.30 Neonatal aspiration of milk and regurgitated food without respiratory symptoms
Neonatal aspiration of milk and regurgitated food NOS

P24.31 Neonatal aspiration of milk and regurgitated food with respiratory symptoms
Neonatal aspiration of milk and regurgitated food with pneumonia
Neonatal aspiration of milk and regurgitated food with pneumonitis
Use additional code to identify any secondary pulmonary hypertension, if applicable (I27.2)

√5ᵗʰ **P24.8 Other neonatal aspiration**

P24.80 Other neonatal aspiration without respiratory symptoms
Neonatal aspiration NEC

P24.81 Other neonatal aspiration with respiratory symptoms
Neonatal aspiration pneumonia NEC
Neonatal aspiration with pneumonitis NEC
Neonatal aspiration with pneumonia NOS
Neonatal aspiration with pneumonitis NOS
Use additional code to identify any secondary pulmonary hypertension, if applicable (I27.2)

P24.9 Neonatal aspiration, unspecified   ▽

√4ᵗʰ **P25 Interstitial emphysema and related conditions originating in the perinatal period**

P25.0 Interstitial emphysema originating in the perinatal period

P25.1 Pneumothorax originating in the perinatal period

P25.2 Pneumomediastinum originating in the perinatal period

P25.3 Pneumopericardium originating in the perinatal period

P25.8 Other conditions related to interstitial emphysema originating in the perinatal period

√4ᵗʰ **P26 Pulmonary hemorrhage originating in the perinatal period**
EXCLUDES 1 acute idiopathic hemorrhage in infants over 28 days old (R04.81)

P26.0 Tracheobronchial hemorrhage originating in the perinatal period

P26.1 Massive pulmonary hemorrhage originating in the perinatal period

P26.8 Other pulmonary hemorrhages originating in the perinatal period

P26.9 Unspecified pulmonary hemorrhage originating in the perinatal period   ▽

√4ᵗʰ **P27 Chronic respiratory disease originating in the perinatal period**
EXCLUDES 1 respiratory distress of newborn (P22.0-P22.9)

P27.0 Wilson-Mikity syndrome
Pulmonary dysmaturity

P27.1 Bronchopulmonary dysplasia originating in the perinatal period

P27.8 Other chronic respiratory diseases originating in the perinatal period
Congenital pulmonary fibrosis
Ventilator lung in newborn

P27.9 Unspecified chronic respiratory disease originating in the perinatal period   ▽

√4ᵗʰ **P28 Other respiratory conditions originating in the perinatal period**
EXCLUDES 1 congenital malformations of the respiratory system (Q30-Q34)

P28.0 Primary atelectasis of newborn
Primary failure to expand terminal respiratory units
Pulmonary hypoplasia associated with short gestation
Pulmonary immaturity NOS

√5ᵗʰ **P28.1 Other and unspecified atelectasis of newborn**

P28.10 Unspecified atelectasis of newborn   ▽
Atelectasis of newborn NOS

P28.11 Resorption atelectasis without respiratory distress syndrome
EXCLUDES 1 resorption atelectasis with respiratory distress syndrome (P22.0)

P28.19 Other atelectasis of newborn
Partial atelectasis of newborn
Secondary atelectasis of newborn

P28.2 Cyanotic attacks of newborn
EXCLUDES 1 apnea of newborn (P28.3-P28.4)

P28.3 Primary sleep apnea of newborn
Central sleep apnea of newborn
Obstructive sleep apnea of newborn
Sleep apnea of newborn NOS
DEF: Unexplained cessation of breathing when a neonate makes no respiratory effort for 20 seconds or longer, or when neonate's breathing cessation is accompanied by cyanosis, bradycardia, or hypotonia.

P28.4 Other apnea of newborn
Apnea of prematurity
Obstructive apnea of newborn
EXCLUDES 1 obstructive sleep apnea of newborn (P28.3)

P28.5 Respiratory failure of newborn
EXCLUDES 1 respiratory arrest of newborn (P28.81)
respiratory distress of newborn (P22.0-)

√5ᵗʰ **P28.8 Other specified respiratory conditions of newborn**

P28.81 Respiratory arrest of newborn

P28.89 Other specified respiratory conditions of newborn
Congenital laryngeal stridor
Sniffles in newborn
Snuffles in newborn
EXCLUDES 1 early congenital syphilitic rhinitis (A50.05)

P28.9 Respiratory condition of newborn, unspecified   ▽
Respiratory depression in newborn

√4ᵗʰ **P29 Cardiovascular disorders originating in the perinatal period**
EXCLUDES 1 congenital malformations of the circulatory system (Q20-Q28)

P29.0 Neonatal cardiac failure

√5ᵗʰ **P29.1 Neonatal cardiac dysrhythmia**

P29.11 Neonatal tachycardia

P29.12 Neonatal bradycardia

P29.2 Neonatal hypertension

P29.3 **Persistent fetal circulation**
  Delayed closure of ductus arteriosus
  (Persistent) pulmonary hypertension of newborn

P29.4 **Transient myocardial ischemia in newborn**

✓5ᵗʰ **P29.8** **Other cardiovascular disorders originating in the perinatal period**

    P29.81 **Cardiac arrest of newborn**

    P29.89 **Other cardiovascular disorders originating in the perinatal period**
        AHA: 2014,4Q,23

P29.9 **Cardiovascular disorder originating in the perinatal period, unspecified** ▽

Infections specific to the perinatal period (P35-P39)

Infections acquired in utero, during birth via the umbilicus, or during the first 28 days after birth

EXCLUDES 2 *asymptomatic human immunodeficiency virus [HIV] infection status (Z21)*
congenital gonococcal infection (A54.-)
congenital pneumonia (P23.-)
congenital syphilis (A50.-)
human immunodeficiency virus [HIV] disease (B20)
infant botulism (A48.51)
infectious diseases not specific to the perinatal period (A00-B99, J09, J10.-)
intestinal infectious disease (A00-A09)
laboratory evidence of human immunodeficiency virus [HIV] (R75)
tetanus neonatorum (A33)

✓4ᵗʰ **P35** **Congenital viral diseases**

    INCLUDES infections acquired in utero or during birth

P35.0 **Congenital rubella syndrome**
  Congenital rubella pneumonitis

P35.1 **Congenital cytomegalovirus infection**

P35.2 **Congenital herpesviral [herpes simplex] infection**

P35.3 **Congenital viral hepatitis**

P35.8 **Other congenital viral diseases**
  Congenital varicella [chickenpox]

P35.9 **Congenital viral disease, unspecified** ▽

✓4ᵗʰ **P36** **Bacterial sepsis of newborn**

    INCLUDES congenital sepsis
    Use additional code(s), if applicable, to identify severe sepsis (R65.2-) and associated acute organ dysfunction(s)

P36.0 **Sepsis of newborn due to streptococcus, group B**

✓5ᵗʰ **P36.1** **Sepsis of newborn due to other and unspecified streptococci**

    P36.10 **Sepsis of newborn due to unspecified streptococci** ▽

    P36.19 **Sepsis of newborn due to other streptococci**

P36.2 **Sepsis of newborn due to Staphylococcus aureus**

✓5ᵗʰ **P36.3** **Sepsis of newborn due to other and unspecified staphylococci**

    P36.30 **Sepsis of newborn due to unspecified staphylococci** ▽

    P36.39 **Sepsis of newborn due to other staphylococci**

P36.4 **Sepsis of newborn due to Escherichia coli**

P36.5 **Sepsis of newborn due to anaerobes**

P36.8 **Other bacterial sepsis of newborn**
  Use additional code from category B96 to identify organism

P36.9 **Bacterial sepsis of newborn, unspecified** ▽

✓4ᵗʰ **P37** **Other congenital infectious and parasitic diseases**

    EXCLUDES 2 *congenital syphilis (A50.-)*
    infectious neonatal diarrhea (A00-A09)
    necrotizing enterocolitis in newborn (P77.-)
    noninfectious neonatal diarrhea (P78.3)
    ophthalmia neonatorum due to gonococcus (A54.31)
    tetanus neonatorum (A33)

P37.0 **Congenital tuberculosis**

P37.1 **Congenital toxoplasmosis**
  Hydrocephalus due to congenital toxoplasmosis

P37.2 **Neonatal (disseminated) listeriosis**

P37.3 **Congenital falciparum malaria**

P37.4 **Other congenital malaria**

P37.5 **Neonatal candidiasis**

P37.8 **Other specified congenital infectious and parasitic diseases**

P37.9 **Congenital infectious or parasitic disease, unspecified** ▽

✓4ᵗʰ **P38** **Omphalitis of newborn**

    EXCLUDES 1 *omphalitis not of newborn (L08.82)*
    tetanus omphalitis (A33)
    umbilical hemorrhage of newborn (P51.-)

P38.1 **Omphalitis with mild hemorrhage**

P38.9 **Omphalitis without hemorrhage**
  Omphalitis of newborn NOS

✓4ᵗʰ **P39** **Other infections specific to the perinatal period**
  Use additional code to identify organism or specific infection

P39.0 **Neonatal infective mastitis**

    EXCLUDES 1 *breast engorgement of newborn (P83.4)*
    noninfective mastitis of newborn (P83.4)

P39.1 **Neonatal conjunctivitis and dacryocystitis**
  Neonatal chlamydial conjunctivitis
  Ophthalmia neonatorum NOS

    EXCLUDES 1 *gonococcal conjunctivitis (A54.31)*

P39.2 **Intra-amniotic infection affecting newborn, not elsewhere classified**

P39.3 **Neonatal urinary tract infection**

P39.4 **Neonatal skin infection**
  Neonatal pyoderma

    EXCLUDES 1 *pemphigus neonatorum (L00)*
    staphylococcal scalded skin syndrome (L00)

P39.8 **Other specified infections specific to the perinatal period**

P39.9 **Infection specific to the perinatal period, unspecified** ▽

Hemorrhagic and hematological disorders of newborn (P50-P61)

EXCLUDES 1 *congenital stenosis and stricture of bile ducts (Q44.3)*
Crigler-Najjar syndrome (E80.5)
Dubin-Johnson syndrome (E80.6)
Gilbert syndrome (E80.4)
hereditary hemolytic anemias (D55-D58)

✓4ᵗʰ **P50** **Newborn affected by intrauterine (fetal) blood loss**

    EXCLUDES 1 *congenital anemia from intrauterine (fetal) blood loss (P61.3)*

P50.0 **Newborn affected by intrauterine (fetal) blood loss from vasa previa**

P50.1 **Newborn affected by intrauterine (fetal) blood loss from ruptured cord**

P50.2 **Newborn affected by intrauterine (fetal) blood loss from placenta**

P50.3 **Newborn affected by hemorrhage into co-twin**

P50.4 **Newborn affected by hemorrhage into maternal circulation**

P50.5 **Newborn affected by intrauterine (fetal) blood loss from cut end of co-twin's cord**

P50.8 **Newborn affected by other intrauterine (fetal) blood loss**

P50.9 **Newborn affected by intrauterine (fetal) blood loss, unspecified** ▽
  Newborn affected by fetal hemorrhage NOS

✓4ᵗʰ **P51** **Umbilical hemorrhage of newborn**

    EXCLUDES 1 *omphalitis with mild hemorrhage (P38.1)*
    umbilical hemorrhage from cut end of co-twins cord (P50.5)

P51.0 **Massive umbilical hemorrhage of newborn**

P51.8 **Other umbilical hemorrhages of newborn**
  Slipped umbilical ligature NOS

P51.9 **Umbilical hemorrhage of newborn, unspecified** ▽

✓4ᵗʰ **P52** **Intracranial nontraumatic hemorrhage of newborn**

    INCLUDES intracranial hemorrhage due to anoxia or hypoxia
    EXCLUDES 1 *intracranial hemorrhage due to birth injury (P10.-)*
    intracranial hemorrhage due to other injury (S06.-)

P52.0 **Intraventricular (nontraumatic) hemorrhage, grade 1, of newborn**
  Subependymal hemorrhage (without intraventricular extension)
  Bleeding into germinal matrix

P52.1 **Intraventricular (nontraumatic) hemorrhage, grade 2, of newborn**
  Subependymal hemorrhage with intraventricular extension
  Bleeding into ventricle

✓5ᵗʰ **P52.2** **Intraventricular (nontraumatic) hemorrhage, grade 3 and grade 4, of newborn**

    P52.21 **Intraventricular (nontraumatic) hemorrhage, grade 3, of newborn**
        Subependymal hemorrhage with intraventricular extension with enlargement of ventricle

EXCLUDES 1 Not coded here   EXCLUDES 2 Not included here   N Newborn Age : 0   P Pediatric Age : 0-17   M Maternity Age : 12-55   A Adult Age : 15-124

842   ICD-10-CM 2017

P52.22 Intraventricular (nontraumatic) hemorrhage, grade 4, of newborn
Bleeding into cerebral cortex
Subependymal hemorrhage with intracerebral extension

P52.3 Unspecified intraventricular (nontraumatic) hemorrhage of newborn ▽

P52.4 Intracerebral (nontraumatic) hemorrhage of newborn

P52.5 Subarachnoid (nontraumatic) hemorrhage of newborn

P52.6 Cerebellar (nontraumatic) and posterior fossa hemorrhage of newborn

P52.8 Other intracranial (nontraumatic) hemorrhages of newborn

P52.9 Intracranial (nontraumatic) hemorrhage of newborn, unspecified ▽

P53 Hemorrhagic disease of newborn
Vitamin K deficiency of newborn

✓4ᵗʰ **P54 Other neonatal hemorrhages**
EXCLUDES 1 *newborn affected by (intrauterine) blood loss (P50.-)*
pulmonary hemorrhage originating in the perinatal period (P26.-)

P54.0 Neonatal hematemesis
EXCLUDES 1 *neonatal hematemesis due to swallowed maternal blood (P78.2)*

P54.1 Neonatal melena
EXCLUDES 1 *neonatal melena due to swallowed maternal blood (P78.2)*

P54.2 Neonatal rectal hemorrhage

P54.3 Other neonatal gastrointestinal hemorrhage

P54.4 Neonatal adrenal hemorrhage

P54.5 Neonatal cutaneous hemorrhage
Neonatal bruising
Neonatal ecchymoses
Neonatal petechiae
Neonatal superficial hematomata
EXCLUDES 2 *bruising of scalp due to birth injury (P12.3)*
cephalhematoma due to birth injury (P12.0)

P54.6 Neonatal vaginal hemorrhage ♀
Neonatal pseudomenses

P54.8 Other specified neonatal hemorrhages

P54.9 Neonatal hemorrhage, unspecified ▽

✓4ᵗʰ **P55 Hemolytic disease of newborn**

P55.0 Rh isoimmunization of newborn

P55.1 ABO isoimmunization of newborn
AHA: 2015,3Q,20

P55.8 Other hemolytic diseases of newborn

P55.9 Hemolytic disease of newborn, unspecified ▽

✓4ᵗʰ **P56 Hydrops fetalis due to hemolytic disease**
EXCLUDES 1 *hydrops fetalis NOS (P83.2)*

P56.0 Hydrops fetalis due to isoimmunization

✓5ᵗʰ **P56.9 Hydrops fetalis due to other and unspecified hemolytic disease**

P56.90 Hydrops fetalis due to unspecified hemolytic disease ▽

P56.99 Hydrops fetalis due to other hemolytic disease

✓4ᵗʰ **P57 Kernicterus**

P57.0 Kernicterus due to isoimmunization
DEF: Complication of erythroblastosis fetalis associated with severe neural symptoms, high blood bilirubin levels and nerve cell destruction; results in bilirubin-pigmented gray matter of central nervous system.

P57.8 Other specified kernicterus
EXCLUDES 1 *Crigler-Najjar syndrome (E80.5)*

P57.9 Kernicterus, unspecified ▽

✓4ᵗʰ **P58 Neonatal jaundice due to other excessive hemolysis**
EXCLUDES 1 *jaundice due to isoimmunization (P55-P57)*

P58.0 Neonatal jaundice due to bruising

P58.1 Neonatal jaundice due to bleeding

P58.2 Neonatal jaundice due to infection

P58.3 Neonatal jaundice due to polycythemia

✓5ᵗʰ **P58.4 Neonatal jaundice due to drugs or toxins transmitted from mother or given to newborn**
Code first poisoning due to drug or toxin, if applicable (T36-T65 with fifth or sixth character 1-4 or 6)
Use additional code for adverse effect, if applicable, to identify drug (T36-T50 with fifth or sixth character 5)

P58.41 Neonatal jaundice due to drugs or toxins transmitted from mother

P58.42 Neonatal jaundice due to drugs or toxins given to newborn

P58.5 Neonatal jaundice due to swallowed maternal blood

P58.8 Neonatal jaundice due to other specified excessive hemolysis

P58.9 Neonatal jaundice due to excessive hemolysis, unspecified ▽

✓4ᵗʰ **P59 Neonatal jaundice from other and unspecified causes**
EXCLUDES 1 *jaundice due to inborn errors of metabolism (E70-E88)*
kernicterus (P57.-)

P59.0 Neonatal jaundice associated with preterm delivery
Hyperbilirubinemia of prematurity
Jaundice due to delayed conjugation associated with preterm delivery

P59.1 Inspissated bile syndrome

✓5ᵗʰ **P59.2 Neonatal jaundice from other and unspecified hepatocellular damage**
EXCLUDES 1 *congenital viral hepatitis (P35.3)*

P59.20 Neonatal jaundice from unspecified hepatocellular damage ▽

P59.29 Neonatal jaundice from other hepatocellular damage
Neonatal giant cell hepatitis
Neonatal (idiopathic) hepatitis

P59.3 Neonatal jaundice from breast milk inhibitor

P59.8 Neonatal jaundice from other specified causes

P59.9 Neonatal jaundice, unspecified ▽
Neonatal physiological jaundice (intense)(prolonged) NOS
AHA: 2015,3Q,20

P60 Disseminated intravascular coagulation of newborn
Defibrination syndrome of newborn

✓4ᵗʰ **P61 Other perinatal hematological disorders**
EXCLUDES 1 *transient hypogammaglobulinemia of infancy (D80.7)*

P61.0 Transient neonatal thrombocytopenia
Neonatal thrombocytopenia due to exchange transfusion
Neonatal thrombocytopenia due to idiopathic maternal thrombocytopenia
Neonatal thrombocytopenia due to isoimmunization

P61.1 Polycythemia neonatorum

P61.2 Anemia of prematurity

P61.3 Congenital anemia from fetal blood loss

P61.4 Other congenital anemias, not elsewhere classified
Congenital anemia NOS

P61.5 Transient neonatal neutropenia
EXCLUDES 1 *congenital neutropenia (nontransient) (D70.0)*

P61.6 Other transient neonatal disorders of coagulation

P61.8 Other specified perinatal hematological disorders

P61.9 Perinatal hematological disorder, unspecified ▽

Transitory endocrine and metabolic disorders specific to newborn (P70-P74)

INCLUDES transitory endocrine and metabolic disturbances caused by the infant's response to maternal endocrine and metabolic factors, or its adjustment to extrauterine environment

✓4ᵗʰ **P70 Transitory disorders of carbohydrate metabolism specific to newborn**

P70.0 Syndrome of infant of mother with gestational diabetes
Newborn (with hypoglycemia) affected by maternal gestational diabetes
EXCLUDES 1 *newborn (with hypoglycemia) affected by maternal (pre-existing) diabetes mellitus (P70.1)*
syndrome of infant of a diabetic mother (P70.1)

P70.1 Syndrome of infant of a diabetic mother
Newborn (with hypoglycemia) affected by maternal (pre-existing) diabetes mellitus
EXCLUDES 1 *newborn (with hypoglycemia) affected by maternal gestational diabetes (P70.0)*
syndrome of infant of mother with gestational diabetes (P70.0)

P70.2 Neonatal diabetes mellitus

✓ Additional Character Required   ✓7ᵗʰ Placeholder Alert   Manifestation Dx   ▽ Unspecified Dx   ►◄ Revised Text   ● New Code   ▲ Revised Code Title

Chapter 16. Certain Conditions Originating in the Perinatal Period

P70.3   Iatrogenic **neonatal** hypoglycemia

P70.4   **Other neonatal hypoglycemia**
Transitory neonatal hypoglycemia

P70.8   **Other transitory disorders of carbohydrate metabolism of newborn**

P70.9   **Transitory disorder of carbohydrate metabolism of newborn, unspecified** ▽

✓4ᵗʰ **P71**   **Transitory neonatal disorders of calcium and magnesium metabolism**

P71.0   **Cow's milk hypocalcemia** in newborn

P71.1   **Other neonatal hypocalcemia**
EXCLUDES 1   *neonatal hypoparathyroidism (P71.4)*

P71.2   **Neonatal hypomagnesemia**

P71.3   **Neonatal tetany without calcium or magnesium deficiency**
Neonatal tetany NOS

P71.4   **Transitory neonatal hypoparathyroidism**

P71.8   **Other transitory neonatal disorders of calcium and magnesium metabolism**

P71.9   **Transitory neonatal disorder of calcium and magnesium metabolism, unspecified** ▽

✓4ᵗʰ **P72**   **Other transitory neonatal endocrine disorders**
EXCLUDES 1   *congenital hypothyroidism with or without goiter (E03.0-E03.1)*
dyshormogenetic goiter (E07.1)
Pendred's syndrome (E07.1)

P72.0   **Neonatal goiter, not elsewhere classified**
Transitory congenital goiter with normal functioning

P72.1   **Transitory neonatal hyperthyroidism**
Neonatal thyrotoxicosis

P72.2   **Other transitory neonatal disorders of thyroid function, not elsewhere classified**
Transitory neonatal hypothyroidism

P72.8   **Other specified transitory neonatal endocrine disorders**

P72.9   **Transitory neonatal endocrine disorder, unspecified** ▽

✓4ᵗʰ **P74**   **Other transitory neonatal electrolyte and metabolic disturbances**

P74.0   **Late metabolic acidosis of newborn**
EXCLUDES 1   *(fetal) metabolic acidosis of newborn (P19)*

P74.1   **Dehydration of newborn**

P74.2   **Disturbances of sodium balance of newborn**

P74.3   **Disturbances of potassium balance of newborn**

P74.4   **Other transitory electrolyte disturbances of newborn**

P74.5   **Transitory tyrosinemia of newborn**

P74.6   **Transitory hyperammonemia of newborn**

P74.8   **Other transitory metabolic disturbances of newborn**
Amino-acid metabolic disorders described as transitory

P74.9   **Transitory metabolic disturbance of newborn, unspecified** ▽

Digestive system disorders of newborn (P76-P78)

✓4ᵗʰ **P76**   **Other intestinal obstruction of newborn**

P76.0   **Meconium plug syndrome**
Meconium ileus NOS
EXCLUDES 1   *meconium ileus in cystic fibrosis (E84.11)*

P76.1   **Transitory ileus of newborn**
EXCLUDES 1   *Hirschsprung's disease (Q43.1)*

P76.2   **Intestinal obstruction due to inspissated milk**

P76.8   **Other specified intestinal obstruction of newborn**
EXCLUDES 1   *intestinal obstruction classifiable to K56.-*

P76.9   **Intestinal obstruction of newborn, unspecified** ▽

✓4ᵗʰ **P77**   **Necrotizing enterocolitis of newborn**
DEF: Serious intestinal infection and inflammation in preterm infants; severity is measured by stages and may progress to life-threatening perforation or peritonitis; resection surgical treatment may be necessary.

P77.1   **Stage 1 necrotizing enterocolitis in newborn**
Necrotizing enterocolitis without pneumatosis, without perforation
DEF: Broad-spectrum symptoms with nonspecific signs, including feeding intolerance, abdominal distention, bradycardia, and metabolic abnormalities.

P77.2   **Stage 2 necrotizing enterocolitis in newborn**
Necrotizing enterocolitis with pneumatosis, without perforation
DEF: Radiographic confirmation of necrotizing enterocolitis showing intestinal dilatation, fixed loops of bowels, pneumatosis intestinalis, metabolic acidosis, and thrombocytopenia.

P77.3   **Stage 3 necrotizing enterocolitis in newborn**
Necrotizing enterocolitis with perforation
Necrotizing enterocolitis with pneumatosis and perforation
DEF: Advanced stage in which infant demonstrates signs of bowel perforation, septic shock, metabolic acidosis, ascites, disseminated intravascular coagulopathy, neutropenia.

P77.9   **Necrotizing enterocolitis in newborn, unspecified**
Necrotizing enterocolitis in newborn, NOS ▽

✓4ᵗʰ **P78**   **Other perinatal digestive system disorders**
EXCLUDES 1   *cystic fibrosis (E84.0-E84.9)*
neonatal gastrointestinal hemorrhages (P54.0-P54.3)

P78.0   **Perinatal intestinal perforation**
Meconium peritonitis

P78.1   **Other neonatal peritonitis**
Neonatal peritonitis NOS

P78.2   **Neonatal hematemesis and melena due to swallowed maternal blood**

P78.3   **Noninfective neonatal diarrhea**
Neonatal diarrhea NOS

✓5ᵗʰ **P78.8**   **Other specified perinatal digestive system disorders**

P78.81   **Congenital cirrhosis (of liver)**

P78.82   **Peptic ulcer of newborn**

P78.83   **Newborn esophageal reflux**
Neonatal esophageal reflux

P78.89   **Other specified perinatal digestive system disorders**

P78.9   **Perinatal digestive system disorder, unspecified** ▽

Conditions involving the integument and temperature regulation of newborn (P80-P83)

✓4ᵗʰ **P80**   **Hypothermia of newborn**

P80.0   **Cold injury syndrome**
Severe and usually chronic hypothermia associated with a pink flushed appearance, edema and neurological and biochemical abnormalities.
EXCLUDES 1   *mild hypothermia of newborn (P80.8)*

P80.8   **Other hypothermia of newborn**
Mild hypothermia of newborn

P80.9   **Hypothermia of newborn, unspecified** ▽

✓4ᵗʰ **P81**   **Other disturbances of temperature regulation of newborn**

P81.0   **Environmental hyperthermia of newborn**

P81.8   **Other specified disturbances of temperature regulation of newborn**

P81.9   **Disturbance of temperature regulation of newborn, unspecified** ▽
Fever of newborn NOS

✓4ᵗʰ **P83**   **Other conditions of integument specific to newborn**
EXCLUDES 1   *congenital malformations of skin and integument (Q80-Q84)*
hydrops fetalis due to hemolytic disease (P56.-)
neonatal skin infection (P39.4)
staphylococcal scalded skin syndrome (L00)
EXCLUDES 2   *cradle cap (L21.0)*
diaper [napkin] dermatitis (L22)

P83.0   **Sclerema neonatorum**
DEF: Diffuse, rapidly progressing white, waxy, nonpitting hardening of tissue, usually of legs and feet that is life-threatening; found in preterm or debilitated infants; unknown etiology.

P83.1   **Neonatal erythema toxicum**

P83.2   **Hydrops fetalis not due to hemolytic disease**
Hydrops fetalis NOS

✓5ᵗʰ **P83.3**   **Other and unspecified edema specific to newborn**

P83.30   **Unspecified edema specific to newborn** ▽

P83.39   **Other edema specific to newborn**

P83.4   **Breast engorgement of newborn**
Noninfective mastitis of newborn

P83.5   **Congenital hydrocele** ♂

P83.6   **Umbilical polyp of newborn**

P83.8   **Other specified conditions of integument specific to newborn**
Bronze baby syndrome
Neonatal scleroderma
Urticaria neonatorum

P83.9   **Condition of the integument specific to newborn, unspecified** ▽

EXCLUDES 1 Not coded here   *EXCLUDES 2* Not included here   N Newborn Age : 0   P Pediatric Age : 0-17   M Maternity Age : 12-55   A Adult Age : 15-124

Other problems with newborn (P84)

P84 Other problems with newborn
Acidemia of newborn
Acidosis of newborn
Anoxia of newborn NOS
Asphyxia of newborn NOS
Hypercapnia of newborn
Hypoxemia of newborn
Hypoxia of newborn NOS
Mixed metabolic and respiratory acidosis of newborn
> EXCLUDES 1   *intracranial hemorrhage due to anoxia or hypoxia (P52.-)*
> *hypoxic ischemic encephalopathy [HIE] (P91.6-)*
> *late metabolic acidosis of newborn (P74.0)*

Other disorders originating in the perinatal period (P90-P96)

P90 Convulsions of newborn
> EXCLUDES 1   *benign myoclonic epilepsy in infancy (G40.3-)*
> *benign neonatal convulsions (familial) (G40.3-)*

✓4th **P91 Other disturbances of cerebral status of newborn**

P91.0 Neonatal cerebral ischemia

P91.1 Acquired periventricular cysts of newborn

P91.2 Neonatal cerebral leukomalacia
Periventricular leukomalacia

P91.3 Neonatal cerebral irritability

P91.4 Neonatal cerebral depression

P91.5 Neonatal coma

✓5th **P91.6 Hypoxic ischemic encephalopathy [HIE]**

     P91.60 Hypoxic ischemic encephalopathy [HIE], unspecified ▽

     P91.61 Mild hypoxic ischemic encephalopathy [HIE]

     P91.62 Moderate hypoxic ischemic encephalopathy [HIE]

     P91.63 Severe hypoxic ischemic encephalopathy [HIE]

P91.8 Other specified disturbances of cerebral status of newborn

P91.9 Disturbance of cerebral status of newborn, unspecified ▽

✓4th **P92 Feeding problems of newborn**
> EXCLUDES 1   *feeding problems in child over 28 days old (R63.3)*

✓5th **P92.0 Vomiting of newborn**
> EXCLUDES 1   *vomiting of child over 28 days old (R11.-)*

     P92.01 Bilious vomiting of newborn
> EXCLUDES 1   *bilious vomiting in child over 28 days old (R11.14)*

     P92.09 Other vomiting of newborn
> EXCLUDES 1   *regurgitation of food in newborn (P92.1)*

P92.1 Regurgitation and rumination of newborn

P92.2 Slow feeding of newborn

P92.3 Underfeeding of newborn

P92.4 Overfeeding of newborn

P92.5 Neonatal difficulty in feeding at breast

P92.6 Failure to thrive in newborn
> EXCLUDES 1   *failure to thrive in child over 28 days old (R62.51)*

P92.8 Other feeding problems of newborn

P92.9 Feeding problem of newborn, unspecified ▽

✓4th **P93 Reactions and intoxications due to drugs administered to newborn**
> INCLUDES   reactions and intoxications due to drugs administered to fetus affecting newborn
> EXCLUDES 1   *jaundice due to drugs or toxins transmitted from mother or given to newborn (P58.4-)*
> *reactions and intoxications from maternal opiates, tranquilizers and other medication (P04.0-P04.1, P04.4)*
> *withdrawal symptoms from maternal use of drugs of addiction (P96.1)*
> *withdrawal symptoms from therapeutic use of drugs in newborn (P96.2)*

P93.0 Grey baby syndrome
Grey syndrome from chloramphenicol administration in newborn

P93.8 Other reactions and intoxications due to drugs administered to newborn
Use additional code for adverse effect, if applicable, to identify drug (T36-T50 with fifth or sixth character 5)

✓4th **P94 Disorders of muscle tone of newborn**

P94.0 Transient neonatal myasthenia gravis
> EXCLUDES 1   *myasthenia gravis (G70.0)*

P94.1 Congenital hypertonia

P94.2 Congenital hypotonia
Floppy baby syndrome, unspecified

P94.8 Other disorders of muscle tone of newborn

P94.9 Disorder of muscle tone of newborn, unspecified ▽

P95 Stillbirth
Deadborn fetus NOS
Fetal death of unspecified cause
Stillbirth NOS
> EXCLUDES 1   *maternal care for intrauterine death (O36.4)*
> *missed abortion (O02.1)*
> *outcome of delivery, stillbirth (Z37.1, Z37.3, Z37.4, Z37.7)*

✓4th **P96 Other conditions originating in the perinatal period**

P96.0 Congenital renal failure
Uremia of newborn

P96.1 Neonatal withdrawal symptoms from maternal use of drugs of addiction
Drug withdrawal syndrome in infant of dependent mother
Neonatal abstinence syndrome
> EXCLUDES 1   *reactions and intoxications from maternal opiates and tranquilizers administered during labor and delivery (P04.0)*

P96.2 Withdrawal symptoms from therapeutic use of drugs in newborn

P96.3 Wide cranial sutures of newborn
Neonatal craniotabes

P96.5 Complication to newborn due to (fetal) intrauterine procedure
> EXCLUDES 2   ►*newborn affected by amniocentesis (P00.6)*◄

✓5th **P96.8 Other specified conditions originating in the perinatal period**

     P96.81 Exposure to (parental) (environmental) tobacco smoke in the perinatal period
> EXCLUDES 2   *newborn affected by in utero exposure to tobacco (P04.2)*
> *exposure to environmental tobacco smoke after the perinatal period (Z77.22)*

     P96.82 Delayed separation of umbilical cord

     P96.83 Meconium staining
> EXCLUDES 1   *meconium aspiration (P24.00, P24.01)*
> *meconium passage during delivery (P03.82)*

     P96.89 Other specified conditions originating in the perinatal period
Use additional code to specify condition

P96.9 Condition originating in the perinatal period, unspecified ▽
Congenital debility NOS

☑ Additional Character Required   ✓x7th Placeholder Alert   Manifestation Dx   ▽ Unspecified Dx   ►◄ Revised Text   ● New Code   ▲ Revised Code Title

Chapter 17. Congenital Malformations, Deformations and Chromosomal Abnormalities (Q00–Q99)

Chapter Specific Guidelines with Coding Examples

The chapter specific guidelines from the ICD-10-CM Official Guidelines for Coding and Reporting have been provided below. Along with these guidelines are coding examples, contained in the shaded boxes, that have been developed to help illustrate the coding and/or sequencing guidance found in these guidelines.

Assign an appropriate code(s) from categories Q00-Q99, Congenital malformations, deformations, and chromosomal abnormalities when a malformation/deformation or chromosomal abnormality is documented. A malformation/deformation/or chromosomal abnormality may be the principal/first-listed diagnosis on a record or a secondary diagnosis.

When a malformation/deformation/or chromosomal abnormality does not have a unique code assignment, assign additional code(s) for any manifestations that may be present.

When the code assignment specifically identifies the malformation/deformation/or chromosomal abnormality, manifestations that are an inherent component of the anomaly should not be coded separately. Additional codes should be assigned for manifestations that are not an inherent component.

8-day-old infant with tetralogy of Fallot and pulmonary stenosis

Q21.3   Tetralogy of Fallot

Explanation: Pulmonary stenosis is inherent in the disease process of tetralogy of Fallot. When the code assignment specifically identifies the malformation/deformation/or chromosomal abnormality, manifestations that are inherent components of the anomaly should not be coded separately.

7-month-old infant with Down syndrome and common atrioventricular canal

Q90.9   Down syndrome, unspecified

Q21.2   Atrioventricular septal defect

Explanation: While a common atrioventricular canal is often associated with patients with Down syndrome, this manifestation is not an inherent component and may be reported separately. When the code assignment specifically identifies the anomaly, manifestations that are inherent components of the condition should not be coded separately. Additional codes should be assigned for manifestations that are not inherent components.

Codes from Chapter 17 may be used throughout the life of the patient. If a congenital malformation or deformity has been corrected, a personal history code should be used to identify the history of the malformation or deformity. Although present at birth, malformation/deformation/or chromosomal abnormality may not be identified until later in life. Whenever the condition is diagnosed by the physician, it is appropriate to assign a code from codes Q00-Q99. For the birth admission, the appropriate code from category Z38, Liveborn infants, according to place of birth and type of delivery, should be sequenced as the principal diagnosis, followed by any congenital anomaly codes, Q00- Q99.

Three-year-old with history of corrected ventricular septal defect

Z87.74   Personal history of (corrected) congenital malformations of heart and circulatory system

Explanation: If a congenital malformation or deformity has been corrected, a personal history code should be used to identify the history of the malformation or deformity.

Forty-year-old man with headaches diagnosed with congenital arteriovenous malformation by brain scan

Q28.2   Arteriovenous malformation of cerebral vessels

Explanation: Although present at birth, malformations may not be identified until later in life. Whenever the condition is diagnosed by the physician, it is appropriate to assign a code from the range Q00–Q99.

Newborn with anencephaly delivered vaginally in hospital

Z38.00   Single liveborn infant, delivered vaginally

Q00.0   Anencephaly

Explanation: For the birth admission, the appropriate code from category Z38 Liveborn infants, according to place of birth and type of delivery, should be sequenced as the principal diagnosis, followed by any congenital anomaly codes, Q00–Q99.

Chapter 17. Congenital Malformations, Deformations and Chromosomal Abnormalities (Q00-Q99)

> **NOTE**   Codes from this chapter are not for use on maternal or fetal records
>
> **EXCLUDES 2** *inborn errors of metabolism (E70-E88)*

This chapter contains the following blocks:

Q00-Q07	Congenital malformations of the nervous system
Q10-Q18	Congenital malformations of eye, ear, face and neck
Q20-Q28	Congenital malformations of the circulatory system
Q30-Q34	Congenital malformations of the respiratory system
Q35-Q37	Cleft lip and cleft palate
Q38-Q45	Other congenital malformations of the digestive system
Q50-Q56	Congenital malformations of genital organs
Q60-Q64	Congenital malformations of the urinary system
Q65-Q79	Congenital malformations and deformations of the musculoskeletal system
Q80-Q89	Other congenital malformations
Q90-Q99	Chromosomal abnormalities, not elsewhere classified

Congenital malformations of the nervous system (Q00-Q07)

☑4ᵗʰ **Q00 Anencephaly and similar malformations**

    Q00.0 Anencephaly
        Acephaly
        Acrania
        Amyelencephaly
        Hemianencephaly
        Hemicephaly

    Q00.1 Craniorachischisis
    Q00.2 Iniencephaly

☑4ᵗʰ **Q01 Encephalocele**

    INCLUDES   Arnold-Chiari syndrome, type III
        encephalocystocele
        encephalomyelocele
        hydroencephalocele
        hydromeningocele, cranial
        meningocele, cerebral
        meningoencephalocele

    EXCLUDES 1 *Meckel-Gruber syndrome (Q61.9)*

    Q01.0 Frontal encephalocele
    Q01.1 Nasofrontal encephalocele
    Q01.2 Occipital encephalocele
    Q01.8 Encephalocele of other sites
    Q01.9 Encephalocele, unspecified   ▽

  Q02 Microcephaly

    INCLUDES   hydromicrocephaly
        micrencephalon
    EXCLUDES 1 *Meckel-Gruber syndrome (Q61.9)*

☑4ᵗʰ **Q03 Congenital hydrocephalus**

    INCLUDES   hydrocephalus in newborn
    EXCLUDES 1 *Arnold-Chiari syndrome, type II (Q07.0-)*
        acquired hydrocephalus (G91.-)
        hydrocephalus due to congenital toxoplasmosis (P37.1)
        hydrocephalus with spina bifida (Q05.0-Q05.4)

    Q03.0 Malformations of aqueduct of Sylvius
        Anomaly of aqueduct of Sylvius
        Obstruction of aqueduct of Sylvius, congenital
        Stenosis of aqueduct of Sylvius

    Q03.1 Atresia of foramina of Magendie and Luschka
        Dandy-Walker syndrome

    Q03.8 Other congenital hydrocephalus
    Q03.9 Congenital hydrocephalus, unspecified   ▽

☑4ᵗʰ **Q04 Other congenital malformations of brain**

    EXCLUDES 1 *cyclopia (Q87.0)*
        macrocephaly (Q75.3)

    Q04.0 Congenital malformations of corpus callosum
        Agenesis of corpus callosum

    Q04.1 Arhinencephaly
    Q04.2 Holoprosencephaly

    Q04.3 Other reduction deformities of brain
        Absence of part of brain
        Agenesis of part of brain
        Agyria
        Aplasia of part of brain
        Hydranencephaly
        Hypoplasia of part of brain
        Lissencephaly
        Microgyria
        Pachygyria
        EXCLUDES 1 *congenital malformations of corpus callosum (Q04.0)*

    Q04.4 Septo-optic dysplasia of brain
    Q04.5 Megalencephaly
    Q04.6 Congenital cerebral cysts
        Porencephaly
        Schizencephaly
        EXCLUDES 1 *acquired porencephalic cyst (G93.0)*

    Q04.8 Other specified congenital malformations of brain
        Arnold-Chiari syndrome, type IV
        Macrogyria

    Q04.9 Congenital malformation of brain, unspecified   ▽
        Congenital anomaly NOS of brain
        Congenital deformity NOS of brain
        Congenital disease or lesion NOS of brain
        Multiple anomalies NOS of brain, congenital

☑4ᵗʰ **Q05 Spina bifida**

    INCLUDES   hydromeningocele (spinal)
        meningocele (spinal)
        meningomyelocele
        myelocele
        myelomeningocele
        rachischisis
        spina bifida (aperta)(cystica)
        syringomyelocele

    Use additional code for any associated paraplegia (paraparesis) (G82.2-)

    EXCLUDES 1 *Arnold-Chiari syndrome, type II (Q07.0-)*
        spina bifida occulta (Q76.0)

Spina Bifida

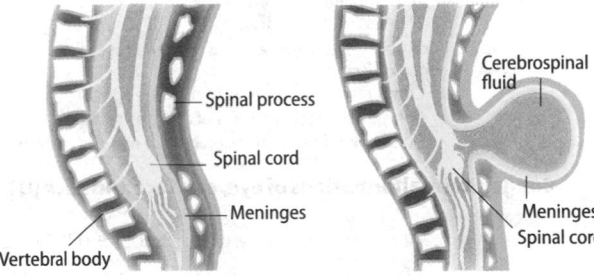

Spinal process — Spinal cord — Meninges — Vertebral body

Cerebrospinal fluid — Meninges — Spinal cord

Spina bifida occulta   **Meningocele**

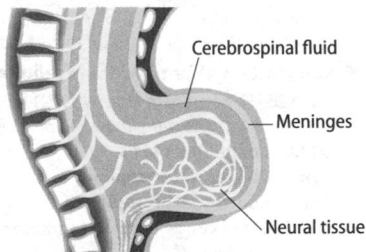

Cerebrospinal fluid — Meninges — Neural tissue

Myelomeningocele

    Q05.0 Cervical spina bifida with hydrocephalus
    Q05.1 Thoracic spina bifida with hydrocephalus
        Dorsal spina bifida with hydrocephalus
        Thoracolumbar spina bifida with hydrocephalus

    Q05.2 Lumbar spina bifida with hydrocephalus
        Lumbosacral spina bifida with hydrocephalus

    Q05.3 Sacral spina bifida with hydrocephalus
    Q05.4 Unspecified spina bifida with hydrocephalus   ▽
    Q05.5 Cervical spina bifida without hydrocephalus

☑ Additional Character Required   ✓x7ᵗʰ Placeholder Alert   Manifestation Dx   ▽ Unspecified Dx   ▶◀ Revised Text   ● New Code   ▲ Revised Code Title

ICD-10-CM 2017   847

Q05.6   **Thoracic spina bifida without hydrocephalus**
    Dorsal spina bifida NOS
    Thoracolumbar spina bifida NOS

Q05.7   **Lumbar spina bifida without hydrocephalus**
    Lumbosacral spina bifida NOS

Q05.8   **Sacral spina bifida without hydrocephalus**

Q05.9   **Spina bifida, unspecified**   ▽

☑4ᵗʰ **Q06**   **Other congenital malformations of spinal cord**

Q06.0   **Amyelia**

Q06.1   **Hypoplasia and dysplasia of spinal cord**
    Atelomyelia
    Myelatelia
    Myelodysplasia of spinal cord

Q06.2   **Diastematomyelia**

Q06.3   **Other congenital cauda equina malformations**

Q06.4   **Hydromyelia**
    Hydrorachis

Q06.8   **Other specified congenital malformations of spinal cord**

Q06.9   **Congenital malformation of spinal cord, unspecified**   ▽
    Congenital anomaly NOS of spinal cord
    Congenital deformity NOS of spinal cord
    Congenital disease or lesion NOS of spinal cord

☑4ᵗʰ **Q07**   **Other congenital malformations of nervous system**
    EXCLUDES 2   *congenital central alveolar hypoventilation syndrome (G47.35)*
       familial dysautonomia [Riley-Day] (G90.1)
       neurofibromatosis (nonmalignant) (Q85.0-)

☑5ᵗʰ **Q07.0**   **Arnold-Chiari syndrome**
    Arnold-Chiari syndrome, type II
     EXCLUDES 1   *Arnold-Chiari syndrome, type III (Q01.-)*
       Arnold-Chiari syndrome, type IV (Q04.8)

Q07.00   **Arnold-Chiari syndrome without spina bifida or hydrocephalus**

Q07.01   **Arnold-Chiari syndrome with spina bifida**

Q07.02   **Arnold-Chiari syndrome with hydrocephalus**

Q07.03   **Arnold-Chiari syndrome with spina bifida and hydrocephalus**

Q07.8   **Other specified congenital malformations of nervous system**
    Agenesis of nerve
    Displacement of brachial plexus
    Jaw-winking syndrome
    Marcus Gunn's syndrome

Q07.9   **Congenital malformation of nervous system, unspecified**   ▽
    Congenital anomaly NOS of nervous system
    Congenital deformity NOS of nervous system
    Congenital disease or lesion NOS of nervous system

Congenital malformations of eye, ear, face and neck (Q10-Q18)

EXCLUDES 2   *cleft lip and cleft palate (Q35-Q37)*
    congenital malformation of cervical spine (Q05.0, Q05.5, Q67.5, Q76.0-Q76.4)
    congenital malformation of larynx (Q31.-)
    congenital malformation of lip NEC (Q38.0)
    congenital malformation of nose (Q30.-)
    congenital malformation of parathyroid gland (Q89.2)
    congenital malformation of thyroid gland (Q89.2)

☑4ᵗʰ **Q10**   **Congenital malformations of eyelid, lacrimal apparatus and orbit**
    EXCLUDES 1   *cryptophthalmos NOS (Q11.2)*
       cryptophthalmos syndrome (Q87.0)

Q10.0   **Congenital ptosis**

Q10.1   **Congenital ectropion**

Q10.2   **Congenital entropion**

Q10.3   **Other congenital malformations of eyelid**
    Ablepharon
    Blepharophimosis, congenital
    Coloboma of eyelid
    Congenital absence or agenesis of cilia
    Congenital absence or agenesis of eyelid
    Congenital accessory eyelid
    Congenital accessory eye muscle
    Congenital malformation of eyelid NOS

Q10.4   **Absence and agenesis of lacrimal apparatus**
    Congenital absence of punctum lacrimale

Q10.5   **Congenital stenosis and stricture of lacrimal duct**

Q10.6   **Other congenital malformations of lacrimal apparatus**
    Congenital malformation of lacrimal apparatus NOS

Q10.7   **Congenital malformation of orbit**

☑4ᵗʰ **Q11**   **Anophthalmos, microphthalmos and macrophthalmos**

Q11.0   **Cystic eyeball**

Q11.1   **Other anophthalmos**
    Anophthalmos NOS
    Agenesis of eye
    Aplasia of eye

Q11.2   **Microphthalmos**
    Cryptophthalmos NOS
    Dysplasia of eye
    Hypoplasia of eye
    Rudimentary eye
     EXCLUDES 1   *cryptophthalmos syndrome (Q87.0)*

Q11.3   **Macrophthalmos**
     EXCLUDES 1   *macrophthalmos in congenital glaucoma (Q15.0)*

☑4ᵗʰ **Q12**   **Congenital lens malformations**

Q12.0   **Congenital cataract**

Q12.1   **Congenital displaced lens**

Q12.2   **Coloboma of lens**

Coloboma of Lens

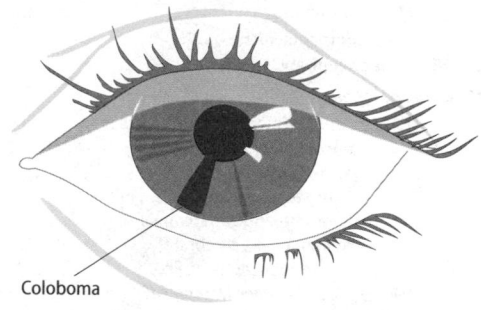

Coloboma

Q12.3   **Congenital aphakia**

Q12.4   **Spherophakia**

Q12.8   **Other congenital lens malformations**
    Microphakia

Q12.9   **Congenital lens malformation, unspecified**   ▽

☑4ᵗʰ **Q13**   **Congenital malformations of anterior segment of eye**

Q13.0   **Coloboma of iris**
    Coloboma NOS

Q13.1   **Absence of iris**
    Aniridia
    Use additional code for associated glaucoma (H42)
    DEF: Incompletely formed or absent iris; affects both eyes; dominant trait.

Q13.2   **Other congenital malformations of iris**
    Anisocoria, congenital
    Atresia of pupil
    Congenital malformation of iris NOS
    Corectopia

Q13.3   **Congenital corneal opacity**

Q13.4   **Other congenital corneal malformations**
    Congenital malformation of cornea NOS
    Microcornea
    Peter's anomaly

Q13.5   **Blue sclera**

☑5ᵗʰ **Q13.8**   **Other congenital malformations of anterior segment of eye**

Q13.81   **Rieger's anomaly**
    Use additional code for associated glaucoma (H42)

Q13.89   **Other congenital malformations of anterior segment of eye**

Q13.9   **Congenital malformation of anterior segment of eye, unspecified**   ▽

☑4ᵗʰ **Q14**   **Congenital malformations of posterior segment of eye**
    EXCLUDES 2   *optic nerve hypoplasia (H47.03-)*

Q14.0   **Congenital malformation of vitreous humor**
    Congenital vitreous opacity

EXCLUDES 1   Not coded here   EXCLUDES 2   Not included here   N Newborn Age : 0   P Pediatric Age : 0-17   M Maternity Age : 12-55   A Adult Age : 15-124

848   ICD-10-CM 2017

Q14.1 Congenital malformation of retina
Congenital retinal aneurysm

Q14.2 Congenital malformation of optic disc
Coloboma of optic disc

Q14.3 Congenital malformation of choroid

Q14.8 Other congenital malformations of posterior segment of eye
Coloboma of the fundus

Q14.9 Congenital malformation of posterior segment of eye, unspecified ▽

✓4ᵗʰ **Q15 Other congenital malformations of eye**
EXCLUDES 1   *congenital nystagmus (H55.01)*
      ocular albinism (E70.31-)
      optic nerve hypoplasia (H47.03-)
      retinitis pigmentosa (H35.52)

Q15.0 Congenital glaucoma
Axenfeld's anomaly
Buphthalmos
Glaucoma of childhood
Glaucoma of newborn
Hydrophthalmos
Keratoglobus, congenital, with glaucoma
Macrocornea with glaucoma
Macrophthalmos in congenital glaucoma
Megalocornea with glaucoma

Q15.8 Other specified congenital malformations of eye

Q15.9 Congenital malformation of eye, unspecified ▽
Congenital anomaly of eye
Congenital deformity of eye

✓4ᵗʰ **Q16 Congenital malformations of ear causing impairment of hearing**
EXCLUDES 1   *congenital deafness (H90.-)*

Q16.0 Congenital absence of (ear) auricle

Q16.1 Congenital absence, atresia and stricture of auditory canal (external)
Congenital atresia or stricture of osseous meatus

Q16.2 Absence of eustachian tube

Q16.3 Congenital malformation of ear ossicles
Congenital fusion of ear ossicles

Q16.4 Other congenital malformations of middle ear
Congenital malformation of middle ear NOS

Q16.5 Congenital malformation of inner ear
Congenital anomaly of membranous labyrinth
Congenital anomaly of organ of Corti

Q16.9 Congenital malformation of ear causing impairment of hearing, unspecified ▽
Congenital absence of ear NOS

✓4ᵗʰ **Q17 Other congenital malformations of ear**
EXCLUDES 1   *congenital malformations of ear with impairment of hearing (Q16.0-Q16.9)*
      preauricular sinus (Q18.1)

Q17.0 Accessory auricle
Accessory tragus
Polyotia
Preauricular appendage or tag
Supernumerary ear
Supernumerary lobule

Q17.1 Macrotia

Q17.2 Microtia

Q17.3 Other misshapen ear
Pointed ear

Q17.4 Misplaced ear
Low-set ears
EXCLUDES 1   *cervical auricle (Q18.2)*

Q17.5 Prominent ear
Bat ear

Q17.8 Other specified congenital malformations of ear
Congenital absence of lobe of ear

Q17.9 Congenital malformation of ear, unspecified ▽
Congenital anomaly of ear NOS

✓4ᵗʰ **Q18 Other congenital malformations of face and neck**
EXCLUDES 1   *cleft lip and cleft palate (Q35-Q37)*
      conditions classified to Q67.0-Q67.4
      congenital malformations of skull and face bones (Q75.-)
      cyclopia (Q87.0)
      dentofacial anomalies [including malocclusion] (M26.-)
      malformation syndromes affecting facial appearance (Q87.0)
      persistent thyroglossal duct (Q89.2)

Q18.0 Sinus, fistula and cyst of branchial cleft
Branchial vestige

Q18.1 Preauricular sinus and cyst
Fistula of auricle, congenital
Cervicoaural fistula

Q18.2 Other branchial cleft malformations
Branchial cleft malformation NOS
Cervical auricle
Otocephaly

Q18.3 Webbing of neck
Pterygium colli

Q18.4 Macrostomia

Q18.5 Microstomia

Q18.6 Macrocheilia
Hypertrophy of lip, congenital

Q18.7 Microcheilia

Q18.8 Other specified congenital malformations of face and neck
Medial cyst of face and neck
Medial fistula of face and neck
Medial sinus of face and neck

Q18.9 Congenital malformation of face and neck, unspecified ▽
Congenital anomaly NOS of face and neck

Congenital malformations of the circulatory system (Q20-Q28)

✓4ᵗʰ **Q20 Congenital malformations of cardiac chambers and connections**
EXCLUDES 1   *dextrocardia with situs inversus (Q89.3)*
      mirror-image atrial arrangement with situs inversus (Q89.3)

Q20.0 Common arterial trunk
Persistent truncus arteriosus
EXCLUDES 1   *aortic septal defect (Q21.4)*

Q20.1 Double outlet right ventricle
Taussig-Bing syndrome

Q20.2 Double outlet left ventricle

Q20.3 Discordant ventriculoarterial connection
Dextrotransposition of aorta
Transposition of great vessels (complete)

Q20.4 Double inlet ventricle
Common ventricle
Cor triloculare biatriatum
Single ventricle

Q20.5 Discordant atrioventricular connection
Corrected transposition
Levotransposition
Ventricular inversion

Q20.6 Isomerism of atrial appendages
Isomerism of atrial appendages with asplenia or polysplenia

Q20.8 Other congenital malformations of cardiac chambers and connections
Cor binoculare

Q20.9 Congenital malformation of cardiac chambers and connections, unspecified ▽

✓4ᵗʰ **Q21 Congenital malformations of cardiac septa**
EXCLUDES 1   *acquired cardiac septal defect (I51.0)*

Q21.0 Ventricular septal defect
Roger's disease

Q21.1 Atrial septal defect
Coronary sinus defect
Patent or persistent foramen ovale
Patent or persistent ostium secundum defect (type II)
Patent or persistent sinus venosus defect

Q21.2 Atrioventricular septal defect
Common atrioventricular canal
Endocardial cushion defect
Ostium primum atrial septal defect (type I)

☑ Additional Character Required   ✓x7ᵗʰ Placeholder Alert   Manifestation Dx   ▽ Unspecified Dx   ▶◀ Revised Text   ● New Code   ▲ Revised Code Title

Q21.3 **Tetralogy of Fallot**
Ventricular septal defect with pulmonary stenosis or atresia, dextroposition of aorta and hypertrophy of right ventricle.
AHA: 2014,3Q,16

Q21.4 **Aortopulmonary septal defect**
Aortic septal defect
Aortopulmonary window

Q21.8 **Other congenital malformations of cardiac septa**
Eisenmenger's defect
Pentalogy of Fallot
EXCLUDES 1 *Eisenmenger's complex (I27.8)*
Eisenmenger's syndrome (I27.8)

Q21.9 **Congenital malformation of cardiac septum, unspecified** ▽
Septal (heart) defect NOS

✓4ᵗʰ **Q22** **Congenital malformations of pulmonary and tricuspid valves**

Q22.0 **Pulmonary valve atresia**

Q22.1 **Congenital pulmonary valve stenosis**
DEF: Stenosis of opening between pulmonary artery and right ventricle; causes obstructed blood outflow from right ventricle.

Q22.2 **Congenital pulmonary valve insufficiency**
Congenital pulmonary valve regurgitation

Q22.3 **Other congenital malformations of pulmonary valve**
Congenital malformation of pulmonary valve NOS
Supernumerary cusps of pulmonary valve

Q22.4 **Congenital tricuspid stenosis**
Congenital tricuspid atresia

Q22.5 **Ebstein's anomaly**

Q22.6 **Hypoplastic right heart syndrome**

Q22.8 **Other congenital malformations of tricuspid valve**

Q22.9 **Congenital malformation of tricuspid valve, unspecified** ▽

✓4ᵗʰ **Q23** **Congenital malformations of aortic and mitral valves**

Q23.0 **Congenital stenosis of aortic valve**
Congenital aortic atresia
Congenital aortic stenosis NOS
EXCLUDES 1 *congenital stenosis of aortic valve in hypoplastic left heart syndrome (Q23.4)*
congenital subaortic stenosis (Q24.4)
supravalvular aortic stenosis (congenital) (Q25.3)

Q23.1 **Congenital insufficiency of aortic valve**
Bicuspid aortic valve
Congenital aortic insufficiency

Q23.2 **Congenital mitral stenosis**
Congenital mitral atresia

Q23.3 **Congenital mitral insufficiency**

Q23.4 **Hypoplastic left heart syndrome**

Q23.8 **Other congenital malformations of aortic and mitral valves**

Q23.9 **Congenital malformation of aortic and mitral valves, unspecified** ▽

✓4ᵗʰ **Q24** **Other congenital malformations of heart**
EXCLUDES 1 *endocardial fibroelastosis (I42.4)*

Q24.0 **Dextrocardia**
EXCLUDES 1 *dextrocardia with situs inversus (Q89.3)*
isomerism of atrial appendages (with asplenia or polysplenia) (Q20.6)
mirror-image atrial arrangement with situs inversus (Q89.3)

Q24.1 **Levocardia**

Q24.2 **Cor triatriatum**

Q24.3 **Pulmonary infundibular stenosis**
Subvalvular pulmonic stenosis

Q24.4 **Congenital subaortic stenosis**

Q24.5 **Malformation of coronary vessels**
Congenital coronary (artery) aneurysm

Q24.6 **Congenital heart block**

Q24.8 **Other specified congenital malformations of heart**
Congenital diverticulum of left ventricle
Congenital malformation of myocardium
Congenital malformation of pericardium
Malposition of heart
Uhl's disease

Q24.9 **Congenital malformation of heart, unspecified** ▽
Congenital anomaly of heart
Congenital disease of heart

✓4ᵗʰ **Q25** **Congenital malformations of great arteries**

Q25.0 **Patent ductus arteriosus**
Patent ductus Botallo
Persistent ductus arteriosus

Q25.1 **Coarctation of aorta**
Coarctation of aorta (preductal) (postductal)
▶Stenosis of aorta◀

✓5ᵗʰ **Q25.2** **Atresia of aorta**
● **Q25.21** **Interruption of aortic arch**
Atresia of aortic arch
● **Q25.29** **Other atresia of aorta**
Atresia of aorta

Q25.3 **Supravalvular aortic stenosis**
EXCLUDES 1 *congenital aortic stenosis NOS (Q23.0)*
congenital stenosis of aortic valve (Q23.0)

✓5ᵗʰ **Q25.4** **Other congenital malformations of aorta**
EXCLUDES 1 *hypoplasia of aorta in hypoplastic left heart syndrome (Q23.4)*
● **Q25.40** **Congenital malformation of aorta unspecified** ▽
● **Q25.41** **Absence and aplasia of aorta**
● **Q25.42** **Hypoplasia of aorta**
● **Q25.43** **Congenital aneurysm of aorta**
Congenital aneurysm of aortic root
Congenital aneurysm of aortic sinus
● **Q25.44** **Congenital dilation of aorta**
● **Q25.45** **Double aortic arch**
Vascular ring of aorta
● **Q25.46** **Tortuous aortic arch**
Persistent convolutions of aortic arch
● **Q25.47** **Right aortic arch**
Persistent right aortic arch
● **Q25.48** **Anomalous origin of subclavian artery**
● **Q25.49** **Other congenital malformations of aorta**

Q25.5 **Atresia of pulmonary artery**

Q25.6 **Stenosis of pulmonary artery**
Supravalvular pulmonary stenosis

✓5ᵗʰ **Q25.7** **Other congenital malformations of pulmonary artery**
Q25.71 **Coarctation of pulmonary artery**
Q25.72 **Congenital pulmonary arteriovenous malformation**
Congenital pulmonary arteriovenous aneurysm
Q25.79 **Other congenital malformations of pulmonary artery**
Aberrant pulmonary artery
Agenesis of pulmonary artery
Congenital aneurysm of pulmonary artery
Congenital anomaly of pulmonary artery
Hypoplasia of pulmonary artery

Q25.8 **Other congenital malformations of other great arteries**

Q25.9 **Congenital malformation of great arteries, unspecified** ▽

✓4ᵗʰ **Q26** **Congenital malformations of great veins**

Q26.0 **Congenital stenosis of vena cava**
Congenital stenosis of vena cava (inferior)(superior)

Q26.1 **Persistent left superior vena cava**

Q26.2 **Total anomalous pulmonary venous connection**
Total anomalous pulmonary venous return [TAPVR], subdiaphragmatic
Total anomalous pulmonary venous return [TAPVR], supradiaphragmatic

Q26.3 **Partial anomalous pulmonary venous connection**
Partial anomalous pulmonary venous return

Q26.4 **Anomalous pulmonary venous connection, unspecified** ▽

Q26.5 **Anomalous portal venous connection**

Q26.6 **Portal vein-hepatic artery fistula**

Q26.8 **Other congenital malformations of great veins**
Absence of vena cava (inferior) (superior)
Azygos continuation of inferior vena cava
Persistent left posterior cardinal vein
Scimitar syndrome

Q26.9 **Congenital malformation of great vein, unspecified** ▽
Congenital anomaly of vena cava (inferior) (superior) NOS

✓4ᵗʰ **Q27** **Other congenital malformations of peripheral vascular system**
     EXCLUDES 2   *anomalies of cerebral and precerebral vessels (Q28.0-Q28.3)*
         anomalies of coronary vessels (Q24.5)
         anomalies of pulmonary artery (Q25.5-Q25.7)
         congenital retinal aneurysm (Q14.1)
         hemangioma and lymphangioma (D18.-)

Q27.0 **Congenital absence and hypoplasia of umbilical artery**
     Single umbilical artery

Q27.1 **Congenital renal artery stenosis**

Q27.2 **Other congenital malformations of renal artery**
     Congenital malformation of renal artery NOS
     Multiple renal arteries

✓5ᵗʰ **Q27.3** **Arteriovenous malformation (peripheral)**
     Arteriovenous aneurysm
     EXCLUDES 1   *acquired arteriovenous aneurysm (I77.0)*
     EXCLUDES 2   *arteriovenous malformation of cerebral vessels (Q28.2)*
         arteriovenous malformation of precerebral vessels (Q28.0)

     Q27.30 **Arteriovenous malformation, site unspecified** ▽

     Q27.31 **Arteriovenous malformation of vessel of upper limb**

     Q27.32 **Arteriovenous malformation of vessel of lower limb**

     Q27.33 **Arteriovenous malformation of digestive system vessel**

     Q27.34 **Arteriovenous malformation of renal vessel**

     Q27.39 **Arteriovenous malformation, other site**

Q27.4 **Congenital phlebectasia**

Q27.8 **Other specified congenital malformations of peripheral vascular system**
     Absence of peripheral vascular system
     Atresia of peripheral vascular system
     Congenital aneurysm (peripheral)
     Congenital stricture, artery
     Congenital varix
     EXCLUDES 1   *arteriovenous malformation (Q27.3-)*

Q27.9 **Congenital malformation of peripheral vascular system, unspecified** ▽
     Anomaly of artery or vein NOS

✓4ᵗʰ **Q28** **Other congenital malformations of circulatory system**
     EXCLUDES 1   *congenital aneurysm NOS (Q27.8)*
         congenital coronary aneurysm (Q24.5)
         ruptured cerebral arteriovenous malformation (I60.8)
         ruptured malformation of precerebral vessels (I72.0)
     EXCLUDES 2   *congenital peripheral aneurysm (Q27.8)*
         congenital pulmonary aneurysm (Q25.79)
         congenital retinal aneurysm (Q14.1)

Q28.0 **Arteriovenous malformation of precerebral vessels**
     Congenital arteriovenous precerebral aneurysm (nonruptured)

Q28.1 **Other malformations of precerebral vessels**
     Congenital malformation of precerebral vessels NOS
     Congenital precerebral aneurysm (nonruptured)

Q28.2 **Arteriovenous malformation of cerebral vessels**
     Arteriovenous malformation of brain NOS
     Congenital arteriovenous cerebral aneurysm (nonruptured)

Q28.3 **Other malformations of cerebral vessels**
     Congenital cerebral aneurysm (nonruptured)
     Congenital malformation of cerebral vessels NOS
     Developmental venous anomaly

Q28.8 **Other specified congenital malformations of circulatory system**
     Congenital aneurysm, specified site NEC
     Spinal vessel anomaly

Q28.9 **Congenital malformation of circulatory system, unspecified** ▽

Congenital malformations of the respiratory system (Q30-Q34)

✓4ᵗʰ **Q30** **Congenital malformations of nose**
     EXCLUDES 1   *congenital deviation of nasal septum (Q67.4)*

Q30.0 **Choanal atresia**
     Atresia of nares (anterior) (posterior)
     Congenital stenosis of nares (anterior) (posterior)

Q30.1 **Agenesis and underdevelopment of nose**
     Congenital absent of nose

Q30.2 **Fissured, notched and cleft nose**

Q30.3 **Congenital perforated nasal septum**

Q30.8 **Other congenital malformations of nose**
     Accessory nose
     Congenital anomaly of nasal sinus wall

Q30.9 **Congenital malformation of nose, unspecified** ▽

✓4ᵗʰ **Q31** **Congenital malformations of larynx**
     EXCLUDES 1   *congenital laryngeal stridor NOS (P28.89)*

Q31.0 **Web of larynx**
     Glottic web of larynx
     Subglottic web of larynx
     Web of larynx NOS

Q31.1 **Congenital subglottic stenosis**

Q31.2 **Laryngeal hypoplasia**

Q31.3 **Laryngocele**

Q31.5 **Congenital laryngomalacia**

Q31.8 **Other congenital malformations of larynx**
     Absence of larynx
     Agenesis of larynx
     Atresia of larynx
     Congenital cleft thyroid cartilage
     Congenital fissure of epiglottis
     Congenital stenosis of larynx NEC
     Posterior cleft of cricoid cartilage

Q31.9 **Congenital malformation of larynx, unspecified** ▽

✓4ᵗʰ **Q32** **Congenital malformations of trachea and bronchus**
     EXCLUDES 1   *congenital bronchiectasis (Q33.4)*

Q32.0 **Congenital tracheomalacia**

Q32.1 **Other congenital malformations of trachea**
     Atresia of trachea
     Congenital anomaly of tracheal cartilage
     Congenital dilatation of trachea
     Congenital malformation of trachea
     Congenital stenosis of trachea
     Congenital tracheocele

Q32.2 **Congenital bronchomalacia**

Q32.3 **Congenital stenosis of bronchus**

Q32.4 **Other congenital malformations of bronchus**
     Absence of bronchus
     Agenesis of bronchus
     Atresia of bronchus
     Congenital diverticulum of bronchus
     Congenital malformation of bronchus NOS

✓4ᵗʰ **Q33** **Congenital malformations of lung**

Q33.0 **Congenital cystic lung**
     Congenital cystic lung disease
     Congenital honeycomb lung
     Congenital polycystic lung disease
     EXCLUDES 1   *cystic fibrosis (E84.0)*
         cystic lung disease, acquired or unspecified (J98.4)

Q33.1 **Accessory lobe of lung**
     Azygos lobe (fissured), lung

Q33.2 **Sequestration of lung**

Q33.3 **Agenesis of lung**
     Congenital absence of lung (lobe)

Q33.4 **Congenital bronchiectasis**

Q33.5 **Ectopic tissue in lung**

Q33.6 **Congenital hypoplasia and dysplasia of lung**
     EXCLUDES 1   *pulmonary hypoplasia associated with short gestation (P28.0)*

Q33.8 **Other congenital malformations of lung**

Q33.9 **Congenital malformation of lung, unspecified** ▽

✓4ᵗʰ **Q34** **Other congenital malformations of respiratory system**
     EXCLUDES 2   *congenital central alveolar hypoventilation syndrome (G47.35)*

Q34.0 **Anomaly of pleura**

Q34.1 **Congenital cyst of mediastinum**

Q34.8 **Other specified congenital malformations of respiratory system**
     Atresia of nasopharynx

Q34.9 **Congenital malformation of respiratory system, unspecified** ▽
     Congenital absence of respiratory system
     Congenital anomaly of respiratory system NOS

✔ Additional Character Required   ✓x7ᵗʰ Placeholder Alert   Manifestation Dx   ▽ Unspecified Dx   ▶◀ Revised Text   ● New Code   ▲ Revised Code Title

Cleft lip and cleft palate (Q35-Q37)

Use additional code to identify associated malformation of the nose (Q30.2)

EXCLUDES 1   Robin syndrome (Q87.0)

✓4ᵗʰ Q35   Cleft palate

INCLUDES   fissure of palate
palatoschisis

EXCLUDES 1   cleft palate with cleft lip (Q37.-)

Q35.1   Cleft hard palate

Q35.3   Cleft soft palate

Q35.5   Cleft hard palate with cleft soft palate

Q35.7   Cleft uvula

Q35.9   Cleft palate, unspecified   ▽
Cleft palate NOS

✓4ᵗʰ Q36   Cleft lip

INCLUDES   cheiloschisis
congenital fissure of lip
harelip
labium leporinum

EXCLUDES 1   cleft lip with cleft palate (Q37.-)

Q36.0   Cleft lip, bilateral

Q36.1   Cleft lip, median

Q36.9   Cleft lip, unilateral
Cleft lip NOS

✓4ᵗʰ Q37   Cleft palate with cleft lip

INCLUDES   cheilopalatoschisis

Q37.0   Cleft hard palate with bilateral cleft lip

Q37.1   Cleft hard palate with unilateral cleft lip
Cleft hard palate with cleft lip NOS

Q37.2   Cleft soft palate with bilateral cleft lip

Q37.3   Cleft soft palate with unilateral cleft lip
Cleft soft palate with cleft lip NOS

Q37.4   Cleft hard and soft palate with bilateral cleft lip

Q37.5   Cleft hard and soft palate with unilateral cleft lip
Cleft hard and soft palate with cleft lip NOS

Q37.8   Unspecified cleft palate with bilateral cleft lip   ▽

Q37.9   Unspecified cleft palate with unilateral cleft lip   ▽
Cleft palate with cleft lip NOS

Other congenital malformations of the digestive system (Q38-Q45)

✓4ᵗʰ Q38   Other congenital malformations of tongue, mouth and pharynx

EXCLUDES 1   dentofacial anomalies (M26.-)
macrostomia (Q18.4)
microstomia (Q18.5)

Q38.0   Congenital malformations of lips, not elsewhere classified
Congenital fistula of lip
Congenital malformation of lip NOS
Van der Woude's syndrome

EXCLUDES 1   cleft lip (Q36.-)
cleft lip with cleft palate (Q37.-)
macrocheilia (Q18.6)
microcheilia (Q18.7)

Q38.1   Ankyloglossia
Tongue tie

Q38.2   Macroglossia
Congenital hypertrophy of tongue

Q38.3   Other congenital malformations of tongue
Aglossia
Bifid tongue
Congenital adhesion of tongue
Congenital fissure of tongue
Congenital malformation of tongue NOS
Double tongue
Hypoglossia
Hypoplasia of tongue
Microglossia

Q38.4   Congenital malformations of salivary glands and ducts
Atresia of salivary glands and ducts
Congenital absence of salivary glands and ducts
Congenital accessory salivary glands and ducts
Congenital fistula of salivary gland

Q38.5   Congenital malformations of palate, not elsewhere classified
Congenital absence of uvula
Congenital malformation of palate NOS
Congenital high arched palate

EXCLUDES 1   cleft palate (Q35.-)
cleft palate with cleft lip (Q37.-)

Q38.6   Other congenital malformations of mouth
Congenital malformation of mouth NOS

Q38.7   Congenital pharyngeal pouch
Congenital diverticulum of pharynx

EXCLUDES 1   pharyngeal pouch syndrome (D82.1)

Q38.8   Other congenital malformations of pharynx
Congenital malformation of pharynx NOS
Imperforate pharynx

✓4ᵗʰ Q39   Congenital malformations of esophagus

Q39.0   Atresia of esophagus without fistula
Atresia of esophagus NOS

Q39.1   Atresia of esophagus with tracheo-esophageal fistula
Atresia of esophagus with broncho-esophageal fistula

Q39.2   Congenital tracheo-esophageal fistula without atresia
Congenital tracheo-esophageal fistula NOS

Q39.3   Congenital stenosis and stricture of esophagus

Q39.4   Esophageal web

Q39.5   Congenital dilatation of esophagus
Congenital cardiospasm

Q39.6   Congenital diverticulum of esophagus
Congenital esophageal pouch

Q39.8   Other congenital malformations of esophagus
Congenital absence of esophagus
Congenital displacement of esophagus
Congenital duplication of esophagus

Q39.9   Congenital malformation of esophagus, unspecified   ▽

✓4ᵗʰ Q40   Other congenital malformations of upper alimentary tract

Q40.0   Congenital hypertrophic pyloric stenosis
Congenital or infantile constriction
Congenital or infantile hypertrophy
Congenital or infantile spasm
Congenital or infantile stenosis
Congenital or infantile stricture

Q40.1   Congenital hiatus hernia
Congenital displacement of cardia through esophageal hiatus

EXCLUDES 1   congenital diaphragmatic hernia (Q79.0)

Q40.2   Other specified congenital malformations of stomach
Congenital displacement of stomach
Congenital diverticulum of stomach
Congenital hourglass stomach
Congenital duplication of stomach
Megalogastria
Microgastria

Q40.3   Congenital malformation of stomach, unspecified   ▽

Q40.8   Other specified congenital malformations of upper alimentary tract

Q40.9   Congenital malformation of upper alimentary tract, unspecified   ▽
Congenital anomaly of upper alimentary tract
Congenital deformity of upper alimentary tract

✓4ᵗʰ Q41   Congenital absence, atresia and stenosis of small intestine

INCLUDES   congenital obstruction, occlusion or stricture of small intestine or intestine NOS

EXCLUDES 1   cystic fibrosis with intestinal manifestation (E84.11)
meconium ileus NOS (without cystic fibrosis) (P76.0)

Q41.0   Congenital absence, atresia and stenosis of duodenum

Q41.1   Congenital absence, atresia and stenosis of jejunum
Apple peel syndrome
Imperforate jejunum

Q41.2   Congenital absence, atresia and stenosis of ileum

Q41.8   Congenital absence, atresia and stenosis of other specified parts of small intestine

Q41.9   Congenital absence, atresia and stenosis of small intestine, part unspecified   ▽
Congenital absence, atresia and stenosis of intestine NOS

✓4ᵗʰ Q42   Congenital absence, atresia and stenosis of large intestine

INCLUDES   congenital obstruction, occlusion and stricture of large intestine

Q42.0   Congenital absence, atresia and stenosis of rectum with fistula

Q42.1   Congenital absence, atresia and stenosis of rectum without fistula
Imperforate rectum

Q42.2   Congenital absence, atresia and stenosis of anus with fistula

---

EXCLUDES 1 Not coded here   EXCLUDES 2 Not included here   N Newborn Age : 0   P Pediatric Age : 0-17   M Maternity Age : 12-55   A Adult Age : 15-124

Q42.3 **Congenital absence, atresia and stenosis of** anus without fistula

    Imperforate anus

Q42.8 **Congenital absence, atresia and stenosis of other parts of large intestine**

Q42.9 **Congenital absence, atresia and stenosis of large intestine, part unspecified** ▽

☑4ᵗʰ **Q43** **Other congenital malformations of** intestine

Q43.0 **Meckel's diverticulum (displaced) (hypertrophic)**

    Persistent omphalomesenteric duct

    Persistent vitelline duct

Q43.1 **Hirschsprung's disease**

    Aganglionosis

    Congenital (aganglionic) megacolon

Q43.2 **Other congenital functional disorders of colon**

    Congenital dilatation of colon

Q43.3 **Congenital malformations of intestinal fixation**

    Congenital omental, anomalous adhesions [bands]

    Congenital peritoneal adhesions [bands]

    Incomplete rotation of cecum and colon

    Insufficient rotation of cecum and colon

    Jackson's membrane

    Malrotation of colon

    Rotation failure of cecum and colon

    Universal mesentery

Q43.4 **Duplication of intestine**

Q43.5 **Ectopic anus**

Q43.6 **Congenital fistula of rectum and anus**

    EXCLUDES 1 *congenital fistula of anus with absence, atresia and stenosis (Q42.2)*

       congenital fistula of rectum with absence, atresia and stenosis (Q42.0)

       congenital rectovaginal fistula (Q52.2)

       congenital urethrorectal fistula (Q64.73)

       pilonidal fistula or sinus (L05.-)

Q43.7 **Persistent cloaca**

    Cloaca NOS

Q43.8 **Other specified congenital malformations of intestine**

    Congenital blind loop syndrome

    Congenital diverticulitis, colon

    Congenital diverticulum, intestine

    Dolichocolon

    Megaloappendix

    Megaloduodenum

    Microcolon

    Transposition of appendix

    Transposition of colon

    Transposition of intestine

    AHA: 2013,2Q,31

Q43.9 **Congenital malformation of intestine, unspecified** ▽

☑4ᵗʰ **Q44** **Congenital malformations of** gallbladder, bile ducts and liver

Q44.0 **Agenesis, aplasia and hypoplasia of gallbladder**

    Congenital absence of gallbladder

Q44.1 **Other congenital malformations of gallbladder**

    Congenital malformation of gallbladder NOS

    Intrahepatic gallbladder

Q44.2 **Atresia** of bile ducts

Q44.3 **Congenital** stenosis and stricture of bile ducts

Q44.4 **Choledochal cyst**

Q44.5 **Other congenital malformations of bile ducts**

    Accessory hepatic duct

    Biliary duct duplication

    Congenital malformation of bile duct NOS

    Cystic duct duplication

Q44.6 **Cystic** disease of liver

    Fibrocystic disease of liver

Q44.7 **Other congenital malformations of liver**

    Accessory liver

    Alagille's syndrome

    Congenital absence of liver

    Congenital hepatomegaly

    Congenital malformation of liver NOS

☑4ᵗʰ **Q45** **Other congenital malformations of** digestive system

    EXCLUDES 2 *congenital diaphragmatic hernia (Q79.0)*

       congenital hiatus hernia (Q40.1)

Q45.0 **Agenesis, aplasia and hypoplasia of pancreas**

    Congenital absence of pancreas

Q45.1 **Annular pancreas**

Q45.2 **Congenital** pancreatic cyst

Q45.3 **Other congenital malformations of pancreas and pancreatic duct**

    Accessory pancreas

    Congenital malformation of pancreas or pancreatic duct NOS

    EXCLUDES 1 *congenital diabetes mellitus (E10.-)*

       cystic fibrosis (E84.0-E84.9)

       fibrocystic disease of pancreas (E84.-)

       neonatal diabetes mellitus (P70.2)

Q45.8 **Other specified congenital malformations of digestive system**

    Absence (complete) (partial) of alimentary tract NOS

    Duplication of digestive system

    Malposition, congenital of digestive system

Q45.9 **Congenital malformation of digestive system, unspecified** ▽

    Congenital anomaly of digestive system

    Congenital deformity of digestive system

Congenital malformations of genital organs (Q50-Q56)

    EXCLUDES 1 *androgen insensitivity syndrome (E34.5-)*

       syndromes associated with anomalies in the number and form of chromosomes (Q90-Q99)

☑4ᵗʰ **Q50** **Congenital malformations of** ovaries, fallopian tubes and broad ligaments

    ☑5ᵗʰ **Q50.0** **Congenital absence of** ovary

       EXCLUDES 1 *Turner's syndrome (Q96.-)*

       Q50.01 **Congenital absence of ovary,** unilateral   ♀

       Q50.02 **Congenital absence of ovary,** bilateral   ♀

    Q50.1 **Developmental ovarian cyst**   ♀

    Q50.2 **Congenital torsion of ovary**   ♀

    ☑5ᵗʰ **Q50.3** **Other congenital malformations of** ovary

       Q50.31 **Accessory ovary**   ♀

       Q50.32 **Ovarian streak**   ♀

          46, XX with streak gonads

       Q50.39 **Other congenital malformation of ovary**   ♀

          Congenital malformation of ovary NOS

    Q50.4 **Embryonic cyst of** fallopian tube   ♀

       Fimbrial cyst

    Q50.5 **Embryonic cyst of** broad ligament   ♀

       Epoophoron cyst

       Parovarian cyst

    Q50.6 **Other congenital malformations of fallopian tube and broad ligament**   ♀

       Absence of fallopian tube and broad ligament

       Accessory fallopian tube and broad ligament

       Atresia of fallopian tube and broad ligament

       Congenital malformation of fallopian tube or broad ligament NOS

☑4ᵗʰ **Q51** **Congenital malformations of** uterus and cervix

    Q51.0 **Agenesis and aplasia of uterus**   ♀

       Congenital absence of uterus

    ☑5ᵗʰ **Q51.1** **Doubling of uterus with doubling of cervix and vagina**

       Q51.10 **Doubling of uterus with doubling of cervix and vagina** without obstruction   ♀

          Doubling of uterus with doubling of cervix and vagina NOS

       Q51.11 **Doubling of uterus with doubling of cervix and vagina** with obstruction   ♀

    Q51.2 **Other doubling of uterus**   ♀

       Doubling of uterus NOS

       Septate uterus, complete or partial

    Q51.3 **Bicornate uterus**   ♀

       Bicornate uterus, complete or partial

    Q51.4 **Unicornate uterus**   ♀

       Unicornate uterus with or without a separate uterine horn

       Uterus with only one functioning horn

    Q51.5 **Agenesis and aplasia of cervix**   ♀

       Congenital absence of cervix

    Q51.6 **Embryonic** cyst of cervix   ♀

    Q51.7 **Congenital** fistulae between uterus and digestive and urinary tracts   ♀

☑ Additional Character Required   ☑7ᵗʰ Placeholder Alert   Manifestation Dx   ▽ Unspecified Dx   ▶◀ Revised Text   ● New Code   ▲ Revised Code Title

ICD-10-CM 2017   **853**

✓5ᵗʰ **Q51.8** **Other congenital malformations of uterus and cervix**

✓6ᵗʰ **Q51.81** **Other congenital malformations of uterus**

Q51.810 **Arcuate uterus** ♀
Arcuatus uterus

Q51.811 **Hypoplasia of uterus** ♀

Q51.818 **Other congenital malformations of uterus** ♀
Müllerian anomaly of uterus NEC

✓6ᵗʰ **Q51.82** **Other congenital malformations of cervix**

Q51.820 **Cervical duplication** ♀

Q51.821 **Hypoplasia of cervix** ♀

Q51.828 **Other congenital malformations of cervix** ♀

Q51.9 **Congenital malformation of uterus and cervix, unspecified** ♀ ▽

✓4ᵗʰ **Q52** **Other congenital malformations of female genitalia**

Q52.0 **Congenital absence of vagina** ♀
Vaginal agenesis, total or partial

✓5ᵗʰ **Q52.1** **Doubling of vagina**
EXCLUDES 1 *doubling of vagina with doubling of uterus and cervix (Q51.1-)*

Q52.10 **Doubling of vagina, unspecified** ♀ ▽
Septate vagina NOS

Q52.11 **Transverse vaginal septum** ♀

✓6ᵗʰ **Q52.12** **Longitudinal vaginal septum**

● **Q52.120** **Longitudinal vaginal septum, nonobstructing**

● **Q52.121** **Longitudinal vaginal septum, obstructing, right side**

● **Q52.122** **Longitudinal vaginal septum, obstructing, left side**

● **Q52.123** **Longitudinal vaginal septum, microperforate, right side**

● **Q52.124** **Longitudinal vaginal septum, microperforate, left side**

● **Q52.129** **Other and unspecified longitudinal vaginal septum** ▽

Q52.2 **Congenital rectovaginal fistula** ♀
EXCLUDES 1 *cloaca (Q43.7)*

Q52.3 **Imperforate hymen** ♀

Q52.4 **Other congenital malformations of vagina** ♀
Canal of Nuck cyst, congenital
Congenital malformation of vagina NOS
Embryonic vaginal cyst
Gartner's duct cyst

Q52.5 **Fusion of labia** ♀

Q52.6 **Congenital malformation of clitoris** ♀

✓5ᵗʰ **Q52.7** **Other and unspecified congenital malformations of vulva**

Q52.70 **Unspecified congenital malformations of vulva** ♀ ▽
Congenital malformation of vulva NOS

Q52.71 **Congenital absence of vulva** ♀

Q52.79 **Other congenital malformations of vulva** ♀
Congenital cyst of vulva

Q52.8 **Other specified congenital malformations of female genitalia** ♀

Q52.9 **Congenital malformation of female genitalia, unspecified** ♀ ▽

✓4ᵗʰ **Q53** **Undescended and ectopic testicle**

✓5ᵗʰ **Q53.0** **Ectopic testis**

Q53.00 **Ectopic testis, unspecified** ♂ ▽

Q53.01 **Ectopic testis, unilateral** ♂

Q53.02 **Ectopic testes, bilateral** ♂

✓5ᵗʰ **Q53.1** **Undescended testicle, unilateral**

Q53.10 **Unspecified undescended testicle, unilateral** ♂ ▽

Q53.11 **Abdominal testis, unilateral** ♂

Q53.12 **Ectopic perineal testis, unilateral** ♂

✓5ᵗʰ **Q53.2** **Undescended testicle, bilateral**

Q53.20 **Undescended testicle, unspecified, bilateral** ♂ ▽

Q53.21 **Abdominal testis, bilateral** ♂

Q53.22 **Ectopic perineal testis, bilateral** ♂

Q53.9 **Undescended testicle, unspecified** ♂ ▽
Cryptorchism NOS

✓4ᵗʰ **Q54** **Hypospadias**
EXCLUDES 1 *epispadias (Q64.0)*
DEF: Abnormal opening of urethra on the ventral (underside) surface of the penis.

Hypospadias and Epispadias

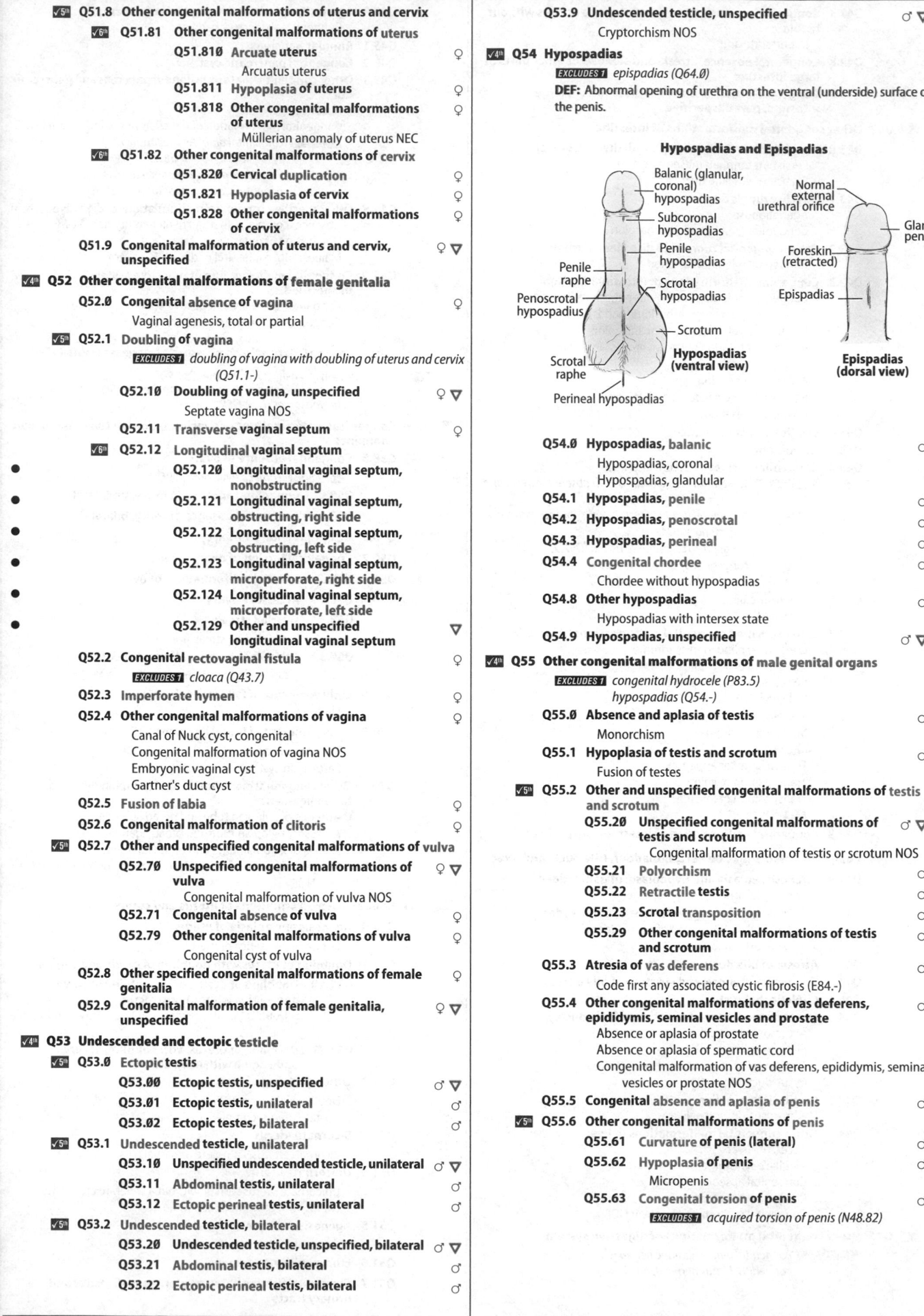

Balanic (glanular, coronal) hypospadias
Subcoronal hypospadias
Penile hypospadias
Penile raphe
Penoscrotal hypospadius
Scrotal raphe
Scrotal hypospadias
Scrotum
Perineal hypospadias
Hypospadias (ventral view)

Normal external urethral orifice
Glans penis
Foreskin (retracted)
Epispadias
Epispadias (dorsal view)

Q54.0 **Hypospadias, balanic** ♂
Hypospadias, coronal
Hypospadias, glandular

Q54.1 **Hypospadias, penile** ♂

Q54.2 **Hypospadias, penoscrotal** ♂

Q54.3 **Hypospadias, perineal** ♂

Q54.4 **Congenital chordee** ♂
Chordee without hypospadias

Q54.8 **Other hypospadias** ♂
Hypospadias with intersex state

Q54.9 **Hypospadias, unspecified** ♂ ▽

✓4ᵗʰ **Q55** **Other congenital malformations of male genital organs**
EXCLUDES 1 *congenital hydrocele (P83.5)*
hypospadias (Q54.-)

Q55.0 **Absence and aplasia of testis** ♂
Monorchism

Q55.1 **Hypoplasia of testis and scrotum** ♂
Fusion of testes

✓5ᵗʰ **Q55.2** **Other and unspecified congenital malformations of testis and scrotum**

Q55.20 **Unspecified congenital malformations of testis and scrotum** ♂ ▽
Congenital malformation of testis or scrotum NOS

Q55.21 **Polyorchism** ♂

Q55.22 **Retractile testis** ♂

Q55.23 **Scrotal transposition** ♂

Q55.29 **Other congenital malformations of testis and scrotum** ♂

Q55.3 **Atresia of vas deferens** ♂
Code first any associated cystic fibrosis (E84.-)

Q55.4 **Other congenital malformations of vas deferens, epididymis, seminal vesicles and prostate** ♂
Absence or aplasia of prostate
Absence or aplasia of spermatic cord
Congenital malformation of vas deferens, epididymis, seminal vesicles or prostate NOS

Q55.5 **Congenital absence and aplasia of penis** ♂

✓5ᵗʰ **Q55.6** **Other congenital malformations of penis**

Q55.61 **Curvature of penis (lateral)** ♂

Q55.62 **Hypoplasia of penis** ♂
Micropenis

Q55.63 **Congenital torsion of penis** ♂
EXCLUDES 1 *acquired torsion of penis (N48.82)*

EXCLUDES 1 Not coded here   EXCLUDES 2 Not included here   N Newborn Age : 0   P Pediatric Age : 0-17   M Maternity Age : 12-55   A Adult Age : 15-124

854   ICD-10-CM 2017

Q55.64   **Hidden penis**   ♂
Buried penis
Concealed penis
EXCLUDES 1 *acquired buried penis (N48.83)*

Q55.69   **Other congenital malformation of penis**   ♂
Congenital malformation of penis NOS

Q55.7   **Congenital vasocutaneous fistula**   ♂

Q55.8   **Other specified congenital malformations of male genital organs**   ♂

Q55.9   **Congenital malformation of male genital organ, unspecified**   ♂ ▽
Congenital anomaly of male genital organ
Congenital deformity of male genital organ

☑4ᵗʰ **Q56**   **Indeterminate sex and pseudohermaphroditism**
EXCLUDES 1 *46, XX true hermaphrodite (Q99.1)*
androgen insensitivity syndrome (E34.5-)
chimera 46, XX/46, XY true hermaphrodite (Q99.0)
female pseudohermaphroditism with adrenocortical disorder (E25.-)
pseudohermaphroditism with specified chromosomal anomaly (Q96-Q99)
pure gonadal dysgenesis (Q99.1)

Q56.0   **Hermaphroditism, not elsewhere classified**
Ovotestis

Q56.1   **Male pseudohermaphroditism, not elsewhere classified**   ♂
46, XY with streak gonads
Male pseudohermaphroditism NOS

Q56.2   **Female pseudohermaphroditism, not elsewhere classified**   ♀
Female pseudohermaphroditism NOS

Q56.3   **Pseudohermaphroditism, unspecified**   ▽

Q56.4   **Indeterminate sex, unspecified**   ▽
Ambiguous genitalia

Congenital malformations of the urinary system (Q60-Q64)

☑4ᵗʰ **Q60**   **Renal agenesis and other reduction defects of kidney**
INCLUDES congenital absence of kidney
congenital atrophy of kidney
infantile atrophy of kidney

Q60.0   **Renal agenesis, unilateral**
Q60.1   **Renal agenesis, bilateral**
Q60.2   **Renal agenesis, unspecified**   ▽
Q60.3   **Renal hypoplasia, unilateral**
Q60.4   **Renal hypoplasia, bilateral**
Q60.5   **Renal hypoplasia, unspecified**   ▽
Q60.6   **Potter's syndrome**

☑4ᵗʰ **Q61**   **Cystic kidney disease**
EXCLUDES 1 *acquired cyst of kidney (N28.1)*
Potter's syndrome (Q60.6)

☑5ᵗʰ **Q61.0**   **Congenital renal cyst**

Q61.00   **Congenital renal cyst, unspecified**   ▽
Cyst of kidney NOS (congenital)

Q61.01   **Congenital single renal cyst**
Q61.02   **Congenital multiple renal cysts**

☑5ᵗʰ **Q61.1**   **Polycystic kidney, infantile type**
Polycystic kidney, autosomal recessive

Q61.11   **Cystic dilatation of collecting ducts**
Q61.19   **Other polycystic kidney, infantile type**

Q61.2   **Polycystic kidney, adult type**
Polycystic kidney, autosomal dominant

Q61.3   **Polycystic kidney, unspecified**   ▽

Q61.4   **Renal dysplasia**
Multicystic dysplastic kidney
Multicystic kidney (development)
Multicystic kidney disease
Multicystic renal dysplasia
EXCLUDES 1 *polycystic kidney disease (Q61.11-Q61.3)*

Q61.5   **Medullary cystic kidney**
Nephronopthisis
Sponge kidney NOS
DEF: Sponge kidney: Dilated collecting tubules; usually asymptomatic but calcinosis in tubules may cause renal insufficiency.

Q61.8   **Other cystic kidney diseases**
Fibrocystic kidney
Fibrocystic renal degeneration or disease

Q61.9   **Cystic kidney disease, unspecified**   ▽
Meckel-Gruber syndrome

☑4ᵗʰ **Q62**   **Congenital obstructive defects of renal pelvis and congenital malformations of ureter**
Q62.0   **Congenital hydronephrosis**

☑5ᵗʰ **Q62.1**   **Congenital occlusion of ureter**
Atresia and stenosis of ureter

Q62.10   **Congenital occlusion of ureter, unspecified**   ▽
Q62.11   **Congenital occlusion of ureteropelvic junction**
Q62.12   **Congenital occlusion of ureterovesical orifice**

Q62.2   **Congenital megaureter**
Congenital dilatation of ureter

☑5ᵗʰ **Q62.3**   **Other obstructive defects of renal pelvis and ureter**

Q62.31   **Congenital ureterocele, orthotopic**
Q62.32   **Cecoureterocele**
Ectopic ureterocele
Q62.39   **Other obstructive defects of renal pelvis and ureter**
Ureteropelvic junction obstruction NOS

Q62.4   **Agenesis of ureter**
Congenital absence ureter

Q62.5   **Duplication of ureter**
Accessory ureter
Double ureter

☑5ᵗʰ **Q62.6**   **Malposition of ureter**

Q62.60   **Malposition of ureter, unspecified**   ▽
Q62.61   **Deviation of ureter**
Q62.62   **Displacement of ureter**
Q62.63   **Anomalous implantation of ureter**
Ectopia of ureter
Ectopic ureter
Q62.69   **Other malposition of ureter**

Q62.7   **Congenital vesico-uretero-renal reflux**
Q62.8   **Other congenital malformations of ureter**
Anomaly of ureter NOS

☑4ᵗʰ **Q63**   **Other congenital malformations of kidney**
EXCLUDES 1 *congenital nephrotic syndrome (N04.-)*

Q63.0   **Accessory kidney**
Q63.1   **Lobulated, fused and horseshoe kidney**
Q63.2   **Ectopic kidney**
Congenital displaced kidney
Malrotation of kidney

Q63.3   **Hyperplastic and giant kidney**
Compensatory hypertrophy of kidney

Q63.8   **Other specified congenital malformations of kidney**
Congenital renal calculi

Q63.9   **Congenital malformation of kidney, unspecified**   ▽

☑4ᵗʰ **Q64**   **Other congenital malformations of urinary system**

Q64.0   **Epispadias**   ♂
EXCLUDES 1 *hypospadias (Q54.-)*

☑5ᵗʰ **Q64.1**   **Exstrophy of urinary bladder**

Q64.10   **Exstrophy of urinary bladder, unspecified**   ▽
Ectopia vesicae
Q64.11   **Supravesical fissure of urinary bladder**
Q64.12   **Cloacal extrophy of urinary bladder**
Q64.19   **Other exstrophy of urinary bladder**
Extroversion of bladder

Q64.2   **Congenital posterior urethral valves**

☑5ᵗʰ **Q64.3**   **Other atresia and stenosis of urethra and bladder neck**

Q64.31   **Congenital bladder neck obstruction**
Congenital obstruction of vesicourethral orifice
Q64.32   **Congenital stricture of urethra**
Q64.33   **Congenital stricture of urinary meatus**

☑ Additional Character Required   ✓x7ᵗʰ Placeholder Alert   Manifestation Dx   ▽ Unspecified Dx   ►◄ Revised Text   ● New Code   ▲ Revised Code Title

Q64.39 **Other atresia and stenosis of urethra and bladder neck**
Atresia and stenosis of urethra and bladder neck NOS

Q64.4 **Malformation of urachus**
Cyst of urachus
Patent urachus
Prolapse of urachus

Q64.5 **Congenital absence of bladder and urethra**

Q64.6 **Congenital diverticulum of bladder**

√5ᵗʰ **Q64.7** **Other and unspecified congenital malformations of bladder and urethra**
EXCLUDES 1   *congenital prolapse of bladder (mucosa) (Q79.4)*

Q64.70 **Unspecified congenital malformation of bladder and urethra** ▽
Malformation of bladder or urethra NOS

Q64.71 **Congenital prolapse of urethra**

Q64.72 **Congenital prolapse of urinary meatus**

Q64.73 **Congenital urethrorectal fistula**

Q64.74 **Double urethra**

Q64.75 **Double urinary meatus**

Q64.79 **Other congenital malformations of bladder and urethra**

Q64.8 **Other specified congenital malformations of urinary system**

Q64.9 **Congenital malformation of urinary system, unspecified** ▽
Congenital anomaly NOS of urinary system
Congenital deformity NOS of urinary system

Congenital malformations and deformations of the musculoskeletal system (Q65-Q79)

√4ᵗʰ **Q65** **Congenital deformities of hip**
EXCLUDES 1   *clicking hip (R29.4)*

√5ᵗʰ **Q65.0** **Congenital dislocation of hip, unilateral**

Q65.00 **Congenital dislocation of unspecified hip, unilateral** ▽

Q65.01 **Congenital dislocation of right hip, unilateral**

Q65.02 **Congenital dislocation of left hip, unilateral**

Q65.1 **Congenital dislocation of hip, bilateral**

Q65.2 **Congenital dislocation of hip, unspecified** ▽

√5ᵗʰ **Q65.3** **Congenital partial dislocation of hip, unilateral**

Q65.30 **Congenital partial dislocation of unspecified hip, unilateral** ▽

Q65.31 **Congenital partial dislocation of right hip, unilateral**

Q65.32 **Congenital partial dislocation of left hip, unilateral**

Q65.4 **Congenital partial dislocation of hip, bilateral**

Q65.5 **Congenital partial dislocation of hip, unspecified** ▽

Q65.6 **Congenital unstable hip**
Congenital dislocatable hip

√5ᵗʰ **Q65.8** **Other congenital deformities of hip**

Q65.81 **Congenital coxa valga**

Q65.82 **Congenital coxa vara**

Q65.89 **Other specified congenital deformities of hip**
Anteversion of femoral neck
Congenital acetabular dysplasia

Q65.9 **Congenital deformity of hip, unspecified** ▽

√4ᵗʰ **Q66** **Congenital deformities of feet**
EXCLUDES 1   *reduction defects of feet (Q72.-)*
valgus deformities (acquired) (M21.0-)
varus deformities (acquired) (M21.1-)

Q66.0 **Congenital talipes equinovarus**

Q66.1 **Congenital talipes calcaneovarus**

√5ᵗʰ **Q66.2** **Congenital metatarsus (primus) varus**

● **Q66.21** **Congenital metatarsus primus varus**

● **Q66.22** **Congenital metatarsus adductus**
Congenital metatarsus varus

Q66.3 **Other congenital varus deformities of feet**
Hallux varus, congenital

Q66.4 **Congenital talipes calcaneovalgus**

√5ᵗʰ **Q66.5** **Congenital pes planus**
Congenital flat foot
Congenital rigid flat foot
Congenital spastic (everted) flat foot
EXCLUDES 1   *pes planus, acquired (M21.4)*

Q66.50 **Congenital pes planus, unspecified foot** ▽

Q66.51 **Congenital pes planus, right foot**

Q66.52 **Congenital pes planus, left foot**

Q66.6 **Other congenital valgus deformities of feet**
Congenital metatarsus valgus

Q66.7 **Congenital pes cavus**

√5ᵗʰ **Q66.8** **Other congenital deformities of feet**

Q66.80 **Congenital vertical talus deformity, unspecified foot** ▽

Q66.81 **Congenital vertical talus deformity, right foot**

Q66.82 **Congenital vertical talus deformity, left foot**

Q66.89 **Other specified congenital deformities of feet**
Congenital asymmetric talipes
Congenital clubfoot NOS
Congenital talipes NOS
Congenital tarsal coalition
Hammer toe, congenital

Q66.9 **Congenital deformity of feet, unspecified** ▽

√4ᵗʰ **Q67** **Congenital musculoskeletal deformities of head, face, spine and chest**
EXCLUDES 1   *congenital malformation syndromes classified to Q87.-*
Potter's syndrome (Q60.6)

Q67.0 **Congenital facial asymmetry**

Q67.1 **Congenital compression facies**

Q67.2 **Dolichocephaly**

Q67.3 **Plagiocephaly**

Q67.4 **Other congenital deformities of skull, face and jaw**
Congenital depressions in skull
Congenital hemifacial atrophy or hypertrophy
Deviation of nasal septum, congenital
Squashed or bent nose, congenital
EXCLUDES 1   *dentofacial anomalies [including malocclusion] (M26.-)*
syphilitic saddle nose (A50.5)

Q67.5 **Congenital deformity of spine**
Congenital postural scoliosis
Congenital scoliosis NOS
EXCLUDES 1   *infantile idiopathic scoliosis (M41.0)*
scoliosis due to congenital bony malformation (Q76.3)
AHA: 2014,4Q,26

Q67.6 **Pectus excavatum**
Congenital funnel chest

Q67.7 **Pectus carinatum**
Congenital pigeon chest

Q67.8 **Other congenital deformities of chest**
Congenital deformity of chest wall NOS

√4ᵗʰ **Q68** **Other congenital musculoskeletal deformities**
EXCLUDES 1   *reduction defects of limb(s) (Q71-Q73)*
EXCLUDES 2   *congenital myotonic chondrodystrophy (G71.13)*

Q68.0 **Congenital deformity of sternocleidomastoid muscle**
Congenital contracture of sternocleidomastoid (muscle)
Congenital (sternomastoid) torticollis
Sternomastoid tumor (congenital)

Q68.1 **Congenital deformity of finger(s) and hand**
Congenital clubfinger
Spade-like hand (congenital)

Q68.2 **Congenital deformity of knee**
Congenital dislocation of knee
Congenital genu recurvatum

Q68.3 **Congenital bowing of femur**
EXCLUDES 1   *anteversion of femur (neck) (Q65.89)*

Q68.4 **Congenital bowing of tibia and fibula**

Q68.5 **Congenital bowing of long bones of leg, unspecified** ▽

Q68.6 **Discoid meniscus**

Q68.8 **Other specified congenital musculoskeletal deformities**
Congenital deformity of clavicle
Congenital deformity of elbow
Congenital deformity of forearm
Congenital deformity of scapula
Congenital deformity of wrist
Congenital dislocation of elbow
Congenital dislocation of shoulder
Congenital dislocation of wrist

√4ᵗʰ **Q69** **Polydactyly**

Q69.0 **Accessory finger(s)**

Q69.1 **Accessory thumb(s)**

EXCLUDES 1 Not coded here   EXCLUDES 2 Not included here   N Newborn Age : 0   P Pediatric Age : 0-17   M Maternity Age : 12-55   A Adult Age : 15-124

Q69.2   **Accessory** toe(s)
Accessory hallux

Q69.9   **Polydactyly, unspecified**   ▽
Supernumerary digit(s) NOS

✓4ᵗʰ **Q70**   **Syndactyly**

   ✓5ᵗʰ **Q70.0**   **Fused fingers**
     Complex syndactyly of fingers with synostosis

     Q70.00   **Fused fingers, unspecified hand**   ▽
     Q70.01   **Fused fingers,** right **hand**
     Q70.02   **Fused fingers,** left **hand**
     Q70.03   **Fused fingers,** bilateral

   ✓5ᵗʰ **Q70.1**   **Webbed fingers**
     Simple syndactyly of fingers without synostosis

     Q70.10   **Webbed fingers, unspecified hand**   ▽
     Q70.11   **Webbed fingers,** right **hand**
     Q70.12   **Webbed fingers,** left **hand**
     Q70.13   **Webbed fingers,** bilateral

   ✓5ᵗʰ **Q70.2**   **Fused toes**
     Complex syndactyly of toes with synostosis

     Q70.20   **Fused toes, unspecified foot**   ▽
     Q70.21   **Fused toes,** right **foot**
     Q70.22   **Fused toes,** left **foot**
     Q70.23   **Fused toes,** bilateral

   ✓5ᵗʰ **Q70.3**   **Webbed toes**
     Simple syndactyly of toes without synostosis

     Q70.30   **Webbed toes, unspecified foot**   ▽
     Q70.31   **Webbed toes,** right **foot**
     Q70.32   **Webbed toes,** left **foot**
     Q70.33   **Webbed toes,** bilateral

   Q70.4   **Polysyndactyly, unspecified**   ▽
     EXCLUDES 1   specified syndactyly of hand and feet - code to specified conditions (Q70.0-Q70.3-)

   Q70.9   **Syndactyly, unspecified**   ▽
     Symphalangy NOS

✓4ᵗʰ **Q71**   **Reduction defects of** upper limb

   ✓5ᵗʰ **Q71.0**   **Congenital** complete absence **of upper limb**

     Q71.00   **Congenital complete absence of unspecified upper limb**   ▽
     Q71.01   **Congenital complete absence of** right **upper limb**
     Q71.02   **Congenital complete absence of** left **upper limb**
     Q71.03   **Congenital complete absence of upper limb, bilateral**

   ✓5ᵗʰ **Q71.1**   **Congenital** absence of upper arm and forearm with hand present

     Q71.10   **Congenital absence of unspecified upper arm and forearm with hand present**   ▽
     Q71.11   **Congenital absence of** right **upper arm and forearm with hand present**
     Q71.12   **Congenital absence of** left **upper arm and forearm with hand present**
     Q71.13   **Congenital absence of upper arm and forearm with hand present,** bilateral

   ✓5ᵗʰ **Q71.2**   **Congenital** absence of both forearm and hand

     Q71.20   **Congenital absence of both forearm and hand, unspecified upper limb**   ▽
     Q71.21   **Congenital absence of both forearm and hand,** right **upper limb**
     Q71.22   **Congenital absence of both forearm and hand,** left **upper limb**
     Q71.23   **Congenital absence of both forearm and hand, bilateral**

   ✓5ᵗʰ **Q71.3**   **Congenital** absence of hand and finger

     Q71.30   **Congenital absence of unspecified hand and finger**
     Q71.31   **Congenital absence of** right **hand and finger**
     Q71.32   **Congenital absence of** left **hand and finger**
     Q71.33   **Congenital absence of hand and finger,** bilateral

   ✓5ᵗʰ **Q71.4**   **Longitudinal reduction defect of** radius
     Clubhand (congenital)
     Radial clubhand

     Q71.40   **Longitudinal reduction defect of unspecified radius**   ▽
     Q71.41   **Longitudinal reduction defect of** right **radius**
     Q71.42   **Longitudinal reduction defect of** left **radius**
     Q71.43   **Longitudinal reduction defect of radius, bilateral**

   ✓5ᵗʰ **Q71.5**   **Longitudinal reduction defect of** ulna

     Q71.50   **Longitudinal reduction defect of unspecified ulna**   ▽
     Q71.51   **Longitudinal reduction defect of** right **ulna**
     Q71.52   **Longitudinal reduction defect of** left **ulna**
     Q71.53   **Longitudinal reduction defect of ulna,** bilateral

   ✓5ᵗʰ **Q71.6**   **Lobster-claw hand**

     Q71.60   **Lobster-claw hand, unspecified hand**
     Q71.61   **Lobster-claw** right **hand**
     Q71.62   **Lobster-claw** left **hand**
     Q71.63   **Lobster-claw hand,** bilateral

   ✓5ᵗʰ **Q71.8**   **Other reduction defects of** upper limb

     ✓6ᵗʰ **Q71.81**   **Congenital** shortening **of upper limb**

       Q71.811   **Congenital shortening of** right **upper limb**
       Q71.812   **Congenital shortening of** left **upper limb**
       Q71.813   **Congenital shortening of upper limb, bilateral**
       Q71.819   **Congenital shortening of unspecified upper limb**   ▽

     ✓6ᵗʰ **Q71.89**   **Other reduction defects of upper limb**

       Q71.891   **Other reduction defects of** right **upper limb**
       Q71.892   **Other reduction defects of** left **upper limb**
       Q71.893   **Other reduction defects of upper limb, bilateral**
       Q71.899   **Other reduction defects of unspecified upper limb**   ▽

   ✓5ᵗʰ **Q71.9**   **Unspecified reduction defect of upper limb**

     Q71.90   **Unspecified reduction defect of unspecified upper limb**   ▽
     Q71.91   **Unspecified reduction defect of** right **upper limb**   ▽
     Q71.92   **Unspecified reduction defect of** left **upper limb**   ▽
     Q71.93   **Unspecified reduction defect of upper limb, bilateral**   ▽

✓4ᵗʰ **Q72**   **Reduction defects of** lower limb

   ✓5ᵗʰ **Q72.0**   **Congenital** complete absence **of lower limb**

     Q72.00   **Congenital complete absence of unspecified lower limb**   ▽
     Q72.01   **Congenital complete absence of** right **lower limb**
     Q72.02   **Congenital complete absence of** left **lower limb**
     Q72.03   **Congenital complete absence of lower limb, bilateral**

   ✓5ᵗʰ **Q72.1**   **Congenital** absence of thigh and lower leg with foot present

     Q72.10   **Congenital absence of unspecified thigh and lower leg with foot present**   ▽
     Q72.11   **Congenital absence of** right **thigh and lower leg with foot present**
     Q72.12   **Congenital absence of** left **thigh and lower leg with foot present**
     Q72.13   **Congenital absence of thigh and lower leg with foot present,** bilateral

   ✓5ᵗʰ **Q72.2**   **Congenital** absence of both lower leg and foot

     Q72.20   **Congenital absence of both lower leg and foot, unspecified lower limb**   ▽
     Q72.21   **Congenital absence of both lower leg and foot,** right **lower limb**
     Q72.22   **Congenital absence of both lower leg and foot,** left **lower limb**
     Q72.23   **Congenital absence of both lower leg and foot, bilateral**

   ✓5ᵗʰ **Q72.3**   **Congenital** absence of foot and toe(s)

     Q72.30   **Congenital absence of unspecified foot and toe(s)**   ▽
     Q72.31   **Congenital absence of** right **foot and toe(s)**
     Q72.32   **Congenital absence of** left **foot and toe(s)**
     Q72.33   **Congenital absence of foot and toe(s),** bilateral

   ✓5ᵗʰ **Q72.4**   **Longitudinal reduction defect of** femur
     Proximal femoral focal deficiency

     Q72.40   **Longitudinal reduction defect of unspecified femur**   ▽
     Q72.41   **Longitudinal reduction defect of** right **femur**
     Q72.42   **Longitudinal reduction defect of** left **femur**
     Q72.43   **Longitudinal reduction defect of femur,** bilateral

☑ Additional Character Required   ✓x7ᵗʰ Placeholder Alert   Manifestation Dx   ▽ Unspecified Dx   ►◄ Revised Text   ● New Code   ▲ Revised Code Title

ICD-10-CM 2017   **857**

Chapter 17. Congenital Malformations, Deformations and Chromosomal Abnormalities

Q69.2–Q72.43

✓5ᵗʰ **Q72.5 Longitudinal reduction defect of tibia**

Q72.50 Longitudinal reduction defect of unspecified tibia ▽

Q72.51 Longitudinal reduction defect of right tibia

Q72.52 Longitudinal reduction defect of left tibia

Q72.53 Longitudinal reduction defect of tibia, bilateral

✓5ᵗʰ **Q72.6 Longitudinal reduction defect of fibula**

Q72.60 Longitudinal reduction defect of unspecified fibula ▽

Q72.61 Longitudinal reduction defect of right fibula

Q72.62 Longitudinal reduction defect of left fibula

Q72.63 Longitudinal reduction defect of fibula, bilateral

✓5ᵗʰ **Q72.7 Split foot**

Q72.70 Split foot, unspecified lower limb ▽

Q72.71 Split foot, right lower limb

Q72.72 Split foot, left lower limb

Q72.73 Split foot, bilateral

✓5ᵗʰ **Q72.8 Other reduction defects of lower limb**

✓6ᵗʰ **Q72.81 Congenital shortening of lower limb**

Q72.811 Congenital shortening of right lower limb

Q72.812 Congenital shortening of left lower limb

Q72.813 Congenital shortening of lower limb, bilateral

Q72.819 Congenital shortening of unspecified lower limb ▽

✓6ᵗʰ **Q72.89 Other reduction defects of lower limb**

Q72.891 Other reduction defects of right lower limb

Q72.892 Other reduction defects of left lower limb

Q72.893 Other reduction defects of lower limb, bilateral

Q72.899 Other reduction defects of unspecified lower limb ▽

✓5ᵗʰ **Q72.9 Unspecified reduction defect of lower limb**

Q72.90 Unspecified reduction defect of unspecified lower limb ▽

Q72.91 Unspecified reduction defect of right lower limb ▽

Q72.92 Unspecified reduction defect of left lower limb ▽

Q72.93 Unspecified reduction defect of lower limb, bilateral ▽

✓4ᵗʰ **Q73 Reduction defects of unspecified limb**

Q73.0 Congenital absence of unspecified limb(s) ▽
Amelia NOS

Q73.1 Phocomelia, unspecified limb(s) ▽
Phocomelia NOS

Q73.8 Other reduction defects of unspecified limb(s) ▽
Longitudinal reduction deformity of unspecified limb(s)
Ectromelia of limb NOS
Hemimelia of limb NOS
Reduction defect of limb NOS

✓4ᵗʰ **Q74 Other congenital malformations of limb(s)**

EXCLUDES 1   *polydactyly (Q69.-)*
reduction defect of limb (Q71-Q73)
syndactyly (Q70.-)

Q74.0 Other congenital malformations of upper limb(s), including shoulder girdle
Accessory carpal bones
Cleidocranial dysostosis
Congenital pseudarthrosis of clavicle
Macrodactylia (fingers)
Madelung's deformity
Radioulnar synostosis
Sprengel's deformity
Triphalangeal thumb

Q74.1 Congenital malformation of knee
Congenital absence of patella
Congenital dislocation of patella
Congenital genu valgum
Congenital genu varum
Rudimentary patella

EXCLUDES 1   *congenital dislocation of knee (Q68.2)*
congenital genu recurvatum (Q68.2)
nail patella syndrome (Q87.2)

Q74.2 Other congenital malformations of lower limb(s), including pelvic girdle
Congenital fusion of sacroiliac joint
Congenital malformation of ankle joint
Congenital malformation of sacroiliac joint

EXCLUDES 1   *anteversion of femur (neck) (Q65.89)*

Q74.3 Arthrogryposis multiplex congenita

Q74.8 Other specified congenital malformations of limb(s)

Q74.9 Unspecified congenital malformation of limb(s) ▽
Congenital anomaly of limb(s) NOS

✓4ᵗʰ **Q75 Other congenital malformations of skull and face bones**

EXCLUDES 1   *congenital malformation of face NOS (Q18.-)*
congenital malformation syndromes classified to Q87.-
dentofacial anomalies [including malocclusion] (M26.-)
musculoskeletal deformities of head and face (Q67.0-Q67.4)
skull defects associated with congenital anomalies of brain such as:
anencephaly (Q00.0)
encephalocele (Q01.-)
hydrocephalus (Q03.-)
microcephaly (Q02)

Q75.0 Craniosynostosis
Acrocephaly
Imperfect fusion of skull
Oxycephaly
Trigonocephaly

Q75.1 Craniofacial dysostosis
Crouzon's disease

Q75.2 Hypertelorism

Q75.3 Macrocephaly

Q75.4 Mandibulofacial dysostosis
Franceschetti syndrome
Treacher Collins syndrome

Q75.5 Oculomandibular dysostosis

Q75.8 Other specified congenital malformations of skull and face bones
Absence of skull bone, congenital
Congenital deformity of forehead
Platybasia

Q75.9 Congenital malformation of skull and face bones, unspecified ▽
Congenital anomaly of face bones NOS
Congenital anomaly of skull NOS

✓4ᵗʰ **Q76 Congenital malformations of spine and bony thorax**

EXCLUDES 1   *congenital musculoskeletal deformities of spine and chest (Q67.5-Q67.8)*

Q76.0 Spina bifida occulta

EXCLUDES 1   *meningocele (spinal) (Q05.-)*
spina bifida (aperta) (cystica) (Q05.-)

Q76.1 Klippel-Feil syndrome
Cervical fusion syndrome

Q76.2 Congenital spondylolisthesis
Congenital spondylolysis

EXCLUDES 1   *spondylolisthesis (acquired) (M43.1-)*
spondylolysis (acquired) (M43.0-)

Q76.3 Congenital scoliosis due to congenital bony malformation
Hemivertebra fusion or failure of segmentation with scoliosis

✓5ᵗʰ **Q76.4 Other congenital malformations of spine, not associated with scoliosis**

✓6ᵗʰ **Q76.41 Congenital kyphosis**

Q76.411 Congenital kyphosis, occipito-atlanto-axial region

Q76.412 Congenital kyphosis, cervical region

Q76.413 Congenital kyphosis, cervicothoracic region

Q76.414 Congenital kyphosis, thoracic region

Q76.415 Congenital kyphosis, thoracolumbar region

Q76.419 Congenital kyphosis, unspecified region ▽

✓6ᵗʰ **Q76.42 Congenital lordosis**

Q76.425 Congenital lordosis, thoracolumbar region

Q76.426 Congenital lordosis, lumbar region

Q76.427 Congenital lordosis, lumbosacral region

Q76.428 Congenital lordosis, sacral and sacrococcygeal region

EXCLUDES 1 Not coded here   EXCLUDES 2 Not included here   N Newborn Age : 0   P Pediatric Age : 0-17   M Maternity Age : 12-55   A Adult Age : 15-124

858   ICD-10-CM 2017

Q76.429 **Congenital lordosis, unspecified region** ▽

Q76.49 **Other congenital malformations of spine, not associated with scoliosis**
Congenital absence of vertebra NOS
Congenital fusion of spine NOS
Congenital malformation of lumbosacral (joint) (region) NOS
Congenital malformation of spine NOS
Hemivertebra NOS
Malformation of spine NOS
Platyspondylisis NOS
Supernumerary vertebra NOS

Q76.5 **Cervical rib**
Supernumerary rib in cervical region

Q76.6 **Other congenital malformations of ribs**
Accessory rib
Congenital absence of rib
Congenital fusion of ribs
Congenital malformation of ribs NOS
EXCLUDES 1 short rib syndrome (Q77.2)

Q76.7 **Congenital malformation of sternum**
Congenital absence of sternum
Sternum bifidum

Q76.8 **Other congenital malformations of bony thorax**

Q76.9 **Congenital malformation of bony thorax, unspecified** ▽

☑4ᵗʰ **Q77 Osteochondrodysplasia with defects of growth of tubular bones and spine**
EXCLUDES 1 mucopolysaccharidosis (E76.0-E76.3)
EXCLUDES 2 congenital myotonic chondrodystrophy (G71.13)

Q77.0 **Achondrogenesis**
Hypochondrogenesis

Q77.1 **Thanatophoric short stature**

Q77.2 **Short rib syndrome**
Asphyxiating thoracic dysplasia [Jeune]

Q77.3 **Chondrodysplasia punctata**
EXCLUDES 1 Rhizomelic chondrodysplasia punctata (E71.43)

Q77.4 **Achondroplasia**
Hypochondroplasia
Osteosclerosis congenita

Q77.5 **Diastrophic dysplasia**

Q77.6 **Chondroectodermal dysplasia**
Ellis-van Creveld syndrome

Q77.7 **Spondyloepiphyseal dysplasia**

Q77.8 **Other osteochondrodysplasia with defects of growth of tubular bones and spine**

Q77.9 **Osteochondrodysplasia with defects of growth of tubular bones and spine, unspecified** ▽

☑4ᵗʰ **Q78 Other osteochondrodysplasias**
EXCLUDES 2 congenital myotonic chondrodystrophy (G71.13)

Q78.0 **Osteogenesis imperfecta**
Fragilitas ossium
Osteopsathyrosis

Q78.1 **Polyostotic fibrous dysplasia**
Albright(-McCune)(-Sternberg) syndrome

Q78.2 **Osteopetrosis**
Albers-Schönberg syndrome
Osteosclerosis NOS

Q78.3 **Progressive diaphyseal dysplasia**
Camurati-Engelmann syndrome

Q78.4 **Enchondromatosis**
Maffucci's syndrome
Ollier's disease

Q78.5 **Metaphyseal dysplasia**
Pyle's syndrome

Q78.6 **Multiple congenital exostoses**
Diaphyseal aclasis

Q78.8 **Other specified osteochondrodysplasias**
Osteopoikilosis

Q78.9 **Osteochondrodysplasia, unspecified** ▽
Chondrodystrophy NOS
Osteodystrophy NOS

☑4ᵗʰ **Q79 Congenital malformations of musculoskeletal system, not elsewhere classified**
EXCLUDES 2 congenital (sternomastoid) torticollis (Q68.0)

Q79.0 **Congenital diaphragmatic hernia**
EXCLUDES 1 congenital hiatus hernia (Q40.1)

Q79.1 **Other congenital malformations of diaphragm**
Absence of diaphragm
Congenital malformation of diaphragm NOS
Eventration of diaphragm

Q79.2 **Exomphalos**
Omphalocele
EXCLUDES 1 umbilical hernia (K42.-)

Q79.3 **Gastroschisis**

Q79.4 **Prune belly syndrome**
Congenital prolapse of bladder mucosa
Eagle-Barrett syndrome

☑5ᵗʰ Q79.5 **Other congenital malformations of abdominal wall**
EXCLUDES 1 umbilical hernia (K42.-)

Q79.51 **Congenital hernia of bladder**

Q79.59 **Other congenital malformations of abdominal wall**

Q79.6 **Ehlers-Danlos syndrome**
DEF: Connective tissue disorder that causes hyperextended skin and joints; results in fragile blood vessels with bleeding, poor wound healing, and subcutaneous pseudotumors.

Q79.8 **Other congenital malformations of musculoskeletal system**
Absence of muscle
Absence of tendon
Accessory muscle
Amyotrophia congenita
Congenital constricting bands
Congenital shortening of tendon
Poland syndrome

Q79.9 **Congenital malformation of musculoskeletal system, unspecified** ▽
Congenital anomaly of musculoskeletal system NOS
Congenital deformity of musculoskeletal system NOS

Other congenital malformations (Q80-Q89)

☑4ᵗʰ **Q80 Congenital ichthyosis**
EXCLUDES 1 Refsum's disease (G60.1)

Q80.0 **Ichthyosis vulgaris**

Q80.1 **X-linked ichthyosis**

Q80.2 **Lamellar ichthyosis**
Collodion baby

Q80.3 **Congenital bullous ichthyosiform erythroderma**

Q80.4 **Harlequin fetus**

Q80.8 **Other congenital ichthyosis**

Q80.9 **Congenital ichthyosis, unspecified** ▽

☑4ᵗʰ **Q81 Epidermolysis bullosa**

Q81.0 **Epidermolysis bullosa simplex**
EXCLUDES 1 Cockayne's syndrome (Q87.1)

Q81.1 **Epidermolysis bullosa letalis**
Herlitz' syndrome

Q81.2 **Epidermolysis bullosa dystrophica**

Q81.8 **Other epidermolysis bullosa**

Q81.9 **Epidermolysis bullosa, unspecified** ▽

☑4ᵗʰ **Q82 Other congenital malformations of skin**
EXCLUDES 1 acrodermatitis enteropathica (E83.2)
congenital erythropoietic porphyria (E80.0)
pilonidal cyst or sinus (L05.-)
Sturge-Weber (-Dimitri) syndrome (Q85.8)

Q82.0 **Hereditary lymphedema**

Q82.1 **Xeroderma pigmentosum**

Q82.2 **Mastocytosis**
Urticaria pigmentosa
EXCLUDES 1 malignant mastocytosis (C96.2)

Q82.3 **Incontinentia pigmenti**

Q82.4 **Ectodermal dysplasia (anhidrotic)**
EXCLUDES 1 Ellis-van Creveld syndrome (Q77.6)

Chapter 17. Congenital Malformations, Deformations and Chromosomal Abnormalities

Q82.5 Congenital non-neoplastic nevus
Birthmark NOS
Flammeus Nevus
Portwine Nevus
Sanguineous Nevus
Strawberry Nevus
Vascular Nevus NOS
Verrucous Nevus
EXCLUDES 2 *araneus nevus (I78.1)*
Café au lait spots (L81.3)
lentigo (L81.4)
melanocytic nevus (D22.-)
nevus NOS (D22.-)
pigmented nevus (D22.-)
spider nevus (I78.1)
stellar nevus (I78.1)

● **Q82.6 Congenital sacral dimple**
Parasacral dimple
EXCLUDES 2 *pilonidal cyst with abscess (L05.01)*
pilonidal cyst without abscess (L05.91)

Q82.8 Other specified congenital malformations of skin
Abnormal palmar creases
Accessory skin tags
Benign familial pemphigus [Hailey-Hailey]
Congenital poikiloderma
Cutis laxa (hyperelastica)
Dermatoglyphic anomalies
Inherited keratosis palmaris et plantaris
Keratosis follicularis [Darier-White]
EXCLUDES 1 *Ehlers-Danlos syndrome (Q79.6)*
AHA: 2016,1Q,17

Q82.9 Congenital malformation of skin, unspecified ▽

✓4ᵗʰ **Q83 Congenital malformations of breast**
EXCLUDES 2 *absence of pectoral muscle (Q79.8)*
hypoplasia of breast (N64.82)
micromastia (N64.82)

Q83.0 Congenital absence of breast with absent nipple
Q83.1 Accessory breast
Supernumerary breast
Q83.2 Absent nipple
Q83.3 Accessory nipple
Supernumerary nipple
Q83.8 Other congenital malformations of breast
Q83.9 Congenital malformation of breast, unspecified ▽

✓4ᵗʰ **Q84 Other congenital malformations of integument**
Q84.0 Congenital alopecia
Congenital atrichosis
Q84.1 Congenital morphological disturbances of hair, not elsewhere classified
Beaded hair
Monilethrix
Pili annulati
EXCLUDES 1 *Menkes' kinky hair syndrome (E83.0)*
Q84.2 Other congenital malformations of hair
Congenital hypertrichosis
Congenital malformation of hair NOS
Persistent lanugo
Q84.3 Anonychia
EXCLUDES 1 *nail patella syndrome (Q87.2)*
Q84.4 Congenital leukonychia
Q84.5 Enlarged and hypertrophic nails
Congenital onychauxis
Pachyonychia
Q84.6 Other congenital malformations of nails
Congenital clubnail
Congenital koilonychia
Congenital malformation of nail NOS
Q84.8 Other specified congenital malformations of integument
Aplasia cutis congenita
Q84.9 Congenital malformation of integument, unspecified ▽
Congenital anomaly of integument NOS
Congenital deformity of integument NOS

✓4ᵗʰ **Q85 Phakomatoses, not elsewhere classified**
EXCLUDES 1 *ataxia telangiectasia [Louis-Bar] (G11.3)*
familial dysautonomia [Riley-Day] (G90.1)

✓5ᵗʰ **Q85.0 Neurofibromatosis (nonmalignant)**
Q85.00 Neurofibromatosis, unspecified ▽
Q85.01 Neurofibromatosis, type 1
Von Recklinghausen disease
Q85.02 Neurofibromatosis, type 2
Acoustic neurofibromatosis
DEF: Inherited condition with cutaneous lesions, benign tumors of peripheral nerves, and bilateral 8th nerve masses.
Q85.03 Schwannomatosis
DEF: A genetic mutation (SMARCB1/INI1) causing multiple benign tumors along nerve pathways; characterized by the exception of 8th cranial nerve involvement.
Q85.09 Other neurofibromatosis
Q85.1 Tuberous sclerosis
Bourneville's disease
Epiloia
Q85.8 Other phakomatoses, not elsewhere classified
Peutz-Jeghers Syndrome
Sturge-Weber(-Dimitri) syndrome
von Hippel-Lindau syndrome
EXCLUDES 1 *Meckel-Gruber syndrome (Q61.9)*
Q85.9 Phakomatosis, unspecified ▽
Hamartosis NOS

✓4ᵗʰ **Q86 Congenital malformation syndromes due to known exogenous causes, not elsewhere classified**
EXCLUDES 2 *iodine-deficiency-related hypothyroidism (E00-E02)*
nonteratogenic effects of substances transmitted via placenta or breast milk (P04.-)

Q86.0 Fetal alcohol syndrome (dysmorphic)
Q86.1 Fetal hydantoin syndrome
Meadow's syndrome
Q86.2 Dysmorphism due to warfarin
Q86.8 Other congenital malformation syndromes due to known exogenous causes

✓4ᵗʰ **Q87 Other specified congenital malformation syndromes affecting multiple systems**
Use additional code(s) to identify all associated manifestations
Q87.0 Congenital malformation syndromes predominantly affecting facial appearance
Acrocephalopolysyndactyly
Acrocephalosyndactyly [Apert]
Cryptophthalmos syndrome
Cyclopia
Goldenhar syndrome
Moebius syndrome
Oro-facial-digital syndrome
Robin syndrome
Whistling face
Q87.1 Congenital malformation syndromes predominantly associated with short stature
Aarskog syndrome
Cockayne syndrome
De Lange syndrome
Dubowitz syndrome
Noonan syndrome
Prader-Willi syndrome
Robinow-Silverman-Smith syndrome
Russell-Silver syndrome
Seckel syndrome
EXCLUDES 1 *Ellis-van Creveld syndrome (Q77.6)*
Smith-Lemli-Opitz syndrome (E78.72)
Q87.2 Congenital malformation syndromes predominantly involving limbs
Holt-Oram syndrome
Klippel-Trenaunay-Weber syndrome
Nail patella syndrome
Rubinstein-Taybi syndrome
Sirenomelia syndrome
Thrombocytopenia with absent radius [TAR] syndrome
VATER syndrome

EXCLUDES 1 Not coded here   EXCLUDES 2 Not included here   N Newborn Age : 0   P Pediatric Age : 0-17   M Maternity Age : 12-55   A Adult Age : 15-124

Q87.3 **Congenital malformation syndromes involving early overgrowth**
Beckwith-Wiedemann syndrome
Sotos syndrome
Weaver syndrome

✓5ᵗʰ Q87.4 **Marfan's syndrome**

Q87.40 **Marfan's syndrome, unspecified** ▽

✓6ᵗʰ Q87.41 **Marfan's syndrome with cardiovascular manifestations**

Q87.410 **Marfan's syndrome with aortic dilation**

Q87.418 **Marfan's syndrome with other cardiovascular manifestations**

Q87.42 **Marfan's syndrome with ocular manifestations**

Q87.43 **Marfan's syndrome with skeletal manifestation**

Q87.5 **Other congenital malformation syndromes with other skeletal changes**

✓5ᵗʰ Q87.8 **Other specified congenital malformation syndromes, not elsewhere classified**
EXCLUDES 1 *Zellweger syndrome (E71.510)*

Q87.81 **Alport syndrome**
Use additional code to identify stage of chronic kidney disease (N18.1-N18.6)

Q87.82 **Arterial tortuosity syndrome**

Q87.89 **Other specified congenital malformation syndromes, not elsewhere classified**
Laurence-Moon (-Bardet)-Biedl syndrome

✓4ᵗʰ Q89 **Other congenital malformations, not elsewhere classified**

✓5ᵗʰ Q89.0 **Congenital absence and malformations of spleen**
EXCLUDES 1 *isomerism of atrial appendages (with asplenia or polysplenia) (Q20.6)*

Q89.01 **Asplenia (congenital)**

Q89.09 **Congenital malformations of spleen**
Congenital splenomegaly

Q89.1 **Congenital malformations of adrenal gland**
EXCLUDES 1 *adrenogenital disorders (E25.-)*
congenital adrenal hyperplasia (E25.0)

Q89.2 **Congenital malformations of other endocrine glands**
Congenital malformation of parathyroid or thyroid gland
Persistent thyroglossal duct
Thyroglossal cyst
EXCLUDES 1 *congenital goiter (E03.0)*
congenital hypothyroidism (E03.1)

Q89.3 **Situs inversus**
Dextrocardia with situs inversus
Mirror-image atrial arrangement with situs inversus
Situs inversus or transversus abdominalis
Situs inversus or transversus thoracis
Transposition of abdominal viscera
Transposition of thoracic viscera
EXCLUDES 1 *dextrocardia NOS (Q24.0)*

Q89.4 **Conjoined twins**
Craniopagus
Dicephaly
Pygopagus
Thoracopagus

Q89.7 **Multiple congenital malformations, not elsewhere classified**
Multiple congenital anomalies NOS
Multiple congenital deformities NOS
EXCLUDES 1 *congenital malformation syndromes affecting multiple systems (Q87.-)*

Q89.8 **Other specified congenital malformations**
Use additional code(s) to identify all associated manifestations

Q89.9 **Congenital malformation, unspecified** ▽
Congenital anomaly NOS
Congenital deformity NOS

Chromosomal abnormalities, not elsewhere classified (Q90-Q99)

EXCLUDES 2 *mitochondrial metabolic disorders (E88.4-)*

✓4ᵗʰ Q90 **Down syndrome**
Use additional code(s) to identify any associated physical conditions and degree of intellectual disabilities (F70-F79)

Q90.0 **Trisomy 21, nonmosaicism (meiotic nondisjunction)**

Q90.1 **Trisomy 21, mosaicism (mitotic nondisjunction)**

Q90.2 **Trisomy 21, translocation**

Q90.9 **Down syndrome, unspecified** ▽
Trisomy 21 NOS

✓4ᵗʰ Q91 **Trisomy 18 and Trisomy 13**

Q91.0 **Trisomy 18, nonmosaicism (meiotic nondisjunction)**

Q91.1 **Trisomy 18, mosaicism (mitotic nondisjunction)**

Q91.2 **Trisomy 18, translocation**

Q91.3 **Trisomy 18, unspecified** ▽

Q91.4 **Trisomy 13, nonmosaicism (meiotic nondisjunction)**

Q91.5 **Trisomy 13, mosaicism (mitotic nondisjunction)**

Q91.6 **Trisomy 13, translocation**

Q91.7 **Trisomy 13, unspecified** ▽

✓4ᵗʰ Q92 **Other trisomies and partial trisomies of the autosomes, not elsewhere classified**
INCLUDES unbalanced translocations and insertions
EXCLUDES 1 *trisomies of chromosomes 13, 18, 21 (Q90-Q91)*

Q92.0 **Whole chromosome trisomy, nonmosaicism (meiotic nondisjunction)**

Q92.1 **Whole chromosome trisomy, mosaicism (mitotic nondisjunction)**

Q92.2 **Partial trisomy**
Less than whole arm duplicated
Whole arm or more duplicated
EXCLUDES 1 *partial trisomy due to unbalanced translocation (Q92.5)*

Q92.5 **Duplications with other complex rearrangements**
Partial trisomy due to unbalanced translocations
Code also any associated deletions due to unbalanced translocations, inversions and insertions (Q93.7)

✓5ᵗʰ Q92.6 **Marker chromosomes**
Trisomies due to dicentrics
Trisomies due to extra rings
Trisomies due to isochromosomes
Individual with marker heterochromatin

Q92.61 **Marker chromosomes in normal individual**

Q92.62 **Marker chromosomes in abnormal individual**

Q92.7 **Triploidy and polyploidy**

Q92.8 **Other specified trisomies and partial trisomies of autosomes**
Duplications identified by fluorescence in situ hybridization (FISH)
Duplications identified by in situ hybridization (ISH)
Duplications seen only at prometaphase

Q92.9 **Trisomy and partial trisomy of autosomes, unspecified** ▽

✓4ᵗʰ Q93 **Monosomies and deletions from the autosomes, not elsewhere classified**

Q93.0 **Whole chromosome monosomy, nonmosaicism (meiotic nondisjunction)**

Q93.1 **Whole chromosome monosomy, mosaicism (mitotic nondisjunction)**

Q93.2 **Chromosome replaced with ring, dicentric or isochromosome**

Q93.3 **Deletion of short arm of chromosome 4**
Wolff-Hirschorn syndrome

Q93.4 **Deletion of short arm of chromosome 5**
Cri-du-chat syndrome

Q93.5 **Other deletions of part of a chromosome**
Angelman syndrome

Q93.7 **Deletions with other complex rearrangements**
Deletions due to unbalanced translocations, inversions and insertions
Code also any associated duplications due to unbalanced translocations, inversions and insertions (Q92.5)

✓5ᵗʰ Q93.8 **Other deletions from the autosomes**

Q93.81 **Velo-cardio-facial syndrome**
Deletion 22q11.2
DEF: Microdeletion syndrome affecting multiple organs; characteristic cleft palate, heart defects, elongated face with almond-shaped eyes, wide nose, small ears, weak musculature, weak immune system, hypothyroidism, short stature, and scoliosis; deletion at q11.2 on the long arm of the chromosome 22.

Q93.88 **Other microdeletions**
Miller-Dieker syndrome
Smith-Magenis syndrome

☑ Additional Character Required   ✓x7ᵗʰ Placeholder Alert   Manifestation Dx   ▽ Unspecified Dx   ►◄ Revised Text   ● New Code   ▲ Revised Code Title

Q93.89   **Other deletions from the autosomes**
Deletions identified by fluorescence in situ hybridization (FISH)
Deletions identified by in situ hybridization (ISH)
Deletions seen only at prometaphase

Q93.9   **Deletion from autosomes, unspecified**   ▽

√4ᵗʰ   **Q95**   **Balanced rearrangements and structural markers, not elsewhere classified**
[INCLUDES]   Robertsonian and balanced reciprocal translocations and insertions

Q95.0   **Balanced translocation and insertion in normal individual**

Q95.1   **Chromosome inversion in normal individual**

Q95.2   **Balanced autosomal rearrangement in abnormal individual**

Q95.3   **Balanced sex/autosomal rearrangement in abnormal individual**

Q95.5   **Individual with autosomal fragile site**

Q95.8   **Other balanced rearrangements and structural markers**

Q95.9   **Balanced rearrangement and structural marker, unspecified**   ▽

√4ᵗʰ   **Q96**   **Turner's syndrome**
[EXCLUDES 1]   Noonan syndrome (Q87.1)

Q96.0   **Karyotype 45, X**   ♀

Q96.1   **Karyotype 46, X iso (Xq)**   ♀
Karyotype 46, isochromosome Xq

Q96.2   **Karyotype 46, X with abnormal sex chromosome, except iso (Xq)**   ♀
Karyotype 46, X with abnormal sex chromosome, except isochromosome Xq

Q96.3   **Mosaicism, 45, X/46, XX or XY**   ♀

Q96.4   **Mosaicism, 45, X/other cell line(s) with abnormal sex chromosome**   ♀

Q96.8   **Other variants of Turner's syndrome**   ♀

Q96.9   **Turner's syndrome, unspecified**   ♀ ▽

√4ᵗʰ   **Q97**   **Other sex chromosome abnormalities, female phenotype, not elsewhere classified**
[EXCLUDES 1]   Turner's syndrome (Q96.-)

Q97.0   **Karyotype 47, XXX**   ♀

Q97.1   **Female with more than three X chromosomes**   ♀

Q97.2   **Mosaicism, lines with various numbers of X chromosomes**   ♀

Q97.3   **Female with 46, XY karyotype**   ♀

Q97.8   **Other specified sex chromosome abnormalities, female phenotype**   ♀

Q97.9   **Sex chromosome abnormality, female phenotype, unspecified**   ♀ ▽

√4ᵗʰ   **Q98**   **Other sex chromosome abnormalities, male phenotype, not elsewhere classified**

Q98.0   **Klinefelter syndrome karyotype 47, XXY**   ♂

Q98.1   **Klinefelter syndrome, male with more than two X chromosomes**   ♂

Q98.3   **Other male with 46, XX karyotype**   ♂

Q98.4   **Klinefelter syndrome, unspecified**   ♂ ▽

Q98.5   **Karyotype 47, XYY**

Q98.6   **Male with structurally abnormal sex chromosome**   ♂

Q98.7   **Male with sex chromosome mosaicism**   ♂

Q98.8   **Other specified sex chromosome abnormalities, male phenotype**   ♂

Q98.9   **Sex chromosome abnormality, male phenotype, unspecified**   ♂ ▽

√4ᵗʰ   **Q99**   **Other chromosome abnormalities, not elsewhere classified**

Q99.0   **Chimera 46, XX/46, XY**
Chimera 46, XX/46, XY true hermaphrodite

Q99.1   **46, XX true hermaphrodite**
46, XX with streak gonads
46, XY with streak gonads
Pure gonadal dysgenesis

Q99.2   **Fragile X chromosome**
Fragile X syndrome

Q99.8   **Other specified chromosome abnormalities**

Q99.9   **Chromosomal abnormality, unspecified**   ▽

[EXCLUDES 1] Not coded here   [EXCLUDES 2] Not included here   N Newborn Age : 0   P Pediatric Age : 0-17   M Maternity Age : 12-55   A Adult Age : 15-124

Chapter 18. Symptoms, Signs and Abnormal Clinical and Laboratory Findings, Not Elsewhere Classified (R00–R99)

Chapter Specific Guidelines with Coding Examples

The chapter specific guidelines from the ICD-10-CM Official Guidelines for Coding and Reporting have been provided below. Along with these guidelines are coding examples, contained in the shaded boxes, that have been developed to help illustrate the coding and/or sequencing guidance found in these guidelines.

Chapter 18 includes symptoms, signs, abnormal results of clinical or other investigative procedures, and ill-defined conditions regarding which no diagnosis classifiable elsewhere is recorded. Signs and symptoms that point to a specific diagnosis have been assigned to a category in other chapters of the classification.

a. Use of symptom codes

Codes that describe symptoms and signs are acceptable for reporting purposes when a related definitive diagnosis has not been established (confirmed) by the provider.

Chest pain of unknown origin

R07.9   Chest pain, unspecified

Explanation: Codes that describe symptoms such as chest pain are acceptable for reporting purposes when the provider has not established (confirmed) a related definitive diagnosis.

---

b. Use of a symptom code with a definitive diagnosis code

Codes for signs and symptoms may be reported in addition to a related definitive diagnosis when the sign or symptom is not routinely associated with that diagnosis, such as the various signs and symptoms associated with complex syndromes. The definitive diagnosis code should be sequenced before the symptom code.

Signs or symptoms that are associated routinely with a disease process should not be assigned as additional codes, unless otherwise instructed by the classification.

Pneumonia with hemoptysis

J18.9   Pneumonia, unspecified organism

R04.2   Hemoptysis

Explanation: Codes for signs and symptoms may be reported in addition to a related definitive diagnosis when the sign or symptom is not routinely associated with that diagnosis.

Abdominal pain due to acute appendicitis

K35.80   Unspecified acute appendicitis

Explanation: Codes for signs or symptoms routinely associated with a disease process should not be assigned unless the classification instructs otherwise.

---

c. Combination codes that include symptoms

ICD-10-CM contains a number of combination codes that identify both the definitive diagnosis and common symptoms of that diagnosis. When using one of these combination codes, an additional code should not be assigned for the symptom.

Acute gastritis with hemorrhage

K29.01   Acute gastritis with bleeding

Explanation: When a combination code identifies both the definitive diagnosis and the symptom, an additional code should not be assigned for the symptom.

---

d. Repeated falls

Code R29.6, Repeated falls, is for use for encounters when a patient has recently fallen and the reason for the fall is being investigated.

Code Z91.81, History of falling, is for use when a patient has fallen in the past and is at risk for future falls. When appropriate, both codes R29.6 and Z91.81 may be assigned together.

e. Coma scale

The coma scale codes (R40.2-) can be used in conjunction with traumatic brain injury codes, acute cerebrovascular disease or sequelae of cerebrovascular disease codes. These codes are primarily for use by trauma registries, but they may be used in any setting where this information is collected. **The coma scale may also be used to assess the status of the central nervous system for other non-trauma conditions, such as monitoring patients in the intensive care unit regardless of medical condition.** The coma scale codes should be sequenced after the diagnosis code(s).

These codes, one from each subcategory, are needed to complete the scale. The 7th character indicates when the scale was recorded. The 7th character should match for all three codes.

At a minimum, report the initial score documented on presentation at your facility. This may be a score from the emergency medicine technician (EMT) or in the emergency department. If desired, a facility may choose to capture multiple coma scale scores.

Assign code R40.24, Glasgow coma scale, total score, when only the total score is documented in the medical record and not the individual score(s).

23-year-old man found down after unknown injury with skull fracture and with concussion and loss of consciousness of unknown duration. EMS evaluated the patient in the field and reported the individual Glasgow coma scores:

Eye opening response—3: eyes open to speech

Verbal response—4: confused but coherent speech

Motor response—6: obeys commands fully

S02.0XXA   Fracture of vault of skull, initial encounter for closed fracture

S06.0X9A   Concussion with loss of consciousness of unspecified duration, initial encounter

R40.2131   Coma scale, eyes open, to sound, in the field [EMT or ambulance]

R40.2241   Coma scale, best verbal response, confused conversation, in the field [EMT or ambulance]

R40.2361   Coma scale, best motor response, obeys commands, in the field [EMT or ambulance]

Explanation: When individual scores for the Glasgow coma scale are documented, one code from each category is needed to complete the scale. The seventh character indicates when the scale was recorded and should match for all three codes. Assign a code from subcategory R40.24-Glasgow coma scale, total score, when only the total and not the individual score(s) is documented.

---

f. Functional quadriplegia

Functional quadriplegia (code R53.2) is the lack of ability to use one's limbs or to ambulate due to extreme debility. It is not associated with neurologic deficit or injury, and code R53.2 should not be used for cases of neurologic quadriplegia. It should only be assigned if functional quadriplegia is specifically documented in the medical record.

g. SIRS due to non-infectious process

The systemic inflammatory response syndrome (SIRS) can develop as a result of certain non-infectious disease processes, such as trauma, malignant neoplasm, or pancreatitis. When SIRS is documented with a noninfectious condition, and no subsequent infection is documented, the code for the underlying condition, such as an injury, should be assigned, followed by code R65.10, Systemic inflammatory response syndrome (SIRS) of non-infectious origin without acute organ dysfunction, or code R65.11, Systemic inflammatory response syndrome (SIRS) of non-infectious origin with acute organ dysfunction. If an associated acute organ dysfunction is documented, the appropriate code(s) for the specific type of organ dysfunction(s) should be assigned in addition to code R65.11. If acute organ dysfunction is documented, but it cannot be determined if the acute organ dysfunction is associated with SIRS or due to another condition (e.g., directly due to the trauma), the provider should be queried.

Systemic inflammatory response syndrome (SIRS) due to acute gallstone pancreatitis

K85.1Ø	**Biliary acute pancreatitis without necrosis or infection**
R65.1Ø	**Systemic inflammatory response syndrome (SIRS) of noninfectious origin without acute organ dysfunction**

Explanation: When SIRS is documented with a noninfectious condition without subsequent infection documented, the code for the underlying condition such as pancreatitis should be assigned followed by the appropriate code for SIRS of noninfectious origin, either with or without associated organ dysfunction.

h. Death NOS

Code R99, Ill-defined and unknown cause of mortality, is only for use in the very limited circumstance when a patient who has already died is brought into an emergency department or other healthcare facility and is pronounced dead upon arrival. It does not represent the discharge disposition of death.

i. NIHSS stroke scale

The NIH stroke scale (NIHSS) codes (R29.7- -) can be used in conjunction with acute stroke codes (I63) to identify the patient's neurological status and the severity of the stroke. The stroke scale codes should be sequenced after the acute stroke diagnosis code(s).

At a minimum, report the initial score documented. If desired, a facility may choose to capture multiple stroke scale scores.

See Section I.B.14. for information concerning the medical record documentation that may be used for assignment of the NIHSS codes.

Chapter 18. Symptoms, Signs and Abnormal Clinical and Laboratory Findings, Not Elsewhere Classified (R00-R99)

NOTE This chapter includes symptoms, signs, abnormal results of clinical or other investigative procedures, and ill-defined conditions regarding which no diagnosis classifiable elsewhere is recorded.

Signs and symptoms that point rather definitely to a given diagnosis have been assigned to a category in other chapters of the classification. In general, categories in this chapter include the less well-defined conditions and symptoms that, without the necessary study of the case to establish a final diagnosis, point perhaps equally to two or more diseases or to two or more systems of the body. Practically all categories in the chapter could be designated 'not otherwise specified', 'unknown etiology' or 'transient'. The Alphabetical Index should be consulted to determine which symptoms and signs are to be allocated here and which to other chapters. The residual subcategories, numbered .8, are generally provided for other relevant symptoms that cannot be allocated elsewhere in the classification.

The conditions and signs or symptoms included in categories R00-R94 consist of:

(a) cases for which no more specific diagnosis can be made even after all the facts bearing on the case have been investigated;

(b) signs or symptoms existing at the time of initial encounter that proved to be transient and whose causes could not be determined;

(c) provisional diagnosis in a patient who failed to return for further investigation or care;

(d) cases referred elsewhere for investigation or treatment before the diagnosis was made;

(e) cases in which a more precise diagnosis was not available for any other reason;

(f) certain symptoms, for which supplementary information is provided, that represent important problems in medical care in their own right.

EXCLUDES 2 *abnormal findings on antenatal screening of mother (O28.-)*
certain conditions originating in the perinatal period (P04-P96)
signs and symptoms classified in the body system chapters
signs and symptoms of breast (N63, N64.5)

This chapter contains the following blocks:

R00-R09 Symptoms and signs involving the circulatory and respiratory systems
R10-R19 Symptoms and signs involving the digestive system and abdomen
R20-R23 Symptoms and signs involving the skin and subcutaneous tissue
R25-R29 Symptoms and signs involving the nervous and musculoskeletal systems
R30-R39 Symptoms and signs involving the genitourinary system
R40-R46 Symptoms and signs involving cognition, perception, emotional state and behavior
R47-R49 Symptoms and signs involving speech and voice
R50-R69 General symptoms and signs
R70-R79 Abnormal findings on examination of blood, without diagnosis
R80-R82 Abnormal findings on examination of urine, without diagnosis
R83-R89 Abnormal findings on examination of other body fluids, substances and tissues, without diagnosis
R90-R94 Abnormal findings on diagnostic imaging and in function studies, without diagnosis
R97   Abnormal tumor markers
R99   Ill-defined and unknown cause of mortality

Symptoms and signs involving the circulatory and respiratory systems (R00-R09)

✓4ᵗʰ R00 Abnormalities of heart beat

EXCLUDES 1 *abnormalities originating in the perinatal period (P29.1-)*
EXCLUDES 2 *▶specified arrhythmias (I47-I49)◀*

R00.0 Tachycardia, unspecified ▽
Rapid heart beat
Sinoauricular tachycardia NOS
Sinus [sinusal] tachycardia NOS
EXCLUDES 1 *neonatal tachycardia (P29.11)*
paroxysmal tachycardia (I47.-)

R00.1 Bradycardia, unspecified ▽
Sinoatrial bradycardia
Sinus bradycardia
Slow heart beat
Vagal bradycardia
Use additional code for adverse effect, if applicable, to identify drug (T36-T50 with fifth or sixth character 5)
EXCLUDES 1 *neonatal bradycardia (P29.12)*

R00.2 Palpitations
Awareness of heart beat

R00.8 Other abnormalities of heart beat

R00.9 Unspecified abnormalities of heart beat ▽

✓4ᵗʰ R01 Cardiac murmurs and other cardiac sounds
EXCLUDES 1 *cardiac murmurs and sounds originating in the perinatal period (P29.8)*

R01.0 Benign and innocent cardiac murmurs
Functional cardiac murmur

R01.1 Cardiac murmur, unspecified ▽
Cardiac bruit NOS
Heart murmur NOS
▶Systolic murmur NOS◀

R01.2 Other cardiac sounds
Cardiac dullness, increased or decreased
Precordial friction

✓4ᵗʰ R03 Abnormal blood-pressure reading, without diagnosis

R03.0 Elevated blood-pressure reading, without diagnosis of hypertension
NOTE This category is to be used to record an episode of elevated blood pressure in a patient in whom no formal diagnosis of hypertension has been made, or as an isolated incidental finding.

R03.1 Nonspecific low blood-pressure reading
EXCLUDES 1 *hypotension (I95.-)*
maternal hypotension syndrome (O26.5-)
neurogenic orthostatic hypotension (G90.3)

✓4ᵗʰ R04 Hemorrhage from respiratory passages

R04.0 Epistaxis
Hemorrhage from nose
Nosebleed

R04.1 Hemorrhage from throat
EXCLUDES 2 *hemoptysis (R04.2)*

R04.2 Hemoptysis
Blood-stained sputum
Cough with hemorrhage
AHA: 2013,4Q,118

✓5ᵗʰ R04.8 Hemorrhage from other sites in respiratory passages

R04.81 Acute idiopathic pulmonary hemorrhage in infants P
AIPHI
Acute idiopathic hemorrhage in infants over 28 days old
EXCLUDES 1 *perinatal pulmonary hemorrhage (P26.-)*
von Willebrand's disease (D68.0)

R04.89 Hemorrhage from other sites in respiratory passages
Pulmonary hemorrhage NOS

R04.9 Hemorrhage from respiratory passages, unspecified ▽

R05 Cough
EXCLUDES 1 *cough with hemorrhage (R04.2)*
smoker's cough (J41.0)
AHA: 2016,2Q,33

✓4ᵗʰ R06 Abnormalities of breathing
EXCLUDES 1 *acute respiratory distress syndrome (J80)*
respiratory arrest (R09.2)
respiratory arrest of newborn (P28.81)
respiratory distress syndrome of newborn (P22.-)
respiratory failure (J96.-)
respiratory failure of newborn (P28.5)

✓5ᵗʰ R06.0 Dyspnea
EXCLUDES 1 *tachypnea NOS (R06.82)*
transient tachypnea of newborn (P22.1)

R06.00 Dyspnea, unspecified ▽
R06.01 Orthopnea
R06.02 Shortness of breath
R06.09 Other forms of dyspnea

R06.1 Stridor
EXCLUDES 1 *congenital laryngeal stridor (P28.89)*
laryngismus (stridulus) (J38.5)

R06.2 Wheezing
EXCLUDES 1 *asthma (J45.-)*
AHA: 2016,2Q,33

☑ Additional Character Required   √x7ᵗʰ Placeholder Alert   Manifestation Dx   ▽ Unspecified Dx   ▶◀ Revised Text   ● New Code   ▲ Revised Code Title

Chapter 18. Symptoms, Signs and Abnormal Clinical and Laboratory Findings

R06.3 Periodic breathing
    Cheyne-Stokes breathing

R06.4 Hyperventilation
    EXCLUDES 1 *psychogenic hyperventilation (F45.8)*

R06.5 Mouth breathing
    EXCLUDES 2 *dry mouth NOS (R68.2)*

R06.6 Hiccough
    EXCLUDES 1 *psychogenic hiccough (F45.8)*

R06.7 Sneezing

✓5th **R06.8 Other abnormalities of breathing**

    R06.81 Apnea, not elsewhere classified
      Apnea NOS
      EXCLUDES 1 *apnea (of) newborn (P28.4)*
          sleep apnea (G47.3-)
          sleep apnea of newborn (primary) (P28.3)

    R06.82 Tachypnea, not elsewhere classified
      Tachypnea NOS
      EXCLUDES 1 *transitory tachypnea of newborn (P22.1)*

    R06.83 Snoring
    R06.89 Other abnormalities of breathing
      Breath-holding (spells)
      Sighing

R06.9 Unspecified abnormalities of breathing ▽

✓4th **R07 Pain in throat and chest**
    EXCLUDES 1 *epidemic myalgia (B33.0)*
    EXCLUDES 2 *jaw pain R68.84*
      pain in breast (N64.4)

R07.0 Pain in throat
    EXCLUDES 1 *chronic sore throat (J31.2)*
      sore throat (acute) NOS (J02.9)
    EXCLUDES 2 *dysphagia (R13.1-)*
      pain in neck (M54.2)

R07.1 Chest pain on breathing
    Painful respiration

R07.2 Precordial pain

✓5th **R07.8 Other chest pain**

    R07.81 Pleurodynia
      Pleurodynia NOS
      EXCLUDES 1 *epidemic pleurodynia (B33.0)*

    R07.82 Intercostal pain
    R07.89 Other chest pain
      Anterior chest-wall pain NOS

R07.9 Chest pain, unspecified ▽

✓4th **R09 Other symptoms and signs involving the circulatory and respiratory system**
    EXCLUDES 1 *acute respiratory distress syndrome (J80)*
      respiratory arrest of newborn (P28.81)
      respiratory distress syndrome of newborn (P22.0)
      respiratory failure (J96.-)
      respiratory failure of newborn (P28.5)

✓5th **R09.0 Asphyxia and hypoxemia**
    EXCLUDES 1 *asphyxia due to carbon monoxide (T58.-)*
      asphyxia due to foreign body in respiratory tract (T17.-)
      birth (intrauterine) asphyxia (P84)
      hypercapnia (R06.4)
      hyperventilation (R06.4)
      traumatic asphyxia (T71.-)

    R09.01 Asphyxia
    R09.02 Hypoxemia

R09.1 Pleurisy
    EXCLUDES 1 *pleurisy with effusion (J90)*

R09.2 Respiratory arrest
    Cardiorespiratory failure
    EXCLUDES 1 *cardiac arrest (I46.-)*
      respiratory arrest of newborn (P28.81)
      respiratory distress of newborn (P22.0)
      respiratory failure (J96.-)
      respiratory failure of newborn (P28.5)
      respiratory insufficiency (R06.89)
      respiratory insufficiency of newborn (P28.5)

R09.3 Abnormal sputum
    Abnormal amount of sputum
    Abnormal color of sputum
    Abnormal odor of sputum
    Excessive sputum
    EXCLUDES 1 *blood-stained sputum (R04.2)*

✓5th **R09.8 Other specified symptoms and signs involving the circulatory and respiratory systems**

    R09.81 Nasal congestion
    R09.82 Postnasal drip
    R09.89 Other specified symptoms and signs involving the circulatory and respiratory systems
      Abnormal chest percussion
      Bruit (arterial)
      Chest tympany
      Choking sensation
      Feeling of foreign body in throat
      Friction sounds in chest
      Rales
      Weak pulse
      EXCLUDES 2 *foreign body in throat (T17.2-)*
          wheezing (R06.2)

Symptoms and signs involving the digestive system and abdomen (R10-R19)

    EXCLUDES 2 ▶*congenital or infantile pylorospasm (Q40.0)*◀
      ▶*gastrointestinal hemorrhage (K92.0-K92.2)*◀
      ▶*intestinal obstruction (K56.-)*◀
      ▶*newborn gastrointestinal hemorrhage (P54.0-P54.3)*◀
      ▶*newborn intestinal obstruction (P76.-)*◀
      ▶*pylorospasm (K31.3)*◀
      ▶*signs and symptoms involving the urinary system (R30-R39)*◀
      ▶*symptoms referable to female genital organs (N94.-)*◀
      ▶*symptoms referable to male genital organs (N48-N50)*◀

✓4th **R10 Abdominal and pelvic pain**
    EXCLUDES 1 *renal colic (N23)*
    EXCLUDES 2 *dorsalgia (M54.-)*
      flatulence and related conditions (R14.-)

R10.0 Acute abdomen
    Severe abdominal pain (generalized) (with abdominal rigidity)
    EXCLUDES 1 *abdominal rigidity NOS (R19.3)*
      generalized abdominal pain NOS (R10.84)
      localized abdominal pain (R10.1-R10.3-)

✓5th **R10.1 Pain localized to upper abdomen**

    R10.10 Upper abdominal pain, unspecified ▽
    R10.11 Right upper quadrant pain
    R10.12 Left upper quadrant pain
    R10.13 Epigastric pain
      Dyspepsia
      EXCLUDES 1 *functional dyspepsia (K30)*

R10.2 Pelvic and perineal pain
    EXCLUDES 1 *vulvodynia (N94.81)*

✓5th **R10.3 Pain localized to other parts of lower abdomen**

    R10.30 Lower abdominal pain, unspecified ▽
    R10.31 Right lower quadrant pain
    R10.32 Left lower quadrant pain
    R10.33 Periumbilical pain

✓5th **R10.8 Other abdominal pain**

    ✓6th **R10.81 Abdominal tenderness**
      Abdominal tenderness NOS
      R10.811 Right upper quadrant abdominal tenderness
      R10.812 Left upper quadrant abdominal tenderness
      R10.813 Right lower quadrant abdominal tenderness
      R10.814 Left lower quadrant abdominal tenderness
      R10.815 Periumbilic abdominal tenderness
      R10.816 Epigastric abdominal tenderness
      R10.817 Generalized abdominal tenderness
      R10.819 Abdominal tenderness, unspecified site ▽

    ✓6th **R10.82 Rebound abdominal tenderness**
      R10.821 Right upper quadrant rebound abdominal tenderness
      R10.822 Left upper quadrant rebound abdominal tenderness

EXCLUDES 1 Not coded here   EXCLUDES 2 Not included here   N Newborn Age : 0   P Pediatric Age : 0-17   M Maternity Age : 12-55   A Adult Age : 15-124

866   ICD-10-CM 2017

R06.3–R10.822

R10.823   **Right lower** quadrant rebound abdominal tenderness

R10.824   **Left lower** quadrant rebound abdominal tenderness

R10.825   **Periumbilic** rebound abdominal tenderness

R10.826   **Epigastric** rebound abdominal tenderness

R10.827   **Generalized** rebound abdominal tenderness

R10.829   **Rebound abdominal tenderness, unspecified site**   ▽

R10.83   **Colic**   P

    Colic NOS

    Infantile colic

    EXCLUDES 1   colic in adult and child over 12 months old (R10.84)

    DEF: Inconsolable crying in an otherwise well-fed and healthy infant for more than three hours a day, three days a week, for more than three weeks.

R10.84   **Generalized abdominal pain**

    EXCLUDES 1   generalized abdominal pain associated with acute abdomen (R10.0)

R10.9   **Unspecified abdominal pain**   ▽

✓4th **R11**   **Nausea and vomiting**

    EXCLUDES 1   cyclical vomiting associated with migraine (G43.A-)

       excessive vomiting in pregnancy (O21.-)

       hematemesis (K92.0)

       neonatal hematemesis (P54.0)

       newborn vomiting (P92.0-)

       psychogenic vomiting ▶(F50.89)◀

       vomiting associated with bulimia nervosa (F50.2)

       vomiting following gastrointestinal surgery (K91.0)

R11.0   **Nausea**

    Nausea NOS

    Nausea without vomiting

✓5th R11.1   **Vomiting**

    R11.10   **Vomiting, unspecified**   ▽

       Vomiting NOS

    R11.11   **Vomiting** without nausea

    R11.12   **Projectile** vomiting

    R11.13   **Vomiting of** fecal matter

    R11.14   **Bilious vomiting**

       Bilious emesis

R11.2   **Nausea with vomiting, unspecified**   ▽

    Persistent nausea with vomiting NOS

R12   **Heartburn**

    EXCLUDES 1   dyspepsia NOS (R10.13)

       functional dyspepsia (K30)

✓4th **R13**   **Aphagia and dysphagia**

R13.0   **Aphagia**

    Inability to swallow

    EXCLUDES 1   psychogenic aphagia (F50.9)

✓5th R13.1   **Dysphagia**

    Code first, if applicable, dysphagia following cerebrovascular disease (I69. with final characters -91)

    EXCLUDES 1   psychogenic dysphagia (F45.8)

Swallowing Function

Oral phase   Oropharyngeal phase

Pharyngeal phase   Pharyngoesophageal phase

    R13.10   **Dysphagia, unspecified**   ▽

       Difficulty in swallowing NOS

    R13.11   **Dysphagia,** oral **phase**

    R13.12   **Dysphagia,** oropharyngeal **phase**

    R13.13   **Dysphagia,** pharyngeal **phase**

    R13.14   **Dysphagia,** pharyngoesophageal **phase**

    R13.19   **Other dysphagia**

       Cervical dysphagia

       Neurogenic dysphagia

✓4th **R14**   **Flatulence and related conditions**

    EXCLUDES 1   psychogenic aerophagy (F45.8)

R14.0   **Abdominal distension (gaseous)**

    Bloating

    Tympanites (abdominal) (intestinal)

R14.1   **Gas pain**

R14.2   **Eructation**

R14.3   **Flatulence**

✓4th **R15**   **Fecal incontinence**

    INCLUDES   encopresis NOS

    EXCLUDES 1   fecal incontinence of nonorganic origin (F98.1)

R15.0   **Incomplete defecation**

    EXCLUDES 1   constipation (K59.0-)

       fecal impaction (K56.41)

R15.1   **Fecal smearing**

    Fecal soiling

R15.2   **Fecal urgency**

R15.9   **Full incontinence of feces**

    Fecal incontinence NOS

✓4th **R16**   **Hepatomegaly and splenomegaly, not elsewhere classified**

R16.0   **Hepatomegaly, not elsewhere classified**

    Hepatomegaly NOS

R16.1   **Splenomegaly, not elsewhere classified**

    Splenomegaly NOS

R16.2   **Hepatomegaly with splenomegaly, not elsewhere classified**

    Hepatosplenomegaly NOS

R17   **Unspecified jaundice**   ▽

    EXCLUDES 1   neonatal jaundice (P55, P57-P59)

✓4th **R18**   **Ascites**

    INCLUDES   fluid in peritoneal cavity

    EXCLUDES 1   ascites in alcoholic cirrhosis (K70.31)

       ascites in alcoholic hepatitis (K70.11)

       ascites in toxic liver disease with chronic active hepatitis (K71.51)

R18.0   **Malignant ascites**

    Code first malignancy, such as:

       malignant neoplasm of ovary (C56.-)

       secondary malignant neoplasm of retroperitoneum and peritoneum (C78.6)

✓ Additional Character Required   ✓x7th Placeholder Alert   Manifestation Dx   ▽ Unspecified Dx   ▶◀ Revised Text   ● New Code   ▲ Revised Code Title

Chapter 18. Symptoms, Signs and Abnormal Clinical and Laboratory Findings

R18.8   Other ascites
Ascites NOS
Peritoneal effusion (chronic)

✓4ᵗʰ **R19   Other symptoms and signs involving the digestive system and abdomen**
    EXCLUDES 1   *acute abdomen (R10.0)*

✓5ᵗʰ **R19.0   Intra-abdominal and pelvic swelling, mass and lump**
    EXCLUDES 1   *abdominal distension (gaseous) (R14.-)*
       ascites (R18.-)

    R19.00   Intra-abdominal and pelvic swelling, mass and lump, unspecified site ▽

    R19.01   Right upper quadrant abdominal swelling, mass and lump

    R19.02   Left upper quadrant abdominal swelling, mass and lump

    R19.03   Right lower quadrant abdominal swelling, mass and lump

    R19.04   Left lower quadrant abdominal swelling, mass and lump

    R19.05   Periumbilic swelling, mass or lump
       Diffuse or generalized umbilical swelling or mass

    R19.06   Epigastric swelling, mass or lump

    R19.07   Generalized intra-abdominal and pelvic swelling, mass and lump
       Diffuse or generalized intra-abdominal swelling or mass NOS
       Diffuse or generalized pelvic swelling or mass NOS

    R19.09   Other intra-abdominal and pelvic swelling, mass and lump

✓5ᵗʰ **R19.1   Abnormal bowel sounds**

    R19.11   Absent bowel sounds

    R19.12   Hyperactive bowel sounds

    R19.15   Other abnormal bowel sounds
       Abnormal bowel sounds NOS

R19.2   Visible peristalsis
Hyperperistalsis

✓5ᵗʰ **R19.3   Abdominal rigidity**
    EXCLUDES 1   *abdominal rigidity with severe abdominal pain (R10.0)*

    R19.30   Abdominal rigidity, unspecified site ▽

    R19.31   Right upper quadrant abdominal rigidity

    R19.32   Left upper quadrant abdominal rigidity

    R19.33   Right lower quadrant abdominal rigidity

    R19.34   Left lower quadrant abdominal rigidity

    R19.35   Periumbilic abdominal rigidity

    R19.36   Epigastric abdominal rigidity

    R19.37   Generalized abdominal rigidity

R19.4   Change in bowel habit
    EXCLUDES 1   *constipation (K59.0-)*
       functional diarrhea (K59.1)

R19.5   Other fecal abnormalities
Abnormal stool color
Bulky stools
Mucus in stools
Occult blood in feces
Occult blood in stools
    EXCLUDES 1   *melena (K92.1)*
       neonatal melena (P54.1)

R19.6   Halitosis

R19.7   Diarrhea, unspecified ▽
Diarrhea NOS
    EXCLUDES 1   *functional diarrhea (K59.1)*
       neonatal diarrhea (P78.3)
       psychogenic diarrhea (F45.8)

R19.8   Other specified symptoms and signs involving the digestive system and abdomen

Symptoms and signs involving the skin and subcutaneous tissue (R20-R23)

EXCLUDES 2   *symptoms relating to breast (N64.4-N64.5)*

✓4ᵗʰ **R20   Disturbances of skin sensation**
    EXCLUDES 1   *dissociative anesthesia and sensory loss (F44.6)*
       psychogenic disturbances (F45.8)

    R20.0   Anesthesia of skin

    R20.1   Hypoesthesia of skin

R20.2   Paresthesia of skin
Formication
Pins and needles
Tingling skin
    EXCLUDES 1   *acroparesthesia (I73.8)*

R20.3   Hyperesthesia

R20.8   Other disturbances of skin sensation

R20.9   Unspecified disturbances of skin sensation ▽

R21   Rash and other nonspecific skin eruption
    INCLUDES   rash NOS
    EXCLUDES 1   *specified type of rash - code to condition*
       vesicular eruption (R23.8)

✓4ᵗʰ **R22   Localized swelling, mass and lump of skin and subcutaneous tissue**
    INCLUDES   subcutaneous nodules (localized)(superficial)
    EXCLUDES 1   *abnormal findings on diagnostic imaging (R90-R93)*
       edema (R60.-)
       enlarged lymph nodes (R59.-)
       localized adiposity (E65)
       swelling of joint (M25.4-)

    R22.0   Localized swelling, mass and lump, head

    R22.1   Localized swelling, mass and lump, neck

    R22.2   Localized swelling, mass and lump, trunk
      EXCLUDES 1   *intra-abdominal or pelvic mass and lump (R19.0-)*
       intra-abdominal or pelvic swelling (R19.0-)
      EXCLUDES 2   *breast mass and lump (N63)*

✓5ᵗʰ   **R22.3   Localized swelling, mass and lump, upper limb**

    R22.30   Localized swelling, mass and lump, unspecified upper limb ▽

    R22.31   Localized swelling, mass and lump, right upper limb

    R22.32   Localized swelling, mass and lump, left upper limb

    R22.33   Localized swelling, mass and lump, upper limb, bilateral

✓5ᵗʰ   **R22.4   Localized swelling, mass and lump, lower limb**

    R22.40   Localized swelling, mass and lump, unspecified lower limb ▽

    R22.41   Localized swelling, mass and lump, right lower limb

    R22.42   Localized swelling, mass and lump, left lower limb

    R22.43   Localized swelling, mass and lump, lower limb, bilateral

    R22.9   Localized swelling, mass and lump, unspecified ▽

✓4ᵗʰ **R23   Other skin changes**

    R23.0   Cyanosis
      EXCLUDES 1   *acrocyanosis (I73.8)*
       cyanotic attacks of newborn (P28.2)

    R23.1   Pallor
      Clammy skin

    R23.2   Flushing
      Excessive blushing
      Code first, if applicable, menopausal and female climacteric states (N95.1)

    R23.3   Spontaneous ecchymoses
      Petechiae
      EXCLUDES 1   *ecchymoses of newborn (P54.5)*
       purpura (D69.-)

    R23.4   Changes in skin texture
      Desquamation of skin
      Induration of skin
      Scaling of skin
      EXCLUDES 1   *epidermal thickening NOS (L85.9)*

    R23.8   Other skin changes

    R23.9   Unspecified skin changes ▽

Symptoms and signs involving the nervous and musculoskeletal systems (R25-R29)

✓4ᵗʰ **R25   Abnormal involuntary movements**
    EXCLUDES 1   *specific movement disorders (G20-G26)*
       stereotyped movement disorders (F98.4)
       tic disorders (F95.-)

    R25.0   Abnormal head movements

R25.1 Tremor, unspecified ▽
EXCLUDES 1   chorea NOS (G25.5)
       essential tremor (G25.0)
       hysterical tremor (F44.4)
       intention tremor (G25.2)

R25.2 Cramp and spasm
EXCLUDES 2   carpopedal spasm (R29.0)
       charley-horse (M62.831)
       infantile spasms (G40.4-)
       muscle spasm of back (M62.830)
       muscle spasm of calf (M62.831)

R25.3 Fasciculation
Twitching NOS

R25.8 Other abnormal involuntary movements

R25.9 Unspecified abnormal involuntary movements ▽

✓4ᵗʰ **R26 Abnormalities of gait and mobility**
EXCLUDES 1   ataxia NOS (R27.0)
       hereditary ataxia (G11.-)
       locomotor (syphilitic) ataxia (A52.11)
       immobility syndrome (paraplegic) (M62.3)

R26.0 Ataxic gait
Staggering gait

R26.1 Paralytic gait
Spastic gait

R26.2 Difficulty in walking, not elsewhere classified
EXCLUDES 1   falling (R29.6)
       unsteadiness on feet (R26.81)
AHA: 2016,2Q,7

✓5ᵗʰ **R26.8 Other abnormalities of gait and mobility**
R26.81 Unsteadiness on feet
R26.89 Other abnormalities of gait and mobility

R26.9 Unspecified abnormalities of gait and mobility ▽

✓4ᵗʰ **R27 Other lack of coordination**
EXCLUDES 1   ataxic gait (R26.0)
       hereditary ataxia (G11.-)
       vertigo NOS (R42)

R27.0 Ataxia, unspecified ▽
EXCLUDES 1   ataxia following cerebrovascular disease (I69, with
         final characters 93)

R27.8 Other lack of coordination

R27.9 Unspecified lack of coordination ▽

✓4ᵗʰ **R29 Other symptoms and signs involving the nervous and musculoskeletal systems**

R29.0 Tetany
Carpopedal spasm
EXCLUDES 1   hysterical tetany (F44.5)
       neonatal tetany (P71.3)
       parathyroid tetany (E20.9)
       post-thyroidectomy tetany (E89.2)

R29.1 Meningismus

R29.2 Abnormal reflex
EXCLUDES 2   abnormal pupillary reflex (H57.0)
       hyperactive gag reflex (J39.2)
       vasovagal reaction or syncope (R55)

R29.3 Abnormal posture

R29.4 Clicking hip
EXCLUDES 1   congenital deformities of hip (Q65.-)

R29.5 Transient paralysis
Code first any associated spinal cord injury (S14.0, S14.1-, S24.0, S24.1-, S34.0-, S34.1-)
EXCLUDES 1   transient ischemic attack (G45.9)

R29.6 Repeated falls
Falling
Tendency to fall
EXCLUDES 2   at risk for falling (Z91.81)
       history of falling (Z91.81)
AHA: 2016,2Q,6

● ✓5ᵗʰ **R29.7 National Institutes of Health Stroke Scale (NIHSS) score**
Code first the type of cerebral infarction (I63.-)

● ✓6ᵗʰ **R29.70 NIHSS score 0-9**
● **R29.700 NIHSS score 0**
● **R29.701 NIHSS score 1**
● **R29.702 NIHSS score 2**
● **R29.703 NIHSS score 3**

● **R29.704 NIHSS score 4**
● **R29.705 NIHSS score 5**
● **R29.706 NIHSS score 6**
● **R29.707 NIHSS score 7**
● **R29.708 NIHSS score 8**
● **R29.709 NIHSS score 9**

✓6ᵗʰ **R29.71 NIHSS score 10-19**
● **R29.710 NIHSS score 10**
● **R29.711 NIHSS score 11**
● **R29.712 NIHSS score 12**
● **R29.713 NIHSS score 13**
● **R29.714 NIHSS score 14**
● **R29.715 NIHSS score 15**
● **R29.716 NIHSS score 16**
● **R29.717 NIHSS score 17**
● **R29.718 NIHSS score 18**
● **R29.719 NIHSS score 19**

✓6ᵗʰ **R29.72 NIHSS score 20-29**
● **R29.720 NIHSS score 20**
● **R29.721 NIHSS score 21**
● **R29.722 NIHSS score 22**
● **R29.723 NIHSS score 23**
● **R29.724 NIHSS score 24**
● **R29.725 NIHSS score 25**
● **R29.726 NIHSS score 26**
● **R29.727 NIHSS score 27**
● **R29.728 NIHSS score 28**
● **R29.729 NIHSS score 29**

✓6ᵗʰ **R29.73 NIHSS score 30-39**
● **R29.730 NIHSS score 30**
● **R29.731 NIHSS score 31**
● **R29.732 NIHSS score 32**
● **R29.733 NIHSS score 33**
● **R29.734 NIHSS score 34**
● **R29.735 NIHSS score 35**
● **R29.736 NIHSS score 36**
● **R29.737 NIHSS score 37**
● **R29.738 NIHSS score 38**
● **R29.739 NIHSS score 39**

✓6ᵗʰ **R29.74 NIHSS score 40-42**
● **R29.740 NIHSS score 40**
● **R29.741 NIHSS score 41**
● **R29.742 NIHSS score 42**

✓5ᵗʰ **R29.8 Other symptoms and signs involving the nervous and musculoskeletal systems**

✓6ᵗʰ **R29.81 Other symptoms and signs involving the nervous system**
R29.810 Facial weakness
Facial droop
EXCLUDES 1   Bell's palsy (G51.0)
       facial weakness following cerebrovascular disease (I69. with final characters -92)

R29.818 Other symptoms and signs involving the nervous system

✓6ᵗʰ **R29.89 Other symptoms and signs involving the musculoskeletal system**
EXCLUDES 2   pain in limb (M79.6-)
R29.890 Loss of height
EXCLUDES 1   osteoporosis (M80-M81)
R29.891 Ocular torticollis
EXCLUDES 1   congenital (sternomastoid) torticollis Q68.0
       psychogenic torticollis (F45.8)
       spasmodic torticollis (G24.3)
       torticollis due to birth injury (P15.8)
       torticollis NOS M43.6
R29.898 Other symptoms and signs involving the musculoskeletal system

---

✅ Additional Character Required   ✓7ᵗʰ Placeholder Alert   Manifestation Dx   ▽ Unspecified Dx   ▶◀ Revised Text   ● New Code   ▲ Revised Code Title

Chapter 18. Symptoms, Signs and Abnormal Clinical and Laboratory Findings

R29.9–R40.221

√5ᵗʰ **R29.9 Unspecified symptoms and signs involving the nervous and musculoskeletal systems**

     R29.90 Unspecified symptoms and signs involving the nervous system ▽

     R29.91 Unspecified symptoms and signs involving the musculoskeletal system ▽

Symptoms and signs involving the genitourinary system (R30-R39)

√4ᵗʰ **R30 Pain associated with micturition**

     EXCLUDES 1 psychogenic pain associated with micturition (F45.8)

     R30.0 Dysuria
       Strangury

     R30.1 Vesical tenesmus

     R30.9 Painful micturition, unspecified ▽
       Painful urination NOS

√4ᵗʰ **R31 Hematuria**

     EXCLUDES 1 hematuria included with underlying conditions, such as:
       acute cystitis with hematuria (N30.01)
       recurrent and persistent hematuria in glomerular diseases (N02.-)

     R31.0 Gross hematuria

     R31.1 Benign essential microscopic hematuria

√5ᵗʰ   **R31.2 Other microscopic hematuria**

       R31.21 Asymptomatic microscopic hematuria
         AMH

       R31.29 Other microscopic hematuria

     R31.9 Hematuria, unspecified ▽

R32 Unspecified urinary incontinence ▽
     Enuresis NOS

     EXCLUDES 1 functional urinary incontinence (R39.81)
       nonorganic enuresis (F98.0)
       stress incontinence and other specified urinary incontinence (N39.3-N39.4-)
       urinary incontinence associated with cognitive impairment (R39.81)

√4ᵗʰ **R33 Retention of urine**

     EXCLUDES 1 psychogenic retention of urine (F45.8)

     R33.0 Drug induced retention of urine
       Use additional code for adverse effect, if applicable, to identify drug (T36-T50 with fifth or sixth character 5)

     R33.8 Other retention of urine
       Code first, if applicable, any causal condition, such as:
       enlarged prostate (N40.1)

     R33.9 Retention of urine, unspecified ▽

R34 Anuria and oliguria

     EXCLUDES 1 anuria and oliguria complicating abortion or ectopic or molar pregnancy (O00-O07, O08.4)
       anuria and oliguria complicating pregnancy (O26.83-)
       anuria and oliguria complicating the puerperium (O90.4)

√4ᵗʰ **R35 Polyuria**
     Code first, if applicable, any causal condition, such as:
     enlarged prostate (N40.1)

     EXCLUDES 1 psychogenic polyuria (F45.8)

     R35.0 Frequency of micturition

     R35.1 Nocturia

     R35.8 Other polyuria
       Polyuria NOS

√4ᵗʰ **R36 Urethral discharge**

     R36.0 Urethral discharge without blood

     R36.1 Hematospermia ♂

     R36.9 Urethral discharge, unspecified ▽
       Penile discharge NOS
       Urethrorrhea

R37 Sexual dysfunction, unspecified ▽

√4ᵗʰ **R39 Other and unspecified symptoms and signs involving the genitourinary system**

     R39.0 Extravasation of urine

√5ᵗʰ   **R39.1 Other difficulties with micturition**
       Code first, if applicable, any causal condition, such as:
       enlarged prostate (N40.1)

       R39.11 Hesitancy of micturition

     R39.12 Poor urinary stream
       Weak urinary steam

     R39.13 Splitting of urinary stream

     R39.14 Feeling of incomplete bladder emptying

     R39.15 Urgency of urination
       EXCLUDES 1 urge incontinence (N39.41, N39.46)

     R39.16 Straining to void

√6ᵗʰ   **R39.19 Other difficulties with micturition**

       R39.191 Need to immediately re-void

       R39.192 Position dependent micturition

       R39.198 Other difficulties with micturition

     R39.2 Extrarenal uremia
       Prerenal uremia
       EXCLUDES 1 uremia NOS (N19)

√5ᵗʰ **R39.8 Other symptoms and signs involving the genitourinary system**

     R39.81 Functional urinary incontinence
       Urinary incontinence due to cognitive impairment, or severe physical disability or immobility
       EXCLUDES 1 stress incontinence and other specified urinary incontinence (N39.3-N39.4-)
       urinary incontinence NOS (R32)

     R39.82 Chronic bladder pain

     R39.89 Other symptoms and signs involving the genitourinary system

     R39.9 Unspecified symptoms and signs involving the genitourinary system ▽

Symptoms and signs involving cognition, perception, emotional state and behavior (R40-R46)

EXCLUDES 2 ▶symptoms and signs constituting part of a pattern of mental disorder (F01-F99)◀

√4ᵗʰ **R40 Somnolence, stupor and coma**

     EXCLUDES 1 neonatal coma (P91.5)
       somnolence, stupor and coma in diabetes (E08-E13)
       somnolence, stupor and coma in hepatic failure (K72.-)
       somnolence, stupor and coma in hypoglycemia (nondiabetic) (E15)

     R40.0 Somnolence
       Drowsiness
       EXCLUDES 1 coma (R40.2-)

     R40.1 Stupor
       Catatonic stupor
       Semicoma
       EXCLUDES 1 catatonic schizophrenia (F20.2)
       coma (R40.2-)
       depressive stupor (F31-F33)
       dissociative stupor (F44.2)
       manic stupor (F30.2)

√5ᵗʰ **R40.2 Coma**
     Code first any associated:
     fracture of skull (S02.-)
     intracranial injury (S06.-)

     NOTE ▶One code from each subcategory, R40.21-R40.23, is required to complete the coma scale◀

     AHA: 2015,2Q,17; 2014,1Q,19

     R40.20 Unspecified coma ▽
       Coma NOS
       Unconsciousness NOS

√6ᵗʰ   **R40.21 Coma scale, eyes open**

       The following appropriate 7th character is to be added to subcategory R40.21-, R40.22-, R40.23-, and R40.24-.
       0   unspecified time
       1   in the field [EMT or ambulance]
       2   at arrival to emergency department
       3   at hospital admission
       4   24 hours or more after hospital admission

       √7ᵗʰ **R40.211 Coma scale, eyes open, never**

       √7ᵗʰ **R40.212 Coma scale, eyes open, to pain**

       √7ᵗʰ **R40.213 Coma scale, eyes open, to sound**

       √7ᵗʰ **R40.214 Coma scale, eyes open, spontaneous**

√6ᵗʰ   **R40.22 Coma scale, best verbal response**

       √7ᵗʰ **R40.221 Coma scale, best verbal response, none**

EXCLUDES 1 Not coded here   *EXCLUDES 2* Not included here   N Newborn Age : 0   P Pediatric Age : 0-17   M Maternity Age : 12-55   A Adult Age : 15-124

870   ICD-10-CM 2017

√7th **R40.222 Coma scale, best verbal response, incomprehensible words**

√7th **R40.223 Coma scale, best verbal response, inappropriate words**

√7th **R40.224 Coma scale, best verbal response, confused conversation**

√7th **R40.225 Coma scale, best verbal response, oriented**

√6th **R40.23 Coma scale, best motor response**

√7th **R40.231 Coma scale, best motor response, none**

√7th **R40.232 Coma scale, best motor response, extension**

√7th **R40.233 Coma scale, best motor response, abnormal**

√7th **R40.234 Coma scale, best motor response, flexion withdrawal**

√7th **R40.235 Coma scale, best motor response, localizes pain**

√7th **R40.236 Coma scale, best motor response, obeys commands**

√6th **R40.24 Glasgow coma scale, total score**

> **NOTE** ►Assign a code from subcategory R40.24, when only the total coma score is documented◄

√7th **R40.241 Glasgow coma scale score 13-15**

√7th **R40.242 Glasgow coma scale score 9-12**

√7th **R40.243 Glasgow coma scale score 3-8**

√7th **R40.244 Other coma, without documented Glasgow coma scale score, or with partial score reported**

R40.3 Persistent vegetative state
DEF: Persistent wakefulness without consciousness due to nonfunctioning cerebral cortex.

R40.4 Transient alteration of awareness

√4th **R41 Other symptoms and signs involving cognitive functions and awareness**
EXCLUDES 1 *dissociative [conversion] disorders (F44.-)*
mild cognitive impairment, so stated (G31.84)

R41.0 Disorientation, unspecified ▽
Confusion NOS
Delirium NOS

R41.1 Anterograde amnesia

R41.2 Retrograde amnesia

R41.3 Other amnesia
Amnesia NOS
Memory loss NOS
EXCLUDES 1 *amnestic disorder due to known physiologic condition (F04)*
amnestic syndrome due to psychoactive substance use (F10-F19 with 5th character .6)
mild memory disturbance due to known physiological condition (F06.8)
transient global amnesia (G45.4)

R41.4 Neurologic neglect syndrome
Asomatognosia
Hemi-akinesia
Hemi-inattention
Hemispatial neglect
Left-sided neglect
Sensory neglect
Visuospatial neglect
EXCLUDES 1 *visuospatial deficit (R41.842)*

√5th **R41.8 Other symptoms and signs involving cognitive functions and awareness**

R41.81 Age-related cognitive decline 🅰
Senility NOS

R41.82 Altered mental status, unspecified ▽
Change in mental status NOS
EXCLUDES 1 *altered level of consciousness (R40.-)*
altered mental status due to known condition - code to condition
delirium NOS (R41.0)
AHA: 2012,4Q,97

R41.83 Borderline intellectual functioning
IQ level 71 to 84
EXCLUDES 1 *intellectual disabilities (F70-F79)*

√6th **R41.84 Other specified cognitive deficit**
EXCLUDES 1 ►*cognitive deficits as sequelae of cerebrovascular disease (I69.01-, I69.11-, I69.21-, I69.31-, I69.81-, I69.91-)*◄

R41.840 Attention and concentration deficit
EXCLUDES 1 *attention-deficit hyperactivity disorders (F90.-)*

R41.841 Cognitive communication deficit

R41.842 Visuospatial deficit

R41.843 Psychomotor deficit

R41.844 Frontal lobe and executive function deficit

R41.89 Other symptoms and signs involving cognitive functions and awareness
Anosognosia

R41.9 Unspecified symptoms and signs involving cognitive functions and awareness ▽

R42 Dizziness and giddiness
Light-headedness
Vertigo NOS
EXCLUDES 1 *vertiginous syndromes (H81.-)*
vertigo from infrasound (T75.23)

√4th **R43 Disturbances of smell and taste**

R43.0 Anosmia

R43.1 Parosmia

R43.2 Parageusia

R43.8 Other disturbances of smell and taste
Mixed disturbance of smell and taste

R43.9 Unspecified disturbances of smell and taste ▽

√4th **R44 Other symptoms and signs involving general sensations and perceptions**
EXCLUDES 1 *alcoholic hallucinations (F1.5)*
hallucinations in drug psychosis (F11-F19 with .5)
hallucinations in mood disorders with psychotic symptoms (F30.2, F31.5, F32.3, F33.3)
hallucinations in schizophrenia, schizotypal and delusional disorders (F20-F29)
EXCLUDES 2 *disturbances of skin sensation (R20.-)*

R44.0 Auditory hallucinations

R44.1 Visual hallucinations

R44.2 Other hallucinations

R44.3 Hallucinations, unspecified ▽

R44.8 Other symptoms and signs involving general sensations and perceptions

R44.9 Unspecified symptoms and signs involving general sensations and perceptions ▽

√4th **R45 Symptoms and signs involving emotional state**

R45.0 Nervousness
Nervous tension

R45.1 Restlessness and agitation

R45.2 Unhappiness

R45.3 Demoralization and apathy
EXCLUDES 1 *anhedonia (R45.84)*

R45.4 Irritability and anger

R45.5 Hostility

R45.6 Violent behavior

R45.7 State of emotional shock and stress, unspecified ▽

√5th **R45.8 Other symptoms and signs involving emotional state**

R45.81 Low self-esteem

R45.82 Worries

R45.83 Excessive crying of child, adolescent or adult
EXCLUDES 1 *excessive crying of infant (baby) R68.11*

R45.84 Anhedonia

√6th **R45.85 Homicidal and suicidal ideations**
EXCLUDES 1 *suicide attempt (T14.91)*

R45.850 Homicidal ideations

R45.851 Suicidal Ideations
DEF: Thoughts of committing suicide; no actual attempt of suicide has been made.

R45.86 Emotional lability

R45.87 Impulsiveness

R45.89 Other symptoms and signs involving emotional state

☑ Additional Character Required   √x7th Placeholder Alert   Manifestation Dx   ▽ Unspecified Dx   ►◄ Revised Text   ● New Code   ▲ Revised Code Title

✓4ᵗʰ R46 Symptoms and signs involving appearance and behavior

> EXCLUDES 1   *appearance and behavior in schizophrenia, schizotypal and delusional disorders (F20-F29)*
> *mental and behavioral disorders (F01-F99)*

R46.0 Very low level of personal hygiene

R46.1 Bizarre personal appearance

R46.2 Strange and inexplicable behavior

R46.3 Overactivity

R46.4 Slowness and poor responsiveness

> EXCLUDES 1   *stupor (R40.1)*

R46.5 Suspiciousness and marked evasiveness

R46.6 Undue concern and preoccupation with stressful events

R46.7 Verbosity and circumstantial detail obscuring reason for contact

✓5ᵗʰ R46.8 Other symptoms and signs involving appearance and behavior

     R46.81 Obsessive-compulsive behavior

> EXCLUDES 1   *obsessive-compulsive disorder ▶(F42-)◀*

     R46.89 Other symptoms and signs involving appearance and behavior

Symptoms and signs involving speech and voice (R47-R49)

✓4ᵗʰ R47 Speech disturbances, not elsewhere classified

> EXCLUDES 1   *autism (F84.0)*
> *cluttering (F80.81)*
> *specific developmental disorders of speech and language (F80.-)*
> *stuttering (F80.81)*

✓5ᵗʰ R47.0 Dysphasia and aphasia

     R47.01 Aphasia

> EXCLUDES 1   *aphasia following cerebrovascular disease (I69. with final characters -20)*
> *progressive isolated aphasia (G31.01)*

     R47.02 Dysphasia

> EXCLUDES 1   *dysphasia following cerebrovascular disease (I69. with final characters -21)*

R47.1 Dysarthria and anarthria

> EXCLUDES 1   *dysarthria following cerebrovascular disease (I69. with final characters -22)*

✓5ᵗʰ R47.8 Other speech disturbances

> EXCLUDES 1   *dysarthria following cerebrovascular disease (I69. with final characters -28)*

     R47.81 Slurred speech

     R47.82 *Fluency disorder in conditions classified elsewhere*

         Stuttering in conditions classified elsewhere

         Code first underlying disease or condition, such as:
         Parkinson's disease (G20)

> EXCLUDES 1   *adult onset fluency disorder (F98.5)*
> *childhood onset fluency disorder (F80.81)*
> *fluency disorder (stuttering) following cerebrovascular disease (I69. with final characters -23)*

     R47.89 Other speech disturbances

R47.9 Unspecified speech disturbances   ▽

✓4ᵗʰ R48 Dyslexia and other symbolic dysfunctions, not elsewhere classified

> EXCLUDES 1   *specific developmental disorders of scholastic skills (F81.-)*

R48.0 Dyslexia and alexia

R48.1 Agnosia

     Astereognosia (astereognosis)

     Autotopagnosia

> EXCLUDES 1   *visual object agnosia (R48.3)*

R48.2 Apraxia

> EXCLUDES 1   *apraxia following cerebrovascular disease (I69. with final characters -90)*

R48.3 Visual agnosia

     Prosopagnosia

     Simultanagnosia (asimultagnosia)

R48.8 Other symbolic dysfunctions

     Acalculia

     Agraphia

R48.9 Unspecified symbolic dysfunctions   ▽

✓4ᵗʰ R49 Voice and resonance disorders

> EXCLUDES 1   *psychogenic voice and resonance disorders (F44.4)*

R49.0 Dysphonia

     Hoarseness

R49.1 Aphonia

     Loss of voice

✓5ᵗʰ R49.2 Hypernasality and hyponasality

     R49.21 Hypernasality

     R49.22 Hyponasality

R49.8 Other voice and resonance disorders

R49.9 Unspecified voice and resonance disorder   ▽

     Change in voice NOS

     Resonance disorder NOS

General symptoms and signs (R50-R69)

✓4ᵗʰ R50 Fever of other and unknown origin

> EXCLUDES 1   *chills without fever (R68.83)*
> *febrile convulsions (R56.0-)*
> *fever of unknown origin during labor (O75.2)*
> *fever of unknown origin in newborn (P81.9)*
> *hypothermia due to illness (R68.0)*
> *malignant hyperthermia due to anesthesia (T88.3)*
> *puerperal pyrexia NOS (O86.4)*

R50.2 Drug induced fever

     Use additional code for adverse effect, if applicable, to identify drug (T36-T50 with fifth or sixth character 5)

> EXCLUDES 1   *postvaccination (postimmunization) fever (R50.83)*

✓5ᵗʰ R50.8 Other specified fever

     R50.81 *Fever presenting with conditions classified elsewhere*

         Code first underlying condition when associated fever is present, such as with:

         leukemia (C91-C95)

         neutropenia (D70.-)

         sickle-cell disease (D57.-)

         AHA: 2014,4Q,22

     R50.82 Postprocedural fever

> EXCLUDES 1   *postprocedural infection ▶(T81.4-)◀*
> *posttransfusion fever (R50.84)*
> *postvaccination (postimmunization) fever (R50.83)*

     R50.83 Postvaccination fever

         Postimmunization fever

     R50.84 Febrile nonhemolytic transfusion reaction

         FNHTR

         Posttransfusion fever

R50.9 Fever, unspecified   ▽

     Fever NOS

     Fever of unknown origin [FUO]

     Fever with chills

     Fever with rigors

     Hyperpyrexia NOS

     Persistent fever

     Pyrexia NOS

R51 Headache

     Facial pain NOS

> EXCLUDES 1   *atypical face pain (G50.1)*
> *migraine and other headache syndromes (G43-G44)*
> *trigeminal neuralgia (G50.0)*

EXCLUDES 1 Not coded here   EXCLUDES 2 Not included here   N Newborn Age : 0   P Pediatric Age : 0-17   M Maternity Age : 12-55   A Adult Age : 15-124

R52 Pain, unspecified ▽

    Acute pain NOS

    Generalized pain NOS

    Pain NOS

    EXCLUDES 1   *acute and chronic pain, not elsewhere classified (G89.-)*

        localized pain, unspecified type - code to pain by site, such as:

          abdomen pain (R10.-)

          back pain (M54.9)

          breast pain (N64.4)

          chest pain (R07.1-R07.9)

          ear pain (H92.0-)

          eye pain (H57.1)

          headache (R51)

          joint pain (M25.5-)

          limb pain (M79.6-)

          lumbar region pain (M54.5)

          pelvic and perineal pain (R10.2)

          renal colic (N23)

          shoulder pain (M25.51-)

          spine pain (M54.-)

          throat pain (R07.0)

          tongue pain (K14.6)

          tooth pain (K08.8)

        pain disorders exclusively related to psychological factors (F45.41)

✓4ᵗʰ R53 Malaise and fatigue

    R53.0 Neoplastic (malignant) related fatigue

        Code first associated neoplasm

    R53.1 Weakness

        Asthenia NOS

        EXCLUDES 1   *age-related weakness (R54)*

            muscle weakness (M62.8-)

            ▶*sarcopenia (M62.84)*◀

            senile asthenia (R54)

        AHA: 2015,1Q,25

    R53.2 Functional quadriplegia

        Complete immobility due to severe physical disability or frailty

        EXCLUDES 1   *frailty NOS (R54)*

            hysterical paralysis (F44.4)

            immobility syndrome (M62.3)

            neurologic quadriplegia (G82.5-)

            quadriplegia (G82.50)

        AHA: 2016,2Q,6

        DEF: Inability to move due to a nonphysiological condition, such as dementia; no mental ability to move independently; typically found in severely demented patients.

    ✓5ᵗʰ R53.8 Other malaise and fatigue

        EXCLUDES 1   *combat exhaustion and fatigue (F43.0)*

            congenital debility (P96.9)

            exhaustion and fatigue due to depressive episode (F32.-)

            exhaustion and fatigue due to excessive exertion (T73.3)

            exhaustion and fatigue due to exposure (T73.2)

            exhaustion and fatigue due to heat (T67.-)

            exhaustion and fatigue due to pregnancy (O26.8-)

            exhaustion and fatigue due to recurrent depressive episode (F33)

            exhaustion and fatigue due to senile debility (R54)

        R53.81 Other malaise

           Chronic debility

           Debility NOS

           General physical deterioration

           Malaise NOS

           Nervous debility

           EXCLUDES 1   *age-related physical debility (R54)*

        R53.82 Chronic fatigue, unspecified ▽

           Chronic fatigue syndrome NOS

           EXCLUDES 1   *postviral fatigue syndrome (G93.3)*

        R53.83 Other fatigue

           Fatigue NOS

           Lack of energy

           Lethargy

           Tiredness

R54 Age-related physical debility Ⓐ

    Frailty

    Old age

    Senescence

    Senile asthenia

    Senile debility

    EXCLUDES 1   *age-related cognitive decline (R41.81)*

        ▶*sarcopenia (M62.84)*◀

        senile psychosis (F03)

        senility NOS (R41.81)

R55 Syncope and collapse

    Blackout

    Fainting

    Vasovagal attack

    EXCLUDES 1   *cardiogenic shock (R57.0)*

        carotid sinus syncope (G90.01)

        heat syncope (T67.1)

        neurocirculatory asthenia (F45.8)

        neurogenic orthostatic hypotension (G90.3)

        orthostatic hypotension (I95.1)

        postprocedural shock (T81.1-)

        psychogenic syncope (F48.8)

        shock NOS (R57.9)

        shock complicating or following abortion or ectopic or molar pregnancy (O00-O07, O08.3)

        shock complicating or following labor and delivery (O75.1)

        Stokes-Adams attack (I45.9)

        unconsciousness NOS (R40.2-)

✓4ᵗʰ R56 Convulsions, not elsewhere classified

    EXCLUDES 1   *dissociative convulsions and seizures (F44.5)*

        epileptic convulsions and seizures (G40.-)

        newborn convulsions and seizures (P90)

    ✓5ᵗʰ R56.0 Febrile convulsions

        R56.00 Simple febrile convulsions

           Febrile convulsion NOS

           Febrile seizure NOS

        R56.01 Complex febrile convulsions

           Atypical febrile seizure

           Complex febrile seizure

           Complicated febrile seizure

           EXCLUDES 1   *status epilepticus (G40.901)*

    R56.1 Post traumatic seizures

        EXCLUDES 1   *post traumatic epilepsy (G40.-)*

    R56.9 Unspecified convulsions ▽

        Convulsion disorder

        Fit NOS

        Recurrent convulsions

        Seizure(s) (convulsive) NOS

✓4ᵗʰ R57 Shock, not elsewhere classified

    EXCLUDES 1   *anaphylactic shock NOS (T78.2)*

        anaphylactic reaction or shock due to adverse food reaction (T78.0-)

        anaphylactic shock due to adverse effect of correct drug or medicament properly administered (T88.6)

        anaphylactic shock due to serum (T80.5-)

        anesthetic shock (T88.3)

        electric shock (T75.4)

        obstetric shock (O75.1)

        postprocedural shock (T81.1-)

        psychic shock (F43.0)

        septic shock (R65.21)

        shock complicating or following ectopic or molar pregnancy (O00-O07, O08.3)

        shock due to lightning (T75.01)

        traumatic shock (T79.4)

        toxic shock syndrome (A48.3)

    R57.0 Cardiogenic shock

        DEF: Associated with myocardial infarction, cardiac tamponade, and massive pulmonary embolism; symptoms include mental confusion, reduced blood pressure, tachycardia, pallor, and cold, clammy skin.

    R57.1 Hypovolemic shock

    R57.8 Other shock

    R57.9 Shock, unspecified ▽

        Failure of peripheral circulation NOS

☑ Additional Character Required   ✓7ᵗʰ Placeholder Alert   Manifestation Dx   ▽ Unspecified Dx   ▶◀ Revised Text   ● New Code   ▲ Revised Code Title

ICD-10-CM 2017   **873**

R58 Hemorrhage, not elsewhere classified
Hemorrhage NOS
EXCLUDES 1 *hemorrhage included with underlying conditions, such as:*
acute duodenal ulcer with hemorrhage (K26.0)
acute gastritis with bleeding (K29.01)
ulcerative enterocolitis with rectal bleeding (K51.01)

√4ᵗʰ **R59 Enlarged lymph nodes**
INCLUDES swollen glands
EXCLUDES 1 *acute lymphadenitis (L04.-)*
chronic lymphadenitis (I88.1)
lymphadenitis NOS (I88.9)
mesenteric (acute) (chronic) lymphadenitis (I88.0)

R59.0 Localized enlarged lymph nodes

R59.1 Generalized enlarged lymph nodes
Lymphadenopathy NOS

R59.9 Enlarged lymph nodes, unspecified ▽

√4ᵗʰ **R60 Edema, not elsewhere classified**
EXCLUDES 1 *angioneurotic edema (T78.3)*
ascites (R18.-)
cerebral edema (G93.6)
cerebral edema due to birth injury (P11.0)
edema of larynx (J38.4)
edema of nasopharynx (J39.2)
edema of pharynx (J39.2)
gestational edema (O12.0-)
hereditary edema (Q82.0)
hydrops fetalis NOS (P83.2)
hydrothorax (J94.8)
nutritional edema (E40-E46)
hydrops fetalis NOS (P83.2)
newborn edema (P83.3)
pulmonary edema (J81.-)

R60.0 Localized edema

R60.1 Generalized edema

R60.9 Edema, unspecified ▽
Fluid retention NOS

R61 Generalized hyperhidrosis
Excessive sweating
Night sweats
Secondary hyperhidrosis
Code first, if applicable, menopausal and female climacteric states
(N95.1)
EXCLUDES 1 *focal (primary) (secondary) hyperhidrosis (L74.5-)*
Frey's syndrome (L74.52)
localized (primary) (secondary) hyperhidrosis (L74.5-)

√4ᵗʰ **R62 Lack of expected normal physiological development in childhood and adults**
EXCLUDES 1 *delayed puberty (E30.0)*
gonadal dysgenesis (Q99.1)
hypopituitarism (E23.0)

R62.0 Delayed milestone in childhood P
Delayed attainment of expected physiological developmental stage
Late talker
Late walker

√5ᵗʰ **R62.5 Other and unspecified lack of expected normal physiological development in childhood**
EXCLUDES 1 *HIV disease resulting in failure to thrive (B20)*
physical retardation due to malnutrition (E45)

R62.50 Unspecified lack of expected normal physiological development in childhood ▽
Infantilism NOS

R62.51 Failure to thrive (child) P
Failure to gain weight
EXCLUDES 1 *failure to thrive in child under 28 days old (P92.6)*
DEF: Organic failure to thrive (FTT): Acute or chronic illness that interferes with nutritional intake, absorption, metabolism excretion, and energy requirements; nonorganic FTT is a symptom of neglect or abuse.

R62.52 Short stature (child)
Lack of growth
Physical retardation
Short stature NOS
EXCLUDES 1 *short stature due to endocrine disorder (E34.3)*

R62.59 Other lack of expected normal physiological development in childhood

R62.7 Adult failure to thrive A

√4ᵗʰ **R63 Symptoms and signs concerning food and fluid intake**
EXCLUDES 1 *bulimia NOS (F50.2)*
eating disorders of nonorganic origin (F50.-)
malnutrition (E40-E46)

R63.0 Anorexia
Loss of appetite
EXCLUDES 1 *anorexia nervosa (F50.0-)*
loss of appetite of nonorganic origin ▶(F50.89)◀

R63.1 Polydipsia
Excessive thirst

R63.2 Polyphagia
Excessive eating
Hyperalimentation NOS

R63.3 Feeding difficulties
Feeding problem (elderly) (infant) NOS
EXCLUDES 1 *feeding problems of newborn (P92.-)*
infant feeding disorder of nonorganic origin (F98.2-)

R63.4 Abnormal weight loss

R63.5 Abnormal weight gain
EXCLUDES 1 *excessive weight gain in pregnancy (O26.0-)*
obesity (E66.-)

R63.6 Underweight
Use additional code to identify body mass index (BMI), if known
(Z68.-)
EXCLUDES 1 *abnormal weight loss (R63.4)*
anorexia nervosa (F50.0-)
malnutrition (E40-E46)

R63.8 Other symptoms and signs concerning food and fluid intake

R64 Cachexia
Wasting syndrome
Code first underlying condition, if known
EXCLUDES 1 *abnormal weight loss (R63.4)*
nutritional marasmus (E41)

√4ᵗʰ **R65 Symptoms and signs specifically associated with systemic inflammation and infection**

√5ᵗʰ **R65.1 Systemic inflammatory response syndrome [SIRS] of non-infectious origin**
Code first underlying condition, such as:
heatstroke (T67.0)
injury and trauma (S00-T88)
EXCLUDES 1 *sepsis - code to infection*
severe sepsis (R65.2)

R65.10 Systemic inflammatory response syndrome [SIRS] of non-infectious origin without acute organ dysfunction
Systemic inflammatory response syndrome (SIRS) NOS

R65.11 Systemic inflammatory response syndrome [SIRS] of non-infectious origin with acute organ dysfunction
Use additional code to identify specific acute organ dysfunction, such as:
acute kidney failure (N17.-)
acute respiratory failure (J96.0-)
critical illness myopathy (G72.81)
critical illness polyneuropathy (G62.81)
disseminated intravascular coagulopathy [DIC] (D65)
encephalopathy (metabolic) (septic) (G93.41)
hepatic failure (K72.0-)

EXCLUDES 1 Not coded here   EXCLUDES 2 Not included here   N Newborn Age : 0   P Pediatric Age : 0-17   M Maternity Age : 12-55   A Adult Age : 15-124

874   ICD-10-CM 2017

R58–R65.11

☑5ᵗʰ **R65.2** **Severe sepsis**

Infection with associated acute organ dysfunction

Sepsis with acute organ dysfunction

Sepsis with multiple organ dysfunction

Systemic inflammatory response syndrome due to infectious process with acute organ dysfunction

Code first underlying infection, such as:

infection following a procedure ▶(T81.4-)◀

infections following infusion, transfusion and therapeutic injection (T80.2-)

puerperal sepsis (O85)

sepsis following complete or unspecified spontaneous abortion (O03.87)

sepsis following ectopic and molar pregnancy (O08.82)

sepsis following incomplete spontaneous abortion (O03.37)

sepsis following (induced) termination of pregnancy (O04.87)

sepsis NOS (A41.9)

Use additional code to identify specific acute organ dysfunction, such as:

acute kidney failure (N17.-)

acute respiratory failure (J96.0-)

critical illness myopathy (G72.81)

critical illness polyneuropathy (G62.81)

disseminated intravascular coagulopathy [DIC] (D65)

encephalopathy (metabolic) (septic) (G93.41)

hepatic failure (K72.0-)

     R65.20 **Severe sepsis without septic shock**

         Severe sepsis NOS

         AHA: 2013,4Q,119

     R65.21 **Severe sepsis with septic shock**

☑4ᵗʰ **R68** **Other general symptoms and signs**

     R68.0 **Hypothermia, not associated with low environmental temperature**

         EXCLUDES 1   *hypothermia NOS (accidental) (T68)*

                 hypothermia due to anesthesia (T88.51)

                 hypothermia due to low environmental temperature (T68)

                 newborn hypothermia (P80.-)

☑5ᵗʰ **R68.1** **Nonspecific symptoms peculiar to infancy**

         EXCLUDES 1   *colic, infantile (R10.83)*

                 neonatal cerebral irritability (P91.3)

                 teething syndrome (K00.7)

     R68.11 **Excessive crying of infant (baby)**   P

         EXCLUDES 1   *excessive crying of child, adolescent, or adult (R45.83)*

     R68.12 **Fussy infant (baby)**   P

         Irritable infant

     R68.13 **Apparent life threatening event in infant [ALTE]**   P

         Apparent life threatening event in newborn

         Code first confirmed diagnosis, if known

         Use additional code(s) for associated signs and symptoms if no confirmed diagnosis established, or if signs and symptoms are not associated routinely with confirmed diagnosis, or provide additional information for cause of ALTE

     R68.19 **Other nonspecific symptoms peculiar to infancy**   P

     R68.2 **Dry mouth, unspecified**   ▽

         EXCLUDES 1   *dry mouth due to dehydration (E86.0)*

                 dry mouth due to sicca syndrome [Sjögren] (M35.0-)

                 salivary gland hyposecretion (K11.7)

     R68.3 **Clubbing of fingers**

         Clubbing of nails

         EXCLUDES 1   *congenital clubfinger (Q68.1)*

☑5ᵗʰ **R68.8** **Other general symptoms and signs**

     R68.81 **Early satiety**

     R68.82 **Decreased libido**   A

         Decreased sexual desire

     R68.83 **Chills (without fever)**

         Chills NOS

         EXCLUDES 1   *chills with fever (R50.9)*

     R68.84 **Jaw pain**

         Mandibular pain

         Maxilla pain

         EXCLUDES 1   *temporomandibular joint arthralgia ▶(M26.62-)◀*

     R68.89 **Other general symptoms and signs**

R69 **Illness, unspecified**   ▽

     Unknown and unspecified cases of morbidity

Abnormal findings on examination of blood, without diagnosis (R70–R79)

     EXCLUDES 2   ▶*abnormal findings on antenatal screening of mother (O28.-)◀*

         ▶*abnormalities of lipids (E78.-)◀*

         ▶*abnormalities of platelets and thrombocytes (D69.-)◀*

         ▶*abnormalities of white blood cells classified elsewhere (D70-D72)◀*

         ▶*coagulation hemorrhagic disorders (D65-D68)◀*

         ▶*diagnostic abnormal findings classified elsewhere - see Alphabetical Index◀*

         ▶*hemorrhagic and hematological disorders of newborn (P50-P61)◀*

☑4ᵗʰ **R70** **Elevated erythrocyte sedimentation rate and abnormality of plasma viscosity**

     R70.0 **Elevated erythrocyte sedimentation rate**

     R70.1 **Abnormal plasma viscosity**

☑4ᵗʰ **R71** **Abnormality of red blood cells**

     EXCLUDES 1   *anemias (D50–D64)*

         anemia of premature infant (P61.2)

         benign (familial) polycythemia (D75.0)

         congenital anemias (P61.2-P61.4)

         newborn anemia due to isoimmunization (P55.-)

         polycythemia neonatorum (P61.1)

         polycythemia NOS (D75.1)

         polycythemia vera (D45)

         secondary polycythemia (D75.1)

     R71.0 **Precipitous drop in hematocrit**

         Drop (precipitous) in hemoglobin

         Drop in hematocrit

     R71.8 **Other abnormality of red blood cells**

         Abnormal red-cell morphology NOS

         Abnormal red-cell volume NOS

         Anisocytosis

         Poikilocytosis

☑4ᵗʰ **R73** **Elevated blood glucose level**

     EXCLUDES 1   *diabetes mellitus (E08-E13)*

         diabetes mellitus in pregnancy, childbirth and the puerperium (O24.-)

         neonatal disorders (P70.0-P70.2)

         postsurgical hypoinsulinemia (E89.1)

☑5ᵗʰ **R73.0** **Abnormal glucose**

         EXCLUDES 1   *abnormal glucose in pregnancy (O99.81-)*

                 diabetes mellitus (E08-E13)

                 dysmetabolic syndrome X (E88.81)

                 gestational diabetes (O24.4-)

                 glycosuria (R81)

                 hypoglycemia (E16.2)

     R73.01 **Impaired fasting glucose**

         Elevated fasting glucose

     R73.02 **Impaired glucose tolerance (oral)**

         Elevated glucose tolerance

    • **R73.03** **Prediabetes**

         Latent diabetes

     R73.09 **Other abnormal glucose**

         Abnormal glucose NOS

         Abnormal non-fasting glucose tolerance

     R73.9 **Hyperglycemia, unspecified**   ▽

☑4ᵗʰ **R74** **Abnormal serum enzyme levels**

     R74.0 **Nonspecific elevation of levels of transaminase and lactic acid dehydrogenase [LDH]**

     R74.8 **Abnormal levels of other serum enzymes**

         Abnormal level of acid phosphatase

         Abnormal level of alkaline phosphatase

         Abnormal level of amylase

         Abnormal level of lipase [triacylglycerol lipase]

     R74.9 **Abnormal serum enzyme level, unspecified**   ▽

☑ Additional Character Required   ✓x7ᵗʰ Placeholder Alert   Manifestation Dx   ▽ Unspecified Dx   ▶◀ Revised Text   ● New Code   ▲ Revised Code Title

ICD-10-CM 2017   875

R75 Inconclusive laboratory evidence of human immunodeficiency virus [HIV]

Nonconclusive HIV-test finding in infants

> EXCLUDES 1   asymptomatic human immunodeficiency virus [HIV] infection status (Z21)
> human immunodeficiency virus [HIV] disease (B20)

✓4th **R76 Other abnormal immunological findings in serum**

R76.0 Raised antibody titer

> EXCLUDES 1   isoimmunization in pregnancy (O36.0-O36.1)
> isoimmunization affecting newborn (P55.-)

✓5th **R76.1 Nonspecific reaction to test for tuberculosis**

R76.11 Nonspecific reaction to tuberculin skin test without active tuberculosis

Abnormal result of Mantoux test

PPD positive

Tuberculin (skin test) positive

Tuberculin (skin test) reactor

> EXCLUDES 1   nonspecific reaction to cell mediated immunity measurement of gamma interferon antigen response without active tuberculosis (R76.12)

R76.12 Nonspecific reaction to cell mediated immunity measurement of gamma interferon antigen response without active tuberculosis

Nonspecific reaction to QuantiFERON-TB test (QFT) without active tuberculosis

> EXCLUDES 1   nonspecific reaction to tuberculin skin test without active tuberculosis (R76.11)
> positive tuberculin skin test (R76.11)

R76.8 Other specified abnormal immunological findings in serum

Raised level of immunoglobulins NOS

R76.9 Abnormal immunological finding in serum, unspecified ▽

✓4th **R77 Other abnormalities of plasma proteins**

> EXCLUDES 1   disorders of plasma-protein metabolism (E88.0)

R77.0 Abnormality of albumin

R77.1 Abnormality of globulin

Hyperglobulinemia NOS

R77.2 Abnormality of alphafetoprotein

R77.8 Other specified abnormalities of plasma proteins

R77.9 Abnormality of plasma protein, unspecified ▽

✓4th **R78 Findings of drugs and other substances, not normally found in blood**

Use additional code to identify the any retained foreign body, if applicable (Z18.-)

> EXCLUDES 1   mental or behavioral disorders due to psychoactive substance use (F10-F19)

R78.0 Finding of alcohol in blood

Use additional external cause code (Y90.-), for detail regarding alcohol level

R78.1 Finding of opiate drug in blood

R78.2 Finding of cocaine in blood

R78.3 Finding of hallucinogen in blood

R78.4 Finding of other drugs of addictive potential in blood

R78.5 Finding of other psychotropic drug in blood

R78.6 Finding of steroid agent in blood

✓5th **R78.7 Finding of abnormal level of heavy metals in blood**

R78.71 Abnormal lead level in blood

> EXCLUDES 1   lead poisoning (T56.0-)

R78.79 Finding of abnormal level of heavy metals in blood

✓5th **R78.8 Finding of other specified substances, not normally found in blood**

R78.81 Bacteremia

> EXCLUDES 1   ►sepsis — code to specified infection◄

R78.89 Finding of other specified substances, not normally found in blood

Finding of abnormal level of lithium in blood

R78.9 Finding of unspecified substance, not normally found in blood ▽

✓4th **R79 Other abnormal findings of blood chemistry**

Use additional code to identify any retained foreign body, if applicable (Z18.-)

> EXCLUDES 1   abnormality of fluid, electrolyte or acid-base balance (E86-E87)
> asymptomatic hyperuricemia (E79.0)
> hyperglycemia NOS (R73.9)
> hypoglycemia NOS (E16.2)
> neonatal hypoglycemia (P70.3-P70.4)
> specific findings indicating disorder of amino-acid metabolism (E70-E72)
> specific findings indicating disorder of carbohydrate metabolism (E73-E74)
> specific findings indicating disorder of lipid metabolism (E75.-)

R79.0 Abnormal level of blood mineral

Abnormal blood level of cobalt

Abnormal blood level of copper

Abnormal blood level of iron

Abnormal blood level of magnesium

Abnormal blood level of mineral NEC

Abnormal blood level of zinc

> EXCLUDES 1   abnormal level of lithium (R78.89)
> disorders of mineral metabolism (E83.-)
> neonatal hypomagnesemia (P71.2)
> nutritional mineral deficiency (E58-E61)

R79.1 Abnormal coagulation profile

Abnormal or prolonged bleeding time

Abnormal or prolonged coagulation time

Abnormal or prolonged partial thromboplastin time [PTT]

Abnormal or prolonged prothrombin time [PT]

> EXCLUDES 1   coagulation defects (D68.-)

✓5th **R79.8 Other specified abnormal findings of blood chemistry**

R79.81 Abnormal blood-gas level

R79.82 Elevated C-reactive protein [CRP]

R79.89 Other specified abnormal findings of blood chemistry

R79.9 Abnormal finding of blood chemistry, unspecified ▽

Abnormal findings on examination of urine, without diagnosis (R80-R82)

> EXCLUDES 1   abnormal findings on antenatal screening of mother (O28.-)
> diagnostic abnormal findings classified elsewhere - see Alphabetical Index
> specific findings indicating disorder of amino-acid metabolism (E70-E72)
> specific findings indicating disorder of carbohydrate metabolism (E73-E74)

✓4th **R80 Proteinuria**

> EXCLUDES 1   gestational proteinuria (O12.1-)

R80.0 Isolated proteinuria

Idiopathic proteinuria

> EXCLUDES 1   isolated proteinuria with specific morphological lesion (N06.-)

R80.1 Persistent proteinuria, unspecified ▽

R80.2 Orthostatic proteinuria, unspecified ▽

Postural proteinuria

R80.3 Bence Jones proteinuria

R80.8 Other proteinuria

R80.9 Proteinuria, unspecified ▽

Albuminuria NOS

R81 Glycosuria

> EXCLUDES 1   renal glycosuria (E74.8)

✓4th **R82 Other and unspecified abnormal findings in urine**

> INCLUDES   chromoabnormalities in urine

Use additional code to identify any retained foreign body, if applicable (Z18.-)

> EXCLUDES 2   hematuria (R31.-)

R82.0 Chyluria

> EXCLUDES 1   filarial chyluria (B74.-)

R82.1 Myoglobinuria

R82.2 Biliuria

R82.3 Hemoglobinuria

> EXCLUDES 1   hemoglobinuria due to hemolysis from external causes NEC (D59.6)
> hemoglobinuria due to paroxysmal nocturnal [Marchiafava-Micheli] (D59.5)

| EXCLUDES 1 Not coded here | EXCLUDES 2 Not included here | N Newborn Age : 0 | P Pediatric Age : 0-17 | M Maternity Age : 12-55 | A Adult Age : 15-124 |

876

ICD-10-CM 2017

R82.4 Acetonuria
Ketonuria

R82.5 Elevated urine levels of drugs, medicaments and biological substances
Elevated urine levels of catecholamines
Elevated urine levels of indoleacetic acid
Elevated urine levels of 17-ketosteroids
Elevated urine levels of steroids

R82.6 Abnormal urine levels of substances chiefly nonmedicinal as to source
Abnormal urine level of heavy metals

✓5ᵗʰ **R82.7 Abnormal findings on microbiological examination of urine**
EXCLUDES 1 *colonization status (Z22.-)*

●   **R82.71 Bacteriuria**

●   **R82.79 Other abnormal findings on microbiological examination of urine**
Positive culture findings of urine

R82.8 Abnormal findings on cytological and histological examination of urine

✓5ᵗʰ **R82.9 Other and unspecified abnormal findings in urine**

R82.90 Unspecified abnormal findings in urine ▽

R82.91 Other chromoabnormalities of urine
Chromoconversion (dipstick)
Idiopathic dipstick converts positive for blood with no cellular forms in sediment
EXCLUDES 1 *hemoglobinuria (R82.3)*
myoglobinuria (R82.1)

R82.99 Other abnormal findings in urine
Cells and casts in urine
Crystalluria
Melanuria

Abnormal findings on examination of other body fluids, substances and tissues, without diagnosis (R83-R89)

EXCLUDES 1 *abnormal findings on antenatal screening of mother (O28.-)*
diagnostic abnormal findings classified elsewhere - see Alphabetical Index
EXCLUDES 2 *abnormal findings on examination of blood, without diagnosis (R70-R79)*
abnormal findings on examination of urine, without diagnosis (R80-R82)
abnormal tumor markers (R97.-)

✓4ᵗʰ **R83 Abnormal findings in cerebrospinal fluid**

R83.0 Abnormal level of enzymes in cerebrospinal fluid

R83.1 Abnormal level of hormones in cerebrospinal fluid

R83.2 Abnormal level of other drugs, medicaments and biological substances in cerebrospinal fluid

R83.3 Abnormal level of substances chiefly nonmedicinal as to source in cerebrospinal fluid

R83.4 Abnormal immunological findings in cerebrospinal fluid

R83.5 Abnormal microbiological findings in cerebrospinal fluid
Positive culture findings in cerebrospinal fluid
EXCLUDES 1 *colonization status (Z22.-)*

R83.6 Abnormal cytological findings in cerebrospinal fluid

R83.8 Other abnormal findings in cerebrospinal fluid
Abnormal chromosomal findings in cerebrospinal fluid

R83.9 Unspecified abnormal finding in cerebrospinal fluid ▽

✓4ᵗʰ **R84 Abnormal findings in specimens from respiratory organs and thorax**
INCLUDES abnormal findings in bronchial washings
abnormal findings in nasal secretions
abnormal findings in pleural fluid
abnormal findings in sputum
abnormal findings in throat scrapings
EXCLUDES 1 *blood-stained sputum (R04.2)*

R84.0 Abnormal level of enzymes in specimens from respiratory organs and thorax

R84.1 Abnormal level of hormones in specimens from respiratory organs and thorax

R84.2 Abnormal level of other drugs, medicaments and biological substances in specimens from respiratory organs and thorax

R84.3 Abnormal level of substances chiefly nonmedicinal as to source in specimens from respiratory organs and thorax

R84.4 Abnormal immunological findings in specimens from respiratory organs and thorax

R84.5 Abnormal microbiological findings in specimens from respiratory organs and thorax
Positive culture findings in specimens from respiratory organs and thorax
EXCLUDES 1 *colonization status (Z22.-)*

R84.6 Abnormal cytological findings in specimens from respiratory organs and thorax

R84.7 Abnormal histological findings in specimens from respiratory organs and thorax

R84.8 Other abnormal findings in specimens from respiratory organs and thorax
Abnormal chromosomal findings in specimens from respiratory organs and thorax

R84.9 Unspecified abnormal finding in specimens from respiratory organs and thorax ▽

✓4ᵗʰ **R85 Abnormal findings in specimens from digestive organs and abdominal cavity**
INCLUDES abnormal findings in peritoneal fluid
abnormal findings in saliva
EXCLUDES 1 *cloudy peritoneal dialysis effluent (R88.0)*
fecal abnormalities (R19.5)

R85.0 Abnormal level of enzymes in specimens from digestive organs and abdominal cavity

R85.1 Abnormal level of hormones in specimens from digestive organs and abdominal cavity

R85.2 Abnormal level of other drugs, medicaments and biological substances in specimens from digestive organs and abdominal cavity

R85.3 Abnormal level of substances chiefly nonmedicinal as to source in specimens from digestive organs and abdominal cavity

R85.4 Abnormal immunological findings in specimens from digestive organs and abdominal cavity

R85.5 Abnormal microbiological findings in specimens from digestive organs and abdominal cavity
Positive culture findings in specimens from digestive organs and abdominal cavity
EXCLUDES 1 *colonization status (Z22.-)*

✓5ᵗʰ **R85.6 Abnormal cytological findings in specimens from digestive organs and abdominal cavity**

✓6ᵗʰ **R85.61 Abnormal cytologic smear of anus**
EXCLUDES 1 *abnormal cytological findings in specimens from other digestive organs and abdominal cavity (R85.69)*
anal intraepithelial neoplasia I [AIN I] (K62.82)
anal intraepithelial neoplasia II [AIN II] (K62.82)
anal intraepithelial neoplasia III [AIN III] (D01.3)
carcinoma in situ of anus (histologically confirmed) (D01.3)
dysplasia (mild) (moderate) of anus (histologically confirmed) (K62.82)
severe dysplasia of anus (histologically confirmed) (D01.3)
EXCLUDES 2 *anal high risk human papillomavirus (HPV) DNA test positive (R85.81)*
anal low risk human papillomavirus (HPV) DNA test positive (R85.82)

R85.610 Atypical squamous cells of undetermined significance on cytologic smear of anus [ASC-US]

R85.611 Atypical squamous cells cannot exclude high grade squamous intraepithelial lesion on cytologic smear of anus [ASC-H]

R85.612 Low grade squamous intraepithelial lesion on cytologic smear of anus [LGSIL]

R85.613 High grade squamous intraepithelial lesion on cytologic smear of anus [HGSIL]

R85.614 Cytologic evidence of malignancy on smear of anus

R85.615 Unsatisfactory cytologic smear of anus
Inadequate sample of cytologic smear of anus

R85.616 Satisfactory anal smear but lacking transformation zone

R85.618 Other abnormal cytological findings on specimens from anus

---

R85.619   **Unspecified abnormal cytological findings in specimens from anus** ▽
Abnormal anal cytology NOS
Atypical glandular cells of anus NOS

R85.69   **Abnormal cytological findings in specimens from other digestive organs and abdominal cavity**

R85.7   **Abnormal histological findings in specimens from digestive organs and abdominal cavity**

✓5ᵗʰ R85.8   **Other abnormal findings in specimens from digestive organs and abdominal cavity**

R85.81   **Anal high risk human papillomavirus [HPV] DNA test positive**
    EXCLUDES 1   *anogenital warts due to human papillomavirus (HPV) (A63.0)*
condyloma acuminatum (A63.0)

R85.82   **Anal low risk human papillomavirus [HPV] DNA test positive**
Use additional code for associated human papillomavirus (B97.7)

R85.89   **Other abnormal findings in specimens from digestive organs and abdominal cavity**
Abnormal chromosomal findings in specimens from digestive organs and abdominal cavity

R85.9   **Unspecified abnormal finding in specimens from digestive organs and abdominal cavity** ▽

✓4ᵗʰ **R86   Abnormal findings in specimens from male genital organs**
   INCLUDES   abnormal findings in prostatic secretions
abnormal findings in semen, seminal fluid
abnormal spermatozoa
    EXCLUDES 1   *azoospermia (N46.0-)*
oligospermia (N46.1-)

R86.0   **Abnormal level of enzymes in specimens from male genital organs** ♂

R86.1   **Abnormal level of hormones in specimens from male genital organs** ♂

R86.2   **Abnormal level of other drugs, medicaments and biological substances in specimens from male genital organs** ♂

R86.3   **Abnormal level of substances chiefly nonmedicinal as to source in specimens from male genital organs** ♂

R86.4   **Abnormal immunological findings in specimens from male genital organs** ♂

R86.5   **Abnormal microbiological findings in specimens from male genital organs** ♂
Positive culture findings in specimens from male genital organs
    EXCLUDES 1   *colonization status (Z22.-)*

R86.6   **Abnormal cytological findings in specimens from male genital organs** ♂

R86.7   **Abnormal histological findings in specimens from male genital organs** ♂

R86.8   **Other abnormal findings in specimens from male genital organs** ♂
Abnormal chromosomal findings in specimens from male genital organs

R86.9   **Unspecified abnormal finding in specimens from male genital organs** ♂ ▽

✓4ᵗʰ **R87   Abnormal findings in specimens from female genital organs**
   INCLUDES   abnormal findings in secretion and smears from cervix uteri
abnormal findings in secretion and smears from vagina
abnormal findings in secretion and smears from vulva

R87.0   **Abnormal level of enzymes in specimens from female genital organs** ♀

R87.1   **Abnormal level of hormones in specimens from female genital organs** ♀

R87.2   **Abnormal level of other drugs, medicaments and biological substances in specimens from female genital organs** ♀

R87.3   **Abnormal level of substances chiefly nonmedicinal as to source in specimens from female genital organs** ♀

R87.4   **Abnormal immunological findings in specimens from female genital organs** ♀

R87.5   **Abnormal microbiological findings in specimens from female genital organs** ♀
Positive culture findings in specimens from female genital organs
    EXCLUDES 1   *colonization status (Z22.-)*

✓5ᵗʰ R87.6   **Abnormal cytological findings in specimens from female genital organs**

✓6ᵗʰ R87.61   **Abnormal cytological findings in specimens from cervix uteri**
    EXCLUDES 1   *abnormal cytological findings in specimens from other female genital organs (R87.69)*
abnormal cytological findings in specimens from vagina (R87.62-)
carcinoma in situ of cervix uteri (histologically confirmed) (D06.-)
cervical intraepithelial neoplasia I [CIN I] (N87.0)
cervical intraepithelial neoplasia II [CIN II] (N87.1)
cervical intraepithelial neoplasia III [CIN III] (D06.-)
dysplasia (mild) (moderate) of cervix uteri (histologically confirmed) (N87.-)
severe dysplasia of cervix uteri (histologically confirmed) (D06.-)
    EXCLUDES 2   *cervical high risk human papillomavirus (HPV) DNA test positive (R87.810)*
cervical low risk human papillomavirus (HPV) DNA test positive (R87.820)

R87.610   **Atypical squamous cells of undetermined significance on cytologic smear of cervix [ASC-US]** ♀

R87.611   **Atypical squamous cells cannot exclude high grade squamous intraepithelial lesion on cytologic smear of cervix [ASC-H]** ♀

R87.612   **Low grade squamous intraepithelial lesion on cytologic smear of cervix [LGSIL]** ♀

R87.613   **High grade squamous intraepithelial lesion on cytologic smear of cervix [HGSIL]** ♀

R87.614   **Cytologic evidence of malignancy on smear of cervix** ♀

R87.615   **Unsatisfactory cytologic smear of cervix** ♀
Inadequate sample of cytologic smear of cervix

R87.616   **Satisfactory cervical smear but lacking transformation zone** ♀

R87.618   **Other abnormal cytological findings on specimens from cervix uteri** ♀

R87.619   **Unspecified abnormal cytological findings in specimens from cervix uteri** ♀ ▽
Abnormal cervical cytology NOS
Abnormal Papanicolaou smear of cervix NOS
Abnormal thin preparation smear of cervix NOS
Atypical endocervical cells of cervix NOS
Atypical endometrial cells of cervix NOS
Atypical glandular cells of cervix NOS

EXCLUDES 1   Not coded here   EXCLUDES 2   Not included here   N Newborn Age : 0   P Pediatric Age : 0-17   M Maternity Age : 12-55   A Adult Age : 15-124

878   ICD-10-CM 2017

✓6ᵗʰ **R87.62 Abnormal cytological findings in specimens from vagina**

Use additional code to identify acquired absence of uterus and cervix, if applicable (Z90.71-)

EXCLUDES 1 *abnormal cytological findings in specimens from cervix uteri (R87.61-)*
abnormal cytological findings in specimens from other female genital organs (R87.69)
carcinoma in situ of vagina (histologically confirmed) (D07.2)
dysplasia (mild) (moderate) of vagina (histologically confirmed) (N89.-)
severe dysplasia of vagina (histologically confirmed) (D07.2)
vaginal intraepithelial neoplasia I [VAIN I] (N89.0)
vaginal intraepithelial neoplasia II [VAIN II] (N89.1)
vaginal intraepithelial neoplasia III [VAIN III] (D07.2)

EXCLUDES 2 *vaginal high risk human papillomavirus (HPV) DNA test positive (R87.811)*
vaginal low risk human papillomavirus (HPV) DNA test positive (R87.821)

R87.620 Atypical squamous cells of undetermined significance on cytologic smear of vagina [ASC-US] ♀

R87.621 Atypical squamous cells cannot exclude high grade squamous intraepithelial lesion on cytologic smear of vagina [ASC-H] ♀

R87.622 Low grade squamous intraepithelial lesion on cytologic smear of vagina [LGSIL] ♀

R87.623 High grade squamous intraepithelial lesion on cytologic smear of vagina [HGSIL] ♀

R87.624 Cytologic evidence of malignancy on smear of vagina ♀

R87.625 Unsatisfactory cytologic smear of vagina ♀

Inadequate sample of cytologic smear of vagina

R87.628 Other abnormal cytological findings on specimens from vagina ♀

R87.629 Unspecified abnormal cytological findings in specimens from vagina ♀ ▽

Abnormal Papanicolaou smear of vagina NOS
Abnormal thin preparation smear of vagina NOS
Abnormal vaginal cytology NOS
Atypical endocervical cells of vagina NOS
Atypical endometrial cells of vagina NOS
Atypical glandular cells of vagina NOS

R87.69 Abnormal cytological findings in specimens from other female genital organs ♀

Abnormal cytological findings in specimens from female genital organs NOS

EXCLUDES 1 *dysplasia of vulva (histologically confirmed) (N90.0-N90.3)*

R87.7 Abnormal histological findings in specimens from female genital organs ♀

EXCLUDES 1 *carcinoma in situ (histologically confirmed) of female genital organs (D06-D07.3)*
cervical intraepithelial neoplasia I [CIN I] (N87.0)
cervical intraepithelial neoplasia II [CIN II] (N87.1)
cervical intraepithelial neoplasia III [CIN III] (D06.-)
dysplasia (mild) (moderate) of cervix uteri (histologically confirmed) (N87.-)
dysplasia (mild) (moderate) of vagina (histologically confirmed) (N89.-)
severe dysplasia of cervix uteri (histologically confirmed) (D06.-)
severe dysplasia of vagina (histologically confirmed) (D07.2)
vaginal intraepithelial neoplasia I [VAIN I] (N89.0)
vaginal intraepithelial neoplasia II [VAIN II] (N89.1)
vaginal intraepithelial neoplasia III [VAIN III] (D07.2)

✓5ᵗʰ **R87.8 Other abnormal findings in specimens from female genital organs**

✓6ᵗʰ **R87.81 High risk human papillomavirus [HPV] DNA test positive from female genital organs**

EXCLUDES 1 *anogenital warts due to human papillomavirus (HPV) (A63.0)*
condyloma acuminatum (A63.0)

R87.810 Cervical high risk human papillomavirus [HPV] DNA test positive ♀

R87.811 Vaginal high risk human papillomavirus [HPV] DNA test positive ♀

✓6ᵗʰ **R87.82 Low risk human papillomavirus [HPV] DNA test positive from female genital organs**

Use additional code for associated human papillomavirus (B97.7)

R87.820 Cervical low risk human papillomavirus [HPV] DNA test positive ♀

R87.821 Vaginal low risk human papillomavirus [HPV] DNA test positive ♀

R87.89 Other abnormal findings in specimens from female genital organs ♀

Abnormal chromosomal findings in specimens from female genital organs

R87.9 Unspecified abnormal finding in specimens from female genital organs ♀ ▽

✓4ᵗʰ **R88 Abnormal findings in other body fluids and substances**

R88.0 Cloudy (hemodialysis) (peritoneal) dialysis effluent

R88.8 Abnormal findings in other body fluids and substances

✓4ᵗʰ **R89 Abnormal findings in specimens from other organs, systems and tissues**

INCLUDES abnormal findings in nipple discharge
abnormal findings in synovial fluid
abnormal findings in wound secretions

R89.0 Abnormal level of enzymes in specimens from other organs, systems and tissues

R89.1 Abnormal level of hormones in specimens from other organs, systems and tissues

R89.2 Abnormal level of other drugs, medicaments and biological substances in specimens from other organs, systems and tissues

R89.3 Abnormal level of substances chiefly nonmedicinal as to source in specimens from other organs, systems and tissues

R89.4 Abnormal immunological findings in specimens from other organs, systems and tissues

R89.5 Abnormal microbiological findings in specimens from other organs, systems and tissues

Positive culture findings in specimens from other organs, systems and tissues

EXCLUDES 1 *colonization status (Z22.-)*

R89.6 Abnormal cytological findings in specimens from other organs, systems and tissues

R89.7 Abnormal histological findings in specimens from other organs, systems and tissues

R89.8 Other abnormal findings in specimens from other organs, systems and tissues

Abnormal chromosomal findings in specimens from other organs, systems and tissues

R89.9 Unspecified abnormal finding in specimens from other organs, systems and tissues ▽

Abnormal findings on diagnostic imaging and in function studies, without diagnosis (R90-R94)

INCLUDES   nonspecific abnormal findings on diagnostic imaging by computerized axial tomography [CAT scan]
nonspecific abnormal findings on diagnostic imaging by magnetic resonance imaging [MRI][NMR]
nonspecific abnormal findings on diagnostic imaging by positron emission tomography [PET scan]
nonspecific abnormal findings on diagnostic imaging by thermography
nonspecific abnormal findings on diagnostic imaging by ultrasound [echogram]
nonspecific abnormal findings on diagnostic imaging by X-ray examination

EXCLUDES 1   *abnormal findings on antenatal screening of mother (O28.-)*
diagnostic abnormal findings classified elsewhere - see Alphabetical Index

✓4ᵗʰ R90   Abnormal findings on diagnostic imaging of central nervous system

     R90.0   Intracranial space-occupying lesion found on diagnostic imaging of central nervous system

     ✓5ᵗʰ R90.8   Other abnormal findings on diagnostic imaging of central nervous system

       R90.81   Abnormal echoencephalogram

       R90.82   White matter disease, unspecified ▽

       R90.89   Other abnormal findings on diagnostic imaging of central nervous system
         Other cerebrovascular abnormality found on diagnostic imaging of central nervous system

✓4ᵗʰ R91   Abnormal findings on diagnostic imaging of lung

     R91.1   Solitary pulmonary nodule
       Coin lesion lung
       Solitary pulmonary nodule, subsegmental branch of the bronchial tree

     R91.8   Other nonspecific abnormal finding of lung field
       Lung mass NOS found on diagnostic imaging of lung
       Pulmonary infiltrate NOS
       Shadow, lung

✓4ᵗʰ R92   Abnormal and inconclusive findings on diagnostic imaging of breast

     R92.0   Mammographic microcalcification found on diagnostic imaging of breast

       EXCLUDES 2   *mammographic calcification (calculus) found on diagnostic imaging of breast (R92.1)*

       DEF: Calcium and cellular debris deposits in the breast that cannot be felt but can be detected on a mammogram; can be a sign of cancer, benign conditions, or changes in the breast tissue as a result of inflammation, injury, or obstructed duct.

     R92.1   Mammographic calcification found on diagnostic imaging of breast
       Mammographic calculus found on diagnostic imaging of breast

     R92.2   Inconclusive mammogram
       Dense breasts NOS
       Inconclusive mammogram NEC
       Inconclusive mammography due to dense breasts
       Inconclusive mammography NEC
       AHA: 2015,1Q,24

     R92.8   Other abnormal and inconclusive findings on diagnostic imaging of breast

✓4ᵗʰ R93   Abnormal findings on diagnostic imaging of other body structures

     R93.0   Abnormal findings on diagnostic imaging of skull and head, not elsewhere classified
       EXCLUDES 1   *intracranial space-occupying lesion found on diagnostic imaging (R90.0)*

     R93.1   Abnormal findings on diagnostic imaging of heart and coronary circulation
       Abnormal echocardiogram NOS
       Abnormal heart shadow

     R93.2   Abnormal findings on diagnostic imaging of liver and biliary tract
       Nonvisualization of gallbladder

     R93.3   Abnormal findings on diagnostic imaging of other parts of digestive tract

✓5ᵗʰ R93.4   Abnormal findings on diagnostic imaging of urinary organs
     EXCLUDES 2   ▶*hypertrophy of kidney (N28.81)*◀

     R93.41   Abnormal radiologic findings on diagnostic imaging of renal pelvis, ureter, or bladder
       Filling defect of bladder found on diagnostic imaging
       Filling defect of renal pelvis found on diagnostic imaging
       Filling defect of ureter found on diagnostic imaging

     R93.42   Abnormal radiologic findings on diagnostic imaging of kidney

       R93.421   Abnormal radiologic findings on diagnostic imaging of right kidney

       R93.422   Abnormal radiologic findings on diagnostic imaging of left kidney

       R93.429   Abnormal radiologic findings on diagnostic imaging of unspecified kidney ▽

     R93.49   Abnormal radiologic findings on diagnostic imaging of other urinary organs

     R93.5   Abnormal findings on diagnostic imaging of other abdominal regions, including retroperitoneum

     R93.6   Abnormal findings on diagnostic imaging of limbs
       EXCLUDES 2   *abnormal finding in skin and subcutaneous tissue (R93.8)*

     R93.7   Abnormal findings on diagnostic imaging of other parts of musculoskeletal system
       EXCLUDES 2   *abnormal findings on diagnostic imaging of skull (R93.0)*

     R93.8   Abnormal findings on diagnostic imaging of other specified body structures
       Abnormal finding by radioisotope localization of placenta
       Abnormal radiological finding in skin and subcutaneous tissue
       Mediastinal shift

     R93.9   Diagnostic imaging inconclusive due to excess body fat of patient

✓4ᵗʰ R94   Abnormal results of function studies
     INCLUDES   abnormal results of radionuclide [radioisotope] uptake studies
       abnormal results of scintigraphy

     ✓5ᵗʰ R94.0   Abnormal results of function studies of central nervous system

       R94.01   Abnormal electroencephalogram [EEG]

       R94.02   Abnormal brain scan

       R94.09   Abnormal results of other function studies of central nervous system

     ✓5ᵗʰ R94.1   Abnormal results of function studies of peripheral nervous system and special senses

       ✓6ᵗʰ R94.11   Abnormal results of function studies of eye

         R94.110   Abnormal electro-oculogram [EOG]

         R94.111   Abnormal electroretinogram [ERG]
           Abnormal retinal function study

         R94.112   Abnormal visually evoked potential [VEP]

         R94.113   Abnormal oculomotor study

         R94.118   Abnormal results of other function studies of eye

       ✓6ᵗʰ R94.12   Abnormal results of function studies of ear and other special senses

         R94.120   Abnormal auditory function study

         R94.121   Abnormal vestibular function study

         R94.128   Abnormal results of other function studies of ear and other special senses

       ✓6ᵗʰ R94.13   Abnormal results of function studies of peripheral nervous system

         R94.130   Abnormal response to nerve stimulation, unspecified ▽

         R94.131   Abnormal electromyogram [EMG]
           EXCLUDES 1   *electromyogram of eye (R94.113)*

         R94.138   Abnormal results of other function studies of peripheral nervous system

     R94.2   Abnormal results of pulmonary function studies
       Reduced ventilatory capacity
       Reduced vital capacity

     ✓5ᵗʰ R94.3   Abnormal results of cardiovascular function studies

       R94.30   Abnormal result of cardiovascular function study, unspecified ▽

       R94.31   Abnormal electrocardiogram [ECG] [EKG]
         EXCLUDES 1   *long QT syndrome (I45.81)*

       R94.39   Abnormal result of other cardiovascular function study
         Abnormal electrophysiological intracardiac studies
         Abnormal phonocardiogram
         Abnormal vectorcardiogram

EXCLUDES 1 Not coded here   **EXCLUDES 2** Not included here   **N** Newborn Age : 0   **P** Pediatric Age : 0-17   **M** Maternity Age : 12-55   **A** Adult Age : 15-124

880   ICD-10-CM 2017

R94.4 **Abnormal results of kidney function studies**
Abnormal renal function test

R94.5 **Abnormal results of liver function studies**

R94.6 **Abnormal results of thyroid function studies**

R94.7 **Abnormal results of other endocrine function studies**
EXCLUDES 2   *abnormal glucose (R73.0-)*

R94.8 **Abnormal results of function studies of other organs and systems**
Abnormal basal metabolic rate [BMR]
Abnormal bladder function test
Abnormal splenic function test

Abnormal tumor markers (R97)

☑4ᵗʰ **R97** **Abnormal tumor markers**
Elevated tumor associated antigens [TAA]
Elevated tumor specific antigens [TSA]

R97.0 **Elevated carcinoembryonic antigen [CEA]**

R97.1 **Elevated cancer antigen 125 [CA 125]**   ♀

☑5ᵗʰ **R97.2** **Elevated prostate specific antigen [PSA]**

●   **R97.20** **Elevated prostate specific antigen [PSA]**

●   **R97.21** **Rising PSA following treatment for malignant neoplasm of prostate**

R97.8 **Other abnormal tumor markers**

Ill-defined and unknown cause of mortality (R99)

R99 **Ill-defined and unknown cause of mortality**   ▽
Death (unexplained) NOS
Unspecified cause of mortality

☑ Additional Character Required   ☑ₓ₇ᵗʰ Placeholder Alert   Manifestation Dx   ▽ Unspecified Dx   ▶◀ Revised Text   ● New Code   ▲ Revised Code Title

Chapter 19. Injury, Poisoning and Certain Other Consequences of External Causes (SØØ–T88)

Chapter Specific Guidelines with Coding Examples

The chapter specific guidelines from the ICD-10-CM Official Guidelines for Coding and Reporting have been provided below. Along with these guidelines are coding examples, contained in the shaded boxes, that have been developed to help illustrate the coding and/or sequencing guidance found in these guidelines.

a. Application of 7th characters in Chapter 19

Most categories in chapter 19 have a 7th character requirement for each applicable code. Most categories in this chapter have three 7th character values (with the exception of fractures): A, initial encounter, D, subsequent encounter and S, sequela. Categories for traumatic fractures have additional 7th character values. While the patient may be seen by a new or different provider over the course of treatment for an injury, assignment of the 7th character is based on whether the patient is undergoing active treatment and not whether the provider is seeing the patient for the first time.

For complication codes, active treatment refers to treatment for the condition described by the code, even though it may be related to an earlier precipitating problem. For example, code T84.50XA, Infection and inflammatory reaction due to unspecified internal joint prosthesis, initial encounter, is used when active treatment is provided for the infection, even though the condition relates to the prosthetic device, implant or graft that was placed at a previous encounter.

7th character "A", initial encounter is used **for each encounter where** the patient is receiving active treatment for the condition.

> Patient admitted after fall from a skateboard onto the sidewalk, x-rays identify a nondisplaced fracture to the distal pole of the right scaphoid bone. The patient is placed in a cast.
>
> | | |
> |---|---|
> | S62.Ø14A | Nondisplaced fracture of distal pole of navicular [scaphoid] bone of right wrist, initial encounter for closed fracture |
> | VØØ.131A | Fall from skateboard, initial encounter |
> | Y92.48Ø | Sidewalk as the place of occurrence of the external cause |
> | Y93.51 | Activity, roller skating (inline) and skateboarding |
> | Y99.8 | Other external cause status |
>
> *Explanation:* This fracture would be coded with a seventh character A for initial encounter because the patient received x-rays to identify the site of the fracture and treatment was rendered; this would be considered active treatment.

7th character "D" subsequent encounter is used for encounters after the patient has **completed** active treatment of the condition and is receiving routine care for the condition during the healing or recovery phase.

> Patient admitted after fall from a skateboard onto the sidewalk resulted in casting of the right arm. X-rays are taken to evaluate how well the nondisplaced fracture to the distal pole of the right scaphoid bone is healing. The physician feels the fracture is healing appropriately; no adjustments to the cast are made.
>
> | | |
> |---|---|
> | S62.Ø14D | Nondisplaced fracture of distal pole of navicular [scaphoid] bone of right wrist, subsequent encounter for fracture with routine healing |
> | VØØ.131D | Fall from skateboard, subsequent encounter |
>
> *Explanation:* This fracture would be coded with a seventh character D for subsequent encounter, whether the same physician who provided the initial cast application or a different physician is now seeing the patient. Although the patient received x-rays, the intent of the x-rays was to assess how the fracture was healing. There was no active treatment rendered and the visit is therefore considered a subsequent encounter.

The aftercare Z codes should not be used for aftercare for conditions such as injuries or poisonings, where 7th characters are provided to identify subsequent care. For example, for aftercare of an injury, assign the acute injury code with the 7th character "D" (subsequent encounter).

7th character "S", sequela, is for use for complications or conditions that arise as a direct result of a condition, such as scar formation after a burn.

The scars are sequelae of the burn. When using 7th character "S", it is necessary to use both the injury code that precipitated the sequela and the code for the sequela itself. The "S" is added only to the injury code, not the sequela code. The 7th character "S" identifies the injury responsible for the sequela. The specific type of sequela (e.g. scar) is sequenced first, followed by the injury code.

See Section I.B.10 Sequelae, (Late Effects)

> Patient with a history of a nondisplaced fracture to the distal pole of the right scaphoid bone due to a fall from a skateboard is admitted for evaluation of arthritis to the right wrist that has developed as a consequence of the traumatic fracture.
>
> | | |
> |---|---|
> | M12.531 | Traumatic arthropathy, right wrist |
> | S62.Ø14S | Nondisplaced fracture of distal pole of navicular [scaphoid] bone of right wrist, sequela |
> | VØØ.131S | Fall from skateboard, sequela |
>
> *Explanation:* The code identifying the specific sequela condition (traumatic arthritis) should be coded first followed by the injury that instigated the development of the sequela (fracture). The scaphoid fracture injury code is given a 7th character S for sequela to represent its role as the inciting injury. The fracture has healed and is not being managed or treated on this admit and therefore is not applicable as a first listed or principal diagnosis. However, it is directly related to the development of the arthritis and should be appended as a secondary code to signify this cause and effect relationship.

b. Coding of injuries

When coding injuries, assign separate codes for each injury unless a combination code is provided, in which case the combination code is assigned. Code T07, Unspecified multiple injuries should not be assigned in the inpatient setting unless information for a more specific code is not available. Traumatic injury codes (S00-T14.9) are not to be used for normal, healing surgical wounds or to identify complications of surgical wounds.

> 11-year-old girl fell from her horse, resulting in a laceration to her right forearm with several large pieces of wooden fragments embedded in the wound as well as abrasions to her right ear; in addition, her right shoulder was dislocated
>
> | | |
> |---|---|
> | S43.ØØ4A | Unspecified dislocation of right shoulder joint, initial encounter |
> | S51.821A | Laceration with foreign body of right forearm, initial encounter |
> | SØØ.411A | Abrasion of right ear, initial encounter |
> | V8Ø.Ø1ØA | Animal-rider injured by fall from or being thrown from horse in noncollision accident, initial encounter |
> | Y93.52 | Activity, horseback riding |
>
> *Explanation:* Each separate injury should be reported. The patient's injury to the forearm is reported with one combination code that captures both the laceration and the foreign body.

The code for the most serious injury, as determined by the provider and the focus of treatment, is sequenced first.

1) Superficial injuries

Superficial injuries such as abrasions or contusions are not coded when associated with more severe injuries of the same site.

2) Primary injury with damage to nerves/blood vessels

When a primary injury results in minor damage to peripheral nerves or blood vessels, the primary injury is sequenced first with additional code(s) for injuries to nerves and spinal cord (such as category SØ4), and/or injury to blood vessels (such as category S15). When the primary injury is to the blood vessels or nerves, that injury should be sequenced first.

c. Coding of traumatic fractures

The principles of multiple coding of injuries should be followed in coding fractures. Fractures of specified sites are coded individually by site in accordance with both the provisions within categories S02, S12, S22, S32, S42, S49, S52, S59, S62, S72, S79, S82, S89, S92 and the level of detail furnished by medical record content.

A fracture not indicated as open or closed should be coded to closed. A fracture not indicated whether displaced or not displaced should be coded to displaced.

More specific guidelines are as follows:

1) Initial vs. subsequent encounter for fractures

Traumatic fractures are coded using the appropriate 7th character for initial encounter (A, B, C) **for each encounter where** the patient is receiving active treatment for the fracture. The appropriate 7th character for initial encounter should also be assigned for a patient who delayed seeking treatment for the fracture or nonunion.

Fractures are coded using the appropriate 7th character for subsequent care for encounters after the patient has completed active treatment of the fracture and is receiving routine care for the fracture during the healing or recovery phase.

Care for complications of surgical treatment for fracture repairs during the healing or recovery phase should be coded with the appropriate complication codes.

Care of complications of fractures, such as malunion and nonunion, should be reported with the appropriate 7th character for subsequent care with nonunion (K, M, N,) or subsequent care with malunion (P, Q, R).

Malunion/nonunion: The appropriate 7th character for initial encounter should also be assigned for a patient who delayed seeking treatment for the fracture or nonunion.

> Female patient fell during a forest hiking excursion almost six months ago and until recently did not feel she needed to seek medical attention for her left ankle pain; x-rays show nonunion of lateral malleolus and surgery has been scheduled
>
> | **S82.62XA** | **Displaced fracture of lateral malleolus of left fibula, initial encounter for closed fracture** |
> |---|---|
> | **W01.0XXA** | **Fall on same level from slipping, tripping and stumbling without subsequent striking against object, initial encounter** |
> | **Y92.821** | **Forest as place of occurrence of the external cause** |
> | **Y93.01** | **Activity, walking, marching and hiking** |
> | **Y99.8** | **Other external cause status** |
>
> *Explanation:* A seventh character of A is used for the lateral malleolus nonunion fracture to signify that the fracture is receiving active treatment. The delayed care for the fracture has resulted in a nonunion, but capturing the nonunion in the seventh character is trumped by the provision of active care.

The open fracture designations in the assignment of the 7th character for fractures of the forearm, femur and lower leg, including ankle are based on the Gustilo open fracture classification. When the Gustilo classification type is not specified for an open fracture, the 7th character for open fracture type I or II should be assigned (B, E, H, M, Q).

A code from category M80, not a traumatic fracture code, should be used for any patient with known osteoporosis who suffers a fracture, even if the patient had a minor fall or trauma, if that fall or trauma would not usually break a normal, healthy bone.

See Section I.C.13. Osteoporosis.

The aftercare Z codes should not be used for aftercare for traumatic fractures. For aftercare of a traumatic fracture, assign the acute fracture code with the appropriate 7th character.

2) Multiple fractures sequencing

Multiple fractures are sequenced in accordance with the severity of the fracture.

d. Coding of burns and corrosions

The ICD-10-CM makes a distinction between burns and corrosions. The burn codes are for thermal burns, except sunburns, that come from a heat source, such as a fire or hot appliance. The burn codes are also for burns resulting from electricity and radiation. Corrosions are burns due to chemicals. The guidelines are the same for burns and corrosions.

Current burns (T20-T25) are classified by depth, extent and by agent (X code). Burns are classified by depth as first degree (erythema), second degree (blistering), and third degree (full-thickness involvement). Burns of the eye and internal organs (T26-T28) are classified by site, but not by degree.

1) Sequencing of burn and related condition codes

Sequence first the code that reflects the highest degree of burn when more than one burn is present.

a. When the reason for the admission or encounter is for treatment of external multiple burns, sequence first the code that reflects the burn of the highest degree.

b. When a patient has both internal and external burns, the circumstances of admission govern the selection of the principal diagnosis or first-listed diagnosis.

c. When a patient is admitted for burn injuries and other related conditions such as smoke inhalation and/or respiratory failure, the circumstances of admission govern the selection of the principal or first-listed diagnosis.

> Patient admitted with minor first-degree burns to multiple sites of her right and left hands as well as severe smoke inhalation. While she was sleeping at home, a candle on her dresser lit the bedroom curtains on fire.
>
> | **T59.811A** | **Toxic effect of smoke, accidental (unintentional), initial encounter** |
> |---|---|
> | **J70.5** | **Respiratory conditions due to smoke inhalation** |
> | **T23.191A** | **Burn of first degree of multiple sites of right wrist and hand, initial encounter** |
> | **T23.192A** | **Burn of first degree of multiple sites of left wrist and hand, initial encounter** |
> | **X08.8XXA** | **Exposure to other specified smoke, fire and flames, initial encounter** |
> | **Y92.003** | **Bedroom of unspecified non-institutional (private) residence as the place of occurrence of the external cause** |
> | **Y93.84** | **Activity, sleeping** |
>
> *Explanation:* Based on the documentation, the inhalation injury is more severe than the first-degree burns and is sequenced first. The burns to the hands are appended as secondary diagnoses.

2) Burns of the same local site

Classify burns of the same local site (three-character category level, T20-T28) but of different degrees to the subcategory identifying the highest degree recorded in the diagnosis.

> 10-year-old male patient is admitted for third-degree burns of his right palm and second degree burns of multiple right fingers; right thumb not affected
>
> | **T23.351A** | **Burn of third degree of right palm, initial encounter** |
> |---|---|
>
> *Explanation:* Although there is a code for second-degree burns of multiple fingers, not including the thumb (T23.131-), this code falls in the same three-digit category that the third-degree burn of the right palm falls under, category T23. Only the subcategory identifying the highest degree is captured when different burn degrees are classified to a single category.

> Patient is admitted with third-degree burns of the scalp as well as second-degree burns to the back of the right hand
>
> | **T20.35XA** | **Burn of third degree of scalp [any part], initial encounter** |
> |---|---|
> | **T23.261A** | **Burn of second degree of back of right hand, initial encounter** |
>
> *Explanation:* Since burns to the hand and scalp are classified to two different three-digit categories, both burns may be reported as they represent distinct sites.

3) Non-healing burns

Non-healing burns are coded as acute burns.

Necrosis of burned skin should be coded as a non-healed burn.

4) Infected burn

For any documented infected burn site, use an additional code for the infection.

5) Assign separate codes for each burn site

When coding burns, assign separate codes for each burn site. Category T30, Burn and corrosion, body region unspecified is extremely vague and should rarely be used.

6) Burns and corrosions classified according to extent of body surface involved

Assign codes from category T31, Burns classified according to extent of body surface involved, or T32, Corrosions classified according to extent of body surface involved, when the site of the burn is not specified or when there is a need for additional data. It is advisable to use category T31 as additional coding when needed to provide data for evaluating burn mortality, such as that needed by burn units. It is also advisable to use category T31 as an additional code for reporting purposes when there is mention of a third-degree burn involving 20 percent or more of the body surface.

Categories T31 and T32 are based on the classic "rule of nines" in estimating body surface involved: head and neck are assigned nine percent, each arm nine percent, each leg 18 percent, the anterior trunk 18 percent, posterior trunk 18 percent, and genitalia one percent. Providers may change these percentage assignments where necessary to accommodate infants and children who have proportionally larger heads than adults, and patients who have large buttocks, thighs, or abdomen that involve burns.

Patient seen for dressing change after he accidentally spilled acetic acid on himself two days ago. The second-degree burns to his right thigh, covering about 3 percent of his body surface, are healing appropriately.

T54.2X1D	**Toxic effect of corrosive acids and acid-like substances, accidental (unintentional), subsequent encounter**
T24.611D	**Corrosion of second degree of right thigh, subsequent encounter**
T32.0	**Corrosions involving less than 10% of body surface**

Explanation: Code T32.0 provides additional information as to how much of the patient's body was affected by the corrosive substance.

---

7) Encounters for treatment of sequela of burns

Encounters for the treatment of the late effects of burns or corrosions (i.e., scars or joint contractures) should be coded with a burn or corrosion code with the 7th character "S" for sequela.

8) Sequelae with a late effect code and current burn

When appropriate, both a code for a current burn or corrosion with 7th character "A" or "D" and a burn or corrosion code with 7th character "S" may be assigned on the same record (when both a current burn and sequelae of an old burn exist). Burns and corrosions do not heal at the same rate and a current healing wound may still exist with sequela of a healed burn or corrosion.

See Section I.B.10 Sequela (Late Effects)

Female patient seen for second-degree burn to the left ear; she also has significant scarring on her left elbow from a third-degree burn from childhood

T20.212A	**Burn of second degree of left ear [any part, except ear drum], initial encounter**
L90.5	**Scar conditions and fibrosis of skin**
T22.322S	**Burn of third degree of left elbow, sequela**

Explanation: The patient is being seen for management of a current second-degree burn, which is reflected in the code by appending the seventh character of A, indicating active treatment or management of this burn. The elbow scarring is a sequela of a previous third-degree burn. The sequela condition precedes the original burn injury, which is appended with a seventh character of S.

---

9) Use of an external cause code with burns and corrosions

An external cause code should be used with burns and corrosions to identify the source and intent of the burn, as well as the place where it occurred.

e. Adverse effects, poisoning, underdosing and toxic effects

Codes in categories T36-T65 are combination codes that include the substance that was taken as well as the intent. No additional external cause code is required for poisonings, toxic effects, adverse effects and underdosing codes.

1) Do not code directly from the Table of Drugs

Do not code directly from the Table of Drugs and Chemicals. Always refer back to the Tabular List.

2) Use as many codes as necessary to describe

Use as many codes as necessary to describe completely all drugs, medicinal or biological substances.

3) If the same code would describe the causative agent

If the same code would describe the causative agent for more than one adverse reaction, poisoning, toxic effect or underdosing, assign the code only once.

4) If two or more drugs, medicinal or biological substances

If two or more drugs, medicinal or biological substances are reported, code each individually unless a combination code is listed in the Table of Drugs and Chemicals.

5) The occurrence of drug toxicity is classified in ICD-10-CM as follows:

(a) Adverse effect

When coding an adverse effect of a drug that has been correctly prescribed and properly administered, assign the appropriate code for the nature of the adverse effect followed by the appropriate code for the adverse effect of the drug (T36-T50). The code for the drug should have a 5th or 6th character "5" (for example T36.0X5-) Examples of the nature of an adverse effect are tachycardia, delirium, gastrointestinal hemorrhaging, vomiting, hypokalemia, hepatitis, renal failure, or respiratory failure.

Patient seen for stomach pain and jaundice, indicated by physician as possible side-effects of Inderal, recently started for hypertension. Inderal was discontinued and the patient switched to Atenolol instead.

R10.9	**Unspecified abdominal pain**
R17	**Unspecified jaundice**
T44.7X5A	**Adverse effect of beta-adrenoreceptor antagonists, initial encounter**
I10	**Essential (primary) hypertension**

Explanation: The side-effects caused by the drug are listed first, followed by the code for the adverse effect of the drug to capture the specific drug that was used.

(b) Poisoning

When coding a poisoning or reaction to the improper use of a medication (e.g., overdose, wrong substance given or taken in error, wrong route of administration), first assign the appropriate code from categories T36-T50. The poisoning codes have an associated intent as their 5th or 6th character (accidental, intentional self-harm, assault and undetermined. **If the intent of the poisoning is unknown or unspecified, code the intent as accidental intent. The undetermined intent is only for use if the documentation in the record specifies that the intent cannot be determined.** Use additional code(s) for all manifestations of poisonings.

If there is also a diagnosis of abuse or dependence of the substance, the abuse or dependence is assigned as an additional code.

Examples of poisoning include:

(i) Error was made in drug prescription

Errors made in drug prescription or in the administration of the drug by provider, nurse, patient, or other person.

(ii Overdose of a drug intentionally taken

If an overdose of a drug was intentionally taken or administered and resulted in drug toxicity, it would be coded as a poisoning.

(iii) Nonprescribed drug taken with correctly prescribed and properly administered drug

If a nonprescribed drug or medicinal agent was taken in combination with a correctly prescribed and properly administered drug, any drug toxicity or other reaction resulting from the interaction of the two drugs would be classified as a poisoning.

(iv) Interaction of drug(s) and alcohol

When a reaction results from the interaction of a drug(s) and alcohol, this would be classified as poisoning.

See Section I.C.4. if poisoning is the result of insulin pump malfunctions.

(c) Underdosing

Underdosing refers to taking less of a medication than is prescribed by a provider or a manufacturer's instruction. For underdosing, assign the code from categories T36-T50 (fifth or sixth character "6").

Codes for underdosing should never be assigned as principal or first-listed codes. If a patient has a relapse or exacerbation of the medical condition for which the drug is prescribed because of the reduction in dose, then the medical condition itself should be coded.

Noncompliance (Z91.12-, Z91.13-) or complication of care (Y63.6-Y63.9) codes are to be used with an underdosing code to indicate intent, if known.

> Patient admitted for atrial fibrillation with history of chronic atrial fibrillation for which she is prescribed amiodarone. Financial concerns have left the patient unable to pay for her prescriptions and she has been skipping her amiodarone dose every other day to offset the cost.
>
> **I48.2**   **Chronic atrial fibrillation**
>
> **T46.2X6A**   **Underdosing of other antidysrhythmic drugs, initial encounter**
>
> **Z91.12Ø**   **Patient's intentional underdosing of medication regimen due to financial hardship**
>
> *Explanation:* By skipping her amiodarone pill every other day, the patient's atrial fibrillation returned. The condition for which the drug was being taken is reported first, followed by an underdosing code to show that the patient was not adhering to her prescription regiment. The Z code helps elaborate on the patient's social and/or economic circumstances that led to the patient taking less then what she was prescribed.

(d) Toxic effects

When a harmful substance is ingested or comes in contact with a person, this is classified as a toxic effect. The toxic effect codes are in categories T51-T65.

Toxic effect codes have an associated intent: accidental, intentional self-harm, assault and undetermined.

f. Adult and child abuse, neglect and other maltreatment

Sequence first the appropriate code from categories T74.- (Adult and child abuse, neglect and other maltreatment, confirmed) or T76.- (Adult and child abuse, neglect and other maltreatment, suspected) for abuse, neglect and other maltreatment, followed by any accompanying mental health or injury code(s).

If the documentation in the medical record states abuse or neglect it is coded as confirmed (T74.-). It is coded as suspected if it is documented as suspected (T76.-).

For cases of confirmed abuse or neglect an external cause code from the assault section (X92-**Y09**) should be added to identify the cause of any physical injuries. A perpetrator code (Y07) should be added when the perpetrator of the abuse is known. For suspected cases of abuse or neglect, do not report external cause or perpetrator code.

If a suspected case of abuse, neglect or mistreatment is ruled out during an encounter code Z04.71, Encounter for examination and observation following alleged physical adult abuse, ruled out, or code Z04.72, Encounter for examination and observation following alleged child physical abuse, ruled out, should be used, not a code from T76.

If a suspected case of alleged rape or sexual abuse is ruled out during an encounter code Z04.41, Encounter for examination and observation following alleged **adult rape** or code Z04.42, Encounter for examination and observation following alleged **child** rape, should be used, not a code from T76.

See Section I.C.15. Abuse in a pregnant patient.

g. Complications of care
1) General guidelines for complications of care
(a) Documentation of complications of care

See Section I.B.16. for information on documentation of complications of care.

2) Pain due to medical devices

Pain associated with devices, implants or grafts left in a surgical site (for example painful hip prosthesis) is assigned to the appropriate code(s) found in Chapter 19, Injury, poisoning, and certain other consequences of external causes. Specific codes for pain due to medical devices are found in the T code section of the ICD-10-CM. Use additional code(s) from category G89 to identify acute or chronic pain due to presence of the device, implant or graft (G89.18 or G89.28).

> Chronic left breast pain secondary to breast implant
>
> **T85.848A**   **Pain due to other internal prosthetic devices, implants and grafts, initial encounter**
>
> **N64.4**   **Mastodynia**
>
> **G89.28**   **Other chronic postprocedural pain**
>
> *Explanation:* As the pain is a complication related to the breast implant, the complication code is sequenced first. The T code does not describe the site or type of pain, so additional codes may be appended to indicate that the patient is experiencing chronic pain in the breast.

3) Transplant complications
(a) Transplant complications other than kidney

Codes under category T86, Complications of transplanted organs and tissues, are for use for both complications and rejection of transplanted organs. A transplant complication code is only assigned if the complication affects the function of the transplanted organ. Two codes are required to fully describe a transplant complication: the appropriate code from category T86 and a secondary code that identifies the complication.

Pre-existing conditions or conditions that develop after the transplant are not coded as complications unless they affect the function of the transplanted organs.

See I.C.21. for transplant organ removal status

See I.C.2. for malignant neoplasm associated with transplanted organ.

(b) Kidney transplant complications

Patients who have undergone kidney transplant may still have some form of chronic kidney disease (CKD) because the kidney transplant may not fully restore kidney function. Code T86.1- should be assigned for documented complications of a kidney transplant, such as transplant failure or rejection or other transplant complication. Code T86.1- should not be assigned for post kidney transplant patients who have chronic kidney (CKD) unless a transplant complication such as transplant failure or rejection is documented. If the documentation is unclear as to whether the patient has a complication of the transplant, query the provider.

Conditions that affect the function of the transplanted kidney, other than CKD, should be assigned a code from subcategory T86.1, Complications of transplanted organ, Kidney, and a secondary code that identifies the complication.

For patients with CKD following a kidney transplant, but who do not have a complication such as failure or rejection, *see section I.C.14. Chronic kidney disease and kidney transplant status.*

> Patient seen for chronic kidney disease stage 2; history of successful kidney transplant with no complications identified
>
> **N18.2**   **Chronic kidney disease, stage 2 (mild)**
>
> **Z94.Ø**   **Kidney transplant status**
>
> *Explanation:* This patient's stage 2 CKD is not indicated as being due to the transplanted kidney but instead is just the residual disease the patient had prior to the transplant.

4) Complication codes that include the external cause

As with certain other T codes, some of the complications of care codes have the external cause included in the code. The code includes the nature of the complication as well as the type of procedure that caused the complication. No external cause code indicating the type of procedure is necessary for these codes.

5) Complications of care codes within the body system chapters

Intraoperative and postprocedural complication codes are found within the body system chapters with codes specific to the organs and structures of that body system. These codes should be sequenced first, followed by a code(s) for the specific complication, if applicable.

> During a spinal fusion procedure, the surgeon inadvertently punctured the dura. The midline durotomy was repaired, and the fusion procedure was completed.
>
> **G97.41**   **Accidental puncture or laceration of dura during a procedure**
>
> *Explanation:* The accidental durotomy is not coded to an injury code in chapter 19 but instead is categorized to the nervous system chapter.

Muscle/Tendon Table

ICD-10-CM categorizes certain muscles and tendons in the upper and lower extremities by their action (e.g., extension, flexion), their anatomical location (e.g., posterior, anterior), and/or whether they are intrinsic or extrinsic to a certain anatomical area. The Muscle/Tendon Table is provided at the beginning of chapters 13 and 19 as a resource to help users when code selection depends on one or more of these characteristics. Please note that this table is not all-inclusive, and proper code assignment should be based on the provider's documentation.

Body Region	Muscle	Extensor Tendon	Flexor Tendon	Other Tendon
Shoulder				
	Deltoid	Posterior deltoid	Anterior deltoid	
	Rotator cuff			
	Infraspinatus			Infraspinatus
	Subscapularis			Subscapularis
	Supraspinatus			Supraspinatus
	Teres minor			Teres minor
	Teres major	Teres major		
Upper arm				
	Anterior muscles			
	Biceps brachii — long head		Biceps brachii — long head	
	Biceps brachii — short head		Biceps brachii — short head	
	Brachialis		Brachialis	
	Coracobrachialis		Coracobrachialis	
	Posterior muscles			
	Triceps brachii	Triceps brachii		
Forearm				
	Anterior muscles			
	Flexors			
	Deep			
	Flexor digitorum profundus		Flexor digitorum profundus	
	Flexor pollicis longus		Flexor pollicis longus	
	Intermediate			
	Flexor digitorum superficialis		Flexor digitorum superficialis	
	Superficial			
	Flexor carpi radialis		Flexor carpi radialis	
	Flexor carpi ulnaris		Flexor carpi ulnaris	
	Palmaris longus		Palmaris longus	
	Pronators			
	Pronator quadratus			Pronator quadratus
	Pronator teres			Pronator teres
	Posterior muscles			
	Extensors			
	Deep			
	Abductor pollicis longus			Abductor pollicis longus
	Extensor indicis	Extensor indicis		
	Extensor pollicis brevis	Extensor pollicis brevis		
	Extensor pollicis longus	Extensor pollicis longus		
	Superficial			
	Brachioradialis			Brachioradialis
	Extensor carpi radialis brevis	Extensor carpi radialis brevis		
	Extensor carpi radialis longus	Extensor carpi radialis longus		
	Extensor carpi ulnaris	Extensor carpi ulnaris		
	Extensor digiti minimi	Extensor digiti minimi		
	Extensor digitorum	Extensor digitorum		
	Anconeus	Anconeus		
	Supinator			Supinator

Body Region	Muscle	Extensor Tendon	Flexor Tendon	Other Tendon
Hand				
Extrinsic — attach to a site in the forearm as well as a site in the hand with action related to hand movement at the wrist				
	Extensor carpi radialis brevis	Extensor carpi radialis brevis		
	Extensor carpi radialis longus	Extensor carpie radialis longus		
	Extensor carpi ulnaris	Extensor carpi ulnaris		
	Flexor carpi radialis		Flexor carpi radialis	
	Flexor carpi ulnaris		Flexor carpi ulnaris	
	Flexor digitorum superficialis		Flexor digitorum superficialis	
	Palmaris longus		Palmaris longus	
Extrinsic — attach to a site in the forearm as well as a site in the hand with action in the hand related to finger movement				
	Adductor pollicis longus			Adductor pollicis longus
	Extensor digiti minimi	Extensor digiti minimi		
	Extensor digitorum	Extensor digitorum		
	Extensor indicis	Extensor indicis		
	Flexor digitorum profundus		Flexor digitorum profundus	
	Flexor digitorum superficialis		Flexor digitorum superficialis	
Extrinsic — attach to a site in the forearm as well as a site in the hand with action in the hand related to thumb movement				
	Extensor pollicis brevis	Extensor pollicis brevis		
	Extensor pollicis longus	Extensor pollicis longus		
	Flexor pollicis longus		Flexor pollicis longus	
Intrinsic — found within the hand only				
	Adductor pollicis			Adductor pollicis
	Dorsal interossei	Dorsal interossei	Dorsal interossei	
	Lumbricals	Lumbricals	Lumbricals	
	Palmaris brevis			Palmaris brevis
	Palmar interossei	Palmar interossei	Palmar interossei	
	Hypothenar muscles			
	Abductor digiti minimi			Abductor digiti minimi
	Flexor digiti minimi brevis		Flexor digiti minimi brevis	
	Oppenens digiti minimi		Oppenens digiti minimi	
	Thenar muscles			
	Abductor pollicis brevis			Abductor pollicis brevis
	Flexor pollicis brevis		Flexor pollicis brevis	
	Oppenens pollicis		Oppenens pollicis	
Thigh				
	Anterior muscles			
	Iliopsoas		Iliopsoas	
	Pectineus		Pectineus	
	Quadriceps	Quadriceps		
	Rectus femoris	Rectus femoris — Extends knee	Rectus femoris — Flexes hip	
	Vastus intermedius	Vastus intermedius		
	Vastus lateralis	Vastus lateralis		
	Vastus medialis	Vastus medialis		
	Sartorius		Sartorius	
	Medial muscles			
	Adductor brevis			Adductor brevis
	Adductor longus			Adductor longus
	Adductor magnus			Adductor magnus
	Gracilis			Gracilis
	Obturator externus			Obturator externus
	Posterior muscles			
	Hamstring	Hamstring — Extends hip	Hamstring — Flexes knee	
	Biceps femoris	Biceps femoris	Biceps femoris	
	Semimembranosus	Semimembranosus	Semimembranosus	
	Semitendinosus	Semitendinosus	Semitendinosus	

Chapter 19. Injury, Poisoning and Certain Other Consequences of External Causes

Body Region	Muscle	Extensor Tendon	Flexor Tendon	Other Tendon
Lower leg				
	Anterior muscles			
	Extensor digitorum longus	Extensor digitorum longus		
	Extensor hallucis longus	Extensor hallucis longus		
	Fibularis (peroneus) tertius	Fibularis (peroneus) tertius		
	Tibialis anterior	Tibialis anterior		Tibialis anterior
	Lateral muscles			
	Fibularis (peroneus) brevis		Fibularis (peroneus) brevis	
	Fibularis (peroneus) longus		Fibularis (peroneus) longus	
	Posterior muscles			
	Deep			
	Flexor digitorum longus		Flexor digitorum longus	
	Flexor hallucis longus		Flexor hallucis longus	
	Popliteus		Popliteus	
	Tibialis posterior		Tibialis posterior	
	Superficial			
	Gastrocnemius		Gastrocnemius	
	Plantaris		Plantaris	
	Soleus		Soleus	
				Calcaneal (Achilles)
Ankle/Foot				
Extrinsic — attach to a site in the lower leg as well as a site in the foot with action related to foot movement at the ankle				
	Plantaris		Plantaris	
	Soleus		Soleus	
	Tibialis anterior	Tibialis anterior		
	Tibialis posterior		Tibialis posterior	
Extrinsic — attach to a site in the lower leg as well as a site in the foot with action in the foot related to toe movement				
	Extensor digitorum longus	Extensor digitorum longus		
	Extensor hallicus longus	Extensor hallicus longus		
	Flexor digitorum longus		Flexor digitorum longus	
	Flexor hallucis longus		Flexor hallucis longus	
Intrinsic — found within the ankle/foot only				
	Dorsal muscles			
	Extensor digitorum brevis	Extensor digitorum brevis		
	Extensor hallucis brevis	Extensor hallicus brevis		
	Plantar muscles			
	Abductor digiti minimi		Abductor digiti minimi	
	Abductor hallucis		Abductor hallucis	
	Dorsal interossei	Dorsal interossei	Dorsal interossei	
	Flexor digiti minimi brevis		Flexor digiti minimi brevis	
	Flexor digitorum brevis		Flexor digitorum brevis	
	Flexor hallucis brevis		Flexor hallucis brevis	
	Lumbricals	Lumbricals	Lumbricals	
	Quadratus plantae		Quadratus plantae	
	Plantar interossei	Plantar interossei	Plantar interossei	

Chapter 19. Injury, Poisoning and Certain Other Consequences of External Causes (S00-T88)

> **NOTE** Use secondary code(s) from Chapter 20, External causes of morbidity, to indicate cause of injury. Codes within the T section that include the external cause do not require an additional external cause code.

Use additional code to identify any retained foreign body, if applicable (Z18.-)

> **EXCLUDES 1** birth trauma (P10-P15)
> obstetric trauma (O70-O71)

> **NOTE** The chapter uses the S-section for coding different types of injuries related to single body regions and the T-section to cover injuries to unspecified body regions as well as poisoning and certain other consequences of external causes.

AHA: 2016,2Q,3-7; 2015,4Q,35-38; 2015,3Q,37-39,40; 2015,2Q,6; 2015,1Q,3-21

This chapter contains the following blocks:

S00-S09	Injuries to the head
S10-S19	Injuries to the neck
S20-S29	Injuries to the thorax
S30-S39	Injuries to the abdomen, lower back, lumbar spine, pelvis and external genitals
S40-S49	Injuries to the shoulder and upper arm
S50-S59	Injuries to the elbow and forearm
S60-S69	Injuries to the wrist, hand and fingers
S70-S79	Injuries to the hip and thigh
S80-S89	Injuries to the knee and lower leg
S90-S99	Injuries to the ankle and foot
T07	Injuries involving multiple body regions
T14	Injury of unspecified body region
T15-T19	Effects of foreign body entering through natural orifice
T20-T25	Burns and corrosions of external body surface, specified by site
T26-T28	Burns and corrosions confined to eye and internal organs
T30-T32	Burns and corrosions of multiple and unspecified body regions
T33-T34	Frostbite
T36-T50	Poisoning by, adverse effect of and underdosing of drugs, medicaments and biological substances
T51-T65	Toxic effects of substances chiefly nonmedicinal as to source
T66-T78	Other and unspecified effects of external causes
T79	Certain early complications of trauma
T80-T88	Complications of surgical and medical care, not elsewhere classified

Injuries to the head (S00-S09)

> **INCLUDES** injuries of ear
> injuries of eye
> injuries of face [any part]
> injuries of gum
> injuries of jaw
> injuries of oral cavity
> injuries of palate
> injuries of periocular area
> injuries of scalp
> injuries of temporomandibular joint area
> injuries of tongue
> injuries of tooth

Code also for any associated infection

> **EXCLUDES 2** burns and corrosions (T20-T32)
> effects of foreign body in ear (T16)
> effects of foreign body in larynx (T17.3)
> effects of foreign body in mouth NOS (T18.0)
> effects of foreign body in nose (T17.0-T17.1)
> effects of foreign body in pharynx (T17.2)
> effects of foreign body on external eye (T15.-)
> frostbite (T33-T34)
> insect bite or sting, venomous (T63.4)

√4th **S00 Superficial injury of head**

> **EXCLUDES 1** diffuse cerebral contusion (S06.2-)
> focal cerebral contusion (S06.3-)
> injury of eye and orbit (S05.-)
> open wound of head (S01.-)

The appropriate 7th character is to be added to each code from category S00.
A   initial encounter
D   subsequent encounter
S   sequela

√5th **S00.0 Superficial injury of scalp**

√x7th   **S00.00 Unspecified superficial injury of scalp** ▽

√x7th   **S00.01 Abrasion** of scalp

√x7th   **S00.02 Blister (nonthermal)** of scalp

√x7th   **S00.03 Contusion** of scalp

     Bruise of scalp
     Hematoma of scalp

√x7th   **S00.04 External constriction** of part of scalp

√x7th   **S00.05 Superficial foreign body** of scalp

     Splinter in the scalp

√x7th   **S00.06 Insect bite (nonvenomous)** of scalp

√x7th   **S00.07 Other superficial bite** of scalp

> **EXCLUDES 1** open bite of scalp (S01.05)

√5th **S00.1 Contusion** of eyelid and periocular area

     Black eye

> **EXCLUDES 2** contusion of eyeball and orbital tissues (S05.1)

√x7th   **S00.10 Contusion of unspecified eyelid and periocular area** ▽

√x7th   **S00.11 Contusion of right eyelid and periocular area**

√x7th   **S00.12 Contusion of left eyelid and periocular area**

√5th **S00.2 Other and unspecified superficial injuries of eyelid and periocular area**

> **EXCLUDES 2** superficial injury of conjunctiva and cornea (S05.0-)

√6th   **S00.20 Unspecified superficial injury of eyelid and periocular area**

     √7th   **S00.201 Unspecified superficial injury of right eyelid and periocular area** ▽

     √7th   **S00.202 Unspecified superficial injury of left eyelid and periocular area** ▽

     √7th   **S00.209 Unspecified superficial injury of unspecified eyelid and periocular area** ▽

√6th   **S00.21 Abrasion** of eyelid and periocular area

     √7th   **S00.211 Abrasion of right eyelid and periocular area**

     √7th   **S00.212 Abrasion of left eyelid and periocular area**

     √7th   **S00.219 Abrasion of unspecified eyelid and periocular area** ▽

√6th   **S00.22 Blister (nonthermal)** of eyelid and periocular area

     √7th   **S00.221 Blister (nonthermal) of right eyelid and periocular area**

     √7th   **S00.222 Blister (nonthermal) of left eyelid and periocular area**

     √7th   **S00.229 Blister (nonthermal) of unspecified eyelid and periocular area**

√6th   **S00.24 External constriction** of eyelid and periocular area

     √7th   **S00.241 External constriction of right eyelid and periocular area**

     √7th   **S00.242 External constriction of left eyelid and periocular area**

     √7th   **S00.249 External constriction of unspecified eyelid and periocular area** ▽

√6th   **S00.25 Superficial foreign body** of eyelid and periocular area

     Splinter of eyelid and periocular area

> **EXCLUDES 2** retained foreign body in eyelid (H02.81-)

     √7th   **S00.251 Superficial foreign body of right eyelid and periocular area**

     √7th   **S00.252 Superficial foreign body of left eyelid and periocular area**

     √7th   **S00.259 Superficial foreign body of unspecified eyelid and periocular area** ▽

√6th   **S00.26 Insect bite (nonvenomous)** of eyelid and periocular area

     √7th   **S00.261 Insect bite (nonvenomous) of right eyelid and periocular area**

     √7th   **S00.262 Insect bite (nonvenomous) of left eyelid and periocular area**

     √7th   **S00.269 Insect bite (nonvenomous) of unspecified eyelid and periocular area** ▽

√6th   **S00.27 Other superficial bite** of eyelid and periocular area

> **EXCLUDES 1** open bite of eyelid and periocular area (S01.15)

     √7th   **S00.271 Other superficial bite of right eyelid and periocular area**

     √7th   **S00.272 Other superficial bite of left eyelid and periocular area**

     √7th   **S00.279 Other superficial bite of unspecified eyelid and periocular area** ▽

√5th **S00.3 Superficial injury of nose**

√x7th   **S00.30 Unspecified superficial injury of nose** ▽

√x7th   **S00.31 Abrasion of nose**

√x7th   **S00.32 Blister (nonthermal) of nose**

☑ Additional Character Required   √x7th Placeholder Alert   Manifestation Dx   ▽ Unspecified Dx   ►◄ Revised Text   ● New Code   ▲ Revised Code Title

√x7ᵗʰ **S00.33** Contusion of nose
> Bruise of nose
> Hematoma of nose

√x7ᵗʰ **S00.34** External constriction of nose

√x7ᵗʰ **S00.35** Superficial foreign body of nose
> Splinter in the nose

√x7ᵗʰ **S00.36** Insect bite (nonvenomous) of nose

√x7ᵗʰ **S00.37** Other superficial bite of nose
> **EXCLUDES 1** open bite of nose (S01.25)

√5ᵗʰ **S00.4** Superficial injury of ear

√6ᵗʰ **S00.40** Unspecified superficial injury of ear

√7ᵗʰ **S00.401** Unspecified superficial injury of right ear ▽

√7ᵗʰ **S00.402** Unspecified superficial injury of left ear ▽

√7ᵗʰ **S00.409** Unspecified superficial injury of unspecified ear ▽

√6ᵗʰ **S00.41** Abrasion of ear

√7ᵗʰ **S00.411** Abrasion of right ear

√7ᵗʰ **S00.412** Abrasion of left ear

√7ᵗʰ **S00.419** Abrasion of unspecified ear ▽

√6ᵗʰ **S00.42** Blister (nonthermal) of ear

√7ᵗʰ **S00.421** Blister (nonthermal) of right ear

√7ᵗʰ **S00.422** Blister (nonthermal) of left ear

√7ᵗʰ **S00.429** Blister (nonthermal) of unspecified ear ▽

√6ᵗʰ **S00.43** Contusion of ear
> Bruise of ear
> Hematoma of ear

√7ᵗʰ **S00.431** Contusion of right ear

√7ᵗʰ **S00.432** Contusion of left ear

√7ᵗʰ **S00.439** Contusion of unspecified ear ▽

√6ᵗʰ **S00.44** External constriction of ear

√7ᵗʰ **S00.441** External constriction of right ear

√7ᵗʰ **S00.442** External constriction of left ear

√7ᵗʰ **S00.449** External constriction of unspecified ear ▽

√6ᵗʰ **S00.45** Superficial foreign body of ear
> Splinter in the ear

√7ᵗʰ **S00.451** Superficial foreign body of right ear

√7ᵗʰ **S00.452** Superficial foreign body of left ear

√7ᵗʰ **S00.459** Superficial foreign body of unspecified ear ▽

√6ᵗʰ **S00.46** Insect bite (nonvenomous) of ear

√7ᵗʰ **S00.461** Insect bite (nonvenomous) of right ear

√7ᵗʰ **S00.462** Insect bite (nonvenomous) of left ear

√7ᵗʰ **S00.469** Insect bite (nonvenomous) of unspecified ear ▽

√6ᵗʰ **S00.47** Other superficial bite of ear
> **EXCLUDES 1** open bite of ear (S01.35)

√7ᵗʰ **S00.471** Other superficial bite of right ear

√7ᵗʰ **S00.472** Other superficial bite of left ear

√7ᵗʰ **S00.479** Other superficial bite of unspecified ear ▽

√5ᵗʰ **S00.5** Superficial injury of lip and oral cavity

√6ᵗʰ **S00.50** Unspecified superficial injury of lip and oral cavity

√7ᵗʰ **S00.501** Unspecified superficial injury of lip ▽

√7ᵗʰ **S00.502** Unspecified superficial injury of oral cavity ▽

√6ᵗʰ **S00.51** Abrasion of lip and oral cavity

√7ᵗʰ **S00.511** Abrasion of lip

√7ᵗʰ **S00.512** Abrasion of oral cavity

√6ᵗʰ **S00.52** Blister (nonthermal) of lip and oral cavity

√7ᵗʰ **S00.521** Blister (nonthermal) of lip

√7ᵗʰ **S00.522** Blister (nonthermal) of oral cavity

√6ᵗʰ **S00.53** Contusion of lip and oral cavity

√7ᵗʰ **S00.531** Contusion of lip
> Bruise of lip
> Hematoma of oral cavity

√7ᵗʰ **S00.532** Contusion of oral cavity
> Bruise of lip
> Hematoma of oral cavity

√6ᵗʰ **S00.54** External constriction of lip and oral cavity

√7ᵗʰ **S00.541** External constriction of lip

√7ᵗʰ **S00.542** External constriction of oral cavity

√6ᵗʰ **S00.55** Superficial foreign body of lip and oral cavity

√7ᵗʰ **S00.551** Superficial foreign body of lip
> Splinter of lip and oral cavity

√7ᵗʰ **S00.552** Superficial foreign body of oral cavity
> Splinter of lip and oral cavity

√6ᵗʰ **S00.56** Insect bite (nonvenomous) of lip and oral cavity

√7ᵗʰ **S00.561** Insect bite (nonvenomous) of lip

√7ᵗʰ **S00.562** Insect bite (nonvenomous) of oral cavity

√6ᵗʰ **S00.57** Other superficial bite of lip and oral cavity

√7ᵗʰ **S00.571** Other superficial bite of lip
> **EXCLUDES 1** open bite of lip (S01.551)

√7ᵗʰ **S00.572** Other superficial bite of oral cavity
> **EXCLUDES 1** open bite of oral cavity (S01.552)

√5ᵗʰ **S00.8** Superficial injury of other parts of head
> ▶Superficial injuries of face [any part]◀

√x7ᵗʰ **S00.80** Unspecified superficial injury of other part of head ▽

√x7ᵗʰ **S00.81** Abrasion of other part of head

√x7ᵗʰ **S00.82** Blister (nonthermal) of other part of head

√x7ᵗʰ **S00.83** Contusion of other part of head
> Bruise of other part of head
> Hematoma of other part of head

√x7ᵗʰ **S00.84** External constriction of other part of head

√x7ᵗʰ **S00.85** Superficial foreign body of other part of head
> Splinter in other part of head

√x7ᵗʰ **S00.86** Insect bite (nonvenomous) of other part of head

√x7ᵗʰ **S00.87** Other superficial bite of other part of head
> **EXCLUDES 1** open bite of other part of head (S01.85)

√5ᵗʰ **S00.9** Superficial injury of unspecified part of head

√x7ᵗʰ **S00.90** Unspecified superficial injury of unspecified part of head ▽

√x7ᵗʰ **S00.91** Abrasion of unspecified part of head ▽

√x7ᵗʰ **S00.92** Blister (nonthermal) of unspecified part of head ▽

√x7ᵗʰ **S00.93** Contusion of unspecified part of head ▽
> Bruise of head
> Hematoma of head

√x7ᵗʰ **S00.94** External constriction of unspecified part of head ▽

√x7ᵗʰ **S00.95** Superficial foreign body of unspecified part of head ▽
> Splinter of head

√x7ᵗʰ **S00.96** Insect bite (nonvenomous) of unspecified part of head ▽

√x7ᵗʰ **S00.97** Other superficial bite of unspecified part of head ▽
> **EXCLUDES 1** open bite of head (S01.95)

√4ᵗʰ **S01** **Open wound of head**
> Code also any associated:
> injury of cranial nerve (S04.-)
> injury of muscle and tendon of head (S09.1-)
> intracranial injury (S06.-)
> wound infection
> **EXCLUDES 1** open skull fracture (S02.- with 7th character B)
> **EXCLUDES 2** injury of eye and orbit (S05.-)
> traumatic amputation of part of head (S08.-)

> The appropriate 7th character is to be added to each code from category S01.
> A initial encounter
> D subsequent encounter
> S sequela

√5ᵗʰ **S01.0** **Open wound of scalp**
> **EXCLUDES 1** avulsion of scalp (S08.0)

√x7ᵗʰ **S01.00** Unspecified open wound of scalp ▽

√x7ᵗʰ **S01.01** Laceration without foreign body of scalp

√x7ᵗʰ **S01.02** Laceration with foreign body of scalp

√x7ᵗʰ **S01.03** Puncture wound without foreign body of scalp

√x7ᵗʰ **S01.04** Puncture wound with foreign body of scalp

√x7ᵗʰ **S01.05** Open bite of scalp

    Bite of scalp NOS

    EXCLUDES 1 *superficial bite of scalp (S00.06, S00.07-)*

√5ᵗʰ **S01.1** Open wound of eyelid and periocular area

    Open wound of eyelid and periocular area with or without involvement of lacrimal passages

  √6ᵗʰ **S01.10** Unspecified open wound of eyelid and periocular area

    √7ᵗʰ **S01.101** Unspecified open wound of right eyelid and periocular area ▽

    √7ᵗʰ **S01.102** Unspecified open wound of left eyelid and periocular area ▽

    √7ᵗʰ **S01.109** Unspecified open wound of unspecified eyelid and periocular area ▽

  √6ᵗʰ **S01.11** Laceration without foreign body of eyelid and periocular area

    √7ᵗʰ **S01.111** Laceration without foreign body of right eyelid and periocular area

    √7ᵗʰ **S01.112** Laceration without foreign body of left eyelid and periocular area

    √7ᵗʰ **S01.119** Laceration without foreign body of unspecified eyelid and periocular area ▽

  √6ᵗʰ **S01.12** Laceration with foreign body of eyelid and periocular area

    √7ᵗʰ **S01.121** Laceration with foreign body of right eyelid and periocular area

    √7ᵗʰ **S01.122** Laceration with foreign body of left eyelid and periocular area

    √7ᵗʰ **S01.129** Laceration with foreign body of unspecified eyelid and periocular area ▽

  √6ᵗʰ **S01.13** Puncture wound without foreign body of eyelid and periocular area

    √7ᵗʰ **S01.131** Puncture wound without foreign body of right eyelid and periocular area

    √7ᵗʰ **S01.132** Puncture wound without foreign body of left eyelid and periocular area

    √7ᵗʰ **S01.139** Puncture wound without foreign body of unspecified eyelid and periocular area ▽

  √6ᵗʰ **S01.14** Puncture wound with foreign body of eyelid and periocular area

    √7ᵗʰ **S01.141** Puncture wound with foreign body of right eyelid and periocular area

    √7ᵗʰ **S01.142** Puncture wound with foreign body of left eyelid and periocular area

    √7ᵗʰ **S01.149** Puncture wound with foreign body of unspecified eyelid and periocular area ▽

  √6ᵗʰ **S01.15** Open bite of eyelid and periocular area

    Bite of eyelid and periocular area NOS

    EXCLUDES 1 *superficial bite of eyelid and periocular area (S00.26, S00.27)*

    √7ᵗʰ **S01.151** Open bite of right eyelid and periocular area

    √7ᵗʰ **S01.152** Open bite of left eyelid and periocular area

    √7ᵗʰ **S01.159** Open bite of unspecified eyelid and periocular area ▽

√5ᵗʰ **S01.2** Open wound of nose

  √x7ᵗʰ **S01.20** Unspecified open wound of nose ▽

  √x7ᵗʰ **S01.21** Laceration without foreign body of nose

  √x7ᵗʰ **S01.22** Laceration with foreign body of nose

  √x7ᵗʰ **S01.23** Puncture wound without foreign body of nose

  √x7ᵗʰ **S01.24** Puncture wound with foreign body of nose

  √x7ᵗʰ **S01.25** Open bite of nose

    Bite of nose NOS

    EXCLUDES 1 *superficial bite of nose (S00.36, S00.37)*

√5ᵗʰ **S01.3** Open wound of ear

  √6ᵗʰ **S01.30** Unspecified open wound of ear

    √7ᵗʰ **S01.301** Unspecified open wound of right ear ▽

    √7ᵗʰ **S01.302** Unspecified open wound of left ear ▽

√7ᵗʰ **S01.309** Unspecified open wound of unspecified ear ▽

√6ᵗʰ **S01.31** Laceration without foreign body of ear

  √7ᵗʰ **S01.311** Laceration without foreign body of right ear

  √7ᵗʰ **S01.312** Laceration without foreign body of left ear

  √7ᵗʰ **S01.319** Laceration without foreign body of unspecified ear ▽

√6ᵗʰ **S01.32** Laceration with foreign body of ear

  √7ᵗʰ **S01.321** Laceration with foreign body of right ear

  √7ᵗʰ **S01.322** Laceration with foreign body of left ear

  √7ᵗʰ **S01.329** Laceration with foreign body of unspecified ear ▽

√6ᵗʰ **S01.33** Puncture wound without foreign body of ear

  √7ᵗʰ **S01.331** Puncture wound without foreign body of right ear

  √7ᵗʰ **S01.332** Puncture wound without foreign body of left ear

  √7ᵗʰ **S01.339** Puncture wound without foreign body of unspecified ear ▽

√6ᵗʰ **S01.34** Puncture wound with foreign body of ear

  √7ᵗʰ **S01.341** Puncture wound with foreign body of right ear

  √7ᵗʰ **S01.342** Puncture wound with foreign body of left ear

  √7ᵗʰ **S01.349** Puncture wound with foreign body of unspecified ear ▽

√6ᵗʰ **S01.35** Open bite of ear

  Bite of ear NOS

  EXCLUDES 1 *superficial bite of ear (S00.46, S00.47)*

  √7ᵗʰ **S01.351** Open bite of right ear

  √7ᵗʰ **S01.352** Open bite of left ear

  √7ᵗʰ **S01.359** Open bite of unspecified ear ▽

√5ᵗʰ **S01.4** Open wound of cheek and temporomandibular area

  √6ᵗʰ **S01.40** Unspecified open wound of cheek and temporomandibular area

    √7ᵗʰ **S01.401** Unspecified open wound of right cheek and temporomandibular area ▽

    √7ᵗʰ **S01.402** Unspecified open wound of left cheek and temporomandibular area ▽

    √7ᵗʰ **S01.409** Unspecified open wound of unspecified cheek and temporomandibular area ▽

  √6ᵗʰ **S01.41** Laceration without foreign body of cheek and temporomandibular area

    √7ᵗʰ **S01.411** Laceration without foreign body of right cheek and temporomandibular area

    √7ᵗʰ **S01.412** Laceration without foreign body of left cheek and temporomandibular area

    √7ᵗʰ **S01.419** Laceration without foreign body of unspecified cheek and temporomandibular area ▽

  √6ᵗʰ **S01.42** Laceration with foreign body of cheek and temporomandibular area

    √7ᵗʰ **S01.421** Laceration with foreign body of right cheek and temporomandibular area

    √7ᵗʰ **S01.422** Laceration with foreign body of left cheek and temporomandibular area

    √7ᵗʰ **S01.429** Laceration with foreign body of unspecified cheek and temporomandibular area ▽

  √6ᵗʰ **S01.43** Puncture wound without foreign body of cheek and temporomandibular area

    √7ᵗʰ **S01.431** Puncture wound without foreign body of right cheek and temporomandibular area

    √7ᵗʰ **S01.432** Puncture wound without foreign body of left cheek and temporomandibular area

    √7ᵗʰ **S01.439** Puncture wound without foreign body of unspecified cheek and temporomandibular area ▽

  √6ᵗʰ **S01.44** Puncture wound with foreign body of cheek and temporomandibular area

    √7ᵗʰ **S01.441** Puncture wound with foreign body of right cheek and temporomandibular area

    √7ᵗʰ **S01.442** Puncture wound with foreign body of left cheek and temporomandibular area

---

☑ Additional Character Required   √x7ᵗʰ Placeholder Alert   Manifestation Dx   ▽ Unspecified Dx   ►◄ Revised Text   ● New Code   ▲ Revised Code Title

✓7ᵗʰ **S01.449** **Puncture wound with foreign body** of unspecified cheek and temporomandibular area ▽

✓6ᵗʰ **S01.45** **Open bite** of cheek and temporomandibular area

Bite of cheek and temporomandibular area NOS

    EXCLUDES 2 *superficial bite of cheek and temporomandibular area (S00.86, S00.87)*

    ✓7ᵗʰ **S01.451** **Open bite of right cheek and temporomandibular area**

    ✓7ᵗʰ **S01.452** **Open bite of left cheek and temporomandibular area**

    ✓7ᵗʰ **S01.459** **Open bite of unspecified cheek and temporomandibular area** ▽

✓5ᵗʰ **S01.5** **Open wound of lip and oral cavity**

    EXCLUDES 2 *tooth dislocation (S03.2)*
              tooth fracture (S02.5)

    ✓6ᵗʰ **S01.50** **Unspecified open wound of lip and oral cavity**

       ✓7ᵗʰ **S01.501** **Unspecified open wound of lip** ▽

       ✓7ᵗʰ **S01.502** **Unspecified open wound of oral cavity** ▽

    ✓6ᵗʰ **S01.51** **Laceration of lip and oral cavity without foreign body** ●

       ✓7ᵗʰ **S01.511** **Laceration without foreign body of lip** ●

       ✓7ᵗʰ **S01.512** **Laceration without foreign body of oral cavity** ●

    ✓6ᵗʰ **S01.52** **Laceration of lip and oral cavity with foreign body** ▲

       ✓7ᵗʰ **S01.521** **Laceration with foreign body of lip**

       ✓7ᵗʰ **S01.522** **Laceration with foreign body of oral cavity**

    ✓6ᵗʰ **S01.53** **Puncture wound of lip and oral cavity without foreign body**

       ✓7ᵗʰ **S01.531** **Puncture wound without foreign body of lip**

       ✓7ᵗʰ **S01.532** **Puncture wound without foreign body of oral cavity** ▲

    ✓6ᵗʰ **S01.54** **Puncture wound of lip and oral cavity with foreign body**

       ✓7ᵗʰ **S01.541** **Puncture wound with foreign body of lip** ●

       ✓7ᵗʰ **S01.542** **Puncture wound with foreign body of oral cavity** ●

    ✓6ᵗʰ **S01.55** **Open bite of lip and oral cavity**

       ✓7ᵗʰ **S01.551** **Open bite of lip** ●

          Bite of lip NOS

          EXCLUDES 1 *superficial bite of lip (S00.571)* ●

       ✓7ᵗʰ **S01.552** **Open bite of oral cavity** ●

          Bite of oral cavity NOS

          EXCLUDES 1 *superficial bite of oral cavity (S00.572)* ●

✓5ᵗʰ **S01.8** **Open wound of other parts of head**

    ✓x7ᵗʰ **S01.80** **Unspecified open wound of other part of head** ▽

    ✓x7ᵗʰ **S01.81** **Laceration without foreign body of other part of head**

    ✓x7ᵗʰ **S01.82** **Laceration with foreign body of other part of head**

    ✓x7ᵗʰ **S01.83** **Puncture wound without foreign body of other part of head**

    ✓x7ᵗʰ **S01.84** **Puncture wound with foreign body of other part of head**

    ✓x7ᵗʰ **S01.85** **Open bite of other part of head**

       Bite of other part of head NOS

       EXCLUDES 1 *superficial bite of other part of head (S00.85)*

✓5ᵗʰ **S01.9** **Open wound of unspecified part of head** ●

    ✓x7ᵗʰ **S01.90** **Unspecified open wound of unspecified part of head** ▽ ●

    ✓x7ᵗʰ **S01.91** **Laceration without foreign body of unspecified part of head** ▽

    ✓x7ᵗʰ **S01.92** **Laceration with foreign body of unspecified part of head** ▽

    ✓x7ᵗʰ **S01.93** **Puncture wound without foreign body of unspecified part of head** ▽

    ✓x7ᵗʰ **S01.94** **Puncture wound with foreign body of unspecified part of head** ▽

    ✓x7ᵗʰ **S01.95** **Open bite of unspecified part of head** ▽ ▲

       Bite of head NOS

       EXCLUDES 1 *superficial bite of head NOS (S00.97)* ▲

✓4ᵗʰ **S02** **Fracture of skull and facial bones**

    NOTE   A fracture not indicated as open or closed should be coded to closed.

    Code also any associated intracranial injury (S06.-)

    The appropriate 7th character is to be added to each code from category S02.
    A   initial encounter for closed fracture
    B   initial encounter for open fracture
    D   subsequent encounter for fracture with routine healing
    G   subsequent encounter for fracture with delayed healing
    K   subsequent encounter for fracture with nonunion
    S   sequela

✓x7ᵗʰ **S02.0** **Fracture of vault of skull**

    Fracture of frontal bone
    Fracture of parietal bone

✓5ᵗʰ **S02.1** **Fracture of base of skull**

    EXCLUDES 1 *orbit NOS (S02.8)*
    EXCLUDES 2 *orbital floor (S02.3-)*

    ✓6ᵗʰ **S02.10** **Unspecified fracture of base of skull**

       ✓7ᵗʰ **S02.101** **Fracture of base of skull, right side** ●

       ✓7ᵗʰ **S02.102** **Fracture of base of skull, left side** ●

       ✓7ᵗʰ **S02.109** **Fracture of base of skull, unspecified side** ▽ ●

    ✓6ᵗʰ **S02.11** **Fracture of occiput**

       ✓7ᵗʰ **S02.110** **Type I occipital condyle fracture, unspecified side** ▽

       ✓7ᵗʰ **S02.111** **Type II occipital condyle fracture, unspecified side** ▽

       ✓7ᵗʰ **S02.112** **Type III occipital condyle fracture, unspecified side** ▽

       ✓7ᵗʰ **S02.113** **Unspecified occipital condyle fracture**

       ✓7ᵗʰ **S02.118** **Other fracture of occiput, unspecified side** ▽

       ✓7ᵗʰ **S02.119** **Unspecified fracture of occiput** ▽

       ✓7ᵗʰ **S02.11A** **Type I occipital condyle fracture, right side** ●

       ✓7ᵗʰ **S02.11B** **Type I occipital condyle fracture, left side** ●

       ✓7ᵗʰ **S02.11C** **Type II occipital condyle fracture, right side** ●

       ✓7ᵗʰ **S02.11D** **Type II occipital condyle fracture, left side** ●

       ✓7ᵗʰ **S02.11E** **Type III occipital condyle fracture, right side** ●

       ✓7ᵗʰ **S02.11F** **Type III occipital condyle fracture, left side** ●

       ✓7ᵗʰ **S02.11G** **Other fracture of occiput, right side** ●

       ✓7ᵗʰ **S02.11H** **Other fracture of occiput, left side** ●

    ✓x7ᵗʰ **S02.19** **Other fracture of base of skull**

       Fracture of anterior fossa of base of skull
       Fracture of ethmoid sinus
       Fracture of frontal sinus
       Fracture of middle fossa of base of skull
       Fracture of orbital roof
       Fracture of posterior fossa of base of skull
       Fracture of sphenoid
       Fracture of temporal bone

✓x7ᵗʰ **S02.2** **Fracture of nasal bones**

✓5ᵗʰ **S02.3** **Fracture of orbital floor**

    EXCLUDES 1 *orbit NOS (S02.8)*
    EXCLUDES 2 *orbital roof (S02.1-)*

    ✓x7ᵗʰ **S02.30** **Fracture of orbital floor, unspecified side** ▽ ●

    ✓x7ᵗʰ **S02.31** **Fracture of orbital floor, right side** ●

    ✓x7ᵗʰ **S02.32** **Fracture of orbital floor, left side** ●

✓5ᵗʰ **S02.4** **Fracture of malar, maxillary and zygoma bones**

    Fracture of superior maxilla
    Fracture of upper jaw (bone)
    Fracture of zygomatic process of temporal bone

    ✓6ᵗʰ **S02.40** **Fracture of malar, maxillary and zygoma bones, unspecified**

       ✓7ᵗʰ **S02.400** **Malar fracture, unspecified side** ▽ ▲

       ✓7ᵗʰ **S02.401** **Maxillary fracture, unspecified side** ▽ ▲

       ✓7ᵗʰ **S02.402** **Zygomatic fracture, unspecified side** ▽ ▲

       ✓7ᵗʰ **S02.40A** **Malar fracture, right side** ●

EXCLUDES 1 Not coded here   EXCLUDES 2 Not included here   N Newborn Age : 0   P Pediatric Age : 0-17   M Maternity Age : 12-55   A Adult Age : 15-124

- ☑7ᵗʰ **S02.40B** Malar fracture, left side
- ☑7ᵗʰ **S02.40C** Maxillary fracture, right side
- ☑7ᵗʰ **S02.40D** Maxillary fracture, left side
- ☑7ᵗʰ **S02.40E** Zygomatic fracture, right side
- ☑7ᵗʰ **S02.40F** Zygomatic fracture, left side
- ☑6ᵗʰ **S02.41** LeFort fracture

LeFort Fracture Types

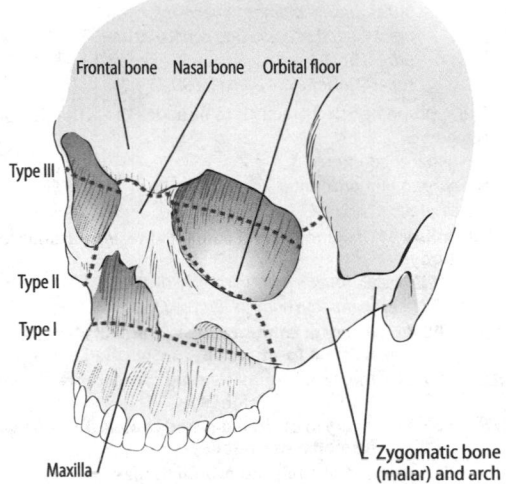

Frontal bone   Nasal bone   Orbital floor

Type III

Type II

Type I

Maxilla

Zygomatic bone (malar) and arch

- ☑7ᵗʰ **S02.411** LeFort I fracture
- ☑7ᵗʰ **S02.412** LeFort II fracture
- ☑7ᵗʰ **S02.413** LeFort III fracture
- ☑ₓ7ᵗʰ **S02.42** Fracture of alveolus of maxilla
- ☑ₓ7ᵗʰ **S02.5** Fracture of tooth (traumatic)

  Broken tooth
  EXCLUDES 1 cracked tooth (nontraumatic) (K03.81)

- ☑5ᵗʰ **S02.6** Fracture of mandible

  Fracture of lower jaw (bone)

  - ☑6ᵗʰ **S02.60** Fracture of mandible, unspecified
    - ▲ ☑7ᵗʰ **S02.600** Fracture of unspecified part of body of mandible, unspecified side ▽
    - ● ☑7ᵗʰ **S02.601** Fracture of unspecified part of body of right mandible ▽
    - ● ☑7ᵗʰ **S02.602** Fracture of unspecified part of body of left mandible ▽
    - ☑7ᵗʰ **S02.609** Fracture of mandible, unspecified ▽
  - ☑6ᵗʰ **S02.61** Fracture of condylar process of mandible
    - ● ☑7ᵗʰ **S02.610** Fracture of condylar process of mandible, unspecified side ▽
    - ● ☑7ᵗʰ **S02.611** Fracture of condylar process of right mandible
    - ● ☑7ᵗʰ **S02.612** Fracture of condylar process of left mandible
  - ☑6ᵗʰ **S02.62** Fracture of subcondylar process of mandible
    - ● ☑7ᵗʰ **S02.620** Fracture of subcondylar process of mandible, unspecified side ▽
    - ● ☑7ᵗʰ **S02.621** Fracture of subcondylar process of right mandible
    - ● ☑7ᵗʰ **S02.622** Fracture of subcondylar process of left mandible
  - ☑6ᵗʰ **S02.63** Fracture of coronoid process of mandible
    - ● ☑7ᵗʰ **S02.630** Fracture of coronoid process of mandible, unspecified side ▽
    - ● ☑7ᵗʰ **S02.631** Fracture of coronoid process of right mandible
    - ● ☑7ᵗʰ **S02.632** Fracture of coronoid process of left mandible
  - ☑6ᵗʰ **S02.64** Fracture of ramus of mandible
    - ● ☑7ᵗʰ **S02.640** Fracture of ramus of mandible, unspecified side ▽
    - ☑7ᵗʰ **S02.641** Fracture of ramus of right mandible
    - ● ☑7ᵗʰ **S02.642** Fracture of ramus of left mandible
  - ☑6ᵗʰ **S02.65** Fracture of angle of mandible

- ● ☑7ᵗʰ **S02.650** Fracture of angle of mandible, unspecified side ▽
- ● ☑7ᵗʰ **S02.651** Fracture of angle of right mandible
- ● ☑7ᵗʰ **S02.652** Fracture of angle of left mandible
- ☑7ᵗʰ **S02.66** Fracture of symphysis of mandible
- ☑6ᵗʰ **S02.67** Fracture of alveolus of mandible
  - ☑7ᵗʰ **S02.670** Fracture of alveolus of mandible, unspecified side ▽
  - ● ☑7ᵗʰ **S02.671** Fracture of alveolus of right mandible
  - ● ☑7ᵗʰ **S02.672** Fracture of alveolus of left mandible
- ☑ₓ7ᵗʰ **S02.69** Fracture of mandible of other specified site
- ☑5ᵗʰ **S02.8** Fractures of other specified skull and facial bones

  Fracture of orbit NOS
  Fracture of palate
  EXCLUDES 1 fracture of orbital floor (S02.3-)
  fracture of orbital roof (S02.1-)

  - ● ☑ₓ7ᵗʰ **S02.80** Fracture of other specified skull and facial bones, unspecified side ▽
  - ● **S02.81** Fracture of other specified skull and facial bones, right side
  - ● **S02.82** Fracture of other specified skull and facial bones, left side
- ☑5ᵗʰ **S02.9** Fracture of unspecified skull and facial bones
  - ☑ₓ7ᵗʰ **S02.91** Unspecified fracture of skull ▽
  - ☑ₓ7ᵗʰ **S02.92** Unspecified fracture of facial bones ▽

☑4ᵗʰ **S03** **Dislocation and sprain of joints and ligaments of head**

INCLUDES avulsion of joint (capsule) or ligament of head
laceration of cartilage, joint (capsule) or ligament of head
sprain of cartilage, joint (capsule) or ligament of head
traumatic hemarthrosis of joint or ligament of head
traumatic rupture of joint or ligament of head
traumatic subluxation of joint or ligament of head
traumatic tear of joint or ligament of head

Code also any associated open wound
EXCLUDES 2 strain of muscle or tendon of head (S09.1)

The appropriate 7th character is to be added to each code from category S03.
A   initial encounter
D   subsequent encounter
S   sequela

- ☑5ᵗʰ **S03.0** Dislocation of jaw

  Dislocation of jaw (cartilage) (meniscus)
  Dislocation of mandible
  Dislocation of temporomandibular (joint)

  - ● ☑ₓ7ᵗʰ **S03.00** Dislocation of jaw, unspecified side ▽
  - ● ☑ₓ7ᵗʰ **S03.01** Dislocation of jaw, right side
  - ● ☑ₓ7ᵗʰ **S03.02** Dislocation of jaw, left side
  - ● ☑ₓ7ᵗʰ **S03.03** Dislocation of jaw, bilateral
- ☑ₓ7ᵗʰ **S03.1** Dislocation of septal cartilage of nose
- ☑ₓ7ᵗʰ **S03.2** Dislocation of tooth
- ☑5ᵗʰ **S03.4** Sprain of jaw

  Sprain of temporomandibular (joint) (ligament)

  - ● ☑ₓ7ᵗʰ **S03.40** Sprain of jaw, unspecified side ▽
  - ● ☑ₓ7ᵗʰ **S03.41** Sprain of jaw, right side
  - ● ☑ₓ7ᵗʰ **S03.42** Sprain of jaw, left side
  - ● ☑ₓ7ᵗʰ **S03.43** Sprain of jaw, bilateral
- ☑ₓ7ᵗʰ **S03.8** Sprain of joints and ligaments of other parts of head
- ☑ₓ7ᵗʰ **S03.9** Sprain of joints and ligaments of unspecified parts of head ▽

☑4ᵗʰ **S04** **Injury of cranial nerve**

The selection of side should be based on the side of the body being affected
Code first any associated intracranial injury (S06.-)
Code also any associated:
open wound of head (S01.-)
skull fracture (S02.-)

The appropriate 7th character is to be added to each code from category S04.
A   initial encounter
D   subsequent encounter
S   sequela

✓6ᵗʰ **S04.0** **Injury of optic nerve and pathways**

    Use additional code to identify any visual field defect or blindness (H53.4-, H54)

  ✓6ᵗʰ **S04.01** **Injury of optic nerve**

    Injury of 2nd cranial nerve

    ✓7ᵗʰ **S04.011** **Injury of optic nerve, right eye**

    ✓7ᵗʰ **S04.012** **Injury of optic nerve, left eye**

    ✓7ᵗʰ **S04.019** **Injury of optic nerve, unspecified eye** ▽

      Injury of optic nerve NOS

  ✓ₓ7ᵗʰ **S04.02** **Injury of optic chiasm**

  ✓6ᵗʰ **S04.03** **Injury of optic tract and pathways**

    Injury of optic radiation

    ✓7ᵗʰ **S04.031** **Injury of optic tract and pathways, right eye**

    ✓7ᵗʰ **S04.032** **Injury of optic tract and pathways, left eye**

    ✓7ᵗʰ **S04.039** **Injury of optic tract and pathways, unspecified eye** ▽

      Injury of optic tract and pathways NOS

  ✓6ᵗʰ **S04.04** **Injury of visual cortex**

    ✓7ᵗʰ **S04.041** **Injury of visual cortex, right eye**

    ✓7ᵗʰ **S04.042** **Injury of visual cortex, left eye**

    ✓7ᵗʰ **S04.049** **Injury of visual cortex, unspecified eye** ▽

      Injury of visual cortex NOS

✓5ᵗʰ **S04.1** **Injury of oculomotor nerve**

  Injury of 3rd cranial nerve

  ✓ₓ7ᵗʰ **S04.10** **Injury of oculomotor nerve, unspecified side** ▽

  ✓ₓ7ᵗʰ **S04.11** **Injury of oculomotor nerve, right side**

  ✓ₓ7ᵗʰ **S04.12** **Injury of oculomotor nerve, left side**

✓5ᵗʰ **S04.2** **Injury of trochlear nerve**

  Injury of 4th cranial nerve

  ✓ₓ7ᵗʰ **S04.20** **Injury of trochlear nerve, unspecified side** ▽

  ✓ₓ7ᵗʰ **S04.21** **Injury of trochlear nerve, right side**

  ✓ₓ7ᵗʰ **S04.22** **Injury of trochlear nerve, left side**

✓5ᵗʰ **S04.3** **Injury of trigeminal nerve**

  Injury of 5th cranial nerve

  ✓ₓ7ᵗʰ **S04.30** **Injury of trigeminal nerve, unspecified side** ▽

  ✓ₓ7ᵗʰ **S04.31** **Injury of trigeminal nerve, right side**

  ✓ₓ7ᵗʰ **S04.32** **Injury of trigeminal nerve, left side**

✓5ᵗʰ **S04.4** **Injury of abducent nerve**

  Injury of 6th cranial nerve

  ✓ₓ7ᵗʰ **S04.40** **Injury of abducent nerve, unspecified side** ▽

  ✓ₓ7ᵗʰ **S04.41** **Injury of abducent nerve, right side**

  ✓ₓ7ᵗʰ **S04.42** **Injury of abducent nerve, left side**

✓5ᵗʰ **S04.5** **Injury of facial nerve**

  Injury of 7th cranial nerve

  ✓ₓ7ᵗʰ **S04.50** **Injury of facial nerve, unspecified side** ▽

  ✓ₓ7ᵗʰ **S04.51** **Injury of facial nerve, right side**

  ✓ₓ7ᵗʰ **S04.52** **Injury of facial nerve, left side**

✓5ᵗʰ **S04.6** **Injury of acoustic nerve**

  Injury of auditory nerve

  Injury of 8th cranial nerve

  ✓ₓ7ᵗʰ **S04.60** **Injury of acoustic nerve, unspecified side** ▽

  ✓ₓ7ᵗʰ **S04.61** **Injury of acoustic nerve, right side**

  ✓ₓ7ᵗʰ **S04.62** **Injury of acoustic nerve, left side**

✓5ᵗʰ **S04.7** **Injury of accessory nerve**

  Injury of 11th cranial nerve

  ✓ₓ7ᵗʰ **S04.70** **Injury of accessory nerve, unspecified side** ▽

  ✓ₓ7ᵗʰ **S04.71** **Injury of accessory nerve, right side**

  ✓ₓ7ᵗʰ **S04.72** **Injury of accessory nerve, left side**

✓6ᵗʰ **S04.8** **Injury of other cranial nerves**

  ✓6ᵗʰ **S04.81** **Injury of olfactory [1st] nerve**

    ✓7ᵗʰ **S04.811** **Injury of olfactory [1st] nerve, right side**

    ✓7ᵗʰ **S04.812** **Injury of olfactory [1st] nerve, left side**

    ✓7ᵗʰ **S04.819** **Injury of olfactory [1st] nerve, unspecified side** ▽

  ✓6ᵗʰ **S04.89** **Injury of other cranial nerves**

    Injury of vagus [10th] nerve

    ✓7ᵗʰ **S04.891** **Injury of other cranial nerves, right side**

    ✓7ᵗʰ **S04.892** **Injury of other cranial nerves, left side**

    ✓7ᵗʰ **S04.899** **Injury of other cranial nerves, unspecified side** ▽

✓ₓ7ᵗʰ **S04.9** **Injury of unspecified cranial nerve** ▽

✓4ᵗʰ **S05** **Injury of eye and orbit**

  INCLUDES open wound of eye and orbit

  EXCLUDES 2 *2nd cranial [optic] nerve injury (S04.0-)*

    3rd cranial [oculomotor] nerve injury (S04.1-)

    open wound of eyelid and periocular area (S01.1-)

    orbital bone fracture (S02.1-, S02.3-, S02.8-)

    superficial injury of eyelid (S00.1-S00.2)

  The appropriate 7th character is to be added to each code from category S05.

  A initial encounter

  D subsequent encounter

  S sequela

  ✓5ᵗʰ **S05.0** **Injury of conjunctiva and corneal abrasion without foreign body**

    EXCLUDES 1 *foreign body in conjunctival sac (T15.1)*

      foreign body in cornea (T15.0)

    ✓ₓ7ᵗʰ **S05.00** **Injury of conjunctiva and corneal abrasion without foreign body, unspecified eye** ▽

    ✓ₓ7ᵗʰ **S05.01** **Injury of conjunctiva and corneal abrasion without foreign body, right eye**

    ✓ₓ7ᵗʰ **S05.02** **Injury of conjunctiva and corneal abrasion without foreign body, left eye**

  ✓5ᵗʰ **S05.1** **Contusion of eyeball and orbital tissues**

    Traumatic hyphema

    EXCLUDES 2 *black eye NOS (S00.1)*

      contusion of eyelid and periocular area (S00.1)

    ✓ₓ7ᵗʰ **S05.10** **Contusion of eyeball and orbital tissues, unspecified eye** ▽

    ✓ₓ7ᵗʰ **S05.11** **Contusion of eyeball and orbital tissues, right eye**

    ✓ₓ7ᵗʰ **S05.12** **Contusion of eyeball and orbital tissues, left eye**

  ✓5ᵗʰ **S05.2** **Ocular laceration and rupture with prolapse or loss of intraocular tissue**

    ✓ₓ7ᵗʰ **S05.20** **Ocular laceration and rupture with prolapse or loss of intraocular tissue, unspecified eye** ▽

    ✓ₓ7ᵗʰ **S05.21** **Ocular laceration and rupture with prolapse or loss of intraocular tissue, right eye**

    ✓ₓ7ᵗʰ **S05.22** **Ocular laceration and rupture with prolapse or loss of intraocular tissue, left eye**

  ✓5ᵗʰ **S05.3** **Ocular laceration without prolapse or loss of intraocular tissue**

    Laceration of eye NOS

    ✓ₓ7ᵗʰ **S05.30** **Ocular laceration without prolapse or loss of intraocular tissue, unspecified eye** ▽

    ✓ₓ7ᵗʰ **S05.31** **Ocular laceration without prolapse or loss of intraocular tissue, right eye**

    ✓ₓ7ᵗʰ **S05.32** **Ocular laceration without prolapse or loss of intraocular tissue, left eye**

  ✓5ᵗʰ **S05.4** **Penetrating wound of orbit with or without foreign body**

    EXCLUDES 2 *retained (old) foreign body following penetrating wound in orbit (H05.5-)*

    ✓ₓ7ᵗʰ **S05.40** **Penetrating wound of orbit with or without foreign body, unspecified eye** ▽

    ✓ₓ7ᵗʰ **S05.41** **Penetrating wound of orbit with or without foreign body, right eye**

    ✓ₓ7ᵗʰ **S05.42** **Penetrating wound of orbit with or without foreign body, left eye**

  ✓5ᵗʰ **S05.5** **Penetrating wound with foreign body of eyeball**

    EXCLUDES 2 *retained (old) intraocular foreign body (H44.6-, H44.7)*

    ✓ₓ7ᵗʰ **S05.50** **Penetrating wound with foreign body of unspecified eyeball** ▽

    ✓ₓ7ᵗʰ **S05.51** **Penetrating wound with foreign body of right eyeball**

    ✓ₓ7ᵗʰ **S05.52** **Penetrating wound with foreign body of left eyeball**

  ✓5ᵗʰ **S05.6** **Penetrating wound without foreign body of eyeball**

    Ocular penetration NOS

    ✓ₓ7ᵗʰ **S05.60** **Penetrating wound without foreign body of unspecified eyeball** ▽

    ✓ₓ7ᵗʰ **S05.61** **Penetrating wound without foreign body of right eyeball**

EXCLUDES 1 Not coded here   **EXCLUDES 2** Not included here   N Newborn Age : 0   P Pediatric Age : 0-17   M Maternity Age : 12-55   A Adult Age : 15-124

894   ICD-10-CM 2017

✓x7ᵗʰ **S05.62** **Penetrating wound without foreign body of** left eyeball

✓5ᵗʰ **S05.7** **Avulsion of eye**
Traumatic enucleation

✓x7ᵗʰ **S05.70** **Avulsion of unspecified eye** ▽
✓x7ᵗʰ **S05.71** **Avulsion of** right **eye**
✓x7ᵗʰ **S05.72** **Avulsion of** left **eye**

✓5ᵗʰ **S05.8** **Other injuries of eye and orbit**
Lacrimal duct injury

✓6ᵗʰ **S05.8X** **Other injuries of eye and orbit**
✓7ᵗʰ **S05.8X1** **Other injuries of** right **eye and orbit**
✓7ᵗʰ **S05.8X2** **Other injuries of** left **eye and orbit**
✓7ᵗʰ **S05.8X9** **Other injuries of unspecified eye and orbit** ▽

✓5ᵗʰ **S05.9** **Unspecified injury of eye and orbit**
Injury of eye NOS

✓x7ᵗʰ **S05.90** **Unspecified injury of unspecified eye and orbit** ▽
✓x7ᵗʰ **S05.91** **Unspecified injury of** right **eye and orbit** ▽
✓x7ᵗʰ **S05.92** **Unspecified injury of** left **eye and orbit** ▽

✓4ᵗʰ **S06** **Intracranial injury**
INCLUDES traumatic brain injury
Code also any associated:
  open wound of head (S01.-)
  skull fracture (S02.-)
EXCLUDES 1 head injury NOS (S09.90)
AHA: 2015,3Q,37

The appropriate 7th character is to be added to each code from category S06.
A   initial encounter
D   subsequent encounter
S   sequela

✓5ᵗʰ **S06.0** **Concussion**
Commotio cerebri
EXCLUDES 1 ►concussion with other intracranial injuries classified in subcategories S06.1- to S06.6-, S06.81- and S06.82- code to specified intracranial injury◄

✓6ᵗʰ **S06.0X** **Concussion**
✓7ᵗʰ **S06.0X0** **Concussion** without loss of consciousness
✓7ᵗʰ **S06.0X1** **Concussion with loss of consciousness of** 30 minutes or less
✓7ᵗʰ **S06.0X9** **Concussion with loss of consciousness of unspecified duration** ▽
Concussion NOS

✓5ᵗʰ **S06.1** **Traumatic cerebral edema**
Diffuse traumatic cerebral edema
Focal traumatic cerebral edema

✓6ᵗʰ **S06.1X** **Traumatic** cerebral edema
✓7ᵗʰ **S06.1X0** **Traumatic cerebral edema** without loss of consciousness
✓7ᵗʰ **S06.1X1** **Traumatic cerebral edema with loss of consciousness of** 30 minutes or less
✓7ᵗʰ **S06.1X2** **Traumatic cerebral edema with loss of consciousness of** 31 minutes to 59 minutes
✓7ᵗʰ **S06.1X3** **Traumatic cerebral edema with loss of consciousness of** 1 hour to 5 hours 59 minutes
✓7ᵗʰ **S06.1X4** **Traumatic cerebral edema with loss of consciousness of** 6 hours to 24 hours
✓7ᵗʰ **S06.1X5** **Traumatic cerebral edema with loss of consciousness** greater than 24 hours with return to pre-existing conscious level
✓7ᵗʰ **S06.1X6** **Traumatic cerebral edema with loss of consciousness** greater than 24 hours without return to pre-existing conscious level with patient surviving
✓7ᵗʰ **S06.1X7** **Traumatic cerebral edema with loss of consciousness of** any duration with death due to brain injury prior to regaining consciousness
✓7ᵗʰ **S06.1X8** **Traumatic cerebral edema with loss of consciousness of** any duration with death due to **other** cause prior to regaining consciousness

✓7ᵗʰ **S06.1X9** **Traumatic cerebral edema with loss of consciousness of unspecified duration** ▽
Traumatic cerebral edema NOS

✓5ᵗʰ **S06.2** **Diffuse traumatic brain injury**
Diffuse axonal brain injury
EXCLUDES 1 traumatic diffuse cerebral edema (S06.1X-)

✓6ᵗʰ **S06.2X** **Diffuse traumatic brain injury**
✓7ᵗʰ **S06.2X0** **Diffuse traumatic brain injury** without loss of consciousness
✓7ᵗʰ **S06.2X1** **Diffuse traumatic brain injury with loss of consciousness of** 30 minutes or less
✓7ᵗʰ **S06.2X2** **Diffuse traumatic brain injury with loss of consciousness of** 31 minutes to 59 minutes
✓7ᵗʰ **S06.2X3** **Diffuse traumatic brain injury with loss of consciousness of** 1 hour to 5 hours 59 minutes
✓7ᵗʰ **S06.2X4** **Diffuse traumatic brain injury with loss of consciousness of** 6 hours to 24 hours
✓7ᵗʰ **S06.2X5** **Diffuse traumatic brain injury with loss of consciousness** greater than 24 hours with return to pre-existing conscious levels
✓7ᵗʰ **S06.2X6** **Diffuse traumatic brain injury with loss of consciousness** greater than 24 hours without return to pre-existing conscious level with patient surviving
✓7ᵗʰ **S06.2X7** **Diffuse traumatic brain injury with loss of consciousness of** any duration with death due to brain injury prior to regaining consciousness
✓7ᵗʰ **S06.2X8** **Diffuse traumatic brain injury with loss of consciousness of** any duration with death due to **other** cause prior to regaining consciousness
✓7ᵗʰ **S06.2X9** **Diffuse traumatic brain injury with loss of consciousness of unspecified duration** ▽
Diffuse traumatic brain injury NOS

✓5ᵗʰ **S06.3** **Focal traumatic brain injury**
EXCLUDES 1 any condition classifiable to S06.4-S06.6 focal cerebral edema (S06.1)

✓6ᵗʰ **S06.30** **Unspecified focal traumatic brain injury**
✓7ᵗʰ **S06.300** **Unspecified focal traumatic brain injury** without loss of consciousness ▽
✓7ᵗʰ **S06.301** **Unspecified focal traumatic brain injury with loss of consciousness of** 30 minutes or less ▽
✓7ᵗʰ **S06.302** **Unspecified focal traumatic brain injury with loss of consciousness of** 31 minutes to 59 minutes ▽
✓7ᵗʰ **S06.303** **Unspecified focal traumatic brain injury with loss of consciousness of** 1 hour to 5 hours 59 minutes ▽
✓7ᵗʰ **S06.304** **Unspecified focal traumatic brain injury with loss of consciousness of** 6 hours to 24 hours ▽
✓7ᵗʰ **S06.305** **Unspecified focal traumatic brain injury with loss of consciousness** greater than 24 hours with return to pre-existing conscious level ▽
✓7ᵗʰ **S06.306** **Unspecified focal traumatic brain injury with loss of consciousness** greater than 24 hours without return to pre-existing conscious level with patient surviving ▽
✓7ᵗʰ **S06.307** **Unspecified focal traumatic brain injury with loss of consciousness of** any duration with death due to brain injury prior to regaining consciousness ▽
✓7ᵗʰ **S06.308** **Unspecified focal traumatic brain injury with loss of consciousness of** any duration with death due to **other** cause prior to regaining consciousness ▽

☑ Additional Character Required   ✓x7ᵗʰ Placeholder Alert   Manifestation Dx   ▽ Unspecified Dx   ►◄ Revised Text   ● New Code   ▲ Revised Code Title

✓7ᵗʰ **S06.309 Unspecified focal traumatic brain injury with loss of consciousness of unspecified duration** ▽
Unspecified focal traumatic brain injury NOS

✓6ᵗʰ **S06.31 Contusion and laceration of** right cerebrum

✓7ᵗʰ **S06.310 Contusion and laceration of right cerebrum** without loss of consciousness

✓7ᵗʰ **S06.311 Contusion and laceration of right cerebrum with loss of consciousness of** 30 minutes or less

✓7ᵗʰ **S06.312 Contusion and laceration of right cerebrum with loss of consciousness of** 31 minutes to 59 minutes

✓7ᵗʰ **S06.313 Contusion and laceration of right cerebrum with loss of consciousness of** 1 hour to 5 hours 59 minutes

✓7ᵗʰ **S06.314 Contusion and laceration of right cerebrum with loss of consciousness of** 6 hours to 24 hours

✓7ᵗʰ **S06.315 Contusion and laceration of right cerebrum with loss of consciousness** greater than 24 hours with return to pre-existing conscious level

✓7ᵗʰ **S06.316 Contusion and laceration of right cerebrum with loss of consciousness** greater than 24 hours without return to pre-existing conscious level with patient surviving

✓7ᵗʰ **S06.317 Contusion and laceration of right cerebrum with loss of consciousness of** any duration with death due to brain injury prior to regaining consciousness

✓7ᵗʰ **S06.318 Contusion and laceration of right cerebrum with loss of consciousness of** any duration with death due to **other** cause prior to regaining consciousness

✓7ᵗʰ **S06.319 Contusion and laceration of right cerebrum with loss of consciousness of unspecified duration** ▽
Contusion and laceration of right cerebrum NOS

✓6ᵗʰ **S06.32 Contusion and laceration of** left cerebrum

✓7ᵗʰ **S06.320 Contusion and laceration of left cerebrum** without loss of consciousness

✓7ᵗʰ **S06.321 Contusion and laceration of left cerebrum with loss of consciousness of** 30 minutes or less

✓7ᵗʰ **S06.322 Contusion and laceration of left cerebrum with loss of consciousness of** 31 minutes to 59 minutes

✓7ᵗʰ **S06.323 Contusion and laceration of left cerebrum with loss of consciousness of** 1 hour to 5 hours 59 minutes

✓7ᵗʰ **S06.324 Contusion and laceration of left cerebrum with loss of consciousness of** 6 hours to 24 hours

✓7ᵗʰ **S06.325 Contusion and laceration of left cerebrum with loss of consciousness** greater than 24 hours with return to pre-existing conscious level

✓7ᵗʰ **S06.326 Contusion and laceration of left cerebrum with loss of consciousness** greater than 24 hours without return to pre-existing conscious level with patient surviving

✓7ᵗʰ **S06.327 Contusion and laceration of left cerebrum with loss of consciousness of** any duration with death due to brain injury prior to regaining consciousness

✓7ᵗʰ **S06.328 Contusion and laceration of left cerebrum with loss of consciousness of** any duration with death due to **other** cause prior to regaining consciousness

✓7ᵗʰ **S06.329 Contusion and laceration of left cerebrum with loss of consciousness of unspecified duration** ▽
Contusion and laceration of left cerebrum NOS

✓6ᵗʰ **S06.33 Contusion and laceration of cerebrum, unspecified**

✓7ᵗʰ **S06.330 Contusion and laceration of cerebrum, unspecified,** without loss of consciousness ▽

✓7ᵗʰ **S06.331 Contusion and laceration of cerebrum, unspecified, with loss of consciousness of** 30 minutes or less ▽

✓7ᵗʰ **S06.332 Contusion and laceration of cerebrum, unspecified, with loss of consciousness of** 31 minutes to 59 minutes ▽

✓7ᵗʰ **S06.333 Contusion and laceration of cerebrum, unspecified, with loss of consciousness of** 1 hour to 5 hours 59 minutes ▽

✓7ᵗʰ **S06.334 Contusion and laceration of cerebrum, unspecified, with loss of consciousness of** 6 hours to 24 hours ▽

✓7ᵗʰ **S06.335 Contusion and laceration of cerebrum, unspecified, with loss of consciousness** greater than 24 hours with return to pre-existing conscious level ▽

✓7ᵗʰ **S06.336 Contusion and laceration of cerebrum, unspecified, with loss of consciousness** greater than 24 hours without return to pre-existing conscious level with patient surviving ▽

✓7ᵗʰ **S06.337 Contusion and laceration of cerebrum, unspecified, with loss of consciousness of** any duration with death due to brain injury prior to regaining consciousness ▽

✓7ᵗʰ **S06.338 Contusion and laceration of cerebrum, unspecified, with loss of consciousness of** any duration with death due to **other** cause prior to regaining consciousness ▽

✓7ᵗʰ **S06.339 Contusion and laceration of cerebrum, unspecified, with loss of consciousness of unspecified duration** ▽
Contusion and laceration of cerebrum NOS

✓6ᵗʰ **S06.34 Traumatic hemorrhage of** right cerebrum
Traumatic intracerebral hemorrhage and hematoma of right cerebrum

✓7ᵗʰ **S06.340 Traumatic hemorrhage of right cerebrum** without loss of consciousness

✓7ᵗʰ **S06.341 Traumatic hemorrhage of right cerebrum with loss of consciousness of** 30 minutes or less

✓7ᵗʰ **S06.342 Traumatic hemorrhage of right cerebrum with loss of consciousness of** 31 minutes to 59 minutes

✓7ᵗʰ **S06.343 Traumatic hemorrhage of right cerebrum with loss of consciousness of** 1 hours to 5 hours 59 minutes

✓7ᵗʰ **S06.344 Traumatic hemorrhage of right cerebrum with loss of consciousness of** 6 hours to 24 hours

✓7ᵗʰ **S06.345 Traumatic hemorrhage of right cerebrum with loss of consciousness** greater than 24 hours with return to pre-existing conscious level

✓7ᵗʰ **S06.346 Traumatic hemorrhage of right cerebrum with loss of consciousness** greater than 24 hours without return to pre-existing conscious level with patient surviving

✓7ᵗʰ **S06.347 Traumatic hemorrhage of right cerebrum with loss of consciousness of** any duration with death due to brain injury prior to regaining consciousness

✓7ᵗʰ **S06.348 Traumatic hemorrhage of right cerebrum with loss of consciousness of** any duration with death due to **other** cause prior to regaining consciousness

✓7ᵗʰ **S06.349 Traumatic hemorrhage of right cerebrum with loss of consciousness of unspecified duration** ▽
Traumatic hemorrhage of right cerebrum NOS

✓6ᵗʰ **S06.35 Traumatic hemorrhage of** left cerebrum
Traumatic intracerebral hemorrhage and hematoma of left cerebrum

✓7ᵗʰ **S06.350 Traumatic hemorrhage of left cerebrum** without loss of consciousness

☑7ᵗʰ **S06.351** **Traumatic hemorrhage of left cerebrum with loss of consciousness of** 30 minutes or less

☑7ᵗʰ **S06.352** **Traumatic hemorrhage of left cerebrum with loss of consciousness of** 31 minutes to 59 minutes

☑7ᵗʰ **S06.353** **Traumatic hemorrhage of left cerebrum with loss of consciousness of** 1 hours to 5 hours 59 minutes

☑7ᵗʰ **S06.354** **Traumatic hemorrhage of left cerebrum with loss of consciousness of** 6 hours to 24 hours

☑7ᵗʰ **S06.355** **Traumatic hemorrhage of left cerebrum with loss of consciousness** greater than 24 hours with return to pre-existing conscious level

☑7ᵗʰ **S06.356** **Traumatic hemorrhage of left cerebrum with loss of consciousness** greater than 24 hours without return to pre-existing conscious level with patient surviving

☑7ᵗʰ **S06.357** **Traumatic hemorrhage of left cerebrum with loss of consciousness of** any duration with death due to brain injury prior to regaining consciousness

☑7ᵗʰ **S06.358** **Traumatic hemorrhage of left cerebrum with loss of consciousness of** any duration with death due to **other** cause prior to regaining consciousness

☑7ᵗʰ **S06.359** **Traumatic hemorrhage of left cerebrum with loss of consciousness of unspecified duration** ▽

Traumatic hemorrhage of left cerebrum NOS

☑6ᵗʰ **S06.36** **Traumatic hemorrhage of cerebrum, unspecified**

Traumatic intracerebral hemorrhage and hematoma, unspecified

☑7ᵗʰ **S06.360** **Traumatic hemorrhage of cerebrum, unspecified,** without loss of consciousness ▽

☑7ᵗʰ **S06.361** **Traumatic hemorrhage of cerebrum, unspecified, with loss of consciousness of** 30 minutes or less ▽

☑7ᵗʰ **S06.362** **Traumatic hemorrhage of cerebrum, unspecified, with loss of consciousness of** 31 minutes to 59 minutes ▽

☑7ᵗʰ **S06.363** **Traumatic hemorrhage of cerebrum, unspecified, with loss of consciousness of** 1 hours to 5 hours 59 minutes ▽

☑7ᵗʰ **S06.364** **Traumatic hemorrhage of cerebrum, unspecified, with loss of consciousness of** 6 hours to 24 hours ▽

☑7ᵗʰ **S06.365** **Traumatic hemorrhage of cerebrum, unspecified, with loss of consciousness** greater than 24 hours with return to pre-existing conscious level ▽

☑7ᵗʰ **S06.366** **Traumatic hemorrhage of cerebrum, unspecified, with loss of consciousness** greater than 24 hours without return to pre-existing conscious level with patient surviving ▽

☑7ᵗʰ **S06.367** **Traumatic hemorrhage of cerebrum, unspecified, with loss of consciousness of** any duration with death due to brain injury prior to regaining consciousness ▽

☑7ᵗʰ **S06.368** **Traumatic hemorrhage of cerebrum, unspecified, with loss of consciousness of** any duration with death due to **other** cause prior to regaining consciousness ▽

☑7ᵗʰ **S06.369** **Traumatic hemorrhage of cerebrum, unspecified, with loss of consciousness of unspecified duration** ▽

Traumatic hemorrhage of cerebrum NOS

☑6ᵗʰ **S06.37** **Contusion, laceration, and hemorrhage of cerebellum**

☑7ᵗʰ **S06.370** **Contusion, laceration, and hemorrhage of cerebellum** without loss of consciousness

☑7ᵗʰ **S06.371** **Contusion, laceration, and hemorrhage of cerebellum with loss of consciousness of** 30 minutes or less

☑7ᵗʰ **S06.372** **Contusion, laceration, and hemorrhage of cerebellum with loss of consciousness of** 31 minutes to 59 minutes

☑7ᵗʰ **S06.373** **Contusion, laceration, and hemorrhage of cerebellum with loss of consciousness of** 1 hour to 5 hours 59 minutes

☑7ᵗʰ **S06.374** **Contusion, laceration, and hemorrhage of cerebellum with loss of consciousness of** 6 hours to 24 hours

☑7ᵗʰ **S06.375** **Contusion, laceration, and hemorrhage of cerebellum with loss of consciousness** greater than 24 hours with return to pre-existing conscious level

☑7ᵗʰ **S06.376** **Contusion, laceration, and hemorrhage of cerebellum with loss of consciousness** greater than 24 hours without return to pre-existing conscious level with patient surviving

☑7ᵗʰ **S06.377** **Contusion, laceration, and hemorrhage of cerebellum with loss of consciousness of** any duration with death due to brain injury prior to regaining consciousness

☑7ᵗʰ **S06.378** **Contusion, laceration, and hemorrhage of cerebellum with loss of consciousness of** any duration with death due to **other** cause prior to regaining consciousness

☑7ᵗʰ **S06.379** **Contusion, laceration, and hemorrhage of cerebellum with loss of consciousness of unspecified duration** ▽

Contusion, laceration, and hemorrhage of cerebellum NOS

☑6ᵗʰ **S06.38** **Contusion, laceration, and hemorrhage of brainstem**

☑7ᵗʰ **S06.380** **Contusion, laceration, and hemorrhage of brainstem** without loss of consciousness

☑7ᵗʰ **S06.381** **Contusion, laceration, and hemorrhage of brainstem with loss of consciousness of** 30 minutes or less

☑7ᵗʰ **S06.382** **Contusion, laceration, and hemorrhage of brainstem with loss of consciousness of** 31 minutes to 59 minutes

☑7ᵗʰ **S06.383** **Contusion, laceration, and hemorrhage of brainstem with loss of consciousness of** 1 hour to 5 hours 59 minutes

☑7ᵗʰ **S06.384** **Contusion, laceration, and hemorrhage of brainstem with loss of consciousness of** 6 hours to 24 hours

☑7ᵗʰ **S06.385** **Contusion, laceration, and hemorrhage of brainstem with loss of consciousness** greater than 24 hours with return to pre-existing conscious level

☑7ᵗʰ **S06.386** **Contusion, laceration, and hemorrhage of brainstem with loss of consciousness** greater than 24 hours without return to pre-existing conscious level with patient surviving

☑7ᵗʰ **S06.387** **Contusion, laceration, and hemorrhage of brainstem with loss of consciousness of** any duration with death due to brain injury prior to regaining consciousness

☑7ᵗʰ **S06.388** **Contusion, laceration, and hemorrhage of brainstem with loss of consciousness of** any duration with death due to **other** cause prior to regaining consciousness

☑7ᵗʰ **S06.389** **Contusion, laceration, and hemorrhage of brainstem with loss of consciousness of unspecified duration** ▽

Contusion, laceration, and hemorrhage of brainstem NOS

☑5ᵗʰ **S06.4** **Epidural hemorrhage**

Extradural hemorrhage NOS

Extradural hemorrhage (traumatic)

☑6ᵗʰ **S06.4X** **Epidural hemorrhage**

☑ Additional Character Required   ☑ⁿ⁷ᵗʰ Placeholder Alert   Manifestation Dx   ▽ Unspecified Dx   ▶◀ Revised Text   ● New Code   ▲ Revised Code Title

ICD-10-CM 2017

897

√7ᵗʰ **S06.4X0 Epidural hemorrhage** without loss of consciousness

√7ᵗʰ **S06.4X1 Epidural hemorrhage with loss of consciousness of** 30 minutes or less

√7ᵗʰ **S06.4X2 Epidural hemorrhage with loss of consciousness of** 31 minutes to 59 minutes

√7ᵗʰ **S06.4X3 Epidural hemorrhage with loss of consciousness of** 1 hour to 5 hours 59 minutes

√7ᵗʰ **S06.4X4 Epidural hemorrhage with loss of consciousness of** 6 hours to 24 hours

√7ᵗʰ **S06.4X5 Epidural hemorrhage with loss of consciousness** greater than 24 hours with return to pre-existing conscious level

√7ᵗʰ **S06.4X6 Epidural hemorrhage with loss of consciousness** greater than 24 hours without return to pre-existing conscious level with patient surviving

√7ᵗʰ **S06.4X7 Epidural hemorrhage with loss of consciousness of** any duration with death due to brain injury prior to regaining consciousness

√7ᵗʰ **S06.4X8 Epidural hemorrhage with loss of consciousness of** any duration with death due to **other** causes prior to regaining consciousness

√7ᵗʰ **S06.4X9 Epidural hemorrhage with loss of consciousness of** unspecified duration   ▽
Epidural hemorrhage NOS

√5ᵗʰ **S06.5 Traumatic** subdural **hemorrhage**

√6ᵗʰ **S06.5X Traumatic subdural hemorrhage**

√7ᵗʰ **S06.5X0 Traumatic subdural hemorrhage** without loss of consciousness

√7ᵗʰ **S06.5X1 Traumatic subdural hemorrhage with loss of consciousness of** 30 minutes or less

√7ᵗʰ **S06.5X2 Traumatic subdural hemorrhage with loss of consciousness of** 31 minutes to 59 minutes

√7ᵗʰ **S06.5X3 Traumatic subdural hemorrhage with loss of consciousness of** 1 hour to 5 hours 59 minutes

√7ᵗʰ **S06.5X4 Traumatic subdural hemorrhage with loss of consciousness of** 6 hours to 24 hours

√7ᵗʰ **S06.5X5 Traumatic subdural hemorrhage with loss of consciousness** greater than 24 hours with return to pre-existing conscious level

√7ᵗʰ **S06.5X6 Traumatic subdural hemorrhage with loss of consciousness** greater than 24 hours without return to pre-existing conscious level with patient surviving

√7ᵗʰ **S06.5X7 Traumatic subdural hemorrhage with loss of consciousness of** any duration with death due to brain injury before regaining consciousness

√7ᵗʰ **S06.5X8 Traumatic subdural hemorrhage with loss of consciousness of** any duration with death due to **other** cause before regaining consciousness

√7ᵗʰ **S06.5X9 Traumatic subdural hemorrhage with loss of consciousness of** unspecified duration   ▽
Traumatic subdural hemorrhage NOS

√5ᵗʰ **S06.6 Traumatic** subarachnoid **hemorrhage**

√6ᵗʰ **S06.6X Traumatic subarachnoid hemorrhage**

√7ᵗʰ **S06.6X0 Traumatic subarachnoid hemorrhage** without loss of consciousness

√7ᵗʰ **S06.6X1 Traumatic subarachnoid hemorrhage with loss of consciousness of** 30 minutes or less

√7ᵗʰ **S06.6X2 Traumatic subarachnoid hemorrhage with loss of consciousness of** 31 minutes to 59 minutes

√7ᵗʰ **S06.6X3 Traumatic subarachnoid hemorrhage with loss of consciousness of** 1 hour to 5 hours 59 minutes

√7ᵗʰ **S06.6X4 Traumatic subarachnoid hemorrhage with loss of consciousness of** 6 hours to 24 hours

√7ᵗʰ **S06.6X5 Traumatic subarachnoid hemorrhage with loss of consciousness** greater than 24 hours with return to pre-existing conscious level

√7ᵗʰ **S06.6X6 Traumatic subarachnoid hemorrhage with loss of consciousness** greater than 24 hours without return to pre-existing conscious level with patient surviving

√7ᵗʰ **S06.6X7 Traumatic subarachnoid hemorrhage with loss of consciousness of** any duration with death due to brain injury prior to regaining consciousness

√7ᵗʰ **S06.6X8 Traumatic subarachnoid hemorrhage with loss of consciousness of** any duration with death due to **other** cause prior to regaining consciousness

√7ᵗʰ **S06.6X9 Traumatic subarachnoid hemorrhage with loss of consciousness of unspecified duration**   ▽
Traumatic subarachnoid hemorrhage NOS

√5ᵗʰ **S06.8 Other specified intracranial injuries**

√6ᵗʰ **S06.81 Injury of** right internal carotid artery, **intracranial portion, not elsewhere classified**

√7ᵗʰ **S06.810 Injury of right internal carotid artery, intracranial portion, not elsewhere classified** without loss of consciousness

√7ᵗʰ **S06.811 Injury of right internal carotid artery, intracranial portion, not elsewhere classified with loss of consciousness of** 30 minutes or less

√7ᵗʰ **S06.812 Injury of right internal carotid artery, intracranial portion, not elsewhere classified with loss of consciousness of** 31 minutes to 59 minutes

√7ᵗʰ **S06.813 Injury of right internal carotid artery, intracranial portion, not elsewhere classified with loss of consciousness of** 1 hour to 5 hours 59 minutes

√7ᵗʰ **S06.814 Injury of right internal carotid artery, intracranial portion, not elsewhere classified with loss of consciousness of** 6 hours to 24 hours

√7ᵗʰ **S06.815 Injury of right internal carotid artery, intracranial portion, not elsewhere classified with loss of consciousness** greater than 24 hours with return to pre-existing conscious level

√7ᵗʰ **S06.816 Injury of right internal carotid artery, intracranial portion, not elsewhere classified with loss of consciousness** greater than 24 hours without return to pre-existing conscious level with patient surviving

√7ᵗʰ **S06.817 Injury of right internal carotid artery, intracranial portion, not elsewhere classified with loss of consciousness of** any duration with death due to brain injury prior to regaining consciousness

√7ᵗʰ **S06.818 Injury of right internal carotid artery, intracranial portion, not elsewhere classified with loss of consciousness of** any duration with death due to **other** cause prior to regaining consciousness

√7ᵗʰ **S06.819 Injury of right internal carotid artery, intracranial portion, not elsewhere classified with loss of consciousness of unspecified duration**   ▽
Injury of right internal carotid artery, intracranial portion, not elsewhere classified NOS

√6ᵗʰ **S06.82 Injury of** left internal carotid artery, **intracranial portion, not elsewhere classified**

√7ᵗʰ **S06.820 Injury of left internal carotid artery, intracranial portion, not elsewhere classified** without loss of consciousness

√7ᵗʰ **S06.821 Injury of left internal carotid artery, intracranial portion, not elsewhere classified with loss of consciousness of** 30 minutes or less

√7ᵗʰ **S06.822 Injury of left internal carotid artery, intracranial portion, not elsewhere classified with loss of consciousness of** 31 minutes to 59 minutes

√7ᵗʰ **S06.823** **Injury of left internal carotid artery, intracranial portion, not elsewhere classified with loss of consciousness of** 1 hour to 5 hours 59 minutes

√7ᵗʰ **S06.824** **Injury of left internal carotid artery, intracranial portion, not elsewhere classified with loss of consciousness of** 6 hours to 24 hours

√7ᵗʰ **S06.825** **Injury of left internal carotid artery, intracranial portion, not elsewhere classified with loss of consciousness** greater than 24 hours with return to pre-existing conscious level

√7ᵗʰ **S06.826** **Injury of left internal carotid artery, intracranial portion, not elsewhere classified with loss of consciousness** greater than 24 hours without return to pre-existing conscious level with patient surviving

√7ᵗʰ **S06.827** **Injury of left internal carotid artery, intracranial portion, not elsewhere classified with loss of consciousness of** any duration with death due to brain injury prior to regaining consciousness

√7ᵗʰ **S06.828** **Injury of left internal carotid artery, intracranial portion, not elsewhere classified with loss of consciousness of** other cause prior to regaining consciousness

√7ᵗʰ **S06.829** **Injury of left internal carotid artery, intracranial portion, not elsewhere classified with loss of consciousness of unspecified duration**   ▽
Injury of left internal carotid artery, intracranial portion, not elsewhere classified NOS

√6ᵗʰ **S06.89** **Other specified intracranial injury**
EXCLUDES 1 ▶concussion (S06.0X-)◀

√7ᵗʰ **S06.890** **Other specified intracranial injury** without loss of consciousness

√7ᵗʰ **S06.891** **Other specified intracranial injury with loss of consciousness of** 30 minutes or less

√7ᵗʰ **S06.892** **Other specified intracranial injury with loss of consciousness of** 31 minutes to 59 minutes

√7ᵗʰ **S06.893** **Other specified intracranial injury with loss of consciousness of** 1 hour to 5 hours 59 minutes

√7ᵗʰ **S06.894** **Other specified intracranial injury with loss of consciousness of** 6 hours to 24 hours

√7ᵗʰ **S06.895** **Other specified intracranial injury with loss of consciousness** greater than 24 hours with return to pre-existing conscious level

√7ᵗʰ **S06.896** **Other specified intracranial injury with loss of consciousness** greater than 24 hours without return to pre-existing conscious level with patient surviving

√7ᵗʰ **S06.897** **Other specified intracranial injury with loss of consciousness of** any duration with death due to brain injury prior to regaining consciousness

√7ᵗʰ **S06.898** **Other specified intracranial injury with loss of consciousness of** any duration with death due to other cause prior to regaining consciousness

√7ᵗʰ **S06.899** **Other specified intracranial injury with loss of consciousness of unspecified duration**   ▽

√5ᵗʰ **S06.9** **Unspecified intracranial injury**
Brain injury NOS
Head injury NOS with loss of consciousness
▶Traumatic brain injury NOS◀
EXCLUDES 1 ▶conditions classifiable to S06.0- to S06.8- code to specified intracranial injury◀
head injury NOS (S09.90)

√6ᵗʰ **S06.9X** **Unspecified intracranial injury**

√7ᵗʰ **S06.9X0** **Unspecified intracranial injury** without loss of consciousness   ▽

√7ᵗʰ **S06.9X1** **Unspecified intracranial injury with loss of consciousness of** 30 minutes or less   ▽

√7ᵗʰ **S06.9X2** **Unspecified intracranial injury with loss of consciousness of** 31 minutes to 59 minutes   ▽

√7ᵗʰ **S06.9X3** **Unspecified intracranial injury with loss of consciousness of** 1 hour to 5 hours 59 minutes   ▽

√7ᵗʰ **S06.9X4** **Unspecified intracranial injury with loss of consciousness of** 6 hours to 24 hours   ▽

√7ᵗʰ **S06.9X5** **Unspecified intracranial injury with loss of consciousness** greater than 24 hours with return to pre-existing conscious level   ▽

√7ᵗʰ **S06.9X6** **Unspecified intracranial injury with loss of consciousness** greater than 24 hours without return to pre-existing conscious level with patient surviving   ▽

√7ᵗʰ **S06.9X7** **Unspecified intracranial injury with loss of consciousness of** any duration with death due to brain injury prior to regaining consciousness   ▽

√7ᵗʰ **S06.9X8** **Unspecified intracranial injury with loss of consciousness of** any duration with death due to other cause prior to regaining consciousness   ▽

√7ᵗʰ **S06.9X9** **Unspecified intracranial injury with loss of consciousness of unspecified duration**   ▽

√4ᵗʰ **S07** **Crushing injury of head**
Use additional code for all associated injuries, such as:
intracranial injuries (S06.-)
skull fractures (S02.-)

The appropriate 7th character is to be added to each code from category S07.
A   initial encounter
D   subsequent encounter
S   sequela

√x7ᵗʰ **S07.0** **Crushing injury of** face

√x7ᵗʰ **S07.1** **Crushing injury of** skull

√x7ᵗʰ **S07.8** **Crushing injury of other parts of head**

√x7ᵗʰ **S07.9** **Crushing injury of head, part unspecified**   ▽

√4ᵗʰ **S08** **Avulsion and traumatic amputation of part of head**
NOTE   An amputation not identified as partial or complete should be coded to complete

The appropriate 7th character is to be added to each code from category S08.
A   initial encounter
D   subsequent encounter
S   sequela

√x7ᵗʰ **S08.0** **Avulsion of** scalp

√5ᵗʰ **S08.1** **Traumatic amputation of** ear

√6ᵗʰ **S08.11** **Complete traumatic amputation of ear**

√7ᵗʰ **S08.111** **Complete traumatic amputation of** right ear

√7ᵗʰ **S08.112** **Complete traumatic amputation of** left ear

√7ᵗʰ **S08.119** **Complete traumatic amputation of unspecified ear**   ▽

√6ᵗʰ **S08.12** **Partial traumatic amputation of ear**

√7ᵗʰ **S08.121** **Partial traumatic amputation of** right ear

√7ᵗʰ **S08.122** **Partial traumatic amputation of** left ear

√7ᵗʰ **S08.129** **Partial traumatic amputation of unspecified ear**   ▽

√5ᵗʰ **S08.8** **Traumatic amputation of other parts of head**

√6ᵗʰ **S08.81** **Traumatic amputation of** nose

√7ᵗʰ **S08.811** **Complete traumatic amputation of nose**

√7ᵗʰ **S08.812** **Partial traumatic amputation of nose**

√x7ᵗʰ **S08.89** **Traumatic amputation of other parts of head**

☑ Additional Character Required   √x7ᵗʰ Placeholder Alert   Manifestation Dx   ▽ Unspecified Dx   ▶◀ Revised Text   ● New Code   ▲ Revised Code Title

✓4th **S09 Other and unspecified injuries of head**

> The appropriate 7th character is to be added to each code from category S09.
> A　initial encounter
> D　subsequent encounter
> S　sequela

✓x7th **S09.0 Injury of blood vessels of head, not elsewhere classified**
> EXCLUDES 1 *injury of cerebral blood vessels (S06.-)*
> *injury of precerebral blood vessels (S15.-)*

✓5th **S09.1 Injury of muscle and tendon of head**
> Code also any associated open wound (S01.-)
> EXCLUDES 2 *sprain to joints and ligament of head (S03.9)*

✓x7th **S09.10 Unspecified injury of muscle and tendon of head** ▽
> Injury of muscle and tendon of head NOS

✓x7th **S09.11 Strain of muscle and tendon of head**

✓x7th **S09.12 Laceration of muscle and tendon of head**

✓x7th **S09.19 Other specified injury of muscle and tendon of head**

✓5th **S09.2 Traumatic rupture of ear drum**
> EXCLUDES 1 *traumatic rupture of ear drum due to blast injury (S09.31-)*

✓x7th **S09.20 Traumatic rupture of unspecified ear drum** ▽

✓x7th **S09.21 Traumatic rupture of right ear drum**

✓x7th **S09.22 Traumatic rupture of left ear drum**

✓5th **S09.3 Other specified and unspecified injury of middle and inner ear**
> EXCLUDES 1 *injury to ear NOS (S09.91-)*
> EXCLUDES 2 *injury to external ear (S00.4-, S01.3-, S08.1-)*

✓6th **S09.30 Unspecified injury of middle and inner ear**

✓7th **S09.301 Unspecified injury of right middle and inner ear** ▽

✓7th **S09.302 Unspecified injury of left middle and inner ear** ▽

✓7th **S09.309 Unspecified injury of unspecified middle and inner ear** ▽

✓6th **S09.31 Primary blast injury of ear**
> Blast injury of ear NOS

✓7th **S09.311 Primary blast injury of right ear**

✓7th **S09.312 Primary blast injury of left ear**

✓7th **S09.313 Primary blast injury of ear, bilateral**

✓7th **S09.319 Primary blast injury of unspecified ear** ▽

✓6th **S09.39 Other specified injury of middle and inner ear**
> Secondary blast injury to ear

✓7th **S09.391 Other specified injury of right middle and inner ear**

✓7th **S09.392 Other specified injury of left middle and inner ear**

✓7th **S09.399 Other specified injury of unspecified middle and inner ear** ▽

✓x7th **S09.8 Other specified injuries of head**

✓5th **S09.9 Unspecified injury of face and head**

✓x7th **S09.90 Unspecified injury of head** ▽
> Head injury NOS
> EXCLUDES 1 *brain injury NOS (S06.9-)*
> *head injury NOS with loss of consciousness (S06.9-)*
> *intracranial injury NOS (S06.9-)*

✓x7th **S09.91 Unspecified injury of ear** ▽
> Injury of ear NOS

✓x7th **S09.92 Unspecified injury of nose** ▽
> Injury of nose NOS

✓x7th **S09.93 Unspecified injury of face** ▽
> Injury of face NOS

Injuries to the neck (S10-S19)

INCLUDES　injuries of nape
　　　　　injuries of supraclavicular region
　　　　　injuries of throat
EXCLUDES 2　*burns and corrosions (T20-T32)*
　　　　　effects of foreign body in esophagus (T18.1)
　　　　　effects of foreign body in larynx (T17.3)
　　　　　effects of foreign body in pharynx (T17.2)
　　　　　effects of foreign body in trachea (T17.4)
　　　　　frostbite (T33-T34)
　　　　　insect bite or sting, venomous (T63.4)

✓4th **S10 Superficial injury of neck**

> The appropriate 7th character is to be added to each code from category S10.
> A　initial encounter
> D　subsequent encounter
> S　sequela

✓x7th **S10.0 Contusion of throat**
> Contusion of cervical esophagus
> Contusion of larynx
> Contusion of pharynx
> Contusion of trachea

✓5th **S10.1 Other and unspecified superficial injuries of throat**

✓x7th **S10.10 Unspecified superficial injuries of throat** ▽

✓x7th **S10.11 Abrasion of throat**

✓x7th **S10.12 Blister (nonthermal) of throat**

✓x7th **S10.14 External constriction of part of throat**

✓x7th **S10.15 Superficial foreign body of throat**
> Splinter in the throat

✓x7th **S10.16 Insect bite (nonvenomous) of throat**

✓x7th **S10.17 Other superficial bite of throat**
> EXCLUDES 1 *open bite of throat (S11.85)*

✓5th **S10.8 Superficial injury of other specified parts of neck**

✓x7th **S10.80 Unspecified superficial injury of other specified part of neck** ▽

✓x7th **S10.81 Abrasion of other specified part of neck**

✓x7th **S10.82 Blister (nonthermal) of other specified part of neck**

✓x7th **S10.83 Contusion of other specified part of neck**

✓x7th **S10.84 External constriction of other specified part of neck**

✓x7th **S10.85 Superficial foreign body of other specified part of neck**
> Splinter in other specified part of neck

✓x7th **S10.86 Insect bite of other specified part of neck**

✓x7th **S10.87 Other superficial bite of other specified part of neck**
> EXCLUDES 1 *open bite of other specified parts of neck (S11.85)*

✓5th **S10.9 Superficial injury of unspecified part of neck**

✓x7th **S10.90 Unspecified superficial injury of unspecified part of neck** ▽

✓x7th **S10.91 Abrasion of unspecified part of neck** ▽

✓x7th **S10.92 Blister (nonthermal) of unspecified part of neck** ▽

✓x7th **S10.93 Contusion of unspecified part of neck** ▽

✓x7th **S10.94 External constriction of unspecified part of neck** ▽

✓x7th **S10.95 Superficial foreign body of unspecified part of neck** ▽

✓x7th **S10.96 Insect bite of unspecified part of neck** ▽

✓x7th **S10.97 Other superficial bite of unspecified part of neck** ▽

✓4th **S11 Open wound of neck**
> Code also any associated:
> spinal cord injury (S14.0, S14.1-)
> wound infection
> EXCLUDES 2 *open fracture of vertebra (S12.- with 7th character B)*

> The appropriate 7th character is to be added to each code from category S11.
> A　initial encounter
> D　subsequent encounter
> S　sequela

✓5th **S11.0 Open wound of larynx and trachea**

✓6th **S11.01 Open wound of larynx**
> EXCLUDES 2 *open wound of vocal cord (S11.03)*

✓7th **S11.011 Laceration without foreign body of larynx**

✓7th **S11.012 Laceration with foreign body of larynx**

✓7th **S11.013 Puncture wound without foreign body of larynx**

✓7th **S11.014 Puncture wound with foreign body of larynx**

✓7th **S11.015 Open bite of larynx**
> Bite of larynx NOS

✓7th **S11.019 Unspecified open wound of larynx** ▽

√6ᵗʰ **S11.02 Open wound of trachea**
Open wound of cervical trachea
Open wound of trachea NOS
EXCLUDES 2 *open wound of thoracic trachea (S27.5-)*

√7ᵗʰ **S11.021 Laceration without foreign body of trachea**

√7ᵗʰ **S11.022 Laceration with foreign body of trachea**

√7ᵗʰ **S11.023 Puncture wound without foreign body of trachea**

√7ᵗʰ **S11.024 Puncture wound with foreign body of trachea**

√7ᵗʰ **S11.025 Open bite of trachea**
Bite of trachea NOS

√7ᵗʰ **S11.029 Unspecified open wound of trachea** ▽

√6ᵗʰ **S11.03 Open wound of vocal cord**

√7ᵗʰ **S11.031 Laceration without foreign body of vocal cord**

√7ᵗʰ **S11.032 Laceration with foreign body of vocal cord**

√7ᵗʰ **S11.033 Puncture wound without foreign body of vocal cord**

√7ᵗʰ **S11.034 Puncture wound with foreign body of vocal cord**

√7ᵗʰ **S11.035 Open bite of vocal cord**
Bite of vocal cord NOS

√7ᵗʰ **S11.039 Unspecified open wound of vocal cord** ▽

√5ᵗʰ **S11.1 Open wound of thyroid gland**

√x7ᵗʰ **S11.10 Unspecified open wound of thyroid gland** ▽

√x7ᵗʰ **S11.11 Laceration without foreign body of thyroid gland**

√x7ᵗʰ **S11.12 Laceration with foreign body of thyroid gland**

√x7ᵗʰ **S11.13 Puncture wound without foreign body of thyroid gland**

√x7ᵗʰ **S11.14 Puncture wound with foreign body of thyroid gland**

√x7ᵗʰ **S11.15 Open bite of thyroid gland**
Bite of thyroid gland NOS

√5ᵗʰ **S11.2 Open wound of pharynx and cervical esophagus**
EXCLUDES 1 *open wound of esophagus NOS (S27.8-)*

√x7ᵗʰ **S11.20 Unspecified open wound of pharynx and cervical esophagus** ▽

√x7ᵗʰ **S11.21 Laceration without foreign body of pharynx and cervical esophagus**

√x7ᵗʰ **S11.22 Laceration with foreign body of pharynx and cervical esophagus**

√x7ᵗʰ **S11.23 Puncture wound without foreign body of pharynx and cervical esophagus**

√x7ᵗʰ **S11.24 Puncture wound with foreign body of pharynx and cervical esophagus**

√x7ᵗʰ **S11.25 Open bite of pharynx and cervical esophagus**
Bite of pharynx and cervical esophagus NOS

√5ᵗʰ **S11.8 Open wound of other specified parts of neck**

√x7ᵗʰ **S11.80 Unspecified open wound of other specified part of neck** ▽

√x7ᵗʰ **S11.81 Laceration without foreign body of other specified part of neck**

√x7ᵗʰ **S11.82 Laceration with foreign body of other specified part of neck**

√x7ᵗʰ **S11.83 Puncture wound without foreign body of other specified part of neck**

√x7ᵗʰ **S11.84 Puncture wound with foreign body of other specified part of neck**

√x7ᵗʰ **S11.85 Open bite of other specified part of neck**
Bite of other specified part of neck NOS
EXCLUDES 1 *superficial bite of other specified part of neck (S10.87)*

√x7ᵗʰ **S11.89 Other open wound of other specified part of neck**

√5ᵗʰ **S11.9 Open wound of unspecified part of neck**

√x7ᵗʰ **S11.90 Unspecified open wound of unspecified part of neck** ▽

√x7ᵗʰ **S11.91 Laceration without foreign body of unspecified part of neck** ▽

√x7ᵗʰ **S11.92 Laceration with foreign body of unspecified part of neck** ▽

√x7ᵗʰ **S11.93 Puncture wound without foreign body of unspecified part of neck** ▽

√x7ᵗʰ **S11.94 Puncture wound with foreign body of unspecified part of neck** ▽

√x7ᵗʰ **S11.95 Open bite of unspecified part of neck** ▽
Bite of neck NOS
EXCLUDES 1 *superficial bite of neck (S10.97)*

√4ᵗʰ **S12 Fracture of cervical vertebra and other parts of neck**

NOTE A fracture not indicated as displaced or nondisplaced should be coded to displaced.
A fracture not indicated as open or closed should be coded to closed.

INCLUDES fracture of cervical neural arch
fracture of cervical spine
fracture of cervical spinous process
fracture of cervical transverse process
fracture of cervical vertebral arch
fracture of neck

Code first any associated cervical spinal cord injury (S14.0, S14.1-)
AHA: 2015,3Q,37-39

The appropriate 7th character is to be added to all codes from subcategories S12.0-S12.6.
A initial encounter for closed fracture
B initial encounter for open fracture
D subsequent encounter for fracture with routine healing
G subsequent encounter for fracture with delayed healing
K subsequent encounter for fracture with nonunion
S sequela

√5ᵗʰ **S12.0 Fracture of first cervical vertebra**
Atlas

√6ᵗʰ **S12.00 Unspecified fracture of first cervical vertebra**

√7ᵗʰ **S12.000 Unspecified displaced fracture of first cervical vertebra** ▽

√7ᵗʰ **S12.001 Unspecified nondisplaced fracture of first cervical vertebra** ▽

√7ᵗʰ **S12.01 Stable burst fracture of first cervical vertebra**

√7ᵗʰ **S12.02 Unstable burst fracture of first cervical vertebra**

√6ᵗʰ **S12.03 Posterior arch fracture of first cervical vertebra**

√7ᵗʰ **S12.030 Displaced posterior arch fracture of first cervical vertebra**

√7ᵗʰ **S12.031 Nondisplaced posterior arch fracture of first cervical vertebra**

√6ᵗʰ **S12.04 Lateral mass fracture of first cervical vertebra**

√7ᵗʰ **S12.040 Displaced lateral mass fracture of first cervical vertebra**

√7ᵗʰ **S12.041 Nondisplaced lateral mass fracture of first cervical vertebra**

√6ᵗʰ **S12.09 Other fracture of first cervical vertebra**

√7ᵗʰ **S12.090 Other displaced fracture of first cervical vertebra**

√7ᵗʰ **S12.091 Other nondisplaced fracture of first cervical vertebra**

√5ᵗʰ **S12.1 Fracture of second cervical vertebra**
Axis

√6ᵗʰ **S12.10 Unspecified fracture of second cervical vertebra**

√7ᵗʰ **S12.100 Unspecified displaced fracture of second cervical vertebra** ▽

√7ᵗʰ **S12.101 Unspecified nondisplaced fracture of second cervical vertebra** ▽

√6ᵗʰ **S12.11 Type II dens fracture**

√7ᵗʰ **S12.110 Anterior displaced Type II dens fracture**

√7ᵗʰ **S12.111 Posterior displaced Type II dens fracture**

√7ᵗʰ **S12.112 Nondisplaced Type II dens fracture**

√6ᵗʰ **S12.12 Other dens fracture**

√7ᵗʰ **S12.120 Other displaced dens fracture**

√7ᵗʰ **S12.121 Other nondisplaced dens fracture**

√6ᵗʰ **S12.13 Unspecified traumatic spondylolisthesis of second cervical vertebra**

√7ᵗʰ **S12.130 Unspecified traumatic displaced spondylolisthesis of second cervical vertebra** ▽

√7ᵗʰ **S12.131 Unspecified traumatic nondisplaced spondylolisthesis of second cervical vertebra** ▽

√x7ᵗʰ **S12.14 Type III traumatic spondylolisthesis of second cervical vertebra**

☑ Additional Character Required   √x7ᵗʰ Placeholder Alert   Manifestation Dx   ▽ Unspecified Dx   ►◄ Revised Text   ● New Code   ▲ Revised Code Title

√6ᵗʰ **S12.15** Other traumatic spondylolisthesis of second cervical vertebra

√7ᵗʰ **S12.150** Other traumatic displaced spondylolisthesis of second cervical vertebra

√7ᵗʰ **S12.151** Other traumatic nondisplaced spondylolisthesis of second cervical vertebra

√6ᵗʰ **S12.19** Other fracture of second cervical vertebra

√7ᵗʰ **S12.190** Other displaced fracture of second cervical vertebra

√7ᵗʰ **S12.191** Other nondisplaced fracture of second cervical vertebra

√5ᵗʰ **S12.2** Fracture of third cervical vertebra

√6ᵗʰ **S12.20** Unspecified fracture of third cervical vertebra

√7ᵗʰ **S12.200** Unspecified displaced fracture of third cervical vertebra ▽

√7ᵗʰ **S12.201** Unspecified nondisplaced fracture of third cervical vertebra ▽

√6ᵗʰ **S12.23** Unspecified traumatic spondylolisthesis of third cervical vertebra

√7ᵗʰ **S12.230** Unspecified traumatic displaced spondylolisthesis of third cervical vertebra ▽

√7ᵗʰ **S12.231** Unspecified traumatic nondisplaced spondylolisthesis of third cervical vertebra ▽

√x7ᵗʰ **S12.24** Type III traumatic spondylolisthesis of third cervical vertebra

√6ᵗʰ **S12.25** Other traumatic spondylolisthesis of third cervical vertebra

√7ᵗʰ **S12.250** Other traumatic displaced spondylolisthesis of third cervical vertebra

√7ᵗʰ **S12.251** Other traumatic nondisplaced spondylolisthesis of third cervical vertebra

√6ᵗʰ **S12.29** Other fracture of third cervical vertebra

√7ᵗʰ **S12.290** Other displaced fracture of third cervical vertebra

√7ᵗʰ **S12.291** Other nondisplaced fracture of third cervical vertebra

√5ᵗʰ **S12.3** Fracture of fourth cervical vertebra

√6ᵗʰ **S12.30** Unspecified fracture of fourth cervical vertebra

√7ᵗʰ **S12.300** Unspecified displaced fracture of fourth cervical vertebra ▽

√7ᵗʰ **S12.301** Unspecified nondisplaced fracture of fourth cervical vertebra ▽

√6ᵗʰ **S12.33** Unspecified traumatic spondylolisthesis of fourth cervical vertebra

√7ᵗʰ **S12.330** Unspecified traumatic displaced spondylolisthesis of fourth cervical vertebra ▽

√7ᵗʰ **S12.331** Unspecified traumatic nondisplaced spondylolisthesis of fourth cervical vertebra ▽

√x7ᵗʰ **S12.34** Type III traumatic spondylolisthesis of fourth cervical vertebra

√6ᵗʰ **S12.35** Other traumatic spondylolisthesis of fourth cervical vertebra

√7ᵗʰ **S12.350** Other traumatic displaced spondylolisthesis of fourth cervical vertebra

√7ᵗʰ **S12.351** Other traumatic nondisplaced spondylolisthesis of fourth cervical vertebra

√6ᵗʰ **S12.39** Other fracture of fourth cervical vertebra

√7ᵗʰ **S12.390** Other displaced fracture of fourth cervical vertebra

√7ᵗʰ **S12.391** Other nondisplaced fracture of fourth cervical vertebra

√5ᵗʰ **S12.4** Fracture of fifth cervical vertebra

√6ᵗʰ **S12.40** Unspecified fracture of fifth cervical vertebra

√7ᵗʰ **S12.400** Unspecified displaced fracture of fifth cervical vertebra ▽

√7ᵗʰ **S12.401** Unspecified nondisplaced fracture of fifth cervical vertebra ▽

√6ᵗʰ **S12.43** Unspecified traumatic spondylolisthesis of fifth cervical vertebra

√7ᵗʰ **S12.430** Unspecified traumatic displaced spondylolisthesis of fifth cervical vertebra ▽

√7ᵗʰ **S12.431** Unspecified traumatic nondisplaced spondylolisthesis of fifth cervical vertebra ▽

√x7ᵗʰ **S12.44** Type III traumatic spondylolisthesis of fifth cervical vertebra

√6ᵗʰ **S12.45** Other traumatic spondylolisthesis of fifth cervical vertebra

√7ᵗʰ **S12.450** Other traumatic displaced spondylolisthesis of fifth cervical vertebra

√7ᵗʰ **S12.451** Other traumatic nondisplaced spondylolisthesis of fifth cervical vertebra

√6ᵗʰ **S12.49** Other fracture of fifth cervical vertebra

√7ᵗʰ **S12.490** Other displaced fracture of fifth cervical vertebra

√7ᵗʰ **S12.491** Other nondisplaced fracture of fifth cervical vertebra

√5ᵗʰ **S12.5** Fracture of sixth cervical vertebra

√6ᵗʰ **S12.50** Unspecified fracture of sixth cervical vertebra

√7ᵗʰ **S12.500** Unspecified displaced fracture of sixth cervical vertebra ▽

√7ᵗʰ **S12.501** Unspecified nondisplaced fracture of sixth cervical vertebra ▽

√6ᵗʰ **S12.53** Unspecified traumatic spondylolisthesis of sixth cervical vertebra

√7ᵗʰ **S12.530** Unspecified traumatic displaced spondylolisthesis of sixth cervical vertebra ▽

√7ᵗʰ **S12.531** Unspecified traumatic nondisplaced spondylolisthesis of sixth cervical vertebra ▽

√x7ᵗʰ **S12.54** Type III traumatic spondylolisthesis of sixth cervical vertebra

√6ᵗʰ **S12.55** Other traumatic spondylolisthesis of sixth cervical vertebra

√7ᵗʰ **S12.550** Other traumatic displaced spondylolisthesis of sixth cervical vertebra

√7ᵗʰ **S12.551** Other traumatic nondisplaced spondylolisthesis of sixth cervical vertebra

√6ᵗʰ **S12.59** Other fracture of sixth cervical vertebra

√7ᵗʰ **S12.590** Other displaced fracture of sixth cervical vertebra

√7ᵗʰ **S12.591** Other nondisplaced fracture of sixth cervical vertebra

√5ᵗʰ **S12.6** Fracture of seventh cervical vertebra

√6ᵗʰ **S12.60** Unspecified fracture of seventh cervical vertebra

√7ᵗʰ **S12.600** Unspecified displaced fracture of seventh cervical vertebra ▽

√7ᵗʰ **S12.601** Unspecified nondisplaced fracture of seventh cervical vertebra ▽

√6ᵗʰ **S12.63** Unspecified traumatic spondylolisthesis of seventh cervical vertebra

√7ᵗʰ **S12.630** Unspecified traumatic displaced spondylolisthesis of seventh cervical vertebra ▽

√7ᵗʰ **S12.631** Unspecified traumatic nondisplaced spondylolisthesis of seventh cervical vertebra ▽

√x7ᵗʰ **S12.64** Type III traumatic spondylolisthesis of seventh cervical vertebra

√6ᵗʰ **S12.65** Other traumatic spondylolisthesis of seventh cervical vertebra

√7ᵗʰ **S12.650** Other traumatic displaced spondylolisthesis of seventh cervical vertebra

√7ᵗʰ **S12.651** Other traumatic nondisplaced spondylolisthesis of seventh cervical vertebra

√6ᵗʰ **S12.69** Other fracture of seventh cervical vertebra

√7ᵗʰ **S12.690** Other displaced fracture of seventh cervical vertebra

√7ᵗʰ **S12.691** Other nondisplaced fracture of seventh cervical vertebra

EXCLUDES 1 Not coded here   **EXCLUDES 2** Not included here   Ⓝ Newborn Age : 0   Ⓟ Pediatric Age : 0-17   Ⓜ Maternity Age : 12-55   Ⓐ Adult Age : 15-124

902

ICD-10-CM 2017

✓x7ᵗʰ **S12.8**   **Fracture of other parts of neck**

Hyoid bone
Larynx
Thyroid cartilage
Trachea

> The appropriate 7th character is to be added to code S12.8.
> A   initial encounter
> D   subsequent encounter
> S   sequela

✓x7ᵗʰ **S12.9**   **Fracture of neck, unspecified**   ▽

Fracture of neck NOS
Fracture of cervical spine NOS
Fracture of cervical vertebra NOS

> The appropriate 7th character is to be added to code S12.9.
> A   initial encounter
> D   subsequent encounter
> S   sequela

✓4ᵗʰ **S13**   **Dislocation and sprain of joints and ligaments at neck level**

> **INCLUDES**   avulsion of joint or ligament at neck level
> laceration of cartilage, joint or ligament at neck level
> sprain of cartilage, joint or ligament at neck level
> traumatic hemarthrosis of joint or ligament at neck level
> traumatic rupture of joint or ligament at neck level
> traumatic subluxation of joint or ligament at neck level
> traumatic tear of joint or ligament at neck level

Code also any associated open wound

> *EXCLUDES 2*   *strain of muscle or tendon at neck level (S16.1)*

> The appropriate 7th character is to be added to each code from category S13.
> A   initial encounter
> D   subsequent encounter
> S   sequela

✓x7ᵗʰ **S13.0**   **Traumatic rupture of cervical intervertebral disc**

> *EXCLUDES 1*   *rupture or displacement (nontraumatic) of cervical intervertebral disc NOS (M50.-)*

✓5ᵗʰ **S13.1**   **Subluxation and dislocation of cervical vertebrae**

Code also any associated:
open wound of neck (S11.-)
spinal cord injury (S14.-)
> *EXCLUDES 2*   *fracture of cervical vertebrae (S12.0-S12.3-)*

✓6ᵗʰ   **S13.10**   **Subluxation and dislocation of unspecified cervical vertebrae**

✓7ᵗʰ   **S13.100**   **Subluxation of unspecified cervical**   ▽
vertebrae

✓7ᵗʰ   **S13.101**   **Dislocation of unspecified cervical**   ▽
vertebrae

✓6ᵗʰ   **S13.11**   **Subluxation and dislocation of C0/C1 cervical vertebrae**

Subluxation and dislocation of atlantooccipital joint
Subluxation and dislocation of atloidooccipital joint
Subluxation and dislocation of occipitoatloid joint

✓7ᵗʰ   **S13.110**   **Subluxation of C0/C1 cervical vertebrae**

✓7ᵗʰ   **S13.111**   **Dislocation of C0/C1 cervical vertebrae**

✓6ᵗʰ   **S13.12**   **Subluxation and dislocation of C1/C2 cervical vertebrae**

Subluxation and dislocation of atlantoaxial joint

✓7ᵗʰ   **S13.120**   **Subluxation of C1/C2 cervical vertebrae**

✓7ᵗʰ   **S13.121**   **Dislocation of C1/C2 cervical vertebrae**

✓6ᵗʰ   **S13.13**   **Subluxation and dislocation of C2/C3 cervical vertebrae**

✓7ᵗʰ   **S13.130**   **Subluxation of C2/C3 cervical vertebrae**

✓7ᵗʰ   **S13.131**   **Dislocation of C2/C3 cervical vertebrae**

✓6ᵗʰ   **S13.14**   **Subluxation and dislocation of C3/C4 cervical vertebrae**

✓7ᵗʰ   **S13.140**   **Subluxation of C3/C4 cervical vertebrae**

✓7ᵗʰ   **S13.141**   **Dislocation of C3/C4 cervical vertebrae**

✓6ᵗʰ   **S13.15**   **Subluxation and dislocation of C4/C5 cervical vertebrae**

✓7ᵗʰ   **S13.150**   **Subluxation of C4/C5 cervical vertebrae**

✓7ᵗʰ   **S13.151**   **Dislocation of C4/C5 cervical vertebrae**

✓6ᵗʰ   **S13.16**   **Subluxation and dislocation of C5/C6 cervical vertebrae**

✓7ᵗʰ   **S13.160**   **Subluxation of C5/C6 cervical vertebrae**

✓7ᵗʰ   **S13.161**   **Dislocation of C5/C6 cervical vertebrae**

✓6ᵗʰ   **S13.17**   **Subluxation and dislocation of C6/C7 cervical vertebrae**

✓7ᵗʰ   **S13.170**   **Subluxation of C6/C7 cervical vertebrae**

✓7ᵗʰ   **S13.171**   **Dislocation of C6/C7 cervical vertebrae**

✓6ᵗʰ   **S13.18**   **Subluxation and dislocation of C7/T1 cervical vertebrae**

✓7ᵗʰ   **S13.180**   **Subluxation of C7/T1 cervical vertebrae**

✓7ᵗʰ   **S13.181**   **Dislocation of C7/T1 cervical vertebrae**

✓5ᵗʰ   **S13.2**   **Dislocation of other and unspecified parts of neck**

✓x7ᵗʰ   **S13.20**   **Dislocation of unspecified parts of neck**   ▽

✓x7ᵗʰ   **S13.29**   **Dislocation of other parts of neck**

✓x7ᵗʰ   **S13.4**   **Sprain of ligaments of cervical spine**

Sprain of anterior longitudinal (ligament), cervical
Sprain of atlanto-axial (joints)
Sprain of atlanto-occipital (joints)
Whiplash injury of cervical spine

✓x7ᵗʰ   **S13.5**   **Sprain of thyroid region**

Sprain of cricoarytenoid (joint) (ligament)
Sprain of cricothyroid (joint) (ligament)
Sprain of thyroid cartilage

✓x7ᵗʰ   **S13.8**   **Sprain of joints and ligaments of other parts of neck**

✓x7ᵗʰ   **S13.9**   **Sprain of joints and ligaments of unspecified parts of neck**   ▽

✓4ᵗʰ **S14**   **Injury of nerves and spinal cord at neck level**

> **NOTE**   Code to highest level of cervical cord injury

Code also any associated:
fracture of cervical vertebra (S12.0- — S12.6.-)
open wound of neck (S11.-)
transient paralysis (R29.5)

> The appropriate 7th character is to be added to each code from category S14.
> A   initial encounter
> D   subsequent encounter
> S   sequela

✓x7ᵗʰ   **S14.0**   **Concussion and edema of cervical spinal cord**

✓5ᵗʰ   **S14.1**   **Other and unspecified injuries of cervical spinal cord**

✓6ᵗʰ   **S14.10**   **Unspecified injury of cervical spinal cord**

✓7ᵗʰ   **S14.101**   **Unspecified injury at C1 level of**   ▽
cervical spinal cord

✓7ᵗʰ   **S14.102**   **Unspecified injury at C2 level of**   ▽
cervical spinal cord

✓7ᵗʰ   **S14.103**   **Unspecified injury at C3 level of**   ▽
cervical spinal cord

✓7ᵗʰ   **S14.104**   **Unspecified injury at C4 level of**   ▽
cervical spinal cord

✓7ᵗʰ   **S14.105**   **Unspecified injury at C5 level of**   ▽
cervical spinal cord

✓7ᵗʰ   **S14.106**   **Unspecified injury at C6 level of**   ▽
cervical spinal cord

✓7ᵗʰ   **S14.107**   **Unspecified injury at C7 level of**   ▽
cervical spinal cord

✓7ᵗʰ   **S14.108**   **Unspecified injury at C8 level of**   ▽
cervical spinal cord

✓7ᵗʰ   **S14.109**   **Unspecified injury at unspecified**   ▽
level of cervical spinal cord
Injury of cervical spinal cord NOS

✓6ᵗʰ   **S14.11**   **Complete lesion of cervical spinal cord**

✓7ᵗʰ   **S14.111**   **Complete lesion at C1 level of cervical spinal cord**

✓7ᵗʰ   **S14.112**   **Complete lesion at C2 level of cervical spinal cord**

✓7ᵗʰ   **S14.113**   **Complete lesion at C3 level of cervical spinal cord**

✓7ᵗʰ   **S14.114**   **Complete lesion at C4 level of cervical spinal cord**

✓7ᵗʰ   **S14.115**   **Complete lesion at C5 level of cervical spinal cord**

✓7ᵗʰ   **S14.116**   **Complete lesion at C6 level of cervical spinal cord**

✓7ᵗʰ   **S14.117**   **Complete lesion at C7 level of cervical spinal cord**

✓7ᵗʰ   **S14.118**   **Complete lesion at C8 level of cervical spinal cord**

✓7ᵗʰ   **S14.119**   **Complete lesion at unspecified**   ▽
level of cervical spinal cord

☑ Additional Character Required   ✓x7ᵗʰ Placeholder Alert   Manifestation Dx   ▽ Unspecified Dx   ►◄ Revised Text   ● New Code   ▲ Revised Code Title

ICD-10-CM 2017   903

√6ᵗʰ **S14.12** Central cord syndrome of cervical spinal cord

    √7ᵗʰ **S14.121** **Central cord syndrome at** C1 level **of cervical spinal cord**

    √7ᵗʰ **S14.122** **Central cord syndrome at** C2 level **of cervical spinal cord**

    √7ᵗʰ **S14.123** **Central cord syndrome at** C3 level **of cervical spinal cord**

    √7ᵗʰ **S14.124** **Central cord syndrome at** C4 level **of cervical spinal cord**

    √7ᵗʰ **S14.125** **Central cord syndrome at** C5 level **of cervical spinal cord**

    √7ᵗʰ **S14.126** **Central cord syndrome at** C6 level **of cervical spinal cord**

    √7ᵗʰ **S14.127** **Central cord syndrome at** C7 level **of cervical spinal cord**

    √7ᵗʰ **S14.128** **Central cord syndrome at** C8 level **of cervical spinal cord**

    √7ᵗʰ **S14.129** **Central cord syndrome at unspecified level of cervical spinal cord** ▽

√6ᵗʰ **S14.13** Anterior cord syndrome of cervical spinal cord

    √7ᵗʰ **S14.131** **Anterior cord syndrome at** C1 level **of cervical spinal cord**

    √7ᵗʰ **S14.132** **Anterior cord syndrome at** C2 level **of cervical spinal cord**

    √7ᵗʰ **S14.133** **Anterior cord syndrome at** C3 level **of cervical spinal cord**

    √7ᵗʰ **S14.134** **Anterior cord syndrome at** C4 level **of cervical spinal cord**

    √7ᵗʰ **S14.135** **Anterior cord syndrome at** C5 level **of cervical spinal cord**

    √7ᵗʰ **S14.136** **Anterior cord syndrome at** C6 level **of cervical spinal cord**

    √7ᵗʰ **S14.137** **Anterior cord syndrome at** C7 level **of cervical spinal cord**

    √7ᵗʰ **S14.138** **Anterior cord syndrome at** C8 level **of cervical spinal cord**

    √7ᵗʰ **S14.139** **Anterior cord syndrome at unspecified level of cervical spinal cord** ▽

√6ᵗʰ **S14.14** Brown-Séquard syndrome of cervical spinal cord

    √7ᵗʰ **S14.141** **Brown-Séquard syndrome at** C1 level **of cervical spinal cord**

    √7ᵗʰ **S14.142** **Brown-Séquard syndrome at** C2 level **of cervical spinal cord**

    √7ᵗʰ **S14.143** **Brown-Séquard syndrome at** C3 level **of cervical spinal cord**

    √7ᵗʰ **S14.144** **Brown-Séquard syndrome at** C4 level **of cervical spinal cord**

    √7ᵗʰ **S14.145** **Brown-Séquard syndrome at** C5 level **of cervical spinal cord**

    √7ᵗʰ **S14.146** **Brown-Séquard syndrome at** C6 level **of cervical spinal cord**

    √7ᵗʰ **S14.147** **Brown-Séquard syndrome at** C7 level **of cervical spinal cord**

    √7ᵗʰ **S14.148** **Brown-Séquard syndrome at** C8 level **of cervical spinal cord**

    √7ᵗʰ **S14.149** **Brown-Séquard syndrome at unspecified level of cervical spinal cord** ▽

√6ᵗʰ **S14.15** Other incomplete lesions of cervical spinal cord

    Incomplete lesion of cervical spinal cord NOS
    Posterior cord syndrome of cervical spinal cord

    √7ᵗʰ **S14.151** **Other incomplete lesion at** C1 level **of cervical spinal cord**

    √7ᵗʰ **S14.152** **Other incomplete lesion at** C2 level **of cervical spinal cord**

    √7ᵗʰ **S14.153** **Other incomplete lesion at** C3 level **of cervical spinal cord**

    √7ᵗʰ **S14.154** **Other incomplete lesion at** C4 level **of cervical spinal cord**

    √7ᵗʰ **S14.155** **Other incomplete lesion at** C5 level **of cervical spinal cord**

    √7ᵗʰ **S14.156** **Other incomplete lesion at** C6 level **of cervical spinal cord**

    √7ᵗʰ **S14.157** **Other incomplete lesion at** C7 level **of cervical spinal cord**

    √7ᵗʰ **S14.158** **Other incomplete lesion at** C8 level **of cervical spinal cord**

    √7ᵗʰ **S14.159** **Other incomplete lesion at unspecified level of cervical spinal cord** ▽

√x7ᵗʰ **S14.2** Injury of nerve root of cervical spine

√x7ᵗʰ **S14.3** Injury of brachial plexus

√x7ᵗʰ **S14.4** Injury of peripheral nerves of neck

√x7ᵗʰ **S14.5** Injury of cervical sympathetic nerves

√x7ᵗʰ **S14.8** Injury of other specified nerves of neck

√x7ᵗʰ **S14.9** Injury of unspecified nerves of neck   ▽

√4ᵗʰ **S15** **Injury of blood vessels at neck level**

    Code also any associated open wound (S11.-)

> The appropriate 7th character is to be added to each code from category S15.
> A   initial encounter
> D   subsequent encounter
> S   sequela

√5ᵗʰ **S15.0** Injury of carotid artery of neck

    Injury of carotid artery (common) (external) (internal, extracranial portion)
    Injury of carotid artery NOS

    EXCLUDES 1   *injury of internal carotid artery, intracranial portion (S06.8)*

    √6ᵗʰ **S15.00** **Unspecified injury of carotid artery**

        √7ᵗʰ **S15.001** **Unspecified injury of** right **carotid artery** ▽

        √7ᵗʰ **S15.002** **Unspecified injury of** left **carotid artery** ▽

        √7ᵗʰ **S15.009** **Unspecified injury of unspecified carotid artery** ▽

    √6ᵗʰ **S15.01** Minor laceration of carotid artery

        Incomplete transection of carotid artery
        Laceration of carotid artery NOS
        Superficial laceration of carotid artery

        √7ᵗʰ **S15.011** **Minor laceration of** right **carotid artery**

        √7ᵗʰ **S15.012** **Minor laceration of** left **carotid artery**

        √7ᵗʰ **S15.019** **Minor laceration of unspecified carotid artery** ▽

    √6ᵗʰ **S15.02** Major laceration of carotid artery

        Complete transection of carotid artery
        Traumatic rupture of carotid artery

        √7ᵗʰ **S15.021** **Major laceration of** right **carotid artery**

        √7ᵗʰ **S15.022** **Major laceration of** left **carotid artery**

        √7ᵗʰ **S15.029** **Major laceration of unspecified carotid artery** ▽

    √6ᵗʰ **S15.09** Other specified injury of carotid artery

        √7ᵗʰ **S15.091** **Other specified injury of** right **carotid artery**

        √7ᵗʰ **S15.092** **Other specified injury of** left **carotid artery**

        √7ᵗʰ **S15.099** **Other specified injury of unspecified carotid artery** ▽

√5ᵗʰ **S15.1** Injury of vertebral artery

    √6ᵗʰ **S15.10** **Unspecified injury of vertebral artery**

        √7ᵗʰ **S15.101** **Unspecified injury of** right **vertebral artery** ▽

        √7ᵗʰ **S15.102** **Unspecified injury of** left **vertebral artery** ▽

        √7ᵗʰ **S15.109** **Unspecified injury of unspecified vertebral artery** ▽

    √6ᵗʰ **S15.11** Minor laceration of vertebral artery

        Incomplete transection of vertebral artery
        Laceration of vertebral artery NOS
        Superficial laceration of vertebral artery

        √7ᵗʰ **S15.111** **Minor laceration of** right **vertebral artery**

        √7ᵗʰ **S15.112** **Minor laceration of** left **vertebral artery**

        √7ᵗʰ **S15.119** **Minor laceration of unspecified vertebral artery** ▽

    √6ᵗʰ **S15.12** Major laceration of vertebral artery

        Complete transection of vertebral artery
        Traumatic rupture of vertebral artery

        √7ᵗʰ **S15.121** **Major laceration of** right **vertebral artery**

        √7ᵗʰ **S15.122** **Major laceration of** left **vertebral artery**

        √7ᵗʰ **S15.129** **Major laceration of unspecified vertebral artery** ▽

    √6ᵗʰ **S15.19** Other specified injury of vertebral artery

        √7ᵗʰ **S15.191** **Other specified injury of** right **vertebral artery**

        √7ᵗʰ **S15.192** **Other specified injury of** left **vertebral artery**

EXCLUDES 1 Not coded here   *EXCLUDES 2* Not included here   N Newborn Age : 0   P Pediatric Age : 0-17   M Maternity Age : 12-55   A Adult Age : 15-124

904   ICD-10-CM 2017

√7th **S15.199** Other specified injury of unspecified vertebral artery ▽

√5th **S15.2** Injury of external jugular vein

√6th **S15.20** Unspecified injury of external jugular vein

√7th **S15.201** Unspecified injury of right external jugular vein ▽

√7th **S15.202** Unspecified injury of left external jugular vein ▽

√7th **S15.209** Unspecified injury of unspecified external jugular vein ▽

√6th **S15.21** Minor laceration of external jugular vein

Incomplete transection of external jugular vein
Laceration of external jugular vein NOS
Superficial laceration of external jugular vein

√7th **S15.211** Minor laceration of right external jugular vein

√7th **S15.212** Minor laceration of left external jugular vein

√7th **S15.219** Minor laceration of unspecified external jugular vein ▽

√6th **S15.22** Major laceration of external jugular vein

Complete transection of external jugular vein
Traumatic rupture of external jugular vein

√7th **S15.221** Major laceration of right external jugular vein

√7th **S15.222** Major laceration of left external jugular vein

√7th **S15.229** Major laceration of unspecified external jugular vein ▽

√6th **S15.29** Other specified injury of external jugular vein

√7th **S15.291** Other specified injury of right external jugular vein

√7th **S15.292** Other specified injury of left external jugular vein

√7th **S15.299** Other specified injury of unspecified external jugular vein ▽

√5th **S15.3** Injury of internal jugular vein

√6th **S15.30** Unspecified injury of internal jugular vein

√7th **S15.301** Unspecified injury of right internal jugular vein ▽

√7th **S15.302** Unspecified injury of left internal jugular vein ▽

√7th **S15.309** Unspecified injury of unspecified internal jugular vein ▽

√6th **S15.31** Minor laceration of internal jugular vein

Incomplete transection of internal jugular vein
Laceration of internal jugular vein NOS
Superficial laceration of internal jugular vein

√7th **S15.311** Minor laceration of right internal jugular vein

√7th **S15.312** Minor laceration of left internal jugular vein

√7th **S15.319** Minor laceration of unspecified internal jugular vein ▽

√6th **S15.32** Major laceration of internal jugular vein

Complete transection of internal jugular vein
Traumatic rupture of internal jugular vein

√7th **S15.321** Major laceration of right internal jugular vein

√7th **S15.322** Major laceration of left internal jugular vein

√7th **S15.329** Major laceration of unspecified internal jugular vein ▽

√6th **S15.39** Other specified injury of internal jugular vein

√7th **S15.391** Other specified injury of right internal jugular vein

√7th **S15.392** Other specified injury of left internal jugular vein

√7th **S15.399** Other specified injury of unspecified internal jugular vein ▽

√x7th **S15.8** Injury of other specified blood vessels at neck level

√x7th **S15.9** Injury of unspecified blood vessel at neck level ▽

√4th **S16** Injury of muscle, fascia and tendon at neck level

Code also any associated open wound (S11.-)

EXCLUDES 2 *sprain of joint or ligament at neck level (S13.9)*

The appropriate 7th character is to be added to each code from category S16.
A   initial encounter
D   subsequent encounter
S   sequela

√x7th **S16.1** Strain of muscle, fascia and tendon at neck level

√x7th **S16.2** Laceration of muscle, fascia and tendon at neck level

√x7th **S16.8** Other specified injury of muscle, fascia and tendon at neck level

√x7th **S16.9** Unspecified injury of muscle, fascia and tendon at neck level ▽

√4th **S17** Crushing injury of neck

Use additional code for all associated injuries, such as:
injury of blood vessels (S15.-)
open wound of neck (S11.-)
spinal cord injury (S14.0, S14.1-)
vertebral fracture (S12.0- — S12.3-)

The appropriate 7th character is to be added to each code from category S17.
A   initial encounter
D   subsequent encounter
S   sequela

√x7th **S17.0** Crushing injury of larynx and trachea

√x7th **S17.8** Crushing injury of other specified parts of neck

√x7th **S17.9** Crushing injury of neck, part unspecified ▽

√4th **S19** Other specified and unspecified injuries of neck

The appropriate 7th character is to be added to each code from category S19.
A   initial encounter
D   subsequent encounter
S   sequela

√5th **S19.8** Other specified injuries of neck

√x7th **S19.80** Other specified injuries of unspecified part of neck ▽

√x7th **S19.81** Other specified injuries of larynx

√x7th **S19.82** Other specified injuries of cervical trachea

EXCLUDES 2 *other specified injury of thoracic trachea (S27.5-)*

√x7th **S19.83** Other specified injuries of vocal cord

√x7th **S19.84** Other specified injuries of thyroid gland

√x7th **S19.85** Other specified injuries of pharynx and cervical esophagus

√x7th **S19.89** Other specified injuries of other specified part of neck

√x7th **S19.9** Unspecified injury of neck ▽

Injuries to the thorax (S20-S29)

INCLUDES   injuries of breast
injuries of chest (wall)
injuries of interscapular area

EXCLUDES 2 *burns and corrosions (T20-T32)*
effects of foreign body in bronchus (T17.5)
effects of foreign body in esophagus (T18.1)
effects of foreign body in lung (T17.8)
effects of foreign body in trachea (T17.4)
frostbite (T33-T34)
injuries of axilla
injuries of clavicle
injuries of scapular region
injuries of shoulder
insect bite or sting, venomous (T63.4)

√4th **S20** Superficial injury of thorax

The appropriate 7th character is to be added to each code from category S20.
A   initial encounter
D   subsequent encounter
S   sequela

√5th **S20.0** Contusion of breast

√x7th **S20.00** Contusion of breast, unspecified breast ▽

√x7th **S20.01** Contusion of right breast

√x7th **S20.02** Contusion of left breast

☑ Additional Character Required   √x7th Placeholder Alert   Manifestation Dx   ▽ Unspecified Dx   ►◄ Revised Text   ● New Code   ▲ Revised Code Title

√5ᵗʰ **S20.1 Other and unspecified superficial injuries of breast**

√6ᵗʰ **S20.10 Unspecified superficial injuries of breast**

- **S20.101** Unspecified superficial injuries of breast, right breast
- **S20.102** Unspecified superficial injuries of breast, left breast
- **S20.109** Unspecified superficial injuries of breast, unspecified breast ▽

√6ᵗʰ **S20.11 Abrasion of breast**

- **S20.111** Abrasion of breast, right breast
- **S20.112** Abrasion of breast, left breast
- **S20.119** Abrasion of breast, unspecified breast ▽

√6ᵗʰ **S20.12 Blister (nonthermal) of breast**

- **S20.121** Blister (nonthermal) of breast, right breast
- **S20.122** Blister (nonthermal) of breast, left breast
- **S20.129** Blister (nonthermal) of breast, unspecified breast ▽

√6ᵗʰ **S20.14 External constriction of part of breast**

- **S20.141** External constriction of part of breast, right breast
- **S20.142** External constriction of part of breast, left breast
- **S20.149** External constriction of part of breast, unspecified breast ▽

√6ᵗʰ **S20.15 Superficial foreign body of breast**

  Splinter in the breast

- **S20.151** Superficial foreign body of breast, right breast
- **S20.152** Superficial foreign body of breast, left breast
- **S20.159** Superficial foreign body of breast, unspecified breast ▽

√6ᵗʰ **S20.16 Insect bite (nonvenomous) of breast**

- **S20.161** Insect bite (nonvenomous) of breast, right breast
- **S20.162** Insect bite (nonvenomous) of breast, left breast
- **S20.169** Insect bite (nonvenomous) of breast, unspecified breast ▽

√6ᵗʰ **S20.17 Other superficial bite of breast**

  EXCLUDES 1 *open bite of breast (S21.05-)*

- **S20.171** Other superficial bite of breast, right breast
- **S20.172** Other superficial bite of breast, left breast
- **S20.179** Other superficial bite of breast, unspecified breast ▽

√5ᵗʰ **S20.2 Contusion of thorax**

√x7ᵗʰ **S20.20 Contusion of thorax, unspecified** ▽

√6ᵗʰ **S20.21 Contusion of front wall of thorax**

- **S20.211** Contusion of right front wall of thorax
- **S20.212** Contusion of left front wall of thorax
- **S20.219** Contusion of unspecified front wall of thorax ▽

√6ᵗʰ **S20.22 Contusion of back wall of thorax**

- **S20.221** Contusion of right back wall of thorax
- **S20.222** Contusion of left back wall of thorax
- **S20.229** Contusion of unspecified back wall of thorax ▽

√5ᵗʰ **S20.3 Other and unspecified superficial injuries of front wall of thorax**

√6ᵗʰ **S20.30 Unspecified superficial injuries of front wall of thorax**

- **S20.301** Unspecified superficial injuries of right front wall of thorax ▽
- **S20.302** Unspecified superficial injuries of left front wall of thorax ▽
- **S20.309** Unspecified superficial injuries of unspecified front wall of thorax ▽

√6ᵗʰ **S20.31 Abrasion of front wall of thorax**

- **S20.311** Abrasion of right front wall of thorax
- **S20.312** Abrasion of left front wall of thorax
- **S20.319** Abrasion of unspecified front wall of thorax ▽

√6ᵗʰ **S20.32 Blister (nonthermal) of front wall of thorax**

- **S20.321** Blister (nonthermal) of right front wall of thorax
- **S20.322** Blister (nonthermal) of left front wall of thorax
- **S20.329** Blister (nonthermal) of unspecified front wall of thorax ▽

√6ᵗʰ **S20.34 External constriction of front wall of thorax**

- **S20.341** External constriction of right front wall of thorax
- **S20.342** External constriction of left front wall of thorax
- **S20.349** External constriction of unspecified front wall of thorax ▽

√6ᵗʰ **S20.35 Superficial foreign body of front wall of thorax**

  Splinter in front wall of thorax

- **S20.351** Superficial foreign body of right front wall of thorax
- **S20.352** Superficial foreign body of left front wall of thorax
- **S20.359** Superficial foreign body of unspecified front wall of thorax ▽

√6ᵗʰ **S20.36 Insect bite (nonvenomous) of front wall of thorax**

- **S20.361** Insect bite (nonvenomous) of right front wall of thorax
- **S20.362** Insect bite (nonvenomous) of left front wall of thorax
- **S20.369** Insect bite (nonvenomous) of unspecified front wall of thorax ▽

√6ᵗʰ **S20.37 Other superficial bite of front wall of thorax**

  EXCLUDES 1 *open bite of front wall of thorax (S21.15)*

- **S20.371** Other superficial bite of right front wall of thorax
- **S20.372** Other superficial bite of left front wall of thorax
- **S20.379** Other superficial bite of unspecified front wall of thorax ▽

√5ᵗʰ **S20.4 Other and unspecified superficial injuries of back wall of thorax**

√6ᵗʰ **S20.40 Unspecified superficial injuries of back wall of thorax**

- **S20.401** Unspecified superficial injuries of right back wall of thorax ▽
- **S20.402** Unspecified superficial injuries of left back wall of thorax ▽
- **S20.409** Unspecified superficial injuries of unspecified back wall of thorax ▽

√6ᵗʰ **S20.41 Abrasion of back wall of thorax**

- **S20.411** Abrasion of right back wall of thorax
- **S20.412** Abrasion of left back wall of thorax
- **S20.419** Abrasion of unspecified back wall of thorax ▽

√6ᵗʰ **S20.42 Blister (nonthermal) of back wall of thorax**

- **S20.421** Blister (nonthermal) of right back wall of thorax
- **S20.422** Blister (nonthermal) of left back wall of thorax
- **S20.429** Blister (nonthermal) of unspecified back wall of thorax ▽

√6ᵗʰ **S20.44 External constriction of back wall of thorax**

- **S20.441** External constriction of right back wall of thorax
- **S20.442** External constriction of left back wall of thorax
- **S20.449** External constriction of unspecified back wall of thorax ▽

√6ᵗʰ **S20.45 Superficial foreign body of back wall of thorax**

  Splinter of back wall of thorax

- **S20.451** Superficial foreign body of right back wall of thorax
- **S20.452** Superficial foreign body of left back wall of thorax
- **S20.459** Superficial foreign body of unspecified back wall of thorax ▽

√6ᵗʰ **S20.46 Insect bite (nonvenomous) of back wall of thorax**

- **S20.461** Insect bite (nonvenomous) of right back wall of thorax
- **S20.462** Insect bite (nonvenomous) of left back wall of thorax
- **S20.469** Insect bite (nonvenomous) of unspecified back wall of thorax ▽

EXCLUDES 1 Not coded here   EXCLUDES 2 Not included here   N Newborn Age : 0   P Pediatric Age : 0-17   M Maternity Age : 12-55   A Adult Age : 15-124

906

ICD-10-CM 2017

√6ᵗʰ **S20.47** **Other superficial bite of back wall of thorax**
     EXCLUDES 1 *open bite of back wall of thorax (S21.25)*
     √7ᵗʰ **S20.471** **Other superficial bite of right back wall of thorax**
     √7ᵗʰ **S20.472** **Other superficial bite of left back wall of thorax**
     √7ᵗʰ **S20.479** **Other superficial bite of unspecified back wall of thorax** ▽

√5ᵗʰ **S20.9** **Superficial injury of unspecified parts of thorax**
     EXCLUDES 1 *contusion of thorax NOS (S20.20)*
     √x7ᵗʰ **S20.90** **Unspecified superficial injury of unspecified parts of thorax** ▽
       Superficial injury of thoracic wall NOS
     √x7ᵗʰ **S20.91** **Abrasion of unspecified parts of thorax** ▽
     √x7ᵗʰ **S20.92** **Blister (nonthermal) of unspecified parts of thorax** ▽
     √x7ᵗʰ **S20.94** **External constriction of unspecified parts of thorax** ▽
     √x7ᵗʰ **S20.95** **Superficial foreign body of unspecified parts of thorax** ▽
       Splinter in thorax NOS
     √x7ᵗʰ **S20.96** **Insect bite (nonvenomous) of unspecified parts of thorax** ▽
     √x7ᵗʰ **S20.97** **Other superficial bite of unspecified parts of thorax** ▽
       EXCLUDES 1 *open bite of thorax NOS (S21.95)*

√4ᵗʰ **S21** **Open wound of thorax**
   Code also any associated injury, such as:
     injury of heart (S26.-)
     injury of intrathoracic organs (S27.-)
     rib fracture (S22.3-, S22.4-)
     spinal cord injury (S24.0-, S24.1-)
     traumatic hemopneumothorax (S27.3)
     traumatic hemothorax (S27.1)
     traumatic pneumothorax (S27.0)
     wound infection
   EXCLUDES 1 *traumatic amputation (partial) of thorax (S28.1)*

   The appropriate 7th character is to be added to each code from category S21.
   A   initial encounter
   D   subsequent encounter
   S   sequela

√5ᵗʰ **S21.0** **Open wound of breast**
     √6ᵗʰ **S21.00** **Unspecified open wound of breast**
       √7ᵗʰ **S21.001** **Unspecified open wound of right breast** ▽
       √7ᵗʰ **S21.002** **Unspecified open wound of left breast** ▽
       √7ᵗʰ **S21.009** **Unspecified open wound of unspecified breast** ▽
     √6ᵗʰ **S21.01** **Laceration without foreign body of breast**
       √7ᵗʰ **S21.011** **Laceration without foreign body of right breast**
       √7ᵗʰ **S21.012** **Laceration without foreign body of left breast**
       √7ᵗʰ **S21.019** **Laceration without foreign body of unspecified breast** ▽
     √6ᵗʰ **S21.02** **Laceration with foreign body of breast**
       √7ᵗʰ **S21.021** **Laceration with foreign body of right breast**
       √7ᵗʰ **S21.022** **Laceration with foreign body of left breast**
       √7ᵗʰ **S21.029** **Laceration with foreign body of unspecified breast** ▽
     √6ᵗʰ **S21.03** **Puncture wound without foreign body of breast**
       √7ᵗʰ **S21.031** **Puncture wound without foreign body of right breast**
       √7ᵗʰ **S21.032** **Puncture wound without foreign body of left breast**
       √7ᵗʰ **S21.039** **Puncture wound without foreign body of unspecified breast** ▽
     √6ᵗʰ **S21.04** **Puncture wound with foreign body of breast**
       √7ᵗʰ **S21.041** **Puncture wound with foreign body of right breast**
       √7ᵗʰ **S21.042** **Puncture wound with foreign body of left breast**
       √7ᵗʰ **S21.049** **Puncture wound with foreign body of unspecified breast** ▽

√6ᵗʰ **S21.05** **Open bite of breast**
     Bite of breast NOS
     EXCLUDES 1 *superficial bite of breast (S20.17)*
     √7ᵗʰ **S21.051** **Open bite of right breast**
     √7ᵗʰ **S21.052** **Open bite of left breast**
     √7ᵗʰ **S21.059** **Open bite of unspecified breast**

√5ᵗʰ **S21.1** **Open wound of front wall of thorax without penetration into thoracic cavity**
   Open wound of chest without penetration into thoracic cavity
     √6ᵗʰ **S21.10** **Unspecified open wound of front wall of thorax without penetration into thoracic cavity**
       √7ᵗʰ **S21.101** **Unspecified open wound of right front wall of thorax without penetration into thoracic cavity** ▽
       √7ᵗʰ **S21.102** **Unspecified open wound of left front wall of thorax without penetration into thoracic cavity** ▽
       √7ᵗʰ **S21.109** **Unspecified open wound of unspecified front wall of thorax without penetration into thoracic cavity** ▽
     √6ᵗʰ **S21.11** **Laceration without foreign body of front wall of thorax without penetration into thoracic cavity**
       √7ᵗʰ **S21.111** **Laceration without foreign body of right front wall of thorax without penetration into thoracic cavity**
       √7ᵗʰ **S21.112** **Laceration without foreign body of left front wall of thorax without penetration into thoracic cavity**
       √7ᵗʰ **S21.119** **Laceration without foreign body of unspecified front wall of thorax without penetration into thoracic cavity** ▽
     √6ᵗʰ **S21.12** **Laceration with foreign body of front wall of thorax without penetration into thoracic cavity**
       √7ᵗʰ **S21.121** **Laceration with foreign body of right front wall of thorax without penetration into thoracic cavity**
       √7ᵗʰ **S21.122** **Laceration with foreign body of left front wall of thorax without penetration into thoracic cavity**
       √7ᵗʰ **S21.129** **Laceration with foreign body of unspecified front wall of thorax without penetration into thoracic cavity** ▽
     √6ᵗʰ **S21.13** **Puncture wound without foreign body of front wall of thorax without penetration into thoracic cavity**
       √7ᵗʰ **S21.131** **Puncture wound without foreign body of right front wall of thorax without penetration into thoracic cavity**
       √7ᵗʰ **S21.132** **Puncture wound without foreign body of left front wall of thorax without penetration into thoracic cavity**
       √7ᵗʰ **S21.139** **Puncture wound without foreign body of unspecified front wall of thorax without penetration into thoracic cavity** ▽
     √6ᵗʰ **S21.14** **Puncture wound with foreign body of front wall of thorax without penetration into thoracic cavity**
       √7ᵗʰ **S21.141** **Puncture wound with foreign body of right front wall of thorax without penetration into thoracic cavity**
       √7ᵗʰ **S21.142** **Puncture wound with foreign body of left front wall of thorax without penetration into thoracic cavity**
       √7ᵗʰ **S21.149** **Puncture wound with foreign body of unspecified front wall of thorax without penetration into thoracic cavity** ▽
     √6ᵗʰ **S21.15** **Open bite of front wall of thorax without penetration into thoracic cavity**
       Bite of front wall of thorax NOS
       EXCLUDES 1 *superficial bite of front wall of thorax (S20.37)*
       √7ᵗʰ **S21.151** **Open bite of right front wall of thorax without penetration into thoracic cavity**
       √7ᵗʰ **S21.152** **Open bite of left front wall of thorax without penetration into thoracic cavity**
       √7ᵗʰ **S21.159** **Open bite of unspecified front wall of thorax without penetration into thoracic cavity** ▽

☑ Additional Character Required   √x7ᵗʰ Placeholder Alert   Manifestation Dx   ▽ Unspecified Dx   ▶◀ Revised Text   ● New Code   ▲ Revised Code Title

☑5ᵗʰ **S21.2 Open wound of back wall of thorax without penetration into thoracic cavity**

  ☑6ᵗʰ **S21.20 Unspecified open wound of back wall of thorax without penetration into thoracic cavity**

    ☑7ᵗʰ **S21.201 Unspecified open wound of right back wall of thorax without penetration into thoracic cavity** ▽

    ☑7ᵗʰ **S21.202 Unspecified open wound of left back wall of thorax without penetration into thoracic cavity** ▽

    ☑7ᵗʰ **S21.209 Unspecified open wound of unspecified back wall of thorax without penetration into thoracic cavity** ▽

  ☑6ᵗʰ **S21.21 Laceration without foreign body of back wall of thorax without penetration into thoracic cavity**

    ☑7ᵗʰ **S21.211 Laceration without foreign body of right back wall of thorax without penetration into thoracic cavity**

    ☑7ᵗʰ **S21.212 Laceration without foreign body of left back wall of thorax without penetration into thoracic cavity**

    ☑7ᵗʰ **S21.219 Laceration without foreign body of unspecified back wall of thorax without penetration into thoracic cavity** ▽

  ☑6ᵗʰ **S21.22 Laceration with foreign body of back wall of thorax without penetration into thoracic cavity**

    ☑7ᵗʰ **S21.221 Laceration with foreign body of right back wall of thorax without penetration into thoracic cavity**

    ☑7ᵗʰ **S21.222 Laceration with foreign body of left back wall of thorax without penetration into thoracic cavity**

    ☑7ᵗʰ **S21.229 Laceration with foreign body of unspecified back wall of thorax without penetration into thoracic cavity** ▽

  ☑6ᵗʰ **S21.23 Puncture wound without foreign body of back wall of thorax without penetration into thoracic cavity**

    ☑7ᵗʰ **S21.231 Puncture wound without foreign body of right back wall of thorax without penetration into thoracic cavity**

    ☑7ᵗʰ **S21.232 Puncture wound without foreign body of left back wall of thorax without penetration into thoracic cavity**

    ☑7ᵗʰ **S21.239 Puncture wound without foreign body of unspecified back wall of thorax without penetration into thoracic cavity** ▽

  ☑6ᵗʰ **S21.24 Puncture wound with foreign body of back wall of thorax without penetration into thoracic cavity**

    ☑7ᵗʰ **S21.241 Puncture wound with foreign body of right back wall of thorax without penetration into thoracic cavity**

    ☑7ᵗʰ **S21.242 Puncture wound with foreign body of left back wall of thorax without penetration into thoracic cavity**

    ☑7ᵗʰ **S21.249 Puncture wound with foreign body of unspecified back wall of thorax without penetration into thoracic cavity** ▽

  ☑6ᵗʰ **S21.25 Open bite of back wall of thorax without penetration into thoracic cavity**

    Bite of back wall of thorax NOS

    EXCLUDES 1   *superficial bite of back wall of thorax (S20.47)*

    ☑7ᵗʰ **S21.251 Open bite of right back wall of thorax without penetration into thoracic cavity**

    ☑7ᵗʰ **S21.252 Open bite of left back wall of thorax without penetration into thoracic cavity**

    ☑7ᵗʰ **S21.259 Open bite of unspecified back wall of thorax without penetration into thoracic cavity** ▽

☑5ᵗʰ **S21.3 Open wound of front wall of thorax with penetration into thoracic cavity**

  Open wound of chest with penetration into thoracic cavity

  ☑6ᵗʰ **S21.30 Unspecified open wound of front wall of thorax with penetration into thoracic cavity**

    ☑7ᵗʰ **S21.301 Unspecified open wound of right front wall of thorax with penetration into thoracic cavity** ▽

    ☑7ᵗʰ **S21.302 Unspecified open wound of left front wall of thorax with penetration into thoracic cavity** ▽

    ☑7ᵗʰ **S21.309 Unspecified open wound of unspecified front wall of thorax with penetration into thoracic cavity** ▽

  ☑6ᵗʰ **S21.31 Laceration without foreign body of front wall of thorax with penetration into thoracic cavity**

    ☑7ᵗʰ **S21.311 Laceration without foreign body of right front wall of thorax with penetration into thoracic cavity**

    ☑7ᵗʰ **S21.312 Laceration without foreign body of left front wall of thorax with penetration into thoracic cavity**

    ☑7ᵗʰ **S21.319 Laceration without foreign body of unspecified front wall of thorax with penetration into thoracic cavity** ▽

  ☑6ᵗʰ **S21.32 Laceration with foreign body of front wall of thorax with penetration into thoracic cavity**

    ☑7ᵗʰ **S21.321 Laceration with foreign body of right front wall of thorax with penetration into thoracic cavity**

    ☑7ᵗʰ **S21.322 Laceration with foreign body of left front wall of thorax with penetration into thoracic cavity**

    ☑7ᵗʰ **S21.329 Laceration with foreign body of unspecified front wall of thorax with penetration into thoracic cavity** ▽

  ☑6ᵗʰ **S21.33 Puncture wound without foreign body of front wall of thorax with penetration into thoracic cavity**

    ☑7ᵗʰ **S21.331 Puncture wound without foreign body of right front wall of thorax with penetration into thoracic cavity**

    ☑7ᵗʰ **S21.332 Puncture wound without foreign body of left front wall of thorax with penetration into thoracic cavity**

    ☑7ᵗʰ **S21.339 Puncture wound without foreign body of unspecified front wall of thorax with penetration into thoracic cavity** ▽

  ☑6ᵗʰ **S21.34 Puncture wound with foreign body of front wall of thorax with penetration into thoracic cavity**

    ☑7ᵗʰ **S21.341 Puncture wound with foreign body of right front wall of thorax with penetration into thoracic cavity**

    ☑7ᵗʰ **S21.342 Puncture wound with foreign body of left front wall of thorax with penetration into thoracic cavity**

    ☑7ᵗʰ **S21.349 Puncture wound with foreign body of unspecified front wall of thorax with penetration into thoracic cavity** ▽

  ☑6ᵗʰ **S21.35 Open bite of front wall of thorax with penetration into thoracic cavity**

    EXCLUDES 1   *superficial bite of front wall of thorax (S20.37)*

    ☑7ᵗʰ **S21.351 Open bite of right front wall of thorax with penetration into thoracic cavity**

    ☑7ᵗʰ **S21.352 Open bite of left front wall of thorax with penetration into thoracic cavity**

    ☑7ᵗʰ **S21.359 Open bite of unspecified front wall of thorax with penetration into thoracic cavity** ▽

☑5ᵗʰ **S21.4 Open wound of back wall of thorax with penetration into thoracic cavity**

  ☑6ᵗʰ **S21.40 Unspecified open wound of back wall of thorax with penetration into thoracic cavity**

    ☑7ᵗʰ **S21.401 Unspecified open wound of right back wall of thorax with penetration into thoracic cavity** ▽

    ☑7ᵗʰ **S21.402 Unspecified open wound of left back wall of thorax with penetration into thoracic cavity** ▽

    ☑7ᵗʰ **S21.409 Unspecified open wound of unspecified back wall of thorax with penetration into thoracic cavity** ▽

  ☑6ᵗʰ **S21.41 Laceration without foreign body of back wall of thorax with penetration into thoracic cavity**

    ☑7ᵗʰ **S21.411 Laceration without foreign body of right back wall of thorax with penetration into thoracic cavity**

    ☑7ᵗʰ **S21.412 Laceration without foreign body of left back wall of thorax with penetration into thoracic cavity**

EXCLUDES 1 Not coded here   *EXCLUDES 2* Not included here   N Newborn Age : 0   P Pediatric Age : 0-17   M Maternity Age : 12-55   A Adult Age : 15-124

908   ICD-10-CM 2017

√7ᵗʰ **S21.419 Laceration without foreign body** of unspecified back wall of thorax with penetration into thoracic cavity ▽

√6ᵗʰ **S21.42 Laceration with foreign body** of back wall of thorax with penetration into thoracic cavity

    √7ᵗʰ **S21.421 Laceration with foreign body of** right back wall of thorax with penetration into thoracic cavity

    √7ᵗʰ **S21.422 Laceration with foreign body of** left back wall of thorax with penetration into thoracic cavity

    √7ᵗʰ **S21.429 Laceration with foreign body of** unspecified back wall of thorax with penetration into thoracic cavity ▽

√6ᵗʰ **S21.43 Puncture wound without foreign body** of back wall of thorax with penetration into thoracic cavity

    √7ᵗʰ **S21.431 Puncture wound without foreign body of** right back wall of thorax with penetration into thoracic cavity

    √7ᵗʰ **S21.432 Puncture wound without foreign body of** left back wall of thorax with penetration into thoracic cavity

    √7ᵗʰ **S21.439 Puncture wound without foreign body of** unspecified back wall of thorax with penetration into thoracic cavity ▽

√6ᵗʰ **S21.44 Puncture wound with foreign body** of back wall of thorax with penetration into thoracic cavity

    √7ᵗʰ **S21.441 Puncture wound with foreign body of** right back wall of thorax with penetration into thoracic cavity

    √7ᵗʰ **S21.442 Puncture wound with foreign body of** left back wall of thorax with penetration into thoracic cavity

    √7ᵗʰ **S21.449 Puncture wound with foreign body of** unspecified back wall of thorax with penetration into thoracic cavity ▽

√6ᵗʰ **S21.45 Open bite** of back wall of thorax with penetration into thoracic cavity

Bite of back wall of thorax NOS

EXCLUDES 1 superficial bite of back wall of thorax (S20.47)

    √7ᵗʰ **S21.451 Open bite of** right back wall of thorax with penetration into thoracic cavity

    √7ᵗʰ **S21.452 Open bite of** left back wall of thorax with penetration into thoracic cavity

    √7ᵗʰ **S21.459 Open bite of unspecified** back wall of thorax with penetration into thoracic cavity ▽

√5ᵗʰ **S21.9 Open wound of unspecified part of thorax**

Open wound of thoracic wall NOS

√x7ᵗʰ **S21.90 Unspecified open wound of unspecified part of thorax** ▽

√x7ᵗʰ **S21.91 Laceration without foreign body of** unspecified part of thorax ▽

√x7ᵗʰ **S21.92 Laceration with foreign body of** unspecified part of thorax ▽

√x7ᵗʰ **S21.93 Puncture wound without foreign body of** unspecified part of thorax ▽

√x7ᵗʰ **S21.94 Puncture wound with foreign body of** unspecified part of thorax ▽

√x7ᵗʰ **S21.95 Open bite of unspecified part of thorax** ▽

EXCLUDES 1 superficial bite of thorax (S20.97)

√4ᵗʰ **S22 Fracture of rib(s), sternum and thoracic spine**

NOTE   A fracture not indicated as displaced or nondisplaced should be coded to displaced

A fracture not indicated as open or closed should be coded to closed

INCLUDES   fracture of thoracic neural arch
fracture of thoracic spinous process
fracture of thoracic transverse process
fracture of thoracic vertebra
fracture of thoracic vertebral arch

Code first any associated:
injury of intrathoracic organ (S27.-)
spinal cord injury (S24.0-, S24.1-)

EXCLUDES 1 transection of thorax (S28.1)

EXCLUDES 2 fracture of clavicle (S42.0-)
fracture of scapula (S42.1-)

AHA: 2015,3Q,37-39

The appropriate 7th character is to be added to each code from category S22.
A   initial encounter for closed fracture
B   initial encounter for open fracture
D   subsequent encounter for fracture with routine healing
G   subsequent encounter for fracture with delayed healing
K   subsequent encounter for fracture with nonunion
S   sequela

√5ᵗʰ **S22.0 Fracture of thoracic vertebra**

√6ᵗʰ **S22.00 Fracture of unspecified thoracic vertebra**

    √7ᵗʰ **S22.000 Wedge compression fracture of** unspecified thoracic vertebra ▽

    √7ᵗʰ **S22.001 Stable burst fracture of** unspecified thoracic vertebra ▽

    √7ᵗʰ **S22.002 Unstable burst fracture of** unspecified thoracic vertebra ▽

    √7ᵗʰ **S22.008 Other fracture of unspecified** thoracic vertebra

    √7ᵗʰ **S22.009 Unspecified fracture of** unspecified thoracic vertebra ▽

√6ᵗʰ **S22.01 Fracture of first thoracic vertebra**

    √7ᵗʰ **S22.010 Wedge compression fracture of first** thoracic vertebra

    √7ᵗʰ **S22.011 Stable burst fracture of first thoracic** vertebra

    √7ᵗʰ **S22.012 Unstable burst fracture of first thoracic** vertebra

    √7ᵗʰ **S22.018 Other fracture of first thoracic vertebra**

    √7ᵗʰ **S22.019 Unspecified fracture of first** thoracic vertebra ▽

√6ᵗʰ **S22.02 Fracture of second thoracic vertebra**

    √7ᵗʰ **S22.020 Wedge compression fracture of second** thoracic vertebra

    √7ᵗʰ **S22.021 Stable burst fracture of second thoracic** vertebra

    √7ᵗʰ **S22.022 Unstable burst fracture of second thoracic** vertebra

    √7ᵗʰ **S22.028 Other fracture of second thoracic vertebra**

    √7ᵗʰ **S22.029 Unspecified fracture of second** thoracic vertebra ▽

√6ᵗʰ **S22.03 Fracture of third thoracic vertebra**

    √7ᵗʰ **S22.030 Wedge compression fracture of third** thoracic vertebra

    √7ᵗʰ **S22.031 Stable burst fracture of third thoracic** vertebra

    √7ᵗʰ **S22.032 Unstable burst fracture of third thoracic** vertebra

    √7ᵗʰ **S22.038 Other fracture of third thoracic vertebra**

    √7ᵗʰ **S22.039 Unspecified fracture of third** thoracic vertebra ▽

√6ᵗʰ **S22.04 Fracture of fourth thoracic vertebra**

    √7ᵗʰ **S22.040 Wedge compression fracture of fourth** thoracic vertebra

    √7ᵗʰ **S22.041 Stable burst fracture of fourth thoracic** vertebra

    √7ᵗʰ **S22.042 Unstable burst fracture of fourth thoracic** vertebra

    √7ᵗʰ **S22.048 Other fracture of fourth thoracic vertebra**

    √7ᵗʰ **S22.049 Unspecified fracture of fourth** thoracic vertebra ▽

☑ Additional Character Required   √x7ᵗʰ Placeholder Alert   Manifestation Dx   ▽ Unspecified Dx   ►◄ Revised Text   ● New Code   ▲ Revised Code Title

ICD-10-CM 2017   909

√6ᵗʰ **S22.05** Fracture of T5-T6 vertebra
- √7ᵗʰ **S22.050** Wedge compression fracture of T5-T6 vertebra
- √7ᵗʰ **S22.051** Stable burst fracture of T5-T6 vertebra
- √7ᵗʰ **S22.052** Unstable burst fracture of T5-T6 vertebra
- √7ᵗʰ **S22.058** Other fracture of T5-T6 vertebra
- √7ᵗʰ **S22.059** Unspecified fracture of T5-T6 vertebra ▽

√6ᵗʰ **S22.06** Fracture of T7-T8 vertebra
- √7ᵗʰ **S22.060** Wedge compression fracture of T7-T8 vertebra
- √7ᵗʰ **S22.061** Stable burst fracture of T7-T8 vertebra
- √7ᵗʰ **S22.062** Unstable burst fracture of T7-T8 vertebra
- √7ᵗʰ **S22.068** Other fracture of T7-T8 thoracic vertebra
- √7ᵗʰ **S22.069** Unspecified fracture of T7-T8 vertebra ▽

√6ᵗʰ **S22.07** Fracture of T9-T10 vertebra
- √7ᵗʰ **S22.070** Wedge compression fracture of T9-T10 vertebra
- √7ᵗʰ **S22.071** Stable burst fracture of T9-T10 vertebra
- √7ᵗʰ **S22.072** Unstable burst fracture of T9-T10 vertebra
- √7ᵗʰ **S22.078** Other fracture of T9-T10 vertebra
- √7ᵗʰ **S22.079** Unspecified fracture of T9-T10 vertebra ▽

√6ᵗʰ **S22.08** Fracture of T11-T12 vertebra
- √7ᵗʰ **S22.080** Wedge compression fracture of T11-T12 vertebra
- √7ᵗʰ **S22.081** Stable burst fracture of T11-T12 vertebra
- √7ᵗʰ **S22.082** Unstable burst fracture of T11-T12 vertebra
- √7ᵗʰ **S22.088** Other fracture of T11-T12 vertebra
- √7ᵗʰ **S22.089** Unspecified fracture of T11-T12 vertebra ▽

√5ᵗʰ **S22.2** Fracture of sternum
- √x7ᵗʰ **S22.20** Unspecified fracture of sternum ▽
- √x7ᵗʰ **S22.21** Fracture of manubrium
- √x7ᵗʰ **S22.22** Fracture of body of sternum
- √x7ᵗʰ **S22.23** Sternal manubrial dissociation
- √x7ᵗʰ **S22.24** Fracture of xiphoid process

√5ᵗʰ **S22.3** Fracture of one rib
- √x7ᵗʰ **S22.31** Fracture of one rib, right side
- √x7ᵗʰ **S22.32** Fracture of one rib, left side
- √x7ᵗʰ **S22.39** Fracture of one rib, unspecified side ▽

√5ᵗʰ **S22.4** Multiple fractures of ribs

    Fractures of two or more ribs

    EXCLUDES 1 flail chest (S22.5-)
- √x7ᵗʰ **S22.41** Multiple fractures of ribs, right side
- √x7ᵗʰ **S22.42** Multiple fractures of ribs, left side
- √x7ᵗʰ **S22.43** Multiple fractures of ribs, bilateral
- √x7ᵗʰ **S22.49** Multiple fractures of ribs, unspecified side ▽

√x7ᵗʰ **S22.5** Flail chest

√x7ᵗʰ **S22.9** Fracture of bony thorax, part unspecified ▽

√4ᵗʰ **S23** Dislocation and sprain of joints and ligaments of thorax

    INCLUDES avulsion of joint or ligament of thorax
       laceration of cartilage, joint or ligament of thorax
       sprain of cartilage, joint or ligament of thorax
       traumatic hemarthrosis of joint or ligament of thorax
       traumatic rupture of joint or ligament of thorax
       traumatic subluxation of joint or ligament of thorax
       traumatic tear of joint or ligament of thorax

    Code also any associated open wound

    EXCLUDES 2 dislocation, sprain of sternoclavicular joint (S43.2, S43.6)
       strain of muscle or tendon of thorax (S29.01-)

    The appropriate 7th character is to be added to each code from category S23.
    A   initial encounter
    D   subsequent encounter
    S   sequela

√x7ᵗʰ **S23.0** Traumatic rupture of thoracic intervertebral disc

    EXCLUDES 1 rupture or displacement (nontraumatic) of thoracic intervertebral disc NOS (M51.- with fifth character 4)

√5ᵗʰ **S23.1** Subluxation and dislocation of thoracic vertebra

    Code also any associated:
       open wound of thorax (S21.-)
       spinal cord injury (S24.0-, S24.1-)

    EXCLUDES 2 fracture of thoracic vertebrae (S22.0-)

√6ᵗʰ **S23.10** Subluxation and dislocation of unspecified thoracic vertebra
- √7ᵗʰ **S23.100** Subluxation of unspecified thoracic vertebra ▽
- √7ᵗʰ **S23.101** Dislocation of unspecified thoracic vertebra ▽

√6ᵗʰ **S23.11** Subluxation and dislocation of T1/T2 thoracic vertebra
- √7ᵗʰ **S23.110** Subluxation of T1/T2 thoracic vertebra
- √7ᵗʰ **S23.111** Dislocation of T1/T2 thoracic vertebra

√6ᵗʰ **S23.12** Subluxation and dislocation of T2/T3-T3/T4 thoracic vertebra
- √7ᵗʰ **S23.120** Subluxation of T2/T3 thoracic vertebra
- √7ᵗʰ **S23.121** Dislocation of T2/T3 thoracic vertebra
- √7ᵗʰ **S23.122** Subluxation of T3/T4 thoracic vertebra
- √7ᵗʰ **S23.123** Dislocation of T3/T4 thoracic vertebra

√6ᵗʰ **S23.13** Subluxation and dislocation of T4/T5-T5/T6 thoracic vertebra
- √7ᵗʰ **S23.130** Subluxation of T4/T5 thoracic vertebra
- √7ᵗʰ **S23.131** Dislocation of T4/T5 thoracic vertebra
- √7ᵗʰ **S23.132** Subluxation of T5/T6 thoracic vertebra
- √7ᵗʰ **S23.133** Dislocation of T5/T6 thoracic vertebra

√6ᵗʰ **S23.14** Subluxation and dislocation of T6/T7-T7/T8 thoracic vertebra
- √7ᵗʰ **S23.140** Subluxation of T6/T7 thoracic vertebra
- √7ᵗʰ **S23.141** Dislocation of T6/T7 thoracic vertebra
- √7ᵗʰ **S23.142** Subluxation of T7/T8 thoracic vertebra
- √7ᵗʰ **S23.143** Dislocation of T7/T8 thoracic vertebra

√6ᵗʰ **S23.15** Subluxation and dislocation of T8/T9-T9/T10 thoracic vertebra
- √7ᵗʰ **S23.150** Subluxation of T8/T9 thoracic vertebra
- √7ᵗʰ **S23.151** Dislocation of T8/T9 thoracic vertebra
- √7ᵗʰ **S23.152** Subluxation of T9/T10 thoracic vertebra
- √7ᵗʰ **S23.153** Dislocation of T9/T10 thoracic vertebra

√6ᵗʰ **S23.16** Subluxation and dislocation of T10/T11-T11/T12 thoracic vertebra
- √7ᵗʰ **S23.160** Subluxation of T10/T11 thoracic vertebra
- √7ᵗʰ **S23.161** Dislocation of T10/T11 thoracic vertebra
- √7ᵗʰ **S23.162** Subluxation of T11/T12 thoracic vertebra
- √7ᵗʰ **S23.163** Dislocation of T11/T12 thoracic vertebra

√6ᵗʰ **S23.17** Subluxation and dislocation of T12/L1 thoracic vertebra
- √7ᵗʰ **S23.170** Subluxation of T12/L1 thoracic vertebra
- √7ᵗʰ **S23.171** Dislocation of T12/L1 thoracic vertebra

√5ᵗʰ **S23.2** Dislocation of other and unspecified parts of thorax
- √x7ᵗʰ **S23.20** Dislocation of unspecified part of thorax ▽
- √x7ᵗʰ **S23.29** Dislocation of other parts of thorax

√x7ᵗʰ **S23.3** Sprain of ligaments of thoracic spine

√5ᵗʰ **S23.4** Sprain of ribs and sternum
- √x7ᵗʰ **S23.41** Sprain of ribs
- √6ᵗʰ **S23.42** Sprain of sternum
  - √7ᵗʰ **S23.420** Sprain of sternoclavicular (joint) (ligament)
  - √7ᵗʰ **S23.421** Sprain of chondrosternal joint
  - √7ᵗʰ **S23.428** Other sprain of sternum
  - √7ᵗʰ **S23.429** Unspecified sprain of sternum ▽

√x7ᵗʰ **S23.8** Sprain of other specified parts of thorax

√x7ᵗʰ **S23.9** Sprain of unspecified parts of thorax ▽

EXCLUDES 1 Not coded here   *EXCLUDES 2* Not included here   N Newborn Age : 0   P Pediatric Age : 0-17   M Maternity Age : 12-55   A Adult Age : 15-124

910   ICD-10-CM 2017

✓4ᵗʰ S24 Injury of nerves and spinal cord at thorax level

> **NOTE** Code to highest level of thoracic spinal cord injury.
>
> Injuries to the spinal cord (S24.0 and S24.1) refer to the cord level and not bone level injury, and can affect nerve roots at and below the level given.

Code also any associated:
   fracture of thoracic vertebra (S22.0-)
   open wound of thorax (S21.-)
   transient paralysis (R29.5)

EXCLUDES 2 injury of brachial plexus (S14.3)

> The appropriate 7th character is to be added to each code from category S24.
> A   initial encounter
> D   subsequent encounter
> S   sequela

✓7ᵗʰ S24.0 Concussion and edema of thoracic spinal cord

✓5ᵗʰ S24.1 Other and unspecified injuries of thoracic spinal cord

    ✓6ᵗʰ S24.10 Unspecified injury of thoracic spinal cord

        ✓7ᵗʰ S24.101 Unspecified injury at T1 level of thoracic spinal cord ▽

        ✓7ᵗʰ S24.102 Unspecified injury at T2-T6 level of thoracic spinal cord ▽

        ✓7ᵗʰ S24.103 Unspecified injury at T7-T10 level of thoracic spinal cord ▽

        ✓7ᵗʰ S24.104 Unspecified injury at T11-T12 level of thoracic spinal cord ▽

        ✓7ᵗʰ S24.109 Unspecified injury at unspecified level of thoracic spinal cord ▽
           Injury of thoracic spinal cord NOS

    ✓6ᵗʰ S24.11 Complete lesion of thoracic spinal cord

        ✓7ᵗʰ S24.111 Complete lesion at T1 level of thoracic spinal cord

        ✓7ᵗʰ S24.112 Complete lesion at T2-T6 level of thoracic spinal cord

        ✓7ᵗʰ S24.113 Complete lesion at T7-T10 level of thoracic spinal cord

        ✓7ᵗʰ S24.114 Complete lesion at T11-T12 level of thoracic spinal cord

        ✓7ᵗʰ S24.119 Complete lesion at unspecified level of thoracic spinal cord ▽

    ✓6ᵗʰ S24.13 Anterior cord syndrome of thoracic spinal cord

        ✓7ᵗʰ S24.131 Anterior cord syndrome at T1 level of thoracic spinal cord

        ✓7ᵗʰ S24.132 Anterior cord syndrome at T2-T6 level of thoracic spinal cord

        ✓7ᵗʰ S24.133 Anterior cord syndrome at T7-T10 level of thoracic spinal cord

        ✓7ᵗʰ S24.134 Anterior cord syndrome at T11-T12 level of thoracic spinal cord

        ✓7ᵗʰ S24.139 Anterior cord syndrome at unspecified level of thoracic spinal cord ▽

    ✓6ᵗʰ S24.14 Brown-Séquard syndrome of thoracic spinal cord

        ✓7ᵗʰ S24.141 Brown-Séquard syndrome at T1 level of thoracic spinal cord

        ✓7ᵗʰ S24.142 Brown-Séquard syndrome at T2-T6 level of thoracic spinal cord

        ✓7ᵗʰ S24.143 Brown-Séquard syndrome at T7-T10 level of thoracic spinal cord

        ✓7ᵗʰ S24.144 Brown-Séquard syndrome at T11-T12 level of thoracic spinal cord

        ✓7ᵗʰ S24.149 Brown-Séquard syndrome at unspecified level of thoracic spinal cord ▽

    ✓6ᵗʰ S24.15 Other incomplete lesions of thoracic spinal cord
         Incomplete lesion of thoracic spinal cord NOS
         Posterior cord syndrome of thoracic spinal cord

        ✓7ᵗʰ S24.151 Other incomplete lesion at T1 level of thoracic spinal cord

        ✓7ᵗʰ S24.152 Other incomplete lesion at T2-T6 level of thoracic spinal cord

        ✓7ᵗʰ S24.153 Other incomplete lesion at T7-T10 level of thoracic spinal cord

        ✓7ᵗʰ S24.154 Other incomplete lesion at T11-T12 level of thoracic spinal cord

        ✓7ᵗʰ S24.159 Other incomplete lesion at unspecified level of thoracic spinal cord ▽

✓7ᵗʰ S24.2 Injury of nerve root of thoracic spine

✓x7ᵗʰ S24.3 Injury of peripheral nerves of thorax

✓x7ᵗʰ S24.4 Injury of thoracic sympathetic nervous system
     Injury of cardiac plexus
     Injury of esophageal plexus
     Injury of pulmonary plexus
     Injury of stellate ganglion
     Injury of thoracic sympathetic ganglion

✓x7ᵗʰ S24.8 Injury of other specified nerves of thorax

✓x7ᵗʰ S24.9 Injury of unspecified nerve of thorax ▽

✓4ᵗʰ S25 Injury of blood vessels of thorax

Code also any associated open wound (S21.-)

> The appropriate 7th character is to be added to each code from category S25.
> A   initial encounter
> D   subsequent encounter
> S   sequela

✓5ᵗʰ S25.0 Injury of thoracic aorta
     Injury of aorta NOS

    ✓x7ᵗʰ S25.00 Unspecified injury of thoracic aorta ▽

    ✓x7ᵗʰ S25.01 Minor laceration of thoracic aorta
         Incomplete transection of thoracic aorta
         Laceration of thoracic aorta NOS
         Superficial laceration of thoracic aorta

    ✓x7ᵗʰ S25.02 Major laceration of thoracic aorta
         Complete transection of thoracic aorta
         Traumatic rupture of thoracic aorta

    ✓x7ᵗʰ S25.09 Other specified injury of thoracic aorta

✓5ᵗʰ S25.1 Injury of innominate or subclavian artery

    ✓6ᵗʰ S25.10 Unspecified injury of innominate or subclavian artery

        ✓7ᵗʰ S25.101 Unspecified injury of right innominate or subclavian artery ▽

        ✓7ᵗʰ S25.102 Unspecified injury of left innominate or subclavian artery ▽

        ✓7ᵗʰ S25.109 Unspecified injury of unspecified innominate or subclavian artery ▽

    ✓6ᵗʰ S25.11 Minor laceration of innominate or subclavian artery
         Incomplete transection of innominate or subclavian artery
         Laceration of innominate or subclavian artery NOS
         Superficial laceration of innominate or subclavian artery

        ✓7ᵗʰ S25.111 Minor laceration of right innominate or subclavian artery

        ✓7ᵗʰ S25.112 Minor laceration of left innominate or subclavian artery

        ✓7ᵗʰ S25.119 Minor laceration of unspecified innominate or subclavian artery ▽

    ✓6ᵗʰ S25.12 Major laceration of innominate or subclavian artery
         Complete transection of innominate or subclavian artery
         Traumatic rupture of innominate or subclavian artery

        ✓7ᵗʰ S25.121 Major laceration of right innominate or subclavian artery

        ✓7ᵗʰ S25.122 Major laceration of left innominate or subclavian artery

        ✓7ᵗʰ S25.129 Major laceration of unspecified innominate or subclavian artery ▽

    ✓6ᵗʰ S25.19 Other specified injury of innominate or subclavian artery

        ✓7ᵗʰ S25.191 Other specified injury of right innominate or subclavian artery

        ✓7ᵗʰ S25.192 Other specified injury of left innominate or subclavian artery

        ✓7ᵗʰ S25.199 Other specified injury of unspecified innominate or subclavian artery ▽

✓5ᵗʰ S25.2 Injury of superior vena cava
     Injury of vena cava NOS

    ✓x7ᵗʰ S25.20 Unspecified injury of superior vena cava ▽

    ✓x7ᵗʰ S25.21 Minor laceration of superior vena cava
         Incomplete transection of superior vena cava
         Laceration of superior vena cava NOS
         Superficial laceration of superior vena cava

✓ Additional Character Required   ✓x7ᵗʰ Placeholder Alert   Manifestation Dx   ▽ Unspecified Dx   ▶◀ Revised Text   ● New Code   ▲ Revised Code Title

√x7ᵗʰ **S25.22** **Major laceration of superior vena cava**

Complete transection of superior vena cava

Traumatic rupture of superior vena cava

√x7ᵗʰ **S25.29** **Other specified injury of superior vena cava**

√5ᵗʰ **S25.3** **Injury of innominate or subclavian vein**

√6ᵗʰ **S25.30** **Unspecified injury of innominate or subclavian vein**

√7ᵗʰ **S25.301** **Unspecified injury of right innominate or subclavian vein** ▽

√7ᵗʰ **S25.302** **Unspecified injury of left innominate or subclavian vein** ▽

√7ᵗʰ **S25.309** **Unspecified injury of unspecified innominate or subclavian vein** ▽

√6ᵗʰ **S25.31** **Minor laceration of innominate or subclavian vein**

Incomplete transection of innominate or subclavian vein

Laceration of innominate or subclavian vein NOS

Superficial laceration of innominate or subclavian vein

√7ᵗʰ **S25.311** **Minor laceration of right innominate or subclavian vein**

√7ᵗʰ **S25.312** **Minor laceration of left innominate or subclavian vein**

√7ᵗʰ **S25.319** **Minor laceration of unspecified innominate or subclavian vein** ▽

√6ᵗʰ **S25.32** **Major laceration of innominate or subclavian vein**

Complete transection of innominate or subclavian vein

Traumatic rupture of innominate or subclavian vein

√7ᵗʰ **S25.321** **Major laceration of right innominate or subclavian vein**

√7ᵗʰ **S25.322** **Major laceration of left innominate or subclavian vein**

√7ᵗʰ **S25.329** **Major laceration of unspecified innominate or subclavian vein** ▽

√6ᵗʰ **S25.39** **Other specified injury of innominate or subclavian vein**

√7ᵗʰ **S25.391** **Other specified injury of right innominate or subclavian vein**

√7ᵗʰ **S25.392** **Other specified injury of left innominate or subclavian vein**

√7ᵗʰ **S25.399** **Other specified injury of unspecified innominate or subclavian vein** ▽

√5ᵗʰ **S25.4** **Injury of pulmonary blood vessels**

√6ᵗʰ **S25.40** **Unspecified injury of pulmonary blood vessels**

√7ᵗʰ **S25.401** **Unspecified injury of right pulmonary blood vessels** ▽

√7ᵗʰ **S25.402** **Unspecified injury of left pulmonary blood vessels** ▽

√7ᵗʰ **S25.409** **Unspecified injury of unspecified pulmonary blood vessels** ▽

√6ᵗʰ **S25.41** **Minor laceration of pulmonary blood vessels**

Incomplete transection of pulmonary blood vessels

Laceration of pulmonary blood vessels NOS

Superficial laceration of pulmonary blood vessels

√7ᵗʰ **S25.411** **Minor laceration of right pulmonary blood vessels**

√7ᵗʰ **S25.412** **Minor laceration of left pulmonary blood vessels**

√7ᵗʰ **S25.419** **Minor laceration of unspecified pulmonary blood vessels** ▽

√6ᵗʰ **S25.42** **Major laceration of pulmonary blood vessels**

Complete transection of pulmonary blood vessels

Traumatic rupture of pulmonary blood vessels

√7ᵗʰ **S25.421** **Major laceration of right pulmonary blood vessels**

√7ᵗʰ **S25.422** **Major laceration of left pulmonary blood vessels**

√7ᵗʰ **S25.429** **Major laceration of unspecified pulmonary blood vessels** ▽

√6ᵗʰ **S25.49** **Other specified injury of pulmonary blood vessels**

√7ᵗʰ **S25.491** **Other specified injury of right pulmonary blood vessels**

√7ᵗʰ **S25.492** **Other specified injury of left pulmonary blood vessels**

√7ᵗʰ **S25.499** **Other specified injury of unspecified pulmonary blood vessels** ▽

√5ᵗʰ **S25.5** **Injury of intercostal blood vessels**

√6ᵗʰ **S25.50** **Unspecified injury of intercostal blood vessels**

√7ᵗʰ **S25.501** **Unspecified injury of intercostal blood vessels, right side** ▽

√7ᵗʰ **S25.502** **Unspecified injury of intercostal blood vessels, left side** ▽

√7ᵗʰ **S25.509** **Unspecified injury of intercostal blood vessels, unspecified side** ▽

√6ᵗʰ **S25.51** **Laceration of intercostal blood vessels**

√7ᵗʰ **S25.511** **Laceration of intercostal blood vessels, right side**

√7ᵗʰ **S25.512** **Laceration of intercostal blood vessels, left side**

√7ᵗʰ **S25.519** **Laceration of intercostal blood vessels, unspecified side** ▽

√6ᵗʰ **S25.59** **Other specified injury of intercostal blood vessels**

√7ᵗʰ **S25.591** **Other specified injury of intercostal blood vessels, right side**

√7ᵗʰ **S25.592** **Other specified injury of intercostal blood vessels, left side**

√7ᵗʰ **S25.599** **Other specified injury of intercostal blood vessels, unspecified side** ▽

√5ᵗʰ **S25.8** **Injury of other blood vessels of thorax**

Injury of azygos vein

Injury of mammary artery or vein

√6ᵗʰ **S25.80** **Unspecified injury of other blood vessels of thorax**

√7ᵗʰ **S25.801** **Unspecified injury of other blood vessels of thorax, right side** ▽

√7ᵗʰ **S25.802** **Unspecified injury of other blood vessels of thorax, left side** ▽

√7ᵗʰ **S25.809** **Unspecified injury of other blood vessels of thorax, unspecified side** ▽

√6ᵗʰ **S25.81** **Laceration of other blood vessels of thorax**

√7ᵗʰ **S25.811** **Laceration of other blood vessels of thorax, right side**

√7ᵗʰ **S25.812** **Laceration of other blood vessels of thorax, left side**

√7ᵗʰ **S25.819** **Laceration of other blood vessels of thorax, unspecified side** ▽

√6ᵗʰ **S25.89** **Other specified injury of other blood vessels of thorax**

√7ᵗʰ **S25.891** **Other specified injury of other blood vessels of thorax, right side**

√7ᵗʰ **S25.892** **Other specified injury of other blood vessels of thorax, left side**

√7ᵗʰ **S25.899** **Other specified injury of other blood vessels of thorax, unspecified side** ▽

√5ᵗʰ **S25.9** **Injury of unspecified blood vessel of thorax**

√x7ᵗʰ **S25.90** **Unspecified injury of unspecified blood vessel of thorax** ▽

√x7ᵗʰ **S25.91** **Laceration of unspecified blood vessel of thorax** ▽

√x7ᵗʰ **S25.99** **Other specified injury of unspecified blood vessel of thorax** ▽

√4ᵗʰ **S26** **Injury of heart**

Code also any associated:

open wound of thorax (S21.-)

traumatic hemopneumothorax (S27.2)

traumatic hemothorax (S27.1)

traumatic pneumothorax (S27.0)

> The appropriate 7th character is to be added to each code from category S26.
> A   initial encounter
> D   subsequent encounter
> S   sequela

√5ᵗʰ **S26.0** **Injury of heart with hemopericardium**

√x7ᵗʰ **S26.00** **Unspecified injury of heart with hemopericardium** ▽

√x7ᵗʰ **S26.01** **Contusion of heart with hemopericardium**

√6ᵗʰ **S26.02** **Laceration of heart with hemopericardium**

√7ᵗʰ **S26.020** **Mild laceration of heart with hemopericardium**

Laceration of heart without penetration of heart chamber

EXCLUDES 1 Not coded here   **EXCLUDES 2** Not included here   N Newborn Age : 0   P Pediatric Age : 0-17   M Maternity Age : 12-55   A Adult Age : 15-124

912   **ICD-10-CM 2017**

√7ᵗʰ **S26.021** Moderate **laceration of heart with hemopericardium**
Laceration of heart with penetration of heart chamber

√7ᵗʰ **S26.022** Major **laceration of heart with hemopericardium**
Laceration of heart with penetration of multiple heart chambers

√x7ᵗʰ **S26.09** **Other injury of heart with hemopericardium**

√5ᵗʰ **S26.1** **Injury of heart** without hemopericardium

√x7ᵗʰ **S26.10** **Unspecified injury of heart without hemopericardium** ▽

√x7ᵗʰ **S26.11** **Contusion** of heart without hemopericardium

√x7ᵗʰ **S26.12** **Laceration** of heart without hemopericardium

√x7ᵗʰ **S26.19** **Other injury of heart without hemopericardium**

√5ᵗʰ **S26.9** **Injury of heart, unspecified with or without hemopericardium**

√x7ᵗʰ **S26.90** **Unspecified injury of heart, unspecified with or without hemopericardium** ▽

√x7ᵗʰ **S26.91** **Contusion** of heart, unspecified with or without hemopericardium ▽

√x7ᵗʰ **S26.92** **Laceration** of heart, unspecified with or without hemopericardium ▽
Laceration of heart NOS

√x7ᵗʰ **S26.99** **Other injury of heart, unspecified with or without hemopericardium** ▽

√4ᵗʰ **S27** **Injury of other and unspecified intrathoracic organs**
Code also any associated open wound of thorax (S21.-)
EXCLUDES 2 *injury of cervical esophagus (S10-S19)*
injury of trachea (cervical) (S10-S19)

The appropriate 7th character is to be added to each code from category S27.
A   initial encounter
D   subsequent encounter
S   sequela

√x7ᵗʰ **S27.0** **Traumatic pneumothorax**
EXCLUDES 1 *spontaneous pneumothorax (J93.-)*

√x7ᵗʰ **S27.1** **Traumatic hemothorax**

√x7ᵗʰ **S27.2** **Traumatic hemopneumothorax**

√5ᵗʰ **S27.3** **Other and unspecified injuries of** lung

√6ᵗʰ **S27.30** **Unspecified injury of lung**

√7ᵗʰ **S27.301** **Unspecified injury of lung, unilateral** ▽

√7ᵗʰ **S27.302** **Unspecified injury of lung, bilateral** ▽

√7ᵗʰ **S27.309** **Unspecified injury of lung, unspecified** ▽

√6ᵗʰ **S27.31** **Primary blast injury of lung**
Blast injury of lung NOS

√7ᵗʰ **S27.311** **Primary blast injury of lung, unilateral**

√7ᵗʰ **S27.312** **Primary blast injury of lung, bilateral**

√7ᵗʰ **S27.319** **Primary blast injury of lung, unspecified** ▽

√6ᵗʰ **S27.32** **Contusion of lung**
DEF: Bruising of lung without mention of open wound.

√7ᵗʰ **S27.321** **Contusion of lung, unilateral**

√7ᵗʰ **S27.322** **Contusion of lung, bilateral**

√7ᵗʰ **S27.329** **Contusion of lung, unspecified** ▽

√6ᵗʰ **S27.33** **Laceration of lung**

√7ᵗʰ **S27.331** **Laceration of lung, unilateral**

√7ᵗʰ **S27.332** **Laceration of lung, bilateral**

√7ᵗʰ **S27.339** **Laceration of lung, unspecified** ▽

√6ᵗʰ **S27.39** **Other injuries of lung**
Secondary blast injury of lung

√7ᵗʰ **S27.391** **Other injuries of lung, unilateral**

√7ᵗʰ **S27.392** **Other injuries of lung, bilateral**

√7ᵗʰ **S27.399** **Other injuries of lung, unspecified** ▽

√6ᵗʰ **S27.4** **Injury of** bronchus

√6ᵗʰ **S27.40** **Unspecified injury of bronchus**

√7ᵗʰ **S27.401** **Unspecified injury of bronchus, unilateral**

√7ᵗʰ **S27.402** **Unspecified injury of bronchus, bilateral** ▽

√7ᵗʰ **S27.409** **Unspecified injury of bronchus, unspecified** ▽

√6ᵗʰ **S27.41** **Primary blast injury of bronchus**
Blast injury of bronchus NOS

√7ᵗʰ **S27.411** **Primary blast injury of bronchus, unilateral**

√7ᵗʰ **S27.412** **Primary blast injury of bronchus, bilateral**

√7ᵗʰ **S27.419** **Primary blast injury of bronchus, unspecified** ▽

√6ᵗʰ **S27.42** **Contusion of bronchus**

√7ᵗʰ **S27.421** **Contusion of bronchus, unilateral**

√7ᵗʰ **S27.422** **Contusion of bronchus, bilateral**

√7ᵗʰ **S27.429** **Contusion of bronchus, unspecified** ▽

√6ᵗʰ **S27.43** **Laceration of bronchus**

√7ᵗʰ **S27.431** **Laceration of bronchus, unilateral**

√7ᵗʰ **S27.432** **Laceration of bronchus, bilateral**

√7ᵗʰ **S27.439** **Laceration of bronchus, unspecified** ▽

√6ᵗʰ **S27.49** **Other injury of bronchus**
Secondary blast injury of bronchus

√7ᵗʰ **S27.491** **Other injury of bronchus, unilateral**

√7ᵗʰ **S27.492** **Other injury of bronchus, bilateral**

√7ᵗʰ **S27.499** **Other injury of bronchus, unspecified** ▽

√5ᵗʰ **S27.5** **Injury of** thoracic trachea

√x7ᵗʰ **S27.50** **Unspecified injury of thoracic trachea** ▽

√x7ᵗʰ **S27.51** **Primary blast injury of thoracic trachea**
Blast injury of thoracic trachea NOS

√x7ᵗʰ **S27.52** **Contusion of thoracic trachea**

√x7ᵗʰ **S27.53** **Laceration of thoracic trachea**

√x7ᵗʰ **S27.59** **Other injury of thoracic trachea**
Secondary blast injury of thoracic trachea

√5ᵗʰ **S27.6** **Injury of** pleura

√x7ᵗʰ **S27.60** **Unspecified injury of pleura** ▽

√x7ᵗʰ **S27.63** **Laceration of pleura**

√x7ᵗʰ **S27.69** **Other injury of pleura**

√5ᵗʰ **S27.8** **Injury of other specified intrathoracic organs**

√6ᵗʰ **S27.80** **Injury of** diaphragm

√7ᵗʰ **S27.802** **Contusion of diaphragm**

√7ᵗʰ **S27.803** **Laceration of diaphragm**

√7ᵗʰ **S27.808** **Other injury of diaphragm**

√7ᵗʰ **S27.809** **Unspecified injury of diaphragm** ▽

√6ᵗʰ **S27.81** **Injury of esophagus (thoracic part)**

√7ᵗʰ **S27.812** **Contusion of esophagus (thoracic part)**

√7ᵗʰ **S27.813** **Laceration of esophagus (thoracic part)**

√7ᵗʰ **S27.818** **Other injury of esophagus (thoracic part)**

√7ᵗʰ **S27.819** **Unspecified injury of esophagus (thoracic part)** ▽

√6ᵗʰ **S27.89** **Injury of other specified intrathoracic organs**
Injury of lymphatic thoracic duct
Injury of thymus gland

√7ᵗʰ **S27.892** **Contusion of other specified intrathoracic organs**

√7ᵗʰ **S27.893** **Laceration of other specified intrathoracic organs**

√7ᵗʰ **S27.898** **Other injury of other specified intrathoracic organs**

√7ᵗʰ **S27.899** **Unspecified injury of other specified intrathoracic organs** ▽

√x7ᵗʰ **S27.9** **Injury of unspecified intrathoracic organ** ▽

√4ᵗʰ **S28** **Crushing injury of thorax, and traumatic amputation of part of thorax**

The appropriate 7th character is to be added to each code from category S28.
A   initial encounter
D   subsequent encounter
S   sequela

√x7ᵗʰ **S28.0** **Crushed chest**
Use additional code for all associated injuries
EXCLUDES 1 *flail chest (S22.5)*

☑ Additional Character Required   √x7ᵗʰ Placeholder Alert   Manifestation Dx   ▽ Unspecified Dx   ▶◀ Revised Text   ● New Code   ▲ Revised Code Title

√x7ᵗʰ **S28.1 Traumatic amputation (partial) of part of thorax, except breast**

√5ᵗʰ **S28.2 Traumatic amputation of breast**

  √6ᵗʰ **S28.21 Complete traumatic amputation of breast**

    Traumatic amputation of breast NOS

    √7ᵗʰ **S28.211 Complete traumatic amputation of right breast**

    √7ᵗʰ **S28.212 Complete traumatic amputation of left breast**

    √7ᵗʰ **S28.219 Complete traumatic amputation of unspecified breast** ▽

  √6ᵗʰ **S28.22 Partial traumatic amputation of breast**

    √7ᵗʰ **S28.221 Partial traumatic amputation of right breast**

    √7ᵗʰ **S28.222 Partial traumatic amputation of left breast**

    √7ᵗʰ **S28.229 Partial traumatic amputation of unspecified breast** ▽

√4ᵗʰ **S29 Other and unspecified injuries of thorax**

  Code also any associated open wound (S21.-)

  The appropriate 7th character is to be added to each code from category S29.
  A initial encounter
  D subsequent encounter
  S sequela

  √5ᵗʰ **S29.0 Injury of muscle and tendon at thorax level**

    √6ᵗʰ **S29.00 Unspecified injury of muscle and tendon of thorax**

      √7ᵗʰ **S29.001 Unspecified injury of muscle and tendon of front wall of thorax** ▽

      √7ᵗʰ **S29.002 Unspecified injury of muscle and tendon of back wall of thorax** ▽

      √7ᵗʰ **S29.009 Unspecified injury of muscle and tendon of unspecified wall of thorax** ▽

    √6ᵗʰ **S29.01 Strain of muscle and tendon of thorax**

      √7ᵗʰ **S29.011 Strain of muscle and tendon of front wall of thorax**

      √7ᵗʰ **S29.012 Strain of muscle and tendon of back wall of thorax**

      √7ᵗʰ **S29.019 Strain of muscle and tendon of unspecified wall of thorax** ▽

    √6ᵗʰ **S29.02 Laceration of muscle and tendon of thorax**

      √7ᵗʰ **S29.021 Laceration of muscle and tendon of front wall of thorax**

      √7ᵗʰ **S29.022 Laceration of muscle and tendon of back wall of thorax**

      √7ᵗʰ **S29.029 Laceration of muscle and tendon of unspecified wall of thorax** ▽

    √6ᵗʰ **S29.09 Other injury of muscle and tendon of thorax**

      √7ᵗʰ **S29.091 Other injury of muscle and tendon of front wall of thorax**

      √7ᵗʰ **S29.092 Other injury of muscle and tendon of back wall of thorax**

      √7ᵗʰ **S29.099 Other injury of muscle and tendon of unspecified wall of thorax** ▽

  √x7ᵗʰ **S29.8 Other specified injuries of thorax**

  √x7ᵗʰ **S29.9 Unspecified injury of thorax** ▽

Injuries to the abdomen, lower back, lumbar spine, pelvis and external genitals (S30-S39)

INCLUDES injuries to the abdominal wall
injuries to the anus
injuries to the buttock
injuries to the external genitalia
injuries to the flank
injuries to the groin
EXCLUDES 2 burns and corrosions (T20-T32)
effects of foreign body in anus and rectum (T18.5)
effects of foreign body in genitourinary tract (T19.-)
effects of foreign body in stomach, small intestine and colon (T18.2-T18.4)
frostbite (T33-T34)
insect bite or sting, venomous (T63.4)

√4ᵗʰ **S30 Superficial injury of abdomen, lower back, pelvis and external genitals**

  EXCLUDES 2 superficial injury of hip (S70.-)

  The appropriate 7th character is to be added to each code from category S30.
  A initial encounter
  D subsequent encounter
  S sequela

  √x7ᵗʰ **S30.0 Contusion of lower back and pelvis**

    Contusion of buttock

  √x7ᵗʰ **S30.1 Contusion of abdominal wall**

    Contusion of flank
    Contusion of groin

  √5ᵗʰ **S30.2 Contusion of external genital organs**

    √6ᵗʰ **S30.20 Contusion of unspecified external genital organ**

      √7ᵗʰ **S30.201 Contusion of unspecified external genital organ, male** ♂ ▽

      √7ᵗʰ **S30.202 Contusion of unspecified external genital organ, female** ♀ ▽

    √x7ᵗʰ **S30.21 Contusion of penis** ♂

    √x7ᵗʰ **S30.22 Contusion of scrotum and testes** ♂

    √x7ᵗʰ **S30.23 Contusion of vagina and vulva** ♀

  √x7ᵗʰ **S30.3 Contusion of anus**

  √5ᵗʰ **S30.8 Other superficial injuries of abdomen, lower back, pelvis and external genitals**

    √6ᵗʰ **S30.81 Abrasion of abdomen, lower back, pelvis and external genitals**

      √7ᵗʰ **S30.810 Abrasion of lower back and pelvis**

      √7ᵗʰ **S30.811 Abrasion of abdominal wall**

      √7ᵗʰ **S30.812 Abrasion of penis** ♂

      √7ᵗʰ **S30.813 Abrasion of scrotum and testes** ♂

      √7ᵗʰ **S30.814 Abrasion of vagina and vulva** ♀

      √7ᵗʰ **S30.815 Abrasion of unspecified external genital organs, male** ♂ ▽

      √7ᵗʰ **S30.816 Abrasion of unspecified external genital organs, female** ♀ ▽

      √7ᵗʰ **S30.817 Abrasion of anus**

    √6ᵗʰ **S30.82 Blister (nonthermal) of abdomen, lower back, pelvis and external genitals**

      √7ᵗʰ **S30.820 Blister (nonthermal) of lower back and pelvis**

      √7ᵗʰ **S30.821 Blister (nonthermal) of abdominal wall**

      √7ᵗʰ **S30.822 Blister (nonthermal) of penis** ♂

      √7ᵗʰ **S30.823 Blister (nonthermal) of scrotum and testes** ♂

      √7ᵗʰ **S30.824 Blister (nonthermal) of vagina and vulva** ♀

      √7ᵗʰ **S30.825 Blister (nonthermal) of unspecified external genital organs, male** ♂ ▽

      √7ᵗʰ **S30.826 Blister (nonthermal) of unspecified external genital organs, female** ♀ ▽

      √7ᵗʰ **S30.827 Blister (nonthermal) of anus**

    √6ᵗʰ **S30.84 External constriction of abdomen, lower back, pelvis and external genitals**

      √7ᵗʰ **S30.840 External constriction of lower back and pelvis**

      √7ᵗʰ **S30.841 External constriction of abdominal wall**

      √7ᵗʰ **S30.842 External constriction of penis** ♂

        Hair tourniquet syndrome of penis
        Use additional cause code to identify the constricting item (W49.0-)

      √7ᵗʰ **S30.843 External constriction of scrotum and testes** ♂

      √7ᵗʰ **S30.844 External constriction of vagina and vulva** ♀

      √7ᵗʰ **S30.845 External constriction of unspecified external genital organs, male** ♂ ▽

      √7ᵗʰ **S30.846 External constriction of unspecified external genital organs, female** ♀ ▽

    √6ᵗʰ **S30.85 Superficial foreign body of abdomen, lower back, pelvis and external genitals**

      Splinter in the abdomen, lower back, pelvis and external genitals

      √7ᵗʰ **S30.850 Superficial foreign body of lower back and pelvis**

EXCLUDES 1 Not coded here   **EXCLUDES 2** Not included here   N Newborn Age : 0   P Pediatric Age : 0-17   M Maternity Age : 12-55   A Adult Age : 15-124

914   ICD-10-CM 2017

√7ᵗʰ **S30.851 Superficial foreign body of** abdominal wall

√7ᵗʰ **S30.852 Superficial foreign body of** penis   ♂

√7ᵗʰ **S30.853 Superficial foreign body of** scrotum and testes   ♂

√7ᵗʰ **S30.854 Superficial foreign body of** vagina and vulva   ♀

√7ᵗʰ **S30.855 Superficial foreign body of** unspecified external genital organs, male   ♂ ▽

√7ᵗʰ **S30.856 Superficial foreign body of** unspecified external genital organs, female   ♀ ▽

√7ᵗʰ **S30.857 Superficial foreign body of** anus

√6ᵗʰ **S30.86 Insect bite (nonvenomous) of abdomen, lower back, pelvis and external genitals**

√7ᵗʰ **S30.860 Insect bite (nonvenomous) of** lower back and pelvis

√7ᵗʰ **S30.861 Insect bite (nonvenomous) of** abdominal wall

√7ᵗʰ **S30.862 Insect bite (nonvenomous) of** penis   ♂

√7ᵗʰ **S30.863 Insect bite (nonvenomous) of** scrotum and testes   ♂

√7ᵗʰ **S30.864 Insect bite (nonvenomous) of** vagina and vulva   ♀

√7ᵗʰ **S30.865 Insect bite (nonvenomous) of** unspecified external genital organs, male   ♂ ▽

√7ᵗʰ **S30.866 Insect bite (nonvenomous) of** unspecified external genital organs, female   ♀ ▽

√7ᵗʰ **S30.867 Insect bite (nonvenomous) of** anus

√6ᵗʰ **S30.87 Other superficial bite of abdomen, lower back, pelvis and external genitals**

    EXCLUDES 1   *open bite of abdomen, lower back, pelvis and external genitals (S31.05, S31.15, S31.25, S31.35, S31.45, S31.55)*

√7ᵗʰ **S30.870 Other superficial bite of** lower back and pelvis

√7ᵗʰ **S30.871 Other superficial bite of** abdominal wall

√7ᵗʰ **S30.872 Other superficial bite of** penis   ♂

√7ᵗʰ **S30.873 Other superficial bite of** scrotum and testes   ♂

√7ᵗʰ **S30.874 Other superficial bite of** vagina and vulva   ♀

√7ᵗʰ **S30.875 Other superficial bite of** unspecified external genital organs, male   ♂ ▽

√7ᵗʰ **S30.876 Other superficial bite of** unspecified external genital organs, female   ♀ ▽

√7ᵗʰ **S30.877 Other superficial bite of** anus

√5ᵗʰ **S30.9 Unspecified superficial injury of abdomen, lower back, pelvis and external genitals**

√x7ᵗʰ **S30.91 Unspecified superficial injury of** lower back and pelvis   ▽

√x7ᵗʰ **S30.92 Unspecified superficial injury of** abdominal wall   ▽

√x7ᵗʰ **S30.93 Unspecified superficial injury of** penis   ♂ ▽

√x7ᵗʰ **S30.94 Unspecified superficial injury of** scrotum and testes   ♂ ▽

√x7ᵗʰ **S30.95 Unspecified superficial injury of** vagina and vulva   ♀ ▽

√x7ᵗʰ **S30.96 Unspecified superficial injury of unspecified** external genital organs, male   ♂ ▽

√x7ᵗʰ **S30.97 Unspecified superficial injury of unspecified** external genital organs, female   ♀ ▽

√x7ᵗʰ **S30.98 Unspecified superficial injury of** anus   ▽

√4ᵗʰ **S31 Open wound of abdomen, lower back, pelvis and external genitals**

Code also any associated:
    spinal cord injury (S24.0, S24.1-, S34.0-, S34.1-)
    wound infection

    EXCLUDES 1   *traumatic amputation of part of abdomen, lower back and pelvis (S38.2-, S38.3)*

    EXCLUDES 2   *open wound of hip (S71.00-S71.02)*
         open fracture of pelvis (S32.1- — S32.9 with 7th character B)

The appropriate 7th character is to be added to each code from category S31.
A   initial encounter
D   subsequent encounter
S   sequela

√5ᵗʰ **S31.0 Open wound of** lower back and pelvis

√6ᵗʰ **S31.00 Unspecified open wound of lower back and pelvis**

√7ᵗʰ **S31.000 Unspecified open wound of lower back and pelvis without penetration into retroperitoneum**   ▽
    Unspecified open wound of lower back and pelvis NOS

√7ᵗʰ **S31.001 Unspecified open wound of lower back and pelvis with penetration into retroperitoneum**   ▽

√6ᵗʰ **S31.01 Laceration without foreign body of lower back and pelvis**

√7ᵗʰ **S31.010 Laceration without foreign body of lower back and pelvis without penetration into retroperitoneum**
    Laceration without foreign body of lower back and pelvis NOS

√7ᵗʰ **S31.011 Laceration without foreign body of lower back and pelvis with penetration into retroperitoneum**

√6ᵗʰ **S31.02 Laceration with foreign body of lower back and pelvis**

√7ᵗʰ **S31.020 Laceration with foreign body of lower back and pelvis without penetration into retroperitoneum**
    Laceration with foreign body of lower back and pelvis NOS

√7ᵗʰ **S31.021 Laceration with foreign body of lower back and pelvis with penetration into retroperitoneum**

√6ᵗʰ **S31.03 Puncture wound without foreign body of lower back and pelvis**

√7ᵗʰ **S31.030 Puncture wound without foreign body of lower back and pelvis without penetration into retroperitoneum**
    Puncture wound without foreign body of lower back and pelvis NOS

√7ᵗʰ **S31.031 Puncture wound without foreign body of lower back and pelvis with penetration into retroperitoneum**

√6ᵗʰ **S31.04 Puncture wound with foreign body of lower back and pelvis**

√7ᵗʰ **S31.040 Puncture wound with foreign body of lower back and pelvis without penetration into retroperitoneum**
    Puncture wound with foreign body of lower back and pelvis NOS

√7ᵗʰ **S31.041 Puncture wound with foreign body of lower back and pelvis with penetration into retroperitoneum**

√6ᵗʰ **S31.05 Open bite of lower back and pelvis**

    Bite of lower back and pelvis NOS

    EXCLUDES 1   *superficial bite of lower back and pelvis (S30.860, S30.870)*

√7ᵗʰ **S31.050 Open bite of lower back and pelvis without penetration into retroperitoneum**
    Open bite of lower back and pelvis NOS

√7ᵗʰ **S31.051 Open bite of lower back and pelvis with penetration into retroperitoneum**

√5ᵗʰ **S31.1 Open wound of** abdominal wall without penetration into peritoneal cavity

    Open wound of abdominal wall NOS

    EXCLUDES 2   *open wound of abdominal wall with penetration into peritoneal cavity (S31.6-)*

√6ᵗʰ **S31.10 Unspecified open wound of abdominal wall without penetration into peritoneal cavity**

☑ Additional Character Required   √x7ᵗʰ Placeholder Alert   Manifestation Dx   ▽ Unspecified Dx   ▶◀ Revised Text   ● New Code   ▲ Revised Code Title

✓7ᵗʰ **S31.100** Unspecified open wound of abdominal wall, **right upper quadrant** without penetration into peritoneal cavity ▽

✓7ᵗʰ **S31.101** Unspecified open wound of abdominal wall, **left upper quadrant** without penetration into peritoneal cavity ▽

✓7ᵗʰ **S31.102** Unspecified open wound of abdominal wall, **epigastric region** without penetration into peritoneal cavity ▽

✓7ᵗʰ **S31.103** Unspecified open wound of abdominal wall, **right lower quadrant** without penetration into peritoneal cavity ▽

✓7ᵗʰ **S31.104** Unspecified open wound of abdominal wall, **left lower quadrant** without penetration into peritoneal cavity ▽

✓7ᵗʰ **S31.105** Unspecified open wound of abdominal wall, **periumbilic region** without penetration into peritoneal cavity ▽

✓7ᵗʰ **S31.109** Unspecified open wound of abdominal wall, unspecified quadrant without penetration into peritoneal cavity ▽

Unspecified open wound of abdominal wall NOS

✓6ᵗʰ **S31.11** **Laceration without foreign body of abdominal wall without penetration into peritoneal cavity**

✓7ᵗʰ **S31.110** Laceration without foreign body of abdominal wall, **right upper quadrant** without penetration into peritoneal cavity

✓7ᵗʰ **S31.111** Laceration without foreign body of abdominal wall, **left upper quadrant** without penetration into peritoneal cavity

✓7ᵗʰ **S31.112** Laceration without foreign body of abdominal wall, **epigastric region** without penetration into peritoneal cavity

✓7ᵗʰ **S31.113** Laceration without foreign body of abdominal wall, **right lower quadrant** without penetration into peritoneal cavity

✓7ᵗʰ **S31.114** Laceration without foreign body of abdominal wall, **left lower quadrant** without penetration into peritoneal cavity

✓7ᵗʰ **S31.115** Laceration without foreign body of abdominal wall, **periumbilic region** without penetration into peritoneal cavity

✓7ᵗʰ **S31.119** Laceration without foreign body of abdominal wall, unspecified quadrant without penetration into peritoneal cavity ▽

✓6ᵗʰ **S31.12** **Laceration with foreign body of abdominal wall without penetration into peritoneal cavity**

✓7ᵗʰ **S31.120** Laceration of abdominal wall with foreign body, **right upper quadrant** without penetration into peritoneal cavity

✓7ᵗʰ **S31.121** Laceration of abdominal wall with foreign body, **left upper quadrant** without penetration into peritoneal cavity

✓7ᵗʰ **S31.122** Laceration of abdominal wall with foreign body, **epigastric region** without penetration into peritoneal cavity

✓7ᵗʰ **S31.123** Laceration of abdominal wall with foreign body, **right lower quadrant** without penetration into peritoneal cavity

✓7ᵗʰ **S31.124** Laceration of abdominal wall with foreign body, **left lower quadrant** without penetration into peritoneal cavity

✓7ᵗʰ **S31.125** Laceration of abdominal wall with foreign body, **periumbilic region** without penetration into peritoneal cavity

✓7ᵗʰ **S31.129** Laceration of abdominal wall with foreign body, unspecified quadrant without penetration into peritoneal cavity ▽

✓6ᵗʰ **S31.13** **Puncture wound of abdominal wall without foreign body without penetration into peritoneal cavity**

✓7ᵗʰ **S31.130** Puncture wound of abdominal wall without foreign body, **right upper quadrant** without penetration into peritoneal cavity

✓7ᵗʰ **S31.131** Puncture wound of abdominal wall without foreign body, **left upper quadrant** without penetration into peritoneal cavity

✓7ᵗʰ **S31.132** Puncture wound of abdominal wall without foreign body, **epigastric region** without penetration into peritoneal cavity

✓7ᵗʰ **S31.133** Puncture wound of abdominal wall without foreign body, **right lower quadrant** without penetration into peritoneal cavity

✓7ᵗʰ **S31.134** Puncture wound of abdominal wall without foreign body, **left lower quadrant** without penetration into peritoneal cavity

✓7ᵗʰ **S31.135** Puncture wound of abdominal wall without foreign body, **periumbilic region** without penetration into peritoneal cavity

✓7ᵗʰ **S31.139** Puncture wound of abdominal wall without foreign body, unspecified quadrant without penetration into peritoneal cavity ▽

✓6ᵗʰ **S31.14** **Puncture wound of abdominal wall with foreign body without penetration into peritoneal cavity**

✓7ᵗʰ **S31.140** Puncture wound of abdominal wall with foreign body, **right upper quadrant** without penetration into peritoneal cavity

✓7ᵗʰ **S31.141** Puncture wound of abdominal wall with foreign body, **left upper quadrant** without penetration into peritoneal cavity

✓7ᵗʰ **S31.142** Puncture wound of abdominal wall with foreign body, **epigastric region** without penetration into peritoneal cavity

✓7ᵗʰ **S31.143** Puncture wound of abdominal wall with foreign body, **right lower quadrant** without penetration into peritoneal cavity

✓7ᵗʰ **S31.144** Puncture wound of abdominal wall with foreign body, **left lower quadrant** without penetration into peritoneal cavity

✓7ᵗʰ **S31.145** Puncture wound of abdominal wall with foreign body, **periumbilic region** without penetration into peritoneal cavity

✓7ᵗʰ **S31.149** Puncture wound of abdominal wall with foreign body, unspecified quadrant without penetration into peritoneal cavity ▽

✓6ᵗʰ **S31.15** **Open bite of abdominal wall without penetration into peritoneal cavity**

Bite of abdominal wall NOS

EXCLUDES 1 *superficial bite of abdominal wall (S30.871)*

✓7ᵗʰ **S31.150** Open bite of abdominal wall, **right upper quadrant** without penetration into peritoneal cavity

✓7ᵗʰ **S31.151** Open bite of abdominal wall, **left upper quadrant** without penetration into peritoneal cavity

✓7ᵗʰ **S31.152** Open bite of abdominal wall, **epigastric region** without penetration into peritoneal cavity

✓7ᵗʰ **S31.153** Open bite of abdominal wall, **right lower quadrant** without penetration into peritoneal cavity

✓7ᵗʰ **S31.154** Open bite of abdominal wall, **left lower quadrant** without penetration into peritoneal cavity

✓7ᵗʰ **S31.155** Open bite of abdominal wall, **periumbilic region** without penetration into peritoneal cavity

✓7ᵗʰ **S31.159** Open bite of abdominal wall, unspecified quadrant without penetration into peritoneal cavity ▽

✓5ᵗʰ **S31.2** **Open wound of penis**

✓x7ᵗʰ **S31.20** **Unspecified open wound of penis** ♂ ▽

✓x7ᵗʰ **S31.21** **Laceration without foreign body of penis** ♂

✓x7ᵗʰ **S31.22** **Laceration with foreign body of penis** ♂

EXCLUDES 1 Not coded here   **EXCLUDES 2** Not included here   **N** Newborn Age : 0   **P** Pediatric Age : 0-17   **M** Maternity Age : 12-55   **A** Adult Age : 15-124

916   ICD-10-CM 2017

√x7th   **S31.23**   **Puncture wound without foreign body of**   ♂
penis

√x7th   **S31.24**   **Puncture wound with foreign body of penis**   ♂

√x7th   **S31.25**   **Open bite of penis**   ♂

Bite of penis NOS
EXCLUDES 1   *superficial bite of penis (S30.862, S30.872)*

√5th   **S31.3**   **Open wound of scrotum and testes**

√x7th   **S31.30**   **Unspecified open wound of scrotum and**   ♂ ▽
testes

√x7th   **S31.31**   **Laceration without foreign body of scrotum**   ♂
and testes

√x7th   **S31.32**   **Laceration with foreign body of scrotum and**   ♂
testes

√x7th   **S31.33**   **Puncture wound without foreign body of**   ♂
scrotum and testes

√x7th   **S31.34**   **Puncture wound with foreign body of**   ♂
scrotum and testes

√x7th   **S31.35**   **Open bite of scrotum and testes**   ♂

Bite of scrotum and testes NOS
EXCLUDES 1   *superficial bite of scrotum and testes*
(S30.863, S30.873)

√5th   **S31.4**   **Open wound of vagina and vulva**

EXCLUDES 1   *injury to vagina and vulva during delivery (O70.-,*
O71.4)

√x7th   **S31.40**   **Unspecified open wound of vagina and vulva**   ♀ ▽

√x7th   **S31.41**   **Laceration without foreign body of vagina**   ♀
and vulva

√x7th   **S31.42**   **Laceration with foreign body of vagina and**   ♀
vulva

√x7th   **S31.43**   **Puncture wound without foreign body of**   ♀
vagina and vulva

√x7th   **S31.44**   **Puncture wound with foreign body of vagina**   ♀
and vulva

√x7th   **S31.45**   **Open bite of vagina and vulva**   ♀

Bite of vagina and vulva NOS
EXCLUDES 1   *superficial bite of vagina and vulva (S30.864,*
S30.874)

√5th   **S31.5**   **Open wound of unspecified external genital organs**

EXCLUDES 1   *traumatic amputation of external genital organs*
(S38.21, S38.22)

√6th   **S31.50**   **Unspecified open wound of unspecified external**
genital organs

√7th   **S31.501**   **Unspecified open wound of**   ♂ ▽
unspecified external genital
organs, male

√7th   **S31.502**   **Unspecified open wound of**   ♀ ▽
unspecified external genital
organs, female

√6th   **S31.51**   **Laceration without foreign body of unspecified**
external genital organs

√7th   **S31.511**   **Laceration without foreign body**   ♂ ▽
of unspecified external genital
organs, male

√7th   **S31.512**   **Laceration without foreign body**   ♀ ▽
of unspecified external genital
organs, female

√6th   **S31.52**   **Laceration with foreign body of unspecified**
external genital organs

√7th   **S31.521**   **Laceration with foreign body of**   ♂ ▽
unspecified external genital
organs, male

√7th   **S31.522**   **Laceration with foreign body of**   ♀ ▽
unspecified external genital
organs, female

√6th   **S31.53**   **Puncture wound without foreign body of**
unspecified external genital organs

√7th   **S31.531**   **Puncture wound without foreign**   ♂ ▽
body of unspecified external
genital organs, male

√7th   **S31.532**   **Puncture wound without foreign**   ♀ ▽
body of unspecified external
genital organs, female

√6th   **S31.54**   **Puncture wound with foreign body of unspecified**
external genital organs

√7th   **S31.541**   **Puncture wound with foreign body**   ♂ ▽
of unspecified external genital
organs, male

√7th   **S31.542**   **Puncture wound with foreign body**   ♀ ▽
of unspecified external genital
organs, female

√6th   **S31.55**   **Open bite of unspecified external genital organs**

Bite of unspecified external genital organs NOS
EXCLUDES 1   *superficial bite of unspecified external*
genital organs (S30.865, S30.866,
S30.875, S30.876)

√7th   **S31.551**   **Open bite of unspecified external**   ♂ ▽
genital organs, male

√7th   **S31.552**   **Open bite of unspecified external**   ♀ ▽
genital organs, female

√5th   **S31.6**   **Open wound of abdominal wall with penetration into**
peritoneal cavity

√6th   **S31.60**   **Unspecified open wound of abdominal wall with**
penetration into peritoneal cavity

√7th   **S31.600**   **Unspecified open wound of**   ▽
abdominal wall, right upper
quadrant with penetration into
peritoneal cavity

√7th   **S31.601**   **Unspecified open wound of**   ▽
abdominal wall, left upper
quadrant with penetration into
peritoneal cavity

√7th   **S31.602**   **Unspecified open wound of**   ▽
abdominal wall, epigastric region
with penetration into peritoneal
cavity

√7th   **S31.603**   **Unspecified open wound of**   ▽
abdominal wall, right lower
quadrant with penetration into
peritoneal cavity

√7th   **S31.604**   **Unspecified open wound of**   ▽
abdominal wall, left lower
quadrant with penetration into
peritoneal cavity

√7th   **S31.605**   **Unspecified open wound of**   ▽
abdominal wall, periumbilic
region with penetration into
peritoneal cavity

√7th   **S31.609**   **Unspecified open wound of**   ▽
abdominal wall, unspecified
quadrant with penetration into
peritoneal cavity

√6th   **S31.61**   **Laceration without foreign body of abdominal wall**
with penetration into peritoneal cavity

√7th   **S31.610**   **Laceration without foreign body of**
abdominal wall, right upper quadrant
with penetration into peritoneal cavity

√7th   **S31.611**   **Laceration without foreign body of**
abdominal wall, left upper quadrant with
penetration into peritoneal cavity

√7th   **S31.612**   **Laceration without foreign body of**
abdominal wall, epigastric region with
penetration into peritoneal cavity

√7th   **S31.613**   **Laceration without foreign body of**
abdominal wall, right lower quadrant
with penetration into peritoneal cavity

√7th   **S31.614**   **Laceration without foreign body of**
abdominal wall, left lower quadrant with
penetration into peritoneal cavity

√7th   **S31.615**   **Laceration without foreign body of**
abdominal wall, periumbilic region with
penetration into peritoneal cavity

√7th   **S31.619**   **Laceration without foreign body**   ▽
of abdominal wall, unspecified
quadrant with penetration into
peritoneal cavity

√6th   **S31.62**   **Laceration with foreign body of abdominal wall**
with penetration into peritoneal cavity

√7th   **S31.620**   **Laceration with foreign body of**
abdominal wall, right upper quadrant
with penetration into peritoneal cavity

√7th   **S31.621**   **Laceration with foreign body of**
abdominal wall, left upper quadrant with
penetration into peritoneal cavity

√7th   **S31.622**   **Laceration with foreign body of**
abdominal wall, epigastric region with
penetration into peritoneal cavity

√7th   **S31.623**   **Laceration with foreign body of**
abdominal wall, right lower quadrant
with penetration into peritoneal cavity

√7th   **S31.624**   **Laceration with foreign body of**
abdominal wall, left lower quadrant with
penetration into peritoneal cavity

√7th   **S31.625**   **Laceration with foreign body of**
abdominal wall, periumbilic region with
penetration into peritoneal cavity

✔️ Additional Character Required   √x7th Placeholder Alert   Manifestation Dx   ▽ Unspecified Dx   ▶◀ Revised Text   ● New Code   ▲ Revised Code Title

√7th **S31.629** **Laceration with foreign body of abdominal wall, unspecified quadrant with penetration into peritoneal cavity** ▽

√6th **S31.63** Puncture wound without foreign body of abdominal wall with penetration into peritoneal cavity

√7th **S31.630** **Puncture wound without foreign body of abdominal wall, right upper quadrant with penetration into peritoneal cavity**

√7th **S31.631** **Puncture wound without foreign body of abdominal wall, left upper quadrant with penetration into peritoneal cavity**

√7th **S31.632** **Puncture wound without foreign body of abdominal wall, epigastric region with penetration into peritoneal cavity**

√7th **S31.633** **Puncture wound without foreign body of abdominal wall, right lower quadrant with penetration into peritoneal cavity**

√7th **S31.634** **Puncture wound without foreign body of abdominal wall, left lower quadrant with penetration into peritoneal cavity**

√7th **S31.635** **Puncture wound without foreign body of abdominal wall, periumbilic region with penetration into peritoneal cavity**

√7th **S31.639** **Puncture wound without foreign body of abdominal wall, unspecified quadrant with penetration into peritoneal cavity** ▽

√6th **S31.64** Puncture wound with foreign body of abdominal wall with penetration into peritoneal cavity

√7th **S31.640** **Puncture wound with foreign body of abdominal wall, right upper quadrant with penetration into peritoneal cavity**

√7th **S31.641** **Puncture wound with foreign body of abdominal wall, left upper quadrant with penetration into peritoneal cavity**

√7th **S31.642** **Puncture wound with foreign body of abdominal wall, epigastric region with penetration into peritoneal cavity**

√7th **S31.643** **Puncture wound with foreign body of abdominal wall, right lower quadrant with penetration into peritoneal cavity**

√7th **S31.644** **Puncture wound with foreign body of abdominal wall, left lower quadrant with penetration into peritoneal cavity**

√7th **S31.645** **Puncture wound with foreign body of abdominal wall, periumbilic region with penetration into peritoneal cavity**

√7th **S31.649** **Puncture wound with foreign body of abdominal wall, unspecified quadrant with penetration into peritoneal cavity** ▽

√6th **S31.65** Open bite of abdominal wall with penetration into peritoneal cavity

EXCLUDES 1 *superficial bite of abdominal wall (S30.861, S30.871)*

√7th **S31.650** **Open bite of abdominal wall, right upper quadrant with penetration into peritoneal cavity**

√7th **S31.651** **Open bite of abdominal wall, left upper quadrant with penetration into peritoneal cavity**

√7th **S31.652** **Open bite of abdominal wall, epigastric region with penetration into peritoneal cavity**

√7th **S31.653** **Open bite of abdominal wall, right lower quadrant with penetration into peritoneal cavity**

√7th **S31.654** **Open bite of abdominal wall, left lower quadrant with penetration into peritoneal cavity**

√7th **S31.655** **Open bite of abdominal wall, periumbilic region with penetration into peritoneal cavity**

√7th **S31.659** **Open bite of abdominal wall, unspecified quadrant with penetration into peritoneal cavity** ▽

√5th **S31.8** **Open wound of other parts of abdomen, lower back and pelvis**

√6th **S31.80** **Open wound of unspecified buttock**

√7th **S31.801** **Laceration without foreign body of unspecified buttock** ▽

√7th **S31.802** **Laceration with foreign body of unspecified buttock** ▽

√7th **S31.803** **Puncture wound without foreign body of unspecified buttock** ▽

√7th **S31.804** **Puncture wound with foreign body of unspecified buttock** ▽

√7th **S31.805** **Open bite of unspecified buttock** ▽

Bite of buttock NOS

EXCLUDES 1 *superficial bite of buttock (S30.870)*

√7th **S31.809** **Unspecified open wound of unspecified buttock** ▽

√6th **S31.81** **Open wound of right buttock**

√7th **S31.811** **Laceration without foreign body of right buttock**

√7th **S31.812** **Laceration with foreign body of right buttock**

√7th **S31.813** **Puncture wound without foreign body of right buttock**

√7th **S31.814** **Puncture wound with foreign body of right buttock**

√7th **S31.815** **Open bite of right buttock**

Bite of right buttock NOS

EXCLUDES 1 *superficial bite of buttock (S30.870)*

√7th **S31.819** **Unspecified open wound of right buttock** ▽

√6th **S31.82** **Open wound of left buttock**

√7th **S31.821** **Laceration without foreign body of left buttock**

√7th **S31.822** **Laceration with foreign body of left buttock**

√7th **S31.823** **Puncture wound without foreign body of left buttock**

√7th **S31.824** **Puncture wound with foreign body of left buttock**

√7th **S31.825** **Open bite of left buttock**

Bite of left buttock NOS

EXCLUDES 1 *superficial bite of buttock (S30.870)*

√7th **S31.829** **Unspecified open wound of left buttock** ▽

√6th **S31.83** **Open wound of anus**

√7th **S31.831** **Laceration without foreign body of anus**

√7th **S31.832** **Laceration with foreign body of anus**

√7th **S31.833** **Puncture wound without foreign body of anus**

√7th **S31.834** **Puncture wound with foreign body of anus**

√7th **S31.835** **Open bite of anus**

Bite of anus NOS

EXCLUDES 1 *superficial bite of anus (S30.877)*

√7th **S31.839** **Unspecified open wound of anus** ▽

√4th **S32** **Fracture of lumbar spine and pelvis**

NOTE A fracture not indicated as displaced or nondisplaced should be coded to displaced.

A fracture not indicated as opened or closed should be coded to closed.

INCLUDES fracture of lumbosacral neural arch
fracture of lumbosacral spinous process
fracture of lumbosacral transverse process
fracture of lumbosacral vertebra
fracture of lumbosacral vertebral arch

Code first any associated spinal cord and spinal nerve injury (S34.-)

EXCLUDES 1 *transection of abdomen (S38.3)*

EXCLUDES 2 *fracture of hip NOS (S72.0-)*

AHA: 2015,3Q,37-39; 2012,4Q,93

The appropriate 7th character is to be added to each code from category S32.
A   initial encounter for closed fracture
B   initial encounter for open fracture
D   subsequent encounter for fracture with routine healing
G   subsequent encounter for fracture with delayed healing
K   subsequent encounter for fracture with nonunion
S   sequela

√5th **S32.0** **Fracture of lumbar vertebra**

Fracture of lumbar spine NOS

√6th **S32.00** **Fracture of unspecified lumbar vertebra**

√7th **S32.000** **Wedge compression fracture of unspecified lumbar vertebra** ▽

EXCLUDES 1 Not coded here   EXCLUDES 2 Not included here   N Newborn Age : 0   P Pediatric Age : 0-17   M Maternity Age : 12-55   A Adult Age : 15-124

918   ICD-10-CM 2017

☑7th **S32.001** Stable burst fracture of unspecified lumbar vertebra ▽

☑7th **S32.002** Unstable burst fracture of unspecified lumbar vertebra ▽

☑7th **S32.008** Other fracture of unspecified lumbar vertebra ▽

☑7th **S32.009** Unspecified fracture of unspecified lumbar vertebra ▽

☑6th **S32.01** Fracture of first lumbar vertebra

  ☑7th **S32.010** Wedge compression fracture of first lumbar vertebra

  ☑7th **S32.011** Stable burst fracture of first lumbar vertebra

  ☑7th **S32.012** Unstable burst fracture of first lumbar vertebra

  ☑7th **S32.018** Other fracture of first lumbar vertebra

  ☑7th **S32.019** Unspecified fracture of first lumbar vertebra ▽

☑6th **S32.02** Fracture of second lumbar vertebra

  ☑7th **S32.020** Wedge compression fracture of second lumbar vertebra

  ☑7th **S32.021** Stable burst fracture of second lumbar vertebra

  ☑7th **S32.022** Unstable burst fracture of second lumbar vertebra

  ☑7th **S32.028** Other fracture of second lumbar vertebra

  ☑7th **S32.029** Unspecified fracture of second lumbar vertebra ▽

☑6th **S32.03** Fracture of third lumbar vertebra

  ☑7th **S32.030** Wedge compression fracture of third lumbar vertebra

  ☑7th **S32.031** Stable burst fracture of third lumbar vertebra

  ☑7th **S32.032** Unstable burst fracture of third lumbar vertebra

  ☑7th **S32.038** Other fracture of third lumbar vertebra

  ☑7th **S32.039** Unspecified fracture of third lumbar vertebra ▽

☑6th **S32.04** Fracture of fourth lumbar vertebra

  ☑7th **S32.040** Wedge compression fracture of fourth lumbar vertebra

  ☑7th **S32.041** Stable burst fracture of fourth lumbar vertebra

  ☑7th **S32.042** Unstable burst fracture of fourth lumbar vertebra

  ☑7th **S32.048** Other fracture of fourth lumbar vertebra

  ☑7th **S32.049** Unspecified fracture of fourth lumbar vertebra ▽

☑6th **S32.05** Fracture of fifth lumbar vertebra

  ☑7th **S32.050** Wedge compression fracture of fifth lumbar vertebra

  ☑7th **S32.051** Stable burst fracture of fifth lumbar vertebra

  ☑7th **S32.052** Unstable burst fracture of fifth lumbar vertebra

  ☑7th **S32.058** Other fracture of fifth lumbar vertebra

  ☑7th **S32.059** Unspecified fracture of fifth lumbar vertebra ▽

☑5th **S32.1** **Fracture of sacrum**

  NOTE For vertical fractures, code to most medial fracture extension

    Use two codes if both a vertical and transverse fracture are present

  Code also any associated fracture of pelvic ring (S32.8-)

☑x7th **S32.10** Unspecified fracture of sacrum ▽

☑6th **S32.11** Zone I fracture of sacrum

    Vertical sacral ala fracture of sacrum

  ☑7th **S32.110** Nondisplaced Zone I fracture of sacrum

  ☑7th **S32.111** Minimally displaced Zone I fracture of sacrum

  ☑7th **S32.112** Severely displaced Zone I fracture of sacrum

  ☑7th **S32.119** Unspecified Zone I fracture of sacrum ▽

☑6th **S32.12** Zone II fracture of sacrum

    Vertical foraminal region fracture of sacrum

  ☑7th **S32.120** Nondisplaced Zone II fracture of sacrum

  ☑7th **S32.121** Minimally displaced Zone II fracture of sacrum

  ☑7th **S32.122** Severely displaced Zone II fracture of sacrum

  ☑7th **S32.129** Unspecified Zone II fracture of sacrum ▽

☑6th **S32.13** Zone III fracture of sacrum

    Vertical fracture into spinal canal region of sacrum

  ☑7th **S32.130** Nondisplaced Zone III fracture of sacrum

  ☑7th **S32.131** Minimally displaced Zone III fracture of sacrum

  ☑7th **S32.132** Severely displaced Zone III fracture of sacrum

  ☑7th **S32.139** Unspecified Zone III fracture of sacrum ▽

☑x7th **S32.14** Type 1 fracture of sacrum

    Transverse flexion fracture of sacrum without displacement

☑x7th **S32.15** Type 2 fracture of sacrum

    Transverse flexion fracture of sacrum with posterior displacement

☑x7th **S32.16** Type 3 fracture of sacrum

    Transverse extension fracture of sacrum with anterior displacement

☑x7th **S32.17** Type 4 fracture of sacrum

    Transverse segmental comminution of upper sacrum

☑x7th **S32.19** Other fracture of sacrum

☑x7th **S32.2** **Fracture of coccyx**

☑5th **S32.3** **Fracture of ilium**

  EXCLUDES 1 *fracture of ilium with associated disruption of pelvic ring (S32.8-)*

☑6th **S32.30** Unspecified fracture of ilium

  ☑7th **S32.301** Unspecified fracture of right ilium ▽

  ☑7th **S32.302** Unspecified fracture of left ilium ▽

  ☑7th **S32.309** Unspecified fracture of unspecified ilium ▽

☑6th **S32.31** Avulsion fracture of ilium

  ☑7th **S32.311** Displaced avulsion fracture of right ilium

  ☑7th **S32.312** Displaced avulsion fracture of left ilium

  ☑7th **S32.313** Displaced avulsion fracture of unspecified ilium ▽

  ☑7th **S32.314** Nondisplaced avulsion fracture of right ilium

  ☑7th **S32.315** Nondisplaced avulsion fracture of left ilium

  ☑7th **S32.316** Nondisplaced avulsion fracture of unspecified ilium ▽

☑6th **S32.39** Other fracture of ilium

  ☑7th **S32.391** Other fracture of right ilium

  ☑7th **S32.392** Other fracture of left ilium

  ☑7th **S32.399** Other fracture of unspecified ilium ▽

☑5th **S32.4** **Fracture of acetabulum**

  Code also any associated fracture of pelvic ring (S32.8-)

☑6th **S32.40** Unspecified fracture of acetabulum

  ☑7th **S32.401** Unspecified fracture of right acetabulum ▽

  ☑7th **S32.402** Unspecified fracture of left acetabulum ▽

  ☑7th **S32.409** Unspecified fracture of unspecified acetabulum ▽

☑6th **S32.41** Fracture of anterior wall of acetabulum

  ☑7th **S32.411** Displaced fracture of anterior wall of right acetabulum

  ☑7th **S32.412** Displaced fracture of anterior wall of left acetabulum

  ☑7th **S32.413** Displaced fracture of anterior wall of unspecified acetabulum ▽

  ☑7th **S32.414** Nondisplaced fracture of anterior wall of right acetabulum

  ☑7th **S32.415** Nondisplaced fracture of anterior wall of left acetabulum

  ☑7th **S32.416** Nondisplaced fracture of anterior wall of unspecified acetabulum ▽

☑ Additional Character Required   ☑x7th Placeholder Alert   Manifestation Dx   ▽ Unspecified Dx   ▶◀ Revised Text   ● New Code   ▲ Revised Code Title

ICD-10-CM 2017   919

Chapter 19. Injury, Poisoning and Certain Other Consequences of External Causes

S32.42–S32.699

√6th **S32.42** Fracture of posterior wall of acetabulum

    √7th **S32.421** Displaced fracture of posterior wall of right acetabulum

    √7th **S32.422** Displaced fracture of posterior wall of left acetabulum

    √7th **S32.423** Displaced fracture of posterior wall of unspecified acetabulum ▽

    √7th **S32.424** Nondisplaced fracture of posterior wall of right acetabulum

    √7th **S32.425** Nondisplaced fracture of posterior wall of left acetabulum

    √7th **S32.426** Nondisplaced fracture of posterior wall of unspecified acetabulum ▽

√6th **S32.43** Fracture of anterior column [iliopubic] of acetabulum

    √7th **S32.431** Displaced fracture of anterior column [iliopubic] of right acetabulum

    √7th **S32.432** Displaced fracture of anterior column [iliopubic] of left acetabulum

    √7th **S32.433** Displaced fracture of anterior column [iliopubic] of unspecified acetabulum ▽

    √7th **S32.434** Nondisplaced fracture of anterior column [iliopubic] of right acetabulum

    √7th **S32.435** Nondisplaced fracture of anterior column [iliopubic] of left acetabulum

    √7th **S32.436** Nondisplaced fracture of anterior column [iliopubic] of unspecified acetabulum ▽

√6th **S32.44** Fracture of posterior column [ilioischial] of acetabulum

    √7th **S32.441** Displaced fracture of posterior column [ilioischial] of right acetabulum

    √7th **S32.442** Displaced fracture of posterior column [ilioischial] of left acetabulum

    √7th **S32.443** Displaced fracture of posterior column [ilioischial] of unspecified acetabulum ▽

    √7th **S32.444** Nondisplaced fracture of posterior column [ilioischial] of right acetabulum

    √7th **S32.445** Nondisplaced fracture of posterior column [ilioischial] of left acetabulum

    √7th **S32.446** Nondisplaced fracture of posterior column [ilioischial] of unspecified acetabulum ▽

√6th **S32.45** Transverse fracture of acetabulum

    √7th **S32.451** Displaced transverse fracture of right acetabulum

    √7th **S32.452** Displaced transverse fracture of left acetabulum

    √7th **S32.453** Displaced transverse fracture of unspecified acetabulum ▽

    √7th **S32.454** Nondisplaced transverse fracture of right acetabulum

    √7th **S32.455** Nondisplaced transverse fracture of left acetabulum

    √7th **S32.456** Nondisplaced transverse fracture of unspecified acetabulum ▽

√6th **S32.46** Associated transverse-posterior fracture of acetabulum

    √7th **S32.461** Displaced associated transverse-posterior fracture of right acetabulum

    √7th **S32.462** Displaced associated transverse-posterior fracture of left acetabulum

    √7th **S32.463** Displaced associated transverse-posterior fracture of unspecified acetabulum ▽

    √7th **S32.464** Nondisplaced associated transverse-posterior fracture of right acetabulum

    √7th **S32.465** Nondisplaced associated transverse-posterior fracture of left acetabulum

    √7th **S32.466** Nondisplaced associated transverse-posterior fracture of unspecified acetabulum ▽

√6th **S32.47** Fracture of medial wall of acetabulum

    √7th **S32.471** Displaced fracture of medial wall of right acetabulum

    √7th **S32.472** Displaced fracture of medial wall of left acetabulum

    √7th **S32.473** Displaced fracture of medial wall of unspecified acetabulum ▽

    √7th **S32.474** Nondisplaced fracture of medial wall of right acetabulum

    √7th **S32.475** Nondisplaced fracture of medial wall of left acetabulum

    √7th **S32.476** Nondisplaced fracture of medial wall of unspecified acetabulum ▽

√6th **S32.48** Dome fracture of acetabulum

    √7th **S32.481** Displaced dome fracture of right acetabulum

    √7th **S32.482** Displaced dome fracture of left acetabulum

    √7th **S32.483** Displaced dome fracture of unspecified acetabulum ▽

    √7th **S32.484** Nondisplaced dome fracture of right acetabulum

    √7th **S32.485** Nondisplaced dome fracture of left acetabulum

    √7th **S32.486** Nondisplaced dome fracture of unspecified acetabulum ▽

√6th **S32.49** Other specified fracture of acetabulum

    √7th **S32.491** Other specified fracture of right acetabulum

    √7th **S32.492** Other specified fracture of left acetabulum

    √7th **S32.499** Other specified fracture of unspecified acetabulum ▽

√5th **S32.5** Fracture of pubis

    EXCLUDES 1 *fracture of pubis with associated disruption of pelvic ring (S32.8-)*

√6th **S32.50** Unspecified fracture of pubis

    √7th **S32.501** Unspecified fracture of right pubis ▽

    √7th **S32.502** Unspecified fracture of left pubis ▽

    √7th **S32.509** Unspecified fracture of unspecified pubis ▽

√6th **S32.51** Fracture of superior rim of pubis

    √7th **S32.511** Fracture of superior rim of right pubis

    √7th **S32.512** Fracture of superior rim of left pubis

    √7th **S32.519** Fracture of superior rim of unspecified pubis ▽

√6th **S32.59** Other specified fracture of pubis

    √7th **S32.591** Other specified fracture of right pubis

    √7th **S32.592** Other specified fracture of left pubis

    √7th **S32.599** Other specified fracture of unspecified pubis ▽

√5th **S32.6** Fracture of ischium

    EXCLUDES 1 *fracture of ischium with associated disruption of pelvic ring (S32.8-)*

√6th **S32.60** Unspecified fracture of ischium

    √7th **S32.601** Unspecified fracture of right ischium ▽

    √7th **S32.602** Unspecified fracture of left ischium ▽

    √7th **S32.609** Unspecified fracture of unspecified ischium ▽

√6th **S32.61** Avulsion fracture of ischium

    √7th **S32.611** Displaced avulsion fracture of right ischium

    √7th **S32.612** Displaced avulsion fracture of left ischium

    √7th **S32.613** Displaced avulsion fracture of unspecified ischium

    √7th **S32.614** Nondisplaced avulsion fracture of right ischium

    √7th **S32.615** Nondisplaced avulsion fracture of left ischium

    √7th **S32.616** Nondisplaced avulsion fracture of unspecified ischium ▽

√6th **S32.69** Other specified fracture of ischium

    √7th **S32.691** Other specified fracture of right ischium

    √7th **S32.692** Other specified fracture of left ischium

    √7th **S32.699** Other specified fracture of unspecified ischium ▽

EXCLUDES 1 Not coded here   EXCLUDES 2 Not included here   N Newborn Age : 0   P Pediatric Age : 0-17   M Maternity Age : 12-55   A Adult Age : 15-124

920   ICD-10-CM 2017

√5ᵗʰ **S32.8**   **Fracture of other parts of pelvis**

Code also any associated:
    fracture of acetabulum (S32.4-)
    sacral fracture (S32.1-)

Fractures Disrupting Pelvic Circle

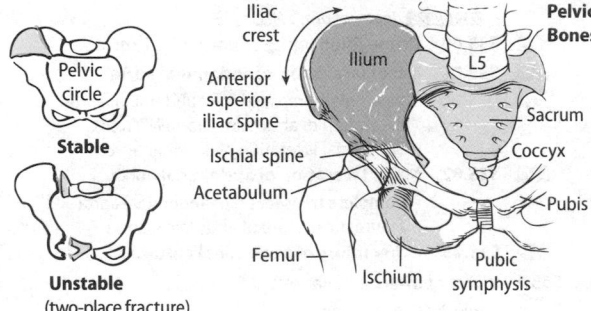

Stable

Unstable
(two-place fracture)

√6ᵗʰ **S32.81**   **Multiple fractures of pelvis with disruption of pelvic ring**

Multiple pelvic fractures with disruption of pelvic circle

√7ᵗʰ **S32.810**   Multiple fractures of pelvis with **stable disruption of pelvic ring**

√7ᵗʰ **S32.811**   Multiple fractures of pelvis with **unstable disruption of pelvic ring**

√x7ᵗʰ **S32.82**   **Multiple fractures of pelvis without disruption of pelvic ring**

Multiple pelvic fractures without disruption of pelvic circle

√x7ᵗʰ **S32.89**   **Fracture of other parts of pelvis**

√x7ᵗʰ **S32.9**   **Fracture of unspecified parts of lumbosacral spine and pelvis** ▽

Fracture of lumbosacral spine NOS
Fracture of pelvis NOS
AHA: 2012,4Q,93

√4ᵗʰ **S33**   **Dislocation and sprain of joints and ligaments of lumbar spine and pelvis**

INCLUDES   avulsion of joint or ligament of lumbar spine and pelvis
     laceration of cartilage, joint or ligament of lumbar spine and pelvis
     sprain of cartilage, joint or ligament of lumbar spine and pelvis
     traumatic hemarthrosis of joint or ligament of lumbar spine and pelvis
     traumatic rupture of joint or ligament of lumbar spine and pelvis
     traumatic subluxation of joint or ligament of lumbar spine and pelvis
     traumatic tear of joint or ligament of lumbar spine and pelvis

Code also any associated open wound

EXCLUDES 1   nontraumatic rupture or displacement of lumbar intervertebral disc NOS (M51.-)
     obstetric damage to pelvic joints and ligaments (O71.6)

EXCLUDES 2   dislocation and sprain of joints and ligaments of hip (S73.-)
     strain of muscle of lower back and pelvis (S39.01-)

The appropriate 7th character is to be added to each code from category S33.
A   initial encounter
D   subsequent encounter
S   sequela

√x7ᵗʰ **S33.0**   **Traumatic rupture of lumbar intervertebral disc**

EXCLUDES 1   rupture or displacement (nontraumatic) of lumbar intervertebral disc NOS (M51.- with fifth character 6)

√5ᵗʰ **S33.1**   **Subluxation and dislocation of lumbar vertebra**

Code also any associated:
    open wound of abdomen, lower back and pelvis (S31)
    spinal cord injury (S24.0, S24.1-, S34.0-, S34.1-)
    EXCLUDES 2   fracture of lumbar vertebrae (S32.0-)

√6ᵗʰ **S33.10**   **Subluxation and dislocation of unspecified lumbar vertebra**

√7ᵗʰ **S33.100**   **Subluxation of unspecified lumbar vertebra**   ▽

√7ᵗʰ **S33.101**   **Dislocation of unspecified lumbar vertebra**   ▽

√6ᵗʰ **S33.11**   **Subluxation and dislocation of L1/L2 lumbar vertebra**

√7ᵗʰ **S33.110**   **Subluxation of L1/L2 lumbar vertebra**

√7ᵗʰ **S33.111**   **Dislocation of L1/L2 lumbar vertebra**

√6ᵗʰ **S33.12**   **Subluxation and dislocation of L2/L3 lumbar vertebra**

√7ᵗʰ **S33.120**   **Subluxation of L2/L3 lumbar vertebra**

√7ᵗʰ **S33.121**   **Dislocation of L2/L3 lumbar vertebra**

√6ᵗʰ **S33.13**   **Subluxation and dislocation of L3/L4 lumbar vertebra**

√7ᵗʰ **S33.130**   **Subluxation of L3/L4 lumbar vertebra**

√7ᵗʰ **S33.131**   **Dislocation of L3/L4 lumbar vertebra**

√6ᵗʰ **S33.14**   **Subluxation and dislocation of L4/L5 lumbar vertebra**

√7ᵗʰ **S33.140**   **Subluxation of L4/L5 lumbar vertebra**

√7ᵗʰ **S33.141**   **Dislocation of L4/L5 lumbar vertebra**

√x7ᵗʰ **S33.2**   **Dislocation of sacroiliac and sacrococcygeal joint**

√5ᵗʰ **S33.3**   **Dislocation of other and unspecified parts of lumbar spine and pelvis**

√x7ᵗʰ **S33.30**   **Dislocation of unspecified parts of lumbar spine and pelvis**   ▽

√x7ᵗʰ **S33.39**   **Dislocation of other parts of lumbar spine and pelvis**

√x7ᵗʰ **S33.4**   **Traumatic rupture of symphysis pubis**

√x7ᵗʰ **S33.5**   **Sprain of ligaments of lumbar spine**

√x7ᵗʰ **S33.6**   **Sprain of sacroiliac joint**

√x7ᵗʰ **S33.8**   **Sprain of other parts of lumbar spine and pelvis**

√x7ᵗʰ **S33.9**   **Sprain of unspecified parts of lumbar spine and pelvis**   ▽

√4ᵗʰ **S34**   **Injury of lumbar and sacral spinal cord and nerves at abdomen, lower back and pelvis level**

NOTE   Code to highest level of lumbar cord injury

Injuries to the spinal cord (S34.0 and S34.1) refer to the cord level and not bone level injury, and can affect nerve roots at and below the level given.

Code also any associated:
    fracture of vertebra (S22.0-, S32.0-)
    open wound of abdomen, lower back and pelvis (S31.-)
    transient paralysis (R29.5)

The appropriate 7th character is to be added to each code from category S34.
A   initial encounter
D   subsequent encounter
S   sequela

√5ᵗʰ **S34.0**   **Concussion and edema of lumbar and sacral spinal cord**

√x7ᵗʰ **S34.01**   **Concussion and edema of lumbar spinal cord**

√x7ᵗʰ **S34.02**   **Concussion and edema of sacral spinal cord**

Concussion and edema of conus medullaris

√5ᵗʰ **S34.1**   **Other and unspecified injury of lumbar and sacral spinal cord**

√6ᵗʰ **S34.10**   **Unspecified injury to lumbar spinal cord**

√7ᵗʰ **S34.101**   **Unspecified injury to L1 level of lumbar spinal cord**   ▽
    ▶Unspecified injury to lumbar spinal cord level 1◀

√7ᵗʰ **S34.102**   **Unspecified injury to L2 level of lumbar spinal cord**   ▽
    ▶Unspecified injury to lumbar spinal cord level 2◀

√7ᵗʰ **S34.103**   **Unspecified injury to L3 level of lumbar spinal cord**   ▽
    ▶Unspecified injury to lumbar spinal cord level 3◀

√7ᵗʰ **S34.104**   **Unspecified injury to L4 level of lumbar spinal cord**   ▽
    ▶Unspecified injury to lumbar spinal cord level 4◀

√7ᵗʰ **S34.105**   **Unspecified injury to L5 level of lumbar spinal cord**   ▽
    ▶Unspecified injury to lumbar spinal cord level 5◀

√7ᵗʰ **S34.109**   **Unspecified injury to unspecified level of lumbar spinal cord**   ▽

☑ Additional Character Required   √x7ᵗʰ Placeholder Alert   Manifestation Dx   ▽ Unspecified Dx   ▶◀ Revised Text   ● New Code   ▲ Revised Code Title

ICD-10-CM 2017   **921**

√6ᵗʰ **S34.11** Complete lesion **of lumbar spinal cord**

 √7ᵗʰ **S34.111** Complete lesion **of** L1 level **of lumbar spinal cord**
  ▶Complete lesion of lumbar spinal cord level 1◀

 √7ᵗʰ **S34.112** Complete lesion **of** L2 level **of lumbar spinal cord**
  ▶Complete lesion of lumbar spinal cord level 2◀

 √7ᵗʰ **S34.113** Complete lesion **of** L3 level **of lumbar spinal cord**
  ▶Complete lesion of lumbar spinal cord level 3◀

 √7ᵗʰ **S34.114** Complete lesion **of** L4 level **of lumbar spinal cord**
  ▶Complete lesion of lumbar spinal cord level 4◀

 √7ᵗʰ **S34.115** Complete lesion **of** L5 level **of lumbar spinal cord**
  ▶Complete lesion of lumbar spinal cord level 5◀

 √7ᵗʰ **S34.119** Complete lesion **of unspecified level of lumbar spinal cord** ▽

√6ᵗʰ **S34.12** Incomplete lesion **of lumbar spinal cord**

 √7ᵗʰ **S34.121** Incomplete lesion **of** L1 level **of lumbar spinal cord**
  ▶Incomplete lesion of lumbar spinal cord level 1◀

 √7ᵗʰ **S34.122** Incomplete lesion **of** L2 level **of lumbar spinal cord**
  ▶Incomplete lesion of lumbar spinal cord level 2◀

 √7ᵗʰ **S34.123** Incomplete lesion **of** L3 level **of lumbar spinal cord**
  ▶Incomplete lesion of lumbar spinal cord level 3◀

 √7ᵗʰ **S34.124** Incomplete lesion **of** L4 level **of lumbar spinal cord**
  ▶Incomplete lesion of lumbar spinal cord level 4◀

 √7ᵗʰ **S34.125** Incomplete lesion **of** L5 level **of lumbar spinal cord**
  ▶Incomplete lesion of lumbar spinal cord level 5◀

 √7ᵗʰ **S34.129** Incomplete lesion **of unspecified level of lumbar spinal cord** ▽

√6ᵗʰ **S34.13** Other and unspecified injury to sacral spinal cord
 Other injury to conus medullaris

 √7ᵗʰ **S34.131** Complete lesion **of sacral spinal cord**
  Complete lesion of conus medullaris

 √7ᵗʰ **S34.132** Incomplete lesion **of sacral spinal cord**
  Incomplete lesion of conus medullaris

 √7ᵗʰ **S34.139** Unspecified injury to sacral spinal cord ▽
  Unspecified injury of conus medullaris

√5ᵗʰ **S34.2** Injury of nerve root of lumbar and sacral spine

 √x7ᵗʰ **S34.21** Injury of nerve root of lumbar spine

 √x7ᵗʰ **S34.22** Injury of nerve root of sacral spine

√x7ᵗʰ **S34.3** Injury of cauda equina

√x7ᵗʰ **S34.4** Injury of lumbosacral plexus

√x7ᵗʰ **S34.5** Injury of lumbar, sacral and pelvic sympathetic nerves
 Injury of celiac ganglion or plexus
 Injury of hypogastric plexus
 Injury of mesenteric plexus (inferior) (superior)
 Injury of splanchnic nerve

√x7ᵗʰ **S34.6** Injury of peripheral nerve(s) at abdomen, lower back and pelvis level

√x7ᵗʰ **S34.8** Injury of other nerves at abdomen, lower back and pelvis level

√x7ᵗʰ **S34.9** Injury of unspecified nerves at abdomen, lower back and pelvis level ▽

√4ᵗʰ **S35** Injury of blood vessels at abdomen, lower back and pelvis level
 Code also any associated open wound (S31.-)

> The appropriate 7th character is to be added to each code from category S35.
> A initial encounter
> D subsequent encounter
> S sequela

√5ᵗʰ **S35.0** Injury of abdominal aorta
 EXCLUDES 1 injury of aorta NOS (S25.0)

 √x7ᵗʰ **S35.00** Unspecified injury of abdominal aorta ▽

 √x7ᵗʰ **S35.01** Minor laceration of abdominal aorta
  Incomplete transection of abdominal aorta
  Laceration of abdominal aorta NOS
  Superficial laceration of abdominal aorta

 √x7ᵗʰ **S35.02** Major laceration of abdominal aorta
  Complete transection of abdominal aorta
  Traumatic rupture of abdominal aorta

 √x7ᵗʰ **S35.09** Other injury of abdominal aorta

√5ᵗʰ **S35.1** Injury of inferior vena cava
 Injury of hepatic vein
 EXCLUDES 1 injury of vena cava NOS (S25.2)

 √x7ᵗʰ **S35.10** Unspecified injury of inferior vena cava ▽

 √x7ᵗʰ **S35.11** Minor laceration of inferior vena cava
  Incomplete transection of inferior vena cava
  Laceration of inferior vena cava NOS
  Superficial laceration of inferior vena cava

 √x7ᵗʰ **S35.12** Major laceration of inferior vena cava
  Complete transection of inferior vena cava
  Traumatic rupture of inferior vena cava

 √x7ᵗʰ **S35.19** Other injury of inferior vena cava

√5ᵗʰ **S35.2** Injury of celiac or mesenteric artery and branches

 √6ᵗʰ **S35.21** Injury of celiac artery

  √7ᵗʰ **S35.211** Minor laceration of celiac artery
   Incomplete transection of celiac artery
   Laceration of celiac artery NOS
   Superficial laceration of celiac artery

  √7ᵗʰ **S35.212** Major laceration of celiac artery
   Complete transection of celiac artery
   Traumatic rupture of celiac artery

  √7ᵗʰ **S35.218** Other injury of celiac artery

  √7ᵗʰ **S35.219** Unspecified injury of celiac artery ▽

 √6ᵗʰ **S35.22** Injury of superior mesenteric artery

  √7ᵗʰ **S35.221** Minor laceration of superior mesenteric artery
   Incomplete transection of superior mesenteric artery
   Laceration of superior mesenteric artery NOS
   Superficial laceration of superior mesenteric artery

  √7ᵗʰ **S35.222** Major laceration of superior mesenteric artery
   Complete transection of superior mesenteric artery
   Traumatic rupture of superior mesenteric artery

  √7ᵗʰ **S35.228** Other injury of superior mesenteric artery

  √7ᵗʰ **S35.229** Unspecified injury of superior mesenteric artery ▽

 √6ᵗʰ **S35.23** Injury of inferior mesenteric artery

  √7ᵗʰ **S35.231** Minor laceration of inferior mesenteric artery
   Incomplete transection of inferior mesenteric artery
   Laceration of inferior mesenteric artery NOS
   Superficial laceration of inferior mesenteric artery

EXCLUDES 1 Not coded here *EXCLUDES 2* Not included here Ⓝ Newborn Age : 0 Ⓟ Pediatric Age : 0-17 Ⓜ Maternity Age : 12-55 Ⓐ Adult Age : 15-124

922 ICD-10-CM 2017

√7ʰ **S35.232** **Major laceration** of inferior mesenteric artery
     Complete transection of inferior mesenteric artery
     Traumatic rupture of inferior mesenteric artery

√7ʰ **S35.238** **Other injury of inferior mesenteric artery**

√7ʰ **S35.239** **Unspecified injury of inferior**   ▽
     mesenteric artery

√6ʰ **S35.29** Injury of **branches of celiac and mesenteric artery**
     Injury of gastric artery
     Injury of gastroduodenal artery
     Injury of hepatic artery
     Injury of splenic artery

√7ʰ **S35.291** **Minor laceration** of branches of celiac and mesenteric artery
     Incomplete transection of branches of celiac and mesenteric artery
     Laceration of branches of celiac and mesenteric artery NOS
     Superficial laceration of branches of celiac and mesenteric artery

√7ʰ **S35.292** **Major laceration** of branches of celiac and mesenteric artery
     Complete transection of branches of celiac and mesenteric artery
     Traumatic rupture of branches of celiac and mesenteric artery

√7ʰ **S35.298** **Other injury of branches of celiac and mesenteric artery**

√7ʰ **S35.299** **Unspecified injury of branches of**   ▽
     celiac and mesenteric artery

√5ʰ **S35.3** Injury of **portal or splenic vein and branches**

√6ʰ **S35.31** Injury of **portal vein**

√7ʰ **S35.311** **Laceration** of portal vein

√7ʰ **S35.318** **Other specified injury of portal vein**

√7ʰ **S35.319** **Unspecified injury of portal vein**   ▽

√6ʰ **S35.32** Injury of **splenic vein**

√7ʰ **S35.321** **Laceration** of splenic vein

√7ʰ **S35.328** **Other specified injury of splenic vein**

√7ʰ **S35.329** **Unspecified injury of splenic vein**   ▽

√6ʰ **S35.33** Injury of **superior mesenteric vein**

√7ʰ **S35.331** **Laceration** of superior mesenteric vein

√7ʰ **S35.338** **Other specified injury of superior mesenteric vein**

√7ʰ **S35.339** **Unspecified injury of superior**   ▽
     mesenteric vein

√6ʰ **S35.34** Injury of **inferior mesenteric vein**

√7ʰ **S35.341** **Laceration** of inferior mesenteric vein

√7ʰ **S35.348** **Other specified injury of inferior mesenteric vein**

√7ʰ **S35.349** **Unspecified injury of inferior**   ▽
     mesenteric vein

√5ʰ **S35.4** Injury of **renal blood vessels**

√6ʰ **S35.40** **Unspecified injury of renal blood vessel**

√7ʰ **S35.401** **Unspecified injury of right renal**   ▽
     artery

√7ʰ **S35.402** **Unspecified injury of left renal**   ▽
     artery

√7ʰ **S35.403** **Unspecified injury of unspecified**   ▽
     renal artery

√7ʰ **S35.404** **Unspecified injury of right renal**   ▽
     vein

√7ʰ **S35.405** **Unspecified injury of left renal**   ▽
     vein

√7ʰ **S35.406** **Unspecified injury of unspecified**   ▽
     renal vein

√6ʰ **S35.41** **Laceration of renal blood vessel**

√7ʰ **S35.411** **Laceration of right renal artery**

√7ʰ **S35.412** **Laceration of left renal artery**

√7ʰ **S35.413** **Laceration of unspecified renal**   ▽
     artery

√7ʰ **S35.414** **Laceration of right renal vein**

√7ʰ **S35.415** **Laceration of left renal vein**

√7ʰ **S35.416** **Laceration of unspecified renal**   ▽
     vein

√6ʰ **S35.49** **Other specified injury of renal blood vessel**

√7ʰ **S35.491** **Other specified injury of right renal artery**

√7ʰ **S35.492** **Other specified injury of left renal artery**

√7ʰ **S35.493** **Other specified injury of**   ▽
     unspecified renal artery

√7ʰ **S35.494** **Other specified injury of right renal vein**

√7ʰ **S35.495** **Other specified injury of left renal vein**

√7ʰ **S35.496** **Other specified injury of**   ▽
     unspecified renal vein

√5ʰ **S35.5** Injury of **iliac blood vessels**

√x7ʰ **S35.50** **Injury of unspecified iliac blood vessel(s)**   ▽

√6ʰ **S35.51** Injury of **iliac artery or vein**
     Injury of hypogastric artery or vein

√7ʰ **S35.511** **Injury of right iliac artery**

√7ʰ **S35.512** **Injury of left iliac artery**

√7ʰ **S35.513** **Injury of unspecified iliac artery**   ▽

√7ʰ **S35.514** **Injury of right iliac vein**

√7ʰ **S35.515** **Injury of left iliac vein**

√7ʰ **S35.516** **Injury of unspecified iliac vein**   ▽

√6ʰ **S35.53** Injury of **uterine artery or vein**

√7ʰ **S35.531** **Injury of right uterine artery**   ♀

√7ʰ **S35.532** **Injury of left uterine artery**   ♀

√7ʰ **S35.533** **Injury of unspecified uterine artery** ♀ ▽

√7ʰ **S35.534** **Injury of right uterine vein**   ♀

√7ʰ **S35.535** **Injury of left uterine vein**   ♀

√7ʰ **S35.536** **Injury of unspecified uterine vein** ♀ ▽

√x7ʰ **S35.59** **Injury of other iliac blood vessels**

√6ʰ **S35.8** Injury of **other blood vessels at abdomen, lower back and pelvis level**
     Injury of ovarian artery or vein

√6ʰ **S35.8X** **Injury of other blood vessels at abdomen, lower back and pelvis level**

√7ʰ **S35.8X1** **Laceration of other blood vessels at abdomen, lower back and pelvis level**

√7ʰ **S35.8X8** **Other specified injury of other blood vessels at abdomen, lower back and pelvis level**

√7ʰ **S35.8X9** **Unspecified injury of other blood**   ▽
     vessels at abdomen, lower back and pelvis level

√5ʰ **S35.9** Injury of **unspecified blood vessel at abdomen, lower back and pelvis level**

√x7ʰ **S35.90** **Unspecified injury of unspecified blood**   ▽
     vessel at abdomen, lower back and pelvis level

√x7ʰ **S35.91** **Laceration of unspecified blood vessel at**   ▽
     abdomen, lower back and pelvis level

√x7ʰ **S35.99** **Other specified injury of unspecified blood**   ▽
     vessel at abdomen, lower back and pelvis level

√4ʰ **S36** **Injury of intra-abdominal organs**
     Code also any associated open wound (S31.-)

> The appropriate 7th character is to be added to each code from category S36.
> A   initial encounter
> D   subsequent encounter
> S   sequela

√5ʰ **S36.0** Injury of **spleen**
     AHA: 2015,2Q,36; 2015,1Q,10

√x7ʰ **S36.00** **Unspecified injury of spleen**   ▽

√6ʰ **S36.02** **Contusion of spleen**

√7ʰ **S36.020** **Minor contusion of spleen**
     Contusion of spleen less than 2 cm

√7ʰ **S36.021** **Major contusion of spleen**
     Contusion of spleen greater than 2 cm

√7ʰ **S36.029** **Unspecified contusion of spleen**   ▽

√6ʰ **S36.03** **Laceration of spleen**

√7ʰ **S36.030** **Superficial (capsular) laceration of spleen**
     Laceration of spleen less than 1 cm
     Minor laceration of spleen

√7ʰ **S36.031** **Moderate laceration of spleen**
     Laceration of spleen 1 to 3 cm

☑ Additional Character Required   √x7ʰ Placeholder Alert   Manifestation Dx   ▽ Unspecified Dx   ▶◀ Revised Text   ● New Code   ▲ Revised Code Title

ICD-10-CM 2017   923

√7ᵗʰ **S36.032** Major **laceration of spleen**
- Avulsion of spleen
- Laceration of spleen greater than 3 cm
- Massive laceration of spleen
- Multiple moderate lacerations of spleen
- Stellate laceration of spleen

√7ᵗʰ **S36.039** **Unspecified laceration of spleen** ▽

√x7ᵗʰ **S36.09** **Other injury of spleen**

√5ᵗʰ **S36.1** **Injury of liver and gallbladder and bile duct**

√6ᵗʰ **S36.11** **Injury of** liver

√7ᵗʰ **S36.112** **Contusion** of **liver**

√7ᵗʰ **S36.113** **Laceration** of **liver, unspecified degree** ▽

√7ᵗʰ **S36.114** **Minor laceration of liver**
- Laceration involving capsule only, or, without significant involvement of hepatic parenchyma [i.e., less than 1 cm deep]

√7ᵗʰ **S36.115** **Moderate laceration of liver**
- Laceration involving parenchyma but without major disruption of parenchyma [i.e., less than 10 cm long and less than 3 cm deep]

√7ᵗʰ **S36.116** **Major laceration of liver**
- Laceration with significant disruption of hepatic parenchyma [i.e., greater than 10 cm long and 3 cm deep]
- Multiple moderate lacerations, with or without hematoma
- Stellate laceration of liver

√7ᵗʰ **S36.118** **Other injury of liver**

√7ᵗʰ **S36.119** **Unspecified injury of liver** ▽

√6ᵗʰ **S36.12** **Injury of** gallbladder

√7ᵗʰ **S36.122** **Contusion of gallbladder**

√7ᵗʰ **S36.123** **Laceration of gallbladder**

√7ᵗʰ **S36.128** **Other injury of gallbladder**

√7ᵗʰ **S36.129** **Unspecified injury of gallbladder** ▽

√x7ᵗʰ **S36.13** **Injury of** bile duct

√5ᵗʰ **S36.2** **Injury of** pancreas

√6ᵗʰ **S36.20** **Unspecified injury of pancreas**

√7ᵗʰ **S36.200** **Unspecified injury of** head of pancreas ▽

√7ᵗʰ **S36.201** **Unspecified injury of** body of pancreas ▽

√7ᵗʰ **S36.202** **Unspecified injury of** tail of pancreas ▽

√7ᵗʰ **S36.209** **Unspecified injury of unspecified part of pancreas** ▽

√6ᵗʰ **S36.22** **Contusion of pancreas**

√7ᵗʰ **S36.220** **Contusion of** head of pancreas

√7ᵗʰ **S36.221** **Contusion of** body of pancreas

√7ᵗʰ **S36.222** **Contusion of** tail of pancreas

√7ᵗʰ **S36.229** **Contusion of unspecified part of pancreas** ▽

√6ᵗʰ **S36.23** **Laceration** of pancreas, unspecified degree

√7ᵗʰ **S36.230** **Laceration of** head of pancreas, unspecified degree ▽

√7ᵗʰ **S36.231** **Laceration of** body of pancreas, unspecified degree ▽

√7ᵗʰ **S36.232** **Laceration of** tail of pancreas, unspecified degree ▽

√7ᵗʰ **S36.239** **Laceration of unspecified part of pancreas, unspecified degree** ▽

√6ᵗʰ **S36.24** **Minor laceration** of pancreas

√7ᵗʰ **S36.240** **Minor laceration of** head of pancreas

√7ᵗʰ **S36.241** **Minor laceration of** body of pancreas

√7ᵗʰ **S36.242** **Minor laceration of** tail of pancreas

√7ᵗʰ **S36.249** **Minor laceration of unspecified part of pancreas** ▽

√6ᵗʰ **S36.25** **Moderate laceration** of pancreas

√7ᵗʰ **S36.250** **Moderate laceration of** head of pancreas

√7ᵗʰ **S36.251** **Moderate laceration of** body of pancreas

√7ᵗʰ **S36.252** **Moderate laceration of** tail of pancreas

√7ᵗʰ **S36.259** **Moderate laceration of unspecified part of pancreas** ▽

√6ᵗʰ **S36.26** **Major laceration** of pancreas

√7ᵗʰ **S36.260** **Major laceration of** head of pancreas

√7ᵗʰ **S36.261** **Major laceration of** body of pancreas

√7ᵗʰ **S36.262** **Major laceration of** tail of pancreas

√7ᵗʰ **S36.269** **Major laceration of unspecified part of pancreas** ▽

√6ᵗʰ **S36.29** **Other injury of pancreas**

√7ᵗʰ **S36.290** **Other injury of** head of pancreas

√7ᵗʰ **S36.291** **Other injury of** body of pancreas

√7ᵗʰ **S36.292** **Other injury of** tail of pancreas

√7ᵗʰ **S36.299** **Other injury of unspecified part of pancreas** ▽

√5ᵗʰ **S36.3** **Injury of** stomach

√x7ᵗʰ **S36.30** **Unspecified injury of stomach** ▽

√x7ᵗʰ **S36.32** **Contusion of stomach**

√x7ᵗʰ **S36.33** **Laceration of stomach**

√x7ᵗʰ **S36.39** **Other injury of stomach**

√5ᵗʰ **S36.4** **Injury of** small intestine

√6ᵗʰ **S36.40** **Unspecified injury of small intestine**

√7ᵗʰ **S36.400** **Unspecified injury of** duodenum ▽

√7ᵗʰ **S36.408** **Unspecified injury of other part of small intestine** ▽

√7ᵗʰ **S36.409** **Unspecified injury of unspecified part of small intestine** ▽

√6ᵗʰ **S36.41** **Primary blast injury of small intestine**
- Blast injury of small intestine NOS

√7ᵗʰ **S36.410** **Primary blast injury of** duodenum

√7ᵗʰ **S36.418** **Primary blast injury of other part of small intestine**

√7ᵗʰ **S36.419** **Primary blast injury of unspecified part of small intestine** ▽

√6ᵗʰ **S36.42** **Contusion of small intestine**

√7ᵗʰ **S36.420** **Contusion of** duodenum

√7ᵗʰ **S36.428** **Contusion of other part of small intestine**

√7ᵗʰ **S36.429** **Contusion of unspecified part of small intestine** ▽

√6ᵗʰ **S36.43** **Laceration of small intestine**

√7ᵗʰ **S36.430** **Laceration of** duodenum

√7ᵗʰ **S36.438** **Laceration of other part of small intestine**

√7ᵗʰ **S36.439** **Laceration of unspecified part of small intestine** ▽

√6ᵗʰ **S36.49** **Other injury of small intestine**

√7ᵗʰ **S36.490** **Other injury of** duodenum

√7ᵗʰ **S36.498** **Other injury of other part of small intestine**

√7ᵗʰ **S36.499** **Other injury of unspecified part of small intestine** ▽

√5ᵗʰ **S36.5** **Injury of** colon

EXCLUDES 2 injury of rectum (S36.6-)

√6ᵗʰ **S36.50** **Unspecified injury of colon**

√7ᵗʰ **S36.500** **Unspecified injury of** ascending [right] colon ▽

√7ᵗʰ **S36.501** **Unspecified injury of** transverse colon ▽

√7ᵗʰ **S36.502** **Unspecified injury of** descending [left] colon ▽

√7ᵗʰ **S36.503** **Unspecified injury of** sigmoid colon ▽

√7ᵗʰ **S36.508** **Unspecified injury of other part of colon** ▽

√7ᵗʰ **S36.509** **Unspecified injury of unspecified part of colon** ▽

√6ᵗʰ **S36.51** **Primary blast injury of colon**
- Blast injury of colon NOS

√7ᵗʰ **S36.510** **Primary blast injury of** ascending [right] colon

√7ᵗʰ **S36.511** **Primary blast injury of** transverse colon

√7ᵗʰ **S36.512** **Primary blast injury of** descending [left] colon

√7ᵗʰ **S36.513** **Primary blast injury of** sigmoid colon

√7ᵗʰ **S36.518** **Primary blast injury of other part of colon**

√6ᵗʰ S36.519 Primary blast injury of unspecified part of colon ▽

√6ᵗʰ **S36.52 Contusion of colon**

   √7ᵗʰ **S36.520 Contusion of ascending [right] colon**

   √7ᵗʰ **S36.521 Contusion of transverse colon**

   √7ᵗʰ **S36.522 Contusion of descending [left] colon**

   √7ᵗʰ **S36.523 Contusion of sigmoid colon**

   √7ᵗʰ **S36.528 Contusion of other part of colon**

   √7ᵗʰ **S36.529 Contusion of unspecified part of colon** ▽

√6ᵗʰ **S36.53 Laceration of colon**

   √7ᵗʰ **S36.530 Laceration of ascending [right] colon**

   √7ᵗʰ **S36.531 Laceration of transverse colon**

   √7ᵗʰ **S36.532 Laceration of descending [left] colon**

   √7ᵗʰ **S36.533 Laceration of sigmoid colon**

   √7ᵗʰ **S36.538 Laceration of other part of colon**

   √7ᵗʰ **S36.539 Laceration of unspecified part of colon** ▽

√6ᵗʰ **S36.59 Other injury of colon**

   Secondary blast injury of colon

   √7ᵗʰ **S36.590 Other injury of ascending [right] colon**

   √7ᵗʰ **S36.591 Other injury of transverse colon**

   √7ᵗʰ **S36.592 Other injury of descending [left] colon**

   √7ᵗʰ **S36.593 Other injury of sigmoid colon**

   √7ᵗʰ **S36.598 Other injury of other part of colon**

   √7ᵗʰ **S36.599 Other injury of unspecified part of colon** ▽

√5ᵗʰ **S36.6 Injury of rectum**

√x7ᵗʰ **S36.60 Unspecified injury of rectum** ▽

√x7ᵗʰ **S36.61 Primary blast injury of rectum**

   Blast injury of rectum NOS

√x7ᵗʰ **S36.62 Contusion of rectum**

√x7ᵗʰ **S36.63 Laceration of rectum**

√x7ᵗʰ **S36.69 Other injury of rectum**

   Secondary blast injury of rectum

√5ᵗʰ **S36.8 Injury of other intra-abdominal organs**

√x7ᵗʰ **S36.81 Injury of peritoneum**

√6ᵗʰ **S36.89 Injury of other intra-abdominal organs**

   Injury of retroperitoneum

   √7ᵗʰ **S36.892 Contusion of other intra-abdominal organs**

   √7ᵗʰ **S36.893 Laceration of other intra-abdominal organs**

   √7ᵗʰ **S36.898 Other injury of other intra-abdominal organs**

   √7ᵗʰ **S36.899 Unspecified injury of other intra-abdominal organs** ▽

√5ᵗʰ **S36.9 Injury of unspecified intra-abdominal organ**

√x7ᵗʰ **S36.90 Unspecified injury of unspecified intra-abdominal organ** ▽

√x7ᵗʰ **S36.92 Contusion of unspecified intra-abdominal organ** ▽

√x7ᵗʰ **S36.93 Laceration of unspecified intra-abdominal organ** ▽

√x7ᵗʰ **S36.99 Other injury of unspecified intra-abdominal organ** ▽

√4ᵗʰ **S37 Injury of urinary and pelvic organs**

Code also any associated open wound (S31.-)

EXCLUDES 1 obstetric trauma to pelvic organs (O71.-)

EXCLUDES 2 injury of peritoneum (S36.81)
        injury of retroperitoneum (S36.89-)

The appropriate 7th character is to be added to each code from category S37.

A   initial encounter

D   subsequent encounter

S   sequela

√5ᵗʰ **S37.0 Injury of kidney**

EXCLUDES 2 acute kidney injury (nontraumatic) (N17.9)

√6ᵗʰ **S37.00 Unspecified injury of kidney**

   √7ᵗʰ **S37.001 Unspecified injury of right kidney** ▽

   √7ᵗʰ **S37.002 Unspecified injury of left kidney** ▽

   √7ᵗʰ **S37.009 Unspecified injury of unspecified kidney** ▽

√6ᵗʰ **S37.01 Minor contusion of kidney**

   Contusion of kidney less than 2 cm
   Contusion of kidney NOS

   √7ᵗʰ **S37.011 Minor contusion of right kidney**

   √7ᵗʰ **S37.012 Minor contusion of left kidney**

   √7ᵗʰ **S37.019 Minor contusion of unspecified kidney** ▽

√6ᵗʰ **S37.02 Major contusion of kidney**

   Contusion of kidney greater than 2 cm

   √7ᵗʰ **S37.021 Major contusion of right kidney**

   √7ᵗʰ **S37.022 Major contusion of left kidney**

   √7ᵗʰ **S37.029 Major contusion of unspecified kidney** ▽

√6ᵗʰ **S37.03 Laceration of kidney, unspecified degree**

   √7ᵗʰ **S37.031 Laceration of right kidney, unspecified degree** ▽

   √7ᵗʰ **S37.032 Laceration of left kidney, unspecified degree** ▽

   √7ᵗʰ **S37.039 Laceration of unspecified kidney, unspecified degree** ▽

√6ᵗʰ **S37.04 Minor laceration of kidney**

   Laceration of kidney less than 1 cm

   √7ᵗʰ **S37.041 Minor laceration of right kidney**

   √7ᵗʰ **S37.042 Minor laceration of left kidney**

   √7ᵗʰ **S37.049 Minor laceration of unspecified kidney** ▽

√6ᵗʰ **S37.05 Moderate laceration of kidney**

   Laceration of kidney 1 to 3 cm

   √7ᵗʰ **S37.051 Moderate laceration of right kidney**

   √7ᵗʰ **S37.052 Moderate laceration of left kidney**

   √7ᵗʰ **S37.059 Moderate laceration of unspecified kidney** ▽

√6ᵗʰ **S37.06 Major laceration of kidney**

   Avulsion of kidney
   Laceration of kidney greater than 3 cm
   Massive laceration of kidney
   Multiple moderate lacerations of kidney
   Stellate laceration of kidney

   √7ᵗʰ **S37.061 Major laceration of right kidney**

   √7ᵗʰ **S37.062 Major laceration of left kidney**

   √7ᵗʰ **S37.069 Major laceration of unspecified kidney** ▽

√6ᵗʰ **S37.09 Other injury of kidney**

   √7ᵗʰ **S37.091 Other injury of right kidney**

   √7ᵗʰ **S37.092 Other injury of left kidney**

   √7ᵗʰ **S37.099 Other injury of unspecified kidney** ▽

√5ᵗʰ **S37.1 Injury of ureter**

√x7ᵗʰ **S37.10 Unspecified injury of ureter** ▽

√x7ᵗʰ **S37.12 Contusion of ureter**

√x7ᵗʰ **S37.13 Laceration of ureter**

√x7ᵗʰ **S37.19 Other injury of ureter**

√5ᵗʰ **S37.2 Injury of bladder**

√x7ᵗʰ **S37.20 Unspecified injury of bladder** ▽

√x7ᵗʰ **S37.22 Contusion of bladder**

√x7ᵗʰ **S37.23 Laceration of bladder**

√x7ᵗʰ **S37.29 Other injury of bladder**

√5ᵗʰ **S37.3 Injury of urethra**

√x7ᵗʰ **S37.30 Unspecified injury of urethra** ▽

√x7ᵗʰ **S37.32 Contusion of urethra**

√x7ᵗʰ **S37.33 Laceration of urethra**

√x7ᵗʰ **S37.39 Other injury of urethra**

√5ᵗʰ **S37.4 Injury of ovary**

√6ᵗʰ **S37.40 Unspecified injury of ovary**

   √7ᵗʰ **S37.401 Unspecified injury of ovary, unilateral** ♀ ▽

   √7ᵗʰ **S37.402 Unspecified injury of ovary, bilateral** ♀ ▽

   √7ᵗʰ **S37.409 Unspecified injury of ovary, unspecified** ♀ ▽

√6ᵗʰ **S37.42 Contusion of ovary**

   √7ᵗʰ **S37.421 Contusion of ovary, unilateral** ♀

☑ Additional Character Required   √x7ᵗʰ Placeholder Alert   Manifestation Dx   ▽ Unspecified Dx   ►◄ Revised Text   ● New Code   ▲ Revised Code Title

√7th **S37.422** Contusion of ovary, **bilateral** ♀

√7th **S37.429** Contusion of ovary, unspecified ♀ ▽

√6th **S37.43** Laceration of ovary

√7th **S37.431** Laceration of ovary, **unilateral** ♀

√7th **S37.432** Laceration of ovary, **bilateral** ♀

√7th **S37.439** Laceration of ovary, unspecified ♀ ▽

√6th **S37.49** Other injury of ovary

√7th **S37.491** Other injury of ovary, **unilateral** ♀

√7th **S37.492** Other injury of ovary, **bilateral** ♀

√7th **S37.499** Other injury of ovary, unspecified ♀ ▽

√5th **S37.5** Injury of **fallopian tube**

√6th **S37.50** Unspecified injury of fallopian tube

√7th **S37.501** Unspecified injury of fallopian tube, **unilateral** ♀ ▽

√7th **S37.502** Unspecified injury of fallopian tube, **bilateral** ♀ ▽

√7th **S37.509** Unspecified injury of fallopian tube, unspecified ♀ ▽

√6th **S37.51** Primary **blast injury of fallopian tube**

Blast injury of fallopian tube NOS

√7th **S37.511** Primary blast injury of fallopian tube, **unilateral** ♀

√7th **S37.512** Primary blast injury of fallopian tube, **bilateral** ♀

√7th **S37.519** Primary blast injury of fallopian tube, unspecified ♀ ▽

√6th **S37.52** Contusion of fallopian tube

√7th **S37.521** Contusion of fallopian tube, **unilateral** ♀

√7th **S37.522** Contusion of fallopian tube, **bilateral** ♀

√7th **S37.529** Contusion of fallopian tube, unspecified ♀ ▽

√6th **S37.53** Laceration of fallopian tube

√7th **S37.531** Laceration of fallopian tube, **unilateral** ♀

√7th **S37.532** Laceration of fallopian tube, **bilateral** ♀

√7th **S37.539** Laceration of fallopian tube, unspecified ♀ ▽

√6th **S37.59** Other injury of fallopian tube

Secondary blast injury of fallopian tube

√7th **S37.591** Other injury of fallopian tube, **unilateral** ♀

√7th **S37.592** Other injury of fallopian tube, **bilateral** ♀

√7th **S37.599** Other injury of fallopian tube, unspecified ♀ ▽

√5th **S37.6** Injury of **uterus**

EXCLUDES 1 *injury to gravid uterus (O9A.2-)*
injury to uterus during delivery (O71.-)

√x 7th **S37.60** Unspecified injury of uterus ♀ ▽

√x 7th **S37.62** Contusion of uterus ♀

√x 7th **S37.63** Laceration of uterus ♀

√x 7th **S37.69** Other injury of uterus ♀

√5th **S37.8** Injury of other urinary and pelvic organs

√6th **S37.81** Injury of **adrenal gland**

√7th **S37.812** Contusion of adrenal gland

√7th **S37.813** Laceration of adrenal gland

√7th **S37.818** Other injury of adrenal gland

√7th **S37.819** Unspecified injury of adrenal gland ▽

√6th **S37.82** Injury of **prostate**

√7th **S37.822** Contusion of prostate ♂

√7th **S37.823** Laceration of prostate ♂

√7th **S37.828** Other injury of prostate ♂

√7th **S37.829** Unspecified injury of prostate ♂ ▽

√6th **S37.89** Injury of other urinary and pelvic organ

√7th **S37.892** Contusion of other urinary and pelvic organ

√7th **S37.893** Laceration of other urinary and pelvic organ

√7th **S37.898** Other injury of other urinary and pelvic organ

√7th **S37.899** Unspecified injury of other urinary and pelvic organ ▽

√5th **S37.9** Injury of unspecified urinary and pelvic organ

√x 7th **S37.90** Unspecified injury of unspecified urinary and pelvic organ ▽

√x 7th **S37.92** Contusion of unspecified urinary and pelvic organ ▽

√x 7th **S37.93** Laceration of unspecified urinary and pelvic organ ▽

√x 7th **S37.99** Other injury of unspecified urinary and pelvic organ ▽

√4th **S38** Crushing injury and traumatic amputation of abdomen, lower back, pelvis and external genitals

NOTE An amputation not identified as partial or complete should be coded to complete

The appropriate 7th character is to be added to each code from category S38.
A   initial encounter
D   subsequent encounter
S   sequela

√5th **S38.0** Crushing injury of **external genital organs**

Use additional code for any associated injuries

√6th **S38.00** Crushing injury of unspecified external genital organs

√7th **S38.001** Crushing injury of unspecified external genital organs, **male** ♂ ▽

√7th **S38.002** Crushing injury of unspecified external genital organs, **female** ♀ ▽

√x 7th **S38.01** Crushing injury of **penis** ♂

√x 7th **S38.02** Crushing injury of **scrotum and testis** ♂

√x 7th **S38.03** Crushing injury of **vulva** ♀

√x 7th **S38.1** Crushing injury of abdomen, lower back, and pelvis

Use additional code for all associated injuries, such as:
fracture of thoracic or lumbar spine and pelvis (S22.0-, S32.-)
injury to intra-abdominal organs (S36.-)
injury to urinary and pelvic organs (S37.-)
open wound of abdominal wall (S31.-)
spinal cord injury (S34.0, S34.1-)

EXCLUDES 2 *crushing injury of external genital organs (S38.0-)*

√5th **S38.2** Traumatic amputation of external genital organs

√6th **S38.21** Traumatic amputation of **female** external genital organs

Traumatic amputation of clitoris
Traumatic amputation of labium (majus) (minus)
Traumatic amputation of vulva

√7th **S38.211** Complete traumatic amputation of female external genital organs ♀

√7th **S38.212** Partial traumatic amputation of female external genital organs ♀

√6th **S38.22** Traumatic amputation of **penis**

√7th **S38.221** Complete traumatic amputation of penis ♂

√7th **S38.222** Partial traumatic amputation of penis ♂

√6th **S38.23** Traumatic amputation of **scrotum and testis**

√7th **S38.231** Complete traumatic amputation of scrotum and testis ♂

√7th **S38.232** Partial traumatic amputation of scrotum and testis ♂

√x 7th **S38.3** Transection (partial) of abdomen

√4th **S39** Other and unspecified injuries of abdomen, lower back, pelvis and external genitals

Code also any associated open wound (S31.-)

EXCLUDES 2 *sprain of joints and ligaments of lumbar spine and pelvis (S33.-)*

The appropriate 7th character is to be added to each code from category S39.
A   initial encounter
D   subsequent encounter
S   sequela

√5th **S39.0** Injury of muscle, fascia and tendon of abdomen, lower back and pelvis

√6th **S39.00** Unspecified injury of muscle, fascia and tendon of abdomen, lower back and pelvis

√7th **S39.001** Unspecified injury of muscle, fascia and tendon of **abdomen** ▽

√7th **S39.002** Unspecified injury of muscle, fascia and tendon of **lower back** ▽

EXCLUDES 1 Not coded here   EXCLUDES 2 Not included here   N Newborn Age : 0   P Pediatric Age : 0-17   M Maternity Age : 12-55   A Adult Age : 15-124

926

ICD-10-CM 2017

√7ᵗʰ **S39.003** Unspecified injury of muscle, fascia and tendon of **pelvis** ▽

√6ᵗʰ **S39.01** Strain of muscle, fascia and tendon of abdomen, lower back and pelvis

　√7ᵗʰ **S39.011** Strain of muscle, fascia and tendon of **abdomen**

　√7ᵗʰ **S39.012** Strain of muscle, fascia and tendon of **lower back**

　√7ᵗʰ **S39.013** Strain of muscle, fascia and tendon of **pelvis**

√6ᵗʰ **S39.02** Laceration of muscle, fascia and tendon of abdomen, lower back and pelvis

　√7ᵗʰ **S39.021** Laceration of muscle, fascia and tendon of **abdomen**

　√7ᵗʰ **S39.022** Laceration of muscle, fascia and tendon of **lower back**

　√7ᵗʰ **S39.023** Laceration of muscle, fascia and tendon of **pelvis**

√6ᵗʰ **S39.09** Other injury of muscle, fascia and tendon of abdomen, lower back and pelvis

　√7ᵗʰ **S39.091** Other injury of muscle, fascia and tendon of **abdomen**

　√7ᵗʰ **S39.092** Other injury of muscle, fascia and tendon of **lower back**

　√7ᵗʰ **S39.093** Other injury of muscle, fascia and tendon of **pelvis**

√6ᵗʰ **S39.8** Other specified injuries of abdomen, lower back, pelvis and external genitals

　√×7ᵗʰ **S39.81** Other specified injuries of **abdomen**

　√×7ᵗʰ **S39.82** Other specified injuries of **lower back**

　√×7ᵗʰ **S39.83** Other specified injuries of **pelvis**

　√6ᵗʰ **S39.84** Other specified injuries of **external genitals**

　　√7ᵗʰ **S39.840** Fracture of **corpus cavernosum penis** ♂

　　√7ᵗʰ **S39.848** Other specified injuries of external genitals

√5ᵗʰ **S39.9** Unspecified injury of abdomen, lower back, pelvis and external genitals

　√×7ᵗʰ **S39.91** Unspecified injury of **abdomen** ▽

　√×7ᵗʰ **S39.92** Unspecified injury of **lower back** ▽

　√×7ᵗʰ **S39.93** Unspecified injury of **pelvis** ▽

　√×7ᵗʰ **S39.94** Unspecified injury of **external genitals** ▽

Injuries to the shoulder and upper arm (S40-S49)

INCLUDES injuries of axilla
injuries of scapular region

EXCLUDES 2 burns and corrosions (T20-T32)
frostbite (T33-T34)
injuries of elbow (S50-S59)
insect bite or sting, venomous (T63.4)

√4ᵗʰ **S40** Superficial injury of shoulder and upper arm

The appropriate 7th character is to be added to each code from category S40.
A　initial encounter
D　subsequent encounter
S　sequela

√5ᵗʰ **S40.0** Contusion of shoulder and upper arm

　√6ᵗʰ **S40.01** Contusion of **shoulder**

　　√7ᵗʰ **S40.011** Contusion of **right** shoulder

　　√7ᵗʰ **S40.012** Contusion of **left** shoulder

　　√7ᵗʰ **S40.019** Contusion of **unspecified** shoulder ▽

　√6ᵗʰ **S40.02** Contusion of **upper arm**

　　√7ᵗʰ **S40.021** Contusion of **right** upper arm

　　√7ᵗʰ **S40.022** Contusion of **left** upper arm

　　√7ᵗʰ **S40.029** Contusion of **unspecified** upper arm ▽

√5ᵗʰ **S40.2** Other superficial injuries of **shoulder**

　√6ᵗʰ **S40.21** Abrasion of **shoulder**

　　√7ᵗʰ **S40.211** Abrasion of **right** shoulder

　　√7ᵗʰ **S40.212** Abrasion of **left** shoulder

　　√7ᵗʰ **S40.219** Abrasion of **unspecified** shoulder ▽

　√6ᵗʰ **S40.22** Blister (nonthermal) of **shoulder**

　　√7ᵗʰ **S40.221** Blister (nonthermal) of **right** shoulder

　　√7ᵗʰ **S40.222** Blister (nonthermal) of **left** shoulder

　　√7ᵗʰ **S40.229** Blister (nonthermal) of unspecified shoulder ▽

　√6ᵗʰ **S40.24** External constriction of shoulder

　　√7ᵗʰ **S40.241** External constriction of **right** shoulder

　　√7ᵗʰ **S40.242** External constriction of **left** shoulder

　　√7ᵗʰ **S40.249** External constriction of unspecified shoulder ▽

　√6ᵗʰ **S40.25** Superficial foreign body of shoulder
　　　Splinter in the shoulder

　　√7ᵗʰ **S40.251** Superficial foreign body of **right** shoulder

　　√7ᵗʰ **S40.252** Superficial foreign body of **left** shoulder

　　√7ᵗʰ **S40.259** Superficial foreign body of unspecified shoulder ▽

　√6ᵗʰ **S40.26** Insect bite (nonvenomous) of shoulder

　　√7ᵗʰ **S40.261** Insect bite (nonvenomous) of **right** shoulder

　　√7ᵗʰ **S40.262** Insect bite (nonvenomous) of **left** shoulder

　　√7ᵗʰ **S40.269** Insect bite (nonvenomous) of unspecified shoulder ▽

　√6ᵗʰ **S40.27** Other superficial bite of shoulder

　　EXCLUDES 1 open bite of shoulder (S41.05)

　　√7ᵗʰ **S40.271** Other superficial bite of **right** shoulder

　　√7ᵗʰ **S40.272** Other superficial bite of **left** shoulder

　　√7ᵗʰ **S40.279** Other superficial bite of unspecified shoulder ▽

√5ᵗʰ **S40.8** Other superficial injuries of **upper arm**

　√6ᵗʰ **S40.81** Abrasion of upper arm

　　√7ᵗʰ **S40.811** Abrasion of **right** upper arm

　　√7ᵗʰ **S40.812** Abrasion of **left** upper arm

　　√7ᵗʰ **S40.819** Abrasion of unspecified upper arm ▽

　√6ᵗʰ **S40.82** Blister (nonthermal) of upper arm

　　√7ᵗʰ **S40.821** Blister (nonthermal) of **right** upper arm

　　√7ᵗʰ **S40.822** Blister (nonthermal) of **left** upper arm

　　√7ᵗʰ **S40.829** Blister (nonthermal) of unspecified upper arm ▽

　√6ᵗʰ **S40.84** External constriction of upper arm

　　√7ᵗʰ **S40.841** External constriction of **right** upper arm

　　√7ᵗʰ **S40.842** External constriction of **left** upper arm

　　√7ᵗʰ **S40.849** External constriction of unspecified upper arm ▽

　√6ᵗʰ **S40.85** Superficial foreign body of upper arm
　　　Splinter in the upper arm

　　√7ᵗʰ **S40.851** Superficial foreign body of **right** upper arm

　　√7ᵗʰ **S40.852** Superficial foreign body of **left** upper arm

　　√7ᵗʰ **S40.859** Superficial foreign body of unspecified upper arm ▽

　√6ᵗʰ **S40.86** Insect bite (nonvenomous) of upper arm

　　√7ᵗʰ **S40.861** Insect bite (nonvenomous) of **right** upper arm

　　√7ᵗʰ **S40.862** Insect bite (nonvenomous) of **left** upper arm

　　√7ᵗʰ **S40.869** Insect bite (nonvenomous) of unspecified upper arm ▽

　√6ᵗʰ **S40.87** Other superficial bite of upper arm

　　EXCLUDES 1 open bite of upper arm (S41.14)
　　EXCLUDES 2 other superficial bite of shoulder (S40.27-)

　　√7ᵗʰ **S40.871** Other superficial bite of **right** upper arm

　　√7ᵗʰ **S40.872** Other superficial bite of **left** upper arm

　　√7ᵗʰ **S40.879** Other superficial bite of unspecified upper arm ▽

√5ᵗʰ **S40.9** Unspecified superficial injury of shoulder and upper arm

　√6ᵗʰ **S40.91** Unspecified superficial injury of **shoulder**

　　√7ᵗʰ **S40.911** Unspecified superficial injury of **right** shoulder ▽

　　√7ᵗʰ **S40.912** Unspecified superficial injury of **left** shoulder ▽

　　√7ᵗʰ **S40.919** Unspecified superficial injury of unspecified shoulder ▽

　√6ᵗʰ **S40.92** Unspecified superficial injury of **upper arm**

　　√7ᵗʰ **S40.921** Unspecified superficial injury of **right** upper arm ▽

　　√7ᵗʰ **S40.922** Unspecified superficial injury of **left** upper arm ▽

☑ Additional Character Required　　√×7ᵗʰ Placeholder Alert　　Manifestation Dx　　▽ Unspecified Dx　　►◄ Revised Text　　● New Code　　▲ Revised Code Title

ICD-10-CM 2017　　　　　　　　　　　　　　　　　　　　　　　　　　**927**

    √7ᵗʰ **S40.929** **Unspecified superficial injury of unspecified upper arm** ▽

√4ᵗʰ **S41 Open wound of shoulder and upper arm**

Code also any associated wound infection

EXCLUDES 1 *traumatic amputation of shoulder and upper arm (S48.-)*

EXCLUDES 2 *open fracture of shoulder and upper arm (S42.- with 7th character B or C)*

The appropriate 7th character is to be added to each code from category S41.
A   initial encounter
D   subsequent encounter
S   sequela

√5ᵗʰ **S41.0 Open wound of shoulder**

  √6ᵗʰ **S41.00 Unspecified open wound of shoulder**

    √7ᵗʰ **S41.001 Unspecified open wound of right shoulder** ▽

    √7ᵗʰ **S41.002 Unspecified open wound of left shoulder** ▽

    √7ᵗʰ **S41.009 Unspecified open wound of unspecified shoulder** ▽

  √6ᵗʰ **S41.01 Laceration without foreign body of shoulder**

    √7ᵗʰ **S41.011 Laceration without foreign body of right shoulder** ▽

    √7ᵗʰ **S41.012 Laceration without foreign body of left shoulder** ▽

    √7ᵗʰ **S41.019 Laceration without foreign body of unspecified shoulder** ▽

  √6ᵗʰ **S41.02 Laceration with foreign body of shoulder**

    √7ᵗʰ **S41.021 Laceration with foreign body of right shoulder** ▽

    √7ᵗʰ **S41.022 Laceration with foreign body of left shoulder** ▽

    √7ᵗʰ **S41.029 Laceration with foreign body of unspecified shoulder** ▽

  √6ᵗʰ **S41.03 Puncture wound without foreign body of shoulder**

    √7ᵗʰ **S41.031 Puncture wound without foreign body of right shoulder** ▽

    √7ᵗʰ **S41.032 Puncture wound without foreign body of left shoulder** ▽

    √7ᵗʰ **S41.039 Puncture wound without foreign body of unspecified shoulder** ▽

  √6ᵗʰ **S41.04 Puncture wound with foreign body of shoulder**

    √7ᵗʰ **S41.041 Puncture wound with foreign body of right shoulder** ▽

    √7ᵗʰ **S41.042 Puncture wound with foreign body of left shoulder** ▽

    √7ᵗʰ **S41.049 Puncture wound with foreign body of unspecified shoulder** ▽

  √6ᵗʰ **S41.05 Open bite of shoulder**

Bite of shoulder NOS

EXCLUDES 1 *superficial bite of shoulder (S40.27)*

    √7ᵗʰ **S41.051 Open bite of right shoulder**

    √7ᵗʰ **S41.052 Open bite of left shoulder**

    √7ᵗʰ **S41.059 Open bite of unspecified shoulder** ▽

√5ᵗʰ **S41.1 Open wound of upper arm**

  √6ᵗʰ **S41.10 Unspecified open wound of upper arm**

    √7ᵗʰ **S41.101 Unspecified open wound of right upper arm** ▽

    √7ᵗʰ **S41.102 Unspecified open wound of left upper arm** ▽

    √7ᵗʰ **S41.109 Unspecified open wound of unspecified upper arm** ▽

  √6ᵗʰ **S41.11 Laceration without foreign body of upper arm**

    √7ᵗʰ **S41.111 Laceration without foreign body of right upper arm** ▽

    √7ᵗʰ **S41.112 Laceration without foreign body of left upper arm** ▽

    √7ᵗʰ **S41.119 Laceration without foreign body of unspecified upper arm** ▽

  √6ᵗʰ **S41.12 Laceration with foreign body of upper arm**

    √7ᵗʰ **S41.121 Laceration with foreign body of right upper arm** ▽

    √7ᵗʰ **S41.122 Laceration with foreign body of left upper arm** ▽

    √7ᵗʰ **S41.129 Laceration with foreign body of unspecified upper arm** ▽

  √6ᵗʰ **S41.13 Puncture wound without foreign body of upper arm**

    √7ᵗʰ **S41.131 Puncture wound without foreign body of right upper arm** ▽

    √7ᵗʰ **S41.132 Puncture wound without foreign body of left upper arm** ▽

    √7ᵗʰ **S41.139 Puncture wound without foreign body of unspecified upper arm** ▽

  √6ᵗʰ **S41.14 Puncture wound with foreign body of upper arm**

    √7ᵗʰ **S41.141 Puncture wound with foreign body of right upper arm** ▽

    √7ᵗʰ **S41.142 Puncture wound with foreign body of left upper arm** ▽

    √7ᵗʰ **S41.149 Puncture wound with foreign body of unspecified upper arm** ▽

  √6ᵗʰ **S41.15 Open bite of upper arm**

Bite of upper arm NOS

EXCLUDES 1 *superficial bite of upper arm (S40.87)*

    √7ᵗʰ **S41.151 Open bite of right upper arm**

    √7ᵗʰ **S41.152 Open bite of left upper arm**

    √7ᵗʰ **S41.159 Open bite of unspecified upper arm** ▽

√4ᵗʰ **S42 Fracture of shoulder and upper arm**

NOTE A fracture not indicated as displaced or nondisplaced should be coded to displaced

A fracture not indicated as open or closed should be coded to closed

EXCLUDES 1 *traumatic amputation of shoulder and upper arm (S48.-)*

AHA: 2015,3Q,37-39

The appropriate 7th character is to be added to all codes from category S42 [unless otherwise indicated].
A   initial encounter for closed fracture
B   initial encounter for open fracture
D   subsequent encounter for fracture with routine healing
G   subsequent encounter for fracture with delayed healing
K   subsequent encounter for fracture with nonunion
P   subsequent encounter for fracture with malunion
S   sequela

√5ᵗʰ **S42.0 Fracture of clavicle**

  √6ᵗʰ **S42.00 Fracture of unspecified part of clavicle**

    √7ᵗʰ **S42.001 Fracture of unspecified part of right clavicle** ▽

    √7ᵗʰ **S42.002 Fracture of unspecified part of left clavicle** ▽

    √7ᵗʰ **S42.009 Fracture of unspecified part of unspecified clavicle** ▽

      AHA: 2012,4Q,93

  √6ᵗʰ **S42.01 Fracture of sternal end of clavicle**

    √7ᵗʰ **S42.011 Anterior displaced fracture of sternal end of right clavicle**

    √7ᵗʰ **S42.012 Anterior displaced fracture of sternal end of left clavicle**

    √7ᵗʰ **S42.013 Anterior displaced fracture of sternal end of unspecified clavicle** ▽

Displaced fracture of sternal end of clavicle NOS

    √7ᵗʰ **S42.014 Posterior displaced fracture of sternal end of right clavicle**

    √7ᵗʰ **S42.015 Posterior displaced fracture of sternal end of left clavicle**

    √7ᵗʰ **S42.016 Posterior displaced fracture of sternal end of unspecified clavicle** ▽

    √7ᵗʰ **S42.017 Nondisplaced fracture of sternal end of right clavicle**

    √7ᵗʰ **S42.018 Nondisplaced fracture of sternal end of left clavicle**

    √7ᵗʰ **S42.019 Nondisplaced fracture of sternal end of unspecified clavicle** ▽

  √6ᵗʰ **S42.02 Fracture of shaft of clavicle**

    √7ᵗʰ **S42.021 Displaced fracture of shaft of right clavicle**

    √7ᵗʰ **S42.022 Displaced fracture of shaft of left clavicle**

    √7ᵗʰ **S42.023 Displaced fracture of shaft of unspecified clavicle** ▽

    √7ᵗʰ **S42.024 Nondisplaced fracture of shaft of right clavicle**

    √7ᵗʰ **S42.025 Nondisplaced fracture of shaft of left clavicle**

    √7ᵗʰ **S42.026 Nondisplaced fracture of shaft of unspecified clavicle** ▽

EXCLUDES 1 Not coded here   *EXCLUDES 2* Not included here   Ⓝ Newborn Age : 0   Ⓟ Pediatric Age : 0-17   Ⓜ Maternity Age : 12-55   Ⓐ Adult Age : 15-124

928   ICD-10-CM 2017

√6ᵗʰ **S42.03**   **Fracture of lateral end of clavicle**
     Fracture of acromial end of clavicle

   √7ᵗʰ **S42.031**   **Displaced fracture of lateral end of right clavicle**

   √7ᵗʰ **S42.032**   **Displaced fracture of lateral end of left clavicle**

   √7ᵗʰ **S42.033**   **Displaced fracture of lateral end of unspecified clavicle** ▽

   √7ᵗʰ **S42.034**   **Nondisplaced fracture of lateral end of right clavicle**

   √7ᵗʰ **S42.035**   **Nondisplaced fracture of lateral end of left clavicle**

   √7ᵗʰ **S42.036**   **Nondisplaced fracture of lateral end of unspecified clavicle** ▽

√5ᵗʰ **S42.1**   **Fracture of scapula**

   √6ᵗʰ **S42.10**   **Fracture of unspecified part of scapula**

     √7ᵗʰ **S42.101**   **Fracture of unspecified part of scapula, right shoulder** ▽

     √7ᵗʰ **S42.102**   **Fracture of unspecified part of scapula, left shoulder** ▽

     √7ᵗʰ **S42.109**   **Fracture of unspecified part of scapula, unspecified shoulder** ▽

   √6ᵗʰ **S42.11**   **Fracture of body of scapula**

     √7ᵗʰ **S42.111**   **Displaced fracture of body of scapula, right shoulder**

     √7ᵗʰ **S42.112**   **Displaced fracture of body of scapula, left shoulder**

     √7ᵗʰ **S42.113**   **Displaced fracture of body of scapula, unspecified shoulder** ▽

     √7ᵗʰ **S42.114**   **Nondisplaced fracture of body of scapula, right shoulder**

     √7ᵗʰ **S42.115**   **Nondisplaced fracture of body of scapula, left shoulder**

     √7ᵗʰ **S42.116**   **Nondisplaced fracture of body of scapula, unspecified shoulder** ▽

   √6ᵗʰ **S42.12**   **Fracture of acromial process**

     √7ᵗʰ **S42.121**   **Displaced fracture of acromial process, right shoulder**

     √7ᵗʰ **S42.122**   **Displaced fracture of acromial process, left shoulder**

     √7ᵗʰ **S42.123**   **Displaced fracture of acromial process, unspecified shoulder** ▽

     √7ᵗʰ **S42.124**   **Nondisplaced fracture of acromial process, right shoulder**

     √7ᵗʰ **S42.125**   **Nondisplaced fracture of acromial process, left shoulder**

     √7ᵗʰ **S42.126**   **Nondisplaced fracture of acromial process, unspecified shoulder** ▽

   √6ᵗʰ **S42.13**   **Fracture of coracoid process**

     √7ᵗʰ **S42.131**   **Displaced fracture of coracoid process, right shoulder**

     √7ᵗʰ **S42.132**   **Displaced fracture of coracoid process, left shoulder**

     √7ᵗʰ **S42.133**   **Displaced fracture of coracoid process, unspecified shoulder** ▽

     √7ᵗʰ **S42.134**   **Nondisplaced fracture of coracoid process, right shoulder**

     √7ᵗʰ **S42.135**   **Nondisplaced fracture of coracoid process, left shoulder**

     √7ᵗʰ **S42.136**   **Nondisplaced fracture of coracoid process, unspecified shoulder** ▽

   √6ᵗʰ **S42.14**   **Fracture of glenoid cavity of scapula**

     √7ᵗʰ **S42.141**   **Displaced fracture of glenoid cavity of scapula, right shoulder**

     √7ᵗʰ **S42.142**   **Displaced fracture of glenoid cavity of scapula, left shoulder**

     √7ᵗʰ **S42.143**   **Displaced fracture of glenoid cavity of scapula, unspecified shoulder** ▽

     √7ᵗʰ **S42.144**   **Nondisplaced fracture of glenoid cavity of scapula, right shoulder**

     √7ᵗʰ **S42.145**   **Nondisplaced fracture of glenoid cavity of scapula, left shoulder**

     √7ᵗʰ **S42.146**   **Nondisplaced fracture of glenoid cavity of scapula, unspecified shoulder** ▽

   √6ᵗʰ **S42.15**   **Fracture of neck of scapula**

     √7ᵗʰ **S42.151**   **Displaced fracture of neck of scapula, right shoulder**

     √7ᵗʰ **S42.152**   **Displaced fracture of neck of scapula, left shoulder**

     √7ᵗʰ **S42.153**   **Displaced fracture of neck of scapula, unspecified shoulder** ▽

     √7ᵗʰ **S42.154**   **Nondisplaced fracture of neck of scapula, right shoulder**

     √7ᵗʰ **S42.155**   **Nondisplaced fracture of neck of scapula, left shoulder**

     √7ᵗʰ **S42.156**   **Nondisplaced fracture of neck of scapula, unspecified shoulder** ▽

   √6ᵗʰ **S42.19**   **Fracture of other part of scapula**

     √7ᵗʰ **S42.191**   **Fracture of other part of scapula, right shoulder**

     √7ᵗʰ **S42.192**   **Fracture of other part of scapula, left shoulder**

     √7ᵗʰ **S42.199**   **Fracture of other part of scapula, unspecified shoulder** ▽

√5ᵗʰ **S42.2**   **Fracture of upper end of humerus**
     Fracture of proximal end of humerus
     EXCLUDES 2   *fracture of shaft of humerus (S42.3-)*
           physeal fracture of upper end of humerus (S49.0-)

   √6ᵗʰ **S42.20**   **Unspecified fracture of upper end of humerus**

     √7ᵗʰ **S42.201**   **Unspecified fracture of upper end of right humerus** ▽

     √7ᵗʰ **S42.202**   **Unspecified fracture of upper end of left humerus** ▽

     √7ᵗʰ **S42.209**   **Unspecified fracture of upper end of unspecified humerus** ▽

   √6ᵗʰ **S42.21**   **Unspecified fracture of surgical neck of humerus**
     Fracture of neck of humerus NOS

     √7ᵗʰ **S42.211**   **Unspecified displaced fracture of surgical neck of right humerus** ▽

     √7ᵗʰ **S42.212**   **Unspecified displaced fracture of surgical neck of left humerus** ▽

     √7ᵗʰ **S42.213**   **Unspecified displaced fracture of surgical neck of unspecified humerus** ▽

     √7ᵗʰ **S42.214**   **Unspecified nondisplaced fracture of surgical neck of right humerus** ▽

     √7ᵗʰ **S42.215**   **Unspecified nondisplaced fracture of surgical neck of left humerus** ▽

     √7ᵗʰ **S42.216**   **Unspecified nondisplaced fracture of surgical neck of unspecified humerus** ▽

   √6ᵗʰ **S42.22**   **2-part fracture of surgical neck of humerus**

     √7ᵗʰ **S42.221**   **2-part displaced fracture of surgical neck of right humerus**

     √7ᵗʰ **S42.222**   **2-part displaced fracture of surgical neck of left humerus**

     √7ᵗʰ **S42.223**   **2-part displaced fracture of surgical neck of unspecified humerus** ▽

     √7ᵗʰ **S42.224**   **2-part nondisplaced fracture of surgical neck of right humerus**

     √7ᵗʰ **S42.225**   **2-part nondisplaced fracture of surgical neck of left humerus**

     √7ᵗʰ **S42.226**   **2-part nondisplaced fracture of surgical neck of unspecified humerus** ▽

   √6ᵗʰ **S42.23**   **3-part fracture of surgical neck of humerus**

     √7ᵗʰ **S42.231**   **3-part fracture of surgical neck of right humerus**

     √7ᵗʰ **S42.232**   **3-part fracture of surgical neck of left humerus**

     √7ᵗʰ **S42.239**   **3-part fracture of surgical neck of unspecified humerus** ▽

   √6ᵗʰ **S42.24**   **4-part fracture of surgical neck of humerus**

     √7ᵗʰ **S42.241**   **4-part fracture of surgical neck of right humerus**

     √7ᵗʰ **S42.242**   **4-part fracture of surgical neck of left humerus**

     √7ᵗʰ **S42.249**   **4-part fracture of surgical neck of unspecified humerus** ▽

   √6ᵗʰ **S42.25**   **Fracture of greater tuberosity of humerus**

     √7ᵗʰ **S42.251**   **Displaced fracture of greater tuberosity of right humerus**

     √7ᵗʰ **S42.252**   **Displaced fracture of greater tuberosity of left humerus**

     √7ᵗʰ **S42.253**   **Displaced fracture of greater tuberosity of unspecified humerus** ▽

     √7ᵗʰ **S42.254**   **Nondisplaced fracture of greater tuberosity of right humerus**

☑ Additional Character Required   ᵛˣ⁷ᵗʰ Placeholder Alert   Manifestation Dx   ▽ Unspecified Dx   ▶◀ Revised Text   ● New Code   ▲ Revised Code Title

√7ᵗʰ **S42.255** Nondisplaced **fracture of greater tuberosity of** left **humerus**

√7ᵗʰ **S42.256** Nondisplaced **fracture of greater tuberosity of unspecified humerus** ▽

√6ᵗʰ **S42.26** **Fracture of** lesser tuberosity of humerus

√7ᵗʰ **S42.261** Displaced **fracture of lesser tuberosity of** right **humerus**

√7ᵗʰ **S42.262** Displaced **fracture of lesser tuberosity of** left **humerus**

√7ᵗʰ **S42.263** Displaced **fracture of lesser tuberosity of unspecified humerus** ▽

√7ᵗʰ **S42.264** Nondisplaced **fracture of lesser tuberosity of** right **humerus**

√7ᵗʰ **S42.265** Nondisplaced **fracture of lesser tuberosity of** left **humerus**

√7ᵗʰ **S42.266** Nondisplaced **fracture of lesser tuberosity of unspecified humerus** ▽

√6ᵗʰ **S42.27** Torus **fracture of upper end of humerus**

> The appropriate 7th character is to be added to all codes in subcategory S42.27
> A   initial encounter for closed fracture
> D   subsequent encounter for fracture with routine healing
> G   subsequent encounter for fracture with delayed healing
> K   subsequent encounter for fracture with nonunion
> P   subsequent encounter for fracture with malunion
> S   sequela

√7ᵗʰ **S42.271** **Torus fracture of upper end of** right **humerus**

√7ᵗʰ **S42.272** **Torus fracture of upper end of** left **humerus**

√7ᵗʰ **S42.279** **Torus fracture of upper end of unspecified humerus** ▽

√6ᵗʰ **S42.29** **Other fracture of upper end of humerus**

Fracture of anatomical neck of humerus
Fracture of articular head of humerus

√7ᵗʰ **S42.291** **Other** displaced **fracture of upper end of** right **humerus**

√7ᵗʰ **S42.292** **Other** displaced **fracture of upper end of** left **humerus**

√7ᵗʰ **S42.293** **Other** displaced **fracture of upper end of unspecified humerus** ▽

√7ᵗʰ **S42.294** **Other** nondisplaced **fracture of upper end of** right **humerus**

√7ᵗʰ **S42.295** **Other** nondisplaced **fracture of upper end of** left **humerus**

√7ᵗʰ **S42.296** **Other** nondisplaced **fracture of upper end of unspecified humerus** ▽

√5ᵗʰ **S42.3** **Fracture of** shaft of **humerus**

Fracture of humerus NOS
Fracture of upper arm NOS
EXCLUDES 2 physeal fractures of upper end of humerus (S49.Ø-)
physeal fractures of lower end of humerus (S49.1-)

√6ᵗʰ **S42.3Ø** **Unspecified fracture of shaft of humerus**

√7ᵗʰ **S42.3Ø1** **Unspecified fracture of shaft of humerus,** right **arm** ▽

√7ᵗʰ **S42.3Ø2** **Unspecified fracture of shaft of humerus,** left **arm** ▽

√7ᵗʰ **S42.3Ø9** **Unspecified fracture of shaft of humerus, unspecified arm** ▽

√6ᵗʰ **S42.31** Greenstick **fracture of shaft of humerus**

> The appropriate 7th character is to be added to all codes in subcategory S42.31
> A   initial encounter for closed fracture
> D   subsequent encounter for fracture with routine healing
> G   subsequent encounter for fracture with delayed healing
> K   subsequent encounter for fracture with nonunion
> P   subsequent encounter for fracture with malunion
> S   sequela

√7ᵗʰ **S42.311** **Greenstick fracture of shaft of humerus,** right **arm**

√7ᵗʰ **S42.312** **Greenstick fracture of shaft of humerus,** left **arm**

√7ᵗʰ **S42.319** **Greenstick fracture of shaft of humerus, unspecified arm** ▽

√6ᵗʰ **S42.32** Transverse **fracture of shaft of humerus**

√7ᵗʰ **S42.321** Displaced **transverse fracture of shaft of humerus,** right **arm**

√7ᵗʰ **S42.322** Displaced **transverse fracture of shaft of humerus,** left **arm**

√7ᵗʰ **S42.323** Displaced **transverse fracture of shaft of humerus, unspecified arm** ▽

√7ᵗʰ **S42.324** Nondisplaced **transverse fracture of shaft of humerus,** right **arm**

√7ᵗʰ **S42.325** Nondisplaced **transverse fracture of shaft of humerus,** left **arm**

√7ᵗʰ **S42.326** Nondisplaced **transverse fracture of shaft of humerus, unspecified arm** ▽

√6ᵗʰ **S42.33** Oblique **fracture of shaft of humerus**

√7ᵗʰ **S42.331** Displaced **oblique fracture of shaft of humerus,** right **arm**

√7ᵗʰ **S42.332** Displaced **oblique fracture of shaft of humerus,** left **arm**

√7ᵗʰ **S42.333** Displaced **oblique fracture of shaft of humerus, unspecified arm** ▽

√7ᵗʰ **S42.334** Nondisplaced **oblique fracture of shaft of humerus,** right **arm**

√7ᵗʰ **S42.335** Nondisplaced **oblique fracture of shaft of humerus,** left **arm**

√7ᵗʰ **S42.336** Nondisplaced **oblique fracture of shaft of humerus, unspecified arm** ▽

√6ᵗʰ **S42.34** Spiral **fracture of shaft of humerus**

√7ᵗʰ **S42.341** Displaced **spiral fracture of shaft of humerus,** right **arm**

√7ᵗʰ **S42.342** Displaced **spiral fracture of shaft of humerus,** left **arm**

√7ᵗʰ **S42.343** Displaced **spiral fracture of shaft of humerus, unspecified arm** ▽

√7ᵗʰ **S42.344** Nondisplaced **spiral fracture of shaft of humerus,** right **arm**

√7ᵗʰ **S42.345** Nondisplaced **spiral fracture of shaft of humerus,** left **arm**

√7ᵗʰ **S42.346** Nondisplaced **spiral fracture of shaft of humerus, unspecified arm** ▽

√6ᵗʰ **S42.35** Comminuted **fracture of shaft of humerus**

√7ᵗʰ **S42.351** Displaced **comminuted fracture of shaft of humerus,** right **arm**

√7ᵗʰ **S42.352** Displaced **comminuted fracture of shaft of humerus,** left **arm**

√7ᵗʰ **S42.353** Displaced **comminuted fracture of shaft of humerus, unspecified arm** ▽

√7ᵗʰ **S42.354** Nondisplaced **comminuted fracture of shaft of humerus,** right **arm**

√7ᵗʰ **S42.355** Nondisplaced **comminuted fracture of shaft of humerus,** left **arm**

√7ᵗʰ **S42.356** Nondisplaced **comminuted fracture of shaft of humerus, unspecified arm** ▽

√6ᵗʰ **S42.36** Segmental **fracture of shaft of humerus**

√7ᵗʰ **S42.361** Displaced **segmental fracture of shaft of humerus,** right **arm**

√7ᵗʰ **S42.362** Displaced **segmental fracture of shaft of humerus,** left **arm**

√7ᵗʰ **S42.363** Displaced **segmental fracture of shaft of humerus, unspecified arm** ▽

√7ᵗʰ **S42.364** Nondisplaced **segmental fracture of shaft of humerus,** right **arm**

√7ᵗʰ **S42.365** Nondisplaced **segmental fracture of shaft of humerus,** left **arm**

√7ᵗʰ **S42.366** Nondisplaced **segmental fracture of shaft of humerus, unspecified arm** ▽

√6ᵗʰ **S42.39** **Other fracture of shaft of humerus**

√7ᵗʰ **S42.391** **Other fracture of shaft of** right **humerus** ▽

√7ᵗʰ **S42.392** **Other fracture of shaft of** left **humerus** ▽

√7ᵗʰ **S42.399** **Other fracture of shaft of unspecified humerus** ▽

EXCLUDES 1 Not coded here   *EXCLUDES 2* Not included here   N Newborn Age : 0   P Pediatric Age : 0-17   M Maternity Age : 12-55   A Adult Age : 15-124

√5ᵗʰ **S42.4 Fracture of lower end of humerus**

Fracture of distal end of humerus

EXCLUDES 2 *fracture of shaft of humerus (S42.3-)*
physeal fracture of lower end of humerus (S49.1-)

√6ᵗʰ **S42.40 Unspecified fracture of lower end of humerus**

Fracture of elbow NOS

√7ᵗʰ **S42.401 Unspecified fracture of lower end of right humerus** ▽

√7ᵗʰ **S42.402 Unspecified fracture of lower end of left humerus** ▽

√7ᵗʰ **S42.409 Unspecified fracture of lower end of unspecified humerus** ▽

√6ᵗʰ **S42.41 Simple supracondylar fracture without intercondylar fracture of humerus**

√7ᵗʰ **S42.411 Displaced simple supracondylar fracture without intercondylar fracture of right humerus**

√7ᵗʰ **S42.412 Displaced simple supracondylar fracture without intercondylar fracture of left humerus**

√7ᵗʰ **S42.413 Displaced simple supracondylar fracture without intercondylar fracture of unspecified humerus** ▽

√7ᵗʰ **S42.414 Nondisplaced simple supracondylar fracture without intercondylar fracture of right humerus**

√7ᵗʰ **S42.415 Nondisplaced simple supracondylar fracture without intercondylar fracture of left humerus**

√7ᵗʰ **S42.416 Nondisplaced simple supracondylar fracture without intercondylar fracture of unspecified humerus** ▽

√6ᵗʰ **S42.42 Comminuted supracondylar fracture without intercondylar fracture of humerus**

√7ᵗʰ **S42.421 Displaced comminuted supracondylar fracture without intercondylar fracture of right humerus**

√7ᵗʰ **S42.422 Displaced comminuted supracondylar fracture without intercondylar fracture of left humerus**

√7ᵗʰ **S42.423 Displaced comminuted supracondylar fracture without intercondylar fracture of unspecified humerus** ▽

√7ᵗʰ **S42.424 Nondisplaced comminuted supracondylar fracture without intercondylar fracture of right humerus**

√7ᵗʰ **S42.425 Nondisplaced comminuted supracondylar fracture without intercondylar fracture of left humerus**

√7ᵗʰ **S42.426 Nondisplaced comminuted supracondylar fracture without intercondylar fracture of unspecified humerus** ▽

√6ᵗʰ **S42.43 Fracture (avulsion) of lateral epicondyle of humerus**

√7ᵗʰ **S42.431 Displaced fracture (avulsion) of lateral epicondyle of right humerus**

√7ᵗʰ **S42.432 Displaced fracture (avulsion) of lateral epicondyle of left humerus**

√7ᵗʰ **S42.433 Displaced fracture (avulsion) of lateral epicondyle of unspecified humerus** ▽

√7ᵗʰ **S42.434 Nondisplaced fracture (avulsion) of lateral epicondyle of right humerus**

√7ᵗʰ **S42.435 Nondisplaced fracture (avulsion) of lateral epicondyle of left humerus**

√7ᵗʰ **S42.436 Nondisplaced fracture (avulsion) of lateral epicondyle of unspecified humerus** ▽

√6ᵗʰ **S42.44 Fracture (avulsion) of medial epicondyle of humerus**

√7ᵗʰ **S42.441 Displaced fracture (avulsion) of medial epicondyle of right humerus**

√7ᵗʰ **S42.442 Displaced fracture (avulsion) of medial epicondyle of left humerus**

√7ᵗʰ **S42.443 Displaced fracture (avulsion) of medial epicondyle of unspecified humerus** ▽

√7ᵗʰ **S42.444 Nondisplaced fracture (avulsion) of medial epicondyle of right humerus**

√7ᵗʰ **S42.445 Nondisplaced fracture (avulsion) of medial epicondyle of left humerus**

√7ᵗʰ **S42.446 Nondisplaced fracture (avulsion) of medial epicondyle of unspecified humerus** ▽

√7ᵗʰ **S42.447 Incarcerated fracture (avulsion) of medial epicondyle of right humerus**

√7ᵗʰ **S42.448 Incarcerated fracture (avulsion) of medial epicondyle of left humerus**

√7ᵗʰ **S42.449 Incarcerated fracture (avulsion) of medial epicondyle of unspecified humerus** ▽

√6ᵗʰ **S42.45 Fracture of lateral condyle of humerus**

Fracture of capitellum of humerus

√7ᵗʰ **S42.451 Displaced fracture of lateral condyle of right humerus**

√7ᵗʰ **S42.452 Displaced fracture of lateral condyle of left humerus**

√7ᵗʰ **S42.453 Displaced fracture of lateral condyle of unspecified humerus** ▽

√7ᵗʰ **S42.454 Nondisplaced fracture of lateral condyle of right humerus**

√7ᵗʰ **S42.455 Nondisplaced fracture of lateral condyle of left humerus**

√7ᵗʰ **S42.456 Nondisplaced fracture of lateral condyle of unspecified humerus** ▽

√6ᵗʰ **S42.46 Fracture of medial condyle of humerus**

Trochlea fracture of humerus

√7ᵗʰ **S42.461 Displaced fracture of medial condyle of right humerus**

√7ᵗʰ **S42.462 Displaced fracture of medial condyle of left humerus**

√7ᵗʰ **S42.463 Displaced fracture of medial condyle of unspecified humerus** ▽

√7ᵗʰ **S42.464 Nondisplaced fracture of medial condyle of right humerus**

√7ᵗʰ **S42.465 Nondisplaced fracture of medial condyle of left humerus**

√7ᵗʰ **S42.466 Nondisplaced fracture of medial condyle of unspecified humerus** ▽

√6ᵗʰ **S42.47 Transcondylar fracture of humerus**

√7ᵗʰ **S42.471 Displaced transcondylar fracture of right humerus**

√7ᵗʰ **S42.472 Displaced transcondylar fracture of left humerus**

√7ᵗʰ **S42.473 Displaced transcondylar fracture of unspecified humerus** ▽

√7ᵗʰ **S42.474 Nondisplaced transcondylar fracture of right humerus**

√7ᵗʰ **S42.475 Nondisplaced transcondylar fracture of left humerus**

√7ᵗʰ **S42.476 Nondisplaced transcondylar fracture of unspecified humerus** ▽

√6ᵗʰ **S42.48 Torus fracture of lower end of humerus**

The appropriate 7th character is to be added to all codes in subcategory S42.48

A initial encounter for closed fracture

D subsequent encounter for fracture with routine healing

G subsequent encounter for fracture with delayed healing

K subsequent encounter for fracture with nonunion

P subsequent encounter for fracture with malunion

S sequela

√7ᵗʰ **S42.481 Torus fracture of lower end of right humerus**

√7ᵗʰ **S42.482 Torus fracture of lower end of left humerus**

√7ᵗʰ **S42.489 Torus fracture of lower end of unspecified humerus** ▽

√6ᵗʰ **S42.49 Other fracture of lower end of humerus**

√7ᵗʰ **S42.491 Other displaced fracture of lower end of right humerus**

√7ᵗʰ **S42.492 Other displaced fracture of lower end of left humerus**

√7ᵗʰ **S42.493 Other displaced fracture of lower end of unspecified humerus** ▽

√7ᵗʰ **S42.494 Other nondisplaced fracture of lower end of right humerus**

√7ᵗʰ **S42.495 Other nondisplaced fracture of lower end of left humerus**

☑ Additional Character Required   √x7ᵗʰ Placeholder Alert   Manifestation Dx   ▽ Unspecified Dx   ►◄ Revised Text   ● New Code   ▲ Revised Code Title

ICD-10-CM 2017   931

√7ᵗʰ **S42.496** Other nondisplaced fracture of lower end of unspecified humerus ▽

√5ᵗʰ **S42.9** Fracture of shoulder girdle, part unspecified

Fracture of shoulder NOS

√x7ᵗʰ **S42.90** Fracture of unspecified shoulder girdle, part unspecified ▽

√x7ᵗʰ **S42.91** Fracture of right shoulder girdle, part unspecified ▽

√x7ᵗʰ **S42.92** Fracture of left shoulder girdle, part unspecified ▽

√4ᵗʰ **S43** Dislocation and sprain of joints and ligaments of shoulder girdle

INCLUDES   avulsion of joint or ligament of shoulder girdle
laceration of cartilage, joint or ligament of shoulder girdle
sprain of cartilage, joint or ligament of shoulder girdle
traumatic hemarthrosis of joint or ligament of shoulder girdle
traumatic rupture of joint or ligament of shoulder girdle
traumatic subluxation of joint or ligament of shoulder girdle
traumatic tear of joint or ligament of shoulder girdle

Code also any associated open wound

EXCLUDES 2   strain of muscle, fascia and tendon of shoulder and upper arm (S46.-)

The appropriate 7th character is to be added to each code from category S43.
A   initial encounter
D   subsequent encounter
S   sequela

√5ᵗʰ **S43.0** Subluxation and dislocation of shoulder joint

Dislocation of glenohumeral joint
Subluxation of glenohumeral joint

√6ᵗʰ **S43.00** Unspecified subluxation and dislocation of shoulder joint

Dislocation of humerus NOS
Subluxation of humerus NOS

√7ᵗʰ **S43.001** Unspecified subluxation of right shoulder joint ▽

√7ᵗʰ **S43.002** Unspecified subluxation of left shoulder joint ▽

√7ᵗʰ **S43.003** Unspecified subluxation of unspecified shoulder joint ▽

√7ᵗʰ **S43.004** Unspecified dislocation of right shoulder joint ▽

√7ᵗʰ **S43.005** Unspecified dislocation of left shoulder joint ▽

√7ᵗʰ **S43.006** Unspecified dislocation of unspecified shoulder joint ▽

√6ᵗʰ **S43.01** Anterior subluxation and dislocation of humerus

√7ᵗʰ **S43.011** Anterior subluxation of right humerus

√7ᵗʰ **S43.012** Anterior subluxation of left humerus

√7ᵗʰ **S43.013** Anterior subluxation of unspecified humerus ▽

√7ᵗʰ **S43.014** Anterior dislocation of right humerus

√7ᵗʰ **S43.015** Anterior dislocation of left humerus

√7ᵗʰ **S43.016** Anterior dislocation of unspecified humerus ▽

√6ᵗʰ **S43.02** Posterior subluxation and dislocation of humerus

√7ᵗʰ **S43.021** Posterior subluxation of right humerus

√7ᵗʰ **S43.022** Posterior subluxation of left humerus

√7ᵗʰ **S43.023** Posterior subluxation of unspecified humerus ▽

√7ᵗʰ **S43.024** Posterior dislocation of right humerus

√7ᵗʰ **S43.025** Posterior dislocation of left humerus

√7ᵗʰ **S43.026** Posterior dislocation of unspecified humerus ▽

√6ᵗʰ **S43.03** Inferior subluxation and dislocation of humerus

√7ᵗʰ **S43.031** Inferior subluxation of right humerus

√7ᵗʰ **S43.032** Inferior subluxation of left humerus

√7ᵗʰ **S43.033** Inferior subluxation of unspecified humerus ▽

√7ᵗʰ **S43.034** Inferior dislocation of right humerus

√7ᵗʰ **S43.035** Inferior dislocation of left humerus

√7ᵗʰ **S43.036** Inferior dislocation of unspecified humerus ▽

√6ᵗʰ **S43.08** Other subluxation and dislocation of shoulder joint

√7ᵗʰ **S43.081** Other subluxation of right shoulder joint

√7ᵗʰ **S43.082** Other subluxation of left shoulder joint

√7ᵗʰ **S43.083** Other subluxation of unspecified shoulder joint ▽

√7ᵗʰ **S43.084** Other dislocation of right shoulder joint

√7ᵗʰ **S43.085** Other dislocation of left shoulder joint

√7ᵗʰ **S43.086** Other dislocation of unspecified shoulder joint ▽

√5ᵗʰ **S43.1** Subluxation and dislocation of acromioclavicular joint

√6ᵗʰ **S43.10** Unspecified dislocation of acromioclavicular joint

√7ᵗʰ **S43.101** Unspecified dislocation of right acromioclavicular joint ▽

√7ᵗʰ **S43.102** Unspecified dislocation of left acromioclavicular joint ▽

√7ᵗʰ **S43.109** Unspecified dislocation of unspecified acromioclavicular joint ▽

√6ᵗʰ **S43.11** Subluxation of acromioclavicular joint

√7ᵗʰ **S43.111** Subluxation of right acromioclavicular joint

√7ᵗʰ **S43.112** Subluxation of left acromioclavicular joint

√7ᵗʰ **S43.119** Subluxation of unspecified acromioclavicular joint ▽

√6ᵗʰ **S43.12** Dislocation of acromioclavicular joint, 100%-200% displacement

√7ᵗʰ **S43.121** Dislocation of right acromioclavicular joint, 100%-200% displacement

√7ᵗʰ **S43.122** Dislocation of left acromioclavicular joint, 100%-200% displacement

√7ᵗʰ **S43.129** Dislocation of unspecified acromioclavicular joint, 100%-200% displacement ▽

√6ᵗʰ **S43.13** Dislocation of acromioclavicular joint, greater than 200% displacement

√7ᵗʰ **S43.131** Dislocation of right acromioclavicular joint, greater than 200% displacement

√7ᵗʰ **S43.132** Dislocation of left acromioclavicular joint, greater than 200% displacement

√7ᵗʰ **S43.139** Dislocation of unspecified acromioclavicular joint, greater than 200% displacement ▽

√6ᵗʰ **S43.14** Inferior dislocation of acromioclavicular joint

√7ᵗʰ **S43.141** Inferior dislocation of right acromioclavicular joint

√7ᵗʰ **S43.142** Inferior dislocation of left acromioclavicular joint

√7ᵗʰ **S43.149** Inferior dislocation of unspecified acromioclavicular joint ▽

√6ᵗʰ **S43.15** Posterior dislocation of acromioclavicular joint

√7ᵗʰ **S43.151** Posterior dislocation of right acromioclavicular joint

√7ᵗʰ **S43.152** Posterior dislocation of left acromioclavicular joint

√7ᵗʰ **S43.159** Posterior dislocation of unspecified acromioclavicular joint ▽

√5ᵗʰ **S43.2** Subluxation and dislocation of sternoclavicular joint

√6ᵗʰ **S43.20** Unspecified subluxation and dislocation of sternoclavicular joint

√7ᵗʰ **S43.201** Unspecified subluxation of right sternoclavicular joint ▽

√7ᵗʰ **S43.202** Unspecified subluxation of left sternoclavicular joint ▽

√7ᵗʰ **S43.203** Unspecified subluxation of unspecified sternoclavicular joint ▽

√7ᵗʰ **S43.204** Unspecified dislocation of right sternoclavicular joint ▽

√7ᵗʰ **S43.205** Unspecified dislocation of left sternoclavicular joint ▽

√7ᵗʰ **S43.206** Unspecified dislocation of unspecified sternoclavicular joint ▽

√6ᵗʰ **S43.21** Anterior subluxation and dislocation of sternoclavicular joint

√7ᵗʰ **S43.211** Anterior subluxation of right sternoclavicular joint

√7ᵗʰ **S43.212** Anterior subluxation of left sternoclavicular joint

√7ᵗʰ **S43.213** Anterior subluxation of unspecified sternoclavicular joint ▽

√7ᵗʰ **S43.214** Anterior dislocation of right sternoclavicular joint

EXCLUDES 1 Not coded here   EXCLUDES 2 Not included here   N Newborn Age : 0   P Pediatric Age : 0-17   M Maternity Age : 12-55   A Adult Age : 15-124

932

ICD-10-CM 2017

√7ᵗʰ **S43.215** Anterior dislocation of left sternoclavicular joint

√7ᵗʰ **S43.216** Anterior dislocation of unspecified sternoclavicular joint ▽

√6ᵗʰ **S43.22** Posterior subluxation and dislocation of sternoclavicular joint

√7ᵗʰ **S43.221** Posterior subluxation of right sternoclavicular joint

√7ᵗʰ **S43.222** Posterior subluxation of left sternoclavicular joint

√7ᵗʰ **S43.223** Posterior subluxation of unspecified sternoclavicular joint ▽

√7ᵗʰ **S43.224** Posterior dislocation of right sternoclavicular joint

√7ᵗʰ **S43.225** Posterior dislocation of left sternoclavicular joint

√7ᵗʰ **S43.226** Posterior dislocation of unspecified sternoclavicular joint ▽

√5ᵗʰ **S43.3** Subluxation and dislocation of other and unspecified parts of shoulder girdle

√6ᵗʰ **S43.30** Subluxation and dislocation of unspecified parts of shoulder girdle

Dislocation of shoulder girdle NOS

Subluxation of shoulder girdle NOS

√7ᵗʰ **S43.301** Subluxation of unspecified parts of right shoulder girdle ▽

√7ᵗʰ **S43.302** Subluxation of unspecified parts of left shoulder girdle ▽

√7ᵗʰ **S43.303** Subluxation of unspecified parts of unspecified shoulder girdle ▽

√7ᵗʰ **S43.304** Dislocation of unspecified parts of right shoulder girdle ▽

√7ᵗʰ **S43.305** Dislocation of unspecified parts of left shoulder girdle ▽

√7ᵗʰ **S43.306** Dislocation of unspecified parts of unspecified shoulder girdle ▽

√6ᵗʰ **S43.31** Subluxation and dislocation of scapula

√7ᵗʰ **S43.311** Subluxation of right scapula

√7ᵗʰ **S43.312** Subluxation of left scapula

√7ᵗʰ **S43.313** Subluxation of unspecified scapula ▽

√7ᵗʰ **S43.314** Dislocation of right scapula

√7ᵗʰ **S43.315** Dislocation of left scapula

√7ᵗʰ **S43.316** Dislocation of unspecified scapula ▽

√6ᵗʰ **S43.39** Subluxation and dislocation of other parts of shoulder girdle

√7ᵗʰ **S43.391** Subluxation of other parts of right shoulder girdle

√7ᵗʰ **S43.392** Subluxation of other parts of left shoulder girdle

√7ᵗʰ **S43.393** Subluxation of other parts of unspecified shoulder girdle ▽

√7ᵗʰ **S43.394** Dislocation of other parts of right shoulder girdle

√7ᵗʰ **S43.395** Dislocation of other parts of left shoulder girdle

√7ᵗʰ **S43.396** Dislocation of other parts of unspecified shoulder girdle ▽

√5ᵗʰ **S43.4** Sprain of shoulder joint

√6ᵗʰ **S43.40** Unspecified sprain of shoulder joint

√7ᵗʰ **S43.401** Unspecified sprain of right shoulder joint ▽

√7ᵗʰ **S43.402** Unspecified sprain of left shoulder joint ▽

√7ᵗʰ **S43.409** Unspecified sprain of unspecified shoulder joint ▽

√6ᵗʰ **S43.41** Sprain of coracohumeral (ligament)

√7ᵗʰ **S43.411** Sprain of right coracohumeral (ligament)

√7ᵗʰ **S43.412** Sprain of left coracohumeral (ligament)

√7ᵗʰ **S43.419** Sprain of unspecified coracohumeral (ligament) ▽

√6ᵗʰ **S43.42** Sprain of rotator cuff capsule

EXCLUDES 1 rotator cuff syndrome (complete) (incomplete), not specified as traumatic (M75.1-)

EXCLUDES 2 injury of tendon of rotator cuff (S46.0-)

√7ᵗʰ **S43.421** Sprain of right rotator cuff capsule

√7ᵗʰ **S43.422** Sprain of left rotator cuff capsule

√7ᵗʰ **S43.429** Sprain of unspecified rotator cuff capsule ▽

√6ᵗʰ **S43.43** Superior glenoid labrum lesion

SLAP lesion

DEF: Detachment injury of the superior aspect of the glenoid labrum, which is the ring of fibrocartilage attached to the rim of the glenoid cavity of the scapula.

√7ᵗʰ **S43.431** Superior glenoid labrum lesion of right shoulder

√7ᵗʰ **S43.432** Superior glenoid labrum lesion of left shoulder

√7ᵗʰ **S43.439** Superior glenoid labrum lesion of unspecified shoulder ▽

√6ᵗʰ **S43.49** Other sprain of shoulder joint

√7ᵗʰ **S43.491** Other sprain of right shoulder joint

√7ᵗʰ **S43.492** Other sprain of left shoulder joint

√7ᵗʰ **S43.499** Other sprain of unspecified shoulder joint ▽

√5ᵗʰ **S43.5** Sprain of acromioclavicular joint

Sprain of acromioclavicular ligament

√x7ᵗʰ **S43.50** Sprain of unspecified acromioclavicular joint ▽

√x7ᵗʰ **S43.51** Sprain of right acromioclavicular joint

√x7ᵗʰ **S43.52** Sprain of left acromioclavicular joint

√5ᵗʰ **S43.6** Sprain of sternoclavicular joint

√x7ᵗʰ **S43.60** Sprain of unspecified sternoclavicular joint ▽

√x7ᵗʰ **S43.61** Sprain of right sternoclavicular joint

√x7ᵗʰ **S43.62** Sprain of left sternoclavicular joint

√5ᵗʰ **S43.8** Sprain of other specified parts of shoulder girdle

√x7ᵗʰ **S43.80** Sprain of other specified parts of unspecified shoulder girdle ▽

√x7ᵗʰ **S43.81** Sprain of other specified parts of right shoulder girdle

√x7ᵗʰ **S43.82** Sprain of other specified parts of left shoulder girdle

√5ᵗʰ **S43.9** Sprain of unspecified parts of shoulder girdle

√x7ᵗʰ **S43.90** Sprain of unspecified parts of unspecified shoulder girdle ▽

Sprain of shoulder girdle NOS

√x7ᵗʰ **S43.91** Sprain of unspecified parts of right shoulder girdle ▽

√x7ᵗʰ **S43.92** Sprain of unspecified parts of left shoulder girdle ▽

√4ᵗʰ **S44** Injury of nerves at shoulder and upper arm level

Code also any associated open wound (S41.-)

EXCLUDES 2 injury of brachial plexus (S14.3-)

The appropriate 7th character is to be added to each code from category S44.

A initial encounter

D subsequent encounter

S sequela

√5ᵗʰ **S44.0** Injury of ulnar nerve at upper arm level

EXCLUDES 1 ulnar nerve NOS (S54.0)

√x7ᵗʰ **S44.00** Injury of ulnar nerve at upper arm level, unspecified arm ▽

√x7ᵗʰ **S44.01** Injury of ulnar nerve at upper arm level, right arm

√x7ᵗʰ **S44.02** Injury of ulnar nerve at upper arm level, left arm

√5ᵗʰ **S44.1** Injury of median nerve at upper arm level

EXCLUDES 1 median nerve NOS (S54.1)

√x7ᵗʰ **S44.10** Injury of median nerve at upper arm level, unspecified arm ▽

√x7ᵗʰ **S44.11** Injury of median nerve at upper arm level, right arm

√x7ᵗʰ **S44.12** Injury of median nerve at upper arm level, left arm

√5ᵗʰ **S44.2** Injury of radial nerve at upper arm level

EXCLUDES 1 radial nerve NOS (S54.2)

√x7ᵗʰ **S44.20** Injury of radial nerve at upper arm level, unspecified arm ▽

√x7ᵗʰ **S44.21** Injury of radial nerve at upper arm level, right arm

√x7ᵗʰ **S44.22** Injury of radial nerve at upper arm level, left arm

√5ᵗʰ **S44.3** Injury of axillary nerve

√x7ᵗʰ **S44.30** Injury of axillary nerve, unspecified arm ▽

√x7ᵗʰ **S44.31** Injury of axillary nerve, right arm

√x7ᵗʰ **S44.32** Injury of axillary nerve, left arm

☑ Additional Character Required   √x7ᵗʰ Placeholder Alert   Manifestation Dx   ▽ Unspecified Dx   ▶◀ Revised Text   ● New Code   ▲ Revised Code Title

Chapter 19. Injury, Poisoning and Certain Other Consequences of External Causes

S44.4–S45.89

✓5th **S44.4**   Injury of musculocutaneous nerve

    ✓x7th **S44.40**   Injury of musculocutaneous nerve, unspecified arm ▽

    ✓x7th **S44.41**   Injury of musculocutaneous nerve, right arm

    ✓x7th **S44.42**   Injury of musculocutaneous nerve, left arm

✓5th **S44.5**   Injury of cutaneous sensory nerve at shoulder and upper arm level

    ✓x7th **S44.50**   Injury of cutaneous sensory nerve at shoulder and upper arm level, unspecified arm ▽

    ✓x7th **S44.51**   Injury of cutaneous sensory nerve at shoulder and upper arm level, right arm

    ✓x7th **S44.52**   Injury of cutaneous sensory nerve at shoulder and upper arm level, left arm

✓5th **S44.8**   Injury of other nerves at shoulder and upper arm level

    ✓6th **S44.8X**   Injury of other nerves at shoulder and upper arm level

       ✓7th **S44.8X1**   Injury of other nerves at shoulder and upper arm level, right arm

       ✓7th **S44.8X2**   Injury of other nerves at shoulder and upper arm level, left arm

       ✓7th **S44.8X9**   Injury of other nerves at shoulder and upper arm level, unspecified arm ▽

✓5th **S44.9**   Injury of unspecified nerve at shoulder and upper arm level

    ✓x7th **S44.90**   Injury of unspecified nerve at shoulder and upper arm level, unspecified arm ▽

    ✓x7th **S44.91**   Injury of unspecified nerve at shoulder and upper arm level, right arm ▽

    ✓x7th **S44.92**   Injury of unspecified nerve at shoulder and upper arm level, left arm ▽

✓4th **S45**   **Injury of blood vessels at shoulder and upper arm level**

    Code also any associated open wound (S41.-)

    EXCLUDES 2   injury of subclavian artery (S25.1)

               injury of subclavian vein (S25.3)

    The appropriate 7th character is to be added to each code from category S45.
    A   initial encounter
    D   subsequent encounter
    S   sequela

✓5th **S45.0**   Injury of axillary artery

    ✓6th **S45.00**   Unspecified injury of axillary artery

       ✓7th **S45.001**   Unspecified injury of axillary artery, right side ▽

       ✓7th **S45.002**   Unspecified injury of axillary artery, left side ▽

       ✓7th **S45.009**   Unspecified injury of axillary artery, unspecified side ▽

    ✓6th **S45.01**   Laceration of axillary artery

       ✓7th **S45.011**   Laceration of axillary artery, right side

       ✓7th **S45.012**   Laceration of axillary artery, left side

       ✓7th **S45.019**   Laceration of axillary artery, unspecified side ▽

    ✓6th **S45.09**   Other specified injury of axillary artery

       ✓7th **S45.091**   Other specified injury of axillary artery, right side

       ✓7th **S45.092**   Other specified injury of axillary artery, left side

       ✓7th **S45.099**   Other specified injury of axillary artery, unspecified side ▽

✓5th **S45.1**   Injury of brachial artery

    ✓6th **S45.10**   Unspecified injury of brachial artery

       ✓7th **S45.101**   Unspecified injury of brachial artery, right side ▽

       ✓7th **S45.102**   Unspecified injury of brachial artery, left side ▽

       ✓7th **S45.109**   Unspecified injury of brachial artery, unspecified side ▽

    ✓6th **S45.11**   Laceration of brachial artery

       ✓7th **S45.111**   Laceration of brachial artery, right side

       ✓7th **S45.112**   Laceration of brachial artery, left side

       ✓7th **S45.119**   Laceration of brachial artery, unspecified side ▽

    ✓6th **S45.19**   Other specified injury of brachial artery

       ✓7th **S45.191**   Other specified injury of brachial artery, right side

       ✓7th **S45.192**   Other specified injury of brachial artery, left side

       ✓7th **S45.199**   Other specified injury of brachial artery, unspecified side ▽

✓5th **S45.2**   Injury of axillary or brachial vein

    ✓6th **S45.20**   Unspecified injury of axillary or brachial vein

       ✓7th **S45.201**   Unspecified injury of axillary or brachial vein, right side ▽

       ✓7th **S45.202**   Unspecified injury of axillary or brachial vein, left side

       ✓7th **S45.209**   Unspecified injury of axillary or brachial vein, unspecified side ▽

    ✓6th **S45.21**   Laceration of axillary or brachial vein

       ✓7th **S45.211**   Laceration of axillary or brachial vein, right side

       ✓7th **S45.212**   Laceration of axillary or brachial vein, left side

       ✓7th **S45.219**   Laceration of axillary or brachial vein, unspecified side ▽

    ✓6th **S45.29**   Other specified injury of axillary or brachial vein

       ✓7th **S45.291**   Other specified injury of axillary or brachial vein, right side

       ✓7th **S45.292**   Other specified injury of axillary or brachial vein, left side

       ✓7th **S45.299**   Other specified injury of axillary or brachial vein, unspecified side ▽

✓5th **S45.3**   Injury of superficial vein at shoulder and upper arm level

    ✓6th **S45.30**   Unspecified injury of superficial vein at shoulder and upper arm level

       ✓7th **S45.301**   Unspecified injury of superficial vein at shoulder and upper arm level, right arm ▽

       ✓7th **S45.302**   Unspecified injury of superficial vein at shoulder and upper arm level, left arm ▽

       ✓7th **S45.309**   Unspecified injury of superficial vein at shoulder and upper arm level, unspecified arm ▽

    ✓6th **S45.31**   Laceration of superficial vein at shoulder and upper arm level

       ✓7th **S45.311**   Laceration of superficial vein at shoulder and upper arm level, right arm

       ✓7th **S45.312**   Laceration of superficial vein at shoulder and upper arm level, left arm

       ✓7th **S45.319**   Laceration of superficial vein at shoulder and upper arm level, unspecified arm ▽

    ✓6th **S45.39**   Other specified injury of superficial vein at shoulder and upper arm level

       ✓7th **S45.391**   Other specified injury of superficial vein at shoulder and upper arm level, right arm

       ✓7th **S45.392**   Other specified injury of superficial vein at shoulder and upper arm level, left arm

       ✓7th **S45.399**   Other specified injury of superficial vein at shoulder and upper arm level, unspecified arm ▽

✓5th **S45.8**   Injury of other specified blood vessels at shoulder and upper arm level

    ✓6th **S45.80**   Unspecified injury of other specified blood vessels at shoulder and upper arm level

       ✓7th **S45.801**   Unspecified injury of other specified blood vessels at shoulder and upper arm level, right arm ▽

       ✓7th **S45.802**   Unspecified injury of other specified blood vessels at shoulder and upper arm level, left arm ▽

       ✓7th **S45.809**   Unspecified injury of other specified blood vessels at shoulder and upper arm level, unspecified arm ▽

    ✓6th **S45.81**   Laceration of other specified blood vessels at shoulder and upper arm level

       ✓7th **S45.811**   Laceration of other specified blood vessels at shoulder and upper arm level, right arm

       ✓7th **S45.812**   Laceration of other specified blood vessels at shoulder and upper arm level, left arm

       ✓7th **S45.819**   Laceration of other specified blood vessels at shoulder and upper arm level, unspecified arm ▽

    ✓6th **S45.89**   Other specified injury of other specified blood vessels at shoulder and upper arm level

EXCLUDES 1 Not coded here   *EXCLUDES 2* Not included here   **N** Newborn Age : 0   **P** Pediatric Age : 0-17   **M** Maternity Age : 12-55   **A** Adult Age : 15-124

934

ICD-10-CM 2017

✓7ᵗʰ **S45.891** Other specified injury of other specified blood vessels at shoulder and upper arm level, right arm

✓7ᵗʰ **S45.892** Other specified injury of other specified blood vessels at shoulder and upper arm level, left arm

✓7ᵗʰ **S45.899** Other specified injury of other specified blood vessels at shoulder and upper arm level, unspecified arm ▽

✓5ᵗʰ **S45.9** Injury of unspecified blood vessel at shoulder and upper arm level

✓6ᵗʰ **S45.90** Unspecified injury of unspecified blood vessel at shoulder and upper arm level

✓7ᵗʰ **S45.901** Unspecified injury of unspecified blood vessel at shoulder and upper arm level, right arm ▽

✓7ᵗʰ **S45.902** Unspecified injury of unspecified blood vessel at shoulder and upper arm level, left arm ▽

✓7ᵗʰ **S45.909** Unspecified injury of unspecified blood vessel at shoulder and upper arm level, unspecified arm ▽

✓6ᵗʰ **S45.91** Laceration of unspecified blood vessel at shoulder and upper arm level

✓7ᵗʰ **S45.911** Laceration of unspecified blood vessel at shoulder and upper arm level, right arm ▽

✓7ᵗʰ **S45.912** Laceration of unspecified blood vessel at shoulder and upper arm level, left arm ▽

✓7ᵗʰ **S45.919** Laceration of unspecified blood vessel at shoulder and upper arm level, unspecified arm ▽

✓6ᵗʰ **S45.99** Other specified injury of unspecified blood vessel at shoulder and upper arm level

✓7ᵗʰ **S45.991** Other specified injury of unspecified blood vessel at shoulder and upper arm level, right arm ▽

✓7ᵗʰ **S45.992** Other specified injury of unspecified blood vessel at shoulder and upper arm level, left arm ▽

✓7ᵗʰ **S45.999** Other specified injury of unspecified blood vessel at shoulder and upper arm level, unspecified arm ▽

✓4ᵗʰ **S46 Injury of muscle, fascia and tendon at shoulder and upper arm level**

Code also any associated open wound (S41.-)

EXCLUDES 2 *injury of muscle, fascia and tendon at elbow (S56.-)*
sprain of joints and ligaments of shoulder girdle (S43.9)

TIP: Refer to the Muscle/Tendon table at the beginning of this chapter

The appropriate 7th character is to be added to each code from category S46.
A   initial encounter
D   subsequent encounter
S   sequela

✓5ᵗʰ **S46.0** Injury of muscle(s) and tendon(s) of the rotator cuff of shoulder

✓6ᵗʰ **S46.00** Unspecified injury of muscle(s) and tendon(s) of the rotator cuff of shoulder

✓7ᵗʰ **S46.001** Unspecified injury of muscle(s) and tendon(s) of the rotator cuff of right shoulder ▽

✓7ᵗʰ **S46.002** Unspecified injury of muscle(s) and tendon(s) of the rotator cuff of left shoulder ▽

✓7ᵗʰ **S46.009** Unspecified injury of muscle(s) and tendon(s) of the rotator cuff of unspecified shoulder ▽

✓6ᵗʰ **S46.01** Strain of muscle(s) and tendon(s) of the rotator cuff of shoulder

✓7ᵗʰ **S46.011** Strain of muscle(s) and tendon(s) of the rotator cuff of right shoulder

✓7ᵗʰ **S46.012** Strain of muscle(s) and tendon(s) of the rotator cuff of left shoulder

✓7ᵗʰ **S46.019** Strain of muscle(s) and tendon(s) of the rotator cuff of unspecified shoulder ▽

✓6ᵗʰ **S46.02** Laceration of muscle(s) and tendon(s) of the rotator cuff of shoulder

✓7ᵗʰ **S46.021** Laceration of muscle(s) and tendon(s) of the rotator cuff of right shoulder

✓7ᵗʰ **S46.022** Laceration of muscle(s) and tendon(s) of the rotator cuff of left shoulder

✓7ᵗʰ **S46.029** Laceration of muscle(s) and tendon(s) of the rotator cuff of unspecified shoulder ▽

✓6ᵗʰ **S46.09** Other injury of muscle(s) and tendon(s) of the rotator cuff of shoulder

✓7ᵗʰ **S46.091** Other injury of muscle(s) and tendon(s) of the rotator cuff of right shoulder

✓7ᵗʰ **S46.092** Other injury of muscle(s) and tendon(s) of the rotator cuff of left shoulder

✓7ᵗʰ **S46.099** Other injury of muscle(s) and tendon(s) of the rotator cuff of unspecified shoulder ▽

✓5ᵗʰ **S46.1** Injury of muscle, fascia and tendon of long head of biceps

✓6ᵗʰ **S46.10** Unspecified injury of muscle, fascia and tendon of long head of biceps

✓7ᵗʰ **S46.101** Unspecified injury of muscle, fascia and tendon of long head of biceps, right arm ▽

✓7ᵗʰ **S46.102** Unspecified injury of muscle, fascia and tendon of long head of biceps, left arm ▽

✓7ᵗʰ **S46.109** Unspecified injury of muscle, fascia and tendon of long head of biceps, unspecified arm ▽

✓6ᵗʰ **S46.11** Strain of muscle, fascia and tendon of long head of biceps

✓7ᵗʰ **S46.111** Strain of muscle, fascia and tendon of long head of biceps, right arm

✓7ᵗʰ **S46.112** Strain of muscle, fascia and tendon of long head of biceps, left arm

✓7ᵗʰ **S46.119** Strain of muscle, fascia and tendon of long head of biceps, unspecified arm ▽

✓6ᵗʰ **S46.12** Laceration of muscle, fascia and tendon of long head of biceps

✓7ᵗʰ **S46.121** Laceration of muscle, fascia and tendon of long head of biceps, right arm

✓7ᵗʰ **S46.122** Laceration of muscle, fascia and tendon of long head of biceps, left arm

✓7ᵗʰ **S46.129** Laceration of muscle, fascia and tendon of long head of biceps, unspecified arm ▽

✓6ᵗʰ **S46.19** Other injury of muscle, fascia and tendon of long head of biceps

✓7ᵗʰ **S46.191** Other injury of muscle, fascia and tendon of long head of biceps, right arm

✓7ᵗʰ **S46.192** Other injury of muscle, fascia and tendon of long head of biceps, left arm

✓7ᵗʰ **S46.199** Other injury of muscle, fascia and tendon of long head of biceps, unspecified arm ▽

✓5ᵗʰ **S46.2** Injury of muscle, fascia and tendon of other parts of biceps

✓6ᵗʰ **S46.20** Unspecified injury of muscle, fascia and tendon of other parts of biceps

✓7ᵗʰ **S46.201** Unspecified injury of muscle, fascia and tendon of other parts of biceps, right arm ▽

✓7ᵗʰ **S46.202** Unspecified injury of muscle, fascia and tendon of other parts of biceps, left arm ▽

✓7ᵗʰ **S46.209** Unspecified injury of muscle, fascia and tendon of other parts of biceps, unspecified arm ▽

✓6ᵗʰ **S46.21** Strain of muscle, fascia and tendon of other parts of biceps

✓7ᵗʰ **S46.211** Strain of muscle, fascia and tendon of other parts of biceps, right arm

✓7ᵗʰ **S46.212** Strain of muscle, fascia and tendon of other parts of biceps, left arm

✓7ᵗʰ **S46.219** Strain of muscle, fascia and tendon of other parts of biceps, unspecified arm ▽

✓6ᵗʰ **S46.22** Laceration of muscle, fascia and tendon of other parts of biceps

✓7ᵗʰ **S46.221** Laceration of muscle, fascia and tendon of other parts of biceps, right arm

✓7ᵗʰ **S46.222** Laceration of muscle, fascia and tendon of other parts of biceps, left arm

☑ Additional Character Required   ✓ₓ7ᵗʰ Placeholder Alert   Manifestation Dx   ▽ Unspecified Dx   ▶◀ Revised Text   ● New Code   ▲ Revised Code Title

ICD-10-CM 2017   **935**

Chapter 19. Injury, Poisoning and Certain Other Consequences of External Causes

      ✓7ᵗʰ **S46.229** Laceration of muscle, fascia and tendon of other parts of biceps, unspecified arm ▽

   ✓6ᵗʰ **S46.29** Other injury of muscle, fascia and tendon of other parts of biceps

      ✓7ᵗʰ **S46.291** Other injury of muscle, fascia and tendon of other parts of biceps, right arm

      ✓7ᵗʰ **S46.292** Other injury of muscle, fascia and tendon of other parts of biceps, left arm

      ✓7ᵗʰ **S46.299** Other injury of muscle, fascia and tendon of other parts of biceps, unspecified arm ▽

✓5ᵗʰ **S46.3** Injury of muscle, fascia and tendon of triceps

   ✓6ᵗʰ **S46.30** Unspecified injury of muscle, fascia and tendon of triceps

      ✓7ᵗʰ **S46.301** Unspecified injury of muscle, fascia and tendon of triceps, right arm ▽

      ✓7ᵗʰ **S46.302** Unspecified injury of muscle, fascia and tendon of triceps, left arm ▽

      ✓7ᵗʰ **S46.309** Unspecified injury of muscle, fascia and tendon of triceps, unspecified arm ▽

   ✓6ᵗʰ **S46.31** Strain of muscle, fascia and tendon of triceps

      ✓7ᵗʰ **S46.311** Strain of muscle, fascia and tendon of triceps, right arm

      ✓7ᵗʰ **S46.312** Strain of muscle, fascia and tendon of triceps, left arm

      ✓7ᵗʰ **S46.319** Strain of muscle, fascia and tendon of triceps, unspecified arm ▽

   ✓6ᵗʰ **S46.32** Laceration of muscle, fascia and tendon of triceps

      ✓7ᵗʰ **S46.321** Laceration of muscle, fascia and tendon of triceps, right arm

      ✓7ᵗʰ **S46.322** Laceration of muscle, fascia and tendon of triceps, left arm

      ✓7ᵗʰ **S46.329** Laceration of muscle, fascia and tendon of triceps, unspecified arm ▽

   ✓6ᵗʰ **S46.39** Other injury of muscle, fascia and tendon of triceps

      ✓7ᵗʰ **S46.391** Other injury of muscle, fascia and tendon of triceps, right arm

      ✓7ᵗʰ **S46.392** Other injury of muscle, fascia and tendon of triceps, left arm

      ✓7ᵗʰ **S46.399** Other injury of muscle, fascia and tendon of triceps, unspecified arm ▽

✓5ᵗʰ **S46.8** Injury of other muscles, fascia and tendons at shoulder and upper arm level

   ✓6ᵗʰ **S46.80** Unspecified injury of other muscles, fascia and tendons at shoulder and upper arm level

      ✓7ᵗʰ **S46.801** Unspecified injury of other muscles, fascia and tendons at shoulder and upper arm level, right arm ▽

      ✓7ᵗʰ **S46.802** Unspecified injury of other muscles, fascia and tendons at shoulder and upper arm level, left arm ▽

      ✓7ᵗʰ **S46.809** Unspecified injury of other muscles, fascia and tendons at shoulder and upper arm level, unspecified arm ▽

   ✓6ᵗʰ **S46.81** Strain of other muscles, fascia and tendons at shoulder and upper arm level

      ✓7ᵗʰ **S46.811** Strain of other muscles, fascia and tendons at shoulder and upper arm level, right arm

      ✓7ᵗʰ **S46.812** Strain of other muscles, fascia and tendons at shoulder and upper arm level, left arm

      ✓7ᵗʰ **S46.819** Strain of other muscles, fascia and tendons at shoulder and upper arm level, unspecified arm ▽

   ✓6ᵗʰ **S46.82** Laceration of other muscles, fascia and tendons at shoulder and upper arm level

      ✓7ᵗʰ **S46.821** Laceration of other muscles, fascia and tendons at shoulder and upper arm level, right arm

      ✓7ᵗʰ **S46.822** Laceration of other muscles, fascia and tendons at shoulder and upper arm level, left arm

      ✓7ᵗʰ **S46.829** Laceration of other muscles, fascia and tendons at shoulder and upper arm level, unspecified arm ▽

   ✓6ᵗʰ **S46.89** Other injury of other muscles, fascia and tendons at shoulder and upper arm level

      ✓7ᵗʰ **S46.891** Other injury of other muscles, fascia and tendons at shoulder and upper arm level, right arm

      ✓7ᵗʰ **S46.892** Other injury of other muscles, fascia and tendons at shoulder and upper arm level, left arm

      ✓7ᵗʰ **S46.899** Other injury of other muscles, fascia and tendons at shoulder and upper arm level, unspecified arm ▽

✓5ᵗʰ **S46.9** Injury of unspecified muscle, fascia and tendon at shoulder and upper arm level

   ✓6ᵗʰ **S46.90** Unspecified injury of unspecified muscle, fascia and tendon at shoulder and upper arm level

      ✓7ᵗʰ **S46.901** Unspecified injury of unspecified muscle, fascia and tendon at shoulder and upper arm level, right arm ▽

      ✓7ᵗʰ **S46.902** Unspecified injury of unspecified muscle, fascia and tendon at shoulder and upper arm level, left arm ▽

      ✓7ᵗʰ **S46.909** Unspecified injury of unspecified muscle, fascia and tendon at shoulder and upper arm level, unspecified arm ▽

   ✓6ᵗʰ **S46.91** Strain of unspecified muscle, fascia and tendon at shoulder and upper arm level

      ✓7ᵗʰ **S46.911** Strain of unspecified muscle, fascia and tendon at shoulder and upper arm level, right arm ▽

      ✓7ᵗʰ **S46.912** Strain of unspecified muscle, fascia and tendon at shoulder and upper arm level, left arm ▽

      ✓7ᵗʰ **S46.919** Strain of unspecified muscle, fascia and tendon at shoulder and upper arm level, unspecified arm ▽

   ✓6ᵗʰ **S46.92** Laceration of unspecified muscle, fascia and tendon at shoulder and upper arm level

      ✓7ᵗʰ **S46.921** Laceration of unspecified muscle, fascia and tendon at shoulder and upper arm level, right arm ▽

      ✓7ᵗʰ **S46.922** Laceration of unspecified muscle, fascia and tendon at shoulder and upper arm level, left arm ▽

      ✓7ᵗʰ **S46.929** Laceration of unspecified muscle, fascia and tendon at shoulder and upper arm level, unspecified arm ▽

   ✓6ᵗʰ **S46.99** Other injury of unspecified muscle, fascia and tendon at shoulder and upper arm level

      ✓7ᵗʰ **S46.991** Other injury of unspecified muscle, fascia and tendon at shoulder and upper arm level, right arm ▽

      ✓7ᵗʰ **S46.992** Other injury of unspecified muscle, fascia and tendon at shoulder and upper arm level, left arm ▽

      ✓7ᵗʰ **S46.999** Other injury of unspecified muscle, fascia and tendon at shoulder and upper arm level, unspecified arm ▽

✓4ᵗʰ **S47 Crushing injury of shoulder and upper arm**

     Use additional code for all associated injuries

     EXCLUDES 2   *crushing injury of elbow (S57.0-)*

     The appropriate 7th character is to be added to each code from category S47.
     A   initial encounter
     D   subsequent encounter
     S   sequela

   ✓x7ᵗʰ **S47.1** Crushing injury of right shoulder and upper arm

   ✓x7ᵗʰ **S47.2** Crushing injury of left shoulder and upper arm

   ✓x7ᵗʰ **S47.9** Crushing injury of shoulder and upper arm, unspecified arm ▽

EXCLUDES 1 Not coded here   EXCLUDES 2 Not included here   N Newborn Age : 0   P Pediatric Age : 0-17   M Maternity Age : 12-55   A Adult Age : 15-124

936   ICD-10-CM 2017

√4ʰ **S48 Traumatic amputation of shoulder and upper arm**

> **NOTE**   An amputation not identified as partial or complete should be coded to complete
>
> **EXCLUDES 1** *traumatic amputation at elbow level (S58.0)*
>
> The appropriate 7th character is to be added to each code from category S48.
> A   initial encounter
> D   subsequent encounter
> S   sequela

√5ʰ **S48.0 Traumatic amputation at** shoulder joint

    √6ʰ **S48.01 Complete** traumatic amputation at shoulder joint

       √7ʰ **S48.011 Complete traumatic amputation at right shoulder joint**

       √7ʰ **S48.012 Complete traumatic amputation at left shoulder joint**

       S48.019 Complete traumatic amputation at unspecified shoulder joint ▽

    √6ʰ **S48.02 Partial** traumatic amputation at shoulder joint

       √7ʰ **S48.021 Partial traumatic amputation at right shoulder joint**

       √7ʰ **S48.022 Partial traumatic amputation at left shoulder joint**

       S48.029 Partial traumatic amputation at unspecified shoulder joint ▽

√5ʰ **S48.1 Traumatic amputation at** level between shoulder and elbow ▲

    √6ʰ **S48.11 Complete** traumatic amputation at level between shoulder and elbow ▲

       √7ʰ **S48.111 Complete traumatic amputation at level between right shoulder and elbow** ▲

       √7ʰ **S48.112 Complete traumatic amputation at level between left shoulder and elbow**

       S48.119 Complete traumatic amputation at level between unspecified shoulder and elbow ▽

    √6ʰ **S48.12 Partial** traumatic amputation at level between shoulder and elbow

       √7ʰ **S48.121 Partial traumatic amputation at level between right shoulder and elbow**

       √7ʰ **S48.122 Partial traumatic amputation at level between left shoulder and elbow**

       S48.129 Partial traumatic amputation at level between unspecified shoulder and elbow ▽

√5ʰ **S48.9 Traumatic amputation of shoulder and upper arm, level unspecified**

    √6ʰ **S48.91 Complete** traumatic amputation of shoulder and upper arm, level unspecified

       √7ʰ **S48.911 Complete traumatic amputation of right shoulder and upper arm, level unspecified** ▽

       √7ʰ **S48.912 Complete traumatic amputation of left shoulder and upper arm, level unspecified** ▽

       √7ʰ **S48.919 Complete traumatic amputation of unspecified shoulder and upper arm, level unspecified** ▽

    √6ʰ **S48.92 Partial** traumatic amputation of shoulder and upper arm, level unspecified

       √7ʰ **S48.921 Partial traumatic amputation of right shoulder and upper arm, level unspecified** ▽

       √7ʰ **S48.922 Partial traumatic amputation of left shoulder and upper arm, level unspecified** ▽

       √7ʰ **S48.929 Partial traumatic amputation of unspecified shoulder and upper arm, level unspecified** ▽

√4ʰ **S49 Other and unspecified injuries of shoulder and upper arm**

> The appropriate 7th character is to be added to each code from subcategories S49.0 and S49.1.
> A   initial encounter for closed fracture
> D   subsequent encounter for fracture with routine healing
> G   subsequent encounter for fracture with delayed healing
> K   subsequent encounter for fracture with nonunion
> P   subsequent encounter for fracture with malunion
> S   sequela

√5ʰ **S49.0 Physeal** fracture of upper end of humerus

    √6ʰ **S49.00 Unspecified physeal fracture of upper end of humerus**

       √7ʰ **S49.001 Unspecified physeal fracture of upper end of humerus, right arm** ▽

       √7ʰ **S49.002 Unspecified physeal fracture of upper end of humerus, left arm** ▽

       √7ʰ **S49.009 Unspecified physeal fracture of upper end of humerus, unspecified arm** ▽

    √6ʰ **S49.01 Salter-Harris Type I** physeal fracture of upper end of humerus

       √7ʰ **S49.011 Salter-Harris Type I physeal fracture of upper end of humerus, right arm**

       √7ʰ **S49.012 Salter-Harris Type I physeal fracture of upper end of humerus, left arm**

       √7ʰ **S49.019 Salter-Harris Type I physeal fracture of upper end of humerus, unspecified arm** ▽

    √6ʰ **S49.02 Salter-Harris Type II** physeal fracture of upper end of humerus

       √7ʰ **S49.021 Salter-Harris Type II physeal fracture of upper end of humerus, right arm**

       √7ʰ **S49.022 Salter-Harris Type II physeal fracture of upper end of humerus, left arm**

       √7ʰ **S49.029 Salter-Harris Type II physeal fracture of upper end of humerus, unspecified arm** ▽

    √6ʰ **S49.03 Salter-Harris Type III** physeal fracture of upper end of humerus

       √7ʰ **S49.031 Salter-Harris Type III physeal fracture of upper end of humerus, right arm**

       √7ʰ **S49.032 Salter-Harris Type III physeal fracture of upper end of humerus, left arm**

       √7ʰ **S49.039 Salter-Harris Type III physeal fracture of upper end of humerus, unspecified arm** ▽

    √6ʰ **S49.04 Salter-Harris Type IV** physeal fracture of upper end of humerus

       √7ʰ **S49.041 Salter-Harris Type IV physeal fracture of upper end of humerus, right arm**

       √7ʰ **S49.042 Salter-Harris Type IV physeal fracture of upper end of humerus, left arm**

       √7ʰ **S49.049 Salter-Harris Type IV physeal fracture of upper end of humerus, unspecified arm** ▽

    √6ʰ **S49.09 Other physeal fracture of upper end of humerus**

       √7ʰ **S49.091 Other physeal fracture of upper end of humerus, right arm**

       √7ʰ **S49.092 Other physeal fracture of upper end of humerus, left arm**

       √7ʰ **S49.099 Other physeal fracture of upper end of humerus, unspecified arm** ▽

√5ʰ **S49.1 Physeal fracture of** lower end of humerus

    √6ʰ **S49.10 Unspecified physeal fracture of lower end of humerus**

       √7ʰ **S49.101 Unspecified physeal fracture of lower end of humerus, right arm** ▽

       √7ʰ **S49.102 Unspecified physeal fracture of lower end of humerus, left arm** ▽

       √7ʰ **S49.109 Unspecified physeal fracture of lower end of humerus, unspecified arm** ▽

    √6ʰ **S49.11 Salter-Harris Type I** physeal fracture of lower end of humerus

       √7ʰ **S49.111 Salter-Harris Type I physeal fracture of lower end of humerus, right arm**

       √7ʰ **S49.112 Salter-Harris Type I physeal fracture of lower end of humerus, left arm**

       √7ʰ **S49.119 Salter-Harris Type I physeal fracture of lower end of humerus, unspecified arm** ▽

    √6ʰ **S49.12 Salter-Harris Type II** physeal fracture of lower end of humerus

       √7ʰ **S49.121 Salter-Harris Type II physeal fracture of lower end of humerus, right arm**

       √7ʰ **S49.122 Salter-Harris Type II physeal fracture of lower end of humerus, left arm**

       √7ʰ **S49.129 Salter-Harris Type II physeal fracture of lower end of humerus, unspecified arm** ▽

    √6ʰ **S49.13 Salter-Harris Type III** physeal fracture of lower end of humerus ▲

       √7ʰ **S49.131 Salter-Harris Type III physeal fracture of lower end of humerus, right arm** ▲

☑ Additional Character Required   √x7ʰ Placeholder Alert   Manifestation Dx   ▽ Unspecified Dx   ▶◀ Revised Text   ● New Code   ▲ Revised Code Title

▲ ✓7ᵗʰ S49.132 Salter-Harris Type III physeal fracture of lower end of humerus, left arm
▲ ✓7ᵗʰ S49.139 Salter-Harris Type III physeal fracture of lower end of humerus, unspecified arm ▽

✓6ᵗʰ S49.14 Salter-Harris Type IV physeal fracture of lower end of humerus
  ✓7ᵗʰ S49.141 Salter-Harris Type IV physeal fracture of lower end of humerus, right arm
  ✓7ᵗʰ S49.142 Salter-Harris Type IV physeal fracture of lower end of humerus, left arm
  ✓7ᵗʰ S49.149 Salter-Harris Type IV physeal fracture of lower end of humerus, unspecified arm ▽

✓6ᵗʰ S49.19 Other physeal fracture of lower end of humerus
  ✓7ᵗʰ S49.191 Other physeal fracture of lower end of humerus, right arm
  ✓7ᵗʰ S49.192 Other physeal fracture of lower end of humerus, left arm
  ✓7ᵗʰ S49.199 Other physeal fracture of lower end of humerus, unspecified arm ▽

✓5ᵗʰ S49.8 Other specified injuries of shoulder and upper arm

The appropriate 7th character is to be added to each code in subcategory S49.8.
A   initial encounter
D   subsequent encounter
S   sequela

  ✓x7ᵗʰ S49.80 Other specified injuries of shoulder and upper arm, unspecified arm ▽
  ✓x7ᵗʰ S49.81 Other specified injuries of right shoulder and upper arm
  ✓x7ᵗʰ S49.82 Other specified injuries of left shoulder and upper arm

✓5ᵗʰ S49.9 Unspecified injury of shoulder and upper arm

The appropriate 7th character is to be added to each code in subcategory S49.9.
A   initial encounter
D   subsequent encounter
S   sequela

  ✓x7ᵗʰ S49.90 Unspecified injury of shoulder and upper arm, unspecified arm ▽
  ✓x7ᵗʰ S49.91 Unspecified injury of right shoulder and upper arm ▽
  ✓x7ᵗʰ S49.92 Unspecified injury of left shoulder and upper arm ▽

Injuries to the elbow and forearm (S50-S59)

EXCLUDES 2 burns and corrosions (T20-T32)
  frostbite (T33-T34)
  injuries of wrist and hand (S60-S69)
  insect bite or sting, venomous (T63.4)

✓4ᵗʰ S50 Superficial injury of elbow and forearm
  EXCLUDES 2 superficial injury of wrist and hand (S60.-)

The appropriate 7th character is to be added to each code from category S50.
A   initial encounter
D   subsequent encounter
S   sequela

✓5ᵗʰ S50.0 Contusion of elbow
  ✓x7ᵗʰ S50.00 Contusion of unspecified elbow ▽
  ✓x7ᵗʰ S50.01 Contusion of right elbow
  ✓x7ᵗʰ S50.02 Contusion of left elbow

✓5ᵗʰ S50.1 Contusion of forearm
  ✓x7ᵗʰ S50.10 Contusion of unspecified forearm ▽
  ✓x7ᵗʰ S50.11 Contusion of right forearm
  ✓x7ᵗʰ S50.12 Contusion of left forearm

✓5ᵗʰ S50.3 Other superficial injuries of elbow
  ✓6ᵗʰ S50.31 Abrasion of elbow
    ✓7ᵗʰ S50.311 Abrasion of right elbow
    ✓7ᵗʰ S50.312 Abrasion of left elbow
    ✓7ᵗʰ S50.319 Abrasion of unspecified elbow ▽
  ✓6ᵗʰ S50.32 Blister (nonthermal) of elbow
    ✓7ᵗʰ S50.321 Blister (nonthermal) of right elbow
    ✓7ᵗʰ S50.322 Blister (nonthermal) of left elbow

  ✓7ᵗʰ S50.329 Blister (nonthermal) of unspecified elbow ▽
✓6ᵗʰ S50.34 External constriction of elbow
  ✓7ᵗʰ S50.341 External constriction of right elbow
  ✓7ᵗʰ S50.342 External constriction of left elbow
  ✓7ᵗʰ S50.349 External constriction of unspecified elbow ▽
✓6ᵗʰ S50.35 Superficial foreign body of elbow
    Splinter in the elbow
  ✓7ᵗʰ S50.351 Superficial foreign body of right elbow
  ✓7ᵗʰ S50.352 Superficial foreign body of left elbow
  ✓7ᵗʰ S50.359 Superficial foreign body of unspecified elbow ▽
✓6ᵗʰ S50.36 Insect bite (nonvenomous) of elbow
  ✓7ᵗʰ S50.361 Insect bite (nonvenomous) of right elbow
  ✓7ᵗʰ S50.362 Insect bite (nonvenomous) of left elbow
  ✓7ᵗʰ S50.369 Insect bite (nonvenomous) of unspecified elbow ▽
✓6ᵗʰ S50.37 Other superficial bite of elbow
    EXCLUDES 1 open bite of elbow (S51.05)
  ✓7ᵗʰ S50.371 Other superficial bite of right elbow
  ✓7ᵗʰ S50.372 Other superficial bite of left elbow
  ✓7ᵗʰ S50.379 Other superficial bite of unspecified elbow ▽

✓5ᵗʰ S50.8 Other superficial injuries of forearm
  ✓6ᵗʰ S50.81 Abrasion of forearm
    ✓7ᵗʰ S50.811 Abrasion of right forearm
    ✓7ᵗʰ S50.812 Abrasion of left forearm
    ✓7ᵗʰ S50.819 Abrasion of unspecified forearm ▽
  ✓6ᵗʰ S50.82 Blister (nonthermal) of forearm
    ✓7ᵗʰ S50.821 Blister (nonthermal) of right forearm
    ✓7ᵗʰ S50.822 Blister (nonthermal) of left forearm
    ✓7ᵗʰ S50.829 Blister (nonthermal) of unspecified forearm ▽
  ✓6ᵗʰ S50.84 External constriction of forearm
    ✓7ᵗʰ S50.841 External constriction of right forearm
    ✓7ᵗʰ S50.842 External constriction of left forearm
    ✓7ᵗʰ S50.849 External constriction of unspecified forearm ▽
  ✓6ᵗʰ S50.85 Superficial foreign body of forearm
      Splinter in the forearm
    ✓7ᵗʰ S50.851 Superficial foreign body of right forearm
    ✓7ᵗʰ S50.852 Superficial foreign body of left forearm
    ✓7ᵗʰ S50.859 Superficial foreign body of unspecified forearm ▽
  ✓6ᵗʰ S50.86 Insect bite (nonvenomous) of forearm
    ✓7ᵗʰ S50.861 Insect bite (nonvenomous) of right forearm
    ✓7ᵗʰ S50.862 Insect bite (nonvenomous) of left forearm
    ✓7ᵗʰ S50.869 Insect bite (nonvenomous) of unspecified forearm ▽
  ✓6ᵗʰ S50.87 Other superficial bite of forearm
      EXCLUDES 1 open bite of forearm (S51.85)
    ✓7ᵗʰ S50.871 Other superficial bite of right forearm
    ✓7ᵗʰ S50.872 Other superficial bite of left forearm
    ✓7ᵗʰ S50.879 Other superficial bite of unspecified forearm ▽

✓5ᵗʰ S50.9 Unspecified superficial injury of elbow and forearm
  ✓6ᵗʰ S50.90 Unspecified superficial injury of elbow
    ✓7ᵗʰ S50.901 Unspecified superficial injury of right elbow ▽
    ✓7ᵗʰ S50.902 Unspecified superficial injury of left elbow ▽
    ✓7ᵗʰ S50.909 Unspecified superficial injury of unspecified elbow ▽
  ✓6ᵗʰ S50.91 Unspecified superficial injury of forearm
    ✓7ᵗʰ S50.911 Unspecified superficial injury of right forearm ▽
    ✓7ᵗʰ S50.912 Unspecified superficial injury of left forearm ▽
    ✓7ᵗʰ S50.919 Unspecified superficial injury of unspecified forearm ▽

√4ᵗʰ **S51**   **Open wound of elbow and forearm**

Code also any associated wound infection

EXCLUDES 1   *open fracture of elbow and forearm (S52.- with open fracture 7th character)*

traumatic amputation of elbow and forearm (S58.-)

EXCLUDES 2   *open wound of wrist and hand (S61.-)*

The appropriate 7th character is to be added to each code from category S51.

A   initial encounter
D   subsequent encounter
S   sequela

√5ᵗʰ   **S51.0**   **Open wound of elbow**

√6ᵗʰ   **S51.00**   **Unspecified open wound of elbow**

√7ᵗʰ   **S51.001**   Unspecified open wound of **right elbow**   ▽
     AHA: 2012,4Q,108

√7ᵗʰ   **S51.002**   Unspecified open wound of **left elbow**   ▽

√7ᵗʰ   **S51.009**   Unspecified open wound of unspecified elbow   ▽
     Open wound of elbow NOS

√6ᵗʰ   **S51.01**   Laceration without foreign body of elbow

√7ᵗʰ   **S51.011**   Laceration without foreign body of **right elbow**

√7ᵗʰ   **S51.012**   Laceration without foreign body of **left elbow**

√7ᵗʰ   **S51.019**   Laceration without foreign body of unspecified elbow   ▽

√6ᵗʰ   **S51.02**   Laceration with foreign body of elbow

√7ᵗʰ   **S51.021**   Laceration with foreign body of **right elbow**

√7ᵗʰ   **S51.022**   Laceration with foreign body of **left elbow**

√7ᵗʰ   **S51.029**   Laceration with foreign body of unspecified elbow   ▽

√6ᵗʰ   **S51.03**   Puncture wound without foreign body of elbow

√7ᵗʰ   **S51.031**   Puncture wound without foreign body of **right elbow**

√7ᵗʰ   **S51.032**   Puncture wound without foreign body of **left elbow**

√7ᵗʰ   **S51.039**   Puncture wound without foreign body of unspecified elbow   ▽

√6ᵗʰ   **S51.04**   Puncture wound with foreign body of elbow

√7ᵗʰ   **S51.041**   Puncture wound with foreign body of **right elbow**

√7ᵗʰ   **S51.042**   Puncture wound with foreign body of **left elbow**

√7ᵗʰ   **S51.049**   Puncture wound with foreign body of unspecified elbow   ▽

√6ᵗʰ   **S51.05**   Open bite of elbow
     Bite of elbow NOS
     EXCLUDES 1   *superficial bite of elbow (S50.36, S50.37)*

√7ᵗʰ   **S51.051**   Open bite, **right elbow**

√7ᵗʰ   **S51.052**   Open bite, **left elbow**

√7ᵗʰ   **S51.059**   Open bite, unspecified elbow   ▽

√5ᵗʰ   **S51.8**   **Open wound of forearm**
     EXCLUDES 2   *open wound of elbow (S51.0-)*

√6ᵗʰ   **S51.80**   Unspecified open wound of forearm

√7ᵗʰ   **S51.801**   Unspecified open wound of **right forearm**   ▽

√7ᵗʰ   **S51.802**   Unspecified open wound of **left forearm**   ▽

√7ᵗʰ   **S51.809**   Unspecified open wound of unspecified forearm   ▽
     Open wound of forearm NOS

√6ᵗʰ   **S51.81**   Laceration without foreign body of forearm

√7ᵗʰ   **S51.811**   Laceration without foreign body of **right forearm**

√7ᵗʰ   **S51.812**   Laceration without foreign body of **left forearm**

√7ᵗʰ   **S51.819**   Laceration without foreign body of unspecified forearm   ▽

√6ᵗʰ   **S51.82**   Laceration with foreign body of forearm

√7ᵗʰ   **S51.821**   Laceration with foreign body of **right forearm**

√7ᵗʰ   **S51.822**   Laceration with foreign body of **left forearm**

√7ᵗʰ   **S51.829**   Laceration with foreign body of unspecified forearm   ▽

√6ᵗʰ   **S51.83**   Puncture wound without foreign body of forearm

√7ᵗʰ   **S51.831**   Puncture wound without foreign body of **right forearm**

√7ᵗʰ   **S51.832**   Puncture wound without foreign body of **left forearm**

√7ᵗʰ   **S51.839**   Puncture wound without foreign body of unspecified forearm

√6ᵗʰ   **S51.84**   Puncture wound with foreign body of forearm

√7ᵗʰ   **S51.841**   Puncture wound with foreign body of **right forearm**

√7ᵗʰ   **S51.842**   Puncture wound with foreign body of **left forearm**

√7ᵗʰ   **S51.849**   Puncture wound with foreign body of unspecified forearm

√6ᵗʰ   **S51.85**   Open bite of forearm
     Bite of forearm NOS
     EXCLUDES 1   *superficial bite of forearm (S50.86, S50.87)*

√7ᵗʰ   **S51.851**   Open bite of **right forearm**

√7ᵗʰ   **S51.852**   Open bite of **left forearm**

√7ᵗʰ   **S51.859**   Open bite of unspecified forearm   ▽

√4ᵗʰ   **S52**   **Fracture of forearm**

NOTE   A fracture not indicated as displaced or nondisplaced should be coded to displaced.

A fracture not indicated as open or closed should be coded to closed.

The open fracture designations are based on the Gustilo open fracture classification.

EXCLUDES 1   *traumatic amputation of forearm (S58.-)*

EXCLUDES 2   *fracture at wrist and hand level (S62.-)*

AHA: 2016,1Q,33; 2015,3Q,37-39

The appropriate 7th character is to be added to all codes from category S52 [unless otherwise indicated].

A   initial encounter for closed fracture
B   initial encounter for open fracture type I or II
     initial encounter for open fracture NOS
C   initial encounter for open fracture type IIIA, IIIB, or IIIC
D   subsequent encounter for closed fracture with routine healing
E   subsequent encounter for open fracture type I or II with routine healing
F   subsequent encounter for open fracture type IIIA, IIIB, or IIIC with routine healing
G   subsequent encounter for closed fracture with delayed healing
H   subsequent encounter for open fracture type I or II with delayed healing
J   subsequent encounter for open fracture type IIIA, IIIB, or IIIC with delayed healing
K   subsequent encounter for closed fracture with nonunion
M   subsequent encounter for open fracture type I or II with nonunion
N   subsequent encounter for open fracture type IIIA, IIIB, or IIIC with nonunion
P   subsequent encounter for closed fracture with malunion
Q   subsequent encounter for open fracture type I or II with malunion
R   subsequent encounter for open fracture type IIIA, IIIB, or IIIC with malunion
S   sequela

√5ᵗʰ   **S52.0**   **Fracture of upper end of ulna**
     Fracture of proximal end of ulna
     EXCLUDES 2   *fracture of elbow NOS (S42.40-)*
               fractures of shaft of ulna (S52.2-)

√6ᵗʰ   **S52.00**   Unspecified fracture of upper end of ulna

√7ᵗʰ   **S52.001**   Unspecified fracture of upper end of **right ulna**   ▽

√7ᵗʰ   **S52.002**   Unspecified fracture of upper end of **left ulna**   ▽

√7ᵗʰ   **S52.009**   Unspecified fracture of upper end of unspecified ulna   ▽

☑ Additional Character Required   √x7ᵗʰ Placeholder Alert   Manifestation Dx   ▽ Unspecified Dx   ▶◀ Revised Text   ● New Code   ▲ Revised Code Title

ICD-10-CM 2017   **939**

Chapter 19. Injury, Poisoning and Certain Other Consequences of External Causes

S52.01–S52.212

√6th **S52.01**   **Torus** fracture of upper end of ulna

> The appropriate 7th character is to be added to all codes in subcategory S52.01
> A   initial encounter for closed fracture
> D   subsequent encounter for fracture with routine healing
> G   subsequent encounter for fracture with delayed healing
> K   subsequent encounter for fracture with nonunion
> P   subsequent encounter for fracture with malunion
> S   sequela

    √7th **S52.011**   Torus fracture of upper end of right ulna
    √7th **S52.012**   Torus fracture of upper end of left ulna
    √7th **S52.019**   Torus fracture of upper end of unspecified ulna ▽

√6th **S52.02**   Fracture of olecranon process without intraarticular extension of ulna

    √7th **S52.021**   Displaced fracture of olecranon process without intraarticular extension of right ulna
    √7th **S52.022**   Displaced fracture of olecranon process without intraarticular extension of left ulna
    √7th **S52.023**   Displaced fracture of olecranon process without intraarticular extension of unspecified ulna ▽
    √7th **S52.024**   Nondisplaced fracture of olecranon process without intraarticular extension of right ulna
    √7th **S52.025**   Nondisplaced fracture of olecranon process without intraarticular extension of left ulna
    √7th **S52.026**   Nondisplaced fracture of olecranon process without intraarticular extension of unspecified ulna ▽

√6th **S52.03**   Fracture of olecranon process with intraarticular extension of ulna

    √7th **S52.031**   Displaced fracture of olecranon process with intraarticular extension of right ulna
    √7th **S52.032**   Displaced fracture of olecranon process with intraarticular extension of left ulna
    √7th **S52.033**   Displaced fracture of olecranon process with intraarticular extension of unspecified ulna ▽
    √7th **S52.034**   Nondisplaced fracture of olecranon process with intraarticular extension of right ulna
    √7th **S52.035**   Nondisplaced fracture of olecranon process with intraarticular extension of left ulna
    √7th **S52.036**   Nondisplaced fracture of olecranon process with intraarticular extension of unspecified ulna ▽

√6th **S52.04**   Fracture of coronoid process of ulna

    √7th **S52.041**   Displaced fracture of coronoid process of right ulna
    √7th **S52.042**   Displaced fracture of coronoid process of left ulna
    √7th **S52.043**   Displaced fracture of coronoid process of unspecified ulna ▽
    √7th **S52.044**   Nondisplaced fracture of coronoid process of right ulna
    √7th **S52.045**   Nondisplaced fracture of coronoid process of left ulna
    √7th **S52.046**   Nondisplaced fracture of coronoid process of unspecified ulna ▽

√6th **S52.09**   Other fracture of upper end of ulna

    √7th **S52.091**   Other fracture of upper end of right ulna
    √7th **S52.092**   Other fracture of upper end of left ulna
    √7th **S52.099**   Other fracture of upper end of unspecified ulna ▽

√5th **S52.1**   Fracture of upper end of radius

> Fracture of proximal end of radius
> EXCLUDES 2   physeal fractures of upper end of radius (S59.2-)
>   fracture of shaft of radius (S52.3-)

√6th **S52.10**   Unspecified fracture of upper end of radius

    √7th **S52.101**   Unspecified fracture of upper end of right radius ▽
    √7th **S52.102**   Unspecified fracture of upper end of left radius ▽
    √7th **S52.109**   Unspecified fracture of upper end of unspecified radius ▽

√6th **S52.11**   **Torus** fracture of upper end of radius

> The appropriate 7th character is to be added to all codes in subcategory S52.11
> A   initial encounter for closed fracture
> D   subsequent encounter for fracture with routine healing
> G   subsequent encounter for fracture with delayed healing
> K   subsequent encounter for fracture with nonunion
> P   subsequent encounter for fracture with malunion
> S   sequela

    √7th **S52.111**   Torus fracture of upper end of right radius
    √7th **S52.112**   Torus fracture of upper end of left radius
    √7th **S52.119**   Torus fracture of upper end of unspecified radius ▽

√6th **S52.12**   Fracture of head of radius

    √7th **S52.121**   Displaced fracture of head of right radius
    √7th **S52.122**   Displaced fracture of head of left radius
    √7th **S52.123**   Displaced fracture of head of unspecified radius ▽
    √7th **S52.124**   Nondisplaced fracture of head of right radius
    √7th **S52.125**   Nondisplaced fracture of head of left radius
    √7th **S52.126**   Nondisplaced fracture of head of unspecified radius ▽

√6th **S52.13**   Fracture of neck of radius

    √7th **S52.131**   Displaced fracture of neck of right radius
    √7th **S52.132**   Displaced fracture of neck of left radius
    √7th **S52.133**   Displaced fracture of neck of unspecified radius ▽
    √7th **S52.134**   Nondisplaced fracture of neck of right radius
    √7th **S52.135**   Nondisplaced fracture of neck of left radius
    √7th **S52.136**   Nondisplaced fracture of neck of unspecified radius ▽

√6th **S52.18**   Other fracture of upper end of radius

    √7th **S52.181**   Other fracture of upper end of right radius
    √7th **S52.182**   Other fracture of upper end of left radius
    √7th **S52.189**   Other fracture of upper end of unspecified radius ▽

√5th **S52.2**   Fracture of shaft of ulna

√6th **S52.20**   Unspecified fracture of shaft of ulna

> Fracture of ulna NOS

    √7th **S52.201**   Unspecified fracture of shaft of right ulna ▽
    √7th **S52.202**   Unspecified fracture of shaft of left ulna ▽
    √7th **S52.209**   Unspecified fracture of shaft of unspecified ulna ▽

√6th **S52.21**   **Greenstick** fracture of shaft of ulna

> The appropriate 7th character is to be added to all codes in subcategory S52.21
> A   initial encounter for closed fracture
> D   subsequent encounter for fracture with routine healing
> G   subsequent encounter for fracture with delayed healing
> K   subsequent encounter for fracture with nonunion
> P   subsequent encounter for fracture with malunion
> S   sequela

    √7th **S52.211**   Greenstick fracture of shaft of right ulna
    √7th **S52.212**   Greenstick fracture of shaft of left ulna

---

EXCLUDES 1 Not coded here   EXCLUDES 2 Not included here   N Newborn Age : 0   P Pediatric Age : 0-17   M Maternity Age : 12-55   A Adult Age : 15-124

940

ICD-10-CM 2017

√7ᵗʰ **S52.219 Greenstick fracture of shaft of unspecified ulna** ▽

√6ᵗʰ **S52.22 Transverse fracture of shaft of ulna**

√7ᵗʰ **S52.221 Displaced transverse fracture of shaft of right ulna**

√7ᵗʰ **S52.222 Displaced transverse fracture of shaft of left ulna**

√7ᵗʰ **S52.223 Displaced transverse fracture of shaft of unspecified ulna** ▽

√7ᵗʰ **S52.224 Nondisplaced transverse fracture of shaft of right ulna**

√7ᵗʰ **S52.225 Nondisplaced transverse fracture of shaft of left ulna**

√7ᵗʰ **S52.226 Nondisplaced transverse fracture of shaft of unspecified ulna** ▽

√6ᵗʰ **S52.23 Oblique fracture of shaft of ulna**

√7ᵗʰ **S52.231 Displaced oblique fracture of shaft of right ulna**

√7ᵗʰ **S52.232 Displaced oblique fracture of shaft of left ulna**

√7ᵗʰ **S52.233 Displaced oblique fracture of shaft of unspecified ulna** ▽

√7ᵗʰ **S52.234 Nondisplaced oblique fracture of shaft of right ulna**

√7ᵗʰ **S52.235 Nondisplaced oblique fracture of shaft of left ulna**

√7ᵗʰ **S52.236 Nondisplaced oblique fracture of shaft of unspecified ulna** ▽

√6ᵗʰ **S52.24 Spiral fracture of shaft of ulna**

√7ᵗʰ **S52.241 Displaced spiral fracture of shaft of ulna, right arm**

√7ᵗʰ **S52.242 Displaced spiral fracture of shaft of ulna, left arm**

√7ᵗʰ **S52.243 Displaced spiral fracture of shaft of ulna, unspecified arm** ▽

√7ᵗʰ **S52.244 Nondisplaced spiral fracture of shaft of ulna, right arm**

√7ᵗʰ **S52.245 Nondisplaced spiral fracture of shaft of ulna, left arm**

√7ᵗʰ **S52.246 Nondisplaced spiral fracture of shaft of ulna, unspecified arm** ▽

√6ᵗʰ **S52.25 Comminuted fracture of shaft of ulna**

√7ᵗʰ **S52.251 Displaced comminuted fracture of shaft of ulna, right arm**

√7ᵗʰ **S52.252 Displaced comminuted fracture of shaft of ulna, left arm**

√7ᵗʰ **S52.253 Displaced comminuted fracture of shaft of ulna, unspecified arm** ▽

√7ᵗʰ **S52.254 Nondisplaced comminuted fracture of shaft of ulna, right arm**

√7ᵗʰ **S52.255 Nondisplaced comminuted fracture of shaft of ulna, left arm**

√7ᵗʰ **S52.256 Nondisplaced comminuted fracture of shaft of ulna, unspecified arm** ▽

√6ᵗʰ **S52.26 Segmental fracture of shaft of ulna**

√7ᵗʰ **S52.261 Displaced segmental fracture of shaft of ulna, right arm**

√7ᵗʰ **S52.262 Displaced segmental fracture of shaft of ulna, left arm**

√7ᵗʰ **S52.263 Displaced segmental fracture of shaft of ulna, unspecified arm** ▽

√7ᵗʰ **S52.264 Nondisplaced segmental fracture of shaft of ulna, right arm**

√7ᵗʰ **S52.265 Nondisplaced segmental fracture of shaft of ulna, left arm**

√7ᵗʰ **S52.266 Nondisplaced segmental fracture of shaft of ulna, unspecified arm** ▽

√6ᵗʰ **S52.27 Monteggia's fracture of ulna**

Fracture of upper shaft of ulna with dislocation of radial head

√7ᵗʰ **S52.271 Monteggia's fracture of right ulna**

√7ᵗʰ **S52.272 Monteggia's fracture of left ulna**

√7ᵗʰ **S52.279 Monteggia's fracture of unspecified ulna** ▽

√6ᵗʰ **S52.28 Bent bone of ulna**

√7ᵗʰ **S52.281 Bent bone of right ulna**

√7ᵗʰ **S52.282 Bent bone of left ulna**

√7ᵗʰ **S52.283 Bent bone of unspecified ulna** ▽

√6ᵗʰ **S52.29 Other fracture of shaft of ulna**

√7ᵗʰ **S52.291 Other fracture of shaft of right ulna**

√7ᵗʰ **S52.292 Other fracture of shaft of left ulna**

√7ᵗʰ **S52.299 Other fracture of shaft of unspecified ulna** ▽

√5ᵗʰ **S52.3 Fracture of shaft of radius**

√6ᵗʰ **S52.30 Unspecified fracture of shaft of radius**

√7ᵗʰ **S52.301 Unspecified fracture of shaft of right radius** ▽

√7ᵗʰ **S52.302 Unspecified fracture of shaft of left radius** ▽

√7ᵗʰ **S52.309 Unspecified fracture of shaft of unspecified radius** ▽

√6ᵗʰ **S52.31 Greenstick fracture of shaft of radius**

The appropriate 7th character is to be added to all codes in subcategory S52.31
A   initial encounter for closed fracture
D   subsequent encounter for fracture with routine healing
G   subsequent encounter for fracture with delayed healing
K   subsequent encounter for fracture with nonunion
P   subsequent encounter for fracture with malunion
S   sequela

√7ᵗʰ **S52.311 Greenstick fracture of shaft of radius, right arm**

√7ᵗʰ **S52.312 Greenstick fracture of shaft of radius, left arm**

√7ᵗʰ **S52.319 Greenstick fracture of shaft of radius, unspecified arm** ▽

√6ᵗʰ **S52.32 Transverse fracture of shaft of radius**

√7ᵗʰ **S52.321 Displaced transverse fracture of shaft of right radius**

√7ᵗʰ **S52.322 Displaced transverse fracture of shaft of left radius**

√7ᵗʰ **S52.323 Displaced transverse fracture of shaft of unspecified radius** ▽

√7ᵗʰ **S52.324 Nondisplaced transverse fracture of shaft of right radius**

√7ᵗʰ **S52.325 Nondisplaced transverse fracture of shaft of left radius**

√7ᵗʰ **S52.326 Nondisplaced transverse fracture of shaft of unspecified radius** ▽

√6ᵗʰ **S52.33 Oblique fracture of shaft of radius**

√7ᵗʰ **S52.331 Displaced oblique fracture of shaft of right radius**

√7ᵗʰ **S52.332 Displaced oblique fracture of shaft of left radius**

√7ᵗʰ **S52.333 Displaced oblique fracture of shaft of unspecified radius** ▽

√7ᵗʰ **S52.334 Nondisplaced oblique fracture of shaft of right radius**

√7ᵗʰ **S52.335 Nondisplaced oblique fracture of shaft of left radius**

√7ᵗʰ **S52.336 Nondisplaced oblique fracture of shaft of unspecified radius** ▽

√6ᵗʰ **S52.34 Spiral fracture of shaft of radius**

√7ᵗʰ **S52.341 Displaced spiral fracture of shaft of radius, right arm**

√7ᵗʰ **S52.342 Displaced spiral fracture of shaft of radius, left arm**

√7ᵗʰ **S52.343 Displaced spiral fracture of shaft of radius, unspecified arm** ▽

√7ᵗʰ **S52.344 Nondisplaced spiral fracture of shaft of radius, right arm**

√7ᵗʰ **S52.345 Nondisplaced spiral fracture of shaft of radius, left arm**

√7ᵗʰ **S52.346 Nondisplaced spiral fracture of shaft of radius, unspecified arm** ▽

√6ᵗʰ **S52.35 Comminuted fracture of shaft of radius**

√7ᵗʰ **S52.351 Displaced comminuted fracture of shaft of radius, right arm**

√7ᵗʰ **S52.352 Displaced comminuted fracture of shaft of radius, left arm**

√7ᵗʰ **S52.353 Displaced comminuted fracture of shaft of radius, unspecified arm** ▽

√7ᵗʰ **S52.354 Nondisplaced comminuted fracture of shaft of radius, right arm**

✔ Additional Character Required   √7ᵗʰ Placeholder Alert   Manifestation Dx   ▽ Unspecified Dx   ►◄ Revised Text   ● New Code   ▲ Revised Code Title

- √7ᵗʰ **S52.355** **Nondisplaced comminuted fracture of shaft of radius, left arm**
- √7ᵗʰ **S52.356** **Nondisplaced comminuted fracture of shaft of radius, unspecified arm** ▽
- √6ᵗʰ **S52.36** **Segmental fracture of shaft of radius**
  - √7ᵗʰ **S52.361** **Displaced segmental fracture of shaft of radius, right arm**
  - √7ᵗʰ **S52.362** **Displaced segmental fracture of shaft of radius, left arm**
  - √7ᵗʰ **S52.363** **Displaced segmental fracture of shaft of radius, unspecified arm** ▽
  - √7ᵗʰ **S52.364** **Nondisplaced segmental fracture of shaft of radius, right arm**
  - √7ᵗʰ **S52.365** **Nondisplaced segmental fracture of shaft of radius, left arm**
  - √7ᵗʰ **S52.366** **Nondisplaced segmental fracture of shaft of radius, unspecified arm** ▽
- √6ᵗʰ **S52.37** **Galeazzi's fracture**

  Fracture of lower shaft of radius with radioulnar joint dislocation
  - √7ᵗʰ **S52.371** **Galeazzi's fracture of right radius**
  - √7ᵗʰ **S52.372** **Galeazzi's fracture of left radius**
  - √7ᵗʰ **S52.379** **Galeazzi's fracture of unspecified radius** ▽
- √6ᵗʰ **S52.38** **Bent bone of radius**
  - √7ᵗʰ **S52.381** **Bent bone of right radius**
  - √7ᵗʰ **S52.382** **Bent bone of left radius**
  - √7ᵗʰ **S52.389** **Bent bone of unspecified radius** ▽
- √6ᵗʰ **S52.39** **Other fracture of shaft of radius**
  - √7ᵗʰ **S52.391** **Other fracture of shaft of radius, right arm**
  - √7ᵗʰ **S52.392** **Other fracture of shaft of radius, left arm**
  - √7ᵗʰ **S52.399** **Other fracture of shaft of radius, unspecified arm** ▽
- √5ᵗʰ **S52.5** **Fracture of lower end of radius**

  Fracture of distal end of radius

  EXCLUDES 2 *physeal fractures of lower end of radius (S59.2-)*
  - √6ᵗʰ **S52.50** **Unspecified fracture of the lower end of radius**
    - √7ᵗʰ **S52.501** **Unspecified fracture of the lower end of right radius** ▽
    - √7ᵗʰ **S52.502** **Unspecified fracture of the lower end of left radius** ▽
    - √7ᵗʰ **S52.509** **Unspecified fracture of the lower end of unspecified radius** ▽
  - √6ᵗʰ **S52.51** **Fracture of radial styloid process**
    - √7ᵗʰ **S52.511** **Displaced fracture of right radial styloid process**
    - √7ᵗʰ **S52.512** **Displaced fracture of left radial styloid process**
    - √7ᵗʰ **S52.513** **Displaced fracture of unspecified radial styloid process** ▽
    - √7ᵗʰ **S52.514** **Nondisplaced fracture of right radial styloid process**
    - √7ᵗʰ **S52.515** **Nondisplaced fracture of left radial styloid process**
    - √7ᵗʰ **S52.516** **Nondisplaced fracture of unspecified radial styloid process** ▽
  - √6ᵗʰ **S52.52** **Torus fracture of lower end of radius**

    The appropriate 7th character is to be added to all codes in subcategory S52.52
    - A   initial encounter for closed fracture
    - D   subsequent encounter for fracture with routine healing
    - G   subsequent encounter for fracture with delayed healing
    - K   subsequent encounter for fracture with nonunion
    - P   subsequent encounter for fracture with malunion
    - S   sequela
    - √7ᵗʰ **S52.521** **Torus fracture of lower end of right radius**
    - √7ᵗʰ **S52.522** **Torus fracture of lower end of left radius**
    - √7ᵗʰ **S52.529** **Torus fracture of lower end of unspecified radius** ▽

- √6ᵗʰ **S52.53** **Colles' fracture**

  AHA: 2016,2Q,4
  - √7ᵗʰ **S52.531** **Colles' fracture of right radius**
  - √7ᵗʰ **S52.532** **Colles' fracture of left radius**
  - √7ᵗʰ **S52.539** **Colles' fracture of unspecified radius** ▽
- √6ᵗʰ **S52.54** **Smith's fracture**
  - √7ᵗʰ **S52.541** **Smith's fracture of right radius**
  - √7ᵗʰ **S52.542** **Smith's fracture of left radius**
  - √7ᵗʰ **S52.549** **Smith's fracture of unspecified radius** ▽
- √6ᵗʰ **S52.55** **Other extraarticular fracture of lower end of radius**
  - √7ᵗʰ **S52.551** **Other extraarticular fracture of lower end of right radius**
  - √7ᵗʰ **S52.552** **Other extraarticular fracture of lower end of left radius**
  - √7ᵗʰ **S52.559** **Other extraarticular fracture of lower end of unspecified radius** ▽
- √6ᵗʰ **S52.56** **Barton's fracture**
  - √7ᵗʰ **S52.561** **Barton's fracture of right radius**
  - √7ᵗʰ **S52.562** **Barton's fracture of left radius**
  - √7ᵗʰ **S52.569** **Barton's fracture of unspecified radius** ▽
- √6ᵗʰ **S52.57** **Other intraarticular fracture of lower end of radius**
  - √7ᵗʰ **S52.571** **Other intraarticular fracture of lower end of right radius**
  - √7ᵗʰ **S52.572** **Other intraarticular fracture of lower end of left radius**
  - √7ᵗʰ **S52.579** **Other intraarticular fracture of lower end of unspecified radius** ▽
- √6ᵗʰ **S52.59** **Other fractures of lower end of radius**
  - √7ᵗʰ **S52.591** **Other fractures of lower end of right radius**
  - √7ᵗʰ **S52.592** **Other fractures of lower end of left radius**
  - √7ᵗʰ **S52.599** **Other fractures of lower end of unspecified radius** ▽
- √5ᵗʰ **S52.6** **Fracture of lower end of ulna**
  - √6ᵗʰ **S52.60** **Unspecified fracture of lower end of ulna**
    - √7ᵗʰ **S52.601** **Unspecified fracture of lower end of right ulna** ▽
    - √7ᵗʰ **S52.602** **Unspecified fracture of lower end of left ulna** ▽
    - √7ᵗʰ **S52.609** **Unspecified fracture of lower end of unspecified ulna** ▽
  - √6ᵗʰ **S52.61** **Fracture of ulna styloid process**
    - √7ᵗʰ **S52.611** **Displaced fracture of right ulna styloid process**
    - √7ᵗʰ **S52.612** **Displaced fracture of left ulna styloid process**
    - √7ᵗʰ **S52.613** **Displaced fracture of unspecified ulna styloid process**
    - √7ᵗʰ **S52.614** **Nondisplaced fracture of right ulna styloid process**
    - √7ᵗʰ **S52.615** **Nondisplaced fracture of left ulna styloid process**
    - √7ᵗʰ **S52.616** **Nondisplaced fracture of unspecified ulna styloid process** ▽
  - √6ᵗʰ **S52.62** **Torus fracture of lower end of ulna**

    The appropriate 7th character is to be added to all codes in subcategory S52.62
    - A   initial encounter for closed fracture
    - D   subsequent encounter for fracture with routine healing
    - G   subsequent encounter for fracture with delayed healing
    - K   subsequent encounter for fracture with nonunion
    - P   subsequent encounter for fracture with malunion
    - S   sequela
    - √7ᵗʰ **S52.621** **Torus fracture of lower end of right ulna**
    - √7ᵗʰ **S52.622** **Torus fracture of lower end of left ulna**
    - √7ᵗʰ **S52.629** **Torus fracture of lower end of unspecified ulna** ▽
  - √6ᵗʰ **S52.69** **Other fracture of lower end of ulna**
    - √7ᵗʰ **S52.691** **Other fracture of lower end of right ulna**

EXCLUDES 1 Not coded here   EXCLUDES 2 Not included here   N Newborn Age : 0   P Pediatric Age : 0-17   M Maternity Age : 12-55   A Adult Age : 15-124

√7ᵗʰ **S52.692** Other fracture of lower end of left ulna

√7ᵗʰ **S52.699** Other fracture of lower end of unspecified ulna ▽

√5ᵗʰ **S52.9** **Unspecified fracture of forearm**

√x7ᵗʰ **S52.90** Unspecified fracture of unspecified forearm ▽

√x7ᵗʰ **S52.91** Unspecified fracture of right forearm ▽

√x7ᵗʰ **S52.92** Unspecified fracture of left forearm ▽

√4ᵗʰ **S53** **Dislocation and sprain of joints and ligaments of elbow**

INCLUDES avulsion of joint or ligament of elbow
laceration of cartilage, joint or ligament of elbow
sprain of cartilage, joint or ligament of elbow
traumatic hemarthrosis of joint or ligament of elbow
traumatic rupture of joint or ligament of elbow
traumatic subluxation of joint or ligament of elbow
traumatic tear of joint or ligament of elbow

Code also any associated open wound

EXCLUDES 2 *strain of muscle, fascia and tendon at forearm level (S56.-)*

The appropriate 7th character is to be added to each code from category S53.
A initial encounter
D subsequent encounter
S sequela

√5ᵗʰ **S53.0** **Subluxation and dislocation of radial head**

Dislocation of radiohumeral joint
Subluxation of radiohumeral joint

EXCLUDES 1 *Monteggia's fracture-dislocation (S52.27-)*

√6ᵗʰ **S53.00** Unspecified subluxation and dislocation of radial head

√7ᵗʰ **S53.001** Unspecified subluxation of right radial head ▽

√7ᵗʰ **S53.002** Unspecified subluxation of left radial head ▽

√7ᵗʰ **S53.003** Unspecified subluxation of unspecified radial head ▽

√7ᵗʰ **S53.004** Unspecified dislocation of right radial head ▽

√7ᵗʰ **S53.005** Unspecified dislocation of left radial head ▽

√7ᵗʰ **S53.006** Unspecified dislocation of unspecified radial head ▽

√6ᵗʰ **S53.01** Anterior subluxation and dislocation of radial head

Anteriomedial subluxation and dislocation of radial head

√7ᵗʰ **S53.011** Anterior subluxation of right radial head

√7ᵗʰ **S53.012** Anterior subluxation of left radial head

√7ᵗʰ **S53.013** Anterior subluxation of unspecified radial head ▽

√7ᵗʰ **S53.014** Anterior dislocation of right radial head

√7ᵗʰ **S53.015** Anterior dislocation of left radial head

√7ᵗʰ **S53.016** Anterior dislocation of unspecified radial head ▽

√6ᵗʰ **S53.02** Posterior subluxation and dislocation of radial head

Posteriolateral subluxation and dislocation of radial head

√7ᵗʰ **S53.021** Posterior subluxation of right radial head

√7ᵗʰ **S53.022** Posterior subluxation of left radial head

√7ᵗʰ **S53.023** Posterior subluxation of unspecified radial head ▽

√7ᵗʰ **S53.024** Posterior dislocation of right radial head

√7ᵗʰ **S53.025** Posterior dislocation of left radial head

√7ᵗʰ **S53.026** Posterior dislocation of unspecified radial head ▽

√6ᵗʰ **S53.03** Nursemaid's elbow

√7ᵗʰ **S53.031** Nursemaid's elbow, right elbow

√7ᵗʰ **S53.032** Nursemaid's elbow, left elbow

√7ᵗʰ **S53.033** Nursemaid's elbow, unspecified elbow ▽

√6ᵗʰ **S53.09** Other subluxation and dislocation of radial head

√7ᵗʰ **S53.091** Other subluxation of right radial head

√7ᵗʰ **S53.092** Other subluxation of left radial head

√7ᵗʰ **S53.093** Other subluxation of unspecified radial head ▽

√7ᵗʰ **S53.094** Other dislocation of right radial head

√7ᵗʰ **S53.095** Other dislocation of left radial head

√7ᵗʰ **S53.096** Other dislocation of unspecified radial head ▽

√5ᵗʰ **S53.1** **Subluxation and dislocation of ulnohumeral joint**

Subluxation and dislocation of elbow NOS

EXCLUDES 1 *dislocation of radial head alone (S53.0-)*

√6ᵗʰ **S53.10** Unspecified subluxation and dislocation of ulnohumeral joint

√7ᵗʰ **S53.101** Unspecified subluxation of right ulnohumeral joint ▽

√7ᵗʰ **S53.102** Unspecified subluxation of left ulnohumeral joint ▽

√7ᵗʰ **S53.103** Unspecified subluxation of unspecified ulnohumeral joint ▽

√7ᵗʰ **S53.104** Unspecified dislocation of right ulnohumeral joint ▽

√7ᵗʰ **S53.105** Unspecified dislocation of left ulnohumeral joint ▽

√7ᵗʰ **S53.106** Unspecified dislocation of unspecified ulnohumeral joint ▽

√6ᵗʰ **S53.11** Anterior subluxation and dislocation of ulnohumeral joint

√7ᵗʰ **S53.111** Anterior subluxation of right ulnohumeral joint

√7ᵗʰ **S53.112** Anterior subluxation of left ulnohumeral joint

√7ᵗʰ **S53.113** Anterior subluxation of unspecified ulnohumeral joint ▽

√7ᵗʰ **S53.114** Anterior dislocation of right ulnohumeral joint

AHA: 2012,4Q,108

√7ᵗʰ **S53.115** Anterior dislocation of left ulnohumeral joint

√7ᵗʰ **S53.116** Anterior dislocation of unspecified ulnohumeral joint ▽

√6ᵗʰ **S53.12** Posterior subluxation and dislocation of ulnohumeral joint

√7ᵗʰ **S53.121** Posterior subluxation of right ulnohumeral joint

√7ᵗʰ **S53.122** Posterior subluxation of left ulnohumeral joint

√7ᵗʰ **S53.123** Posterior subluxation of unspecified ulnohumeral joint ▽

√7ᵗʰ **S53.124** Posterior dislocation of right ulnohumeral joint

√7ᵗʰ **S53.125** Posterior dislocation of left ulnohumeral joint

√7ᵗʰ **S53.126** Posterior dislocation of unspecified ulnohumeral joint ▽

√6ᵗʰ **S53.13** Medial subluxation and dislocation of ulnohumeral joint

√7ᵗʰ **S53.131** Medial subluxation of right ulnohumeral joint

√7ᵗʰ **S53.132** Medial subluxation of left ulnohumeral joint

√7ᵗʰ **S53.133** Medial subluxation of unspecified ulnohumeral joint ▽

√7ᵗʰ **S53.134** Medial dislocation of right ulnohumeral joint

√7ᵗʰ **S53.135** Medial dislocation of left ulnohumeral joint

√7ᵗʰ **S53.136** Medial dislocation of unspecified ulnohumeral joint ▽

√6ᵗʰ **S53.14** Lateral subluxation and dislocation of ulnohumeral joint

√7ᵗʰ **S53.141** Lateral subluxation of right ulnohumeral joint

√7ᵗʰ **S53.142** Lateral subluxation of left ulnohumeral joint

√7ᵗʰ **S53.143** Lateral subluxation of unspecified ulnohumeral joint ▽

√7ᵗʰ **S53.144** Lateral dislocation of right ulnohumeral joint

√7ᵗʰ **S53.145** Lateral dislocation of left ulnohumeral joint

√7ᵗʰ **S53.146** Lateral dislocation of unspecified ulnohumeral joint ▽

√6ᵗʰ **S53.19** Other subluxation and dislocation of ulnohumeral joint

√7ᵗʰ **S53.191** Other subluxation of right ulnohumeral joint

√7ᵗʰ **S53.192** Other subluxation of left ulnohumeral joint

☑ Additional Character Required   √x7ᵗʰ Placeholder Alert   Manifestation Dx   ▽Unspecified Dx   ▶◀ Revised Text   ● New Code   ▲ Revised Code Title

√7th **S53.193**   Other subluxation of unspecified ulnohumeral joint

√7th **S53.194**   Other dislocation of right ulnohumeral joint

√7th **S53.195**   Other dislocation of left ulnohumeral joint

√7th **S53.196**   Other dislocation of unspecified ulnohumeral joint

√5th **S53.2**   **Traumatic rupture of radial collateral ligament**

    EXCLUDES 1   *sprain of radial collateral ligament NOS (S53.43-)*

√x7th **S53.20**   Traumatic rupture of unspecified radial collateral ligament

√x7th **S53.21**   Traumatic rupture of right radial collateral ligament

√x7th **S53.22**   Traumatic rupture of left radial collateral ligament

√5th **S53.3**   **Traumatic rupture of ulnar collateral ligament**

    EXCLUDES 1   *sprain of ulnar collateral ligament (S53.44-)*

√x7th **S53.30**   Traumatic rupture of unspecified ulnar collateral ligament

√x7th **S53.31**   Traumatic rupture of right ulnar collateral ligament

√x7th **S53.32**   Traumatic rupture of left ulnar collateral ligament

√5th **S53.4**   **Sprain of elbow**

    EXCLUDES 2   *traumatic rupture of radial collateral ligament (S53.2-)* ▲

            traumatic rupture of ulnar collateral ligament (S53.3-) ▲

√6th **S53.40**   Unspecified sprain of elbow

    √7th **S53.401**   Unspecified sprain of right elbow

    √7th **S53.402**   Unspecified sprain of left elbow ▲

    √7th **S53.409**   Unspecified sprain of unspecified elbow

              Sprain of elbow NOS

√6th **S53.41**   Radiohumeral (joint) sprain

    √7th **S53.411**   Radiohumeral (joint) sprain of right elbow

    √7th **S53.412**   Radiohumeral (joint) sprain of left elbow

    √7th **S53.419**   Radiohumeral (joint) sprain of unspecified elbow

√6th **S53.42**   Ulnohumeral (joint) sprain

    √7th **S53.421**   Ulnohumeral (joint) sprain of right elbow

    √7th **S53.422**   Ulnohumeral (joint) sprain of left elbow

    √7th **S53.429**   Ulnohumeral (joint) sprain of unspecified elbow

√6th **S53.43**   Radial collateral ligament sprain

    √7th **S53.431**   Radial collateral ligament sprain of right elbow

    √7th **S53.432**   Radial collateral ligament sprain of left elbow

    √7th **S53.439**   Radial collateral ligament sprain of unspecified elbow

√6th **S53.44**   Ulnar collateral ligament sprain

    √7th **S53.441**   Ulnar collateral ligament sprain of right elbow

    √7th **S53.442**   Ulnar collateral ligament sprain of left elbow

    √7th **S53.449**   Ulnar collateral ligament sprain of unspecified elbow

√6th **S53.49**   Other sprain of elbow

    √7th **S53.491**   Other sprain of right elbow

    √7th **S53.492**   Other sprain of left elbow

    √7th **S53.499**   Other sprain of unspecified elbow

√4th **S54**   **Injury of nerves at forearm level**

    Code also any associated open wound (S51.-)

    EXCLUDES 2   *injury of nerves at wrist and hand level (S64.-)*

    The appropriate 7th character is to be added to each code from category S54.
    A   initial encounter
    D   subsequent encounter
    S   sequela

√5th **S54.0**   **Injury of ulnar nerve at forearm level**

    Injury of ulnar nerve NOS

√x7th **S54.00**   Injury of ulnar nerve at forearm level, unspecified arm

√x7th **S54.01**   Injury of ulnar nerve at forearm level, right arm

√x7th **S54.02**   Injury of ulnar nerve at forearm level, left arm

√5th **S54.1**   **Injury of median nerve at forearm level**

    Injury of median nerve NOS

√x7th **S54.10**   Injury of median nerve at forearm level, unspecified arm

√x7th **S54.11**   Injury of median nerve at forearm level, right arm

√x7th **S54.12**   Injury of median nerve at forearm level, left arm

√5th **S54.2**   **Injury of radial nerve at forearm level**

    Injury of radial nerve NOS

√x7th **S54.20**   Injury of radial nerve at forearm level, unspecified arm

√x7th **S54.21**   Injury of radial nerve at forearm level, right arm

√x7th **S54.22**   Injury of radial nerve at forearm level, left arm

√5th **S54.3**   **Injury of cutaneous sensory nerve at forearm level**

√x7th **S54.30**   Injury of cutaneous sensory nerve at forearm level, unspecified arm

√x7th **S54.31**   Injury of cutaneous sensory nerve at forearm level, right arm

√x7th **S54.32**   Injury of cutaneous sensory nerve at forearm level, left arm

√5th **S54.8**   **Injury of other nerves at forearm level**

√6th **S54.8X**   Injury of other nerves at forearm level

    √7th **S54.8X1**   Injury of other nerves at forearm level, right arm

    √7th **S54.8X2**   Injury of other nerves at forearm level, left arm

    √7th **S54.8X9**   Injury of other nerves at forearm level, unspecified arm

√5th **S54.9**   **Injury of unspecified nerve at forearm level**

√x7th **S54.90**   Injury of unspecified nerve at forearm level, unspecified arm

√x7th **S54.91**   Injury of unspecified nerve at forearm level, right arm

√x7th **S54.92**   Injury of unspecified nerve at forearm level, left arm

√4th **S55**   **Injury of blood vessels at forearm level**

    Code also any associated open wound (S51.-)

    EXCLUDES 2   *injury of blood vessels at wrist and hand level (S65.-)*

           injury of brachial vessels (S45.1-S45.2)

    The appropriate 7th character is to be added to each code from category S55.
    A   initial encounter
    D   subsequent encounter
    S   sequela

√5th **S55.0**   **Injury of ulnar artery at forearm level**

√6th **S55.00**   Unspecified injury of ulnar artery at forearm level

    √7th **S55.001**   Unspecified injury of ulnar artery at forearm level, right arm

    √7th **S55.002**   Unspecified injury of ulnar artery at forearm level, left arm

    √7th **S55.009**   Unspecified injury of ulnar artery at forearm level, unspecified arm

√6th **S55.01**   Laceration of ulnar artery at forearm level

    √7th **S55.011**   Laceration of ulnar artery at forearm level, right arm

    √7th **S55.012**   Laceration of ulnar artery at forearm level, left arm

    √7th **S55.019**   Laceration of ulnar artery at forearm level, unspecified arm

√6th **S55.09**   Other specified injury of ulnar artery at forearm level

    √7th **S55.091**   Other specified injury of ulnar artery at forearm level, right arm

    √7th **S55.092**   Other specified injury of ulnar artery at forearm level, left arm

    √7th **S55.099**   Other specified injury of ulnar artery at forearm level, unspecified arm

√5th **S55.1**   **Injury of radial artery at forearm level**

√6th **S55.10**   Unspecified injury of radial artery at forearm level

    √7th **S55.101**   Unspecified injury of radial artery at forearm level, right arm

    √7th **S55.102**   Unspecified injury of radial artery at forearm level, left arm

    √7th **S55.109**   Unspecified injury of radial artery at forearm level, unspecified arm

EXCLUDES 1 Not coded here   EXCLUDES 2 Not included here   N Newborn Age : 0   P Pediatric Age : 0-17   M Maternity Age : 12-55   A Adult Age : 15-124

944   ICD-10-CM 2017

√6ᵗʰ **S55.11** Laceration of radial artery at forearm level

    √7ᵗʰ **S55.111** Laceration of radial artery at forearm level, right arm

    √7ᵗʰ **S55.112** Laceration of radial artery at forearm level, left arm

    √7ᵗʰ **S55.119** Laceration of radial artery at forearm level, unspecified arm ▽

√6ᵗʰ **S55.19** Other specified injury of radial artery at forearm level

    √7ᵗʰ **S55.191** Other specified injury of radial artery at forearm level, right arm

    √7ᵗʰ **S55.192** Other specified injury of radial artery at forearm level, left arm

    √7ᵗʰ **S55.199** Other specified injury of radial artery at forearm level, unspecified arm ▽

√5ᵗʰ **S55.2** Injury of vein at forearm level

  √6ᵗʰ **S55.20** Unspecified injury of vein at forearm level

    √7ᵗʰ **S55.201** Unspecified injury of vein at forearm level, right arm ▽

    √7ᵗʰ **S55.202** Unspecified injury of vein at forearm level, left arm ▽

    √7ᵗʰ **S55.209** Unspecified injury of vein at forearm level, unspecified arm ▽

  √6ᵗʰ **S55.21** Laceration of vein at forearm level

    √7ᵗʰ **S55.211** Laceration of vein at forearm level, right arm

    √7ᵗʰ **S55.212** Laceration of vein at forearm level, left arm

    √7ᵗʰ **S55.219** Laceration of vein at forearm level, unspecified arm ▽

  √6ᵗʰ **S55.29** Other specified injury of vein at forearm level

    √7ᵗʰ **S55.291** Other specified injury of vein at forearm level, right arm

    √7ᵗʰ **S55.292** Other specified injury of vein at forearm level, left arm

    √7ᵗʰ **S55.299** Other specified injury of vein at forearm level, unspecified arm ▽

√5ᵗʰ **S55.8** Injury of other blood vessels at forearm level

  √6ᵗʰ **S55.80** Unspecified injury of other blood vessels at forearm level

    √7ᵗʰ **S55.801** Unspecified injury of other blood vessels at forearm level, right arm ▽

    √7ᵗʰ **S55.802** Unspecified injury of other blood vessels at forearm level, left arm ▽

    √7ᵗʰ **S55.809** Unspecified injury of other blood vessels at forearm level, unspecified arm ▽

  √6ᵗʰ **S55.81** Laceration of other blood vessels at forearm level

    √7ᵗʰ **S55.811** Laceration of other blood vessels at forearm level, right arm

    √7ᵗʰ **S55.812** Laceration of other blood vessels at forearm level, left arm

    √7ᵗʰ **S55.819** Laceration of other blood vessels at forearm level, unspecified arm ▽

  √6ᵗʰ **S55.89** Other specified injury of other blood vessels at forearm level

    √7ᵗʰ **S55.891** Other specified injury of other blood vessels at forearm level, right arm

    √7ᵗʰ **S55.892** Other specified injury of other blood vessels at forearm level, left arm

    √7ᵗʰ **S55.899** Other specified injury of other blood vessels at forearm level, unspecified arm ▽

√5ᵗʰ **S55.9** Injury of unspecified blood vessel at forearm level

  √6ᵗʰ **S55.90** Unspecified injury of unspecified blood vessel at forearm level

    √7ᵗʰ **S55.901** Unspecified injury of unspecified blood vessel at forearm level, right arm ▽

    √7ᵗʰ **S55.902** Unspecified injury of unspecified blood vessel at forearm level, left arm ▽

    √7ᵗʰ **S55.909** Unspecified injury of unspecified blood vessel at forearm level, unspecified arm ▽

  √6ᵗʰ **S55.91** Laceration of unspecified blood vessel at forearm level

    √7ᵗʰ **S55.911** Laceration of unspecified blood vessel at forearm level, right arm ▽

    √7ᵗʰ **S55.912** Laceration of unspecified blood vessel at forearm level, left arm ▽

    √7ᵗʰ **S55.919** Laceration of unspecified blood vessel at forearm level, unspecified arm ▽

  √6ᵗʰ **S55.99** Other specified injury of unspecified blood vessel at forearm level

    √7ᵗʰ **S55.991** Other specified injury of unspecified blood vessel at forearm level, right arm ▽

    √7ᵗʰ **S55.992** Other specified injury of unspecified blood vessel at forearm level, left arm ▽

    √7ᵗʰ **S55.999** Other specified injury of unspecified blood vessel at forearm level, unspecified arm ▽

√4ᵗʰ **S56 Injury of muscle, fascia and tendon at forearm level**

  Code also any associated open wound (S51.-)

  EXCLUDES 2 injury of muscle, fascia and tendon at or below wrist (S66.-)
    sprain of joints and ligaments of elbow (S53.4-)

  TIP: Refer to the Muscle/Tendon table at the beginning of this chapter

  The appropriate 7th character is to be added to each code from category S56.
  A initial encounter
  D subsequent encounter
  S sequela

√5ᵗʰ **S56.0** Injury of flexor muscle, fascia and tendon of thumb at forearm level

  √6ᵗʰ **S56.00** Unspecified injury of flexor muscle, fascia and tendon of thumb at forearm level

    √7ᵗʰ **S56.001** Unspecified injury of flexor muscle, fascia and tendon of right thumb at forearm level ▽

    √7ᵗʰ **S56.002** Unspecified injury of flexor muscle, fascia and tendon of left thumb at forearm level ▽

    √7ᵗʰ **S56.009** Unspecified injury of flexor muscle, fascia and tendon of unspecified thumb at forearm level ▽

  √6ᵗʰ **S56.01** Strain of flexor muscle, fascia and tendon of thumb at forearm level

    √7ᵗʰ **S56.011** Strain of flexor muscle, fascia and tendon of right thumb at forearm level

    √7ᵗʰ **S56.012** Strain of flexor muscle, fascia and tendon of left thumb at forearm level

    √7ᵗʰ **S56.019** Strain of flexor muscle, fascia and tendon of unspecified thumb at forearm level ▽

  √6ᵗʰ **S56.02** Laceration of flexor muscle, fascia and tendon of thumb at forearm level

    √7ᵗʰ **S56.021** Laceration of flexor muscle, fascia and tendon of right thumb at forearm level

    √7ᵗʰ **S56.022** Laceration of flexor muscle, fascia and tendon of left thumb at forearm level

    √7ᵗʰ **S56.029** Laceration of flexor muscle, fascia and tendon of unspecified thumb at forearm level ▽

  √6ᵗʰ **S56.09** Other injury of flexor muscle, fascia and tendon of thumb at forearm level

    √7ᵗʰ **S56.091** Other injury of flexor muscle, fascia and tendon of right thumb at forearm level

    √7ᵗʰ **S56.092** Other injury of flexor muscle, fascia and tendon of left thumb at forearm level

    √7ᵗʰ **S56.099** Other injury of flexor muscle, fascia and tendon of unspecified thumb at forearm level ▽

√5ᵗʰ **S56.1** Injury of flexor muscle, fascia and tendon of other and unspecified finger at forearm level

  √6ᵗʰ **S56.10** Unspecified injury of flexor muscle, fascia and tendon of other and unspecified finger at forearm level

    √7ᵗʰ **S56.101** Unspecified injury of flexor muscle, fascia and tendon of right index finger at forearm level ▽

    √7ᵗʰ **S56.102** Unspecified injury of flexor muscle, fascia and tendon of left index finger at forearm level ▽

    √7ᵗʰ **S56.103** Unspecified injury of flexor muscle, fascia and tendon of right middle finger at forearm level ▽

    √7ᵗʰ **S56.104** Unspecified injury of flexor muscle, fascia and tendon of left middle finger at forearm level ▽

☑ Additional Character Required √ₓ7ᵗʰ Placeholder Alert Manifestation Dx ▽ Unspecified Dx ►◄ Revised Text ● New Code ▲ Revised Code Title

ICD-10-CM 2017   945

√7ᵗʰ **S56.105** Unspecified injury of flexor muscle, fascia and tendon of right ring finger at forearm level ▽

√7ᵗʰ **S56.106** Unspecified injury of flexor muscle, fascia and tendon of left ring finger at forearm level ▽

√7ᵗʰ **S56.107** Unspecified injury of flexor muscle, fascia and tendon of right little finger at forearm level ▽

√7ᵗʰ **S56.108** Unspecified injury of flexor muscle, fascia and tendon of left little finger at forearm level ▽

√7ᵗʰ **S56.109** Unspecified injury of flexor muscle, fascia and tendon of unspecified finger at forearm level ▽

√6ᵗʰ **S56.11** Strain of flexor muscle, fascia and tendon of other and unspecified finger at forearm level

√7ᵗʰ **S56.111** Strain of flexor muscle, fascia and tendon of right index finger at forearm level

√7ᵗʰ **S56.112** Strain of flexor muscle, fascia and tendon of left index finger at forearm level

√7ᵗʰ **S56.113** Strain of flexor muscle, fascia and tendon of right middle finger at forearm level

√7ᵗʰ **S56.114** Strain of flexor muscle, fascia and tendon of left middle finger at forearm level

√7ᵗʰ **S56.115** Strain of flexor muscle, fascia and tendon of right ring finger at forearm level

√7ᵗʰ **S56.116** Strain of flexor muscle, fascia and tendon of left ring finger at forearm level

√7ᵗʰ **S56.117** Strain of flexor muscle, fascia and tendon of right little finger at forearm level

√7ᵗʰ **S56.118** Strain of flexor muscle, fascia and tendon of left little finger at forearm level

√7ᵗʰ **S56.119** Strain of flexor muscle, fascia and tendon of finger of unspecified finger at forearm level ▽

√6ᵗʰ **S56.12** Laceration of flexor muscle, fascia and tendon of other and unspecified finger at forearm level

√7ᵗʰ **S56.121** Laceration of flexor muscle, fascia and tendon of right index finger at forearm level

√7ᵗʰ **S56.122** Laceration of flexor muscle, fascia and tendon of left index finger at forearm level

√7ᵗʰ **S56.123** Laceration of flexor muscle, fascia and tendon of right middle finger at forearm level

√7ᵗʰ **S56.124** Laceration of flexor muscle, fascia and tendon of left middle finger at forearm level

√7ᵗʰ **S56.125** Laceration of flexor muscle, fascia and tendon of right ring finger at forearm level

√7ᵗʰ **S56.126** Laceration of flexor muscle, fascia and tendon of left ring finger at forearm level

√7ᵗʰ **S56.127** Laceration of flexor muscle, fascia and tendon of right little finger at forearm level

√7ᵗʰ **S56.128** Laceration of flexor muscle, fascia and tendon of left little finger at forearm level

√7ᵗʰ **S56.129** Laceration of flexor muscle, fascia and tendon of unspecified finger at forearm level ▽

√6ᵗʰ **S56.19** Other injury of flexor muscle, fascia and tendon of other and unspecified finger at forearm level

√7ᵗʰ **S56.191** Other injury of flexor muscle, fascia and tendon of right index finger at forearm level

√7ᵗʰ **S56.192** Other injury of flexor muscle, fascia and tendon of left index finger at forearm level

√7ᵗʰ **S56.193** Other injury of flexor muscle, fascia and tendon of right middle finger at forearm level

√7ᵗʰ **S56.194** Other injury of flexor muscle, fascia and tendon of left middle finger at forearm level

√7ᵗʰ **S56.195** Other injury of flexor muscle, fascia and tendon of right ring finger at forearm level

√7ᵗʰ **S56.196** Other injury of flexor muscle, fascia and tendon of left ring finger at forearm level

√7ᵗʰ **S56.197** Other injury of flexor muscle, fascia and tendon of right little finger at forearm level

√7ᵗʰ **S56.198** Other injury of flexor muscle, fascia and tendon of left little finger at forearm level

√7ᵗʰ **S56.199** Other injury of flexor muscle, fascia and tendon of unspecified finger at forearm level ▽

√5ᵗʰ **S56.2** Injury of other flexor muscle, fascia and tendon at forearm level

√6ᵗʰ **S56.20** Unspecified injury of other flexor muscle, fascia and tendon at forearm level

√7ᵗʰ **S56.201** Unspecified injury of other flexor muscle, fascia and tendon at forearm level, right arm ▽

√7ᵗʰ **S56.202** Unspecified injury of other flexor muscle, fascia and tendon at forearm level, left arm ▽

√7ᵗʰ **S56.209** Unspecified injury of other flexor muscle, fascia and tendon at forearm level, unspecified arm ▽

√6ᵗʰ **S56.21** Strain of other flexor muscle, fascia and tendon at forearm level

√7ᵗʰ **S56.211** Strain of other flexor muscle, fascia and tendon at forearm level, right arm

√7ᵗʰ **S56.212** Strain of other flexor muscle, fascia and tendon at forearm level, left arm

√7ᵗʰ **S56.219** Strain of other flexor muscle, fascia and tendon at forearm level, unspecified arm ▽

√6ᵗʰ **S56.22** Laceration of other flexor muscle, fascia and tendon at forearm level

√7ᵗʰ **S56.221** Laceration of other flexor muscle, fascia and tendon at forearm level, right arm

√7ᵗʰ **S56.222** Laceration of other flexor muscle, fascia and tendon at forearm level, left arm

√7ᵗʰ **S56.229** Laceration of other flexor muscle, fascia and tendon at forearm level, unspecified arm ▽

√6ᵗʰ **S56.29** Other injury of other flexor muscle, fascia and tendon at forearm level

√7ᵗʰ **S56.291** Other injury of other flexor muscle, fascia and tendon at forearm level, right arm

√7ᵗʰ **S56.292** Other injury of other flexor muscle, fascia and tendon at forearm level, left arm

√7ᵗʰ **S56.299** Other injury of other flexor muscle, fascia and tendon at forearm level, unspecified arm ▽

√5ᵗʰ **S56.3** Injury of extensor or abductor muscles, fascia and tendons of thumb at forearm level

√6ᵗʰ **S56.30** Unspecified injury of extensor or abductor muscles, fascia and tendons of thumb at forearm level

√7ᵗʰ **S56.301** Unspecified injury of extensor or abductor muscles, fascia and tendons of right thumb at forearm level ▽

√7ᵗʰ **S56.302** Unspecified injury of extensor or abductor muscles, fascia and tendons of left thumb at forearm level ▽

√7ᵗʰ **S56.309** Unspecified injury of extensor or abductor muscles, fascia and tendons of unspecified thumb at forearm level ▽

√6ᵗʰ **S56.31** Strain of extensor or abductor muscles, fascia and tendons of thumb at forearm level

√7ᵗʰ **S56.311** Strain of extensor or abductor muscles, fascia and tendons of right thumb at forearm level

√7ᵗʰ **S56.312** Strain of extensor or abductor muscles, fascia and tendons of left thumb at forearm level

√7ᵗʰ **S56.319** Strain of extensor or abductor muscles, fascia and tendons of unspecified thumb at forearm level ▽

√6ᵗʰ **S56.32** Laceration of extensor or abductor muscles, fascia and tendons of thumb at forearm level

√7ᵗʰ **S56.321** Laceration of extensor or abductor muscles, fascia and tendons of right thumb at forearm level

√7ᵗʰ **S56.322** Laceration of extensor or abductor muscles, fascia and tendons of left thumb at forearm level

√7ᵗʰ **S56.329** Laceration of extensor or abductor muscles, fascia and tendons of unspecified thumb at forearm level ▽

EXCLUDES 1 Not coded here   **EXCLUDES 2** Not included here   **N** Newborn Age : 0   **P** Pediatric Age : 0-17   **M** Maternity Age : 12-55   **A** Adult Age : 15-124

√6ᵗʰ **S56.39** Other injury of extensor or abductor muscles, fascia and tendons of thumb at forearm level

    √7ᵗʰ **S56.391** Other injury of extensor or abductor muscles, fascia and tendons of right thumb at forearm level

    √7ᵗʰ **S56.392** Other injury of extensor or abductor muscles, fascia and tendons of left thumb at forearm level

    √7ᵗʰ **S56.399** Other injury of extensor or abductor muscles, fascia and tendons of unspecified thumb at forearm level   ▽

√5ᵗʰ **S56.4** Injury of extensor muscle, fascia and tendon of other and unspecified finger at forearm level

   √6ᵗʰ **S56.40** Unspecified injury of extensor muscle, fascia and tendon of other and unspecified finger at forearm level

    √7ᵗʰ **S56.401** Unspecified injury of extensor muscle, fascia and tendon of right index finger at forearm level   ▽

    √7ᵗʰ **S56.402** Unspecified injury of extensor muscle, fascia and tendon of left index finger at forearm level   ▽

    √7ᵗʰ **S56.403** Unspecified injury of extensor muscle, fascia and tendon of right middle finger at forearm level   ▽

    √7ᵗʰ **S56.404** Unspecified injury of extensor muscle, fascia and tendon of left middle finger at forearm level   ▽

    √7ᵗʰ **S56.405** Unspecified injury of extensor muscle, fascia and tendon of right ring finger at forearm level   ▽

    √7ᵗʰ **S56.406** Unspecified injury of extensor muscle, fascia and tendon of left ring finger at forearm level   ▽

    √7ᵗʰ **S56.407** Unspecified injury of extensor muscle, fascia and tendon of right little finger at forearm level   ▽

    √7ᵗʰ **S56.408** Unspecified injury of extensor muscle, fascia and tendon of left little finger at forearm level   ▽

    √7ᵗʰ **S56.409** Unspecified injury of extensor muscle, fascia and tendon of unspecified finger at forearm level   ▽

   √6ᵗʰ **S56.41** Strain of extensor muscle, fascia and tendon of other and unspecified finger at forearm level

    √7ᵗʰ **S56.411** Strain of extensor muscle, fascia and tendon of right index finger at forearm level

    √7ᵗʰ **S56.412** Strain of extensor muscle, fascia and tendon of left index finger at forearm level

    √7ᵗʰ **S56.413** Strain of extensor muscle, fascia and tendon of right middle finger at forearm level

    √7ᵗʰ **S56.414** Strain of extensor muscle, fascia and tendon of left middle finger at forearm level

    √7ᵗʰ **S56.415** Strain of extensor muscle, fascia and tendon of right ring finger at forearm level

    √7ᵗʰ **S56.416** Strain of extensor muscle, fascia and tendon of left ring finger at forearm level

    √7ᵗʰ **S56.417** Strain of extensor muscle, fascia and tendon of right little finger at forearm level

    √7ᵗʰ **S56.418** Strain of extensor muscle, fascia and tendon of left little finger at forearm level

    √7ᵗʰ **S56.419** Strain of extensor muscle, fascia and tendon of finger, unspecified finger at forearm level   ▽

   √6ᵗʰ **S56.42** Laceration of extensor muscle, fascia and tendon of other and unspecified finger at forearm level

    √7ᵗʰ **S56.421** Laceration of extensor muscle, fascia and tendon of right index finger at forearm level

    √7ᵗʰ **S56.422** Laceration of extensor muscle, fascia and tendon of left index finger at forearm level

    √7ᵗʰ **S56.423** Laceration of extensor muscle, fascia and tendon of right middle finger at forearm level

    √7ᵗʰ **S56.424** Laceration of extensor muscle, fascia and tendon of left middle finger at forearm level

√7ᵗʰ **S56.425** Laceration of extensor muscle, fascia and tendon of right ring finger at forearm level

√7ᵗʰ **S56.426** Laceration of extensor muscle, fascia and tendon of left ring finger at forearm level

√7ᵗʰ **S56.427** Laceration of extensor muscle, fascia and tendon of right little finger at forearm level

√7ᵗʰ **S56.428** Laceration of extensor muscle, fascia and tendon of left little finger at forearm level

√7ᵗʰ **S56.429** Laceration of extensor muscle, fascia and tendon of unspecified finger at forearm level   ▽

√6ᵗʰ **S56.49** Other injury of extensor muscle, fascia and tendon of other and unspecified finger at forearm level

   √7ᵗʰ **S56.491** Other injury of extensor muscle, fascia and tendon of right index finger at forearm level

   √7ᵗʰ **S56.492** Other injury of extensor muscle, fascia and tendon of left index finger at forearm level

   √7ᵗʰ **S56.493** Other injury of extensor muscle, fascia and tendon of right middle finger at forearm level

   √7ᵗʰ **S56.494** Other injury of extensor muscle, fascia and tendon of left middle finger at forearm level

   √7ᵗʰ **S56.495** Other injury of extensor muscle, fascia and tendon of right ring finger at forearm level

   √7ᵗʰ **S56.496** Other injury of extensor muscle, fascia and tendon of left ring finger at forearm level

   √7ᵗʰ **S56.497** Other injury of extensor muscle, fascia and tendon of right little finger at forearm level

   √7ᵗʰ **S56.498** Other injury of extensor muscle, fascia and tendon of left little finger at forearm level

   √7ᵗʰ **S56.499** Other injury of extensor muscle, fascia and tendon of unspecified finger at forearm level   ▽

√5ᵗʰ **S56.5** Injury of other extensor muscle, fascia and tendon at forearm level

   √6ᵗʰ **S56.50** Unspecified injury of other extensor muscle, fascia and tendon at forearm level

    √7ᵗʰ **S56.501** Unspecified injury of other extensor muscle, fascia and tendon at forearm level, right arm   ▽

    √7ᵗʰ **S56.502** Unspecified injury of other extensor muscle, fascia and tendon at forearm level, left arm   ▽

    √7ᵗʰ **S56.509** Unspecified injury of other extensor muscle, fascia and tendon at forearm level, unspecified arm   ▽

   √6ᵗʰ **S56.51** Strain of other extensor muscle, fascia and tendon at forearm level

    √7ᵗʰ **S56.511** Strain of other extensor muscle, fascia and tendon at forearm level, right arm

    √7ᵗʰ **S56.512** Strain of other extensor muscle, fascia and tendon at forearm level, left arm

    √7ᵗʰ **S56.519** Strain of other extensor muscle, fascia and tendon at forearm level, unspecified arm   ▽

   √6ᵗʰ **S56.52** Laceration of other extensor muscle, fascia and tendon at forearm level

    √7ᵗʰ **S56.521** Laceration of other extensor muscle, fascia and tendon at forearm level, right arm

    √7ᵗʰ **S56.522** Laceration of other extensor muscle, fascia and tendon at forearm level, left arm

    √7ᵗʰ **S56.529** Laceration of other extensor muscle, fascia and tendon at forearm level, unspecified arm   ▽

   √6ᵗʰ **S56.59** Other injury of other extensor muscle, fascia and tendon at forearm level

    √7ᵗʰ **S56.591** Other injury of other extensor muscle, fascia and tendon at forearm level, right arm

    √7ᵗʰ **S56.592** Other injury of other extensor muscle, fascia and tendon at forearm level, left arm

---

✔ Additional Character Required   √x7ᵗʰ Placeholder Alert   Manifestation Dx   ▽ Unspecified Dx   ▶◀ Revised Text   ● New Code   ▲ Revised Code Title

√7ᵗʰ **S56.599** Other injury of other extensor muscle, fascia and tendon at forearm level, unspecified arm ▽

√5ᵗʰ **S56.8** Injury of other muscles, fascia and tendons at forearm level

√6ᵗʰ   **S56.80** Unspecified injury of other muscles, fascia and tendons at forearm level

√7ᵗʰ   **S56.801** Unspecified injury of other muscles, fascia and tendon at forearm level, right arm ▽

√7ᵗʰ   **S56.802** Unspecified injury of other muscles, fascia and tendon at forearm level, left arm ▽

√7ᵗʰ   **S56.809** Unspecified injury of other muscles, fascia and tendon at forearm level, unspecified arm ▽

√6ᵗʰ   **S56.81** Strain of other muscles, fascia and tendons at forearm level

√7ᵗʰ   **S56.811** Strain of other muscles, fascia and tendons at forearm level, right arm

√7ᵗʰ   **S56.812** Strain of other muscles, fascia and tendons at forearm level, left arm

√7ᵗʰ   **S56.819** Strain of other muscles, fascia and tendons at forearm level, unspecified arm ▽

√6ᵗʰ   **S56.82** Laceration of other muscles, fascia and tendons at forearm level

√7ᵗʰ   **S56.821** Laceration of other muscles, fascia and tendons at forearm level, right arm

√7ᵗʰ   **S56.822** Laceration of other muscles, fascia and tendons at forearm level, left arm

√7ᵗʰ   **S56.829** Laceration of other muscles, fascia and tendons at forearm level, unspecified arm ▽

√6ᵗʰ   **S56.89** Other injury of other muscles, fascia and tendons at forearm level

√7ᵗʰ   **S56.891** Other injury of other muscles, fascia and tendons at forearm level, right arm

√7ᵗʰ   **S56.892** Other injury of other muscles, fascia and tendons at forearm level, left arm

√7ᵗʰ   **S56.899** Other injury of other muscles, fascia and tendons at forearm level, unspecified arm ▽

√5ᵗʰ **S56.9** Injury of unspecified muscles, fascia and tendons at forearm level

√6ᵗʰ   **S56.90** Unspecified injury of unspecified muscles, fascia and tendons at forearm level

√7ᵗʰ   **S56.901** Unspecified injury of unspecified muscles, fascia and tendons at forearm level, right arm ▽

√7ᵗʰ   **S56.902** Unspecified injury of unspecified muscles, fascia and tendons at forearm level, left arm ▽

√7ᵗʰ   **S56.909** Unspecified injury of unspecified muscles, fascia and tendons at forearm level, unspecified arm ▽

√6ᵗʰ   **S56.91** Strain of unspecified muscles, fascia and tendons at forearm level

√7ᵗʰ   **S56.911** Strain of unspecified muscles, fascia and tendons at forearm level, right arm ▽

√7ᵗʰ   **S56.912** Strain of unspecified muscles, fascia and tendons at forearm level, left arm ▽

√7ᵗʰ   **S56.919** Strain of unspecified muscles, fascia and tendons at forearm level, unspecified arm ▽

√6ᵗʰ   **S56.92** Laceration of unspecified muscles, fascia and tendons at forearm level

√7ᵗʰ   **S56.921** Laceration of unspecified muscles, fascia and tendons at forearm level, right arm ▽

√7ᵗʰ   **S56.922** Laceration of unspecified muscles, fascia and tendons at forearm level, left arm ▽

√7ᵗʰ   **S56.929** Laceration of unspecified muscles, fascia and tendons at forearm level, unspecified arm ▽

√6ᵗʰ   **S56.99** Other injury of unspecified muscles, fascia and tendons at forearm level

√7ᵗʰ   **S56.991** Other injury of unspecified muscles, fascia and tendons at forearm level, right arm ▽

√7ᵗʰ   **S56.992** Other injury of unspecified muscles, fascia and tendons at forearm level, left arm ▽

√7ᵗʰ   **S56.999** Other injury of unspecified muscles, fascia and tendons at forearm level, unspecified arm ▽

√4ᵗʰ **S57** Crushing injury of elbow and forearm

Use additional code(s) for all associated injuries

EXCLUDES 2 *crushing injury of wrist and hand (S67.-)*

The appropriate 7th character is to be added to each code from category S57.
A   initial encounter
D   subsequent encounter
S   sequela

√5ᵗʰ   **S57.0** Crushing injury of elbow

√×7ᵗʰ   **S57.00** Crushing injury of unspecified elbow ▽

√×7ᵗʰ   **S57.01** Crushing injury of right elbow

√×7ᵗʰ   **S57.02** Crushing injury of left elbow

√5ᵗʰ   **S57.8** Crushing injury of forearm

√×7ᵗʰ   **S57.80** Crushing injury of unspecified forearm ▽

√×7ᵗʰ   **S57.81** Crushing injury of right forearm

√×7ᵗʰ   **S57.82** Crushing injury of left forearm

√4ᵗʰ **S58** Traumatic amputation of elbow and forearm

NOTE An amputation not identified as partial or complete should be coded to complete

EXCLUDES 1 *traumatic amputation of wrist and hand (S68.-)*

The appropriate 7th character is to be added to each code from category S58.
A   initial encounter
D   subsequent encounter
S   sequela

√5ᵗʰ   **S58.0** Traumatic amputation at elbow level

√6ᵗʰ   **S58.01** Complete traumatic amputation at elbow level

√7ᵗʰ   **S58.011** Complete traumatic amputation at elbow level, right arm

√7ᵗʰ   **S58.012** Complete traumatic amputation at elbow level, left arm

√7ᵗʰ   **S58.019** Complete traumatic amputation at elbow level, unspecified arm ▽

√6ᵗʰ   **S58.02** Partial traumatic amputation at elbow level

√7ᵗʰ   **S58.021** Partial traumatic amputation at elbow level, right arm

√7ᵗʰ   **S58.022** Partial traumatic amputation at elbow level, left arm

√7ᵗʰ   **S58.029** Partial traumatic amputation at elbow level, unspecified arm ▽

√5ᵗʰ   **S58.1** Traumatic amputation at level between elbow and wrist

√6ᵗʰ   **S58.11** Complete traumatic amputation at level between elbow and wrist

√7ᵗʰ   **S58.111** Complete traumatic amputation at level between elbow and wrist, right arm

√7ᵗʰ   **S58.112** Complete traumatic amputation at level between elbow and wrist, left arm

√7ᵗʰ   **S58.119** Complete traumatic amputation at level between elbow and wrist, unspecified arm ▽

√6ᵗʰ   **S58.12** Partial traumatic amputation at level between elbow and wrist

√7ᵗʰ   **S58.121** Partial traumatic amputation at level between elbow and wrist, right arm

√7ᵗʰ   **S58.122** Partial traumatic amputation at level between elbow and wrist, left arm

√7ᵗʰ   **S58.129** Partial traumatic amputation at level between elbow and wrist, unspecified arm ▽

√5ᵗʰ   **S58.9** Traumatic amputation of forearm, level unspecified

EXCLUDES 1 *traumatic amputation of wrist (S68.-)*

√6ᵗʰ   **S58.91** Complete traumatic amputation of forearm, level unspecified

√7ᵗʰ   **S58.911** Complete traumatic amputation of right forearm, level unspecified ▽

√7ᵗʰ   **S58.912** Complete traumatic amputation of left forearm, level unspecified

√7ᵗʰ   **S58.919** Complete traumatic amputation of unspecified forearm, level unspecified ▽

EXCLUDES 1 Not coded here   EXCLUDES 2 Not included here   N Newborn Age : 0   P Pediatric Age : 0-17   M Maternity Age : 12-55   A Adult Age : 15-124

948   ICD-10-CM 2017

✓6ᵗʰ **S58.92** Partial traumatic amputation of forearm, level unspecified

    ✓7ᵗʰ **S58.921** Partial traumatic amputation of right forearm, level unspecified ▽

    ✓7ᵗʰ **S58.922** Partial traumatic amputation of left forearm, level unspecified ▽

    ✓7ᵗʰ **S58.929** Partial traumatic amputation of unspecified forearm, level unspecified ▽

✓4ᵗʰ **S59** Other and unspecified injuries of elbow and forearm

   EXCLUDES 2   *other and unspecified injuries of wrist and hand (S69.-)*

   AHA: 2015,3Q,37-39

> The appropriate 7th character is to be added to each code from subcategories S59.0, S59.1, and S59.2.
> A   initial encounter for closed fracture
> D   subsequent encounter for fracture with routine healing
> G   subsequent encounter for fracture with delayed healing
> K   subsequent encounter for fracture with nonunion
> P   subsequent encounter for fracture with malunion
> S   sequela

✓5ᵗʰ **S59.0** Physeal fracture of lower end of ulna

  ✓6ᵗʰ **S59.00** Unspecified physeal fracture of lower end of ulna

    ✓7ᵗʰ **S59.001** Unspecified physeal fracture of lower end of ulna, right arm ▽

    ✓7ᵗʰ **S59.002** Unspecified physeal fracture of lower end of ulna, left arm ▽

    ✓7ᵗʰ **S59.009** Unspecified physeal fracture of lower end of ulna, unspecified arm ▽

  ✓6ᵗʰ **S59.01** Salter-Harris Type I physeal fracture of lower end of ulna

    ✓7ᵗʰ **S59.011** Salter-Harris Type I physeal fracture of lower end of ulna, right arm

    ✓7ᵗʰ **S59.012** Salter-Harris Type I physeal fracture of lower end of ulna, left arm

    ✓7ᵗʰ **S59.019** Salter-Harris Type I physeal fracture of lower end of ulna, unspecified arm ▽

  ✓6ᵗʰ **S59.02** Salter-Harris Type II physeal fracture of lower end of ulna

    ✓7ᵗʰ **S59.021** Salter-Harris Type II physeal fracture of lower end of ulna, right arm

    ✓7ᵗʰ **S59.022** Salter-Harris Type II physeal fracture of lower end of ulna, left arm

    ✓7ᵗʰ **S59.029** Salter-Harris Type II physeal fracture of lower end of ulna, unspecified arm ▽

  ✓6ᵗʰ **S59.03** Salter-Harris Type III physeal fracture of lower end of ulna

    ✓7ᵗʰ **S59.031** Salter-Harris Type III physeal fracture of lower end of ulna, right arm

    ✓7ᵗʰ **S59.032** Salter-Harris Type III physeal fracture of lower end of ulna, left arm

    ✓7ᵗʰ **S59.039** Salter-Harris Type III physeal fracture of lower end of ulna, unspecified arm ▽

  ✓6ᵗʰ **S59.04** Salter-Harris Type IV physeal fracture of lower end of ulna

    ✓7ᵗʰ **S59.041** Salter-Harris Type IV physeal fracture of lower end of ulna, right arm

    ✓7ᵗʰ **S59.042** Salter-Harris Type IV physeal fracture of lower end of ulna, left arm

    ✓7ᵗʰ **S59.049** Salter-Harris Type IV physeal fracture of lower end of ulna, unspecified arm ▽

  ✓6ᵗʰ **S59.09** Other physeal fracture of lower end of ulna

    ✓7ᵗʰ **S59.091** Other physeal fracture of lower end of ulna, right arm

    ✓7ᵗʰ **S59.092** Other physeal fracture of lower end of ulna, left arm

    ✓7ᵗʰ **S59.099** Other physeal fracture of lower end of ulna, unspecified arm ▽

✓5ᵗʰ **S59.1** Physeal fracture of upper end of radius

  ✓6ᵗʰ **S59.10** Unspecified physeal fracture of upper end of radius

    ✓7ᵗʰ **S59.101** Unspecified physeal fracture of upper end of radius, right arm ▽

    ✓7ᵗʰ **S59.102** Unspecified physeal fracture of upper end of radius, left arm ▽

    ✓7ᵗʰ **S59.109** Unspecified physeal fracture of upper end of radius, unspecified arm ▽

  ✓6ᵗʰ **S59.11** Salter-Harris Type I physeal fracture of upper end of radius

    ✓7ᵗʰ **S59.111** Salter-Harris Type I physeal fracture of upper end of radius, right arm

    ✓7ᵗʰ **S59.112** Salter-Harris Type I physeal fracture of upper end of radius, left arm

    ✓7ᵗʰ **S59.119** Salter-Harris Type I physeal fracture of upper end of radius, unspecified arm ▽

  ✓6ᵗʰ **S59.12** Salter-Harris Type II physeal fracture of upper end of radius

    ✓7ᵗʰ **S59.121** Salter-Harris Type II physeal fracture of upper end of radius, right arm

    ✓7ᵗʰ **S59.122** Salter-Harris Type II physeal fracture of upper end of radius, left arm

    ✓7ᵗʰ **S59.129** Salter-Harris Type II physeal fracture of upper end of radius, unspecified arm ▽

  ✓6ᵗʰ **S59.13** Salter-Harris Type III physeal fracture of upper end of radius

    ✓7ᵗʰ **S59.131** Salter-Harris Type III physeal fracture of upper end of radius, right arm

    ✓7ᵗʰ **S59.132** Salter-Harris Type III physeal fracture of upper end of radius, left arm

    ✓7ᵗʰ **S59.139** Salter-Harris Type III physeal fracture of upper end of radius, unspecified arm ▽

  ✓6ᵗʰ **S59.14** Salter-Harris Type IV physeal fracture of upper end of radius

    ✓7ᵗʰ **S59.141** Salter-Harris Type IV physeal fracture of upper end of radius, right arm

    ✓7ᵗʰ **S59.142** Salter-Harris Type IV physeal fracture of upper end of radius, left arm

    ✓7ᵗʰ **S59.149** Salter-Harris Type IV physeal fracture of upper end of radius, unspecified arm ▽

  ✓6ᵗʰ **S59.19** Other physeal fracture of upper end of radius

    ✓7ᵗʰ **S59.191** Other physeal fracture of upper end of radius, right arm

    ✓7ᵗʰ **S59.192** Other physeal fracture of upper end of radius, left arm

    ✓7ᵗʰ **S59.199** Other physeal fracture of upper end of radius, unspecified arm ▽

✓5ᵗʰ **S59.2** Physeal fracture of lower end of radius

  ✓6ᵗʰ **S59.20** Unspecified physeal fracture of lower end of radius

    ✓7ᵗʰ **S59.201** Unspecified physeal fracture of lower end of radius, right arm ▽

    ✓7ᵗʰ **S59.202** Unspecified physeal fracture of lower end of radius, left arm ▽

    ✓7ᵗʰ **S59.209** Unspecified physeal fracture of lower end of radius, unspecified arm ▽

  ✓6ᵗʰ **S59.21** Salter-Harris Type I physeal fracture of lower end of radius

    ✓7ᵗʰ **S59.211** Salter-Harris Type I physeal fracture of lower end of radius, right arm

    ✓7ᵗʰ **S59.212** Salter-Harris Type I physeal fracture of lower end of radius, left arm

    ✓7ᵗʰ **S59.219** Salter-Harris Type I physeal fracture of lower end of radius, unspecified arm ▽

  ✓6ᵗʰ **S59.22** Salter-Harris Type II physeal fracture of lower end of radius

    ✓7ᵗʰ **S59.221** Salter-Harris Type II physeal fracture of lower end of radius, right arm

    ✓7ᵗʰ **S59.222** Salter-Harris Type II physeal fracture of lower end of radius, left arm

    ✓7ᵗʰ **S59.229** Salter-Harris Type II physeal fracture of lower end of radius, unspecified arm ▽

  ✓6ᵗʰ **S59.23** Salter-Harris Type III physeal fracture of lower end of radius

    ✓7ᵗʰ **S59.231** Salter-Harris Type III physeal fracture of lower end of radius, right arm

    ✓7ᵗʰ **S59.232** Salter-Harris Type III physeal fracture of lower end of radius, left arm

    ✓7ᵗʰ **S59.239** Salter-Harris Type III physeal fracture of lower end of radius, unspecified arm ▽

  ✓6ᵗʰ **S59.24** Salter-Harris Type IV physeal fracture of lower end of radius

    ✓7ᵗʰ **S59.241** Salter-Harris Type IV physeal fracture of lower end of radius, right arm

---

☑ Additional Character Required   ✓x7ᵗʰ Placeholder Alert   Manifestation Dx   ▽ Unspecified Dx   ▶◀ Revised Text   ● New Code   ▲ Revised Code Title

√7th **S59.242** Salter-Harris Type IV physeal fracture of lower end of radius, left arm

√7th **S59.249** Salter-Harris Type IV physeal fracture of lower end of radius, unspecified arm ▽

√6th **S59.29** Other physeal fracture of lower end of radius

√7th **S59.291** Other physeal fracture of lower end of radius, right arm

√7th **S59.292** Other physeal fracture of lower end of radius, left arm

√7th **S59.299** Other physeal fracture of lower end of radius, unspecified arm ▽

√5th **S59.8 Other specified injuries of elbow and forearm**

> The appropriate 7th character is to be added to each code in subcategory S59.8.
> A   initial encounter
> D   subsequent encounter
> S   sequela

√6th **S59.80 Other specified injuries of elbow**

√7th **S59.801** Other specified injuries of right elbow

√7th **S59.802** Other specified injuries of left elbow

√7th **S59.809** Other specified injuries of unspecified elbow ▽

√6th **S59.81 Other specified injuries of forearm**

√7th **S59.811** Other specified injuries right forearm

√7th **S59.812** Other specified injuries left forearm

√7th **S59.819** Other specified injuries unspecified forearm ▽

√5th **S59.9 Unspecified injury of elbow and forearm**

> The appropriate 7th character is to be added to each code in subcategory S59.9.
> A   initial encounter
> D   subsequent encounter
> S   sequela

√6th **S59.90 Unspecified injury of elbow**

√7th **S59.901** Unspecified injury of right elbow ▽

√7th **S59.902** Unspecified injury of left elbow ▽

√7th **S59.909** Unspecified injury of unspecified elbow ▽

√6th **S59.91 Unspecified injury of forearm**

√7th **S59.911** Unspecified injury of right forearm ▽

√7th **S59.912** Unspecified injury of left forearm ▽

√7th **S59.919** Unspecified injury of unspecified forearm ▽

Injuries to the wrist, hand and fingers (S60-S69)

EXCLUDES 2   burns and corrosions (T20-T32)
frostbite (T33-T34)
insect bite or sting, venomous (T63.4)

√4th **S60 Superficial injury of wrist, hand and fingers**

> The appropriate 7th character is to be added to each code from category S60.
> A   initial encounter
> D   subsequent encounter
> S   sequela

√5th **S60.0 Contusion of finger without damage to nail**

> EXCLUDES 1   contusion involving nail (matrix) (S60.1)

√x7th **S60.00 Contusion of unspecified finger without damage to nail** ▽
Contusion of finger(s) NOS

√6th **S60.01 Contusion of thumb without damage to nail**

√7th **S60.011** Contusion of right thumb without damage to nail

√7th **S60.012** Contusion of left thumb without damage to nail

√7th **S60.019** Contusion of unspecified thumb without damage to nail ▽

√6th **S60.02 Contusion of index finger without damage to nail**

√7th **S60.021** Contusion of right index finger without damage to nail

√7th **S60.022** Contusion of left index finger without damage to nail

√7th **S60.029** Contusion of unspecified index finger without damage to nail ▽

√6th **S60.03 Contusion of middle finger without damage to nail**

√7th **S60.031** Contusion of right middle finger without damage to nail

√7th **S60.032** Contusion of left middle finger without damage to nail

√7th **S60.039** Contusion of unspecified middle finger without damage to nail ▽

√6th **S60.04 Contusion of ring finger without damage to nail**

√7th **S60.041** Contusion of right ring finger without damage to nail

√7th **S60.042** Contusion of left ring finger without damage to nail

√7th **S60.049** Contusion of unspecified ring finger without damage to nail ▽

√6th **S60.05 Contusion of little finger without damage to nail**

√7th **S60.051** Contusion of right little finger without damage to nail

√7th **S60.052** Contusion of left little finger without damage to nail

√7th **S60.059** Contusion of unspecified little finger without damage to nail ▽

√5th **S60.1 Contusion of finger with damage to nail**

√x7th **S60.10 Contusion of unspecified finger with damage to nail** ▽

√6th **S60.11 Contusion of thumb with damage to nail**

√7th **S60.111** Contusion of right thumb with damage to nail

√7th **S60.112** Contusion of left thumb with damage to nail

√7th **S60.119** Contusion of unspecified thumb with damage to nail ▽

√6th **S60.12 Contusion of index finger with damage to nail**

√7th **S60.121** Contusion of right index finger with damage to nail

√7th **S60.122** Contusion of left index finger with damage to nail

√7th **S60.129** Contusion of unspecified index finger with damage to nail ▽

√6th **S60.13 Contusion of middle finger with damage to nail**

√7th **S60.131** Contusion of right middle finger with damage to nail

√7th **S60.132** Contusion of left middle finger with damage to nail

√7th **S60.139** Contusion of unspecified middle finger with damage to nail ▽

√6th **S60.14 Contusion of ring finger with damage to nail**

√7th **S60.141** Contusion of right ring finger with damage to nail

√7th **S60.142** Contusion of left ring finger with damage to nail

√7th **S60.149** Contusion of unspecified ring finger with damage to nail ▽

√6th **S60.15 Contusion of little finger with damage to nail**

√7th **S60.151** Contusion of right little finger with damage to nail

√7th **S60.152** Contusion of left little finger with damage to nail

√7th **S60.159** Contusion of unspecified little finger with damage to nail ▽

√5th **S60.2 Contusion of wrist and hand**

> EXCLUDES 2   contusion of fingers (S60.0-, S60.1-)

√6th **S60.21 Contusion of wrist**

√7th **S60.211** Contusion of right wrist

√7th **S60.212** Contusion of left wrist

√7th **S60.219** Contusion of unspecified wrist ▽

√6th **S60.22 Contusion of hand**

√7th **S60.221** Contusion of right hand

√7th **S60.222** Contusion of left hand

√7th **S60.229** Contusion of unspecified hand ▽

√5th **S60.3 Other superficial injuries of thumb**

√6th **S60.31 Abrasion of thumb**

√7th **S60.311** Abrasion of right thumb

√7th **S60.312** Abrasion of left thumb

√7th **S60.319** Abrasion of unspecified thumb ▽

√6th **S60.32 Blister (nonthermal) of thumb**

√7th **S60.321** Blister (nonthermal) of right thumb

√7th **S60.322** Blister (nonthermal) of left thumb

EXCLUDES 1 Not coded here   EXCLUDES 2 Not included here   N Newborn Age : 0   P Pediatric Age : 0-17   M Maternity Age : 12-55   A Adult Age : 15-124

950   ICD-10-CM 2017

√7ᵗʰ **S60.329 Blister (nonthermal) of unspecified thumb** ▽

√6ᵗʰ **S60.34 External constriction of thumb**
    Hair tourniquet syndrome of thumb
    Use additional cause code to identify the constricting item (W49.0-)

   √7ᵗʰ **S60.341 External constriction of right thumb**
   √7ᵗʰ **S60.342 External constriction of left thumb**
   √7ᵗʰ **S60.349 External constriction of unspecified thumb** ▽

√6ᵗʰ **S60.35 Superficial foreign body of thumb**
    Splinter in the thumb

   √7ᵗʰ **S60.351 Superficial foreign body of right thumb**
   √7ᵗʰ **S60.352 Superficial foreign body of left thumb**
   √7ᵗʰ **S60.359 Superficial foreign body of unspecified thumb** ▽

√6ᵗʰ **S60.36 Insect bite (nonvenomous) of thumb**

   √7ᵗʰ **S60.361 Insect bite (nonvenomous) of right thumb**
   √7ᵗʰ **S60.362 Insect bite (nonvenomous) of left thumb**
   √7ᵗʰ **S60.369 Insect bite (nonvenomous) of unspecified thumb** ▽

√6ᵗʰ **S60.37 Other superficial bite of thumb**
    EXCLUDES 1 *open bite of thumb (S61.05-, S61.15-)*

   √7ᵗʰ **S60.371 Other superficial bite of right thumb**
   √7ᵗʰ **S60.372 Other superficial bite of left thumb**
   √7ᵗʰ **S60.379 Other superficial bite of unspecified thumb** ▽

√6ᵗʰ **S60.39 Other superficial injuries of thumb**

   √7ᵗʰ **S60.391 Other superficial injuries of right thumb**
   √7ᵗʰ **S60.392 Other superficial injuries of left thumb**
   √7ᵗʰ **S60.399 Other superficial injuries of unspecified thumb** ▽

√5ᵗʰ **S60.4 Other superficial injuries of other fingers**

√6ᵗʰ **S60.41 Abrasion of fingers**

   √7ᵗʰ **S60.410 Abrasion of right index finger**
   √7ᵗʰ **S60.411 Abrasion of left index finger**
   √7ᵗʰ **S60.412 Abrasion of right middle finger**
   √7ᵗʰ **S60.413 Abrasion of left middle finger**
   √7ᵗʰ **S60.414 Abrasion of right ring finger**
   √7ᵗʰ **S60.415 Abrasion of left ring finger**
   √7ᵗʰ **S60.416 Abrasion of right little finger**
   √7ᵗʰ **S60.417 Abrasion of left little finger**
   √7ᵗʰ **S60.418 Abrasion of other finger**
     Abrasion of specified finger with unspecified laterality
   √7ᵗʰ **S60.419 Abrasion of unspecified finger** ▽

√6ᵗʰ **S60.42 Blister (nonthermal) of fingers**

   √7ᵗʰ **S60.420 Blister (nonthermal) of right index finger**
   √7ᵗʰ **S60.421 Blister (nonthermal) of left index finger**
   √7ᵗʰ **S60.422 Blister (nonthermal) of right middle finger**
   √7ᵗʰ **S60.423 Blister (nonthermal) of left middle finger**
   √7ᵗʰ **S60.424 Blister (nonthermal) of right ring finger**
   √7ᵗʰ **S60.425 Blister (nonthermal) of left ring finger**
   √7ᵗʰ **S60.426 Blister (nonthermal) of right little finger**
   √7ᵗʰ **S60.427 Blister (nonthermal) of left little finger**
   √7ᵗʰ **S60.428 Blister (nonthermal) of other finger**
     Blister (nonthermal) of specified finger with unspecified laterality
   √7ᵗʰ **S60.429 Blister (nonthermal) of unspecified finger** ▽

√6ᵗʰ **S60.44 External constriction of fingers**
    Hair tourniquet syndrome of finger
    Use additional cause code to identify the constricting item (W49.0-)

   √7ᵗʰ **S60.440 External constriction of right index finger**
   √7ᵗʰ **S60.441 External constriction of left index finger**
   √7ᵗʰ **S60.442 External constriction of right middle finger**
   √7ᵗʰ **S60.443 External constriction of left middle finger**
   √7ᵗʰ **S60.444 External constriction of right ring finger**

   √7ᵗʰ **S60.445 External constriction of left ring finger**
   √7ᵗʰ **S60.446 External constriction of right little finger**
   √7ᵗʰ **S60.447 External constriction of left little finger**
   √7ᵗʰ **S60.448 External constriction of other finger**
     External constriction of specified finger with unspecified laterality
   √7ᵗʰ **S60.449 External constriction of unspecified finger** ▽

√6ᵗʰ **S60.45 Superficial foreign body of fingers**
    Splinter in the finger(s)

   √7ᵗʰ **S60.450 Superficial foreign body of right index finger**
   √7ᵗʰ **S60.451 Superficial foreign body of left index finger**
   √7ᵗʰ **S60.452 Superficial foreign body of right middle finger**
   √7ᵗʰ **S60.453 Superficial foreign body of left middle finger**
   √7ᵗʰ **S60.454 Superficial foreign body of right ring finger**
   √7ᵗʰ **S60.455 Superficial foreign body of left ring finger**
   √7ᵗʰ **S60.456 Superficial foreign body of right little finger**
   √7ᵗʰ **S60.457 Superficial foreign body of left little finger**
   √7ᵗʰ **S60.458 Superficial foreign body of other finger**
     Superficial foreign body of specified finger with unspecified laterality
   √7ᵗʰ **S60.459 Superficial foreign body of unspecified finger** ▽

√6ᵗʰ **S60.46 Insect bite (nonvenomous) of fingers**

   √7ᵗʰ **S60.460 Insect bite (nonvenomous) of right index finger**
   √7ᵗʰ **S60.461 Insect bite (nonvenomous) of left index finger**
   √7ᵗʰ **S60.462 Insect bite (nonvenomous) of right middle finger**
   √7ᵗʰ **S60.463 Insect bite (nonvenomous) of left middle finger**
   √7ᵗʰ **S60.464 Insect bite (nonvenomous) of right ring finger**
   √7ᵗʰ **S60.465 Insect bite (nonvenomous) of left ring finger**
   √7ᵗʰ **S60.466 Insect bite (nonvenomous) of right little finger**
   √7ᵗʰ **S60.467 Insect bite (nonvenomous) of left little finger**
   √7ᵗʰ **S60.468 Insect bite (nonvenomous) of other finger**
     Insect bite (nonvenomous) of specified finger with unspecified laterality
   √7ᵗʰ **S60.469 Insect bite (nonvenomous) of unspecified finger** ▽

√6ᵗʰ **S60.47 Other superficial bite of fingers**
    EXCLUDES 1 *open bite of fingers (S61.25-, S61.35-)*

   √7ᵗʰ **S60.470 Other superficial bite of right index finger**
   √7ᵗʰ **S60.471 Other superficial bite of left index finger**
   √7ᵗʰ **S60.472 Other superficial bite of right middle finger**
   √7ᵗʰ **S60.473 Other superficial bite of left middle finger**
   √7ᵗʰ **S60.474 Other superficial bite of right ring finger**
   √7ᵗʰ **S60.475 Other superficial bite of left ring finger**
   √7ᵗʰ **S60.476 Other superficial bite of right little finger**
   √7ᵗʰ **S60.477 Other superficial bite of left little finger**
   √7ᵗʰ **S60.478 Other superficial bite of other finger**
     Other superficial bite of specified finger with unspecified laterality
   √7ᵗʰ **S60.479 Other superficial bite of unspecified finger** ▽

√5ᵗʰ **S60.5 Other superficial injuries of hand**
    EXCLUDES 2 *superficial injuries of fingers (S60.3-, S60.4-)*

√6ᵗʰ **S60.51 Abrasion of hand**

   √7ᵗʰ **S60.511 Abrasion of right hand**
   √7ᵗʰ **S60.512 Abrasion of left hand**
   √7ᵗʰ **S60.519 Abrasion of unspecified hand** ▽

√6ᵗʰ **S60.52 Blister (nonthermal) of hand**

   √7ᵗʰ **S60.521 Blister (nonthermal) of right hand**

☑ Additional Character Required   √x7ᵗʰ Placeholder Alert   Manifestation Dx   ▽ Unspecified Dx   ►◄ Revised Text   ● New Code   ▲ Revised Code Title

ICD-10-CM 2017   **951**

√7ᵗʰ **S60.522** Blister (nonthermal) of **left** hand

√7ᵗʰ **S60.529** Blister (nonthermal) of unspecified hand ▽

√6ᵗʰ **S60.54** External constriction of hand

√7ᵗʰ **S60.541** External constriction of **right** hand

√7ᵗʰ **S60.542** External constriction of **left** hand

√7ᵗʰ **S60.549** External constriction of unspecified hand ▽

√6ᵗʰ **S60.55** Superficial **foreign body** of hand

Splinter in the hand

√7ᵗʰ **S60.551** Superficial foreign body of **right** hand

√7ᵗʰ **S60.552** Superficial foreign body of **left** hand

√7ᵗʰ **S60.559** Superficial foreign body of unspecified hand ▽

√6ᵗʰ **S60.56** Insect bite (nonvenomous) of hand

√7ᵗʰ **S60.561** Insect bite (nonvenomous) of **right** hand

√7ᵗʰ **S60.562** Insect bite (nonvenomous) of **left** hand

√7ᵗʰ **S60.569** Insect bite (nonvenomous) of unspecified hand ▽

√6ᵗʰ **S60.57** Other superficial **bite** of hand

EXCLUDES 1 *open bite of hand (S61.45-)*

√7ᵗʰ **S60.571** Other superficial bite of hand of **right** hand

√7ᵗʰ **S60.572** Other superficial bite of hand of **left** hand

√7ᵗʰ **S60.579** Other superficial bite of hand of unspecified hand ▽

√5ᵗʰ **S60.8** Other superficial injuries of **wrist**

√6ᵗʰ **S60.81** **Abrasion** of wrist

√7ᵗʰ **S60.811** Abrasion of **right** wrist

√7ᵗʰ **S60.812** Abrasion of **left** wrist

√7ᵗʰ **S60.819** Abrasion of unspecified wrist ▽

√6ᵗʰ **S60.82** Blister (nonthermal) of wrist

√7ᵗʰ **S60.821** Blister (nonthermal) of **right** wrist

√7ᵗʰ **S60.822** Blister (nonthermal) of **left** wrist

√7ᵗʰ **S60.829** Blister (nonthermal) of unspecified wrist ▽

√6ᵗʰ **S60.84** External constriction of wrist

√7ᵗʰ **S60.841** External constriction of **right** wrist

√7ᵗʰ **S60.842** External constriction of **left** wrist

√7ᵗʰ **S60.849** External constriction of unspecified wrist ▽

√6ᵗʰ **S60.85** Superficial **foreign body** of wrist

Splinter in the wrist

√7ᵗʰ **S60.851** Superficial foreign body of **right** wrist

√7ᵗʰ **S60.852** Superficial foreign body of **left** wrist

√7ᵗʰ **S60.859** Superficial foreign body of unspecified wrist ▽

√6ᵗʰ **S60.86** Insect bite (nonvenomous) of wrist

√7ᵗʰ **S60.861** Insect bite (nonvenomous) of **right** wrist

√7ᵗʰ **S60.862** Insect bite (nonvenomous) of **left** wrist

√7ᵗʰ **S60.869** Insect bite (nonvenomous) of unspecified wrist ▽

√6ᵗʰ **S60.87** Other superficial **bite** of wrist

EXCLUDES 1 *open bite of wrist (S61.55)*

√7ᵗʰ **S60.871** Other superficial bite of **right** wrist

√7ᵗʰ **S60.872** Other superficial bite of **left** wrist

√7ᵗʰ **S60.879** Other superficial bite of unspecified wrist ▽

√5ᵗʰ **S60.9** Unspecified superficial injury of wrist, hand and fingers

√6ᵗʰ **S60.91** Unspecified superficial injury of **wrist**

√7ᵗʰ **S60.911** Unspecified superficial injury of **right** wrist ▽

√7ᵗʰ **S60.912** Unspecified superficial injury of **left** wrist ▽

√7ᵗʰ **S60.919** Unspecified superficial injury of unspecified wrist ▽

√6ᵗʰ **S60.92** Unspecified superficial injury of **hand**

√7ᵗʰ **S60.921** Unspecified superficial injury of **right** hand ▽

√7ᵗʰ **S60.922** Unspecified superficial injury of **left** hand ▽

√7ᵗʰ **S60.929** Unspecified superficial injury of unspecified hand ▽

√6ᵗʰ **S60.93** Unspecified superficial injury of **thumb**

√7ᵗʰ **S60.931** Unspecified superficial injury of **right** thumb ▽

√7ᵗʰ **S60.932** Unspecified superficial injury of **left** thumb ▽

√7ᵗʰ **S60.939** Unspecified superficial injury of unspecified thumb ▽

√6ᵗʰ **S60.94** Unspecified superficial injury of other **fingers**

√7ᵗʰ **S60.940** Unspecified superficial injury of **right** index **finger** ▽

√7ᵗʰ **S60.941** Unspecified superficial injury of **left** index **finger** ▽

√7ᵗʰ **S60.942** Unspecified superficial injury of **right** middle **finger** ▽

√7ᵗʰ **S60.943** Unspecified superficial injury of **left** middle **finger** ▽

√7ᵗʰ **S60.944** Unspecified superficial injury of **right** ring **finger** ▽

√7ᵗʰ **S60.945** Unspecified superficial injury of **left** ring **finger** ▽

√7ᵗʰ **S60.946** Unspecified superficial injury of **right** little **finger** ▽

√7ᵗʰ **S60.947** Unspecified superficial injury of **left** little **finger** ▽

√7ᵗʰ **S60.948** Unspecified superficial injury of other **finger** ▽

Unspecified superficial injury of specified finger with unspecified laterality

√7ᵗʰ **S60.949** Unspecified superficial injury of unspecified finger ▽

√4ᵗʰ **S61** **Open wound of wrist, hand and fingers**

Code also any associated wound infection

EXCLUDES 1 *open fracture of wrist, hand and finger (S62.- with 7th character B)*

traumatic amputation of wrist and hand (S68.-)

The appropriate 7th character is to be added to each code from category S61.
A   initial encounter
D   subsequent encounter
S   sequela

√5ᵗʰ **S61.0** **Open wound of thumb without damage to nail**

EXCLUDES 1 *open wound of thumb with damage to nail (S61.1-)*

√6ᵗʰ **S61.00** Unspecified open wound of thumb without damage to nail

√7ᵗʰ **S61.001** Unspecified open wound of **right** thumb without damage to nail ▽

√7ᵗʰ **S61.002** Unspecified open wound of **left** thumb without damage to nail ▽

√7ᵗʰ **S61.009** Unspecified open wound of unspecified thumb without damage to nail ▽

√6ᵗʰ **S61.01** Laceration without foreign body of thumb without damage to nail

√7ᵗʰ **S61.011** Laceration without foreign body of **right** thumb without damage to nail ▽

√7ᵗʰ **S61.012** Laceration without foreign body of **left** thumb without damage to nail ▽

√7ᵗʰ **S61.019** Laceration without foreign body of unspecified thumb without damage to nail ▽

√6ᵗʰ **S61.02** Laceration with foreign body of thumb without damage to nail

√7ᵗʰ **S61.021** Laceration with foreign body of **right** thumb without damage to nail ▽

√7ᵗʰ **S61.022** Laceration with foreign body of **left** thumb without damage to nail ▽

√7ᵗʰ **S61.029** Laceration with foreign body of unspecified thumb without damage to nail ▽

√6ᵗʰ **S61.03** Puncture wound without foreign body of thumb without damage to nail

√7ᵗʰ **S61.031** Puncture wound without foreign body of **right** thumb without damage to nail ▽

√7ᵗʰ **S61.032** Puncture wound without foreign body of **left** thumb without damage to nail ▽

√7ᵗʰ **S61.039** Puncture wound without foreign body of unspecified thumb without damage to nail ▽

√6ᵗʰ **S61.04** Puncture wound with foreign body of thumb without damage to nail

√7ᵗʰ **S61.041** Puncture wound with foreign body of **right** thumb without damage to nail

EXCLUDES 1 Not coded here   EXCLUDES 2 Not included here   N Newborn Age : 0   P Pediatric Age : 0-17   M Maternity Age : 12-55   A Adult Age : 15-124

√7ᵗʰ **S61.042** Puncture wound with foreign body of left thumb without damage to nail

√7ᵗʰ **S61.049** Puncture wound with foreign body of unspecified thumb without damage to nail ▽

√6ᵗʰ **S61.05** Open bite of thumb without damage to nail

Bite of thumb NOS

EXCLUDES 1 *superficial bite of thumb (S60.36-, S60.37-)*

√7ᵗʰ **S61.051** Open bite of right thumb without damage to nail

√7ᵗʰ **S61.052** Open bite of left thumb without damage to nail

√7ᵗʰ **S61.059** Open bite of unspecified thumb without damage to nail ▽

√5ᵗʰ **S61.1** Open wound of thumb with damage to nail

√6ᵗʰ **S61.10** Unspecified open wound of thumb with damage to nail

√7ᵗʰ **S61.101** Unspecified open wound of right thumb with damage to nail ▽

√7ᵗʰ **S61.102** Unspecified open wound of left thumb with damage to nail ▽

√7ᵗʰ **S61.109** Unspecified open wound of unspecified thumb with damage to nail ▽

√6ᵗʰ **S61.11** Laceration without foreign body of thumb with damage to nail

√7ᵗʰ **S61.111** Laceration without foreign body of right thumb with damage to nail

√7ᵗʰ **S61.112** Laceration without foreign body of left thumb with damage to nail

√7ᵗʰ **S61.119** Laceration without foreign body of unspecified thumb with damage to nail ▽

√6ᵗʰ **S61.12** Laceration with foreign body of thumb with damage to nail

√7ᵗʰ **S61.121** Laceration with foreign body of right thumb with damage to nail

√7ᵗʰ **S61.122** Laceration with foreign body of left thumb with damage to nail

√7ᵗʰ **S61.129** Laceration with foreign body of unspecified thumb with damage to nail ▽

√6ᵗʰ **S61.13** Puncture wound without foreign body of thumb with damage to nail

√7ᵗʰ **S61.131** Puncture wound without foreign body of right thumb with damage to nail

√7ᵗʰ **S61.132** Puncture wound without foreign body of left thumb with damage to nail

√7ᵗʰ **S61.139** Puncture wound without foreign body of unspecified thumb with damage to nail ▽

√6ᵗʰ **S61.14** Puncture wound with foreign body of thumb with damage to nail

√7ᵗʰ **S61.141** Puncture wound with foreign body of right thumb with damage to nail

√7ᵗʰ **S61.142** Puncture wound with foreign body of left thumb with damage to nail

√7ᵗʰ **S61.149** Puncture wound with foreign body of unspecified thumb with damage to nail ▽

√6ᵗʰ **S61.15** Open bite of thumb with damage to nail

Bite of thumb with damage to nail NOS

EXCLUDES 1 *superficial bite of thumb (S60.36-, S60.37-)*

√7ᵗʰ **S61.151** Open bite of right thumb with damage to nail

√7ᵗʰ **S61.152** Open bite of left thumb with damage to nail

√7ᵗʰ **S61.159** Open bite of unspecified thumb with damage to nail ▽

√5ᵗʰ **S61.2** Open wound of other finger without damage to nail

EXCLUDES 1 *open wound of finger involving nail (matrix) (S61.3-)*

EXCLUDES 2 *open wound of thumb without damage to nail (S61.0-)*

√6ᵗʰ **S61.20** Unspecified open wound of other finger without damage to nail

√7ᵗʰ **S61.200** Unspecified open wound of right index finger without damage to nail ▽

√7ᵗʰ **S61.201** Unspecified open wound of left index finger without damage to nail ▽

√7ᵗʰ **S61.202** Unspecified open wound of right middle finger without damage to nail ▽

√7ᵗʰ **S61.203** Unspecified open wound of left middle finger without damage to nail ▽

√7ᵗʰ **S61.204** Unspecified open wound of right ring finger without damage to nail ▽

√7ᵗʰ **S61.205** Unspecified open wound of left ring finger without damage to nail ▽

√7ᵗʰ **S61.206** Unspecified open wound of right little finger without damage to nail ▽

√7ᵗʰ **S61.207** Unspecified open wound of left little finger without damage to nail ▽

√7ᵗʰ **S61.208** Unspecified open wound of other finger without damage to nail ▽

Unspecified open wound of specified finger with unspecified laterality without damage to nail

√7ᵗʰ **S61.209** Unspecified open wound of unspecified finger without damage to nail ▽

√6ᵗʰ **S61.21** Laceration without foreign body of finger without damage to nail

√7ᵗʰ **S61.210** Laceration without foreign body of right index finger without damage to nail

√7ᵗʰ **S61.211** Laceration without foreign body of left index finger without damage to nail

√7ᵗʰ **S61.212** Laceration without foreign body of right middle finger without damage to nail

√7ᵗʰ **S61.213** Laceration without foreign body of left middle finger without damage to nail

√7ᵗʰ **S61.214** Laceration without foreign body of right ring finger without damage to nail

√7ᵗʰ **S61.215** Laceration without foreign body of left ring finger without damage to nail

√7ᵗʰ **S61.216** Laceration without foreign body of right little finger without damage to nail

√7ᵗʰ **S61.217** Laceration without foreign body of left little finger without damage to nail

√7ᵗʰ **S61.218** Laceration without foreign body of other finger without damage to nail

Laceration without foreign body of specified finger with unspecified laterality without damage to nail

√7ᵗʰ **S61.219** Laceration without foreign body of unspecified finger without damage to nail ▽

√8ᵗʰ **S61.22** Laceration with foreign body of finger without damage to nail

√7ᵗʰ **S61.220** Laceration with foreign body of right index finger without damage to nail

√7ᵗʰ **S61.221** Laceration with foreign body of left index finger without damage to nail

√7ᵗʰ **S61.222** Laceration with foreign body of right middle finger without damage to nail

√7ᵗʰ **S61.223** Laceration with foreign body of left middle finger without damage to nail

√7ᵗʰ **S61.224** Laceration with foreign body of right ring finger without damage to nail

√7ᵗʰ **S61.225** Laceration with foreign body of left ring finger without damage to nail

√7ᵗʰ **S61.226** Laceration with foreign body of right little finger without damage to nail

√7ᵗʰ **S61.227** Laceration with foreign body of left little finger without damage to nail

√7ᵗʰ **S61.228** Laceration with foreign body of other finger without damage to nail

Laceration with foreign body of specified finger with unspecified laterality without damage to nail

√7ᵗʰ **S61.229** Laceration with foreign body of unspecified finger without damage to nail ▽

√6ᵗʰ **S61.23** Puncture wound without foreign body of finger without damage to nail

√7ᵗʰ **S61.230** Puncture wound without foreign body of right index finger without damage to nail

√7ᵗʰ **S61.231** Puncture wound without foreign body of left index finger without damage to nail

☑ Additional Character Required   √×7ᵗʰ Placeholder Alert   Manifestation Dx   ▽ Unspecified Dx   ▶◀ Revised Text   ● New Code   ▲ Revised Code Title

ICD-10-CM 2017   953

Chapter 19. Injury, Poisoning and Certain Other Consequences of External Causes

S61.042–S61.231

Chapter 19. Injury, Poisoning and Certain Other Consequences of External Causes

S61.232–S61.333

√7ᵗʰ **S61.232 Puncture wound without foreign body of right middle finger without damage to nail**

√7ᵗʰ **S61.233 Puncture wound without foreign body of left middle finger without damage to nail**

√7ᵗʰ **S61.234 Puncture wound without foreign body of right ring finger without damage to nail**

√7ᵗʰ **S61.235 Puncture wound without foreign body of left ring finger without damage to nail**

√7ᵗʰ **S61.236 Puncture wound without foreign body of right little finger without damage to nail**

√7ᵗʰ **S61.237 Puncture wound without foreign body of left little finger without damage to nail**

√7ᵗʰ **S61.238 Puncture wound without foreign body of other finger without damage to nail**

Puncture wound without foreign body of specified finger with unspecified laterality without damage to nail

√7ᵗʰ **S61.239 Puncture wound without foreign body of unspecified finger without damage to nail** ▽

√6ᵗʰ **S61.24 Puncture wound with foreign body of finger without damage to nail**

√7ᵗʰ **S61.240 Puncture wound with foreign body of right index finger without damage to nail**

√7ᵗʰ **S61.241 Puncture wound with foreign body of left index finger without damage to nail**

√7ᵗʰ **S61.242 Puncture wound with foreign body of right middle finger without damage to nail**

√7ᵗʰ **S61.243 Puncture wound with foreign body of left middle finger without damage to nail**

√7ᵗʰ **S61.244 Puncture wound with foreign body of right ring finger without damage to nail**

√7ᵗʰ **S61.245 Puncture wound with foreign body of left ring finger without damage to nail**

√7ᵗʰ **S61.246 Puncture wound with foreign body of right little finger without damage to nail**

√7ᵗʰ **S61.247 Puncture wound with foreign body of left little finger without damage to nail**

√7ᵗʰ **S61.248 Puncture wound with foreign body of other finger without damage to nail**

Puncture wound with foreign body of specified finger with unspecified laterality without damage to nail

√7ᵗʰ **S61.249 Puncture wound with foreign body of unspecified finger without damage to nail** ▽

√6ᵗʰ **S61.25 Open bite of finger without damage to nail**

Bite of finger without damage to nail NOS

EXCLUDES 1 *superficial bite of finger (S60.46-, S60.47-)*

√7ᵗʰ **S61.250 Open bite of right index finger without damage to nail**

√7ᵗʰ **S61.251 Open bite of left index finger without damage to nail**

√7ᵗʰ **S61.252 Open bite of right middle finger without damage to nail**

√7ᵗʰ **S61.253 Open bite of left middle finger without damage to nail**

√7ᵗʰ **S61.254 Open bite of right ring finger without damage to nail**

√7ᵗʰ **S61.255 Open bite of left ring finger without damage to nail**

√7ᵗʰ **S61.256 Open bite of right little finger without damage to nail**

√7ᵗʰ **S61.257 Open bite of left little finger without damage to nail**

√7ᵗʰ **S61.258 Open bite of other finger without damage to nail**

Open bite of specified finger with unspecified laterality without damage to nail

√7ᵗʰ **S61.259 Open bite of unspecified finger without damage to nail** ▽

√5ᵗʰ **S61.3 Open wound of other finger with damage to nail**

√6ᵗʰ **S61.30 Unspecified open wound of finger with damage to nail**

√7ᵗʰ **S61.300 Unspecified open wound of right index finger with damage to nail** ▽

√7ᵗʰ **S61.301 Unspecified open wound of left index finger with damage to nail** ▽

√7ᵗʰ **S61.302 Unspecified open wound of right middle finger with damage to nail** ▽

√7ᵗʰ **S61.303 Unspecified open wound of left middle finger with damage to nail** ▽

√7ᵗʰ **S61.304 Unspecified open wound of right ring finger with damage to nail** ▽

√7ᵗʰ **S61.305 Unspecified open wound of left ring finger with damage to nail** ▽

√7ᵗʰ **S61.306 Unspecified open wound of right little finger with damage to nail** ▽

√7ᵗʰ **S61.307 Unspecified open wound of left little finger with damage to nail** ▽

√7ᵗʰ **S61.308 Unspecified open wound of other finger with damage to nail** ▽

Unspecified open wound of specified finger with unspecified laterality with damage to nail

√7ᵗʰ **S61.309 Unspecified open wound of unspecified finger with damage to nail** ▽

√6ᵗʰ **S61.31 Laceration without foreign body of finger with damage to nail**

√7ᵗʰ **S61.310 Laceration without foreign body of right index finger with damage to nail**

√7ᵗʰ **S61.311 Laceration without foreign body of left index finger with damage to nail**

√7ᵗʰ **S61.312 Laceration without foreign body of right middle finger with damage to nail**

√7ᵗʰ **S61.313 Laceration without foreign body of left middle finger with damage to nail**

√7ᵗʰ **S61.314 Laceration without foreign body of right ring finger with damage to nail**

√7ᵗʰ **S61.315 Laceration without foreign body of left ring finger with damage to nail**

√7ᵗʰ **S61.316 Laceration without foreign body of right little finger with damage to nail**

√7ᵗʰ **S61.317 Laceration without foreign body of left little finger with damage to nail**

√7ᵗʰ **S61.318 Laceration without foreign body of other finger with damage to nail**

Laceration without foreign body of specified finger with unspecified laterality with damage to nail

√7ᵗʰ **S61.319 Laceration without foreign body of unspecified finger with damage to nail** ▽

√6ᵗʰ **S61.32 Laceration with foreign body of finger with damage to nail**

√7ᵗʰ **S61.320 Laceration with foreign body of right index finger with damage to nail**

√7ᵗʰ **S61.321 Laceration with foreign body of left index finger with damage to nail**

√7ᵗʰ **S61.322 Laceration with foreign body of right middle finger with damage to nail**

√7ᵗʰ **S61.323 Laceration with foreign body of left middle finger with damage to nail**

√7ᵗʰ **S61.324 Laceration with foreign body of right ring finger with damage to nail**

√7ᵗʰ **S61.325 Laceration with foreign body of left ring finger with damage to nail**

√7ᵗʰ **S61.326 Laceration with foreign body of right little finger with damage to nail**

√7ᵗʰ **S61.327 Laceration with foreign body of left little finger with damage to nail**

√7ᵗʰ **S61.328 Laceration with foreign body of other finger with damage to nail**

Laceration with foreign body of specified finger with unspecified laterality with damage to nail

√7ᵗʰ **S61.329 Laceration with foreign body of unspecified finger with damage to nail** ▽

√6ᵗʰ **S61.33 Puncture wound without foreign body of finger with damage to nail**

√7ᵗʰ **S61.330 Puncture wound without foreign body of right index finger with damage to nail**

√7ᵗʰ **S61.331 Puncture wound without foreign body of left index finger with damage to nail**

√7ᵗʰ **S61.332 Puncture wound without foreign body of right middle finger with damage to nail**

√7ᵗʰ **S61.333 Puncture wound without foreign body of left middle finger with damage to nail**

EXCLUDES 1 Not coded here   EXCLUDES 2 Not included here   N Newborn Age : 0   P Pediatric Age : 0-17   M Maternity Age : 12-55   A Adult Age : 15-124

954   ICD-10-CM 2017

√7ᵗʰ **S61.334 Puncture wound without foreign body of right ring finger with damage to nail**

√7ᵗʰ **S61.335 Puncture wound without foreign body of left ring finger with damage to nail**

√7ᵗʰ **S61.336 Puncture wound without foreign body of right little finger with damage to nail**

√7ᵗʰ **S61.337 Puncture wound without foreign body of left little finger with damage to nail**

√7ᵗʰ **S61.338 Puncture wound without foreign body of other finger with damage to nail**

> Puncture wound without foreign body of specified finger with unspecified laterality with damage to nail

√7ᵗʰ **S61.339 Puncture wound without foreign body of unspecified finger with damage to nail** ▽

√6ᵗʰ **S61.34 Puncture wound with foreign body of finger with damage to nail**

√7ᵗʰ **S61.340 Puncture wound with foreign body of right index finger with damage to nail**

√7ᵗʰ **S61.341 Puncture wound with foreign body of left index finger with damage to nail**

√7ᵗʰ **S61.342 Puncture wound with foreign body of right middle finger with damage to nail**

√7ᵗʰ **S61.343 Puncture wound with foreign body of left middle finger with damage to nail**

√7ᵗʰ **S61.344 Puncture wound with foreign body of right ring finger with damage to nail**

√7ᵗʰ **S61.345 Puncture wound with foreign body of left ring finger with damage to nail**

√7ᵗʰ **S61.346 Puncture wound with foreign body of right little finger with damage to nail**

√7ᵗʰ **S61.347 Puncture wound with foreign body of left little finger with damage to nail**

√7ᵗʰ **S61.348 Puncture wound with foreign body of other finger with damage to nail**

> Puncture wound with foreign body of specified finger with unspecified laterality with damage to nail

√7ᵗʰ **S61.349 Puncture wound with foreign body of unspecified finger with damage to nail** ▽

√6ᵗʰ **S61.35 Open bite of finger with damage to nail**

> Bite of finger with damage to nail NOS
> **EXCLUDES 1** *superficial bite of finger (S60.46-, S60.47-)*

√7ᵗʰ **S61.350 Open bite of right index finger with damage to nail**

√7ᵗʰ **S61.351 Open bite of left index finger with damage to nail**

√7ᵗʰ **S61.352 Open bite of right middle finger with damage to nail**

√7ᵗʰ **S61.353 Open bite of left middle finger with damage to nail**

√7ᵗʰ **S61.354 Open bite of right ring finger with damage to nail**

√7ᵗʰ **S61.355 Open bite of left ring finger with damage to nail**

√7ᵗʰ **S61.356 Open bite of right little finger with damage to nail**

√7ᵗʰ **S61.357 Open bite of left little finger with damage to nail**

√7ᵗʰ **S61.358 Open bite of other finger with damage to nail**

> Open bite of specified finger with unspecified laterality with damage to nail

√7ᵗʰ **S61.359 Open bite of unspecified finger with damage to nail** ▽

√5ᵗʰ **S61.4 Open wound of hand**

√6ᵗʰ **S61.40 Unspecified open wound of hand**

√7ᵗʰ **S61.401 Unspecified open wound of right hand** ▽

√7ᵗʰ **S61.402 Unspecified open wound of left hand** ▽

√7ᵗʰ **S61.409 Unspecified open wound of unspecified hand** ▽

√6ᵗʰ **S61.41 Laceration without foreign body of hand**

√7ᵗʰ **S61.411 Laceration without foreign body of right hand**

√7ᵗʰ **S61.412 Laceration without foreign body of left hand**

√7ᵗʰ **S61.419 Laceration without foreign body of unspecified hand** ▽

√6ᵗʰ **S61.42 Laceration with foreign body of hand**

√7ᵗʰ **S61.421 Laceration with foreign body of right hand**

√7ᵗʰ **S61.422 Laceration with foreign body of left hand**

√7ᵗʰ **S61.429 Laceration with foreign body of unspecified hand** ▽

√6ᵗʰ **S61.43 Puncture wound without foreign body of hand**

√7ᵗʰ **S61.431 Puncture wound without foreign body of right hand**

√7ᵗʰ **S61.432 Puncture wound without foreign body of left hand**

√7ᵗʰ **S61.439 Puncture wound without foreign body of unspecified hand** ▽

√6ᵗʰ **S61.44 Puncture wound with foreign body of hand**

√7ᵗʰ **S61.441 Puncture wound with foreign body of right hand**

√7ᵗʰ **S61.442 Puncture wound with foreign body of left hand**

√7ᵗʰ **S61.449 Puncture wound with foreign body of unspecified hand** ▽

√6ᵗʰ **S61.45 Open bite of hand**

> Bite of hand NOS
> **EXCLUDES 1** *superficial bite of hand (S60.56-, S60.57-)*

√7ᵗʰ **S61.451 Open bite of right hand**

√7ᵗʰ **S61.452 Open bite of left hand**

√7ᵗʰ **S61.459 Open bite of unspecified hand** ▽

√5ᵗʰ **S61.5 Open wound of wrist**

√6ᵗʰ **S61.50 Unspecified open wound of wrist**

√7ᵗʰ **S61.501 Unspecified open wound of right wrist** ▽

√7ᵗʰ **S61.502 Unspecified open wound of left wrist** ▽

√7ᵗʰ **S61.509 Unspecified open wound of unspecified wrist** ▽

√6ᵗʰ **S61.51 Laceration without foreign body of wrist**

√7ᵗʰ **S61.511 Laceration without foreign body of right wrist**

√7ᵗʰ **S61.512 Laceration without foreign body of left wrist**

√7ᵗʰ **S61.519 Laceration without foreign body of unspecified wrist** ▽

√6ᵗʰ **S61.52 Laceration with foreign body of wrist**

√7ᵗʰ **S61.521 Laceration with foreign body of right wrist**

√7ᵗʰ **S61.522 Laceration with foreign body of left wrist**

√7ᵗʰ **S61.529 Laceration with foreign body of unspecified wrist** ▽

√6ᵗʰ **S61.53 Puncture wound without foreign body of wrist**

√7ᵗʰ **S61.531 Puncture wound without foreign body of right wrist**

√7ᵗʰ **S61.532 Puncture wound without foreign body of left wrist**

√7ᵗʰ **S61.539 Puncture wound without foreign body of unspecified wrist** ▽

√6ᵗʰ **S61.54 Puncture wound with foreign body of wrist**

√7ᵗʰ **S61.541 Puncture wound with foreign body of right wrist**

√7ᵗʰ **S61.542 Puncture wound with foreign body of left wrist**

√7ᵗʰ **S61.549 Puncture wound with foreign body of unspecified wrist** ▽

√6ᵗʰ **S61.55 Open bite of wrist**

> Bite of wrist NOS
> **EXCLUDES 1** *superficial bite of wrist (S60.86-, S60.87-)*

√7ᵗʰ **S61.551 Open bite of right wrist**

√7ᵗʰ **S61.552 Open bite of left wrist**

√7ᵗʰ **S61.559 Open bite of unspecified wrist** ▽

☑ Additional Character Required   √√7ᵗʰ Placeholder Alert   Manifestation Dx   ▽ Unspecified Dx   ▶◀ Revised Text   ● New Code   ▲ Revised Code Title

ICD-10-CM 2017   955

Chapter 19. Injury, Poisoning and Certain Other Consequences of External Causes

S62–S62.155

✓4ᵗʰ S62 Fracture at wrist and hand level

> **NOTE** A fracture not indicated as displaced or nondisplaced should be coded to displaced
>
> A fracture not indicated as open or closed should be coded to closed

> **EXCLUDES 1** *traumatic amputation of wrist and hand (S68.-)*
> **EXCLUDES 2** *fracture of distal parts of ulna and radius (S52.-)*

AHA: 2015,3Q,37-39

> The appropriate 7th character is to be added to each code from category S62.
> A   initial encounter for closed fracture
> B   initial encounter for open fracture
> D   subsequent encounter for fracture with routine healing
> G   subsequent encounter for fracture with delayed healing
> K   subsequent encounter for fracture with nonunion
> P   subsequent encounter for fracture with malunion
> S   sequela

✓5ᵗʰ S62.0 Fracture of navicular [scaphoid] bone of wrist

  ✓6ᵗʰ S62.00 Unspecified fracture of navicular [scaphoid] bone of wrist

    ✓7ᵗʰ S62.001 Unspecified fracture of navicular [scaphoid] bone of right wrist ▽

    ✓7ᵗʰ S62.002 Unspecified fracture of navicular [scaphoid] bone of left wrist ▽

        AHA: 2012,4Q,106

    ✓7ᵗʰ S62.009 Unspecified fracture of navicular [scaphoid] bone of unspecified wrist ▽

  ✓6ᵗʰ S62.01 Fracture of distal pole of navicular [scaphoid] bone of wrist

    Fracture of volar tuberosity of navicular [scaphoid] bone of wrist

    ✓7ᵗʰ S62.011 Displaced fracture of distal pole of navicular [scaphoid] bone of right wrist

    ✓7ᵗʰ S62.012 Displaced fracture of distal pole of navicular [scaphoid] bone of left wrist

    ✓7ᵗʰ S62.013 Displaced fracture of distal pole of navicular [scaphoid] bone of unspecified wrist ▽

    ✓7ᵗʰ S62.014 Nondisplaced fracture of distal pole of navicular [scaphoid] bone of right wrist

    ✓7ᵗʰ S62.015 Nondisplaced fracture of distal pole of navicular [scaphoid] bone of left wrist

    ✓7ᵗʰ S62.016 Nondisplaced fracture of distal pole of navicular [scaphoid] bone of unspecified wrist ▽

  ✓6ᵗʰ S62.02 Fracture of middle third of navicular [scaphoid] bone of wrist

    ✓7ᵗʰ S62.021 Displaced fracture of middle third of navicular [scaphoid] bone of right wrist

    ✓7ᵗʰ S62.022 Displaced fracture of middle third of navicular [scaphoid] bone of left wrist

    ✓7ᵗʰ S62.023 Displaced fracture of middle third of navicular [scaphoid] bone of unspecified wrist ▽

    ✓7ᵗʰ S62.024 Nondisplaced fracture of middle third of navicular [scaphoid] bone of right wrist

    ✓7ᵗʰ S62.025 Nondisplaced fracture of middle third of navicular [scaphoid] bone of left wrist

    ✓7ᵗʰ S62.026 Nondisplaced fracture of middle third of navicular [scaphoid] bone of unspecified wrist ▽

  ✓6ᵗʰ S62.03 Fracture of proximal third of navicular [scaphoid] bone of wrist

    ✓7ᵗʰ S62.031 Displaced fracture of proximal third of navicular [scaphoid] bone of right wrist

    ✓7ᵗʰ S62.032 Displaced fracture of proximal third of navicular [scaphoid] bone of left wrist

    ✓7ᵗʰ S62.033 Displaced fracture of proximal third of navicular [scaphoid] bone of unspecified wrist ▽

    ✓7ᵗʰ S62.034 Nondisplaced fracture of proximal third of navicular [scaphoid] bone of right wrist

    ✓7ᵗʰ S62.035 Nondisplaced fracture of proximal third of navicular [scaphoid] bone of left wrist

    ✓7ᵗʰ S62.036 Nondisplaced fracture of proximal third of navicular [scaphoid] bone of unspecified wrist ▽

✓5ᵗʰ S62.1 Fracture of other and unspecified carpal bone(s)

> **EXCLUDES 2** *fracture of scaphoid of wrist (S62.0-)*

✓6ᵗʰ S62.10 Fracture of unspecified carpal bone

  Fracture of wrist NOS

  ✓7ᵗʰ S62.101 Fracture of unspecified carpal bone, right wrist ▽

  ✓7ᵗʰ S62.102 Fracture of unspecified carpal bone, left wrist ▽

    AHA: 2012,4Q,95

  ✓7ᵗʰ S62.109 Fracture of unspecified carpal bone, unspecified wrist ▽

✓6ᵗʰ S62.11 Fracture of triquetrum [cuneiform] bone of wrist

  ✓7ᵗʰ S62.111 Displaced fracture of triquetrum [cuneiform] bone, right wrist

  ✓7ᵗʰ S62.112 Displaced fracture of triquetrum [cuneiform] bone, left wrist

  ✓7ᵗʰ S62.113 Displaced fracture of triquetrum [cuneiform] bone, unspecified wrist ▽

  ✓7ᵗʰ S62.114 Nondisplaced fracture of triquetrum [cuneiform] bone, right wrist

  ✓7ᵗʰ S62.115 Nondisplaced fracture of triquetrum [cuneiform] bone, left wrist

  ✓7ᵗʰ S62.116 Nondisplaced fracture of triquetrum [cuneiform] bone, unspecified wrist ▽

✓6ᵗʰ S62.12 Fracture of lunate [semilunar]

  ✓7ᵗʰ S62.121 Displaced fracture of lunate [semilunar], right wrist

  ✓7ᵗʰ S62.122 Displaced fracture of lunate [semilunar], left wrist

  ✓7ᵗʰ S62.123 Displaced fracture of lunate [semilunar], unspecified wrist ▽

  ✓7ᵗʰ S62.124 Nondisplaced fracture of lunate [semilunar], right wrist

  ✓7ᵗʰ S62.125 Nondisplaced fracture of lunate [semilunar], left wrist

  ✓7ᵗʰ S62.126 Nondisplaced fracture of lunate [semilunar], unspecified wrist ▽

✓6ᵗʰ S62.13 Fracture of capitate [os magnum] bone

  ✓7ᵗʰ S62.131 Displaced fracture of capitate [os magnum] bone, right wrist

  ✓7ᵗʰ S62.132 Displaced fracture of capitate [os magnum] bone, left wrist

  ✓7ᵗʰ S62.133 Displaced fracture of capitate [os magnum] bone, unspecified wrist ▽

  ✓7ᵗʰ S62.134 Nondisplaced fracture of capitate [os magnum] bone, right wrist

  ✓7ᵗʰ S62.135 Nondisplaced fracture of capitate [os magnum] bone, left wrist

  ✓7ᵗʰ S62.136 Nondisplaced fracture of capitate [os magnum] bone, unspecified wrist ▽

✓6ᵗʰ S62.14 Fracture of body of hamate [unciform] bone

  Fracture of hamate [unciform] bone NOS

  ✓7ᵗʰ S62.141 Displaced fracture of body of hamate [unciform] bone, right wrist

  ✓7ᵗʰ S62.142 Displaced fracture of body of hamate [unciform] bone, left wrist

  ✓7ᵗʰ S62.143 Displaced fracture of body of hamate [unciform] bone, unspecified wrist ▽

  ✓7ᵗʰ S62.144 Nondisplaced fracture of body of hamate [unciform] bone, right wrist

  ✓7ᵗʰ S62.145 Nondisplaced fracture of body of hamate [unciform] bone, left wrist

  ✓7ᵗʰ S62.146 Nondisplaced fracture of body of hamate [unciform] bone, unspecified wrist ▽

✓6ᵗʰ S62.15 Fracture of hook process of hamate [unciform] bone

  Fracture of unciform process of hamate [unciform] bone

  ✓7ᵗʰ S62.151 Displaced fracture of hook process of hamate [unciform] bone, right wrist

  ✓7ᵗʰ S62.152 Displaced fracture of hook process of hamate [unciform] bone, left wrist

  ✓7ᵗʰ S62.153 Displaced fracture of hook process of hamate [unciform] bone, unspecified wrist ▽

  ✓7ᵗʰ S62.154 Nondisplaced fracture of hook process of hamate [unciform] bone, right wrist

  ✓7ᵗʰ S62.155 Nondisplaced fracture of hook process of hamate [unciform] bone, left wrist

---

EXCLUDES 1 Not coded here   **EXCLUDES 2** Not included here   **N** Newborn Age : 0   **P** Pediatric Age : 0-17   **M** Maternity Age : 12-55   **A** Adult Age : 15-124

956   ICD-10-CM 2017

√7ᵗʰ **S62.156** Nondisplaced fracture of hook process of hamate [unciform] bone, unspecified wrist

√6ᵗʰ **S62.16** Fracture of pisiform

√7ᵗʰ **S62.161** Displaced fracture of pisiform, right wrist

√7ᵗʰ **S62.162** Displaced fracture of pisiform, left wrist

√7ᵗʰ **S62.163** Displaced fracture of pisiform, unspecified wrist ▽

√7ᵗʰ **S62.164** Nondisplaced fracture of pisiform, right wrist

√7ᵗʰ **S62.165** Nondisplaced fracture of pisiform, left wrist

√7ᵗʰ **S62.166** Nondisplaced fracture of pisiform, unspecified wrist ▽

√6ᵗʰ **S62.17** Fracture of trapezium [larger multangular]

√7ᵗʰ **S62.171** Displaced fracture of trapezium [larger multangular], right wrist

√7ᵗʰ **S62.172** Displaced fracture of trapezium [larger multangular], left wrist

√7ᵗʰ **S62.173** Displaced fracture of trapezium [larger multangular], unspecified wrist ▽

√7ᵗʰ **S62.174** Nondisplaced fracture of trapezium [larger multangular], right wrist

√7ᵗʰ **S62.175** Nondisplaced fracture of trapezium [larger multangular], left wrist

√7ᵗʰ **S62.176** Nondisplaced fracture of trapezium [larger multangular], unspecified wrist ▽

√6ᵗʰ **S62.18** Fracture of trapezoid [smaller multangular]

√7ᵗʰ **S62.181** Displaced fracture of trapezoid [smaller multangular], right wrist

√7ᵗʰ **S62.182** Displaced fracture of trapezoid [smaller multangular], left wrist

√7ᵗʰ **S62.183** Displaced fracture of trapezoid [smaller multangular], unspecified wrist ▽

√7ᵗʰ **S62.184** Nondisplaced fracture of trapezoid [smaller multangular], right wrist

√7ᵗʰ **S62.185** Nondisplaced fracture of trapezoid [smaller multangular], left wrist

√7ᵗʰ **S62.186** Nondisplaced fracture of trapezoid [smaller multangular], unspecified wrist ▽

√5ᵗʰ **S62.2** Fracture of first metacarpal bone

√6ᵗʰ **S62.20** Unspecified fracture of first metacarpal bone

√7ᵗʰ **S62.201** Unspecified fracture of first metacarpal bone, right hand ▽

√7ᵗʰ **S62.202** Unspecified fracture of first metacarpal bone, left hand ▽

√7ᵗʰ **S62.209** Unspecified fracture of first metacarpal bone, unspecified hand ▽

√6ᵗʰ **S62.21** Bennett's fracture

√7ᵗʰ **S62.211** Bennett's fracture, right hand

√7ᵗʰ **S62.212** Bennett's fracture, left hand

√7ᵗʰ **S62.213** Bennett's fracture, unspecified hand ▽

√6ᵗʰ **S62.22** Rolando's fracture

√7ᵗʰ **S62.221** Displaced Rolando's fracture, right hand

√7ᵗʰ **S62.222** Displaced Rolando's fracture, left hand

√7ᵗʰ **S62.223** Displaced Rolando's fracture, unspecified hand ▽

√7ᵗʰ **S62.224** Nondisplaced Rolando's fracture, right hand

√7ᵗʰ **S62.225** Nondisplaced Rolando's fracture, left hand

√7ᵗʰ **S62.226** Nondisplaced Rolando's fracture, unspecified hand ▽

√6ᵗʰ **S62.23** Other fracture of base of first metacarpal bone

√7ᵗʰ **S62.231** Other displaced fracture of base of first metacarpal bone, right hand

√7ᵗʰ **S62.232** Other displaced fracture of base of first metacarpal bone, left hand

√7ᵗʰ **S62.233** Other displaced fracture of base of first metacarpal bone, unspecified hand ▽

√7ᵗʰ **S62.234** Other nondisplaced fracture of base of first metacarpal bone, right hand

√7ᵗʰ **S62.235** Other nondisplaced fracture of base of first metacarpal bone, left hand

√7ᵗʰ **S62.236** Other nondisplaced fracture of base of first metacarpal bone, unspecified hand ▽

√6ᵗʰ **S62.24** Fracture of shaft of first metacarpal bone

√7ᵗʰ **S62.241** Displaced fracture of shaft of first metacarpal bone, right hand

√7ᵗʰ **S62.242** Displaced fracture of shaft of first metacarpal bone, left hand

√7ᵗʰ **S62.243** Displaced fracture of shaft of first metacarpal bone, unspecified hand ▽

√7ᵗʰ **S62.244** Nondisplaced fracture of shaft of first metacarpal bone, right hand

√7ᵗʰ **S62.245** Nondisplaced fracture of shaft of first metacarpal bone, left hand

√7ᵗʰ **S62.246** Nondisplaced fracture of shaft of first metacarpal bone, unspecified hand ▽

√6ᵗʰ **S62.25** Fracture of neck of first metacarpal bone

√7ᵗʰ **S62.251** Displaced fracture of neck of first metacarpal bone, right hand

√7ᵗʰ **S62.252** Displaced fracture of neck of first metacarpal bone, left hand

√7ᵗʰ **S62.253** Displaced fracture of neck of first metacarpal bone, unspecified hand ▽

√7ᵗʰ **S62.254** Nondisplaced fracture of neck of first metacarpal bone, right hand

√7ᵗʰ **S62.255** Nondisplaced fracture of neck of first metacarpal bone, left hand

√7ᵗʰ **S62.256** Nondisplaced fracture of neck of first metacarpal bone, unspecified hand ▽

√6ᵗʰ **S62.29** Other fracture of first metacarpal bone

√7ᵗʰ **S62.291** Other fracture of first metacarpal bone, right hand

√7ᵗʰ **S62.292** Other fracture of first metacarpal bone, left hand

√7ᵗʰ **S62.299** Other fracture of first metacarpal bone, unspecified hand ▽

√5ᵗʰ **S62.3** Fracture of other and unspecified metacarpal bone

EXCLUDES 2 fracture of first metacarpal bone (S62.2-)

√6ᵗʰ **S62.30** Unspecified fracture of other metacarpal bone

√7ᵗʰ **S62.300** Unspecified fracture of second metacarpal bone, right hand ▽

√7ᵗʰ **S62.301** Unspecified fracture of second metacarpal bone, left hand ▽

√7ᵗʰ **S62.302** Unspecified fracture of third metacarpal bone, right hand ▽

√7ᵗʰ **S62.303** Unspecified fracture of third metacarpal bone, left hand ▽

√7ᵗʰ **S62.304** Unspecified fracture of fourth metacarpal bone, right hand ▽

√7ᵗʰ **S62.305** Unspecified fracture of fourth metacarpal bone, left hand ▽

√7ᵗʰ **S62.306** Unspecified fracture of fifth metacarpal bone, right hand ▽

√7ᵗʰ **S62.307** Unspecified fracture of fifth metacarpal bone, left hand ▽

√7ᵗʰ **S62.308** Unspecified fracture of other metacarpal bone ▽

Unspecified fracture of specified metacarpal bone with unspecified laterality

√7ᵗʰ **S62.309** Unspecified fracture of unspecified metacarpal bone ▽

√6ᵗʰ **S62.31** Displaced fracture of base of other metacarpal bone

√7ᵗʰ **S62.310** Displaced fracture of base of second metacarpal bone, right hand

√7ᵗʰ **S62.311** Displaced fracture of base of second metacarpal bone, left hand

√7ᵗʰ **S62.312** Displaced fracture of base of third metacarpal bone, right hand

√7ᵗʰ **S62.313** Displaced fracture of base of third metacarpal bone, left hand

√7ᵗʰ **S62.314** Displaced fracture of base of fourth metacarpal bone, right hand

√7ᵗʰ **S62.315** Displaced fracture of base of fourth metacarpal bone, left hand

☑ Additional Character Required   ✓ₓ7ᵗʰ Placeholder Alert   Manifestation Dx   ▽ Unspecified Dx   ▶◀ Revised Text   ● New Code   ▲ Revised Code Title

ICD-10-CM 2017

957

☑7ᵗʰ **S62.316 Displaced fracture of base of fifth metacarpal bone, right hand**

☑7ᵗʰ **S62.317 Displaced fracture of base of fifth metacarpal bone, left hand**

☑7ᵗʰ **S62.318 Displaced fracture of base of other metacarpal bone**

Displaced fracture of base of specified metacarpal bone with unspecified laterality

☑7ᵗʰ **S62.319 Displaced fracture of base of ▽ unspecified metacarpal bone**

√6ᵗʰ **S62.32 Displaced fracture of shaft of other metacarpal bone**

☑7ᵗʰ **S62.320 Displaced fracture of shaft of second metacarpal bone, right hand**

☑7ᵗʰ **S62.321 Displaced fracture of shaft of second metacarpal bone, left hand**

☑7ᵗʰ **S62.322 Displaced fracture of shaft of third metacarpal bone, right hand**

☑7ᵗʰ **S62.323 Displaced fracture of shaft of third metacarpal bone, left hand**

☑7ᵗʰ **S62.324 Displaced fracture of shaft of fourth metacarpal bone, right hand**

☑7ᵗʰ **S62.325 Displaced fracture of shaft of fourth metacarpal bone, left hand**

☑7ᵗʰ **S62.326 Displaced fracture of shaft of fifth metacarpal bone, right hand**

☑7ᵗʰ **S62.327 Displaced fracture of shaft of fifth metacarpal bone, left hand**

☑7ᵗʰ **S62.328 Displaced fracture of shaft of other metacarpal bone**

Displaced fracture of shaft of specified metacarpal bone with unspecified laterality

☑7ᵗʰ **S62.329 Displaced fracture of shaft of ▽ unspecified metacarpal bone**

√6ᵗʰ **S62.33 Displaced fracture of neck of other metacarpal bone**

☑7ᵗʰ **S62.330 Displaced fracture of neck of second metacarpal bone, right hand**

☑7ᵗʰ **S62.331 Displaced fracture of neck of second metacarpal bone, left hand**

☑7ᵗʰ **S62.332 Displaced fracture of neck of third metacarpal bone, right hand**

☑7ᵗʰ **S62.333 Displaced fracture of neck of third metacarpal bone, left hand**

☑7ᵗʰ **S62.334 Displaced fracture of neck of fourth metacarpal bone, right hand**

☑7ᵗʰ **S62.335 Displaced fracture of neck of fourth metacarpal bone, left hand**

☑7ᵗʰ **S62.336 Displaced fracture of neck of fifth metacarpal bone, right hand**

☑7ᵗʰ **S62.337 Displaced fracture of neck of fifth metacarpal bone, left hand**

☑7ᵗʰ **S62.338 Displaced fracture of neck of other metacarpal bone**

Displaced fracture of neck of specified metacarpal bone with unspecified laterality

☑7ᵗʰ **S62.339 Displaced fracture of neck of ▽ unspecified metacarpal bone**

√6ᵗʰ **S62.34 Nondisplaced fracture of base of other metacarpal bone**

☑7ᵗʰ **S62.340 Nondisplaced fracture of base of second metacarpal bone, right hand**

☑7ᵗʰ **S62.341 Nondisplaced fracture of base of second metacarpal bone. left hand**

☑7ᵗʰ **S62.342 Nondisplaced fracture of base of third metacarpal bone, right hand**

☑7ᵗʰ **S62.343 Nondisplaced fracture of base of third metacarpal bone, left hand**

☑7ᵗʰ **S62.344 Nondisplaced fracture of base of fourth metacarpal bone, right hand**

☑7ᵗʰ **S62.345 Nondisplaced fracture of base of fourth metacarpal bone, left hand**

☑7ᵗʰ **S62.346 Nondisplaced fracture of base of fifth metacarpal bone, right hand**

☑7ᵗʰ **S62.347 Nondisplaced fracture of base of fifth metacarpal bone, left hand**

☑7ᵗʰ **S62.348 Nondisplaced fracture of base of other metacarpal bone**

Nondisplaced fracture of base of specified metacarpal bone with unspecified laterality

☑7ᵗʰ **S62.349 Nondisplaced fracture of base of ▽ unspecified metacarpal bone**

√6ᵗʰ **S62.35 Nondisplaced fracture of shaft of other metacarpal bone**

☑7ᵗʰ **S62.350 Nondisplaced fracture of shaft of second metacarpal bone, right hand**

☑7ᵗʰ **S62.351 Nondisplaced fracture of shaft of second metacarpal bone, left hand**

☑7ᵗʰ **S62.352 Nondisplaced fracture of shaft of third metacarpal bone, right hand**

☑7ᵗʰ **S62.353 Nondisplaced fracture of shaft of third metacarpal bone, left hand**

☑7ᵗʰ **S62.354 Nondisplaced fracture of shaft of fourth metacarpal bone, right hand**

☑7ᵗʰ **S62.355 Nondisplaced fracture of shaft of fourth metacarpal bone, left hand**

☑7ᵗʰ **S62.356 Nondisplaced fracture of shaft of fifth metacarpal bone, right hand**

☑7ᵗʰ **S62.357 Nondisplaced fracture of shaft of fifth metacarpal bone, left hand**

☑7ᵗʰ **S62.358 Nondisplaced fracture of shaft of other metacarpal bone**

Nondisplaced fracture of shaft of specified metacarpal bone with unspecified laterality

☑7ᵗʰ **S62.359 Nondisplaced fracture of shaft of ▽ unspecified metacarpal bone**

√6ᵗʰ **S62.36 Nondisplaced fracture of neck of other metacarpal bone**

☑7ᵗʰ **S62.360 Nondisplaced fracture of neck of second metacarpal bone, right hand**

☑7ᵗʰ **S62.361 Nondisplaced fracture of neck of second metacarpal bone, left hand**

☑7ᵗʰ **S62.362 Nondisplaced fracture of neck of third metacarpal bone, right hand**

☑7ᵗʰ **S62.363 Nondisplaced fracture of neck of third metacarpal bone, left hand**

☑7ᵗʰ **S62.364 Nondisplaced fracture of neck of fourth metacarpal bone, right hand**

☑7ᵗʰ **S62.365 Nondisplaced fracture of neck of fourth metacarpal bone, left hand**

☑7ᵗʰ **S62.366 Nondisplaced fracture of neck of fifth metacarpal bone, right hand**

☑7ᵗʰ **S62.367 Nondisplaced fracture of neck of fifth metacarpal bone, left hand**

☑7ᵗʰ **S62.368 Nondisplaced fracture of neck of other metacarpal bone**

Nondisplaced fracture of neck of specified metacarpal bone with unspecified laterality

☑7ᵗʰ **S62.369 Nondisplaced fracture of neck of ▽ unspecified metacarpal bone**

√6ᵗʰ **S62.39 Other fracture of other metacarpal bone**

☑7ᵗʰ **S62.390 Other fracture of second metacarpal bone, right hand**

☑7ᵗʰ **S62.391 Other fracture of second metacarpal bone, left hand**

☑7ᵗʰ **S62.392 Other fracture of third metacarpal bone, right hand**

☑7ᵗʰ **S62.393 Other fracture of third metacarpal bone, left hand**

☑7ᵗʰ **S62.394 Other fracture of fourth metacarpal bone, right hand**

☑7ᵗʰ **S62.395 Other fracture of fourth metacarpal bone, left hand**

☑7ᵗʰ **S62.396 Other fracture of fifth metacarpal bone, right hand**

☑7ᵗʰ **S62.397 Other fracture of fifth metacarpal bone, left hand**

☑7ᵗʰ **S62.398 Other fracture of other metacarpal bone**

Other fracture of specified metacarpal bone with unspecified laterality

☑7ᵗʰ **S62.399 Other fracture of unspecified ▽ metacarpal bone**

√5ᵗʰ **S62.5 Fracture of thumb**

√6ᵗʰ **S62.50 Fracture of unspecified phalanx of thumb**

☑7ᵗʰ **S62.501 Fracture of unspecified phalanx of ▽ right thumb**

EXCLUDES 1 Not coded here   **EXCLUDES 2** Not included here   N Newborn Age : 0   P Pediatric Age : 0-17   M Maternity Age : 12-55   A Adult Age : 15-124

958   ICD-10-CM 2017

√7ᵗʰ **S62.502** Fracture of unspecified phalanx of left thumb ▽

√7ᵗʰ **S62.509** Fracture of unspecified phalanx of unspecified thumb ▽

√6ᵗʰ **S62.51** Fracture of proximal phalanx of thumb

√7ᵗʰ **S62.511** Displaced fracture of proximal phalanx of right thumb

√7ᵗʰ **S62.512** Displaced fracture of proximal phalanx of left thumb

√7ᵗʰ **S62.513** Displaced fracture of proximal phalanx of unspecified thumb ▽

√7ᵗʰ **S62.514** Nondisplaced fracture of proximal phalanx of right thumb

√7ᵗʰ **S62.515** Nondisplaced fracture of proximal phalanx of left thumb

√7ᵗʰ **S62.516** Nondisplaced fracture of proximal phalanx of unspecified thumb ▽

√6ᵗʰ **S62.52** Fracture of distal phalanx of thumb

√7ᵗʰ **S62.521** Displaced fracture of distal phalanx of right thumb

√7ᵗʰ **S62.522** Displaced fracture of distal phalanx of left thumb

√7ᵗʰ **S62.523** Displaced fracture of distal phalanx of unspecified thumb ▽

√7ᵗʰ **S62.524** Nondisplaced fracture of distal phalanx of right thumb

√7ᵗʰ **S62.525** Nondisplaced fracture of distal phalanx of left thumb

√7ᵗʰ **S62.526** Nondisplaced fracture of distal phalanx of unspecified thumb ▽

√5ᵗʰ **S62.6** Fracture of other and unspecified finger(s)

EXCLUDES 2 fracture of thumb (S62.5-)

√6ᵗʰ **S62.60** Fracture of unspecified phalanx of finger

√7ᵗʰ **S62.600** Fracture of unspecified phalanx of right index finger ▽

√7ᵗʰ **S62.601** Fracture of unspecified phalanx of left index finger ▽

√7ᵗʰ **S62.602** Fracture of unspecified phalanx of right middle finger ▽

√7ᵗʰ **S62.603** Fracture of unspecified phalanx of left middle finger ▽

√7ᵗʰ **S62.604** Fracture of unspecified phalanx of right ring finger ▽

√7ᵗʰ **S62.605** Fracture of unspecified phalanx of left ring finger ▽

√7ᵗʰ **S62.606** Fracture of unspecified phalanx of right little finger ▽

√7ᵗʰ **S62.607** Fracture of unspecified phalanx of left little finger ▽

√7ᵗʰ **S62.608** Fracture of unspecified phalanx of other finger ▽

Fracture of unspecified phalanx of specified finger with unspecified laterality

√7ᵗʰ **S62.609** Fracture of unspecified phalanx of unspecified finger ▽

√6ᵗʰ **S62.61** Displaced fracture of proximal phalanx of finger

√7ᵗʰ **S62.610** Displaced fracture of proximal phalanx of right index finger

√7ᵗʰ **S62.611** Displaced fracture of proximal phalanx of left index finger

√7ᵗʰ **S62.612** Displaced fracture of proximal phalanx of right middle finger

√7ᵗʰ **S62.613** Displaced fracture of proximal phalanx of left middle finger

√7ᵗʰ **S62.614** Displaced fracture of proximal phalanx of right ring finger

√7ᵗʰ **S62.615** Displaced fracture of proximal phalanx of left ring finger

√7ᵗʰ **S62.616** Displaced fracture of proximal phalanx of right little finger

√7ᵗʰ **S62.617** Displaced fracture of proximal phalanx of left little finger

√7ᵗʰ **S62.618** Displaced fracture of proximal phalanx of other finger

Displaced fracture of proximal phalanx of specified finger with unspecified laterality

√7ᵗʰ **S62.619** Displaced fracture of proximal phalanx of unspecified finger ▽

√6ᵗʰ **S62.62** Displaced fracture of medial phalanx of finger

√7ᵗʰ **S62.620** Displaced fracture of medial phalanx of right index finger

√7ᵗʰ **S62.621** Displaced fracture of medial phalanx of left index finger

√7ᵗʰ **S62.622** Displaced fracture of medial phalanx of right middle finger

√7ᵗʰ **S62.623** Displaced fracture of medial phalanx of left middle finger

√7ᵗʰ **S62.624** Displaced fracture of medial phalanx of right ring finger

√7ᵗʰ **S62.625** Displaced fracture of medial phalanx of left ring finger

√7ᵗʰ **S62.626** Displaced fracture of medial phalanx of right little finger

√7ᵗʰ **S62.627** Displaced fracture of medial phalanx of left little finger

√7ᵗʰ **S62.628** Displaced fracture of medial phalanx of other finger

Displaced fracture of medial phalanx of specified finger with unspecified laterality

√7ᵗʰ **S62.629** Displaced fracture of medial phalanx of unspecified finger ▽

√6ᵗʰ **S62.63** Displaced fracture of distal phalanx of finger

√7ᵗʰ **S62.630** Displaced fracture of distal phalanx of right index finger

√7ᵗʰ **S62.631** Displaced fracture of distal phalanx of left index finger

√7ᵗʰ **S62.632** Displaced fracture of distal phalanx of right middle finger

√7ᵗʰ **S62.633** Displaced fracture of distal phalanx of left middle finger

√7ᵗʰ **S62.634** Displaced fracture of distal phalanx of right ring finger

√7ᵗʰ **S62.635** Displaced fracture of distal phalanx of left ring finger

√7ᵗʰ **S62.636** Displaced fracture of distal phalanx of right little finger

√7ᵗʰ **S62.637** Displaced fracture of distal phalanx of left little finger

√7ᵗʰ **S62.638** Displaced fracture of distal phalanx of other finger

Displaced fracture of distal phalanx of specified finger with unspecified laterality

√7ᵗʰ **S62.639** Displaced fracture of distal phalanx of unspecified finger ▽

√6ᵗʰ **S62.64** Nondisplaced fracture of proximal phalanx of finger

√7ᵗʰ **S62.640** Nondisplaced fracture of proximal phalanx of right index finger

√7ᵗʰ **S62.641** Nondisplaced fracture of proximal phalanx of left index finger

√7ᵗʰ **S62.642** Nondisplaced fracture of proximal phalanx of right middle finger

√7ᵗʰ **S62.643** Nondisplaced fracture of proximal phalanx of left middle finger

√7ᵗʰ **S62.644** Nondisplaced fracture of proximal phalanx of right ring finger

√7ᵗʰ **S62.645** Nondisplaced fracture of proximal phalanx of left ring finger

√7ᵗʰ **S62.646** Nondisplaced fracture of proximal phalanx of right little finger

√7ᵗʰ **S62.647** Nondisplaced fracture of proximal phalanx of left little finger

√7ᵗʰ **S62.648** Nondisplaced fracture of proximal phalanx of other finger

Nondisplaced fracture of proximal phalanx of specified finger with unspecified laterality

√7ᵗʰ **S62.649** Nondisplaced fracture of proximal phalanx of unspecified finger ▽

√6ᵗʰ **S62.65** Nondisplaced fracture of medial phalanx of finger

√7ᵗʰ **S62.650** Nondisplaced fracture of medial phalanx of right index finger

√7ᵗʰ **S62.651** Nondisplaced fracture of medial phalanx of left index finger

√7ᵗʰ **S62.652** Nondisplaced fracture of medial phalanx of right middle finger

√7ᵗʰ **S62.653** Nondisplaced fracture of medial phalanx of left middle finger

Chapter 19. Injury, Poisoning and Certain Other Consequences of External Causes

S62.654–S63.062

√7ᵗʰ **S62.654** **Nondisplaced fracture of medial phalanx of right ring finger**

√7ᵗʰ **S62.655** **Nondisplaced fracture of medial phalanx of left ring finger**

√7ᵗʰ **S62.656** **Nondisplaced fracture of medial phalanx of right little finger**

√7ᵗʰ **S62.657** **Nondisplaced fracture of medial phalanx of left little finger**

√7ᵗʰ **S62.658** **Nondisplaced fracture of medial phalanx of other finger**
Nondisplaced fracture of medial phalanx of specified finger with unspecified laterality

√7ᵗʰ **S62.659** **Nondisplaced fracture of medial phalanx of unspecified finger** ▽

√6ᵗʰ **S62.66** **Nondisplaced fracture of distal phalanx of finger**

√7ᵗʰ **S62.660** **Nondisplaced fracture of distal phalanx of right index finger**

√7ᵗʰ **S62.661** **Nondisplaced fracture of distal phalanx of left index finger**

√7ᵗʰ **S62.662** **Nondisplaced fracture of distal phalanx of right middle finger**

√7ᵗʰ **S62.663** **Nondisplaced fracture of distal phalanx of left middle finger**

√7ᵗʰ **S62.664** **Nondisplaced fracture of distal phalanx of right ring finger**

√7ᵗʰ **S62.665** **Nondisplaced fracture of distal phalanx of left ring finger**

√7ᵗʰ **S62.666** **Nondisplaced fracture of distal phalanx of right little finger**

√7ᵗʰ **S62.667** **Nondisplaced fracture of distal phalanx of left little finger**

√7ᵗʰ **S62.668** **Nondisplaced fracture of distal phalanx of other finger**
Nondisplaced fracture of distal phalanx of specified finger with unspecified laterality

√7ᵗʰ **S62.669** **Nondisplaced fracture of distal phalanx of unspecified finger** ▽

√5ᵗʰ **S62.9** **Unspecified fracture of wrist and hand**

√ₓ7ᵗʰ **S62.90** **Unspecified fracture of unspecified wrist and hand** ▽

√ₓ7ᵗʰ **S62.91** **Unspecified fracture of right wrist and hand** ▽

√ₓ7ᵗʰ **S62.92** **Unspecified fracture of left wrist and hand** ▽

√4ᵗʰ **S63** **Dislocation and sprain of joints and ligaments at wrist and hand level**

INCLUDES avulsion of joint or ligament at wrist and hand level
laceration of cartilage, joint or ligament at wrist and hand level
sprain of cartilage, joint or ligament at wrist and hand level
traumatic hemarthrosis of joint or ligament at wrist and hand level
traumatic rupture of joint or ligament at wrist and hand level
traumatic subluxation of joint or ligament at wrist and hand level
traumatic tear of joint or ligament at wrist and hand level

Code also any associated open wound

EXCLUDES 2 *strain of muscle, fascia and tendon of wrist and hand (S66.-)*

The appropriate 7th character is to be added to each code from category S63.
A initial encounter
D subsequent encounter
S sequela

√5ᵗʰ **S63.0** **Subluxation and dislocation of wrist and hand joints**

√6ᵗʰ **S63.00** **Unspecified subluxation and dislocation of wrist and hand**
Dislocation of carpal bone NOS
Dislocation of distal end of radius NOS
Subluxation of carpal bone NOS
Subluxation of distal end of radius NOS

√7ᵗʰ **S63.001** **Unspecified subluxation of right wrist and hand** ▽

√7ᵗʰ **S63.002** **Unspecified subluxation of left wrist and hand** ▽

√7ᵗʰ **S63.003** **Unspecified subluxation of unspecified wrist and hand** ▽

√7ᵗʰ **S63.004** **Unspecified dislocation of right wrist and hand** ▽

√7ᵗʰ **S63.005** **Unspecified dislocation of left wrist and hand** ▽

√7ᵗʰ **S63.006** **Unspecified dislocation of unspecified wrist and hand** ▽

√6ᵗʰ **S63.01** **Subluxation and dislocation of distal radioulnar joint**

√7ᵗʰ **S63.011** **Subluxation of distal radioulnar joint of right wrist**

√7ᵗʰ **S63.012** **Subluxation of distal radioulnar joint of left wrist**

√7ᵗʰ **S63.013** **Subluxation of distal radioulnar joint of unspecified wrist** ▽

√7ᵗʰ **S63.014** **Dislocation of distal radioulnar joint of right wrist**

√7ᵗʰ **S63.015** **Dislocation of distal radioulnar joint of left wrist**

√7ᵗʰ **S63.016** **Dislocation of distal radioulnar joint of unspecified wrist** ▽

√6ᵗʰ **S63.02** **Subluxation and dislocation of radiocarpal joint**

√7ᵗʰ **S63.021** **Subluxation of radiocarpal joint of right wrist**

√7ᵗʰ **S63.022** **Subluxation of radiocarpal joint of left wrist**

√7ᵗʰ **S63.023** **Subluxation of radiocarpal joint of unspecified wrist** ▽

√7ᵗʰ **S63.024** **Dislocation of radiocarpal joint of right wrist**

√7ᵗʰ **S63.025** **Dislocation of radiocarpal joint of left wrist**

√7ᵗʰ **S63.026** **Dislocation of radiocarpal joint of unspecified wrist** ▽

√6ᵗʰ **S63.03** **Subluxation and dislocation of midcarpal joint**

√7ᵗʰ **S63.031** **Subluxation of midcarpal joint of right wrist**

√7ᵗʰ **S63.032** **Subluxation of midcarpal joint of left wrist**

√7ᵗʰ **S63.033** **Subluxation of midcarpal joint of unspecified wrist** ▽

√7ᵗʰ **S63.034** **Dislocation of midcarpal joint of right wrist**

√7ᵗʰ **S63.035** **Dislocation of midcarpal joint of left wrist**

√7ᵗʰ **S63.036** **Dislocation of midcarpal joint of unspecified wrist** ▽

√6ᵗʰ **S63.04** **Subluxation and dislocation of carpometacarpal joint of thumb**
EXCLUDES 2 *interphalangeal subluxation and dislocation of thumb (S63.1-)*

√7ᵗʰ **S63.041** **Subluxation of carpometacarpal joint of right thumb**

√7ᵗʰ **S63.042** **Subluxation of carpometacarpal joint of left thumb**

√7ᵗʰ **S63.043** **Subluxation of carpometacarpal joint of unspecified thumb** ▽

√7ᵗʰ **S63.044** **Dislocation of carpometacarpal joint of right thumb**

√7ᵗʰ **S63.045** **Dislocation of carpometacarpal joint of left thumb**

√7ᵗʰ **S63.046** **Dislocation of carpometacarpal joint of unspecified thumb** ▽

√6ᵗʰ **S63.05** **Subluxation and dislocation of other carpometacarpal joint**
EXCLUDES 2 *subluxation and dislocation of carpometacarpal joint of thumb (S63.04-)*

√7ᵗʰ **S63.051** **Subluxation of other carpometacarpal joint of right hand**

√7ᵗʰ **S63.052** **Subluxation of other carpometacarpal joint of left hand**

√7ᵗʰ **S63.053** **Subluxation of other carpometacarpal joint of unspecified hand** ▽

√7ᵗʰ **S63.054** **Dislocation of other carpometacarpal joint of right hand**

√7ᵗʰ **S63.055** **Dislocation of other carpometacarpal joint of left hand**

√7ᵗʰ **S63.056** **Dislocation of other carpometacarpal joint of unspecified hand** ▽

√6ᵗʰ **S63.06** **Subluxation and dislocation of metacarpal (bone), proximal end**

√7ᵗʰ **S63.061** **Subluxation of metacarpal (bone), proximal end of right hand**

√7ᵗʰ **S63.062** **Subluxation of metacarpal (bone), proximal end of left hand**

☑6ᵗʰ **S63.063** Subluxation of metacarpal (bone), proximal end of unspecified hand ▽

☑7ᵗʰ **S63.064** Dislocation of metacarpal (bone), proximal end of right hand

☑7ᵗʰ **S63.065** Dislocation of metacarpal (bone), proximal end of left hand

☑7ᵗʰ **S63.066** Dislocation of metacarpal (bone), proximal end of unspecified hand

☑6ᵗʰ **S63.07** Subluxation and dislocation of distal end of ulna

☑7ᵗʰ **S63.071** Subluxation of distal end of right ulna

☑7ᵗʰ **S63.072** Subluxation of distal end of left ulna

☑7ᵗʰ **S63.073** Subluxation of distal end of unspecified ulna ▽

☑7ᵗʰ **S63.074** Dislocation of distal end of right ulna

☑7ᵗʰ **S63.075** Dislocation of distal end of left ulna

☑7ᵗʰ **S63.076** Dislocation of distal end of unspecified ulna ▽

☑6ᵗʰ **S63.09** Other subluxation and dislocation of wrist and hand

☑7ᵗʰ **S63.091** Other subluxation of right wrist and hand

☑7ᵗʰ **S63.092** Other subluxation of left wrist and hand

☑7ᵗʰ **S63.093** Other subluxation of unspecified wrist and hand ▽

☑7ᵗʰ **S63.094** Other dislocation of right wrist and hand

☑7ᵗʰ **S63.095** Other dislocation of left wrist and hand

☑7ᵗʰ **S63.096** Other dislocation of unspecified wrist and hand ▽

☑5ᵗʰ **S63.1** Subluxation and dislocation of thumb

☑6ᵗʰ **S63.10** Unspecified subluxation and dislocation of thumb

☑7ᵗʰ **S63.101** Unspecified subluxation of right thumb ▽

☑7ᵗʰ **S63.102** Unspecified subluxation of left thumb ▽

☑7ᵗʰ **S63.103** Unspecified subluxation of unspecified thumb ▽

☑7ᵗʰ **S63.104** Unspecified dislocation of right thumb ▽

☑7ᵗʰ **S63.105** Unspecified dislocation of left thumb ▽

☑7ᵗʰ **S63.106** Unspecified dislocation of unspecified thumb ▽

☑6ᵗʰ **S63.11** Subluxation and dislocation of metacarpophalangeal joint of thumb

☑7ᵗʰ **S63.111** Subluxation of metacarpophalangeal joint of right thumb

☑7ᵗʰ **S63.112** Subluxation of metacarpophalangeal joint of left thumb

☑7ᵗʰ **S63.113** Subluxation of metacarpophalangeal joint of unspecified thumb ▽

☑7ᵗʰ **S63.114** Dislocation of metacarpophalangeal joint of right thumb

☑7ᵗʰ **S63.115** Dislocation of metacarpophalangeal joint of left thumb

☑7ᵗʰ **S63.116** Dislocation of metacarpophalangeal joint of unspecified thumb ▽

☑6ᵗʰ **S63.12** Subluxation and dislocation of unspecified interphalangeal joint of thumb

☑7ᵗʰ **S63.121** Subluxation of unspecified interphalangeal joint of right thumb ▽

☑7ᵗʰ **S63.122** Subluxation of unspecified interphalangeal joint of left thumb ▽

☑7ᵗʰ **S63.123** Subluxation of unspecified interphalangeal joint of unspecified thumb ▽

☑7ᵗʰ **S63.124** Dislocation of unspecified interphalangeal joint of right thumb ▽

☑7ᵗʰ **S63.125** Dislocation of unspecified interphalangeal joint of left thumb ▽

☑7ᵗʰ **S63.126** Dislocation of unspecified interphalangeal joint of unspecified thumb ▽

☑6ᵗʰ **S63.13** Subluxation and dislocation of proximal interphalangeal joint of thumb

☑7ᵗʰ **S63.131** Subluxation of proximal interphalangeal joint of right thumb

☑7ᵗʰ **S63.132** Subluxation of proximal interphalangeal joint of left thumb

☑7ᵗʰ **S63.133** Subluxation of proximal interphalangeal joint of unspecified thumb ▽

☑7ᵗʰ **S63.134** Dislocation of proximal interphalangeal joint of right thumb

☑7ᵗʰ **S63.135** Dislocation of proximal interphalangeal joint of left thumb

☑7ᵗʰ **S63.136** Dislocation of proximal interphalangeal joint of unspecified thumb ▽

☑6ᵗʰ **S63.14** Subluxation and dislocation of distal interphalangeal joint of thumb

☑7ᵗʰ **S63.141** Subluxation of distal interphalangeal joint of right thumb

☑7ᵗʰ **S63.142** Subluxation of distal interphalangeal joint of left thumb

☑7ᵗʰ **S63.143** Subluxation of distal interphalangeal joint of unspecified thumb ▽

☑7ᵗʰ **S63.144** Dislocation of distal interphalangeal joint of right thumb

☑7ᵗʰ **S63.145** Dislocation of distal interphalangeal joint of left thumb

☑7ᵗʰ **S63.146** Dislocation of distal interphalangeal joint of unspecified thumb ▽

☑5ᵗʰ **S63.2** Subluxation and dislocation of other finger(s)

EXCLUDES 2 subluxation and dislocation of thumb (S63.1-)

☑6ᵗʰ **S63.20** Unspecified subluxation of other finger

☑7ᵗʰ **S63.200** Unspecified subluxation of right index finger ▽

☑7ᵗʰ **S63.201** Unspecified subluxation of left index finger ▽

☑7ᵗʰ **S63.202** Unspecified subluxation of right middle finger ▽

☑7ᵗʰ **S63.203** Unspecified subluxation of left middle finger ▽

☑7ᵗʰ **S63.204** Unspecified subluxation of right ring finger ▽

☑7ᵗʰ **S63.205** Unspecified subluxation of left ring finger ▽

☑7ᵗʰ **S63.206** Unspecified subluxation of right little finger ▽

☑7ᵗʰ **S63.207** Unspecified subluxation of left little finger ▽

☑7ᵗʰ **S63.208** Unspecified subluxation of other finger ▽
Unspecified subluxation of specified finger with unspecified laterality

☑7ᵗʰ **S63.209** Unspecified subluxation of unspecified finger ▽

☑6ᵗʰ **S63.21** Subluxation of metacarpophalangeal joint of finger

☑7ᵗʰ **S63.210** Subluxation of metacarpophalangeal joint of right index finger

☑7ᵗʰ **S63.211** Subluxation of metacarpophalangeal joint of left index finger

☑7ᵗʰ **S63.212** Subluxation of metacarpophalangeal joint of right middle finger

☑7ᵗʰ **S63.213** Subluxation of metacarpophalangeal joint of left middle finger

☑7ᵗʰ **S63.214** Subluxation of metacarpophalangeal joint of right ring finger

☑7ᵗʰ **S63.215** Subluxation of metacarpophalangeal joint of left ring finger

☑7ᵗʰ **S63.216** Subluxation of metacarpophalangeal joint of right little finger

☑7ᵗʰ **S63.217** Subluxation of metacarpophalangeal joint of left little finger

☑7ᵗʰ **S63.218** Subluxation of metacarpophalangeal joint of other finger
Subluxation of metacarpophalangeal joint of specified finger with unspecified laterality

☑7ᵗʰ **S63.219** Subluxation of metacarpophalangeal joint of unspecified finger ▽

☑6ᵗʰ **S63.22** Subluxation of unspecified interphalangeal joint of finger

☑7ᵗʰ **S63.220** Subluxation of unspecified interphalangeal joint of right index finger ▽

☑ Additional Character Required   ☑×7ᵗʰ Placeholder Alert   Manifestation Dx   ▽ Unspecified Dx   ▶◀ Revised Text   ● New Code   ▲ Revised Code Title

√7ᵗʰ **S63.221 Subluxation of unspecified interphalangeal joint of** left index finger ▽

√7ᵗʰ **S63.222 Subluxation of unspecified interphalangeal joint of** right middle **finger** ▽

√7ᵗʰ **S63.223 Subluxation of unspecified interphalangeal joint of** left middle **finger** ▽

√7ᵗʰ **S63.224 Subluxation of unspecified interphalangeal joint of** right ring **finger** ▽

√7ᵗʰ **S63.225 Subluxation of unspecified interphalangeal joint of** left ring **finger** ▽

√7ᵗʰ **S63.226 Subluxation of unspecified interphalangeal joint of** right little **finger** ▽

√7ᵗʰ **S63.227 Subluxation of unspecified interphalangeal joint of** left little **finger** ▽

√7ᵗʰ **S63.228 Subluxation of unspecified interphalangeal joint of other finger** ▽

Subluxation of unspecified interphalangeal joint of specified finger with unspecified laterality

√7ᵗʰ **S63.229 Subluxation of unspecified interphalangeal joint of unspecified finger** ▽

√6ᵗʰ **S63.23 Subluxation of proximal interphalangeal** joint of **finger**

√7ᵗʰ **S63.230 Subluxation of proximal interphalangeal joint of** right index **finger**

√7ᵗʰ **S63.231 Subluxation of proximal interphalangeal joint of** left index **finger**

√7ᵗʰ **S63.232 Subluxation of proximal interphalangeal joint of** right middle **finger**

√7ᵗʰ **S63.233 Subluxation of proximal interphalangeal joint of** left middle **finger**

√7ᵗʰ **S63.234 Subluxation of proximal interphalangeal joint of** right ring **finger**

√7ᵗʰ **S63.235 Subluxation of proximal interphalangeal joint of** left ring **finger**

√7ᵗʰ **S63.236 Subluxation of proximal interphalangeal joint of** right little **finger**

√7ᵗʰ **S63.237 Subluxation of proximal interphalangeal joint of** left little **finger**

√7ᵗʰ **S63.238 Subluxation of proximal interphalangeal joint of other finger**

Subluxation of proximal interphalangeal joint of specified finger with unspecified laterality

√7ᵗʰ **S63.239 Subluxation of proximal interphalangeal joint of unspecified finger** ▽

√6ᵗʰ **S63.24 Subluxation of** distal interphalangeal **joint of finger**

√7ᵗʰ **S63.240 Subluxation of distal interphalangeal joint of** right index **finger**

√7ᵗʰ **S63.241 Subluxation of distal interphalangeal joint of** left index **finger**

√7ᵗʰ **S63.242 Subluxation of distal interphalangeal joint of** right middle **finger**

√7ᵗʰ **S63.243 Subluxation of distal interphalangeal joint of** left middle **finger**

√7ᵗʰ **S63.244 Subluxation of distal interphalangeal joint of** right ring **finger**

√7ᵗʰ **S63.245 Subluxation of distal interphalangeal joint of** left ring **finger**

√7ᵗʰ **S63.246 Subluxation of distal interphalangeal joint of** right little **finger**

√7ᵗʰ **S63.247 Subluxation of distal interphalangeal joint of** left little **finger**

√7ᵗʰ **S63.248 Subluxation of distal interphalangeal joint of other finger**

Subluxation of distal interphalangeal joint of specified finger with unspecified laterality

√7ᵗʰ **S63.249 Subluxation of distal interphalangeal joint of unspecified finger** ▽

√6ᵗʰ **S63.25 Unspecified dislocation of other finger**

√7ᵗʰ **S63.250 Unspecified dislocation of** right index **finger** ▽

√7ᵗʰ **S63.251 Unspecified dislocation of** left index **finger** ▽

√7ᵗʰ **S63.252 Unspecified dislocation of** right middle **finger** ▽

√7ᵗʰ **S63.253 Unspecified dislocation of** left middle **finger** ▽

√7ᵗʰ **S63.254 Unspecified dislocation of** right ring **finger** ▽

√7ᵗʰ **S63.255 Unspecified dislocation of** left ring **finger** ▽

√7ᵗʰ **S63.256 Unspecified dislocation of** right little **finger** ▽

√7ᵗʰ **S63.257 Unspecified dislocation of** left little **finger** ▽

√7ᵗʰ **S63.258 Unspecified dislocation of other finger** ▽

Unspecified dislocation of specified finger with unspecified laterality

√7ᵗʰ **S63.259 Unspecified dislocation of unspecified finger** ▽

Unspecified dislocation of specified finger with unspecified laterality

√6ᵗʰ **S63.26 Dislocation of** metacarpophalangeal joint **of finger**

√7ᵗʰ **S63.260 Dislocation of metacarpophalangeal joint of** right index **finger**

√7ᵗʰ **S63.261 Dislocation of metacarpophalangeal joint of** left index **finger**

√7ᵗʰ **S63.262 Dislocation of metacarpophalangeal joint of** right middle **finger**

√7ᵗʰ **S63.263 Dislocation of metacarpophalangeal joint of** left middle **finger**

√7ᵗʰ **S63.264 Dislocation of metacarpophalangeal joint of** right ring **finger**

√7ᵗʰ **S63.265 Dislocation of metacarpophalangeal joint of** left ring **finger**

√7ᵗʰ **S63.266 Dislocation of metacarpophalangeal joint of** right little **finger**

√7ᵗʰ **S63.267 Dislocation of metacarpophalangeal joint of** left little **finger**

√7ᵗʰ **S63.268 Dislocation of metacarpophalangeal joint of other finger**

Dislocation of metacarpophalangeal joint of specified finger with unspecified laterality

√7ᵗʰ **S63.269 Dislocation of metacarpophalangeal joint of unspecified finger** ▽

√6ᵗʰ **S63.27 Dislocation of unspecified interphalangeal joint of finger**

√7ᵗʰ **S63.270 Dislocation of unspecified interphalangeal joint of** right index **finger** ▽

√7ᵗʰ **S63.271 Dislocation of unspecified interphalangeal joint of** left index **finger** ▽

√7ᵗʰ **S63.272 Dislocation of unspecified interphalangeal joint of** right middle **finger** ▽

√7ᵗʰ **S63.273 Dislocation of unspecified interphalangeal joint of** left middle **finger** ▽

√7ᵗʰ **S63.274 Dislocation of unspecified interphalangeal joint of** right ring **finger** ▽

√7ᵗʰ **S63.275 Dislocation of unspecified interphalangeal joint of** left ring **finger** ▽

√7ᵗʰ **S63.276 Dislocation of unspecified interphalangeal joint of** right little **finger** ▽

√7ᵗʰ **S63.277 Dislocation of unspecified interphalangeal joint of** left little **finger** ▽

√7ᵗʰ **S63.278 Dislocation of unspecified interphalangeal joint of other finger** ▽

Dislocation of unspecified interphalangeal joint of specified finger with unspecified laterality

EXCLUDES 1 Not coded here   EXCLUDES 2 Not included here   N Newborn Age : 0   P Pediatric Age : 0-17   M Maternity Age : 12-55   A Adult Age : 15-124

962

ICD-10-CM 2017

√7ᵗʰ **S63.279** **Dislocation of unspecified interphalangeal joint of unspecified finger** ▽
Dislocation of unspecified interphalangeal joint of specified finger without specified laterality

√6ᵗʰ **S63.28** **Dislocation of proximal interphalangeal joint of finger**

√7ᵗʰ **S63.280** **Dislocation of proximal interphalangeal joint of right index finger**

√7ᵗʰ **S63.281** **Dislocation of proximal interphalangeal joint of left index finger**

√7ᵗʰ **S63.282** **Dislocation of proximal interphalangeal joint of right middle finger**

√7ᵗʰ **S63.283** **Dislocation of proximal interphalangeal joint of left middle finger**

√7ᵗʰ **S63.284** **Dislocation of proximal interphalangeal joint of right ring finger**

√7ᵗʰ **S63.285** **Dislocation of proximal interphalangeal joint of left ring finger**

√7ᵗʰ **S63.286** **Dislocation of proximal interphalangeal joint of right little finger**

√7ᵗʰ **S63.287** **Dislocation of proximal interphalangeal joint of left little finger**

√7ᵗʰ **S63.288** **Dislocation of proximal interphalangeal joint of other finger**
Dislocation of proximal interphalangeal joint of specified finger with unspecified laterality

√7ᵗʰ **S63.289** **Dislocation of proximal interphalangeal joint of unspecified finger** ▽

√6ᵗʰ **S63.29** **Dislocation of distal interphalangeal joint of finger**

√7ᵗʰ **S63.290** **Dislocation of distal interphalangeal joint of right index finger**

√7ᵗʰ **S63.291** **Dislocation of distal interphalangeal joint of left index finger**

√7ᵗʰ **S63.292** **Dislocation of distal interphalangeal joint of right middle finger**

√7ᵗʰ **S63.293** **Dislocation of distal interphalangeal joint of left middle finger**

√7ᵗʰ **S63.294** **Dislocation of distal interphalangeal joint of right ring finger**

√7ᵗʰ **S63.295** **Dislocation of distal interphalangeal joint of left ring finger**

√7ᵗʰ **S63.296** **Dislocation of distal interphalangeal joint of right little finger**

√7ᵗʰ **S63.297** **Dislocation of distal interphalangeal joint of left little finger**

√7ᵗʰ **S63.298** **Dislocation of distal interphalangeal joint of other finger**
Dislocation of distal interphalangeal joint of specified finger with unspecified laterality

√7ᵗʰ **S63.299** **Dislocation of distal interphalangeal joint of unspecified finger** ▽

√5ᵗʰ **S63.3** **Traumatic rupture of ligament of wrist**

√6ᵗʰ **S63.30** **Traumatic rupture of unspecified ligament of wrist**

√7ᵗʰ **S63.301** **Traumatic rupture of unspecified ligament of right wrist** ▽

√7ᵗʰ **S63.302** **Traumatic rupture of unspecified ligament of left wrist** ▽

√7ᵗʰ **S63.309** **Traumatic rupture of unspecified ligament of unspecified wrist** ▽

√6ᵗʰ **S63.31** **Traumatic rupture of collateral ligament of wrist**

√7ᵗʰ **S63.311** **Traumatic rupture of collateral ligament of right wrist**

√7ᵗʰ **S63.312** **Traumatic rupture of collateral ligament of left wrist**

√7ᵗʰ **S63.319** **Traumatic rupture of collateral ligament of unspecified wrist** ▽

√6ᵗʰ **S63.32** **Traumatic rupture of radiocarpal ligament**

√7ᵗʰ **S63.321** **Traumatic rupture of right radiocarpal ligament**

√7ᵗʰ **S63.322** **Traumatic rupture of left radiocarpal ligament**

√7ᵗʰ **S63.329** **Traumatic rupture of unspecified radiocarpal ligament** ▽

√6ᵗʰ **S63.33** **Traumatic rupture of ulnocarpal (palmar) ligament**

√7ᵗʰ **S63.331** **Traumatic rupture of right ulnocarpal (palmar) ligament**

√7ᵗʰ **S63.332** **Traumatic rupture of left ulnocarpal (palmar) ligament**

√7ᵗʰ **S63.339** **Traumatic rupture of unspecified ulnocarpal (palmar) ligament** ▽

√6ᵗʰ **S63.39** **Traumatic rupture of other ligament of wrist**

√7ᵗʰ **S63.391** **Traumatic rupture of other ligament of right wrist**

√7ᵗʰ **S63.392** **Traumatic rupture of other ligament of left wrist**

√7ᵗʰ **S63.399** **Traumatic rupture of other ligament of unspecified wrist** ▽

√5ᵗʰ **S63.4** **Traumatic rupture of ligament of finger at metacarpophalangeal and interphalangeal joint(s)**

√6ᵗʰ **S63.40** **Traumatic rupture of unspecified ligament of finger at metacarpophalangeal and interphalangeal joint**

√7ᵗʰ **S63.400** **Traumatic rupture of unspecified ligament of right index finger at metacarpophalangeal and interphalangeal joint** ▽

√7ᵗʰ **S63.401** **Traumatic rupture of unspecified ligament of left index finger at metacarpophalangeal and interphalangeal joint** ▽

√7ᵗʰ **S63.402** **Traumatic rupture of unspecified ligament of right middle finger at metacarpophalangeal and interphalangeal joint** ▽

√7ᵗʰ **S63.403** **Traumatic rupture of unspecified ligament of left middle finger at metacarpophalangeal and interphalangeal joint** ▽

√7ᵗʰ **S63.404** **Traumatic rupture of unspecified ligament of right ring finger at metacarpophalangeal and interphalangeal joint** ▽

√7ᵗʰ **S63.405** **Traumatic rupture of unspecified ligament of left ring finger at metacarpophalangeal and interphalangeal joint** ▽

√7ᵗʰ **S63.406** **Traumatic rupture of unspecified ligament of right little finger at metacarpophalangeal and interphalangeal joint** ▽

√7ᵗʰ **S63.407** **Traumatic rupture of unspecified ligament of left little finger at metacarpophalangeal and interphalangeal joint** ▽

√7ᵗʰ **S63.408** **Traumatic rupture of unspecified ligament of other finger at metacarpophalangeal and interphalangeal joint** ▽
Traumatic rupture of unspecified ligament of specified finger with unspecified laterality at metacarpophalangeal and interphalangeal joint

√7ᵗʰ **S63.409** **Traumatic rupture of unspecified ligament of unspecified finger at metacarpophalangeal and interphalangeal joint** ▽

√6ᵗʰ **S63.41** **Traumatic rupture of collateral ligament of finger at metacarpophalangeal and interphalangeal joint**

√7ᵗʰ **S63.410** **Traumatic rupture of collateral ligament of right index finger at metacarpophalangeal and interphalangeal joint**

√7ᵗʰ **S63.411** **Traumatic rupture of collateral ligament of left index finger at metacarpophalangeal and interphalangeal joint**

√7ᵗʰ **S63.412** **Traumatic rupture of collateral ligament of right middle finger at metacarpophalangeal and interphalangeal joint**

√7ᵗʰ **S63.413** **Traumatic rupture of collateral ligament of left middle finger at metacarpophalangeal and interphalangeal joint**

√7ᵗʰ **S63.414** **Traumatic rupture of collateral ligament of right ring finger at metacarpophalangeal and interphalangeal joint**

☑ Additional Character Required   ✓ₓ7ᵗʰ Placeholder Alert   Manifestation Dx   ▽ Unspecified Dx   ►◄ Revised Text   ● New Code   ▲ Revised Code Title

ICD-10-CM 2017

963

✓7ᵗʰ **S63.415** **Traumatic rupture of collateral ligament of left ring finger at metacarpophalangeal and interphalangeal joint**

✓7ᵗʰ **S63.416** **Traumatic rupture of collateral ligament of right little finger at metacarpophalangeal and interphalangeal joint**

✓7ᵗʰ **S63.417** **Traumatic rupture of collateral ligament of left little finger at metacarpophalangeal and interphalangeal joint**

✓7ᵗʰ **S63.418** **Traumatic rupture of collateral ligament of other finger at metacarpophalangeal and interphalangeal joint**

Traumatic rupture of collateral ligament of specified finger with unspecified laterality at metacarpophalangeal and interphalangeal joint

✓7ᵗʰ **S63.419** **Traumatic rupture of collateral ligament of unspecified finger at metacarpophalangeal and interphalangeal joint** ▽

✓6ᵗʰ **S63.42** **Traumatic rupture of palmar ligament of finger at metacarpophalangeal and interphalangeal joint**

✓7ᵗʰ **S63.420** **Traumatic rupture of palmar ligament of right index finger at metacarpophalangeal and interphalangeal joint**

✓7ᵗʰ **S63.421** **Traumatic rupture of palmar ligament of left index finger at metacarpophalangeal and interphalangeal joint**

✓7ᵗʰ **S63.422** **Traumatic rupture of palmar ligament of right middle finger at metacarpophalangeal and interphalangeal joint**

✓7ᵗʰ **S63.423** **Traumatic rupture of palmar ligament of left middle finger at metacarpophalangeal and interphalangeal joint**

✓7ᵗʰ **S63.424** **Traumatic rupture of palmar ligament of right ring finger at metacarpophalangeal and interphalangeal joint**

✓7ᵗʰ **S63.425** **Traumatic rupture of palmar ligament of left ring finger at metacarpophalangeal and interphalangeal joint**

✓7ᵗʰ **S63.426** **Traumatic rupture of palmar ligament of right little finger at metacarpophalangeal and interphalangeal joint**

✓7ᵗʰ **S63.427** **Traumatic rupture of palmar ligament of left little finger at metacarpophalangeal and interphalangeal joint**

✓7ᵗʰ **S63.428** **Traumatic rupture of palmar ligament of other finger at metacarpophalangeal and interphalangeal joint**

Traumatic rupture of palmar ligament of specified finger with unspecified laterality at metacarpophalangeal and interphalangeal joint

✓7ᵗʰ **S63.429** **Traumatic rupture of palmar ligament of unspecified finger at metacarpophalangeal and interphalangeal joint** ▽

✓6ᵗʰ **S63.43** **Traumatic rupture of volar plate of finger at metacarpophalangeal and interphalangeal joint**

✓7ᵗʰ **S63.430** **Traumatic rupture of volar plate of right index finger at metacarpophalangeal and interphalangeal joint**

✓7ᵗʰ **S63.431** **Traumatic rupture of volar plate of left index finger at metacarpophalangeal and interphalangeal joint**

✓7ᵗʰ **S63.432** **Traumatic rupture of volar plate of right middle finger at metacarpophalangeal and interphalangeal joint**

✓7ᵗʰ **S63.433** **Traumatic rupture of volar plate of left middle finger at metacarpophalangeal and interphalangeal joint**

✓7ᵗʰ **S63.434** **Traumatic rupture of volar plate of right ring finger at metacarpophalangeal and interphalangeal joint**

✓7ᵗʰ **S63.435** **Traumatic rupture of volar plate of left ring finger at metacarpophalangeal and interphalangeal joint**

✓7ᵗʰ **S63.436** **Traumatic rupture of volar plate of right little finger at metacarpophalangeal and interphalangeal joint**

✓7ᵗʰ **S63.437** **Traumatic rupture of volar plate of left little finger at metacarpophalangeal and interphalangeal joint**

✓7ᵗʰ **S63.438** **Traumatic rupture of volar plate of other finger at metacarpophalangeal and interphalangeal joint**

Traumatic rupture of volar plate of specified finger with unspecified laterality at metacarpophalangeal and interphalangeal joint

✓7ᵗʰ **S63.439** **Traumatic rupture of volar plate of unspecified finger at metacarpophalangeal and interphalangeal joint** ▽

✓6ᵗʰ **S63.49** **Traumatic rupture of other ligament of finger at metacarpophalangeal and interphalangeal joint**

✓7ᵗʰ **S63.490** **Traumatic rupture of other ligament of right index finger at metacarpophalangeal and interphalangeal joint**

✓7ᵗʰ **S63.491** **Traumatic rupture of other ligament of left index finger at metacarpophalangeal and interphalangeal joint**

✓7ᵗʰ **S63.492** **Traumatic rupture of other ligament of right middle finger at metacarpophalangeal and interphalangeal joint**

✓7ᵗʰ **S63.493** **Traumatic rupture of other ligament of left middle finger at metacarpophalangeal and interphalangeal joint**

✓7ᵗʰ **S63.494** **Traumatic rupture of other ligament of right ring finger at metacarpophalangeal and interphalangeal joint**

✓7ᵗʰ **S63.495** **Traumatic rupture of other ligament of left ring finger at metacarpophalangeal and interphalangeal joint**

✓7ᵗʰ **S63.496** **Traumatic rupture of other ligament of right little finger at metacarpophalangeal and interphalangeal joint**

✓7ᵗʰ **S63.497** **Traumatic rupture of other ligament of left little finger at metacarpophalangeal and interphalangeal joint**

✓7ᵗʰ **S63.498** **Traumatic rupture of other ligament of other finger at metacarpophalangeal and interphalangeal joint**

Traumatic rupture of ligament of specified finger with unspecified laterality at metacarpophalangeal and interphalangeal joint

✓7ᵗʰ **S63.499** **Traumatic rupture of other ligament of unspecified finger at metacarpophalangeal and interphalangeal joint** ▽

✓5ᵗʰ **S63.5** **Other and unspecified sprain of wrist**

✓6ᵗʰ **S63.50** **Unspecified sprain of wrist**

✓7ᵗʰ **S63.501** **Unspecified sprain of right wrist** ▽

✓7ᵗʰ **S63.502** **Unspecified sprain of left wrist** ▽

✓7ᵗʰ **S63.509** **Unspecified sprain of unspecified wrist** ▽

✓6ᵗʰ **S63.51** **Sprain of carpal (joint)**

✓7ᵗʰ **S63.511** **Sprain of carpal joint of right wrist**

✓7ᵗʰ **S63.512** **Sprain of carpal joint of left wrist**

✓7ᵗʰ **S63.519** **Sprain of carpal joint of unspecified wrist** ▽

✓6ᵗʰ **S63.52** **Sprain of radiocarpal joint**

EXCLUDES 1 *traumatic rupture of radiocarpal ligament (S63.32-)*

✓7ᵗʰ **S63.521** **Sprain of radiocarpal joint of right wrist**

✓7ᵗʰ **S63.522** **Sprain of radiocarpal joint of left wrist**

✓7ᵗʰ **S63.529** **Sprain of radiocarpal joint of unspecified wrist** ▽

✓6ᵗʰ **S63.59** **Other specified sprain of wrist**

✓7ᵗʰ **S63.591** **Other specified sprain of right wrist**

✓7ᵗʰ **S63.592** **Other specified sprain of left wrist**

✓7ᵗʰ **S63.599** **Other specified sprain of unspecified wrist** ▽

EXCLUDES 1 Not coded here   **EXCLUDES 2** Not included here   **N** Newborn Age : 0   **P** Pediatric Age : 0-17   **M** Maternity Age : 12-55   **A** Adult Age : 15-124

✓5ᵗʰ **S63.6**   **Other and unspecified sprain of finger(s)**

     EXCLUDES 1   *traumatic rupture of ligament of finger at metacarpophalangeal and interphalangeal joint(s) (S63.4-)*

    ✓6ᵗʰ **S63.60**   **Unspecified sprain of** thumb

       ✓7ᵗʰ **S63.601**   **Unspecified sprain of** right **thumb** ▽

       ✓7ᵗʰ **S63.602**   **Unspecified sprain of** left **thumb** ▽

       ✓7ᵗʰ **S63.609**   **Unspecified sprain of unspecified thumb** ▽

    ✓6ᵗʰ **S63.61**   **Unspecified sprain of other and unspecified** finger(s)

       ✓7ᵗʰ **S63.610**   **Unspecified sprain of** right index **finger** ▽

       ✓7ᵗʰ **S63.611**   **Unspecified sprain of** left index **finger** ▽

       ✓7ᵗʰ **S63.612**   **Unspecified sprain of** right middle **finger** ▽

       ✓7ᵗʰ **S63.613**   **Unspecified sprain of** left middle **finger** ▽

       ✓7ᵗʰ **S63.614**   **Unspecified sprain of** right ring **finger** ▽

       ✓7ᵗʰ **S63.615**   **Unspecified sprain of** left ring **finger** ▽

       ✓7ᵗʰ **S63.616**   **Unspecified sprain of** right little **finger** ▽

       ✓7ᵗʰ **S63.617**   **Unspecified sprain of** left little **finger** ▽

       ✓7ᵗʰ **S63.618**   **Unspecified sprain of other finger** ▽

         Unspecified sprain of specified finger with unspecified laterality

       ✓7ᵗʰ **S63.619**   **Unspecified sprain of unspecified finger** ▽

    ✓6ᵗʰ **S63.62**   **Sprain of** interphalangeal joint of thumb

       ✓7ᵗʰ **S63.621**   **Sprain of interphalangeal joint of** right **thumb**

       ✓7ᵗʰ **S63.622**   **Sprain of interphalangeal joint of** left **thumb**

       ✓7ᵗʰ **S63.629**   **Sprain of interphalangeal joint of unspecified thumb** ▽

    ✓6ᵗʰ **S63.63**   **Sprain of interphalangeal joint of other and unspecified** finger(s)

       ✓7ᵗʰ **S63.630**   **Sprain of interphalangeal joint of** right index **finger**

       ✓7ᵗʰ **S63.631**   **Sprain of interphalangeal joint of** left index **finger**

       ✓7ᵗʰ **S63.632**   **Sprain of interphalangeal joint of** right middle **finger**

       ✓7ᵗʰ **S63.633**   **Sprain of interphalangeal joint of** left middle **finger**

       ✓7ᵗʰ **S63.634**   **Sprain of interphalangeal joint of** right ring **finger**

       ✓7ᵗʰ **S63.635**   **Sprain of interphalangeal joint of** left ring **finger**

       ✓7ᵗʰ **S63.636**   **Sprain of interphalangeal joint of** right little **finger**

       ✓7ᵗʰ **S63.637**   **Sprain of interphalangeal joint of** left little **finger**

       ✓7ᵗʰ **S63.638**   **Sprain of interphalangeal joint of other finger**

       ✓7ᵗʰ **S63.639**   **Sprain of interphalangeal joint of unspecified finger** ▽

    ✓6ᵗʰ **S63.64**   **Sprain of** metacarpophalangeal joint of thumb

       ✓7ᵗʰ **S63.641**   **Sprain of metacarpophalangeal joint of** right **thumb**

       ✓7ᵗʰ **S63.642**   **Sprain of metacarpophalangeal joint of** left **thumb**

       ✓7ᵗʰ **S63.649**   **Sprain of metacarpophalangeal joint of unspecified thumb** ▽

    ✓6ᵗʰ **S63.65**   **Sprain of metacarpophalangeal joint of other and unspecified** finger(s)

       ✓7ᵗʰ **S63.650**   **Sprain of metacarpophalangeal joint of** right index **finger**

       ✓7ᵗʰ **S63.651**   **Sprain of metacarpophalangeal joint of** left index **finger**

       ✓7ᵗʰ **S63.652**   **Sprain of metacarpophalangeal joint of** right middle **finger**

       ✓7ᵗʰ **S63.653**   **Sprain of metacarpophalangeal joint of** left middle **finger**

       ✓7ᵗʰ **S63.654**   **Sprain of metacarpophalangeal joint of** right ring **finger**

       ✓7ᵗʰ **S63.655**   **Sprain of metacarpophalangeal joint of** left ring **finger**

       ✓7ᵗʰ **S63.656**   **Sprain of metacarpophalangeal joint of** right little **finger**

       ✓7ᵗʰ **S63.657**   **Sprain of metacarpophalangeal joint of** left little **finger**

       ✓7ᵗʰ **S63.658**   **Sprain of metacarpophalangeal joint of other finger**

         Sprain of metacarpophalangeal joint of specified finger with unspecified laterality

       ✓7ᵗʰ **S63.659**   **Sprain of metacarpophalangeal joint of unspecified finger** ▽

    ✓6ᵗʰ **S63.68**   **Other sprain of** thumb

       ✓7ᵗʰ **S63.681**   **Other sprain of** right **thumb**

       ✓7ᵗʰ **S63.682**   **Other sprain of** left **thumb**

       ✓7ᵗʰ **S63.689**   **Other sprain of unspecified thumb** ▽

    ✓6ᵗʰ **S63.69**   **Other sprain of other and unspecified** finger(s)

       ✓7ᵗʰ **S63.690**   **Other sprain of** right index **finger**

       ✓7ᵗʰ **S63.691**   **Other sprain of** left index **finger**

       ✓7ᵗʰ **S63.692**   **Other sprain of** right middle **finger**

       ✓7ᵗʰ **S63.693**   **Other sprain of** left middle **finger**

       ✓7ᵗʰ **S63.694**   **Other sprain of** right ring **finger**

       ✓7ᵗʰ **S63.695**   **Other sprain of** left ring **finger**

       ✓7ᵗʰ **S63.696**   **Other sprain of** right little **finger**

       ✓7ᵗʰ **S63.697**   **Other sprain of** left little **finger**

       ✓7ᵗʰ **S63.698**   **Other sprain of other finger**

         Other sprain of specified finger with unspecified laterality

       ✓7ᵗʰ **S63.699**   **Other sprain of unspecified finger** ▽

✓5ᵗʰ **S63.8**   **Sprain of other part of wrist and hand**

    ✓6ᵗʰ **S63.8X**   **Sprain of other part of wrist and hand**

       ✓7ᵗʰ **S63.8X1**   **Sprain of other part of** right **wrist and hand**

       ✓7ᵗʰ **S63.8X2**   **Sprain of other part of** left **wrist and hand**

       ✓7ᵗʰ **S63.8X9**   **Sprain of other part of unspecified wrist and hand** ▽

✓5ᵗʰ **S63.9**   **Sprain of unspecified part of wrist and hand**

    ✓×7ᵗʰ **S63.90**   **Sprain of unspecified part of unspecified wrist and hand** ▽

    ✓×7ᵗʰ **S63.91**   **Sprain of unspecified part of** right **wrist and hand** ▽

    ✓×7ᵗʰ **S63.92**   **Sprain of unspecified part of** left **wrist and hand** ▽

✓4ᵗʰ **S64**   **Injury of nerves at wrist and hand level**

     Code also any associated open wound (S61.-)

     The appropriate 7th character is to be added to each code from category S64.
     A   initial encounter
     D   subsequent encounter
     S   sequela

    ✓5ᵗʰ **S64.0**   **Injury of** ulnar **nerve at wrist and hand level**

       ✓×7ᵗʰ **S64.00**   **Injury of ulnar nerve at wrist and hand level of unspecified arm** ▽

       ✓×7ᵗʰ **S64.01**   **Injury of ulnar nerve at wrist and hand level of** right **arm**

       ✓×7ᵗʰ **S64.02**   **Injury of ulnar nerve at wrist and hand level of** left **arm**

    ✓5ᵗʰ **S64.1**   **Injury of** median **nerve at wrist and hand level**

       ✓×7ᵗʰ **S64.10**   **Injury of median nerve at wrist and hand level of unspecified arm** ▽

       ✓×7ᵗʰ **S64.11**   **Injury of median nerve at wrist and hand level of** right **arm**

       ✓×7ᵗʰ **S64.12**   **Injury of median nerve at wrist and hand level of** left **arm**

    ✓5ᵗʰ **S64.2**   **Injury of** radial **nerve at wrist and hand level**

       ✓×7ᵗʰ **S64.20**   **Injury of radial nerve at wrist and hand level of unspecified arm** ▽

       ✓×7ᵗʰ **S64.21**   **Injury of radial nerve at wrist and hand level of** right **arm**

       ✓×7ᵗʰ **S64.22**   **Injury of radial nerve at wrist and hand level of** left **arm**

    ✓5ᵗʰ **S64.3**   **Injury of** digital **nerve of thumb**

       ✓×7ᵗʰ **S64.30**   **Injury of digital nerve of unspecified thumb** ▽

☑ Additional Character Required   ✓×7ᵗʰ Placeholder Alert   Manifestation Dx   ▽ Unspecified Dx   ▶◀ Revised Text   ● New Code   ▲ Revised Code Title

ICD-10-CM 2017   **965**

√x7ᵗʰ **S64.31**   Injury of digital nerve of right thumb

√x7ᵗʰ **S64.32**   Injury of digital nerve of left thumb

√5ᵗʰ **S64.4**   Injury of digital nerve of other and unspecified finger

    √x7ᵗʰ **S64.40**   Injury of digital nerve of unspecified finger   ▽

    √6ᵗʰ **S64.49**   Injury of digital nerve of other finger

       √7ᵗʰ **S64.490**   Injury of digital nerve of right index finger

       √7ᵗʰ **S64.491**   Injury of digital nerve of left index finger

       √7ᵗʰ **S64.492**   Injury of digital nerve of right middle finger

       √7ᵗʰ **S64.493**   Injury of digital nerve of left middle finger

       √7ᵗʰ **S64.494**   Injury of digital nerve of right ring finger

       √7ᵗʰ **S64.495**   Injury of digital nerve of left ring finger

       √7ᵗʰ **S64.496**   Injury of digital nerve of right little finger

       √7ᵗʰ **S64.497**   Injury of digital nerve of left little finger

       √7ᵗʰ **S64.498**   Injury of digital nerve of other finger

          Injury of digital nerve of specified finger with unspecified laterality

√5ᵗʰ **S64.8**   Injury of other nerves at wrist and hand level

    √6ᵗʰ **S64.8X**   Injury of other nerves at wrist and hand level

       √7ᵗʰ **S64.8X1**   Injury of other nerves at wrist and hand level of right arm

       √7ᵗʰ **S64.8X2**   Injury of other nerves at wrist and hand level of left arm

       √7ᵗʰ **S64.8X9**   Injury of other nerves at wrist and hand level of unspecified arm   ▽

√5ᵗʰ **S64.9**   Injury of unspecified nerve at wrist and hand level

    √x7ᵗʰ **S64.90**   Injury of unspecified nerve at wrist and hand level of unspecified arm   ▽

    √x7ᵗʰ **S64.91**   Injury of unspecified nerve at wrist and hand level of right arm   ▽

    √x7ᵗʰ **S64.92**   Injury of unspecified nerve at wrist and hand level of left arm   ▽

√4ᵗʰ **S65**   **Injury of blood vessels at wrist and hand level**

    Code also any associated open wound (S61.-)

> The appropriate 7th character is to be added to each code from category S65.
> A   initial encounter
> D   subsequent encounter
> S   sequela

√5ᵗʰ **S65.0**   Injury of ulnar artery at wrist and hand level

    √6ᵗʰ **S65.00**   Unspecified injury of ulnar artery at wrist and hand level

       √7ᵗʰ **S65.001**   Unspecified injury of ulnar artery at wrist and hand level of right arm   ▽

       √7ᵗʰ **S65.002**   Unspecified injury of ulnar artery at wrist and hand level of left arm   ▽

       √7ᵗʰ **S65.009**   Unspecified injury of ulnar artery at wrist and hand level of unspecified arm   ▽

    √6ᵗʰ **S65.01**   Laceration of ulnar artery at wrist and hand level

       √7ᵗʰ **S65.011**   Laceration of ulnar artery at wrist and hand level of right arm

       √7ᵗʰ **S65.012**   Laceration of ulnar artery at wrist and hand level of left arm

       √7ᵗʰ **S65.019**   Laceration of ulnar artery at wrist and hand level of unspecified arm   ▽

    √6ᵗʰ **S65.09**   Other specified injury of ulnar artery at wrist and hand level

       √7ᵗʰ **S65.091**   Other specified injury of ulnar artery at wrist and hand level of right arm

       √7ᵗʰ **S65.092**   Other specified injury of ulnar artery at wrist and hand level of left arm

       √7ᵗʰ **S65.099**   Other specified injury of ulnar artery at wrist and hand level of unspecified arm   ▽

√5ᵗʰ **S65.1**   Injury of radial artery at wrist and hand level

    √6ᵗʰ **S65.10**   Unspecified injury of radial artery at wrist and hand level

       √7ᵗʰ **S65.101**   Unspecified injury of radial artery at wrist and hand level of right arm   ▽

       √7ᵗʰ **S65.102**   Unspecified injury of radial artery at wrist and hand level of left arm   ▽

       √7ᵗʰ **S65.109**   Unspecified injury of radial artery at wrist and hand level of unspecified arm   ▽

    √6ᵗʰ **S65.11**   Laceration of radial artery at wrist and hand level

       √7ᵗʰ **S65.111**   Laceration of radial artery at wrist and hand level of right arm

       √7ᵗʰ **S65.112**   Laceration of radial artery at wrist and hand level of left arm

       √7ᵗʰ **S65.119**   Laceration of radial artery at wrist and hand level of unspecified arm   ▽

    √6ᵗʰ **S65.19**   Other specified injury of radial artery at wrist and hand level

       √7ᵗʰ **S65.191**   Other specified injury of radial artery at wrist and hand level of right arm

       √7ᵗʰ **S65.192**   Other specified injury of radial artery at wrist and hand level of left arm

       √7ᵗʰ **S65.199**   Other specified injury of radial artery at wrist and hand level of unspecified arm   ▽

√5ᵗʰ **S65.2**   Injury of superficial palmar arch

    √6ᵗʰ **S65.20**   Unspecified injury of superficial palmar arch

       √7ᵗʰ **S65.201**   Unspecified injury of superficial palmar arch of right hand   ▽

       √7ᵗʰ **S65.202**   Unspecified injury of superficial palmar arch of left hand   ▽

       √7ᵗʰ **S65.209**   Unspecified injury of superficial palmar arch of unspecified hand   ▽

    √6ᵗʰ **S65.21**   Laceration of superficial palmar arch

       √7ᵗʰ **S65.211**   Laceration of superficial palmar arch of right hand

       √7ᵗʰ **S65.212**   Laceration of superficial palmar arch of left hand

       √7ᵗʰ **S65.219**   Laceration of superficial palmar arch of unspecified hand   ▽

    √6ᵗʰ **S65.29**   Other specified injury of superficial palmar arch

       √7ᵗʰ **S65.291**   Other specified injury of superficial palmar arch of right hand

       √7ᵗʰ **S65.292**   Other specified injury of superficial palmar arch of left hand

       √7ᵗʰ **S65.299**   Other specified injury of superficial palmar arch of unspecified hand   ▽

√5ᵗʰ **S65.3**   Injury of deep palmar arch

    √6ᵗʰ **S65.30**   Unspecified injury of deep palmar arch

       √7ᵗʰ **S65.301**   Unspecified injury of deep palmar arch of right hand   ▽

       √7ᵗʰ **S65.302**   Unspecified injury of deep palmar arch of left hand   ▽

       √7ᵗʰ **S65.309**   Unspecified injury of deep palmar arch of unspecified hand   ▽

    √6ᵗʰ **S65.31**   Laceration of deep palmar arch

       √7ᵗʰ **S65.311**   Laceration of deep palmar arch of right hand

       √7ᵗʰ **S65.312**   Laceration of deep palmar arch of left hand

       √7ᵗʰ **S65.319**   Laceration of deep palmar arch of unspecified hand   ▽

    √6ᵗʰ **S65.39**   Other specified injury of deep palmar arch

       √7ᵗʰ **S65.391**   Other specified injury of deep palmar arch of right hand

       √7ᵗʰ **S65.392**   Other specified injury of deep palmar arch of left hand

       √7ᵗʰ **S65.399**   Other specified injury of deep palmar arch of unspecified hand   ▽

√5ᵗʰ **S65.4**   Injury of blood vessel of thumb

    √6ᵗʰ **S65.40**   Unspecified injury of blood vessel of thumb

       √7ᵗʰ **S65.401**   Unspecified injury of blood vessel of right thumb   ▽

       √7ᵗʰ **S65.402**   Unspecified injury of blood vessel of left thumb   ▽

       √7ᵗʰ **S65.409**   Unspecified injury of blood vessel of unspecified thumb   ▽

    √6ᵗʰ **S65.41**   Laceration of blood vessel of thumb

       √7ᵗʰ **S65.411**   Laceration of blood vessel of right thumb

       √7ᵗʰ **S65.412**   Laceration of blood vessel of left thumb

       √7ᵗʰ **S65.419**   Laceration of blood vessel of unspecified thumb   ▽

    √6ᵗʰ **S65.49**   Other specified injury of blood vessel of thumb

       √7ᵗʰ **S65.491**   Other specified injury of blood vessel of right thumb

EXCLUDES 1 Not coded here   EXCLUDES 2 Not included here   N Newborn Age : 0   P Pediatric Age : 0-17   M Maternity Age : 12-55   A Adult Age : 15-124

966   ICD-10-CM 2017

√7ᵗʰ **S65.492** **Other specified injury of blood vessel of left thumb**

√7ᵗʰ **S65.499** **Other specified injury of blood vessel of unspecified thumb** ▽

√5ᵗʰ **S65.5** **Injury of blood vessel of other and unspecified finger**

√6ᵗʰ **S65.50** **Unspecified injury of blood vessel of other and unspecified finger**

√7ᵗʰ **S65.500** **Unspecified injury of blood vessel of right index finger** ▽

√7ᵗʰ **S65.501** **Unspecified injury of blood vessel of left index finger** ▽

√7ᵗʰ **S65.502** **Unspecified injury of blood vessel of right middle finger** ▽

√7ᵗʰ **S65.503** **Unspecified injury of blood vessel of left middle finger** ▽

√7ᵗʰ **S65.504** **Unspecified injury of blood vessel of right ring finger** ▽

√7ᵗʰ **S65.505** **Unspecified injury of blood vessel of left ring finger** ▽

√7ᵗʰ **S65.506** **Unspecified injury of blood vessel of right little finger** ▽

√7ᵗʰ **S65.507** **Unspecified injury of blood vessel of left little finger** ▽

√7ᵗʰ **S65.508** **Unspecified injury of blood vessel of other finger** ▽
    Unspecified injury of blood vessel of specified finger with unspecified laterality

√7ᵗʰ **S65.509** **Unspecified injury of blood vessel of unspecified finger** ▽

√6ᵗʰ **S65.51** **Laceration of blood vessel of other and unspecified finger**

√7ᵗʰ **S65.510** **Laceration of blood vessel of right index finger**

√7ᵗʰ **S65.511** **Laceration of blood vessel of left index finger**

√7ᵗʰ **S65.512** **Laceration of blood vessel of right middle finger**

√7ᵗʰ **S65.513** **Laceration of blood vessel of left middle finger**

√7ᵗʰ **S65.514** **Laceration of blood vessel of right ring finger**

√7ᵗʰ **S65.515** **Laceration of blood vessel of left ring finger**

√7ᵗʰ **S65.516** **Laceration of blood vessel of right little finger**

√7ᵗʰ **S65.517** **Laceration of blood vessel of left little finger**

√7ᵗʰ **S65.518** **Laceration of blood vessel of other finger**
    Laceration of blood vessel of specified finger with unspecified laterality

√7ᵗʰ **S65.519** **Laceration of blood vessel of unspecified finger** ▽

√6ᵗʰ **S65.59** **Other specified injury of blood vessel of other and unspecified finger**

√7ᵗʰ **S65.590** **Other specified injury of blood vessel of right index finger**

√7ᵗʰ **S65.591** **Other specified injury of blood vessel of left index finger**

√7ᵗʰ **S65.592** **Other specified injury of blood vessel of right middle finger**

√7ᵗʰ **S65.593** **Other specified injury of blood vessel of left middle finger**

√7ᵗʰ **S65.594** **Other specified injury of blood vessel of right ring finger**

√7ᵗʰ **S65.595** **Other specified injury of blood vessel of left ring finger**

√7ᵗʰ **S65.596** **Other specified injury of blood vessel of right little finger**

√7ᵗʰ **S65.597** **Other specified injury of blood vessel of left little finger**

√7ᵗʰ **S65.598** **Other specified injury of blood vessel of other finger**
    Other specified injury of blood vessel of specified finger with unspecified laterality

√7ᵗʰ **S65.599** **Other specified injury of blood vessel of unspecified finger** ▽

√5ᵗʰ **S65.8** **Injury of other blood vessels at wrist and hand level**

√6ᵗʰ **S65.80** **Unspecified injury of other blood vessels at wrist and hand level**

√7ᵗʰ **S65.801** **Unspecified injury of other blood vessels at wrist and hand level of right arm** ▽

√7ᵗʰ **S65.802** **Unspecified injury of other blood vessels at wrist and hand level of left arm** ▽

√7ᵗʰ **S65.809** **Unspecified injury of other blood vessels at wrist and hand level of unspecified arm** ▽

√6ᵗʰ **S65.81** **Laceration of other blood vessels at wrist and hand level**

√7ᵗʰ **S65.811** **Laceration of other blood vessels at wrist and hand level of right arm**

√7ᵗʰ **S65.812** **Laceration of other blood vessels at wrist and hand level of left arm**

√7ᵗʰ **S65.819** **Laceration of other blood vessels at wrist and hand level of unspecified arm** ▽

√6ᵗʰ **S65.89** **Other specified injury of other blood vessels at wrist and hand level**

√7ᵗʰ **S65.891** **Other specified injury of other blood vessels at wrist and hand level of right arm**

√7ᵗʰ **S65.892** **Other specified injury of other blood vessels at wrist and hand level of left arm**

√7ᵗʰ **S65.899** **Other specified injury of other blood vessels at wrist and hand level of unspecified arm** ▽

√5ᵗʰ **S65.9** **Injury of unspecified blood vessel at wrist and hand level**

√6ᵗʰ **S65.90** **Unspecified injury of unspecified blood vessel at wrist and hand level**

√7ᵗʰ **S65.901** **Unspecified injury of unspecified blood vessel at wrist and hand level of right arm** ▽

√7ᵗʰ **S65.902** **Unspecified injury of unspecified blood vessel at wrist and hand level of left arm** ▽

√7ᵗʰ **S65.909** **Unspecified injury of unspecified blood vessel at wrist and hand level of unspecified arm** ▽

√6ᵗʰ **S65.91** **Laceration of unspecified blood vessel at wrist and hand level**

√7ᵗʰ **S65.911** **Laceration of unspecified blood vessel at wrist and hand level of right arm** ▽

√7ᵗʰ **S65.912** **Laceration of unspecified blood vessel at wrist and hand level of left arm** ▽

√7ᵗʰ **S65.919** **Laceration of unspecified blood vessel at wrist and hand level of unspecified arm** ▽

√6ᵗʰ **S65.99** **Other specified injury of unspecified blood vessel at wrist and hand level**

√7ᵗʰ **S65.991** **Other specified injury of unspecified blood vessel at wrist and hand of right arm** ▽

√7ᵗʰ **S65.992** **Other specified injury of unspecified blood vessel at wrist and hand of left arm** ▽

√7ᵗʰ **S65.999** **Other specified injury of unspecified blood vessel at wrist and hand of unspecified arm** ▽

√4ᵗʰ **S66** **Injury of muscle, fascia and tendon at wrist and hand level**
Code also any associated open wound (S61.-)
EXCLUDES 2 *sprain of joints and ligaments of wrist and hand (S63.-)*
TIP: Refer to the Muscle/Tendon table at the beginning of this chapter

The appropriate 7th character is to be added to each code from category S66.
A initial encounter
D subsequent encounter
S sequela

√5ᵗʰ **S66.0** **Injury of long flexor muscle, fascia and tendon of thumb at wrist and hand level**

√6ᵗʰ **S66.00** **Unspecified injury of long flexor muscle, fascia and tendon of thumb at wrist and hand level**

√7ᵗʰ **S66.001** **Unspecified injury of long flexor muscle, fascia and tendon of right thumb at wrist and hand level** ▽

√7ᵗʰ **S66.002** **Unspecified injury of long flexor muscle, fascia and tendon of left thumb at wrist and hand level** ▽

Chapter 19. Injury, Poisoning and Certain Other Consequences of External Causes

S66.009–S66.194

√7ᵗʰ **S66.009** Unspecified injury of long flexor muscle, fascia and tendon of unspecified thumb at wrist and hand level ▽

√6ᵗʰ **S66.01** Strain of long flexor muscle, fascia and tendon of thumb at wrist and hand level

√7ᵗʰ **S66.011** Strain of long flexor muscle, fascia and tendon of right thumb at wrist and hand level

√7ᵗʰ **S66.012** Strain of long flexor muscle, fascia and tendon of left thumb at wrist and hand level

√7ᵗʰ **S66.019** Strain of long flexor muscle, fascia and tendon of unspecified thumb at wrist and hand level ▽

√6ᵗʰ **S66.02** Laceration of long flexor muscle, fascia and tendon of thumb at wrist and hand level

√7ᵗʰ **S66.021** Laceration of long flexor muscle, fascia and tendon of right thumb at wrist and hand level

√7ᵗʰ **S66.022** Laceration of long flexor muscle, fascia and tendon of left thumb at wrist and hand level

√7ᵗʰ **S66.029** Laceration of long flexor muscle, fascia and tendon of unspecified thumb at wrist and hand level ▽

√6ᵗʰ **S66.09** Other specified injury of long flexor muscle, fascia and tendon of thumb at wrist and hand level

√7ᵗʰ **S66.091** Other specified injury of long flexor muscle, fascia and tendon of right thumb at wrist and hand level

√7ᵗʰ **S66.092** Other specified injury of long flexor muscle, fascia and tendon of left thumb at wrist and hand level

√7ᵗʰ **S66.099** Other specified injury of long flexor muscle, fascia and tendon of unspecified thumb at wrist and hand level ▽

√5ᵗʰ **S66.1** Injury of flexor muscle, fascia and tendon of other and unspecified finger at wrist and hand level

EXCLUDES 2   *Injury of long flexor muscle, fascia and tendon of thumb at wrist and hand level (S66.0-)*

√6ᵗʰ **S66.10** Unspecified injury of flexor muscle, fascia and tendon of other and unspecified finger at wrist and hand level

√7ᵗʰ **S66.100** Unspecified injury of flexor muscle, fascia and tendon of right index finger at wrist and hand level ▽

√7ᵗʰ **S66.101** Unspecified injury of flexor muscle, fascia and tendon of left index finger at wrist and hand level ▽

√7ᵗʰ **S66.102** Unspecified injury of flexor muscle, fascia and tendon of right middle finger at wrist and hand level ▽

√7ᵗʰ **S66.103** Unspecified injury of flexor muscle, fascia and tendon of left middle finger at wrist and hand level ▽

√7ᵗʰ **S66.104** Unspecified injury of flexor muscle, fascia and tendon of right ring finger at wrist and hand level ▽

√7ᵗʰ **S66.105** Unspecified injury of flexor muscle, fascia and tendon of left ring finger at wrist and hand level ▽

√7ᵗʰ **S66.106** Unspecified injury of flexor muscle, fascia and tendon of right little finger at wrist and hand level ▽

√7ᵗʰ **S66.107** Unspecified injury of flexor muscle, fascia and tendon of left little finger at wrist and hand level ▽

√7ᵗʰ **S66.108** Unspecified injury of flexor muscle, fascia and tendon of other finger at wrist and hand level ▽

Unspecified injury of flexor muscle, fascia and tendon of specified finger with unspecified laterality at wrist and hand level

√7ᵗʰ **S66.109** Unspecified injury of flexor muscle, fascia and tendon of unspecified finger at wrist and hand level ▽

√6ᵗʰ **S66.11** Strain of flexor muscle, fascia and tendon of other and unspecified finger at wrist and hand level

√7ᵗʰ **S66.110** Strain of flexor muscle, fascia and tendon of right index finger at wrist and hand level

√7ᵗʰ **S66.111** Strain of flexor muscle, fascia and tendon of left index finger at wrist and hand level

√7ᵗʰ **S66.112** Strain of flexor muscle, fascia and tendon of right middle finger at wrist and hand level

√7ᵗʰ **S66.113** Strain of flexor muscle, fascia and tendon of left middle finger at wrist and hand level

√7ᵗʰ **S66.114** Strain of flexor muscle, fascia and tendon of right ring finger at wrist and hand level

√7ᵗʰ **S66.115** Strain of flexor muscle, fascia and tendon of left ring finger at wrist and hand level

√7ᵗʰ **S66.116** Strain of flexor muscle, fascia and tendon of right little finger at wrist and hand level

√7ᵗʰ **S66.117** Strain of flexor muscle, fascia and tendon of left little finger at wrist and hand level

√7ᵗʰ **S66.118** Strain of flexor muscle, fascia and tendon of other finger at wrist and hand level

Strain of flexor muscle, fascia and tendon of specified finger with unspecified laterality at wrist and hand level

√7ᵗʰ **S66.119** Strain of flexor muscle, fascia and tendon of unspecified finger at wrist and hand level ▽

√6ᵗʰ **S66.12** Laceration of flexor muscle, fascia and tendon of other and unspecified finger at wrist and hand level

√7ᵗʰ **S66.120** Laceration of flexor muscle, fascia and tendon of right index finger at wrist and hand level

√7ᵗʰ **S66.121** Laceration of flexor muscle, fascia and tendon of left index finger at wrist and hand level

√7ᵗʰ **S66.122** Laceration of flexor muscle, fascia and tendon of right middle finger at wrist and hand level

√7ᵗʰ **S66.123** Laceration of flexor muscle, fascia and tendon of left middle finger at wrist and hand level

√7ᵗʰ **S66.124** Laceration of flexor muscle, fascia and tendon of right ring finger at wrist and hand level

√7ᵗʰ **S66.125** Laceration of flexor muscle, fascia and tendon of left ring finger at wrist and hand level

√7ᵗʰ **S66.126** Laceration of flexor muscle, fascia and tendon of right little finger at wrist and hand level

√7ᵗʰ **S66.127** Laceration of flexor muscle, fascia and tendon of left little finger at wrist and hand level

√7ᵗʰ **S66.128** Laceration of flexor muscle, fascia and tendon of other finger at wrist and hand level

Laceration of flexor muscle, fascia and tendon of specified finger with unspecified laterality at wrist and hand level

√7ᵗʰ **S66.129** Laceration of flexor muscle, fascia and tendon of unspecified finger at wrist and hand level ▽

√6ᵗʰ **S66.19** Other injury of flexor muscle, fascia and tendon of other and unspecified finger at wrist and hand level

√7ᵗʰ **S66.190** Other injury of flexor muscle, fascia and tendon of right index finger at wrist and hand level

√7ᵗʰ **S66.191** Other injury of flexor muscle, fascia and tendon of left index finger at wrist and hand level

√7ᵗʰ **S66.192** Other injury of flexor muscle, fascia and tendon of right middle finger at wrist and hand level

√7ᵗʰ **S66.193** Other injury of flexor muscle, fascia and tendon of left middle finger at wrist and hand level

√7ᵗʰ **S66.194** Other injury of flexor muscle, fascia and tendon of right ring finger at wrist and hand level

EXCLUDES 1   Not coded here   EXCLUDES 2   Not included here   N Newborn Age : 0   P Pediatric Age : 0-17   M Maternity Age : 12-55   A Adult Age : 15-124

968   ICD-10-CM 2017

√7ᵗʰ **S66.195** Other injury of flexor muscle, fascia and tendon of left ring finger at wrist and hand level

√7ᵗʰ **S66.196** Other injury of flexor muscle, fascia and tendon of right little finger at wrist and hand level

√7ᵗʰ **S66.197** Other injury of flexor muscle, fascia and tendon of left little finger at wrist and hand level

√7ᵗʰ **S66.198** Other injury of flexor muscle, fascia and tendon of other finger at wrist and hand level

     Other injury of flexor muscle, fascia and tendon of specified finger with unspecified laterality at wrist and hand level

√7ᵗʰ **S66.199** Other injury of flexor muscle, fascia and tendon of unspecified finger at wrist and hand level   ▽

√5ᵗʰ **S66.2** **Injury of extensor muscle, fascia and tendon of thumb at wrist and hand level**

   √6ᵗʰ **S66.20** Unspecified injury of extensor muscle, fascia and tendon of thumb at wrist and hand level

     √7ᵗʰ **S66.201** Unspecified injury of extensor muscle, fascia and tendon of right thumb at wrist and hand level   ▽

     √7ᵗʰ **S66.202** Unspecified injury of extensor muscle, fascia and tendon of left thumb at wrist and hand level   ▽

     √7ᵗʰ **S66.209** Unspecified injury of extensor muscle, fascia and tendon of unspecified thumb at wrist and hand level   ▽

   √6ᵗʰ **S66.21** Strain of extensor muscle, fascia and tendon of thumb at wrist and hand level

     √7ᵗʰ **S66.211** Strain of extensor muscle, fascia and tendon of right thumb at wrist and hand level

     √7ᵗʰ **S66.212** Strain of extensor muscle, fascia and tendon of left thumb at wrist and hand level

     √7ᵗʰ **S66.219** Strain of extensor muscle, fascia and tendon of unspecified thumb at wrist and hand level   ▽

   √6ᵗʰ **S66.22** Laceration of extensor muscle, fascia and tendon of thumb at wrist and hand level

     √7ᵗʰ **S66.221** Laceration of extensor muscle, fascia and tendon of right thumb at wrist and hand level

     √7ᵗʰ **S66.222** Laceration of extensor muscle, fascia and tendon of left thumb at wrist and hand level

     √7ᵗʰ **S66.229** Laceration of extensor muscle, fascia and tendon of unspecified thumb at wrist and hand level   ▽

   √6ᵗʰ **S66.29** Other specified injury of extensor muscle, fascia and tendon of thumb at wrist and hand level

     √7ᵗʰ **S66.291** Other specified injury of extensor muscle, fascia and tendon of right thumb at wrist and hand level

     √7ᵗʰ **S66.292** Other specified injury of extensor muscle, fascia and tendon of left thumb at wrist and hand level

     √7ᵗʰ **S66.299** Other specified injury of extensor muscle, fascia and tendon of unspecified thumb at wrist and hand level   ▽

√5ᵗʰ **S66.3** **Injury of extensor muscle, fascia and tendon of other and unspecified finger at wrist and hand level**

   EXCLUDES 2 *Injury of extensor muscle, fascia and tendon of thumb at wrist and hand level (S66.2-)*

   √6ᵗʰ **S66.30** Unspecified injury of extensor muscle, fascia and tendon of other and unspecified finger at wrist and hand level

     √7ᵗʰ **S66.300** Unspecified injury of extensor muscle, fascia and tendon of right index finger at wrist and hand level   ▽

     √7ᵗʰ **S66.301** Unspecified injury of extensor muscle, fascia and tendon of left index finger at wrist and hand level   ▽

     √7ᵗʰ **S66.302** Unspecified injury of extensor muscle, fascia and tendon of right middle finger at wrist and hand level   ▽

     √7ᵗʰ **S66.303** Unspecified injury of extensor muscle, fascia and tendon of left middle finger at wrist and hand level   ▽

     √7ᵗʰ **S66.304** Unspecified injury of extensor muscle, fascia and tendon of right ring finger at wrist and hand level   ▽

     √7ᵗʰ **S66.305** Unspecified injury of extensor muscle, fascia and tendon of left ring finger at wrist and hand level   ▽

     √7ᵗʰ **S66.306** Unspecified injury of extensor muscle, fascia and tendon of right little finger at wrist and hand level   ▽

     √7ᵗʰ **S66.307** Unspecified injury of extensor muscle, fascia and tendon of left little finger at wrist and hand level   ▽

     √7ᵗʰ **S66.308** Unspecified injury of extensor muscle, fascia and tendon of other finger at wrist and hand level   ▽

     Unspecified injury of extensor muscle, fascia and tendon of specified finger with unspecified laterality at wrist and hand level

     √7ᵗʰ **S66.309** Unspecified injury of extensor muscle, fascia and tendon of unspecified finger at wrist and hand level   ▽

   √6ᵗʰ **S66.31** Strain of extensor muscle, fascia and tendon of other and unspecified finger at wrist and hand level

     √7ᵗʰ **S66.310** Strain of extensor muscle, fascia and tendon of right index finger at wrist and hand level

     √7ᵗʰ **S66.311** Strain of extensor muscle, fascia and tendon of left index finger at wrist and hand level

     √7ᵗʰ **S66.312** Strain of extensor muscle, fascia and tendon of right middle finger at wrist and hand level

     √7ᵗʰ **S66.313** Strain of extensor muscle, fascia and tendon of left middle finger at wrist and hand level

     √7ᵗʰ **S66.314** Strain of extensor muscle, fascia and tendon of right ring finger at wrist and hand level

     √7ᵗʰ **S66.315** Strain of extensor muscle, fascia and tendon of left ring finger at wrist and hand level

     √7ᵗʰ **S66.316** Strain of extensor muscle, fascia and tendon of right little finger at wrist and hand level

     √7ᵗʰ **S66.317** Strain of extensor muscle, fascia and tendon of left little finger at wrist and hand level

     √7ᵗʰ **S66.318** Strain of extensor muscle, fascia and tendon of other finger at wrist and hand level

     Strain of extensor muscle, fascia and tendon of specified finger with unspecified laterality at wrist and hand level

     √7ᵗʰ **S66.319** Strain of extensor muscle, fascia and tendon of unspecified finger at wrist and hand level   ▽

   √6ᵗʰ **S66.32** Laceration of extensor muscle, fascia and tendon of other and unspecified finger at wrist and hand level

     √7ᵗʰ **S66.320** Laceration of extensor muscle, fascia and tendon of right index finger at wrist and hand level

     √7ᵗʰ **S66.321** Laceration of extensor muscle, fascia and tendon of left index finger at wrist and hand level

     √7ᵗʰ **S66.322** Laceration of extensor muscle, fascia and tendon of right middle finger at wrist and hand level

     √7ᵗʰ **S66.323** Laceration of extensor muscle, fascia and tendon of left middle finger at wrist and hand level

     √7ᵗʰ **S66.324** Laceration of extensor muscle, fascia and tendon of right ring finger at wrist and hand level

☑ Additional Character Required   √x7ᵗʰ Placeholder Alert   Manifestation Dx   ▽ Unspecified Dx   ►◄ Revised Text   ● New Code   ▲ Revised Code Title

ICD-10-CM 2017   **969**

√7ᵗʰ **S66.325** **Laceration of extensor muscle, fascia and tendon of** left ring **finger at wrist and hand level**

√7ᵗʰ **S66.326** **Laceration of extensor muscle, fascia and tendon of** right little **finger at wrist and hand level**

√7ᵗʰ **S66.327** **Laceration of extensor muscle, fascia and tendon of** left little **finger at wrist and hand level**

√7ᵗʰ **S66.328** **Laceration of extensor muscle, fascia and tendon of other finger at wrist and hand level**

Laceration of extensor muscle, fascia and tendon of specified finger with unspecified laterality at wrist and hand level

√7ᵗʰ **S66.329** **Laceration of extensor muscle, fascia and tendon of unspecified finger at wrist and hand level** ▽

√6ᵗʰ **S66.39** **Other injury of extensor muscle, fascia and tendon of other and unspecified finger at wrist and hand level**

√7ᵗʰ **S66.390** **Other injury of extensor muscle, fascia and tendon of** right index **finger at wrist and hand level**

√7ᵗʰ **S66.391** **Other injury of extensor muscle, fascia and tendon of** left index **finger at wrist and hand level**

√7ᵗʰ **S66.392** **Other injury of extensor muscle, fascia and tendon of** right middle **finger at wrist and hand level**

√7ᵗʰ **S66.393** **Other injury of extensor muscle, fascia and tendon of** left middle **finger at wrist and hand level**

√7ᵗʰ **S66.394** **Other injury of extensor muscle, fascia and tendon of** right ring **finger at wrist and hand level**

√7ᵗʰ **S66.395** **Other injury of extensor muscle, fascia and tendon of** left ring **finger at wrist and hand level**

√7ᵗʰ **S66.396** **Other injury of extensor muscle, fascia and tendon of** right little **finger at wrist and hand level**

√7ᵗʰ **S66.397** **Other injury of extensor muscle, fascia and tendon of** left little **finger at wrist and hand level**

√7ᵗʰ **S66.398** **Other injury of extensor muscle, fascia and tendon of other finger at wrist and hand level**

Other injury of extensor muscle, fascia and tendon of specified finger with unspecified laterality at wrist and hand level

√7ᵗʰ **S66.399** **Other injury of extensor muscle, fascia and tendon of unspecified finger at wrist and hand level** ▽

√5ᵗʰ **S66.4** **Injury of** intrinsic muscle, fascia and tendon of thumb **at wrist and hand level**

√6ᵗʰ **S66.40** **Unspecified injury of intrinsic muscle, fascia and tendon of thumb at wrist and hand level**

√7ᵗʰ **S66.401** **Unspecified injury of intrinsic muscle, fascia and tendon of** right **thumb at wrist and hand level** ▽

√7ᵗʰ **S66.402** **Unspecified injury of intrinsic muscle, fascia and tendon of** left **thumb at wrist and hand level** ▽

√7ᵗʰ **S66.409** **Unspecified injury of intrinsic muscle, fascia and tendon of unspecified thumb at wrist and hand level** ▽

√6ᵗʰ **S66.41** **Strain of intrinsic muscle, fascia and tendon of thumb at wrist and hand level**

√7ᵗʰ **S66.411** **Strain of intrinsic muscle, fascia and tendon of** right **thumb at wrist and hand level**

√7ᵗʰ **S66.412** **Strain of intrinsic muscle, fascia and tendon of** left **thumb at wrist and hand level**

√7ᵗʰ **S66.419** **Strain of intrinsic muscle, fascia and tendon of unspecified thumb at wrist and hand level** ▽

√6ᵗʰ **S66.42** **Laceration of intrinsic muscle, fascia and tendon of thumb at wrist and hand level**

√7ᵗʰ **S66.421** **Laceration of intrinsic muscle, fascia and tendon of** right **thumb at wrist and hand level**

√7ᵗʰ **S66.422** **Laceration of intrinsic muscle, fascia and tendon of** left **thumb at wrist and hand level**

√7ᵗʰ **S66.429** **Laceration of intrinsic muscle, fascia and tendon of unspecified thumb at wrist and hand level** ▽

√6ᵗʰ **S66.49** **Other specified injury of intrinsic muscle, fascia and tendon of thumb at wrist and hand level**

√7ᵗʰ **S66.491** **Other specified injury of intrinsic muscle, fascia and tendon of** right **thumb at wrist and hand level**

√7ᵗʰ **S66.492** **Other specified injury of intrinsic muscle, fascia and tendon of** left **thumb at wrist and hand level**

√7ᵗʰ **S66.499** **Other specified injury of intrinsic muscle, fascia and tendon of unspecified thumb at wrist and hand level** ▽

√5ᵗʰ **S66.5** **Injury of** intrinsic muscle, fascia and tendon of other and unspecified finger **at wrist and hand level**

EXCLUDES 2 injury of intrinsic muscle, fascia and tendon of thumb at wrist and hand level (S66.4-)

√6ᵗʰ **S66.50** **Unspecified injury of intrinsic muscle, fascia and tendon of other and unspecified finger at wrist and hand level**

√7ᵗʰ **S66.500** **Unspecified injury of intrinsic muscle, fascia and tendon of** right index **finger at wrist and hand level** ▽

√7ᵗʰ **S66.501** **Unspecified injury of intrinsic muscle, fascia and tendon of** left index **finger at wrist and hand level** ▽

√7ᵗʰ **S66.502** **Unspecified injury of intrinsic muscle, fascia and tendon of** right middle **finger at wrist and hand level** ▽

√7ᵗʰ **S66.503** **Unspecified injury of intrinsic muscle, fascia and tendon of** left middle **finger at wrist and hand level** ▽

√7ᵗʰ **S66.504** **Unspecified injury of intrinsic muscle, fascia and tendon of** right ring **finger at wrist and hand level** ▽

√7ᵗʰ **S66.505** **Unspecified injury of intrinsic muscle, fascia and tendon of** left ring **finger at wrist and hand level** ▽

√7ᵗʰ **S66.506** **Unspecified injury of intrinsic muscle, fascia and tendon of** right little **finger at wrist and hand level** ▽

√7ᵗʰ **S66.507** **Unspecified injury of intrinsic muscle, fascia and tendon of** left little **finger at wrist and hand level** ▽

√7ᵗʰ **S66.508** **Unspecified injury of intrinsic muscle, fascia and tendon of other finger at wrist and hand level** ▽

Unspecified injury of intrinsic muscle, fascia and tendon of specified finger with unspecified laterality at wrist and hand level

√7ᵗʰ **S66.509** **Unspecified injury of intrinsic muscle, fascia and tendon of unspecified finger at wrist and hand level** ▽

√6ᵗʰ **S66.51** **Strain of intrinsic muscle, fascia and tendon of other and unspecified finger at wrist and hand level**

√7ᵗʰ **S66.510** **Strain of intrinsic muscle, fascia and tendon of** right index **finger at wrist and hand level**

√7ᵗʰ **S66.511** **Strain of intrinsic muscle, fascia and tendon of** left index **finger at wrist and hand level**

√7ᵗʰ **S66.512** **Strain of intrinsic muscle, fascia and tendon of** right middle **finger at wrist and hand level**

√7ᵗʰ **S66.513** **Strain of intrinsic muscle, fascia and tendon of** left middle **finger at wrist and hand level**

√7ᵗʰ **S66.514** **Strain of intrinsic muscle, fascia and tendon of** right ring **finger at wrist and hand level**

√7ᵗʰ **S66.515 Strain** of intrinsic muscle, fascia and tendon of **left ring** finger at wrist and hand level

√7ᵗʰ **S66.516 Strain** of intrinsic muscle, fascia and tendon of **right little** finger at wrist and hand level

√7ᵗʰ **S66.517 Strain** of intrinsic muscle, fascia and tendon of **left little** finger at wrist and hand level

√7ᵗʰ **S66.518 Strain** of intrinsic muscle, fascia and tendon of **other** finger at wrist and hand level

Strain of intrinsic muscle, fascia and tendon of specified finger with unspecified laterality at wrist and hand level

√7ᵗʰ **S66.519 Strain** of intrinsic muscle, fascia and tendon of **unspecified** finger at wrist and hand level ▽

√6ᵗʰ **S66.52 Laceration** of intrinsic muscle, fascia and tendon of other and unspecified finger at wrist and hand level

√7ᵗʰ **S66.520 Laceration** of intrinsic muscle, fascia and tendon of **right index** finger at wrist and hand level

√7ᵗʰ **S66.521 Laceration** of intrinsic muscle, fascia and tendon of **left index** finger at wrist and hand level

√7ᵗʰ **S66.522 Laceration** of intrinsic muscle, fascia and tendon of **right middle** finger at wrist and hand level

√7ᵗʰ **S66.523 Laceration** of intrinsic muscle, fascia and tendon of **left middle** finger at wrist and hand level

√7ᵗʰ **S66.524 Laceration** of intrinsic muscle, fascia and tendon of **right ring** finger at wrist and hand level

√7ᵗʰ **S66.525 Laceration** of intrinsic muscle, fascia and tendon of **left ring** finger at wrist and hand level

√7ᵗʰ **S66.526 Laceration** of intrinsic muscle, fascia and tendon of **right little** finger at wrist and hand level

√7ᵗʰ **S66.527 Laceration** of intrinsic muscle, fascia and tendon of **left little** finger at wrist and hand level

√7ᵗʰ **S66.528 Laceration** of intrinsic muscle, fascia and tendon of **other** finger at wrist and hand level

Laceration of intrinsic muscle, fascia and tendon of specified finger with unspecified laterality at wrist and hand level

√7ᵗʰ **S66.529 Laceration** of intrinsic muscle, fascia and tendon of **unspecified** finger at wrist and hand level ▽

√6ᵗʰ **S66.59 Other injury** of intrinsic muscle, fascia and tendon of other and unspecified finger at wrist and hand level

√7ᵗʰ **S66.590 Other injury** of intrinsic muscle, fascia and tendon of **right index** finger at wrist and hand level

√7ᵗʰ **S66.591 Other injury** of intrinsic muscle, fascia and tendon of **left index** finger at wrist and hand level

√7ᵗʰ **S66.592 Other injury** of intrinsic muscle, fascia and tendon of **right middle** finger at wrist and hand level

√7ᵗʰ **S66.593 Other injury** of intrinsic muscle, fascia and tendon of **left middle** finger at wrist and hand level

√7ᵗʰ **S66.594 Other injury** of intrinsic muscle, fascia and tendon of **right ring** finger at wrist and hand level

√7ᵗʰ **S66.595 Other injury** of intrinsic muscle, fascia and tendon of **left ring** finger at wrist and hand level

√7ᵗʰ **S66.596 Other injury** of intrinsic muscle, fascia and tendon of **right little** finger at wrist and hand level

√7ᵗʰ **S66.597 Other injury** of intrinsic muscle, fascia and tendon of **left little** finger at wrist and hand level

√7ᵗʰ **S66.598 Other injury** of intrinsic muscle, fascia and tendon of **other** finger at wrist and hand level

Other injury of intrinsic muscle, fascia and tendon of specified finger with unspecified laterality at wrist and hand level

√7ᵗʰ **S66.599 Other injury** of intrinsic muscle, fascia and tendon of **unspecified** finger at wrist and hand level ▽

√5ᵗʰ **S66.8 Injury of other specified muscles, fascia and tendons at wrist and hand level**

√6ᵗʰ **S66.80 Unspecified injury** of other specified muscles, fascia and tendons at wrist and hand level

√7ᵗʰ **S66.801 Unspecified injury** of other specified muscles, fascia and tendons at wrist and hand level, **right hand** ▽

√7ᵗʰ **S66.802 Unspecified injury** of other specified muscles, fascia and tendons at wrist and hand level, **left hand** ▽

√7ᵗʰ **S66.809 Unspecified injury** of other specified muscles, fascia and tendons at wrist and hand level, **unspecified hand** ▽

√6ᵗʰ **S66.81 Strain** of other specified muscles, fascia and tendons at wrist and hand level

√7ᵗʰ **S66.811 Strain** of other specified muscles, fascia and tendons at wrist and hand level, **right hand**

√7ᵗʰ **S66.812 Strain** of other specified muscles, fascia and tendons at wrist and hand level, **left hand**

√7ᵗʰ **S66.819 Strain** of other specified muscles, fascia and tendons at wrist and hand level, **unspecified hand** ▽

√6ᵗʰ **S66.82 Laceration** of other specified muscles, fascia and tendons at wrist and hand level

√7ᵗʰ **S66.821 Laceration** of other specified muscles, fascia and tendons at wrist and hand level, **right hand**

√7ᵗʰ **S66.822 Laceration** of other specified muscles, fascia and tendons at wrist and hand level, **left hand**

√7ᵗʰ **S66.829 Laceration** of other specified muscles, fascia and tendons at wrist and hand level, **unspecified hand** ▽

√6ᵗʰ **S66.89 Other injury** of other specified muscles, fascia and tendons at wrist and hand level

√7ᵗʰ **S66.891 Other injury** of other specified muscles, fascia and tendons at wrist and hand level, **right hand**

√7ᵗʰ **S66.892 Other injury** of other specified muscles, fascia and tendons at wrist and hand level, **left hand**

√7ᵗʰ **S66.899 Other injury** of other specified muscles, fascia and tendons at wrist and hand level, **unspecified hand** ▽

√5ᵗʰ **S66.9 Injury of unspecified muscle, fascia and tendon at wrist and hand level**

√6ᵗʰ **S66.90 Unspecified injury** of unspecified muscle, fascia and tendon at wrist and hand level

√7ᵗʰ **S66.901 Unspecified injury** of unspecified muscle, fascia and tendon at wrist and hand level, **right hand** ▽

√7ᵗʰ **S66.902 Unspecified injury** of unspecified muscle, fascia and tendon at wrist and hand level, **left hand** ▽

√7ᵗʰ **S66.909 Unspecified injury** of unspecified muscle, fascia and tendon at wrist and hand level, **unspecified hand** ▽

√6ᵗʰ **S66.91 Strain** of unspecified muscle, fascia and tendon at wrist and hand level

√7ᵗʰ **S66.911 Strain** of unspecified muscle, fascia and tendon at wrist and hand level, **right hand** ▽

√7ᵗʰ **S66.912 Strain** of unspecified muscle, fascia and tendon at wrist and hand level, **left hand** ▽

√7ᵗʰ **S66.919 Strain** of unspecified muscle, fascia and tendon at wrist and hand level, **unspecified hand** ▽

☑ Additional Character Required   Placeholder Alert   Manifestation Dx   ▽ Unspecified Dx   ▶◀ Revised Text   ● New Code   ▲ Revised Code Title

ICD-10-CM 2017   971

✓6ᵗʰ S66.92 Laceration of unspecified muscle, fascia and tendon at wrist and hand level

     ✓7ᵗʰ **S66.921** Laceration of unspecified muscle, fascia and tendon at wrist and hand level, right hand ▽

     ✓7ᵗʰ **S66.922** Laceration of unspecified muscle, fascia and tendon at wrist and hand level, left hand ▽

     ✓7ᵗʰ **S66.929** Laceration of unspecified muscle, fascia and tendon at wrist and hand level, unspecified hand ▽

✓6ᵗʰ S66.99 Other injury of unspecified muscle, fascia and tendon at wrist and hand level

     ✓7ᵗʰ **S66.991** Other injury of unspecified muscle, fascia and tendon at wrist and hand level, right hand ▽

     ✓7ᵗʰ **S66.992** Other injury of unspecified muscle, fascia and tendon at wrist and hand level, left hand ▽

     ✓7ᵗʰ **S66.999** Other injury of unspecified muscle, fascia and tendon at wrist and hand level, unspecified hand ▽

✓4ᵗʰ S67 Crushing injury of wrist, hand and fingers

Use additional code for all associated injuries, such as:
    fracture of wrist and hand (S62.-)
    open wound of wrist and hand (S61.-)

The appropriate 7th character is to be added to each code from category S67.
   A   initial encounter
   D   subsequent encounter
   S   sequela

✓5ᵗʰ S67.0 Crushing injury of thumb

   ✓x7ᵗʰ **S67.00** Crushing injury of unspecified thumb ▽

   ✓x7ᵗʰ **S67.01** Crushing injury of right thumb

   ✓x7ᵗʰ **S67.02** Crushing injury of left thumb

✓5ᵗʰ S67.1 Crushing injury of other and unspecified finger(s)

     EXCLUDES 2   crushing injury of thumb (S67.0-)

   ✓x7ᵗʰ **S67.10** Crushing injury of unspecified finger(s) ▽

   ✓6ᵗʰ **S67.19** Crushing injury of other finger(s)

     ✓7ᵗʰ **S67.190** Crushing injury of right index finger

     ✓7ᵗʰ **S67.191** Crushing injury of left index finger

     ✓7ᵗʰ **S67.192** Crushing injury of right middle finger

     ✓7ᵗʰ **S67.193** Crushing injury of left middle finger

     ✓7ᵗʰ **S67.194** Crushing injury of right ring finger

     ✓7ᵗʰ **S67.195** Crushing injury of left ring finger

     ✓7ᵗʰ **S67.196** Crushing injury of right little finger

     ✓7ᵗʰ **S67.197** Crushing injury of left little finger

     ✓7ᵗʰ **S67.198** Crushing injury of other finger

       Crushing injury of specified finger with unspecified laterality

✓5ᵗʰ S67.2 Crushing injury of hand

     EXCLUDES 2   crushing injury of fingers (S67.1-)
             crushing injury of thumb (S67.0-)

   ✓x7ᵗʰ **S67.20** Crushing injury of unspecified hand ▽

   ✓x7ᵗʰ **S67.21** Crushing injury of right hand

   ✓x7ᵗʰ **S67.22** Crushing injury of left hand

✓5ᵗʰ S67.3 Crushing injury of wrist

   ✓x7ᵗʰ **S67.30** Crushing injury of unspecified wrist ▽

   ✓x7ᵗʰ **S67.31** Crushing injury of right wrist

   ✓x7ᵗʰ **S67.32** Crushing injury of left wrist

✓5ᵗʰ S67.4 Crushing injury of wrist and hand

     EXCLUDES 1   crushing injury of hand alone (S67.2-)
             crushing injury of wrist alone (S67.3-)
     EXCLUDES 2   crushing injury of fingers (S67.1-)
             crushing injury of thumb (S67.0-)

   ✓x7ᵗʰ **S67.40** Crushing injury of unspecified wrist and hand ▽

   ✓x7ᵗʰ **S67.41** Crushing injury of right wrist and hand

   ✓x7ᵗʰ **S67.42** Crushing injury of left wrist and hand

✓5ᵗʰ S67.9 Crushing injury of unspecified part(s) of wrist, hand and fingers

   ✓x7ᵗʰ **S67.90** Crushing injury of unspecified part(s) of unspecified wrist, hand and fingers ▽

   ✓x7ᵗʰ **S67.91** Crushing injury of unspecified part(s) of right wrist, hand and fingers ▽

   ✓x7ᵗʰ **S67.92** Crushing injury of unspecified part(s) of left wrist, hand and fingers ▽

✓4ᵗʰ S68 Traumatic amputation of wrist, hand and fingers

NOTE   An amputation not identified as partial or complete should be coded to complete

The appropriate 7th character is to be added to each code from category S68.
   A   initial encounter
   D   subsequent encounter
   S   sequela

✓5ᵗʰ S68.0 Traumatic metacarpophalangeal amputation of thumb

     Traumatic amputation of thumb NOS

   ✓6ᵗʰ **S68.01** Complete traumatic metacarpophalangeal amputation of thumb

     ✓7ᵗʰ **S68.011** Complete traumatic metacarpophalangeal amputation of right thumb

     ✓7ᵗʰ **S68.012** Complete traumatic metacarpophalangeal amputation of left thumb

     ✓7ᵗʰ **S68.019** Complete traumatic metacarpophalangeal amputation of unspecified thumb ▽

   ✓6ᵗʰ **S68.02** Partial traumatic metacarpophalangeal amputation of thumb

     ✓7ᵗʰ **S68.021** Partial traumatic metacarpophalangeal amputation of right thumb

     ✓7ᵗʰ **S68.022** Partial traumatic metacarpophalangeal amputation of left thumb

     ✓7ᵗʰ **S68.029** Partial traumatic metacarpophalangeal amputation of unspecified thumb ▽

✓5ᵗʰ S68.1 Traumatic metacarpophalangeal amputation of other and unspecified finger

     Traumatic amputation of finger NOS

     EXCLUDES 2   traumatic metacarpophalangeal amputation of thumb (S68.0-)

   ✓6ᵗʰ **S68.11** Complete traumatic metacarpophalangeal amputation of other and unspecified finger

     ✓7ᵗʰ **S68.110** Complete traumatic metacarpophalangeal amputation of right index finger

     ✓7ᵗʰ **S68.111** Complete traumatic metacarpophalangeal amputation of left index finger

     ✓7ᵗʰ **S68.112** Complete traumatic metacarpophalangeal amputation of right middle finger

     ✓7ᵗʰ **S68.113** Complete traumatic metacarpophalangeal amputation of left middle finger

     ✓7ᵗʰ **S68.114** Complete traumatic metacarpophalangeal amputation of right ring finger

     ✓7ᵗʰ **S68.115** Complete traumatic metacarpophalangeal amputation of left ring finger

     ✓7ᵗʰ **S68.116** Complete traumatic metacarpophalangeal amputation of right little finger

     ✓7ᵗʰ **S68.117** Complete traumatic metacarpophalangeal amputation of left little finger

     ✓7ᵗʰ **S68.118** Complete traumatic metacarpophalangeal amputation of other finger

       Complete traumatic metacarpophalangeal amputation of specified finger with unspecified laterality

     ✓7ᵗʰ **S68.119** Complete traumatic metacarpophalangeal amputation of unspecified finger ▽

   ✓6ᵗʰ **S68.12** Partial traumatic metacarpophalangeal amputation of other and unspecified finger

     ✓7ᵗʰ **S68.120** Partial traumatic metacarpophalangeal amputation of right index finger

     ✓7ᵗʰ **S68.121** Partial traumatic metacarpophalangeal amputation of left index finger

     ✓7ᵗʰ **S68.122** Partial traumatic metacarpophalangeal amputation of right middle finger

EXCLUDES 1 Not coded here   EXCLUDES 2 Not included here   N Newborn Age : 0   P Pediatric Age : 0-17   M Maternity Age : 12-55   A Adult Age : 15-124

972

ICD-10-CM 2017

√7ᵗʰ **S68.123** Partial traumatic metacarpophalangeal amputation of left middle finger

√7ᵗʰ **S68.124** Partial traumatic metacarpophalangeal amputation of right ring finger

√7ᵗʰ **S68.125** Partial traumatic metacarpophalangeal amputation of left ring finger

√7ᵗʰ **S68.126** Partial traumatic metacarpophalangeal amputation of right little finger

√7ᵗʰ **S68.127** Partial traumatic metacarpophalangeal amputation of left little finger

√7ᵗʰ **S68.128** Partial traumatic metacarpophalangeal amputation of other finger

Partial traumatic metacarpophalangeal amputation of specified finger with unspecified laterality

√7ᵗʰ **S68.129** Partial traumatic metacarpophalangeal amputation of unspecified finger ▽

√5ᵗʰ **S68.4 Traumatic amputation of hand at wrist level**

Traumatic amputation of hand NOS
Traumatic amputation of wrist

√6ᵗʰ **S68.41** Complete traumatic amputation of hand at wrist level

√7ᵗʰ **S68.411** Complete traumatic amputation of right hand at wrist level

√7ᵗʰ **S68.412** Complete traumatic amputation of left hand at wrist level

√7ᵗʰ **S68.419** Complete traumatic amputation of unspecified hand at wrist level ▽

√6ᵗʰ **S68.42** Partial traumatic amputation of hand at wrist level

√7ᵗʰ **S68.421** Partial traumatic amputation of right hand at wrist level

√7ᵗʰ **S68.422** Partial traumatic amputation of left hand at wrist level

√7ᵗʰ **S68.429** Partial traumatic amputation of unspecified hand at wrist level ▽

√5ᵗʰ **S68.5 Traumatic transphalangeal amputation of thumb**

Traumatic interphalangeal joint amputation of thumb

√6ᵗʰ **S68.51** Complete traumatic transphalangeal amputation of thumb

√7ᵗʰ **S68.511** Complete traumatic transphalangeal amputation of right thumb

√7ᵗʰ **S68.512** Complete traumatic transphalangeal amputation of left thumb

√7ᵗʰ **S68.519** Complete traumatic transphalangeal amputation of unspecified thumb ▽

√6ᵗʰ **S68.52** Partial traumatic transphalangeal amputation of thumb

√7ᵗʰ **S68.521** Partial traumatic transphalangeal amputation of right thumb

√7ᵗʰ **S68.522** Partial traumatic transphalangeal amputation of left thumb

√7ᵗʰ **S68.529** Partial traumatic transphalangeal amputation of unspecified thumb ▽

√5ᵗʰ **S68.6 Traumatic transphalangeal amputation of other and unspecified finger**

√6ᵗʰ **S68.61** Complete traumatic transphalangeal amputation of other and unspecified finger(s)

√7ᵗʰ **S68.610** Complete traumatic transphalangeal amputation of right index finger

√7ᵗʰ **S68.611** Complete traumatic transphalangeal amputation of left index finger

√7ᵗʰ **S68.612** Complete traumatic transphalangeal amputation of right middle finger

√7ᵗʰ **S68.613** Complete traumatic transphalangeal amputation of left middle finger

√7ᵗʰ **S68.614** Complete traumatic transphalangeal amputation of right ring finger

√7ᵗʰ **S68.615** Complete traumatic transphalangeal amputation of left ring finger

√7ᵗʰ **S68.616** Complete traumatic transphalangeal amputation of right little finger

√7ᵗʰ **S68.617** Complete traumatic transphalangeal amputation of left little finger

√7ᵗʰ **S68.618** Complete traumatic transphalangeal amputation of other finger

Complete traumatic transphalangeal amputation of specified finger with unspecified laterality

√7ᵗʰ **S68.619** Complete traumatic transphalangeal amputation of unspecified finger ▽

√6ᵗʰ **S68.62** Partial traumatic transphalangeal amputation of other and unspecified finger

√7ᵗʰ **S68.620** Partial traumatic transphalangeal amputation of right index finger

√7ᵗʰ **S68.621** Partial traumatic transphalangeal amputation of left index finger

√7ᵗʰ **S68.622** Partial traumatic transphalangeal amputation of right middle finger

√7ᵗʰ **S68.623** Partial traumatic transphalangeal amputation of left middle finger

√7ᵗʰ **S68.624** Partial traumatic transphalangeal amputation of right ring finger

√7ᵗʰ **S68.625** Partial traumatic transphalangeal amputation of left ring finger

√7ᵗʰ **S68.626** Partial traumatic transphalangeal amputation of right little finger

√7ᵗʰ **S68.627** Partial traumatic transphalangeal amputation of left little finger

√7ᵗʰ **S68.628** Partial traumatic transphalangeal amputation of other finger

Partial traumatic transphalangeal amputation of specified finger with unspecified laterality

√7ᵗʰ **S68.629** Partial traumatic transphalangeal amputation of unspecified finger ▽

√5ᵗʰ **S68.7 Traumatic transmetacarpal amputation of hand**

√6ᵗʰ **S68.71** Complete traumatic transmetacarpal amputation of hand

√7ᵗʰ **S68.711** Complete traumatic transmetacarpal amputation of right hand

√7ᵗʰ **S68.712** Complete traumatic transmetacarpal amputation of left hand

√7ᵗʰ **S68.719** Complete traumatic transmetacarpal amputation of unspecified hand ▽

√6ᵗʰ **S68.72** Partial traumatic transmetacarpal amputation of hand

√7ᵗʰ **S68.721** Partial traumatic transmetacarpal amputation of right hand

√7ᵗʰ **S68.722** Partial traumatic transmetacarpal amputation of left hand

√7ᵗʰ **S68.729** Partial traumatic transmetacarpal amputation of unspecified hand ▽

√4ᵗʰ **S69 Other and unspecified injuries of wrist, hand and finger(s)**

> The appropriate 7th character is to be added to each code from category S69.
> A   initial encounter
> D   subsequent encounter
> S   sequela

√5ᵗʰ **S69.8 Other specified injuries of wrist, hand and finger(s)**

√x7ᵗʰ **S69.80** Other specified injuries of unspecified wrist, hand and finger(s) ▽

√x7ᵗʰ **S69.81** Other specified injuries of right wrist, hand and finger(s)

√x7ᵗʰ **S69.82** Other specified injuries of left wrist, hand and finger(s)

√5ᵗʰ **S69.9 Unspecified injury of wrist, hand and finger(s)**

√x7ᵗʰ **S69.90** Unspecified injury of unspecified wrist, hand and finger(s) ▽

√x7ᵗʰ **S69.91** Unspecified injury of right wrist, hand and finger(s) ▽

√x7ᵗʰ **S69.92** Unspecified injury of left wrist, hand and finger(s) ▽

Injuries to the hip and thigh (S70-S79)

EXCLUDES 2   *burns and corrosions (T20-T32)*
frostbite (T33-T34)
snake bite (T63.0-)
venomous insect bite or sting (T63.4-)

√4ᵗʰ **S70 Superficial injury of hip and thigh**

> The appropriate 7th character is to be added to each code from category S70.
> A   initial encounter
> D   subsequent encounter
> S   sequela

√5ᵗʰ **S70.0 Contusion of hip**

√x7ᵗʰ **S70.00** Contusion of unspecified hip ▽

☑ Additional Character Required   √x7ᵗʰ Placeholder Alert   Manifestation Dx   ▽ Unspecified Dx   ►◄ Revised Text   ● New Code   ▲ Revised Code Title

ICD-10-CM 2017   973

☑x7ᵗʰ **S70.01** Contusion of **right hip**

☑x7ᵗʰ **S70.02** Contusion of **left hip**

☑5ᵗʰ **S70.1** **Contusion of thigh**

☑x7ᵗʰ **S70.10** Contusion of **unspecified thigh** ▽

☑x7ᵗʰ **S70.11** Contusion of **right thigh**

☑x7ᵗʰ **S70.12** Contusion of **left thigh**

☑5ᵗʰ **S70.2** **Other superficial injuries of hip**

☑6ᵗʰ **S70.21** **Abrasion of hip**

☑7ᵗʰ **S70.211** Abrasion, **right hip**

☑7ᵗʰ **S70.212** Abrasion, **left hip**

☑7ᵗʰ **S70.219** Abrasion, **unspecified hip** ▽

☑6ᵗʰ **S70.22** **Blister (nonthermal) of hip**

☑7ᵗʰ **S70.221** Blister (nonthermal), **right hip**

☑7ᵗʰ **S70.222** Blister (nonthermal), **left hip**

☑7ᵗʰ **S70.229** Blister (nonthermal), **unspecified hip** ▽

☑6ᵗʰ **S70.24** **External constriction of hip**

☑7ᵗʰ **S70.241** External constriction, **right hip**

☑7ᵗʰ **S70.242** External constriction, **left hip**

☑7ᵗʰ **S70.249** External constriction, **unspecified hip** ▽

☑6ᵗʰ **S70.25** **Superficial foreign body of hip**

Splinter in the hip

☑7ᵗʰ **S70.251** Superficial foreign body, **right hip**

☑7ᵗʰ **S70.252** Superficial foreign body, **left hip**

☑7ᵗʰ **S70.259** Superficial foreign body, **unspecified hip** ▽

☑6ᵗʰ **S70.26** **Insect bite (nonvenomous) of hip**

☑7ᵗʰ **S70.261** Insect bite (nonvenomous), **right hip**

☑7ᵗʰ **S70.262** Insect bite (nonvenomous), **left hip**

☑7ᵗʰ **S70.269** Insect bite (nonvenomous), **unspecified hip** ▽

☑6ᵗʰ **S70.27** **Other superficial bite of hip**

EXCLUDES 1 open bite of hip (S71.05-)

☑7ᵗʰ **S70.271** Other superficial bite of hip, **right hip**

☑7ᵗʰ **S70.272** Other superficial bite of hip, **left hip**

☑7ᵗʰ **S70.279** Other superficial bite of hip, **unspecified hip** ▽

☑5ᵗʰ **S70.3** **Other superficial injuries of thigh**

☑6ᵗʰ **S70.31** **Abrasion of thigh**

☑7ᵗʰ **S70.311** Abrasion, **right thigh**

☑7ᵗʰ **S70.312** Abrasion, **left thigh**

☑7ᵗʰ **S70.319** Abrasion, **unspecified thigh** ▽

☑6ᵗʰ **S70.32** **Blister (nonthermal) of thigh**

☑7ᵗʰ **S70.321** Blister (nonthermal), **right thigh**

☑7ᵗʰ **S70.322** Blister (nonthermal), **left thigh**

☑7ᵗʰ **S70.329** Blister (nonthermal), **unspecified thigh** ▽

☑6ᵗʰ **S70.34** **External constriction of thigh**

☑7ᵗʰ **S70.341** External constriction, **right thigh**

☑7ᵗʰ **S70.342** External constriction, **left thigh**

☑7ᵗʰ **S70.349** External constriction, **unspecified thigh** ▽

☑6ᵗʰ **S70.35** **Superficial foreign body of thigh**

Splinter in the thigh

☑7ᵗʰ **S70.351** Superficial foreign body, **right thigh**

☑7ᵗʰ **S70.352** Superficial foreign body, **left thigh**

☑7ᵗʰ **S70.359** Superficial foreign body, **unspecified thigh** ▽

☑6ᵗʰ **S70.36** **Insect bite (nonvenomous) of thigh**

☑7ᵗʰ **S70.361** Insect bite (nonvenomous), **right thigh**

☑7ᵗʰ **S70.362** Insect bite (nonvenomous), **left thigh**

☑7ᵗʰ **S70.369** Insect bite (nonvenomous), **unspecified thigh** ▽

☑6ᵗʰ **S70.37** **Other superficial bite of thigh**

EXCLUDES 1 open bite of thigh (S71.15)

☑7ᵗʰ **S70.371** Other superficial bite of **right thigh**

☑7ᵗʰ **S70.372** Other superficial bite of **left thigh**

☑7ᵗʰ **S70.379** Other superficial bite of **unspecified thigh** ▽

☑5ᵗʰ **S70.9** **Unspecified superficial injury of hip and thigh**

☑6ᵗʰ **S70.91** **Unspecified superficial injury of hip**

☑7ᵗʰ **S70.911** Unspecified superficial injury of **right hip** ▽

☑7ᵗʰ **S70.912** Unspecified superficial injury of **left hip** ▽

☑7ᵗʰ **S70.919** Unspecified superficial injury of **unspecified hip** ▽

☑6ᵗʰ **S70.92** **Unspecified superficial injury of thigh**

☑7ᵗʰ **S70.921** Unspecified superficial injury of **right thigh** ▽

☑7ᵗʰ **S70.922** Unspecified superficial injury of **left thigh** ▽

☑7ᵗʰ **S70.929** Unspecified superficial injury of **unspecified thigh** ▽

☑4ᵗʰ **S71** **Open wound of hip and thigh**

Code also any associated wound infection

EXCLUDES 1 open fracture of hip and thigh (S72.-)

traumatic amputation of hip and thigh (S78.-)

EXCLUDES 2 bite of venomous animal (T63.-)

open wound of ankle, foot and toes (S91.-)

open wound of knee and lower leg (S81.-)

The appropriate 7th character is to be added to each code from category S71.

A initial encounter

D subsequent encounter

S sequela

☑5ᵗʰ **S71.0** **Open wound of hip**

☑6ᵗʰ **S71.00** **Unspecified open wound of hip**

☑7ᵗʰ **S71.001** Unspecified open wound, **right hip** ▽

☑7ᵗʰ **S71.002** Unspecified open wound, **left hip** ▽

☑7ᵗʰ **S71.009** Unspecified open wound, **unspecified hip** ▽

☑6ᵗʰ **S71.01** **Laceration without foreign body of hip**

☑7ᵗʰ **S71.011** Laceration without foreign body, **right hip**

☑7ᵗʰ **S71.012** Laceration without foreign body, **left hip**

☑7ᵗʰ **S71.019** Laceration without foreign body, **unspecified hip** ▽

☑6ᵗʰ **S71.02** **Laceration with foreign body of hip**

☑7ᵗʰ **S71.021** Laceration with foreign body, **right hip**

☑7ᵗʰ **S71.022** Laceration with foreign body, **left hip**

☑7ᵗʰ **S71.029** Laceration with foreign body, **unspecified hip** ▽

☑6ᵗʰ **S71.03** **Puncture wound without foreign body of hip**

☑7ᵗʰ **S71.031** Puncture wound without foreign body, **right hip**

☑7ᵗʰ **S71.032** Puncture wound without foreign body, **left hip**

☑7ᵗʰ **S71.039** Puncture wound without foreign body, **unspecified hip** ▽

☑6ᵗʰ **S71.04** **Puncture wound with foreign body of hip**

☑7ᵗʰ **S71.041** Puncture wound with foreign body, **right hip**

☑7ᵗʰ **S71.042** Puncture wound with foreign body, **left hip**

☑7ᵗʰ **S71.049** Puncture wound with foreign body, **unspecified hip** ▽

☑6ᵗʰ **S71.05** **Open bite of hip**

Bite of hip NOS

EXCLUDES 1 superficial bite of hip (S70.26, S70.27)

☑7ᵗʰ **S71.051** Open bite, **right hip**

☑7ᵗʰ **S71.052** Open bite, **left hip**

☑7ᵗʰ **S71.059** Open bite, **unspecified hip** ▽

☑5ᵗʰ **S71.1** **Open wound of thigh**

☑6ᵗʰ **S71.10** **Unspecified open wound of thigh**

☑7ᵗʰ **S71.101** Unspecified open wound, **right thigh** ▽

☑7ᵗʰ **S71.102** Unspecified open wound, **left thigh** ▽

☑7ᵗʰ **S71.109** Unspecified open wound, **unspecified thigh** ▽

EXCLUDES 1 Not coded here   *EXCLUDES 2* Not included here   Ⓝ Newborn Age : 0   Ⓟ Pediatric Age : 0-17   Ⓜ Maternity Age : 12-55   Ⓐ Adult Age : 15-124

974   ICD-10-CM 2017

√6ᵗʰ **S71.11**   **Laceration without foreign body** of thigh

    √7ᵗʰ **S71.111**   **Laceration without foreign body, right thigh**

    √7ᵗʰ **S71.112**   **Laceration without foreign body, left thigh**

    √7ᵗʰ **S71.119**   **Laceration without foreign body, unspecified thigh** ▽

√6ᵗʰ **S71.12**   **Laceration with foreign body** of thigh

    √7ᵗʰ **S71.121**   **Laceration with foreign body, right thigh**

    √7ᵗʰ **S71.122**   **Laceration with foreign body, left thigh**

    √7ᵗʰ **S71.129**   **Laceration with foreign body, unspecified thigh** ▽

√6ᵗʰ **S71.13**   **Puncture wound without foreign body** of thigh

    √7ᵗʰ **S71.131**   **Puncture wound without foreign body, right thigh**

    √7ᵗʰ **S71.132**   **Puncture wound without foreign body, left thigh**

    √7ᵗʰ **S71.139**   **Puncture wound without foreign body, unspecified thigh** ▽

√6ᵗʰ **S71.14**   **Puncture wound with foreign body** of thigh

    √7ᵗʰ **S71.141**   **Puncture wound with foreign body, right thigh**

    √7ᵗʰ **S71.142**   **Puncture wound with foreign body, left thigh**

    √7ᵗʰ **S71.149**   **Puncture wound with foreign body, unspecified thigh** ▽

√6ᵗʰ **S71.15**   **Open bite** of thigh

    Bite of thigh NOS

    EXCLUDES 1   *superficial bite of thigh (S70.37-)*

    √7ᵗʰ **S71.151**   **Open bite, right thigh**

    √7ᵗʰ **S71.152**   **Open bite, left thigh**

    √7ᵗʰ **S71.159**   **Open bite, unspecified thigh** ▽

√4ᵗʰ **S72**   **Fracture of femur**

> **NOTE**   A fracture not indicated as displaced or nondisplaced should be coded to displaced.
>
> A fracture not indicated as open or closed should be coded to closed.
>
> The open fracture designations are based on the Gustilo open fracture classification.

    EXCLUDES 1   *traumatic amputation of hip and thigh (S78.-)*

    EXCLUDES 2   *fracture of lower leg and ankle (S82.-)*
              fracture of foot (S92.-)
              periprosthetic fracture of prosthetic implant of hip (T84.040, T84.041)

    AHA: 2016,1Q,33; 2015,3Q,37-39; 2015,1Q,17; 2013,4Q,128

The appropriate 7th character is to be added to all codes from category S72 [unless otherwise indicated].

A   initial encounter for closed fracture

B   initial encounter for open fracture type I or II
    initial encounter for open fracture NOS

C   initial encounter for open fracture type IIIA, IIIB, or IIIC

D   subsequent encounter for closed fracture with routine healing

E   subsequent encounter for open fracture type I or II with routine healing

F   subsequent encounter for open fracture type IIIA, IIIB, or IIIC with routine healing

G   subsequent encounter for closed fracture with delayed healing

H   subsequent encounter for open fracture type I or II with delayed healing

J   subsequent encounter for open fracture type IIIA, IIIB, or IIIC with delayed healing

K   subsequent encounter for closed fracture with nonunion

M   subsequent encounter for open fracture type I or II with nonunion

N   subsequent encounter for open fracture type IIIA, IIIB, or IIIC with nonunion

P   subsequent encounter for closed fracture with malunion

Q   subsequent encounter for open fracture type I or II with malunion

R   subsequent encounter for open fracture type IIIA, IIIB, or IIIC with malunion

S   sequela

√5ᵗʰ **S72.0**   **Fracture of head and neck of femur**

    EXCLUDES 2   *physeal fracture of upper end of femur (S79.0-)*

√6ᵗʰ **S72.00**   **Fracture of unspecified part of neck of femur**

    Fracture of hip NOS

    Fracture of neck of femur NOS

    √7ᵗʰ **S72.001**   **Fracture of unspecified part of neck of right femur** ▽

    √7ᵗʰ **S72.002**   **Fracture of unspecified part of neck of left femur** ▽

    √7ᵗʰ **S72.009**   **Fracture of unspecified part of neck of unspecified femur** ▽

√6ᵗʰ **S72.01**   **Unspecified intracapsular fracture of femur**

    Subcapital fracture of femur

    √7ᵗʰ **S72.011**   **Unspecified intracapsular fracture of right femur** ▽

    √7ᵗʰ **S72.012**   **Unspecified intracapsular fracture of left femur** ▽

    √7ᵗʰ **S72.019**   **Unspecified intracapsular fracture of unspecified femur** ▽

√6ᵗʰ **S72.02**   **Fracture of epiphysis (separation) (upper) of femur**

    Transepiphyseal fracture of femur

    EXCLUDES 1   *capital femoral epiphyseal fracture (pediatric) of femur (S79.01-)*
                Salter-Harris Type I physeal fracture of upper end of femur (S79.01-)

    √7ᵗʰ **S72.021**   **Displaced fracture of epiphysis (separation) (upper) of right femur**

    √7ᵗʰ **S72.022**   **Displaced fracture of epiphysis (separation) (upper) of left femur**

    √7ᵗʰ **S72.023**   **Displaced fracture of epiphysis (separation) (upper) of unspecified femur** ▽

    √7ᵗʰ **S72.024**   **Nondisplaced fracture of epiphysis (separation) (upper) of right femur**

    √7ᵗʰ **S72.025**   **Nondisplaced fracture of epiphysis (separation) (upper) of left femur**

    √7ᵗʰ **S72.026**   **Nondisplaced fracture of epiphysis (separation) (upper) of unspecified femur** ▽

√8ᵗʰ **S72.03**   **Midcervical fracture of femur**

    Transcervical fracture of femur NOS

    √7ᵗʰ **S72.031**   **Displaced midcervical fracture of right femur**

    √7ᵗʰ **S72.032**   **Displaced midcervical fracture of left femur**

    √7ᵗʰ **S72.033**   **Displaced midcervical fracture of unspecified femur** ▽

    √7ᵗʰ **S72.034**   **Nondisplaced midcervical fracture of right femur**

    √7ᵗʰ **S72.035**   **Nondisplaced midcervical fracture of left femur**

    √7ᵗʰ **S72.036**   **Nondisplaced midcervical fracture of unspecified femur** ▽

√6ᵗʰ **S72.04**   **Fracture of base of neck of femur**

    Cervicotrochanteric fracture of femur

    √7ᵗʰ **S72.041**   **Displaced fracture of base of neck of right femur**

    √7ᵗʰ **S72.042**   **Displaced fracture of base of neck of left femur**

    √7ᵗʰ **S72.043**   **Displaced fracture of base of neck of unspecified femur** ▽

    √7ᵗʰ **S72.044**   **Nondisplaced fracture of base of neck of right femur**

    √7ᵗʰ **S72.045**   **Nondisplaced fracture of base of neck of left femur**

    √7ᵗʰ **S72.046**   **Nondisplaced fracture of base of neck of unspecified femur** ▽

√6ᵗʰ **S72.05**   **Unspecified fracture of head of femur**

    Fracture of head of femur NOS

    √7ᵗʰ **S72.051**   **Unspecified fracture of head of right femur** ▽

    √7ᵗʰ **S72.052**   **Unspecified fracture of head of left femur** ▽

    √7ᵗʰ **S72.059**   **Unspecified fracture of head of unspecified femur** ▽

√6ᵗʰ **S72.06**   **Articular fracture of head of femur**

    √7ᵗʰ **S72.061**   **Displaced articular fracture of head of right femur**

    √7ᵗʰ **S72.062**   **Displaced articular fracture of head of left femur**

    √7ᵗʰ **S72.063**   **Displaced articular fracture of head of unspecified femur** ▽

    √7ᵗʰ **S72.064**   **Nondisplaced articular fracture of head of right femur**

    √7ᵗʰ **S72.065**   **Nondisplaced articular fracture of head of left femur**

    √7ᵗʰ **S72.066**   **Nondisplaced articular fracture of head of unspecified femur** ▽

☑ Additional Character Required   √x7ᵗʰ Placeholder Alert   Manifestation Dx   ▽ Unspecified Dx   ▶◀ Revised Text   ● New Code   ▲ Revised Code Title

√6ᵗʰ **S72.09** **Other fracture of** head and neck **of femur**

- √7ᵗʰ **S72.091** **Other fracture of head and neck of** right **femur**
- √7ᵗʰ **S72.092** **Other fracture of head and neck of** left **femur**
- √7ᵗʰ **S72.099** **Other fracture of head and neck of unspecified femur** ▽

√5ᵗʰ **S72.1** **Pertrochanteric fracture**

√6ᵗʰ **S72.10** **Unspecified trochanteric fracture of femur**

Fracture of trochanter NOS

- √7ᵗʰ **S72.101** **Unspecified trochanteric fracture of** right **femur** ▽
- √7ᵗʰ **S72.102** **Unspecified trochanteric fracture of** left **femur** ▽
- √7ᵗʰ **S72.109** **Unspecified trochanteric fracture of unspecified femur** ▽

√6ᵗʰ **S72.11** **Fracture of** greater trochanter **of femur**

- √7ᵗʰ **S72.111** **Displaced fracture of greater trochanter of** right **femur**
- √7ᵗʰ **S72.112** **Displaced fracture of greater trochanter of** left **femur**
- √7ᵗʰ **S72.113** **Displaced fracture of greater trochanter of unspecified femur** ▽
- √7ᵗʰ **S72.114** **Nondisplaced fracture of greater trochanter of** right **femur**
- √7ᵗʰ **S72.115** **Nondisplaced fracture of greater trochanter of** left **femur**
- √7ᵗʰ **S72.116** **Nondisplaced fracture of greater trochanter of unspecified femur** ▽

√6ᵗʰ **S72.12** **Fracture of** lesser trochanter **of femur**

- √7ᵗʰ **S72.121** **Displaced fracture of lesser trochanter of** right **femur**
- √7ᵗʰ **S72.122** **Displaced fracture of lesser trochanter of** left **femur**
- √7ᵗʰ **S72.123** **Displaced fracture of lesser trochanter of unspecified femur** ▽
- √7ᵗʰ **S72.124** **Nondisplaced fracture of lesser trochanter of** right **femur**
- √7ᵗʰ **S72.125** **Nondisplaced fracture of lesser trochanter of** left **femur**
- √7ᵗʰ **S72.126** **Nondisplaced fracture of lesser trochanter of unspecified femur** ▽

√6ᵗʰ **S72.13** **Apophyseal fracture of femur**

EXCLUDES 1 *chronic (nontraumatic) slipped upper femoral epiphysis (M93.0-)*

- √7ᵗʰ **S72.131** **Displaced apophyseal fracture of** right **femur**
- √7ᵗʰ **S72.132** **Displaced apophyseal fracture of** left **femur**
- √7ᵗʰ **S72.133** **Displaced apophyseal fracture of unspecified femur** ▽
- √7ᵗʰ **S72.134** **Nondisplaced apophyseal fracture of** right **femur**
- √7ᵗʰ **S72.135** **Nondisplaced apophyseal fracture of** left **femur**
- √7ᵗʰ **S72.136** **Nondisplaced apophyseal fracture of unspecified femur** ▽

√6ᵗʰ **S72.14** **Intertrochanteric fracture of femur**

- √7ᵗʰ **S72.141** **Displaced intertrochanteric fracture of** right **femur**
- √7ᵗʰ **S72.142** **Displaced intertrochanteric fracture of** left **femur**
- √7ᵗʰ **S72.143** **Displaced intertrochanteric fracture of unspecified femur** ▽
- √7ᵗʰ **S72.144** **Nondisplaced intertrochanteric fracture of** right **femur**
- √7ᵗʰ **S72.145** **Nondisplaced intertrochanteric fracture of** left **femur**
- √7ᵗʰ **S72.146** **Nondisplaced intertrochanteric fracture of unspecified femur** ▽

√5ᵗʰ **S72.2** **Subtrochanteric fracture of femur**

- √x7ᵗʰ **S72.21** **Displaced subtrochanteric fracture of** right **femur**
- √x7ᵗʰ **S72.22** **Displaced subtrochanteric fracture of** left **femur**
- √x7ᵗʰ **S72.23** **Displaced subtrochanteric fracture of unspecified femur** ▽
- √x7ᵗʰ **S72.24** **Nondisplaced subtrochanteric fracture of** right **femur**
- √x7ᵗʰ **S72.25** **Nondisplaced subtrochanteric fracture of** left **femur**
- √x7ᵗʰ **S72.26** **Nondisplaced subtrochanteric fracture of unspecified femur** ▽

√5ᵗʰ **S72.3** **Fracture of** shaft **of femur**

√6ᵗʰ **S72.30** **Unspecified fracture of shaft of femur**

- √7ᵗʰ **S72.301** **Unspecified fracture of shaft of** right **femur** ▽
- √7ᵗʰ **S72.302** **Unspecified fracture of shaft of** left **femur** ▽
- √7ᵗʰ **S72.309** **Unspecified fracture of shaft of unspecified femur** ▽

√6ᵗʰ **S72.32** **Transverse fracture of shaft of femur**

- √7ᵗʰ **S72.321** **Displaced transverse fracture of shaft of** right **femur**
- √7ᵗʰ **S72.322** **Displaced transverse fracture of shaft of** left **femur**
- √7ᵗʰ **S72.323** **Displaced transverse fracture of shaft of unspecified femur**
- √7ᵗʰ **S72.324** **Nondisplaced transverse fracture of shaft of** right **femur**
- √7ᵗʰ **S72.325** **Nondisplaced transverse fracture of shaft of** left **femur**
- √7ᵗʰ **S72.326** **Nondisplaced transverse fracture of shaft of unspecified femur**

√6ᵗʰ **S72.33** **Oblique fracture of shaft of femur**

- √7ᵗʰ **S72.331** **Displaced oblique fracture of shaft of** right **femur**
- √7ᵗʰ **S72.332** **Displaced oblique fracture of shaft of** left **femur**
- √7ᵗʰ **S72.333** **Displaced oblique fracture of shaft of unspecified femur** ▽
- √7ᵗʰ **S72.334** **Nondisplaced oblique fracture of shaft of** right **femur**
- √7ᵗʰ **S72.335** **Nondisplaced oblique fracture of shaft of** left **femur**
- √7ᵗʰ **S72.336** **Nondisplaced oblique fracture of shaft of unspecified femur** ▽

√6ᵗʰ **S72.34** **Spiral fracture of shaft of femur**

- √7ᵗʰ **S72.341** **Displaced spiral fracture of shaft of** right **femur**
- √7ᵗʰ **S72.342** **Displaced spiral fracture of shaft of** left **femur**
- √7ᵗʰ **S72.343** **Displaced spiral fracture of shaft of unspecified femur** ▽
- √7ᵗʰ **S72.344** **Nondisplaced spiral fracture of shaft of** right **femur**
- √7ᵗʰ **S72.345** **Nondisplaced spiral fracture of shaft of** left **femur**
- √7ᵗʰ **S72.346** **Nondisplaced spiral fracture of shaft of unspecified femur** ▽

√6ᵗʰ **S72.35** **Comminuted fracture of shaft of femur**

- √7ᵗʰ **S72.351** **Displaced comminuted fracture of shaft of** right **femur**
- √7ᵗʰ **S72.352** **Displaced comminuted fracture of shaft of** left **femur**
- √7ᵗʰ **S72.353** **Displaced comminuted fracture of shaft of unspecified femur** ▽
- √7ᵗʰ **S72.354** **Nondisplaced comminuted fracture of shaft of** right **femur**
- √7ᵗʰ **S72.355** **Nondisplaced comminuted fracture of shaft of** left **femur**
- √7ᵗʰ **S72.356** **Nondisplaced comminuted fracture of shaft of unspecified femur** ▽

√6ᵗʰ **S72.36** **Segmental fracture of shaft of femur**

- √7ᵗʰ **S72.361** **Displaced segmental fracture of shaft of** right **femur**
- √7ᵗʰ **S72.362** **Displaced segmental fracture of shaft of** left **femur**
- √7ᵗʰ **S72.363** **Displaced segmental fracture of shaft of unspecified femur** ▽
- √7ᵗʰ **S72.364** **Nondisplaced segmental fracture of shaft of** right **femur**
- √7ᵗʰ **S72.365** **Nondisplaced segmental fracture of shaft of** left **femur**
- √7ᵗʰ **S72.366** **Nondisplaced segmental fracture of shaft of unspecified femur** ▽

√6ᵗʰ **S72.39** **Other fracture of shaft of femur**

- √7ᵗʰ **S72.391** **Other fracture of shaft of** right **femur**
- √7ᵗʰ **S72.392** **Other fracture of shaft of** left **femur**
- √7ᵗʰ **S72.399** **Other fracture of shaft of unspecified femur** ▽

√5ᵗʰ **S72.4 Fracture of lower end of femur**
     Fracture of distal end of femur
     EXCLUDES 2 *fracture of shaft of femur (S72.3-)*
                  physeal fracture of lower end of femur (S79.1-)

√6ᵗʰ **S72.40 Unspecified fracture of lower end of femur**
   √7ᵗʰ **S72.401 Unspecified fracture of lower end of**   ▽
              right femur
   √7ᵗʰ **S72.402 Unspecified fracture of lower end**   ▽
              of left femur
   √7ᵗʰ **S72.409 Unspecified fracture of lower end**   ▽
              of unspecified femur

√6ᵗʰ **S72.41 Unspecified condyle fracture of lower end of femur**
         Condyle fracture of femur NOS
   √7ᵗʰ **S72.411 Displaced unspecified condyle**   ▽
              fracture of lower end of right
              femur
   √7ᵗʰ **S72.412 Displaced unspecified condyle**   ▽
              fracture of lower end of left femur
   √7ᵗʰ **S72.413 Displaced unspecified condyle**   ▽
              fracture of lower end of
              unspecified femur
   √7ᵗʰ **S72.414 Nondisplaced unspecified condyle**   ▽
              fracture of lower end of right
              femur
   √7ᵗʰ **S72.415 Nondisplaced unspecified condyle**   ▽
              fracture of lower end of left femur
   √7ᵗʰ **S72.416 Nondisplaced unspecified condyle**   ▽
              fracture of lower end of
              unspecified femur

√6ᵗʰ **S72.42 Fracture of lateral condyle of femur**
   √7ᵗʰ **S72.421 Displaced fracture of lateral condyle of**
              right femur
   √7ᵗʰ **S72.422 Displaced fracture of lateral condyle of**
              left femur
   √7ᵗʰ **S72.423 Displaced fracture of lateral**   ▽
              condyle of unspecified femur
   √7ᵗʰ **S72.424 Nondisplaced fracture of lateral condyle**
              of right femur
   √7ᵗʰ **S72.425 Nondisplaced fracture of lateral condyle**
              of left femur
   √7ᵗʰ **S72.426 Nondisplaced fracture of lateral**   ▽
              condyle of unspecified femur

√6ᵗʰ **S72.43 Fracture of medial condyle of femur**
   √7ᵗʰ **S72.431 Displaced fracture of medial condyle of**
              right femur
   √7ᵗʰ **S72.432 Displaced fracture of medial condyle of**
              left femur
   √7ᵗʰ **S72.433 Displaced fracture of medial**   ▽
              condyle of unspecified femur
   √7ᵗʰ **S72.434 Nondisplaced fracture of medial condyle**
              of right femur
   √7ᵗʰ **S72.435 Nondisplaced fracture of medial condyle**
              of left femur
   √7ᵗʰ **S72.436 Nondisplaced fracture of medial**   ▽
              condyle of unspecified femur

√6ᵗʰ **S72.44 Fracture of lower epiphysis (separation) of femur**
         EXCLUDES 1 *Salter-Harris Type I physeal fracture of lower*
                      end of femur (S79.11-)
   √7ᵗʰ **S72.441 Displaced fracture of lower epiphysis**
              (separation) of right femur
   √7ᵗʰ **S72.442 Displaced fracture of lower epiphysis**
              (separation) of left femur
   √7ᵗʰ **S72.443 Displaced fracture of lower**   ▽
              epiphysis (separation) of
              unspecified femur
   √7ᵗʰ **S72.444 Nondisplaced fracture of lower epiphysis**
              (separation) of right femur
   √7ᵗʰ **S72.445 Nondisplaced fracture of lower epiphysis**
              (separation) of left femur
   √7ᵗʰ **S72.446 Nondisplaced fracture of lower**   ▽
              epiphysis (separation) of
              unspecified femur

√6ᵗʰ **S72.45 Supracondylar fracture without intracondylar**
         extension of lower end of femur
         Supracondylar fracture of lower end of femur NOS
         EXCLUDES 1 *supracondylar fracture with intracondylar*
                      extension of lower end of femur
                      (S72.46-)
   √7ᵗʰ **S72.451 Displaced supracondylar fracture without**
              intracondylar extension of lower end of
              right femur

   √7ᵗʰ **S72.452 Displaced supracondylar fracture without**
              intracondylar extension of lower end of
              left femur
   √7ᵗʰ **S72.453 Displaced supracondylar fracture**   ▽
              without intracondylar extension
              of lower end of unspecified femur
   √7ᵗʰ **S72.454 Nondisplaced supracondylar fracture**
              without intracondylar extension of lower
              end of right femur
   √7ᵗʰ **S72.455 Nondisplaced supracondylar fracture**
              without intracondylar extension of lower
              end of left femur
   √7ᵗʰ **S72.456 Nondisplaced supracondylar**   ▽
              fracture without intracondylar
              extension of lower end of
              unspecified femur

√6ᵗʰ **S72.46 Supracondylar fracture with intracondylar**
         extension of lower end of femur
         EXCLUDES 1 *supracondylar fracture without*
                      intracondylar extension of lower end
                      of femur (S72.45-)
   √7ᵗʰ **S72.461 Displaced supracondylar fracture with**
              intracondylar extension of lower end of
              right femur
   √7ᵗʰ **S72.462 Displaced supracondylar fracture with**
              intracondylar extension of lower end of
              left femur
   √7ᵗʰ **S72.463 Displaced supracondylar fracture**   ▽
              with intracondylar extension of
              lower end of unspecified femur
   √7ᵗʰ **S72.464 Nondisplaced supracondylar fracture**
              with intracondylar extension of lower end
              of right femur
   √7ᵗʰ **S72.465 Nondisplaced supracondylar fracture**
              with intracondylar extension of lower end
              of left femur
   √7ᵗʰ **S72.466 Nondisplaced supracondylar**   ▽
              fracture with intracondylar
              extension of lower end of
              unspecified femur

√6ᵗʰ **S72.47 Torus fracture of lower end of femur**

         The appropriate 7th character is to be added to all
         codes in subcategory S72.47
         A   initial encounter for closed fracture
         D   subsequent encounter for fracture with routine
              healing
         G   subsequent encounter for fracture with delayed
              healing
         K   subsequent encounter for fracture with
              nonunion
         P   subsequent encounter for fracture with
              malunion
         S   sequela

   √7ᵗʰ **S72.471 Torus fracture of lower end of right femur**
   √7ᵗʰ **S72.472 Torus fracture of lower end of left femur**
   √7ᵗʰ **S72.479 Torus fracture of lower end of**   ▽
              unspecified femur

√6ᵗʰ **S72.49 Other fracture of lower end of femur**
   √7ᵗʰ **S72.491 Other fracture of lower end of right femur**
   √7ᵗʰ **S72.492 Other fracture of lower end of left femur**
   √7ᵗʰ **S72.499 Other fracture of lower end of**   ▽
              unspecified femur

√5ᵗʰ **S72.8 Other fracture of femur**
   √6ᵗʰ **S72.8X Other fracture of femur**
      √7ᵗʰ **S72.8X1 Other fracture of right femur**
      √7ᵗʰ **S72.8X2 Other fracture of left femur**
      √7ᵗʰ **S72.8X9 Other fracture of unspecified**   ▽
                 femur

√5ᵗʰ **S72.9 Unspecified fracture of femur**
     Fracture of thigh NOS
     Fracture of upper leg NOS
     EXCLUDES 1 *fracture of hip NOS (S72.00-, S72.01-)*
   √x7ᵗʰ **S72.90 Unspecified fracture of unspecified femur**   ▽
              AHA: 2012,4Q,93
   √x7ᵗʰ **S72.91 Unspecified fracture of right femur**   ▽
   √x7ᵗʰ **S72.92 Unspecified fracture of left femur**   ▽

☑ Additional Character Required   √x7ᵗʰ Placeholder Alert   Manifestation Dx   ▽Unspecified Dx   ►◄ Revised Text   ● New Code   ▲ Revised Code Title

✓4ᵗʰ **S73 Dislocation and sprain of joint and ligaments of hip**

INCLUDES avulsion of joint or ligament of hip
laceration of cartilage, joint or ligament of hip
sprain of cartilage, joint or ligament of hip
traumatic hemarthrosis of joint or ligament of hip
traumatic rupture of joint or ligament of hip
traumatic subluxation of joint or ligament of hip
traumatic tear of joint or ligament of hip

Code also any associated open wound

EXCLUDES 2 *strain of muscle, fascia and tendon of hip and thigh (S76.-)*

The appropriate 7th character is to be added to each code from category S73.
A   initial encounter
D   subsequent encounter
S   sequela

✓5ᵗʰ **S73.0 Subluxation and dislocation of hip**

EXCLUDES 2 *dislocation and subluxation of hip prosthesis (T84.020, T84.021)*

✓6ᵗʰ **S73.00 Unspecified subluxation and dislocation of hip**

Dislocation of hip NOS
Subluxation of hip NOS

✓7ᵗʰ **S73.001 Unspecified** subluxation of **right hip** ▽

✓7ᵗʰ **S73.002 Unspecified** subluxation of **left hip** ▽

✓7ᵗʰ **S73.003 Unspecified** subluxation of **unspecified hip** ▽

✓7ᵗʰ **S73.004 Unspecified** dislocation of **right hip** ▽

✓7ᵗʰ **S73.005 Unspecified** dislocation of **left hip** ▽

✓7ᵗʰ **S73.006 Unspecified** dislocation of **unspecified hip** ▽

✓6ᵗʰ **S73.01 Posterior subluxation and dislocation of hip**

✓7ᵗʰ **S73.011 Posterior** subluxation of **right hip**

✓7ᵗʰ **S73.012 Posterior** subluxation of **left hip**

✓7ᵗʰ **S73.013 Posterior** subluxation of **unspecified hip** ▽

✓7ᵗʰ **S73.014 Posterior** dislocation of **right hip**

✓7ᵗʰ **S73.015 Posterior** dislocation of **left hip**

✓7ᵗʰ **S73.016 Posterior** dislocation of **unspecified hip** ▽

✓6ᵗʰ **S73.02 Obturator subluxation and dislocation of hip**

✓7ᵗʰ **S73.021 Obturator** subluxation of **right hip**

✓7ᵗʰ **S73.022 Obturator** subluxation of **left hip**

✓7ᵗʰ **S73.023 Obturator** subluxation of **unspecified hip** ▽

✓7ᵗʰ **S73.024 Obturator** dislocation of **right hip**

✓7ᵗʰ **S73.025 Obturator** dislocation of **left hip**

✓7ᵗʰ **S73.026 Obturator** dislocation of **unspecified hip** ▽

✓6ᵗʰ **S73.03 Other anterior dislocation of hip**

✓7ᵗʰ **S73.031 Other anterior** subluxation of **right hip**

✓7ᵗʰ **S73.032 Other anterior** subluxation of **left hip**

✓7ᵗʰ **S73.033 Other anterior** subluxation of **unspecified hip** ▽

✓7ᵗʰ **S73.034 Other anterior** dislocation of **right hip**

✓7ᵗʰ **S73.035 Other anterior** dislocation of **left hip**

✓7ᵗʰ **S73.036 Other anterior** dislocation of **unspecified hip** ▽

✓6ᵗʰ **S73.04 Central dislocation of hip**

✓7ᵗʰ **S73.041 Central** subluxation of **right hip**

✓7ᵗʰ **S73.042 Central** subluxation of **left hip**

✓7ᵗʰ **S73.043 Central** subluxation of **unspecified hip** ▽

✓7ᵗʰ **S73.044 Central** dislocation of **right hip**

✓7ᵗʰ **S73.045 Central** dislocation of **left hip**

✓7ᵗʰ **S73.046 Central** dislocation of **unspecified hip** ▽

✓5ᵗʰ **S73.1 Sprain of hip**

AHA: 2014,4Q,25

✓6ᵗʰ **S73.10 Unspecified sprain of hip**

✓7ᵗʰ **S73.101 Unspecified sprain of right hip** ▽

✓7ᵗʰ **S73.102 Unspecified sprain of left hip** ▽

✓7ᵗʰ **S73.109 Unspecified sprain of unspecified hip** ▽

✓6ᵗʰ **S73.11 Iliofemoral ligament sprain of hip**

✓7ᵗʰ **S73.111 Iliofemoral ligament sprain of right hip**

✓7ᵗʰ **S73.112 Iliofemoral ligament sprain of left hip**

✓7ᵗʰ **S73.119 Iliofemoral ligament sprain of unspecified hip** ▽

✓6ᵗʰ **S73.12 Ischiocapsular (ligament) sprain of hip**

✓7ᵗʰ **S73.121 Ischiocapsular ligament sprain of right hip**

✓7ᵗʰ **S73.122 Ischiocapsular ligament sprain of left hip**

✓7ᵗʰ **S73.129 Ischiocapsular ligament sprain of unspecified hip** ▽

✓6ᵗʰ **S73.19 Other sprain of hip**

✓7ᵗʰ **S73.191 Other sprain of right hip**

✓7ᵗʰ **S73.192 Other sprain of left hip**

✓7ᵗʰ **S73.199 Other sprain of unspecified hip** ▽

✓4ᵗʰ **S74 Injury of nerves at hip and thigh level**

Code also any associated open wound (S71.-)

EXCLUDES 2 *injury of nerves at ankle and foot level (S94.-)*
injury of nerves at lower leg level (S84.-)

The appropriate 7th character is to be added to each code from category S74.
A   initial encounter
D   subsequent encounter
S   sequela

✓5ᵗʰ **S74.0 Injury of sciatic nerve at hip and thigh level**

✓x7ᵗʰ **S74.00 Injury of sciatic nerve at hip and thigh level, unspecified leg** ▽

✓x7ᵗʰ **S74.01 Injury of sciatic nerve at hip and thigh level, right leg** ▽

✓x7ᵗʰ **S74.02 Injury of sciatic nerve at hip and thigh level, left leg**

✓5ᵗʰ **S74.1 Injury of femoral nerve at hip and thigh level**

✓x7ᵗʰ **S74.10 Injury of femoral nerve at hip and thigh level, unspecified leg** ▽

✓x7ᵗʰ **S74.11 Injury of femoral nerve at hip and thigh level, right leg**

✓x7ᵗʰ **S74.12 Injury of femoral nerve at hip and thigh level, left leg**

✓5ᵗʰ **S74.2 Injury of cutaneous sensory nerve at hip and thigh level**

✓x7ᵗʰ **S74.20 Injury of cutaneous sensory nerve at hip and thigh level, unspecified leg** ▽

✓x7ᵗʰ **S74.21 Injury of cutaneous sensory nerve at hip and high level, right leg**

✓x7ᵗʰ **S74.22 Injury of cutaneous sensory nerve at hip and thigh level, left leg**

✓5ᵗʰ **S74.8 Injury of other nerves at hip and thigh level**

✓6ᵗʰ **S74.8X Injury of other nerves at hip and thigh level**

✓7ᵗʰ **S74.8X1 Injury of other nerves at hip and thigh level, right leg**

✓7ᵗʰ **S74.8X2 Injury of other nerves at hip and thigh level, left leg**

✓7ᵗʰ **S74.8X9 Injury of other nerves at hip and thigh level, unspecified leg** ▽

✓5ᵗʰ **S74.9 Injury of unspecified nerve at hip and thigh level**

✓x7ᵗʰ **S74.90 Injury of unspecified nerve at hip and thigh level, unspecified leg** ▽

✓x7ᵗʰ **S74.91 Injury of unspecified nerve at hip and thigh level, right leg** ▽

✓x7ᵗʰ **S74.92 Injury of unspecified nerve at hip and thigh level, left leg**

✓4ᵗʰ **S75 Injury of blood vessels at hip and thigh level**

Code also any associated open wound (S71.-)

EXCLUDES 2 *injury of blood vessels at lower leg level (S85.-)*
injury of popliteal artery (S85.0)

The appropriate 7th character is to be added to each code from category S75.
A   initial encounter
D   subsequent encounter
S   sequela

✓5ᵗʰ **S75.0 Injury of femoral artery**

✓6ᵗʰ **S75.00 Unspecified injury of femoral artery**

✓7ᵗʰ **S75.001 Unspecified injury of femoral artery, right leg** ▽

✓7ᵗʰ **S75.002 Unspecified injury of femoral artery, left leg** ▽

EXCLUDES 1 Not coded here   EXCLUDES 2 Not included here   N Newborn Age : 0   P Pediatric Age : 0-17   M Maternity Age : 12-55   A Adult Age : 15-124

√7ᵗʰ **S75.009** **Unspecified injury of femoral** ▽
artery, unspecified leg

√6ᵗʰ **S75.01** **Minor laceration of femoral artery**

Incomplete transection of femoral artery
Laceration of femoral artery NOS
Superficial laceration of femoral artery

√7ᵗʰ **S75.011** **Minor laceration of femoral artery, right**
leg

√7ᵗʰ **S75.012** **Minor laceration of femoral artery, left**
leg

√7ᵗʰ **S75.019** **Minor laceration of femoral artery,** ▽
unspecified leg

√6ᵗʰ **S75.02** **Major laceration of femoral artery**

Complete transection of femoral artery
Traumatic rupture of femoral artery

√7ᵗʰ **S75.021** **Major laceration of femoral artery, right**
leg

√7ᵗʰ **S75.022** **Major laceration of femoral artery, left**
leg

√7ᵗʰ **S75.029** **Major laceration of femoral artery,** ▽
unspecified leg

√6ᵗʰ **S75.09** **Other specified injury of femoral artery**

√7ᵗʰ **S75.091** **Other specified injury of femoral artery,**
right leg

√7ᵗʰ **S75.092** **Other specified injury of femoral artery,**
left leg

√7ᵗʰ **S75.099** **Other specified injury of femoral** ▽
artery, unspecified leg

√5ᵗʰ **S75.1** **Injury of femoral vein at hip and thigh level**

√6ᵗʰ **S75.10** **Unspecified injury of femoral vein at hip and thigh**
level

√7ᵗʰ **S75.101** **Unspecified injury of femoral vein** ▽
at hip and thigh level, right leg

√7ᵗʰ **S75.102** **Unspecified injury of femoral vein** ▽
at hip and thigh level, left leg

√7ᵗʰ **S75.109** **Unspecified injury of femoral vein** ▽
at hip and thigh level, unspecified
leg

√6ᵗʰ **S75.11** **Minor laceration of femoral vein at hip and thigh**
level

Incomplete transection of femoral vein at hip and
thigh level
Laceration of femoral vein at hip and thigh level NOS
Superficial laceration of femoral vein at hip and thigh
level

√7ᵗʰ **S75.111** **Minor laceration of femoral vein at hip**
and thigh level, right leg

√7ᵗʰ **S75.112** **Minor laceration of femoral vein at hip**
and thigh level, left leg

√7ᵗʰ **S75.119** **Minor laceration of femoral vein** ▽
at hip and thigh level, unspecified
leg

√6ᵗʰ **S75.12** **Major laceration of femoral vein at hip and thigh**
level

Complete transection of femoral vein at hip and thigh
level
Traumatic rupture of femoral vein at hip and thigh
level

√7ᵗʰ **S75.121** **Major laceration of femoral vein at hip**
and thigh level, right leg

√7ᵗʰ **S75.122** **Major laceration of femoral vein at hip**
and thigh level, left leg

√7ᵗʰ **S75.129** **Major laceration of femoral vein** ▽
at hip and thigh level, unspecified
leg

√6ᵗʰ **S75.19** **Other specified injury of femoral vein at hip and**
thigh level

√7ᵗʰ **S75.191** **Other specified injury of femoral vein at**
hip and thigh level, right leg

√7ᵗʰ **S75.192** **Other specified injury of femoral vein at**
hip and thigh level, left leg

√7ᵗʰ **S75.199** **Other specified injury of femoral** ▽
vein at hip and thigh level,
unspecified leg

√5ᵗʰ **S75.2** **Injury of greater saphenous vein at hip and thigh level**

EXCLUDES 1 *greater saphenous vein NOS (S85.3)*

√6ᵗʰ **S75.20** **Unspecified injury of greater saphenous vein at hip**
and thigh level

√7ᵗʰ **S75.201** **Unspecified injury of greater** ▽
saphenous vein at hip and thigh
level, right leg

√7ᵗʰ **S75.202** **Unspecified injury of greater** ▽
saphenous vein at hip and thigh
level, left leg

√7ᵗʰ **S75.209** **Unspecified injury of greater** ▽
saphenous vein at hip and thigh
level, unspecified leg

√6ᵗʰ **S75.21** **Minor laceration of greater saphenous vein at hip**
and thigh level

Incomplete transection of greater saphenous vein at
hip and thigh level
Laceration of greater saphenous vein at hip and thigh
level NOS
Superficial laceration of greater saphenous vein at
hip and thigh level

√7ᵗʰ **S75.211** **Minor laceration of greater saphenous**
vein at hip and thigh level, right leg

√7ᵗʰ **S75.212** **Minor laceration of greater saphenous**
vein at hip and thigh level, left leg

√7ᵗʰ **S75.219** **Minor laceration of greater** ▽
saphenous vein at hip and thigh
level, unspecified leg

√6ᵗʰ **S75.22** **Major laceration of greater saphenous vein at hip**
and thigh level

Complete transection of greater saphenous vein at
hip and thigh level
Traumatic rupture of greater saphenous vein at hip
and thigh level

√7ᵗʰ **S75.221** **Major laceration of greater saphenous**
vein at hip and thigh level, right leg

√7ᵗʰ **S75.222** **Major laceration of greater saphenous**
vein at hip and thigh level, left leg

√7ᵗʰ **S75.229** **Major laceration of greater** ▽
saphenous vein at hip and thigh
level, unspecified leg

√6ᵗʰ **S75.29** **Other specified injury of greater saphenous vein at**
hip and thigh level

√7ᵗʰ **S75.291** **Other specified injury of greater**
saphenous vein at hip and thigh level,
right leg

√7ᵗʰ **S75.292** **Other specified injury of greater**
saphenous vein at hip and thigh level,
left leg

√7ᵗʰ **S75.299** **Other specified injury of greater** ▽
saphenous vein at hip and thigh
level, unspecified leg

√5ᵗʰ **S75.8** **Injury of other blood vessels at hip and thigh level**

√6ᵗʰ **S75.80** **Unspecified injury of other blood vessels at hip and**
thigh level

√7ᵗʰ **S75.801** **Unspecified injury of other blood** ▽
vessels at hip and thigh level, right
leg

√7ᵗʰ **S75.802** **Unspecified injury of other blood** ▽
vessels at hip and thigh level, left
leg

√7ᵗʰ **S75.809** **Unspecified injury of other blood** ▽
vessels at hip and thigh level,
unspecified leg

√6ᵗʰ **S75.81** **Laceration of other blood vessels at hip and thigh**
level

√7ᵗʰ **S75.811** **Laceration of other blood vessels at hip**
and thigh level, right leg

√7ᵗʰ **S75.812** **Laceration of other blood vessels at hip**
and thigh level, left leg

√7ᵗʰ **S75.819** **Laceration of other blood vessels** ▽
at hip and thigh level, unspecified
leg

√6ᵗʰ **S75.89** **Other specified injury of other blood vessels at hip**
and thigh level

√7ᵗʰ **S75.891** **Other specified injury of other blood**
vessels at hip and thigh level, right leg

√7ᵗʰ **S75.892** **Other specified injury of other blood**
vessels at hip and thigh level, left leg

√7ᵗʰ **S75.899** **Other specified injury of other** ▽
blood vessels at hip and thigh
level, unspecified leg

√5ᵗʰ **S75.9** **Injury of unspecified blood vessel at hip and thigh level**

√6ᵗʰ **S75.90** **Unspecified injury of unspecified blood vessel at**
hip and thigh level

√7ᵗʰ **S75.901** **Unspecified injury of unspecified** ▽
blood vessel at hip and thigh level,
right leg

✓7th **S75.902** Unspecified injury of unspecified blood vessel at hip and thigh level, **left** leg ▽

✓7th **S75.909** Unspecified injury of unspecified blood vessel at hip and thigh level, unspecified leg

✓6th **S75.91** Laceration of unspecified blood vessel at hip and thigh level

    ✓7th **S75.911** Laceration of unspecified blood vessel at hip and thigh level, **right** leg ▽

    ✓7th **S75.912** Laceration of unspecified blood vessel at hip and thigh level, **left** leg ▽

    ✓7th **S75.919** Laceration of unspecified blood vessel at hip and thigh level, unspecified leg ▽

✓6th **S75.99** Other specified injury of unspecified blood vessel at hip and thigh level

    ✓7th **S75.991** Other specified injury of unspecified blood vessel at hip and thigh level, **right** leg ▽

    ✓7th **S75.992** Other specified injury of unspecified blood vessel at hip and thigh level, **left** leg ▽

    ✓7th **S75.999** Other specified injury of unspecified blood vessel at hip and thigh level, unspecified leg ▽

✓4th **S76** **Injury of muscle, fascia and tendon at hip and thigh level**

Code also any associated open wound (S71.-)

EXCLUDES 2   *injury of muscle, fascia and tendon at lower leg level (S86)*
           sprain of joint and ligament of hip (S73.1)

TIP: Refer to the Muscle/Tendon table at the beginning of this chapter

The appropriate 7th character is to be added to each code from category S76.
A   initial encounter
D   subsequent encounter
S   sequela

✓5th **S76.0** **Injury of muscle, fascia and tendon of hip**

  ✓6th **S76.00** Unspecified injury of muscle, fascia and tendon of hip

    ✓7th **S76.001** Unspecified injury of muscle, fascia and tendon of **right** hip ▽

    ✓7th **S76.002** Unspecified injury of muscle, fascia and tendon of **left** hip ▽

    ✓7th **S76.009** Unspecified injury of muscle, fascia and tendon of unspecified hip ▽

  ✓6th **S76.01** Strain of muscle, fascia and tendon of hip

    ✓7th **S76.011** Strain of muscle, fascia and tendon of **right** hip

    ✓7th **S76.012** Strain of muscle, fascia and tendon of **left** hip

    ✓7th **S76.019** Strain of muscle, fascia and tendon of unspecified hip ▽

  ✓6th **S76.02** Laceration of muscle, fascia and tendon of hip

    ✓7th **S76.021** Laceration of muscle, fascia and tendon of **right** hip

    ✓7th **S76.022** Laceration of muscle, fascia and tendon of **left** hip

    ✓7th **S76.029** Laceration of muscle, fascia and tendon of unspecified hip ▽

  ✓6th **S76.09** Other specified injury of muscle, fascia and tendon of hip

    ✓7th **S76.091** Other specified injury of muscle, fascia and tendon of **right** hip

    ✓7th **S76.092** Other specified injury of muscle, fascia and tendon of **left** hip

    ✓7th **S76.099** Other specified injury of muscle, fascia and tendon of unspecified hip ▽

✓5th **S76.1** **Injury of quadriceps muscle, fascia and tendon**

Injury of patellar ligament (tendon)

  ✓6th **S76.10** Unspecified injury of quadriceps muscle, fascia and tendon

    ✓7th **S76.101** Unspecified injury of **right** quadriceps muscle, fascia and tendon ▽

    ✓7th **S76.102** Unspecified injury of **left** quadriceps muscle, fascia and tendon ▽

    ✓7th **S76.109** Unspecified injury of unspecified quadriceps muscle, fascia and tendon ▽

  ✓6th **S76.11** Strain of quadriceps muscle, fascia and tendon

    ✓7th **S76.111** Strain of **right** quadriceps muscle, fascia and tendon

    ✓7th **S76.112** Strain of **left** quadriceps muscle, fascia and tendon

    ✓7th **S76.119** Strain of unspecified quadriceps muscle, fascia and tendon ▽

  ✓6th **S76.12** Laceration of quadriceps muscle, fascia and tendon

    ✓7th **S76.121** Laceration of **right** quadriceps muscle, fascia and tendon

    ✓7th **S76.122** Laceration of **left** quadriceps muscle, fascia and tendon

    ✓7th **S76.129** Laceration of unspecified quadriceps muscle, fascia and tendon ▽

  ✓6th **S76.19** Other specified injury of quadriceps muscle, fascia and tendon

    ✓7th **S76.191** Other specified injury of **right** quadriceps muscle, fascia and tendon

    ✓7th **S76.192** Other specified injury of **left** quadriceps muscle, fascia and tendon

    ✓7th **S76.199** Other specified injury of unspecified quadriceps muscle, fascia and tendon ▽

✓5th **S76.2** **Injury of adductor muscle, fascia and tendon of thigh**

  ✓6th **S76.20** Unspecified injury of adductor muscle, fascia and tendon of thigh

    ✓7th **S76.201** Unspecified injury of adductor muscle, fascia and tendon of **right** thigh ▽

    ✓7th **S76.202** Unspecified injury of adductor muscle, fascia and tendon of **left** thigh ▽

    ✓7th **S76.209** Unspecified injury of adductor muscle, fascia and tendon of unspecified thigh ▽

  ✓6th **S76.21** Strain of adductor muscle, fascia and tendon of thigh

    ✓7th **S76.211** Strain of adductor muscle, fascia and tendon of **right** thigh

    ✓7th **S76.212** Strain of adductor muscle, fascia and tendon of **left** thigh

    ✓7th **S76.219** Strain of adductor muscle, fascia and tendon of unspecified thigh ▽

  ✓6th **S76.22** Laceration of adductor muscle, fascia and tendon of thigh

    ✓7th **S76.221** Laceration of adductor muscle, fascia and tendon of **right** thigh

    ✓7th **S76.222** Laceration of adductor muscle, fascia and tendon of **left** thigh

    ✓7th **S76.229** Laceration of adductor muscle, fascia and tendon of unspecified thigh ▽

  ✓6th **S76.29** Other injury of adductor muscle, fascia and tendon of thigh

    ✓7th **S76.291** Other injury of adductor muscle, fascia and tendon of **right** thigh

    ✓7th **S76.292** Other injury of adductor muscle, fascia and tendon of **left** thigh

    ✓7th **S76.299** Other injury of adductor muscle, fascia and tendon of unspecified thigh ▽

✓5th **S76.3** **Injury of muscle, fascia and tendon of the posterior muscle group at thigh level**

  ✓6th **S76.30** Unspecified injury of muscle, fascia and tendon of the posterior muscle group at thigh level

    ✓7th **S76.301** Unspecified injury of muscle, fascia and tendon of the posterior muscle group at thigh level, **right** thigh ▽

    ✓7th **S76.302** Unspecified injury of muscle, fascia and tendon of the posterior muscle group at thigh level, **left** thigh ▽

    ✓7th **S76.309** Unspecified injury of muscle, fascia and tendon of the posterior muscle group at thigh level, unspecified thigh ▽

  ✓6th **S76.31** Strain of muscle, fascia and tendon of the posterior muscle group at thigh level

    ✓7th **S76.311** Strain of muscle, fascia and tendon of the posterior muscle group at thigh level, **right** thigh

EXCLUDES 1 Not coded here   *EXCLUDES 2* Not included here   N Newborn Age : 0   P Pediatric Age : 0-17   M Maternity Age : 12-55   A Adult Age : 15-124

980   ICD-10-CM 2017

☑7ᵗʰ **S76.312** Strain of muscle, fascia and tendon of the posterior muscle group at thigh level, left thigh

☑7ᵗʰ **S76.319** Strain of muscle, fascia and tendon of the posterior muscle group at thigh level, unspecified thigh ▽

☑6ᵗʰ **S76.32** **Laceration** of muscle, fascia and tendon of the posterior muscle group at thigh level

☑7ᵗʰ **S76.321** Laceration of muscle, fascia and tendon of the posterior muscle group at thigh level, right thigh

☑7ᵗʰ **S76.322** Laceration of muscle, fascia and tendon of the posterior muscle group at thigh level, left thigh

☑7ᵗʰ **S76.329** Laceration of muscle, fascia and tendon of the posterior muscle group at thigh level, unspecified thigh ▽

☑6ᵗʰ **S76.39** Other specified injury of muscle, fascia and tendon of the posterior muscle group at thigh level

☑7ᵗʰ **S76.391** Other specified injury of muscle, fascia and tendon of the posterior muscle group at thigh level, right thigh

☑7ᵗʰ **S76.392** Other specified injury of muscle, fascia and tendon of the posterior muscle group at thigh level, left thigh

☑7ᵗʰ **S76.399** Other specified injury of muscle, fascia and tendon of the posterior muscle group at thigh level, unspecified thigh ▽

☑5ᵗʰ **S76.8** Injury of other specified muscles, fascia and tendons at thigh level

☑6ᵗʰ **S76.80** Unspecified injury of other specified muscles, fascia and tendons at thigh level

☑7ᵗʰ **S76.801** Unspecified injury of other specified muscles, fascia and tendons at thigh level, right thigh ▽

☑7ᵗʰ **S76.802** Unspecified injury of other specified muscles, fascia and tendons at thigh level, left thigh ▽

☑7ᵗʰ **S76.809** Unspecified injury of other specified muscles, fascia and tendons at thigh level, unspecified thigh ▽

☑6ᵗʰ **S76.81** Strain of other specified muscles, fascia and tendons at thigh level

☑7ᵗʰ **S76.811** Strain of other specified muscles, fascia and tendons at thigh level, right thigh

☑7ᵗʰ **S76.812** Strain of other specified muscles, fascia and tendons at thigh level, left thigh

☑7ᵗʰ **S76.819** Strain of other specified muscles, fascia and tendons at thigh level, unspecified thigh ▽

☑6ᵗʰ **S76.82** **Laceration** of other specified muscles, fascia and tendons at thigh level

☑7ᵗʰ **S76.821** Laceration of other specified muscles, fascia and tendons at thigh level, right thigh

☑7ᵗʰ **S76.822** Laceration of other specified muscles, fascia and tendons at thigh level, left thigh

☑7ᵗʰ **S76.829** Laceration of other specified muscles, fascia and tendons at thigh level, unspecified thigh ▽

☑6ᵗʰ **S76.89** Other injury of other specified muscles, fascia and tendons at thigh level

☑7ᵗʰ **S76.891** Other injury of other specified muscles, fascia and tendons at thigh level, right thigh

☑7ᵗʰ **S76.892** Other injury of other specified muscles, fascia and tendons at thigh level, left thigh

☑7ᵗʰ **S76.899** Other injury of other specified muscles, fascia and tendons at thigh level, unspecified thigh ▽

☑5ᵗʰ **S76.9** Injury of unspecified muscles, fascia and tendons at thigh level

☑6ᵗʰ **S76.90** Unspecified injury of unspecified muscles, fascia and tendons at thigh level

☑7ᵗʰ **S76.901** Unspecified injury of unspecified muscles, fascia and tendons at thigh level, right thigh ▽

☑7ᵗʰ **S76.902** Unspecified injury of unspecified muscles, fascia and tendons at thigh level, left thigh ▽

☑7ᵗʰ **S76.909** Unspecified injury of unspecified muscles, fascia and tendons at thigh level, unspecified thigh ▽

☑6ᵗʰ **S76.91** **Strain** of unspecified muscles, fascia and tendons at thigh level

☑7ᵗʰ **S76.911** Strain of unspecified muscles, fascia and tendons at thigh level, right thigh ▽

☑7ᵗʰ **S76.912** Strain of unspecified muscles, fascia and tendons at thigh level, left thigh ▽

☑7ᵗʰ **S76.919** Strain of unspecified muscles, fascia and tendons at thigh level, unspecified thigh ▽

☑6ᵗʰ **S76.92** **Laceration** of unspecified muscles, fascia and tendons at thigh level

☑7ᵗʰ **S76.921** Laceration of unspecified muscles, fascia and tendons at thigh level, right thigh ▽

☑7ᵗʰ **S76.922** Laceration of unspecified muscles, fascia and tendons at thigh level, left thigh ▽

☑7ᵗʰ **S76.929** Laceration of unspecified muscles, fascia and tendons at thigh level, unspecified thigh ▽

☑6ᵗʰ **S76.99** Other specified injury of unspecified muscles, fascia and tendons at thigh level

☑7ᵗʰ **S76.991** Other specified injury of unspecified muscles, fascia and tendons at thigh level, right thigh ▽

☑7ᵗʰ **S76.992** Other specified injury of unspecified muscles, fascia and tendons at thigh level, left thigh ▽

☑7ᵗʰ **S76.999** Other specified injury of unspecified muscles, fascia and tendons at thigh level, unspecified thigh ▽

☑4ᵗʰ **S77** **Crushing injury of hip and thigh**

Use additional code(s) for all associated injuries

EXCLUDES 2 crushing injury of ankle and foot (S97.-)
crushing injury of lower leg (S87.-)

The appropriate 7th character is to be added to each code from category S77.
A initial encounter
D subsequent encounter
S sequela

☑5ᵗʰ **S77.0** **Crushing injury of hip**

☑x7ᵗʰ **S77.00** Crushing injury of unspecified hip ▽

☑x7ᵗʰ **S77.01** Crushing injury of right hip

☑x7ᵗʰ **S77.02** Crushing injury of left hip

☑5ᵗʰ **S77.1** **Crushing injury of thigh**

☑x7ᵗʰ **S77.10** Crushing injury of unspecified thigh ▽

☑x7ᵗʰ **S77.11** Crushing injury of right thigh

☑x7ᵗʰ **S77.12** Crushing injury of left thigh

☑5ᵗʰ **S77.2** **Crushing injury of hip with thigh**

☑x7ᵗʰ **S77.20** Crushing injury of unspecified hip with thigh ▽

☑x7ᵗʰ **S77.21** Crushing injury of right hip with thigh

☑x7ᵗʰ **S77.22** Crushing injury of left hip with thigh

☑4ᵗʰ **S78** **Traumatic amputation of hip and thigh**

An amputation not identified as partial or complete should be coded to complete

EXCLUDES 1 traumatic amputation of knee (S88.0-)

The appropriate 7th character is to be added to each code from category S78.
A initial encounter
D subsequent encounter
S sequela

☑6ᵗʰ **S78.0** **Traumatic amputation at hip joint**

☑6ᵗʰ **S78.01** **Complete** traumatic amputation at hip joint

☑7ᵗʰ **S78.011** Complete traumatic amputation at right hip joint

☑7ᵗʰ **S78.012** Complete traumatic amputation at left hip joint

☑ Additional Character Required ☑x7ᵗʰ Placeholder Alert Manifestation Dx ▽Unspecified Dx ▶◀ Revised Text ● New Code ▲ Revised Code Title

ICD-10-CM 2017 **981**

- ✓7ᵗʰ **S78.019** Complete traumatic amputation at unspecified hip joint ▽
- ✓6ᵗʰ **S78.02** **Partial** traumatic amputation at hip joint
  - ✓7ᵗʰ **S78.021** Partial traumatic amputation at **right** hip joint
  - ✓7ᵗʰ **S78.022** Partial traumatic amputation at **left** hip joint
  - ✓7ᵗʰ **S78.029** Partial traumatic amputation at unspecified hip joint ▽
- ✓5ᵗʰ **S78.1** Traumatic amputation at level between hip and knee
  - EXCLUDES 1 *traumatic amputation of knee (S88.0-)*
  - ✓6ᵗʰ **S78.11** **Complete** traumatic amputation at level between hip and knee
    - ✓7ᵗʰ **S78.111** Complete traumatic amputation at level between **right** hip and knee
    - ✓7ᵗʰ **S78.112** Complete traumatic amputation at level between **left** hip and knee
    - ✓7ᵗʰ **S78.119** Complete traumatic amputation at level between unspecified hip and knee ▽
  - ✓6ᵗʰ **S78.12** **Partial** traumatic amputation at level between hip and knee
    - ✓7ᵗʰ **S78.121** Partial traumatic amputation at level between **right** hip and knee
    - ✓7ᵗʰ **S78.122** Partial traumatic amputation at level between **left** hip and knee
    - ✓7ᵗʰ **S78.129** Partial traumatic amputation at level between unspecified hip and knee ▽
- ✓5ᵗʰ **S78.9** Traumatic amputation of hip and thigh, level unspecified
  - ✓6ᵗʰ **S78.91** **Complete** traumatic amputation of hip and thigh, level unspecified
    - ✓7ᵗʰ **S78.911** Complete traumatic amputation of **right** hip and thigh, level unspecified ▽
    - ✓7ᵗʰ **S78.912** Complete traumatic amputation of **left** hip and thigh, level unspecified ▽
    - ✓7ᵗʰ **S78.919** Complete traumatic amputation of unspecified hip and thigh, level unspecified ▽
  - ✓6ᵗʰ **S78.92** **Partial** traumatic amputation of hip and thigh, level unspecified
    - ✓7ᵗʰ **S78.921** Partial traumatic amputation of **right** hip and thigh, level unspecified ▽
    - ✓7ᵗʰ **S78.922** Partial traumatic amputation of **left** hip and thigh, level unspecified ▽
    - ✓7ᵗʰ **S78.929** Partial traumatic amputation of unspecified hip and thigh, level unspecified ▽

✓4ᵗʰ **S79** **Other and unspecified injuries of hip and thigh**

> **NOTE** A fracture not indicated as open or closed should be coded to closed

AHA: 2015,3Q,37-39

> The appropriate 7th character is to be added to each code from subcategories S79.0 and S79.1.
> A   initial encounter for closed fracture
> D   subsequent encounter for fracture with routine healing
> G   subsequent encounter for fracture with delayed healing
> K   subsequent encounter for fracture with nonunion
> P   subsequent encounter for fracture with malunion
> S   sequela

- ✓5ᵗʰ **S79.0** **Physeal** fracture of upper end of femur
  - EXCLUDES 1 *apophyseal fracture of upper end of femur (S72.13-)*
  - *nontraumatic slipped upper femoral epiphysis (M93.0-)*
  - ✓6ᵗʰ **S79.00** Unspecified physeal fracture of upper end of femur
    - ✓7ᵗʰ **S79.001** Unspecified physeal fracture of upper end of **right** femur ▽
    - ✓7ᵗʰ **S79.002** Unspecified physeal fracture of upper end of **left** femur ▽
    - ✓7ᵗʰ **S79.009** Unspecified physeal fracture of upper end of unspecified femur ▽
  - ✓6ᵗʰ **S79.01** **Salter-Harris Type I** physeal fracture of upper end of femur
    - Acute on chronic slipped capital femoral epiphysis (traumatic)
    - Acute slipped capital femoral epiphysis (traumatic)
    - Capital femoral epiphyseal fracture
    - EXCLUDES 1 *chronic slipped upper femoral epiphysis (nontraumatic) (M93.02-)*
    - ✓7ᵗʰ **S79.011** Salter-Harris Type I physeal fracture of upper end of **right** femur
    - ✓7ᵗʰ **S79.012** Salter-Harris Type I physeal fracture of upper end of **left** femur
    - ✓7ᵗʰ **S79.019** Salter-Harris Type I physeal fracture of upper end of unspecified femur ▽
  - ✓6ᵗʰ **S79.09** Other physeal fracture of upper end of femur
    - ✓7ᵗʰ **S79.091** Other physeal fracture of upper end of **right** femur
    - ✓7ᵗʰ **S79.092** Other physeal fracture of upper end of **left** femur
    - ✓7ᵗʰ **S79.099** Other physeal fracture of upper end of unspecified femur ▽
- ✓5ᵗʰ **S79.1** **Physeal** fracture of lower end of femur
  - ✓6ᵗʰ **S79.10** Unspecified physeal fracture of lower end of femur
    - ✓7ᵗʰ **S79.101** Unspecified physeal fracture of lower end of **right** femur ▽
    - ✓7ᵗʰ **S79.102** Unspecified physeal fracture of lower end of **left** femur ▽
    - ✓7ᵗʰ **S79.109** Unspecified physeal fracture of lower end of unspecified femur ▽
  - ✓6ᵗʰ **S79.11** **Salter-Harris Type I** physeal fracture of lower end of femur
    - ✓7ᵗʰ **S79.111** Salter-Harris Type I physeal fracture of lower end of **right** femur
    - ✓7ᵗʰ **S79.112** Salter-Harris Type I physeal fracture of lower end of **left** femur
    - ✓7ᵗʰ **S79.119** Salter-Harris Type I physeal fracture of lower end of unspecified femur ▽
  - ✓6ᵗʰ **S79.12** **Salter-Harris Type II** physeal fracture of lower end of femur
    - ✓7ᵗʰ **S79.121** Salter-Harris Type II physeal fracture of lower end of **right** femur
    - ✓7ᵗʰ **S79.122** Salter-Harris Type II physeal fracture of lower end of **left** femur
    - ✓7ᵗʰ **S79.129** Salter-Harris Type II physeal fracture of lower end of unspecified femur ▽
  - ✓6ᵗʰ **S79.13** **Salter-Harris Type III** physeal fracture of lower end of femur
    - ✓7ᵗʰ **S79.131** Salter-Harris Type III physeal fracture of lower end of **right** femur
    - ✓7ᵗʰ **S79.132** Salter-Harris Type III physeal fracture of lower end of **left** femur
    - ✓7ᵗʰ **S79.139** Salter-Harris Type III physeal fracture of lower end of unspecified femur ▽
  - ✓6ᵗʰ **S79.14** **Salter-Harris Type IV** physeal fracture of lower end of femur
    - ✓7ᵗʰ **S79.141** Salter-Harris Type IV physeal fracture of lower end of **right** femur
    - ✓7ᵗʰ **S79.142** Salter-Harris Type IV physeal fracture of lower end of **left** femur
    - ✓7ᵗʰ **S79.149** Salter-Harris Type IV physeal fracture of lower end of unspecified femur ▽
  - ✓6ᵗʰ **S79.19** Other physeal fracture of lower end of femur
    - ✓7ᵗʰ **S79.191** Other physeal fracture of lower end of **right** femur
    - ✓7ᵗʰ **S79.192** Other physeal fracture of lower end of **left** femur
    - ✓7ᵗʰ **S79.199** Other physeal fracture of lower end of unspecified femur ▽
- ✓5ᵗʰ **S79.8** **Other specified injuries of hip and thigh**

> The appropriate 7th character is to be added to each code in subcategory S79.8.
> A   initial encounter
> D   subsequent encounter
> S   sequela

  - ✓6ᵗʰ **S79.81** Other specified injuries of hip
    - ✓7ᵗʰ **S79.811** Other specified injuries of **right** hip

---

EXCLUDES 1 Not coded here   EXCLUDES 2 Not included here   N Newborn Age : 0   P Pediatric Age : 0-17   M Maternity Age : 12-55   A Adult Age : 15-124

√7ᵗʰ **S79.812** Other specified injuries of left hip

√7ᵗʰ **S79.819** Other specified injuries of unspecified hip ▽

√6ᵗʰ **S79.82** Other specified injuries of thigh

√7ᵗʰ **S79.821** Other specified injuries of right thigh

√7ᵗʰ **S79.822** Other specified injuries of left thigh

√7ᵗʰ **S79.829** Other specified injuries of unspecified thigh ▽

√5ᵗʰ **S79.9** Unspecified injury of hip and thigh

> The appropriate 7th character is to be added to each code in subcategory S79.9.
> A   initial encounter
> D   subsequent encounter
> S   sequela

√6ᵗʰ **S79.91** Unspecified injury of hip

√7ᵗʰ **S79.911** Unspecified injury of right hip ▽

√7ᵗʰ **S79.912** Unspecified injury of left hip ▽

√7ᵗʰ **S79.919** Unspecified injury of unspecified hip ▽

√6ᵗʰ **S79.92** Unspecified injury of thigh

√7ᵗʰ **S79.921** Unspecified injury of right thigh ▽

√7ᵗʰ **S79.922** Unspecified injury of left thigh ▽

√7ᵗʰ **S79.929** Unspecified injury of unspecified thigh ▽

Injuries to the knee and lower leg (S80-S89)

EXCLUDES 2 burns and corrosions (T20-T32)
frostbite (T33-T34)
injuries of ankle and foot, except fracture of ankle and malleolus (S90-S99)
insect bite or sting, venomous (T63.4)

√4ᵗʰ **S80** Superficial injury of knee and lower leg

EXCLUDES 2 superficial injury of ankle and foot (S90.-)

> The appropriate 7th character is to be added to each code from category S80.
> A   initial encounter
> D   subsequent encounter
> S   sequela

√5ᵗʰ **S80.0** Contusion of knee

√x7ᵗʰ **S80.00** Contusion of unspecified knee ▽

√x7ᵗʰ **S80.01** Contusion of right knee

√x7ᵗʰ **S80.02** Contusion of left knee

√5ᵗʰ **S80.1** Contusion of lower leg

√x7ᵗʰ **S80.10** Contusion of unspecified lower leg ▽

√x7ᵗʰ **S80.11** Contusion of right lower leg

√x7ᵗʰ **S80.12** Contusion of left lower leg

√5ᵗʰ **S80.2** Other superficial injuries of knee

√6ᵗʰ **S80.21** Abrasion of knee

√7ᵗʰ **S80.211** Abrasion, right knee

√7ᵗʰ **S80.212** Abrasion, left knee

√7ᵗʰ **S80.219** Abrasion, unspecified knee ▽

√6ᵗʰ **S80.22** Blister (nonthermal) of knee

√7ᵗʰ **S80.221** Blister (nonthermal), right knee

√7ᵗʰ **S80.222** Blister (nonthermal), left knee

√7ᵗʰ **S80.229** Blister (nonthermal), unspecified knee ▽

√6ᵗʰ **S80.24** External constriction of knee

√7ᵗʰ **S80.241** External constriction, right knee

√7ᵗʰ **S80.242** External constriction, left knee

√7ᵗʰ **S80.249** External constriction, unspecified knee ▽

√6ᵗʰ **S80.25** Superficial foreign body of knee

> Splinter in the knee

√7ᵗʰ **S80.251** Superficial foreign body, right knee

√7ᵗʰ **S80.252** Superficial foreign body, left knee

√7ᵗʰ **S80.259** Superficial foreign body, unspecified knee ▽

√6ᵗʰ **S80.26** Insect bite (nonvenomous) of knee

√7ᵗʰ **S80.261** Insect bite (nonvenomous), right knee

√7ᵗʰ **S80.262** Insect bite (nonvenomous), left knee

√7ᵗʰ **S80.269** Insect bite (nonvenomous), unspecified knee ▽

√6ᵗʰ **S80.27** Other superficial bite of knee

EXCLUDES 1 open bite of knee (S81.05-)

√7ᵗʰ **S80.271** Other superficial bite of right knee

√7ᵗʰ **S80.272** Other superficial bite of left knee

√7ᵗʰ **S80.279** Other superficial bite of unspecified knee ▽

√5ᵗʰ **S80.8** Other superficial injuries of lower leg

√6ᵗʰ **S80.81** Abrasion of lower leg

√7ᵗʰ **S80.811** Abrasion, right lower leg

√7ᵗʰ **S80.812** Abrasion, left lower leg

√7ᵗʰ **S80.819** Abrasion, unspecified lower leg ▽

√6ᵗʰ **S80.82** Blister (nonthermal) of lower leg

√7ᵗʰ **S80.821** Blister (nonthermal), right lower leg

√7ᵗʰ **S80.822** Blister (nonthermal), left lower leg

√7ᵗʰ **S80.829** Blister (nonthermal), unspecified lower leg ▽

√6ᵗʰ **S80.84** External constriction of lower leg

√7ᵗʰ **S80.841** External constriction, right lower leg

√7ᵗʰ **S80.842** External constriction, left lower leg

√7ᵗʰ **S80.849** External constriction, unspecified lower leg ▽

√6ᵗʰ **S80.85** Superficial foreign body of lower leg

> Splinter in the lower leg

√7ᵗʰ **S80.851** Superficial foreign body, right lower leg

√7ᵗʰ **S80.852** Superficial foreign body, left lower leg

√7ᵗʰ **S80.859** Superficial foreign body, unspecified lower leg ▽

√6ᵗʰ **S80.86** Insect bite (nonvenomous) of lower leg

√7ᵗʰ **S80.861** Insect bite (nonvenomous), right lower leg

√7ᵗʰ **S80.862** Insect bite (nonvenomous), left lower leg

√7ᵗʰ **S80.869** Insect bite (nonvenomous), unspecified lower leg ▽

√6ᵗʰ **S80.87** Other superficial bite of lower leg

EXCLUDES 1 open bite of lower leg (S81.85-)

√7ᵗʰ **S80.871** Other superficial bite, right lower leg

√7ᵗʰ **S80.872** Other superficial bite, left lower leg

√7ᵗʰ **S80.879** Other superficial bite, unspecified lower leg ▽

√6ᵗʰ **S80.9** Unspecified superficial injury of knee and lower leg

√6ᵗʰ **S80.91** Unspecified superficial injury of knee

√7ᵗʰ **S80.911** Unspecified superficial injury of right knee ▽

√7ᵗʰ **S80.912** Unspecified superficial injury of left knee ▽

√7ᵗʰ **S80.919** Unspecified superficial injury of unspecified knee ▽

√6ᵗʰ **S80.92** Unspecified superficial injury of lower leg

√7ᵗʰ **S80.921** Unspecified superficial injury of right lower leg ▽

√7ᵗʰ **S80.922** Unspecified superficial injury of left lower leg ▽

√7ᵗʰ **S80.929** Unspecified superficial injury of unspecified lower leg ▽

√4ᵗʰ **S81** Open wound of knee and lower leg

> Code also any associated wound infection

EXCLUDES 1 open fracture of knee and lower leg (S82.-)
traumatic amputation of lower leg (S88.-)

EXCLUDES 2 open wound of ankle and foot (S91.-)

> The appropriate 7th character is to be added to each code from category S81.
> A   initial encounter
> D   subsequent encounter
> S   sequela

√5ᵗʰ **S81.0** Open wound of knee

√6ᵗʰ **S81.00** Unspecified open wound of knee

√7ᵗʰ **S81.001** Unspecified open wound, right knee ▽

√7ᵗʰ **S81.002** Unspecified open wound, left knee ▽

√7ᵗʰ **S81.009** Unspecified open wound, unspecified knee ▽

☑ Additional Character Required   √x7ᵗʰ Placeholder Alert   Manifestation Dx   ▽ Unspecified Dx   ►◄ Revised Text   ● New Code   ▲ Revised Code Title

ICD-10-CM 2017   **983**

√6ᵗʰ **S81.01** Laceration without foreign body of knee

   √7ᵗʰ **S81.011** Laceration without foreign body, right knee

   √7ᵗʰ **S81.012** Laceration without foreign body, left knee

   √7ᵗʰ **S81.019** Laceration without foreign body, unspecified knee ▽

√6ᵗʰ **S81.02** Laceration with foreign body of knee

   √7ᵗʰ **S81.021** Laceration with foreign body, right knee

   √7ᵗʰ **S81.022** Laceration with foreign body, left knee

   √7ᵗʰ **S81.029** Laceration with foreign body, unspecified knee ▽

√6ᵗʰ **S81.03** Puncture wound without foreign body of knee

   √7ᵗʰ **S81.031** Puncture wound without foreign body, right knee

   √7ᵗʰ **S81.032** Puncture wound without foreign body, left knee

   √7ᵗʰ **S81.039** Puncture wound without foreign body, unspecified knee ▽

√6ᵗʰ **S81.04** Puncture wound with foreign body of knee

   √7ᵗʰ **S81.041** Puncture wound with foreign body, right knee

   √7ᵗʰ **S81.042** Puncture wound with foreign body, left knee

   √7ᵗʰ **S81.049** Puncture wound with foreign body, unspecified knee ▽

√6ᵗʰ **S81.05** Open bite of knee

   Bite of knee NOS

   EXCLUDES 1 superficial bite of knee (S80.27-)

   √7ᵗʰ **S81.051** Open bite, right knee

   √7ᵗʰ **S81.052** Open bite, left knee

   √7ᵗʰ **S81.059** Open bite, unspecified knee ▽

√5ᵗʰ **S81.8** Open wound of lower leg

√6ᵗʰ **S81.80** Unspecified open wound of lower leg

   √7ᵗʰ **S81.801** Unspecified open wound, right lower leg ▽

   √7ᵗʰ **S81.802** Unspecified open wound, left lower leg ▽

   √7ᵗʰ **S81.809** Unspecified open wound, unspecified lower leg ▽

√6ᵗʰ **S81.81** Laceration without foreign body of lower leg

   √7ᵗʰ **S81.811** Laceration without foreign body, right lower leg

   √7ᵗʰ **S81.812** Laceration without foreign body, left lower leg

   √7ᵗʰ **S81.819** Laceration without foreign body, unspecified lower leg ▽

√6ᵗʰ **S81.82** Laceration with foreign body of lower leg

   √7ᵗʰ **S81.821** Laceration with foreign body, right lower leg

   √7ᵗʰ **S81.822** Laceration with foreign body, left lower leg

   √7ᵗʰ **S81.829** Laceration with foreign body, unspecified lower leg ▽

√6ᵗʰ **S81.83** Puncture wound without foreign body of lower leg

   √7ᵗʰ **S81.831** Puncture wound without foreign body, right lower leg

   √7ᵗʰ **S81.832** Puncture wound without foreign body, left lower leg

   √7ᵗʰ **S81.839** Puncture wound without foreign body, unspecified lower leg ▽

√6ᵗʰ **S81.84** Puncture wound with foreign body of lower leg

   √7ᵗʰ **S81.841** Puncture wound with foreign body, right lower leg

   √7ᵗʰ **S81.842** Puncture wound with foreign body, left lower leg

   √7ᵗʰ **S81.849** Puncture wound with foreign body, unspecified lower leg ▽

√6ᵗʰ **S81.85** Open bite of lower leg

   Bite of lower leg NOS

   EXCLUDES 1 superficial bite of lower leg (S80.86-, S80.87-)

   √7ᵗʰ **S81.851** Open bite, right lower leg

   √7ᵗʰ **S81.852** Open bite, left lower leg

   √7ᵗʰ **S81.859** Open bite, unspecified lower leg ▽

√4ᵗʰ **S82** Fracture of lower leg, including ankle

NOTE A fracture not indicated as displaced or nondisplaced should be coded to displaced

A fracture not indicated as open or closed should be coded to closed

The open fracture designations are based on the Gustilo open fracture classification.

INCLUDES fracture of malleolus

EXCLUDES 1 traumatic amputation of lower leg (S88.-)

EXCLUDES 2 fracture of foot, except ankle (S92.-)

periprosthetic fracture of prosthetic implant of knee (T84.042, T84.043)

AHA: 2016,1Q,33; 2015,3Q,37-39

The appropriate 7th character is to be added to all codes from category S82 [unless otherwise indicated].

A   initial encounter for closed fracture

B   initial encounter for open fracture type I or II

    initial encounter for open fracture NOS

C   initial encounter for open fracture type IIIA, IIIB, or IIIC

D   subsequent encounter for closed fracture with routine healing

E   subsequent encounter for open fracture type I or II with routine healing

F   subsequent encounter for open fracture type IIIA, IIIB, or IIIC with routine healing

G   subsequent encounter for closed fracture with delayed healing

H   subsequent encounter for open fracture type I or II with delayed healing

J   subsequent encounter for open fracture type IIIA, IIIB, or IIIC with delayed healing

K   subsequent encounter for closed fracture with nonunion

M   subsequent encounter for open fracture type I or II with nonunion

N   subsequent encounter for open fracture type IIIA, IIIB, or IIIC with nonunion

P   subsequent encounter for closed fracture with malunion

Q   subsequent encounter for open fracture type I or II with malunion

R   subsequent encounter for open fracture type IIIA, IIIB, or IIIC with malunion

S   sequela

√5ᵗʰ **S82.0** Fracture of patella

   Knee cap

√6ᵗʰ **S82.00** Unspecified fracture of patella

   √7ᵗʰ **S82.001** Unspecified fracture of right patella ▽

   √7ᵗʰ **S82.002** Unspecified fracture of left patella ▽

   √7ᵗʰ **S82.009** Unspecified fracture of unspecified patella ▽

√6ᵗʰ **S82.01** Osteochondral fracture of patella

   √7ᵗʰ **S82.011** Displaced osteochondral fracture of right patella

   √7ᵗʰ **S82.012** Displaced osteochondral fracture of left patella

   √7ᵗʰ **S82.013** Displaced osteochondral fracture of unspecified patella ▽

   √7ᵗʰ **S82.014** Nondisplaced osteochondral fracture of right patella

   √7ᵗʰ **S82.015** Nondisplaced osteochondral fracture of left patella

   √7ᵗʰ **S82.016** Nondisplaced osteochondral fracture of unspecified patella ▽

√6ᵗʰ **S82.02** Longitudinal fracture of patella

   √7ᵗʰ **S82.021** Displaced longitudinal fracture of right patella

   √7ᵗʰ **S82.022** Displaced longitudinal fracture of left patella

   √7ᵗʰ **S82.023** Displaced longitudinal fracture of unspecified patella ▽

   √7ᵗʰ **S82.024** Nondisplaced longitudinal fracture of right patella

   √7ᵗʰ **S82.025** Nondisplaced longitudinal fracture of left patella

   √7ᵗʰ **S82.026** Nondisplaced longitudinal fracture of unspecified patella ▽

√6ᵗʰ **S82.03** Transverse fracture of patella

   √7ᵗʰ **S82.031** Displaced transverse fracture of right patella

   √7ᵗʰ **S82.032** Displaced transverse fracture of left patella

EXCLUDES 1 Not coded here   *EXCLUDES 2* Not included here   N Newborn Age : 0   P Pediatric Age : 0-17   M Maternity Age : 12-55   A Adult Age : 15-124

984   ICD-10-CM 2017

✓7ᵗʰ **S82.033** Displaced **transverse** fracture of **unspecified** patella ▽

✓7ᵗʰ **S82.034** Nondisplaced **transverse** fracture of **right** patella

✓7ᵗʰ **S82.035** Nondisplaced **transverse** fracture of **left** patella

✓7ᵗʰ **S82.036** Nondisplaced **transverse** fracture of **unspecified** patella ▽

✓6ᵗʰ **S82.04** Comminuted **fracture of patella**

✓7ᵗʰ **S82.041** Displaced **comminuted** fracture of **right** patella

✓7ᵗʰ **S82.042** Displaced **comminuted** fracture of **left** patella

✓7ᵗʰ **S82.043** Displaced **comminuted** fracture of **unspecified** patella ▽

✓7ᵗʰ **S82.044** Nondisplaced **comminuted** fracture of **right** patella

✓7ᵗʰ **S82.045** Nondisplaced **comminuted** fracture of **left** patella

✓7ᵗʰ **S82.046** Nondisplaced **comminuted fracture of unspecified patella** ▽

✓6ᵗʰ **S82.09** Other **fracture of patella**

✓7ᵗʰ **S82.091** Other **fracture of** right **patella**

✓7ᵗʰ **S82.092** Other **fracture of** left **patella**

✓7ᵗʰ **S82.099** Other **fracture of unspecified patella** ▽

✓5ᵗʰ **S82.1** Fracture of upper end of tibia

    Fracture of proximal end of tibia

    EXCLUDES 2   *fracture of shaft of tibia (S82.2-)*

        physeal fracture of upper end of tibia (S89.0-)

✓6ᵗʰ **S82.10** Unspecified fracture of upper end of tibia

✓7ᵗʰ **S82.101** Unspecified fracture of upper end of **right tibia** ▽

✓7ᵗʰ **S82.102** Unspecified fracture of upper end of **left tibia** ▽

✓7ᵗʰ **S82.109** Unspecified fracture of upper end of **unspecified tibia** ▽

✓6ᵗʰ **S82.11** Fracture of tibial spine

✓7ᵗʰ **S82.111** Displaced **fracture of** right **tibial spine**

✓7ᵗʰ **S82.112** Displaced **fracture of** left **tibial spine**

✓7ᵗʰ **S82.113** Displaced **fracture of unspecified tibial spine** ▽

✓7ᵗʰ **S82.114** Nondisplaced **fracture of right tibial spine**

✓7ᵗʰ **S82.115** Nondisplaced **fracture of left tibial spine**

✓7ᵗʰ **S82.116** Nondisplaced **fracture of unspecified tibial spine** ▽

✓6ᵗʰ **S82.12** Fracture of lateral condyle of tibia

✓7ᵗʰ **S82.121** Displaced **fracture of lateral condyle of** right **tibia**

✓7ᵗʰ **S82.122** Displaced **fracture of lateral condyle of** left **tibia**

✓7ᵗʰ **S82.123** Displaced **fracture of lateral condyle of unspecified tibia** ▽

✓7ᵗʰ **S82.124** Nondisplaced **fracture of lateral condyle of** right **tibia**

✓7ᵗʰ **S82.125** Nondisplaced **fracture of lateral condyle of** left **tibia**

✓7ᵗʰ **S82.126** Nondisplaced **fracture of lateral condyle of unspecified tibia** ▽

✓6ᵗʰ **S82.13** Fracture of medial condyle of tibia

✓7ᵗʰ **S82.131** Displaced **fracture of medial condyle of** right **tibia**

✓7ᵗʰ **S82.132** Displaced **fracture of medial condyle of** left **tibia**

✓7ᵗʰ **S82.133** Displaced **fracture of medial condyle of unspecified tibia** ▽

✓7ᵗʰ **S82.134** Nondisplaced **fracture of medial condyle of** right **tibia**

✓7ᵗʰ **S82.135** Nondisplaced **fracture of medial condyle of** left **tibia**

✓7ᵗʰ **S82.136** Nondisplaced **fracture of medial condyle of unspecified tibia** ▽

✓6ᵗʰ **S82.14** Bicondylar **fracture of tibia**

    Fracture of tibial plateau NOS

✓7ᵗʰ **S82.141** Displaced **bicondylar** fracture of **right** tibia

✓7ᵗʰ **S82.142** Displaced **bicondylar** fracture of **left tibia**

✓7ᵗʰ **S82.143** Displaced **bicondylar** fracture of **unspecified tibia** ▽

✓7ᵗʰ **S82.144** Nondisplaced **bicondylar** fracture of **right tibia**

✓7ᵗʰ **S82.145** Nondisplaced **bicondylar** fracture of **left tibia**

✓7ᵗʰ **S82.146** Nondisplaced **bicondylar fracture of unspecified tibia** ▽

✓6ᵗʰ **S82.15** Fracture of tibial tuberosity

✓7ᵗʰ **S82.151** Displaced **fracture of** right **tibial tuberosity**

✓7ᵗʰ **S82.152** Displaced **fracture of** left **tibial tuberosity**

✓7ᵗʰ **S82.153** Displaced **fracture of unspecified tibial tuberosity** ▽

✓7ᵗʰ **S82.154** Nondisplaced **fracture of** right **tibial tuberosity**

✓7ᵗʰ **S82.155** Nondisplaced **fracture of** left **tibial tuberosity**

✓7ᵗʰ **S82.156** Nondisplaced **fracture of unspecified tibial tuberosity** ▽

✓6ᵗʰ **S82.16** Torus **fracture of upper end of tibia**

> The appropriate 7th character is to be added to all codes in subcategory S82.16
> A   initial encounter for closed fracture
> D   subsequent encounter for fracture with routine healing
> G   subsequent encounter for fracture with delayed healing
> K   subsequent encounter for fracture with nonunion
> P   subsequent encounter for fracture with malunion
> S   sequela

✓7ᵗʰ **S82.161** Torus **fracture of upper end of** right **tibia**

✓7ᵗʰ **S82.162** Torus **fracture of upper end of** left **tibia**

✓7ᵗʰ **S82.169** Torus **fracture of upper end of unspecified tibia** ▽

✓6ᵗʰ **S82.19** Other **fracture of upper end of tibia**

✓7ᵗʰ **S82.191** Other **fracture of upper end of** right **tibia**

✓7ᵗʰ **S82.192** Other **fracture of upper end of** left **tibia**

✓7ᵗʰ **S82.199** Other **fracture of upper end of unspecified tibia** ▽

✓5ᵗʰ **S82.2** Fracture of shaft of tibia

✓6ᵗʰ **S82.20** Unspecified fracture of shaft of tibia

    Fracture of tibia NOS

✓7ᵗʰ **S82.201** Unspecified fracture of shaft of **right tibia** ▽

✓7ᵗʰ **S82.202** Unspecified fracture of shaft of **left tibia** ▽

✓7ᵗʰ **S82.209** Unspecified fracture of shaft of **unspecified tibia** ▽

✓6ᵗʰ **S82.22** Transverse **fracture of shaft of tibia**

✓7ᵗʰ **S82.221** Displaced **transverse** fracture of shaft of **right tibia**

✓7ᵗʰ **S82.222** Displaced **transverse** fracture of shaft of **left tibia**

✓7ᵗʰ **S82.223** Displaced **transverse** fracture of **shaft of unspecified tibia**

✓7ᵗʰ **S82.224** Nondisplaced **transverse** fracture of shaft of **right tibia**

✓7ᵗʰ **S82.225** Nondisplaced **transverse** fracture of shaft of **left tibia**

✓7ᵗʰ **S82.226** Nondisplaced **transverse** fracture of shaft of **unspecified tibia** ▽

✓6ᵗʰ **S82.23** Oblique **fracture of shaft of tibia**

✓7ᵗʰ **S82.231** Displaced **oblique** fracture of shaft of **right tibia**

✓7ᵗʰ **S82.232** Displaced **oblique** fracture of shaft of **left tibia**

✓7ᵗʰ **S82.233** Displaced **oblique** fracture of **shaft of unspecified tibia** ▽

✓7ᵗʰ **S82.234** Nondisplaced **oblique** fracture of shaft of **right tibia**

✓7ᵗʰ **S82.235** Nondisplaced **oblique** fracture of shaft of **left tibia**

✓7ᵗʰ **S82.236** Nondisplaced **oblique** fracture of **shaft of unspecified tibia** ▽

✓6ᵗʰ **S82.24** Spiral **fracture of shaft of tibia**

    Toddler fracture

✓7ᵗʰ **S82.241** Displaced **spiral** fracture of shaft of **right tibia**

☑ Additional Character Required   ✓7ᵗʰ Placeholder Alert   Manifestation Dx   ▽ Unspecified Dx   ▶◀ Revised Text   ● New Code   ▲ Revised Code Title

ICD-10-CM 2017   985

Chapter 19. Injury, Poisoning and Certain Other Consequences of External Causes

√7ᵗʰ **S82.242** Displaced spiral fracture of shaft of left tibia

√7ᵗʰ **S82.243** Displaced spiral fracture of shaft of unspecified tibia ▽

√7ᵗʰ **S82.244** Nondisplaced spiral fracture of shaft of right tibia

√7ᵗʰ **S82.245** Nondisplaced spiral fracture of shaft of left tibia

√7ᵗʰ **S82.246** Nondisplaced spiral fracture of shaft of unspecified tibia ▽

√6ᵗʰ **S82.25** Comminuted fracture of shaft of tibia

√7ᵗʰ **S82.251** Displaced comminuted fracture of shaft of right tibia

√7ᵗʰ **S82.252** Displaced comminuted fracture of shaft of left tibia

√7ᵗʰ **S82.253** Displaced comminuted fracture of shaft of unspecified tibia ▽

√7ᵗʰ **S82.254** Nondisplaced comminuted fracture of shaft of right tibia

√7ᵗʰ **S82.255** Nondisplaced comminuted fracture of shaft of left tibia

√7ᵗʰ **S82.256** Nondisplaced comminuted fracture of shaft of unspecified tibia ▽

√6ᵗʰ **S82.26** Segmental fracture of shaft of tibia

√7ᵗʰ **S82.261** Displaced segmental fracture of shaft of right tibia

√7ᵗʰ **S82.262** Displaced segmental fracture of shaft of left tibia

√7ᵗʰ **S82.263** Displaced segmental fracture of shaft of unspecified tibia ▽

√7ᵗʰ **S82.264** Nondisplaced segmental fracture of shaft of right tibia

√7ᵗʰ **S82.265** Nondisplaced segmental fracture of shaft of left tibia

√7ᵗʰ **S82.266** Nondisplaced segmental fracture of shaft of unspecified tibia ▽

√6ᵗʰ **S82.29** Other fracture of shaft of tibia

√7ᵗʰ **S82.291** Other fracture of shaft of right tibia

√7ᵗʰ **S82.292** Other fracture of shaft of left tibia

√7ᵗʰ **S82.299** Other fracture of shaft of unspecified tibia ▽

√5ᵗʰ **S82.3** Fracture of lower end of tibia

EXCLUDES 1 bimalleolar fracture of lower leg (S82.84-)
fracture of medial malleolus alone (S82.5-)
Maisonneuve's fracture (S82.86-)
pilon fracture of distal tibia (S82.87-)
trimalleolar fractures of lower leg (S82.85-)

√6ᵗʰ **S82.30** Unspecified fracture of lower end of tibia

√7ᵗʰ **S82.301** Unspecified fracture of lower end of right tibia ▽

√7ᵗʰ **S82.302** Unspecified fracture of lower end of left tibia ▽

√7ᵗʰ **S82.309** Unspecified fracture of lower end of unspecified tibia ▽

√6ᵗʰ **S82.31** Torus fracture of lower end of tibia

> The appropriate 7th character is to be added to all codes in subcategory S82.31
> A initial encounter for closed fracture
> D subsequent encounter for fracture with routine healing
> G subsequent encounter for fracture with delayed healing
> K subsequent encounter for fracture with nonunion
> P subsequent encounter for fracture with malunion
> S sequela

√7ᵗʰ **S82.311** Torus fracture of lower end of right tibia

√7ᵗʰ **S82.312** Torus fracture of lower end of left tibia

√7ᵗʰ **S82.319** Torus fracture of lower end of unspecified tibia ▽

√6ᵗʰ **S82.39** Other fracture of lower end of tibia

AHA: 2015,1Q,25

√7ᵗʰ **S82.391** Other fracture of lower end of right tibia

√7ᵗʰ **S82.392** Other fracture of lower end of left tibia

√7ᵗʰ **S82.399** Other fracture of lower end of unspecified tibia ▽

√5ᵗʰ **S82.4** Fracture of shaft of fibula

EXCLUDES 2 fracture of lateral malleolus alone (S82.6-)

√6ᵗʰ **S82.40** Unspecified fracture of shaft of fibula

√7ᵗʰ **S82.401** Unspecified fracture of shaft of right fibula ▽

√7ᵗʰ **S82.402** Unspecified fracture of shaft of left fibula ▽

√7ᵗʰ **S82.409** Unspecified fracture of shaft of unspecified fibula ▽

√6ᵗʰ **S82.42** Transverse fracture of shaft of fibula

√7ᵗʰ **S82.421** Displaced transverse fracture of shaft of right fibula

√7ᵗʰ **S82.422** Displaced transverse fracture of shaft of left fibula

√7ᵗʰ **S82.423** Displaced transverse fracture of shaft of unspecified fibula ▽

√7ᵗʰ **S82.424** Nondisplaced transverse fracture of shaft of right fibula

√7ᵗʰ **S82.425** Nondisplaced transverse fracture of shaft of left fibula

√7ᵗʰ **S82.426** Nondisplaced transverse fracture of shaft of unspecified fibula ▽

√6ᵗʰ **S82.43** Oblique fracture of shaft of fibula

√7ᵗʰ **S82.431** Displaced oblique fracture of shaft of right fibula

√7ᵗʰ **S82.432** Displaced oblique fracture of shaft of left fibula

√7ᵗʰ **S82.433** Displaced oblique fracture of shaft of unspecified fibula ▽

√7ᵗʰ **S82.434** Nondisplaced oblique fracture of shaft of right fibula

√7ᵗʰ **S82.435** Nondisplaced oblique fracture of shaft of left fibula

√7ᵗʰ **S82.436** Nondisplaced oblique fracture of shaft of unspecified fibula ▽

√6ᵗʰ **S82.44** Spiral fracture of shaft of fibula

√7ᵗʰ **S82.441** Displaced spiral fracture of shaft of right fibula

√7ᵗʰ **S82.442** Displaced spiral fracture of shaft of left fibula

√7ᵗʰ **S82.443** Displaced spiral fracture of shaft of unspecified fibula ▽

√7ᵗʰ **S82.444** Nondisplaced spiral fracture of shaft of right fibula

√7ᵗʰ **S82.445** Nondisplaced spiral fracture of shaft of left fibula

√7ᵗʰ **S82.446** Nondisplaced spiral fracture of shaft of unspecified fibula ▽

√6ᵗʰ **S82.45** Comminuted fracture of shaft of fibula

√7ᵗʰ **S82.451** Displaced comminuted fracture of shaft of right fibula

√7ᵗʰ **S82.452** Displaced comminuted fracture of shaft of left fibula

√7ᵗʰ **S82.453** Displaced comminuted fracture of shaft of unspecified fibula ▽

√7ᵗʰ **S82.454** Nondisplaced comminuted fracture of shaft of right fibula

√7ᵗʰ **S82.455** Nondisplaced comminuted fracture of shaft of left fibula

√7ᵗʰ **S82.456** Nondisplaced comminuted fracture of shaft of unspecified fibula ▽

√6ᵗʰ **S82.46** Segmental fracture of shaft of fibula

√7ᵗʰ **S82.461** Displaced segmental fracture of shaft of right fibula

√7ᵗʰ **S82.462** Displaced segmental fracture of shaft of left fibula

√7ᵗʰ **S82.463** Displaced segmental fracture of shaft of unspecified fibula ▽

√7ᵗʰ **S82.464** Nondisplaced segmental fracture of shaft of right fibula

√7ᵗʰ **S82.465** Nondisplaced segmental fracture of shaft of left fibula

√7ᵗʰ **S82.466** Nondisplaced segmental fracture of shaft of unspecified fibula ▽

√6ᵗʰ **S82.49** Other fracture of shaft of fibula

√7ᵗʰ **S82.491** Other fracture of shaft of right fibula

√7ᵗʰ **S82.492** Other fracture of shaft of left fibula

√7ᵗʰ **S82.499** Other fracture of shaft of unspecified fibula ▽

EXCLUDES 1 Not coded here   *EXCLUDES 2* Not included here   N Newborn Age : 0   P Pediatric Age : 0-17   M Maternity Age : 12-55   A Adult Age : 15-124

986   ICD-10-CM 2017

✓5ᵗʰ **S82.5** **Fracture of medial malleolus**

> **EXCLUDES 1** *pilon fracture of distal tibia (S82.87-)*
> *Salter-Harris type III of lower end of tibia (S89.13-)*
> *Salter-Harris type IV of lower end of tibia (S89.14-)*

✓x7ᵗʰ **S82.51** Displaced **fracture of medial malleolus of** right **tibia**

✓x7ᵗʰ **S82.52** Displaced **fracture of medial malleolus of** left **tibia**

✓x7ᵗʰ **S82.53** Displaced **fracture of medial malleolus of unspecified tibia** ▽

✓x7ᵗʰ **S82.54** Nondisplaced **fracture of medial malleolus of** right **tibia**

✓x7ᵗʰ **S82.55** Nondisplaced **fracture of medial malleolus of** left **tibia**

✓x7ᵗʰ **S82.56** Nondisplaced **fracture of medial malleolus of unspecified tibia** ▽

✓5ᵗʰ **S82.6** **Fracture of lateral malleolus**

> **EXCLUDES 1** *pilon fracture of distal tibia (S82.87-)*

✓x7ᵗʰ **S82.61** Displaced **fracture of lateral malleolus of** right **fibula**

✓x7ᵗʰ **S82.62** Displaced **fracture of lateral malleolus of** left **fibula**

✓x7ᵗʰ **S82.63** Displaced **fracture of lateral malleolus of unspecified fibula** ▽

✓x7ᵗʰ **S82.64** Nondisplaced **fracture of lateral malleolus of** right **fibula**

✓x7ᵗʰ **S82.65** Nondisplaced **fracture of lateral malleolus of** left **fibula**

✓x7ᵗʰ **S82.66** Nondisplaced **fracture of lateral malleolus of unspecified fibula** ▽

✓5ᵗʰ **S82.8** **Other fractures of** lower leg

✓6ᵗʰ **S82.81** Torus **fracture of upper end of fibula**

> The appropriate 7th character is to be added to all codes in subcategory S82.81
> A initial encounter for closed fracture
> D subsequent encounter for fracture with routine healing
> G subsequent encounter for fracture with delayed healing
> K subsequent encounter for fracture with nonunion
> P subsequent encounter for fracture with malunion
> S sequela

✓7ᵗʰ **S82.811** Torus fracture of upper end of right fibula

✓7ᵗʰ **S82.812** Torus fracture of upper end of left fibula

✓7ᵗʰ **S82.819** Torus fracture of upper end of unspecified fibula ▽

✓6ᵗʰ **S82.82** Torus **fracture of** lower end of fibula

> The appropriate 7th character is to be added to all codes in subcategory S82.82
> A initial encounter for closed fracture
> D subsequent encounter for fracture with routine healing
> G subsequent encounter for fracture with delayed healing
> K subsequent encounter for fracture with nonunion
> P subsequent encounter for fracture with malunion
> S sequela

✓7ᵗʰ **S82.821** Torus fracture of lower end of right fibula

✓7ᵗʰ **S82.822** Torus fracture of lower end of left fibula

✓7ᵗʰ **S82.829** Torus fracture of lower end of unspecified fibula ▽

✓6ᵗʰ **S82.83** **Other fracture of upper and lower end of fibula**

> **AHA:** 2015,1Q,25

✓7ᵗʰ **S82.831** Other fracture of upper and lower end of right **fibula**

✓7ᵗʰ **S82.832** Other fracture of upper and lower end of left **fibula**

✓7ᵗʰ **S82.839** Other fracture of upper and lower end of unspecified **fibula** ▽

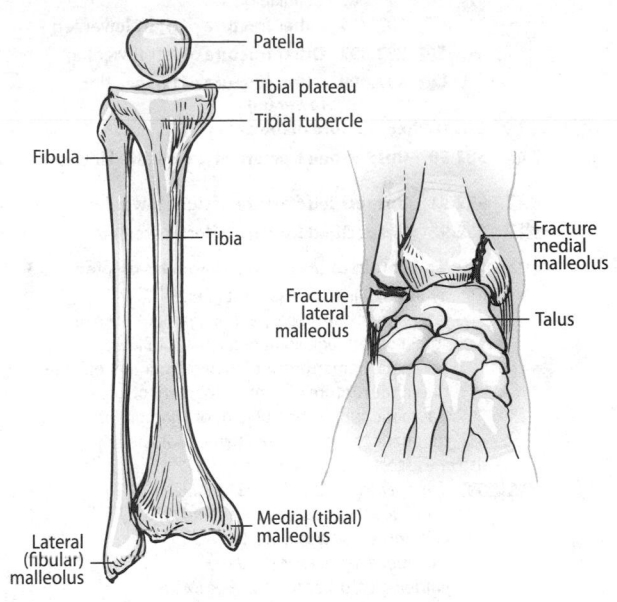

Right Bimalleolar Fracture

Labels: Patella, Tibial plateau, Tibial tubercle, Fibula, Tibia, Fracture medial malleolus, Fracture lateral malleolus, Talus, Medial (tibial) malleolus, Lateral (fibular) malleolus

✓6ᵗʰ **S82.84** **Bimalleolar fracture of lower leg**

✓7ᵗʰ **S82.841** Displaced **bimalleolar fracture of** right **lower leg**

✓7ᵗʰ **S82.842** Displaced **bimalleolar fracture of** left **lower leg**

✓7ᵗʰ **S82.843** Displaced **bimalleolar fracture of unspecified lower leg** ▽

✓7ᵗʰ **S82.844** Nondisplaced **bimalleolar fracture of** right **lower leg**

✓7ᵗʰ **S82.845** Nondisplaced **bimalleolar fracture of** left **lower leg**

✓7ᵗʰ **S82.846** Nondisplaced **bimalleolar fracture of unspecified lower leg** ▽

✓6ᵗʰ **S82.85** **Trimalleolar fracture of lower leg**

✓7ᵗʰ **S82.851** Displaced **trimalleolar fracture of** right **lower leg**

✓7ᵗʰ **S82.852** Displaced **trimalleolar fracture of** left **lower leg**

✓7ᵗʰ **S82.853** Displaced **trimalleolar fracture of unspecified lower leg** ▽

✓7ᵗʰ **S82.854** Nondisplaced **trimalleolar fracture of** right **lower leg**

✓7ᵗʰ **S82.855** Nondisplaced **trimalleolar fracture of** left **lower leg**

✓7ᵗʰ **S82.856** Nondisplaced **trimalleolar fracture of unspecified lower leg** ▽

✓6ᵗʰ **S82.86** **Maisonneuve's fracture**

✓7ᵗʰ **S82.861** Displaced **Maisonneuve's fracture of** right **leg**

✓7ᵗʰ **S82.862** Displaced **Maisonneuve's fracture of** left **leg**

✓7ᵗʰ **S82.863** Displaced **Maisonneuve's fracture of unspecified leg** ▽

✓7ᵗʰ **S82.864** Nondisplaced **Maisonneuve's fracture of** right **leg**

✓7ᵗʰ **S82.865** Nondisplaced **Maisonneuve's fracture of** left **leg**

✓7ᵗʰ **S82.866** Nondisplaced **Maisonneuve's fracture of unspecified leg** ▽

✓6ᵗʰ **S82.87** **Pilon fracture of tibia**

✓7ᵗʰ **S82.871** Displaced **pilon fracture of** right **tibia**

✓7ᵗʰ **S82.872** Displaced **pilon fracture of** left **tibia**

✓7ᵗʰ **S82.873** Displaced **pilon fracture of unspecified tibia** ▽

✓7ᵗʰ **S82.874** Nondisplaced **pilon fracture of** right **tibia**

✓7ᵗʰ **S82.875** Nondisplaced **pilon fracture of** left **tibia**

✓7ᵗʰ **S82.876** Nondisplaced **pilon fracture of unspecified tibia** ▽

✓ Additional Character Required   ✓x7ᵗʰ Placeholder Alert   Manifestation Dx   ▽ Unspecified Dx   ►◄ Revised Text   ● New Code   ▲ Revised Code Title

√6th **S82.89** **Other fractures of lower leg**
Fracture of ankle NOS

√7th **S82.891** **Other fracture of right lower leg**

√7th **S82.892** **Other fracture of left lower leg**

√7th **S82.899** **Other fracture of unspecified lower leg** ▽

√5th **S82.9** **Unspecified fracture of lower leg**

√x7th **S82.90** **Unspecified fracture of unspecified lower leg** ▽

√x7th **S82.91** **Unspecified fracture of right lower leg** ▽

√x7th **S82.92** **Unspecified fracture of left lower leg** ▽

√4th **S83** **Dislocation and sprain of joints and ligaments of knee**

INCLUDES   avulsion of joint or ligament of knee
laceration of cartilage, joint or ligament of knee
sprain of cartilage, joint or ligament of knee
traumatic hemarthrosis of joint or ligament of knee
traumatic rupture of joint or ligament of knee
traumatic subluxation of joint or ligament of knee
traumatic tear of joint or ligament of knee

Code also any associated open wound

EXCLUDES 1   derangement of patella (M22.0-M22.3)
injury of patellar ligament (tendon) (S76.1-)
internal derangement of knee (M23.-)
old dislocation of knee (M23.8X)
pathological dislocation of knee (M24.36)
recurrent dislocation of knee (M22.0)

EXCLUDES 2   strain of muscle, fascia and tendon of lower leg (S86.-)

The appropriate 7th character is to be added to each code from category S83.
A   initial encounter
D   subsequent encounter
S   sequela

√5th **S83.0** **Subluxation and dislocation of patella**

√6th **S83.00** **Unspecified subluxation and dislocation of patella**

√7th **S83.001** **Unspecified subluxation of right patella** ▽

√7th **S83.002** **Unspecified subluxation of left patella** ▽

√7th **S83.003** **Unspecified subluxation of unspecified patella** ▽

√7th **S83.004** **Unspecified dislocation of right patella** ▽

√7th **S83.005** **Unspecified dislocation of left patella** ▽

√7th **S83.006** **Unspecified dislocation of unspecified patella** ▽

√6th **S83.01** **Lateral subluxation and dislocation of patella**

√7th **S83.011** **Lateral subluxation of right patella**

√7th **S83.012** **Lateral subluxation of left patella**

√7th **S83.013** **Lateral subluxation of unspecified patella** ▽

√7th **S83.014** **Lateral dislocation of right patella**

√7th **S83.015** **Lateral dislocation of left patella**

√7th **S83.016** **Lateral dislocation of unspecified patella** ▽

√6th **S83.09** **Other subluxation and dislocation of patella**

√7th **S83.091** **Other subluxation of right patella**

√7th **S83.092** **Other subluxation of left patella**

√7th **S83.093** **Other subluxation of unspecified patella** ▽

√7th **S83.094** **Other dislocation of right patella**

√7th **S83.095** **Other dislocation of left patella**

√7th **S83.096** **Other dislocation of unspecified patella** ▽

√5th **S83.1** **Subluxation and dislocation of knee**

EXCLUDES 2   instability of knee prosthesis (T84.022, T84.023)

√6th **S83.10** **Unspecified subluxation and dislocation of knee**

√7th **S83.101** **Unspecified subluxation of right knee** ▽

√7th **S83.102** **Unspecified subluxation of left knee** ▽

√7th **S83.103** **Unspecified subluxation of unspecified knee** ▽

√7th **S83.104** **Unspecified dislocation of right knee** ▽

√7th **S83.105** **Unspecified dislocation of left knee** ▽

√7th **S83.106** **Unspecified dislocation of unspecified knee** ▽

√6th **S83.11** **Anterior subluxation and dislocation of proximal end of tibia**
Posterior subluxation and dislocation of distal end of femur

√7th **S83.111** **Anterior subluxation of proximal end of tibia, right knee**

√7th **S83.112** **Anterior subluxation of proximal end of tibia, left knee**

√7th **S83.113** **Anterior subluxation of proximal end of tibia, unspecified knee** ▽

√7th **S83.114** **Anterior dislocation of proximal end of tibia, right knee**

√7th **S83.115** **Anterior dislocation of proximal end of tibia, left knee**

√7th **S83.116** **Anterior dislocation of proximal end of tibia, unspecified knee** ▽

√6th **S83.12** **Posterior subluxation and dislocation of proximal end of tibia**
Anterior dislocation of distal end of femur

√7th **S83.121** **Posterior subluxation of proximal end of tibia, right knee**

√7th **S83.122** **Posterior subluxation of proximal end of tibia, left knee**

√7th **S83.123** **Posterior subluxation of proximal end of tibia, unspecified knee** ▽

√7th **S83.124** **Posterior dislocation of proximal end of tibia, right knee**

√7th **S83.125** **Posterior dislocation of proximal end of tibia, left knee**

√7th **S83.126** **Posterior dislocation of proximal end of tibia, unspecified knee** ▽

√6th **S83.13** **Medial subluxation and dislocation of proximal end of tibia**

√7th **S83.131** **Medial subluxation of proximal end of tibia, right knee**

√7th **S83.132** **Medial subluxation of proximal end of tibia, left knee**

√7th **S83.133** **Medial subluxation of proximal end of tibia, unspecified knee** ▽

√7th **S83.134** **Medial dislocation of proximal end of tibia, right knee**

√7th **S83.135** **Medial dislocation of proximal end of tibia, left knee**

√7th **S83.136** **Medial dislocation of proximal end of tibia, unspecified knee** ▽

√6th **S83.14** **Lateral subluxation and dislocation of proximal end of tibia**

√7th **S83.141** **Lateral subluxation of proximal end of tibia, right knee**

√7th **S83.142** **Lateral subluxation of proximal end of tibia, left knee**

√7th **S83.143** **Lateral subluxation of proximal end of tibia, unspecified knee** ▽

√7th **S83.144** **Lateral dislocation of proximal end of tibia, right knee**

√7th **S83.145** **Lateral dislocation of proximal end of tibia, left knee**

√7th **S83.146** **Lateral dislocation of proximal end of tibia, unspecified knee** ▽

√6th **S83.19** **Other subluxation and dislocation of knee**

√7th **S83.191** **Other subluxation of right knee**

√7th **S83.192** **Other subluxation of left knee**

√7th **S83.193** **Other subluxation of unspecified knee** ▽

√7th **S83.194** **Other dislocation of right knee**

√7th **S83.195** **Other dislocation of left knee**

√7th **S83.196** **Other dislocation of unspecified knee** ▽

√5th **S83.2** **Tear of meniscus, current injury**

EXCLUDES 1   old bucket-handle tear (M23.2)

√6th **S83.20** **Tear of unspecified meniscus, current injury**
Tear of meniscus of knee NOS

√7th **S83.200** **Bucket-handle tear of unspecified meniscus, current injury, right knee** ▽

√7th **S83.201** **Bucket-handle tear of unspecified meniscus, current injury, left knee** ▽

EXCLUDES 1 Not coded here   EXCLUDES 2 Not included here   N Newborn Age : 0   P Pediatric Age : 0-17   M Maternity Age : 12-55   A Adult Age : 15-124

✓7ᵗʰ	**S83.202**	**Bucket-handle** tear of unspecified meniscus, current injury, unspecified knee ▽
✓7ᵗʰ	**S83.203**	**Other tear of unspecified meniscus, current injury, right knee** ▽
✓7ᵗʰ	**S83.204**	**Other tear of unspecified meniscus, current injury, left knee** ▽
✓7ᵗʰ	**S83.205**	**Other tear of unspecified meniscus, current injury, unspecified knee** ▽
✓7ᵗʰ	**S83.206**	**Unspecified tear of unspecified meniscus, current injury, right knee** ▽
✓7ᵗʰ	**S83.207**	**Unspecified tear of unspecified meniscus, current injury, left knee** ▽
✓7ᵗʰ	**S83.209**	**Unspecified tear of unspecified meniscus, current injury, unspecified knee** ▽

✓6ᵗʰ **S83.21** **Bucket-handle** tear of **medial** meniscus, current injury

✓7ᵗʰ	**S83.211**	**Bucket-handle tear of medial meniscus, current injury, right knee**
✓7ᵗʰ	**S83.212**	**Bucket-handle tear of medial meniscus, current injury, left knee**
✓7ᵗʰ	**S83.219**	**Bucket-handle tear of medial meniscus, current injury, unspecified knee** ▽

✓6ᵗʰ **S83.22** **Peripheral** tear of **medial** meniscus, current injury

✓7ᵗʰ	**S83.221**	**Peripheral tear of medial meniscus, current injury, right knee**
✓7ᵗʰ	**S83.222**	**Peripheral tear of medial meniscus, current injury, left knee**
✓7ᵗʰ	**S83.229**	**Peripheral tear of medial meniscus, current injury, unspecified knee** ▽

✓6ᵗʰ **S83.23** **Complex** tear of **medial** meniscus, current injury

✓7ᵗʰ	**S83.231**	**Complex tear of medial meniscus, current injury, right knee**
✓7ᵗʰ	**S83.232**	**Complex tear of medial meniscus, current injury, left knee**
✓7ᵗʰ	**S83.239**	**Complex tear of medial meniscus, current injury, unspecified knee** ▽

✓6ᵗʰ **S83.24** **Other tear of medial** meniscus, current injury

✓7ᵗʰ	**S83.241**	**Other tear of medial meniscus, current injury, right knee**
✓7ᵗʰ	**S83.242**	**Other tear of medial meniscus, current injury, left knee**
✓7ᵗʰ	**S83.249**	**Other tear of medial meniscus, current injury, unspecified knee** ▽

✓6ᵗʰ **S83.25** **Bucket-handle** tear of **lateral** meniscus, current injury

✓7ᵗʰ	**S83.251**	**Bucket-handle tear of lateral meniscus, current injury, right knee**
✓7ᵗʰ	**S83.252**	**Bucket-handle tear of lateral meniscus, current injury, left knee**
✓7ᵗʰ	**S83.259**	**Bucket-handle tear of lateral meniscus, current injury, unspecified knee** ▽

✓6ᵗʰ **S83.26** **Peripheral** tear of **lateral** meniscus, current injury

✓7ᵗʰ	**S83.261**	**Peripheral tear of lateral meniscus, current injury, right knee**
✓7ᵗʰ	**S83.262**	**Peripheral tear of lateral meniscus, current injury, left knee**
✓7ᵗʰ	**S83.269**	**Peripheral tear of lateral meniscus, current injury, unspecified knee** ▽

✓6ᵗʰ **S83.27** **Complex** tear of **lateral** meniscus, current injury

✓7ᵗʰ	**S83.271**	**Complex tear of lateral meniscus, current injury, right knee**
✓7ᵗʰ	**S83.272**	**Complex tear of lateral meniscus, current injury, left knee**
✓7ᵗʰ	**S83.279**	**Complex tear of lateral meniscus, current injury, unspecified knee** ▽

✓6ᵗʰ **S83.28** **Other tear of lateral** meniscus, current injury

✓7ᵗʰ	**S83.281**	**Other tear of lateral meniscus, current injury, right knee**
✓7ᵗʰ	**S83.282**	**Other tear of lateral meniscus, current injury, left knee**
✓7ᵗʰ	**S83.289**	**Other tear of lateral meniscus, current injury, unspecified knee** ▽

✓5ᵗʰ **S83.3** Tear of articular cartilage of knee, current

✓ₓ7ᵗʰ	**S83.30**	**Tear of articular cartilage of unspecified knee, current** ▽
✓ₓ7ᵗʰ	**S83.31**	**Tear of articular cartilage of right knee, current**
✓ₓ7ᵗʰ	**S83.32**	**Tear of articular cartilage of left knee, current**

✓5ᵗʰ **S83.4** Sprain of **collateral ligament** of knee

✓6ᵗʰ **S83.40** Sprain of unspecified collateral ligament of knee

✓7ᵗʰ	**S83.401**	**Sprain of unspecified collateral ligament of right knee** ▽
✓7ᵗʰ	**S83.402**	**Sprain of unspecified collateral ligament of left knee** ▽
✓7ᵗʰ	**S83.409**	**Sprain of unspecified collateral ligament of unspecified knee** ▽

✓6ᵗʰ **S83.41** Sprain of **medial** collateral ligament of knee

Sprain of tibial collateral ligament

✓7ᵗʰ	**S83.411**	**Sprain of medial collateral ligament of right knee**
✓7ᵗʰ	**S83.412**	**Sprain of medial collateral ligament of left knee**
✓7ᵗʰ	**S83.419**	**Sprain of medial collateral ligament of unspecified knee** ▽

✓6ᵗʰ **S83.42** Sprain of **lateral** collateral ligament of knee

Sprain of fibular collateral ligament

✓7ᵗʰ	**S83.421**	**Sprain of lateral collateral ligament of right knee**
✓7ᵗʰ	**S83.422**	**Sprain of lateral collateral ligament of left knee**
✓7ᵗʰ	**S83.429**	**Sprain of lateral collateral ligament of unspecified knee** ▽

✓5ᵗʰ **S83.5** Sprain of **cruciate ligament** of knee

AHA: 2016,2Q,3

✓6ᵗʰ **S83.50** Sprain of unspecified cruciate ligament of knee

✓7ᵗʰ	**S83.501**	**Sprain of unspecified cruciate ligament of right knee** ▽
✓7ᵗʰ	**S83.502**	**Sprain of unspecified cruciate ligament of left knee** ▽
✓7ᵗʰ	**S83.509**	**Sprain of unspecified cruciate ligament of unspecified knee** ▽

✓6ᵗʰ **S83.51** Sprain of **anterior** cruciate ligament of knee

✓7ᵗʰ	**S83.511**	**Sprain of anterior cruciate ligament of right knee**
✓7ᵗʰ	**S83.512**	**Sprain of anterior cruciate ligament of left knee**
✓7ᵗʰ	**S83.519**	**Sprain of anterior cruciate ligament of unspecified knee** ▽

✓6ᵗʰ **S83.52** Sprain of **posterior** cruciate ligament of knee

✓7ᵗʰ	**S83.521**	**Sprain of posterior cruciate ligament of right knee**
✓7ᵗʰ	**S83.522**	**Sprain of posterior cruciate ligament of left knee**
✓7ᵗʰ	**S83.529**	**Sprain of posterior cruciate ligament of unspecified knee** ▽

✓5ᵗʰ **S83.6** Sprain of the **superior tibiofibular** joint and ligament

✓ₓ7ᵗʰ	**S83.60**	**Sprain of the superior tibiofibular joint and ligament, unspecified knee** ▽
✓ₓ7ᵗʰ	**S83.61**	**Sprain of the superior tibiofibular joint and ligament, right knee**
✓ₓ7ᵗʰ	**S83.62**	**Sprain of the superior tibiofibular joint and ligament, left knee**

✓5ᵗʰ **S83.8** Sprain of other specified parts of knee

✓6ᵗʰ **S83.8X** Sprain of other specified parts of knee

✓7ᵗʰ	**S83.8X1**	**Sprain of other specified parts of right knee**
✓7ᵗʰ	**S83.8X2**	**Sprain of other specified parts of left knee**
✓7ᵗʰ	**S83.8X9**	**Sprain of other specified parts of unspecified knee** ▽

✓5ᵗʰ **S83.9** Sprain of unspecified site of knee

✓ₓ7ᵗʰ	**S83.90**	**Sprain of unspecified site of unspecified knee** ▽
✓ₓ7ᵗʰ	**S83.91**	**Sprain of unspecified site of right knee** ▽
✓ₓ7ᵗʰ	**S83.92**	**Sprain of unspecified site of left knee** ▽

☑ Additional Character Required	✓ₓ7ᵗʰ Placeholder Alert	Manifestation Dx	▽ Unspecified Dx	▶◀ Revised Text	● New Code	▲ Revised Code Title

✓4ᵗʰ **S84 Injury of nerves at lower leg level**

Code also any associated open wound (S81.-)

EXCLUDES 2 *injury of nerves at ankle and foot level (S94.-)*

> The appropriate 7th character is to be added to each code from category S84.
> A   initial encounter
> D   subsequent encounter
> S   sequela

✓5ᵗʰ **S84.0 Injury of tibial nerve at lower leg level**

   ✓x7ᵗʰ **S84.00 Injury of tibial nerve at lower leg level, unspecified leg** ▽

   ✓x7ᵗʰ **S84.01 Injury of tibial nerve at lower leg level, right leg**

   ✓x7ᵗʰ **S84.02 Injury of tibial nerve at lower leg level, left leg**

✓5ᵗʰ **S84.1 Injury of peroneal nerve at lower leg level**

   ✓x7ᵗʰ **S84.10 Injury of peroneal nerve at lower leg level, unspecified leg** ▽

   ✓x7ᵗʰ **S84.11 Injury of peroneal nerve at lower leg level, right leg**

   ✓x7ᵗʰ **S84.12 Injury of peroneal nerve at lower leg level, left leg**

✓5ᵗʰ **S84.2 Injury of cutaneous sensory nerve at lower leg level**

   ✓x7ᵗʰ **S84.20 Injury of cutaneous sensory nerve at lower leg level, unspecified leg** ▽

   ✓x7ᵗʰ **S84.21 Injury of cutaneous sensory nerve at lower leg level, right leg**

   ✓x7ᵗʰ **S84.22 Injury of cutaneous sensory nerve at lower leg level, left leg**

✓5ᵗʰ **S84.8 Injury of other nerves at lower leg level**

   ✓6ᵗʰ **S84.80 Injury of other nerves at lower leg level**

     ✓7ᵗʰ **S84.801 Injury of other nerves at lower leg level, right leg**

     ✓7ᵗʰ **S84.802 Injury of other nerves at lower leg level, left leg**

     ✓7ᵗʰ **S84.809 Injury of other nerves at lower leg level, unspecified leg** ▽

✓5ᵗʰ **S84.9 Injury of unspecified nerve at lower leg level**

   ✓x7ᵗʰ **S84.90 Injury of unspecified nerve at lower leg level, unspecified leg** ▽

   ✓x7ᵗʰ **S84.91 Injury of unspecified nerve at lower leg level, right leg** ▽

   ✓x7ᵗʰ **S84.92 Injury of unspecified nerve at lower leg level, left leg** ▽

✓4ᵗʰ **S85 Injury of blood vessels at lower leg level**

Code also any associated open wound (S81.-)

EXCLUDES 2 *injury of blood vessels at ankle and foot level (S95.-)*

> The appropriate 7th character is to be added to each code from category S85.
> A   initial encounter
> D   subsequent encounter
> S   sequela

✓5ᵗʰ **S85.0 Injury of popliteal artery**

   ✓6ᵗʰ **S85.00 Unspecified injury of popliteal artery**

     ✓7ᵗʰ **S85.001 Unspecified injury of popliteal artery, right leg** ▽

     ✓7ᵗʰ **S85.002 Unspecified injury of popliteal artery, left leg** ▽

     ✓7ᵗʰ **S85.009 Unspecified injury of popliteal artery, unspecified leg** ▽

   ✓6ᵗʰ **S85.01 Laceration of popliteal artery**

     ✓7ᵗʰ **S85.011 Laceration of popliteal artery, right leg**

     ✓7ᵗʰ **S85.012 Laceration of popliteal artery, left leg**

     ✓7ᵗʰ **S85.019 Laceration of popliteal artery, unspecified leg** ▽

   ✓6ᵗʰ **S85.09 Other specified injury of popliteal artery**

     ✓7ᵗʰ **S85.091 Other specified injury of popliteal artery, right leg**

     ✓7ᵗʰ **S85.092 Other specified injury of popliteal artery, left leg**

     ✓7ᵗʰ **S85.099 Other specified injury of popliteal artery, unspecified leg** ▽

✓5ᵗʰ **S85.1 Injury of tibial artery**

   ✓6ᵗʰ **S85.10 Unspecified injury of unspecified tibial artery**

     Injury of tibial artery NOS

     ✓7ᵗʰ **S85.101 Unspecified injury of unspecified tibial artery, right leg** ▽

     ✓7ᵗʰ **S85.102 Unspecified injury of unspecified tibial artery, left leg** ▽

     ✓7ᵗʰ **S85.109 Unspecified injury of unspecified tibial artery, unspecified leg** ▽

   ✓6ᵗʰ **S85.11 Laceration of unspecified tibial artery**

     ✓7ᵗʰ **S85.111 Laceration of unspecified tibial artery, right leg** ▽

     ✓7ᵗʰ **S85.112 Laceration of unspecified tibial artery, left leg** ▽

     ✓7ᵗʰ **S85.119 Laceration of unspecified tibial artery, unspecified leg** ▽

   ✓6ᵗʰ **S85.12 Other specified injury of unspecified tibial artery**

     ✓7ᵗʰ **S85.121 Other specified injury of unspecified tibial artery, right leg** ▽

     ✓7ᵗʰ **S85.122 Other specified injury of unspecified tibial artery, left leg** ▽

     ✓7ᵗʰ **S85.129 Other specified injury of unspecified tibial artery, unspecified leg** ▽

   ✓6ᵗʰ **S85.13 Unspecified injury of anterior tibial artery**

     ✓7ᵗʰ **S85.131 Unspecified injury of anterior tibial artery, right leg** ▽

     ✓7ᵗʰ **S85.132 Unspecified injury of anterior tibial artery, left leg** ▽

     ✓7ᵗʰ **S85.139 Unspecified injury of anterior tibial artery, unspecified leg** ▽

   ✓6ᵗʰ **S85.14 Laceration of anterior tibial artery**

     ✓7ᵗʰ **S85.141 Laceration of anterior tibial artery, right leg**

     ✓7ᵗʰ **S85.142 Laceration of anterior tibial artery, left leg**

     ✓7ᵗʰ **S85.149 Laceration of anterior tibial artery, unspecified leg** ▽

   ✓6ᵗʰ **S85.15 Other specified injury of anterior tibial artery**

     ✓7ᵗʰ **S85.151 Other specified injury of anterior tibial artery, right leg**

     ✓7ᵗʰ **S85.152 Other specified injury of anterior tibial artery, left leg**

     ✓7ᵗʰ **S85.159 Other specified injury of anterior tibial artery, unspecified leg** ▽

   ✓6ᵗʰ **S85.16 Unspecified injury of posterior tibial artery**

     ✓7ᵗʰ **S85.161 Unspecified injury of posterior tibial artery, right leg** ▽

     ✓7ᵗʰ **S85.162 Unspecified injury of posterior tibial artery, left leg** ▽

     ✓7ᵗʰ **S85.169 Unspecified injury of posterior tibial artery, unspecified leg** ▽

   ✓6ᵗʰ **S85.17 Laceration of posterior tibial artery**

     ✓7ᵗʰ **S85.171 Laceration of posterior tibial artery, right leg**

     ✓7ᵗʰ **S85.172 Laceration of posterior tibial artery, left leg**

     ✓7ᵗʰ **S85.179 Laceration of posterior tibial artery, unspecified leg** ▽

   ✓6ᵗʰ **S85.18 Other specified injury of posterior tibial artery**

     ✓7ᵗʰ **S85.181 Other specified injury of posterior tibial artery, right leg**

     ✓7ᵗʰ **S85.182 Other specified injury of posterior tibial artery, left leg**

     ✓7ᵗʰ **S85.189 Other specified injury of posterior tibial artery, unspecified leg** ▽

✓5ᵗʰ **S85.2 Injury of peroneal artery**

   ✓6ᵗʰ **S85.20 Unspecified injury of peroneal artery**

     ✓7ᵗʰ **S85.201 Unspecified injury of peroneal artery, right leg** ▽

     ✓7ᵗʰ **S85.202 Unspecified injury of peroneal artery, left leg** ▽

     ✓7ᵗʰ **S85.209 Unspecified injury of peroneal artery, unspecified leg** ▽

   ✓6ᵗʰ **S85.21 Laceration of peroneal artery**

     ✓7ᵗʰ **S85.211 Laceration of peroneal artery, right leg** ▽

     ✓7ᵗʰ **S85.212 Laceration of peroneal artery, left leg** ▽

     ✓7ᵗʰ **S85.219 Laceration of peroneal artery, unspecified leg** ▽

   ✓6ᵗʰ **S85.29 Other specified injury of peroneal artery**

     ✓7ᵗʰ **S85.291 Other specified injury of peroneal artery, right leg**

     ✓7ᵗʰ **S85.292 Other specified injury of peroneal artery, left leg**

     ✓7ᵗʰ **S85.299 Other specified injury of peroneal artery, unspecified leg** ▽

EXCLUDES 1 Not coded here   EXCLUDES 2 Not included here   N Newborn Age : 0   P Pediatric Age : 0-17   M Maternity Age : 12-55   A Adult Age : 15-124

990   ICD-10-CM 2017

✓5ᵗʰ S85.3 **Injury of** greater saphenous vein **at lower leg level**
Injury of greater saphenous vein NOS
Injury of saphenous vein NOS

     ✓6ᵗʰ S85.30 **Unspecified injury of greater saphenous vein at lower leg level**

         ✓7ᵗʰ S85.301 **Unspecified injury of greater saphenous vein at lower leg level, right leg** ▽

         ✓7ᵗʰ S85.302 **Unspecified injury of greater saphenous vein at lower leg level, left leg** ▽

         ✓7ᵗʰ S85.309 **Unspecified injury of greater saphenous vein at lower leg level, unspecified leg** ▽

     ✓6ᵗʰ S85.31 **Laceration of greater saphenous vein at lower leg level**

         ✓7ᵗʰ S85.311 **Laceration of greater saphenous vein at lower leg level, right leg**

         ✓7ᵗʰ S85.312 **Laceration of greater saphenous vein at lower leg level, left leg**

         ✓7ᵗʰ S85.319 **Laceration of greater saphenous vein at lower leg level, unspecified leg** ▽

     ✓6ᵗʰ S85.39 **Other specified injury of greater saphenous vein at lower leg level**

         ✓7ᵗʰ S85.391 **Other specified injury of greater saphenous vein at lower leg level, right leg**

         ✓7ᵗʰ S85.392 **Other specified injury of greater saphenous vein at lower leg level, left leg**

         ✓7ᵗʰ S85.399 **Other specified injury of greater saphenous vein at lower leg level, unspecified leg** ▽

✓5ᵗʰ S85.4 **Injury of** lesser saphenous vein **at lower leg level**

     ✓6ᵗʰ S85.40 **Unspecified injury of lesser saphenous vein at lower leg level**

         ✓7ᵗʰ S85.401 **Unspecified injury of lesser saphenous vein at lower leg level, right leg** ▽

         ✓7ᵗʰ S85.402 **Unspecified injury of lesser saphenous vein at lower leg level, left leg** ▽

         ✓7ᵗʰ S85.409 **Unspecified injury of lesser saphenous vein at lower leg level, unspecified leg** ▽

     ✓6ᵗʰ S85.41 **Laceration of lesser saphenous vein at lower leg level**

         ✓7ᵗʰ S85.411 **Laceration of lesser saphenous vein at lower leg level, right leg**

         ✓7ᵗʰ S85.412 **Laceration of lesser saphenous vein at lower leg level, left leg**

         ✓7ᵗʰ S85.419 **Laceration of lesser saphenous vein at lower leg level, unspecified leg** ▽

     ✓6ᵗʰ S85.49 **Other specified injury of lesser saphenous vein at lower leg level**

         ✓7ᵗʰ S85.491 **Other specified injury of lesser saphenous vein at lower leg level, right leg**

         ✓7ᵗʰ S85.492 **Other specified injury of lesser saphenous vein at lower leg level, left leg**

         ✓7ᵗʰ S85.499 **Other specified injury of lesser saphenous vein at lower leg level, unspecified leg** ▽

✓5ᵗʰ S85.5 **Injury of** popliteal vein

     ✓6ᵗʰ S85.50 **Unspecified injury of popliteal vein**

         ✓7ᵗʰ S85.501 **Unspecified injury of popliteal vein, right leg** ▽

         ✓7ᵗʰ S85.502 **Unspecified injury of popliteal vein, left leg** ▽

         ✓7ᵗʰ S85.509 **Unspecified injury of popliteal vein, unspecified leg** ▽

     ✓6ᵗʰ S85.51 **Laceration of popliteal vein**

         ✓7ᵗʰ S85.511 **Laceration of popliteal vein, right leg**

         ✓7ᵗʰ S85.512 **Laceration of popliteal vein, left leg**

         ✓7ᵗʰ S85.519 **Laceration of popliteal vein, unspecified leg** ▽

     ✓6ᵗʰ S85.59 **Other specified injury of popliteal vein**

         ✓7ᵗʰ S85.591 **Other specified injury of popliteal vein, right leg**

         ✓7ᵗʰ S85.592 **Other specified injury of popliteal vein, left leg**

         ✓7ᵗʰ S85.599 **Other specified injury of popliteal vein, unspecified leg** ▽

✓5ᵗʰ S85.8 **Injury of other blood vessels at lower leg level**

     ✓6ᵗʰ S85.80 **Unspecified injury of other blood vessels at lower leg level**

         ✓7ᵗʰ S85.801 **Unspecified injury of other blood vessels at lower leg level, right leg** ▽

         ✓7ᵗʰ S85.802 **Unspecified injury of other blood vessels at lower leg level, left leg** ▽

         ✓7ᵗʰ S85.809 **Unspecified injury of other blood vessels at lower leg level, unspecified leg** ▽

     ✓6ᵗʰ S85.81 **Laceration of other blood vessels at lower leg level**

         ✓7ᵗʰ S85.811 **Laceration of other blood vessels at lower leg level, right leg**

         ✓7ᵗʰ S85.812 **Laceration of other blood vessels at lower leg level, left leg**

         ✓7ᵗʰ S85.819 **Laceration of other blood vessels at lower leg level, unspecified leg** ▽

     ✓6ᵗʰ S85.89 **Other specified injury of other blood vessels at lower leg level**

         ✓7ᵗʰ S85.891 **Other specified injury of other blood vessels at lower leg level, right leg**

         ✓7ᵗʰ S85.892 **Other specified injury of other blood vessels at lower leg level, left leg**

         ✓7ᵗʰ S85.899 **Other specified injury of other blood vessels at lower leg level, unspecified leg** ▽

✓5ᵗʰ S85.9 **Injury of unspecified blood vessel at lower leg level**

     ✓6ᵗʰ S85.90 **Unspecified injury of unspecified blood vessel at lower leg level**

         ✓7ᵗʰ S85.901 **Unspecified injury of unspecified blood vessel at lower leg level, right leg** ▽

         ✓7ᵗʰ S85.902 **Unspecified injury of unspecified blood vessel at lower leg level, left leg** ▽

         ✓7ᵗʰ S85.909 **Unspecified injury of unspecified blood vessel at lower leg level, unspecified leg** ▽

     ✓6ᵗʰ S85.91 **Laceration of unspecified blood vessel at lower leg level**

         ✓7ᵗʰ S85.911 **Laceration of unspecified blood vessel at lower leg level, right leg** ▽

         ✓7ᵗʰ S85.912 **Laceration of unspecified blood vessel at lower leg level, left leg** ▽

         ✓7ᵗʰ S85.919 **Laceration of unspecified blood vessel at lower leg level, unspecified leg** ▽

     ✓6ᵗʰ S85.99 **Other specified injury of unspecified blood vessel at lower leg level**

         ✓7ᵗʰ S85.991 **Other specified injury of unspecified blood vessel at lower leg level, right leg** ▽

         ✓7ᵗʰ S85.992 **Other specified injury of unspecified blood vessel at lower leg level, left leg** ▽

         ✓7ᵗʰ S85.999 **Other specified injury of unspecified blood vessel at lower leg level, unspecified leg** ▽

✓4ᵗʰ S86 **Injury of muscle, fascia and tendon at lower leg level**

Code also any associated open wound (S81.-)

EXCLUDES 2 injury of muscle, fascia and tendon at ankle (S96.-)
injury of patellar ligament (tendon) (S76.1-)
sprain of joints and ligaments of knee (S83.-)

TIP: Refer to the Muscle/Tendon table at the beginning of this chapter

The appropriate 7th character is to be added to each code from category S86.
A   initial encounter
D   subsequent encounter
S   sequela

     ✓5ᵗʰ S86.0 **Injury of** Achilles tendon

         ✓6ᵗʰ S86.00 **Unspecified injury of Achilles tendon**

             ✓7ᵗʰ S86.001 **Unspecified injury of right Achilles tendon** ▽

             ✓7ᵗʰ S86.002 **Unspecified injury of left Achilles tendon** ▽

             ✓7ᵗʰ S86.009 **Unspecified injury of unspecified Achilles tendon** ▽

         ✓6ᵗʰ S86.01 **Strain of Achilles tendon**

             ✓7ᵗʰ S86.011 **Strain of right Achilles tendon**

☑ Additional Character Required   ✓ₓ7ᵗʰ Placeholder Alert   Manifestation Dx   ▽ Unspecified Dx   ▶◀ Revised Text   ● New Code   ▲ Revised Code Title

√7ᵗʰ   **S86.012**   Strain of left Achilles tendon

√7ᵗʰ   **S86.019**   Strain of unspecified Achilles tendon ▽

√6ᵗʰ   **S86.02**   Laceration of Achilles tendon

√7ᵗʰ   **S86.021**   Laceration of right Achilles tendon

√7ᵗʰ   **S86.022**   Laceration of left Achilles tendon

√7ᵗʰ   **S86.029**   Laceration of unspecified Achilles tendon ▽

√6ᵗʰ   **S86.09**   Other specified injury of Achilles tendon

√7ᵗʰ   **S86.091**   Other specified injury of right Achilles tendon

√7ᵗʰ   **S86.092**   Other specified injury of left Achilles tendon

√7ᵗʰ   **S86.099**   Other specified injury of unspecified Achilles tendon ▽

√5ᵗʰ   **S86.1**   Injury of other muscle(s) and tendon(s) of posterior muscle group at lower leg level

√6ᵗʰ   **S86.10**   Unspecified injury of other muscle(s) and tendon(s) of posterior muscle group at lower leg level

√7ᵗʰ   **S86.101**   Unspecified injury of other muscle(s) and tendon(s) of posterior muscle group at lower leg level, right leg ▽

√7ᵗʰ   **S86.102**   Unspecified injury of other muscle(s) and tendon(s) of posterior muscle group at lower leg level, left leg ▽

√7ᵗʰ   **S86.109**   Unspecified injury of other muscle(s) and tendon(s) of posterior muscle group at lower leg level, unspecified leg ▽

√6ᵗʰ   **S86.11**   Strain of other muscle(s) and tendon(s) of posterior muscle group at lower leg level

√7ᵗʰ   **S86.111**   Strain of other muscle(s) and tendon(s) of posterior muscle group at lower leg level, right leg

√7ᵗʰ   **S86.112**   Strain of other muscle(s) and tendon(s) of posterior muscle group at lower leg level, left leg

√7ᵗʰ   **S86.119**   Strain of other muscle(s) and tendon(s) of posterior muscle group at lower leg level, unspecified leg ▽

√6ᵗʰ   **S86.12**   Laceration of other muscle(s) and tendon(s) of posterior muscle group at lower leg level

√7ᵗʰ   **S86.121**   Laceration of other muscle(s) and tendon(s) of posterior muscle group at lower leg level, right leg

√7ᵗʰ   **S86.122**   Laceration of other muscle(s) and tendon(s) of posterior muscle group at lower leg level, left leg

√7ᵗʰ   **S86.129**   Laceration of other muscle(s) and tendon(s) of posterior muscle group at lower leg level, unspecified leg ▽

√6ᵗʰ   **S86.19**   Other injury of other muscle(s) and tendon(s) of posterior muscle group at lower leg level

√7ᵗʰ   **S86.191**   Other injury of other muscle(s) and tendon(s) of posterior muscle group at lower leg level, right leg

√7ᵗʰ   **S86.192**   Other injury of other muscle(s) and tendon(s) of posterior muscle group at lower leg level, left leg

√7ᵗʰ   **S86.199**   Other injury of other muscle(s) and tendon(s) of posterior muscle group at lower leg level, unspecified leg ▽

√5ᵗʰ   **S86.2**   Injury of muscle(s) and tendon(s) of anterior muscle group at lower leg level

√6ᵗʰ   **S86.20**   Unspecified injury of muscle(s) and tendon(s) of anterior muscle group at lower leg level

√7ᵗʰ   **S86.201**   Unspecified injury of muscle(s) and tendon(s) of anterior muscle group at lower leg level, right leg ▽

√7ᵗʰ   **S86.202**   Unspecified injury of muscle(s) and tendon(s) of anterior muscle group at lower leg level, left leg ▽

√7ᵗʰ   **S86.209**   Unspecified injury of muscle(s) and tendon(s) of anterior muscle group at lower leg level, unspecified leg ▽

√6ᵗʰ   **S86.21**   Strain of muscle(s) and tendon(s) of anterior muscle group at lower leg level

√7ᵗʰ   **S86.211**   Strain of muscle(s) and tendon(s) of anterior muscle group at lower leg level, right leg

√7ᵗʰ   **S86.212**   Strain of muscle(s) and tendon(s) of anterior muscle group at lower leg level, left leg

√7ᵗʰ   **S86.219**   Strain of muscle(s) and tendon(s) of anterior muscle group at lower leg level, unspecified leg ▽

√6ᵗʰ   **S86.22**   Laceration of muscle(s) and tendon(s) of anterior muscle group at lower leg level

√7ᵗʰ   **S86.221**   Laceration of muscle(s) and tendon(s) of anterior muscle group at lower leg level, right leg

√7ᵗʰ   **S86.222**   Laceration of muscle(s) and tendon(s) of anterior muscle group at lower leg level, left leg

√7ᵗʰ   **S86.229**   Laceration of muscle(s) and tendon(s) of anterior muscle group at lower leg level, unspecified leg ▽

√6ᵗʰ   **S86.29**   Other injury of muscle(s) and tendon(s) of anterior muscle group at lower leg level

√7ᵗʰ   **S86.291**   Other injury of muscle(s) and tendon(s) of anterior muscle group at lower leg level, right leg

√7ᵗʰ   **S86.292**   Other injury of muscle(s) and tendon(s) of anterior muscle group at lower leg level, left leg

√7ᵗʰ   **S86.299**   Other injury of muscle(s) and tendon(s) of anterior muscle group at lower leg level, unspecified leg ▽

√5ᵗʰ   **S86.3**   Injury of muscle(s) and tendon(s) of peroneal muscle group at lower leg level

√6ᵗʰ   **S86.30**   Unspecified injury of muscle(s) and tendon(s) of peroneal muscle group at lower leg level

√7ᵗʰ   **S86.301**   Unspecified injury of muscle(s) and tendon(s) of peroneal muscle group at lower leg level, right leg ▽

√7ᵗʰ   **S86.302**   Unspecified injury of muscle(s) and tendon(s) of peroneal muscle group at lower leg level, left leg ▽

√7ᵗʰ   **S86.309**   Unspecified injury of muscle(s) and tendon(s) of peroneal muscle group at lower leg level, unspecified leg ▽

√6ᵗʰ   **S86.31**   Strain of muscle(s) and tendon(s) of peroneal muscle group at lower leg level

√7ᵗʰ   **S86.311**   Strain of muscle(s) and tendon(s) of peroneal muscle group at lower leg level, right leg

√7ᵗʰ   **S86.312**   Strain of muscle(s) and tendon(s) of peroneal muscle group at lower leg level, left leg

√7ᵗʰ   **S86.319**   Strain of muscle(s) and tendon(s) of peroneal muscle group at lower leg level, unspecified leg ▽

√6ᵗʰ   **S86.32**   Laceration of muscle(s) and tendon(s) of peroneal muscle group at lower leg level

√7ᵗʰ   **S86.321**   Laceration of muscle(s) and tendon(s) of peroneal muscle group at lower leg level, right leg

√7ᵗʰ   **S86.322**   Laceration of muscle(s) and tendon(s) of peroneal muscle group at lower leg level, left leg

√7ᵗʰ   **S86.329**   Laceration of muscle(s) and tendon(s) of peroneal muscle group at lower leg level, unspecified leg ▽

√6ᵗʰ   **S86.39**   Other injury of muscle(s) and tendon(s) of peroneal muscle group at lower leg level

√7ᵗʰ   **S86.391**   Other injury of muscle(s) and tendon(s) of peroneal muscle group at lower leg level, right leg

√7ᵗʰ   **S86.392**   Other injury of muscle(s) and tendon(s) of peroneal muscle group at lower leg level, left leg

√7ᵗʰ   **S86.399**   Other injury of muscle(s) and tendon(s) of peroneal muscle group at lower leg level, unspecified leg ▽

√5ᵗʰ   **S86.8**   Injury of other muscles and tendons at lower leg level

√6ᵗʰ   **S86.80**   Unspecified injury of other muscles and tendons at lower leg level

√7ᵗʰ   **S86.801**   Unspecified injury of other muscle(s) and tendon(s) at lower leg level, right leg ▽

√7ᵗʰ **S86.802** Unspecified injury of other muscle(s) and tendon(s) at lower leg level, left leg ▽

√7ᵗʰ **S86.809** Unspecified injury of other muscle(s) and tendon(s) at lower leg level, unspecified leg ▽

√6ᵗʰ **S86.81** Strain of other muscles and tendons at lower leg level

√7ᵗʰ **S86.811** Strain of other muscle(s) and tendon(s) at lower leg level, right leg

√7ᵗʰ **S86.812** Strain of other muscle(s) and tendon(s) at lower leg level, left leg

√7ᵗʰ **S86.819** Strain of other muscle(s) and tendon(s) at lower leg level, unspecified leg ▽

√6ᵗʰ **S86.82** Laceration of other muscles and tendons at lower leg level

√7ᵗʰ **S86.821** Laceration of other muscle(s) and tendon(s) at lower leg level, right leg

√7ᵗʰ **S86.822** Laceration of other muscle(s) and tendon(s) at lower leg level, left leg

√7ᵗʰ **S86.829** Laceration of other muscle(s) and tendon(s) at lower leg level, unspecified leg ▽

√6ᵗʰ **S86.89** Other injury of other muscles and tendons at lower leg level

√7ᵗʰ **S86.891** Other injury of other muscle(s) and tendon(s) at lower leg level, right leg

√7ᵗʰ **S86.892** Other injury of other muscle(s) and tendon(s) at lower leg level, left leg

√7ᵗʰ **S86.899** Other injury of other muscle(s) and tendon(s) at lower leg level, unspecified leg ▽

√5ᵗʰ **S86.9** Injury of unspecified muscle and tendon at lower leg level

√6ᵗʰ **S86.90** Unspecified injury of unspecified muscle and tendon at lower leg level

√7ᵗʰ **S86.901** Unspecified injury of unspecified muscle(s) and tendon(s) at lower leg level, right ▽

√7ᵗʰ **S86.902** Unspecified injury of unspecified muscle(s) and tendon(s) at lower leg level, left ▽

√7ᵗʰ **S86.909** Unspecified injury of unspecified muscle(s) and tendon(s) at lower leg level, unspecified ▽

√6ᵗʰ **S86.91** Strain of unspecified muscle and tendon at lower leg level

√7ᵗʰ **S86.911** Strain of unspecified muscle(s) and tendon(s) at lower leg level, right leg ▽

√7ᵗʰ **S86.912** Strain of unspecified muscle(s) and tendon(s) at lower leg level, left leg ▽

√7ᵗʰ **S86.919** Strain of unspecified muscle(s) and tendon(s) at lower leg level, unspecified leg ▽

√6ᵗʰ **S86.92** Laceration of unspecified muscle and tendon at lower leg level

√7ᵗʰ **S86.921** Laceration of unspecified muscle(s) and tendon(s) at lower leg level, right leg ▽

√7ᵗʰ **S86.922** Laceration of unspecified muscle(s) and tendon(s) at lower leg level, left leg ▽

√7ᵗʰ **S86.929** Laceration of unspecified muscle(s) and tendon(s) at lower leg level, unspecified leg ▽

√6ᵗʰ **S86.99** Other injury of unspecified muscle and tendon at lower leg level

√7ᵗʰ **S86.991** Other injury of unspecified muscle(s) and tendon(s) at lower leg level, right leg ▽

√7ᵗʰ **S86.992** Other injury of unspecified muscle(s) and tendon(s) at lower leg level, left leg ▽

√7ᵗʰ **S86.999** Other injury of unspecified muscle(s) and tendon(s) at lower leg level, unspecified leg ▽

√4ᵗʰ **S87** Crushing injury of lower leg

Use additional code(s) for all associated injuries

EXCLUDES 2 *crushing injury of ankle and foot (S97.-)*

The appropriate 7th character is to be added to each code from category S87.
A   initial encounter
D   subsequent encounter
S   sequela

√5ᵗʰ **S87.0** Crushing injury of knee

√x7ᵗʰ **S87.00** Crushing injury of unspecified knee ▽

√x7ᵗʰ **S87.01** Crushing injury of right knee

√x7ᵗʰ **S87.02** Crushing injury of left knee

√5ᵗʰ **S87.8** Crushing injury of lower leg

√x7ᵗʰ **S87.80** Crushing injury of unspecified lower leg ▽

√x7ᵗʰ **S87.81** Crushing injury of right lower leg

√x7ᵗʰ **S87.82** Crushing injury of left lower leg

√4ᵗʰ **S88** Traumatic amputation of lower leg

NOTE An amputation not identified as partial or complete should be coded to complete

EXCLUDES 1 *traumatic amputation of ankle and foot (S98.-)*

The appropriate 7th character is to be added to each code from category S88.
A   initial encounter
D   subsequent encounter
S   sequela

√5ᵗʰ **S88.0** Traumatic amputation at knee level

√6ᵗʰ **S88.01** Complete traumatic amputation at knee level

√7ᵗʰ **S88.011** Complete traumatic amputation at knee level, right lower leg

√7ᵗʰ **S88.012** Complete traumatic amputation at knee level, left lower leg

√7ᵗʰ **S88.019** Complete traumatic amputation at knee level, unspecified lower leg ▽

√6ᵗʰ **S88.02** Partial traumatic amputation at knee level

√7ᵗʰ **S88.021** Partial traumatic amputation at knee level, right lower leg

√7ᵗʰ **S88.022** Partial traumatic amputation at knee level, left lower leg

√7ᵗʰ **S88.029** Partial traumatic amputation at knee level, unspecified lower leg ▽

√5ᵗʰ **S88.1** Traumatic amputation at level between knee and ankle

√6ᵗʰ **S88.11** Complete traumatic amputation at level between knee and ankle

√7ᵗʰ **S88.111** Complete traumatic amputation at level between knee and ankle, right lower leg

√7ᵗʰ **S88.112** Complete traumatic amputation at level between knee and ankle, left lower leg

√7ᵗʰ **S88.119** Complete traumatic amputation at level between knee and ankle, unspecified lower leg ▽

√6ᵗʰ **S88.12** Partial traumatic amputation at level between knee and ankle

√7ᵗʰ **S88.121** Partial traumatic amputation at level between knee and ankle, right lower leg

√7ᵗʰ **S88.122** Partial traumatic amputation at level between knee and ankle, left lower leg

√7ᵗʰ **S88.129** Partial traumatic amputation at level between knee and ankle, unspecified lower leg ▽

√5ᵗʰ **S88.9** Traumatic amputation of lower leg, level unspecified

√6ᵗʰ **S88.91** Complete traumatic amputation of lower leg, level unspecified

√7ᵗʰ **S88.911** Complete traumatic amputation of right lower leg, level unspecified ▽

√7ᵗʰ **S88.912** Complete traumatic amputation of left lower leg, level unspecified ▽

√7ᵗʰ **S88.919** Complete traumatic amputation of unspecified lower leg, level unspecified ▽

√6ᵗʰ **S88.92** Partial traumatic amputation of lower leg, level unspecified

√7ᵗʰ **S88.921** Partial traumatic amputation of right lower leg, level unspecified ▽

√7ᵗʰ **S88.922** Partial traumatic amputation of left lower leg, level unspecified ▽

☑ Additional Character Required   √x7ᵗʰ Placeholder Alert   Manifestation Dx   ▽ Unspecified Dx   ►◄ Revised Text   ● New Code   ▲ Revised Code Title

ICD-10-CM 2017   **993**

☑7th **S88.929** **Partial traumatic amputation of unspecified lower leg, level unspecified** ▽

☑4th **S89** **Other and unspecified injuries of lower leg**

> **NOTE** A fracture not indicated as open or closed should be coded to closed.

> *EXCLUDES 2* *other and unspecified injuries of ankle and foot (S99.-)*
>
> **AHA:** 2015,3Q,37-39

> The appropriate 7th character is to be added to each code from subcategories S89.0, S89.1, S89.2, and S89.3.
> A   initial encounter for closed fracture
> D   subsequent encounter for fracture with routine healing
> G   subsequent encounter for fracture with delayed healing
> K   subsequent encounter for fracture with nonunion
> P   subsequent encounter for fracture with malunion
> S   sequela

☑5th **S89.0** **Physeal fracture of upper end of tibia**

   ☑6th **S89.00** **Unspecified physeal fracture of upper end of tibia**

     ☑7th **S89.001** **Unspecified physeal fracture of upper end of right tibia** ▽

     ☑7th **S89.002** **Unspecified physeal fracture of upper end of left tibia** ▽

     ☑7th **S89.009** **Unspecified physeal fracture of upper end of unspecified tibia** ▽

   ☑6th **S89.01** Salter-Harris Type I **physeal fracture of upper end of tibia**

     ☑7th **S89.011** **Salter-Harris Type I physeal fracture of upper end of right tibia**

     ☑7th **S89.012** **Salter-Harris Type I physeal fracture of upper end of left tibia**

     ☑7th **S89.019** **Salter-Harris Type I physeal fracture of upper end of unspecified tibia** ▽

   ☑6th **S89.02** Salter-Harris Type II **physeal fracture of upper end of tibia**

     ☑7th **S89.021** **Salter-Harris Type II physeal fracture of upper end of right tibia**

     ☑7th **S89.022** **Salter-Harris Type II physeal fracture of upper end of left tibia**

     ☑7th **S89.029** **Salter-Harris Type II physeal fracture of upper end of unspecified tibia** ▽

   ☑6th **S89.03** Salter-Harris Type III **physeal fracture of upper end of tibia**

     ☑7th **S89.031** **Salter-Harris Type III physeal fracture of upper end of right tibia**

     ☑7th **S89.032** **Salter-Harris Type III physeal fracture of upper end of left tibia**

     ☑7th **S89.039** **Salter-Harris Type III physeal fracture of upper end of unspecified tibia** ▽

   ☑6th **S89.04** Salter-Harris Type IV **physeal fracture of upper end of tibia**

     ☑7th **S89.041** **Salter-Harris Type IV physeal fracture of upper end of right tibia**

     ☑7th **S89.042** **Salter-Harris Type IV physeal fracture of upper end of left tibia**

     ☑7th **S89.049** **Salter-Harris Type IV physeal fracture of upper end of unspecified tibia** ▽

   ☑6th **S89.09** **Other physeal fracture of upper end of tibia**

     ☑7th **S89.091** **Other physeal fracture of upper end of right tibia**

     ☑7th **S89.092** **Other physeal fracture of upper end of left tibia**

     ☑7th **S89.099** **Other physeal fracture of upper end of unspecified tibia** ▽

☑5th **S89.1** **Physeal fracture of lower end of tibia**

   ☑6th **S89.10** **Unspecified physeal fracture of lower end of tibia**

     ☑7th **S89.101** **Unspecified physeal fracture of lower end of right tibia** ▽

     ☑7th **S89.102** **Unspecified physeal fracture of lower end of left tibia** ▽

     ☑7th **S89.109** **Unspecified physeal fracture of lower end of unspecified tibia** ▽

   ☑6th **S89.11** Salter-Harris Type I **physeal fracture of lower end of tibia**

     ☑7th **S89.111** **Salter-Harris Type I physeal fracture of lower end of right tibia**

     ☑7th **S89.112** **Salter-Harris Type I physeal fracture of lower end of left tibia**

     ☑7th **S89.119** **Salter-Harris Type I physeal fracture of lower end of unspecified tibia** ▽

   ☑6th **S89.12** Salter-Harris Type II **physeal fracture of lower end of tibia**

     ☑7th **S89.121** **Salter-Harris Type II physeal fracture of lower end of right tibia**

     ☑7th **S89.122** **Salter-Harris Type II physeal fracture of lower end of left tibia**

     ☑7th **S89.129** **Salter-Harris Type II physeal fracture of lower end of unspecified tibia** ▽

   ☑6th **S89.13** Salter-Harris Type III **physeal fracture of lower end of tibia**

> *EXCLUDES 1* *fracture of medial malleolus (adult) (S82.5-)*

     ☑7th **S89.131** **Salter-Harris Type III physeal fracture of lower end of right tibia**

     ☑7th **S89.132** **Salter-Harris Type III physeal fracture of lower end of left tibia**

     ☑7th **S89.139** **Salter-Harris Type III physeal fracture of lower end of unspecified tibia** ▽

   ☑6th **S89.14** Salter-Harris Type IV **physeal fracture of lower end of tibia**

> *EXCLUDES 1* *fracture of medial malleolus (adult) (S82.5-)*

     ☑7th **S89.141** **Salter-Harris Type IV physeal fracture of lower end of right tibia**

     ☑7th **S89.142** **Salter-Harris Type IV physeal fracture of lower end of left tibia**

     ☑7th **S89.149** **Salter-Harris Type IV physeal fracture of lower end of unspecified tibia** ▽

   ☑6th **S89.19** **Other physeal fracture of lower end of tibia**

     ☑7th **S89.191** **Other physeal fracture of lower end of right tibia**

     ☑7th **S89.192** **Other physeal fracture of lower end of left tibia**

     ☑7th **S89.199** **Other physeal fracture of lower end of unspecified tibia** ▽

☑5th **S89.2** **Physeal fracture of upper end of fibula**

   ☑6th **S89.20** **Unspecified physeal fracture of upper end of fibula**

     ☑7th **S89.201** **Unspecified physeal fracture of upper end of right fibula** ▽

     ☑7th **S89.202** **Unspecified physeal fracture of upper end of left fibula** ▽

     ☑7th **S89.209** **Unspecified physeal fracture of upper end of unspecified fibula** ▽

   ☑6th **S89.21** Salter-Harris Type I **physeal fracture of upper end of fibula**

     ☑7th **S89.211** **Salter-Harris Type I physeal fracture of upper end of right fibula**

     ☑7th **S89.212** **Salter-Harris Type I physeal fracture of upper end of left fibula**

     ☑7th **S89.219** **Salter-Harris Type I physeal fracture of upper end of unspecified fibula** ▽

   ☑6th **S89.22** Salter-Harris Type II **physeal fracture of upper end of fibula**

     ☑7th **S89.221** **Salter-Harris Type II physeal fracture of upper end of right fibula**

     ☑7th **S89.222** **Salter-Harris Type II physeal fracture of upper end of left fibula**

     ☑7th **S89.229** **Salter-Harris Type II physeal fracture of upper end of unspecified fibula** ▽

   ☑6th **S89.29** **Other physeal fracture of upper end of fibula**

     ☑7th **S89.291** **Other physeal fracture of upper end of right fibula**

     ☑7th **S89.292** **Other physeal fracture of upper end of left fibula**

     ☑7th **S89.299** **Other physeal fracture of upper end of unspecified fibula** ▽

☑5th **S89.3** **Physeal fracture of lower end of fibula**

   ☑6th **S89.30** **Unspecified physeal fracture of lower end of fibula**

     ☑7th **S89.301** **Unspecified physeal fracture of lower end of right fibula** ▽

     ☑7th **S89.302** **Unspecified physeal fracture of lower end of left fibula** ▽

     ☑7th **S89.309** **Unspecified physeal fracture of lower end of unspecified fibula** ▽

EXCLUDES 1 Not coded here   *EXCLUDES 2* Not included here   N Newborn Age : 0   P Pediatric Age : 0-17   M Maternity Age : 12-55   A Adult Age : 15-124

994   ICD-10-CM 2017

☑6ᵗʰ **S89.31** Salter-Harris Type I physeal fracture of lower end of fibula

    ☑7ᵗʰ **S89.311** Salter-Harris Type I physeal fracture of lower end of right fibula

    ☑7ᵗʰ **S89.312** Salter-Harris Type I physeal fracture of lower end of left fibula

    ☑7ᵗʰ **S89.319** Salter-Harris Type I physeal fracture of lower end of unspecified fibula ▽

☑6ᵗʰ **S89.32** Salter-Harris Type II physeal fracture of lower end of fibula

    ☑7ᵗʰ **S89.321** Salter-Harris Type II physeal fracture of lower end of right fibula

    ☑7ᵗʰ **S89.322** Salter-Harris Type II physeal fracture of lower end of left fibula

    ☑7ᵗʰ **S89.329** Salter-Harris Type II physeal fracture of lower end of unspecified fibula ▽

☑6ᵗʰ **S89.39** Other physeal fracture of lower end of fibula

    ☑7ᵗʰ **S89.391** Other physeal fracture of lower end of right fibula

    ☑7ᵗʰ **S89.392** Other physeal fracture of lower end of left fibula

    ☑7ᵗʰ **S89.399** Other physeal fracture of lower end of unspecified fibula ▽

☑5ᵗʰ **S89.8** Other specified injuries of lower leg

> The appropriate 7th character is to be added to each code in subcategory S89.8
> A   initial encounter
> D   subsequent encounter
> S   sequela

☑x7ᵗʰ **S89.80** Other specified injuries of unspecified lower leg ▽

☑x7ᵗʰ **S89.81** Other specified injuries of right lower leg

☑x7ᵗʰ **S89.82** Other specified injuries of left lower leg

☑5ᵗʰ **S89.9** Unspecified injury of lower leg

> The appropriate 7th character is to be added to each code in subcategory S89.9
> A   initial encounter
> D   subsequent encounter
> S   sequela

☑x7ᵗʰ **S89.90** Unspecified injury of unspecified lower leg ▽

☑x7ᵗʰ **S89.91** Unspecified injury of right lower leg ▽

☑x7ᵗʰ **S89.92** Unspecified injury of left lower leg ▽

Injuries to the ankle and foot (S90-S99)

EXCLUDES 2   burns and corrosions (T20-T32)
     fracture of ankle and malleolus (S82.-)
     frostbite (T33-T34)
     insect bite or sting, venomous (T63.4)

☑4ᵗʰ **S90** Superficial injury of ankle, foot and toes

> The appropriate 7th character is to be added to each code from category S90.
> A   initial encounter
> D   subsequent encounter
> S   sequela

☑5ᵗʰ **S90.0** Contusion of ankle

☑x7ᵗʰ **S90.00** Contusion of unspecified ankle ▽

☑x7ᵗʰ **S90.01** Contusion of right ankle

☑x7ᵗʰ **S90.02** Contusion of left ankle

☑5ᵗʰ **S90.1** Contusion of toe without damage to nail

☑6ᵗʰ **S90.11** Contusion of great toe without damage to nail

    ☑7ᵗʰ **S90.111** Contusion of right great toe without damage to nail

    ☑7ᵗʰ **S90.112** Contusion of left great toe without damage to nail

    ☑7ᵗʰ **S90.119** Contusion of unspecified great toe without damage to nail ▽

☑6ᵗʰ **S90.12** Contusion of lesser toe without damage to nail

    ☑7ᵗʰ **S90.121** Contusion of right lesser toe(s) without damage to nail

    ☑7ᵗʰ **S90.122** Contusion of left lesser toe(s) without damage to nail

    ☑7ᵗʰ **S90.129** Contusion of unspecified lesser toe(s) without damage to nail ▽
     Contusion of toe NOS

☑5ᵗʰ **S90.2** Contusion of toe with damage to nail

☑6ᵗʰ **S90.21** Contusion of great toe with damage to nail

    ☑7ᵗʰ **S90.211** Contusion of right great toe with damage to nail

    ☑7ᵗʰ **S90.212** Contusion of left great toe with damage to nail

    ☑7ᵗʰ **S90.219** Contusion of unspecified great toe with damage to nail ▽

☑6ᵗʰ **S90.22** Contusion of lesser toe with damage to nail

    ☑7ᵗʰ **S90.221** Contusion of right lesser toe(s) with damage to nail

    ☑7ᵗʰ **S90.222** Contusion of left lesser toe(s) with damage to nail

    ☑7ᵗʰ **S90.229** Contusion of unspecified lesser toe(s) with damage to nail ▽

☑5ᵗʰ **S90.3** Contusion of foot

> EXCLUDES 2   contusion of toes (S90.1-, S90.2-)

☑x7ᵗʰ **S90.30** Contusion of unspecified foot ▽
     Contusion of foot NOS

☑x7ᵗʰ **S90.31** Contusion of right foot

☑x7ᵗʰ **S90.32** Contusion of left foot

☑5ᵗʰ **S90.4** Other superficial injuries of toe

☑6ᵗʰ **S90.41** Abrasion of toe

    ☑7ᵗʰ **S90.411** Abrasion, right great toe

    ☑7ᵗʰ **S90.412** Abrasion, left great toe

    ☑7ᵗʰ **S90.413** Abrasion, unspecified great toe ▽

    ☑7ᵗʰ **S90.414** Abrasion, right lesser toe(s)

    ☑7ᵗʰ **S90.415** Abrasion, left lesser toe(s)

    ☑7ᵗʰ **S90.416** Abrasion, unspecified lesser toe(s) ▽

☑6ᵗʰ **S90.42** Blister (nonthermal) of toe

    ☑7ᵗʰ **S90.421** Blister (nonthermal), right great toe

    ☑7ᵗʰ **S90.422** Blister (nonthermal), left great toe

    ☑7ᵗʰ **S90.423** Blister (nonthermal), unspecified great toe ▽

    ☑7ᵗʰ **S90.424** Blister (nonthermal), right lesser toe(s)

    ☑7ᵗʰ **S90.425** Blister (nonthermal), left lesser toe(s)

    ☑7ᵗʰ **S90.426** Blister (nonthermal), unspecified lesser toe(s) ▽

☑6ᵗʰ **S90.44** External constriction of toe
     Hair tourniquet syndrome of toe

    ☑7ᵗʰ **S90.441** External constriction, right great toe

    ☑7ᵗʰ **S90.442** External constriction, left great toe

    ☑7ᵗʰ **S90.443** External constriction, unspecified great toe ▽

    ☑7ᵗʰ **S90.444** External constriction, right lesser toe(s)

    ☑7ᵗʰ **S90.445** External constriction, left lesser toe(s)

    ☑7ᵗʰ **S90.446** External constriction, unspecified lesser toe(s) ▽

☑6ᵗʰ **S90.45** Superficial foreign body of toe
     Splinter in the toe

    ☑7ᵗʰ **S90.451** Superficial foreign body, right great toe

    ☑7ᵗʰ **S90.452** Superficial foreign body, left great toe

    ☑7ᵗʰ **S90.453** Superficial foreign body, unspecified great toe ▽

    ☑7ᵗʰ **S90.454** Superficial foreign body, right lesser toe(s)

    ☑7ᵗʰ **S90.455** Superficial foreign body, left lesser toe(s)

    ☑7ᵗʰ **S90.456** Superficial foreign body, unspecified lesser toe(s) ▽

☑6ᵗʰ **S90.46** Insect bite (nonvenomous) of toe

    ☑7ᵗʰ **S90.461** Insect bite (nonvenomous), right great toe

    ☑7ᵗʰ **S90.462** Insect bite (nonvenomous), left great toe

    ☑7ᵗʰ **S90.463** Insect bite (nonvenomous), unspecified great toe ▽

    ☑7ᵗʰ **S90.464** Insect bite (nonvenomous), right lesser toe(s)

    ☑7ᵗʰ **S90.465** Insect bite (nonvenomous), left lesser toe(s)

    ☑7ᵗʰ **S90.466** Insect bite (nonvenomous), unspecified lesser toe(s) ▽

✓6ᵗʰ **S90.47** Other superficial bite of toe
     EXCLUDES 1 *open bite of toe (S91.15-, S91.25-)*
- ✓7ᵗʰ **S90.471** Other superficial bite of right great toe
- ✓7ᵗʰ **S90.472** Other superficial bite of left great toe
- ✓7ᵗʰ **S90.473** Other superficial bite of unspecified great toe ▽
- ✓7ᵗʰ **S90.474** Other superficial bite of right lesser toe(s)
- ✓7ᵗʰ **S90.475** Other superficial bite of left lesser toe(s)
- ✓7ᵗʰ **S90.476** Other superficial bite of unspecified lesser toe(s) ▽

✓5ᵗʰ **S90.5** Other superficial injuries of ankle
- ✓6ᵗʰ **S90.51** Abrasion of ankle
  - ✓7ᵗʰ **S90.511** Abrasion, right ankle
  - ✓7ᵗʰ **S90.512** Abrasion, left ankle
  - ✓7ᵗʰ **S90.519** Abrasion, unspecified ankle ▽
- ✓6ᵗʰ **S90.52** Blister (nonthermal) of ankle
  - ✓7ᵗʰ **S90.521** Blister (nonthermal), right ankle
  - ✓7ᵗʰ **S90.522** Blister (nonthermal), left ankle
  - ✓7ᵗʰ **S90.529** Blister (nonthermal), unspecified ankle ▽
- ✓6ᵗʰ **S90.54** External constriction of ankle
  - ✓7ᵗʰ **S90.541** External constriction, right ankle
  - ✓7ᵗʰ **S90.542** External constriction, left ankle
  - ✓7ᵗʰ **S90.549** External constriction, unspecified ankle ▽
- ✓6ᵗʰ **S90.55** Superficial foreign body of ankle
  - Splinter in the ankle
  - ✓7ᵗʰ **S90.551** Superficial foreign body, right ankle
  - ✓7ᵗʰ **S90.552** Superficial foreign body, left ankle
  - ✓7ᵗʰ **S90.559** Superficial foreign body, unspecified ankle ▽
- ✓6ᵗʰ **S90.56** Insect bite (nonvenomous) of ankle
  - ✓7ᵗʰ **S90.561** Insect bite (nonvenomous), right ankle
  - ✓7ᵗʰ **S90.562** Insect bite (nonvenomous), left ankle
  - ✓7ᵗʰ **S90.569** Insect bite (nonvenomous), unspecified ankle ▽
- ✓6ᵗʰ **S90.57** Other superficial bite of ankle
  - **EXCLUDES 1** *open bite of ankle (S91.05-)*
  - ✓7ᵗʰ **S90.571** Other superficial bite of ankle, right ankle
  - ✓7ᵗʰ **S90.572** Other superficial bite of ankle, left ankle
  - ✓7ᵗʰ **S90.579** Other superficial bite of ankle, unspecified ankle ▽

✓5ᵗʰ **S90.8** Other superficial injuries of foot
- ✓6ᵗʰ **S90.81** Abrasion of foot
  - ✓7ᵗʰ **S90.811** Abrasion, right foot
  - ✓7ᵗʰ **S90.812** Abrasion, left foot
  - ✓7ᵗʰ **S90.819** Abrasion, unspecified foot ▽
- ✓6ᵗʰ **S90.82** Blister (nonthermal) of foot
  - ✓7ᵗʰ **S90.821** Blister (nonthermal), right foot
  - ✓7ᵗʰ **S90.822** Blister (nonthermal), left foot
  - ✓7ᵗʰ **S90.829** Blister (nonthermal), unspecified foot ▽
- ✓6ᵗʰ **S90.84** External constriction of foot
  - ✓7ᵗʰ **S90.841** External constriction, right foot
  - ✓7ᵗʰ **S90.842** External constriction, left foot
  - ✓7ᵗʰ **S90.849** External constriction, unspecified foot ▽
- ✓6ᵗʰ **S90.85** Superficial foreign body of foot
  - Splinter in the foot
  - ✓7ᵗʰ **S90.851** Superficial foreign body, right foot
  - ✓7ᵗʰ **S90.852** Superficial foreign body, left foot
  - ✓7ᵗʰ **S90.859** Superficial foreign body, unspecified foot ▽
- ✓6ᵗʰ **S90.86** Insect bite (nonvenomous) of foot
  - ✓7ᵗʰ **S90.861** Insect bite (nonvenomous), right foot
  - ✓7ᵗʰ **S90.862** Insect bite (nonvenomous), left foot
  - ✓7ᵗʰ **S90.869** Insect bite (nonvenomous), unspecified foot ▽
- ✓6ᵗʰ **S90.87** Other superficial bite of foot
  - **EXCLUDES 1** *open bite of foot (S91.35-)*
  - ✓7ᵗʰ **S90.871** Other superficial bite of right foot

- ✓7ᵗʰ **S90.872** Other superficial bite of left foot
- ✓7ᵗʰ **S90.879** Other superficial bite of unspecified foot ▽

✓5ᵗʰ **S90.9** Unspecified superficial injury of ankle, foot and toe
- ✓6ᵗʰ **S90.91** Unspecified superficial injury of ankle
  - ✓7ᵗʰ **S90.911** Unspecified superficial injury of right ankle ▽
  - ✓7ᵗʰ **S90.912** Unspecified superficial injury of left ankle ▽
  - ✓7ᵗʰ **S90.919** Unspecified superficial injury of unspecified ankle ▽
- ✓6ᵗʰ **S90.92** Unspecified superficial injury of foot
  - ✓7ᵗʰ **S90.921** Unspecified superficial injury of right foot ▽
  - ✓7ᵗʰ **S90.922** Unspecified superficial injury of left foot ▽
  - ✓7ᵗʰ **S90.929** Unspecified superficial injury of unspecified foot ▽
- ✓6ᵗʰ **S90.93** Unspecified superficial injury of toes
  - ✓7ᵗʰ **S90.931** Unspecified superficial injury of right great toe ▽
  - ✓7ᵗʰ **S90.932** Unspecified superficial injury of left great toe ▽
  - ✓7ᵗʰ **S90.933** Unspecified superficial injury of unspecified great toe ▽
  - ✓7ᵗʰ **S90.934** Unspecified superficial injury of right lesser toe(s) ▽
  - ✓7ᵗʰ **S90.935** Unspecified superficial injury of left lesser toe(s) ▽
  - ✓7ᵗʰ **S90.936** Unspecified superficial injury of unspecified lesser toe(s) ▽

✓4ᵗʰ **S91** Open wound of ankle, foot and toes
     Code also any associated wound infection
     EXCLUDES 1 *open fracture of ankle, foot and toes (S92.- with 7th character B)*
         traumatic amputation of ankle and foot (S98.-)

> The appropriate 7th character is to be added to each code from category S91.
> A   initial encounter
> D   subsequent encounter
> S   sequela

✓5ᵗʰ **S91.0** Open wound of ankle
- ✓6ᵗʰ **S91.00** Unspecified open wound of ankle
  - ✓7ᵗʰ **S91.001** Unspecified open wound, right ankle ▽
  - ✓7ᵗʰ **S91.002** Unspecified open wound, left ankle ▽
  - ✓7ᵗʰ **S91.009** Unspecified open wound, unspecified ankle ▽
- ✓6ᵗʰ **S91.01** Laceration without foreign body of ankle
  - ✓7ᵗʰ **S91.011** Laceration without foreign body, right ankle ▽
  - ✓7ᵗʰ **S91.012** Laceration without foreign body, left ankle ▽
  - ✓7ᵗʰ **S91.019** Laceration without foreign body, unspecified ankle ▽
- ✓6ᵗʰ **S91.02** Laceration with foreign body of ankle
  - ✓7ᵗʰ **S91.021** Laceration with foreign body, right ankle
  - ✓7ᵗʰ **S91.022** Laceration with foreign body, left ankle
  - ✓7ᵗʰ **S91.029** Laceration with foreign body, unspecified ankle ▽
- ✓6ᵗʰ **S91.03** Puncture wound without foreign body of ankle
  - ✓7ᵗʰ **S91.031** Puncture wound without foreign body, right ankle
  - ✓7ᵗʰ **S91.032** Puncture wound without foreign body, left ankle
  - ✓7ᵗʰ **S91.039** Puncture wound without foreign body, unspecified ankle ▽
- ✓6ᵗʰ **S91.04** Puncture wound with foreign body of ankle
  - ✓7ᵗʰ **S91.041** Puncture wound with foreign body, right ankle
  - ✓7ᵗʰ **S91.042** Puncture wound with foreign body, left ankle
  - ✓7ᵗʰ **S91.049** Puncture wound with foreign body, unspecified ankle ▽
- ✓6ᵗʰ **S91.05** Open bite of ankle
  - **EXCLUDES 1** *superficial bite of ankle (S90.56-, S90.57-)*
  - ✓7ᵗʰ **S91.051** Open bite, right ankle

EXCLUDES 1 Not coded here   **EXCLUDES 2** Not included here   **N** Newborn Age : 0   **P** Pediatric Age : 0-17   **M** Maternity Age : 12-55   **A** Adult Age : 15-124

996   ICD-10-CM 2017

√7ᵗʰ **S91.052** Open bite, left ankle

√7ᵗʰ **S91.059** Open bite, unspecified ankle ▽

✓5ᵗʰ **S91.1** **Open wound of toe without damage to nail**

✓6ᵗʰ **S91.10** **Unspecified open wound of toe without damage to nail**

√7ᵗʰ **S91.101** Unspecified open wound of right great toe without damage to nail ▽

√7ᵗʰ **S91.102** Unspecified open wound of left great toe without damage to nail ▽

√7ᵗʰ **S91.103** Unspecified open wound of unspecified great toe without damage to nail ▽

√7ᵗʰ **S91.104** Unspecified open wound of right lesser toe(s) without damage to nail ▽

√7ᵗʰ **S91.105** Unspecified open wound of left lesser toe(s) without damage to nail ▽

√7ᵗʰ **S91.106** Unspecified open wound of unspecified lesser toe(s) without damage to nail ▽

√7ᵗʰ **S91.109** Unspecified open wound of unspecified toe(s) without damage to nail ▽

✓6ᵗʰ **S91.11** **Laceration without foreign body of toe without damage to nail**

√7ᵗʰ **S91.111** Laceration without foreign body of right great toe without damage to nail

√7ᵗʰ **S91.112** Laceration without foreign body of left great toe without damage to nail

√7ᵗʰ **S91.113** Laceration without foreign body of unspecified great toe without damage to nail ▽

√7ᵗʰ **S91.114** Laceration without foreign body of right lesser toe(s) without damage to nail

√7ᵗʰ **S91.115** Laceration without foreign body of left lesser toe(s) without damage to nail

√7ᵗʰ **S91.116** Laceration without foreign body of unspecified lesser toe(s) without damage to nail ▽

√7ᵗʰ **S91.119** Laceration without foreign body of unspecified toe without damage to nail ▽

✓6ᵗʰ **S91.12** **Laceration with foreign body of toe without damage to nail**

√7ᵗʰ **S91.121** Laceration with foreign body of right great toe without damage to nail

√7ᵗʰ **S91.122** Laceration with foreign body of left great toe without damage to nail

√7ᵗʰ **S91.123** Laceration with foreign body of unspecified great toe without damage to nail ▽

√7ᵗʰ **S91.124** Laceration with foreign body of right lesser toe(s) without damage to nail

√7ᵗʰ **S91.125** Laceration with foreign body of left lesser toe(s) without damage to nail

√7ᵗʰ **S91.126** Laceration with foreign body of unspecified lesser toe(s) without damage to nail ▽

√7ᵗʰ **S91.129** Laceration with foreign body of unspecified toe(s) without damage to nail ▽

✓6ᵗʰ **S91.13** **Puncture wound without foreign body of toe without damage to nail**

√7ᵗʰ **S91.131** Puncture wound without foreign body of right great toe without damage to nail

√7ᵗʰ **S91.132** Puncture wound without foreign body of left great toe without damage to nail

√7ᵗʰ **S91.133** Puncture wound without foreign body of unspecified great toe without damage to nail ▽

√7ᵗʰ **S91.134** Puncture wound without foreign body of right lesser toe(s) without damage to nail

√7ᵗʰ **S91.135** Puncture wound without foreign body of left lesser toe(s) without damage to nail

√7ᵗʰ **S91.136** Puncture wound without foreign body of unspecified lesser toe(s) without damage to nail ▽

√7ᵗʰ **S91.139** Puncture wound without foreign body of unspecified toe(s) without damage to nail ▽

✓6ᵗʰ **S91.14** **Puncture wound with foreign body of toe without damage to nail**

√7ᵗʰ **S91.141** Puncture wound with foreign body of right great toe without damage to nail

√7ᵗʰ **S91.142** Puncture wound with foreign body of left great toe without damage to nail

√7ᵗʰ **S91.143** Puncture wound with foreign body of unspecified great toe without damage to nail ▽

√7ᵗʰ **S91.144** Puncture wound with foreign body of right lesser toe(s) without damage to nail

√7ᵗʰ **S91.145** Puncture wound with foreign body of left lesser toe(s) without damage to nail

√7ᵗʰ **S91.146** Puncture wound with foreign body of unspecified lesser toe(s) without damage to nail ▽

√7ᵗʰ **S91.149** Puncture wound with foreign body of unspecified toe(s) without damage to nail ▽

✓6ᵗʰ **S91.15** **Open bite of toe without damage to nail**

Bite of toe NOS

EXCLUDES 1 *superficial bite of toe (S90.46-, S90.47-)*

√7ᵗʰ **S91.151** Open bite of right great toe without damage to nail

√7ᵗʰ **S91.152** Open bite of left great toe without damage to nail

√7ᵗʰ **S91.153** Open bite of unspecified great toe without damage to nail ▽

√7ᵗʰ **S91.154** Open bite of right lesser toe(s) without damage to nail

√7ᵗʰ **S91.155** Open bite of left lesser toe(s) without damage to nail

√7ᵗʰ **S91.156** Open bite of unspecified lesser toe(s) without damage to nail ▽

√7ᵗʰ **S91.159** Open bite of unspecified toe(s) without damage to nail ▽

✓5ᵗʰ **S91.2** **Open wound of toe with damage to nail**

✓6ᵗʰ **S91.20** **Unspecified open wound of toe with damage to nail**

√7ᵗʰ **S91.201** Unspecified open wound of right great toe with damage to nail ▽

√7ᵗʰ **S91.202** Unspecified open wound of left great toe with damage to nail ▽

√7ᵗʰ **S91.203** Unspecified open wound of unspecified great toe with damage to nail ▽

√7ᵗʰ **S91.204** Unspecified open wound of right lesser toe(s) with damage to nail ▽

√7ᵗʰ **S91.205** Unspecified open wound of left lesser toe(s) with damage to nail ▽

√7ᵗʰ **S91.206** Unspecified open wound of unspecified lesser toe(s) with damage to nail ▽

√7ᵗʰ **S91.209** Unspecified open wound of unspecified toe(s) with damage to nail ▽

✓6ᵗʰ **S91.21** **Laceration without foreign body of toe with damage to nail**

√7ᵗʰ **S91.211** Laceration without foreign body of right great toe with damage to nail

√7ᵗʰ **S91.212** Laceration without foreign body of left great toe with damage to nail

√7ᵗʰ **S91.213** Laceration without foreign body of unspecified great toe with damage to nail ▽

√7ᵗʰ **S91.214** Laceration without foreign body of right lesser toe(s) with damage to nail

√7ᵗʰ **S91.215** Laceration without foreign body of left lesser toe(s) with damage to nail

√7ᵗʰ **S91.216** Laceration without foreign body of unspecified lesser toe(s) with damage to nail ▽

√7ᵗʰ **S91.219** Laceration without foreign body of unspecified toe(s) with damage to nail ▽

✓6ᵗʰ **S91.22** **Laceration with foreign body of toe with damage to nail**

√7ᵗʰ **S91.221** Laceration with foreign body of right great toe with damage to nail

√7ᵗʰ **S91.222** Laceration with foreign body of left great toe with damage to nail

√7ᵗʰ **S91.223** Laceration with foreign body of unspecified great toe with damage to nail ▽

√7ᵗʰ **S91.224** Laceration with foreign body of right lesser toe(s) with damage to nail

☑ Additional Character Required   √x7ᵗʰ Placeholder Alert   Manifestation Dx   ▽ Unspecified Dx   ▶◀ Revised Text   ● New Code   ▲ Revised Code Title

ICD-10-CM 2017   **997**

√7ᵗʰ **S91.225** Laceration with foreign body of left lesser toe(s) with damage to nail

√7ᵗʰ **S91.226** Laceration with foreign body of unspecified lesser toe(s) with damage to nail ▽

√7ᵗʰ **S91.229** Laceration with foreign body of unspecified toe(s) with damage to nail ▽

√6ᵗʰ **S91.23** Puncture wound without foreign body of toe with damage to nail

√7ᵗʰ **S91.231** Puncture wound without foreign body of right great toe with damage to nail

√7ᵗʰ **S91.232** Puncture wound without foreign body of left great toe with damage to nail

√7ᵗʰ **S91.233** Puncture wound without foreign body of unspecified great toe with damage to nail ▽

√7ᵗʰ **S91.234** Puncture wound without foreign body of right lesser toe(s) with damage to nail

√7ᵗʰ **S91.235** Puncture wound without foreign body of left lesser toe(s) with damage to nail

√7ᵗʰ **S91.236** Puncture wound without foreign body of unspecified lesser toe(s) with damage to nail ▽

√7ᵗʰ **S91.239** Puncture wound without foreign body of unspecified toe(s) with damage to nail ▽

√6ᵗʰ **S91.24** Puncture wound with foreign body of toe with damage to nail

√7ᵗʰ **S91.241** Puncture wound with foreign body of right great toe with damage to nail

√7ᵗʰ **S91.242** Puncture wound with foreign body of left great toe with damage to nail

√7ᵗʰ **S91.243** Puncture wound with foreign body of unspecified great toe with damage to nail ▽

√7ᵗʰ **S91.244** Puncture wound with foreign body of right lesser toe(s) with damage to nail

√7ᵗʰ **S91.245** Puncture wound with foreign body of left lesser toe(s) with damage to nail

√7ᵗʰ **S91.246** Puncture wound with foreign body of unspecified lesser toe(s) with damage to nail ▽

√7ᵗʰ **S91.249** Puncture wound with foreign body of unspecified toe(s) with damage to nail ▽

√6ᵗʰ **S91.25** Open bite of toe with damage to nail

Bite of toe with damage to nail NOS

EXCLUDES 1 superficial bite of toe (S90.46-, S90.47-)

√7ᵗʰ **S91.251** Open bite of right great toe with damage to nail

√7ᵗʰ **S91.252** Open bite of left great toe with damage to nail

√7ᵗʰ **S91.253** Open bite of unspecified great toe with damage to nail ▽

√7ᵗʰ **S91.254** Open bite of right lesser toe(s) with damage to nail

√7ᵗʰ **S91.255** Open bite of left lesser toe(s) with damage to nail

√7ᵗʰ **S91.256** Open bite of unspecified lesser toe(s) with damage to nail ▽

√7ᵗʰ **S91.259** Open bite of unspecified toe(s) with damage to nail ▽

√5ᵗʰ **S91.3** Open wound of foot

√6ᵗʰ **S91.30** Unspecified open wound of foot

√7ᵗʰ **S91.301** Unspecified open wound, right foot ▽

√7ᵗʰ **S91.302** Unspecified open wound, left foot ▽

√7ᵗʰ **S91.309** Unspecified open wound, unspecified foot ▽

√6ᵗʰ **S91.31** Laceration without foreign body of foot

√7ᵗʰ **S91.311** Laceration without foreign body, right foot

√7ᵗʰ **S91.312** Laceration without foreign body, left foot

√7ᵗʰ **S91.319** Laceration without foreign body, unspecified foot ▽

√6ᵗʰ **S91.32** Laceration with foreign body of foot

√7ᵗʰ **S91.321** Laceration with foreign body, right foot

√7ᵗʰ **S91.322** Laceration with foreign body, left foot

√7ᵗʰ **S91.329** Laceration with foreign body, unspecified foot ▽

√6ᵗʰ **S91.33** Puncture wound without foreign body of foot

√7ᵗʰ **S91.331** Puncture wound without foreign body, right foot

√7ᵗʰ **S91.332** Puncture wound without foreign body, left foot

√7ᵗʰ **S91.339** Puncture wound without foreign body, unspecified foot ▽

√6ᵗʰ **S91.34** Puncture wound with foreign body of foot

√7ᵗʰ **S91.341** Puncture wound with foreign body, right foot

√7ᵗʰ **S91.342** Puncture wound with foreign body, left foot

√7ᵗʰ **S91.349** Puncture wound with foreign body, unspecified foot ▽

√6ᵗʰ **S91.35** Open bite of foot

EXCLUDES 1 superficial bite of foot (S90.86-, S90.87-)

√7ᵗʰ **S91.351** Open bite, right foot

√7ᵗʰ **S91.352** Open bite, left foot

√7ᵗʰ **S91.359** Open bite, unspecified foot ▽

√4ᵗʰ **S92** Fracture of foot and toe, except ankle

NOTE A fracture not indicated as displaced or nondisplaced should be coded to displaced

A fracture not indicated as open or closed should be coded to closed.

EXCLUDES 1 traumatic amputation of ankle and foot (S98.-)

EXCLUDES 2 fracture of ankle (S82.-)

fracture of malleolus (S82.-)

AHA: 2015,3Q,37-39

The appropriate 7th character is to be added to each code from category S92.

A initial encounter for closed fracture

B initial encounter for open fracture

D subsequent encounter for fracture with routine healing

G subsequent encounter for fracture with delayed healing

K subsequent encounter for fracture with nonunion

P subsequent encounter for fracture with malunion

S sequela

√5ᵗʰ **S92.0** Fracture of calcaneus

Heel bone

Os calcis

EXCLUDES 2 ▶physeal fracture of calcaneus (S99.0-)◀

√6ᵗʰ **S92.00** Unspecified fracture of calcaneus

√7ᵗʰ **S92.001** Unspecified fracture of right calcaneus ▽

√7ᵗʰ **S92.002** Unspecified fracture of left calcaneus ▽

√7ᵗʰ **S92.009** Unspecified fracture of unspecified calcaneus ▽

√6ᵗʰ **S92.01** Fracture of body of calcaneus

√7ᵗʰ **S92.011** Displaced fracture of body of right calcaneus

√7ᵗʰ **S92.012** Displaced fracture of body of left calcaneus

√7ᵗʰ **S92.013** Displaced fracture of body of unspecified calcaneus ▽

√7ᵗʰ **S92.014** Nondisplaced fracture of body of right calcaneus

√7ᵗʰ **S92.015** Nondisplaced fracture of body of left calcaneus

√7ᵗʰ **S92.016** Nondisplaced fracture of body of unspecified calcaneus ▽

√6ᵗʰ **S92.02** Fracture of anterior process of calcaneus

√7ᵗʰ **S92.021** Displaced fracture of anterior process of right calcaneus

√7ᵗʰ **S92.022** Displaced fracture of anterior process of left calcaneus

√7ᵗʰ **S92.023** Displaced fracture of anterior process of unspecified calcaneus ▽

√7ᵗʰ **S92.024** Nondisplaced fracture of anterior process of right calcaneus

√7ᵗʰ **S92.025** Nondisplaced fracture of anterior process of left calcaneus

√7ᵗʰ **S92.026** Nondisplaced fracture of anterior process of unspecified calcaneus ▽

√6ᵗʰ **S92.03** Avulsion fracture of tuberosity of calcaneus

√7ᵗʰ **S92.031** Displaced avulsion fracture of tuberosity of right calcaneus

EXCLUDES 1 Not coded here   *EXCLUDES 2* Not included here   N Newborn Age : 0   P Pediatric Age : 0-17   M Maternity Age : 12-55   A Adult Age : 15-124

998

ICD-10-CM 2017

√7ᵗʰ **S92.032** Displaced avulsion fracture of tuberosity of left calcaneus

√7ᵗʰ **S92.033** Displaced avulsion fracture of tuberosity of unspecified calcaneus ▽

√7ᵗʰ **S92.034** Nondisplaced avulsion fracture of tuberosity of right calcaneus

√7ᵗʰ **S92.035** Nondisplaced avulsion fracture of tuberosity of left calcaneus

√7ᵗʰ **S92.036** Nondisplaced avulsion fracture of tuberosity of unspecified calcaneus ▽

√6ᵗʰ **S92.04** Other fracture of tuberosity of calcaneus

√7ᵗʰ **S92.041** Displaced other fracture of tuberosity of right calcaneus

√7ᵗʰ **S92.042** Displaced other fracture of tuberosity of left calcaneus

√7ᵗʰ **S92.043** Displaced other fracture of tuberosity of unspecified calcaneus ▽

√7ᵗʰ **S92.044** Nondisplaced other fracture of tuberosity of right calcaneus

√7ᵗʰ **S92.045** Nondisplaced other fracture of tuberosity of left calcaneus

√7ᵗʰ **S92.046** Nondisplaced other fracture of tuberosity of unspecified calcaneus ▽

√6ᵗʰ **S92.05** Other extraarticular fracture of calcaneus

√7ᵗʰ **S92.051** Displaced other extraarticular fracture of right calcaneus

√7ᵗʰ **S92.052** Displaced other extraarticular fracture of left calcaneus

√7ᵗʰ **S92.053** Displaced other extraarticular fracture of unspecified calcaneus ▽

√7ᵗʰ **S92.054** Nondisplaced other extraarticular fracture of right calcaneus

√7ᵗʰ **S92.055** Nondisplaced other extraarticular fracture of left calcaneus

√7ᵗʰ **S92.056** Nondisplaced other extraarticular fracture of unspecified calcaneus ▽

√6ᵗʰ **S92.06** Intraarticular fracture of calcaneus

√7ᵗʰ **S92.061** Displaced intraarticular fracture of right calcaneus

√7ᵗʰ **S92.062** Displaced intraarticular fracture of left calcaneus

√7ᵗʰ **S92.063** Displaced intraarticular fracture of unspecified calcaneus ▽

√7ᵗʰ **S92.064** Nondisplaced intraarticular fracture of right calcaneus

√7ᵗʰ **S92.065** Nondisplaced intraarticular fracture of left calcaneus

√7ᵗʰ **S92.066** Nondisplaced intraarticular fracture of unspecified calcaneus ▽

√5ᵗʰ **S92.1** Fracture of talus
Astragalus

√6ᵗʰ **S92.10** Unspecified fracture of talus

√7ᵗʰ **S92.101** Unspecified fracture of right talus ▽

√7ᵗʰ **S92.102** Unspecified fracture of left talus ▽

√7ᵗʰ **S92.109** Unspecified fracture of unspecified talus ▽

√6ᵗʰ **S92.11** Fracture of neck of talus

√7ᵗʰ **S92.111** Displaced fracture of neck of right talus

√7ᵗʰ **S92.112** Displaced fracture of neck of left talus

√7ᵗʰ **S92.113** Displaced fracture of neck of unspecified talus ▽

√7ᵗʰ **S92.114** Nondisplaced fracture of neck of right talus

√7ᵗʰ **S92.115** Nondisplaced fracture of neck of left talus

√7ᵗʰ **S92.116** Nondisplaced fracture of neck of unspecified talus ▽

√6ᵗʰ **S92.12** Fracture of body of talus

√7ᵗʰ **S92.121** Displaced fracture of body of right talus

√7ᵗʰ **S92.122** Displaced fracture of body of left talus

√7ᵗʰ **S92.123** Displaced fracture of body of unspecified talus ▽

√7ᵗʰ **S92.124** Nondisplaced fracture of body of right talus

√7ᵗʰ **S92.125** Nondisplaced fracture of body of left talus

√7ᵗʰ **S92.126** Nondisplaced fracture of body of unspecified talus ▽

√6ᵗʰ **S92.13** Fracture of posterior process of talus

√7ᵗʰ **S92.131** Displaced fracture of posterior process of right talus

√7ᵗʰ **S92.132** Displaced fracture of posterior process of left talus

√7ᵗʰ **S92.133** Displaced fracture of posterior process of unspecified talus

√7ᵗʰ **S92.134** Nondisplaced fracture of posterior process of right talus

√7ᵗʰ **S92.135** Nondisplaced fracture of posterior process of left talus

√7ᵗʰ **S92.136** Nondisplaced fracture of posterior process of unspecified talus ▽

√6ᵗʰ **S92.14** Dome fracture of talus

EXCLUDES 1 osteochondritis dissecans (M93.2)

√7ᵗʰ **S92.141** Displaced dome fracture of right talus

√7ᵗʰ **S92.142** Displaced dome fracture of left talus

√7ᵗʰ **S92.143** Displaced dome fracture of unspecified talus ▽

√7ᵗʰ **S92.144** Nondisplaced dome fracture of right talus

√7ᵗʰ **S92.145** Nondisplaced dome fracture of left talus

√7ᵗʰ **S92.146** Nondisplaced dome fracture of unspecified talus ▽

√6ᵗʰ **S92.15** Avulsion fracture (chip fracture) of talus

√7ᵗʰ **S92.151** Displaced avulsion fracture (chip fracture) of right talus

√7ᵗʰ **S92.152** Displaced avulsion fracture (chip fracture) of left talus

√7ᵗʰ **S92.153** Displaced avulsion fracture (chip fracture) of unspecified talus ▽

√7ᵗʰ **S92.154** Nondisplaced avulsion fracture (chip fracture) of right talus

√7ᵗʰ **S92.155** Nondisplaced avulsion fracture (chip fracture) of left talus

√7ᵗʰ **S92.156** Nondisplaced avulsion fracture (chip fracture) of unspecified talus ▽

√6ᵗʰ **S92.19** Other fracture of talus

√7ᵗʰ **S92.191** Other fracture of right talus

√7ᵗʰ **S92.192** Other fracture of left talus

√7ᵗʰ **S92.199** Other fracture of unspecified talus ▽

√6ᵗʰ **S92.2** Fracture of other and unspecified tarsal bone(s)

√6ᵗʰ **S92.20** Fracture of unspecified tarsal bone(s)

√7ᵗʰ **S92.201** Fracture of unspecified tarsal bone(s) of right foot ▽

√7ᵗʰ **S92.202** Fracture of unspecified tarsal bone(s) of left foot ▽

√7ᵗʰ **S92.209** Fracture of unspecified tarsal bone(s) of unspecified foot ▽

√6ᵗʰ **S92.21** Fracture of cuboid bone

√7ᵗʰ **S92.211** Displaced fracture of cuboid bone of right foot

√7ᵗʰ **S92.212** Displaced fracture of cuboid bone of left foot

√7ᵗʰ **S92.213** Displaced fracture of cuboid bone of unspecified foot ▽

√7ᵗʰ **S92.214** Nondisplaced fracture of cuboid bone of right foot

√7ᵗʰ **S92.215** Nondisplaced fracture of cuboid bone of left foot

√7ᵗʰ **S92.216** Nondisplaced fracture of cuboid bone of unspecified foot ▽

√6ᵗʰ **S92.22** Fracture of lateral cuneiform

√7ᵗʰ **S92.221** Displaced fracture of lateral cuneiform of right foot

√7ᵗʰ **S92.222** Displaced fracture of lateral cuneiform of left foot

√7ᵗʰ **S92.223** Displaced fracture of lateral cuneiform of unspecified foot ▽

√7ᵗʰ **S92.224** Nondisplaced fracture of lateral cuneiform of right foot

√7ᵗʰ **S92.225** Nondisplaced fracture of lateral cuneiform of left foot

√7ᵗʰ **S92.226** Nondisplaced fracture of lateral cuneiform of unspecified foot ▽

√6ᵗʰ **S92.23** Fracture of intermediate cuneiform

√7ᵗʰ **S92.231** Displaced fracture of intermediate cuneiform of right foot

---

☑ Additional Character Required   √₇ₜₕ Placeholder Alert   Manifestation Dx   ▽ Unspecified Dx   ►◄ Revised Text   ● New Code   ▲ Revised Code Title

√7ᵗʰ **S92.232** Displaced **fracture of intermediate cuneiform of left foot**

√7ᵗʰ **S92.233** Displaced **fracture of intermediate cuneiform of unspecified foot** ▽

√7ᵗʰ **S92.234** Nondisplaced **fracture of intermediate cuneiform of right foot**

√7ᵗʰ **S92.235** Nondisplaced **fracture of intermediate cuneiform of left foot**

√7ᵗʰ **S92.236** Nondisplaced **fracture of intermediate cuneiform of unspecified foot** ▽

√6ᵗʰ **S92.24** Fracture of medial cuneiform

√7ᵗʰ **S92.241** Displaced **fracture of medial cuneiform of right foot**

√7ᵗʰ **S92.242** Displaced **fracture of medial cuneiform of left foot**

√7ᵗʰ **S92.243** Displaced **fracture of medial cuneiform of unspecified foot** ▽

√7ᵗʰ **S92.244** Nondisplaced **fracture of medial cuneiform of right foot**

√7ᵗʰ **S92.245** Nondisplaced **fracture of medial cuneiform of left foot**

√7ᵗʰ **S92.246** Nondisplaced **fracture of medial cuneiform of unspecified foot** ▽

√6ᵗʰ **S92.25** Fracture of navicular [scaphoid] of foot

√7ᵗʰ **S92.251** Displaced **fracture of navicular [scaphoid] of right foot**

√7ᵗʰ **S92.252** Displaced **fracture of navicular [scaphoid] of left foot**

√7ᵗʰ **S92.253** Displaced **fracture of navicular [scaphoid] of unspecified foot** ▽

√7ᵗʰ **S92.254** Nondisplaced **fracture of navicular [scaphoid] of right foot**

√7ᵗʰ **S92.255** Nondisplaced **fracture of navicular [scaphoid] of left foot**

√7ᵗʰ **S92.256** Nondisplaced **fracture of navicular [scaphoid] of unspecified foot** ▽

√5ᵗʰ **S92.3** Fracture of metatarsal bone(s)

EXCLUDES 2 ▶*physeal fracture of metatarsal (S99.1-)*◀

√6ᵗʰ **S92.30** Fracture of unspecified metatarsal bone(s)

√7ᵗʰ **S92.301** Fracture of unspecified metatarsal bone(s), right foot ▽

√7ᵗʰ **S92.302** Fracture of unspecified metatarsal bone(s), left foot ▽

√7ᵗʰ **S92.309** Fracture of unspecified metatarsal bone(s), unspecified foot ▽

√6ᵗʰ **S92.31** Fracture of first metatarsal bone

√7ᵗʰ **S92.311** Displaced **fracture of first metatarsal bone, right foot**

√7ᵗʰ **S92.312** Displaced **fracture of first metatarsal bone, left foot**

√7ᵗʰ **S92.313** Displaced **fracture of first metatarsal bone, unspecified foot** ▽

√7ᵗʰ **S92.314** Nondisplaced **fracture of first metatarsal bone, right foot**

√7ᵗʰ **S92.315** Nondisplaced **fracture of first metatarsal bone, left foot**

√7ᵗʰ **S92.316** Nondisplaced **fracture of first metatarsal bone, unspecified foot** ▽

√6ᵗʰ **S92.32** Fracture of second metatarsal bone

√7ᵗʰ **S92.321** Displaced **fracture of second metatarsal bone, right foot**

√7ᵗʰ **S92.322** Displaced **fracture of second metatarsal bone, left foot**

√7ᵗʰ **S92.323** Displaced **fracture of second metatarsal bone, unspecified foot** ▽

√7ᵗʰ **S92.324** Nondisplaced **fracture of second metatarsal bone, right foot**

√7ᵗʰ **S92.325** Nondisplaced **fracture of second metatarsal bone, left foot**

√7ᵗʰ **S92.326** Nondisplaced **fracture of second metatarsal bone, unspecified foot** ▽

√6ᵗʰ **S92.33** Fracture of third metatarsal bone

√7ᵗʰ **S92.331** Displaced **fracture of third metatarsal bone, right foot**

√7ᵗʰ **S92.332** Displaced **fracture of third metatarsal bone, left foot**

√7ᵗʰ **S92.333** Displaced **fracture of third metatarsal bone, unspecified foot** ▽

√7ᵗʰ **S92.334** Nondisplaced **fracture of third metatarsal bone, right foot**

√7ᵗʰ **S92.335** Nondisplaced **fracture of third metatarsal bone, left foot**

√7ᵗʰ **S92.336** Nondisplaced **fracture of third metatarsal bone, unspecified foot** ▽

√6ᵗʰ **S92.34** Fracture of fourth metatarsal bone

√7ᵗʰ **S92.341** Displaced **fracture of fourth metatarsal bone, right foot**

√7ᵗʰ **S92.342** Displaced **fracture of fourth metatarsal bone, left foot**

√7ᵗʰ **S92.343** Displaced **fracture of fourth metatarsal bone, unspecified foot** ▽

√7ᵗʰ **S92.344** Nondisplaced **fracture of fourth metatarsal bone, right foot**

√7ᵗʰ **S92.345** Nondisplaced **fracture of fourth metatarsal bone, left foot**

√7ᵗʰ **S92.346** Nondisplaced **fracture of fourth metatarsal bone, unspecified foot** ▽

√6ᵗʰ **S92.35** Fracture of fifth metatarsal bone

√7ᵗʰ **S92.351** Displaced **fracture of fifth metatarsal bone, right foot**

√7ᵗʰ **S92.352** Displaced **fracture of fifth metatarsal bone, left foot**

√7ᵗʰ **S92.353** Displaced **fracture of fifth metatarsal bone, unspecified foot** ▽

√7ᵗʰ **S92.354** Nondisplaced **fracture of fifth metatarsal bone, right foot**

√7ᵗʰ **S92.355** Nondisplaced **fracture of fifth metatarsal bone, left foot**

√7ᵗʰ **S92.356** Nondisplaced **fracture of fifth metatarsal bone, unspecified foot** ▽

√5ᵗʰ **S92.4** Fracture of great toe

EXCLUDES 2 ▶*physeal fracture of phalanx of toe (S99.2-)*◀

√6ᵗʰ **S92.40** Unspecified fracture of great toe

√7ᵗʰ **S92.401** Displaced **unspecified fracture of right great toe** ▽

√7ᵗʰ **S92.402** Displaced **unspecified fracture of left great toe** ▽

√7ᵗʰ **S92.403** Displaced **unspecified fracture of unspecified great toe** ▽

√7ᵗʰ **S92.404** Nondisplaced **unspecified fracture of right great toe** ▽

√7ᵗʰ **S92.405** Nondisplaced **unspecified fracture of left great toe** ▽

√7ᵗʰ **S92.406** Nondisplaced **unspecified fracture of unspecified great toe** ▽

√6ᵗʰ **S92.41** Fracture of proximal phalanx of great toe

√7ᵗʰ **S92.411** Displaced **fracture of proximal phalanx of right great toe**

√7ᵗʰ **S92.412** Displaced **fracture of proximal phalanx of left great toe**

√7ᵗʰ **S92.413** Displaced **fracture of proximal phalanx of unspecified great toe** ▽

√7ᵗʰ **S92.414** Nondisplaced **fracture of proximal phalanx of right great toe**

√7ᵗʰ **S92.415** Nondisplaced **fracture of proximal phalanx of left great toe**

√7ᵗʰ **S92.416** Nondisplaced **fracture of proximal phalanx of unspecified great toe** ▽

√6ᵗʰ **S92.42** Fracture of distal phalanx of great toe

√7ᵗʰ **S92.421** Displaced **fracture of distal phalanx of right great toe**

√7ᵗʰ **S92.422** Displaced **fracture of distal phalanx of left great toe**

√7ᵗʰ **S92.423** Displaced **fracture of distal phalanx of unspecified great toe** ▽

√7ᵗʰ **S92.424** Nondisplaced **fracture of distal phalanx of right great toe**

√7ᵗʰ **S92.425** Nondisplaced **fracture of distal phalanx of left great toe**

√7ᵗʰ **S92.426** Nondisplaced **fracture of distal phalanx of unspecified great toe** ▽

√6ᵗʰ **S92.49** Other fracture of great toe

√7ᵗʰ **S92.491** Other fracture of right great toe

√7ᵗʰ **S92.492** Other fracture of left great toe

√7ᵗʰ **S92.499** Other fracture of unspecified great toe ▽

√5ᵗʰ **S92.5** Fracture of lesser toe(s)

EXCLUDES 2 ▶*physeal fracture of phalanx of toe (S99.2-)*◀

√6ᵗʰ **S92.50** Unspecified fracture of lesser toe(s)

√7ᵗʰ **S92.501** Displaced **unspecified fracture of right lesser toe(s)** ▽

EXCLUDES 1 Not coded here   *EXCLUDES 2* Not included here   Ⓝ Newborn Age : 0   Ⓟ Pediatric Age : 0-17   Ⓜ Maternity Age : 12-55   Ⓐ Adult Age : 15-124

1000

ICD-10-CM 2017

☑7ᵗʰ **S92.502** Displaced unspecified fracture of left lesser toe(s) ▽

☑7ᵗʰ **S92.503** Displaced unspecified fracture of unspecified lesser toe(s) ▽

☑7ᵗʰ **S92.504** Nondisplaced unspecified fracture of right lesser toe(s) ▽

☑7ᵗʰ **S92.505** Nondisplaced unspecified fracture of left lesser toe(s) ▽

☑7ᵗʰ **S92.506** Nondisplaced unspecified fracture of unspecified lesser toe(s) ▽

☑6ᵗʰ **S92.51** Fracture of proximal phalanx of lesser toe(s)

☑7ᵗʰ **S92.511** Displaced fracture of proximal phalanx of right lesser toe(s)

☑7ᵗʰ **S92.512** Displaced fracture of proximal phalanx of left lesser toe(s)

☑7ᵗʰ **S92.513** Displaced fracture of proximal phalanx of unspecified lesser toe(s) ▽

☑7ᵗʰ **S92.514** Nondisplaced fracture of proximal phalanx of right lesser toe(s)

☑7ᵗʰ **S92.515** Nondisplaced fracture of proximal phalanx of left lesser toe(s))

☑7ᵗʰ **S92.516** Nondisplaced fracture of proximal phalanx of unspecified lesser toe(s) ▽

☑6ᵗʰ **S92.52** Fracture of medial phalanx of lesser toe(s)

☑7ᵗʰ **S92.521** Displaced fracture of medial phalanx of right lesser toe(s)

☑7ᵗʰ **S92.522** Displaced fracture of medial phalanx of left lesser toe(s)

☑7ᵗʰ **S92.523** Displaced fracture of medial phalanx of unspecified lesser toe(s) ▽

☑7ᵗʰ **S92.524** Nondisplaced fracture of medial phalanx of right lesser toe(s)

☑7ᵗʰ **S92.525** Nondisplaced fracture of medial phalanx of left lesser toe(s)

☑7ᵗʰ **S92.526** Nondisplaced fracture of medial phalanx of unspecified lesser toe(s) ▽

☑6ᵗʰ **S92.53** Fracture of distal phalanx of lesser toe(s)

☑7ᵗʰ **S92.531** Displaced fracture of distal phalanx of right lesser toe(s)

☑7ᵗʰ **S92.532** Displaced fracture of distal phalanx of left lesser toe(s)

☑7ᵗʰ **S92.533** Displaced fracture of distal phalanx of unspecified lesser toe(s) ▽

☑7ᵗʰ **S92.534** Nondisplaced fracture of distal phalanx of right lesser toe(s)

☑7ᵗʰ **S92.535** Nondisplaced fracture of distal phalanx of left lesser toe(s)

☑7ᵗʰ **S92.536** Nondisplaced fracture of distal phalanx of unspecified lesser toe(s) ▽

☑6ᵗʰ **S92.59** Other fracture of lesser toe(s)

☑7ᵗʰ **S92.591** Other fracture of right lesser toe(s)

☑7ᵗʰ **S92.592** Other fracture of left lesser toe(s)

☑7ᵗʰ **S92.599** Other fracture of unspecified lesser toe(s) ▽

● ☑5ᵗʰ **S92.8** Other fracture of foot, except ankle

● ☑6ᵗʰ **S92.81** Other fracture of foot
Sesamoid fracture of foot

● ☑7ᵗʰ **S92.811** Other fracture of right foot

● ☑7ᵗʰ **S92.812** Other fracture of left foot

● ☑7ᵗʰ **S92.819** Other fracture of unspecified foot ▽

☑5ᵗʰ **S92.9** Unspecified fracture of foot and toe

☑6ᵗʰ **S92.90** Unspecified fracture of foot

☑7ᵗʰ **S92.901** Unspecified fracture of right foot ▽

☑7ᵗʰ **S92.902** Unspecified fracture of left foot ▽

☑7ᵗʰ **S92.909** Unspecified fracture of unspecified foot ▽

☑6ᵗʰ **S92.91** Unspecified fracture of toe

☑7ᵗʰ **S92.911** Unspecified fracture of right toe(s) ▽

☑7ᵗʰ **S92.912** Unspecified fracture of left toe(s) ▽

☑7ᵗʰ **S92.919** Unspecified fracture of unspecified toe(s) ▽

☑4ᵗʰ **S93** Dislocation and sprain of joints and ligaments at ankle, foot and toe level

INCLUDES avulsion of joint or ligament of ankle, foot and toe
laceration of cartilage, joint or ligament of ankle, foot and toe
sprain of cartilage, joint or ligament of ankle, foot and toe
traumatic hemarthrosis of joint or ligament of ankle, foot and toe
traumatic rupture of joint or ligament of ankle, foot and toe
traumatic subluxation of joint or ligament of ankle, foot and toe
traumatic tear of joint or ligament of ankle, foot and toe

Code also any associated open wound

EXCLUDES 2 strain of muscle and tendon of ankle and foot (S96.-)

The appropriate 7th character is to be added to each code from category S93.
A initial encounter
D subsequent encounter
S sequela

☑5ᵗʰ **S93.0** Subluxation and dislocation of ankle joint
Subluxation and dislocation of astragalus
Subluxation and dislocation of fibula, lower end
Subluxation and dislocation of talus
Subluxation and dislocation of tibia, lower end

☑×7ᵗʰ **S93.01** Subluxation of right ankle joint

☑×7ᵗʰ **S93.02** Subluxation of left ankle joint

☑×7ᵗʰ **S93.03** Subluxation of unspecified ankle joint ▽

☑×7ᵗʰ **S93.04** Dislocation of right ankle joint

☑×7ᵗʰ **S93.05** Dislocation of left ankle joint

☑×7ᵗʰ **S93.06** Dislocation of unspecified ankle joint ▽

☑5ᵗʰ **S93.1** Subluxation and dislocation of toe

☑6ᵗʰ **S93.10** Unspecified subluxation and dislocation of toe
Dislocation of toe NOS
Subluxation of toe NOS

☑7ᵗʰ **S93.101** Unspecified subluxation of right toe(s) ▽

☑7ᵗʰ **S93.102** Unspecified subluxation of left toe(s) ▽

☑7ᵗʰ **S93.103** Unspecified subluxation of unspecified toe(s) ▽

☑7ᵗʰ **S93.104** Unspecified dislocation of right toe(s) ▽

☑7ᵗʰ **S93.105** Unspecified dislocation of left toe(s) ▽

☑7ᵗʰ **S93.106** Unspecified dislocation of unspecified toe(s) ▽

☑6ᵗʰ **S93.11** Dislocation of interphalangeal joint

☑7ᵗʰ **S93.111** Dislocation of interphalangeal joint of right great toe

☑7ᵗʰ **S93.112** Dislocation of interphalangeal joint of left great toe

☑7ᵗʰ **S93.113** Dislocation of interphalangeal joint of unspecified great toe ▽

☑7ᵗʰ **S93.114** Dislocation of interphalangeal joint of right lesser toe(s)

☑7ᵗʰ **S93.115** Dislocation of interphalangeal joint of left lesser toe(s)

☑7ᵗʰ **S93.116** Dislocation of interphalangeal joint of unspecified lesser toe(s) ▽

☑7ᵗʰ **S93.119** Dislocation of interphalangeal joint of unspecified toe(s) ▽

☑6ᵗʰ **S93.12** Dislocation of metatarsophalangeal joint

☑7ᵗʰ **S93.121** Dislocation of metatarsophalangeal joint of right great toe

☑7ᵗʰ **S93.122** Dislocation of metatarsophalangeal joint of left great toe

☑7ᵗʰ **S93.123** Dislocation of metatarsophalangeal joint of unspecified great toe ▽

☑7ᵗʰ **S93.124** Dislocation of metatarsophalangeal joint of right lesser toe(s)

☑7ᵗʰ **S93.125** Dislocation of metatarsophalangeal joint of left lesser toe(s)

☑7ᵗʰ **S93.126** Dislocation of metatarsophalangeal joint of unspecified lesser toe(s) ▽

☑7ᵗʰ **S93.129** Dislocation of metatarsophalangeal joint of unspecified toe(s) ▽

☑ Additional Character Required   ☑×7ᵗʰ Placeholder Alert   Manifestation Dx   ▽ Unspecified Dx   ►◄ Revised Text   ● New Code   ▲ Revised Code Title

Chapter 19. Injury, Poisoning and Certain Other Consequences of External Causes

S93.13–S93.524

√6ᵗʰ **S93.13** **Subluxation of interphalangeal joint**

√7ᵗʰ **S93.131** **Subluxation of interphalangeal joint of right great toe**

√7ᵗʰ **S93.132** **Subluxation of interphalangeal joint of left great toe**

√7ᵗʰ **S93.133** **Subluxation of interphalangeal joint of unspecified great toe** ▽

√7ᵗʰ **S93.134** **Subluxation of interphalangeal joint of right lesser toe(s)**

√7ᵗʰ **S93.135** **Subluxation of interphalangeal joint of left lesser toe(s)**

√7ᵗʰ **S93.136** **Subluxation of interphalangeal joint of unspecified lesser toe(s)** ▽

√7ᵗʰ **S93.139** **Subluxation of interphalangeal joint of unspecified toe(s)** ▽

√6ᵗʰ **S93.14** **Subluxation of metatarsophalangeal joint**

√7ᵗʰ **S93.141** **Subluxation of metatarsophalangeal joint of right great toe**

√7ᵗʰ **S93.142** **Subluxation of metatarsophalangeal joint of left great toe**

√7ᵗʰ **S93.143** **Subluxation of metatarsophalangeal joint of unspecified great toe** ▽

√7ᵗʰ **S93.144** **Subluxation of metatarsophalangeal joint of right lesser toe(s)**

√7ᵗʰ **S93.145** **Subluxation of metatarsophalangeal joint of left lesser toe(s)**

√7ᵗʰ **S93.146** **Subluxation of metatarsophalangeal joint of unspecified lesser toe(s)** ▽

√7ᵗʰ **S93.149** **Subluxation of metatarsophalangeal joint of unspecified toe(s)** ▽

√5ᵗʰ **S93.3** **Subluxation and dislocation of foot**

EXCLUDES 2 *dislocation of toe (S93.1-)*

√6ᵗʰ **S93.30** **Unspecified subluxation and dislocation of foot**

Dislocation of foot NOS
Subluxation of foot NOS

√7ᵗʰ **S93.301** **Unspecified subluxation of right foot** ▽

√7ᵗʰ **S93.302** **Unspecified subluxation of left foot** ▽

√7ᵗʰ **S93.303** **Unspecified subluxation of unspecified foot** ▽

√7ᵗʰ **S93.304** **Unspecified dislocation of right foot** ▽

√7ᵗʰ **S93.305** **Unspecified dislocation of left foot** ▽

√7ᵗʰ **S93.306** **Unspecified dislocation of unspecified foot** ▽

√6ᵗʰ **S93.31** **Subluxation and dislocation of tarsal joint**

√7ᵗʰ **S93.311** **Subluxation of tarsal joint of right foot**

√7ᵗʰ **S93.312** **Subluxation of tarsal joint of left foot**

√7ᵗʰ **S93.313** **Subluxation of tarsal joint of unspecified foot** ▽

√7ᵗʰ **S93.314** **Dislocation of tarsal joint of right foot**

√7ᵗʰ **S93.315** **Dislocation of tarsal joint of left foot**

√7ᵗʰ **S93.316** **Dislocation of tarsal joint of unspecified foot** ▽

√6ᵗʰ **S93.32** **Subluxation and dislocation of tarsometatarsal joint**

√7ᵗʰ **S93.321** **Subluxation of tarsometatarsal joint of right foot**

√7ᵗʰ **S93.322** **Subluxation of tarsometatarsal joint of left foot**

√7ᵗʰ **S93.323** **Subluxation of tarsometatarsal joint of unspecified foot** ▽

√7ᵗʰ **S93.324** **Dislocation of tarsometatarsal joint of right foot**

√7ᵗʰ **S93.325** **Dislocation of tarsometatarsal joint of left foot**

√7ᵗʰ **S93.326** **Dislocation of tarsometatarsal joint of unspecified foot** ▽

√6ᵗʰ **S93.33** **Other subluxation and dislocation of foot**

√7ᵗʰ **S93.331** **Other subluxation of right foot**

√7ᵗʰ **S93.332** **Other subluxation of left foot**

√7ᵗʰ **S93.333** **Other subluxation of unspecified foot** ▽

√7ᵗʰ **S93.334** **Other dislocation of right foot**

√7ᵗʰ **S93.335** **Other dislocation of left foot**

√7ᵗʰ **S93.336** **Other dislocation of unspecified foot** ▽

√5ᵗʰ **S93.4** **Sprain of ankle**

EXCLUDES 2 *injury of Achilles tendon (S86.0-)*

√6ᵗʰ **S93.40** **Sprain of unspecified ligament of ankle**

Sprain of ankle NOS
Sprained ankle NOS

√7ᵗʰ **S93.401** **Sprain of unspecified ligament of right ankle** ▽

√7ᵗʰ **S93.402** **Sprain of unspecified ligament of left ankle** ▽

√7ᵗʰ **S93.409** **Sprain of unspecified ligament of unspecified ankle** ▽

√6ᵗʰ **S93.41** **Sprain of calcaneofibular ligament**

√7ᵗʰ **S93.411** **Sprain of calcaneofibular ligament of right ankle**

√7ᵗʰ **S93.412** **Sprain of calcaneofibular ligament of left ankle**

√7ᵗʰ **S93.419** **Sprain of calcaneofibular ligament of unspecified ankle** ▽

√6ᵗʰ **S93.42** **Sprain of deltoid ligament**

√7ᵗʰ **S93.421** **Sprain of deltoid ligament of right ankle**

√7ᵗʰ **S93.422** **Sprain of deltoid ligament of left ankle**

√7ᵗʰ **S93.429** **Sprain of deltoid ligament of unspecified ankle** ▽

√6ᵗʰ **S93.43** **Sprain of tibiofibular ligament**

√7ᵗʰ **S93.431** **Sprain of tibiofibular ligament of right ankle**

√7ᵗʰ **S93.432** **Sprain of tibiofibular ligament of left ankle**

√7ᵗʰ **S93.439** **Sprain of tibiofibular ligament of unspecified ankle** ▽

√6ᵗʰ **S93.49** **Sprain of other ligament of ankle**

Sprain of internal collateral ligament
Sprain of talofibular ligament

√7ᵗʰ **S93.491** **Sprain of other ligament of right ankle**

√7ᵗʰ **S93.492** **Sprain of other ligament of left ankle**

√7ᵗʰ **S93.499** **Sprain of other ligament of unspecified ankle** ▽

√5ᵗʰ **S93.5** **Sprain of toe**

√6ᵗʰ **S93.50** **Unspecified sprain of toe**

√7ᵗʰ **S93.501** **Unspecified sprain of right great toe** ▽

√7ᵗʰ **S93.502** **Unspecified sprain of left great toe** ▽

√7ᵗʰ **S93.503** **Unspecified sprain of unspecified great toe** ▽

√7ᵗʰ **S93.504** **Unspecified sprain of right lesser toe(s)** ▽

√7ᵗʰ **S93.505** **Unspecified sprain of left lesser toe(s)** ▽

√7ᵗʰ **S93.506** **Unspecified sprain of unspecified lesser toe(s)** ▽

√7ᵗʰ **S93.509** **Unspecified sprain of unspecified toe(s)** ▽

√6ᵗʰ **S93.51** **Sprain of interphalangeal joint of toe**

√7ᵗʰ **S93.511** **Sprain of interphalangeal joint of right great toe**

√7ᵗʰ **S93.512** **Sprain of interphalangeal joint of left great toe**

√7ᵗʰ **S93.513** **Sprain of interphalangeal joint of unspecified great toe** ▽

√7ᵗʰ **S93.514** **Sprain of interphalangeal joint of right lesser toe(s)**

√7ᵗʰ **S93.515** **Sprain of interphalangeal joint of left lesser toe(s)**

√7ᵗʰ **S93.516** **Sprain of interphalangeal joint of unspecified lesser toe(s)** ▽

√7ᵗʰ **S93.519** **Sprain of interphalangeal joint of unspecified toe(s)** ▽

√6ᵗʰ **S93.52** **Sprain of metatarsophalangeal joint of toe**

√7ᵗʰ **S93.521** **Sprain of metatarsophalangeal joint of right great toe**

√7ᵗʰ **S93.522** **Sprain of metatarsophalangeal joint of left great toe**

√7ᵗʰ **S93.523** **Sprain of metatarsophalangeal joint of unspecified great toe** ▽

√7ᵗʰ **S93.524** **Sprain of metatarsophalangeal joint of right lesser toe(s)**

EXCLUDES 1 Not coded here   EXCLUDES 2 Not included here   N Newborn Age : 0   P Pediatric Age : 0-17   M Maternity Age : 12-55   A Adult Age : 15-124

1002

ICD-10-CM 2017

    ✓7ᵗʰ **S93.525**   Sprain of metatarsophalangeal joint of left lesser toe(s)

    ✓7ᵗʰ **S93.526**   Sprain of metatarsophalangeal joint of unspecified lesser toe(s)   ▽

    ✓7ᵗʰ **S93.529**   Sprain of metatarsophalangeal joint of unspecified toe(s)   ▽

✓5ᵗʰ **S93.6**   **Sprain of** foot

   EXCLUDES 2   *sprain of metatarsophalangeal joint of toe (S93.52-)*
             sprain of toe (S93.5-)

   ✓6ᵗʰ **S93.60**   **Unspecified sprain of foot**

     ✓7ᵗʰ **S93.601**   Unspecified sprain of right foot   ▽

     ✓7ᵗʰ **S93.602**   Unspecified sprain of left foot   ▽

     ✓7ᵗʰ **S93.609**   Unspecified sprain of unspecified foot   ▽

   ✓6ᵗʰ **S93.61**   **Sprain of** tarsal ligament **of foot**

     ✓7ᵗʰ **S93.611**   Sprain of tarsal ligament of right foot

     ✓7ᵗʰ **S93.612**   Sprain of tarsal ligament of left foot

     ✓7ᵗʰ **S93.619**   Sprain of tarsal ligament of unspecified foot

   ✓6ᵗʰ **S93.62**   **Sprain of** tarsometatarsal ligament **of foot**

     ✓7ᵗʰ **S93.621**   Sprain of tarsometatarsal ligament of right foot

     ✓7ᵗʰ **S93.622**   Sprain of tarsometatarsal ligament of left foot

     ✓7ᵗʰ **S93.629**   Sprain of tarsometatarsal ligament of unspecified foot   ▽

   ✓6ᵗʰ **S93.69**   **Other sprain of foot**

     ✓7ᵗʰ **S93.691**   Other sprain of right foot

     ✓7ᵗʰ **S93.692**   Other sprain of left foot

     ✓7ᵗʰ **S93.699**   Other sprain of unspecified foot   ▽

✓4ᵗʰ **S94**   **Injury of nerves at ankle and foot level**

   Code also any associated open wound (S91.-)

   The appropriate 7th character is to be added to each code from category S94.
   A   initial encounter
   D   subsequent encounter
   S   sequela

  ✓5ᵗʰ **S94.0**   **Injury of** lateral plantar **nerve**

    ✓ˣ7ᵗʰ **S94.00**   Injury of lateral plantar nerve, unspecified leg   ▽

    ✓ˣ7ᵗʰ **S94.01**   Injury of lateral plantar nerve, right leg

    ✓ˣ7ᵗʰ **S94.02**   Injury of lateral plantar nerve, left leg

  ✓5ᵗʰ **S94.1**   **Injury of** medial plantar **nerve**

    ✓ˣ7ᵗʰ **S94.10**   Injury of medial plantar nerve, unspecified leg   ▽

    ✓ˣ7ᵗʰ **S94.11**   Injury of medial plantar nerve, right leg

    ✓ˣ7ᵗʰ **S94.12**   Injury of medial plantar nerve, left leg

  ✓5ᵗʰ **S94.2**   **Injury of** deep peroneal **nerve at ankle and foot level**

     Injury of terminal, lateral branch of deep peroneal nerve

    ✓ˣ7ᵗʰ **S94.20**   Injury of deep peroneal nerve at ankle and foot level, unspecified leg   ▽

    ✓ˣ7ᵗʰ **S94.21**   Injury of deep peroneal nerve at ankle and foot level, right leg

    ✓ˣ7ᵗʰ **S94.22**   Injury of deep peroneal nerve at ankle and foot level, left leg

  ✓5ᵗʰ **S94.3**   **Injury of** cutaneous sensory **nerve at ankle and foot level**

    ✓ˣ7ᵗʰ **S94.30**   Injury of cutaneous sensory nerve at ankle and foot level, unspecified leg   ▽

    ✓ˣ7ᵗʰ **S94.31**   Injury of cutaneous sensory nerve at ankle and foot level, right leg

    ✓ˣ7ᵗʰ **S94.32**   Injury of cutaneous sensory nerve at ankle and foot level, left leg

  ✓5ᵗʰ **S94.8**   **Injury of other nerves at ankle and foot level**

   ✓6ᵗʰ **S94.8X**   **Injury of other nerves at ankle and foot level**

     ✓7ᵗʰ **S94.8X1**   Injury of other nerves at ankle and foot level, right leg

     ✓7ᵗʰ **S94.8X2**   Injury of other nerves at ankle and foot level, left leg

     ✓7ᵗʰ **S94.8X9**   Injury of other nerves at ankle and foot level, unspecified leg   ▽

  ✓5ᵗʰ **S94.9**   **Injury of unspecified nerve at ankle and foot level**

    ✓ˣ7ᵗʰ **S94.90**   Injury of unspecified nerve at ankle and foot level, unspecified leg   ▽

    ✓ˣ7ᵗʰ **S94.91**   Injury of unspecified nerve at ankle and foot level, right leg

  ✓ˣ7ᵗʰ **S94.92**   Injury of unspecified nerve at ankle and foot level, left leg   ▽

✓4ᵗʰ **S95**   **Injury of blood vessels at ankle and foot level**

   Code also any associated open wound (S91.-)

   EXCLUDES 2   *injury of posterior tibial artery and vein (S85.1-, S85.8-)*

   The appropriate 7th character is to be added to each code from category S95.
   A   initial encounter
   D   subsequent encounter
   S   sequela

  ✓5ᵗʰ **S95.0**   **Injury of** dorsal artery **of foot**

   ✓6ᵗʰ **S95.00**   **Unspecified injury of dorsal artery of foot**

     ✓7ᵗʰ **S95.001**   Unspecified injury of dorsal artery of right foot   ▽

     ✓7ᵗʰ **S95.002**   Unspecified injury of dorsal artery of left foot   ▽

     ✓7ᵗʰ **S95.009**   Unspecified injury of dorsal artery of unspecified foot   ▽

   ✓6ᵗʰ **S95.01**   **Laceration of dorsal artery of foot**

     ✓7ᵗʰ **S95.011**   Laceration of dorsal artery of right foot

     ✓7ᵗʰ **S95.012**   Laceration of dorsal artery of left foot

     ✓7ᵗʰ **S95.019**   Laceration of dorsal artery of unspecified foot   ▽

   ✓6ᵗʰ **S95.09**   **Other specified injury of dorsal artery of foot**

     ✓7ᵗʰ **S95.091**   Other specified injury of dorsal artery of right foot

     ✓7ᵗʰ **S95.092**   Other specified injury of dorsal artery of left foot

     ✓7ᵗʰ **S95.099**   Other specified injury of dorsal artery of unspecified foot   ▽

  ✓5ᵗʰ **S95.1**   **Injury of** plantar artery **of foot**

   ✓6ᵗʰ **S95.10**   **Unspecified injury of plantar artery of foot**

     ✓7ᵗʰ **S95.101**   Unspecified injury of plantar artery of right foot   ▽

     ✓7ᵗʰ **S95.102**   Unspecified injury of plantar artery of left foot   ▽

     ✓7ᵗʰ **S95.109**   Unspecified injury of plantar artery of unspecified foot   ▽

   ✓6ᵗʰ **S95.11**   **Laceration of plantar artery of foot**

     ✓7ᵗʰ **S95.111**   Laceration of plantar artery of right foot

     ✓7ᵗʰ **S95.112**   Laceration of plantar artery of left foot

     ✓7ᵗʰ **S95.119**   Laceration of plantar artery of unspecified foot   ▽

   ✓6ᵗʰ **S95.19**   **Other specified injury of plantar artery of foot**

     ✓7ᵗʰ **S95.191**   Other specified injury of plantar artery of right foot

     ✓7ᵗʰ **S95.192**   Other specified injury of plantar artery of left foot

     ✓7ᵗʰ **S95.199**   Other specified injury of plantar artery of unspecified foot   ▽

  ✓5ᵗʰ **S95.2**   **Injury of** dorsal vein **of foot**

   ✓6ᵗʰ **S95.20**   **Unspecified injury of dorsal vein of foot**

     ✓7ᵗʰ **S95.201**   Unspecified injury of dorsal vein of right foot   ▽

     ✓7ᵗʰ **S95.202**   Unspecified injury of dorsal vein of left foot   ▽

     ✓7ᵗʰ **S95.209**   Unspecified injury of dorsal vein of unspecified foot   ▽

   ✓6ᵗʰ **S95.21**   **Laceration of dorsal vein of foot**

     ✓7ᵗʰ **S95.211**   Laceration of dorsal vein of right foot

     ✓7ᵗʰ **S95.212**   Laceration of dorsal vein of left foot

     ✓7ᵗʰ **S95.219**   Laceration of dorsal vein of unspecified foot   ▽

   ✓6ᵗʰ **S95.29**   **Other specified injury of dorsal vein of foot**

     ✓7ᵗʰ **S95.291**   Other specified injury of dorsal vein of right foot

     ✓7ᵗʰ **S95.292**   Other specified injury of dorsal vein of left foot

     ✓7ᵗʰ **S95.299**   Other specified injury of dorsal vein of unspecified foot   ▽

  ✓5ᵗʰ **S95.8**   **Injury of other blood vessels at ankle and foot level**

   ✓6ᵗʰ **S95.80**   **Unspecified injury of other blood vessels at ankle and foot level**

     ✓7ᵗʰ **S95.801**   Unspecified injury of other blood vessels at ankle and foot level, right leg   ▽

☑ Additional Character Required   ✓ˣ7ᵗʰ Placeholder Alert   Manifestation Dx   ▽ Unspecified Dx   ►◄ Revised Text   ● New Code   ▲ Revised Code Title

ICD-10-CM 2017   **1003**

√7ᵗʰ **S95.802** Unspecified injury of other blood vessels at ankle and foot level, left leg ▽

√7ᵗʰ **S95.809** Unspecified injury of other blood vessels at ankle and foot level, unspecified leg ▽

√6ᵗʰ **S95.81** Laceration of other blood vessels at ankle and foot level

√7ᵗʰ **S95.811** Laceration of other blood vessels at ankle and foot level, right leg

√7ᵗʰ **S95.812** Laceration of other blood vessels at ankle and foot level, left leg

√7ᵗʰ **S95.819** Laceration of other blood vessels at ankle and foot level, unspecified leg ▽

√6ᵗʰ **S95.89** Other specified injury of other blood vessels at ankle and foot level

√7ᵗʰ **S95.891** Other specified injury of other blood vessels at ankle and foot level, right leg

√7ᵗʰ **S95.892** Other specified injury of other blood vessels at ankle and foot level, left leg

√7ᵗʰ **S95.899** Other specified injury of other blood vessels at ankle and foot level, unspecified leg ▽

√5ᵗʰ **S95.9** Injury of unspecified blood vessel at ankle and foot level

√6ᵗʰ **S95.90** Unspecified injury of unspecified blood vessel at ankle and foot level

√7ᵗʰ **S95.901** Unspecified injury of unspecified blood vessel at ankle and foot level, right leg ▽

√7ᵗʰ **S95.902** Unspecified injury of unspecified blood vessel at ankle and foot level, left leg ▽

√7ᵗʰ **S95.909** Unspecified injury of unspecified blood vessel at ankle and foot level, unspecified leg ▽

√6ᵗʰ **S95.91** Laceration of unspecified blood vessel at ankle and foot level

√7ᵗʰ **S95.911** Laceration of unspecified blood vessel at ankle and foot level, right leg ▽

√7ᵗʰ **S95.912** Laceration of unspecified blood vessel at ankle and foot level, left leg ▽

√7ᵗʰ **S95.919** Laceration of unspecified blood vessel at ankle and foot level, unspecified leg ▽

√6ᵗʰ **S95.99** Other specified injury of unspecified blood vessel at ankle and foot level

√7ᵗʰ **S95.991** Other specified injury of unspecified blood vessel at ankle and foot level, right leg ▽

√7ᵗʰ **S95.992** Other specified injury of unspecified blood vessel at ankle and foot level, left leg ▽

√7ᵗʰ **S95.999** Other specified injury of unspecified blood vessel at ankle and foot level, unspecified leg ▽

√4ᵗʰ **S96 Injury of muscle and tendon at ankle and foot level**

Code also any associated open wound (S91.-)

EXCLUDES 2   *injury of Achilles tendon (S86.0-)*
    sprain of joints and ligaments of ankle and foot (S93.-)

TIP: Refer to the Muscle/Tendon table at the beginning of this chapter

The appropriate 7th character is to be added to each code from category S96.
- A   initial encounter
- D   subsequent encounter
- S   sequela

√5ᵗʰ **S96.0** Injury of muscle and tendon of long flexor muscle of toe at ankle and foot level

√6ᵗʰ **S96.00** Unspecified injury of muscle and tendon of long flexor muscle of toe at ankle and foot level

√7ᵗʰ **S96.001** Unspecified injury of muscle and tendon of long flexor muscle of toe at ankle and foot level, right foot ▽

√7ᵗʰ **S96.002** Unspecified injury of muscle and tendon of long flexor muscle of toe at ankle and foot level, left foot ▽

√7ᵗʰ **S96.009** Unspecified injury of muscle and tendon of long flexor muscle of toe at ankle and foot level, unspecified foot ▽

√6ᵗʰ **S96.01** Strain of muscle and tendon of long flexor muscle of toe at ankle and foot level

√7ᵗʰ **S96.011** Strain of muscle and tendon of long flexor muscle of toe at ankle and foot level, right foot

√7ᵗʰ **S96.012** Strain of muscle and tendon of long flexor muscle of toe at ankle and foot level, left foot

√7ᵗʰ **S96.019** Strain of muscle and tendon of long flexor muscle of toe at ankle and foot level, unspecified foot ▽

√6ᵗʰ **S96.02** Laceration of muscle and tendon of long flexor muscle of toe at ankle and foot level

√7ᵗʰ **S96.021** Laceration of muscle and tendon of long flexor muscle of toe at ankle and foot level, right foot

√7ᵗʰ **S96.022** Laceration of muscle and tendon of long flexor muscle of toe at ankle and foot level, left foot

√7ᵗʰ **S96.029** Laceration of muscle and tendon of long flexor muscle of toe at ankle and foot level, unspecified foot ▽

√6ᵗʰ **S96.09** Other injury of muscle and tendon of long flexor muscle of toe at ankle and foot level

√7ᵗʰ **S96.091** Other injury of muscle and tendon of long flexor muscle of toe at ankle and foot level, right foot

√7ᵗʰ **S96.092** Other injury of muscle and tendon of long flexor muscle of toe at ankle and foot level, left foot

√7ᵗʰ **S96.099** Other injury of muscle and tendon of long flexor muscle of toe at ankle and foot level, unspecified foot ▽

√5ᵗʰ **S96.1** Injury of muscle and tendon of long extensor muscle of toe at ankle and foot level

√6ᵗʰ **S96.10** Unspecified injury of muscle and tendon of long extensor muscle of toe at ankle and foot level

√7ᵗʰ **S96.101** Unspecified injury of muscle and tendon of long extensor muscle of toe at ankle and foot level, right foot ▽

√7ᵗʰ **S96.102** Unspecified injury of muscle and tendon of long extensor muscle of toe at ankle and foot level, left foot ▽

√7ᵗʰ **S96.109** Unspecified injury of muscle and tendon of long extensor muscle of toe at ankle and foot level, unspecified foot ▽

√6ᵗʰ **S96.11** Strain of muscle and tendon of long extensor muscle of toe at ankle and foot level

√7ᵗʰ **S96.111** Strain of muscle and tendon of long extensor muscle of toe at ankle and foot level, right foot

√7ᵗʰ **S96.112** Strain of muscle and tendon of long extensor muscle of toe at ankle and foot level, left foot

√7ᵗʰ **S96.119** Strain of muscle and tendon of long extensor muscle of toe at ankle and foot level, unspecified foot ▽

√6ᵗʰ **S96.12** Laceration of muscle and tendon of long extensor muscle of toe at ankle and foot level

√7ᵗʰ **S96.121** Laceration of muscle and tendon of long extensor muscle of toe at ankle and foot level, right foot

√7ᵗʰ **S96.122** Laceration of muscle and tendon of long extensor muscle of toe at ankle and foot level, left foot

√7ᵗʰ **S96.129** Laceration of muscle and tendon of long extensor muscle of toe at ankle and foot level, unspecified foot ▽

√6ᵗʰ **S96.19** Other specified injury of muscle and tendon of long extensor muscle of toe at ankle and foot level

√7ᵗʰ **S96.191** Other specified injury of muscle and tendon of long extensor muscle of toe at ankle and foot level, right foot

√7ᵗʰ **S96.192** Other specified injury of muscle and tendon of long extensor muscle of toe at ankle and foot level, left foot

---

EXCLUDES 1 Not coded here   *EXCLUDES 2* Not included here   **N** Newborn Age : 0   **P** Pediatric Age : 0-17   **M** Maternity Age : 12-55   **A** Adult Age : 15-124

1004   ICD-10-CM 2017

√7ᵗʰ **S96.199** Other specified injury of muscle and tendon of long extensor muscle of toe at ankle and foot level, unspecified foot ▽

√5ᵗʰ **S96.2** Injury of intrinsic muscle and tendon at ankle and foot level

    √6ᵗʰ **S96.20** Unspecified injury of intrinsic muscle and tendon at ankle and foot level

       √7ᵗʰ **S96.201** Unspecified injury of intrinsic muscle and tendon at ankle and foot level, **right** foot ▽

       √7ᵗʰ **S96.202** Unspecified injury of intrinsic muscle and tendon at ankle and foot level, **left** foot ▽

       √7ᵗʰ **S96.209** Unspecified injury of intrinsic muscle and tendon at ankle and foot level, unspecified foot ▽

    √6ᵗʰ **S96.21** Strain of intrinsic muscle and tendon at ankle and foot level

       √7ᵗʰ **S96.211** Strain of intrinsic muscle and tendon at ankle and foot level, **right** foot ▽

       √7ᵗʰ **S96.212** Strain of intrinsic muscle and tendon at ankle and foot level, **left** foot ▽

       √7ᵗʰ **S96.219** Strain of intrinsic muscle and tendon at ankle and foot level, unspecified foot ▽

    √6ᵗʰ **S96.22** Laceration of intrinsic muscle and tendon at ankle and foot level

       √7ᵗʰ **S96.221** Laceration of intrinsic muscle and tendon at ankle and foot level, **right** foot ▽

       √7ᵗʰ **S96.222** Laceration of intrinsic muscle and tendon at ankle and foot level, **left** foot ▽

       √7ᵗʰ **S96.229** Laceration of intrinsic muscle and tendon at ankle and foot level, unspecified foot ▽

    √6ᵗʰ **S96.29** Other specified injury of intrinsic muscle and tendon at ankle and foot level

       √7ᵗʰ **S96.291** Other specified injury of intrinsic muscle and tendon at ankle and foot level, **right** foot ▽

       √7ᵗʰ **S96.292** Other specified injury of intrinsic muscle and tendon at ankle and foot level, **left** foot ▽

       √7ᵗʰ **S96.299** Other specified injury of intrinsic muscle and tendon at ankle and foot level, unspecified foot ▽

√5ᵗʰ **S96.8** Injury of other specified muscles and tendons at ankle and foot level

    √6ᵗʰ **S96.80** Unspecified injury of other specified muscles and tendons at ankle and foot level

       √7ᵗʰ **S96.801** Unspecified injury of other specified muscles and tendons at ankle and foot level, **right** foot ▽

       √7ᵗʰ **S96.802** Unspecified injury of other specified muscles and tendons at ankle and foot level, **left** foot ▽

       √7ᵗʰ **S96.809** Unspecified injury of other specified muscles and tendons at ankle and foot level, unspecified foot ▽

    √6ᵗʰ **S96.81** Strain of other specified muscles and tendons at ankle and foot level

       √7ᵗʰ **S96.811** Strain of other specified muscles and tendons at ankle and foot level, **right** foot ▽

       √7ᵗʰ **S96.812** Strain of other specified muscles and tendons at ankle and foot level, **left** foot ▽

       √7ᵗʰ **S96.819** Strain of other specified muscles and tendons at ankle and foot level, unspecified foot ▽

    √6ᵗʰ **S96.82** Laceration of other specified muscles and tendons at ankle and foot level

       √7ᵗʰ **S96.821** Laceration of other specified muscles and tendons at ankle and foot level, **right** foot ▽

       √7ᵗʰ **S96.822** Laceration of other specified muscles and tendons at ankle and foot level, **left** foot ▽

       √7ᵗʰ **S96.829** Laceration of other specified muscles and tendons at ankle and foot level, unspecified foot ▽

    √6ᵗʰ **S96.89** Other specified injury of other specified muscles and tendons at ankle and foot level

       √7ᵗʰ **S96.891** Other specified injury of other specified muscles and tendons at ankle and foot level, **right** foot ▽

       √7ᵗʰ **S96.892** Other specified injury of other specified muscles and tendons at ankle and foot level, **left** foot ▽

       √7ᵗʰ **S96.899** Other specified injury of other specified muscles and tendons at ankle and foot level, unspecified foot ▽

√6ᵗʰ **S96.9** Injury of unspecified muscle and tendon at ankle and foot level

    √6ᵗʰ **S96.90** Unspecified injury of unspecified muscle and tendon at ankle and foot level

       √7ᵗʰ **S96.901** Unspecified injury of unspecified muscle and tendon at ankle and foot level, **right** foot ▽

       √7ᵗʰ **S96.902** Unspecified injury of unspecified muscle and tendon at ankle and foot level, **left** foot ▽

       √7ᵗʰ **S96.909** Unspecified injury of unspecified muscle and tendon at ankle and foot level, unspecified foot ▽

    √6ᵗʰ **S96.91** Strain of unspecified muscle and tendon at ankle and foot level

       √7ᵗʰ **S96.911** Strain of unspecified muscle and tendon at ankle and foot level, **right** foot ▽

       √7ᵗʰ **S96.912** Strain of unspecified muscle and tendon at ankle and foot level, **left** foot ▽

       √7ᵗʰ **S96.919** Strain of unspecified muscle and tendon at ankle and foot level, unspecified foot ▽

    √6ᵗʰ **S96.92** Laceration of unspecified muscle and tendon at ankle and foot level

       √7ᵗʰ **S96.921** Laceration of unspecified muscle and tendon at ankle and foot level, **right** foot ▽

       √7ᵗʰ **S96.922** Laceration of unspecified muscle and tendon at ankle and foot level, **left** foot ▽

       √7ᵗʰ **S96.929** Laceration of unspecified muscle and tendon at ankle and foot level, unspecified foot ▽

    √6ᵗʰ **S96.99** Other specified injury of unspecified muscle and tendon at ankle and foot level

       √7ᵗʰ **S96.991** Other specified injury of unspecified muscle and tendon at ankle and foot level, **right** foot ▽

       √7ᵗʰ **S96.992** Other specified injury of unspecified muscle and tendon at ankle and foot level, **left** foot ▽

       √7ᵗʰ **S96.999** Other specified injury of unspecified muscle and tendon at ankle and foot level, unspecified foot ▽

√4ᵗʰ **S97** **Crushing injury of ankle and foot**

    Use additional code(s) for all associated injuries

    The appropriate 7th character is to be added to each code from category S97.
    A   initial encounter
    D   subsequent encounter
    S   sequela

√5ᵗʰ **S97.0** Crushing injury of ankle

    √×7ᵗʰ **S97.00** Crushing injury of unspecified ankle ▽

    √×7ᵗʰ **S97.01** Crushing injury of **right** ankle

    √×7ᵗʰ **S97.02** Crushing injury of **left** ankle

√5ᵗʰ **S97.1** Crushing injury of toe

    √6ᵗʰ **S97.10** Crushing injury of unspecified toe(s)

       √7ᵗʰ **S97.101** Crushing injury of unspecified **right** toe(s) ▽

       √7ᵗʰ **S97.102** Crushing injury of unspecified **left** toe(s) ▽

       √7ᵗʰ **S97.109** Crushing injury of unspecified toe(s) ▽
             Crushing injury of toe NOS

    √6ᵗʰ **S97.11** Crushing injury of great toe

       √7ᵗʰ **S97.111** Crushing injury of **right** great toe

       √7ᵗʰ **S97.112** Crushing injury of **left** great toe

       √7ᵗʰ **S97.119** Crushing injury of unspecified great toe ▽

☑ Additional Character Required   √×7ᵗʰ Placeholder Alert   Manifestation Dx   ▽ Unspecified Dx   ▶◀ Revised Text   ● New Code   ▲ Revised Code Title

ICD-10-CM 2017   **1005**

✓6ᵗʰ **S97.12**   Crushing injury of lesser toe(s)

    ✓7ᵗʰ **S97.121** Crushing injury of right lesser toe(s)

    ✓7ᵗʰ **S97.122** Crushing injury of left lesser toe(s)

    ✓7ᵗʰ **S97.129** Crushing injury of unspecified lesser toe(s) ▽

✓5ᵗʰ **S97.8**   Crushing injury of foot

    ✓x7ᵗʰ **S97.80** Crushing injury of unspecified foot ▽

        Crushing injury of foot NOS

    ✓x7ᵗʰ **S97.81** Crushing injury of right foot

    ✓x7ᵗʰ **S97.82** Crushing injury of left foot

✓4ᵗʰ **S98**   **Traumatic amputation of ankle and foot**

    An amputation not identified as partial or complete should be coded to complete

    The appropriate 7th character is to be added to each code from category S98.
    A   initial encounter
    D   subsequent encounter
    S   sequela

✓5ᵗʰ **S98.0**   Traumatic amputation of foot at ankle level

    ✓6ᵗʰ **S98.01** Complete traumatic amputation of foot at ankle level

       ✓7ᵗʰ **S98.011** Complete traumatic amputation of right foot at ankle level

       ✓7ᵗʰ **S98.012** Complete traumatic amputation of left foot at ankle level

       ✓7ᵗʰ **S98.019** Complete traumatic amputation of unspecified foot at ankle level ▽

    ✓6ᵗʰ **S98.02** Partial traumatic amputation of foot at ankle level

       ✓7ᵗʰ **S98.021** Partial traumatic amputation of right foot at ankle level

       ✓7ᵗʰ **S98.022** Partial traumatic amputation of left foot at ankle level

       ✓7ᵗʰ **S98.029** Partial traumatic amputation of unspecified foot at ankle level ▽

✓5ᵗʰ **S98.1**   Traumatic amputation of one toe

    ✓6ᵗʰ **S98.11** Complete traumatic amputation of great toe

       ✓7ᵗʰ **S98.111** Complete traumatic amputation of right great toe

       ✓7ᵗʰ **S98.112** Complete traumatic amputation of left great toe

       ✓7ᵗʰ **S98.119** Complete traumatic amputation of unspecified great toe ▽

    ✓6ᵗʰ **S98.12** Partial traumatic amputation of great toe

       ✓7ᵗʰ **S98.121** Partial traumatic amputation of right great toe

       ✓7ᵗʰ **S98.122** Partial traumatic amputation of left great toe

       ✓7ᵗʰ **S98.129** Partial traumatic amputation of unspecified great toe ▽

    ✓6ᵗʰ **S98.13** Complete traumatic amputation of one lesser toe

       Traumatic amputation of toe NOS

       ✓7ᵗʰ **S98.131** Complete traumatic amputation of one right lesser toe

       ✓7ᵗʰ **S98.132** Complete traumatic amputation of one left lesser toe

       ✓7ᵗʰ **S98.139** Complete traumatic amputation of one unspecified lesser toe ▽

    ✓6ᵗʰ **S98.14** Partial traumatic amputation of one lesser toe

       ✓7ᵗʰ **S98.141** Partial traumatic amputation of one right lesser toe

       ✓7ᵗʰ **S98.142** Partial traumatic amputation of one left lesser toe

       ✓7ᵗʰ **S98.149** Partial traumatic amputation of one unspecified lesser toe ▽

✓5ᵗʰ **S98.2**   Traumatic amputation of two or more lesser toes

    ✓6ᵗʰ **S98.21** Complete traumatic amputation of two or more lesser toes

       ✓7ᵗʰ **S98.211** Complete traumatic amputation of two or more right lesser toes

       ✓7ᵗʰ **S98.212** Complete traumatic amputation of two or more left lesser toes

       ✓7ᵗʰ **S98.219** Complete traumatic amputation of two or more unspecified lesser toes ▽

    ✓6ᵗʰ **S98.22** Partial traumatic amputation of two or more lesser toes

       ✓7ᵗʰ **S98.221** Partial traumatic amputation of two or more right lesser toes

       ✓7ᵗʰ **S98.222** Partial traumatic amputation of two or more left lesser toes

       ✓7ᵗʰ **S98.229** Partial traumatic amputation of two or more unspecified lesser toes ▽

✓5ᵗʰ **S98.3**   Traumatic amputation of midfoot

    ✓6ᵗʰ **S98.31** Complete traumatic amputation of midfoot

       ✓7ᵗʰ **S98.311** Complete traumatic amputation of right midfoot

       ✓7ᵗʰ **S98.312** Complete traumatic amputation of left midfoot

       ✓7ᵗʰ **S98.319** Complete traumatic amputation of unspecified midfoot ▽

    ✓6ᵗʰ **S98.32** Partial traumatic amputation of midfoot

       ✓7ᵗʰ **S98.321** Partial traumatic amputation of right midfoot

       ✓7ᵗʰ **S98.322** Partial traumatic amputation of left midfoot

       ✓7ᵗʰ **S98.329** Partial traumatic amputation of unspecified midfoot ▽

✓5ᵗʰ **S98.9**   Traumatic amputation of foot, level unspecified

    ✓6ᵗʰ **S98.91** Complete traumatic amputation of foot, level unspecified

       ✓7ᵗʰ **S98.911** Complete traumatic amputation of right foot, level unspecified ▽

       ✓7ᵗʰ **S98.912** Complete traumatic amputation of left foot, level unspecified ▽

       ✓7ᵗʰ **S98.919** Complete traumatic amputation of unspecified foot, level unspecified ▽

    ✓6ᵗʰ **S98.92** Partial traumatic amputation of foot, level unspecified

       ✓7ᵗʰ **S98.921** Partial traumatic amputation of right foot, level unspecified ▽

       ✓7ᵗʰ **S98.922** Partial traumatic amputation of left foot, level unspecified ▽

       ✓7ᵗʰ **S98.929** Partial traumatic amputation of unspecified foot, level unspecified ▽

✓4ᵗʰ **S99**   **Other and unspecified injuries of ankle and foot**

● ✓5ᵗʰ **S99.0**   Physeal fracture of calcaneus

    The appropriate 7th character is to be added to each code from subcategory S99.0.
    A   initial encounter for closed fracture
    B   initial encounter for open fracture
    D   subsequent encounter for fracture with routine healing
    G   subsequent encounter for fracture with delayed healing
    K   subsequent encounter for fracture with nonunion
    P   subsequent encounter for fracture with malunion
    S   sequela

●   ✓6ᵗʰ **S99.00** Unspecified physeal fracture of calcaneus

●   ✓7ᵗʰ **S99.001** Unspecified physeal fracture of right calcaneus ▽

●   ✓7ᵗʰ **S99.002** Unspecified physeal fracture of left calcaneus ▽

●   ✓7ᵗʰ **S99.009** Unspecified physeal fracture of unspecified calcaneus ▽

●   ✓6ᵗʰ **S99.01** Salter-Harris Type I physeal fracture of calcaneus

●   ✓7ᵗʰ **S99.011** Salter-Harris Type I physeal fracture of right calcaneus

●   ✓7ᵗʰ **S99.012** Salter-Harris Type I physeal fracture of left calcaneus

●   ✓7ᵗʰ **S99.019** Salter-Harris Type I physeal fracture of unspecified calcaneus ▽

●   ✓6ᵗʰ **S99.02** Salter-Harris Type II physeal fracture of calcaneus

●   ✓7ᵗʰ **S99.021** Salter-Harris Type II physeal fracture of right calcaneus

●   ✓7ᵗʰ **S99.022** Salter-Harris Type II physeal fracture of left calcaneus

●   ✓7ᵗʰ **S99.029** Salter-Harris Type II physeal fracture of unspecified calcaneus ▽

●   ✓6ᵗʰ **S99.03** Salter-Harris Type III physeal fracture of calcaneus

●   ✓7ᵗʰ **S99.031** Salter-Harris Type III physeal fracture of right calcaneus

●   ✓7ᵗʰ **S99.032** Salter-Harris Type III physeal fracture of left calcaneus

●   ✓7ᵗʰ **S99.039** Salter-Harris Type III physeal fracture of unspecified calcaneus ▽

●   ✓6ᵗʰ **S99.04** Salter-Harris Type IV physeal fracture of calcaneus

---

EXCLUDES 1   Not coded here   EXCLUDES 2   Not included here   N Newborn Age : 0   P Pediatric Age : 0-17   M Maternity Age : 12-55   A Adult Age : 15-124

● ✓7ᵗʰ S99.041 Salter-Harris Type IV physeal fracture of right calcaneus

● ✓7ᵗʰ S99.042 Salter-Harris Type IV physeal fracture of left calcaneus

● ✓7ᵗʰ S99.049 Salter-Harris Type IV physeal fracture of unspecified calcaneus ▽

● ✓6ᵗʰ S99.09 Other physeal fracture of calcaneus

● ✓7ᵗʰ S99.091 Other physeal fracture of right calcaneus

● ✓7ᵗʰ S99.092 Other physeal fracture of left calcaneus

● ✓7ᵗʰ S99.099 Other physeal fracture of unspecified calcaneus ▽

● ✓5ᵗʰ S99.1 Physeal fracture of metatarsal

> The appropriate 7th character is to be added to each code from subcategory S99.1.
> A initial encounter for closed fracture
> B initial encounter for open fracture
> D subsequent encounter for fracture with routine healing
> G subsequent encounter for fracture with delayed healing
> K subsequent encounter for fracture with nonunion
> P subsequent encounter for fracture with malunion
> S sequela

● ✓6ᵗʰ S99.10 Unspecified physeal fracture of metatarsal

● ✓7ᵗʰ S99.101 Unspecified physeal fracture of right metatarsal ▽

● ✓7ᵗʰ S99.102 Unspecified physeal fracture of left metatarsal ▽

● ✓7ᵗʰ S99.109 Unspecified physeal fracture of unspecified metatarsal ▽

● ✓6ᵗʰ S99.11 Salter-Harris Type I physeal fracture of metatarsal

● ✓7ᵗʰ S99.111 Salter-Harris Type I physeal fracture of right metatarsal

● ✓7ᵗʰ S99.112 Salter-Harris Type I physeal fracture of left metatarsal

● ✓7ᵗʰ S99.119 Salter-Harris Type I physeal fracture of unspecified metatarsal ▽

● ✓6ᵗʰ S99.12 Salter-Harris Type II physeal fracture of metatarsal

● ✓7ᵗʰ S99.121 Salter-Harris Type II physeal fracture of right metatarsal

● ✓7ᵗʰ S99.122 Salter-Harris Type II physeal fracture of left metatarsal

● ✓7ᵗʰ S99.129 Salter-Harris Type II physeal fracture of unspecified metatarsal ▽

● ✓6ᵗʰ S99.13 Salter-Harris Type III physeal fracture of metatarsal

● ✓7ᵗʰ S99.131 Salter-Harris Type III physeal fracture of right metatarsal

● ✓7ᵗʰ S99.132 Salter-Harris Type III physeal fracture of left metatarsal

● ✓7ᵗʰ S99.139 Salter-Harris Type III physeal fracture of unspecified metatarsal ▽

● ✓6ᵗʰ S99.14 Salter-Harris Type IV physeal fracture of metatarsal

● ✓7ᵗʰ S99.141 Salter-Harris Type IV physeal fracture of right metatarsal

● ✓7ᵗʰ S99.142 Salter-Harris Type IV physeal fracture of left metatarsal

● ✓7ᵗʰ S99.149 Salter-Harris Type IV physeal fracture of unspecified metatarsal ▽

● ✓6ᵗʰ S99.19 Other physeal fracture of metatarsal

● ✓7ᵗʰ S99.191 Other physeal fracture of right metatarsal

● ✓7ᵗʰ S99.192 Other physeal fracture of left metatarsal

● ✓7ᵗʰ S99.199 Other physeal fracture of unspecified metatarsal ▽

● ✓5ᵗʰ S99.2 Physeal fracture of phalanx of toe

> The appropriate 7th character is to be added to each code from subcategories S99.2.
> A initial encounter for closed fracture
> B initial encounter for open fracture
> D subsequent encounter for fracture with routine healing
> G subsequent encounter for fracture with delayed healing
> K subsequent encounter for fracture with nonunion
> P subsequent encounter for fracture with malunion
> S sequela

● ✓6ᵗʰ S99.20 Unspecified physeal fracture of phalanx of toe

● ✓7ᵗʰ S99.201 Unspecified physeal fracture of right toe ▽

● ✓7ᵗʰ S99.202 Unspecified physeal fracture of phalanx of left toe ▽

● ✓7ᵗʰ S99.209 Unspecified physeal fracture of phalanx of unspecified toe ▽

● ✓6ᵗʰ S99.21 Salter-Harris Type I physeal fracture of phalanx of toe

● ✓7ᵗʰ S99.211 Salter-Harris Type I physeal fracture of phalanx of right toe

● ✓7ᵗʰ S99.212 Salter-Harris Type I physeal fracture of phalanx of left toe

● ✓7ᵗʰ S99.219 Salter-Harris Type I physeal fracture of phalanx of unspecified toe ▽

● ✓6ᵗʰ S99.22 Salter-Harris Type II physeal fracture of phalanx of toe

● ✓7ᵗʰ S99.221 Salter-Harris Type II physeal fracture of phalanx of right toe

● ✓7ᵗʰ S99.222 Salter-Harris Type II physeal fracture of phalanx of left toe

● ✓7ᵗʰ S99.229 Salter-Harris Type II physeal fracture of phalanx of unspecified toe ▽

● ✓6ᵗʰ S99.23 Salter-Harris Type III physeal fracture of phalanx of toe

● ✓7ᵗʰ S99.231 Salter-Harris Type III physeal fracture of phalanx of right toe

● ✓7ᵗʰ S99.232 Salter-Harris Type III physeal fracture of phalanx of left toe

● ✓7ᵗʰ S99.239 Salter-Harris Type III physeal fracture of phalanx of unspecified toe ▽

● ✓6ᵗʰ S99.24 Salter-Harris Type IV physeal fracture of phalanx of toe

● ✓7ᵗʰ S99.241 Salter-Harris Type IV physeal fracture of phalanx of right toe

● ✓7ᵗʰ S99.242 Salter-Harris Type IV physeal fracture of phalanx of left toe

● ✓7ᵗʰ S99.249 Salter-Harris Type IV physeal fracture of phalanx of unspecified toe ▽

● ✓6ᵗʰ S99.29 Other physeal fracture of phalanx of toe

● ✓7ᵗʰ S99.291 Other physeal fracture of phalanx of right toe

● ✓7ᵗʰ S99.292 Other physeal fracture of phalanx of left toe

● ✓7ᵗʰ S99.299 Other physeal fracture of phalanx of unspecified toe ▽

✓5ᵗʰ S99.8 Other specified injuries of ankle and foot

> The appropriate 7th character is to be added to each code from subcategory S99.8.
> A initial encounter
> D subsequent encounter
> S sequela

● ✓6ᵗʰ S99.81 Other specified injuries of ankle

● ✓7ᵗʰ S99.811 Other specified injuries of right ankle

● ✓7ᵗʰ S99.812 Other specified injuries of left ankle

● ✓7ᵗʰ S99.819 Other specified injuries of unspecified ankle ▽

● ✓6ᵗʰ S99.82 Other specified injuries of foot

● ✓7ᵗʰ S99.821 Other specified injuries of right foot

● ✓7ᵗʰ S99.822 Other specified injuries of left foot

● ✓7ᵗʰ S99.829 Other specified injuries of unspecified foot ▽

✓5ᵗʰ S99.9 Unspecified injury of ankle and foot

> The appropriate 7th character is to be added to each code from subcategory S99.9.
> A initial encounter
> D subsequent encounter
> S sequela

● ✓6ᵗʰ S99.91 Unspecified injury of ankle

● ✓7ᵗʰ S99.911 Unspecified injury of right ankle ▽

● ✓7ᵗʰ S99.912 Unspecified injury of left ankle ▽

● ✓7ᵗʰ S99.919 Unspecified injury of unspecified ankle ▽

● ✓6ᵗʰ S99.92 Unspecified injury of foot

● ✓7ᵗʰ S99.921 Unspecified injury of right foot ▽

● ✓7ᵗʰ S99.922 Unspecified injury of left foot ▽

● ✓7ᵗʰ S99.929 Unspecified injury of unspecified foot ▽

☑ Additional Character Required   ✓ₓ7ᵗʰ Placeholder Alert   Manifestation Dx   ▽ Unspecified Dx   ▶◀ Revised Text   ● New Code   ▲ Revised Code Title

Injury, Poisoning and Certain Other Consequences of External Causes (T07-T88)

Injuries involving multiple body regions (T07)

EXCLUDES 1   burns and corrosions (T20-T32)
frostbite (T33-T34)
insect bite or sting, venomous (T63.4)
sunburn (L55.-)

T07   **Unspecified multiple injuries**   ▽
     EXCLUDES 1   injury NOS (T14)

Injury of unspecified body region (T14)

√4ᵗʰ **T14**   **Injury of unspecified body region**
     EXCLUDES 1   multiple unspecified injuries (T07)

   T14.8   **Other injury of unspecified body region**   ▽
       Abrasion NOS
       Contusion NOS
       Crush injury NOS
       Fracture NOS
       Skin injury NOS
       Vascular injury NOS

   √5ᵗʰ **T14.9**   **Unspecified injury**
       T14.90   **Injury, unspecified**   ▽
            Injury NOS
       T14.91   **Suicide attempt**
            Attempted suicide NOS

Effects of foreign body entering through natural orifice (T15-T19)

EXCLUDES 2   foreign body accidentally left in operation wound (T81.5-)
foreign body in penetrating wound - See open wound by body region
residual foreign body in soft tissue (M79.5)
splinter, without open wound - See superficial injury by body region

√4ᵗʰ **T15**   **Foreign body on external eye**
     EXCLUDES 2   foreign body in penetrating wound of orbit and eye ball (S05.4-, S05.5-)
            open wound of eyelid and periocular area (S01.1-)
            retained foreign body in eyelid (H02.8-)
            retained (old) foreign body in penetrating wound of orbit and eye ball (H05.5-, H44.6-, H44.7-)
            superficial foreign body of eyelid and periocular area (S00.25-)

> The appropriate 7th character is to be added to each code from category T15.
> A   initial encounter
> D   subsequent encounter
> S   sequela

   √5ᵗʰ **T15.0**   **Foreign body in cornea**
       √x7ᵗʰ **T15.00**   **Foreign body in cornea, unspecified eye**   ▽
       √x7ᵗʰ **T15.01**   **Foreign body in cornea, right eye**
       √x7ᵗʰ **T15.02**   **Foreign body in cornea, left eye**

   √5ᵗʰ **T15.1**   **Foreign body in conjunctival sac**
       √x7ᵗʰ **T15.10**   **Foreign body in conjunctival sac, unspecified eye**   ▽
       √x7ᵗʰ **T15.11**   **Foreign body in conjunctival sac, right eye**
       √x7ᵗʰ **T15.12**   **Foreign body in conjunctival sac, left eye**

   √5ᵗʰ **T15.8**   **Foreign body in other and multiple parts of external eye**
       Foreign body in lacrimal punctum
       √x7ᵗʰ **T15.80**   **Foreign body in other and multiple parts of external eye, unspecified eye**   ▽
       √x7ᵗʰ **T15.81**   **Foreign body in other and multiple parts of external eye, right eye**
       √x7ᵗʰ **T15.82**   **Foreign body in other and multiple parts of external eye, left eye**

   √5ᵗʰ **T15.9**   **Foreign body on external eye, part unspecified**
       √x7ᵗʰ **T15.90**   **Foreign body on external eye, part unspecified, unspecified eye**   ▽
       √x7ᵗʰ **T15.91**   **Foreign body on external eye, part unspecified, right eye**   ▽
       √x7ᵗʰ **T15.92**   **Foreign body on external eye, part unspecified, left eye**   ▽

√4ᵗʰ **T16**   **Foreign body in ear**
     INCLUDES   foreign body in auditory canal

> The appropriate 7th character is to be added to each code from category T16.
> A   initial encounter
> D   subsequent encounter
> S   sequela

   √x7ᵗʰ **T16.1**   **Foreign body in right ear**
   √x7ᵗʰ **T16.2**   **Foreign body in left ear**
   √x7ᵗʰ **T16.9**   **Foreign body in ear, unspecified ear**   ▽

√4ᵗʰ **T17**   **Foreign body in respiratory tract**

> The appropriate 7th character is to be added to each code from category T17.
> A   initial encounter
> D   subsequent encounter
> S   sequela

   √x7ᵗʰ **T17.0**   **Foreign body in nasal sinus**
   √x7ᵗʰ **T17.1**   **Foreign body in nostril**
       Foreign body in nose NOS

   √5ᵗʰ **T17.2**   **Foreign body in pharynx**
       Foreign body in nasopharynx
       Foreign body in throat NOS
       √6ᵗʰ **T17.20**   **Unspecified foreign body in pharynx**
            √7ᵗʰ **T17.200**   **Unspecified foreign body in pharynx causing asphyxiation**   ▽
            √7ᵗʰ **T17.208**   **Unspecified foreign body in pharynx causing other injury**   ▽
       √6ᵗʰ **T17.21**   **Gastric contents in pharynx**
            Aspiration of gastric contents into pharynx
            Vomitus in pharynx
            √7ᵗʰ **T17.210**   **Gastric contents in pharynx causing asphyxiation**
            √7ᵗʰ **T17.218**   **Gastric contents in pharynx causing other injury**
       √6ᵗʰ **T17.22**   **Food in pharynx**
            Bones in pharynx
            Seeds in pharynx
            √7ᵗʰ **T17.220**   **Food in pharynx causing asphyxiation**
            √7ᵗʰ **T17.228**   **Food in pharynx causing other injury**
       √6ᵗʰ **T17.29**   **Other foreign object in pharynx**
            √7ᵗʰ **T17.290**   **Other foreign object in pharynx causing asphyxiation**
            √7ᵗʰ **T17.298**   **Other foreign object in pharynx causing other injury**

   √5ᵗʰ **T17.3**   **Foreign body in larynx**
       √6ᵗʰ **T17.30**   **Unspecified foreign body in larynx**
            √7ᵗʰ **T17.300**   **Unspecified foreign body in larynx causing asphyxiation**   ▽
            √7ᵗʰ **T17.308**   **Unspecified foreign body in larynx causing other injury**   ▽
       √6ᵗʰ **T17.31**   **Gastric contents in larynx**
            Aspiration of gastric contents into larynx
            Vomitus in larynx
            √7ᵗʰ **T17.310**   **Gastric contents in larynx causing asphyxiation**
            √7ᵗʰ **T17.318**   **Gastric contents in larynx causing other injury**
       √6ᵗʰ **T17.32**   **Food in larynx**
            ▶Bones in larynx◀
            Seeds in larynx
            √7ᵗʰ **T17.320**   **Food in larynx causing asphyxiation**
            √7ᵗʰ **T17.328**   **Food in larynx causing other injury**
       √6ᵗʰ **T17.39**   **Other foreign object in larynx**
            √7ᵗʰ **T17.390**   **Other foreign object in larynx causing asphyxiation**
            √7ᵗʰ **T17.398**   **Other foreign object in larynx causing other injury**

   √5ᵗʰ **T17.4**   **Foreign body in trachea**
       √6ᵗʰ **T17.40**   **Unspecified foreign body in trachea**
            √7ᵗʰ **T17.400**   **Unspecified foreign body in trachea causing asphyxiation**   ▽
            √7ᵗʰ **T17.408**   **Unspecified foreign body in trachea causing other injury**   ▽

EXCLUDES 1 Not coded here   **EXCLUDES 2** Not included here   N Newborn Age : 0   P Pediatric Age : 0-17   M Maternity Age : 12-55   A Adult Age : 15-124

1008   ICD-10-CM 2017

√6ᵗʰ **T17.41** Gastric contents in trachea
> Aspiration of gastric contents into trachea
> Vomitus in trachea

     √7ᵗʰ **T17.410** Gastric contents in trachea causing asphyxiation

     √7ᵗʰ **T17.418** Gastric contents in trachea causing other injury

√6ᵗʰ **T17.42** Food in trachea
> Bones in trachea
> Seeds in trachea

     √7ᵗʰ **T17.420** Food in trachea causing asphyxiation

     √7ᵗʰ **T17.428** Food in trachea causing other injury

√6ᵗʰ **T17.49** Other foreign object in trachea

     √7ᵗʰ **T17.490** Other foreign object in trachea causing asphyxiation

     √7ᵗʰ **T17.498** Other foreign object in trachea causing other injury

√5ᵗʰ **T17.5** Foreign body in bronchus

√6ᵗʰ **T17.50** Unspecified foreign body in bronchus

     √7ᵗʰ **T17.500** Unspecified foreign body in bronchus causing asphyxiation   ▽

     √7ᵗʰ **T17.508** Unspecified foreign body in bronchus causing other injury   ▽

√6ᵗʰ **T17.51** Gastric contents in bronchus
> Aspiration of gastric contents into bronchus
> Vomitus in bronchus

     √7ᵗʰ **T17.510** Gastric contents in bronchus causing asphyxiation

     √7ᵗʰ **T17.518** Gastric contents in bronchus causing other injury

√6ᵗʰ **T17.52** Food in bronchus
> Bones in bronchus
> Seeds in bronchus

     √7ᵗʰ **T17.520** Food in bronchus causing asphyxiation

     √7ᵗʰ **T17.528** Food in bronchus causing other injury

√6ᵗʰ **T17.59** Other foreign object in bronchus

     √7ᵗʰ **T17.590** Other foreign object in bronchus causing asphyxiation

     √7ᵗʰ **T17.598** Other foreign object in bronchus causing other injury

√5ᵗʰ **T17.8** Foreign body in other parts of respiratory tract
> Foreign body in bronchioles
> Foreign body in lung

√6ᵗʰ **T17.80** Unspecified foreign body in other parts of respiratory tract

     √7ᵗʰ **T17.800** Unspecified foreign body in other parts of respiratory tract causing asphyxiation   ▽

     √7ᵗʰ **T17.808** Unspecified foreign body in other parts of respiratory tract causing other injury   ▽

√6ᵗʰ **T17.81** Gastric contents in other parts of respiratory tract
> Aspiration of gastric contents into other parts of respiratory tract
> Vomitus in other parts of respiratory tract

     √7ᵗʰ **T17.810** Gastric contents in other parts of respiratory tract causing asphyxiation

     √7ᵗʰ **T17.818** Gastric contents in other parts of respiratory tract causing other injury

√6ᵗʰ **T17.82** Food in other parts of respiratory tract
> Bones in other parts of respiratory tract
> Seeds in other parts of respiratory tract

     √7ᵗʰ **T17.820** Food in other parts of respiratory tract causing asphyxiation

     √7ᵗʰ **T17.828** Food in other parts of respiratory tract causing other injury

√6ᵗʰ **T17.89** Other foreign object in other parts of respiratory tract

     √7ᵗʰ **T17.890** Other foreign object in other parts of respiratory tract causing asphyxiation

     √7ᵗʰ **T17.898** Other foreign object in other parts of respiratory tract causing other injury

√5ᵗʰ **T17.9** Foreign body in respiratory tract, part unspecified

√6ᵗʰ **T17.90** Unspecified foreign body in respiratory tract, part unspecified

     √7ᵗʰ **T17.900** Unspecified foreign body in respiratory tract, part unspecified causing asphyxiation   ▽

     √7ᵗʰ **T17.908** Unspecified foreign body in respiratory tract, part unspecified causing other injury   ▽

√6ᵗʰ **T17.91** Gastric contents in respiratory tract, part unspecified
> Aspiration of gastric contents into respiratory tract, part unspecified
> Vomitus in trachea respiratory tract, part unspecified

     √7ᵗʰ **T17.910** Gastric contents in respiratory tract, part unspecified causing asphyxiation   ▽

     √7ᵗʰ **T17.918** Gastric contents in respiratory tract, part unspecified causing other injury   ▽

√6ᵗʰ **T17.92** Food in respiratory tract, part unspecified
> Bones in respiratory tract, part unspecified
> Seeds in respiratory tract, part unspecified

     √7ᵗʰ **T17.920** Food in respiratory tract, part unspecified causing asphyxiation   ▽

     √7ᵗʰ **T17.928** Food in respiratory tract, part unspecified causing other injury   ▽

√6ᵗʰ **T17.99** Other foreign object in respiratory tract, part unspecified

     √7ᵗʰ **T17.990** Other foreign object in respiratory tract, part unspecified in causing asphyxiation   ▽

     √7ᵗʰ **T17.998** Other foreign object in respiratory tract, part unspecified causing other injury   ▽

√4ᵗʰ **T18** Foreign body in alimentary tract
> EXCLUDES 2   foreign body in pharynx (T17.2-)

> The appropriate 7th character is to be added to each code from category T18.
> A   initial encounter
> D   subsequent encounter
> S   sequela

√x7ᵗʰ **T18.0** Foreign body in mouth

√5ᵗʰ **T18.1** Foreign body in esophagus
> EXCLUDES 2   foreign body in respiratory tract (T17.-)

√6ᵗʰ **T18.10** Unspecified foreign body in esophagus

     √7ᵗʰ **T18.100** Unspecified foreign body in esophagus causing compression of trachea   ▽
> Unspecified foreign body in esophagus causing obstruction of respiration

     √7ᵗʰ **T18.108** Unspecified foreign body in esophagus causing other injury   ▽

√6ᵗʰ **T18.11** Gastric contents in esophagus
> Vomitus in esophagus

     √7ᵗʰ **T18.110** Gastric contents in esophagus causing compression of trachea
> Gastric contents in esophagus causing obstruction of respiration

     √7ᵗʰ **T18.118** Gastric contents in esophagus causing other injury

√6ᵗʰ **T18.12** Food in esophagus
> Bones in esophagus
> Seeds in esophagus

     √7ᵗʰ **T18.120** Food in esophagus causing compression of trachea
> Food in esophagus causing obstruction of respiration

     √7ᵗʰ **T18.128** Food in esophagus causing other injury

√6ᵗʰ **T18.19** Other foreign object in esophagus
> **AHA:** 2015,1Q,23

     √7ᵗʰ **T18.190** Other foreign object in esophagus causing compression of trachea
> Other foreign body in esophagus causing obstruction of respiration

     √7ᵗʰ **T18.198** Other foreign object in esophagus causing other injury

√x7ᵗʰ **T18.2** Foreign body in stomach

√x7ᵗʰ **T18.3** Foreign body in small intestine

√x7ᵗʰ **T18.4** Foreign body in colon

√x7ᵗʰ **T18.5** Foreign body in anus and rectum
> Foreign body in rectosigmoid (junction)

√x7ᵗʰ **T18.8** Foreign body in other parts of alimentary tract

☑ Additional Character Required   √x7ᵗʰ Placeholder Alert   Manifestation Dx   ▽ Unspecified Dx   ▶◀ Revised Text   ● New Code   ▲ Revised Code Title

ICD-10-CM 2017   **1009**

√x7ᵗʰ **T18.9 Foreign body of alimentary tract, part unspecified**   ▽
Foreign body in digestive system NOS
Swallowed foreign body NOS

√4ᵗʰ **T19 Foreign body in genitourinary tract**
EXCLUDES 2 *complications due to implanted mesh (T83.7-)*
mechanical complications of contraceptive device (intrauterine)
(vaginal) (T83.3-)
presence of contraceptive device (intrauterine) (vaginal) (Z97.5)

The appropriate 7th character is to be added to each code from
category T19.
A   initial encounter
D   subsequent encounter
S   sequela

√x7ᵗʰ **T19.0 Foreign body in urethra**
√x7ᵗʰ **T19.1 Foreign body in bladder**
√x7ᵗʰ **T19.2 Foreign body in vulva and vagina**   ♀
√x7ᵗʰ **T19.3 Foreign body in uterus**   ♀
√x7ᵗʰ **T19.4 Foreign body in penis**   ♂
√x7ᵗʰ **T19.8 Foreign body in other parts of genitourinary tract**
√x7ᵗʰ **T19.9 Foreign body in genitourinary tract, part unspecified**   ▽

Burns and corrosions (T20-T32)

INCLUDES   burns (thermal) from electrical heating appliances
burns (thermal) from electricity
burns (thermal) from flame
burns (thermal) from friction
burns (thermal) from hot air and hot gases
burns (thermal) from hot objects
burns (thermal) from lightning
burns (thermal) from radiation
chemical burn [corrosion] (external) (internal)
scalds
EXCLUDES 2 *erythema [dermatitis] ab igne (L59.0)*
radiation-related disorders of the skin and subcutaneous tissue (L55-L59)
sunburn (L55.-)
AHA: 2016,2Q,4

Burns and corrosions of external body surface, specified by site (T20-T25)

INCLUDES   burns and corrosions of first degree [erythema]
burns and corrosions of second degree [blisters] [epidermal loss]
burns and corrosions of third degree [deep necrosis of underlying
tissue] [full-thickness skin loss]
Use additional code from category T31 or T32 to identify extent of body surface
involved

√4ᵗʰ **T20 Burn and corrosion of head, face, and neck**
EXCLUDES 2 *burn and corrosion of ear drum (T28.41, T28.91)*
burn and corrosion of eye and adnexa (T26.-)
burn and corrosion of mouth and pharynx (T28.0)
AHA: 2015,1Q,18-19

The appropriate 7th character is to be added to each code from
category T20.
A   initial encounter
D   subsequent encounter
S   sequela

Rule of Nines Estimation of Total Body Surface Burned

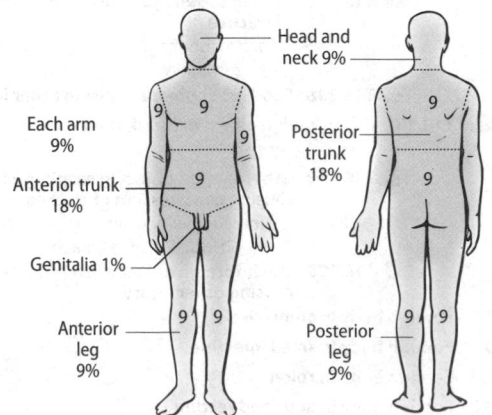

Head and neck 9%
Each arm 9%
Posterior trunk 18%
Anterior trunk 18%
Genitalia 1%
Anterior leg 9%
Posterior leg 9%

√5ᵗʰ **T20.0 Burn of unspecified degree of head, face, and neck**
Use additional external cause code to identify the source, place
and intent of the burn (X00-X19, X75-X77, X96-X98, Y92)

√x7ᵗʰ **T20.00 Burn of unspecified degree of head, face, and neck, unspecified site**   ▽
√6ᵗʰ **T20.01 Burn of unspecified degree of ear [any part, except ear drum]**
EXCLUDES 2 *burn of ear drum (T28.41-)*
√7ᵗʰ **T20.011 Burn of unspecified degree of right ear [any part, except ear drum]**   ▽
√7ᵗʰ **T20.012 Burn of unspecified degree of left ear [any part, except ear drum]**   ▽
√7ᵗʰ **T20.019 Burn of unspecified degree of unspecified ear [any part, except ear drum]**   ▽
√x7ᵗʰ **T20.02 Burn of unspecified degree of lip(s)**   ▽
√x7ᵗʰ **T20.03 Burn of unspecified degree of chin**   ▽
√x7ᵗʰ **T20.04 Burn of unspecified degree of nose (septum)**   ▽
√x7ᵗʰ **T20.05 Burn of unspecified degree of scalp [any part]**   ▽
√x7ᵗʰ **T20.06 Burn of unspecified degree of forehead and cheek**   ▽
√x7ᵗʰ **T20.07 Burn of unspecified degree of neck**   ▽
√x7ᵗʰ **T20.09 Burn of unspecified degree of multiple sites of head, face, and neck**   ▽

√5ᵗʰ **T20.1 Burn of first degree of head, face, and neck**
Use additional external cause code to identify the source, place
and intent of the burn (X00-X19, X75-X77, X96-X98, Y92)

Degree of Burns

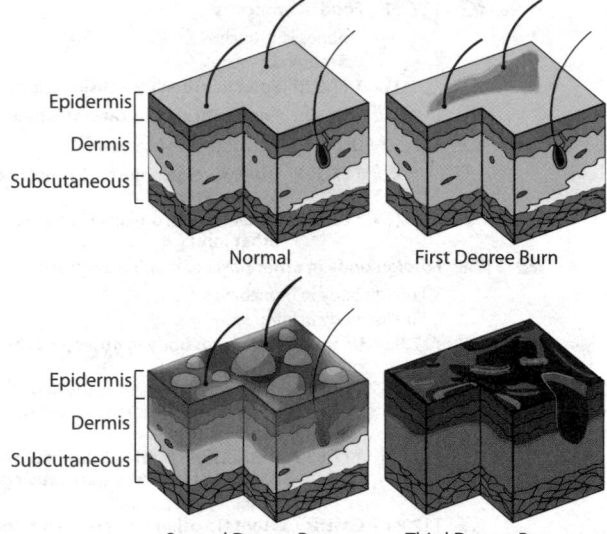

Epidermis
Dermis
Subcutaneous

Normal   First Degree Burn

Second Degree Burn   Third Degree Burn

√x7ᵗʰ **T20.10 Burn of first degree of head, face, and neck, unspecified site**   ▽
√6ᵗʰ **T20.11 Burn of first degree of ear [any part, except ear drum]**
EXCLUDES 2 *burn of ear drum (T28.41-)*
√7ᵗʰ **T20.111 Burn of first degree of right ear [any part, except ear drum]**
√7ᵗʰ **T20.112 Burn of first degree of left ear [any part, except ear drum]**
√7ᵗʰ **T20.119 Burn of first degree of unspecified ear [any part, except ear drum]**   ▽
√x7ᵗʰ **T20.12 Burn of first degree of lip(s)**
√x7ᵗʰ **T20.13 Burn of first degree of chin**
√x7ᵗʰ **T20.14 Burn of first degree of nose (septum)**
√x7ᵗʰ **T20.15 Burn of first degree of scalp [any part]**
√x7ᵗʰ **T20.16 Burn of first degree of forehead and cheek**
√x7ᵗʰ **T20.17 Burn of first degree of neck**
√x7ᵗʰ **T20.19 Burn of first degree of multiple sites of head, face, and neck**

√5ᵗʰ **T20.2** **Burn of second degree of head, face, and neck**

Use additional external cause code to identify the source, place and intent of the burn (X00-X19, X75-X77, X96-X98, Y92)

√x7ᵗʰ **T20.20** **Burn of second degree of head, face, and neck, unspecified site** ▽

√6ᵗʰ **T20.21** **Burn of second degree of ear [any part, except ear drum]**

     EXCLUDES 2   *burn of ear drum (T28.41-)*

√7ᵗʰ **T20.211** **Burn of second degree of right ear [any part, except ear drum]**

√7ᵗʰ **T20.212** **Burn of second degree of left ear [any part, except ear drum]**

√7ᵗʰ **T20.219** **Burn of second degree of unspecified ear [any part, except ear drum]** ▽

√x7ᵗʰ **T20.22** **Burn of second degree of lip(s)**

√x7ᵗʰ **T20.23** **Burn of second degree of chin**

√x7ᵗʰ **T20.24** **Burn of second degree of nose (septum)**

√x7ᵗʰ **T20.25** **Burn of second degree of scalp [any part]**

√x7ᵗʰ **T20.26** **Burn of second degree of forehead and cheek**

√x7ᵗʰ **T20.27** **Burn of second degree of neck**

√x7ᵗʰ **T20.29** **Burn of second degree of multiple sites of head, face, and neck**

√5ᵗʰ **T20.3** **Burn of third degree of head, face, and neck**

Use additional external cause code to identify the source, place and intent of the burn (X00-X19, X75-X77, X96-X98, Y92)

√x7ᵗʰ **T20.30** **Burn of third degree of head, face, and neck, unspecified site** ▽

√6ᵗʰ **T20.31** **Burn of third degree of ear [any part, except ear drum]**

     EXCLUDES 2   *burn of ear drum (T28.41-)*

     AHA: 2015,1Q,18

√7ᵗʰ **T20.311** **Burn of third degree of right ear [any part, except ear drum]**

√7ᵗʰ **T20.312** **Burn of third degree of left ear [any part, except ear drum]**

√7ᵗʰ **T20.319** **Burn of third degree of unspecified ear [any part, except ear drum]** ▽

√x7ᵗʰ **T20.32** **Burn of third degree of lip(s)**

√x7ᵗʰ **T20.33** **Burn of third degree of chin**

√x7ᵗʰ **T20.34** **Burn of third degree of nose (septum)**

√x7ᵗʰ **T20.35** **Burn of third degree of scalp [any part]**

√x7ᵗʰ **T20.36** **Burn of third degree of forehead and cheek**

√x7ᵗʰ **T20.37** **Burn of third degree of neck**

√x7ᵗʰ **T20.39** **Burn of third degree of multiple sites of head, face, and neck**

√5ᵗʰ **T20.4** **Corrosion of unspecified degree of head, face, and neck**

Code first (T51-T65) to identify chemical and intent

Use additional external cause code to identify place (Y92)

√x7ᵗʰ **T20.40** **Corrosion of unspecified degree of head, face, and neck, unspecified site** ▽

√6ᵗʰ **T20.41** **Corrosion of unspecified degree of ear [any part, except ear drum]**

     EXCLUDES 2   *corrosion of ear drum (T28.91-)*

√7ᵗʰ **T20.411** **Corrosion of unspecified degree of right ear [any part, except ear drum]** ▽

√7ᵗʰ **T20.412** **Corrosion of unspecified degree of left ear [any part, except ear drum]** ▽

√7ᵗʰ **T20.419** **Corrosion of unspecified degree of unspecified ear [any part, except ear drum]** ▽

√x7ᵗʰ **T20.42** **Corrosion of unspecified degree of lip(s)** ▽

√x7ᵗʰ **T20.43** **Corrosion of unspecified degree of chin** ▽

√x7ᵗʰ **T20.44** **Corrosion of unspecified degree of nose (septum)** ▽

√x7ᵗʰ **T20.45** **Corrosion of unspecified degree of scalp [any part]** ▽

√x7ᵗʰ **T20.46** **Corrosion of unspecified degree of forehead and cheek** ▽

√x7ᵗʰ **T20.47** **Corrosion of unspecified degree of neck** ▽

√x7ᵗʰ **T20.49** **Corrosion of unspecified degree of multiple sites of head, face, and neck** ▽

√5ᵗʰ **T20.5** **Corrosion of first degree of head, face, and neck**

Code first (T51-T65) to identify chemical and intent

Use additional external cause code to identify place (Y92)

√x7ᵗʰ **T20.50** **Corrosion of first degree of head, face, and neck, unspecified site** ▽

√6ᵗʰ **T20.51** **Corrosion of first degree of ear [any part, except ear drum]**

     EXCLUDES 2   *corrosion of ear drum (T28.91-)*

√7ᵗʰ **T20.511** **Corrosion of first degree of right ear [any part, except ear drum]**

√7ᵗʰ **T20.512** **Corrosion of first degree of left ear [any part, except ear drum]**

√7ᵗʰ **T20.519** **Corrosion of first degree of unspecified ear [any part, except ear drum]** ▽

√x7ᵗʰ **T20.52** **Corrosion of first degree of lip(s)**

√x7ᵗʰ **T20.53** **Corrosion of first degree of chin**

√x7ᵗʰ **T20.54** **Corrosion of first degree of nose (septum)**

√x7ᵗʰ **T20.55** **Corrosion of first degree of scalp [any part]**

√x7ᵗʰ **T20.56** **Corrosion of first degree of forehead and cheek**

√x7ᵗʰ **T20.57** **Corrosion of first degree of neck**

√x7ᵗʰ **T20.59** **Corrosion of first degree of multiple sites of head, face, and neck**

√5ᵗʰ **T20.6** **Corrosion of second degree of head, face, and neck**

Code first (T51-T65) to identify chemical and intent

Use additional external cause code to identify place (Y92)

√x7ᵗʰ **T20.60** **Corrosion of second degree of head, face, and neck, unspecified site** ▽

√6ᵗʰ **T20.61** **Corrosion of second degree of ear [any part, except ear drum]**

     EXCLUDES 2   *corrosion of ear drum (T28.91-)*

√7ᵗʰ **T20.611** **Corrosion of second degree of right ear [any part, except ear drum]**

√7ᵗʰ **T20.612** **Corrosion of second degree of left ear [any part, except ear drum]**

√7ᵗʰ **T20.619** **Corrosion of second degree of unspecified ear [any part, except ear drum]** ▽

√x7ᵗʰ **T20.62** **Corrosion of second degree of lip(s)**

√x7ᵗʰ **T20.63** **Corrosion of second degree of chin**

√x7ᵗʰ **T20.64** **Corrosion of second degree of nose (septum)**

√x7ᵗʰ **T20.65** **Corrosion of second degree of scalp [any part]**

√x7ᵗʰ **T20.66** **Corrosion of second degree of forehead and cheek**

√x7ᵗʰ **T20.67** **Corrosion of second degree of neck**

√x7ᵗʰ **T20.69** **Corrosion of second degree of multiple sites of head, face, and neck**

√5ᵗʰ **T20.7** **Corrosion of third degree of head, face, and neck**

Code first (T51-T65) to identify chemical and intent

Use additional external cause code to identify place (Y92)

√x7ᵗʰ **T20.70** **Corrosion of third degree of head, face, and neck, unspecified site** ▽

√6ᵗʰ **T20.71** **Corrosion of third degree of ear [any part, except ear drum]**

     EXCLUDES 2   *corrosion of ear drum (T28.91-)*

√7ᵗʰ **T20.711** **Corrosion of third degree of right ear [any part, except ear drum]**

√7ᵗʰ **T20.712** **Corrosion of third degree of left ear [any part, except ear drum]**

√7ᵗʰ **T20.719** **Corrosion of third degree of unspecified ear [any part, except ear drum]** ▽

√x7ᵗʰ **T20.72** **Corrosion of third degree of lip(s)**

√x7ᵗʰ **T20.73** **Corrosion of third degree of chin**

√x7ᵗʰ **T20.74** **Corrosion of third degree of nose (septum)**

√x7ᵗʰ **T20.75** **Corrosion of third degree of scalp [any part]**

√x7ᵗʰ **T20.76** **Corrosion of third degree of forehead and cheek**

√x7ᵗʰ **T20.77** **Corrosion of third degree of neck**

√x7ᵗʰ **T20.79** **Corrosion of third degree of multiple sites of head, face, and neck**

☑ Additional Character Required   √x7ᵗʰ Placeholder Alert   Manifestation Dx   ▽ Unspecified Dx   ▶◀ Revised Text   ● New Code   ▲ Revised Code Title

✓4ᵗʰ T21 Burn and corrosion of trunk

> INCLUDES   burns and corrosion of hip region
> EXCLUDES 2   *burns and corrosion of axilla (T22.- with fifth character 4)*
> *burns and corrosion of scapular region (T22.- with fifth character 6)*
> *burns and corrosion of shoulder (T22.- with fifth character 5)*

> The appropriate 7th character is to be added to each code from category T21.
> A   initial encounter
> D   subsequent encounter
> S   sequela

✓5ᵗʰ T21.0   Burn of unspecified degree of trunk

> Use additional external cause code to identify the source, place and intent of the burn (X00-X19, X75-X77, X96-X98, Y92)

   ✓x7ᵗʰ **T21.00   Burn of unspecified degree of trunk, unspecified site** ▽

   ✓x7ᵗʰ **T21.01   Burn of unspecified degree of chest wall** ▽
> Burn of of unspecified degree of breast

   ✓x7ᵗʰ **T21.02   Burn of unspecified degree of abdominal wall** ▽
> Burn of unspecified degree of flank
> Burn of unspecified degree of groin

   ✓x7ᵗʰ **T21.03   Burn of unspecified degree of upper back** ▽
> Burn of unspecified degree of interscapular region

   ✓x7ᵗʰ **T21.04   Burn of unspecified degree of lower back** ▽

   ✓x7ᵗʰ **T21.05   Burn of unspecified degree of buttock** ▽
> Burn of unspecified degree of anus

   ✓x7ᵗʰ **T21.06   Burn of unspecified degree of male genital region** ♂ ▽
> Burn of unspecified degree of penis
> Burn of unspecified degree of scrotum
> Burn of unspecified degree of testis

   ✓x7ᵗʰ **T21.07   Burn of unspecified degree of female genital region** ♀ ▽
> Burn of unspecified degree of labium (majus) (minus)
> Burn of unspecified degree of perineum
> Burn of unspecified degree of vulva
> EXCLUDES 2   *burn of vagina (T28.3)*

   ✓x7ᵗʰ **T21.09   Burn of unspecified degree of other site of trunk** ▽

✓5ᵗʰ T21.1   Burn of first degree of trunk

> Use additional external cause code to identify the source, place and intent of the burn (X00-X19, X75-X77, X96-X98, Y92)

   ✓x7ᵗʰ **T21.10   Burn of first degree of trunk, unspecified site** ▽

   ✓x7ᵗʰ **T21.11   Burn of first degree of chest wall**
> Burn of first degree of breast

   ✓x7ᵗʰ **T21.12   Burn of first degree of abdominal wall**
> Burn of first degree of flank
> Burn of first degree of groin

   ✓x7ᵗʰ **T21.13   Burn of first degree of upper back**
> Burn of first degree of interscapular region

   ✓x7ᵗʰ **T21.14   Burn of first degree of lower back**

   ✓x7ᵗʰ **T21.15   Burn of first degree of buttock**
> Burn of first degree of anus

   ✓x7ᵗʰ **T21.16   Burn of first degree of male genital region** ♂
> Burn of first degree of penis
> Burn of first degree of scrotum
> Burn of first degree of testis

   ✓x7ᵗʰ **T21.17   Burn of first degree of female genital region** ♀
> Burn of first degree of labium (majus) (minus)
> Burn of first degree of perineum
> Burn of first degree of vulva
> EXCLUDES 2   *burn of vagina (T28.3)*

   ✓x7ᵗʰ **T21.19   Burn of first degree of other site of trunk**

✓5ᵗʰ T21.2   Burn of second degree of trunk

> Use additional external cause code to identify the source, place and intent of the burn (X00-X19, X75-X77, X96-X98, Y92)

   ✓x7ᵗʰ **T21.20   Burn of second degree of trunk, unspecified site** ▽

   ✓x7ᵗʰ **T21.21   Burn of second degree of chest wall**
> Burn of second degree of breast

   ✓x7ᵗʰ **T21.22   Burn of second degree of abdominal wall**
> Burn of second degree of flank
> Burn of second degree of groin

   ✓x7ᵗʰ **T21.23   Burn of second degree of upper back**
> Burn of second degree of interscapular region

   ✓x7ᵗʰ **T21.24   Burn of second degree of lower back**

   ✓x7ᵗʰ **T21.25   Burn of second degree of buttock**
> Burn of second degree of anus

   ✓x7ᵗʰ **T21.26   Burn of second degree of male genital region** ♂
> Burn of second degree of penis
> Burn of second degree of scrotum
> Burn of second degree of testis

   ✓x7ᵗʰ **T21.27   Burn of second degree of female genital region** ♀
> Burn of second degree of labium (majus) (minus)
> Burn of second degree of perineum
> Burn of second degree of vulva
> EXCLUDES 2   *burn of vagina (T28.3)*

   ✓x7ᵗʰ **T21.29   Burn of second degree of other site of trunk**

✓5ᵗʰ T21.3   Burn of third degree of trunk

> Use additional external cause code to identify the source, place and intent of the burn (X00-X19, X75-X77, X96-X98, Y92)

   ✓x7ᵗʰ **T21.30   Burn of third degree of trunk, unspecified site** ▽

   ✓x7ᵗʰ **T21.31   Burn of third degree of chest wall**
> Burn of third degree of breast
> **AHA:** 2016,2Q,5

   ✓x7ᵗʰ **T21.32   Burn of third degree of abdominal wall**
> Burn of third degree of flank
> Burn of third degree of groin

   ✓x7ᵗʰ **T21.33   Burn of third degree of upper back**
> Burn of third degree of interscapular region

   ✓x7ᵗʰ **T21.34   Burn of third degree of lower back**

   ✓x7ᵗʰ **T21.35   Burn of third degree of buttock**
> Burn of third degree of anus

   ✓x7ᵗʰ **T21.36   Burn of third degree of male genital region** ♂
> Burn of third degree of penis
> Burn of third degree of scrotum
> Burn of third degree of testis

   ✓x7ᵗʰ **T21.37   Burn of third degree of female genital region** ♀
> Burn of third degree of labium (majus) (minus)
> Burn of third degree of perineum
> Burn of third degree of vulva
> EXCLUDES 2   *burn of vagina (T28.3)*

   ✓x7ᵗʰ **T21.39   Burn of third degree of other site of trunk**

✓5ᵗʰ T21.4   Corrosion of unspecified degree of trunk

> Code first (T51-T65) to identify chemical and intent
> Use additional external cause code to identify place (Y92)

   ✓x7ᵗʰ **T21.40   Corrosion of unspecified degree of trunk, unspecified site** ▽

   ✓x7ᵗʰ **T21.41   Corrosion of unspecified degree of chest wall** ▽
> Corrosion of unspecified degree of breast

   ✓x7ᵗʰ **T21.42   Corrosion of unspecified degree of abdominal wall** ▽
> Corrosion of unspecified degree of flank
> Corrosion of unspecified degree of groin

   ✓x7ᵗʰ **T21.43   Corrosion of unspecified degree of upper back** ▽
> Corrosion of unspecified degree of interscapular region

   ✓x7ᵗʰ **T21.44   Corrosion of unspecified degree of lower back** ▽

   ✓x7ᵗʰ **T21.45   Corrosion of unspecified degree of buttock** ▽
> Corrosion of unspecified degree of anus

   ✓x7ᵗʰ **T21.46   Corrosion of unspecified degree of male genital region** ♂ ▽
> Corrosion of unspecified degree of penis
> Corrosion of unspecified degree of scrotum
> Corrosion of unspecified degree of testis

   ✓x7ᵗʰ **T21.47   Corrosion of unspecified degree of female genital region** ♀ ▽
> Corrosion of unspecified degree of labium (majus) (minus)
> Corrosion of unspecified degree of perineum
> Corrosion of unspecified degree of vulva
> EXCLUDES 2   *corrosion of vagina (T28.8)*

   ✓x7ᵗʰ **T21.49   Corrosion of unspecified degree of other site of trunk** ▽

EXCLUDES 1 Not coded here   EXCLUDES 2 Not included here   Ⓝ Newborn Age : 0   Ⓟ Pediatric Age : 0-17   Ⓜ Maternity Age : 12-55   Ⓐ Adult Age : 15-124

1012

ICD-10-CM 2017

√5ᵗʰ **T21.5** **Corrosion of** first degree **of trunk**

Code first (T51-T65) to identify chemical and intent
Use additional external cause code to identify place (Y92)

√x7ᵗʰ **T21.50** **Corrosion of first degree of trunk, unspecified site** ▽

√x7ᵗʰ **T21.51** **Corrosion of first degree of** chest wall

Corrosion of first degree of breast

√x7ᵗʰ **T21.52** **Corrosion of first degree of** abdominal wall

Corrosion of first degree of flank
Corrosion of first degree of groin

√x7ᵗʰ **T21.53** **Corrosion of first degree of** upper back

Corrosion of first degree of interscapular region

√x7ᵗʰ **T21.54** **Corrosion of first degree of** lower back

√x7ᵗʰ **T21.55** **Corrosion of first degree of** buttock

Corrosion of first degree of anus

√x7ᵗʰ **T21.56** **Corrosion of first degree of** male genital region ♂

Corrosion of first degree of penis
Corrosion of first degree of scrotum
Corrosion of first degree of testis

√x7ᵗʰ **T21.57** **Corrosion of first degree of** female genital region ♀

Corrosion of first degree of labium (majus) (minus)
Corrosion of first degree of perineum
Corrosion of first degree of vulva

EXCLUDES 2 *corrosion of vagina (T28.8)*

√x7ᵗʰ **T21.59** **Corrosion of first degree of other site of trunk**

√5ᵗʰ **T21.6** **Corrosion of** second degree **of trunk**

Code first (T51-T65) to identify chemical and intent
Use additional external cause code to identify place (Y92)

√x7ᵗʰ **T21.60** **Corrosion of second degree of trunk, unspecified site** ▽

√x7ᵗʰ **T21.61** **Corrosion of second degree of** chest wall

Corrosion of second degree of breast

√x7ᵗʰ **T21.62** **Corrosion of second degree of** abdominal wall

Corrosion of second degree of flank
Corrosion of second degree of groin

√x7ᵗʰ **T21.63** **Corrosion of second degree of** upper back

Corrosion of second degree of interscapular region

√x7ᵗʰ **T21.64** **Corrosion of second degree of** lower back

√x7ᵗʰ **T21.65** **Corrosion of second degree of** buttock

Corrosion of second degree of anus

√x7ᵗʰ **T21.66** **Corrosion of second degree of** male genital region ♂

Corrosion of second degree of penis
Corrosion of second degree of scrotum
Corrosion of second degree of testis

√x7ᵗʰ **T21.67** **Corrosion of second degree of** female genital region ♀

Corrosion of second degree of labium (majus) (minus)
Corrosion of second degree of perineum
Corrosion of second degree of vulva

EXCLUDES 2 *corrosion of vagina (T28.8)*

√x7ᵗʰ **T21.69** **Corrosion of second degree of other site of trunk**

√5ᵗʰ **T21.7** **Corrosion of** third degree **of trunk**

Code first (T51-T65) to identify chemical and intent
Use additional external cause code to identify place (Y92)

√x7ᵗʰ **T21.70** **Corrosion of third degree of trunk, unspecified site** ▽

√x7ᵗʰ **T21.71** **Corrosion of third degree of** chest wall

Corrosion of third degree of breast

√x7ᵗʰ **T21.72** **Corrosion of third degree of** abdominal wall

Corrosion of third degree of flank
Corrosion of third degree of groin

√x7ᵗʰ **T21.73** **Corrosion of third degree of** upper back

Corrosion of third degree of interscapular region

√x7ᵗʰ **T21.74** **Corrosion of third degree of** lower back

√x7ᵗʰ **T21.75** **Corrosion of third degree of** buttock

Corrosion of third degree of anus

√x7ᵗʰ **T21.76** **Corrosion of third degree of** male genital region ♂

Corrosion of third degree of penis
Corrosion of third degree of scrotum
Corrosion of third degree of testis

√x7ᵗʰ **T21.77** **Corrosion of third degree of** female genital region ♀

Corrosion of third degree of labium (majus) (minus)
Corrosion of third degree of perineum
Corrosion of third degree of vulva

EXCLUDES 2 *corrosion of vagina (T28.8)*

√x7ᵗʰ **T21.79** **Corrosion of third degree of other site of trunk**

√4ᵗʰ **T22** **Burn and corrosion of shoulder and upper limb, except wrist and hand**

EXCLUDES 2 *burn and corrosion of interscapular region (T21.-)*
burn and corrosion of wrist and hand (T23.-)

The appropriate 7th character is to be added to each code from category T22.
A   initial encounter
D   subsequent encounter
S   sequela

√5ᵗʰ **T22.0** **Burn of unspecified degree of shoulder and upper limb, except wrist and hand**

Use additional external cause code to identify the source, place and intent of the burn (X00-X19, X75-X77, X96-X98, Y92)

√x7ᵗʰ **T22.00** **Burn of unspecified degree of shoulder and upper limb, except wrist and hand, unspecified site** ▽

√6ᵗʰ **T22.01** **Burn of unspecified degree of** forearm

√7ᵗʰ **T22.011** **Burn of unspecified degree of** right forearm ▽

√7ᵗʰ **T22.012** **Burn of unspecified degree of** left forearm ▽

√7ᵗʰ **T22.019** **Burn of unspecified degree of** unspecified forearm ▽

√6ᵗʰ **T22.02** **Burn of unspecified degree of** elbow

√7ᵗʰ **T22.021** **Burn of unspecified degree of** right elbow ▽

√7ᵗʰ **T22.022** **Burn of unspecified degree of** left elbow ▽

√7ᵗʰ **T22.029** **Burn of unspecified degree of** unspecified elbow ▽

√6ᵗʰ **T22.03** **Burn of unspecified degree of** upper arm

√7ᵗʰ **T22.031** **Burn of unspecified degree of** right upper arm ▽

√7ᵗʰ **T22.032** **Burn of unspecified degree of** left upper arm ▽

√7ᵗʰ **T22.039** **Burn of unspecified degree of** unspecified upper arm ▽

√6ᵗʰ **T22.04** **Burn of unspecified degree of** axilla

√7ᵗʰ **T22.041** **Burn of unspecified degree of** right axilla ▽

√7ᵗʰ **T22.042** **Burn of unspecified degree of** left axilla ▽

√7ᵗʰ **T22.049** **Burn of unspecified degree of** unspecified axilla ▽

√6ᵗʰ **T22.05** **Burn of unspecified degree of** shoulder

√7ᵗʰ **T22.051** **Burn of unspecified degree of** right shoulder ▽

√7ᵗʰ **T22.052** **Burn of unspecified degree of** left shoulder ▽

√7ᵗʰ **T22.059** **Burn of unspecified degree of** unspecified shoulder ▽

√6ᵗʰ **T22.06** **Burn of unspecified degree of** scapular region

√7ᵗʰ **T22.061** **Burn of unspecified degree of** right scapular region ▽

√7ᵗʰ **T22.062** **Burn of unspecified degree of** left scapular region ▽

√7ᵗʰ **T22.069** **Burn of unspecified degree of** unspecified scapular region ▽

√6ᵗʰ **T22.09** **Burn of unspecified degree of** multiple sites **of shoulder and upper limb, except wrist and hand**

√7ᵗʰ **T22.091** **Burn of unspecified degree of multiple sites of** right shoulder **and upper limb, except wrist and hand** ▽

√7ᵗʰ **T22.092** **Burn of unspecified degree of multiple sites of** left shoulder **and upper limb, except wrist and hand** ▽

√7ᵗʰ **T22.099** **Burn of unspecified degree of multiple sites of** unspecified **shoulder and upper limb, except wrist and hand** ▽

☑ Additional Character Required   √x7ᵗʰ Placeholder Alert   Manifestation Dx   ▽ Unspecified Dx   ►◄ Revised Text   ● New Code   ▲ Revised Code Title

✓5th **T22.1 Burn of first degree of shoulder and upper limb, except wrist and hand**

> Use additional external cause code to identify the source, place and intent of the burn (X00-X19, X75-X77, X96-X98, Y92)

✓x7th **T22.10 Burn of first degree of shoulder and upper limb, except wrist and hand, unspecified site** ▽

✓6th **T22.11 Burn of first degree of forearm**

   ✓7th **T22.111 Burn of first degree of right forearm**

   ✓7th **T22.112 Burn of first degree of left forearm**

   ✓7th **T22.119 Burn of first degree of unspecified forearm** ▽

✓6th **T22.12 Burn of first degree of elbow**

   ✓7th **T22.121 Burn of first degree of right elbow**

   ✓7th **T22.122 Burn of first degree of left elbow**

   ✓7th **T22.129 Burn of first degree of unspecified elbow** ▽

✓6th **T22.13 Burn of first degree of upper arm**

   ✓7th **T22.131 Burn of first degree of right upper arm**

   ✓7th **T22.132 Burn of first degree of left upper arm**

   ✓7th **T22.139 Burn of first degree of unspecified upper arm** ▽

✓6th **T22.14 Burn of first degree of axilla**

   ✓7th **T22.141 Burn of first degree of right axilla**

   ✓7th **T22.142 Burn of first degree of left axilla**

   ✓7th **T22.149 Burn of first degree of unspecified axilla** ▽

✓6th **T22.15 Burn of first degree of shoulder**

   ✓7th **T22.151 Burn of first degree of right shoulder**

   ✓7th **T22.152 Burn of first degree of left shoulder**

   ✓7th **T22.159 Burn of first degree of unspecified shoulder** ▽

✓6th **T22.16 Burn of first degree of scapular region**

   ✓7th **T22.161 Burn of first degree of right scapular region**

   ✓7th **T22.162 Burn of first degree of left scapular region**

   ✓7th **T22.169 Burn of first degree of unspecified scapular region** ▽

✓6th **T22.19 Burn of first degree of multiple sites of shoulder and upper limb, except wrist and hand**

   ✓7th **T22.191 Burn of first degree of multiple sites of right shoulder and upper limb, except wrist and hand**

   ✓7th **T22.192 Burn of first degree of multiple sites of left shoulder and upper limb, except wrist and hand**

   ✓7th **T22.199 Burn of first degree of multiple sites of unspecified shoulder and upper limb, except wrist and hand** ▽

✓5th **T22.2 Burn of second degree of shoulder and upper limb, except wrist and hand**

> Use additional external cause code to identify the source, place and intent of the burn (X00-X19, X75-X77, X96-X98, Y92)

✓x7th **T22.20 Burn of second degree of shoulder and upper limb, except wrist and hand, unspecified site** ▽

✓6th **T22.21 Burn of second degree of forearm**

   ✓7th **T22.211 Burn of second degree of right forearm**

   ✓7th **T22.212 Burn of second degree of left forearm**

   ✓7th **T22.219 Burn of second degree of unspecified forearm** ▽

✓6th **T22.22 Burn of second degree of elbow**

   ✓7th **T22.221 Burn of second degree of right elbow**

   ✓7th **T22.222 Burn of second degree of left elbow**

   ✓7th **T22.229 Burn of second degree of unspecified elbow** ▽

✓6th **T22.23 Burn of second degree of upper arm**

   ✓7th **T22.231 Burn of second degree of right upper arm**

   ✓7th **T22.232 Burn of second degree of left upper arm**

   ✓7th **T22.239 Burn of second degree of unspecified upper arm** ▽

✓6th **T22.24 Burn of second degree of axilla**

   ✓7th **T22.241 Burn of second degree of right axilla**

   ✓7th **T22.242 Burn of second degree of left axilla**

   ✓7th **T22.249 Burn of second degree of unspecified axilla** ▽

✓6th **T22.25 Burn of second degree of shoulder**

✓7th **T22.251 Burn of second degree of right shoulder**

✓7th **T22.252 Burn of second degree of left shoulder**

✓7th **T22.259 Burn of second degree of unspecified shoulder** ▽

✓6th **T22.26 Burn of second degree of scapular region**

   ✓7th **T22.261 Burn of second degree of right scapular region**

   ✓7th **T22.262 Burn of second degree of left scapular region**

   ✓7th **T22.269 Burn of second degree of unspecified scapular region** ▽

✓6th **T22.29 Burn of second degree of multiple sites of shoulder and upper limb, except wrist and hand**

   ✓7th **T22.291 Burn of second degree of multiple sites of right shoulder and upper limb, except wrist and hand**

   ✓7th **T22.292 Burn of second degree of multiple sites of left shoulder and upper limb, except wrist and hand**

   ✓7th **T22.299 Burn of second degree of multiple sites of unspecified shoulder and upper limb, except wrist and hand** ▽

✓5th **T22.3 Burn of third degree of shoulder and upper limb, except wrist and hand**

> Use additional external cause code to identify the source, place and intent of the burn (X00-X19, X75-X77, X96-X98, Y92)

✓x7th **T22.30 Burn of third degree of shoulder and upper limb, except wrist and hand, unspecified site** ▽

✓6th **T22.31 Burn of third degree of forearm**

   ✓7th **T22.311 Burn of third degree of right forearm**

   ✓7th **T22.312 Burn of third degree of left forearm**

   ✓7th **T22.319 Burn of third degree of unspecified forearm** ▽

✓6th **T22.32 Burn of third degree of elbow**

   ✓7th **T22.321 Burn of third degree of right elbow**

   ✓7th **T22.322 Burn of third degree of left elbow**

   ✓7th **T22.329 Burn of third degree of unspecified elbow** ▽

✓6th **T22.33 Burn of third degree of upper arm**

   ✓7th **T22.331 Burn of third degree of right upper arm**

   ✓7th **T22.332 Burn of third degree of left upper arm**

   ✓7th **T22.339 Burn of third degree of unspecified upper arm** ▽

✓6th **T22.34 Burn of third degree of axilla**

   ✓7th **T22.341 Burn of third degree of right axilla**

   ✓7th **T22.342 Burn of third degree of left axilla**

   ✓7th **T22.349 Burn of third degree of unspecified axilla** ▽

✓6th **T22.35 Burn of third degree of shoulder**

   ✓7th **T22.351 Burn of third degree of right shoulder**

   ✓7th **T22.352 Burn of third degree of left shoulder**

   ✓7th **T22.359 Burn of third degree of unspecified shoulder** ▽

✓6th **T22.36 Burn of third degree of scapular region**

   ✓7th **T22.361 Burn of third degree of right scapular region**

   ✓7th **T22.362 Burn of third degree of left scapular region**

   ✓7th **T22.369 Burn of third degree of unspecified scapular region** ▽

✓6th **T22.39 Burn of third degree of multiple sites of shoulder and upper limb, except wrist and hand**

   ✓7th **T22.391 Burn of third degree of multiple sites of right shoulder and upper limb, except wrist and hand**

   ✓7th **T22.392 Burn of third degree of multiple sites of left shoulder and upper limb, except wrist and hand**

   ✓7th **T22.399 Burn of third degree of multiple sites of unspecified shoulder and upper limb, except wrist and hand** ▽

✓5th **T22.4 Corrosion of unspecified degree of shoulder and upper limb, except wrist and hand**

> Code first (T51-T65) to identify chemical and intent
> Use additional external cause code to identify place (Y92)

✓x7th **T22.40 Corrosion of unspecified degree of shoulder and upper limb, except wrist and hand, unspecified site** ▽

EXCLUDES 1 Not coded here   EXCLUDES 2 Not included here   N Newborn Age : 0   P Pediatric Age : 0-17   M Maternity Age : 12-55   A Adult Age : 15-124

1014   ICD-10-CM 2017

√6ᵗʰ **T22.41** Corrosion of unspecified degree of forearm

   √7ᵗʰ **T22.411** Corrosion of unspecified degree of right forearm ▽

   √7ᵗʰ **T22.412** Corrosion of unspecified degree of left forearm ▽

   √7ᵗʰ **T22.419** Corrosion of unspecified degree of unspecified forearm ▽

√6ᵗʰ **T22.42** Corrosion of unspecified degree of elbow

   √7ᵗʰ **T22.421** Corrosion of unspecified degree of right elbow ▽

   √7ᵗʰ **T22.422** Corrosion of unspecified degree of left elbow ▽

   √7ᵗʰ **T22.429** Corrosion of unspecified degree of unspecified elbow ▽

√6ᵗʰ **T22.43** Corrosion of unspecified degree of upper arm

   √7ᵗʰ **T22.431** Corrosion of unspecified degree of right upper arm ▽

   √7ᵗʰ **T22.432** Corrosion of unspecified degree of left upper arm ▽

   √7ᵗʰ **T22.439** Corrosion of unspecified degree of unspecified upper arm ▽

√6ᵗʰ **T22.44** Corrosion of unspecified degree of axilla

   √7ᵗʰ **T22.441** Corrosion of unspecified degree of right axilla ▽

   √7ᵗʰ **T22.442** Corrosion of unspecified degree of left axilla ▽

   √7ᵗʰ **T22.449** Corrosion of unspecified degree of unspecified axilla ▽

√6ᵗʰ **T22.45** Corrosion of unspecified degree of shoulder

   √7ᵗʰ **T22.451** Corrosion of unspecified degree of right shoulder ▽

   √7ᵗʰ **T22.452** Corrosion of unspecified degree of left shoulder ▽

   √7ᵗʰ **T22.459** Corrosion of unspecified degree of unspecified shoulder ▽

√6ᵗʰ **T22.46** Corrosion of unspecified degree of scapular region

   √7ᵗʰ **T22.461** Corrosion of unspecified degree of right scapular region ▽

   √7ᵗʰ **T22.462** Corrosion of unspecified degree of left scapular region ▽

   √7ᵗʰ **T22.469** Corrosion of unspecified degree of unspecified scapular region ▽

√6ᵗʰ **T22.49** Corrosion of unspecified degree of multiple sites of shoulder and upper limb, except wrist and hand

   √7ᵗʰ **T22.491** Corrosion of unspecified degree of multiple sites of right shoulder and upper limb, except wrist and hand ▽

   √7ᵗʰ **T22.492** Corrosion of unspecified degree of multiple sites of left shoulder and upper limb, except wrist and hand ▽

   √7ᵗʰ **T22.499** Corrosion of unspecified degree of multiple sites of unspecified shoulder and upper limb, except wrist and hand ▽

√5ᵗʰ **T22.5** Corrosion of first degree of shoulder and upper limb, except wrist and hand

   Code first (T51-T65) to identify chemical and intent

   Use additional external cause code to identify place (Y92)

√x7ᵗʰ **T22.50** Corrosion of first degree of shoulder and upper limb, except wrist and hand unspecified site ▽

√6ᵗʰ **T22.51** Corrosion of first degree of forearm

   √7ᵗʰ **T22.511** Corrosion of first degree of right forearm

   √7ᵗʰ **T22.512** Corrosion of first degree of left forearm

   √7ᵗʰ **T22.519** Corrosion of first degree of unspecified forearm ▽

√6ᵗʰ **T22.52** Corrosion of first degree of elbow

   √7ᵗʰ **T22.521** Corrosion of first degree of right elbow

   √7ᵗʰ **T22.522** Corrosion of first degree of left elbow

   √7ᵗʰ **T22.529** Corrosion of first degree of unspecified elbow ▽

√6ᵗʰ **T22.53** Corrosion of first degree of upper arm

   √7ᵗʰ **T22.531** Corrosion of first degree of right upper arm

   √7ᵗʰ **T22.532** Corrosion of first degree of left upper arm

   √7ᵗʰ **T22.539** Corrosion of first degree of unspecified upper arm ▽

√6ᵗʰ **T22.54** Corrosion of first degree of axilla

   √7ᵗʰ **T22.541** Corrosion of first degree of right axilla

   √7ᵗʰ **T22.542** Corrosion of first degree of left axilla

   √7ᵗʰ **T22.549** Corrosion of first degree of unspecified axilla ▽

√6ᵗʰ **T22.55** Corrosion of first degree of shoulder

   √7ᵗʰ **T22.551** Corrosion of first degree of right shoulder

   √7ᵗʰ **T22.552** Corrosion of first degree of left shoulder

   √7ᵗʰ **T22.559** Corrosion of first degree of unspecified shoulder ▽

√6ᵗʰ **T22.56** Corrosion of first degree of scapular region

   √7ᵗʰ **T22.561** Corrosion of first degree of right scapular region

   √7ᵗʰ **T22.562** Corrosion of first degree of left scapular region

   √7ᵗʰ **T22.569** Corrosion of first degree of unspecified scapular region ▽

√6ᵗʰ **T22.59** Corrosion of first degree of multiple sites of shoulder and upper limb, except wrist and hand

   √7ᵗʰ **T22.591** Corrosion of first degree of multiple sites of right shoulder and upper limb, except wrist and hand

   √7ᵗʰ **T22.592** Corrosion of first degree of multiple sites of left shoulder and upper limb, except wrist and hand

   √7ᵗʰ **T22.599** Corrosion of first degree of multiple sites of unspecified shoulder and upper limb, except wrist and hand ▽

√5ᵗʰ **T22.6** Corrosion of second degree of shoulder and upper limb, except wrist and hand

   Code first (T51-T65) to identify chemical and intent

   Use additional external cause code to identify place (Y92)

√x7ᵗʰ **T22.60** Corrosion of second degree of shoulder and upper limb, except wrist and hand, unspecified site ▽

√6ᵗʰ **T22.61** Corrosion of second degree of forearm

   √7ᵗʰ **T22.611** Corrosion of second degree of right forearm

   √7ᵗʰ **T22.612** Corrosion of second degree of left forearm

   √7ᵗʰ **T22.619** Corrosion of second degree of unspecified forearm ▽

√6ᵗʰ **T22.62** Corrosion of second degree of elbow

   √7ᵗʰ **T22.621** Corrosion of second degree of right elbow

   √7ᵗʰ **T22.622** Corrosion of second degree of left elbow

   √7ᵗʰ **T22.629** Corrosion of second degree of unspecified elbow ▽

√6ᵗʰ **T22.63** Corrosion of second degree of upper arm

   √7ᵗʰ **T22.631** Corrosion of second degree of right upper arm

   √7ᵗʰ **T22.632** Corrosion of second degree of left upper arm

   √7ᵗʰ **T22.639** Corrosion of second degree of unspecified upper arm ▽

√6ᵗʰ **T22.64** Corrosion of second degree of axilla

   √7ᵗʰ **T22.641** Corrosion of second degree of right axilla

   √7ᵗʰ **T22.642** Corrosion of second degree of left axilla

   √7ᵗʰ **T22.649** Corrosion of second degree of unspecified axilla ▽

√6ᵗʰ **T22.65** Corrosion of second degree of shoulder

   √7ᵗʰ **T22.651** Corrosion of second degree of right shoulder

   √7ᵗʰ **T22.652** Corrosion of second degree of left shoulder

   √7ᵗʰ **T22.659** Corrosion of second degree of unspecified shoulder ▽

√6ᵗʰ **T22.66** Corrosion of second degree of scapular region

   √7ᵗʰ **T22.661** Corrosion of second degree of right scapular region

   √7ᵗʰ **T22.662** Corrosion of second degree of left scapular region

   √7ᵗʰ **T22.669** Corrosion of second degree of unspecified scapular region

√6ᵗʰ **T22.69** Corrosion of second degree of multiple sites of shoulder and upper limb, except wrist and hand

   √7ᵗʰ **T22.691** Corrosion of second degree of multiple sites of right shoulder and upper limb, except wrist and hand

---

☑ Additional Character Required   √x7ᵗʰ Placeholder Alert   Manifestation Dx   ▽ Unspecified Dx   ►◄ Revised Text   ● New Code   ▲ Revised Code Title

Chapter 19. Injury, Poisoning and Certain Other Consequences of External Causes

T22.692–T23.102

✓7ᵗʰ **T22.692** Corrosion of second degree of multiple sites of left shoulder and upper limb, except wrist and hand

✓7ᵗʰ **T22.699** Corrosion of second degree of multiple sites of unspecified shoulder and upper limb, except wrist and hand ▽

✓5ᵗʰ **T22.7** **Corrosion of third degree of shoulder and upper limb, except wrist and hand**

Code first (T51-T65) to identify chemical and intent

Use additional external cause code to identify place (Y92)

✓x7ᵗʰ **T22.70** Corrosion of third degree of shoulder and upper limb, except wrist and hand, unspecified site ▽

✓6ᵗʰ **T22.71** Corrosion of third degree of forearm

✓7ᵗʰ **T22.711** Corrosion of third degree of right forearm

✓7ᵗʰ **T22.712** Corrosion of third degree of left forearm

✓7ᵗʰ **T22.719** Corrosion of third degree of unspecified forearm

✓6ᵗʰ **T22.72** Corrosion of third degree of elbow

✓7ᵗʰ **T22.721** Corrosion of third degree of right elbow

✓7ᵗʰ **T22.722** Corrosion of third degree of left elbow

✓7ᵗʰ **T22.729** Corrosion of third degree of unspecified elbow ▽

✓6ᵗʰ **T22.73** Corrosion of third degree of upper arm

✓7ᵗʰ **T22.731** Corrosion of third degree of right upper arm

✓7ᵗʰ **T22.732** Corrosion of third degree of left upper arm

✓7ᵗʰ **T22.739** Corrosion of third degree of unspecified upper arm ▽

✓6ᵗʰ **T22.74** Corrosion of third degree of axilla

✓7ᵗʰ **T22.741** Corrosion of third degree of right axilla

✓7ᵗʰ **T22.742** Corrosion of third degree of left axilla

✓7ᵗʰ **T22.749** Corrosion of third degree of unspecified axilla ▽

✓6ᵗʰ **T22.75** Corrosion of third degree of shoulder

✓7ᵗʰ **T22.751** Corrosion of third degree of right shoulder

✓7ᵗʰ **T22.752** Corrosion of third degree of left shoulder

✓7ᵗʰ **T22.759** Corrosion of third degree of unspecified shoulder ▽

✓6ᵗʰ **T22.76** Corrosion of third degree of scapular region

✓7ᵗʰ **T22.761** Corrosion of third degree of right scapular region

✓7ᵗʰ **T22.762** Corrosion of third degree of left scapular region

✓7ᵗʰ **T22.769** Corrosion of third degree of unspecified scapular region ▽

✓6ᵗʰ **T22.79** Corrosion of third degree of multiple sites of shoulder and upper limb, except wrist and hand

✓7ᵗʰ **T22.791** Corrosion of third degree of multiple sites of right shoulder and upper limb, except wrist and hand

✓7ᵗʰ **T22.792** Corrosion of third degree of multiple sites of left shoulder and upper limb, except wrist and hand

✓7ᵗʰ **T22.799** Corrosion of third degree of multiple sites of unspecified shoulder and upper limb, except wrist and hand ▽

✓4ᵗʰ **T23** **Burn and corrosion of wrist and hand**

AHA: 2015,1Q,19

The appropriate 7th character is to be added to each code from category T23.

A initial encounter
D subsequent encounter
S sequela

✓5ᵗʰ **T23.0** **Burn of unspecified degree of wrist and hand**

Use additional external cause code to identify the source, place and intent of the burn (X00-X19, X75-X77, X96-X98, Y92)

✓6ᵗʰ **T23.00** Burn of unspecified degree of hand, unspecified site

✓7ᵗʰ **T23.001** Burn of unspecified degree of right hand, unspecified site ▽

✓7ᵗʰ **T23.002** Burn of unspecified degree of left hand, unspecified site ▽

✓7ᵗʰ **T23.009** Burn of unspecified degree of unspecified hand, unspecified site ▽

✓6ᵗʰ **T23.01** Burn of unspecified degree of thumb (nail)

✓7ᵗʰ **T23.011** Burn of unspecified degree of right thumb (nail) ▽

✓7ᵗʰ **T23.012** Burn of unspecified degree of left thumb (nail) ▽

✓7ᵗʰ **T23.019** Burn of unspecified degree of unspecified thumb (nail) ▽

✓6ᵗʰ **T23.02** Burn of unspecified degree of single finger (nail) except thumb

✓7ᵗʰ **T23.021** Burn of unspecified degree of single right finger (nail) except thumb ▽

✓7ᵗʰ **T23.022** Burn of unspecified degree of single left finger (nail) except thumb ▽

✓7ᵗʰ **T23.029** Burn of unspecified degree of unspecified single finger (nail) except thumb ▽

✓6ᵗʰ **T23.03** Burn of unspecified degree of multiple fingers (nail), not including thumb

✓7ᵗʰ **T23.031** Burn of unspecified degree of multiple right fingers (nail), not including thumb ▽

✓7ᵗʰ **T23.032** Burn of unspecified degree of multiple left fingers (nail), not including thumb ▽

✓7ᵗʰ **T23.039** Burn of unspecified degree of unspecified multiple fingers (nail), not including thumb ▽

✓6ᵗʰ **T23.04** Burn of unspecified degree of multiple fingers (nail), including thumb

✓7ᵗʰ **T23.041** Burn of unspecified degree of multiple right fingers (nail), including thumb ▽

✓7ᵗʰ **T23.042** Burn of unspecified degree of multiple left fingers (nail), including thumb ▽

✓7ᵗʰ **T23.049** Burn of unspecified degree of unspecified multiple fingers (nail), including thumb ▽

✓6ᵗʰ **T23.05** Burn of unspecified degree of palm

✓7ᵗʰ **T23.051** Burn of unspecified degree of right palm ▽

✓7ᵗʰ **T23.052** Burn of unspecified degree of left palm ▽

✓7ᵗʰ **T23.059** Burn of unspecified degree of unspecified palm ▽

✓6ᵗʰ **T23.06** Burn of unspecified degree of back of hand

✓7ᵗʰ **T23.061** Burn of unspecified degree of back of right hand ▽

✓7ᵗʰ **T23.062** Burn of unspecified degree of back of left hand ▽

✓7ᵗʰ **T23.069** Burn of unspecified degree of back of unspecified hand ▽

✓6ᵗʰ **T23.07** Burn of unspecified degree of wrist

✓7ᵗʰ **T23.071** Burn of unspecified degree of right wrist ▽

✓7ᵗʰ **T23.072** Burn of unspecified degree of left wrist ▽

✓7ᵗʰ **T23.079** Burn of unspecified degree of unspecified wrist ▽

✓6ᵗʰ **T23.09** Burn of unspecified degree of multiple sites of wrist and hand

✓7ᵗʰ **T23.091** Burn of unspecified degree of multiple sites of right wrist and hand ▽

✓7ᵗʰ **T23.092** Burn of unspecified degree of multiple sites of left wrist and hand ▽

✓7ᵗʰ **T23.099** Burn of unspecified degree of multiple sites of unspecified wrist and hand ▽

✓5ᵗʰ **T23.1** **Burn of first degree of wrist and hand**

Use additional external cause code to identify the source, place and intent of the burn (X00-X19, X75-X77, X96-X98, Y92)

✓6ᵗʰ **T23.10** Burn of first degree of hand, unspecified site

✓7ᵗʰ **T23.101** Burn of first degree of right hand, unspecified site ▽

✓7ᵗʰ **T23.102** Burn of first degree of left hand, unspecified site ▽

EXCLUDES 1 Not coded here   EXCLUDES 2 Not included here   N Newborn Age : 0   P Pediatric Age : 0-17   M Maternity Age : 12-55   A Adult Age : 15-124

1016   ICD-10-CM 2017

√7ᵗʰ **T23.109** Burn of first degree of unspecified ▽
hand, unspecified site

√6ᵗʰ **T23.11** Burn of first degree of **thumb** (nail)

√7ᵗʰ **T23.111** Burn of first degree of **right** thumb (nail)

√7ᵗʰ **T23.112** Burn of first degree of **left** thumb (nail)

√7ᵗʰ **T23.119** Burn of first degree of unspecified ▽
thumb (nail)

√6ᵗʰ **T23.12** Burn of first degree of **single finger** (nail) except
thumb

√7ᵗʰ **T23.121** Burn of first degree of single **right** finger
(nail) except thumb

√7ᵗʰ **T23.122** Burn of first degree of single **left** finger
(nail) except thumb

√7ᵗʰ **T23.129** Burn of first degree of unspecified ▽
single finger (nail) except thumb

√6ᵗʰ **T23.13** Burn of first degree of **multiple fingers** (nail), not
including thumb

√7ᵗʰ **T23.131** Burn of first degree of multiple **right**
fingers (nail), not including thumb

√7ᵗʰ **T23.132** Burn of first degree of multiple **left**
fingers (nail), not including thumb

√7ᵗʰ **T23.139** Burn of first degree of unspecified ▽
multiple fingers (nail), not
including thumb

√6ᵗʰ **T23.14** Burn of first degree of **multiple fingers** (nail),
including thumb

√7ᵗʰ **T23.141** Burn of first degree of multiple **right**
fingers (nail), including thumb

√7ᵗʰ **T23.142** Burn of first degree of multiple **left**
fingers (nail), including thumb

√7ᵗʰ **T23.149** Burn of first degree of unspecified ▽
multiple fingers (nail), including
thumb

√6ᵗʰ **T23.15** Burn of first degree of **palm**

√7ᵗʰ **T23.151** Burn of first degree of **right** palm

√7ᵗʰ **T23.152** Burn of first degree of **left** palm

√7ᵗʰ **T23.159** Burn of first degree of unspecified ▽
palm

√6ᵗʰ **T23.16** Burn of first degree of **back of hand**

√7ᵗʰ **T23.161** Burn of first degree of back of **right** hand

√7ᵗʰ **T23.162** Burn of first degree of back of **left** hand

√7ᵗʰ **T23.169** Burn of first degree of back of ▽
unspecified hand

√6ᵗʰ **T23.17** Burn of first degree of **wrist**

√7ᵗʰ **T23.171** Burn of first degree of **right** wrist

√7ᵗʰ **T23.172** Burn of first degree of **left** wrist

√7ᵗʰ **T23.179** Burn of first degree of unspecified ▽
wrist

√6ᵗʰ **T23.19** Burn of first degree of **multiple sites** of wrist and
hand

√7ᵗʰ **T23.191** Burn of first degree of multiple sites of
right wrist and hand

√7ᵗʰ **T23.192** Burn of first degree of multiple sites of
left wrist and hand

√7ᵗʰ **T23.199** Burn of first degree of multiple ▽
sites of unspecified wrist and hand

√5ᵗʰ **T23.2** Burn of **second degree** of wrist and hand

Use additional external cause code to identify the source, place
and intent of the burn (X00-X19, X75-X77, X96-X98, Y92)

√6ᵗʰ **T23.20** Burn of second degree of hand, unspecified site

√7ᵗʰ **T23.201** Burn of second degree of **right**
hand, unspecified site ▽

√7ᵗʰ **T23.202** Burn of second degree of **left**
hand, unspecified site ▽

√7ᵗʰ **T23.209** Burn of second degree of ▽
unspecified hand, unspecified site

√6ᵗʰ **T23.21** Burn of second degree of **thumb** (nail)

√7ᵗʰ **T23.211** Burn of second degree of **right** thumb
(nail)

√7ᵗʰ **T23.212** Burn of second degree of **left** thumb (nail)

√7ᵗʰ **T23.219** Burn of second degree of ▽
unspecified thumb (nail)

√6ᵗʰ **T23.22** Burn of second degree of **single finger** (nail) except
thumb

√7ᵗʰ **T23.221** Burn of second degree of single **right**
finger (nail) except thumb

√7ᵗʰ **T23.222** Burn of second degree of single **left** finger
(nail) except thumb

√7ᵗʰ **T23.229** Burn of second degree of ▽
unspecified single finger (nail)
except thumb

√6ᵗʰ **T23.23** Burn of second degree of **multiple fingers** (nail),
not including thumb

√7ᵗʰ **T23.231** Burn of second degree of multiple **right**
fingers (nail), not including thumb

√7ᵗʰ **T23.232** Burn of second degree of multiple **left**
fingers (nail), not including thumb

√7ᵗʰ **T23.239** Burn of second degree of
unspecified multiple fingers (nail),
not including thumb

√6ᵗʰ **T23.24** Burn of second degree of **multiple fingers** (nail),
including thumb

√7ᵗʰ **T23.241** Burn of second degree of multiple **right**
fingers (nail), including thumb

√7ᵗʰ **T23.242** Burn of second degree of multiple **left**
fingers (nail), including thumb

√7ᵗʰ **T23.249** Burn of second degree of ▽
unspecified multiple fingers (nail),
including thumb

√6ᵗʰ **T23.25** Burn of second degree of **palm**

√7ᵗʰ **T23.251** Burn of second degree of **right** palm

√7ᵗʰ **T23.252** Burn of second degree of **left** palm

√7ᵗʰ **T23.259** Burn of second degree of ▽
unspecified palm

√6ᵗʰ **T23.26** Burn of second degree of **back of hand**

√7ᵗʰ **T23.261** Burn of second degree of back of **right**
hand

√7ᵗʰ **T23.262** Burn of second degree of back of **left**
hand

√7ᵗʰ **T23.269** Burn of second degree of back of ▽
unspecified hand

√6ᵗʰ **T23.27** Burn of second degree of **wrist**

√7ᵗʰ **T23.271** Burn of second degree of **right** wrist

√7ᵗʰ **T23.272** Burn of second degree of **left** wrist

√7ᵗʰ **T23.279** Burn of second degree of ▽
unspecified wrist

√6ᵗʰ **T23.29** Burn of second degree of **multiple sites** of wrist and
hand

√7ᵗʰ **T23.291** Burn of second degree of multiple sites
of **right** wrist and hand

√7ᵗʰ **T23.292** Burn of second degree of multiple sites
of **left** wrist and hand

√7ᵗʰ **T23.299** Burn of second degree of multiple ▽
sites of unspecified wrist and hand

√5ᵗʰ **T23.3** Burn of **third degree** of wrist and hand

Use additional external cause code to identify the source, place
and intent of the burn (X00-X19, X75-X77, X96-X98, Y92)

√6ᵗʰ **T23.30** Burn of third degree of hand, unspecified site

AHA: 2016,2Q,5

√7ᵗʰ **T23.301** Burn of third degree of **right** hand, ▽
unspecified site

√7ᵗʰ **T23.302** Burn of third degree of **left** hand, ▽
unspecified site

√7ᵗʰ **T23.309** Burn of third degree of unspecified ▽
hand, unspecified site

√6ᵗʰ **T23.31** Burn of third degree of **thumb** (nail)

√7ᵗʰ **T23.311** Burn of third degree of **right** thumb (nail)

√7ᵗʰ **T23.312** Burn of third degree of **left** thumb (nail)

√7ᵗʰ **T23.319** Burn of third degree of unspecified ▽
thumb (nail)

√6ᵗʰ **T23.32** Burn of third degree of **single finger** (nail) except
thumb

√7ᵗʰ **T23.321** Burn of third degree of single **right** finger
(nail) except thumb

√7ᵗʰ **T23.322** Burn of third degree of single **left** finger
(nail) except thumb

√7ᵗʰ **T23.329** Burn of third degree of unspecified ▽
single finger (nail) except thumb

√6ᵗʰ **T23.33** Burn of third degree of **multiple fingers** (nail), not
including thumb

√7ᵗʰ **T23.331** Burn of third degree of multiple **right**
fingers (nail), not including thumb

√7ᵗʰ **T23.332** Burn of third degree of multiple **left**
fingers (nail), not including thumb

√7ᵗʰ **T23.339** Burn of third degree of unspecified ▽
multiple fingers (nail), not
including thumb

☑ Additional Character Required   √x7ᵗʰ Placeholder Alert   Manifestation Dx   ▽ Unspecified Dx   ►◄ Revised Text   ● New Code   ▲ Revised Code Title

√6ᵗʰ **T23.34** **Burn of third degree of** multiple fingers (nail), **including thumb**

  √7ᵗʰ **T23.341** **Burn of third degree of multiple** right **fingers (nail), including thumb**

  √7ᵗʰ **T23.342** **Burn of third degree of multiple** left **fingers (nail), including thumb**

  √7ᵗʰ **T23.349** **Burn of third degree of unspecified multiple fingers (nail), including thumb** ▽

√6ᵗʰ **T23.35** **Burn of third degree of** palm

  √7ᵗʰ **T23.351** **Burn of third degree of** right **palm**

  √7ᵗʰ **T23.352** **Burn of third degree of** left **palm**

  √7ᵗʰ **T23.359** **Burn of third degree of unspecified palm** ▽

√6ᵗʰ **T23.36** **Burn of third degree of** back of hand

  √7ᵗʰ **T23.361** **Burn of third degree of back of** right **hand**

  √7ᵗʰ **T23.362** **Burn of third degree of back of** left **hand**

  √7ᵗʰ **T23.369** **Burn of third degree of back of unspecified hand** ▽

√6ᵗʰ **T23.37** **Burn of third degree of** wrist

  √7ᵗʰ **T23.371** **Burn of third degree of** right **wrist**

  √7ᵗʰ **T23.372** **Burn of third degree of** left **wrist**

  √7ᵗʰ **T23.379** **Burn of third degree of unspecified wrist** ▽

√6ᵗʰ **T23.39** **Burn of third degree of multiple sites of** wrist and hand

  √7ᵗʰ **T23.391** **Burn of third degree of multiple sites of** right **wrist and hand**

  √7ᵗʰ **T23.392** **Burn of third degree of multiple sites of** left **wrist and hand**

  √7ᵗʰ **T23.399** **Burn of third degree of multiple sites of unspecified wrist and hand** ▽

✅5ᵗʰ **T23.4** **Corrosion of unspecified degree of wrist and hand**

  Code first (T51-T65) to identify chemical and intent
  Use additional external cause code to identify place (Y92)

√6ᵗʰ **T23.40** **Corrosion of unspecified degree of hand, unspecified site**

  √7ᵗʰ **T23.401** **Corrosion of unspecified degree of** right **hand, unspecified site** ▽

  √7ᵗʰ **T23.402** **Corrosion of unspecified degree of** left **hand, unspecified site** ▽

  √7ᵗʰ **T23.409** **Corrosion of unspecified degree of unspecified hand, unspecified site** ▽

√6ᵗʰ **T23.41** **Corrosion of unspecified degree of** thumb (nail)

  √7ᵗʰ **T23.411** **Corrosion of unspecified degree of** right **thumb (nail)** ▽

  √7ᵗʰ **T23.412** **Corrosion of unspecified degree of** left **thumb (nail)** ▽

  √7ᵗʰ **T23.419** **Corrosion of unspecified degree of unspecified thumb (nail)** ▽

√6ᵗʰ **T23.42** **Corrosion of unspecified degree of** single finger (nail) except thumb

  √7ᵗʰ **T23.421** **Corrosion of unspecified degree of single** right **finger (nail) except thumb** ▽

  √7ᵗʰ **T23.422** **Corrosion of unspecified degree of single** left **finger (nail) except thumb** ▽

  √7ᵗʰ **T23.429** **Corrosion of unspecified degree of unspecified single finger (nail) except thumb** ▽

√6ᵗʰ **T23.43** **Corrosion of unspecified degree of** multiple fingers (nail), not including thumb

  √7ᵗʰ **T23.431** **Corrosion of unspecified degree of multiple** right **fingers (nail), not including thumb** ▽

  √7ᵗʰ **T23.432** **Corrosion of unspecified degree of multiple** left **fingers (nail), not including thumb** ▽

  √7ᵗʰ **T23.439** **Corrosion of unspecified degree of unspecified multiple fingers (nail), not including thumb** ▽

√6ᵗʰ **T23.44** **Corrosion of unspecified degree of** multiple fingers (nail), including thumb

  √7ᵗʰ **T23.441** **Corrosion of unspecified degree of multiple** right **fingers (nail), including thumb** ▽

  √7ᵗʰ **T23.442** **Corrosion of unspecified degree of multiple** left **fingers (nail), including thumb** ▽

  √7ᵗʰ **T23.449** **Corrosion of unspecified degree of unspecified multiple fingers (nail), including thumb** ▽

√6ᵗʰ **T23.45** **Corrosion of unspecified degree of** palm

  √7ᵗʰ **T23.451** **Corrosion of unspecified degree of** right **palm**

  √7ᵗʰ **T23.452** **Corrosion of unspecified degree of** left **palm**

  √7ᵗʰ **T23.459** **Corrosion of unspecified degree of unspecified palm**

√6ᵗʰ **T23.46** **Corrosion of unspecified degree of** back of hand

  √7ᵗʰ **T23.461** **Corrosion of unspecified degree of back of** right **hand**

  √7ᵗʰ **T23.462** **Corrosion of unspecified degree of back of** left **hand**

  √7ᵗʰ **T23.469** **Corrosion of unspecified degree of back of unspecified hand**

√6ᵗʰ **T23.47** **Corrosion of unspecified degree of** wrist

  √7ᵗʰ **T23.471** **Corrosion of unspecified degree of** right **wrist** ▽

  √7ᵗʰ **T23.472** **Corrosion of unspecified degree of** left **wrist** ▽

  √7ᵗʰ **T23.479** **Corrosion of unspecified degree of unspecified wrist** ▽

√6ᵗʰ **T23.49** **Corrosion of unspecified degree of** multiple sites of wrist and hand

  √7ᵗʰ **T23.491** **Corrosion of unspecified degree of multiple sites of** right **wrist and hand** ▽

  √7ᵗʰ **T23.492** **Corrosion of unspecified degree of multiple sites of** left **wrist and hand** ▽

  √7ᵗʰ **T23.499** **Corrosion of unspecified degree of multiple sites of unspecified wrist and hand** ▽

✅5ᵗʰ **T23.5** **Corrosion of** first degree **of wrist and hand**

  Code first (T51-T65) to identify chemical and intent
  Use additional external cause code to identify place (Y92)

√6ᵗʰ **T23.50** **Corrosion of first degree of hand, unspecified site**

  √7ᵗʰ **T23.501** **Corrosion of first degree of** right **hand, unspecified site** ▽

  √7ᵗʰ **T23.502** **Corrosion of first degree of** left **hand, unspecified site**

  √7ᵗʰ **T23.509** **Corrosion of first degree of unspecified hand, unspecified site** ▽

√6ᵗʰ **T23.51** **Corrosion of first degree of** thumb (nail)

  √7ᵗʰ **T23.511** **Corrosion of first degree of** right **thumb (nail)**

  √7ᵗʰ **T23.512** **Corrosion of first degree of** left **thumb (nail)**

  √7ᵗʰ **T23.519** **Corrosion of first degree of unspecified thumb (nail)** ▽

√6ᵗʰ **T23.52** **Corrosion of first degree of** single finger (nail) except thumb

  √7ᵗʰ **T23.521** **Corrosion of first degree of single** right **finger (nail) except thumb**

  √7ᵗʰ **T23.522** **Corrosion of first degree of single** left **finger (nail) except thumb**

  √7ᵗʰ **T23.529** **Corrosion of first degree of unspecified single finger (nail) except thumb** ▽

√6ᵗʰ **T23.53** **Corrosion of first degree of** multiple fingers (nail), not including thumb

  √7ᵗʰ **T23.531** **Corrosion of first degree of multiple** right **fingers (nail), not including thumb**

  √7ᵗʰ **T23.532** **Corrosion of first degree of multiple** left **fingers (nail), not including thumb**

  √7ᵗʰ **T23.539** **Corrosion of first degree of unspecified multiple fingers (nail), not including thumb** ▽

√6ᵗʰ **T23.54** **Corrosion of first degree of** multiple fingers (nail), including thumb

  √7ᵗʰ **T23.541** **Corrosion of first degree of multiple** right **fingers (nail), including thumb**

  √7ᵗʰ **T23.542** **Corrosion of first degree of multiple** left **fingers (nail), including thumb**

  √7ᵗʰ **T23.549** **Corrosion of first degree of unspecified multiple fingers (nail), including thumb** ▽

√6ᵗʰ **T23.55** **Corrosion of first degree of** palm

  √7ᵗʰ **T23.551** **Corrosion of first degree of** right **palm**

EXCLUDES 1 Not coded here   EXCLUDES 2 Not included here   N Newborn Age : 0   P Pediatric Age : 0-17   M Maternity Age : 12-55   A Adult Age : 15-124

1018

ICD-10-CM 2017

√7th **T23.552** Corrosion of first degree of left palm

√7th **T23.559** Corrosion of first degree of unspecified palm ▽

√6th **T23.56** Corrosion of first degree of back of hand

    √7th **T23.561** Corrosion of first degree of back of right hand

    √7th **T23.562** Corrosion of first degree of back of left hand

    √7th **T23.569** Corrosion of first degree of back of unspecified hand ▽

√6th **T23.57** Corrosion of first degree of wrist

    √7th **T23.571** Corrosion of first degree of right wrist

    √7th **T23.572** Corrosion of first degree of left wrist

    √7th **T23.579** Corrosion of first degree of unspecified wrist ▽

√6th **T23.59** Corrosion of first degree of multiple sites of wrist and hand

    √7th **T23.591** Corrosion of first degree of multiple sites of right wrist and hand

    √7th **T23.592** Corrosion of first degree of multiple sites of left wrist and hand

    √7th **T23.599** Corrosion of first degree of multiple sites of unspecified wrist and hand ▽

√5th **T23.6** Corrosion of second degree of wrist and hand

    Code first (T51-T65) to identify chemical and intent
    Use additional external cause code to identify place (Y92)

√6th **T23.60** Corrosion of second degree of hand, unspecified site

    √7th **T23.601** Corrosion of second degree of right hand, unspecified site ▽

    √7th **T23.602** Corrosion of second degree of left hand, unspecified site ▽

    √7th **T23.609** Corrosion of second degree of unspecified hand, unspecified site ▽

√6th **T23.61** Corrosion of second degree of thumb (nail)

    √7th **T23.611** Corrosion of second degree of right thumb (nail)

    √7th **T23.612** Corrosion of second degree of left thumb (nail)

    √7th **T23.619** Corrosion of second degree of unspecified thumb (nail) ▽

√6th **T23.62** Corrosion of second degree of single finger (nail) except thumb

    √7th **T23.621** Corrosion of second degree of single right finger (nail) except thumb

    √7th **T23.622** Corrosion of second degree of single left finger (nail) except thumb

    √7th **T23.629** Corrosion of second degree of unspecified single finger (nail) except thumb ▽

√6th **T23.63** Corrosion of second degree of multiple fingers (nail), not including thumb

    √7th **T23.631** Corrosion of second degree of multiple right fingers (nail), not including thumb

    √7th **T23.632** Corrosion of second degree of multiple left fingers (nail), not including thumb

    √7th **T23.639** Corrosion of second degree of unspecified multiple fingers (nail), not including thumb ▽

√6th **T23.64** Corrosion of second degree of multiple fingers (nail), including thumb

    √7th **T23.641** Corrosion of second degree of multiple right fingers (nail), including thumb

    √7th **T23.642** Corrosion of second degree of multiple left fingers (nail), including thumb

    √7th **T23.649** Corrosion of second degree of unspecified multiple fingers (nail), including thumb ▽

√6th **T23.65** Corrosion of second degree of palm

    √7th **T23.651** Corrosion of second degree of right palm

    √7th **T23.652** Corrosion of second degree of left palm

    √7th **T23.659** Corrosion of second degree of unspecified palm ▽

√6th **T23.66** Corrosion of second degree of back of hand

    √7th **T23.661** Corrosion of second degree back of right hand

    √7th **T23.662** Corrosion of second degree back of left hand

    √7th **T23.669** Corrosion of second degree back of unspecified hand ▽

√6th **T23.67** Corrosion of second degree of wrist

    √7th **T23.671** Corrosion of second degree of right wrist

    √7th **T23.672** Corrosion of second degree of left wrist

    √7th **T23.679** Corrosion of second degree of unspecified wrist ▽

√6th **T23.69** Corrosion of second degree of multiple sites of wrist and hand

    √7th **T23.691** Corrosion of second degree of multiple sites of right wrist and hand

    √7th **T23.692** Corrosion of second degree of multiple sites of left wrist and hand

    √7th **T23.699** Corrosion of second degree of multiple sites of unspecified wrist and hand ▽

√5th **T23.7** Corrosion of third degree of wrist and hand

    Code first (T51-T65) to identify chemical and intent
    Use additional external cause code to identify place (Y92)

√6th **T23.70** Corrosion of third degree of hand, unspecified site

    √7th **T23.701** Corrosion of third degree of right hand, unspecified site ▽

    √7th **T23.702** Corrosion of third degree of left hand, unspecified site ▽

    √7th **T23.709** Corrosion of third degree of unspecified hand, unspecified site ▽

√6th **T23.71** Corrosion of third degree of thumb (nail)

    √7th **T23.711** Corrosion of third degree of right thumb (nail)

    √7th **T23.712** Corrosion of third degree of left thumb (nail)

    √7th **T23.719** Corrosion of third degree of unspecified thumb (nail) ▽

√6th **T23.72** Corrosion of third degree of single finger (nail) except thumb

    √7th **T23.721** Corrosion of third degree of single right finger (nail) except thumb

    √7th **T23.722** Corrosion of third degree of single left finger (nail) except thumb

    √7th **T23.729** Corrosion of third degree of unspecified single finger (nail) except thumb ▽

√6th **T23.73** Corrosion of third degree of multiple fingers (nail), not including thumb

    √7th **T23.731** Corrosion of third degree of multiple right fingers (nail), not including thumb

    √7th **T23.732** Corrosion of third degree of multiple left fingers (nail), not including thumb

    √7th **T23.739** Corrosion of third degree of unspecified multiple fingers (nail), not including thumb ▽

√6th **T23.74** Corrosion of third degree of multiple fingers (nail), including thumb

    √7th **T23.741** Corrosion of third degree of multiple right fingers (nail), including thumb

    √7th **T23.742** Corrosion of third degree of multiple left fingers (nail), including thumb

    √7th **T23.749** Corrosion of third degree of unspecified multiple fingers (nail), including thumb ▽

√6th **T23.75** Corrosion of third degree of palm

    √7th **T23.751** Corrosion of third degree of right palm

    √7th **T23.752** Corrosion of third degree of left palm

    √7th **T23.759** Corrosion of third degree of unspecified palm ▽

√6th **T23.76** Corrosion of third degree of back of hand

    √7th **T23.761** Corrosion of third degree of back of right hand

    √7th **T23.762** Corrosion of third degree of back of left hand

    √7th **T23.769** Corrosion of third degree back of unspecified hand ▽

√6th **T23.77** Corrosion of third degree of wrist

    √7th **T23.771** Corrosion of third degree of right wrist

    √7th **T23.772** Corrosion of third degree of left wrist

    √7th **T23.779** Corrosion of third degree of unspecified wrist ▽

√6ᵗʰ **T23.79** **Corrosion of third degree of** multiple sites **of wrist and hand**

    √7ᵗʰ **T23.791** **Corrosion of third degree of multiple sites of** right **wrist and hand**

    √7ᵗʰ **T23.792** **Corrosion of third degree of multiple sites of** left **wrist and hand**

    √7ᵗʰ **T23.799** **Corrosion of third degree of multiple sites of unspecified wrist and hand** ▽

√4ᵗʰ **T24** **Burn and corrosion of lower limb, except ankle and foot**

    EXCLUDES 2 burn and corrosion of ankle and foot (T25.-)
              burn and corrosion of hip region (T21.-)

    The appropriate 7th character is to be added to each code from category T24.
    A   initial encounter
    D   subsequent encounter
    S   sequela

√5ᵗʰ **T24.0** **Burn of unspecified degree of lower limb, except ankle and foot**

    Use additional external cause code to identify the source, place and intent of the burn (X00-X19, X75-X77, X96-X98, Y92)

    √6ᵗʰ **T24.00** **Burn of unspecified degree of unspecified site of lower limb, except ankle and foot**

       √7ᵗʰ **T24.001** **Burn of unspecified degree of unspecified site of** right **lower limb, except ankle and foot** ▽

       √7ᵗʰ **T24.002** **Burn of unspecified degree of unspecified site of** left **lower limb, except ankle and foot** ▽

       √7ᵗʰ **T24.009** **Burn of unspecified degree of unspecified site of unspecified lower limb, except ankle and foot**

    √6ᵗʰ **T24.01** **Burn of unspecified degree of** thigh

       √7ᵗʰ **T24.011** **Burn of unspecified degree of** right **thigh** ▽

       √7ᵗʰ **T24.012** **Burn of unspecified degree of** left **thigh** ▽

       √7ᵗʰ **T24.019** **Burn of unspecified degree of unspecified thigh** ▽

    √6ᵗʰ **T24.02** **Burn of unspecified degree of** knee

       √7ᵗʰ **T24.021** **Burn of unspecified degree of** right **knee** ▽

       √7ᵗʰ **T24.022** **Burn of unspecified degree of** left **knee** ▽

       √7ᵗʰ **T24.029** **Burn of unspecified degree of unspecified knee** ▽

    √6ᵗʰ **T24.03** **Burn of unspecified degree of** lower leg

       √7ᵗʰ **T24.031** **Burn of unspecified degree of** right **lower leg** ▽

       √7ᵗʰ **T24.032** **Burn of unspecified degree of** left **lower leg** ▽

       √7ᵗʰ **T24.039** **Burn of unspecified degree of unspecified lower leg** ▽

    √6ᵗʰ **T24.09** **Burn of unspecified degree of** multiple sites **of lower limb, except ankle and foot**

       √7ᵗʰ **T24.091** **Burn of unspecified degree of multiple sites of** right **lower limb, except ankle and foot** ▽

       √7ᵗʰ **T24.092** **Burn of unspecified degree of multiple sites of** left **lower limb, except ankle and foot** ▽

       √7ᵗʰ **T24.099** **Burn of unspecified degree of multiple sites of unspecified lower limb, except ankle and foot** ▽

√5ᵗʰ **T24.1** **Burn of** first degree **of lower limb, except ankle and foot**

    Use additional external cause code to identify the source, place and intent of the burn (X00-X19, X75-X77, X96-X98, Y92)

    √6ᵗʰ **T24.10** **Burn of first degree of unspecified site of lower limb, except ankle and foot**

       √7ᵗʰ **T24.101** **Burn of first degree of unspecified site of** right **lower limb, except ankle and foot** ▽

       √7ᵗʰ **T24.102** **Burn of first degree of unspecified site of** left **lower limb, except ankle and foot** ▽

       √7ᵗʰ **T24.109** **Burn of first degree of unspecified site of unspecified lower limb, except ankle and foot** ▽

    √6ᵗʰ **T24.11** **Burn of first degree of** thigh

       √7ᵗʰ **T24.111** **Burn of first degree of** right **thigh**

       √7ᵗʰ **T24.112** **Burn of first degree of** left **thigh**

       √7ᵗʰ **T24.119** **Burn of first degree of unspecified thigh** ▽

    √6ᵗʰ **T24.12** **Burn of first degree of** knee

       √7ᵗʰ **T24.121** **Burn of first degree of** right **knee**

       √7ᵗʰ **T24.122** **Burn of first degree of** left **knee**

       √7ᵗʰ **T24.129** **Burn of first degree of unspecified knee** ▽

    √6ᵗʰ **T24.13** **Burn of first degree of** lower leg

       √7ᵗʰ **T24.131** **Burn of first degree of** right **lower leg**

       √7ᵗʰ **T24.132** **Burn of first degree of** left **lower leg**

       √7ᵗʰ **T24.139** **Burn of first degree of unspecified lower leg** ▽

    √6ᵗʰ **T24.19** **Burn of first degree of** multiple sites **of lower limb, except ankle and foot**

       √7ᵗʰ **T24.191** **Burn of first degree of multiple sites of** right **lower limb, except ankle and foot**

       √7ᵗʰ **T24.192** **Burn of first degree of multiple sites of** left **lower limb, except ankle and foot**

       √7ᵗʰ **T24.199** **Burn of first degree of multiple sites of unspecified lower limb, except ankle and foot** ▽

√5ᵗʰ **T24.2** **Burn of** second degree **of lower limb, except ankle and foot**

    Use additional external cause code to identify the source, place and intent of the burn (X00-X19, X75-X77, X96-X98, Y92)

    √6ᵗʰ **T24.20** **Burn of second degree of unspecified site of lower limb, except ankle and foot**

       √7ᵗʰ **T24.201** **Burn of second degree of unspecified site of** right **lower limb, except ankle and foot** ▽

       √7ᵗʰ **T24.202** **Burn of second degree of unspecified site of** left **lower limb, except ankle and foot** ▽

       √7ᵗʰ **T24.209** **Burn of second degree of unspecified site of unspecified lower limb, except ankle and foot** ▽

    √6ᵗʰ **T24.21** **Burn of second degree of** thigh

       √7ᵗʰ **T24.211** **Burn of second degree of** right **thigh**

       √7ᵗʰ **T24.212** **Burn of second degree of** left **thigh**

       √7ᵗʰ **T24.219** **Burn of second degree of unspecified thigh** ▽

    √6ᵗʰ **T24.22** **Burn of second degree of** knee

       √7ᵗʰ **T24.221** **Burn of second degree of** right **knee**

       √7ᵗʰ **T24.222** **Burn of second degree of** left **knee**

       √7ᵗʰ **T24.229** **Burn of second degree of unspecified knee** ▽

    √6ᵗʰ **T24.23** **Burn of second degree of** lower leg

       √7ᵗʰ **T24.231** **Burn of second degree of** right **lower leg**

       √7ᵗʰ **T24.232** **Burn of second degree of** left **lower leg**

       √7ᵗʰ **T24.239** **Burn of second degree of unspecified lower leg** ▽

    √6ᵗʰ **T24.29** **Burn of second degree of** multiple sites **of lower limb, except ankle and foot**

       √7ᵗʰ **T24.291** **Burn of second degree of multiple sites of** right **lower limb, except ankle and foot**

       √7ᵗʰ **T24.292** **Burn of second degree of multiple sites of** left **lower limb, except ankle and foot**

       √7ᵗʰ **T24.299** **Burn of second degree of multiple sites of unspecified lower limb, except ankle and foot** ▽

√5ᵗʰ **T24.3** **Burn of** third degree **of lower limb, except ankle and foot**

    Use additional external cause code to identify the source, place and intent of the burn (X00-X19, X75-X77, X96-X98, Y92)

    √6ᵗʰ **T24.30** **Burn of third degree of unspecified site of lower limb, except ankle and foot**

       √7ᵗʰ **T24.301** **Burn of third degree of unspecified site of** right **lower limb, except ankle and foot** ▽

       √7ᵗʰ **T24.302** **Burn of third degree of unspecified site of** left **lower limb, except ankle and foot** ▽

       √7ᵗʰ **T24.309** **Burn of third degree of unspecified site of unspecified lower limb, except ankle and foot** ▽

    √6ᵗʰ **T24.31** **Burn of third degree of** thigh

       √7ᵗʰ **T24.311** **Burn of third degree of** right **thigh**

       √7ᵗʰ **T24.312** **Burn of third degree of** left **thigh**

       √7ᵗʰ **T24.319** **Burn of third degree of unspecified thigh** ▽

EXCLUDES 1   Not coded here   EXCLUDES 2   Not included here   N Newborn Age : 0   P Pediatric Age : 0-17   M Maternity Age : 12-55   A Adult Age : 15-124

1020   ICD-10-CM 2017

√6ᵗʰ **T24.32**   **Burn of third degree of** knee

   √7ᵗʰ **T24.321**   Burn of third degree of right knee

   √7ᵗʰ **T24.322**   Burn of third degree of left knee

   √7ᵗʰ **T24.329**   Burn of third degree of unspecified knee ▽

√6ᵗʰ **T24.33**   **Burn of third degree of** lower leg

   √7ᵗʰ **T24.331**   Burn of third degree of right lower leg

   √7ᵗʰ **T24.332**   Burn of third degree of left lower leg

   √7ᵗʰ **T24.339**   Burn of third degree of unspecified lower leg ▽

√6ᵗʰ **T24.39**   **Burn of third degree of** multiple sites **of lower limb, except ankle and foot**

    AHA: 2016,2Q,4

   √7ᵗʰ **T24.391**   Burn of third degree of multiple sites of right lower limb, except ankle and foot

   √7ᵗʰ **T24.392**   Burn of third degree of multiple sites of left lower limb, except ankle and foot

   √7ᵗʰ **T24.399**   Burn of third degree of multiple sites of unspecified lower limb, except ankle and foot ▽

√5ᵗʰ **T24.4**   **Corrosion of unspecified degree of lower limb, except ankle and foot**

    Code first (T51-T65) to identify chemical and intent
    Use additional external cause code to identify place (Y92)

√6ᵗʰ **T24.40**   **Corrosion of unspecified degree of unspecified site of lower limb, except ankle and foot**

   √7ᵗʰ **T24.401**   Corrosion of unspecified degree of unspecified site of right lower limb, except ankle and foot ▽

   √7ᵗʰ **T24.402**   Corrosion of unspecified degree of unspecified site of left lower limb, except ankle and foot ▽

   √7ᵗʰ **T24.409**   Corrosion of unspecified degree of unspecified site of unspecified lower limb, except ankle and foot ▽

√6ᵗʰ **T24.41**   **Corrosion of unspecified degree of** thigh

   √7ᵗʰ **T24.411**   Corrosion of unspecified degree of right thigh ▽

   √7ᵗʰ **T24.412**   Corrosion of unspecified degree of left thigh ▽

   √7ᵗʰ **T24.419**   Corrosion of unspecified degree of unspecified thigh ▽

√6ᵗʰ **T24.42**   **Corrosion of unspecified degree of** knee

   √7ᵗʰ **T24.421**   Corrosion of unspecified degree of right knee ▽

   √7ᵗʰ **T24.422**   Corrosion of unspecified degree of left knee ▽

   √7ᵗʰ **T24.429**   Corrosion of unspecified degree of unspecified knee ▽

√6ᵗʰ **T24.43**   **Corrosion of unspecified degree of** lower leg

   √7ᵗʰ **T24.431**   Corrosion of unspecified degree of right lower leg ▽

   √7ᵗʰ **T24.432**   Corrosion of unspecified degree of left lower leg ▽

   √7ᵗʰ **T24.439**   Corrosion of unspecified degree of unspecified lower leg ▽

√6ᵗʰ **T24.49**   **Corrosion of unspecified degree of** multiple sites **of lower limb, except ankle and foot**

   √7ᵗʰ **T24.491**   Corrosion of unspecified degree of multiple sites of right lower limb, except ankle and foot

   √7ᵗʰ **T24.492**   Corrosion of unspecified degree of multiple sites of left lower limb, except ankle and foot ▽

   √7ᵗʰ **T24.499**   Corrosion of unspecified degree of multiple sites of unspecified lower limb, except ankle and foot ▽

√5ᵗʰ **T24.5**   **Corrosion of** first degree **of lower limb, except ankle and foot**

    Code first (T51-T65) to identify chemical and intent
    Use additional external cause code to identify place (Y92)

√6ᵗʰ **T24.50**   **Corrosion of first degree of unspecified site of lower limb, except ankle and foot**

   √7ᵗʰ **T24.501**   Corrosion of first degree of unspecified site of right lower limb, except ankle and foot ▽

   √7ᵗʰ **T24.502**   Corrosion of first degree of unspecified site of left lower limb, except ankle and foot ▽

   √7ᵗʰ **T24.509**   Corrosion of first degree of unspecified site of unspecified lower limb, except ankle and foot ▽

√6ᵗʰ **T24.51**   **Corrosion of first degree of** thigh

   √7ᵗʰ **T24.511**   Corrosion of first degree of right thigh

   √7ᵗʰ **T24.512**   Corrosion of first degree of left thigh

   √7ᵗʰ **T24.519**   Corrosion of first degree of unspecified thigh ▽

√6ᵗʰ **T24.52**   **Corrosion of first degree of** knee

   √7ᵗʰ **T24.521**   Corrosion of first degree of right knee

   √7ᵗʰ **T24.522**   Corrosion of first degree of left knee

   √7ᵗʰ **T24.529**   Corrosion of first degree of unspecified knee ▽

√6ᵗʰ **T24.53**   **Corrosion of first degree of** lower leg

   √7ᵗʰ **T24.531**   Corrosion of first degree of right lower leg

   √7ᵗʰ **T24.532**   Corrosion of first degree of left lower leg

   √7ᵗʰ **T24.539**   Corrosion of first degree of unspecified lower leg ▽

√6ᵗʰ **T24.59**   **Corrosion of first degree of** multiple sites **of lower limb, except ankle and foot**

   √7ᵗʰ **T24.591**   Corrosion of first degree of multiple sites of right lower limb, except ankle and foot

   √7ᵗʰ **T24.592**   Corrosion of first degree of multiple sites of left lower limb, except ankle and foot

   √7ᵗʰ **T24.599**   Corrosion of first degree of multiple sites of unspecified lower limb, except ankle and foot ▽

√5ᵗʰ **T24.6**   **Corrosion of second degree of lower limb, except ankle and foot**

    Code first (T51-T65) to identify chemical and intent
    Use additional external cause code to identify place (Y92)

√6ᵗʰ **T24.60**   **Corrosion of second degree of unspecified site of lower limb, except ankle and foot**

   √7ᵗʰ **T24.601**   Corrosion of second degree of unspecified site of right lower limb, except ankle and foot ▽

   √7ᵗʰ **T24.602**   Corrosion of second degree of unspecified site of left lower limb, except ankle and foot ▽

   √7ᵗʰ **T24.609**   Corrosion of second degree of unspecified site of unspecified lower limb, except ankle and foot ▽

√6ᵗʰ **T24.61**   **Corrosion of second degree of** thigh

   √7ᵗʰ **T24.611**   Corrosion of second degree of right thigh

   √7ᵗʰ **T24.612**   Corrosion of second degree of left thigh

   √7ᵗʰ **T24.619**   Corrosion of second degree of unspecified thigh ▽

√6ᵗʰ **T24.62**   **Corrosion of second degree of** knee

   √7ᵗʰ **T24.621**   Corrosion of second degree of right knee

   √7ᵗʰ **T24.622**   Corrosion of second degree of left knee

   √7ᵗʰ **T24.629**   Corrosion of second degree of unspecified knee ▽

√6ᵗʰ **T24.63**   **Corrosion of second degree of** lower leg

   √7ᵗʰ **T24.631**   Corrosion of second degree of right lower leg

   √7ᵗʰ **T24.632**   Corrosion of second degree of left lower leg

   √7ᵗʰ **T24.639**   Corrosion of second degree of unspecified lower leg ▽

√6ᵗʰ **T24.69**   **Corrosion of second degree of** multiple sites **of lower limb, except ankle and foot**

   √7ᵗʰ **T24.691**   Corrosion of second degree of multiple sites of right lower limb, except ankle and foot

   √7ᵗʰ **T24.692**   Corrosion of second degree of multiple sites of left lower limb, except ankle and foot

   √7ᵗʰ **T24.699**   Corrosion of second degree of multiple sites of unspecified lower limb, except ankle and foot ▽

√5ᵗʰ **T24.7**   **Corrosion of third degree of lower limb, except ankle and foot**

    Code first (T51-T65) to identify chemical and intent
    Use additional external cause code to identify place (Y92)

√6ᵗʰ **T24.70**   **Corrosion of third degree of unspecified site of lower limb, except ankle and foot**

   √7ᵗʰ **T24.701**   Corrosion of third degree of unspecified site of right lower limb, except ankle and foot ▽

☑ Additional Character Required   √✗7ᵗʰ Placeholder Alert   Manifestation Dx   ▽ Unspecified Dx   ►◄ Revised Text   ● New Code   ▲ Revised Code Title

ICD-10-CM 2017   **1021**

√7ᵗʰ **T24.702** Corrosion of third degree of unspecified site of left lower limb, except ankle and foot ▽

√7ᵗʰ **T24.709** Corrosion of third degree of unspecified site of unspecified lower limb, except ankle and foot ▽

√6ᵗʰ **T24.71** Corrosion of third degree of thigh

  √7ᵗʰ **T24.711** Corrosion of third degree of right thigh

  √7ᵗʰ **T24.712** Corrosion of third degree of left thigh

  √7ᵗʰ **T24.719** Corrosion of third degree of unspecified thigh ▽

√6ᵗʰ **T24.72** Corrosion of third degree of knee

  √7ᵗʰ **T24.721** Corrosion of third degree of right knee

  √7ᵗʰ **T24.722** Corrosion of third degree of left knee

  √7ᵗʰ **T24.729** Corrosion of third degree of unspecified knee ▽

√6ᵗʰ **T24.73** Corrosion of third degree of lower leg

  √7ᵗʰ **T24.731** Corrosion of third degree of right lower leg

  √7ᵗʰ **T24.732** Corrosion of third degree of left lower leg

  √7ᵗʰ **T24.739** Corrosion of third degree of unspecified lower leg ▽

√6ᵗʰ **T24.79** Corrosion of third degree of multiple sites of lower limb, except ankle and foot

  √7ᵗʰ **T24.791** Corrosion of third degree of multiple sites of right lower limb, except ankle and foot

  √7ᵗʰ **T24.792** Corrosion of third degree of multiple sites of left lower limb, except ankle and foot

  √7ᵗʰ **T24.799** Corrosion of third degree of multiple sites of unspecified lower limb, except ankle and foot ▽

√4ᵗʰ **T25 Burn and corrosion of ankle and foot**

> The appropriate 7th character is to be added to each code from category T25.
> A   initial encounter
> D   subsequent encounter
> S   sequela

√5ᵗʰ **T25.0 Burn of unspecified degree of ankle and foot**

> Use additional external cause code to identify the source, place and intent of the burn (X00-X19, X75-X77, X96-X98, Y92)

√6ᵗʰ **T25.01** Burn of unspecified degree of ankle

  √7ᵗʰ **T25.011** Burn of unspecified degree of right ankle ▽

  √7ᵗʰ **T25.012** Burn of unspecified degree of left ankle ▽

  √7ᵗʰ **T25.019** Burn of unspecified degree of unspecified ankle ▽

√6ᵗʰ **T25.02** Burn of unspecified degree of foot

  EXCLUDES 2   *burn of unspecified degree of toe(s) (nail) (T25.03-)*

  √7ᵗʰ **T25.021** Burn of unspecified degree of right foot ▽

  √7ᵗʰ **T25.022** Burn of unspecified degree of left foot ▽

  √7ᵗʰ **T25.029** Burn of unspecified degree of unspecified foot ▽

√6ᵗʰ **T25.03** Burn of unspecified degree of toe(s) (nail)

  √7ᵗʰ **T25.031** Burn of unspecified degree of right toe(s) (nail) ▽

  √7ᵗʰ **T25.032** Burn of unspecified degree of left toe(s) (nail) ▽

  √7ᵗʰ **T25.039** Burn of unspecified degree of unspecified toe(s) (nail) ▽

√6ᵗʰ **T25.09** Burn of unspecified degree of multiple sites of ankle and foot

  √7ᵗʰ **T25.091** Burn of unspecified degree of multiple sites of right ankle and foot ▽

  √7ᵗʰ **T25.092** Burn of unspecified degree of multiple sites of left ankle and foot ▽

  √7ᵗʰ **T25.099** Burn of unspecified degree of multiple sites of unspecified ankle and foot ▽

√5ᵗʰ **T25.1 Burn of first degree of ankle and foot**

> Use additional external cause code to identify the source, place and intent of the burn (X00-X19, X75-X77, X96-X98, Y92)

√6ᵗʰ **T25.11** Burn of first degree of ankle

  √7ᵗʰ **T25.111** Burn of first degree of right ankle

  √7ᵗʰ **T25.112** Burn of first degree of left ankle

  √7ᵗʰ **T25.119** Burn of first degree of unspecified ankle ▽

√6ᵗʰ **T25.12** Burn of first degree of foot

  EXCLUDES 2   *burn of first degree of toe(s) (nail) (T25.13-)*

  √7ᵗʰ **T25.121** Burn of first degree of right foot

  √7ᵗʰ **T25.122** Burn of first degree of left foot

  √7ᵗʰ **T25.129** Burn of first degree of unspecified foot ▽

√6ᵗʰ **T25.13** Burn of first degree of toe(s) (nail)

  √7ᵗʰ **T25.131** Burn of first degree of right toe(s) (nail)

  √7ᵗʰ **T25.132** Burn of first degree of left toe(s) (nail)

  √7ᵗʰ **T25.139** Burn of first degree of unspecified toe(s) (nail) ▽

√6ᵗʰ **T25.19** Burn of first degree of multiple sites of ankle and foot

  √7ᵗʰ **T25.191** Burn of first degree of multiple sites of right ankle and foot

  √7ᵗʰ **T25.192** Burn of first degree of multiple sites of left ankle and foot

  √7ᵗʰ **T25.199** Burn of first degree of multiple sites of unspecified ankle and foot ▽

√5ᵗʰ **T25.2 Burn of second degree of ankle and foot**

> Use additional external cause code to identify the source, place and intent of the burn (X00-X19, X75-X77, X96-X98, Y92)

√6ᵗʰ **T25.21** Burn of second degree of ankle

  √7ᵗʰ **T25.211** Burn of second degree of right ankle

  √7ᵗʰ **T25.212** Burn of second degree of left ankle

  √7ᵗʰ **T25.219** Burn of second degree of unspecified ankle ▽

√6ᵗʰ **T25.22** Burn of second degree of foot

  EXCLUDES 2   *burn of second degree of toe(s) (nail) (T25.23-)*

  √7ᵗʰ **T25.221** Burn of second degree of right foot

  √7ᵗʰ **T25.222** Burn of second degree of left foot

  √7ᵗʰ **T25.229** Burn of second degree of unspecified foot ▽

√6ᵗʰ **T25.23** Burn of second degree of toe(s) (nail)

  √7ᵗʰ **T25.231** Burn of second degree of right toe(s) (nail)

  √7ᵗʰ **T25.232** Burn of second degree of left toe(s) (nail)

  √7ᵗʰ **T25.239** Burn of second degree of unspecified toe(s) (nail) ▽

√6ᵗʰ **T25.29** Burn of second degree of multiple sites of ankle and foot

  √7ᵗʰ **T25.291** Burn of second degree of multiple sites of right ankle and foot

  √7ᵗʰ **T25.292** Burn of second degree of multiple sites of left ankle and foot

  √7ᵗʰ **T25.299** Burn of second degree of multiple sites of unspecified ankle and foot ▽

√5ᵗʰ **T25.3 Burn of third degree of ankle and foot**

> Use additional external cause code to identify the source, place and intent of the burn (X00-X19, X75-X77, X96-X98, Y92)

√6ᵗʰ **T25.31** Burn of third degree of ankle

  √7ᵗʰ **T25.311** Burn of third degree of right ankle

  √7ᵗʰ **T25.312** Burn of third degree of left ankle

  √7ᵗʰ **T25.319** Burn of third degree of unspecified ankle ▽

√6ᵗʰ **T25.32** Burn of third degree of foot

  EXCLUDES 2   *burn of third degree of toe(s) (nail) (T25.33-)*

  √7ᵗʰ **T25.321** Burn of third degree of right foot

  √7ᵗʰ **T25.322** Burn of third degree of left foot

  √7ᵗʰ **T25.329** Burn of third degree of unspecified foot ▽

√6ᵗʰ **T25.33** Burn of third degree of toe(s) (nail)

  √7ᵗʰ **T25.331** Burn of third degree of right toe(s) (nail)

  √7ᵗʰ **T25.332** Burn of third degree of left toe(s) (nail)

  √7ᵗʰ **T25.339** Burn of third degree of unspecified toe(s) (nail) ▽

√6ᵗʰ **T25.39** Burn of third degree of multiple sites of ankle and foot

  √7ᵗʰ **T25.391** Burn of third degree of multiple sites of right ankle and foot

  √7ᵗʰ **T25.392** Burn of third degree of multiple sites of left ankle and foot

---

EXCLUDES 1   Not coded here   EXCLUDES 2   Not included here   N Newborn Age : 0   P Pediatric Age : 0-17   M Maternity Age : 12-55   A Adult Age : 15-124

1022   ICD-10-CM 2017

√7ᵗʰ **T25.399** Burn of third degree of multiple sites of unspecified ankle and foot ▽

√5ᵗʰ **T25.4** Corrosion of unspecified degree of ankle and foot

  Code first (T51-T65) to identify chemical and intent
  Use additional external cause code to identify place (Y92)

√6ᵗʰ **T25.41** Corrosion of unspecified degree of ankle

  √7ᵗʰ **T25.411** Corrosion of unspecified degree of right ankle ▽

  √7ᵗʰ **T25.412** Corrosion of unspecified degree of left ankle ▽

  √7ᵗʰ **T25.419** Corrosion of unspecified degree of unspecified ankle ▽

√6ᵗʰ **T25.42** Corrosion of unspecified degree of foot

  EXCLUDES 2 corrosion of unspecified degree of toe(s) (nail) (T25.43-)

  √7ᵗʰ **T25.421** Corrosion of unspecified degree of right foot ▽

  √7ᵗʰ **T25.422** Corrosion of unspecified degree of left foot ▽

  √7ᵗʰ **T25.429** Corrosion of unspecified degree of unspecified foot ▽

√6ᵗʰ **T25.43** Corrosion of unspecified degree of toe(s) (nail)

  √7ᵗʰ **T25.431** Corrosion of unspecified degree of right toe(s) (nail) ▽

  √7ᵗʰ **T25.432** Corrosion of unspecified degree of left toe(s) (nail) ▽

  √7ᵗʰ **T25.439** Corrosion of unspecified degree of unspecified toe(s) (nail) ▽

√6ᵗʰ **T25.49** Corrosion of unspecified degree of multiple sites of ankle and foot

  √7ᵗʰ **T25.491** Corrosion of unspecified degree of multiple sites of right ankle and foot ▽

  √7ᵗʰ **T25.492** Corrosion of unspecified degree of multiple sites of left ankle and foot ▽

  √7ᵗʰ **T25.499** Corrosion of unspecified degree of multiple sites of unspecified ankle and foot ▽

√5ᵗʰ **T25.5** Corrosion of first degree of ankle and foot

  Code first (T51-T65) to identify chemical and intent
  Use additional external cause code to identify place (Y92)

√6ᵗʰ **T25.51** Corrosion of first degree of ankle

  √7ᵗʰ **T25.511** Corrosion of first degree of right ankle

  √7ᵗʰ **T25.512** Corrosion of first degree of left ankle

  √7ᵗʰ **T25.519** Corrosion of first degree of unspecified ankle ▽

√6ᵗʰ **T25.52** Corrosion of first degree of foot

  EXCLUDES 2 corrosion of first degree of toe(s) (nail) (T25.53-)

  √7ᵗʰ **T25.521** Corrosion of first degree of right foot

  √7ᵗʰ **T25.522** Corrosion of first degree of left foot

  √7ᵗʰ **T25.529** Corrosion of first degree of unspecified foot ▽

√6ᵗʰ **T25.53** Corrosion of first degree of toe(s) (nail)

  √7ᵗʰ **T25.531** Corrosion of first degree of right toe(s) (nail)

  √7ᵗʰ **T25.532** Corrosion of first degree of left toe(s) (nail)

  √7ᵗʰ **T25.539** Corrosion of first degree of unspecified toe(s) (nail) ▽

√6ᵗʰ **T25.59** Corrosion of first degree of multiple sites of ankle and foot

  √7ᵗʰ **T25.591** Corrosion of first degree of multiple sites of right ankle and foot

  √7ᵗʰ **T25.592** Corrosion of first degree of multiple sites of left ankle and foot

  √7ᵗʰ **T25.599** Corrosion of first degree of multiple sites of unspecified ankle and foot ▽

√5ᵗʰ **T25.6** Corrosion of second degree of ankle and foot

  Code first (T51-T65) to identify chemical and intent
  Use additional external cause code to identify place (Y92)

√6ᵗʰ **T25.61** Corrosion of second degree of ankle

  √7ᵗʰ **T25.611** Corrosion of second degree of right ankle

  √7ᵗʰ **T25.612** Corrosion of second degree of left ankle

  √7ᵗʰ **T25.619** Corrosion of second degree of unspecified ankle ▽

√6ᵗʰ **T25.62** Corrosion of second degree of foot

  EXCLUDES 2 corrosion of second degree of toe(s) (nail) (T25.63-)

  √7ᵗʰ **T25.621** Corrosion of second degree of right foot

  √7ᵗʰ **T25.622** Corrosion of second degree of left foot

  √7ᵗʰ **T25.629** Corrosion of second degree of unspecified foot

√6ᵗʰ **T25.63** Corrosion of second degree of toe(s) (nail)

  √7ᵗʰ **T25.631** Corrosion of second degree of right toe(s) (nail)

  √7ᵗʰ **T25.632** Corrosion of second degree of left toe(s) (nail)

  √7ᵗʰ **T25.639** Corrosion of second degree of unspecified toe(s) (nail) ▽

√6ᵗʰ **T25.69** Corrosion of second degree of multiple sites of ankle and foot

  √7ᵗʰ **T25.691** Corrosion of second degree of right ankle and foot

  √7ᵗʰ **T25.692** Corrosion of second degree of left ankle and foot

  √7ᵗʰ **T25.699** Corrosion of second degree of unspecified ankle and foot ▽

√5ᵗʰ **T25.7** Corrosion of third degree of ankle and foot

  Code first (T51-T65) to identify chemical and intent
  Use additional external cause code to identify place (Y92)

√6ᵗʰ **T25.71** Corrosion of third degree of ankle

  √7ᵗʰ **T25.711** Corrosion of third degree of right ankle

  √7ᵗʰ **T25.712** Corrosion of third degree of left ankle

  √7ᵗʰ **T25.719** Corrosion of third degree of unspecified ankle ▽

√6ᵗʰ **T25.72** Corrosion of third degree of foot

  EXCLUDES 2 corrosion of third degree of toe(s) (nail) (T25.73-)

  √7ᵗʰ **T25.721** Corrosion of third degree of right foot

  √7ᵗʰ **T25.722** Corrosion of third degree of left foot

  √7ᵗʰ **T25.729** Corrosion of third degree of unspecified foot ▽

√6ᵗʰ **T25.73** Corrosion of third degree of toe(s) (nail)

  √7ᵗʰ **T25.731** Corrosion of third degree of right toe(s) (nail)

  √7ᵗʰ **T25.732** Corrosion of third degree of left toe(s) (nail)

  √7ᵗʰ **T25.739** Corrosion of third degree of unspecified toe(s) (nail) ▽

√6ᵗʰ **T25.79** Corrosion of third degree of multiple sites of ankle and foot

  √7ᵗʰ **T25.791** Corrosion of third degree of multiple sites of right ankle and foot

  √7ᵗʰ **T25.792** Corrosion of third degree of multiple sites of left ankle and foot

  √7ᵗʰ **T25.799** Corrosion of third degree of multiple sites of unspecified ankle and foot ▽

Burns and corrosions confined to eye and internal organs (T26-T28)

√4ᵗʰ **T26** Burn and corrosion confined to eye and adnexa

  The appropriate 7th character is to be added to each code from category T26.
  A   initial encounter
  D   subsequent encounter
  S   sequela

√5ᵗʰ **T26.0** Burn of eyelid and periocular area

  Use additional external cause code to identify the source, place and intent of the burn (X00-X19, X75-X77, X96-X98, Y92)

  √x7ᵗʰ **T26.00** Burn of unspecified eyelid and periocular area ▽

  √x7ᵗʰ **T26.01** Burn of right eyelid and periocular area

  √x7ᵗʰ **T26.02** Burn of left eyelid and periocular area

√5ᵗʰ **T26.1** Burn of cornea and conjunctival sac

  Use additional external cause code to identify the source, place and intent of the burn (X00-X19, X75-X77, X96-X98, Y92)

  √x7ᵗʰ **T26.10** Burn of cornea and conjunctival sac, unspecified eye ▽

  √x7ᵗʰ **T26.11** Burn of cornea and conjunctival sac, right eye

  √x7ᵗʰ **T26.12** Burn of cornea and conjunctival sac, left eye

☑ Additional Character Required   √x7ᵗʰ Placeholder Alert   Manifestation Dx   ▽ Unspecified Dx   ▶◀ Revised Text   ● New Code   ▲ Revised Code Title

ICD-10-CM 2017   **1023**

√5th **T26.2**   **Burn with resulting rupture and destruction of eyeball**

Use additional external cause code to identify the source, place and intent of the burn (X00-X19, X75-X77, X96-X98, Y92)

√x7th **T26.20**   Burn with resulting rupture and destruction of unspecified eyeball ▽

√x7th **T26.21**   Burn with resulting rupture and destruction of right eyeball

√x7th **T26.22**   Burn with resulting rupture and destruction of left eyeball

√5th **T26.3**   **Burns of other specified parts of eye and adnexa**

Use additional external cause code to identify the source, place and intent of the burn (X00-X19, X75-X77, X96-X98, Y92)

√x7th **T26.30**   Burns of other specified parts of unspecified eye and adnexa ▽

√x7th **T26.31**   Burns of other specified parts of right eye and adnexa

√x7th **T26.32**   Burns of other specified parts of left eye and adnexa

√5th **T26.4**   **Burn of eye and adnexa, part unspecified**

Use additional external cause code to identify the source, place and intent of the burn (X00-X19, X75-X77, X96-X98, Y92)

√x7th **T26.40**   Burn of unspecified eye and adnexa, part unspecified ▽

√x7th **T26.41**   Burn of right eye and adnexa, part unspecified ▽

√x7th **T26.42**   Burn of left eye and adnexa, part unspecified ▽

√5th **T26.5**   **Corrosion of eyelid and periocular area**

Code first (T51-T65) to identify chemical and intent
Use additional external cause code to identify place (Y92)

√x7th **T26.50**   Corrosion of unspecified eyelid and periocular area ▽

√x7th **T26.51**   Corrosion of right eyelid and periocular area

√x7th **T26.52**   Corrosion of left eyelid and periocular area

√5th **T26.6**   **Corrosion of cornea and conjunctival sac**

Code first (T51-T65) to identify chemical and intent
Use additional external cause code to identify place (Y92)

√x7th **T26.60**   Corrosion of cornea and conjunctival sac, unspecified eye ▽

√x7th **T26.61**   Corrosion of cornea and conjunctival sac, right eye

√x7th **T26.62**   Corrosion of cornea and conjunctival sac, left eye

√5th **T26.7**   **Corrosion with resulting rupture and destruction of eyeball**

Code first (T51-T65) to identify chemical and intent
Use additional external cause code to identify place (Y92)

√x7th **T26.70**   Corrosion with resulting rupture and destruction of unspecified eyeball ▽

√x7th **T26.71**   Corrosion with resulting rupture and destruction of right eyeball

√x7th **T26.72**   Corrosion with resulting rupture and destruction of left eyeball

√5th **T26.8**   **Corrosions of other specified parts of eye and adnexa**

Code first (T51-T65) to identify chemical and intent
Use additional external cause code to identify place (Y92)

√x7th **T26.80**   Corrosions of other specified parts of unspecified eye and adnexa ▽

√x7th **T26.81**   Corrosions of other specified parts of right eye and adnexa

√x7th **T26.82**   Corrosions of other specified parts of left eye and adnexa

√5th **T26.9**   **Corrosion of eye and adnexa, part unspecified**

Code first (T51-T65) to identify chemical and intent
Use additional external cause code to identify place (Y92)

√x7th **T26.90**   Corrosion of unspecified eye and adnexa, part unspecified ▽

√x7th **T26.91**   Corrosion of right eye and adnexa, part unspecified ▽

√x7th **T26.92**   Corrosion of left eye and adnexa, part unspecified ▽

√4th **T27**   **Burn and corrosion of respiratory tract**

Use additional external cause code to identify the source and intent of the burn (X00-X19, X75-X77, X96-X98)
Use additional external cause code to identify place (Y92)

The appropriate 7th character is to be added to each code from category T27.
A   initial encounter
D   subsequent encounter
S   sequela

√x7th **T27.0**   **Burn of larynx and trachea**

√x7th **T27.1**   **Burn involving larynx and trachea with lung**

√x7th **T27.2**   **Burn of other parts of respiratory tract**

Burn of thoracic cavity

√x7th **T27.3**   **Burn of respiratory tract, part unspecified** ▽

Code first (T51-T65) to identify chemical and intent for codes T27.4-T27.7

√x7th **T27.4**   **Corrosion of larynx and trachea**

√x7th **T27.5**   **Corrosion involving larynx and trachea with lung**

√x7th **T27.6**   **Corrosion of other parts of respiratory tract**

√x7th **T27.7**   **Corrosion of respiratory tract, part unspecified** ▽

√4th **T28**   **Burn and corrosion of other internal organs**

Use additional external cause code to identify the source and intent of the burn (X00-X19, X75-X77, X96-X98)
Use additional external cause code to identify place (Y92)

The appropriate 7th character is to be added to each code from category T28.
A   initial encounter
D   subsequent encounter
S   sequela

√x7th **T28.0**   **Burn of mouth and pharynx**

√x7th **T28.1**   **Burn of esophagus**

√x7th **T28.2**   **Burn of other parts of alimentary tract**

√x7th **T28.3**   **Burn of internal genitourinary organs**

√5th **T28.4**   **Burns of other and unspecified internal organs**

√x7th **T28.40**   Burn of unspecified internal organ ▽

√6th **T28.41**   Burn of ear drum

√7th **T28.411**   Burn of right ear drum

√7th **T28.412**   Burn of left ear drum

√7th **T28.419**   Burn of unspecified ear drum ▽

√x7th **T28.49**   Burn of other internal organ

Code first (T51-T65) to identify chemical and intent for T28.5-T28.9-

√x7th **T28.5**   **Corrosion of mouth and pharynx**

√x7th **T28.6**   **Corrosion of esophagus**

√x7th **T28.7**   **Corrosion of other parts of alimentary tract**

√x7th **T28.8**   **Corrosion of internal genitourinary organs**

√5th **T28.9**   **Corrosions of other and unspecified internal organs**

√x7th **T28.90**   Corrosions of unspecified internal organs ▽

√6th **T28.91**   Corrosions of ear drum

√7th **T28.911**   Corrosions of right ear drum

√7th **T28.912**   Corrosions of left ear drum

√7th **T28.919**   Corrosions of unspecified ear drum ▽

√x7th **T28.99**   Corrosions of other internal organs

Burns and corrosions of multiple and unspecified body regions (T30-T32)

√4th **T30**   **Burn and corrosion, body region unspecified**

T30.0   **Burn of unspecified body region, unspecified degree** ▽

NOTE   This code is not for inpatient use. Code to specified site and degree of burns

Burn NOS
Multiple burns NOS

T30.4   **Corrosion of unspecified body region, unspecified degree** ▽

NOTE   This code is not for inpatient use. Code to specified site and degree of corrosion

Corrosion NOS
Multiple corrosion NOS

√4th **T31**   **Burns classified according to extent of body surface involved**

NOTE   This category is to be used as the primary code only when the site of the burn is unspecified. It should be used as a supplementary code with categories T20-T25 when the site is specified.

T31.0   **Burns involving less than 10% of body surface**

√5th **T31.1**   **Burns involving 10-19% of body surface**

T31.10   **Burns involving 10-19% of body surface with 0% to 9% third degree burns**

Burns involving 10-19% of body surface NOS

EXCLUDES 1 Not coded here   EXCLUDES 2 Not included here   N Newborn Age : 0   P Pediatric Age : 0-17   M Maternity Age : 12-55   A Adult Age : 15-124

1024   ICD-10-CM 2017

    T31.11   **Burns involving 10-19% of body surface with 10-19% third degree burns**

✓5ᵗʰ   **T31.2**   **Burns involving 20-29% of body surface**

    T31.20   **Burns involving 20-29% of body surface with 0% to 9% third degree burns**
         Burns involving 20-29% of body surface NOS

    T31.21   **Burns involving 20-29% of body surface with 10-19% third degree burns**

    T31.22   **Burns involving 20-29% of body surface with 20-29% third degree burns**

✓5ᵗʰ   **T31.3**   **Burns involving 30-39% of body surface**

    T31.30   **Burns involving 30-39% of body surface with 0% to 9% third degree burns**
         Burns involving 30-39% of body surface NOS

    T31.31   **Burns involving 30-39% of body surface with 10-19% third degree burns**

    T31.32   **Burns involving 30-39% of body surface with 20-29% third degree burns**

    T31.33   **Burns involving 30-39% of body surface with 30-39% third degree burns**

✓5ᵗʰ   **T31.4**   **Burns involving 40-49% of body surface**

    T31.40   **Burns involving 40-49% of body surface with 0% to 9% third degree burns**
         Burns involving 40-49% of body surface NOS

    T31.41   **Burns involving 40-49% of body surface with 10-19% third degree burns**

    T31.42   **Burns involving 40-49% of body surface with 20-29% third degree burns**

    T31.43   **Burns involving 40-49% of body surface with 30-39% third degree burns**

    T31.44   **Burns involving 40-49% of body surface with 40-49% third degree burns**

✓5ᵗʰ   **T31.5**   **Burns involving 50-59% of body surface**

    T31.50   **Burns involving 50-59% of body surface with 0% to 9% third degree burns**
         Burns involving 50-59% of body surface NOS

    T31.51   **Burns involving 50-59% of body surface with 10-19% third degree burns**

    T31.52   **Burns involving 50-59% of body surface with 20-29% third degree burns**

    T31.53   **Burns involving 50-59% of body surface with 30-39% third degree burns**

    T31.54   **Burns involving 50-59% of body surface with 40-49% third degree burns**

    T31.55   **Burns involving 50-59% of body surface with 50-59% third degree burns**

✓5ᵗʰ   **T31.6**   **Burns involving 60-69% of body surface**

    T31.60   **Burns involving 60-69% of body surface with 0% to 9% third degree burns**
         Burns involving 60-69% of body surface NOS

    T31.61   **Burns involving 60-69% of body surface with 10-19% third degree burns**

    T31.62   **Burns involving 60-69% of body surface with 20-29% third degree burns**

    T31.63   **Burns involving 60-69% of body surface with 30-39% third degree burns**

    T31.64   **Burns involving 60-69% of body surface with 40-49% third degree burns**

    T31.65   **Burns involving 60-69% of body surface with 50-59% third degree burns**

    T31.66   **Burns involving 60-69% of body surface with 60-69% third degree burns**

✓5ᵗʰ   **T31.7**   **Burns involving 70-79% of body surface**

    T31.70   **Burns involving 70-79% of body surface with 0% to 9% third degree burns**
         Burns involving 70-79% of body surface NOS

    T31.71   **Burns involving 70-79% of body surface with 10-19% third degree burns**

    T31.72   **Burns involving 70-79% of body surface with 20-29% third degree burns**

    T31.73   **Burns involving 70-79% of body surface with 30-39% third degree burns**

    T31.74   **Burns involving 70-79% of body surface with 40-49% third degree burns**

    T31.75   **Burns involving 70-79% of body surface with 50-59% third degree burns**

    T31.76   **Burns involving 70-79% of body surface with 60-69% third degree burns**

    T31.77   **Burns involving 70-79% of body surface with 70-79% third degree burns**

✓5ᵗʰ   **T31.8**   **Burns involving 80-89% of body surface**

    T31.80   **Burns involving 80-89% of body surface with 0% to 9% third degree burns**
         Burns involving 80-89% of body surface NOS

    T31.81   **Burns involving 80-89% of body surface with 10-19% third degree burns**

    T31.82   **Burns involving 80-89% of body surface with 20-29% third degree burns**

    T31.83   **Burns involving 80-89% of body surface with 30-39% third degree burns**

    T31.84   **Burns involving 80-89% of body surface with 40-49% third degree burns**

    T31.85   **Burns involving 80-89% of body surface with 50-59% third degree burns**

    T31.86   **Burns involving 80-89% of body surface with 60-69% third degree burns**

    T31.87   **Burns involving 80-89% of body surface with 70-79% third degree burns**

    T31.88   **Burns involving 80-89% of body surface with 80-89% third degree burns**

✓5ᵗʰ   **T31.9**   **Burns involving 90% or more of body surface**

    T31.90   **Burns involving 90% or more of body surface with 0% to 9% third degree burns**
         Burns involving 90% or more of body surface NOS

    T31.91   **Burns involving 90% or more of body surface with 10-19% third degree burns**

    T31.92   **Burns involving 90% or more of body surface with 20-29% third degree burns**

    T31.93   **Burns involving 90% or more of body surface with 30-39% third degree burns**

    T31.94   **Burns involving 90% or more of body surface with 40-49% third degree burns**

    T31.95   **Burns involving 90% or more of body surface with 50-59% third degree burns**

    T31.96   **Burns involving 90% or more of body surface with 60-69% third degree burns**

    T31.97   **Burns involving 90% or more of body surface with 70-79% third degree burns**

    T31.98   **Burns involving 90% or more of body surface with 80-89% third degree burns**

    T31.99   **Burns involving 90% or more of body surface with 90% or more third degree burns**

✓4ᵗʰ   **T32**   **Corrosions classified according to extent of body surface involved**

     NOTE   This category is to be used as the primary code only when the site of the corrosion is unspecified. It may be used as a supplementary code with categories T20-T25 when the site is specified.

     T32.0   **Corrosions involving less than 10% of body surface**

✓5ᵗʰ   **T32.1**   **Corrosions involving 10-19% of body surface**

    T32.10   **Corrosions involving 10-19% of body surface with 0% to 9% third degree corrosion**
         Corrosions involving 10-19% of body surface NOS

    T32.11   **Corrosions involving 10-19% of body surface with 10-19% third degree corrosion**

✓5ᵗʰ   **T32.2**   **Corrosions involving 20-29% of body surface**

    T32.20   **Corrosions involving 20-29% of body surface with 0% to 9% third degree corrosion**

    T32.21   **Corrosions involving 20-29% of body surface with 10-19% third degree corrosion**

    T32.22   **Corrosions involving 20-29% of body surface with 20-29% third degree corrosion**

✓5ᵗʰ   **T32.3**   **Corrosions involving 30-39% of body surface**

    T32.30   **Corrosions involving 30-39% of body surface with 0% to 9% third degree corrosion**

    T32.31   **Corrosions involving 30-39% of body surface with 10-19% third degree corrosion**

    T32.32   **Corrosions involving 30-39% of body surface with 20-29% third degree corrosion**

    T32.33   **Corrosions involving 30-39% of body surface with 30-39% third degree corrosion**

✓5ᵗʰ   **T32.4**   **Corrosions involving 40-49% of body surface**

    T32.40   **Corrosions involving 40-49% of body surface with 0% to 9% third degree corrosion**

    T32.41   **Corrosions involving 40-49% of body surface with 10-19% third degree corrosion**

✔ Additional Character Required   ✔×7ᵗʰ Placeholder Alert   Manifestation Dx   ▽ Unspecified Dx   ▶◀ Revised Text   ● New Code   ▲ Revised Code Title

T32.42 Corrosions involving 40-49% of body surface with 20-29% third degree corrosion

T32.43 Corrosions involving 40-49% of body surface with 30-39% third degree corrosion

T32.44 Corrosions involving 40-49% of body surface with 40-49% third degree corrosion

√5th **T32.5** Corrosions involving 50-59% of body surface

T32.50 Corrosions involving 50-59% of body surface with 0% to 9% third degree corrosion

T32.51 Corrosions involving 50-59% of body surface with 10-19% third degree corrosion

T32.52 Corrosions involving 50-59% of body surface with 20-29% third degree corrosion

T32.53 Corrosions involving 50-59% of body surface with 30-39% third degree corrosion

T32.54 Corrosions involving 50-59% of body surface with 40-49% third degree corrosion

T32.55 Corrosions involving 50-59% of body surface with 50-59% third degree corrosion

√5th **T32.6** Corrosions involving 60-69% of body surface

T32.60 Corrosions involving 60-69% of body surface with 0% to 9% third degree corrosion

T32.61 Corrosions involving 60-69% of body surface with 10-19% third degree corrosion

T32.62 Corrosions involving 60-69% of body surface with 20-29% third degree corrosion

T32.63 Corrosions involving 60-69% of body surface with 30-39% third degree corrosion

T32.64 Corrosions involving 60-69% of body surface with 40-49% third degree corrosion

T32.65 Corrosions involving 60-69% of body surface with 50-59% third degree corrosion

T32.66 Corrosions involving 60-69% of body surface with 60-69% third degree corrosion

√5th **T32.7** Corrosions involving 70-79% of body surface

T32.70 Corrosions involving 70-79% of body surface with 0% to 9% third degree corrosion

T32.71 Corrosions involving 70-79% of body surface with 10-19% third degree corrosion

T32.72 Corrosions involving 70-79% of body surface with 20-29% third degree corrosion

T32.73 Corrosions involving 70-79% of body surface with 30-39% third degree corrosion

T32.74 Corrosions involving 70-79% of body surface with 40-49% third degree corrosion

T32.75 Corrosions involving 70-79% of body surface with 50-59% third degree corrosion

T32.76 Corrosions involving 70-79% of body surface with 60-69% third degree corrosion

T32.77 Corrosions involving 70-79% of body surface with 70-79% third degree corrosion

√5th **T32.8** Corrosions involving 80-89% of body surface

T32.80 Corrosions involving 80-89% of body surface with 0% to 9% third degree corrosion

T32.81 Corrosions involving 80-89% of body surface with 10-19% third degree corrosion

T32.82 Corrosions involving 80-89% of body surface with 20-29% third degree corrosion

T32.83 Corrosions involving 80-89% of body surface with 30-39% third degree corrosion

T32.84 Corrosions involving 80-89% of body surface with 40-49% third degree corrosion

T32.85 Corrosions involving 80-89% of body surface with 50-59% third degree corrosion

T32.86 Corrosions involving 80-89% of body surface with 60-69% third degree corrosion

T32.87 Corrosions involving 80-89% of body surface with 70-79% third degree corrosion

T32.88 Corrosions involving 80-89% of body surface with 80-89% third degree corrosion

√5th **T32.9** Corrosions involving 90% or more of body surface

T32.90 Corrosions involving 90% or more of body surface with 0% to 9% third degree corrosion

T32.91 Corrosions involving 90% or more of body surface with 10-19% third degree corrosion

T32.92 Corrosions involving 90% or more of body surface with 20-29% third degree corrosion

T32.93 Corrosions involving 90% or more of body surface with 30-39% third degree corrosion

T32.94 Corrosions involving 90% or more of body surface with 40-49% third degree corrosion

T32.95 Corrosions involving 90% or more of body surface with 50-59% third degree corrosion

T32.96 Corrosions involving 90% or more of body surface with 60-69% third degree corrosion

T32.97 Corrosions involving 90% or more of body surface with 70-79% third degree corrosion

T32.98 Corrosions involving 90% or more of body surface with 80-89% third degree corrosion

T32.99 Corrosions involving 90% or more of body surface with 90% or more third degree corrosion

Frostbite (T33-T34)

EXCLUDES 2   *hypothermia and other effects of reduced temperature (T68, T69.-)*

√4th **T33** Superficial frostbite

     INCLUDES   frostbite with partial thickness skin loss

> The appropriate 7th character is to be added to each code from category T33.
> A   initial encounter
> D   subsequent encounter
> S   sequela

√5th **T33.0** Superficial frostbite of head

√6th **T33.01** Superficial frostbite of ear

√7th **T33.011** Superficial frostbite of right ear

√7th **T33.012** Superficial frostbite of left ear

√7th **T33.019** Superficial frostbite of unspecified ear ▽

√x7th **T33.02** Superficial frostbite of nose

√x7th **T33.09** Superficial frostbite of other part of head

√x7th **T33.1** Superficial frostbite of neck

√x7th **T33.2** Superficial frostbite of thorax

√x7th **T33.3** Superficial frostbite of abdominal wall, lower back and pelvis

√5th **T33.4** Superficial frostbite of arm

     EXCLUDES 2   *superficial frostbite of wrist and hand (T33.5-)*

√x7th **T33.40** Superficial frostbite of unspecified arm ▽

√x7th **T33.41** Superficial frostbite of right arm

√x7th **T33.42** Superficial frostbite of left arm

√5th **T33.5** Superficial frostbite of wrist, hand, and fingers

√6th **T33.51** Superficial frostbite of wrist

√7th **T33.511** Superficial frostbite of right wrist

√7th **T33.512** Superficial frostbite of left wrist

√7th **T33.519** Superficial frostbite of unspecified wrist ▽

√6th **T33.52** Superficial frostbite of hand

     EXCLUDES 2   *superficial frostbite of fingers (T33.53-)*

√7th **T33.521** Superficial frostbite of right hand

√7th **T33.522** Superficial frostbite of left hand

√7th **T33.529** Superficial frostbite of unspecified hand ▽

√6th **T33.53** Superficial frostbite of finger(s)

√7th **T33.531** Superficial frostbite of right finger(s)

√7th **T33.532** Superficial frostbite of left finger(s)

√7th **T33.539** Superficial frostbite of unspecified finger(s) ▽

√5th **T33.6** Superficial frostbite of hip and thigh

√x7th **T33.60** Superficial frostbite of unspecified hip and thigh ▽

√x7th **T33.61** Superficial frostbite of right hip and thigh

√x7th **T33.62** Superficial frostbite of left hip and thigh

√5th **T33.7** Superficial frostbite of knee and lower leg

     EXCLUDES 2   *superficial frostbite of ankle and foot (T33.8-)*

√x7th **T33.70** Superficial frostbite of unspecified knee and lower leg ▽

√x7th **T33.71** Superficial frostbite of right knee and lower leg

√x7th **T33.72** Superficial frostbite of left knee and lower leg

√5th **T33.8** Superficial frostbite of ankle, foot, and toe(s)

√6th **T33.81** Superficial frostbite of ankle

√7th **T33.811** Superficial frostbite of right ankle

√7th **T33.812** Superficial frostbite of left ankle

√7th **T33.819** Superficial frostbite of unspecified ankle ▽

√6th **T33.82** Superficial frostbite of foot

√7th **T33.821** Superficial frostbite of right foot

EXCLUDES 1   Not coded here   EXCLUDES 2   Not included here   N   Newborn Age : 0   P   Pediatric Age : 0-17   M   Maternity Age : 12-55   A   Adult Age : 15-124

1026

ICD-10-CM 2017

√7ᵗʰ **T33.822** Superficial frostbite of left **foot**

√7ᵗʰ **T33.829** Superficial frostbite of unspecified **foot** ▽

√6ᵗʰ **T33.83** Superficial frostbite of toe(s)

√7ᵗʰ **T33.831** Superficial frostbite of right **toe(s)**

√7ᵗʰ **T33.832** Superficial frostbite of left **toe(s)**

√7ᵗʰ **T33.839** Superficial frostbite of unspecified **toe(s)** ▽

√5ᵗʰ **T33.9** Superficial frostbite of other and unspecified sites

√x7ᵗʰ **T33.90** Superficial frostbite of unspecified **sites** ▽

Superficial frostbite NOS

√x7ᵗʰ **T33.99** Superficial frostbite of other sites

Superficial frostbite of leg NOS

Superficial frostbite of trunk NOS

√4ᵗʰ **T34** **Frostbite** with tissue necrosis

The appropriate 7th character is to be added to each code from category T34.
A   initial encounter
D   subsequent encounter
S   sequela

√5ᵗʰ **T34.0** Frostbite with tissue necrosis of head

√6ᵗʰ **T34.01** Frostbite with tissue necrosis of ear

√7ᵗʰ **T34.011** Frostbite with tissue necrosis of right **ear**

√7ᵗʰ **T34.012** Frostbite with tissue necrosis of left **ear**

√7ᵗʰ **T34.019** Frostbite with tissue necrosis of unspecified **ear** ▽

√x7ᵗʰ **T34.02** Frostbite with tissue necrosis of nose

√x7ᵗʰ **T34.09** Frostbite with tissue necrosis of other part of head

√x7ᵗʰ **T34.1** Frostbite with tissue necrosis of neck

√x7ᵗʰ **T34.2** Frostbite with tissue necrosis of thorax

√x7ᵗʰ **T34.3** Frostbite with tissue necrosis of abdominal wall, lower back and pelvis

√5ᵗʰ **T34.4** Frostbite with tissue necrosis of arm

EXCLUDES 2 *frostbite with tissue necrosis of wrist and hand (T34.5-)*

√x7ᵗʰ **T34.40** Frostbite with tissue necrosis of unspecified **arm** ▽

√x7ᵗʰ **T34.41** Frostbite with tissue necrosis of right **arm**

√x7ᵗʰ **T34.42** Frostbite with tissue necrosis of left **arm**

√5ᵗʰ **T34.5** Frostbite with tissue necrosis of wrist, hand, and finger(s)

√6ᵗʰ **T34.51** Frostbite with tissue necrosis of wrist

√7ᵗʰ **T34.511** Frostbite with tissue necrosis of right **wrist**

√7ᵗʰ **T34.512** Frostbite with tissue necrosis of left **wrist**

√7ᵗʰ **T34.519** Frostbite with tissue necrosis of unspecified **wrist** ▽

√6ᵗʰ **T34.52** Frostbite with tissue necrosis of hand

EXCLUDES 2 *frostbite with tissue necrosis of finger(s) (T34.53-)*

√7ᵗʰ **T34.521** Frostbite with tissue necrosis of right **hand**

√7ᵗʰ **T34.522** Frostbite with tissue necrosis of left **hand**

√7ᵗʰ **T34.529** Frostbite with tissue necrosis of unspecified **hand** ▽

√6ᵗʰ **T34.53** Frostbite with tissue necrosis of finger(s)

√7ᵗʰ **T34.531** Frostbite with tissue necrosis of right **finger(s)**

√7ᵗʰ **T34.532** Frostbite with tissue necrosis of left **finger(s)**

√7ᵗʰ **T34.539** Frostbite with tissue necrosis of unspecified **finger(s)** ▽

√5ᵗʰ **T34.6** Frostbite with tissue necrosis of hip and thigh

√x7ᵗʰ **T34.60** Frostbite with tissue necrosis of unspecified **hip and thigh** ▽

√x7ᵗʰ **T34.61** Frostbite with tissue necrosis of right **hip and thigh**

√x7ᵗʰ **T34.62** Frostbite with tissue necrosis of left **hip and thigh**

√5ᵗʰ **T34.7** Frostbite with tissue necrosis of knee and lower leg

EXCLUDES 2 *frostbite with tissue necrosis of ankle and foot (T34.8-)*

√x7ᵗʰ **T34.70** Frostbite with tissue necrosis of unspecified **knee and lower leg** ▽

√x7ᵗʰ **T34.71** Frostbite with tissue necrosis of right **knee and lower leg**

√x7ᵗʰ **T34.72** Frostbite with tissue necrosis of left **knee and lower leg**

√5ᵗʰ **T34.8** Frostbite with tissue necrosis of ankle, foot, and toe(s)

√6ᵗʰ **T34.81** Frostbite with tissue necrosis of ankle

√7ᵗʰ **T34.811** Frostbite with tissue necrosis of right **ankle**

√7ᵗʰ **T34.812** Frostbite with tissue necrosis of left **ankle**

√7ᵗʰ **T34.819** Frostbite with tissue necrosis of unspecified **ankle** ▽

√6ᵗʰ **T34.82** Frostbite with tissue necrosis of foot

√7ᵗʰ **T34.821** Frostbite with tissue necrosis of right **foot**

√7ᵗʰ **T34.822** Frostbite with tissue necrosis of left **foot**

√7ᵗʰ **T34.829** Frostbite with tissue necrosis of unspecified **foot** ▽

√6ᵗʰ **T34.83** Frostbite with tissue necrosis of toe(s)

√7ᵗʰ **T34.831** Frostbite with tissue necrosis of right **toe(s)**

√7ᵗʰ **T34.832** Frostbite with tissue necrosis of left **toe(s)**

√7ᵗʰ **T34.839** Frostbite with tissue necrosis of unspecified **toe(s)** ▽

√5ᵗʰ **T34.9** Frostbite with tissue necrosis of other and unspecified sites

√x7ᵗʰ **T34.90** Frostbite with tissue necrosis of unspecified **sites** ▽

Frostbite with tissue necrosis NOS

√x7ᵗʰ **T34.99** Frostbite with tissue necrosis of other sites

Frostbite with tissue necrosis of leg NOS

Frostbite with tissue necrosis of trunk NOS

Poisoning by, adverse effects of and underdosing of drugs, medicaments and biological substances (T36-T50)

INCLUDES   adverse effect of correct substance properly administered
poisoning by overdose of substance
poisoning by wrong substance given or taken in error
underdosing by (inadvertently) (deliberately) taking less substance than prescribed or instructed

Code first, for adverse effects, the nature of the adverse effect, such as:
adverse effect NOS (T88.7)
aspirin gastritis (K29.-)
blood disorders (D56-D76)
contact dermatitis (L23-L25)
dermatitis due to substances taken internally (L27.-)
nephropathy (N14.0-N14.2)

NOTE   The drug giving rise to the adverse effect should be identified by use of codes from categories T36-T50 with fifth or sixth character 5.

Use additional code(s) to specify:
manifestations of poisoning
underdosing or failure in dosage during medical and surgical care (Y63.6, Y63.8-Y63.9)
underdosing of medication regimen (Z91.12-, Z91.13-)

EXCLUDES 1 *toxic reaction to local anesthesia in pregnancy (O29.3-)*
EXCLUDES 2 *abuse and dependence of psychoactive substances (F10-F19)*
abuse of non-dependence-producing substances (F55.-)
drug reaction and poisoning affecting newborn (P00-P96)
pathological drug intoxication (inebriation) (F10-F19)

AHA: 2016,2Q,8; 2015,3Q,22

√4ᵗʰ **T36** Poisoning by, adverse effect of and underdosing of systemic antibiotics

EXCLUDES 1 *antineoplastic antibiotics (T45.1-)*
locally applied antibiotic NEC (T49.0)
topically used antibiotic for ear, nose and throat (T49.6)
topically used antibiotic for eye (T49.5)

The appropriate 7th character is to be added to each code from category T36.
A   initial encounter
D   subsequent encounter
S   sequela

√5ᵗʰ **T36.0** Poisoning by, adverse effect of and underdosing of penicillins

√6ᵗʰ **T36.0X** Poisoning by, adverse effect of and underdosing of penicillins

√7ᵗʰ **T36.0X1** Poisoning by penicillins, accidental (unintentional)

Poisoning by penicillins NOS

√7ᵗʰ **T36.0X2** Poisoning by penicillins, intentional self-harm

√7ᵗʰ **T36.0X3** Poisoning by penicillins, assault

√7ᵗʰ **T36.0X4** Poisoning by penicillins, undetermined

√7ᵗʰ **T36.0X5** Adverse effect of penicillins

√7ᵗʰ **T36.0X6** Underdosing of penicillins

☑ Additional Character Required   √x7ᵗʰ Placeholder Alert   Manifestation Dx   ▽ Unspecified Dx   ►◄ Revised Text   ● New Code   ▲ Revised Code Title

ICD-10-CM 2017   **1027**

✓5ᵗʰ **T36.1** **Poisoning by, adverse effect of and underdosing of cephalosporins and other beta-lactam antibiotics**

  ✓6ᵗʰ **T36.1X** **Poisoning by, adverse effect of and underdosing of cephalosporins and other beta-lactam antibiotics**

    ✓7ᵗʰ **T36.1X1** **Poisoning by cephalosporins and other beta-lactam antibiotics, accidental (unintentional)**
      Poisoning by cephalosporins and other beta-lactam antibiotics NOS

    ✓7ᵗʰ **T36.1X2** **Poisoning by cephalosporins and other beta-lactam antibiotics, intentional self-harm**

    ✓7ᵗʰ **T36.1X3** **Poisoning by cephalosporins and other beta-lactam antibiotics, assault**

    ✓7ᵗʰ **T36.1X4** **Poisoning by cephalosporins and other beta-lactam antibiotics, undetermined**

    ✓7ᵗʰ **T36.1X5** **Adverse effect of cephalosporins and other beta-lactam antibiotics**

    ✓7ᵗʰ **T36.1X6** **Underdosing of cephalosporins and other beta-lactam antibiotics**

✓5ᵗʰ **T36.2** **Poisoning by, adverse effect of and underdosing of chloramphenicol group**

  ✓6ᵗʰ **T36.2X** **Poisoning by, adverse effect of and underdosing of chloramphenicol group**

    ✓7ᵗʰ **T36.2X1** **Poisoning by chloramphenicol group, accidental (unintentional)**
      Poisoning by chloramphenicol group NOS

    ✓7ᵗʰ **T36.2X2** **Poisoning by chloramphenicol group, intentional self-harm**

    ✓7ᵗʰ **T36.2X3** **Poisoning by chloramphenicol group, assault**

    ✓7ᵗʰ **T36.2X4** **Poisoning by chloramphenicol group, undetermined**

    ✓7ᵗʰ **T36.2X5** **Adverse effect of chloramphenicol group**

    ✓7ᵗʰ **T36.2X6** **Underdosing of chloramphenicol group**

✓5ᵗʰ **T36.3** **Poisoning by, adverse effect of and underdosing of macrolides**

  ✓6ᵗʰ **T36.3X** **Poisoning by, adverse effect of and underdosing of macrolides**

    ✓7ᵗʰ **T36.3X1** **Poisoning by macrolides, accidental (unintentional)**
      Poisoning by macrolides NOS

    ✓7ᵗʰ **T36.3X2** **Poisoning by macrolides, intentional self-harm**

    ✓7ᵗʰ **T36.3X3** **Poisoning by macrolides, assault**

    ✓7ᵗʰ **T36.3X4** **Poisoning by macrolides, undetermined**

    ✓7ᵗʰ **T36.3X5** **Adverse effect of macrolides**

    ✓7ᵗʰ **T36.3X6** **Underdosing of macrolides**

✓5ᵗʰ **T36.4** **Poisoning by, adverse effect of and underdosing of tetracyclines**

  ✓6ᵗʰ **T36.4X** **Poisoning by, adverse effect of and underdosing of tetracyclines**

    ✓7ᵗʰ **T36.4X1** **Poisoning by tetracyclines, accidental (unintentional)**
      Poisoning by tetracyclines NOS

    ✓7ᵗʰ **T36.4X2** **Poisoning by tetracyclines, intentional self-harm**

    ✓7ᵗʰ **T36.4X3** **Poisoning by tetracyclines, assault**

    ✓7ᵗʰ **T36.4X4** **Poisoning by tetracyclines, undetermined**

    ✓7ᵗʰ **T36.4X5** **Adverse effect of tetracyclines**

    ✓7ᵗʰ **T36.4X6** **Underdosing of tetracyclines**

✓5ᵗʰ **T36.5** **Poisoning by, adverse effect of and underdosing of aminoglycosides**
  Poisoning by, adverse effect of and underdosing of streptomycin

  ✓6ᵗʰ **T36.5X** **Poisoning by, adverse effect of and underdosing of aminoglycosides**

    ✓7ᵗʰ **T36.5X1** **Poisoning by aminoglycosides, accidental (unintentional)**
      Poisoning by aminoglycosides NOS

    ✓7ᵗʰ **T36.5X2** **Poisoning by aminoglycosides, intentional self-harm**

    ✓7ᵗʰ **T36.5X3** **Poisoning by aminoglycosides, assault**

    ✓7ᵗʰ **T36.5X4** **Poisoning by aminoglycosides, undetermined**

    ✓7ᵗʰ **T36.5X5** **Adverse effect of aminoglycosides**

    ✓7ᵗʰ **T36.5X6** **Underdosing of aminoglycosides**

✓5ᵗʰ **T36.6** **Poisoning by, adverse effect of and underdosing of rifampicins**

  ✓6ᵗʰ **T36.6X** **Poisoning by, adverse effect of and underdosing of rifampicins**

    ✓7ᵗʰ **T36.6X1** **Poisoning by rifampicins, accidental (unintentional)**
      Poisoning by rifampicins NOS

    ✓7ᵗʰ **T36.6X2** **Poisoning by rifampicins, intentional self-harm**

    ✓7ᵗʰ **T36.6X3** **Poisoning by rifampicins, assault**

    ✓7ᵗʰ **T36.6X4** **Poisoning by rifampicins, undetermined**

    ✓7ᵗʰ **T36.6X5** **Adverse effect of rifampicins**

    ✓7ᵗʰ **T36.6X6** **Underdosing of rifampicins**

✓5ᵗʰ **T36.7** **Poisoning by, adverse effect of and underdosing of antifungal antibiotics, systemically used**

  ✓6ᵗʰ **T36.7X** **Poisoning by, adverse effect of and underdosing of antifungal antibiotics, systemically used**

    ✓7ᵗʰ **T36.7X1** **Poisoning by antifungal antibiotics, systemically used, accidental (unintentional)**
      Poisoning by antifungal antibiotics, systemically used NOS

    ✓7ᵗʰ **T36.7X2** **Poisoning by antifungal antibiotics, systemically used, intentional self-harm**

    ✓7ᵗʰ **T36.7X3** **Poisoning by antifungal antibiotics, systemically used, assault**

    ✓7ᵗʰ **T36.7X4** **Poisoning by antifungal antibiotics, systemically used, undetermined**

    ✓7ᵗʰ **T36.7X5** **Adverse effect of antifungal antibiotics, systemically used**

    ✓7ᵗʰ **T36.7X6** **Underdosing of antifungal antibiotics, systemically used**

✓5ᵗʰ **T36.8** **Poisoning by, adverse effect of and underdosing of other systemic antibiotics**

  ✓6ᵗʰ **T36.8X** **Poisoning by, adverse effect of and underdosing of other systemic antibiotics**

    ✓7ᵗʰ **T36.8X1** **Poisoning by other systemic antibiotics, accidental (unintentional)**
      Poisoning by other systemic antibiotics NOS

    ✓7ᵗʰ **T36.8X2** **Poisoning by other systemic antibiotics, intentional self-harm**

    ✓7ᵗʰ **T36.8X3** **Poisoning by other systemic antibiotics, assault**

    ✓7ᵗʰ **T36.8X4** **Poisoning by other systemic antibiotics, undetermined**

    ✓7ᵗʰ **T36.8X5** **Adverse effect of other systemic antibiotics**

    ✓7ᵗʰ **T36.8X6** **Underdosing of other systemic antibiotics**

✓5ᵗʰ **T36.9** **Poisoning by, adverse effect of and underdosing of unspecified systemic antibiotic**

  ✓x7ᵗʰ **T36.91** **Poisoning by unspecified systemic antibiotic, accidental (unintentional)** ▽
    Poisoning by systemic antibiotic NOS

  ✓x7ᵗʰ **T36.92** **Poisoning by unspecified systemic antibiotic, intentional self-harm** ▽

  ✓x7ᵗʰ **T36.93** **Poisoning by unspecified systemic antibiotic, assault** ▽

  ✓x7ᵗʰ **T36.94** **Poisoning by unspecified systemic antibiotic, undetermined** ▽

  ✓x7ᵗʰ **T36.95** **Adverse effect of unspecified systemic antibiotic** ▽

  ✓x7ᵗʰ **T36.96** **Underdosing of unspecified systemic antibiotic** ▽

✓4ᵗʰ **T37** **Poisoning by, adverse effect of and underdosing of other systemic anti-infectives and antiparasitics**
  EXCLUDES 1 *anti-infectives topically used for ear, nose and throat (T49.6-)*
    anti-infectives topically used for eye (T49.5-)
    locally applied anti-infectives NEC (T49.0-)

> The appropriate 7th character is to be added to each code from category T37.
> A   initial encounter
> D   subsequent encounter
> S   sequela

✓5ᵗʰ **T37.0** **Poisoning by, adverse effect of and underdosing of sulfonamides**

  ✓6ᵗʰ **T37.0X** **Poisoning by, adverse effect of and underdosing of sulfonamides**

    ✓7ᵗʰ **T37.0X1** **Poisoning by sulfonamides, accidental (unintentional)**
      Poisoning by sulfonamides NOS

EXCLUDES 1 Not coded here   **EXCLUDES 2** Not included here   **N** Newborn Age : 0   **P** Pediatric Age : 0-17   **M** Maternity Age : 12-55   **A** Adult Age : 15-124

1028   ICD-10-CM 2017

✓7ᵗʰ **T37.0X2** **Poisoning by sulfonamides, intentional self-harm**

✓7ᵗʰ **T37.0X3** **Poisoning by sulfonamides, assault**

✓7ᵗʰ **T37.0X4** **Poisoning by sulfonamides, undetermined**

✓7ᵗʰ **T37.0X5** **Adverse effect of sulfonamides**

✓7ᵗʰ **T37.0X6** **Underdosing of sulfonamides**

✓5ᵗʰ **T37.1** **Poisoning by, adverse effect of and underdosing of antimycobacterial drugs**
> EXCLUDES 1 *rifampicins (T36.6-)*
> *streptomycin (T36.5-)*

  ✓6ᵗʰ **T37.1X** **Poisoning by, adverse effect of and underdosing of antimycobacterial drugs**

    ✓7ᵗʰ **T37.1X1** **Poisoning by antimycobacterial drugs, accidental (unintentional)**
> Poisoning by antimycobacterial drugs NOS

    ✓7ᵗʰ **T37.1X2** **Poisoning by antimycobacterial drugs, intentional self-harm**

    ✓7ᵗʰ **T37.1X3** **Poisoning by antimycobacterial drugs, assault**

    ✓7ᵗʰ **T37.1X4** **Poisoning by antimycobacterial drugs, undetermined**

    ✓7ᵗʰ **T37.1X5** **Adverse effect of antimycobacterial drugs**

    ✓7ᵗʰ **T37.1X6** **Underdosing of antimycobacterial drugs**

✓5ᵗʰ **T37.2** **Poisoning by, adverse effect of and underdosing of antimalarials and drugs acting on other blood protozoa**
> EXCLUDES 1 *hydroxyquinoline derivatives (T37.8-)*

  ✓6ᵗʰ **T37.2X** **Poisoning by, adverse effect of and underdosing of antimalarials and drugs acting on other blood protozoa**

    ✓7ᵗʰ **T37.2X1** **Poisoning by antimalarials and drugs acting on other blood protozoa, accidental (unintentional)**
> Poisoning by antimalarials and drugs acting on other blood protozoa NOS

    ✓7ᵗʰ **T37.2X2** **Poisoning by antimalarials and drugs acting on other blood protozoa, intentional self-harm**

    ✓7ᵗʰ **T37.2X3** **Poisoning by antimalarials and drugs acting on other blood protozoa, assault**

    ✓7ᵗʰ **T37.2X4** **Poisoning by antimalarials and drugs acting on other blood protozoa, undetermined**

    ✓7ᵗʰ **T37.2X5** **Adverse effect of antimalarials and drugs acting on other blood protozoa**

    ✓7ᵗʰ **T37.2X6** **Underdosing of antimalarials and drugs acting on other blood protozoa**

✓6ᵗʰ **T37.3** **Poisoning by, adverse effect of and underdosing of other antiprotozoal drugs**

  ✓6ᵗʰ **T37.3X** **Poisoning by, adverse effect of and underdosing of other antiprotozoal drugs**

    ✓7ᵗʰ **T37.3X1** **Poisoning by other antiprotozoal drugs, accidental (unintentional)**
> Poisoning by other antiprotozoal drugs NOS

    ✓7ᵗʰ **T37.3X2** **Poisoning by other antiprotozoal drugs, intentional self-harm**

    ✓7ᵗʰ **T37.3X3** **Poisoning by other antiprotozoal drugs, assault**

    ✓7ᵗʰ **T37.3X4** **Poisoning by other antiprotozoal drugs, undetermined**

    ✓7ᵗʰ **T37.3X5** **Adverse effect of other antiprotozoal drugs**

    ✓7ᵗʰ **T37.3X6** **Underdosing of other antiprotozoal drugs**

✓5ᵗʰ **T37.4** **Poisoning by, adverse effect of and underdosing of anthelminthics**

  ✓6ᵗʰ **T37.4X** **Poisoning by, adverse effect of and underdosing of anthelminthics**

    ✓7ᵗʰ **T37.4X1** **Poisoning by anthelminthics, accidental (unintentional)**
> Poisoning by anthelminthics NOS

    ✓7ᵗʰ **T37.4X2** **Poisoning by anthelminthics, intentional self-harm**

    ✓7ᵗʰ **T37.4X3** **Poisoning by anthelminthics, assault**

    ✓7ᵗʰ **T37.4X4** **Poisoning by anthelminthics, undetermined**

    ✓7ᵗʰ **T37.4X5** **Adverse effect of anthelminthics**

    ✓7ᵗʰ **T37.4X6** **Underdosing of anthelminthics**

✓5ᵗʰ **T37.5** **Poisoning by, adverse effect of and underdosing of antiviral drugs**
> EXCLUDES 1 *amantadine (T42.8-)*
> *cytarabine (T45.1-)*

  ✓6ᵗʰ **T37.5X** **Poisoning by, adverse effect of and underdosing of antiviral drugs**

    ✓7ᵗʰ **T37.5X1** **Poisoning by antiviral drugs, accidental (unintentional)**
> Poisoning by antiviral drugs NOS

    ✓7ᵗʰ **T37.5X2** **Poisoning by antiviral drugs, intentional self-harm**

    ✓7ᵗʰ **T37.5X3** **Poisoning by antiviral drugs, assault**

    ✓7ᵗʰ **T37.5X4** **Poisoning by antiviral drugs, undetermined**

    ✓7ᵗʰ **T37.5X5** **Adverse effect of antiviral drugs**

    ✓7ᵗʰ **T37.5X6** **Underdosing of antiviral drugs**

✓5ᵗʰ **T37.8** **Poisoning by, adverse effect of and underdosing of other specified systemic anti-infectives and antiparasitics**
> Poisoning by, adverse effect of and underdosing of hydroxyquinoline derivatives
> EXCLUDES 1 *antimalarial drugs (T37.2-)*

  ✓6ᵗʰ **T37.8X** **Poisoning by, adverse effect of and underdosing of other specified systemic anti-infectives and antiparasitics**

    ✓7ᵗʰ **T37.8X1** **Poisoning by other specified systemic anti-infectives and antiparasitics, accidental (unintentional)**
> Poisoning by other specified systemic anti-infectives and antiparasitics NOS

    ✓7ᵗʰ **T37.8X2** **Poisoning by other specified systemic anti-infectives and antiparasitics, intentional self-harm**

    ✓7ᵗʰ **T37.8X3** **Poisoning by other specified systemic anti-infectives and antiparasitics, assault**

    ✓7ᵗʰ **T37.8X4** **Poisoning by other specified systemic anti-infectives and antiparasitics, undetermined**

    ✓7ᵗʰ **T37.8X5** **Adverse effect of other specified systemic anti-infectives and antiparasitics**

    ✓7ᵗʰ **T37.8X6** **Underdosing of other specified systemic anti-infectives and antiparasitics**

✓5ᵗʰ **T37.9** **Poisoning by, adverse effect of and underdosing of unspecified systemic anti-infective and antiparasitics**

  ✓x7ᵗʰ **T37.91** **Poisoning by unspecified systemic anti-infective and antiparasitics, accidental (unintentional)** ▽
> Poisoning by, adverse effect of and underdosing of systemic anti-infective and antiparasitics NOS

  ✓x7ᵗʰ **T37.92** **Poisoning by unspecified systemic anti-infective and antiparasitics, intentional self-harm** ▽

  ✓x7ᵗʰ **T37.93** **Poisoning by unspecified systemic anti-infective and antiparasitics, assault** ▽

  ✓x7ᵗʰ **T37.94** **Poisoning by unspecified systemic anti-infective and antiparasitics, undetermined** ▽

  ✓x7ᵗʰ **T37.95** **Adverse effect of unspecified systemic anti-infective and antiparasitic** ▽

  ✓x7ᵗʰ **T37.96** **Underdosing of unspecified systemic anti-infectives and antiparasitics** ▽

✓4ᵗʰ **T38** **Poisoning by, adverse effect of and underdosing of hormones and their synthetic substitutes and antagonists, not elsewhere classified**
> EXCLUDES 1 *mineralocorticoids and their antagonists (T50.0-)*
> *oxytocic hormones (T48.0-)*
> *parathyroid hormones and derivatives (T50.9-)*

> The appropriate 7th character is to be added to each code from category T38.
> A   initial encounter
> D   subsequent encounter
> S   sequela

✓5ᵗʰ **T38.0** **Poisoning by, adverse effect of and underdosing of glucocorticoids and synthetic analogues**
> EXCLUDES 1 *glucocorticoids, topically used (T49.-)*

  ✓6ᵗʰ **T38.0X** **Poisoning by, adverse effect of and underdosing of glucocorticoids and synthetic analogues**

☑ Additional Character Required   ✓x7ᵗʰ Placeholder Alert   Manifestation Dx   ▽ Unspecified Dx   ▶◀ Revised Text   ● New Code   ▲ Revised Code Title

ICD-10-CM 2017   **1029**

Chapter 19. Injury, Poisoning and Certain Other Consequences of External Causes

T37.0X2–T38.0X

√7th **T38.0X1** **Poisoning by glucocorticoids and synthetic analogues, accidental (unintentional)**
Poisoning by glucocorticoids and synthetic analogues NOS

√7th **T38.0X2** **Poisoning by glucocorticoids and synthetic analogues, intentional self-harm**

√7th **T38.0X3** **Poisoning by glucocorticoids and synthetic analogues, assault**

√7th **T38.0X4** **Poisoning by glucocorticoids and synthetic analogues, undetermined**

√7th **T38.0X5** **Adverse effect of glucocorticoids and synthetic analogues**

√7th **T38.0X6** **Underdosing of glucocorticoids and synthetic analogues**

√5th **T38.1** **Poisoning by, adverse effect of and underdosing of thyroid hormones and substitutes**

√6th **T38.1X** **Poisoning by, adverse effect of and underdosing of thyroid hormones and substitutes**

√7th **T38.1X1** **Poisoning by thyroid hormones and substitutes, accidental (unintentional)**
Poisoning by thyroid hormones and substitutes NOS

√7th **T38.1X2** **Poisoning by thyroid hormones and substitutes, intentional self-harm**

√7th **T38.1X3** **Poisoning by thyroid hormones and substitutes, assault**

√7th **T38.1X4** **Poisoning by thyroid hormones and substitutes, undetermined**

√7th **T38.1X5** **Adverse effect of thyroid hormones and substitutes**

√7th **T38.1X6** **Underdosing of thyroid hormones and substitutes**

√5th **T38.2** **Poisoning by, adverse effect of and underdosing of antithyroid drugs**

√6th **T38.2X** **Poisoning by, adverse effect of and underdosing of antithyroid drugs**

√7th **T38.2X1** **Poisoning by antithyroid drugs, accidental (unintentional)**
Poisoning by antithyroid drugs NOS

√7th **T38.2X2** **Poisoning by antithyroid drugs, intentional self-harm**

√7th **T38.2X3** **Poisoning by antithyroid drugs, assault**

√7th **T38.2X4** **Poisoning by antithyroid drugs, undetermined**

√7th **T38.2X5** **Adverse effect of antithyroid drugs**

√7th **T38.2X6** **Underdosing of antithyroid drugs**

√5th **T38.3** **Poisoning by, adverse effect of and underdosing of insulin and oral hypoglycemic [antidiabetic] drugs**

√6th **T38.3X** **Poisoning by, adverse effect of and underdosing of insulin and oral hypoglycemic [antidiabetic] drugs**

√7th **T38.3X1** **Poisoning by insulin and oral hypoglycemic [antidiabetic] drugs, accidental (unintentional)**
Poisoning by insulin and oral hypoglycemic [antidiabetic] drugs NOS

√7th **T38.3X2** **Poisoning by insulin and oral hypoglycemic [antidiabetic] drugs, intentional self-harm**

√7th **T38.3X3** **Poisoning by insulin and oral hypoglycemic [antidiabetic] drugs, assault**

√7th **T38.3X4** **Poisoning by insulin and oral hypoglycemic [antidiabetic] drugs, undetermined**

√7th **T38.3X5** **Adverse effect of insulin and oral hypoglycemic [antidiabetic] drugs**

√7th **T38.3X6** **Underdosing of insulin and oral hypoglycemic [antidiabetic] drugs**

√5th **T38.4** **Poisoning by, adverse effect of and underdosing of oral contraceptives**
Poisoning by, adverse effect of and underdosing of multiple- and single-ingredient oral contraceptive preparations

√6th **T38.4X** **Poisoning by, adverse effect of and underdosing of oral contraceptives**

√7th **T38.4X1** **Poisoning by oral contraceptives, accidental (unintentional)**
Poisoning by oral contraceptives NOS

√7th **T38.4X2** **Poisoning by oral contraceptives, intentional self-harm**

√7th **T38.4X3** **Poisoning by oral contraceptives, assault**

√7th **T38.4X4** **Poisoning by oral contraceptives, undetermined**

√7th **T38.4X5** **Adverse effect of oral contraceptives**

√7th **T38.4X6** **Underdosing of oral contraceptives**

√5th **T38.5** **Poisoning by, adverse effect of and underdosing of other estrogens and progestogens**
Poisoning by, adverse effect of and underdosing of estrogens and progestogens mixtures and substitutes

√6th **T38.5X** **Poisoning by, adverse effect of and underdosing of other estrogens and progestogens**

√7th **T38.5X1** **Poisoning by other estrogens and progestogens, accidental (unintentional)**
Poisoning by other estrogens and progestogens NOS

√7th **T38.5X2** **Poisoning by other estrogens and progestogens, intentional self-harm**

√7th **T38.5X3** **Poisoning by other estrogens and progestogens, assault**

√7th **T38.5X4** **Poisoning by other estrogens and progestogens, undetermined**

√7th **T38.5X5** **Adverse effect of other estrogens and progestogens**

√7th **T38.5X6** **Underdosing of other estrogens and progestogens**

√5th **T38.6** **Poisoning by, adverse effect of and underdosing of antigonadotrophins, antiestrogens, antiandrogens, not elsewhere classified**
Poisoning by, adverse effect of and underdosing of tamoxifen

√6th **T38.6X** **Poisoning by, adverse effect of and underdosing of antigonadotrophins, antiestrogens, antiandrogens, not elsewhere classified**

√7th **T38.6X1** **Poisoning by antigonadotrophins, antiestrogens, antiandrogens, not elsewhere classified, accidental (unintentional)**
Poisoning by antigonadotrophins, antiestrogens, antiandrogens, not elsewhere classified NOS

√7th **T38.6X2** **Poisoning by antigonadotrophins, antiestrogens, antiandrogens, not elsewhere classified, intentional self-harm**

√7th **T38.6X3** **Poisoning by antigonadotrophins, antiestrogens, antiandrogens, not elsewhere classified, assault**

√7th **T38.6X4** **Poisoning by antigonadotrophins, antiestrogens, antiandrogens, not elsewhere classified, undetermined**

√7th **T38.6X5** **Adverse effect of antigonadotrophins, antiestrogens, antiandrogens, not elsewhere classified**

√7th **T38.6X6** **Underdosing of antigonadotrophins, antiestrogens, antiandrogens, not elsewhere classified**

√5th **T38.7** **Poisoning by, adverse effect of and underdosing of androgens and anabolic congeners**

√6th **T38.7X** **Poisoning by, adverse effect of and underdosing of androgens and anabolic congeners**

√7th **T38.7X1** **Poisoning by androgens and anabolic congeners, accidental (unintentional)**
Poisoning by androgens and anabolic congeners NOS

√7th **T38.7X2** **Poisoning by androgens and anabolic congeners, intentional self-harm**

√7th **T38.7X3** **Poisoning by androgens and anabolic congeners, assault**

√7th **T38.7X4** **Poisoning by androgens and anabolic congeners, undetermined**

√7th **T38.7X5** **Adverse effect of androgens and anabolic congeners**

√7th **T38.7X6** **Underdosing of androgens and anabolic congeners**

√5th **T38.8** **Poisoning by, adverse effect of and underdosing of other and unspecified hormones and synthetic substitutes**

√6th **T38.80** **Poisoning by, adverse effect of and underdosing of unspecified hormones and synthetic substitutes**

EXCLUDES 1 Not coded here   EXCLUDES 2 Not included here   N Newborn Age : 0   P Pediatric Age : 0-17   M Maternity Age : 12-55   A Adult Age : 15-124

1030

ICD-10-CM 2017

✓7ᵗʰ **T38.801 Poisoning by unspecified hormones and synthetic substitutes, accidental (unintentional)** ▽
Poisoning by unspecified hormones and synthetic substitutes NOS

✓7ᵗʰ **T38.802 Poisoning by unspecified hormones and synthetic substitutes, intentional self-harm** ▽

✓7ᵗʰ **T38.803 Poisoning by unspecified hormones and synthetic substitutes, assault** ▽

✓7ᵗʰ **T38.804 Poisoning by unspecified hormones and synthetic substitutes, undetermined** ▽

✓7ᵗʰ **T38.805 Adverse effect of unspecified hormones and synthetic substitutes** ▽

✓7ᵗʰ **T38.806 Underdosing of unspecified hormones and synthetic substitutes** ▽

✓6ᵗʰ **T38.81 Poisoning by, adverse effect of and underdosing of anterior pituitary [adenohypophyseal] hormones**

✓7ᵗʰ **T38.811 Poisoning by anterior pituitary [adenohypophyseal] hormones, accidental (unintentional)**
Poisoning by anterior pituitary [adenohypophyseal] hormones NOS

✓7ᵗʰ **T38.812 Poisoning by anterior pituitary [adenohypophyseal] hormones, intentional self-harm**

✓7ᵗʰ **T38.813 Poisoning by anterior pituitary [adenohypophyseal] hormones, assault**

✓7ᵗʰ **T38.814 Poisoning by anterior pituitary [adenohypophyseal] hormones, undetermined**

✓7ᵗʰ **T38.815 Adverse effect of anterior pituitary [adenohypophyseal] hormones**

✓7ᵗʰ **T38.816 Underdosing of anterior pituitary [adenohypophyseal] hormones**

✓6ᵗʰ **T38.89 Poisoning by, adverse effect of and underdosing of other hormones and synthetic substitutes**

✓7ᵗʰ **T38.891 Poisoning by other hormones and synthetic substitutes, accidental (unintentional)**
Poisoning by other hormones and synthetic substitutes NOS

✓7ᵗʰ **T38.892 Poisoning by other hormones and synthetic substitutes, intentional self-harm**

✓7ᵗʰ **T38.893 Poisoning by other hormones and synthetic substitutes, assault**

✓7ᵗʰ **T38.894 Poisoning by other hormones and synthetic substitutes, undetermined**

✓7ᵗʰ **T38.895 Adverse effect of other hormones and synthetic substitutes**

✓7ᵗʰ **T38.896 Underdosing of other hormones and synthetic substitutes**

✓5ᵗʰ **T38.9 Poisoning by, adverse effect of and underdosing of other and unspecified hormone antagonists**

✓6ᵗʰ **T38.90 Poisoning by, adverse effect of and underdosing of unspecified hormone antagonists**

✓7ᵗʰ **T38.901 Poisoning by unspecified hormone antagonists, accidental (unintentional)** ▽
Poisoning by unspecified hormone antagonists NOS

✓7ᵗʰ **T38.902 Poisoning by unspecified hormone antagonists, intentional self-harm** ▽

✓7ᵗʰ **T38.903 Poisoning by unspecified hormone antagonists, assault** ▽

✓7ᵗʰ **T38.904 Poisoning by unspecified hormone antagonists, undetermined** ▽

✓7ᵗʰ **T38.905 Adverse effect of unspecified hormone antagonists** ▽

✓7ᵗʰ **T38.906 Underdosing of unspecified hormone antagonists** ▽

✓6ᵗʰ **T38.99 Poisoning by, adverse effect of and underdosing of other hormone antagonists**

✓7ᵗʰ **T38.991 Poisoning by other hormone antagonists, accidental (unintentional)**
Poisoning by other hormone antagonists NOS

✓7ᵗʰ **T38.992 Poisoning by other hormone antagonists, intentional self-harm**

✓7ᵗʰ **T38.993 Poisoning by other hormone antagonists, assault**

✓7ᵗʰ **T38.994 Poisoning by other hormone antagonists, undetermined**

✓7ᵗʰ **T38.995 Adverse effect of other hormone antagonists**

✓7ᵗʰ **T38.996 Underdosing of other hormone antagonists**

✓4ᵗʰ **T39 Poisoning by, adverse effect of and underdosing of nonopioid analgesics, antipyretics and antirheumatics**

The appropriate 7th character is to be added to each code from category T39.
A   initial encounter
D   subsequent encounter
S   sequela

✓5ᵗʰ **T39.0 Poisoning by, adverse effect of and underdosing of salicylates**

✓6ᵗʰ **T39.01 Poisoning by, adverse effect of and underdosing of aspirin**
Poisoning by, adverse effect of and underdosing of acetylsalicylic acid

✓7ᵗʰ **T39.011 Poisoning by aspirin, accidental (unintentional)**

✓7ᵗʰ **T39.012 Poisoning by aspirin, intentional self-harm**

✓7ᵗʰ **T39.013 Poisoning by aspirin, assault**

✓7ᵗʰ **T39.014 Poisoning by aspirin, undetermined**

✓7ᵗʰ **T39.015 Adverse effect of aspirin**

     AHA: 2016,1Q,15

✓7ᵗʰ **T39.016 Underdosing of aspirin**

✓6ᵗʰ **T39.09 Poisoning by, adverse effect of and underdosing of other salicylates**

✓7ᵗʰ **T39.091 Poisoning by salicylates, accidental (unintentional)**
Poisoning by salicylates NOS

✓7ᵗʰ **T39.092 Poisoning by salicylates, intentional self-harm**

✓7ᵗʰ **T39.093 Poisoning by salicylates, assault**

✓7ᵗʰ **T39.094 Poisoning by salicylates, undetermined**

✓7ᵗʰ **T39.095 Adverse effect of salicylates**

✓7ᵗʰ **T39.096 Underdosing of salicylates**

✓5ᵗʰ **T39.1 Poisoning by, adverse effect of and underdosing of 4-Aminophenol derivatives**

✓6ᵗʰ **T39.1X Poisoning by, adverse effect of and underdosing of 4-Aminophenol derivatives**

✓7ᵗʰ **T39.1X1 Poisoning by 4-Aminophenol derivatives, accidental (unintentional)**
Poisoning by 4-Aminophenol derivatives NOS

✓7ᵗʰ **T39.1X2 Poisoning by 4-Aminophenol derivatives, intentional self-harm**

✓7ᵗʰ **T39.1X3 Poisoning by 4-Aminophenol derivatives, assault**

✓7ᵗʰ **T39.1X4 Poisoning by 4-Aminophenol derivatives, undetermined**

✓7ᵗʰ **T39.1X5 Adverse effect of 4-Aminophenol derivatives**

✓7ᵗʰ **T39.1X6 Underdosing of 4-Aminophenol derivatives**

✓5ᵗʰ **T39.2 Poisoning by, adverse effect of and underdosing of pyrazolone derivatives**

✓6ᵗʰ **T39.2X Poisoning by, adverse effect of and underdosing of pyrazolone derivatives**

✓7ᵗʰ **T39.2X1 Poisoning by pyrazolone derivatives, accidental (unintentional)**
Poisoning by pyrazolone derivatives NOS

✓7ᵗʰ **T39.2X2 Poisoning by pyrazolone derivatives, intentional self-harm**

✓7ᵗʰ **T39.2X3 Poisoning by pyrazolone derivatives, assault**

✓7ᵗʰ **T39.2X4 Poisoning by pyrazolone derivatives, undetermined**

✓7ᵗʰ **T39.2X5 Adverse effect of pyrazolone derivatives**

√7ᵗʰ **T39.2X6** Underdosing of pyrazolone derivatives

√5ᵗʰ **T39.3** **Poisoning by, adverse effect of and underdosing of other nonsteroidal anti-inflammatory drugs [NSAID]**

√6ᵗʰ **T39.31** **Poisoning by, adverse effect of and underdosing of propionic acid derivatives**

Poisoning by, adverse effect of and underdosing of fenoprofen

Poisoning by, adverse effect of and underdosing of flurbiprofen

Poisoning by, adverse effect of and underdosing of ibuprofen

Poisoning by, adverse effect of and underdosing of ketoprofen

Poisoning by, adverse effect of and underdosing of naproxen

Poisoning by, adverse effect of and underdosing of oxaprozin

√7ᵗʰ **T39.311** **Poisoning by propionic acid derivatives, accidental (unintentional)**

√7ᵗʰ **T39.312** **Poisoning by propionic acid derivatives, intentional self-harm**

√7ᵗʰ **T39.313** **Poisoning by propionic acid derivatives, assault**

√7ᵗʰ **T39.314** **Poisoning by propionic acid derivatives, undetermined**

√7ᵗʰ **T39.315** **Adverse effect of propionic acid derivatives**

√7ᵗʰ **T39.316** Underdosing of propionic acid derivatives

√6ᵗʰ **T39.39** **Poisoning by, adverse effect of and underdosing of other nonsteroidal anti-inflammatory drugs [NSAID]**

√7ᵗʰ **T39.391** **Poisoning by other nonsteroidal anti-inflammatory drugs [NSAID], accidental (unintentional)**

Poisoning by other nonsteroidal anti-inflammatory drugs NOS

√7ᵗʰ **T39.392** **Poisoning by other nonsteroidal anti-inflammatory drugs [NSAID], intentional self-harm**

√7ᵗʰ **T39.393** **Poisoning by other nonsteroidal anti-inflammatory drugs [NSAID], assault**

√7ᵗʰ **T39.394** **Poisoning by other nonsteroidal anti-inflammatory drugs [NSAID], undetermined**

√7ᵗʰ **T39.395** **Adverse effect of other nonsteroidal anti-inflammatory drugs [NSAID]**

√7ᵗʰ **T39.396** Underdosing of other nonsteroidal anti-inflammatory drugs [NSAID]

√5ᵗʰ **T39.4** **Poisoning by, adverse effect of and underdosing of antirheumatics, not elsewhere classified**

EXCLUDES 1 poisoning by, adverse effect of and underdosing of glucocorticoids (T38.0-)

poisoning by, adverse effect of and underdosing of salicylates (T39.0-)

√6ᵗʰ **T39.4X** **Poisoning by, adverse effect of and underdosing of antirheumatics, not elsewhere classified**

√7ᵗʰ **T39.4X1** **Poisoning by antirheumatics, not elsewhere classified, accidental (unintentional)**

Poisoning by antirheumatics, not elsewhere classified NOS

√7ᵗʰ **T39.4X2** **Poisoning by antirheumatics, not elsewhere classified, intentional self-harm**

√7ᵗʰ **T39.4X3** **Poisoning by antirheumatics, not elsewhere classified, assault**

√7ᵗʰ **T39.4X4** **Poisoning by antirheumatics, not elsewhere classified, undetermined**

√7ᵗʰ **T39.4X5** **Adverse effect of antirheumatics, not elsewhere classified**

√7ᵗʰ **T39.4X6** Underdosing of antirheumatics, not elsewhere classified

√5ᵗʰ **T39.8** **Poisoning by, adverse effect of and underdosing of other nonopioid analgesics and antipyretics, not elsewhere classified**

√6ᵗʰ **T39.8X** **Poisoning by, adverse effect of and underdosing of other nonopioid analgesics and antipyretics, not elsewhere classified**

√7ᵗʰ **T39.8X1** **Poisoning by other nonopioid analgesics and antipyretics, not elsewhere classified, accidental (unintentional)**

Poisoning by other nonopioid analgesics and antipyretics, not elsewhere classified NOS

√7ᵗʰ **T39.8X2** **Poisoning by other nonopioid analgesics and antipyretics, not elsewhere classified, intentional self-harm**

√7ᵗʰ **T39.8X3** **Poisoning by other nonopioid analgesics and antipyretics, not elsewhere classified, assault**

√7ᵗʰ **T39.8X4** **Poisoning by other nonopioid analgesics and antipyretics, not elsewhere classified, undetermined**

√7ᵗʰ **T39.8X5** **Adverse effect of other nonopioid analgesics and antipyretics, not elsewhere classified**

√7ᵗʰ **T39.8X6** Underdosing of other nonopioid analgesics and antipyretics, not elsewhere classified

√5ᵗʰ **T39.9** **Poisoning by, adverse effect of and underdosing of unspecified nonopioid analgesic, antipyretic and antirheumatic**

√x7ᵗʰ **T39.91** **Poisoning by unspecified nonopioid analgesic, antipyretic and antirheumatic, accidental (unintentional)** ▽

Poisoning by nonopioid analgesic, antipyretic and antirheumatic NOS

√x7ᵗʰ **T39.92** **Poisoning by unspecified nonopioid analgesic, antipyretic and antirheumatic, intentional self-harm** ▽

√x7ᵗʰ **T39.93** **Poisoning by unspecified nonopioid analgesic, antipyretic and antirheumatic, assault** ▽

√x7ᵗʰ **T39.94** **Poisoning by unspecified nonopioid analgesic, antipyretic and antirheumatic, undetermined** ▽

√x7ᵗʰ **T39.95** **Adverse effect of unspecified nonopioid analgesic, antipyretic and antirheumatic** ▽

√x7ᵗʰ **T39.96** Underdosing of unspecified nonopioid analgesic, antipyretic and antirheumatic ▽

√4ᵗʰ **T40** **Poisoning by, adverse effect of and underdosing of narcotics and psychodysleptics [hallucinogens]**

EXCLUDES 2 drug dependence and related mental and behavioral disorders due to psychoactive substance use (F10.-F19.-)

The appropriate 7th character is to be added to each code from category T40.
A   initial encounter
D   subsequent encounter
S   sequela

√5ᵗʰ **T40.0** **Poisoning by, adverse effect of and underdosing of opium**

√6ᵗʰ **T40.0X** **Poisoning by, adverse effect of and underdosing of opium**

√7ᵗʰ **T40.0X1** **Poisoning by opium, accidental (unintentional)**

Poisoning by opium NOS

√7ᵗʰ **T40.0X2** **Poisoning by opium, intentional self-harm**

√7ᵗʰ **T40.0X3** **Poisoning by opium, assault**

√7ᵗʰ **T40.0X4** **Poisoning by opium, undetermined**

√7ᵗʰ **T40.0X5** **Adverse effect of opium**

√7ᵗʰ **T40.0X6** Underdosing of opium

√5ᵗʰ **T40.1** **Poisoning by and adverse effect of heroin**

√6ᵗʰ **T40.1X** **Poisoning by and adverse effect of heroin**

√7ᵗʰ **T40.1X1** **Poisoning by heroin, accidental (unintentional)**

Poisoning by heroin NOS

√7ᵗʰ **T40.1X2** **Poisoning by heroin, intentional self-harm**

√7ᵗʰ **T40.1X3** **Poisoning by heroin, assault**

√7ᵗʰ **T40.1X4** **Poisoning by heroin, undetermined**

√5ᵗʰ **T40.2** **Poisoning by, adverse effect of and underdosing of other opioids**

√6ᵗʰ **T40.2X** **Poisoning by, adverse effect of and underdosing of other opioids**

√7ᵗʰ **T40.2X1** **Poisoning by other opioids, accidental (unintentional)**

Poisoning by other opioids NOS

EXCLUDES 1 Not coded here   EXCLUDES 2 Not included here   N Newborn Age : 0   P Pediatric Age : 0-17   M Maternity Age : 12-55   A Adult Age : 15-124

1032

ICD-10-CM 2017

√7ᵗʰ **T40.2X2 Poisoning by other opioids, intentional self-harm**

√7ᵗʰ **T40.2X3 Poisoning by other opioids, assault**

√7ᵗʰ **T40.2X4 Poisoning by other opioids, undetermined**

√7ᵗʰ **T40.2X5 Adverse effect of other opioids**

√7ᵗʰ **T40.2X6 Underdosing of other opioids**

√5ᵗʰ **T40.3 Poisoning by, adverse effect of and underdosing of methadone**

√6ᵗʰ **T40.3X Poisoning by, adverse effect of and underdosing of methadone**

√7ᵗʰ **T40.3X1 Poisoning by methadone, accidental (unintentional)**
Poisoning by methadone NOS

√7ᵗʰ **T40.3X2 Poisoning by methadone, intentional self-harm**

√7ᵗʰ **T40.3X3 Poisoning by methadone, assault**

√7ᵗʰ **T40.3X4 Poisoning by methadone, undetermined**

√7ᵗʰ **T40.3X5 Adverse effect of methadone**

√7ᵗʰ **T40.3X6 Underdosing of methadone**

√5ᵗʰ **T40.4 Poisoning by, adverse effect of and underdosing of other synthetic narcotics**

√6ᵗʰ **T40.4X Poisoning by, adverse effect of and underdosing of other synthetic narcotics**

√7ᵗʰ **T40.4X1 Poisoning by other synthetic narcotics, accidental (unintentional)**
Poisoning by other synthetic narcotics NOS

√7ᵗʰ **T40.4X2 Poisoning by other synthetic narcotics, intentional self-harm**

√7ᵗʰ **T40.4X3 Poisoning by other synthetic narcotics, assault**

√7ᵗʰ **T40.4X4 Poisoning by other synthetic narcotics, undetermined**

√7ᵗʰ **T40.4X5 Adverse effect of other synthetic narcotics**

√7ᵗʰ **T40.4X6 Underdosing of other synthetic narcotics**

√5ᵗʰ **T40.5 Poisoning by, adverse effect of and underdosing of cocaine**

√6ᵗʰ **T40.5X Poisoning by, adverse effect of and underdosing of cocaine**

√7ᵗʰ **T40.5X1 Poisoning by cocaine, accidental (unintentional)**
Poisoning by cocaine NOS
AHA: 2016,2Q,8

√7ᵗʰ **T40.5X2 Poisoning by cocaine, intentional self-harm**

√7ᵗʰ **T40.5X3 Poisoning by cocaine, assault**

√7ᵗʰ **T40.5X4 Poisoning by cocaine, undetermined**

√7ᵗʰ **T40.5X5 Adverse effect of cocaine**

√7ᵗʰ **T40.5X6 Underdosing of cocaine**

√5ᵗʰ **T40.6 Poisoning by, adverse effect of and underdosing of other and unspecified narcotics**

√6ᵗʰ **T40.60 Poisoning by, adverse effect of and underdosing of unspecified narcotics**

√7ᵗʰ **T40.601 Poisoning by unspecified narcotics, accidental (unintentional)** ▽
Poisoning by narcotics NOS

√7ᵗʰ **T40.602 Poisoning by unspecified narcotics, intentional self-harm** ▽

√7ᵗʰ **T40.603 Poisoning by unspecified narcotics, assault** ▽

√7ᵗʰ **T40.604 Poisoning by unspecified narcotics, undetermined** ▽

√7ᵗʰ **T40.605 Adverse effect of unspecified narcotics** ▽

√7ᵗʰ **T40.606 Underdosing of unspecified narcotics** ▽

√6ᵗʰ **T40.69 Poisoning by, adverse effect of and underdosing of other narcotics**

√7ᵗʰ **T40.691 Poisoning by other narcotics, accidental (unintentional)**
Poisoning by other narcotics NOS

√7ᵗʰ **T40.692 Poisoning by other narcotics, intentional self-harm**

√7ᵗʰ **T40.693 Poisoning by other narcotics, assault**

√7ᵗʰ **T40.694 Poisoning by other narcotics, undetermined**

√7ᵗʰ **T40.695 Adverse effect of other narcotics**

√7ᵗʰ **T40.696 Underdosing of other narcotics**

√5ᵗʰ **T40.7 Poisoning by, adverse effect of and underdosing of cannabis (derivatives)**

√6ᵗʰ **T40.7X Poisoning by, adverse effect of and underdosing of cannabis (derivatives)**

√7ᵗʰ **T40.7X1 Poisoning by cannabis (derivatives), accidental (unintentional)**
Poisoning by cannabis NOS

√7ᵗʰ **T40.7X2 Poisoning by cannabis (derivatives), intentional self-harm**

√7ᵗʰ **T40.7X3 Poisoning by cannabis (derivatives), assault**

√7ᵗʰ **T40.7X4 Poisoning by cannabis (derivatives), undetermined**

√7ᵗʰ **T40.7X5 Adverse effect of cannabis (derivatives)**

√7ᵗʰ **T40.7X6 Underdosing of cannabis (derivatives)**

√5ᵗʰ **T40.8 Poisoning by and adverse effect of lysergide [LSD]**

√6ᵗʰ **T40.8X Poisoning by and adverse effect of lysergide [LSD]**

√7ᵗʰ **T40.8X1 Poisoning by lysergide [LSD], accidental (unintentional)**
Poisoning by lysergide [LSD]NOS

√7ᵗʰ **T40.8X2 Poisoning by lysergide [LSD], intentional self-harm**

√7ᵗʰ **T40.8X3 Poisoning by lysergide [LSD], assault**

√7ᵗʰ **T40.8X4 Poisoning by lysergide [LSD], undetermined**

√5ᵗʰ **T40.9 Poisoning by, adverse effect of and underdosing of other and unspecified psychodysleptics [hallucinogens]**

√6ᵗʰ **T40.90 Poisoning by, adverse effect of and underdosing of unspecified psychodysleptics [hallucinogens]**

√7ᵗʰ **T40.901 Poisoning by unspecified psychodysleptics [hallucinogens], accidental (unintentional)** ▽

√7ᵗʰ **T40.902 Poisoning by unspecified psychodysleptics [hallucinogens], intentional self-harm** ▽

√7ᵗʰ **T40.903 Poisoning by unspecified psychodysleptics [hallucinogens], assault** ▽

√7ᵗʰ **T40.904 Poisoning by unspecified psychodysleptics [hallucinogens], undetermined** ▽

√7ᵗʰ **T40.905 Adverse effect of unspecified psychodysleptics [hallucinogens]** ▽

√7ᵗʰ **T40.906 Underdosing of unspecified psychodysleptics** ▽

√6ᵗʰ **T40.99 Poisoning by, adverse effect of and underdosing of other psychodysleptics [hallucinogens]**

√7ᵗʰ **T40.991 Poisoning by other psychodysleptics [hallucinogens], accidental (unintentional)**
Poisoning by other psychodysleptics [hallucinogens] NOS

√7ᵗʰ **T40.992 Poisoning by other psychodysleptics [hallucinogens], intentional self-harm**

√7ᵗʰ **T40.993 Poisoning by other psychodysleptics [hallucinogens], assault**

√7ᵗʰ **T40.994 Poisoning by other psychodysleptics [hallucinogens], undetermined**

√7ᵗʰ **T40.995 Adverse effect of other psychodysleptics [hallucinogens]**

√7ᵗʰ **T40.996 Underdosing of other psychodysleptics**

√4ᵗʰ **T41 Poisoning by, adverse effect of and underdosing of anesthetics and therapeutic gases**

EXCLUDES 1 *benzodiazepines (T42.4-)*
cocaine (T40.5-)
complications of anesthesia during labor and delivery (O74.-)
complications of anesthesia during pregnancy (O29.-)
complications of anesthesia during the puerperium (O89.-)
opioids (T40.0-T40.2-)

The appropriate 7th character is to be added to each code from category T41.
A   initial encounter
D   subsequent encounter
S   sequela

√5ᵗʰ **T41.0 Poisoning by, adverse effect of and underdosing of inhaled anesthetics**

EXCLUDES 1 *oxygen (T41.5-)*

√6ᵗʰ **T41.0X Poisoning by, adverse effect of and underdosing of inhaled anesthetics**

☑ Additional Character Required   √x7ᵗʰ Placeholder Alert   Manifestation Dx   ▽ Unspecified Dx   ▶◀ Revised Text   ● New Code   ▲ Revised Code Title

√7ᵗʰ **T41.0X1 Poisoning by inhaled anesthetics, accidental (unintentional)**
Poisoning by inhaled anesthetics NOS

√7ᵗʰ **T41.0X2 Poisoning by inhaled anesthetics, intentional self-harm**

√7ᵗʰ **T41.0X3 Poisoning by inhaled anesthetics, assault**

√7ᵗʰ **T41.0X4 Poisoning by inhaled anesthetics, undetermined**

√7ᵗʰ **T41.0X5 Adverse effect of inhaled anesthetics**

√7ᵗʰ **T41.0X6 Underdosing of inhaled anesthetics**

√5ᵗʰ **T41.1 Poisoning by, adverse effect of and underdosing of intravenous anesthetics**
Poisoning by, adverse effect of and underdosing of thiobarbiturates

√6ᵗʰ **T41.1X Poisoning by, adverse effect of and underdosing of intravenous anesthetics**

√7ᵗʰ **T41.1X1 Poisoning by intravenous anesthetics, accidental (unintentional)**
Poisoning by intravenous anesthetics NOS

√7ᵗʰ **T41.1X2 Poisoning by intravenous anesthetics, intentional self-harm**

√7ᵗʰ **T41.1X3 Poisoning by intravenous anesthetics, assault**

√7ᵗʰ **T41.1X4 Poisoning by intravenous anesthetics, undetermined**

√7ᵗʰ **T41.1X5 Adverse effect of intravenous anesthetics**

√7ᵗʰ **T41.1X6 Underdosing of intravenous anesthetics**

√5ᵗʰ **T41.2 Poisoning by, adverse effect of and underdosing of other and unspecified general anesthetics**

√6ᵗʰ **T41.20 Poisoning by, adverse effect of and underdosing of unspecified general anesthetics**

√7ᵗʰ **T41.201 Poisoning by unspecified general anesthetics, accidental (unintentional)** ▽
Poisoning by general anesthetics NOS

√7ᵗʰ **T41.202 Poisoning by unspecified general anesthetics, intentional self-harm** ▽

√7ᵗʰ **T41.203 Poisoning by unspecified general anesthetics, assault** ▽

√7ᵗʰ **T41.204 Poisoning by unspecified general anesthetics, undetermined** ▽

√7ᵗʰ **T41.205 Adverse effect of unspecified general anesthetics** ▽

√7ᵗʰ **T41.206 Underdosing of unspecified general anesthetics** ▽

√6ᵗʰ **T41.29 Poisoning by, adverse effect of and underdosing of other general anesthetics**

√7ᵗʰ **T41.291 Poisoning by other general anesthetics, accidental (unintentional)**
Poisoning by other general anesthetics NOS

√7ᵗʰ **T41.292 Poisoning by other general anesthetics, intentional self-harm**

√7ᵗʰ **T41.293 Poisoning by other general anesthetics, assault**

√7ᵗʰ **T41.294 Poisoning by other general anesthetics, undetermined**

√7ᵗʰ **T41.295 Adverse effect of other general anesthetics**

√7ᵗʰ **T41.296 Underdosing of other general anesthetics**

√5ᵗʰ **T41.3 Poisoning by, adverse effect of and underdosing of local anesthetics**
Cocaine (topical)

EXCLUDES 2 *poisoning by cocaine used as a central nervous system stimulant (T40.5X1-T40.5X4)*

√6ᵗʰ **T41.3X Poisoning by, adverse effect of and underdosing of local anesthetics**

√7ᵗʰ **T41.3X1 Poisoning by local anesthetics, accidental (unintentional)**
Poisoning by local anesthetics NOS

√7ᵗʰ **T41.3X2 Poisoning by local anesthetics, intentional self-harm**

√7ᵗʰ **T41.3X3 Poisoning by local anesthetics, assault**

√7ᵗʰ **T41.3X4 Poisoning by local anesthetics, undetermined**

√7ᵗʰ **T41.3X5 Adverse effect of local anesthetics**

√7ᵗʰ **T41.3X6 Underdosing of local anesthetics**

√5ᵗʰ **T41.4 Poisoning by, adverse effect of and underdosing of unspecified anesthetic**

√x7ᵗʰ **T41.41 Poisoning by unspecified anesthetic, accidental (unintentional)** ▽
Poisoning by anesthetic NOS

√x7ᵗʰ **T41.42 Poisoning by unspecified anesthetic, intentional self-harm** ▽

√x7ᵗʰ **T41.43 Poisoning by unspecified anesthetic, assault** ▽

√x7ᵗʰ **T41.44 Poisoning by unspecified anesthetic, undetermined** ▽

√x7ᵗʰ **T41.45 Adverse effect of unspecified anesthetic** ▽

√x7ᵗʰ **T41.46 Underdosing of unspecified anesthetics** ▽

√5ᵗʰ **T41.5 Poisoning by, adverse effect of and underdosing of therapeutic gases**

√6ᵗʰ **T41.5X Poisoning by, adverse effect of and underdosing of therapeutic gases**

√7ᵗʰ **T41.5X1 Poisoning by therapeutic gases, accidental (unintentional)**
Poisoning by therapeutic gases NOS

√7ᵗʰ **T41.5X2 Poisoning by therapeutic gases, intentional self-harm**

√7ᵗʰ **T41.5X3 Poisoning by therapeutic gases, assault**

√7ᵗʰ **T41.5X4 Poisoning by therapeutic gases, undetermined**

√7ᵗʰ **T41.5X5 Adverse effect of therapeutic gases**

√7ᵗʰ **T41.5X6 Underdosing of therapeutic gases**

√4ᵗʰ **T42 Poisoning by, adverse effect of and underdosing of antiepileptic, sedative- hypnotic and antiparkinsonism drugs**

EXCLUDES 2 *drug dependence and related mental and behavioral disorders due to psychoactive substance use (F10.- — F19.-)*

The appropriate 7th character is to be added to each code from category T42.
A initial encounter
D subsequent encounter
S sequela

√5ᵗʰ **T42.0 Poisoning by, adverse effect of and underdosing of hydantoin derivatives**

√6ᵗʰ **T42.0X Poisoning by, adverse effect of and underdosing of hydantoin derivatives**

√7ᵗʰ **T42.0X1 Poisoning by hydantoin derivatives, accidental (unintentional)**
Poisoning by hydantoin derivatives NOS

√7ᵗʰ **T42.0X2 Poisoning by hydantoin derivatives, intentional self-harm**

√7ᵗʰ **T42.0X3 Poisoning by hydantoin derivatives, assault**

√7ᵗʰ **T42.0X4 Poisoning by hydantoin derivatives, undetermined**

√7ᵗʰ **T42.0X5 Adverse effect of hydantoin derivatives**

√7ᵗʰ **T42.0X6 Underdosing of hydantoin derivatives**

√5ᵗʰ **T42.1 Poisoning by, adverse effect of and underdosing of iminostilbenes**
Poisoning by, adverse effect of and underdosing of carbamazepine

√6ᵗʰ **T42.1X Poisoning by, adverse effect of and underdosing of iminostilbenes**

√7ᵗʰ **T42.1X1 Poisoning by iminostilbenes, accidental (unintentional)**
Poisoning by iminostilbenes NOS

√7ᵗʰ **T42.1X2 Poisoning by iminostilbenes, intentional self-harm**

√7ᵗʰ **T42.1X3 Poisoning by iminostilbenes, assault**

√7ᵗʰ **T42.1X4 Poisoning by iminostilbenes, undetermined**

√7ᵗʰ **T42.1X5 Adverse effect of iminostilbenes**

√7ᵗʰ **T42.1X6 Underdosing of iminostilbenes**

√5ᵗʰ **T42.2 Poisoning by, adverse effect of and underdosing of succinimides and oxazolidinediones**

√6ᵗʰ **T42.2X Poisoning by, adverse effect of and underdosing of succinimides and oxazolidinediones**

√7ᵗʰ **T42.2X1 Poisoning by succinimides and oxazolidinediones, accidental (unintentional)**
Poisoning by succinimides and oxazolidinediones NOS

√7ᵗʰ **T42.2X2 Poisoning by succinimides and oxazolidinediones, intentional self-harm**

√7ᵗʰ **T42.2X3 Poisoning by succinimides and oxazolidinediones, assault**

√7ᵗʰ **T42.2X4 Poisoning by succinimides and oxazolidinediones, undetermined**

EXCLUDES 1 Not coded here   EXCLUDES 2 Not included here   N Newborn Age : 0   P Pediatric Age : 0-17   M Maternity Age : 12-55   A Adult Age : 15-124

1034   ICD-10-CM 2017

✓7ᵗʰ **T42.2X5** Adverse effect of succinimides and oxazolidinediones

✓7ᵗʰ **T42.2X6** Underdosing of succinimides and oxazolidinediones

✓5ᵗʰ **T42.3** Poisoning by, adverse effect of and underdosing of barbiturates

> **EXCLUDES 1** *poisoning by, adverse effect of and underdosing of thiobarbiturates (T41.1-)*

    ✓6ᵗʰ **T42.3X** Poisoning by, adverse effect of and underdosing of barbiturates

        ✓7ᵗʰ **T42.3X1** Poisoning by barbiturates, accidental (unintentional)

               Poisoning by barbiturates NOS

        ✓7ᵗʰ **T42.3X2** Poisoning by barbiturates, intentional self-harm

        ✓7ᵗʰ **T42.3X3** Poisoning by barbiturates, assault

        ✓7ᵗʰ **T42.3X4** Poisoning by barbiturates, undetermined

        ✓7ᵗʰ **T42.3X5** Adverse effect of barbiturates

        ✓7ᵗʰ **T42.3X6** Underdosing of barbiturates

✓5ᵗʰ **T42.4** Poisoning by, adverse effect of and underdosing of benzodiazepines

    ✓6ᵗʰ **T42.4X** Poisoning by, adverse effect of and underdosing of benzodiazepines

        ✓7ᵗʰ **T42.4X1** Poisoning by benzodiazepines, accidental (unintentional)

               Poisoning by benzodiazepines NOS

        ✓7ᵗʰ **T42.4X2** Poisoning by benzodiazepines, intentional self-harm

        ✓7ᵗʰ **T42.4X3** Poisoning by benzodiazepines, assault

        ✓7ᵗʰ **T42.4X4** Poisoning by benzodiazepines, undetermined

        ✓7ᵗʰ **T42.4X5** Adverse effect of benzodiazepines

        ✓7ᵗʰ **T42.4X6** Underdosing of benzodiazepines

✓5ᵗʰ **T42.5** Poisoning by, adverse effect of and underdosing of mixed antiepileptics

    ✓6ᵗʰ **T42.5X** Poisoning by, adverse effect of and underdosing of antiepileptics

        ✓7ᵗʰ **T42.5X1** Poisoning by mixed antiepileptics, accidental (unintentional)

               Poisoning by mixed antiepileptics NOS

        ✓7ᵗʰ **T42.5X2** Poisoning by mixed antiepileptics, intentional self-harm

        ✓7ᵗʰ **T42.5X3** Poisoning by mixed antiepileptics, assault

        ✓7ᵗʰ **T42.5X4** Poisoning by mixed antiepileptics, undetermined

        ✓7ᵗʰ **T42.5X5** Adverse effect of mixed antiepileptics

        ✓7ᵗʰ **T42.5X6** Underdosing of mixed antiepileptics

✓5ᵗʰ **T42.6** Poisoning by, adverse effect of and underdosing of other antiepileptic and sedative-hypnotic drugs

> Poisoning by, adverse effect of and underdosing of methaqualone
>
> Poisoning by, adverse effect of and underdosing of valproic acid
>
> **EXCLUDES 1** *poisoning by, adverse effect of and underdosing of carbamazepine (T42.1-)*

    ✓6ᵗʰ **T42.6X** Poisoning by, adverse effect of and underdosing of other antiepileptic and sedative-hypnotic drugs

        ✓7ᵗʰ **T42.6X1** Poisoning by other antiepileptic and sedative-hypnotic drugs, accidental (unintentional)

               Poisoning by other antiepileptic and sedative-hypnotic drugs NOS

        ✓7ᵗʰ **T42.6X2** Poisoning by other antiepileptic and sedative-hypnotic drugs, intentional self-harm

        ✓7ᵗʰ **T42.6X3** Poisoning by other antiepileptic and sedative-hypnotic drugs, assault

        ✓7ᵗʰ **T42.6X4** Poisoning by other antiepileptic and sedative-hypnotic drugs, undetermined

        ✓7ᵗʰ **T42.6X5** Adverse effect of other antiepileptic and sedative-hypnotic drugs

        ✓7ᵗʰ **T42.6X6** Underdosing of other antiepileptic and sedative-hypnotic drugs

✓5ᵗʰ **T42.7** Poisoning by, adverse effect of and underdosing of unspecified antiepileptic and sedative-hypnotic drugs

✓×7ᵗʰ **T42.71** Poisoning by unspecified antiepileptic and sedative-hypnotic drugs, accidental (unintentional) ▽

> Poisoning by antiepileptic and sedative-hypnotic drugs NOS

✓×7ᵗʰ **T42.72** Poisoning by unspecified antiepileptic and sedative-hypnotic drugs, intentional self-harm ▽

✓×7ᵗʰ **T42.73** Poisoning by unspecified antiepileptic and sedative-hypnotic drugs, assault ▽

✓×7ᵗʰ **T42.74** Poisoning by unspecified antiepileptic and sedative-hypnotic drugs, undetermined ▽

✓×7ᵗʰ **T42.75** Adverse effect of unspecified antiepileptic and sedative-hypnotic drugs ▽

✓×7ᵗʰ **T42.76** Underdosing of unspecified antiepileptic and sedative-hypnotic drugs ▽

✓5ᵗʰ **T42.8** Poisoning by, adverse effect of and underdosing of antiparkinsonism drugs and other central muscle-tone depressants

> Poisoning by, adverse effect of and underdosing of amantadine

    ✓6ᵗʰ **T42.8X** Poisoning by, adverse effect of and underdosing of antiparkinsonism drugs and other central muscle-tone depressants

        ✓7ᵗʰ **T42.8X1** Poisoning by antiparkinsonism drugs and other central muscle-tone depressants, accidental (unintentional)

               Poisoning by antiparkinsonism drugs and other central muscle-tone depressants NOS

        ✓7ᵗʰ **T42.8X2** Poisoning by antiparkinsonism drugs and other central muscle-tone depressants, intentional self-harm

        ✓7ᵗʰ **T42.8X3** Poisoning by antiparkinsonism drugs and other central muscle-tone depressants, assault

        ✓7ᵗʰ **T42.8X4** Poisoning by antiparkinsonism drugs and other central muscle-tone depressants, undetermined

        ✓7ᵗʰ **T42.8X5** Adverse effect of antiparkinsonism drugs and other central muscle-tone depressants

        ✓7ᵗʰ **T42.8X6** Underdosing of antiparkinsonism drugs and other central muscle-tone depressants

✓4ᵗʰ **T43** Poisoning by, adverse effect of and underdosing of psychotropic drugs, not elsewhere classified

> **EXCLUDES 1** *appetite depressants (T50.5-)*
> *barbiturates (T42.3-)*
> *benzodiazepines (T42.4-)*
> *methaqualone (T42.6-)*
> *psychodysleptics [hallucinogens] (T40.7-T40.9-)*
>
> **EXCLUDES 2** *drug dependence and related mental and behavioral disorders due to psychoactive substance use (F10.- — F19.-)*

The appropriate 7th character is to be added to each code from category T43.

A   initial encounter
D   subsequent encounter
S   sequela

✓5ᵗʰ **T43.0** Poisoning by, adverse effect of and underdosing of tricyclic and tetracyclic antidepressants

    ✓6ᵗʰ **T43.01** Poisoning by, adverse effect of and underdosing of tricyclic antidepressants

        ✓7ᵗʰ **T43.011** Poisoning by tricyclic antidepressants, accidental (unintentional)

               Poisoning by tricyclic antidepressants NOS

        ✓7ᵗʰ **T43.012** Poisoning by tricyclic antidepressants, intentional self-harm

        ✓7ᵗʰ **T43.013** Poisoning by tricyclic antidepressants, assault

        ✓7ᵗʰ **T43.014** Poisoning by tricyclic antidepressants, undetermined

        ✓7ᵗʰ **T43.015** Adverse effect of tricyclic antidepressants

        ✓7ᵗʰ **T43.016** Underdosing of tricyclic antidepressants

    ✓6ᵗʰ **T43.02** Poisoning by, adverse effect of and underdosing of tetracyclic antidepressants

        ✓7ᵗʰ **T43.021** Poisoning by tetracyclic antidepressants, accidental (unintentional)

               Poisoning by tetracyclic antidepressants NOS

        ✓7ᵗʰ **T43.022** Poisoning by tetracyclic antidepressants, intentional self-harm

☑ Additional Character Required   ✓×7ᵗʰ Placeholder Alert   Manifestation Dx   ▽ Unspecified Dx   ▶◀ Revised Text   ● New Code   ▲ Revised Code Title

ICD-10-CM 2017   1035

√7ᵗʰ **T43.023** Poisoning by tetracyclic antidepressants, **assault**

√7ᵗʰ **T43.024** Poisoning by tetracyclic antidepressants, **undetermined**

√7ᵗʰ **T43.025** Adverse effect of tetracyclic antidepressants

√7ᵗʰ **T43.026** Underdosing of tetracyclic antidepressants

√5ᵗʰ **T43.1** Poisoning by, adverse effect of and underdosing of monoamine-oxidase-inhibitor antidepressants

√6ᵗʰ **T43.1X** Poisoning by, adverse effect of and underdosing of monoamine-oxidase-inhibitor antidepressants

√7ᵗʰ **T43.1X1** Poisoning by monoamine-oxidase-inhibitor antidepressants, **accidental (unintentional)**

Poisoning by monoamine-oxidase-inhibitor antidepressants NOS

√7ᵗʰ **T43.1X2** Poisoning by monoamine-oxidase-inhibitor antidepressants, **intentional self-harm**

√7ᵗʰ **T43.1X3** Poisoning by monoamine-oxidase-inhibitor antidepressants, **assault**

√7ᵗʰ **T43.1X4** Poisoning by monoamine-oxidase-inhibitor antidepressants, **undetermined**

√7ᵗʰ **T43.1X5** Adverse effect of monoamine-oxidase-inhibitor antidepressants

√7ᵗʰ **T43.1X6** Underdosing of monoamine-oxidase-inhibitor antidepressants

√5ᵗʰ **T43.2** Poisoning by, adverse effect of and underdosing of other and unspecified antidepressants

√6ᵗʰ **T43.20** Poisoning by, adverse effect of and underdosing of unspecified antidepressants

√7ᵗʰ **T43.201** Poisoning by unspecified antidepressants, **accidental (unintentional)** ▽

Poisoning by antidepressants NOS

√7ᵗʰ **T43.202** Poisoning by unspecified antidepressants, **intentional self-harm** ▽

√7ᵗʰ **T43.203** Poisoning by unspecified antidepressants, **assault** ▽

√7ᵗʰ **T43.204** Poisoning by unspecified antidepressants, **undetermined** ▽

√7ᵗʰ **T43.205** Adverse effect of unspecified antidepressants ▽

√7ᵗʰ **T43.206** Underdosing of unspecified antidepressants ▽

√6ᵗʰ **T43.21** Poisoning by, adverse effect of and underdosing of selective serotonin and norepinephrine reuptake inhibitors

Poisoning by, adverse effect of and underdosing of SSNRI antidepressants

√7ᵗʰ **T43.211** Poisoning by selective serotonin and norepinephrine reuptake inhibitors, **accidental (unintentional)**

√7ᵗʰ **T43.212** Poisoning by selective serotonin and norepinephrine reuptake inhibitors, **intentional self-harm**

√7ᵗʰ **T43.213** Poisoning by selective serotonin and norepinephrine reuptake inhibitors, **assault**

√7ᵗʰ **T43.214** Poisoning by selective serotonin and norepinephrine reuptake inhibitors, **undetermined**

√7ᵗʰ **T43.215** Adverse effect of selective serotonin and norepinephrine reuptake inhibitors

√7ᵗʰ **T43.216** Underdosing of selective serotonin and norepinephrine reuptake inhibitors

√6ᵗʰ **T43.22** Poisoning by, adverse effect of and underdosing of selective serotonin reuptake inhibitors

Poisoning by, adverse effect of and underdosing of SSRI antidepressants

√7ᵗʰ **T43.221** Poisoning by selective serotonin reuptake inhibitors, **accidental (unintentional)**

√7ᵗʰ **T43.222** Poisoning by selective serotonin reuptake inhibitors, **intentional self-harm**

√7ᵗʰ **T43.223** Poisoning by selective serotonin reuptake inhibitors, **assault**

√7ᵗʰ **T43.224** Poisoning by selective serotonin reuptake inhibitors, **undetermined**

√7ᵗʰ **T43.225** Adverse effect of selective serotonin reuptake inhibitors

√7ᵗʰ **T43.226** Underdosing of selective serotonin reuptake inhibitors

√6ᵗʰ **T43.29** Poisoning by, adverse effect of and underdosing of other antidepressants

√7ᵗʰ **T43.291** Poisoning by other antidepressants, **accidental (unintentional)**

Poisoning by other antidepressants NOS

√7ᵗʰ **T43.292** Poisoning by other antidepressants, **intentional self-harm**

√7ᵗʰ **T43.293** Poisoning by other antidepressants, **assault**

√7ᵗʰ **T43.294** Poisoning by other antidepressants, **undetermined**

√7ᵗʰ **T43.295** Adverse effect of other antidepressants

√7ᵗʰ **T43.296** Underdosing of other antidepressants

√5ᵗʰ **T43.3** Poisoning by, adverse effect of and underdosing of phenothiazine antipsychotics and neuroleptics

√6ᵗʰ **T43.3X** Poisoning by, adverse effect of and underdosing of phenothiazine antipsychotics and neuroleptics

√7ᵗʰ **T43.3X1** Poisoning by phenothiazine antipsychotics and neuroleptics, **accidental (unintentional)**

Poisoning by phenothiazine antipsychotics and neuroleptics NOS

√7ᵗʰ **T43.3X2** Poisoning by phenothiazine antipsychotics and neuroleptics, **intentional self-harm**

√7ᵗʰ **T43.3X3** Poisoning by phenothiazine antipsychotics and neuroleptics, **assault**

√7ᵗʰ **T43.3X4** Poisoning by phenothiazine antipsychotics and neuroleptics, **undetermined**

√7ᵗʰ **T43.3X5** Adverse effect of phenothiazine antipsychotics and neuroleptics

√7ᵗʰ **T43.3X6** Underdosing of phenothiazine antipsychotics and neuroleptics

√5ᵗʰ **T43.4** Poisoning by, adverse effect of and underdosing of butyrophenone and thiothixene neuroleptics

√6ᵗʰ **T43.4X** Poisoning by, adverse effect of and underdosing of butyrophenone and thiothixene neuroleptics

√7ᵗʰ **T43.4X1** Poisoning by butyrophenone and thiothixene neuroleptics, **accidental (unintentional)**

Poisoning by butyrophenone and thiothixene neuroleptics NOS

√7ᵗʰ **T43.4X2** Poisoning by butyrophenone and thiothixene neuroleptics, **intentional self-harm**

√7ᵗʰ **T43.4X3** Poisoning by butyrophenone and thiothixene neuroleptics, **assault**

√7ᵗʰ **T43.4X4** Poisoning by butyrophenone and thiothixene neuroleptics, **undetermined**

√7ᵗʰ **T43.4X5** Adverse effect of butyrophenone and thiothixene neuroleptics

√7ᵗʰ **T43.4X6** Underdosing of butyrophenone and thiothixene neuroleptics

√5ᵗʰ **T43.5** Poisoning by, adverse effect of and underdosing of other and unspecified antipsychotics and neuroleptics

EXCLUDES 1 *poisoning by, adverse effect of and underdosing of rauwolfia (T46.5-)*

√6ᵗʰ **T43.50** Poisoning by, adverse effect of and underdosing of unspecified antipsychotics and neuroleptics

√7ᵗʰ **T43.501** Poisoning by unspecified antipsychotics and neuroleptics, **accidental (unintentional)** ▽

Poisoning by antipsychotics and neuroleptics NOS

√7ᵗʰ **T43.502** Poisoning by unspecified antipsychotics and neuroleptics, **intentional self-harm** ▽

√7ᵗʰ **T43.503** Poisoning by unspecified antipsychotics and neuroleptics, **assault** ▽

√7ᵗʰ **T43.504** Poisoning by unspecified antipsychotics and neuroleptics, **undetermined** ▽

√7ᵗʰ **T43.505** Adverse effect of unspecified antipsychotics and neuroleptics ▽

EXCLUDES 1 Not coded here   **EXCLUDES 2** Not included here   **N** Newborn Age : 0   **P** Pediatric Age : 0-17   **M** Maternity Age : 12-55   **A** Adult Age : 15-124

√7ᵗʰ **T43.506** Underdosing of unspecified antipsychotics and neuroleptics ▽

√6ᵗʰ **T43.59** **Poisoning by, adverse effect of and underdosing of** other antipsychotics and neuroleptics

    √7ᵗʰ **T43.591** **Poisoning by other antipsychotics and neuroleptics, accidental (unintentional)**
       Poisoning by other antipsychotics and neuroleptics NOS

    √7ᵗʰ **T43.592** **Poisoning by other antipsychotics and neuroleptics,** intentional self-harm

    √7ᵗʰ **T43.593** **Poisoning by other antipsychotics and neuroleptics,** assault

    √7ᵗʰ **T43.594** **Poisoning by other antipsychotics and neuroleptics,** undetermined

    √7ᵗʰ **T43.595** Adverse effect of other antipsychotics and neuroleptics

    √7ᵗʰ **T43.596** Underdosing of other antipsychotics and neuroleptics

√5ᵗʰ **T43.6** **Poisoning by, adverse effect of and underdosing of psychostimulants**
    EXCLUDES 1 *poisoning by, adverse effect of and underdosing of cocaine (T40.5-)*

    √6ᵗʰ **T43.60** **Poisoning by, adverse effect of and underdosing of** unspecified psychostimulant

       √7ᵗʰ **T43.601** **Poisoning by unspecified psychostimulants, accidental (unintentional)** ▽
          Poisoning by psychostimulants NOS

       √7ᵗʰ **T43.602** **Poisoning by unspecified psychostimulants, intentional self-harm** ▽

       √7ᵗʰ **T43.603** **Poisoning by unspecified psychostimulants, assault** ▽

       √7ᵗʰ **T43.604** **Poisoning by unspecified psychostimulants, undetermined** ▽

       √7ᵗʰ **T43.605** Adverse effect of unspecified psychostimulants ▽

       √7ᵗʰ **T43.606** Underdosing of unspecified psychostimulants ▽

    √6ᵗʰ **T43.61** **Poisoning by, adverse effect of and underdosing of** caffeine

       √7ᵗʰ **T43.611** **Poisoning by caffeine, accidental (unintentional)**
          Poisoning by caffeine NOS

       √7ᵗʰ **T43.612** **Poisoning by caffeine, intentional self-harm**

       √7ᵗʰ **T43.613** **Poisoning by caffeine, assault**

       √7ᵗʰ **T43.614** **Poisoning by caffeine, undetermined**

       √7ᵗʰ **T43.615** Adverse effect of caffeine

       √7ᵗʰ **T43.616** Underdosing of caffeine

    √6ᵗʰ **T43.62** **Poisoning by, adverse effect of and underdosing of** amphetamines
       Poisoning by, adverse effect of and underdosing of methamphetamines

       √7ᵗʰ **T43.621** **Poisoning by amphetamines, accidental (unintentional)**
          Poisoning by amphetamines NOS

       √7ᵗʰ **T43.622** **Poisoning by amphetamines, intentional self-harm**

       √7ᵗʰ **T43.623** **Poisoning by amphetamines, assault**

       √7ᵗʰ **T43.624** **Poisoning by amphetamines, undetermined**

       √7ᵗʰ **T43.625** Adverse effect of amphetamines

       √7ᵗʰ **T43.626** Underdosing of amphetamines

    √6ᵗʰ **T43.63** **Poisoning by, adverse effect of and underdosing of** methylphenidate

       √7ᵗʰ **T43.631** **Poisoning by methylphenidate, accidental (unintentional)**
          Poisoning by methylphenidate NOS

       √7ᵗʰ **T43.632** **Poisoning by methylphenidate, intentional self-harm**

       √7ᵗʰ **T43.633** **Poisoning by methylphenidate, assault**

       √7ᵗʰ **T43.634** **Poisoning by methylphenidate, undetermined**

       √7ᵗʰ **T43.635** Adverse effect of methylphenidate

       √7ᵗʰ **T43.636** Underdosing of methylphenidate

√6ᵗʰ **T43.69** **Poisoning by, adverse effect of and underdosing of** other psychostimulants

    √7ᵗʰ **T43.691** **Poisoning by other psychostimulants, accidental (unintentional)**
       Poisoning by other psychostimulants NOS

    √7ᵗʰ **T43.692** **Poisoning by other psychostimulants, intentional self-harm**

    √7ᵗʰ **T43.693** **Poisoning by other psychostimulants, assault**

    √7ᵗʰ **T43.694** **Poisoning by other psychostimulants, undetermined**

    √7ᵗʰ **T43.695** Adverse effect of other psychostimulants

    √7ᵗʰ **T43.696** Underdosing of other psychostimulants

√5ᵗʰ **T43.8** **Poisoning by, adverse effect of and underdosing of other psychotropic drugs**

    √6ᵗʰ **T43.8X** **Poisoning by, adverse effect of and underdosing of** other psychotropic drugs

       √7ᵗʰ **T43.8X1** **Poisoning by other psychotropic drugs, accidental (unintentional)**
          Poisoning by other psychotropic drugs NOS

       √7ᵗʰ **T43.8X2** **Poisoning by other psychotropic drugs, intentional self-harm**

       √7ᵗʰ **T43.8X3** **Poisoning by other psychotropic drugs, assault**

       √7ᵗʰ **T43.8X4** **Poisoning by other psychotropic drugs, undetermined**

       √7ᵗʰ **T43.8X5** Adverse effect of other psychotropic drugs

       √7ᵗʰ **T43.8X6** Underdosing of other psychotropic drugs

√5ᵗʰ **T43.9** **Poisoning by, adverse effect of and underdosing of unspecified psychotropic drug**

    √x7ᵗʰ **T43.91** **Poisoning by unspecified psychotropic drug, accidental (unintentional)** ▽
       Poisoning by psychotropic drug NOS

    √x7ᵗʰ **T43.92** **Poisoning by unspecified psychotropic drug, intentional self-harm** ▽

    √x7ᵗʰ **T43.93** **Poisoning by unspecified psychotropic drug, assault** ▽

    √x7ᵗʰ **T43.94** **Poisoning by unspecified psychotropic drug, undetermined** ▽

    √x7ᵗʰ **T43.95** Adverse effect of unspecified psychotropic drug ▽

    √x7ᵗʰ **T43.96** Underdosing of unspecified psychotropic drug ▽

√4ᵗʰ **T44** **Poisoning by, adverse effect of and underdosing of drugs primarily affecting the autonomic nervous system**

> The appropriate 7th character is to be added to each code from category T44.
> A   initial encounter
> D   subsequent encounter
> S   sequela

    √5ᵗʰ **T44.0** **Poisoning by, adverse effect of and underdosing of anticholinesterase agents**

       √6ᵗʰ **T44.0X** **Poisoning by, adverse effect of and underdosing of** anticholinesterase agents

          √7ᵗʰ **T44.0X1** **Poisoning by anticholinesterase agents, accidental (unintentional)**
             Poisoning by anticholinesterase agents NOS

          √7ᵗʰ **T44.0X2** **Poisoning by anticholinesterase agents, intentional self-harm**

          √7ᵗʰ **T44.0X3** **Poisoning by anticholinesterase agents, assault**

          √7ᵗʰ **T44.0X4** **Poisoning by anticholinesterase agents, undetermined**

          √7ᵗʰ **T44.0X5** Adverse effect of anticholinesterase agents

          √7ᵗʰ **T44.0X6** Underdosing of anticholinesterase agents

    √5ᵗʰ **T44.1** **Poisoning by, adverse effect of and underdosing of other parasympathomimetics [cholinergics]**

       √6ᵗʰ **T44.1X** **Poisoning by, adverse effect of and underdosing of** other parasympathomimetics [cholinergics]

          √7ᵗʰ **T44.1X1** **Poisoning by other parasympathomimetics [cholinergics], accidental (unintentional)**
             Poisoning by other parasympathomimetics [cholinergics] NOS

          √7ᵗʰ **T44.1X2** **Poisoning by other parasympathomimetics [cholinergics], intentional self-harm**

☑ Additional Character Required   √x7ᵗʰ Placeholder Alert   Manifestation Dx   ▽ Unspecified Dx   ►◄ Revised Text   ● New Code   ▲ Revised Code Title

√7th **T44.1X3** **Poisoning by other parasympathomimetics [cholinergics], assault**

√7th **T44.1X4** **Poisoning by other parasympathomimetics [cholinergics], undetermined**

√7th **T44.1X5** **Adverse effect of other parasympathomimetics [cholinergics]**

√7th **T44.1X6** **Underdosing of other parasympathomimetics**

√5th **T44.2** **Poisoning by, adverse effect of and underdosing of ganglionic blocking drugs**

√6th **T44.2X** **Poisoning by, adverse effect of and underdosing of ganglionic blocking drugs**

√7th **T44.2X1** **Poisoning by ganglionic blocking drugs, accidental (unintentional)**
Poisoning by ganglionic blocking drugs NOS

√7th **T44.2X2** **Poisoning by ganglionic blocking drugs, intentional self-harm**

√7th **T44.2X3** **Poisoning by ganglionic blocking drugs, assault**

√7th **T44.2X4** **Poisoning by ganglionic blocking drugs, undetermined**

√7th **T44.2X5** **Adverse effect of ganglionic blocking drugs**

√7th **T44.2X6** **Underdosing of ganglionic blocking drugs**

√5th **T44.3** **Poisoning by, adverse effect of and underdosing of other parasympatholytics [anticholinergics and antimuscarinics] and spasmolytics**
Poisoning by, adverse effect of and underdosing of papaverine

√6th **T44.3X** **Poisoning by, adverse effect of and underdosing of other parasympatholytics [anticholinergics and antimuscarinics] and spasmolytics**

√7th **T44.3X1** **Poisoning by other parasympatholytics [anticholinergics and antimuscarinics] and spasmolytics, accidental (unintentional)**
Poisoning by other parasympatholytics [anticholinergics and antimuscarinics] and spasmolytics NOS

√7th **T44.3X2** **Poisoning by other parasympatholytics [anticholinergics and antimuscarinics] and spasmolytics, intentional self-harm**

√7th **T44.3X3** **Poisoning by other parasympatholytics [anticholinergics and antimuscarinics] and spasmolytics, assault**

√7th **T44.3X4** **Poisoning by other parasympatholytics [anticholinergics and antimuscarinics] and spasmolytics, undetermined**

√7th **T44.3X5** **Adverse effect of other parasympatholytics [anticholinergics and antimuscarinics] and spasmolytics**

√7th **T44.3X6** **Underdosing of other parasympatholytics [anticholinergics and antimuscarinics] and spasmolytics**

√5th **T44.4** **Poisoning by, adverse effect of and underdosing of predominantly alpha-adrenoreceptor agonists**
Poisoning by, adverse effect of and underdosing of metaraminol

√6th **T44.4X** **Poisoning by, adverse effect of and underdosing of predominantly alpha-adrenoreceptor agonists**

√7th **T44.4X1** **Poisoning by predominantly alpha-adrenoreceptor agonists, accidental (unintentional)**
Poisoning by predominantly alpha-adrenoreceptor agonists NOS

√7th **T44.4X2** **Poisoning by predominantly alpha-adrenoreceptor agonists, intentional self-harm**

√7th **T44.4X3** **Poisoning by predominantly alpha-adrenoreceptor agonists, assault**

√7th **T44.4X4** **Poisoning by predominantly alpha-adrenoreceptor agonists, undetermined**

√7th **T44.4X5** **Adverse effect of predominantly alpha-adrenoreceptor agonists**

√7th **T44.4X6** **Underdosing of predominantly alpha-adrenoreceptor agonists**

√5th **T44.5** **Poisoning by, adverse effect of and underdosing of predominantly beta-adrenoreceptor agonists**
EXCLUDES 1 *poisoning by, adverse effect of and underdosing of beta-adrenoreceptor agonists used in asthma therapy (T48.6-)*

√6th **T44.5X** **Poisoning by, adverse effect of and underdosing of predominantly beta-adrenoreceptor agonists**

√7th **T44.5X1** **Poisoning by predominantly beta-adrenoreceptor agonists, accidental (unintentional)**
Poisoning by predominantly beta-adrenoreceptor agonists NOS

√7th **T44.5X2** **Poisoning by predominantly beta-adrenoreceptor agonists, intentional self-harm**

√7th **T44.5X3** **Poisoning by predominantly beta-adrenoreceptor agonists, assault**

√7th **T44.5X4** **Poisoning by predominantly beta-adrenoreceptor agonists, undetermined**

√7th **T44.5X5** **Adverse effect of predominantly beta-adrenoreceptor agonists**

√7th **T44.5X6** **Underdosing of predominantly beta-adrenoreceptor agonists**

√5th **T44.6** **Poisoning by, adverse effect of and underdosing of alpha-adrenoreceptor antagonists**
EXCLUDES 1 *poisoning by, adverse effect of and underdosing of ergot alkaloids (T48.0)*

√6th **T44.6X** **Poisoning by, adverse effect of and underdosing of alpha-adrenoreceptor antagonists**

√7th **T44.6X1** **Poisoning by alpha-adrenoreceptor antagonists, accidental (unintentional)**
Poisoning by alpha-adrenoreceptor antagonists NOS

√7th **T44.6X2** **Poisoning by alpha-adrenoreceptor antagonists, intentional self-harm**

√7th **T44.6X3** **Poisoning by alpha-adrenoreceptor antagonists, assault**

√7th **T44.6X4** **Poisoning by alpha-adrenoreceptor antagonists, undetermined**

√7th **T44.6X5** **Adverse effect of alpha-adrenoreceptor antagonists**

√7th **T44.6X6** **Underdosing of alpha-adrenoreceptor antagonists**

√5th **T44.7** **Poisoning by, adverse effect of and underdosing of beta-adrenoreceptor antagonists**

√6th **T44.7X** **Poisoning by, adverse effect of and underdosing of beta-adrenoreceptor antagonists**

√7th **T44.7X1** **Poisoning by beta-adrenoreceptor antagonists, accidental (unintentional)**
Poisoning by beta-adrenoreceptor antagonists NOS

√7th **T44.7X2** **Poisoning by beta-adrenoreceptor antagonists, intentional self-harm**

√7th **T44.7X3** **Poisoning by beta-adrenoreceptor antagonists, assault**

√7th **T44.7X4** **Poisoning by beta-adrenoreceptor antagonists, undetermined**

√7th **T44.7X5** **Adverse effect of beta-adrenoreceptor antagonists**

√7th **T44.7X6** **Underdosing of beta-adrenoreceptor antagonists**

√5th **T44.8** **Poisoning by, adverse effect of and underdosing of centrally-acting and adrenergic-neuron- blocking agents**
EXCLUDES 1 *poisoning by, adverse effect of and underdosing of clonidine (T46.5)*
poisoning by, adverse effect of and underdosing of guanethidine (T46.5)

√6th **T44.8X** **Poisoning by, adverse effect of and underdosing of centrally-acting and adrenergic- neuron-blocking agents**

√7th **T44.8X1** **Poisoning by centrally-acting and adrenergic-neuron-blocking agents, accidental (unintentional)**
Poisoning by centrally-acting and adrenergic-neuron-blocking agents NOS

√7th **T44.8X2** **Poisoning by centrally-acting and adrenergic-neuron-blocking agents, intentional self-harm**

√7th **T44.8X3** **Poisoning by centrally-acting and adrenergic-neuron-blocking agents, assault**

EXCLUDES 1 Not coded here   EXCLUDES 2 Not included here   N Newborn Age : 0   P Pediatric Age : 0-17   M Maternity Age : 12-55   A Adult Age : 15-124

1038
ICD-10-CM 2017

☑7ᵗʰ **T44.8X4** **Poisoning by centrally-acting and adrenergic-neuron-blocking agents, undetermined**

☑7ᵗʰ **T44.8X5** **Adverse effect** of centrally-acting and adrenergic-neuron-blocking agents

☑7ᵗʰ **T44.8X6** **Underdosing** of centrally-acting and adrenergic-neuron-blocking agents

☑5ᵗʰ **T44.9** **Poisoning by, adverse effect of and underdosing of other and unspecified drugs primarily affecting the autonomic nervous system**

Poisoning by, adverse effect of and underdosing of drug stimulating both alpha and beta-adrenoreceptors

☑6ᵗʰ **T44.90** **Poisoning by, adverse effect of and underdosing of** unspecified drugs primarily affecting the autonomic nervous system

☑7ᵗʰ **T44.901** **Poisoning by unspecified drugs primarily affecting the autonomic nervous system, accidental (unintentional)** ▽

Poisoning by unspecified drugs primarily affecting the autonomic nervous system NOS

☑7ᵗʰ **T44.902** **Poisoning by unspecified drugs primarily affecting the autonomic nervous system, intentional self-harm** ▽

☑7ᵗʰ **T44.903** **Poisoning by unspecified drugs primarily affecting the autonomic nervous system, assault** ▽

☑7ᵗʰ **T44.904** **Poisoning by unspecified drugs primarily affecting the autonomic nervous system, undetermined** ▽

☑7ᵗʰ **T44.905** **Adverse effect** of unspecified drugs primarily affecting the autonomic nervous system ▽

☑7ᵗʰ **T44.906** **Underdosing** of unspecified drugs primarily affecting the autonomic nervous system ▽

☑6ᵗʰ **T44.99** **Poisoning by, adverse effect of and underdosing of** other drugs primarily affecting the autonomic nervous system

☑7ᵗʰ **T44.991** **Poisoning by other drug primarily affecting the autonomic nervous system, accidental (unintentional)**

Poisoning by other drugs primarily affecting the autonomic nervous system NOS

☑7ᵗʰ **T44.992** **Poisoning by other drug primarily affecting the autonomic nervous system, intentional self-harm**

☑7ᵗʰ **T44.993** **Poisoning by other drug primarily affecting the autonomic nervous system, assault**

☑7ᵗʰ **T44.994** **Poisoning by other drug primarily affecting the autonomic nervous system, undetermined**

☑7ᵗʰ **T44.995** **Adverse effect** of other drug primarily affecting the autonomic nervous system

☑7ᵗʰ **T44.996** **Underdosing** of other drug primarily affecting the autonomic nervous system

☑4ᵗʰ **T45** **Poisoning by, adverse effect of and underdosing of primarily systemic and hematological agents, not elsewhere classified**

The appropriate 7th character is to be added to each code from category T45.
A   initial encounter
D   subsequent encounter
S   sequela

☑5ᵗʰ **T45.0** **Poisoning by, adverse effect of and underdosing of antiallergic and antiemetic drugs**

EXCLUDES 1   *poisoning by, adverse effect of and underdosing of phenothiazine-based neuroleptics (T43.3)*

☑6ᵗʰ **T45.0X** **Poisoning by, adverse effect of and underdosing of** antiallergic and antiemetic drugs

☑7ᵗʰ **T45.0X1** **Poisoning by antiallergic and antiemetic drugs, accidental (unintentional)**

Poisoning by antiallergic and antiemetic drugs NOS

☑7ᵗʰ **T45.0X2** **Poisoning by antiallergic and antiemetic drugs, intentional self-harm**

☑7ᵗʰ **T45.0X3** **Poisoning by antiallergic and antiemetic drugs, assault**

☑7ᵗʰ **T45.0X4** **Poisoning by antiallergic and antiemetic drugs, undetermined**

☑7ᵗʰ **T45.0X5** **Adverse effect** of antiallergic and antiemetic drugs

☑7ᵗʰ **T45.0X6** **Underdosing** of antiallergic and antiemetic drugs

☑5ᵗʰ **T45.1** **Poisoning by, adverse effect of and underdosing of antineoplastic and immunosuppressive drugs**

EXCLUDES 1   *poisoning by, adverse effect of and underdosing of tamoxifen (T38.6)*

AHA: 2014,4Q,22

☑6ᵗʰ **T45.1X** **Poisoning by, adverse effect of and underdosing of antineoplastic and immunosuppressive drugs**

☑7ᵗʰ **T45.1X1** **Poisoning by antineoplastic and immunosuppressive drugs, accidental (unintentional)**

Poisoning by antineoplastic and immunosuppressive drugs NOS

☑7ᵗʰ **T45.1X2** **Poisoning by antineoplastic and immunosuppressive drugs, intentional self-harm**

☑7ᵗʰ **T45.1X3** **Poisoning by antineoplastic and immunosuppressive drugs, assault**

☑7ᵗʰ **T45.1X4** **Poisoning by antineoplastic and immunosuppressive drugs, undetermined**

☑7ᵗʰ **T45.1X5** **Adverse effect** of antineoplastic and immunosuppressive drugs

☑7ᵗʰ **T45.1X6** **Underdosing** of antineoplastic and immunosuppressive drugs

☑5ᵗʰ **T45.2** **Poisoning by, adverse effect of and underdosing of vitamins**

EXCLUDES 2   *poisoning by, adverse effect of and underdosing of iron (T45.4)*

poisoning by, adverse effect of and underdosing of nicotinic acid (derivatives) (T46.7)

poisoning by, adverse effect of and underdosing of vitamin K (T45.7)

☑6ᵗʰ **T45.2X** **Poisoning by, adverse effect of and underdosing of vitamins**

☑7ᵗʰ **T45.2X1** **Poisoning by vitamins, accidental (unintentional)**

Poisoning by vitamins NOS

☑7ᵗʰ **T45.2X2** **Poisoning by vitamins, intentional self-harm**

☑7ᵗʰ **T45.2X3** **Poisoning by vitamins, assault**

☑7ᵗʰ **T45.2X4** **Poisoning by vitamins, undetermined**

☑7ᵗʰ **T45.2X5** **Adverse effect** of vitamins

☑7ᵗʰ **T45.2X6** **Underdosing** of vitamins

EXCLUDES 1   *vitamin deficiencies (E50-E56)*

☑5ᵗʰ **T45.3** **Poisoning by, adverse effect of and underdosing of enzymes**

☑6ᵗʰ **T45.3X** **Poisoning by, adverse effect of and underdosing of enzymes**

☑7ᵗʰ **T45.3X1** **Poisoning by enzymes, accidental (unintentional)**

Poisoning by enzymes NOS

☑7ᵗʰ **T45.3X2** **Poisoning by enzymes, intentional self-harm**

☑7ᵗʰ **T45.3X3** **Poisoning by enzymes, assault**

☑7ᵗʰ **T45.3X4** **Poisoning by enzymes, undetermined**

☑7ᵗʰ **T45.3X5** **Adverse effect** of enzymes

☑7ᵗʰ **T45.3X6** **Underdosing** of enzymes

☑5ᵗʰ **T45.4** **Poisoning by, adverse effect of and underdosing of iron and its compounds**

☑6ᵗʰ **T45.4X** **Poisoning by, adverse effect of and underdosing of iron and its compounds**

☑7ᵗʰ **T45.4X1** **Poisoning by iron and its compounds, accidental (unintentional)**

Poisoning by iron and its compounds NOS

☑7ᵗʰ **T45.4X2** **Poisoning by iron and its compounds, intentional self-harm**

☑7ᵗʰ **T45.4X3** **Poisoning by iron and its compounds, assault**

☑7ᵗʰ **T45.4X4** **Poisoning by iron and its compounds, undetermined**

☑7ᵗʰ **T45.4X5** **Adverse effect** of iron and its compounds

☑7ᵗʰ **T45.4X6** **Underdosing** of iron and its compounds

EXCLUDES 1   *iron deficiency (E61.1)*

☑5ᵗʰ **T45.5** **Poisoning by, adverse effect of and underdosing of anticoagulants and antithrombotic drugs**

☑6ᵗʰ **T45.51** **Poisoning by, adverse effect of and underdosing of anticoagulants**

☑ Additional Character Required   ☑×7ᵗʰ Placeholder Alert   Manifestation Dx   ▽ Unspecified Dx   ►◄ Revised Text   ● New Code   ▲ Revised Code Title

ICD-10-CM 2017   1039

√7th **T45.511 Poisoning by anticoagulants, accidental (unintentional)**

Poisoning by anticoagulants NOS

√7th **T45.512 Poisoning by anticoagulants, intentional self-harm**

√7th **T45.513 Poisoning by anticoagulants, assault**

√7th **T45.514 Poisoning by anticoagulants, undetermined**

√7th **T45.515 Adverse effect of anticoagulants**

AHA: 2016,1Q,14; 2013,2Q,34

√7th **T45.516 Underdosing of anticoagulants**

√6th **T45.52 Poisoning by, adverse effect of and underdosing of antithrombotic drugs**

Poisoning by, adverse effect of and underdosing of antiplatelet drugs

EXCLUDES 2 *poisoning by, adverse effect of and underdosing of aspirin (T39.Ø1-)*

poisoning by, adverse effect of and underdosing of acetylsalicylic acid (T39.Ø1-)

√7th **T45.521 Poisoning by antithrombotic drugs, accidental (unintentional)**

Poisoning by antithrombotic drug NOS

√7th **T45.522 Poisoning by antithrombotic drugs, intentional self-harm**

√7th **T45.523 Poisoning by antithrombotic drugs, assault**

√7th **T45.524 Poisoning by antithrombotic drugs, undetermined**

√7th **T45.525 Adverse effect of antithrombotic drugs**

AHA: 2016,1Q,15

√7th **T45.526 Underdosing of antithrombotic drugs**

√5th **T45.6 Poisoning by, adverse effect of and underdosing of fibrinolysis-affecting drugs**

√6th **T45.6Ø Poisoning by, adverse effect of and underdosing of unspecified fibrinolysis-affecting drugs**

√7th **T45.6Ø1 Poisoning by unspecified fibrinolysis-affecting drugs, accidental (unintentional)** ▽

Poisoning by fibrinolysis-affecting drug NOS

√7th **T45.6Ø2 Poisoning by unspecified fibrinolysis-affecting drugs, intentional self-harm** ▽

√7th **T45.6Ø3 Poisoning by unspecified fibrinolysis-affecting drugs, assault** ▽

√7th **T45.6Ø4 Poisoning by unspecified fibrinolysis-affecting drugs, undetermined** ▽

√7th **T45.6Ø5 Adverse effect of unspecified fibrinolysis-affecting drugs** ▽

√7th **T45.6Ø6 Underdosing of unspecified fibrinolysis-affecting drugs** ▽

√6th **T45.61 Poisoning by, adverse effect of and underdosing of thrombolytic drugs**

√7th **T45.611 Poisoning by thrombolytic drug, accidental (unintentional)**

Poisoning by thrombolytic drug NOS

√7th **T45.612 Poisoning by thrombolytic drug, intentional self-harm**

√7th **T45.613 Poisoning by thrombolytic drug, assault**

√7th **T45.614 Poisoning by thrombolytic drug, undetermined**

√7th **T45.615 Adverse effect of thrombolytic drugs**

√7th **T45.616 Underdosing of thrombolytic drugs**

√6th **T45.62 Poisoning by, adverse effect of and underdosing of hemostatic drugs**

√7th **T45.621 Poisoning by hemostatic drug, accidental (unintentional)**

Poisoning by hemostatic drug NOS

√7th **T45.622 Poisoning by hemostatic drug, intentional self-harm**

√7th **T45.623 Poisoning by hemostatic drug, assault**

√7th **T45.624 Poisoning by hemostatic drug, undetermined**

√7th **T45.625 Adverse effect of hemostatic drug**

√7th **T45.626 Underdosing of hemostatic drugs**

√6th **T45.69 Poisoning by, adverse effect of and underdosing of other fibrinolysis-affecting drugs**

√7th **T45.691 Poisoning by other fibrinolysis-affecting drugs, accidental (unintentional)**

Poisoning by other fibrinolysis-affecting drug NOS

√7th **T45.692 Poisoning by other fibrinolysis-affecting drugs, intentional self-harm**

√7th **T45.693 Poisoning by other fibrinolysis-affecting drugs, assault**

√7th **T45.694 Poisoning by other fibrinolysis-affecting drugs, undetermined**

√7th **T45.695 Adverse effect of other fibrinolysis-affecting drugs**

√7th **T45.696 Underdosing of other fibrinolysis-affecting drugs**

√5th **T45.7 Poisoning by, adverse effect of and underdosing of anticoagulant antagonists, vitamin K and other coagulants**

√6th **T45.7X Poisoning by, adverse effect of and underdosing of anticoagulant antagonists, vitamin K and other coagulants**

√7th **T45.7X1 Poisoning by anticoagulant antagonists, vitamin K and other coagulants, accidental (unintentional)**

Poisoning by anticoagulant antagonists, vitamin K and other coagulants NOS

√7th **T45.7X2 Poisoning by anticoagulant antagonists, vitamin K and other coagulants, intentional self-harm**

√7th **T45.7X3 Poisoning by anticoagulant antagonists, vitamin K and other coagulants, assault**

√7th **T45.7X4 Poisoning by anticoagulant antagonists, vitamin K and other coagulants, undetermined**

√7th **T45.7X5 Adverse effect of anticoagulant antagonists, vitamin K and other coagulants**

√7th **T45.7X6 Underdosing of anticoagulant antagonist, vitamin K and other coagulants**

EXCLUDES 1 *vitamin K deficiency (E56.1)*

√5th **T45.8 Poisoning by, adverse effect of and underdosing of other primarily systemic and hematological agents**

Poisoning by, adverse effect of and underdosing of liver preparations and other antianemic agents

Poisoning by, adverse effect of and underdosing of natural blood and blood products

Poisoning by, adverse effect of and underdosing of plasma substitute

EXCLUDES 2 *poisoning by, adverse effect of and underdosing of immunoglobulin (T5Ø.Z1)*

poisoning by, adverse effect of and underdosing of iron (T45.4)

transfusion reactions (T8Ø.-)

√6th **T45.8X Poisoning by, adverse effect of and underdosing of other primarily systemic and hematological agents**

√7th **T45.8X1 Poisoning by other primarily systemic and hematological agents, accidental (unintentional)**

Poisoning by other primarily systemic and hematological agents NOS

√7th **T45.8X2 Poisoning by other primarily systemic and hematological agents, intentional self-harm**

√7th **T45.8X3 Poisoning by other primarily systemic and hematological agents, assault**

√7th **T45.8X4 Poisoning by other primarily systemic and hematological agents, undetermined**

√7th **T45.8X5 Adverse effect of other primarily systemic and hematological agents**

√7th **T45.8X6 Underdosing of other primarily systemic and hematological agents**

√5th **T45.9 Poisoning by, adverse effect of and underdosing of unspecified primarily systemic and hematological agent**

√x7th **T45.91 Poisoning by unspecified primarily systemic and hematological agent, accidental (unintentional)** ▽

Poisoning by primarily systemic and hematological agent NOS

√x7th **T45.92 Poisoning by unspecified primarily systemic and hematological agent, intentional self-harm** ▽

√x7th **T45.93 Poisoning by unspecified primarily systemic and hematological agent, assault** ▽

EXCLUDES 1 Not coded here   EXCLUDES 2 Not included here   N Newborn Age : 0   P Pediatric Age : 0-17   M Maternity Age : 12-55   A Adult Age : 15-124

1Ø4Ø

ICD-10-CM 2017

√x7ᵗʰ **T45.94** **Poisoning by unspecified primarily systemic and hematological agent,** undetermined ▽

√x7ᵗʰ **T45.95** Adverse effect of unspecified primarily systemic and hematological agent ▽

√x7ᵗʰ **T45.96** Underdosing of unspecified primarily systemic and hematological agent ▽

√4ᵗʰ **T46** **Poisoning by, adverse effect of and underdosing of agents primarily affecting the cardiovascular system**

> EXCLUDES 1   *poisoning by, adverse effect of and underdosing of metaraminol (T44.4)*

> The appropriate 7th character is to be added to each code from category T46.
> A   initial encounter
> D   subsequent encounter
> S   sequela

√5ᵗʰ **T46.Ø** **Poisoning by, adverse effect of and underdosing of cardiac-stimulant glycosides and drugs of similar action**

√6ᵗʰ **T46.ØX** **Poisoning by, adverse effect of and underdosing of cardiac-stimulant glycosides and drugs of similar action**

√7ᵗʰ **T46.ØX1** **Poisoning by cardiac-stimulant glycosides and drugs of similar action,** accidental (unintentional)
Poisoning by cardiac-stimulant glycosides and drugs of similar action NOS

√7ᵗʰ **T46.ØX2** **Poisoning by cardiac-stimulant glycosides and drugs of similar action,** intentional self-harm

√7ᵗʰ **T46.ØX3** **Poisoning by cardiac-stimulant glycosides and drugs of similar action,** assault

√7ᵗʰ **T46.ØX4** **Poisoning by cardiac-stimulant glycosides and drugs of similar action,** undetermined

√7ᵗʰ **T46.ØX5** Adverse effect of cardiac-stimulant glycosides and drugs of similar action

√7ᵗʰ **T46.ØX6** Underdosing of cardiac-stimulant glycosides and drugs of similar action

√5ᵗʰ **T46.1** **Poisoning by, adverse effect of and underdosing of calcium-channel blockers**

√6ᵗʰ **T46.1X** **Poisoning by, adverse effect of and underdosing of calcium-channel blockers**

√7ᵗʰ **T46.1X1** **Poisoning by calcium-channel blockers,** accidental (unintentional)
Poisoning by calcium-channel blockers NOS

√7ᵗʰ **T46.1X2** **Poisoning by calcium-channel blockers,** intentional self-harm

√7ᵗʰ **T46.1X3** **Poisoning by calcium-channel blockers,** assault

√7ᵗʰ **T46.1X4** **Poisoning by calcium-channel blockers,** undetermined

√7ᵗʰ **T46.1X5** Adverse effect of calcium-channel blockers

√7ᵗʰ **T46.1X6** Underdosing of calcium-channel blockers

√5ᵗʰ **T46.2** **Poisoning by, adverse effect of and underdosing of other antidysrhythmic drugs, not elsewhere classified**

> EXCLUDES 1   *poisoning by, adverse effect of and underdosing of beta-adrenoreceptor antagonists (T44.7-)*

√6ᵗʰ **T46.2X** **Poisoning by, adverse effect of and underdosing of other antidysrhythmic drugs**

√7ᵗʰ **T46.2X1** **Poisoning by other antidysrhythmic drugs,** accidental (unintentional)
Poisoning by other antidysrhythmic drugs NOS

√7ᵗʰ **T46.2X2** **Poisoning by other antidysrhythmic drugs,** intentional self-harm

√7ᵗʰ **T46.2X3** **Poisoning by other antidysrhythmic drugs,** assault

√7ᵗʰ **T46.2X4** **Poisoning by other antidysrhythmic drugs,** undetermined

√7ᵗʰ **T46.2X5** Adverse effect of other antidysrhythmic drugs

√7ᵗʰ **T46.2X6** Underdosing of other antidysrhythmic drugs

√5ᵗʰ **T46.3** **Poisoning by, adverse effect of and underdosing of coronary vasodilators**
Poisoning by, adverse effect of and underdosing of dipyridamole

> EXCLUDES 1   *poisoning by, adverse effect of and underdosing of calcium-channel blockers (T46.1)*

√6ᵗʰ **T46.3X** **Poisoning by, adverse effect of and underdosing of coronary vasodilators**

√7ᵗʰ **T46.3X1** **Poisoning by coronary vasodilators,** accidental (unintentional)
Poisoning by coronary vasodilators NOS

√7ᵗʰ **T46.3X2** **Poisoning by coronary vasodilators,** intentional self-harm

√7ᵗʰ **T46.3X3** **Poisoning by coronary vasodilators,** assault

√7ᵗʰ **T46.3X4** **Poisoning by coronary vasodilators,** undetermined

√7ᵗʰ **T46.3X5** Adverse effect of coronary vasodilators

√7ᵗʰ **T46.3X6** Underdosing of coronary vasodilators

√5ᵗʰ **T46.4** **Poisoning by, adverse effect of and underdosing of angiotensin-converting-enzyme inhibitors**

√6ᵗʰ **T46.4X** **Poisoning by, adverse effect of and underdosing of angiotensin-converting-enzyme inhibitors**

√7ᵗʰ **T46.4X1** **Poisoning by angiotensin-converting-enzyme inhibitors,** accidental (unintentional)
Poisoning by angiotensin-converting-enzyme inhibitors NOS

√7ᵗʰ **T46.4X2** **Poisoning by angiotensin-converting-enzyme inhibitors,** intentional self-harm

√7ᵗʰ **T46.4X3** **Poisoning by angiotensin-converting-enzyme inhibitors,** assault

√7ᵗʰ **T46.4X4** **Poisoning by angiotensin-converting-enzyme inhibitors,** undetermined

√7ᵗʰ **T46.4X5** Adverse effect of angiotensin-converting-enzyme inhibitors

√7ᵗʰ **T46.4X6** Underdosing of angiotensin-converting-enzyme inhibitors

√5ᵗʰ **T46.5** **Poisoning by, adverse effect of and underdosing of other antihypertensive drugs**

> EXCLUDES 2   *poisoning by, adverse effect of and underdosing of beta-adrenoreceptor antagonists (T44.7)*
> *poisoning by, adverse effect of and underdosing of calcium-channel blockers (T46.1)*
> *poisoning by, adverse effect of and underdosing of diuretics (T50.0-I50.2)*

√6ᵗʰ **T46.5X** **Poisoning by, adverse effect of and underdosing of other antihypertensive drugs**

√7ᵗʰ **T46.5X1** **Poisoning by other antihypertensive drugs,** accidental (unintentional)
Poisoning by other antihypertensive drugs NOS

√7ᵗʰ **T46.5X2** **Poisoning by other antihypertensive drugs,** intentional self-harm

√7ᵗʰ **T46.5X3** **Poisoning by other antihypertensive drugs,** assault

√7ᵗʰ **T46.5X4** **Poisoning by other antihypertensive drugs,** undetermined

√7ᵗʰ **T46.5X5** Adverse effect of other antihypertensive drugs

√7ᵗʰ **T46.5X6** Underdosing of other antihypertensive drugs

√5ᵗʰ **T46.6** **Poisoning by, adverse effect of and underdosing of antihyperlipidemic and antiarteriosclerotic drugs**

√6ᵗʰ **T46.6X** **Poisoning by, adverse effect of and underdosing of antihyperlipidemic and antiarteriosclerotic drugs**

√7ᵗʰ **T46.6X1** **Poisoning by antihyperlipidemic and antiarteriosclerotic drugs,** accidental (unintentional)
Poisoning by antihyperlipidemic and antiarteriosclerotic drugs NOS

√7ᵗʰ **T46.6X2** **Poisoning by antihyperlipidemic and antiarteriosclerotic drugs,** intentional self-harm

√7ᵗʰ **T46.6X3** **Poisoning by antihyperlipidemic and antiarteriosclerotic drugs,** assault

√7ᵗʰ **T46.6X4** **Poisoning by antihyperlipidemic and antiarteriosclerotic drugs,** undetermined

√7ᵗʰ **T46.6X5** Adverse effect of antihyperlipidemic and antiarteriosclerotic drugs

√7ᵗʰ **T46.6X6** Underdosing of antihyperlipidemic and antiarteriosclerotic drugs

✓5ᵗʰ **T46.7 Poisoning by, adverse effect of and underdosing of peripheral vasodilators**

Poisoning by, adverse effect of and underdosing of nicotinic acid (derivatives)

> EXCLUDES 1 *poisoning by, adverse effect of and underdosing of papaverine (T44.3)*

✓6ᵗʰ **T46.7X Poisoning by, adverse effect of and underdosing of peripheral vasodilators**

✓7ᵗʰ **T46.7X1 Poisoning by peripheral vasodilators, accidental (unintentional)**

Poisoning by peripheral vasodilators NOS

✓7ᵗʰ **T46.7X2 Poisoning by peripheral vasodilators, intentional self-harm**

✓7ᵗʰ **T46.7X3 Poisoning by peripheral vasodilators, assault**

✓7ᵗʰ **T46.7X4 Poisoning by peripheral vasodilators, undetermined**

✓7ᵗʰ **T46.7X5 Adverse effect of peripheral vasodilators**

✓7ᵗʰ **T46.7X6 Underdosing of peripheral vasodilators**

✓5ᵗʰ **T46.8 Poisoning by, adverse effect of and underdosing of antivaricose drugs, including sclerosing agents**

✓6ᵗʰ **T46.8X Poisoning by, adverse effect of and underdosing of antivaricose drugs, including sclerosing agents**

✓7ᵗʰ **T46.8X1 Poisoning by antivaricose drugs, including sclerosing agents, accidental (unintentional)**

Poisoning by antivaricose drugs, including sclerosing agents NOS

✓7ᵗʰ **T46.8X2 Poisoning by antivaricose drugs, including sclerosing agents, intentional self-harm**

✓7ᵗʰ **T46.8X3 Poisoning by antivaricose drugs, including sclerosing agents, assault**

✓7ᵗʰ **T46.8X4 Poisoning by antivaricose drugs, including sclerosing agents, undetermined**

✓7ᵗʰ **T46.8X5 Adverse effect of antivaricose drugs, including sclerosing agents**

✓7ᵗʰ **T46.8X6 Underdosing of antivaricose drugs, including sclerosing agents**

✓5ᵗʰ **T46.9 Poisoning by, adverse effect of and underdosing of other and unspecified agents primarily affecting the cardiovascular system**

✓6ᵗʰ **T46.90 Poisoning by, adverse effect of and underdosing of unspecified agents primarily affecting the cardiovascular system**

✓7ᵗʰ **T46.901 Poisoning by unspecified agents primarily affecting the cardiovascular system, accidental (unintentional)** ▽

✓7ᵗʰ **T46.902 Poisoning by unspecified agents primarily affecting the cardiovascular system, intentional self-harm** ▽

✓7ᵗʰ **T46.903 Poisoning by unspecified agents primarily affecting the cardiovascular system, assault** ▽

✓7ᵗʰ **T46.904 Poisoning by unspecified agents primarily affecting the cardiovascular system, undetermined** ▽

✓7ᵗʰ **T46.905 Adverse effect of unspecified agents primarily affecting the cardiovascular system** ▽

✓7ᵗʰ **T46.906 Underdosing of unspecified agents primarily affecting the cardiovascular system** ▽

✓6ᵗʰ **T46.99 Poisoning by, adverse effect of and underdosing of other agents primarily affecting the cardiovascular system**

✓7ᵗʰ **T46.991 Poisoning by other agents primarily affecting the cardiovascular system, accidental (unintentional)**

✓7ᵗʰ **T46.992 Poisoning by other agents primarily affecting the cardiovascular system, intentional self-harm**

✓7ᵗʰ **T46.993 Poisoning by other agents primarily affecting the cardiovascular system, assault**

✓7ᵗʰ **T46.994 Poisoning by other agents primarily affecting the cardiovascular system, undetermined**

✓7ᵗʰ **T46.995 Adverse effect of other agents primarily affecting the cardiovascular system**

✓7ᵗʰ **T46.996 Underdosing of other agents primarily affecting the cardiovascular system**

✓4ᵗʰ **T47 Poisoning by, adverse effect of and underdosing of agents primarily affecting the gastrointestinal system**

The appropriate 7th character is to be added to each code from category T47.
A   initial encounter
D   subsequent encounter
S   sequela

✓5ᵗʰ **T47.0 Poisoning by, adverse effect of and underdosing of histamine H2-receptor blockers**

✓6ᵗʰ **T47.0X Poisoning by, adverse effect of and underdosing of histamine H2-receptor blockers**

✓7ᵗʰ **T47.0X1 Poisoning by histamine H2-receptor blockers, accidental (unintentional)**

Poisoning by histamine H2-receptor blockers NOS

✓7ᵗʰ **T47.0X2 Poisoning by histamine H2-receptor blockers, intentional self-harm**

✓7ᵗʰ **T47.0X3 Poisoning by histamine H2-receptor blockers, assault**

✓7ᵗʰ **T47.0X4 Poisoning by histamine H2-receptor blockers, undetermined**

✓7ᵗʰ **T47.0X5 Adverse effect of histamine H2-receptor blockers**

✓7ᵗʰ **T47.0X6 Underdosing of histamine H2-receptor blockers**

✓5ᵗʰ **T47.1 Poisoning by, adverse effect of and underdosing of other antacids and anti-gastric-secretion drugs**

✓6ᵗʰ **T47.1X Poisoning by, adverse effect of and underdosing of other antacids and anti-gastric-secretion drugs**

✓7ᵗʰ **T47.1X1 Poisoning by other antacids and anti-gastric-secretion drugs, accidental (unintentional)**

Poisoning by other antacids and anti-gastric-secretion drugs NOS

✓7ᵗʰ **T47.1X2 Poisoning by other antacids and anti-gastric-secretion drugs, intentional self-harm**

✓7ᵗʰ **T47.1X3 Poisoning by other antacids and anti-gastric-secretion drugs, assault**

✓7ᵗʰ **T47.1X4 Poisoning by other antacids and anti-gastric-secretion drugs, undetermined**

✓7ᵗʰ **T47.1X5 Adverse effect of other antacids and anti-gastric-secretion drugs**

✓7ᵗʰ **T47.1X6 Underdosing of other antacids and anti-gastric-secretion drugs**

✓5ᵗʰ **T47.2 Poisoning by, adverse effect of and underdosing of stimulant laxatives**

✓6ᵗʰ **T47.2X Poisoning by, adverse effect of and underdosing of stimulant laxatives**

✓7ᵗʰ **T47.2X1 Poisoning by stimulant laxatives, accidental (unintentional)**

Poisoning by stimulant laxatives NOS

✓7ᵗʰ **T47.2X2 Poisoning by stimulant laxatives, intentional self-harm**

✓7ᵗʰ **T47.2X3 Poisoning by stimulant laxatives, assault**

✓7ᵗʰ **T47.2X4 Poisoning by stimulant laxatives, undetermined**

✓7ᵗʰ **T47.2X5 Adverse effect of stimulant laxatives**

✓7ᵗʰ **T47.2X6 Underdosing of stimulant laxatives**

✓5ᵗʰ **T47.3 Poisoning by, adverse effect of and underdosing of saline and osmotic laxatives**

✓6ᵗʰ **T47.3X Poisoning by and adverse effect of saline and osmotic laxatives**

✓7ᵗʰ **T47.3X1 Poisoning by saline and osmotic laxatives, accidental (unintentional)**

Poisoning by saline and osmotic laxatives NOS

✓7ᵗʰ **T47.3X2 Poisoning by saline and osmotic laxatives, intentional self-harm**

✓7ᵗʰ **T47.3X3 Poisoning by saline and osmotic laxatives, assault**

✓7ᵗʰ **T47.3X4 Poisoning by saline and osmotic laxatives, undetermined**

✓7ᵗʰ **T47.3X5 Adverse effect of saline and osmotic laxatives**

✓7ᵗʰ **T47.3X6 Underdosing of saline and osmotic laxatives**

EXCLUDES 1 Not coded here   **EXCLUDES 2** Not included here   N Newborn Age : 0   P Pediatric Age : 0-17   M Maternity Age : 12-55   A Adult Age : 15-124

1042

ICD-10-CM 2017

✓5th **T47.4**   **Poisoning by, adverse effect of and underdosing of other laxatives**

   ✓6th **T47.4X**   **Poisoning by, adverse effect of and underdosing of** other laxatives

     ✓7th **T47.4X1**   **Poisoning by other laxatives, accidental (unintentional)**
       Poisoning by other laxatives NOS

     ✓7th **T47.4X2**   **Poisoning by other laxatives, intentional self-harm**

     ✓7th **T47.4X3**   **Poisoning by other laxatives, assault**

     ✓7th **T47.4X4**   **Poisoning by other laxatives, undetermined**

     ✓7th **T47.4X5**   **Adverse effect of other laxatives**

     ✓7th **T47.4X6**   **Underdosing of other laxatives**

✓5th **T47.5**   **Poisoning by, adverse effect of and underdosing of digestants**

   ✓6th **T47.5X**   **Poisoning by, adverse effect of and underdosing of** digestants

     ✓7th **T47.5X1**   **Poisoning by digestants, accidental (unintentional)**
       Poisoning by digestants NOS

     ✓7th **T47.5X2**   **Poisoning by digestants, intentional self-harm**

     ✓7th **T47.5X3**   **Poisoning by digestants, assault**

     ✓7th **T47.5X4**   **Poisoning by digestants, undetermined**

     ✓7th **T47.5X5**   **Adverse effect of digestants**

     ✓7th **T47.5X6**   **Underdosing of digestants**

✓5th **T47.6**   **Poisoning by, adverse effect of and underdosing of antidiarrheal drugs**

     EXCLUDES 2   *poisoning by, adverse effect of and underdosing of systemic antibiotics and other anti-infectives (T36-T37)*

   ✓6th **T47.6X**   **Poisoning by, adverse effect of and underdosing of** antidiarrheal drugs

     ✓7th **T47.6X1**   **Poisoning by antidiarrheal drugs, accidental (unintentional)**
       Poisoning by antidiarrheal drugs NOS

     ✓7th **T47.6X2**   **Poisoning by antidiarrheal drugs, intentional self-harm**

     ✓7th **T47.6X3**   **Poisoning by antidiarrheal drugs, assault**

     ✓7th **T47.6X4**   **Poisoning by antidiarrheal drugs, undetermined**

     ✓7th **T47.6X5**   **Adverse effect of antidiarrheal drugs**

     ✓7th **T47.6X6**   **Underdosing of antidiarrheal drugs**

✓5th **T47.7**   **Poisoning by, adverse effect of and underdosing of emetics**

   ✓6th **T47.7X**   **Poisoning by, adverse effect of and underdosing of** emetics

     ✓7th **T47.7X1**   **Poisoning by emetics, accidental (unintentional)**
       Poisoning by emetics NOS

     ✓7th **T47.7X2**   **Poisoning by emetics, intentional self-harm**

     ✓7th **T47.7X3**   **Poisoning by emetics, assault**

     ✓7th **T47.7X4**   **Poisoning by emetics, undetermined**

     ✓7th **T47.7X5**   **Adverse effect of emetics**

     ✓7th **T47.7X6**   **Underdosing of emetics**

✓5th **T47.8**   **Poisoning by, adverse effect of and underdosing of other agents primarily affecting gastrointestinal system**

   ✓6th **T47.8X**   **Poisoning by, adverse effect of and underdosing of** other agents primarily affecting gastrointestinal system

     ✓7th **T47.8X1**   **Poisoning by other agents primarily affecting gastrointestinal system, accidental (unintentional)**
       Poisoning by other agents primarily affecting gastrointestinal system NOS

     ✓7th **T47.8X2**   **Poisoning by other agents primarily affecting gastrointestinal system, intentional self-harm**

     ✓7th **T47.8X3**   **Poisoning by other agents primarily affecting gastrointestinal system, assault**

     ✓7th **T47.8X4**   **Poisoning by other agents primarily affecting gastrointestinal system, undetermined**

     ✓7th **T47.8X5**   **Adverse effect of other agents primarily affecting gastrointestinal system**

     ✓7th **T47.8X6**   **Underdosing of other agents primarily affecting gastrointestinal system**

✓5th **T47.9**   **Poisoning by, adverse effect of and underdosing of unspecified agents primarily affecting the gastrointestinal system**

     ✓x7th **T47.91**   **Poisoning by unspecified agents primarily affecting the gastrointestinal system, accidental (unintentional)**   ▽
       Poisoning by agents primarily affecting the gastrointestinal system NOS

     ✓x7th **T47.92**   **Poisoning by unspecified agents primarily affecting the gastrointestinal system, intentional self-harm**   ▽

     ✓x7th **T47.93**   **Poisoning by unspecified agents primarily affecting the gastrointestinal system, assault**   ▽

     ✓x7th **T47.94**   **Poisoning by unspecified agents primarily affecting the gastrointestinal system, undetermined**   ▽

     ✓x7th **T47.95**   **Adverse effect of unspecified agents primarily affecting the gastrointestinal system**   ▽

     ✓x7th **T47.96**   **Underdosing of unspecified agents primarily affecting the gastrointestinal system**   ▽

✓4th **T48**   **Poisoning by, adverse effect of and underdosing of agents primarily acting on smooth and skeletal muscles and the respiratory system**

> The appropriate 7th character is to be added to each code from category T48.
> A   initial encounter
> D   subsequent encounter
> S   sequela

   ✓5th **T48.0**   **Poisoning by, adverse effect of and underdosing of oxytocic drugs**

     EXCLUDES 1   *poisoning by, adverse effect of and underdosing of estrogens, progestogens and antagonists (T38.4-T38.6)*

     ✓6th **T48.0X**   **Poisoning by, adverse effect of and underdosing of** oxytocic drugs

       ✓7th **T48.0X1**   **Poisoning by oxytocic drugs, accidental (unintentional)**
         Poisoning by oxytocic drugs NOS

       ✓7th **T48.0X2**   **Poisoning by oxytocic drugs, intentional self-harm**

       ✓7th **T48.0X3**   **Poisoning by oxytocic drugs, assault**

       ✓7th **T48.0X4**   **Poisoning by oxytocic drugs, undetermined**

       ✓7th **T48.0X5**   **Adverse effect of oxytocic drugs**

       ✓7th **T48.0X6**   **Underdosing of oxytocic drugs**

   ✓5th **T48.1**   **Poisoning by, adverse effect of and underdosing of skeletal muscle relaxants [neuromuscular blocking agents]**

     ✓6th **T48.1X**   **Poisoning by, adverse effect of and underdosing of** skeletal muscle relaxants [neuromuscular blocking agents]

       ✓7th **T48.1X1**   **Poisoning by skeletal muscle relaxants [neuromuscular blocking agents], accidental (unintentional)**
         Poisoning by skeletal muscle relaxants [neuromuscular blocking agents] NOS

       ✓7th **T48.1X2**   **Poisoning by skeletal muscle relaxants [neuromuscular blocking agents], intentional self-harm**

       ✓7th **T48.1X3**   **Poisoning by skeletal muscle relaxants [neuromuscular blocking agents], assault**

       ✓7th **T48.1X4**   **Poisoning by skeletal muscle relaxants [neuromuscular blocking agents], undetermined**

       ✓7th **T48.1X5**   **Adverse effect of skeletal muscle relaxants [neuromuscular blocking agents]**

       ✓7th **T48.1X6**   **Underdosing of skeletal muscle relaxants [neuromuscular blocking agents]**

   ✓5th **T48.2**   **Poisoning by, adverse effect of and underdosing of other and unspecified drugs acting on muscles**

     ✓6th **T48.20**   **Poisoning by, adverse effect of and underdosing of** unspecified drugs acting on muscles

       ✓7th **T48.201**   **Poisoning by unspecified drugs acting on muscles, accidental (unintentional)**   ▽
         Poisoning by unspecified drugs acting on muscles NOS

       ✓7th **T48.202**   **Poisoning by unspecified drugs acting on muscles, intentional self-harm**   ▽

☑ Additional Character Required   ✓x7th Placeholder Alert   Manifestation Dx   ▽ Unspecified Dx   ▶◀ Revised Text   ● New Code   ▲ Revised Code Title

ICD-10-CM 2017   **1043**

✓7ᵗʰ **T48.203** Poisoning by unspecified drugs acting on muscles, assault ▽

✓7ᵗʰ **T48.204** Poisoning by unspecified drugs acting on muscles, undetermined ▽

✓7ᵗʰ **T48.205** Adverse effect of unspecified drugs acting on muscles ▽

✓7ᵗʰ **T48.206** Underdosing of unspecified drugs acting on muscles ▽

✓6ᵗʰ **T48.29** Poisoning by, adverse effect of and underdosing of other drugs acting on muscles

✓7ᵗʰ **T48.291** Poisoning by other drugs acting on muscles, accidental (unintentional)

Poisoning by other drugs acting on muscles NOS

✓7ᵗʰ **T48.292** Poisoning by other drugs acting on muscles, intentional self-harm

✓7ᵗʰ **T48.293** Poisoning by other drugs acting on muscles, assault

✓7ᵗʰ **T48.294** Poisoning by other drugs acting on muscles, undetermined

✓7ᵗʰ **T48.295** Adverse effect of other drugs acting on muscles

✓7ᵗʰ **T48.296** Underdosing of other drugs acting on muscles

✓5ᵗʰ **T48.3** Poisoning by, adverse effect of and underdosing of antitussives

✓6ᵗʰ **T48.3X** Poisoning by, adverse effect of and underdosing of antitussives

✓7ᵗʰ **T48.3X1** Poisoning by antitussives, accidental (unintentional)

Poisoning by antitussives NOS

✓7ᵗʰ **T48.3X2** Poisoning by antitussives, intentional self-harm

✓7ᵗʰ **T48.3X3** Poisoning by antitussives, assault

✓7ᵗʰ **T48.3X4** Poisoning by antitussives, undetermined

✓7ᵗʰ **T48.3X5** Adverse effect of antitussives

✓7ᵗʰ **T48.3X6** Underdosing of antitussives

✓5ᵗʰ **T48.4** Poisoning by, adverse effect of and underdosing of expectorants

✓6ᵗʰ **T48.4X** Poisoning by, adverse effect of and underdosing of expectorants

✓7ᵗʰ **T48.4X1** Poisoning by expectorants, accidental (unintentional)

Poisoning by expectorants NOS

✓7ᵗʰ **T48.4X2** Poisoning by expectorants, intentional self-harm

✓7ᵗʰ **T48.4X3** Poisoning by expectorants, assault

✓7ᵗʰ **T48.4X4** Poisoning by expectorants, undetermined

✓7ᵗʰ **T48.4X5** Adverse effect of expectorants

✓7ᵗʰ **T48.4X6** Underdosing of expectorants

✓5ᵗʰ **T48.5** Poisoning by, adverse effect of and underdosing of other anti-common-cold drugs

Poisoning by, adverse effect of and underdosing of decongestants

EXCLUDES 2 *poisoning by, adverse effect of and underdosing of antipyretics, NEC (T39.9-)*

poisoning by, adverse effect of and underdosing of non-steroidal antiinflammatory drugs (T39.3-)

poisoning by, adverse effect of and underdosing of salicylates (T39.0-)

✓6ᵗʰ **T48.5X** Poisoning by, adverse effect of and underdosing of other anti-common-cold drugs

✓7ᵗʰ **T48.5X1** Poisoning by other anti-common-cold drugs, accidental (unintentional)

Poisoning by other anti-common-cold drugs NOS

✓7ᵗʰ **T48.5X2** Poisoning by other anti-common-cold drugs, intentional self-harm

✓7ᵗʰ **T48.5X3** Poisoning by other anti-common-cold drugs, assault

✓7ᵗʰ **T48.5X4** Poisoning by other anti-common-cold drugs, undetermined

✓7ᵗʰ **T48.5X5** Adverse effect of other anti-common-cold drugs

✓7ᵗʰ **T48.5X6** Underdosing of other anti-common-cold drugs

✓5ᵗʰ **T48.6** Poisoning by, adverse effect of and underdosing of antiasthmatics, not elsewhere classified

Poisoning by, adverse effect of and underdosing of beta-adrenoreceptor agonists used in asthma therapy

EXCLUDES 1 *poisoning by, adverse effect of and underdosing of anterior pituitary [adenohypophyseal] hormones (T38.8)*

poisoning by, adverse effect of and underdosing of beta-adrenoreceptor agonists not used in asthma therapy (T44.5)

✓6ᵗʰ **T48.6X** Poisoning by, adverse effect of and underdosing of antiasthmatics

✓7ᵗʰ **T48.6X1** Poisoning by antiasthmatics, accidental (unintentional)

Poisoning by antiasthmatics NOS

✓7ᵗʰ **T48.6X2** Poisoning by antiasthmatics, intentional self-harm

✓7ᵗʰ **T48.6X3** Poisoning by antiasthmatics, assault

✓7ᵗʰ **T48.6X4** Poisoning by antiasthmatics, undetermined

✓7ᵗʰ **T48.6X5** Adverse effect of antiasthmatics

✓7ᵗʰ **T48.6X6** Underdosing of antiasthmatics

✓5ᵗʰ **T48.9** Poisoning by, adverse effect of and underdosing of other and unspecified agents primarily acting on the respiratory system

✓6ᵗʰ **T48.90** Poisoning by, adverse effect of and underdosing of unspecified agents primarily acting on the respiratory system

✓7ᵗʰ **T48.901** Poisoning by unspecified agents primarily acting on the respiratory system, accidental (unintentional) ▽

✓7ᵗʰ **T48.902** Poisoning by unspecified agents primarily acting on the respiratory system, intentional self-harm ▽

✓7ᵗʰ **T48.903** Poisoning by unspecified agents primarily acting on the respiratory system, assault ▽

✓7ᵗʰ **T48.904** Poisoning by unspecified agents primarily acting on the respiratory system, undetermined ▽

✓7ᵗʰ **T48.905** Adverse effect of unspecified agents primarily acting on the respiratory system ▽

✓7ᵗʰ **T48.906** Underdosing of unspecified agents primarily acting on the respiratory system ▽

✓6ᵗʰ **T48.99** Poisoning by, adverse effect of and underdosing of other agents primarily acting on the respiratory system

✓7ᵗʰ **T48.991** Poisoning by other agents primarily acting on the respiratory system, accidental (unintentional)

✓7ᵗʰ **T48.992** Poisoning by other agents primarily acting on the respiratory system, intentional self-harm

✓7ᵗʰ **T48.993** Poisoning by other agents primarily acting on the respiratory system, assault

✓7ᵗʰ **T48.994** Poisoning by other agents primarily acting on the respiratory system, undetermined

✓7ᵗʰ **T48.995** Adverse effect of other agents primarily acting on the respiratory system

✓7ᵗʰ **T48.996** Underdosing of other agents primarily acting on the respiratory system

✓4ᵗʰ **T49** Poisoning by, adverse effect of and underdosing of topical agents primarily affecting skin and mucous membrane and by ophthalmological, otorhinolaryngological and dental drugs

INCLUDES poisoning by, adverse effect of and underdosing of glucocorticoids, topically used

The appropriate 7th character is to be added to each code from category T49.
A initial encounter
D subsequent encounter
S sequela

✓5ᵗʰ **T49.0** Poisoning by, adverse effect of and underdosing of local antifungal, anti-infective and anti-inflammatory drugs

✓6ᵗʰ **T49.0X** Poisoning by, adverse effect of and underdosing of local antifungal, anti-infective and anti-inflammatory drugs

---

EXCLUDES 1 Not coded here   **EXCLUDES 2** Not included here   ℕ Newborn Age : 0   ℙ Pediatric Age : 0-17   ⓂMaternity Age : 12-55   🅰 Adult Age : 15-124

1044

ICD-10-CM 2017

√7ᵗʰ **T49.0X1** Poisoning by local antifungal, anti-infective and anti-inflammatory drugs, **accidental (unintentional)**
Poisoning by local antifungal, anti-infective and anti-inflammatory drugs NOS

√7ᵗʰ **T49.0X2** Poisoning by local antifungal, anti-infective and anti-inflammatory drugs, **intentional self-harm**

√7ᵗʰ **T49.0X3** Poisoning by local antifungal, anti-infective and anti-inflammatory drugs, **assault**

√7ᵗʰ **T49.0X4** Poisoning by local antifungal, anti-infective and anti-inflammatory drugs, **undetermined**

√7ᵗʰ **T49.0X5** **Adverse effect** of local antifungal, anti-infective and anti-inflammatory drugs

√7ᵗʰ **T49.0X6** **Underdosing** of local antifungal, anti-infective and anti-inflammatory drugs

√5ᵗʰ **T49.1** Poisoning by, adverse effect of and underdosing of antipruritics

√6ᵗʰ **T49.1X** Poisoning by, adverse effect of and underdosing of antipruritics

√7ᵗʰ **T49.1X1** Poisoning by antipruritics, **accidental (unintentional)**
Poisoning by antipruritics NOS

√7ᵗʰ **T49.1X2** Poisoning by antipruritics, **intentional self-harm**

√7ᵗʰ **T49.1X3** Poisoning by antipruritics, **assault**

√7ᵗʰ **T49.1X4** Poisoning by antipruritics, **undetermined**

√7ᵗʰ **T49.1X5** **Adverse effect** of antipruritics

√7ᵗʰ **T49.1X6** **Underdosing** of antipruritics

√5ᵗʰ **T49.2** Poisoning by, adverse effect of and underdosing of local astringents and local detergents

√6ᵗʰ **T49.2X** Poisoning by, adverse effect of and underdosing of local astringents and local detergents

√7ᵗʰ **T49.2X1** Poisoning by local astringents and local detergents, **accidental (unintentional)**
Poisoning by local astringents and local detergents NOS

√7ᵗʰ **T49.2X2** Poisoning by local astringents and local detergents, **intentional self-harm**

√7ᵗʰ **T49.2X3** Poisoning by local astringents and local detergents, **assault**

√7ᵗʰ **T49.2X4** Poisoning by local astringents and local detergents, **undetermined**

√7ᵗʰ **T49.2X5** **Adverse effect** of local astringents and local detergents

√7ᵗʰ **T49.2X6** **Underdosing** of local astringents and local detergents

√5ᵗʰ **T49.3** Poisoning by, adverse effect of and underdosing of emollients, demulcents and protectants

√6ᵗʰ **T49.3X** Poisoning by, adverse effect of and underdosing of emollients, demulcents and protectants

√7ᵗʰ **T49.3X1** Poisoning by emollients, demulcents and protectants, **accidental (unintentional)**
Poisoning by emollients, demulcents and protectants NOS

√7ᵗʰ **T49.3X2** Poisoning by emollients, demulcents and protectants, **intentional self-harm**

√7ᵗʰ **T49.3X3** Poisoning by emollients, demulcents and protectants, **assault**

√7ᵗʰ **T49.3X4** Poisoning by emollients, demulcents and protectants, **undetermined**

√7ᵗʰ **T49.3X5** **Adverse effect** of emollients, demulcents and protectants

√7ᵗʰ **T49.3X6** **Underdosing** of emollients, demulcents and protectants

√5ᵗʰ **T49.4** Poisoning by, adverse effect of and underdosing of keratolytics, keratoplastics, and other hair treatment drugs and preparations

√6ᵗʰ **T49.4X** Poisoning by, adverse effect of and underdosing of keratolytics, keratoplastics, and other hair treatment drugs and preparations

√7ᵗʰ **T49.4X1** Poisoning by keratolytics, keratoplastics, and other hair treatment drugs and preparations, **accidental (unintentional)**
Poisoning by keratolytics, keratoplastics, and other hair treatment drugs and preparations NOS

√7ᵗʰ **T49.4X2** Poisoning by keratolytics, keratoplastics, and other hair treatment drugs and preparations, **intentional self-harm**

√7ᵗʰ **T49.4X3** Poisoning by keratolytics, keratoplastics, and other hair treatment drugs and preparations, **assault**

√7ᵗʰ **T49.4X4** Poisoning by keratolytics, keratoplastics, and other hair treatment drugs and preparations, **undetermined**

√7ᵗʰ **T49.4X5** **Adverse effect** of keratolytics, keratoplastics, and other hair treatment drugs and preparations

√7ᵗʰ **T49.4X6** **Underdosing** of keratolytics, keratoplastics, and other hair treatment drugs and preparations

√5ᵗʰ **T49.5** Poisoning by, adverse effect of and underdosing of ophthalmological drugs and preparations

√6ᵗʰ **T49.5X** Poisoning by, adverse effect of and underdosing of ophthalmological drugs and preparations

√7ᵗʰ **T49.5X1** Poisoning by ophthalmological drugs and preparations, **accidental (unintentional)**
Poisoning by ophthalmological drugs and preparations NOS

√7ᵗʰ **T49.5X2** Poisoning by ophthalmological drugs and preparations, **intentional self-harm**

√7ᵗʰ **T49.5X3** Poisoning by ophthalmological drugs and preparations, **assault**

√7ᵗʰ **T49.5X4** Poisoning by ophthalmological drugs and preparations, **undetermined**

√7ᵗʰ **T49.5X5** **Adverse effect** of ophthalmological drugs and preparations

√7ᵗʰ **T49.5X6** **Underdosing** of ophthalmological drugs and preparations

√5ᵗʰ **T49.6** Poisoning by, adverse effect of and underdosing of otorhinolaryngological drugs and preparations

√6ᵗʰ **T49.6X** Poisoning by, adverse effect of and underdosing of otorhinolaryngological drugs and preparations

√7ᵗʰ **T49.6X1** Poisoning by otorhinolaryngological drugs and preparations, **accidental (unintentional)**
Poisoning by otorhinolaryngological drugs and preparations NOS

√7ᵗʰ **T49.6X2** Poisoning by otorhinolaryngological drugs and preparations, **intentional self-harm**

√7ᵗʰ **T49.6X3** Poisoning by otorhinolaryngological drugs and preparations, **assault**

√7ᵗʰ **T49.6X4** Poisoning by otorhinolaryngological drugs and preparations, **undetermined**

√7ᵗʰ **T49.6X5** **Adverse effect** of otorhinolaryngological drugs and preparations

√7ᵗʰ **T49.6X6** **Underdosing** of otorhinolaryngological drugs and preparations

√5ᵗʰ **T49.7** Poisoning by, adverse effect of and underdosing of dental drugs, topically applied

√6ᵗʰ **T49.7X** Poisoning by, adverse effect of and underdosing of dental drugs, topically applied

√7ᵗʰ **T49.7X1** Poisoning by dental drugs, topically applied, **accidental (unintentional)**
Poisoning by dental drugs, topically applied NOS

√7ᵗʰ **T49.7X2** Poisoning by dental drugs, topically applied, **intentional self-harm**

√7ᵗʰ **T49.7X3** Poisoning by dental drugs, topically applied, **assault**

√7ᵗʰ **T49.7X4** Poisoning by dental drugs, topically applied, **undetermined**

√7ᵗʰ **T49.7X5** **Adverse effect** of dental drugs, topically applied

√7ᵗʰ **T49.7X6** **Underdosing** of dental drugs, topically applied

√5ᵗʰ **T49.8** Poisoning by, adverse effect of and underdosing of other topical agents
Poisoning by, adverse effect of and underdosing of spermicides

√6ᵗʰ **T49.8X** Poisoning by, adverse effect of and underdosing of other topical agents

√7ᵗʰ **T49.8X1** Poisoning by other topical agents, **accidental (unintentional)**
Poisoning by other topical agents NOS

√7ᵗʰ **T49.8X2** Poisoning by other topical agents, **intentional self-harm**

√7ᵗʰ **T49.8X3** Poisoning by other topical agents, **assault**

☑ Additional Character Required   √ₓ₇ Placeholder Alert   Manifestation Dx   ▽ Unspecified Dx   ►◄ Revised Text   ● New Code   ▲ Revised Code Title

☑7ᵗʰ **T49.8X4 Poisoning by other topical agents, undetermined**

☑7ᵗʰ **T49.8X5 Adverse effect of other topical agents**

☑7ᵗʰ **T49.8X6 Underdosing of other topical agents**

☑5ᵗʰ **T49.9 Poisoning by, adverse effect of and underdosing of unspecified topical agent**

☑x7ᵗʰ **T49.91 Poisoning by unspecified topical agent, accidental (unintentional)** ▽

☑x7ᵗʰ **T49.92 Poisoning by unspecified topical agent, intentional self-harm** ▽

☑x7ᵗʰ **T49.93 Poisoning by unspecified topical agent, assault** ▽

☑x7ᵗʰ **T49.94 Poisoning by unspecified topical agent, undetermined** ▽

☑x7ᵗʰ **T49.95 Adverse effect of unspecified topical agent** ▽

☑x7ᵗʰ **T49.96 Underdosing of unspecified topical agent** ▽

☑4ᵗʰ **T50 Poisoning by, adverse effect of and underdosing of diuretics and other and unspecified drugs, medicaments and biological substances**

The appropriate 7th character is to be added to each code from category T50.
A   initial encounter
D   subsequent encounter
S   sequela

☑5ᵗʰ **T50.0 Poisoning by, adverse effect of and underdosing of mineralocorticoids and their antagonists**

☑6ᵗʰ **T50.0X Poisoning by, adverse effect of and underdosing of mineralocorticoids and their antagonists**

☑7ᵗʰ **T50.0X1 Poisoning by mineralocorticoids and their antagonists, accidental (unintentional)**
Poisoning by mineralocorticoids and their antagonists NOS

☑7ᵗʰ **T50.0X2 Poisoning by mineralocorticoids and their antagonists, intentional self-harm**

☑7ᵗʰ **T50.0X3 Poisoning by mineralocorticoids and their antagonists, assault**

☑7ᵗʰ **T50.0X4 Poisoning by mineralocorticoids and their antagonists, undetermined**

☑7ᵗʰ **T50.0X5 Adverse effect of mineralocorticoids and their antagonists**

☑7ᵗʰ **T50.0X6 Underdosing of mineralocorticoids and their antagonists**

☑5ᵗʰ **T50.1 Poisoning by, adverse effect of and underdosing of loop [high-ceiling] diuretics**

☑6ᵗʰ **T50.1X Poisoning by, adverse effect of and underdosing of loop [high-ceiling] diuretics**

☑7ᵗʰ **T50.1X1 Poisoning by loop [high-ceiling] diuretics, accidental (unintentional)**
Poisoning by loop [high-ceiling] diuretics NOS

☑7ᵗʰ **T50.1X2 Poisoning by loop [high-ceiling] diuretics, intentional self-harm**

☑7ᵗʰ **T50.1X3 Poisoning by loop [high-ceiling] diuretics, assault**

☑7ᵗʰ **T50.1X4 Poisoning by loop [high-ceiling] diuretics, undetermined**

☑7ᵗʰ **T50.1X5 Adverse effect of loop [high-ceiling] diuretics**

☑7ᵗʰ **T50.1X6 Underdosing of loop [high-ceiling] diuretics**

☑5ᵗʰ **T50.2 Poisoning by, adverse effect of and underdosing of carbonic-anhydrase inhibitors, benzothiadiazides and other diuretics**
Poisoning by, adverse effect of and underdosing of acetazolamide

☑6ᵗʰ **T50.2X Poisoning by, adverse effect of and underdosing of carbonic-anhydrase inhibitors, benzothiadiazides and other diuretics**

☑7ᵗʰ **T50.2X1 Poisoning by carbonic-anhydrase inhibitors, benzothiadiazides and other diuretics, accidental (unintentional)**
Poisoning by carbonic-anhydrase inhibitors, benzothiadiazides and other diuretics NOS

☑7ᵗʰ **T50.2X2 Poisoning by carbonic-anhydrase inhibitors, benzothiadiazides and other diuretics, intentional self-harm**

☑7ᵗʰ **T50.2X3 Poisoning by carbonic-anhydrase inhibitors, benzothiadiazides and other diuretics, assault**

☑7ᵗʰ **T50.2X4 Poisoning by carbonic-anhydrase inhibitors, benzothiadiazides and other diuretics, undetermined**

☑7ᵗʰ **T50.2X5 Adverse effect of carbonic-anhydrase inhibitors, benzothiadiazides and other diuretics**

☑7ᵗʰ **T50.2X6 Underdosing of carbonic-anhydrase inhibitors, benzothiadiazides and other diuretics**

☑5ᵗʰ **T50.3 Poisoning by, adverse effect of and underdosing of electrolytic, caloric and water-balance agents**
Poisoning by, adverse effect of and underdosing of oral rehydration salts

☑6ᵗʰ **T50.3X Poisoning by, adverse effect of and underdosing of electrolytic, caloric and water-balance agents**

☑7ᵗʰ **T50.3X1 Poisoning by electrolytic, caloric and water-balance agents, accidental (unintentional)**
Poisoning by electrolytic, caloric and water-balance agents NOS

☑7ᵗʰ **T50.3X2 Poisoning by electrolytic, caloric and water-balance agents, intentional self-harm**

☑7ᵗʰ **T50.3X3 Poisoning by electrolytic, caloric and water-balance agents, assault**

☑7ᵗʰ **T50.3X4 Poisoning by electrolytic, caloric and water-balance agents, undetermined**

☑7ᵗʰ **T50.3X5 Adverse effect of electrolytic, caloric and water-balance agents**

☑7ᵗʰ **T50.3X6 Underdosing of electrolytic, caloric and water-balance agents**

☑5ᵗʰ **T50.4 Poisoning by, adverse effect of and underdosing of drugs affecting uric acid metabolism**

☑6ᵗʰ **T50.4X Poisoning by, adverse effect of and underdosing of drugs affecting uric acid metabolism**

☑7ᵗʰ **T50.4X1 Poisoning by drugs affecting uric acid metabolism, accidental (unintentional)**
Poisoning by drugs affecting uric acid metabolism NOS

☑7ᵗʰ **T50.4X2 Poisoning by drugs affecting uric acid metabolism, intentional self-harm**

☑7ᵗʰ **T50.4X3 Poisoning by drugs affecting uric acid metabolism, assault**

☑7ᵗʰ **T50.4X4 Poisoning by drugs affecting uric acid metabolism, undetermined**

☑7ᵗʰ **T50.4X5 Adverse effect of drugs affecting uric acid metabolism**

☑7ᵗʰ **T50.4X6 Underdosing of drugs affecting uric acid metabolism**

☑5ᵗʰ **T50.5 Poisoning by, adverse effect of and underdosing of appetite depressants**

☑6ᵗʰ **T50.5X Poisoning by, adverse effect of and underdosing of appetite depressants**

☑7ᵗʰ **T50.5X1 Poisoning by appetite depressants, accidental (unintentional)**
Poisoning by appetite depressants NOS

☑7ᵗʰ **T50.5X2 Poisoning by appetite depressants, intentional self-harm**

☑7ᵗʰ **T50.5X3 Poisoning by appetite depressants, assault**

☑7ᵗʰ **T50.5X4 Poisoning by appetite depressants, undetermined**

☑7ᵗʰ **T50.5X5 Adverse effect of appetite depressants**

☑7ᵗʰ **T50.5X6 Underdosing of appetite depressants**

☑5ᵗʰ **T50.6 Poisoning by, adverse effect of and underdosing of antidotes and chelating agents**
Poisoning by, adverse effect of and underdosing of alcohol deterrents

☑6ᵗʰ **T50.6X Poisoning by, adverse effect of and underdosing of antidotes and chelating agents**

☑7ᵗʰ **T50.6X1 Poisoning by antidotes and chelating agents, accidental (unintentional)**
Poisoning by antidotes and chelating agents NOS

☑7ᵗʰ **T50.6X2 Poisoning by antidotes and chelating agents, intentional self-harm**

☑7ᵗʰ **T50.6X3 Poisoning by antidotes and chelating agents, assault**

☑7ᵗʰ **T50.6X4 Poisoning by antidotes and chelating agents, undetermined**

☑7ᵗʰ **T50.6X5 Adverse effect of antidotes and chelating agents**

✓7ᵗʰ **T50.6X6** Underdosing of antidotes and chelating agents

✓5ᵗʰ **T50.7** Poisoning by, adverse effect of and underdosing of analeptics and opioid receptor antagonists

✓6ᵗʰ **T50.7X** Poisoning by, adverse effect of and underdosing of analeptics and opioid receptor antagonists

✓7ᵗʰ **T50.7X1** Poisoning by analeptics and opioid receptor antagonists, accidental (unintentional)
Poisoning by analeptics and opioid receptor antagonists NOS

✓7ᵗʰ **T50.7X2** Poisoning by analeptics and opioid receptor antagonists, intentional self-harm

✓7ᵗʰ **T50.7X3** Poisoning by analeptics and opioid receptor antagonists, assault

✓7ᵗʰ **T50.7X4** Poisoning by analeptics and opioid receptor antagonists, undetermined

✓7ᵗʰ **T50.7X5** Adverse effect of analeptics and opioid receptor antagonists

✓7ᵗʰ **T50.7X6** Underdosing of analeptics and opioid receptor antagonists

✓5ᵗʰ **T50.8** Poisoning by, adverse effect of and underdosing of diagnostic agents

✓6ᵗʰ **T50.8X** Poisoning by, adverse effect of and underdosing of diagnostic agents

✓7ᵗʰ **T50.8X1** Poisoning by diagnostic agents, accidental (unintentional)
Poisoning by diagnostic agents NOS

✓7ᵗʰ **T50.8X2** Poisoning by diagnostic agents, intentional self-harm

✓7ᵗʰ **T50.8X3** Poisoning by diagnostic agents, assault

✓7ᵗʰ **T50.8X4** Poisoning by diagnostic agents, undetermined

✓7ᵗʰ **T50.8X5** Adverse effect of diagnostic agents

✓7ᵗʰ **T50.8X6** Underdosing of diagnostic agents

✓5ᵗʰ **T50.A** Poisoning by, adverse effect of and underdosing of bacterial vaccines

✓6ᵗʰ **T50.A1** Poisoning by, adverse effect of and underdosing of pertussis vaccine, including combinations with a pertussis component

✓7ᵗʰ **T50.A11** Poisoning by pertussis vaccine, including combinations with a pertussis component, accidental (unintentional)

✓7ᵗʰ **T50.A12** Poisoning by pertussis vaccine, including combinations with a pertussis component, intentional self-harm

✓7ᵗʰ **T50.A13** Poisoning by pertussis vaccine, including combinations with a pertussis component, assault

✓7ᵗʰ **T50.A14** Poisoning by pertussis vaccine, including combinations with a pertussis component, undetermined

✓7ᵗʰ **T50.A15** Adverse effect of pertussis vaccine, including combinations with a pertussis component

✓7ᵗʰ **T50.A16** Underdosing of pertussis vaccine, including combinations with a pertussis component

✓6ᵗʰ **T50.A2** Poisoning by, adverse effect of and underdosing of mixed bacterial vaccines without a pertussis component

✓7ᵗʰ **T50.A21** Poisoning by mixed bacterial vaccines without a pertussis component, accidental (unintentional)

✓7ᵗʰ **T50.A22** Poisoning by mixed bacterial vaccines without a pertussis component, intentional self-harm

✓7ᵗʰ **T50.A23** Poisoning by mixed bacterial vaccines without a pertussis component, assault

✓7ᵗʰ **T50.A24** Poisoning by mixed bacterial vaccines without a pertussis component, undetermined

✓7ᵗʰ **T50.A25** Adverse effect of mixed bacterial vaccines without a pertussis component

✓7ᵗʰ **T50.A26** Underdosing of mixed bacterial vaccines without a pertussis component

✓6ᵗʰ **T50.A9** Poisoning by, adverse effect of and underdosing of other bacterial vaccines

✓7ᵗʰ **T50.A91** Poisoning by other bacterial vaccines, accidental (unintentional)

✓7ᵗʰ **T50.A92** Poisoning by other bacterial vaccines, intentional self-harm

✓7ᵗʰ **T50.A93** Poisoning by other bacterial vaccines, assault

✓7ᵗʰ **T50.A94** Poisoning by other bacterial vaccines, undetermined

✓7ᵗʰ **T50.A95** Adverse effect of other bacterial vaccines

✓7ᵗʰ **T50.A96** Underdosing of other bacterial vaccines

✓5ᵗʰ **T50.B** Poisoning by, adverse effect of and underdosing of viral vaccines

✓6ᵗʰ **T50.B1** Poisoning by, adverse effect of and underdosing of smallpox vaccines

✓7ᵗʰ **T50.B11** Poisoning by smallpox vaccines, accidental (unintentional)

✓7ᵗʰ **T50.B12** Poisoning by smallpox vaccines, intentional self-harm

✓7ᵗʰ **T50.B13** Poisoning by smallpox vaccines, assault

✓7ᵗʰ **T50.B14** Poisoning by smallpox vaccines, undetermined

✓7ᵗʰ **T50.B15** Adverse effect of smallpox vaccines

✓7ᵗʰ **T50.B16** Underdosing of smallpox vaccines

✓6ᵗʰ **T50.B9** Poisoning by, adverse effect of and underdosing of other viral vaccines

✓7ᵗʰ **T50.B91** Poisoning by other viral vaccines, accidental (unintentional)

✓7ᵗʰ **T50.B92** Poisoning by other viral vaccines, intentional self-harm

✓7ᵗʰ **T50.B93** Poisoning by other viral vaccines, assault

✓7ᵗʰ **T50.B94** Poisoning by other viral vaccines, undetermined

✓7ᵗʰ **T50.B95** Adverse effect of other viral vaccines

✓7ᵗʰ **T50.B96** Underdosing of other viral vaccines

✓5ᵗʰ **T50.Z** Poisoning by, adverse effect of and underdosing of other vaccines and biological substances

✓6ᵗʰ **T50.Z1** Poisoning by, adverse effect of and underdosing of immunoglobulin

✓7ᵗʰ **T50.Z11** Poisoning by immunoglobulin, accidental (unintentional)

✓7ᵗʰ **T50.Z12** Poisoning by immunoglobulin, intentional self-harm

✓7ᵗʰ **T50.Z13** Poisoning by immunoglobulin, assault

✓7ᵗʰ **T50.Z14** Poisoning by immunoglobulin, undetermined

✓7ᵗʰ **T50.Z15** Adverse effect of immunoglobulin

✓7ᵗʰ **T50.Z16** Underdosing of immunoglobulin

✓6ᵗʰ **T50.Z9** Poisoning by, adverse effect of and underdosing of other vaccines and biological substances

✓7ᵗʰ **T50.Z91** Poisoning by other vaccines and biological substances, accidental (unintentional)

✓7ᵗʰ **T50.Z92** Poisoning by other vaccines and biological substances, intentional self-harm

✓7ᵗʰ **T50.Z93** Poisoning by other vaccines and biological substances, assault

✓7ᵗʰ **T50.Z94** Poisoning by other vaccines and biological substances, undetermined

✓7ᵗʰ **T50.Z95** Adverse effect of other vaccines and biological substances

✓7ᵗʰ **T50.Z96** Underdosing of other vaccines and biological substances

✓5ᵗʰ **T50.9** Poisoning by, adverse effect of and underdosing of other and unspecified drugs, medicaments and biological substances
AHA: 2016,1Q,38; 2015,1Q,21

✓6ᵗʰ **T50.90** Poisoning by, adverse effect of and underdosing of unspecified drugs, medicaments and biological substances

✓7ᵗʰ **T50.901** Poisoning by unspecified drugs, medicaments and biological substances, accidental (unintentional) ▽

✓7ᵗʰ **T50.902** Poisoning by unspecified drugs, medicaments and biological substances, intentional self-harm ▽

✓7ᵗʰ **T50.903** Poisoning by unspecified drugs, medicaments and biological substances, assault ▽

✓7ᵗʰ **T50.904** Poisoning by unspecified drugs, medicaments and biological substances, undetermined ▽

☑ Additional Character Required   ✓ˣ7ᵗʰ Placeholder Alert   Manifestation Dx   ▽ Unspecified Dx   ►◄ Revised Text   ● New Code   ▲ Revised Code Title

√7ᵗʰ **T50.905** **Adverse effect of unspecified drugs, medicaments and biological substances** ▽

√7ᵗʰ **T50.906** **Underdosing of unspecified drugs, medicaments and biological substances** ▽

√6ᵗʰ **T50.99** **Poisoning by, adverse effect of and underdosing of other drugs, medicaments and biological substances**

√7ᵗʰ **T50.991** **Poisoning by other drugs, medicaments and biological substances, accidental (unintentional)**

√7ᵗʰ **T50.992** **Poisoning by other drugs, medicaments and biological substances, intentional self-harm**

√7ᵗʰ **T50.993** **Poisoning by other drugs, medicaments and biological substances, assault**

√7ᵗʰ **T50.994** **Poisoning by other drugs, medicaments and biological substances, undetermined**

√7ᵗʰ **T50.995** **Adverse effect of other drugs, medicaments and biological substances**

√7ᵗʰ **T50.996** **Underdosing of other drugs, medicaments and biological substances**

Toxic effects of substances chiefly nonmedicinal as to source (T51-T65)

NOTE When no intent is indicated code to accidental. Undetermined intent is only for use when there is specific documentation in the record that the intent of the toxic effect cannot be determined.

Use additional code(s) for all associated manifestations of toxic effect, such as:
personal history of foreign body fully removed (Z87.821)
respiratory conditions due to external agents (J60-J70)
to identify any retained foreign body, if applicable (Z18.-)

EXCLUDES 1 *contact with and (suspected) exposure to toxic substances (Z77.-)*

√4ᵗʰ **T51** **Toxic effect of alcohol**

The appropriate 7th character is to be added to each code from category T51.
A initial encounter
D subsequent encounter
S sequela

√5ᵗʰ **T51.0** **Toxic effect of ethanol**

Toxic effect of ethyl alcohol

EXCLUDES 2 *acute alcohol intoxication or "hangover" effects (F10.129, F10.229, F10.929)*
drunkenness (F10.129, F10.229, F10.929)
pathological alcohol intoxication (F10.129, F10.229, F10.929)

√6ᵗʰ **T51.0X** **Toxic effect of ethanol**

√7ᵗʰ **T51.0X1** **Toxic effect of ethanol, accidental (unintentional)**
Toxic effect of ethanol NOS

√7ᵗʰ **T51.0X2** **Toxic effect of ethanol, intentional self-harm**

√7ᵗʰ **T51.0X3** **Toxic effect of ethanol, assault**

√7ᵗʰ **T51.0X4** **Toxic effect of ethanol, undetermined**

√5ᵗʰ **T51.1** **Toxic effect of methanol**

Toxic effect of methyl alcohol

√6ᵗʰ **T51.1X** **Toxic effect of methanol**

√7ᵗʰ **T51.1X1** **Toxic effect of methanol, accidental (unintentional)**
Toxic effect of methanol NOS

√7ᵗʰ **T51.1X2** **Toxic effect of methanol, intentional self-harm**

√7ᵗʰ **T51.1X3** **Toxic effect of methanol, assault**

√7ᵗʰ **T51.1X4** **Toxic effect of methanol, undetermined**

√5ᵗʰ **T51.2** **Toxic effect of 2-Propanol**

Toxic effect of isopropyl alcohol

√6ᵗʰ **T51.2X** **Toxic effect of 2-Propanol**

√7ᵗʰ **T51.2X1** **Toxic effect of 2-Propanol, accidental (unintentional)**
Toxic effect of 2-Propanol NOS

√7ᵗʰ **T51.2X2** **Toxic effect of 2-Propanol, intentional self-harm**

√7ᵗʰ **T51.2X3** **Toxic effect of 2-Propanol, assault**

√7ᵗʰ **T51.2X4** **Toxic effect of 2-Propanol, undetermined**

√5ᵗʰ **T51.3** **Toxic effect of fusel oil**

Toxic effect of amyl alcohol
Toxic effect of butyl [1-butanol] alcohol
Toxic effect of propyl [1-propanol] alcohol

√6ᵗʰ **T51.3X** **Toxic effect of fusel oil**

√7ᵗʰ **T51.3X1** **Toxic effect of fusel oil, accidental (unintentional)**
Toxic effect of fusel oil NOS

√7ᵗʰ **T51.3X2** **Toxic effect of fusel oil, intentional self-harm**

√7ᵗʰ **T51.3X3** **Toxic effect of fusel oil, assault**

√7ᵗʰ **T51.3X4** **Toxic effect of fusel oil, undetermined**

√5ᵗʰ **T51.8** **Toxic effect of other alcohols**

√6ᵗʰ **T51.8X** **Toxic effect of other alcohols**

√7ᵗʰ **T51.8X1** **Toxic effect of other alcohols, accidental (unintentional)**
Toxic effect of other alcohols NOS

√7ᵗʰ **T51.8X2** **Toxic effect of other alcohols, intentional self-harm**

√7ᵗʰ **T51.8X3** **Toxic effect of other alcohols, assault**

√7ᵗʰ **T51.8X4** **Toxic effect of other alcohols, undetermined**

√5ᵗʰ **T51.9** **Toxic effect of unspecified alcohol**

√x7ᵗʰ **T51.91** **Toxic effect of unspecified alcohol, accidental (unintentional)** ▽

√x7ᵗʰ **T51.92** **Toxic effect of unspecified alcohol, intentional self-harm** ▽

√x7ᵗʰ **T51.93** **Toxic effect of unspecified alcohol, assault** ▽

√x7ᵗʰ **T51.94** **Toxic effect of unspecified alcohol, undetermined** ▽

√4ᵗʰ **T52** **Toxic effect of organic solvents**

EXCLUDES 1 *halogen derivatives of aliphatic and aromatic hydrocarbons (T53.-)*

The appropriate 7th character is to be added to each code from category T52.
A initial encounter
D subsequent encounter
S sequela

√5ᵗʰ **T52.0** **Toxic effects of petroleum products**

Toxic effects of ether petroleum
Toxic effects of gasoline [petrol]
Toxic effects of kerosene [paraffin oil]
Toxic effects of naphtha petroleum
Toxic effects of paraffin wax
Toxic effects of spirit petroleum

√6ᵗʰ **T52.0X** **Toxic effects of petroleum products**

√7ᵗʰ **T52.0X1** **Toxic effect of petroleum products, accidental (unintentional)**
Toxic effects of petroleum products NOS

√7ᵗʰ **T52.0X2** **Toxic effect of petroleum products, intentional self-harm**

√7ᵗʰ **T52.0X3** **Toxic effect of petroleum products, assault**

√7ᵗʰ **T52.0X4** **Toxic effect of petroleum products, undetermined**

√5ᵗʰ **T52.1** **Toxic effects of benzene**

EXCLUDES 1 *homologues of benzene (T52.2)*
nitroderivatives and aminoderivatives of benzene and its homologues (T65.3)

√6ᵗʰ **T52.1X** **Toxic effects of benzene**

√7ᵗʰ **T52.1X1** **Toxic effect of benzene, accidental (unintentional)**
Toxic effects of benzene NOS

√7ᵗʰ **T52.1X2** **Toxic effect of benzene, intentional self-harm**

√7ᵗʰ **T52.1X3** **Toxic effect of benzene, assault**

√7ᵗʰ **T52.1X4** **Toxic effect of benzene, undetermined**

√5ᵗʰ **T52.2** **Toxic effects of homologues of benzene**

Toxic effects of toluene [methylbenzene]
Toxic effects of xylene [dimethylbenzene]

√6ᵗʰ **T52.2X** **Toxic effects of homologues of benzene**

√7ᵗʰ **T52.2X1** **Toxic effect of homologues of benzene, accidental (unintentional)**
Toxic effects of homologues of benzene NOS

EXCLUDES 1 Not coded here   **EXCLUDES 2** Not included here   N Newborn Age : 0   P Pediatric Age : 0-17   M Maternity Age : 12-55   A Adult Age : 15-124

1048   ICD-10-CM 2017

☑7th **T52.2X2** **Toxic effect of homologues of benzene,** intentional self-harm

☑7th **T52.2X3** **Toxic effect of homologues of benzene,** assault

☑7th **T52.2X4** **Toxic effect of homologues of benzene,** undetermined

☑5th **T52.3** **Toxic effects of glycols**

  ☑6th **T52.3X** **Toxic effects of** glycols

    ☑7th **T52.3X1** **Toxic effect of glycols,** accidental (unintentional)
         Toxic effects of glycols NOS

    ☑7th **T52.3X2** **Toxic effect of glycols,** intentional self-harm

    ☑7th **T52.3X3** **Toxic effect of glycols,** assault

    ☑7th **T52.3X4** **Toxic effect of glycols,** undetermined

☑5th **T52.4** **Toxic effects of ketones**

  ☑6th **T52.4X** **Toxic effects of** ketones

    ☑7th **T52.4X1** **Toxic effect of ketones,** accidental (unintentional)
         Toxic effects of ketones NOS

    ☑7th **T52.4X2** **Toxic effect of ketones,** intentional self-harm

    ☑7th **T52.4X3** **Toxic effect of ketones,** assault

    ☑7th **T52.4X4** **Toxic effect of ketones,** undetermined

☑5th **T52.8** **Toxic effects of other organic solvents**

  ☑6th **T52.8X** **Toxic effects of** other organic solvents

    ☑7th **T52.8X1** **Toxic effect of other organic solvents,** accidental (unintentional)
         Toxic effects of other organic solvents NOS

    ☑7th **T52.8X2** **Toxic effect of other organic solvents,** intentional self-harm

    ☑7th **T52.8X3** **Toxic effect of other organic solvents,** assault

    ☑7th **T52.8X4** **Toxic effect of other organic solvents,** undetermined

☑5th **T52.9** **Toxic effects of** unspecified organic solvent

  √x7th **T52.91** **Toxic effect of unspecified organic solvent,** accidental (unintentional)   ▽

  √x7th **T52.92** **Toxic effect of unspecified organic solvent,** intentional self-harm   ▽

  √x7th **T52.93** **Toxic effect of unspecified organic solvent,** assault   ▽

  √x7th **T52.94** **Toxic effect of unspecified organic solvent,** undetermined   ▽

☑4th **T53** **Toxic effect of halogen derivatives of aliphatic and aromatic hydrocarbons**

> The appropriate 7th character is to be added to each code from category T53.
> A   initial encounter
> D   subsequent encounter
> S   sequela

☑5th **T53.0** **Toxic effects of carbon tetrachloride**
     Toxic effects of tetrachloromethane

  ☑6th **T53.0X** **Toxic effects of** carbon tetrachloride

    ☑7th **T53.0X1** **Toxic effect of carbon tetrachloride,** accidental (unintentional)
         Toxic effects of carbon tetrachloride NOS

    ☑7th **T53.0X2** **Toxic effect of carbon tetrachloride,** intentional self-harm

    ☑7th **T53.0X3** **Toxic effect of carbon tetrachloride,** assault

    ☑7th **T53.0X4** **Toxic effect of carbon tetrachloride,** undetermined

☑5th **T53.1** **Toxic effects of chloroform**
     Toxic effects of trichloromethane

  ☑6th **T53.1X** **Toxic effects of** chloroform

    ☑7th **T53.1X1** **Toxic effect of chloroform,** accidental (unintentional)
         Toxic effects of chloroform NOS

    ☑7th **T53.1X2** **Toxic effect of chloroform,** intentional self-harm

    ☑7th **T53.1X3** **Toxic effect of chloroform,** assault

    ☑7th **T53.1X4** **Toxic effect of chloroform,** undetermined

☑5th **T53.2** **Toxic effects of trichloroethylene**
     Toxic effects of trichloroethene

  ☑6th **T53.2X** **Toxic effects of** trichloroethylene

    ☑7th **T53.2X1** **Toxic effect of trichloroethylene,** accidental (unintentional)
         Toxic effects of trichloroethylene NOS

    ☑7th **T53.2X2** **Toxic effect of trichloroethylene,** intentional self-harm

    ☑7th **T53.2X3** **Toxic effect of trichloroethylene,** assault

    ☑7th **T53.2X4** **Toxic effect of trichloroethylene,** undetermined

☑5th **T53.3** **Toxic effects of tetrachloroethylene**
     Toxic effects of perchloroethylene
     Toxic effect of tetrachloroethene

  ☑6th **T53.3X** **Toxic effects of** tetrachloroethylene

    ☑7th **T53.3X1** **Toxic effect of tetrachloroethylene,** accidental (unintentional)
         Toxic effects of tetrachloroethylene NOS

    ☑7th **T53.3X2** **Toxic effect of tetrachloroethylene,** intentional self-harm

    ☑7th **T53.3X3** **Toxic effect of tetrachloroethylene,** assault

    ☑7th **T53.3X4** **Toxic effect of tetrachloroethylene,** undetermined

☑5th **T53.4** **Toxic effects of dichloromethane**
     Toxic effects of methylene chloride

  ☑6th **T53.4X** **Toxic effects of** dichloromethane

    ☑7th **T53.4X1** **Toxic effect of dichloromethane,** accidental (unintentional)
         Toxic effects of dichloromethane NOS

    ☑7th **T53.4X2** **Toxic effect of dichloromethane,** intentional self-harm

    ☑7th **T53.4X3** **Toxic effect of dichloromethane,** assault

    ☑7th **T53.4X4** **Toxic effect of dichloromethane,** undetermined

☑5th **T53.5** **Toxic effects of chlorofluorocarbons**

  ☑6th **T53.5X** **Toxic effects of** chlorofluorocarbons

    ☑7th **T53.5X1** **Toxic effect of chlorofluorocarbons,** accidental (unintentional)
         Toxic effects of chlorofluorocarbons NOS

    ☑7th **T53.5X2** **Toxic effect of chlorofluorocarbons,** intentional self-harm

    ☑7th **T53.5X3** **Toxic effect of chlorofluorocarbons,** assault

    ☑7th **T53.5X4** **Toxic effect of chlorofluorocarbons,** undetermined

☑6th **T53.6** **Toxic effects of other halogen derivatives of aliphatic hydrocarbons**

  ☑6th **T53.6X** **Toxic effects of** other halogen derivatives of aliphatic hydrocarbons

    ☑7th **T53.6X1** **Toxic effect of other halogen derivatives of aliphatic hydrocarbons,** accidental (unintentional)
         Toxic effects of other halogen derivatives of aliphatic hydrocarbons NOS

    ☑7th **T53.6X2** **Toxic effect of other halogen derivatives of aliphatic hydrocarbons,** intentional self-harm

    ☑7th **T53.6X3** **Toxic effect of other halogen derivatives of aliphatic hydrocarbons,** assault

    ☑7th **T53.6X4** **Toxic effect of other halogen derivatives of aliphatic hydrocarbons,** undetermined

☑5th **T53.7** **Toxic effects of other halogen derivatives of aromatic hydrocarbons**

  ☑6th **T53.7X** **Toxic effects of** other halogen derivatives of aromatic hydrocarbons

    ☑7th **T53.7X1** **Toxic effect of other halogen derivatives of aromatic hydrocarbons,** accidental (unintentional)
         Toxic effects of other halogen derivatives of aromatic hydrocarbons NOS

    ☑7th **T53.7X2** **Toxic effect of other halogen derivatives of aromatic hydrocarbons,** intentional self-harm

    ☑7th **T53.7X3** **Toxic effect of other halogen derivatives of aromatic hydrocarbons,** assault

    ☑7th **T53.7X4** **Toxic effect of other halogen derivatives of aromatic hydrocarbons,** undetermined

☑5th **T53.9** **Toxic effects of unspecified halogen derivatives of aliphatic and aromatic hydrocarbons**

  √x7th **T53.91** **Toxic effect of unspecified halogen derivatives of aliphatic and aromatic hydrocarbons,** accidental (unintentional)   ▽

☑ Additional Character Required   √x7th Placeholder Alert   Manifestation Dx   ▽Unspecified Dx   ►◄ Revised Text   ● New Code   ▲ Revised Code Title

√x7ᵗʰ **T53.92** **Toxic effect of unspecified halogen derivatives of aliphatic and aromatic hydrocarbons, intentional self-harm** ▽

√x7ᵗʰ **T53.93** **Toxic effect of unspecified halogen derivatives of aliphatic and aromatic hydrocarbons, assault** ▽

√x7ᵗʰ **T53.94** **Toxic effect of unspecified halogen derivatives of aliphatic and aromatic hydrocarbons, undetermined** ▽

√4ᵗʰ **T54 Toxic effect of corrosive substances**

> The appropriate 7th character is to be added to each code from category T54.
> A   initial encounter
> D   subsequent encounter
> S   sequela

√5ᵗʰ **T54.0 Toxic effects of phenol and phenol homologues**

√6ᵗʰ **T54.0X** **Toxic effects of phenol and phenol homologues**

√7ᵗʰ **T54.0X1** **Toxic effect of phenol and phenol homologues, accidental (unintentional)**
Toxic effects of phenol and phenol homologues NOS

√7ᵗʰ **T54.0X2** **Toxic effect of phenol and phenol homologues, intentional self-harm**

√7ᵗʰ **T54.0X3** **Toxic effect of phenol and phenol homologues, assault**

√7ᵗʰ **T54.0X4** **Toxic effect of phenol and phenol homologues, undetermined**

√5ᵗʰ **T54.1 Toxic effects of other corrosive organic compounds**

√6ᵗʰ **T54.1X** **Toxic effects of other corrosive organic compounds**

√7ᵗʰ **T54.1X1** **Toxic effect of other corrosive organic compounds, accidental (unintentional)**
Toxic effects of other corrosive organic compounds NOS

√7ᵗʰ **T54.1X2** **Toxic effect of other corrosive organic compounds, intentional self-harm**

√7ᵗʰ **T54.1X3** **Toxic effect of other corrosive organic compounds, assault**

√7ᵗʰ **T54.1X4** **Toxic effect of other corrosive organic compounds, undetermined**

√5ᵗʰ **T54.2 Toxic effects of corrosive acids and acid-like substances**

Toxic effects of hydrochloric acid
Toxic effects of sulfuric acid

√6ᵗʰ **T54.2X** **Toxic effects of corrosive acids and acid-like substances**

√7ᵗʰ **T54.2X1** **Toxic effect of corrosive acids and acid-like substances, accidental (unintentional)**
Toxic effects of corrosive acids and acid-like substances NOS

√7ᵗʰ **T54.2X2** **Toxic effect of corrosive acids and acid-like substances, intentional self-harm**

√7ᵗʰ **T54.2X3** **Toxic effect of corrosive acids and acid-like substances, assault**

√7ᵗʰ **T54.2X4** **Toxic effect of corrosive acids and acid-like substances, undetermined**

√5ᵗʰ **T54.3 Toxic effects of corrosive alkalis and alkali-like substances**

Toxic effects of potassium hydroxide
Toxic effects of sodium hydroxide

√6ᵗʰ **T54.3X** **Toxic effects of corrosive alkalis and alkali-like substances**

√7ᵗʰ **T54.3X1** **Toxic effect of corrosive alkalis and alkali-like substances, accidental (unintentional)**
Toxic effects of corrosive alkalis and alkali-like substances NOS

√7ᵗʰ **T54.3X2** **Toxic effect of corrosive alkalis and alkali-like substances, intentional self-harm**

√7ᵗʰ **T54.3X3** **Toxic effect of corrosive alkalis and alkali-like substances, assault**

√7ᵗʰ **T54.3X4** **Toxic effect of corrosive alkalis and alkali-like substances, undetermined**

√5ᵗʰ **T54.9 Toxic effects of unspecified corrosive substance**

√x7ᵗʰ **T54.91** **Toxic effect of unspecified corrosive substance, accidental (unintentional)** ▽

√x7ᵗʰ **T54.92** **Toxic effect of unspecified corrosive substance, intentional self-harm** ▽

√x7ᵗʰ **T54.93** **Toxic effect of unspecified corrosive substance, assault** ▽

√x7ᵗʰ **T54.94** **Toxic effect of unspecified corrosive substance, undetermined** ▽

√4ᵗʰ **T55 Toxic effect of soaps and detergents**

> The appropriate 7th character is to be added to each code from category T55.
> A   initial encounter
> D   subsequent encounter
> S   sequela

√5ᵗʰ **T55.0 Toxic effect of soaps**

√6ᵗʰ **T55.0X** **Toxic effect of soaps**

√7ᵗʰ **T55.0X1** **Toxic effect of soaps, accidental (unintentional)**
Toxic effect of soaps NOS

√7ᵗʰ **T55.0X2** **Toxic effect of soaps, intentional self-harm**

√7ᵗʰ **T55.0X3** **Toxic effect of soaps, assault**

√7ᵗʰ **T55.0X4** **Toxic effect of soaps, undetermined**

√5ᵗʰ **T55.1 Toxic effect of detergents**

√6ᵗʰ **T55.1X** **Toxic effect of detergents**

√7ᵗʰ **T55.1X1** **Toxic effect of detergents, accidental (unintentional)**
Toxic effect of detergents NOS

√7ᵗʰ **T55.1X2** **Toxic effect of detergents, intentional self-harm**

√7ᵗʰ **T55.1X3** **Toxic effect of detergents, assault**

√7ᵗʰ **T55.1X4** **Toxic effect of detergents, undetermined**

√4ᵗʰ **T56 Toxic effect of metals**

INCLUDES toxic effects of fumes and vapors of metals
toxic effects of metals from all sources, except medicinal substances
Use additional code to identify any retained metal foreign body, if applicable (Z18.0-, T18.1-)
EXCLUDES 1 arsenic and its compounds (T57.0)
manganese and its compounds (T57.2)

> The appropriate 7th character is to be added to each code from category T56.
> A   initial encounter
> D   subsequent encounter
> S   sequela

√5ᵗʰ **T56.0 Toxic effects of lead and its compounds**

√6ᵗʰ **T56.0X** **Toxic effects of lead and its compounds**

√7ᵗʰ **T56.0X1** **Toxic effect of lead and its compounds, accidental (unintentional)**
Toxic effects of lead and its compounds NOS

√7ᵗʰ **T56.0X2** **Toxic effect of lead and its compounds, intentional self-harm**

√7ᵗʰ **T56.0X3** **Toxic effect of lead and its compounds, assault**

√7ᵗʰ **T56.0X4** **Toxic effect of lead and its compounds, undetermined**

√5ᵗʰ **T56.1 Toxic effects of mercury and its compounds**

√6ᵗʰ **T56.1X** **Toxic effects of mercury and its compounds**

√7ᵗʰ **T56.1X1** **Toxic effect of mercury and its compounds, accidental (unintentional)**
Toxic effects of mercury and its compounds NOS

√7ᵗʰ **T56.1X2** **Toxic effect of mercury and its compounds, intentional self-harm**

√7ᵗʰ **T56.1X3** **Toxic effect of mercury and its compounds, assault**

√7ᵗʰ **T56.1X4** **Toxic effect of mercury and its compounds, undetermined**

√5ᵗʰ **T56.2 Toxic effects of chromium and its compounds**

√6ᵗʰ **T56.2X** **Toxic effects of chromium and its compounds**

√7ᵗʰ **T56.2X1** **Toxic effect of chromium and its compounds, accidental (unintentional)**
Toxic effects of chromium and its compounds NOS

√7ᵗʰ **T56.2X2** **Toxic effect of chromium and its compounds, intentional self-harm**

√7ᵗʰ **T56.2X3** **Toxic effect of chromium and its compounds, assault**

√7ᵗʰ **T56.2X4** **Toxic effect of chromium and its compounds, undetermined**

√5ᵗʰ **T56.3 Toxic effects of cadmium and its compounds**

EXCLUDES 1 Not coded here   **EXCLUDES 2** Not included here   N Newborn Age : 0   P Pediatric Age : 0-17   M Maternity Age : 12-55   A Adult Age : 15-124

1050

ICD-10-CM 2017

√6ᵗʰ **T56.3X**   **Toxic effects of cadmium and its compounds**

    √7ᵗʰ **T56.3X1** **Toxic effect of cadmium and its compounds, accidental (unintentional)**
Toxic effects of cadmium and its compounds NOS

    √7ᵗʰ **T56.3X2** **Toxic effect of cadmium and its compounds, intentional self-harm**

    √7ᵗʰ **T56.3X3** **Toxic effect of cadmium and its compounds, assault**

    √7ᵗʰ **T56.3X4** **Toxic effect of cadmium and its compounds, undetermined**

√5ᵗʰ **T56.4**   **Toxic effects of copper and its compounds**

   √6ᵗʰ **T56.4X**   **Toxic effects of copper and its compounds**

    √7ᵗʰ **T56.4X1** **Toxic effect of copper and its compounds, accidental (unintentional)**
Toxic effects of copper and its compounds NOS

    √7ᵗʰ **T56.4X2** **Toxic effect of copper and its compounds, intentional self-harm**

    √7ᵗʰ **T56.4X3** **Toxic effect of copper and its compounds, assault**

    √7ᵗʰ **T56.4X4** **Toxic effect of copper and its compounds, undetermined**

√5ᵗʰ **T56.5**   **Toxic effects of zinc and its compounds**

   √6ᵗʰ **T56.5X**   **Toxic effects of zinc and its compounds**

    √7ᵗʰ **T56.5X1** **Toxic effect of zinc and its compounds, accidental (unintentional)**
Toxic effects of zinc and its compounds NOS

    √7ᵗʰ **T56.5X2** **Toxic effect of zinc and its compounds, intentional self-harm**

    √7ᵗʰ **T56.5X3** **Toxic effect of zinc and its compounds, assault**

    √7ᵗʰ **T56.5X4** **Toxic effect of zinc and its compounds, undetermined**

√5ᵗʰ **T56.6**   **Toxic effects of tin and its compounds**

   √6ᵗʰ **T56.6X**   **Toxic effects of tin and its compounds**

    √7ᵗʰ **T56.6X1** **Toxic effect of tin and its compounds, accidental (unintentional)**
Toxic effects of tin and its compounds NOS

    √7ᵗʰ **T56.6X2** **Toxic effect of tin and its compounds, intentional self-harm**

    √7ᵗʰ **T56.6X3** **Toxic effect of tin and its compounds, assault**

    √7ᵗʰ **T56.6X4** **Toxic effect of tin and its compounds, undetermined**

√5ᵗʰ **T56.7**   **Toxic effects of beryllium and its compounds**

   √6ᵗʰ **T56.7X**   **Toxic effects of beryllium and its compounds**

    √7ᵗʰ **T56.7X1** **Toxic effect of beryllium and its compounds, accidental (unintentional)**
Toxic effects of beryllium and its compounds NOS

    √7ᵗʰ **T56.7X2** **Toxic effect of beryllium and its compounds, intentional self-harm**

    √7ᵗʰ **T56.7X3** **Toxic effect of beryllium and its compounds, assault**

    √7ᵗʰ **T56.7X4** **Toxic effect of beryllium and its compounds, undetermined**

√5ᵗʰ **T56.8**   **Toxic effects of other metals**

   √6ᵗʰ **T56.81**   **Toxic effect of thallium**

    √7ᵗʰ **T56.811** **Toxic effect of thallium, accidental (unintentional)**
Toxic effect of thallium NOS

    √7ᵗʰ **T56.812** **Toxic effect of thallium, intentional self-harm**

    √7ᵗʰ **T56.813** **Toxic effect of thallium, assault**

    √7ᵗʰ **T56.814** **Toxic effect of thallium, undetermined**

   √6ᵗʰ **T56.89**   **Toxic effects of other metals**

    √7ᵗʰ **T56.891** **Toxic effect of other metals, accidental (unintentional)**
Toxic effects of other metals NOS

    √7ᵗʰ **T56.892** **Toxic effect of other metals, intentional self-harm**

    √7ᵗʰ **T56.893** **Toxic effect of other metals, assault**

    √7ᵗʰ **T56.894** **Toxic effect of other metals, undetermined**

√5ᵗʰ **T56.9**   **Toxic effects of unspecified metal**

   √x7ᵗʰ **T56.91** **Toxic effect of unspecified metal, accidental (unintentional)** ▽

   √x7ᵗʰ **T56.92** **Toxic effect of unspecified metal, intentional self-harm** ▽

   √x7ᵗʰ **T56.93** **Toxic effect of unspecified metal, assault** ▽

   √x7ᵗʰ **T56.94** **Toxic effect of unspecified metal, undetermined** ▽

√4ᵗʰ **T57**   **Toxic effect of other inorganic substances**

> The appropriate 7th character is to be added to each code from category T57.
> A   initial encounter
> D   subsequent encounter
> S   sequela

√5ᵗʰ **T57.0**   **Toxic effect of arsenic and its compounds**

   √6ᵗʰ **T57.0X**   **Toxic effect of arsenic and its compounds**

    √7ᵗʰ **T57.0X1** **Toxic effect of arsenic and its compounds, accidental (unintentional)**
Toxic effect of arsenic and its compounds NOS

    √7ᵗʰ **T57.0X2** **Toxic effect of arsenic and its compounds, intentional self-harm**

    √7ᵗʰ **T57.0X3** **Toxic effect of arsenic and its compounds, assault**

    √7ᵗʰ **T57.0X4** **Toxic effect of arsenic and its compounds, undetermined**

√5ᵗʰ **T57.1**   **Toxic effect of phosphorus and its compounds**

   EXCLUDES 1 *organophosphate insecticides (T60.0)*

   √6ᵗʰ **T57.1X**   **Toxic effect of phosphorus and its compounds**

    √7ᵗʰ **T57.1X1** **Toxic effect of phosphorus and its compounds, accidental (unintentional)**
Toxic effect of phosphorus and its compounds NOS

    √7ᵗʰ **T57.1X2** **Toxic effect of phosphorus and its compounds, intentional self-harm**

    √7ᵗʰ **T57.1X3** **Toxic effect of phosphorus and its compounds, assault**

    √7ᵗʰ **T57.1X4** **Toxic effect of phosphorus and its compounds, undetermined**

√5ᵗʰ **T57.2**   **Toxic effect of manganese and its compounds**

   √6ᵗʰ **T57.2X**   **Toxic effect of manganese and its compounds**

    √7ᵗʰ **T57.2X1** **Toxic effect of manganese and its compounds, accidental (unintentional)**
Toxic effect of manganese and its compounds NOS

    √7ᵗʰ **T57.2X2** **Toxic effect of manganese and its compounds, intentional self-harm**

    √7ᵗʰ **T57.2X3** **Toxic effect of manganese and its compounds, assault**

    √7ᵗʰ **T57.2X4** **Toxic effect of manganese and its compounds, undetermined**

√5ᵗʰ **T57.3**   **Toxic effect of hydrogen cyanide**

   √6ᵗʰ **T57.3X**   **Toxic effect of hydrogen cyanide**

    √7ᵗʰ **T57.3X1** **Toxic effect of hydrogen cyanide, accidental (unintentional)**
Toxic effect of hydrogen cyanide NOS

    √7ᵗʰ **T57.3X2** **Toxic effect of hydrogen cyanide, intentional self-harm**

    √7ᵗʰ **T57.3X3** **Toxic effect of hydrogen cyanide, assault**

    √7ᵗʰ **T57.3X4** **Toxic effect of hydrogen cyanide, undetermined**

√5ᵗʰ **T57.8**   **Toxic effect of other specified inorganic substances**

   √6ᵗʰ **T57.8X**   **Toxic effect of other specified inorganic substances**

    √7ᵗʰ **T57.8X1** **Toxic effect of other specified inorganic substances, accidental (unintentional)**
Toxic effect of other specified inorganic substances NOS

    √7ᵗʰ **T57.8X2** **Toxic effect of other specified inorganic substances, intentional self-harm**

    √7ᵗʰ **T57.8X3** **Toxic effect of other specified inorganic substances, assault**

    √7ᵗʰ **T57.8X4** **Toxic effect of other specified inorganic substances, undetermined**

√5ᵗʰ **T57.9**   **Toxic effect of unspecified inorganic substance**

   √x7ᵗʰ **T57.91** **Toxic effect of unspecified inorganic substance, accidental (unintentional)** ▽

   √x7ᵗʰ **T57.92** **Toxic effect of unspecified inorganic substance, intentional self-harm** ▽

☑ Additional Character Required   √x7ᵗʰ Placeholder Alert   Manifestation Dx   ▽ Unspecified Dx   ►◄ Revised Text   ● New Code   ▲ Revised Code Title

ICD-10-CM 2017   **1051**

√x7ᵗʰ   **T57.93**   **Toxic effect of unspecified inorganic substance, assault** ▽

√x7ᵗʰ   **T57.94**   **Toxic effect of unspecified inorganic substance, undetermined** ▽

√4ᵗʰ   **T58**   **Toxic effect of carbon monoxide**

> INCLUDES   asphyxiation from carbon monoxide
> toxic effect of carbon monoxide from all sources

> The appropriate 7th character is to be added to each code from category T58.
> A   initial encounter
> D   subsequent encounter
> S   sequela

√5ᵗʰ   **T58.0**   **Toxic effect of carbon monoxide from motor vehicle exhaust**

> Toxic effect of exhaust gas from gas engine
> Toxic effect of exhaust gas from motor pump

√x7ᵗʰ   **T58.01**   **Toxic effect of carbon monoxide from motor vehicle exhaust, accidental (unintentional)**

√x7ᵗʰ   **T58.02**   **Toxic effect of carbon monoxide from motor vehicle exhaust, intentional self-harm**

√x7ᵗʰ   **T58.03**   **Toxic effect of carbon monoxide from motor vehicle exhaust, assault**

√x7ᵗʰ   **T58.04**   **Toxic effect of carbon monoxide from motor vehicle exhaust, undetermined**

√5ᵗʰ   **T58.1**   **Toxic effect of carbon monoxide from utility gas**

> Toxic effect of acetylene
> Toxic effect of gas NOS used for lighting, heating, cooking
> Toxic effect of water gas

√x7ᵗʰ   **T58.11**   **Toxic effect of carbon monoxide from utility gas, accidental (unintentional)**

√x7ᵗʰ   **T58.12**   **Toxic effect of carbon monoxide from utility gas, intentional self-harm**

√x7ᵗʰ   **T58.13**   **Toxic effect of carbon monoxide from utility gas, assault**

√x7ᵗʰ   **T58.14**   **Toxic effect of carbon monoxide from utility gas, undetermined**

√5ᵗʰ   **T58.2**   **Toxic effect of carbon monoxide from incomplete combustion of other domestic fuels**

> Toxic effect of carbon monoxide from incomplete combustion of coal, coke, kerosene, wood

√6ᵗʰ   **T58.2X**   **Toxic effect of carbon monoxide from incomplete combustion of other domestic fuels**

7ᵗʰ   **T58.2X1**   **Toxic effect of carbon monoxide from incomplete combustion of other domestic fuels, accidental (unintentional)**

7ᵗʰ   **T58.2X2**   **Toxic effect of carbon monoxide from incomplete combustion of other domestic fuels, intentional self-harm**

7ᵗʰ   **T58.2X3**   **Toxic effect of carbon monoxide from incomplete combustion of other domestic fuels, assault**

7ᵗʰ   **T58.2X4**   **Toxic effect of carbon monoxide from incomplete combustion of other domestic fuels, undetermined**

√5ᵗʰ   **T58.8**   **Toxic effect of carbon monoxide from other source**

> Toxic effect of carbon monoxide from blast furnace gas
> Toxic effect of carbon monoxide from fuels in industrial use
> Toxic effect of carbon monoxide from kiln vapor

√6ᵗʰ   **T58.8X**   **Toxic effect of carbon monoxide from other source**

7ᵗʰ   **T58.8X1**   **Toxic effect of carbon monoxide from other source, accidental (unintentional)**

7ᵗʰ   **T58.8X2**   **Toxic effect of carbon monoxide from other source, intentional self-harm**

7ᵗʰ   **T58.8X3**   **Toxic effect of carbon monoxide from other source, assault**

7ᵗʰ   **T58.8X4**   **Toxic effect of carbon monoxide from other source, undetermined**

√5ᵗʰ   **T58.9**   **Toxic effect of carbon monoxide from unspecified source**

√x7ᵗʰ   **T58.91**   **Toxic effect of carbon monoxide from unspecified source, accidental (unintentional)** ▽

√x7ᵗʰ   **T58.92**   **Toxic effect of carbon monoxide from unspecified source, intentional self-harm** ▽

√x7ᵗʰ   **T58.93**   **Toxic effect of carbon monoxide from unspecified source, assault** ▽

√x7ᵗʰ   **T58.94**   **Toxic effect of carbon monoxide from unspecified source, undetermined** ▽

√4ᵗʰ   **T59**   **Toxic effect of other gases, fumes and vapors**

> INCLUDES   aerosol propellants
> EXCLUDES 1   *chlorofluorocarbons (T53.5)*

> The appropriate 7th character is to be added to each code from category T59.
> A   initial encounter
> D   subsequent encounter
> S   sequela

√5ᵗʰ   **T59.0**   **Toxic effect of nitrogen oxides**

√6ᵗʰ   **T59.0X**   **Toxic effect of nitrogen oxides**

7ᵗʰ   **T59.0X1**   **Toxic effect of nitrogen oxides, accidental (unintentional)**
> Toxic effect of nitrogen oxides NOS

7ᵗʰ   **T59.0X2**   **Toxic effect of nitrogen oxides, intentional self-harm**

7ᵗʰ   **T59.0X3**   **Toxic effect of nitrogen oxides, assault**

7ᵗʰ   **T59.0X4**   **Toxic effect of nitrogen oxides, undetermined**

√5ᵗʰ   **T59.1**   **Toxic effect of sulfur dioxide**

√6ᵗʰ   **T59.1X**   **Toxic effect of sulfur dioxide**

7ᵗʰ   **T59.1X1**   **Toxic effect of sulfur dioxide, accidental (unintentional)**
> Toxic effect of sulfur dioxide NOS

7ᵗʰ   **T59.1X2**   **Toxic effect of sulfur dioxide, intentional self-harm**

7ᵗʰ   **T59.1X3**   **Toxic effect of sulfur dioxide, assault**

7ᵗʰ   **T59.1X4**   **Toxic effect of sulfur dioxide, undetermined**

√5ᵗʰ   **T59.2**   **Toxic effect of formaldehyde**

√6ᵗʰ   **T59.2X**   **Toxic effect of formaldehyde**

7ᵗʰ   **T59.2X1**   **Toxic effect of formaldehyde, accidental (unintentional)**
> Toxic effect of formaldehyde NOS

7ᵗʰ   **T59.2X2**   **Toxic effect of formaldehyde, intentional self-harm**

7ᵗʰ   **T59.2X3**   **Toxic effect of formaldehyde, assault**

7ᵗʰ   **T59.2X4**   **Toxic effect of formaldehyde, undetermined**

√5ᵗʰ   **T59.3**   **Toxic effect of lacrimogenic gas**

> Toxic effect of tear gas

√6ᵗʰ   **T59.3X**   **Toxic effect of lacrimogenic gas**

7ᵗʰ   **T59.3X1**   **Toxic effect of lacrimogenic gas, accidental (unintentional)**
> Toxic effect of lacrimogenic gas NOS

7ᵗʰ   **T59.3X2**   **Toxic effect of lacrimogenic gas, intentional self-harm**

7ᵗʰ   **T59.3X3**   **Toxic effect of lacrimogenic gas, assault**

7ᵗʰ   **T59.3X4**   **Toxic effect of lacrimogenic gas, undetermined**

√5ᵗʰ   **T59.4**   **Toxic effect of chlorine gas**

√6ᵗʰ   **T59.4X**   **Toxic effect of chlorine gas**

7ᵗʰ   **T59.4X1**   **Toxic effect of chlorine gas, accidental (unintentional)**
> Toxic effect of chlorine gas NOS

7ᵗʰ   **T59.4X2**   **Toxic effect of chlorine gas, intentional self-harm**

7ᵗʰ   **T59.4X3**   **Toxic effect of chlorine gas, assault**

7ᵗʰ   **T59.4X4**   **Toxic effect of chlorine gas, undetermined**

√5ᵗʰ   **T59.5**   **Toxic effect of fluorine gas and hydrogen fluoride**

√6ᵗʰ   **T59.5X**   **Toxic effect of fluorine gas and hydrogen fluoride**

7ᵗʰ   **T59.5X1**   **Toxic effect of fluorine gas and hydrogen fluoride, accidental (unintentional)**
> Toxic effect of fluorine gas and hydrogen fluoride NOS

7ᵗʰ   **T59.5X2**   **Toxic effect of fluorine gas and hydrogen fluoride, intentional self-harm**

7ᵗʰ   **T59.5X3**   **Toxic effect of fluorine gas and hydrogen fluoride, assault**

7ᵗʰ   **T59.5X4**   **Toxic effect of fluorine gas and hydrogen fluoride, undetermined**

√5ᵗʰ   **T59.6**   **Toxic effect of hydrogen sulfide**

√6ᵗʰ   **T59.6X**   **Toxic effect of hydrogen sulfide**

7ᵗʰ   **T59.6X1**   **Toxic effect of hydrogen sulfide, accidental (unintentional)**
> Toxic effect of hydrogen sulfide NOS

EXCLUDES 1 Not coded here   EXCLUDES 2 Not included here   N Newborn Age : 0   P Pediatric Age : 0-17   M Maternity Age : 12-55   A Adult Age : 15-124

1052

ICD-10-CM 2017

√7ᵗʰ **T59.6X2 Toxic effect of hydrogen sulfide, intentional self-harm**

√7ᵗʰ **T59.6X3 Toxic effect of hydrogen sulfide, assault**

√7ᵗʰ **T59.6X4 Toxic effect of hydrogen sulfide, undetermined**

√5ᵗʰ **T59.7 Toxic effect of carbon dioxide**

    √6ᵗʰ **T59.7X Toxic effect of carbon dioxide**

       √7ᵗʰ **T59.7X1 Toxic effect of carbon dioxide, accidental (unintentional)**
Toxic effect of carbon dioxide NOS

       √7ᵗʰ **T59.7X2 Toxic effect of carbon dioxide, intentional self-harm**

       √7ᵗʰ **T59.7X3 Toxic effect of carbon dioxide, assault**

       √7ᵗʰ **T59.7X4 Toxic effect of carbon dioxide, undetermined**

√5ᵗʰ **T59.8 Toxic effect of other specified gases, fumes and vapors**

    √6ᵗʰ **T59.81 Toxic effect of smoke**
Smoke inhalation
EXCLUDES 2   *toxic effect of cigarette (tobacco) smoke (T65.22-)*

       √7ᵗʰ **T59.811 Toxic effect of smoke, accidental (unintentional)**
Toxic effect of smoke NOS
AHA: 2013,4Q,121

       √7ᵗʰ **T59.812 Toxic effect of smoke, intentional self-harm**

       √7ᵗʰ **T59.813 Toxic effect of smoke, assault**

       √7ᵗʰ **T59.814 Toxic effect of smoke, undetermined**

    √6ᵗʰ **T59.89 Toxic effect of other specified gases, fumes and vapors**

       √7ᵗʰ **T59.891 Toxic effect of other specified gases, fumes and vapors, accidental (unintentional)**

       √7ᵗʰ **T59.892 Toxic effect of other specified gases, fumes and vapors, intentional self-harm**

       √7ᵗʰ **T59.893 Toxic effect of other specified gases, fumes and vapors, assault**

       √7ᵗʰ **T59.894 Toxic effect of other specified gases, fumes and vapors, undetermined**

√5ᵗʰ **T59.9 Toxic effect of unspecified gases, fumes and vapors**

    √x7ᵗʰ **T59.91 Toxic effect of unspecified gases, fumes and vapors, accidental (unintentional)** ▽

    √x7ᵗʰ **T59.92 Toxic effect of unspecified gases, fumes and vapors, intentional self-harm** ▽

    √x7ᵗʰ **T59.93 Toxic effect of unspecified gases, fumes and vapors, assault** ▽

    √x7ᵗʰ **T59.94 Toxic effect of unspecified gases, fumes and vapors, undetermined** ▽

T60 Toxic effect of pesticides

    INCLUDES   toxic effect of wood preservatives

√4ᵗʰ   The appropriate 7th character is to be added to each code from category T60.
A   initial encounter
D   subsequent encounter
S   sequela

√5ᵗʰ **T60.0 Toxic effect of organophosphate and carbamate insecticides**

    √6ᵗʰ **T60.0X Toxic effect of organophosphate and carbamate insecticides**

       √7ᵗʰ **T60.0X1 Toxic effect of organophosphate and carbamate insecticides, accidental (unintentional)**
Toxic effect of organophosphate and carbamate insecticides NOS

       √7ᵗʰ **T60.0X2 Toxic effect of organophosphate and carbamate insecticides, intentional self-harm**

       √7ᵗʰ **T60.0X3 Toxic effect of organophosphate and carbamate insecticides, assault**

       √7ᵗʰ **T60.0X4 Toxic effect of organophosphate and carbamate insecticides, undetermined**

√5ᵗʰ **T60.1 Toxic effect of halogenated insecticides**
EXCLUDES 1   *chlorinated hydrocarbon (T53.-)*

    √6ᵗʰ **T60.1X Toxic effect of halogenated insecticides**

       √7ᵗʰ **T60.1X1 Toxic effect of halogenated insecticides, accidental (unintentional)**
Toxic effect of halogenated insecticides NOS

       √7ᵗʰ **T60.1X2 Toxic effect of halogenated insecticides, intentional self-harm**

       √7ᵗʰ **T60.1X3 Toxic effect of halogenated insecticides, assault**

       √7ᵗʰ **T60.1X4 Toxic effect of halogenated insecticides, undetermined**

√5ᵗʰ **T60.2 Toxic effect of other insecticides**

    √6ᵗʰ **T60.2X Toxic effect of other insecticides**

       √7ᵗʰ **T60.2X1 Toxic effect of other insecticides, accidental (unintentional)**
Toxic effect of other insecticides NOS

       √7ᵗʰ **T60.2X2 Toxic effect of other insecticides, intentional self-harm**

       √7ᵗʰ **T60.2X3 Toxic effect of other insecticides, assault**

       √7ᵗʰ **T60.2X4 Toxic effect of other insecticides, undetermined**

√5ᵗʰ **T60.3 Toxic effect of herbicides and fungicides**

    √6ᵗʰ **T60.3X Toxic effect of herbicides and fungicides**

       √7ᵗʰ **T60.3X1 Toxic effect of herbicides and fungicides, accidental (unintentional)**
Toxic effect of herbicides and fungicides NOS

       √7ᵗʰ **T60.3X2 Toxic effect of herbicides and fungicides, intentional self-harm**

       √7ᵗʰ **T60.3X3 Toxic effect of herbicides and fungicides, assault**

       √7ᵗʰ **T60.3X4 Toxic effect of herbicides and fungicides, undetermined**

√5ᵗʰ **T60.4 Toxic effect of rodenticides**
EXCLUDES 1   *strychnine and its salts (T65.1)*
thallium (T56.81-)

    √6ᵗʰ **T60.4X Toxic effect of rodenticides**

       √7ᵗʰ **T60.4X1 Toxic effect of rodenticides, accidental (unintentional)**
Toxic effect of rodenticides NOS

       √7ᵗʰ **T60.4X2 Toxic effect of rodenticides, intentional self-harm**

       √7ᵗʰ **T60.4X3 Toxic effect of rodenticides, assault**

       √7ᵗʰ **T60.4X4 Toxic effect of rodenticides, undetermined**

√5ᵗʰ **T60.8 Toxic effect of other pesticides**

    √6ᵗʰ **T60.8X Toxic effect of other pesticides**

       √7ᵗʰ **T60.8X1 Toxic effect of other pesticides, accidental (unintentional)**
Toxic effect of other pesticides NOS

       √7ᵗʰ **T60.8X2 Toxic effect of other pesticides, intentional self-harm**

       √7ᵗʰ **T60.8X3 Toxic effect of other pesticides, assault**

       √7ᵗʰ **T60.8X4 Toxic effect of other pesticides, undetermined**

√5ᵗʰ **T60.9 Toxic effect of unspecified pesticide**

    √x7ᵗʰ **T60.91 Toxic effect of unspecified pesticide, accidental (unintentional)** ▽

    √x7ᵗʰ **T60.92 Toxic effect of unspecified pesticide, intentional self-harm** ▽

    √x7ᵗʰ **T60.93 Toxic effect of unspecified pesticide, assault** ▽

    √x7ᵗʰ **T60.94 Toxic effect of unspecified pesticide, undetermined** ▽

Chapter 19. Injury, Poisoning and Certain Other Consequences of External Causes

T61–T62.94

✓4th **T61 Toxic effect of noxious substances eaten as seafood**

> EXCLUDES 1   *allergic reaction to food, such as:*
> > *anaphylactic reaction or shock due to adverse food reaction (T78.0-)*
> > *bacterial foodborne intoxications (A05.-)*
> > *dermatitis (L23.6, L25.4, L27.2)*
> > ▶*food protein-induced enterocolitis syndrome (K52.21)*◀
> > ▶*food protein-induced enteropathy (K52.22)*◀
> > *gastroenteritis (noninfective)* ▶*(K52.29)*◀
> *toxic effect of aflatoxin and other mycotoxins (T64)*
> *toxic effect of cyanides (T65.0-)*
> *toxic effect of harmful algae bloom (T65.82-)*
> *toxic effect of hydrogen cyanide (T57.3-)*
> *toxic effect of mercury (T56.1-)*
> *toxic effect of red tide (T65.82-)*

> The appropriate 7th character is to be added to each code from category T61.
> A   initial encounter
> D   subsequent encounter
> S   sequela

✓5th **T61.0 Ciguatera fish poisoning**

> ✓x7th **T61.01 Ciguatera fish poisoning, accidental (unintentional)**
> ✓x7th **T61.02 Ciguatera fish poisoning, intentional self-harm**
> ✓x7th **T61.03 Ciguatera fish poisoning, assault**
> ✓x7th **T61.04 Ciguatera fish poisoning, undetermined**

✓5th **T61.1 Scombroid fish poisoning**
> Histamine-like syndrome

> ✓x7th **T61.11 Scombroid fish poisoning, accidental (unintentional)**
> ✓x7th **T61.12 Scombroid fish poisoning, intentional self-harm**
> ✓x7th **T61.13 Scombroid fish poisoning, assault**
> ✓x7th **T61.14 Scombroid fish poisoning, undetermined**

✓5th **T61.7 Other fish and shellfish poisoning**

> ✓6th **T61.77 Other fish poisoning**
> > ✓7th **T61.771 Other fish poisoning, accidental (unintentional)**
> > ✓7th **T61.772 Other fish poisoning, intentional self-harm**
> > ✓7th **T61.773 Other fish poisoning, assault**
> > ✓7th **T61.774 Other fish poisoning, undetermined**

> ✓6th **T61.78 Other shellfish poisoning**
> > ✓7th **T61.781 Other shellfish poisoning, accidental (unintentional)**
> > ✓7th **T61.782 Other shellfish poisoning, intentional self-harm**
> > ✓7th **T61.783 Other shellfish poisoning, assault**
> > ✓7th **T61.784 Other shellfish poisoning, undetermined**

✓5th **T61.8 Toxic effect of other seafood**

> ✓6th **T61.8X Toxic effect of other seafood**
> > ✓7th **T61.8X1 Toxic effect of other seafood, accidental (unintentional)**
> > ✓7th **T61.8X2 Toxic effect of other seafood, intentional self-harm**
> > ✓7th **T61.8X3 Toxic effect of other seafood, assault**
> > ✓7th **T61.8X4 Toxic effect of other seafood, undetermined**

✓5th **T61.9 Toxic effect of unspecified seafood**

> ✓x7th **T61.91 Toxic effect of unspecified seafood, accidental (unintentional)**   ▽
> ✓x7th **T61.92 Toxic effect of unspecified seafood, intentional self-harm**   ▽
> ✓x7th **T61.93 Toxic effect of unspecified seafood, assault**   ▽
> ✓x7th **T61.94 Toxic effect of unspecified seafood, undetermined**   ▽

✓4th **T62 Toxic effect of other noxious substances eaten as food**

> EXCLUDES 1   *allergic reaction to food, such as:*
> > *anaphylactic shock (reaction) due to adverse food reaction (T78.0-)*
> > *bacterial food borne intoxications (A05.-)*
> > *dermatitis (L23.6, L25.4, L27.2)*
> > ▶*food protein-induced enterocolitis syndrome (K52.21)*◀
> > ▶*food protein-induced enteropathy (K52.22)*◀
> > *gastroenteritis (noninfective)* ▶*(K52.29)*◀
> *toxic effect of aflatoxin and other mycotoxins (T64)*
> *toxic effect of cyanides (T65.0-)*
> *toxic effect of hydrogen cyanide (T57.3-)*
> *toxic effect of mercury (T56.1-)*

> The appropriate 7th character is to be added to each code from category T62.
> A   initial encounter
> D   subsequent encounter
> S   sequela

✓5th **T62.0 Toxic effect of ingested mushrooms**

> ✓6th **T62.0X Toxic effect of ingested mushrooms**
> > ✓7th **T62.0X1 Toxic effect of ingested mushrooms, accidental (unintentional)**
> > > Toxic effect of ingested mushrooms NOS
> > ✓7th **T62.0X2 Toxic effect of ingested mushrooms, intentional self-harm**
> > ✓7th **T62.0X3 Toxic effect of ingested mushrooms, assault**
> > ✓7th **T62.0X4 Toxic effect of ingested mushrooms, undetermined**

✓5th **T62.1 Toxic effect of ingested berries**

> ✓6th **T62.1X Toxic effect of ingested berries**
> > ✓7th **T62.1X1 Toxic effect of ingested berries, accidental (unintentional)**
> > > Toxic effect of ingested berries NOS
> > ✓7th **T62.1X2 Toxic effect of ingested berries, intentional self-harm**
> > ✓7th **T62.1X3 Toxic effect of ingested berries, assault**
> > ✓7th **T62.1X4 Toxic effect of ingested berries, undetermined**

✓5th **T62.2 Toxic effect of other ingested (parts of) plant(s)**

> ✓6th **T62.2X Toxic effect of other ingested (parts of) plant(s)**
> > ✓7th **T62.2X1 Toxic effect of other ingested (parts of) plant(s), accidental (unintentional)**
> > > Toxic effect of other ingested (parts of) plant(s) NOS
> > ✓7th **T62.2X2 Toxic effect of other ingested (parts of) plant(s), intentional self-harm**
> > ✓7th **T62.2X3 Toxic effect of other ingested (parts of) plant(s), assault**
> > ✓7th **T62.2X4 Toxic effect of other ingested (parts of) plant(s), undetermined**

✓5th **T62.8 Toxic effect of other specified noxious substances eaten as food**

> ✓6th **T62.8X Toxic effect of other specified noxious substances eaten as food**
> > ✓7th **T62.8X1 Toxic effect of other specified noxious substances eaten as food, accidental (unintentional)**
> > > Toxic effect of other specified noxious substances eaten as food NOS
> > ✓7th **T62.8X2 Toxic effect of other specified noxious substances eaten as food, intentional self-harm**
> > ✓7th **T62.8X3 Toxic effect of other specified noxious substances eaten as food, assault**
> > ✓7th **T62.8X4 Toxic effect of other specified noxious substances eaten as food, undetermined**

✓5th **T62.9 Toxic effect of unspecified noxious substance eaten as food**

> ✓x7th **T62.91 Toxic effect of unspecified noxious substance eaten as food, accidental (unintentional)**   ▽
> > Toxic effect of unspecified noxious substance eaten as food NOS
> ✓x7th **T62.92 Toxic effect of unspecified noxious substance eaten as food, intentional self-harm**   ▽
> ✓x7th **T62.93 Toxic effect of unspecified noxious substance eaten as food, assault**   ▽
> ✓x7th **T62.94 Toxic effect of unspecified noxious substance eaten as food, undetermined**   ▽

EXCLUDES 1 Not coded here   EXCLUDES 2 Not included here   N Newborn Age : 0   P Pediatric Age : 0-17   M Maternity Age : 12-55   A Adult Age : 15-124

1054   ICD-10-CM 2017

✓4ᵗʰ **T63 Toxic effect of contact with venomous animals and plants**

     INCLUDES   bite or touch of venomous animal

                    pricked or stuck by thorn or leaf

     EXCLUDES 2   *ingestion of toxic animal or plant (T61.-, T62.-)*

     The appropriate 7th character is to be added to each code from category T63.
     A   initial encounter
     D   subsequent encounter
     S   sequela

✓5ᵗʰ **T63.0 Toxic effect of snake venom**

   ✓6ᵗʰ **T63.00 Toxic effect of unspecified snake venom**

     ✓7ᵗʰ **T63.001 Toxic effect of unspecified snake venom, accidental (unintentional)** ▽
                 Toxic effect of unspecified snake venom NOS

     ✓7ᵗʰ **T63.002 Toxic effect of unspecified snake venom, intentional self-harm** ▽

     ✓7ᵗʰ **T63.003 Toxic effect of unspecified snake venom, assault** ▽

     ✓7ᵗʰ **T63.004 Toxic effect of unspecified snake venom, undetermined** ▽

   ✓6ᵗʰ **T63.01 Toxic effect of rattlesnake venom**

     ✓7ᵗʰ **T63.011 Toxic effect of rattlesnake venom, accidental (unintentional)**
                 Toxic effect of rattlesnake venom NOS

     ✓7ᵗʰ **T63.012 Toxic effect of rattlesnake venom, intentional self-harm**

     ✓7ᵗʰ **T63.013 Toxic effect of rattlesnake venom, assault**

     ✓7ᵗʰ **T63.014 Toxic effect of rattlesnake venom, undetermined**

   ✓6ᵗʰ **T63.02 Toxic effect of coral snake venom**

     ✓7ᵗʰ **T63.021 Toxic effect of coral snake venom, accidental (unintentional)**
                 Toxic effect of coral snake venom NOS

     ✓7ᵗʰ **T63.022 Toxic effect of coral snake venom, intentional self-harm**

     ✓7ᵗʰ **T63.023 Toxic effect of coral snake venom, assault**

     ✓7ᵗʰ **T63.024 Toxic effect of coral snake venom, undetermined**

   ✓6ᵗʰ **T63.03 Toxic effect of taipan venom**

     ✓7ᵗʰ **T63.031 Toxic effect of taipan venom, accidental (unintentional)**
                 Toxic effect of taipan venom NOS

     ✓7ᵗʰ **T63.032 Toxic effect of taipan venom, intentional self-harm**

     ✓7ᵗʰ **T63.033 Toxic effect of taipan venom, assault**

     ✓7ᵗʰ **T63.034 Toxic effect of taipan venom, undetermined**

   ✓6ᵗʰ **T63.04 Toxic effect of cobra venom**

     ✓7ᵗʰ **T63.041 Toxic effect of cobra venom, accidental (unintentional)**
                 Toxic effect of cobra venom NOS

     ✓7ᵗʰ **T63.042 Toxic effect of cobra venom, intentional self-harm**

     ✓7ᵗʰ **T63.043 Toxic effect of cobra venom, assault**

     ✓7ᵗʰ **T63.044 Toxic effect of cobra venom, undetermined**

   ✓6ᵗʰ **T63.06 Toxic effect of venom of other North and South American snake**

     ✓7ᵗʰ **T63.061 Toxic effect of venom of other North and South American snake, accidental (unintentional)**
                 Toxic effect of venom of other North and South American snake NOS

     ✓7ᵗʰ **T63.062 Toxic effect of venom of other North and South American snake, intentional self-harm**

     ✓7ᵗʰ **T63.063 Toxic effect of venom of other North and South American snake, assault**

     ✓7ᵗʰ **T63.064 Toxic effect of venom of other North and South American snake, undetermined**

   ✓6ᵗʰ **T63.07 Toxic effect of venom of other Australian snake**

     ✓7ᵗʰ **T63.071 Toxic effect of venom of other Australian snake, accidental (unintentional)**
                 Toxic effect of venom of other Australian snake NOS

     ✓7ᵗʰ **T63.072 Toxic effect of venom of other Australian snake, intentional self-harm**

     ✓7ᵗʰ **T63.073 Toxic effect of venom of other Australian snake, assault**

     ✓7ᵗʰ **T63.074 Toxic effect of venom of other Australian snake, undetermined**

   ✓6ᵗʰ **T63.08 Toxic effect of venom of other African and Asian snake**

     ✓7ᵗʰ **T63.081 Toxic effect of venom of other African and Asian snake, accidental (unintentional)**
                 Toxic effect of venom of other African and Asian snake NOS

     ✓7ᵗʰ **T63.082 Toxic effect of venom of other African and Asian snake, intentional self-harm**

     ✓7ᵗʰ **T63.083 Toxic effect of venom of other African and Asian snake, assault**

     ✓7ᵗʰ **T63.084 Toxic effect of venom of other African and Asian snake, undetermined**

   ✓6ᵗʰ **T63.09 Toxic effect of venom of other snake**

     ✓7ᵗʰ **T63.091 Toxic effect of venom of other snake, accidental (unintentional)**
                 Toxic effect of venom of other snake NOS

     ✓7ᵗʰ **T63.092 Toxic effect of venom of other snake, intentional self-harm**

     ✓7ᵗʰ **T63.093 Toxic effect of venom of other snake, assault**

     ✓7ᵗʰ **T63.094 Toxic effect of venom of other snake, undetermined**

✓5ᵗʰ **T63.1 Toxic effect of venom of other reptiles**

   ✓6ᵗʰ **T63.11 Toxic effect of venom of gila monster**

     ✓7ᵗʰ **T63.111 Toxic effect of venom of gila monster, accidental (unintentional)**
                 Toxic effect of venom of gila monster NOS

     ✓7ᵗʰ **T63.112 Toxic effect of venom of gila monster, intentional self-harm**

     ✓7ᵗʰ **T63.113 Toxic effect of venom of gila monster, assault**

     ✓7ᵗʰ **T63.114 Toxic effect of venom of gila monster, undetermined**

   ✓6ᵗʰ **T63.12 Toxic effect of venom of other venomous lizard**

     ✓7ᵗʰ **T63.121 Toxic effect of venom of other venomous lizard, accidental (unintentional)**
                 Toxic effect of venom of other venomous lizard NOS

     ✓7ᵗʰ **T63.122 Toxic effect of venom of other venomous lizard, intentional self-harm**

     ✓7ᵗʰ **T63.123 Toxic effect of venom of other venomous lizard, assault**

     ✓7ᵗʰ **T63.124 Toxic effect of venom of other venomous lizard, undetermined**

   ✓6ᵗʰ **T63.19 Toxic effect of venom of other reptiles**

     ✓7ᵗʰ **T63.191 Toxic effect of venom of other reptiles, accidental (unintentional)**
                 Toxic effect of venom of other reptiles NOS

     ✓7ᵗʰ **T63.192 Toxic effect of venom of other reptiles, intentional self-harm**

     ✓7ᵗʰ **T63.193 Toxic effect of venom of other reptiles, assault**

     ✓7ᵗʰ **T63.194 Toxic effect of venom of other reptiles, undetermined**

✓5ᵗʰ **T63.2 Toxic effect of venom of scorpion**

   ✓6ᵗʰ **T63.2X Toxic effect of venom of scorpion**

     ✓7ᵗʰ **T63.2X1 Toxic effect of venom of scorpion, accidental (unintentional)**
                 Toxic effect of venom of scorpion NOS

     ✓7ᵗʰ **T63.2X2 Toxic effect of venom of scorpion, intentional self-harm**

     ✓7ᵗʰ **T63.2X3 Toxic effect of venom of scorpion, assault**

     ✓7ᵗʰ **T63.2X4 Toxic effect of venom of scorpion, undetermined**

✓5ᵗʰ **T63.3 Toxic effect of venom of spider**

   ✓6ᵗʰ **T63.30 Toxic effect of unspecified spider venom**

     ✓7ᵗʰ **T63.301 Toxic effect of unspecified spider venom, accidental (unintentional)** ▽

     ✓7ᵗʰ **T63.302 Toxic effect of unspecified spider venom, intentional self-harm** ▽

     ✓7ᵗʰ **T63.303 Toxic effect of unspecified spider venom, assault** ▽

     ✓7ᵗʰ **T63.304 Toxic effect of unspecified spider venom, undetermined** ▽

✓ Additional Character Required   ✓x7ᵗʰ Placeholder Alert   Manifestation Dx   ▽ Unspecified Dx   ▶◀ Revised Text   ● New Code   ▲ Revised Code Title

ICD-10-CM 2017   **1055**

√6ᵗʰ **T63.31** Toxic effect of venom of black widow spider
- √7ᵗʰ **T63.311** Toxic effect of venom of black widow spider, accidental (unintentional)
- √7ᵗʰ **T63.312** Toxic effect of venom of black widow spider, intentional self-harm
- √7ᵗʰ **T63.313** Toxic effect of venom of black widow spider, assault
- √7ᵗʰ **T63.314** Toxic effect of venom of black widow spider, undetermined

√6ᵗʰ **T63.32** Toxic effect of venom of tarantula
- √7ᵗʰ **T63.321** Toxic effect of venom of tarantula, accidental (unintentional)
- √7ᵗʰ **T63.322** Toxic effect of venom of tarantula, intentional self-harm
- √7ᵗʰ **T63.323** Toxic effect of venom of tarantula, assault
- √7ᵗʰ **T63.324** Toxic effect of venom of tarantula, undetermined

√6ᵗʰ **T63.33** Toxic effect of venom of brown recluse spider
- √7ᵗʰ **T63.331** Toxic effect of venom of brown recluse spider, accidental (unintentional)
- √7ᵗʰ **T63.332** Toxic effect of venom of brown recluse spider, intentional self-harm
- √7ᵗʰ **T63.333** Toxic effect of venom of brown recluse spider, assault
- √7ᵗʰ **T63.334** Toxic effect of venom of brown recluse spider, undetermined

√6ᵗʰ **T63.39** Toxic effect of venom of other spider
- √7ᵗʰ **T63.391** Toxic effect of venom of other spider, accidental (unintentional)
- √7ᵗʰ **T63.392** Toxic effect of venom of other spider, intentional self-harm
- √7ᵗʰ **T63.393** Toxic effect of venom of other spider, assault
- √7ᵗʰ **T63.394** Toxic effect of venom of other spider, undetermined

√5ᵗʰ **T63.4** Toxic effect of venom of other arthropods

√6ᵗʰ **T63.41** Toxic effect of venom of centipedes and venomous millipedes
- √7ᵗʰ **T63.411** Toxic effect of venom of centipedes and venomous millipedes, accidental (unintentional)
- √7ᵗʰ **T63.412** Toxic effect of venom of centipedes and venomous millipedes, intentional self-harm
- √7ᵗʰ **T63.413** Toxic effect of venom of centipedes and venomous millipedes, assault
- √7ᵗʰ **T63.414** Toxic effect of venom of centipedes and venomous millipedes, undetermined

√6ᵗʰ **T63.42** Toxic effect of venom of ants
- √7ᵗʰ **T63.421** Toxic effect of venom of ants, accidental (unintentional)
- √7ᵗʰ **T63.422** Toxic effect of venom of ants, intentional self-harm
- √7ᵗʰ **T63.423** Toxic effect of venom of ants, assault
- √7ᵗʰ **T63.424** Toxic effect of venom of ants, undetermined

√6ᵗʰ **T63.43** Toxic effect of venom of caterpillars
- √7ᵗʰ **T63.431** Toxic effect of venom of caterpillars, accidental (unintentional)
- √7ᵗʰ **T63.432** Toxic effect of venom of caterpillars, intentional self-harm
- √7ᵗʰ **T63.433** Toxic effect of venom of caterpillars, assault
- √7ᵗʰ **T63.434** Toxic effect of venom of caterpillars, undetermined

√6ᵗʰ **T63.44** Toxic effect of venom of bees
- √7ᵗʰ **T63.441** Toxic effect of venom of bees, accidental (unintentional)
- √7ᵗʰ **T63.442** Toxic effect of venom of bees, intentional self-harm
- √7ᵗʰ **T63.443** Toxic effect of venom of bees, assault
- √7ᵗʰ **T63.444** Toxic effect of venom of bees, undetermined

√6ᵗʰ **T63.45** Toxic effect of venom of hornets
- √7ᵗʰ **T63.451** Toxic effect of venom of hornets, accidental (unintentional)
- √7ᵗʰ **T63.452** Toxic effect of venom of hornets, intentional self-harm
- √7ᵗʰ **T63.453** Toxic effect of venom of hornets, assault
- √7ᵗʰ **T63.454** Toxic effect of venom of hornets, undetermined

√6ᵗʰ **T63.46** Toxic effect of venom of wasps
  Toxic effect of yellow jacket
- √7ᵗʰ **T63.461** Toxic effect of venom of wasps, accidental (unintentional)
- √7ᵗʰ **T63.462** Toxic effect of venom of wasps, intentional self-harm
- √7ᵗʰ **T63.463** Toxic effect of venom of wasps, assault
- √7ᵗʰ **T63.464** Toxic effect of venom of wasps, undetermined

√6ᵗʰ **T63.48** Toxic effect of venom of other arthropod
- √7ᵗʰ **T63.481** Toxic effect of venom of other arthropod, accidental (unintentional)
- √7ᵗʰ **T63.482** Toxic effect of venom of other arthropod, intentional self-harm
- √7ᵗʰ **T63.483** Toxic effect of venom of other arthropod, assault
- √7ᵗʰ **T63.484** Toxic effect of venom of other arthropod, undetermined

√5ᵗʰ **T63.5** Toxic effect of contact with venomous fish
  EXCLUDES 2 poisoning by ingestion of fish (T61.-)

√6ᵗʰ **T63.51** Toxic effect of contact with stingray
- √7ᵗʰ **T63.511** Toxic effect of contact with stingray, accidental (unintentional)
- √7ᵗʰ **T63.512** Toxic effect of contact with stingray, intentional self-harm
- √7ᵗʰ **T63.513** Toxic effect of contact with stingray, assault
- √7ᵗʰ **T63.514** Toxic effect of contact with stingray, undetermined

√6ᵗʰ **T63.59** Toxic effect of contact with other venomous fish
- √7ᵗʰ **T63.591** Toxic effect of contact with other venomous fish, accidental (unintentional)
- √7ᵗʰ **T63.592** Toxic effect of contact with other venomous fish, intentional self-harm
- √7ᵗʰ **T63.593** Toxic effect of contact with other venomous fish, assault
- √7ᵗʰ **T63.594** Toxic effect of contact with other venomous fish, undetermined

√5ᵗʰ **T63.6** Toxic effect of contact with other venomous marine animals
  EXCLUDES 1 sea-snake venom (T63.09)
  EXCLUDES 2 poisoning by ingestion of shellfish (T61.78-)

√6ᵗʰ **T63.61** Toxic effect of contact with Portugese Man-o-war
  Toxic effect of contact with bluebottle
- √7ᵗʰ **T63.611** Toxic effect of contact with Portugese Man-o-war, accidental (unintentional)
- √7ᵗʰ **T63.612** Toxic effect of contact with Portugese Man-o-war, intentional self-harm
- √7ᵗʰ **T63.613** Toxic effect of contact with Portugese Man-o-war, assault
- √7ᵗʰ **T63.614** Toxic effect of contact with Portugese Man-o-war, undetermined

√6ᵗʰ **T63.62** Toxic effect of contact with other jellyfish
- √7ᵗʰ **T63.621** Toxic effect of contact with other jellyfish, accidental (unintentional)
- √7ᵗʰ **T63.622** Toxic effect of contact with other jellyfish, intentional self-harm
- √7ᵗʰ **T63.623** Toxic effect of contact with other jellyfish, assault
- √7ᵗʰ **T63.624** Toxic effect of contact with other jellyfish, undetermined

√6ᵗʰ **T63.63** Toxic effect of contact with sea anemone
- √7ᵗʰ **T63.631** Toxic effect of contact with sea anemone, accidental (unintentional)
- √7ᵗʰ **T63.632** Toxic effect of contact with sea anemone, intentional self-harm
- √7ᵗʰ **T63.633** Toxic effect of contact with sea anemone, assault
- √7ᵗʰ **T63.634** Toxic effect of contact with sea anemone, undetermined

√6ᵗʰ **T63.69** Toxic effect of contact with other venomous marine animals
- √7ᵗʰ **T63.691** Toxic effect of contact with other venomous marine animals, accidental (unintentional)
- √7ᵗʰ **T63.692** Toxic effect of contact with other venomous marine animals, intentional self-harm
- √7ᵗʰ **T63.693** Toxic effect of contact with other venomous marine animals, assault

EXCLUDES 1 Not coded here   EXCLUDES 2 Not included here   N Newborn Age : 0   P Pediatric Age : 0-17   M Maternity Age : 12-55   A Adult Age : 15-124

1056   ICD-10-CM 2017

✓7ᵗʰ **T63.694** Toxic effect of contact with other venomous marine animals, undetermined

✓5ᵗʰ **T63.7** Toxic effect of contact with venomous plant

✓6ᵗʰ **T63.71** Toxic effect of contact with venomous marine plant

✓7ᵗʰ **T63.711** Toxic effect of contact with venomous marine plant, accidental (unintentional)

✓7ᵗʰ **T63.712** Toxic effect of contact with venomous marine plant, intentional self-harm

✓7ᵗʰ **T63.713** Toxic effect of contact with venomous marine plant, assault

✓7ᵗʰ **T63.714** Toxic effect of contact with venomous marine plant, undetermined

✓6ᵗʰ **T63.79** Toxic effect of contact with other venomous plant

✓7ᵗʰ **T63.791** Toxic effect of contact with other venomous plant, accidental (unintentional)

✓7ᵗʰ **T63.792** Toxic effect of contact with other venomous plant, intentional self-harm

✓7ᵗʰ **T63.793** Toxic effect of contact with other venomous plant, assault

✓7ᵗʰ **T63.794** Toxic effect of contact with other venomous plant, undetermined

✓5ᵗʰ **T63.8** Toxic effect of contact with other venomous animals

✓6ᵗʰ **T63.81** Toxic effect of contact with venomous frog

> EXCLUDES 1 *contact with nonvenomous frog (W62.0)*

✓7ᵗʰ **T63.811** Toxic effect of contact with venomous frog, accidental (unintentional)

✓7ᵗʰ **T63.812** Toxic effect of contact with venomous frog, intentional self-harm

✓7ᵗʰ **T63.813** Toxic effect of contact with venomous frog, assault

✓7ᵗʰ **T63.814** Toxic effect of contact with venomous frog, undetermined

✓6ᵗʰ **T63.82** Toxic effect of contact with venomous toad

> EXCLUDES 1 *contact with nonvenomous toad (W62.1)*

✓7ᵗʰ **T63.821** Toxic effect of contact with venomous toad, accidental (unintentional)

✓7ᵗʰ **T63.822** Toxic effect of contact with venomous toad, intentional self-harm

✓7ᵗʰ **T63.823** Toxic effect of contact with venomous toad, assault

✓7ᵗʰ **T63.824** Toxic effect of contact with venomous toad, undetermined

✓6ᵗʰ **T63.83** Toxic effect of contact with other venomous amphibian

> EXCLUDES 1 *contact with nonvenomous amphibian (W62.9)*

✓7ᵗʰ **T63.831** Toxic effect of contact with other venomous amphibian, accidental (unintentional)

✓7ᵗʰ **T63.832** Toxic effect of contact with other venomous amphibian, intentional self-harm

✓7ᵗʰ **T63.833** Toxic effect of contact with other venomous amphibian, assault

✓7ᵗʰ **T63.834** Toxic effect of contact with other venomous amphibian, undetermined

✓6ᵗʰ **T63.89** Toxic effect of contact with other venomous animals

✓7ᵗʰ **T63.891** Toxic effect of contact with other venomous animals, accidental (unintentional)

✓7ᵗʰ **T63.892** Toxic effect of contact with other venomous animals, intentional self-harm

✓7ᵗʰ **T63.893** Toxic effect of contact with other venomous animals, assault

✓7ᵗʰ **T63.894** Toxic effect of contact with other venomous animals, undetermined

✓5ᵗʰ **T63.9** Toxic effect of contact with unspecified venomous animal

✓x7ᵗʰ **T63.91** Toxic effect of contact with unspecified venomous animal, accidental (unintentional) ▽

✓x7ᵗʰ **T63.92** Toxic effect of contact with unspecified venomous animal, intentional self-harm ▽

✓x7ᵗʰ **T63.93** Toxic effect of contact with unspecified venomous animal, assault ▽

✓x7ᵗʰ **T63.94** Toxic effect of contact with unspecified venomous animal, undetermined ▽

✓4ᵗʰ **T64** Toxic effect of aflatoxin and other mycotoxin food contaminants

> The appropriate 7th character is to be added to each code from category T64.
> A initial encounter
> D subsequent encounter
> S sequela

✓5ᵗʰ **T64.0** Toxic effect of aflatoxin

✓x7ᵗʰ **T64.01** Toxic effect of aflatoxin, accidental (unintentional)

✓x7ᵗʰ **T64.02** Toxic effect of aflatoxin, intentional self-harm

✓x7ᵗʰ **T64.03** Toxic effect of aflatoxin, assault

✓x7ᵗʰ **T64.04** Toxic effect of aflatoxin, undetermined

✓5ᵗʰ **T64.8** Toxic effect of other mycotoxin food contaminants

✓x7ᵗʰ **T64.81** Toxic effect of other mycotoxin food contaminants, accidental (unintentional)

✓x7ᵗʰ **T64.82** Toxic effect of other mycotoxin food contaminants, intentional self-harm

✓x7ᵗʰ **T64.83** Toxic effect of other mycotoxin food contaminants, assault

✓x7ᵗʰ **T64.84** Toxic effect of other mycotoxin food contaminants, undetermined

✓4ᵗʰ **T65** Toxic effect of other and unspecified substances

> The appropriate 7th character is to be added to each code from category T65.
> A initial encounter
> D subsequent encounter
> S sequela

✓5ᵗʰ **T65.0** Toxic effect of cyanides

> EXCLUDES 1 *hydrogen cyanide (T57.3-)*

✓6ᵗʰ **T65.0X** Toxic effect of cyanides

✓7ᵗʰ **T65.0X1** Toxic effect of cyanides, accidental (unintentional)
Toxic effect of cyanides NOS

✓7ᵗʰ **T65.0X2** Toxic effect of cyanides, intentional self-harm

✓7ᵗʰ **T65.0X3** Toxic effect of cyanides, assault

✓7ᵗʰ **T65.0X4** Toxic effect of cyanides, undetermined

✓5ᵗʰ **T65.1** Toxic effect of strychnine and its salts

✓6ᵗʰ **T65.1X** Toxic effect of strychnine and its salts

✓7ᵗʰ **T65.1X1** Toxic effect of strychnine and its salts, accidental (unintentional)
Toxic effect of strychnine and its salts NOS

✓7ᵗʰ **T65.1X2** Toxic effect of strychnine and its salts, intentional self-harm

✓7ᵗʰ **T65.1X3** Toxic effect of strychnine and its salts, assault

✓7ᵗʰ **T65.1X4** Toxic effect of strychnine and its salts, undetermined

✓5ᵗʰ **T65.2** Toxic effect of tobacco and nicotine

> EXCLUDES 2 *nicotine dependence (F17.-)*

✓6ᵗʰ **T65.21** Toxic effect of chewing tobacco

✓7ᵗʰ **T65.211** Toxic effect of chewing tobacco, accidental (unintentional)
Toxic effect of chewing tobacco NOS

✓7ᵗʰ **T65.212** Toxic effect of chewing tobacco, intentional self-harm

✓7ᵗʰ **T65.213** Toxic effect of chewing tobacco, assault

✓7ᵗʰ **T65.214** Toxic effect of chewing tobacco, undetermined

✓6ᵗʰ **T65.22** Toxic effect of tobacco cigarettes

Toxic effect of tobacco smoke
Use additional code for exposure to second hand tobacco smoke (Z57.31, Z77.22)

✓7ᵗʰ **T65.221** Toxic effect of tobacco cigarettes, accidental (unintentional)
Toxic effect of tobacco cigarettes NOS

✓7ᵗʰ **T65.222** Toxic effect of tobacco cigarettes, intentional self-harm

✓7ᵗʰ **T65.223** Toxic effect of tobacco cigarettes, assault

✓7ᵗʰ **T65.224** Toxic effect of tobacco cigarettes, undetermined

✓6ᵗʰ **T65.29** Toxic effect of other tobacco and nicotine

✓7ᵗʰ **T65.291** Toxic effect of other tobacco and nicotine, accidental (unintentional)
Toxic effect of other tobacco and nicotine NOS

    ☑7ᵗʰ **T65.292 Toxic effect of other tobacco and nicotine, intentional self-harm**

    ☑7ᵗʰ **T65.293 Toxic effect of other tobacco and nicotine, assault**

    ☑7ᵗʰ **T65.294 Toxic effect of other tobacco and nicotine, undetermined**

☑5ᵗʰ **T65.3 Toxic effect of nitroderivatives and aminoderivatives of benzene and its homologues**
Toxic effect of anilin [benzenamine]
Toxic effect of nitrobenzene
Toxic effect of trinitrotoluene

  ☑6ᵗʰ **T65.3X Toxic effect of nitroderivatives and aminoderivatives of benzene and its homologues**

    ☑7ᵗʰ **T65.3X1 Toxic effect of nitroderivatives and aminoderivatives of benzene and its homologues, accidental (unintentional)**
Toxic effect of nitroderivatives and aminoderivatives of benzene and its homologues NOS

    ☑7ᵗʰ **T65.3X2 Toxic effect of nitroderivatives and aminoderivatives of benzene and its homologues, intentional self-harm**

    ☑7ᵗʰ **T65.3X3 Toxic effect of nitroderivatives and aminoderivatives of benzene and its homologues, assault**

    ☑7ᵗʰ **T65.3X4 Toxic effect of nitroderivatives and aminoderivatives of benzene and its homologues, undetermined**

☑5ᵗʰ **T65.4 Toxic effect of carbon disulfide**

  ☑6ᵗʰ **T65.4X Toxic effect of carbon disulfide**

    ☑7ᵗʰ **T65.4X1 Toxic effect of carbon disulfide, accidental (unintentional)**
Toxic effect of carbon disulfide NOS

    ☑7ᵗʰ **T65.4X2 Toxic effect of carbon disulfide, intentional self-harm**

    ☑7ᵗʰ **T65.4X3 Toxic effect of carbon disulfide, assault**

    ☑7ᵗʰ **T65.4X4 Toxic effect of carbon disulfide, undetermined**

☑5ᵗʰ **T65.5 Toxic effect of nitroglycerin and other nitric acids and esters**
Toxic effect of 1,2,3-Propanetriol trinitrate

  ☑6ᵗʰ **T65.5X Toxic effect of nitroglycerin and other nitric acids and esters**

    ☑7ᵗʰ **T65.5X1 Toxic effect of nitroglycerin and other nitric acids and esters, accidental (unintentional)**
Toxic effect of nitroglycerin and other nitric acids and esters NOS

    ☑7ᵗʰ **T65.5X2 Toxic effect of nitroglycerin and other nitric acids and esters, intentional self-harm**

    ☑7ᵗʰ **T65.5X3 Toxic effect of nitroglycerin and other nitric acids and esters, assault**

    ☑7ᵗʰ **T65.5X4 Toxic effect of nitroglycerin and other nitric acids and esters, undetermined**

☑5ᵗʰ **T65.6 Toxic effect of paints and dyes, not elsewhere classified**

  ☑6ᵗʰ **T65.6X Toxic effect of paints and dyes, not elsewhere classified**

    ☑7ᵗʰ **T65.6X1 Toxic effect of paints and dyes, not elsewhere classified, accidental (unintentional)**
Toxic effect of paints and dyes NOS

    ☑7ᵗʰ **T65.6X2 Toxic effect of paints and dyes, not elsewhere classified, intentional self-harm**

    ☑7ᵗʰ **T65.6X3 Toxic effect of paints and dyes, not elsewhere classified, assault**

    ☑7ᵗʰ **T65.6X4 Toxic effect of paints and dyes, not elsewhere classified, undetermined**

☑5ᵗʰ **T65.8 Toxic effect of other specified substances**

  ☑6ᵗʰ **T65.81 Toxic effect of latex**

    ☑7ᵗʰ **T65.811 Toxic effect of latex, accidental (unintentional)**
Toxic effect of latex NOS

    ☑7ᵗʰ **T65.812 Toxic effect of latex, intentional self-harm**

    ☑7ᵗʰ **T65.813 Toxic effect of latex, assault**

    ☑7ᵗʰ **T65.814 Toxic effect of latex, undetermined**

  ☑6ᵗʰ **T65.82 Toxic effect of harmful algae and algae toxins**
Toxic effect of (harmful) algae bloom NOS
Toxic effect of blue-green algae bloom
Toxic effect of brown tide
Toxic effect of cyanobacteria bloom
Toxic effect of Florida red tide
Toxic effect of pfiesteria piscicida
Toxic effect of red tide

    ☑7ᵗʰ **T65.821 Toxic effect of harmful algae and algae toxins, accidental (unintentional)**
Toxic effect of harmful algae and algae toxins NOS

    ☑7ᵗʰ **T65.822 Toxic effect of harmful algae and algae toxins, intentional self-harm**

    ☑7ᵗʰ **T65.823 Toxic effect of harmful algae and algae toxins, assault**

    ☑7ᵗʰ **T65.824 Toxic effect of harmful algae and algae toxins, undetermined**

  ☑6ᵗʰ **T65.83 Toxic effect of fiberglass**

    ☑7ᵗʰ **T65.831 Toxic effect of fiberglass, accidental (unintentional)**
Toxic effect of fiberglass NOS

    ☑7ᵗʰ **T65.832 Toxic effect of fiberglass, intentional self-harm**

    ☑7ᵗʰ **T65.833 Toxic effect of fiberglass, assault**

    ☑7ᵗʰ **T65.834 Toxic effect of fiberglass, undetermined**

  ☑6ᵗʰ **T65.89 Toxic effect of other specified substances**

    ☑7ᵗʰ **T65.891 Toxic effect of other specified substances, accidental (unintentional)**
Toxic effect of other specified substances NOS

    ☑7ᵗʰ **T65.892 Toxic effect of other specified substances, intentional self-harm**

    ☑7ᵗʰ **T65.893 Toxic effect of other specified substances, assault**

    ☑7ᵗʰ **T65.894 Toxic effect of other specified substances, undetermined**

☑5ᵗʰ **T65.9 Toxic effect of unspecified substance**

  ☑ₓ7ᵗʰ **T65.91 Toxic effect of unspecified substance, accidental (unintentional)**   ▽
Poisoning NOS

  ☑ₓ7ᵗʰ **T65.92 Toxic effect of unspecified substance, intentional self-harm**   ▽

  ☑ₓ7ᵗʰ **T65.93 Toxic effect of unspecified substance, assault**   ▽

  ☑ₓ7ᵗʰ **T65.94 Toxic effect of unspecified substance, undetermined**   ▽

Other and unspecified effects of external causes (T66-T78)

☑4ᵗʰ **T66 Radiation sickness, unspecified**   ▽

  EXCLUDES 1   specified adverse effects of radiation, such as:
    burns (T20-T31)
    leukemia (C91-C95)
    radiation gastroenteritis and colitis (K52.0)
    radiation pneumonitis (J70.0)
    radiation related disorders of the skin and subcutaneous tissue (L55-L59)
    radiation sunburn (L55.-)

> The appropriate 7th character is to be added to code T66.
> A   initial encounter
> D   subsequent encounter
> S   sequela

☑4ᵗʰ **T67 Effects of heat and light**

  EXCLUDES 1   erythema [dermatitis] ab igne (L59.0)
    malignant hyperpyrexia due to anesthesia (T88.3)
    radiation-related disorders of the skin and subcutaneous tissue (L55-L59)

  EXCLUDES 2   burns (T20-T31)
    sunburn (L55.-)
    sweat disorder due to heat (L74-L75)

> The appropriate 7th character is to be added to each code from category T67.
> A   initial encounter
> D   subsequent encounter
> S   sequela

EXCLUDES 1 Not coded here   **EXCLUDES 2** Not included here   ℕ Newborn Age : 0   ℙ Pediatric Age : 0-17   𝕄 Maternity Age : 12-55   𝔸 Adult Age : 15-124

1058   ICD-10-CM 2017

√x7ᵗʰ **T67.0** **Heatstroke and sunstroke**

Heat apoplexy
Heat pyrexia
Siriasis
Thermoplegia
Use additional code(s) to identify any associated complications of heatstroke, such as:
   coma and stupor (R40.-)
   systemic inflammatory response syndrome (R65.1-)

√x7ᵗʰ **T67.1** **Heat syncope**

Heat collapse

√x7ᵗʰ **T67.2** **Heat cramp**

√x7ᵗʰ **T67.3** **Heat exhaustion, anhydrotic**

Heat prostration due to water depletion
  EXCLUDES 1 *heat exhaustion due to salt depletion (T67.4)*

√x7ᵗʰ **T67.4** **Heat exhaustion due to salt depletion**

Heat prostration due to salt (and water) depletion

√x7ᵗʰ **T67.5** **Heat exhaustion, unspecified** ▽

Heat prostration NOS

√x7ᵗʰ **T67.6** **Heat fatigue, transient**

√x7ᵗʰ **T67.7** **Heat edema**

√x7ᵗʰ **T67.8** **Other effects of heat and light**

√x7ᵗʰ **T67.9** **Effect of heat and light, unspecified** ▽

√4ᵗʰ **T68** **Hypothermia**

Accidental hypothermia
Hypothermia NOS
Use additional code to identify source of exposure:
  exposure to excessive cold of man-made origin (W93)
  exposure to excessive cold of natural origin (X31)
  EXCLUDES 1 *hypothermia following anesthesia (T88.51)*
         hypothermia not associated with low environmental
           temperature (R68.0)
         hypothermia of newborn (P80.-)
  EXCLUDES 2 *frostbite (T33-T34)*

The appropriate 7th character is to be added to code T68.
A   initial encounter
D subsequent encounter
S   sequela

√4ᵗʰ **T69** **Other effects of reduced temperature**

Use additional code to identify source of exposure:
  exposure to excessive cold of man-made origin (W93)
  exposure to excessive cold of natural origin (X31)
  EXCLUDES 2 *frostbite (T33-T34)*

The appropriate 7th character is to be added to each code from category T69.
A   initial encounter
D subsequent encounter
S   sequela

√5ᵗʰ **T69.0** **Immersion hand and foot**

√6ᵗʰ **T69.01** **Immersion hand**

√7ᵗʰ **T69.011** **Immersion hand, right hand**

√7ᵗʰ **T69.012** **Immersion hand, left hand**

√7ᵗʰ **T69.019** **Immersion hand, unspecified hand** ▽

√6ᵗʰ **T69.02** **Immersion foot**

Trench foot

√7ᵗʰ **T69.021** **Immersion foot, right foot**

√7ᵗʰ **T69.022** **Immersion foot, left foot**

√7ᵗʰ **T69.029** **Immersion foot, unspecified foot** ▽

√x7ᵗʰ **T69.1** **Chilblains**

DEF: Red, swollen, itchy skin primarily affecting the fingers and toes, nose and ears, and legs; follows damp-cold exposure; can also be associated with pruritus and a burning feeling.

√x7ᵗʰ **T69.8** **Other specified effects of reduced temperature**

√x7ᵗʰ **T69.9** **Effect of reduced temperature, unspecified** ▽

√4ᵗʰ **T70** **Effects of air pressure and water pressure**

The appropriate 7th character is to be added to each code from category T70.
A   initial encounter
D subsequent encounter
S   sequela

√x7ᵗʰ **T70.0** **Otitic barotrauma**

Aero-otitis media
Effects of change in ambient atmospheric pressure or water pressure on ears

√x7ᵗʰ **T70.1** **Sinus barotrauma**

Aerosinusitis
Effects of change in ambient atmospheric pressure on sinuses

√5ᵗʰ **T70.2** **Other and unspecified effects of high altitude**

  EXCLUDES 2 *polycythemia due to high altitude (D75.1)*

√7ᵗʰ **T70.20** **Unspecified effects of high altitude** ▽

√7ᵗʰ **T70.29** **Other effects of high altitude**

Alpine sickness
Anoxia due to high altitude
Barotrauma NOS
Hypobaropathy
Mountain sickness

√x7ᵗʰ **T70.3** **Caisson disease [decompression sickness]**

Compressed-air disease
Diver's palsy or paralysis

√x7ᵗʰ **T70.4** **Effects of high-pressure fluids**

Hydraulic jet injection (industrial)
Pneumatic jet injection (industrial)
Traumatic jet injection (industrial)

√x7ᵗʰ **T70.8** **Other effects of air pressure and water pressure**

√x7ᵗʰ **T70.9** **Effect of air pressure and water pressure, unspecified** ▽

√4ᵗʰ **T71** **Asphyxiation**

Mechanical suffocation
Traumatic suffocation
  EXCLUDES 1 *acute respiratory distress (syndrome) (J80)*
         anoxia due to high altitude (T70.2)
         asphyxia NOS (R09.01)
         asphyxia from carbon monoxide (T58.-)
         asphyxia from inhalation of food or foreign body (T17.-)
         asphyxia from other gases, fumes and vapors (T59.-)
         respiratory distress (syndrome) in newborn (P22.-)

The appropriate 7th character is to be added to each code from category T71.
A   initial encounter
D subsequent encounter
S   sequela

√5ᵗʰ **T71.1** **Asphyxiation due to mechanical threat to breathing**

Suffocation due to mechanical threat to breathing

√6ᵗʰ **T71.11** **Asphyxiation due to smothering under pillow**

√7ᵗʰ **T71.111** **Asphyxiation due to smothering under pillow, accidental**

Asphyxiation due to smothering under pillow NOS

√7ᵗʰ **T71.112** **Asphyxiation due to smothering under pillow, intentional self-harm**

√7ᵗʰ **T71.113** **Asphyxiation due to smothering under pillow, assault**

√7ᵗʰ **T71.114** **Asphyxiation due to smothering under pillow, undetermined**

√6ᵗʰ **T71.12** **Asphyxiation due to plastic bag**

√7ᵗʰ **T71.121** **Asphyxiation due to plastic bag, accidental**

Asphyxiation due to plastic bag NOS

√7ᵗʰ **T71.122** **Asphyxiation due to plastic bag, intentional self-harm**

√7ᵗʰ **T71.123** **Asphyxiation due to plastic bag, assault**

√7ᵗʰ **T71.124** **Asphyxiation due to plastic bag, undetermined**

√6ᵗʰ **T71.13** **Asphyxiation due to being trapped in bed linens**

√7ᵗʰ **T71.131** **Asphyxiation due to being trapped in bed linens, accidental**

Asphyxiation due to being trapped in bed linens NOS

√7ᵗʰ **T71.132** **Asphyxiation due to being trapped in bed linens, intentional self-harm**

√7ᵗʰ **T71.133** **Asphyxiation due to being trapped in bed linens, assault**

√7ᵗʰ **T71.134** **Asphyxiation due to being trapped in bed linens, undetermined**

√6ᵗʰ **T71.14** **Asphyxiation due to smothering under another person's body (in bed)**

☑ Additional Character Required   √x7ᵗʰ Placeholder Alert   Manifestation Dx   ▽ Unspecified Dx   ▶◀ Revised Text   ● New Code   ▲ Revised Code Title

ICD-10-CM 2017   **1059**

√7ᵗʰ **T71.141 Asphyxiation due to smothering under another person's body (in bed), accidental**

Asphyxiation due to smothering under another person's body (in bed) NOS

√7ᵗʰ **T71.143 Asphyxiation due to smothering under another person's body (in bed), assault**

√7ᵗʰ **T71.144 Asphyxiation due to smothering under another person's body (in bed), undetermined**

√6ᵗʰ **T71.15 Asphyxiation due to smothering in furniture**

√7ᵗʰ **T71.151 Asphyxiation due to smothering in furniture, accidental**

Asphyxiation due to smothering in furniture NOS

√7ᵗʰ **T71.152 Asphyxiation due to smothering in furniture, intentional self-harm**

√7ᵗʰ **T71.153 Asphyxiation due to smothering in furniture, assault**

√7ᵗʰ **T71.154 Asphyxiation due to smothering in furniture, undetermined**

√6ᵗʰ **T71.16 Asphyxiation due to hanging**

Hanging by window shade cord

Use additional code for any associated injuries, such as:

crushing injury of neck (S17.-)
fracture of cervical vertebrae (S12.0-S12.2-)
open wound of neck (S11.-)

√7ᵗʰ **T71.161 Asphyxiation due to hanging, accidental**

Asphyxiation due to hanging NOS
Hanging NOS

√7ᵗʰ **T71.162 Asphyxiation due to hanging, intentional self-harm**

√7ᵗʰ **T71.163 Asphyxiation due to hanging, assault**

√7ᵗʰ **T71.164 Asphyxiation due to hanging, undetermined**

√6ᵗʰ **T71.19 Asphyxiation due to mechanical threat to breathing due to other causes**

√7ᵗʰ **T71.191 Asphyxiation due to mechanical threat to breathing due to other causes, accidental**

Asphyxiation due to other causes NOS

√7ᵗʰ **T71.192 Asphyxiation due to mechanical threat to breathing due to other causes, intentional self-harm**

√7ᵗʰ **T71.193 Asphyxiation due to mechanical threat to breathing due to other causes, assault**

√7ᵗʰ **T71.194 Asphyxiation due to mechanical threat to breathing due to other causes, undetermined**

√5ᵗʰ **T71.2 Asphyxiation due to systemic oxygen deficiency due to low oxygen content in ambient air**

Suffocation due to systemic oxygen deficiency due to low oxygen content in ambient air

√x7ᵗʰ **T71.20 Asphyxiation due to systemic oxygen deficiency due to low oxygen content in ambient air due to unspecified cause** ▽

√x7ᵗʰ **T71.21 Asphyxiation due to cave-in or falling earth**

Use additional code for any associated cataclysm (X34-X38)

√6ᵗʰ **T71.22 Asphyxiation due to being trapped in a car trunk**

√7ᵗʰ **T71.221 Asphyxiation due to being trapped in a car trunk, accidental**

√7ᵗʰ **T71.222 Asphyxiation due to being trapped in a car trunk, intentional self-harm**

√7ᵗʰ **T71.223 Asphyxiation due to being trapped in a car trunk, assault**

√7ᵗʰ **T71.224 Asphyxiation due to being trapped in a car trunk, undetermined**

√6ᵗʰ **T71.23 Asphyxiation due to being trapped in a (discarded) refrigerator**

√7ᵗʰ **T71.231 Asphyxiation due to being trapped in a (discarded) refrigerator, accidental**

√7ᵗʰ **T71.232 Asphyxiation due to being trapped in a (discarded) refrigerator, intentional self-harm**

√7ᵗʰ **T71.233 Asphyxiation due to being trapped in a (discarded) refrigerator, assault**

√7ᵗʰ **T71.234 Asphyxiation due to being trapped in a (discarded) refrigerator, undetermined**

√x7ᵗʰ **T71.29 Asphyxiation due to being trapped in other low oxygen environment**

√x7ᵗʰ **T71.9 Asphyxiation due to unspecified cause** ▽

Suffocation (by strangulation) due to unspecified cause
Suffocation NOS
Systemic oxygen deficiency due to low oxygen content in ambient air due to unspecified cause
Systemic oxygen deficiency due to mechanical threat to breathing due to unspecified cause
Traumatic asphyxia NOS

√4ᵗʰ **T73 Effects of other deprivation**

The appropriate 7th character is to be added to each code from category T73.
A   initial encounter
D   subsequent encounter
S   sequela

√x7ᵗʰ **T73.0 Starvation**

Deprivation of food

√x7ᵗʰ **T73.1 Deprivation of water**

√x7ᵗʰ **T73.2 Exhaustion due to exposure**

√x7ᵗʰ **T73.3 Exhaustion due to excessive exertion**

Exhaustion due to overexertion

√x7ᵗʰ **T73.8 Other effects of deprivation**

√x7ᵗʰ **T73.9 Effect of deprivation, unspecified** ▽

√4ᵗʰ **T74 Adult and child abuse, neglect and other maltreatment, confirmed**

Use additional code, if applicable, to identify any associated current injury
Use additional external cause code to identify perpetrator, if known (Y07.-)

EXCLUDES 1 *abuse and maltreatment in pregnancy (O9A.3-, O9A.4-, O9A.5-)*
adult and child maltreatment, suspected (T76.-)

The appropriate 7th character is to be added to each code from category T74.
A   initial encounter
D   subsequent encounter
S   sequela

√5ᵗʰ **T74.0 Neglect or abandonment, confirmed**

√x7ᵗʰ **T74.01 Adult neglect or abandonment, confirmed** A

√x7ᵗʰ **T74.02 Child neglect or abandonment, confirmed** P

√5ᵗʰ **T74.1 Physical abuse, confirmed**

EXCLUDES 2 *sexual abuse (T74.2-)*

√x7ᵗʰ **T74.11 Adult physical abuse, confirmed** A

√x7ᵗʰ **T74.12 Child physical abuse, confirmed** P

EXCLUDES 2 *shaken infant syndrome (T74.4)*

√5ᵗʰ **T74.2 Sexual abuse, confirmed**

Rape, confirmed
Sexual assault, confirmed

√x7ᵗʰ **T74.21 Adult sexual abuse, confirmed** A

√x7ᵗʰ **T74.22 Child sexual abuse, confirmed** P

√5ᵗʰ **T74.3 Psychological abuse, confirmed**

√x7ᵗʰ **T74.31 Adult psychological abuse, confirmed** A

√x7ᵗʰ **T74.32 Child psychological abuse, confirmed** P

√x7ᵗʰ **T74.4 Shaken infant syndrome** P

√5ᵗʰ **T74.9 Unspecified maltreatment, confirmed**

√x7ᵗʰ **T74.91 Unspecified adult maltreatment, confirmed** A ▽

√x7ᵗʰ **T74.92 Unspecified child maltreatment, confirmed** P ▽

√4ᵗʰ **T75 Other and unspecified effects of other external causes**

EXCLUDES 1 *adverse effects NEC (T78.-)*
EXCLUDES 2 *burns (electric) (T20-T31)*

The appropriate 7th character is to be added to each code from category T75.
A   initial encounter
D   subsequent encounter
S   sequela

√5ᵗʰ **T75.0 Effects of lightning**

Struck by lightning

√x7ᵗʰ **T75.00 Unspecified effects of lightning** ▽

Struck by lightning NOS

√x7ᵗʰ **T75.01 Shock due to being struck by lightning**

√x7ᵗʰ **T75.09 Other effects of lightning**

Use additional code for other effects of lightning

EXCLUDES 1 Not coded here   **EXCLUDES 2** Not included here   N Newborn Age : 0   P Pediatric Age : 0-17   M Maternity Age : 12-55   A Adult Age : 15-124

✓x7ᵗʰ **T75.1** **Unspecified effects of drowning and nonfatal submersion** ▽

     Immersion

     EXCLUDES 1 *specified effects of drowning - code to effects*

✓5ᵗʰ **T75.2** **Effects of vibration**

   ✓x7ᵗʰ **T75.20** **Unspecified effects of vibration** ▽

   ✓x7ᵗʰ **T75.21** **Pneumatic hammer syndrome**

   ✓x7ᵗʰ **T75.22** **Traumatic vasospastic syndrome**

   ✓x7ᵗʰ **T75.23** **Vertigo from infrasound**

     EXCLUDES 1 *vertigo NOS (R42)*

   ✓x7ᵗʰ **T75.29** **Other effects of vibration**

✓x7ᵗʰ **T75.3** **Motion sickness**

     Airsickness

     Seasickness

     Travel sickness

     Use additional external cause code to identify vehicle or type of motion (Y92.81-, Y93.5-)

✓x7ᵗʰ **T75.4** **Electrocution**

     Shock from electric current

     Shock from electroshock gun (taser)

✓5ᵗʰ **T75.8** **Other specified effects of external causes**

   ✓x7ᵗʰ **T75.81** **Effects of abnormal gravitation [G] forces**

   ✓x7ᵗʰ **T75.82** **Effects of weightlessness**

   ✓x7ᵗʰ **T75.89** **Other specified effects of external causes**

✓4ᵗʰ **T76 Adult and child abuse, neglect and other maltreatment, suspected**

     Use additional code, if applicable, to identify any associated current injury

     EXCLUDES 1 *adult and child maltreatment, confirmed (T74.-)*

         suspected abuse and maltreatment in pregnancy (O9A.3-, O9A.4-, O9A.5-)

         suspected adult physical abuse, ruled out (Z04.71)

         suspected adult sexual abuse, ruled out (Z04.41)

         suspected child physical abuse, ruled out (Z04.72)

         suspected child sexual abuse, ruled out (Z04.42)

     The appropriate 7th character is to be added to each code from category T76.

     A   initial encounter

     D   subsequent encounter

     S   sequela

✓5ᵗʰ **T76.0** **Neglect or abandonment, suspected**

   ✓x7ᵗʰ **T76.01** **Adult neglect or abandonment, suspected** Ⓐ

   ✓x7ᵗʰ **T76.02** **Child neglect or abandonment, suspected** Ⓟ

✓5ᵗʰ **T76.1** **Physical abuse, suspected**

   ✓x7ᵗʰ **T76.11** **Adult physical abuse, suspected** Ⓐ

   ✓x7ᵗʰ **T76.12** **Child physical abuse, suspected** Ⓟ

✓5ᵗʰ **T76.2** **Sexual abuse, suspected**

     Rape, suspected

     Sexual abuse, suspected

     EXCLUDES 1 *alleged abuse, ruled out (Z04.7)*

   ✓x7ᵗʰ **T76.21** **Adult sexual abuse, suspected** Ⓐ

   ✓x7ᵗʰ **T76.22** **Child sexual abuse, suspected** Ⓟ

✓5ᵗʰ **T76.3** **Psychological abuse, suspected**

   ✓x7ᵗʰ **T76.31** **Adult psychological abuse, suspected** Ⓐ

   ✓x7ᵗʰ **T76.32** **Child psychological abuse, suspected** Ⓟ

✓5ᵗʰ **T76.9** **Unspecified maltreatment, suspected**

   ✓x7ᵗʰ **T76.91** **Unspecified adult maltreatment, suspected** Ⓐ ▽

   ✓x7ᵗʰ **T76.92** **Unspecified child maltreatment, suspected** Ⓟ ▽

✓4ᵗʰ **T78 Adverse effects, not elsewhere classified**

     EXCLUDES 2 *complications of surgical and medical care NEC (T80-T88)*

     The appropriate 7th character is to be added to each code from category T78.

     A   initial encounter

     D   subsequent encounter

     S   sequela

✓5ᵗʰ **T78.0** **Anaphylactic reaction due to food**

     Anaphylactic reaction due to adverse food reaction

     Anaphylactic shock or reaction due to nonpoisonous foods

     Anaphylactoid reaction due to food

   ✓x7ᵗʰ **T78.00** **Anaphylactic reaction due to unspecified food** ▽

   ✓x7ᵗʰ **T78.01** **Anaphylactic reaction due to peanuts**

   ✓x7ᵗʰ **T78.02** **Anaphylactic reaction due to shellfish (crustaceans)**

   ✓x7ᵗʰ **T78.03** **Anaphylactic reaction due to other fish**

   ✓x7ᵗʰ **T78.04** **Anaphylactic reaction due to fruits and vegetables**

   ✓x7ᵗʰ **T78.05** **Anaphylactic reaction due to tree nuts and seeds**

     EXCLUDES 2 ►*anaphylactic reaction due to peanuts (T78.01)*◄

   ✓x7ᵗʰ **T78.06** **Anaphylactic reaction due to food additives**

   ✓x7ᵗʰ **T78.07** **Anaphylactic reaction due to milk and dairy products**

   ✓x7ᵗʰ **T78.08** **Anaphylactic reaction due to eggs**

   ✓x7ᵗʰ **T78.09** **Anaphylactic reaction due to other food products**

✓x7ᵗʰ **T78.1** **Other adverse food reactions, not elsewhere classified**

     ►Use additional code to identify the type of reaction, if applicable◄

     EXCLUDES 1 *anaphylactic reaction or shock due to adverse food reaction (T78.0-)*

         anaphylactic reaction due to food (T78.0-)

         bacterial food borne intoxications (A05.-)

     EXCLUDES 2 *allergic and dietetic gastroenteritis and colitis ►(K52.29)◄*

         allergic rhinitis due to food (J30.5)

         dermatitis due to food in contact with skin (L23.6, L24.6, L25.4)

         dermatitis due to ingested food (L27.2)

         ►*food protein-induced enterocolitis syndrome (K52.21)*◄

         ►*food protein-induced enteropathy (K52.22)*◄

✓x7ᵗʰ **T78.2** **Anaphylactic shock, unspecified** ▽

     Allergic shock

     Anaphylactic reaction

     Anaphylaxis

     EXCLUDES 1 *anaphylactic reaction or shock due to adverse effect of correct medicinal substance properly administered (T88.6)*

         anaphylactic reaction or shock due to adverse food reaction (T78.0-)

         anaphylactic reaction or shock due to serum (T80.5-)

✓x7ᵗʰ **T78.3** **Angioneurotic edema**

     Allergic angioedema

     Giant urticaria

     Quincke's edema

     EXCLUDES 1 *serum urticaria (T80.6-)*

         urticaria (L50.-)

✓5ᵗʰ **T78.4** **Other and unspecified allergy**

     EXCLUDES 1 *specified types of allergic reaction such as:*

         allergic diarrhea ►(K52.29)◄

         allergic gastroenteritis and colitis ►(K52.29)◄

         dermatitis (L23-L25, L27.-)

         ►*food protein-induced enterocolitis syndrome (K52.21)*◄

         ►*food protein-induced enteropathy (K52.22)*◄

         hay fever (J30.1)

   ✓x7ᵗʰ **T78.40** **Allergy, unspecified** ▽

     Allergic reaction NOS

     Hypersensitivity NOS

   ✓x7ᵗʰ **T78.41** **Arthus phenomenon**

     Arthus reaction

   ✓x7ᵗʰ **T78.49** **Other allergy**

✓x7ᵗʰ **T78.8** **Other adverse effects, not elsewhere classified**

Certain early complications of trauma (T79)

✓4ᵗʰ **T79 Certain early complications of trauma, not elsewhere classified**

     EXCLUDES 2 *acute respiratory distress syndrome (J80)*

         complications occurring during or following medical procedures (T80-T88)

         complications of surgical and medical care NEC (T80-T88)

         newborn respiratory distress syndrome (P22.0)

     The appropriate 7th character is to be added to each code from category T79.

     A   initial encounter

     D   subsequent encounter

     S   sequela

☑ Additional Character Required   ✓x7ᵗʰ Placeholder Alert   Manifestation Dx   ▽ Unspecified Dx   ►◄ Revised Text   ● New Code   ▲ Revised Code Title

√x7ᵗʰ **T79.0 Air embolism (traumatic)**

> EXCLUDES 1   *air embolism complicating abortion or ectopic or molar pregnancy (O00-O07, O08.2)*
> *air embolism complicating pregnancy, childbirth and the puerperium (O88.0)*
> *air embolism following infusion, transfusion, and therapeutic injection (T80.0)*
> *air embolism following procedure NEC (T81.7-)*
>
> **DEF:** Arterial or venous obstruction due to introduction of air bubbles into the blood vessels following surgery or trauma.

√x7ᵗʰ **T79.1 Fat embolism (traumatic)**

> EXCLUDES 1   *fat embolism complicating:*
> *abortion or ectopic or molar pregnancy (O00-O07, O08.2)*
> *pregnancy, childbirth and the puerperium (O88.8)*

√x7ᵗʰ **T79.2 Traumatic secondary and recurrent hemorrhage and seroma**

√x7ᵗʰ **T79.4 Traumatic shock**

> Shock (immediate) (delayed) following injury
>
> EXCLUDES 1   *anaphylactic shock due to adverse food reaction (T78.0-)*
> *anaphylactic shock due to correct medicinal substance properly administered (T88.6)*
> *anaphylactic shock due to serum (T80.5-)*
> *anaphylactic shock NOS (T78.2)*
> *anesthetic shock (T88.2)*
> *electric shock (T75.4)*
> *nontraumatic shock NEC (R57.-)*
> *obstetric shock (O75.1)*
> *postprocedural shock (T81.1-)*
> *septic shock (R65.21)*
> *shock complicating abortion or ectopic or molar pregnancy (O00-O07, O08.3)*
> *shock due to lightning (T75.01)*
> *shock NOS (R57.9)*

√x7ᵗʰ **T79.5 Traumatic anuria**

> Crush syndrome
> Renal failure following crushing

√x7ᵗʰ **T79.6 Traumatic ischemia of muscle**

> Traumatic rhabdomyolysis
> Volkmann's ischemic contracture
>
> EXCLUDES 2   *anterior tibial syndrome (M76.8)*
> *compartment syndrome (traumatic) (T79.A-)*
> *nontraumatic ischemia of muscle (M62.2-)*

√x7ᵗʰ **T79.7 Traumatic subcutaneous emphysema**

> EXCLUDES 1   *emphysema NOS (J43)*
> *emphysema (subcutaneous) resulting from a procedure (T81.82)*

√5ᵗʰ **T79.A Traumatic compartment syndrome**

> EXCLUDES 1   *fibromyalgia (M79.7)*
> *nontraumatic compartment syndrome (M79.A-)*
> *traumatic ischemic infarction of muscle (T79.6)*

  √x7ᵗʰ **T79.A0 Compartment syndrome, unspecified** ▽

> Compartment syndrome NOS

  √6ᵗʰ **T79.A1 Traumatic compartment syndrome of upper extremity**

> Traumatic compartment syndrome of shoulder, arm, forearm, wrist, hand, and fingers

    √7ᵗʰ **T79.A11 Traumatic compartment syndrome of right upper extremity**

    √7ᵗʰ **T79.A12 Traumatic compartment syndrome of left upper extremity**

    √7ᵗʰ **T79.A19 Traumatic compartment syndrome of unspecified upper extremity** ▽

  √6ᵗʰ **T79.A2 Traumatic compartment syndrome of lower extremity**

> Traumatic compartment syndrome of hip, buttock, thigh, leg, foot, and toes

    √7ᵗʰ **T79.A21 Traumatic compartment syndrome of right lower extremity**

    √7ᵗʰ **T79.A22 Traumatic compartment syndrome of left lower extremity**

    √7ᵗʰ **T79.A29 Traumatic compartment syndrome of unspecified lower extremity** ▽

  √x7ᵗʰ **T79.A3 Traumatic compartment syndrome of abdomen**

  √x7ᵗʰ **T79.A9 Traumatic compartment syndrome of other sites**

√x7ᵗʰ **T79.8 Other early complications of trauma**

√x7ᵗʰ **T79.9 Unspecified early complication of trauma** ▽

Complications of surgical and medical care, not elsewhere classified (T80-T88)

Use additional code for adverse effect, if applicable, to identify drug (T36-T50 with fifth or sixth character 5)

Use additional code(s) to identify the specified condition resulting from the complication

Use additional code to identify devices involved and details of circumstances (Y62-Y82)

> EXCLUDES 2   *any encounters with medical care for postprocedural conditions in which no complications are present, such as:*
> *artificial opening status (Z93.-)*
> *closure of external stoma (Z43.-)*
> *fitting and adjustment of external prosthetic device (Z44.-)*
> *burns and corrosions from local applications and irradiation (T20-T32)*
> *complications of surgical procedures during pregnancy, childbirth and the puerperium (O00-O9A)*
> *mechanical complication of respirator [ventilator] (J95.850)*
> *poisoning and toxic effects of drugs and chemicals (T36-T65 with fifth or sixth character 1-4 or 6)*
> *postprocedural fever (R50.82)*
> *specified complications classified elsewhere, such as:*
> *cerebrospinal fluid leak from spinal puncture (G97.0)*
> *colostomy malfunction (K94.0-)*
> *disorders of fluid and electrolyte imbalance (E86-E87)*
> *functional disturbances following cardiac surgery (I97.0-I97.1)*
> *intraoperative and postprocedural complications of specified body systems (D78.-, E36.-, E89.-, G97.3-, G97.4, H59.3-, H59.-, H95.2-, H95.3, I97.4-, I97.5, J95.6-, J95.7, K91.6-, L76.-, M96.-, N99.-)*
> *ostomy complications (J95.0-, K94.-, N99.5-)*
> *postgastric surgery syndromes (K91.1)*
> *postlaminectomy syndrome NEC (M96.1)*
> *postmastectomy lymphedema syndrome (I97.2)*
> *postsurgical blind-loop syndrome (K91.2)*
> *ventilator associated pneumonia (J95.851)*

AHA: 2015,1Q,15

√4ᵗʰ **T80 Complications following infusion, transfusion and therapeutic injection**

> INCLUDES   complications following perfusion
>
> EXCLUDES 2   *bone marrow transplant rejection (T86.01)*
> *febrile nonhemolytic transfusion reaction (R50.84)*
> *fluid overload due to transfusion (E87.71)*
> *posttransfusion purpura (D69.51)*
> *transfusion associated circulatory overload (TACO) (E87.71)*
> *transfusion (red blood cell) associated hemochromatosis (E83.111)*
> *transfusion related acute lung injury (TRALI) (J95.84)*

> The appropriate 7th character is to be added to each code from category T80.
> A   initial encounter
> D   subsequent encounter
> S   sequela

√x7ᵗʰ **T80.0 Air embolism following infusion, transfusion and therapeutic injection**

√x7ᵗʰ **T80.1 Vascular complications following infusion, transfusion and therapeutic injection**

> Use additional code to identify the vascular complication
>
> EXCLUDES 2   *extravasation of vesicant agent (T80.81-)*
> *infiltration of vesicant agent (T80.81-)*
> *postprocedural vascular complications (T81.7-)*
> *vascular complications specified as due to prosthetic devices, implants and grafts ▶(T82.8-, T83.8-, T84.8-, T85.8-)◀*

√5ᵗʰ **T80.2 Infections following infusion, transfusion and therapeutic injection**

> Use additional code to identify the specific infection, such as: sepsis (A41.9)
> Use additional code (R65.2-) to identify severe sepsis, if applicable
>
> EXCLUDES 2   *infections specified as due to prosthetic devices, implants and grafts (T82.6-T82.7, T83.5-T83.6, T84.5-T84.7, T85.7)*
> *postprocedural infections ▶(T81.4-)◀*

  √6ᵗʰ **T80.21 Infection due to central venous catheter**

> ▶Infection due to pulmonary artery catheter (Swan-Ganz catheter)◀

EXCLUDES 1   Not coded here   EXCLUDES 2   Not included here   N   Newborn Age : 0   P   Pediatric Age : 0-17   M   Maternity Age : 12-55   A   Adult Age : 15-124

1062   ICD-10-CM 2017

✓7ᵗʰ **T80.211** **Bloodstream infection** **due to central venous catheter**
Catheter-related bloodstream infection (CRBSI) NOS
Central line-associated bloodstream infection (CLABSI)
Bloodstream infection due to Hickman catheter
Bloodstream infection due to peripherally inserted central catheter (PICC)
Bloodstream infection due to portacath (port-a-cath)
▶Bloodstream infection due to pulmonary artery catheter◄
Bloodstream infection due to triple lumen catheter
Bloodstream infection due to umbilical venous catheter

✓7ᵗʰ **T80.212** **Local infection** **due to central venous catheter**
Exit or insertion site infection
Local infection due to Hickman catheter
Local infection due to peripherally inserted central catheter (PICC)
Local infection due to portacath (port-a-cath)
▶Local infection due to pulmonary artery catheter◄
Local infection due to triple lumen catheter
Local infection due to umbilical venous catheter
Port or reservoir infection
Tunnel infection

✓7ᵗʰ **T80.218** **Other infection due to central venous catheter**
Other central line-associated infection
Other infection due to Hickman catheter
Other infection due to peripherally inserted central catheter (PICC)
Other infection due to portacath (port-a-cath)
▶Other infection due to pulmonary artery catheter◄
Other infection due to triple lumen catheter
Other infection due to umbilical venous catheter

✓7ᵗʰ **T80.219** **Unspecified infection due to central venous catheter**   ▽
Central line-associated infection NOS
Unspecified infection due to Hickman catheter
Unspecified infection due to peripherally inserted central catheter (PICC)
Unspecified infection due to portacath (port-a-cath)
▶Unspecified infection due to pulmonary artery catheter◄
Unspecified infection due to triple lumen catheter
Unspecified infection due to umbilical venous catheter

✓x7ᵗʰ **T80.22** **Acute infection following transfusion, infusion, or injection of blood and blood products**

✓x7ᵗʰ **T80.29** **Infection following other infusion, transfusion and therapeutic injection**

✓5ᵗʰ **T80.3** **ABO incompatibility** **reaction due to transfusion of blood or blood products**
EXCLUDES 1 *minor blood group antigens reactions (Duffy) (E) (K(ell)) (Kidd) (Lewis) (M) (N) (P) (S) (T80.A)*

✓x7ᵗʰ **T80.30** **ABO incompatibility reaction due to transfusion of blood or blood products, unspecified**   ▽
ABO incompatibility blood transfusion NOS
Reaction to ABO incompatibility from transfusion NOS

✓6ᵗʰ **T80.31** **ABO incompatibility** **with hemolytic transfusion reaction**

✓7ᵗʰ **T80.310** **ABO incompatibility with** **acute** **hemolytic transfusion reaction**
ABO incompatibility with hemolytic transfusion reaction less than 24 hours after transfusion
Acute hemolytic transfusion reaction (AHTR) due to ABO incompatibility

✓7ᵗʰ **T80.311** **ABO incompatibility with** **delayed** **hemolytic transfusion reaction**
ABO incompatibility with hemolytic transfusion reaction 24 hours or more after transfusion
Delayed hemolytic transfusion reaction (DHTR) due to ABO incompatibility

✓7ᵗʰ **T80.319** **ABO incompatibility with hemolytic transfusion reaction, unspecified**   ▽
ABO incompatibility with hemolytic transfusion reaction at unspecified time after transfusion
Hemolytic transfusion reaction (HTR) due to ABO incompatibility NOS

✓x7ᵗʰ **T80.39** **Other ABO incompatibility reaction due to transfusion of blood or blood products**
Delayed serologic transfusion reaction (DSTR) from ABO incompatibility
Other ABO incompatible blood transfusion
Other reaction to ABO incompatible blood transfusion

✓5ᵗʰ **T80.4** **Rh incompatibility** **reaction due to transfusion of blood or blood products**
Reaction due to incompatibility of Rh antigens (C) (c) (D) (E) (e)

✓x7ᵗʰ **T80.40** **Rh incompatibility reaction due to transfusion** **of blood or blood products, unspecified**   ▽
Reaction due to Rh factor in transfusion NOS
Rh incompatible blood transfusion NOS

✓6ᵗʰ **T80.41** **Rh incompatibility** **with hemolytic transfusion reaction**

✓7ᵗʰ **T80.410** **Rh incompatibility with** **acute** **hemolytic transfusion reaction**
Acute hemolytic transfusion reaction (AHTR) due to Rh incompatibility
Rh incompatibility with hemolytic transfusion reaction less than 24 hours after transfusion

✓7ᵗʰ **T80.411** **Rh incompatibility with** **delayed** **hemolytic transfusion reaction**
Delayed hemolytic transfusion reaction (DHTR) due to Rh incompatibility
Rh incompatibility with hemolytic transfusion reaction 24 hours or more after transfusion

✓7ᵗʰ **T80.419** **Rh incompatibility with hemolytic transfusion reaction, unspecified**   ▽
Rh incompatibility with hemolytic transfusion reaction at unspecified time after transfusion
Hemolytic transfusion reaction (HTR) due to Rh incompatibility NOS

✓x7ᵗʰ **T80.49** **Other Rh incompatibility reaction due to transfusion of blood or blood products**
Delayed serologic transfusion reaction (DSTR) from Rh incompatibility
Other reaction to Rh incompatible blood transfusion

✓5ᵗʰ **T80.A** **Non-ABO incompatibility** **reaction due to transfusion of blood or blood products**
Reaction due to incompatibility of minor antigens (Duffy) (Kell) (Kidd) (Lewis) (M) (N) (P) (S)

✓x7ᵗʰ **T80.A0** **Non-ABO incompatibility reaction due to transfusion of blood or blood products, unspecified**   ▽
Non-ABO antigen incompatibility reaction from transfusion NOS

✓6ᵗʰ **T80.A1** **Non-ABO incompatibility with hemolytic transfusion reaction**

✓7ᵗʰ **T80.A10** **Non-ABO incompatibility with acute hemolytic transfusion reaction**
Acute hemolytic transfusion reaction (AHTR) due to non-ABO incompatibility
Non-ABO incompatibility with hemolytic transfusion reaction less than 24 hours after transfusion

☑7ᵗʰ **T80.A11 Non-ABO incompatibility with delayed hemolytic transfusion reaction**

　　Delayed hemolytic transfusion reaction (DHTR) due to non-ABO incompatibility

　　Non-ABO incompatibility with hemolytic transfusion reaction 24 or more hours after transfusion

☑7ᵗʰ **T80.A19 Non-ABO incompatibility with hemolytic transfusion reaction, unspecified**　　　▽

　　Hemolytic transfusion reaction (HTR) due to non-ABO incompatibility NOS

　　Non-ABO incompatibility with hemolytic transfusion reaction at unspecified time after transfusion

☑x7ᵗʰ **T80.A9 Other non-ABO incompatibility reaction due to transfusion of blood or blood products**

　　Delayed serologic transfusion reaction (DSTR) from non-ABO incompatibility

　　Other reaction to non-ABO incompatible blood transfusion

☑5ᵗʰ **T80.5 Anaphylactic reaction due to serum**

Allergic shock due to serum

Anaphylactic shock due to serum

Anaphylactoid reaction due to serum

Anaphylaxis due to serum

EXCLUDES 1 *ABO incompatibility reaction due to transfusion of blood or blood products (T80.3-)*

allergic reaction or shock NOS (T78.2)

anaphylactic reaction or shock NOS (T78.2)

anaphylactic reaction or shock due to adverse effect of correct medicinal substance properly administered (T88.6)

other serum reaction (T80.6-)

☑x7ᵗʰ **T80.51 Anaphylactic reaction due to administration of blood and blood products**

☑x7ᵗʰ **T80.52 Anaphylactic reaction due to vaccination**

☑x7ᵗʰ **T80.59 Anaphylactic reaction due to other serum**

☑5ᵗʰ **T80.6 Other serum reactions**

Intoxication by serum

Protein sickness

Serum rash

Serum sickness

Serum urticaria

EXCLUDES 2 *serum hepatitis ▶(B16-B19)◀*

DEF: Serum sickness: Hypersensitivity to foreign serum; causes fever, hives, swelling, and lymphadenopathy.

☑x7ᵗʰ **T80.61 Other serum reaction due to administration of blood and blood products**

☑x7ᵗʰ **T80.62 Other serum reaction due to vaccination**

☑x7ᵗʰ **T80.69 Other serum reaction due to other serum**

☑5ᵗʰ **T80.8 Other complications following infusion, transfusion and therapeutic injection**

☑6ᵗʰ **T80.81 Extravasation of vesicant agent**

　　Infiltration of vesicant agent

☑7ᵗʰ **T80.810 Extravasation of vesicant antineoplastic chemotherapy**

　　Infiltration of vesicant antineoplastic chemotherapy

☑7ᵗʰ **T80.818 Extravasation of other vesicant agent**

　　Infiltration of other vesicant agent

☑x7ᵗʰ **T80.89 Other complications following infusion, transfusion and therapeutic injection**

　　Delayed serologic transfusion reaction (DSTR), unspecified incompatibility

　　Use additional code to identify graft-versus-host reaction, if applicable, (D89.81-)

☑5ᵗʰ **T80.9 Unspecified complication following infusion, transfusion and therapeutic injection**

☑x7ᵗʰ **T80.90 Unspecified complication following infusion and therapeutic injection**　　▽

☑6ᵗʰ **T80.91 Hemolytic transfusion reaction, unspecified incompatibility**

EXCLUDES 1 *ABO incompatibility with hemolytic transfusion reaction (T80.31-)*

non-ABO incompatibility with hemolytic transfusion reaction (T80.A1-)

Rh incompatibility with hemolytic transfusion reaction (T80.41-)

☑7ᵗʰ **T80.910 Acute hemolytic transfusion reaction, unspecified incompatibility**　　▽

☑7ᵗʰ **T80.911 Delayed hemolytic transfusion reaction, unspecified incompatibility**　　▽

☑7ᵗʰ **T80.919 Hemolytic transfusion reaction, unspecified incompatibility, unspecified as acute or delayed**　　▽

　　Hemolytic transfusion reaction NOS

☑x7ᵗʰ **T80.92 Unspecified transfusion reaction**　　▽

　　Transfusion reaction NOS

☑4ᵗʰ **T81 Complications of procedures, not elsewhere classified**

Use additional code for adverse effect, if applicable, to identify drug (T36-T50 with fifth or sixth character 5)

EXCLUDES 2 *complications following immunization (T88.0-T88.1)*

complications following infusion, transfusion and therapeutic injection (T80.-)

complications of transplanted organs and tissue (T86.-)

specified complications classified elsewhere, such as:

complication of prosthetic devices, implants and grafts (T82-T85)

dermatitis due to drugs and medicaments (L23.3, L24.4, L25.1, L27.0-L27.1)

endosseous dental implant failure (M27.6-)

floppy iris syndrome (IFIS) (intraoperative) (H21.81)

intraoperative and postprocedural complications of specific body system (D78.-, E36.-, E89.-, G97.3-, G97.4, H59.3-, H59.-, H95.2-, H95.3, I97.4-, I97.5, J95, K91.-, L76.-, M96.-, N99.-)

ostomy complications (J95.0-, K94.-, N99.5-)

plateau iris syndrome (post-iridectomy) (postprocedural) H21.82

poisoning and toxic effects of drugs and chemicals (T36-T65 with fifth or sixth character 1-4 or 6)

The appropriate 7th character is to be added to each code from category T81.

A　initial encounter

D　subsequent encounter

S　sequela

☑5ᵗʰ **T81.1 Postprocedural shock**

Shock during or resulting from a procedure, not elsewhere classified

EXCLUDES 1 *anaphylactic shock due to correct substance properly administered (T88.6)*

anaphylactic shock due to serum (T80.5-)

anaphylactic shock NOS (T78.2)

anesthetic shock (T88.2)

electric shock (T75.4)

obstetric shock (O75.1)

septic shock (R65.21)

shock following abortion or ectopic or molar pregnancy (O00-O07, O08.3)

traumatic shock (T79.4)

☑x7ᵗʰ **T81.10 Postprocedural shock unspecified**　　▽

　　Collapse NOS during or resulting from a procedure, not elsewhere classified

　　Postprocedural failure of peripheral circulation

　　Postprocedural shock NOS

☑x7ᵗʰ **T81.11 Postprocedural cardiogenic shock**

☑x7ᵗʰ **T81.12 Postprocedural septic shock**

　　▶Postprocedural endotoxic shock resulting from a procedure, not elsewhere classified◀

　　▶Postprocedural gram-negative shock resulting from a procedure, not elsewhere classified◀

　　Code first underlying infection

　　Use additional code, to identify any associated acute organ dysfunction, if applicable

---

EXCLUDES 1 Not coded here　　*EXCLUDES 2* Not included here　　Ⓝ Newborn Age : 0　　Ⓟ Pediatric Age : 0-17　　Ⓜ Maternity Age : 12-55　　Ⓐ Adult Age : 15-124

1064　　　　　　　　　　　　　　　　　　　　　　　　　　　　　　　　　　　　　ICD-10-CM 2017

√x7ᵗʰ **T81.19** **Other postprocedural shock**

Postprocedural hypovolemic shock

√5ᵗʰ **T81.3** **Disruption of wound, not elsewhere classified**

Disruption of any suture materials or other closure methods

EXCLUDES 1 *breakdown (mechanical) of permanent sutures (T85.612)*

displacement of permanent sutures (T85.622)

disruption of cesarean delivery wound (O90.0)

disruption of perineal obstetric wound (O90.1)

mechanical complication of permanent sutures NEC (T85.692)

AHA: 2014,1Q,23

√x7ᵗʰ **T81.30** **Disruption of wound, unspecified**   ▽

Disruption of wound NOS

√x7ᵗʰ **T81.31** **Disruption of external operation (surgical) wound, not elsewhere classified**

Dehiscence of operation wound NOS

Disruption of operation wound NOS

Disruption or dehiscence of closure of cornea

Disruption or dehiscence of closure of mucosa

Disruption or dehiscence of closure of skin and subcutaneous tissue

Full-thickness skin disruption or dehiscence

Superficial disruption or dehiscence of operation wound

EXCLUDES 1 *dehiscence of amputation stump (T87.81)*

√x7ᵗʰ **T81.32** **Disruption of internal operation (surgical) wound, not elsewhere classified**

Deep disruption or dehiscence of operation wound NOS

Disruption or dehiscence of closure of internal organ or other internal tissue

Disruption or dehiscence of closure of muscle or muscle flap

Disruption or dehiscence of closure of ribs or rib cage

Disruption or dehiscence of closure of skull or craniotomy

Disruption or dehiscence of closure of sternum or sternotomy

Disruption or dehiscence of closure of tendon or ligament

Disruption or dehiscence of closure of superficial or muscular fascia

√x7ᵗʰ **T81.33** **Disruption of traumatic injury wound repair**

Disruption or dehiscence of closure of traumatic laceration (external) (internal)

√x7ᵗʰ **T81.4** **Infection following a procedure**

Intra-abdominal abscess following a procedure

Postprocedural infection, not elsewhere classified

Sepsis following a procedure

Stitch abscess following a procedure

Subphrenic abscess following a procedure

Wound abscess following a procedure

Use additional code to identify infection

Use additional code (R65.2-) to identify severe sepsis, if applicable

EXCLUDES 1 *obstetric surgical wound infection (O86.0)*

postprocedural fever NOS (R50.82)

postprocedural retroperitoneal abscess (K68.11)

EXCLUDES 2 *bleb associated endophthalmitis (H59.4-)*

infection due to infusion, transfusion and therapeutic injection (T80.2-)

infection due to prosthetic devices, implants and grafts (T82.6-T82.7, T83.5-T83.6, T84.5-T84.7, T85.7)

AHA: 2014,1Q,23

√5ᵗʰ **T81.5** **Complications of foreign body accidentally left in body following procedure**

AHA: 2014,4Q,24

√6ᵗʰ **T81.50** **Unspecified complication of foreign body accidentally left in body following procedure**

√7ᵗʰ **T81.500** **Unspecified complication of foreign body accidentally left in body following surgical operation**   ▽

√7ᵗʰ **T81.501** **Unspecified complication of foreign body accidentally left in body following infusion or transfusion**   ▽

√7ᵗʰ **T81.502** **Unspecified complication of foreign body accidentally left in body following kidney dialysis**   ▽

√7ᵗʰ **T81.503** **Unspecified complication of foreign body accidentally left in body following injection or immunization**   ▽

√7ᵗʰ **T81.504** **Unspecified complication of foreign body accidentally left in body following endoscopic examination**   ▽

√7ᵗʰ **T81.505** **Unspecified complication of foreign body accidentally left in body following heart catheterization**   ▽

√7ᵗʰ **T81.506** **Unspecified complication of foreign body accidentally left in body following aspiration, puncture or other catheterization**   ▽

√7ᵗʰ **T81.507** **Unspecified complication of foreign body accidentally left in body following removal of catheter or packing**   ▽

√7ᵗʰ **T81.508** **Unspecified complication of foreign body accidentally left in body following other procedure**   ▽

√7ᵗʰ **T81.509** **Unspecified complication of foreign body accidentally left in body following unspecified procedure**   ▽

√6ᵗʰ **T81.51** **Adhesions due to foreign body accidentally left in body following procedure**

√7ᵗʰ **T81.510** **Adhesions due to foreign body accidentally left in body following surgical operation**

√7ᵗʰ **T81.511** **Adhesions due to foreign body accidentally left in body following infusion or transfusion**

√7ᵗʰ **T81.512** **Adhesions due to foreign body accidentally left in body following kidney dialysis**

√7ᵗʰ **T81.513** **Adhesions due to foreign body accidentally left in body following injection or immunization**

√7ᵗʰ **T81.514** **Adhesions due to foreign body accidentally left in body following endoscopic examination**

√7ᵗʰ **T81.515** **Adhesions due to foreign body accidentally left in body following heart catheterization**

√7ᵗʰ **T81.516** **Adhesions due to foreign body accidentally left in body following aspiration, puncture or other catheterization**

√7ᵗʰ **T81.517** **Adhesions due to foreign body accidentally left in body following removal of catheter or packing**

√7ᵗʰ **T81.518** **Adhesions due to foreign body accidentally left in body following other procedure**

√7ᵗʰ **T81.519** **Adhesions due to foreign body accidentally left in body following unspecified procedure**   ▽

√6ᵗʰ **T81.52** **Obstruction due to foreign body accidentally left in body following procedure**

√7ᵗʰ **T81.520** **Obstruction due to foreign body accidentally left in body following surgical operation**

√7ᵗʰ **T81.521** **Obstruction due to foreign body accidentally left in body following infusion or transfusion**

√7ᵗʰ **T81.522** **Obstruction due to foreign body accidentally left in body following kidney dialysis**

√7ᵗʰ **T81.523** **Obstruction due to foreign body accidentally left in body following injection or immunization**

√7ᵗʰ **T81.524** **Obstruction due to foreign body accidentally left in body following endoscopic examination**

√7ᵗʰ **T81.525** **Obstruction due to foreign body accidentally left in body following heart catheterization**

☑ Additional Character Required   √x7ᵗʰ Placeholder Alert   Manifestation Dx   ▽ Unspecified Dx   ►◄ Revised Text   ● New Code   ▲ Revised Code Title

ICD-10-CM 2017   **1065**

Chapter 19. Injury, Poisoning and Certain Other Consequences of External Causes

√7ᵗʰ **T81.526 Obstruction due to foreign body accidentally left in body following** aspiration, puncture or other catheterization

√7ᵗʰ **T81.527 Obstruction due to foreign body accidentally left in body following** removal of catheter or packing

√7ᵗʰ **T81.528 Obstruction due to foreign body accidentally left in body following other** procedure

√7ᵗʰ **T81.529 Obstruction due to foreign body accidentally left in body following** unspecified procedure ▽

√6ᵗʰ **T81.53 Perforation** due to foreign body accidentally left in body following procedure

√7ᵗʰ **T81.530 Perforation due to foreign body accidentally left in body following** surgical operation

√7ᵗʰ **T81.531 Perforation due to foreign body accidentally left in body following** infusion or transfusion

√7ᵗʰ **T81.532 Perforation due to foreign body accidentally left in body following** kidney dialysis

√7ᵗʰ **T81.533 Perforation due to foreign body accidentally left in body following** injection or immunization

√7ᵗʰ **T81.534 Perforation due to foreign body accidentally left in body following** endoscopic examination

√7ᵗʰ **T81.535 Perforation due to foreign body accidentally left in body following** heart catheterization

√7ᵗʰ **T81.536 Perforation due to foreign body accidentally left in body following** aspiration, puncture or other catheterization

√7ᵗʰ **T81.537 Perforation due to foreign body accidentally left in body following** removal of catheter or packing

√7ᵗʰ **T81.538 Perforation due to foreign body accidentally left in body following other** procedure

√7ᵗʰ **T81.539 Perforation due to foreign body accidentally left in body following** unspecified procedure ▽

√6ᵗʰ **T81.59 Other complications of foreign body accidentally left in body following procedure**

EXCLUDES 2 *obstruction or perforation due to prosthetic devices and implants intentionally left in body (T82.0-T82.5, T83.0-T83.4, T83.7, T84.0-T84.4, T85.0-T85.6)*

√7ᵗʰ **T81.590 Other complications of foreign body accidentally left in body following** surgical operation

√7ᵗʰ **T81.591 Other complications of foreign body accidentally left in body following** infusion or transfusion

√7ᵗʰ **T81.592 Other complications of foreign body accidentally left in body following** kidney dialysis

√7ᵗʰ **T81.593 Other complications of foreign body accidentally left in body following** injection or immunization

√7ᵗʰ **T81.594 Other complications of foreign body accidentally left in body following** endoscopic examination

√7ᵗʰ **T81.595 Other complications of foreign body accidentally left in body following** heart catheterization

√7ᵗʰ **T81.596 Other complications of foreign body accidentally left in body following** aspiration, puncture or other catheterization

√7ᵗʰ **T81.597 Other complications of foreign body accidentally left in body following** removal of catheter or packing

√7ᵗʰ **T81.598 Other complications of foreign body accidentally left in body following other** procedure

√7ᵗʰ **T81.599 Other complications of foreign body accidentally left in body following unspecified procedure** ▽

√5ᵗʰ **T81.6 Acute reaction to foreign substance accidentally left during a procedure**

EXCLUDES 2 *complications of foreign body accidentally left in body cavity or operation wound following procedure (T81.5-)*

√x7ᵗʰ **T81.60 Unspecified acute reaction to foreign substance accidentally left during a procedure** ▽

√x7ᵗʰ **T81.61 Aseptic peritonitis due to foreign substance accidentally left during a procedure**
Chemical peritonitis

√x7ᵗʰ **T81.69 Other acute reaction to foreign substance accidentally left during a procedure**

√5ᵗʰ **T81.7 Vascular complications following a procedure, not elsewhere classified**
Air embolism following procedure NEC
Phlebitis or thrombophlebitis resulting from a procedure

EXCLUDES 1 *embolism complicating abortion or ectopic or molar pregnancy (O00-O07, O08.2)*
embolism complicating pregnancy, childbirth and the puerperium (O88.-)
traumatic embolism (T79.0)

EXCLUDES 2 *embolism due to prosthetic devices, implants and grafts ▶(T82.8-, T83.81, T84.8-, T85.81-)◀*
embolism following infusion, transfusion and therapeutic injection (T80.0)

√6ᵗʰ **T81.71 Complication of artery following a procedure, not elsewhere classified**

√7ᵗʰ **T81.710 Complication of** mesenteric **artery following a procedure, not elsewhere classified**

√7ᵗʰ **T81.711 Complication of** renal **artery following a procedure, not elsewhere classified**

√7ᵗʰ **T81.718 Complication of other artery following a procedure, not elsewhere classified**

√7ᵗʰ **T81.719 Complication of unspecified artery following a procedure, not elsewhere classified** ▽

√x7ᵗʰ **T81.72 Complication of** vein **following a procedure, not elsewhere classified**

√5ᵗʰ **T81.8 Other complications of procedures, not elsewhere classified**

EXCLUDES 2 *hypothermia following anesthesia (T88.51)*
malignant hyperpyrexia due to anesthesia (T88.3)

√x7ᵗʰ **T81.81 Complication of inhalation therapy**

√x7ᵗʰ **T81.82 Emphysema (subcutaneous) resulting from a procedure**

√x7ᵗʰ **T81.83 Persistent postprocedural fistula**

√x7ᵗʰ **T81.89 Other complications of procedures, not elsewhere classified**
Use additional code to specify complication, such as:
postprocedural delirium (F05)
AHA: 2014,1Q,23

√x7ᵗʰ **T81.9 Unspecified complication of procedure** ▽

√4ᵗʰ **T82 Complications of cardiac and vascular prosthetic devices, implants and grafts**

EXCLUDES 2 *failure and rejection of transplanted organs and tissue (T86.-)*

The appropriate 7th character is to be added to each code from category T82.
A   initial encounter
D   subsequent encounter
S   sequela

√5ᵗʰ **T82.0 Mechanical complication of** heart valve prosthesis
Mechanical complication of artificial heart valve

EXCLUDES 1 *mechanical complication of biological heart valve graft (T82.22-)*

√x7ᵗʰ **T82.01 Breakdown (mechanical) of heart valve prosthesis**

√x7ᵗʰ **T82.02 Displacement of heart valve prosthesis**
Malposition of heart valve prosthesis

√x7ᵗʰ **T82.03 Leakage of heart valve prosthesis**

√x7ᵗʰ **T82.09 Other mechanical complication of heart valve prosthesis**
Obstruction (mechanical) of heart valve prosthesis
Perforation of heart valve prosthesis
Protrusion of heart valve prosthesis

√5ᵗʰ **T82.1 Mechanical complication of** cardiac electronic device

√6ᵗʰ **T82.11 Breakdown (mechanical) of cardiac electronic device**

√7ᵗʰ **T82.110 Breakdown (mechanical) of cardiac electrode**

EXCLUDES 1 Not coded here   EXCLUDES 2 Not included here   N Newborn Age : 0   P Pediatric Age : 0-17   M Maternity Age : 12-55   A Adult Age : 15-124

1066   ICD-10-CM 2017

√7ᵗʰ **T82.111** **Breakdown (mechanical) of cardiac** pulse generator (battery)

√7ᵗʰ **T82.118** **Breakdown (mechanical) of other cardiac** electronic device

√7ᵗʰ **T82.119** **Breakdown (mechanical) of** unspecified cardiac electronic device ▽

√6ᵗʰ **T82.12** **Displacement** of cardiac electronic device
Malposition of cardiac electronic device

√7ᵗʰ **T82.120** **Displacement of** cardiac electrode

√7ᵗʰ **T82.121** **Displacement of cardiac** pulse generator (battery)

√7ᵗʰ **T82.128** **Displacement of other cardiac electronic** device

√7ᵗʰ **T82.129** **Displacement of unspecified** cardiac electronic device ▽

√6ᵗʰ **T82.19** **Other** mechanical complication of cardiac electronic device
Leakage of cardiac electronic device
Obstruction of cardiac electronic device
Perforation of cardiac electronic device
Protrusion of cardiac electronic device

√7ᵗʰ **T82.190** **Other mechanical complication of** cardiac electrode

√7ᵗʰ **T82.191** **Other mechanical complication of cardiac** pulse generator (battery)

√7ᵗʰ **T82.198** **Other mechanical complication of other** cardiac electronic device

√7ᵗʰ **T82.199** **Other mechanical complication of** unspecified cardiac device ▽

√5ᵗʰ **T82.2** **Mechanical complication of coronary artery bypass graft and biological heart valve graft**
EXCLUDES 1 *mechanical complication of artificial heart valve prosthesis (T82.0-)*

√6ᵗʰ **T82.21** **Mechanical complication of** coronary artery bypass graft

√7ᵗʰ **T82.211** **Breakdown (mechanical) of coronary artery bypass graft**

√7ᵗʰ **T82.212** **Displacement of coronary artery bypass graft**
Malposition of coronary artery bypass graft

√7ᵗʰ **T82.213** **Leakage of coronary artery bypass graft**

√7ᵗʰ **T82.218** **Other mechanical complication of coronary artery bypass graft**
Obstruction, mechanical of coronary artery bypass graft
Perforation of coronary artery bypass graft
Protrusion of coronary artery bypass graft

√6ᵗʰ **T82.22** **Mechanical complication of biological heart valve graft**

√7ᵗʰ **T82.221** **Breakdown (mechanical) of biological heart valve graft**

√7ᵗʰ **T82.222** **Displacement of biological heart valve graft**
Malposition of biological heart valve graft

√7ᵗʰ **T82.223** **Leakage of biological heart valve graft**

√7ᵗʰ **T82.228** **Other mechanical complication of biological heart valve graft**
Obstruction of biological heart valve graft
Perforation of biological heart valve graft
Protrusion of biological heart valve graft

√5ᵗʰ **T82.3** **Mechanical complication of** other vascular grafts

√6ᵗʰ **T82.31** **Breakdown (mechanical) of other vascular grafts**

√7ᵗʰ **T82.310** **Breakdown (mechanical) of** aortic (bifurcation) graft (replacement)

√7ᵗʰ **T82.311** **Breakdown (mechanical) of** carotid arterial graft (bypass)

√7ᵗʰ **T82.312** **Breakdown (mechanical) of** femoral arterial graft (bypass)

√7ᵗʰ **T82.318** **Breakdown (mechanical) of other** vascular grafts

√7ᵗʰ **T82.319** **Breakdown (mechanical) of** unspecified vascular grafts ▽

√6ᵗʰ **T82.32** **Displacement** of other vascular grafts
Malposition of other vascular grafts

√7ᵗʰ **T82.320** **Displacement of** aortic (bifurcation) graft (replacement)

√7ᵗʰ **T82.321** **Displacement of** carotid arterial graft (bypass)

√7ᵗʰ **T82.322** **Displacement of** femoral arterial graft (bypass)

√7ᵗʰ **T82.328** **Displacement of other vascular grafts**

√7ᵗʰ **T82.329** **Displacement of unspecified** vascular grafts ▽

√6ᵗʰ **T82.33** **Leakage of other vascular grafts**

√7ᵗʰ **T82.330** **Leakage of** aortic (bifurcation) graft (replacement)

√7ᵗʰ **T82.331** **Leakage of** carotid arterial graft (bypass)

√7ᵗʰ **T82.332** **Leakage of** femoral arterial graft (bypass)

√7ᵗʰ **T82.338** **Leakage of other vascular grafts**

√7ᵗʰ **T82.339** **Leakage of unspecified vascular** graft ▽

√6ᵗʰ **T82.39** **Other mechanical complication of other vascular grafts**
Obstruction (mechanical) of other vascular grafts
Perforation of other vascular grafts
Protrusion of other vascular grafts

√7ᵗʰ **T82.390** **Other mechanical complication of** aortic (bifurcation) graft (replacement)

√7ᵗʰ **T82.391** **Other mechanical complication of** carotid arterial graft (bypass)

√7ᵗʰ **T82.392** **Other mechanical complication of** femoral arterial graft (bypass)

√7ᵗʰ **T82.398** **Other mechanical complication of other vascular grafts**

√7ᵗʰ **T82.399** **Other mechanical complication of** unspecified vascular grafts ▽

√5ᵗʰ **T82.4** **Mechanical complication of** vascular dialysis catheter
Mechanical complication of hemodialysis catheter
EXCLUDES 1 *mechanical complication of intraperitoneal dialysis catheter (T85.62)*

√x7ᵗʰ **T82.41** **Breakdown (mechanical) of vascular dialysis catheter**

√x7ᵗʰ **T82.42** **Displacement of vascular dialysis catheter**
Malposition of vascular dialysis catheter

√x7ᵗʰ **T82.43** **Leakage of vascular dialysis catheter**

√x7ᵗʰ **T82.49** **Other complication of vascular dialysis catheter**
Obstruction (mechanical) of vascular dialysis catheter
Perforation of vascular dialysis catheter
Protrusion of vascular dialysis catheter

√5ᵗʰ **T82.5** **Mechanical complication of** other cardiac and vascular devices and implants
EXCLUDES 2 *mechanical complication of epidural and subdural infusion catheter (T85.61)*

√6ᵗʰ **T82.51** **Breakdown (mechanical) of other cardiac and vascular devices and implants**

√7ᵗʰ **T82.510** **Breakdown (mechanical) of** surgically created arteriovenous fistula

√7ᵗʰ **T82.511** **Breakdown (mechanical) of** surgically created arteriovenous shunt

√7ᵗʰ **T82.512** **Breakdown (mechanical) of** artificial heart

√7ᵗʰ **T82.513** **Breakdown (mechanical) of** balloon (counterpulsation) device

√7ᵗʰ **T82.514** **Breakdown (mechanical) of** infusion catheter

√7ᵗʰ **T82.515** **Breakdown (mechanical) of** umbrella device

√7ᵗʰ **T82.518** **Breakdown (mechanical) of other cardiac and vascular devices and implants**

√7ᵗʰ **T82.519** **Breakdown (mechanical) of** unspecified cardiac and vascular devices and implants ▽

√6ᵗʰ **T82.52** **Displacement of other cardiac and vascular devices and implants**
Malposition of other cardiac and vascular devices and implants

√7ᵗʰ **T82.520** **Displacement of** surgically created arteriovenous fistula

√7ᵗʰ **T82.521** **Displacement of** surgically created arteriovenous shunt

√7ᵗʰ **T82.522** **Displacement of** artificial heart

√7ᵗʰ **T82.523** **Displacement of** balloon (counterpulsation) device

√7ᵗʰ **T82.524** **Displacement of** infusion catheter

√7ᵗʰ **T82.525** **Displacement of** umbrella device

√7ᵗʰ **T82.528** **Displacement of other cardiac and vascular devices and implants**

√7ᵗʰ **T82.529** **Displacement of unspecified cardiac and vascular devices and implants** ▽

√6ᵗʰ **T82.53** **Leakage** of other cardiac and vascular devices and implants

√7ᵗʰ **T82.530** **Leakage of** surgically created arteriovenous fistula

√7ᵗʰ **T82.531** **Leakage of** surgically created arteriovenous shunt

√7ᵗʰ **T82.532** **Leakage of** artificial heart

√7ᵗʰ **T82.533** **Leakage of** balloon (counterpulsation) device

√7ᵗʰ **T82.534** **Leakage of** infusion catheter

√7ᵗʰ **T82.535** **Leakage of** umbrella device

√7ᵗʰ **T82.538** **Leakage of other cardiac and vascular devices and implants**

√7ᵗʰ **T82.539** **Leakage of unspecified cardiac and vascular devices and implants** ▽

√6ᵗʰ **T82.59** **Other mechanical complication of other cardiac and vascular devices and implants**

Obstruction (mechanical) of other cardiac and vascular devices and implants

Perforation of other cardiac and vascular devices and implants

Protrusion of other cardiac and vascular devices and implants

√7ᵗʰ **T82.590** **Other mechanical complication of** surgically created arteriovenous fistula

√7ᵗʰ **T82.591** **Other mechanical complication of** surgically created arteriovenous shunt

√7ᵗʰ **T82.592** **Other mechanical complication of** artificial heart

√7ᵗʰ **T82.593** **Other mechanical complication of** balloon (counterpulsation) device

√7ᵗʰ **T82.594** **Other mechanical complication of** infusion catheter

√7ᵗʰ **T82.595** **Other mechanical complication of** umbrella device

√7ᵗʰ **T82.598** **Other mechanical complication of other cardiac and vascular devices and implants**

√7ᵗʰ **T82.599** **Other mechanical complication of unspecified cardiac and vascular devices and implants** ▽

√x7ᵗʰ **T82.6** **Infection and inflammatory reaction due to** cardiac valve prosthesis

Use additional code to identify infection

√x7ᵗʰ **T82.7** **Infection and inflammatory reaction due to** other cardiac and vascular devices, implants and grafts

Use additional code to identify infection

√5ᵗʰ **T82.8** **Other specified complications of cardiac and vascular prosthetic devices, implants and grafts**

▲ √6ᵗʰ **T82.81** **Embolism due to cardiac and vascular prosthetic devices, implants and grafts**

▲ √7ᵗʰ **T82.817** **Embolism due to** cardiac prosthetic devices, implants and grafts

▲ √7ᵗʰ **T82.818** **Embolism due to** vascular prosthetic devices, implants and grafts

▲ √6ᵗʰ **T82.82** **Fibrosis due to cardiac and vascular prosthetic devices, implants and grafts**

▲ √7ᵗʰ **T82.827** **Fibrosis due to** cardiac prosthetic devices, implants and grafts

▲ √7ᵗʰ **T82.828** **Fibrosis due** vascular prosthetic devices, implants and grafts

▲ √6ᵗʰ **T82.83** **Hemorrhage due to cardiac and vascular prosthetic devices, implants and grafts**

▲ √7ᵗʰ **T82.837** **Hemorrhage due to** cardiac prosthetic devices, implants and grafts

▲ √7ᵗʰ **T82.838** **Hemorrhage due to** vascular prosthetic devices, implants and grafts

▲ √6ᵗʰ **T82.84** **Pain due to cardiac and vascular prosthetic devices, implants and grafts**

▲ √7ᵗʰ **T82.847** **Pain due to** cardiac prosthetic devices, implants and grafts

▲ √7ᵗʰ **T82.848** **Pain due to** vascular prosthetic devices, implants and grafts

▲ √6ᵗʰ **T82.85** **Stenosis due to cardiac and vascular prosthetic devices, implants and grafts**

● √7ᵗʰ **T82.855** **Stenosis of** coronary artery stent

In-stent stenosis (restenosis) of coronary artery stent

Restenosis of coronary artery stent

● √7ᵗʰ **T82.856** **Stenosis of** peripheral vascular stent

In-stent stenosis (restenosis) of peripheral vascular stent

Restenosis of peripheral vascular stent

▲ √7ᵗʰ **T82.857** **Stenosis of other** cardiac prosthetic devices, implants and grafts

▲ √7ᵗʰ **T82.858** **Stenosis of other** vascular prosthetic devices, implants and grafts

√6ᵗʰ **T82.86** **Thrombosis of cardiac and vascular prosthetic devices, implants and grafts**

▲ √7ᵗʰ **T82.867** **Thrombosis due to** cardiac prosthetic devices, implants and grafts

▲ √7ᵗʰ **T82.868** **Thrombosis due to** vascular prosthetic devices, implants and grafts

√6ᵗʰ **T82.89** **Other specified complication of cardiac and vascular prosthetic devices, implants and grafts**

√7ᵗʰ **T82.897** **Other specified complication of** cardiac prosthetic devices, implants and grafts

√7ᵗʰ **T82.898** **Other specified complication of** vascular prosthetic devices, implants and grafts

√x7ᵗʰ **T82.9** **Unspecified complication of cardiac and vascular prosthetic device, implant and graft** ▽

√4ᵗʰ **T83** **Complications of genitourinary prosthetic devices, implants and grafts**

EXCLUDES 2 *failure and rejection of transplanted organs and tissue (T86.-)*

The appropriate 7th character is to be added to each code from category T83.

A   initial encounter
D   subsequent encounter
S   sequela

▲ √5ᵗʰ **T83.0** **Mechanical complication of** urinary catheter

EXCLUDES 2 *complications of stoma of urinary tract (N99.5-)*

▲ √6ᵗʰ **T83.01** **Breakdown (mechanical) of** urinary catheter

√7ᵗʰ **T83.010** **Breakdown (mechanical) of** cystostomy catheter

● √7ᵗʰ **T83.011** **Breakdown (mechanical) of** indwelling urethral catheter

● √7ᵗʰ **T83.012** **Breakdown (mechanical) of** nephrostomy catheter

▲ √7ᵗʰ **T83.018** **Breakdown (mechanical) of other** urinary catheter

▶Breakdown (mechanical) of Hopkins catheter◀

▶Breakdown (mechanical) of ileostomy catheter◀

▶Breakdown (mechanical) urostomy catheter◀

▲ √6ᵗʰ **T83.02** **Displacement of** urinary catheter

▶Malposition of urinary catheter◀

√7ᵗʰ **T83.020** **Displacement of** cystostomy catheter

● √7ᵗʰ **T83.021** **Displacement of** indwelling urethral catheter

● √7ᵗʰ **T83.022** **Displacement of** nephrostomy catheter

▲ √7ᵗʰ **T83.028** **Displacement of other** urinary catheter

▶Displacement of Hopkins catheter◀

▶Displacement of ileostomy catheter◀

▶Displacement of urostomy catheter◀

▲ √6ᵗʰ **T83.03** **Leakage of** urinary catheter

√7ᵗʰ **T83.030** **Leakage of** cystostomy catheter

● √7ᵗʰ **T83.031** **Leakage of** indwelling urethral catheter

√7ᵗʰ **T83.032** **Leakage of** nephrostomy catheter

√7ᵗʰ **T83.038** **Leakage of other** urinary catheter

▶Leakage of Hopkins catheter◀

▶Leakage of ileostomy catheter◀

▶Leakage of urostomy catheter◀

▲ √6ᵗʰ **T83.09** **Other mechanical complication of urinary catheter**

▶Obstruction (mechanical) of urinary catheter◀

▶Perforation of urinary catheter◀

▶Protrusion of urinary catheter◀

√7ᵗʰ **T83.090** **Other mechanical complication of** cystostomy catheter

● √7ᵗʰ **T83.091** **Other mechanical complication of** indwelling urethral catheter

---

EXCLUDES 1 Not coded here   **EXCLUDES 2** Not included here   Ⓝ Newborn Age : 0   Ⓟ Pediatric Age : 0-17   Ⓜ Maternity Age : 12-55   Ⓐ Adult Age : 15-124

●   √7ᵗʰ **T83.092 Other mechanical complication of** nephrostomy **catheter**

▲   √7ᵗʰ **T83.098 Other mechanical complication of** other urinary **catheter**
  - ▶Other mechanical complication of Hopkins catheter◀
  - ▶Other mechanical complication of ileostomy catheter◀
  - ▶Other mechanical complication of urostomy catheter◀

√5ᵗʰ **T83.1 Mechanical complication of** other urinary devices and implants

√6ᵗʰ **T83.11 Breakdown (mechanical) of** other urinary devices and implants

√7ᵗʰ **T83.110 Breakdown (mechanical) of** urinary electronic stimulator device

     EXCLUDES 2 ▶*breakdown (mechanical) of electrode (lead) for sacral nerve neurostimulator (T85.111)◀*
     ▶*breakdown (mechanical) of implanted electronic sacral neurostimulator, pulse generator or receiver (T85.113)◀*

▲   √7ᵗʰ **T83.111 Breakdown (mechanical) of** implanted urinary sphincter

▲   √7ᵗʰ **T83.112 Breakdown (mechanical) of** indwelling ureteral stent

●   √7ᵗʰ **T83.113 Breakdown (mechanical) of** other urinary stents
     Breakdown (mechanical) of ileal conduit stent
     Breakdown (mechanical) of nephroureteral stent

√7ᵗʰ **T83.118 Breakdown (mechanical) of** other urinary devices and implants

√6ᵗʰ **T83.12 Displacement** of other urinary devices and implants
     Malposition of other urinary devices and implants

√7ᵗʰ **T83.120 Displacement of** urinary electronic stimulator device

     EXCLUDES 2 ▶*displacement of electrode (lead) for sacral nerve neurostimulator (T85.121)◀*
     ▶*displacement of implanted electronic sacral neurostimulator, pulse generator or receiver (T85.123)◀*

▲   √7ᵗʰ **T83.121 Displacement of** implanted urinary sphincter

▲   √7ᵗʰ **T83.122 Displacement of** indwelling ureteral stent

●   √7ᵗʰ **T83.123 Displacement of** other urinary stents
     Displacement of ileal conduit stent
     Displacement of nephroureteral stent

√7ᵗʰ **T83.128 Displacement of** other urinary devices and implants

√6ᵗʰ **T83.19 Other mechanical complication of** other urinary devices and implants
     Leakage of other urinary devices and implants
     Obstruction (mechanical) of other urinary devices and implants
     Perforation of other urinary devices and implants
     Protrusion of other urinary devices and implants

√7ᵗʰ **T83.190 Other mechanical complication of** urinary electronic stimulator device

     EXCLUDES 2 ▶*other mechanical complication of electrode (lead) for sacral nerve neurostimulator (T85.191)◀*
     ▶*other mechanical complication of implanted electronic sacral neurostimulator, pulse generator or receiver (T85.193)◀*

▲   √7ᵗʰ **T83.191 Other mechanical complication of** implanted urinary sphincter

▲   √7ᵗʰ **T83.192 Other mechanical complication of** indwelling ureteral stent

●   √7ᵗʰ **T83.193 Other mechanical complication of** other urinary stent
     Other mechanical complication of ileal conduit stent
     Other mechanical complication of nephroureteral stent

√7ᵗʰ **T83.198 Other mechanical complication of** other urinary devices and implants

√5ᵗʰ **T83.2 Mechanical complication of graft of urinary organ**

√x7ᵗʰ **T83.21 Breakdown (mechanical) of graft of urinary organ**

√x7ᵗʰ **T83.22 Displacement of graft of urinary organ**
     Malposition of graft of urinary organ

√x7ᵗʰ **T83.23 Leakage of graft of urinary organ**

●   √x7ᵗʰ **T83.24 Erosion of graft of urinary organ**

●   √x7ᵗʰ **T83.25 Exposure of graft of urinary organ**

√x7ᵗʰ **T83.29 Other mechanical complication of graft of urinary organ**
     Obstruction (mechanical) of graft of urinary organ
     Perforation of graft of urinary organ
     Protrusion of graft of urinary organ

√5ᵗʰ **T83.3 Mechanical complication of intrauterine contraceptive device**

√x7ᵗʰ **T83.31 Breakdown (mechanical) of intrauterine contraceptive device** ♀

√x7ᵗʰ **T83.32 Displacement of intrauterine contraceptive device** ♀
     Malposition of intrauterine contraceptive device
     ▶Missing string of intrauterine contraceptive device◀

√x7ᵗʰ **T83.39 Other mechanical complication of intrauterine contraceptive device** ♀
     Leakage of intrauterine contraceptive device
     Obstruction (mechanical) of intrauterine contraceptive device
     Perforation of intrauterine contraceptive device
     Protrusion of intrauterine contraceptive device

√5ᵗʰ **T83.4 Mechanical complication of** other prosthetic devices, implants and grafts of genital tract

√6ᵗʰ **T83.41 Breakdown (mechanical) of other prosthetic devices, implants and grafts of genital tract**

▲   √7ᵗʰ **T83.410 Breakdown (mechanical) of** implanted penile prosthesis ♂
  - ▶Breakdown (mechanical) of penile prosthesis cylinder◀
  - ▶Breakdown (mechanical) of penile prosthesis pump◀
  - ▶Breakdown (mechanical) of penile prosthesis reservoir◀

●   √7ᵗʰ **T83.411 Breakdown (mechanical) of** implanted testicular prosthesis

√7ᵗʰ **T83.418 Breakdown (mechanical) of other prosthetic devices, implants and grafts of genital tract**

√6ᵗʰ **T83.42 Displacement of other prosthetic devices, implants and grafts of genital tract**
     Malposition of other prosthetic devices, implants and grafts of genital tract

▲   √7ᵗʰ **T83.420 Displacement of** implanted penile prosthesis ♂
  - ▶Displacement of penile prosthesis cylinder◀
  - ▶Displacement of penile prosthesis pump◀
  - ▶Displacement of penile prosthesis reservoir◀

●   √7ᵗʰ **T83.421 Displacement of** implanted testicular prosthesis

√7ᵗʰ **T83.428 Displacement of other prosthetic devices, implants and grafts of genital tract**

√6ᵗʰ **T83.49 Other mechanical complication of other prosthetic devices, implants and grafts of genital tract**
     Leakage of other prosthetic devices, implants and grafts of genital tract
     Obstruction, mechanical of other prosthetic devices, implants and grafts of genital tract
     Perforation of other prosthetic devices, implants and grafts of genital tract
     Protrusion of other prosthetic devices, implants and grafts of genital tract

☑ Additional Character Required   √x7ᵗʰ Placeholder Alert   Manifestation Dx   ▽ Unspecified Dx   ▶◀ Revised Text   ● New Code   ▲ Revised Code Title

ICD-10-CM 2017   **1069**

▲   ✓7ᵗʰ **T83.490 Other mechanical complication of** ♂ **implanted penile prosthesis**
▶Other mechanical complication of penile prosthesis cylinder◀
▶Other mechanical complication of penile prosthesis pump◀
▶Other mechanical complication of penile prosthesis reservoir◀

●   ✓7ᵗʰ **T83.491 Other mechanical complication of implanted testicular prosthesis**

    ✓7ᵗʰ **T83.498 Other mechanical complication of other prosthetic devices, implants and grafts of genital tract**

✓5ᵗʰ **T83.5 Infection and inflammatory reaction due to prosthetic device, implant and graft in urinary system**
Use additional code to identify infection

▲   ✓6ᵗʰ **T83.51 Infection and inflammatory reaction due to** urinary **catheter**
EXCLUDES 2   complications of stoma of urinary tract (N99.5-)

●   ✓7ᵗʰ **T83.510 Infection and inflammatory reaction due to cystostomy catheter**

●   ✓7ᵗʰ **T83.511 Infection and inflammatory reaction due to indwelling urethral catheter**

●   ✓7ᵗʰ **T83.512 Infection and inflammatory reaction due to nephrostomy catheter**

●   ✓7ᵗʰ **T83.518 Infection and inflammatory reaction due to other urinary catheter**
Infection and inflammatory reaction due to Hopkins catheter
Infection and inflammatory reaction due to ileostomy catheter
Infection and inflammatory reaction due to urostomy catheter

✓6ᵗʰ **T83.59 Infection and inflammatory reaction due to prosthetic device, implant and graft in urinary system**

●   ✓7ᵗʰ **T83.590 Infection and inflammatory reaction due to implanted urinary neurostimulation device**
EXCLUDES 2   Infection and inflammatory reaction due to electrode lead of sacral nerve neurostimulator (T85.732)
Infection and inflammatory reaction due to pulse generator or receiver of sacral nerve neurostimulator (T85.734)

●   ✓7ᵗʰ **T83.591 Infection and inflammatory reaction due to implanted urinary sphincter**

●   ✓7ᵗʰ **T83.592 Infection and inflammatory reaction due to indwelling ureteral stent**

●   ✓7ᵗʰ **T83.593 Infection and inflammatory reaction due to other urinary stents**
Infection and inflammatory reaction due to ileal conduit stents
Infection and inflammatory reaction due to nephroureteral stent

●   ✓7ᵗʰ **T83.598 Infection and inflammatory reaction due to other prosthetic device, implant and graft in urinary system**

✓5ᵗʰ **T83.6 Infection and inflammatory reaction due to prosthetic device, implant and graft in** genital **tract**
Use additional code to identify infection

●   ✓x7ᵗʰ **T83.61 Infection and inflammatory reaction due to implanted penile prosthesis**
Infection and inflammatory reaction due to penile prosthesis cylinder
Infection and inflammatory reaction due to penile prosthesis pump
Infection and inflammatory reaction due to penile prosthesis reservoir

●   ✓x7ᵗʰ **T83.62 Infection and inflammatory reaction due to implanted testicular prosthesis**

●   ✓x7ᵗʰ **T83.69 Infection and inflammatory reaction due to** other **prosthetic device, implant and graft in genital tract**

✓6ᵗʰ **T83.7 Complications due to** implanted mesh and other prosthetic **materials**

    ✓6ᵗʰ **T83.71 Erosion of implanted** mesh and other prosthetic **materials**

▲   ✓7ᵗʰ **T83.711 Erosion of implanted vaginal mesh** ♀ **to surrounding organ or tissue**
▶Erosion of implanted vaginal mesh into pelvic floor muscles◀

●   ✓7ᵗʰ **T83.712 Erosion of implanted urethral mesh to surrounding organ or tissue**
Erosion of implanted female urethral sling
Erosion of implanted male urethral sling
Erosion of implanted urethral mesh into pelvic floor muscles

●   ✓7ᵗʰ **T83.713 Erosion of implanted urethral bulking agent to surrounding organ or tissue**

●   ✓7ᵗʰ **T83.714 Erosion of implanted ureteral bulking agent to surrounding organ or tissue**

▲   ✓7ᵗʰ **T83.718 Erosion of other implanted mesh to organ or tissue**

●   ✓7ᵗʰ **T83.719 Erosion of other prosthetic materials to surrounding organ or tissue**

✓6ᵗʰ **T83.72 Exposure of implanted mesh and other prosthetic materials into surrounding organ or tissue**
▶Extrusion of implanted mesh◀

▲   ✓7ᵗʰ **T83.721 Exposure of implanted vaginal** ♀ **mesh into vagina**
▶Exposure of implanted vaginal mesh through vaginal wall◀

    ✓7ᵗʰ **T83.722 Exposure of implanted urethral mesh into urethra**
Exposure of implanted female urethral sling
Exposure of implanted male urethral sling
Exposure of implanted urethral mesh through urethral wall

    ✓7ᵗʰ **T83.723 Exposure of implanted urethral bulking agent into urethra**

    ✓7ᵗʰ **T83.724 Exposure of implanted ureteral bulking agent into ureter**

▲   ✓7ᵗʰ **T83.728 Exposure of other implanted mesh into organ or tissue**

●   ✓7ᵗʰ **T83.729 Exposure of other prosthetic materials into organ or tissue**

●   ✓x7ᵗʰ **T83.79 Other specified complications due to other genitourinary prosthetic materials**

✓5ᵗʰ **T83.8 Other specified complications of genitourinary prosthetic devices, implants and grafts**

▲   ✓x7ᵗʰ **T83.81 Embolism due to genitourinary prosthetic devices, implants and grafts**

▲   ✓x7ᵗʰ **T83.82 Fibrosis due to genitourinary prosthetic devices, implants and grafts**

▲   ✓x7ᵗʰ **T83.83 Hemorrhage due to genitourinary prosthetic devices, implants and grafts**

▲   ✓x7ᵗʰ **T83.84 Pain due to genitourinary prosthetic devices, implants and grafts**

▲   ✓x7ᵗʰ **T83.85 Stenosis due to genitourinary prosthetic devices, implants and grafts**

▲   ✓x7ᵗʰ **T83.86 Thrombosis due to genitourinary prosthetic devices, implants and grafts**

    ✓x7ᵗʰ **T83.89 Other specified complication of genitourinary prosthetic devices, implants and grafts**

✓x7ᵗʰ **T83.9 Unspecified complication of genitourinary prosthetic** ▽ **device, implant and graft**

✓4ᵗʰ **T84 Complications of internal orthopedic prosthetic devices, implants and grafts**
EXCLUDES 2   failure and rejection of transplanted organs and tissues (T86.-)
fracture of bone following insertion of orthopedic implant, joint prosthesis or bone plate (M96.6)

The appropriate 7th character is to be added to each code from category T84.
A   initial encounter
D   subsequent encounter
S   sequela

✓5ᵗʰ **T84.0 Mechanical complication of internal joint prosthesis**

    ✓6ᵗʰ **T84.01 Broken internal joint prosthesis**
Breakage (fracture) of prosthetic joint
Broken prosthetic joint implant
EXCLUDES 1   periprosthetic joint implant fracture (T84.04)

    ✓7ᵗʰ **T84.010 Broken internal right hip prosthesis**

    ✓7ᵗʰ **T84.011 Broken internal left hip prosthesis**

    ✓7ᵗʰ **T84.012 Broken internal right knee prosthesis**

    ✓7ᵗʰ **T84.013 Broken internal left knee prosthesis**

EXCLUDES 1   Not coded here   EXCLUDES 2   Not included here   N   Newborn Age : 0   P   Pediatric Age : 0-17   M   Maternity Age : 12-55   A   Adult Age : 15-124

1070   ICD-10-CM 2017

√7ᵗʰ **T84.018** **Broken internal joint prosthesis, other site**
　　　Use additional code to identify the joint (Z96.6-)

√7ᵗʰ **T84.019** **Broken internal joint prosthesis, unspecified site**　▽

√6ᵗʰ **T84.02** **Dislocation of internal joint prosthesis**
　　Instability of internal joint prosthesis
　　Subluxation of internal joint prosthesis

√7ᵗʰ **T84.020** **Dislocation of internal right hip prosthesis**

√7ᵗʰ **T84.021** **Dislocation of internal left hip prosthesis**

√7ᵗʰ **T84.022** **Instability of internal right knee prosthesis**

√7ᵗʰ **T84.023** **Instability of internal left knee prosthesis**

√7ᵗʰ **T84.028** **Dislocation of other internal joint prosthesis**
　　　Use additional code to identify the joint (Z96.6-)

√7ᵗʰ **T84.029** **Dislocation of unspecified internal joint prosthesis**　▽

√6ᵗʰ **T84.03** **Mechanical loosening of internal prosthetic joint**
　　Aseptic loosening of prosthetic joint

√7ᵗʰ **T84.030** **Mechanical loosening of internal right hip prosthetic joint**

√7ᵗʰ **T84.031** **Mechanical loosening of internal left hip prosthetic joint**

√7ᵗʰ **T84.032** **Mechanical loosening of internal right knee prosthetic joint**

√7ᵗʰ **T84.033** **Mechanical loosening of internal left knee prosthetic joint**

√7ᵗʰ **T84.038** **Mechanical loosening of other internal prosthetic joint**
　　　Use additional code to identify the joint (Z96.6-)

√7ᵗʰ **T84.039** **Mechanical loosening of unspecified internal prosthetic joint**　▽

√6ᵗʰ **T84.05** **Periprosthetic osteolysis of internal prosthetic joint**
　　Use additional code to identify major osseous defect, if applicable (M89.7-)

√7ᵗʰ **T84.050** **Periprosthetic osteolysis of internal prosthetic right hip joint**

√7ᵗʰ **T84.051** **Periprosthetic osteolysis of internal prosthetic left hip joint**

√7ᵗʰ **T84.052** **Periprosthetic osteolysis of internal prosthetic right knee joint**

√7ᵗʰ **T84.053** **Periprosthetic osteolysis of internal prosthetic left knee joint**

√7ᵗʰ **T84.058** **Periprosthetic osteolysis of other internal prosthetic joint**
　　　Use additional code to identify the joint (Z96.6-)

√7ᵗʰ **T84.059** **Periprosthetic osteolysis of unspecified internal prosthetic joint**　▽

√6ᵗʰ **T84.06** **Wear of articular bearing surface of internal prosthetic joint**

√7ᵗʰ **T84.060** **Wear of articular bearing surface of internal prosthetic right hip joint**

√7ᵗʰ **T84.061** **Wear of articular bearing surface of internal prosthetic left hip joint**

√7ᵗʰ **T84.062** **Wear of articular bearing surface of internal prosthetic right knee joint**

√7ᵗʰ **T84.063** **Wear of articular bearing surface of internal prosthetic left knee joint**

√7ᵗʰ **T84.068** **Wear of articular bearing surface of other internal prosthetic joint**
　　　Use additional code to identify the joint (Z96.6-)

√7ᵗʰ **T84.069** **Wear of articular bearing surface of unspecified internal prosthetic joint**　▽

√6ᵗʰ **T84.09** **Other mechanical complication of internal joint prosthesis**
　　Prosthetic joint implant failure NOS

√7ᵗʰ **T84.090** **Other mechanical complication of internal right hip prosthesis**

√7ᵗʰ **T84.091** **Other mechanical complication of internal left hip prosthesis**

√7ᵗʰ **T84.092** **Other mechanical complication of internal right knee prosthesis**

√7ᵗʰ **T84.093** **Other mechanical complication of internal left knee prosthesis**

√7ᵗʰ **T84.098** **Other mechanical complication of other internal joint prosthesis**
　　　Use additional code to identify the joint (Z96.6-)

√7ᵗʰ **T84.099** **Other mechanical complication of unspecified internal joint prosthesis**　▽

√5ᵗʰ **T84.1** **Mechanical complication of internal fixation device of bones of limb**
　　EXCLUDES 2　*mechanical complication of internal fixation device of bones of feet (T84.2-)*
　　　mechanical complication of internal fixation device of bones of fingers (T84.2-)
　　　mechanical complication of internal fixation device of bones of hands (T84.2-)
　　　mechanical complication of internal fixation device of bones of toes (T84.2-)

√6ᵗʰ **T84.11** **Breakdown (mechanical) of internal fixation device of bones of limb**

√7ᵗʰ **T84.110** **Breakdown (mechanical) of internal fixation device of right humerus**

√7ᵗʰ **T84.111** **Breakdown (mechanical) of internal fixation device of left humerus**

√7ᵗʰ **T84.112** **Breakdown (mechanical) of internal fixation device of bone of right forearm**

√7ᵗʰ **T84.113** **Breakdown (mechanical) of internal fixation device of bone of left forearm**

√7ᵗʰ **T84.114** **Breakdown (mechanical) of internal fixation device of right femur**

√7ᵗʰ **T84.115** **Breakdown (mechanical) of internal fixation device of left femur**

√7ᵗʰ **T84.116** **Breakdown (mechanical) of internal fixation device of bone of right lower leg**

√7ᵗʰ **T84.117** **Breakdown (mechanical) of internal fixation device of bone of left lower leg**

√7ᵗʰ **T84.119** **Breakdown (mechanical) of internal fixation device of unspecified bone of limb**　▽

√6ᵗʰ **T84.12** **Displacement of internal fixation device of bones of limb**
　　Malposition of internal fixation device of bones of limb

√7ᵗʰ **T84.120** **Displacement of internal fixation device of right humerus**

√7ᵗʰ **T84.121** **Displacement of internal fixation device of left humerus**

√7ᵗʰ **T84.122** **Displacement of internal fixation device of bone of right forearm**

√7ᵗʰ **T84.123** **Displacement of internal fixation device of bone of left forearm**

√7ᵗʰ **T84.124** **Displacement of internal fixation device of right femur**

√7ᵗʰ **T84.125** **Displacement of internal fixation device of left femur**

√7ᵗʰ **T84.126** **Displacement of internal fixation device of bone of right lower leg**

√7ᵗʰ **T84.127** **Displacement of internal fixation device of bone of left lower leg**

√7ᵗʰ **T84.129** **Displacement of internal fixation device of unspecified bone of limb**　▽

√6ᵗʰ **T84.19** **Other mechanical complication of internal fixation device of bones of limb**
　　Obstruction (mechanical) of internal fixation device of bones of limb
　　Perforation of internal fixation device of bones of limb
　　Protrusion of internal fixation device of bones of limb

√7ᵗʰ **T84.190** **Other mechanical complication of internal fixation device of right humerus**

√7ᵗʰ **T84.191** **Other mechanical complication of internal fixation device of left humerus**

√7ᵗʰ **T84.192** **Other mechanical complication of internal fixation device of bone of right forearm**

√7ᵗʰ **T84.193** **Other mechanical complication of internal fixation device of bone of left forearm**

√7ᵗʰ **T84.194** **Other mechanical complication of internal fixation device of right femur**

☑ Additional Character Required　　√ₓ7ᵗʰ Placeholder Alert　　Manifestation Dx　　▽ Unspecified Dx　　▶◀ Revised Text　　● New Code　　▲ Revised Code Title

ICD-10-CM 2017　　**1071**

☑7ᵗʰ **T84.195** **Other mechanical complication of internal fixation device of** left femur

☑7ᵗʰ **T84.196** **Other mechanical complication of internal fixation device of bone of** right lower leg

☑7ᵗʰ **T84.197** **Other mechanical complication of internal fixation device of bone of** left lower leg

☑7ᵗʰ **T84.199** **Other mechanical complication of internal fixation device of unspecified bone of limb** ▽

☑5ᵗʰ **T84.2** **Mechanical complication of** internal fixation device **of** other bones

☑6ᵗʰ **T84.21** **Breakdown (mechanical) of internal fixation device of other bones**

☑7ᵗʰ **T84.210** **Breakdown (mechanical) of internal fixation device of bones of** hand and fingers

☑7ᵗʰ **T84.213** **Breakdown (mechanical) of internal fixation device of bones of** foot and toes

☑7ᵗʰ **T84.216** **Breakdown (mechanical) of internal fixation device of** vertebrae

☑7ᵗʰ **T84.218** **Breakdown (mechanical) of internal fixation device of other bones**

☑6ᵗʰ **T84.22** **Displacement of internal fixation device of other bones**

Malposition of internal fixation device of other bones

☑7ᵗʰ **T84.220** **Displacement of internal fixation device of bones of** hand and fingers

☑7ᵗʰ **T84.223** **Displacement of internal fixation device of bones of** foot and toes

☑7ᵗʰ **T84.226** **Displacement of internal fixation device of** vertebrae

☑7ᵗʰ **T84.228** **Displacement of internal fixation device of other bones**

☑6ᵗʰ **T84.29** **Other mechanical complication of internal fixation device of other bones**

Obstruction (mechanical) of internal fixation device of other bones

Perforation of internal fixation device of other bones

Protrusion of internal fixation device of other bones

☑7ᵗʰ **T84.290** **Other mechanical complication of internal fixation device of bones of** hand and fingers

☑7ᵗʰ **T84.293** **Other mechanical complication of internal fixation device of bones of** foot and toes

☑7ᵗʰ **T84.296** **Other mechanical complication of internal fixation device of** vertebrae

☑7ᵗʰ **T84.298** **Other mechanical complication of internal fixation device of other bones**

☑5ᵗʰ **T84.3** **Mechanical complication of** other bone devices, implants and grafts

EXCLUDES 2   *other complications of bone graft (T86.83-)*

☑6ᵗʰ **T84.31** **Breakdown (mechanical) of other bone devices, implants and grafts**

☑7ᵗʰ **T84.310** **Breakdown (mechanical) of** electronic bone stimulator

☑7ᵗʰ **T84.318** **Breakdown (mechanical) of other bone devices, implants and grafts**

☑6ᵗʰ **T84.32** **Displacement of other bone devices, implants and grafts**

Malposition of other bone devices, implants and grafts

☑7ᵗʰ **T84.320** **Displacement of** electronic bone stimulator

☑7ᵗʰ **T84.328** **Displacement of other bone devices, implants and grafts**

AHA: 2014,4Q,28

☑6ᵗʰ **T84.39** **Other mechanical complication of other bone devices, implants and grafts**

Obstruction (mechanical) of other bone devices, implants and grafts

Perforation of other bone devices, implants and grafts

Protrusion of other bone devices, implants and grafts

☑7ᵗʰ **T84.390** **Other mechanical complication of** electronic bone stimulator

☑7ᵗʰ **T84.398** **Other mechanical complication of other bone devices, implants and grafts**

☑5ᵗʰ **T84.4** **Mechanical complication of** other internal orthopedic devices, implants and grafts

☑6ᵗʰ **T84.41** **Breakdown (mechanical) of other internal orthopedic devices, implants and grafts**

☑7ᵗʰ **T84.410** **Breakdown (mechanical) of** muscle and tendon graft

☑7ᵗʰ **T84.418** **Breakdown (mechanical) of other internal orthopedic devices, implants and grafts**

☑6ᵗʰ **T84.42** **Displacement of other internal orthopedic devices, implants and grafts**

Malposition of other internal orthopedic devices, implants and grafts

☑7ᵗʰ **T84.420** **Displacement of** muscle and tendon graft

☑7ᵗʰ **T84.428** **Displacement of other internal orthopedic devices, implants and grafts**

☑6ᵗʰ **T84.49** **Other mechanical complication of other internal orthopedic devices, implants and grafts**

Mechanical complication of other internal orthopedic devices, implants and grafts NOS

Obstruction (mechanical) of other internal orthopedic devices, implants and grafts

Perforation of other internal orthopedic devices, implants and grafts

Protrusion of other internal orthopedic devices, implants and grafts

☑7ᵗʰ **T84.490** **Other mechanical complication of** muscle and tendon graft

☑7ᵗʰ **T84.498** **Other mechanical complication of other internal orthopedic devices, implants and grafts**

☑5ᵗʰ **T84.5** **Infection and inflammatory reaction due to** internal joint prosthesis

Use additional code to identify infection

AHA: 2015,1Q,16

☑x7ᵗʰ **T84.50** **Infection and inflammatory reaction due to unspecified internal joint prosthesis** ▽

☑x7ᵗʰ **T84.51** **Infection and inflammatory reaction due to internal** right hip **prosthesis**

☑x7ᵗʰ **T84.52** **Infection and inflammatory reaction due to internal** left hip **prosthesis**

☑x7ᵗʰ **T84.53** **Infection and inflammatory reaction due to internal** right knee **prosthesis**

☑x7ᵗʰ **T84.54** **Infection and inflammatory reaction due to internal** left knee **prosthesis**

☑x7ᵗʰ **T84.59** **Infection and inflammatory reaction due to other internal joint prosthesis**

☑5ᵗʰ **T84.6** **Infection and inflammatory reaction due to** internal fixation device

Use additional code to identify infection

☑x7ᵗʰ **T84.60** **Infection and inflammatory reaction due to internal fixation device of unspecified site** ▽

☑6ᵗʰ **T84.61** **Infection and inflammatory reaction due to internal fixation device of** arm

☑7ᵗʰ **T84.610** **Infection and inflammatory reaction due to internal fixation device of** right humerus

☑7ᵗʰ **T84.611** **Infection and inflammatory reaction due to internal fixation device of** left humerus

☑7ᵗʰ **T84.612** **Infection and inflammatory reaction due to internal fixation device of** right radius

☑7ᵗʰ **T84.613** **Infection and inflammatory reaction due to internal fixation device of** left radius

☑7ᵗʰ **T84.614** **Infection and inflammatory reaction due to internal fixation device of** right ulna

☑7ᵗʰ **T84.615** **Infection and inflammatory reaction due to internal fixation device of** left ulna

☑7ᵗʰ **T84.619** **Infection and inflammatory reaction due to internal fixation device of unspecified bone of arm** ▽

☑6ᵗʰ **T84.62** **Infection and inflammatory reaction due to internal fixation device of** leg

☑7ᵗʰ **T84.620** **Infection and inflammatory reaction due to internal fixation device of** right femur

☑7ᵗʰ **T84.621** **Infection and inflammatory reaction due to internal fixation device of** left femur

☑7ᵗʰ **T84.622** **Infection and inflammatory reaction due to internal fixation device of** right tibia

☑7ᵗʰ **T84.623** **Infection and inflammatory reaction due to internal fixation device of** left tibia

☑7ᵗʰ **T84.624** **Infection and inflammatory reaction due to internal fixation device of** right fibula

☑7ᵗʰ **T84.625** **Infection and inflammatory reaction due to internal fixation device of** left fibula

☑7ᵗʰ **T84.629** **Infection and inflammatory reaction due to internal fixation device of unspecified bone of leg** ▽

EXCLUDES 1 Not coded here   *EXCLUDES 2* Not included here   N Newborn Age : 0   P Pediatric Age : 0-17   M Maternity Age : 12-55   A Adult Age : 15-124

1072   ICD-10-CM 2017

☑x7ᵗʰ **T84.63** **Infection and inflammatory reaction due to internal fixation device of** spine

☑x7ᵗʰ **T84.69** **Infection and inflammatory reaction due to internal fixation device of other site**

✓5ᵗʰ **T84.7** **Infection and inflammatory reaction due to other internal orthopedic prosthetic devices, implants and grafts**
  Use additional code to identify infection

✓5ᵗʰ **T84.8** **Other specified complications of internal orthopedic prosthetic devices, implants and grafts**

  ☑x7ᵗʰ **T84.81** **Embolism** **due to internal orthopedic prosthetic devices, implants and grafts**

  ☑x7ᵗʰ **T84.82** **Fibrosis** **due to internal orthopedic prosthetic devices, implants and grafts**

  ☑x7ᵗʰ **T84.83** **Hemorrhage** **due to internal orthopedic prosthetic devices, implants and grafts**

  ☑x7ᵗʰ **T84.84** **Pain** **due to internal orthopedic prosthetic devices, implants and grafts**

  ☑x7ᵗʰ **T84.85** **Stenosis** **due to internal orthopedic prosthetic devices, implants and grafts**

  ☑x7ᵗʰ **T84.86** **Thrombosis** **due to internal orthopedic prosthetic devices, implants and grafts**

  ☑x7ᵗʰ **T84.89** **Other specified complication of internal orthopedic prosthetic devices, implants and grafts**

☑x7ᵗʰ **T84.9** **Unspecified complication of internal orthopedic** ▽ ●
  prosthetic device, implant and graft

✓4ᵗʰ **T85** **Complications of other internal prosthetic devices, implants and grafts**

  ~~EXCLUDES 2~~ *failure and rejection of transplanted organs and tissue (T86.-)*

  The appropriate 7th character is to be added to each code from category T85.
  A   initial encounter
  D   subsequent encounter
  S   sequela

✓5ᵗʰ **T85.0** **Mechanical complication of** ventricular intracranial **(communicating)** shunt

  ☑x7ᵗʰ **T85.01** **Breakdown (mechanical) of ventricular intracranial (communicating) shunt**

  ☑x7ᵗʰ **T85.02** **Displacement of ventricular intracranial (communicating) shunt**
    Malposition of ventricular intracranial (communicating) shunt

  ☑x7ᵗʰ **T85.03** **Leakage of ventricular intracranial (communicating) shunt**

  ☑7ᵗʰ **T85.09** **Other mechanical complication of ventricular intracranial (communicating) shunt** ▲
    Obstruction (mechanical) of ventricular intracranial (communicating) shunt
    Perforation of ventricular intracranial (communicating) shunt ▲
    Protrusion of ventricular intracranial (communicating) shunt

✓5ᵗʰ **T85.1** **Mechanical complication of** implanted electronic stimulator **of nervous system**

  ✓6ᵗʰ **T85.11** **Breakdown (mechanical) of implanted electronic stimulator of nervous system**

  ▲ ☑7ᵗʰ **T85.110** **Breakdown (mechanical) of implanted electronic neurostimulator of brain electrode (lead)**

  ▲ ☑7ᵗʰ **T85.111** **Breakdown (mechanical) of implanted electronic neurostimulator** **of peripheral nerve electrode (lead)**
      ►Breakdown of electrode (lead) for cranial nerve neurostimulators◄ ▲
      ►Breakdown of electrode (lead) for gastric neurostimulator◄
      ►Breakdown of electrode (lead) for sacral nerve neurostimulator◄
      ►Breakdown of electrode (lead) for vagal nerve neurostimulators◄

  ▲ ☑7ᵗʰ **T85.112** **Breakdown (mechanical) of implanted electronic neurostimulator of spinal cord electrode (lead)**

  ● ☑7ᵗʰ **T85.113** **Breakdown (mechanical) of implanted electronic neurostimulator, generator**
      Breakdown (mechanical) of Implanted electronic neurostimuator generator, brain, peripheral, gastric, spinal
      Breakdown (mechanical) of implanted electronic sacral neurostimulator, pulse generator or receiver

☑7ᵗʰ **T85.118** **Breakdown (mechanical) of other implanted electronic stimulator of nervous system**

✓6ᵗʰ **T85.12** **Displacement of implanted electronic stimulator of nervous system**
  Malposition of implanted electronic stimulator of nervous system

  ▲ ☑7ᵗʰ **T85.120** **Displacement of implanted electronic neurostimulator of brain electrode (lead)**

  ☑7ᵗʰ **T85.121** **Displacement of implanted electronic neurostimulator of peripheral nerve electrode (lead)**
      ►Displacement of electrode (lead) for cranial nerve neurostimulators◄
      ►Displacement of electrode (lead) for gastric neurostimulator◄
      ►Displacement of electrode (lead) for sacral nerve neurostimulator◄
      ►Displacement of electrode (lead) for vagal nerve neurostimulators◄

  ▲ ☑7ᵗʰ **T85.122** **Displacement of implanted electronic neurostimulator of spinal cord electrode (lead)**

  ☑7ᵗʰ **T85.123** **Displacement of implanted electronic neurostimulator, generator**
      Displacement of implanted electronic neurostimulator generator, brain, peripheral, gastric, spinal
      Displacement of implanted electronic sacral neurostimulator, pulse generator or receiver

  ☑7ᵗʰ **T85.128** **Displacement of other implanted electronic stimulator of** nervous system

✓6ᵗʰ **T85.19** **Other mechanical complication of implanted electronic stimulator of nervous system**
  Leakage of implanted electronic stimulator of nervous system
  Obstruction (mechanical) of implanted electronic stimulator of nervous system
  Perforation of implanted electronic stimulator of nervous system
  Protrusion of implanted electronic stimulator of nervous system

  ☑7ᵗʰ **T85.190** **Other mechanical complication of implanted electronic neurostimulator of brain electrode (lead)**

  ▲ ☑7ᵗʰ **T85.191** **Other mechanical complication of implanted electronic neurostimulator of peripheral nerve electrode (lead)**
      ►Other mechanical complication of electrode (lead) for cranial nerve neurostimulators◄
      ►Other mechanical complication of electrode (lead) for gastric neurostimulator◄
      ►Other mechanical complication of electrode (lead) for sacral nerve neurostimulator◄
      ►Other mechanical complication of electrode (lead) for vagal nerve neurostimulators◄

  ☑7ᵗʰ **T85.192** **Other mechanical complication of implanted electronic neurostimulator of spinal cord electrode (lead)**

  ● ☑7ᵗʰ **T85.193** **Other mechanical complication of implanted electronic neurostimulator, generator**
      Other mechanical complication of implanted electronic neurostimulator generator, brain, peripheral, gastric, spinal
      Other mechanical complication of implanted electronic sacral neurostimulator, pulse generator or receiver

  ☑7ᵗʰ **T85.199** **Other mechanical complication of other implanted electronic stimulator of nervous system**

✓5ᵗʰ **T85.2** **Mechanical complication of** intraocular lens

  ☑x7ᵗʰ **T85.21** **Breakdown (mechanical) of intraocular lens**

√x7ᵗʰ **T85.22 Displacement** of intraocular lens

Malposition of intraocular lens

√x7ᵗʰ **T85.29 Other mechanical complication of intraocular lens**

Obstruction (mechanical) of intraocular lens

Perforation of intraocular lens

Protrusion of intraocular lens

√5ᵗʰ **T85.3 Mechanical complication of** other ocular prosthetic devices, implants and grafts

> EXCLUDES 2 *other complications of corneal graft (T86.84-)*

√6ᵗʰ **T85.31 Breakdown (mechanical) of other ocular prosthetic devices, implants and grafts**

√7ᵗʰ **T85.310 Breakdown (mechanical) of prosthetic orbit of** right eye

√7ᵗʰ **T85.311 Breakdown (mechanical) of prosthetic orbit of** left eye

√7ᵗʰ **T85.318 Breakdown (mechanical) of other ocular prosthetic devices, implants and grafts**

√6ᵗʰ **T85.32 Displacement** of other ocular prosthetic devices, implants and grafts

Malposition of other ocular prosthetic devices, implants and grafts

√7ᵗʰ **T85.320 Displacement of prosthetic orbit of** right eye

√7ᵗʰ **T85.321 Displacement of prosthetic orbit of** left eye

√7ᵗʰ **T85.328 Displacement of other ocular prosthetic devices, implants and grafts**

√6ᵗʰ **T85.39 Other mechanical complication of other ocular prosthetic devices, implants and grafts**

Obstruction (mechanical) of other ocular prosthetic devices, implants and grafts

Perforation of other ocular prosthetic devices, implants and grafts

Protrusion of other ocular prosthetic devices, implants and grafts

√7ᵗʰ **T85.390 Other mechanical complication of prosthetic orbit of** right eye

√7ᵗʰ **T85.391 Other mechanical complication of prosthetic orbit of** left eye

√7ᵗʰ **T85.398 Other mechanical complication of other ocular prosthetic devices, implants and grafts**

√5ᵗʰ **T85.4 Mechanical complication of** breast prosthesis and implant

√x7ᵗʰ **T85.41 Breakdown (mechanical) of breast prosthesis and implant**

√x7ᵗʰ **T85.42 Displacement of breast prosthesis and implant**

Malposition of breast prosthesis and implant

√x7ᵗʰ **T85.43 Leakage of breast prosthesis and implant**

√x7ᵗʰ **T85.44 Capsular contracture of breast implant**

√x7ᵗʰ **T85.49 Other mechanical complication of breast prosthesis and implant**

Obstruction (mechanical) of breast prosthesis and implant

Perforation of breast prosthesis and implant

Protrusion of breast prosthesis and implant

√5ᵗʰ **T85.5 Mechanical complication of** gastrointestinal prosthetic devices, implants and grafts

√6ᵗʰ **T85.51 Breakdown (mechanical) of gastrointestinal prosthetic devices, implants and grafts**

√7ᵗʰ **T85.510 Breakdown (mechanical) of** bile duct prosthesis

√7ᵗʰ **T85.511 Breakdown (mechanical) of** esophageal anti-reflux device

√7ᵗʰ **T85.518 Breakdown (mechanical) of other gastrointestinal prosthetic devices, implants and grafts**

√6ᵗʰ **T85.52 Displacement of gastrointestinal prosthetic devices, implants and grafts**

Malposition of gastrointestinal prosthetic devices, implants and grafts

√7ᵗʰ **T85.520 Displacement of** bile duct prosthesis

√7ᵗʰ **T85.521 Displacement of** esophageal anti-reflux device

√7ᵗʰ **T85.528 Displacement of other gastrointestinal prosthetic devices, implants and grafts**

√6ᵗʰ **T85.59 Other mechanical complication of gastrointestinal prosthetic devices, implants and**

Obstruction, mechanical of gastrointestinal prosthetic devices, implants and grafts

Perforation of gastrointestinal prosthetic devices, implants and grafts

Protrusion of gastrointestinal prosthetic devices, implants and grafts

√7ᵗʰ **T85.590 Other mechanical complication of** bile duct **prosthesis**

√7ᵗʰ **T85.591 Other mechanical complication of** esophageal anti-reflux **device**

√7ᵗʰ **T85.598 Other mechanical complication of other gastrointestinal prosthetic devices, implants and grafts**

√5ᵗʰ **T85.6 Mechanical complication of** other specified internal and external prosthetic devices, implants and grafts

√6ᵗʰ **T85.61 Breakdown (mechanical) of other specified internal prosthetic devices, implants and grafts**

√7ᵗʰ **T85.610 Breakdown (mechanical) of** cranial or spinal infusion catheter

▶Breakdown (mechanical) of epidural infusion catheter◀

▶Breakdown (mechanical) of intrathecal infusion catheter◀

▶Breakdown (mechanical) of subarachnoid infusion catheter◀

▶Breakdown (mechanical) of subdural infusion catheter ◀

√7ᵗʰ **T85.611 Breakdown (mechanical) of intraperitoneal dialysis catheter**

> EXCLUDES 1 *mechanical complication of vascular dialysis catheter (T82.4-)*

√7ᵗʰ **T85.612 Breakdown (mechanical) of** permanent sutures

> EXCLUDES 1 *mechanical complication of permanent (wire) suture used in bone repair (T84.1-T84.2)*

√7ᵗʰ **T85.613 Breakdown (mechanical) of** artificial skin graft and decellularized allodermis

Failure of artificial skin graft and decellularized allodermis

Non-adherence of artificial skin graft and decellularized allodermis

Poor incorporation of artificial skin graft and decellularized allodermis

Shearing of artificial skin graft and decellularized allodermis

√7ᵗʰ **T85.614 Breakdown (mechanical) of** insulin pump

√7ᵗʰ **T85.615 Breakdown (mechanical) of** other nervous system device, implant or graft

Breakdown (mechanical) of intrathecal infusion pump

√7ᵗʰ **T85.618 Breakdown (mechanical) of other specified internal prosthetic devices, implants and grafts**

√6ᵗʰ **T85.62 Displacement of other specified internal prosthetic devices, implants and grafts**

Malposition of other specified internal prosthetic devices, implants and grafts

√7ᵗʰ **T85.620 Displacement of** cranial or spinal infusion catheter

▶Displacement of epidural infusion catheter◀

▶Displacement of intrathecal infusion catheter◀

▶Displacement of subarachnoid infusion catheter◀

▶Displacement of subdural infusion catheter◀

√7ᵗʰ **T85.621 Displacement of** intraperitoneal dialysis catheter

> EXCLUDES 1 *mechanical complication of vascular dialysis catheter (T82.4-)*

EXCLUDES 1 Not coded here   EXCLUDES 2 Not included here   N Newborn Age : 0   P Pediatric Age : 0-17   M Maternity Age : 12-55   A Adult Age : 15-124

1074   ICD-10-CM 2017

√7ᵗʰ **T85.622 Displacement of** permanent sutures

EXCLUDES 1 mechanical complication of permanent (wire) suture used in bone repair (T84.1-T84.2)

√7ᵗʰ **T85.623 Displacement of** artificial skin graft and decellularized allodermis

Dislodgement of artificial skin graft and decellularized allodermis

Displacement of artificial skin graft and decellularized allodermis

√7ᵗʰ **T85.624 Displacement of** insulin pump

√7ᵗʰ **T85.625 Displacement of** other **nervous system device, implant or graft**

Displacement of intrathecal infusion pump

√7ᵗʰ **T85.628 Displacement of other specified internal prosthetic devices, implants and grafts**

√6ᵗʰ **T85.63** Leakage **of other specified internal prosthetic devices, implants and grafts**

√7ᵗʰ **T85.630 Leakage of** cranial or spinal infusion catheter

▶Leakage of epidural infusion catheter◀

▶Leakage of intrathecal infusion catheter infusion catheter◀

▶Leakage of subdural infusion catheter◀

▶Leakage of subarachnoid infusion catheter◀

√7ᵗʰ **T85.631 Leakage of** intraperitoneal dialysis catheter

EXCLUDES 1 mechanical complication of vascular dialysis catheter (T82.4)

√7ᵗʰ **T85.633 Leakage of** insulin pump

√7ᵗʰ **T85.635 Leakage of** other **nervous system device, implant or graft**

Leakage of intrathecal infusion pump

√7ᵗʰ **T85.638 Leakage of other specified internal prosthetic devices, implants and grafts**

√6ᵗʰ **T85.69 Other mechanical complication of other specified internal prosthetic devices, implants and grafts**

Obstruction, mechanical of other specified internal prosthetic devices, implants and grafts

Perforation of other specified internal prosthetic devices, implants and grafts

Protrusion of other specified internal prosthetic devices, implants and grafts

√7ᵗʰ **T85.690 Other mechanical complication of** cranial or spinal infusion catheter

▶Other mechanical complication of epidural infusion catheter◀

▶Other mechanical complication of intrathecal infusion catheter◀

▶Other mechanical complication of subarachnoid infusion catheter◀

▶Other mechanical complication of subdural infusion catheter◀

√7ᵗʰ **T85.691 Other mechanical complication of** intraperitoneal dialysis catheter

EXCLUDES 1 mechanical complication of vascular dialysis catheter (T82.4)

√7ᵗʰ **T85.692 Other mechanical complication of** permanent sutures

EXCLUDES 1 mechanical complication of permanent (wire) suture used in bone repair (T84.1-T84.2)

√7ᵗʰ **T85.693 Other mechanical complication of** artificial skin graft and decellularized allodermis

√7ᵗʰ **T85.694 Other mechanical complication of** insulin pump

√7ᵗʰ **T85.695 Other mechanical complication of** other **nervous system device, implant or graft**

Other mechanical complication of intrathecal infusion pump

√7ᵗʰ **T85.698 Other mechanical complication of other specified internal prosthetic devices, implants and grafts**

Mechanical complication of nonabsorbable surgical material NOS

√5ᵗʰ **T85.7 Infection and inflammatory reaction due to other internal prosthetic devices, implants and grafts**

Use additional code to identify infection

√x7ᵗʰ **T85.71 Infection and inflammatory reaction due to peritoneal dialysis catheter**

√x7ᵗʰ **T85.72 Infection and inflammatory reaction due to** insulin pump

√6ᵗʰ **T85.73 Infection and inflammatory reaction due to** nervous system **devices, implants and graft**

√7ᵗʰ **T85.730 Infection and inflammatory reaction due to** ventricular intracranial (communicating) shunt

√7ᵗʰ **T85.731 Infection and inflammatory reaction due to** implanted electronic neurostimulator of brain, electrode (lead)

√7ᵗʰ **T85.732 Infection and inflammatory reaction due to implanted electronic neurostimulator of peripheral nerve, electrode (lead)**

Infection and inflammatory reaction due to electrode (lead) for cranial nerve neurostimulators

Infection and inflammatory reaction due to electrode (lead) for gastric neurostimulator

Infection and inflammatory reaction due to electrode (lead) for sacral nerve neurostimulator

Infection and inflammatory reaction due to electrode (lead) for vagal nerve neurostimulators

√7ᵗʰ **T85.733 Infection and inflammatory reaction due to implanted electronic neurostimulator of spinal cord, electrode (lead)**

√7ᵗʰ **T85.734 Infection and inflammatory reaction due to implanted electronic neurostimulator, generator**

Generator pocket infection|

√7ᵗʰ **T85.735 Infection and inflammatory reaction due to cranial or spinal infusion catheter**

Infection and inflammatory reaction due to epidural catheter

Infection and inflammatory reaction due to intrathecal infusion catheter

Infection and inflammatory reaction due to subarachnoid catheter

Infection and inflammatory reaction due to subdural catheter

√7ᵗʰ **T85.738 Infection and inflammatory reaction due to** other **nervous system device, implant or graft**

Infection and inflammatory reaction due to intrathecal infusion pump

√x7ᵗʰ **T85.79 Infection and inflammatory reaction due to other internal prosthetic devices, implants and grafts**

√5ᵗʰ **T85.8 Other specified complications of internal prosthetic devices, implants and grafts, not elsewhere classified**

√6ᵗʰ **T85.81 Embolism due to internal prosthetic devices, implants and grafts, not elsewhere classified**

√7ᵗʰ **T85.810 Embolism due to** nervous system **prosthetic devices, implants and grafts**

√7ᵗʰ **T85.818 Embolism due to** other **internal prosthetic devices, implants and grafts**

√6ᵗʰ **T85.82 Fibrosis due to** internal prosthetic devices, implants **and grafts, not elsewhere classified**

√7ᵗʰ **T85.820 Fibrosis due to** nervous system **prosthetic devices, implants and grafts**

√7ᵗʰ **T85.828 Fibrosis due to** other **internal prosthetic devices, implants and grafts**

√6ᵗʰ **T85.83 Hemorrhage due to internal prosthetic devices, implants and grafts, not elsewhere classified**

√7ᵗʰ **T85.830 Hemorrhage due to** nervous system **prosthetic devices, implants and grafts**

√7ᵗʰ **T85.838 Hemorrhage due to** other **internal prosthetic devices, implants and grafts**

☑ Additional Character Required   √x7ᵗʰ Placeholder Alert   Manifestation Dx   ▽ Unspecified Dx   ▶◀ Revised Text   ● New Code   ▲ Revised Code Title

ICD-10-CM 2017   1075

Chapter 19. Injury, Poisoning and Certain Other Consequences of External Causes

T85.84–T86.92

√6th T85.84   **Pain due to internal prosthetic devices, implants and grafts, not elsewhere classified**

-   **√7th T85.840**   **Pain due to** nervous system **prosthetic devices, implants and grafts**
-   **√7th T85.848**   **Pain due to** other **internal prosthetic devices, implants and grafts**

√6th T85.85   **Stenosis due to internal prosthetic devices, implants and grafts, not elsewhere classified**

-   **√7th T85.850**   **Stenosis due to** nervous system **prosthetic devices, implants and grafts**
-   **√7th T85.858**   **Stenosis due to** other **internal prosthetic devices, implants and grafts**

√6th T85.86   **Thrombosis due to internal prosthetic devices, implants and grafts, not elsewhere classified**

-   **√7th T85.860**   **Thrombosis due to** nervous system **prosthetic devices, implants and grafts**
-   **√7th T85.868**   **Thrombosis due to** other **internal prosthetic devices, implants and grafts**

√6th T85.89   **Other** specified complication of internal prosthetic **devices, implants and grafts, not elsewhere classified**

     ▶Erosion or breakdown of subcutaneous device pocket◀

-   **√7th T85.890**   **Other specified complication of** nervous system **prosthetic devices, implants and grafts**
-   **√7th T85.898**   **Other specified complication of** other **internal prosthetic devices, implants and grafts**

√x7th T85.9   **Unspecified complication of internal prosthetic device, implant and graft**   ▽

     Complication of internal prosthetic device, implant and graft NOS

√4th T86   **Complications of transplanted organs and tissue**

     Use additional code to identify other transplant complications, such as:
     graft-versus-host disease (D89.81-)
     malignancy associated with organ transplant (C80.2)
     post-transplant lymphoproliferative disorders (PTLD) (D47.Z1)

√5th T86.0   **Complications of** bone marrow **transplant**

   T86.00   **Unspecified complication of bone marrow transplant**   ▽

   T86.01   **Bone marrow transplant** rejection

   T86.02   **Bone marrow transplant** failure

   T86.03   **Bone marrow transplant** infection

   T86.09   **Other complications of bone marrow transplant**

√5th T86.1   **Complications of** kidney **transplant**

   T86.10   **Unspecified complication of kidney transplant**   ▽

   T86.11   **Kidney transplant** rejection

   T86.12   **Kidney transplant** failure

     AHA: 2013,1Q,24

   T86.13   **Kidney transplant** infection

     Use additional code to specify infection

   T86.19   **Other complication of kidney transplant**

√5th T86.2   **Complications of** heart **transplant**

     EXCLUDES 1   complication of:
       artificial heart device (T82.5)
       heart-lung transplant (T86.3)

   T86.20   **Unspecified complication of heart transplant**   ▽

   T86.21   **Heart transplant** rejection

   T86.22   **Heart transplant** failure

   T86.23   **Heart transplant** infection

     Use additional code to specify infection

   √6th T86.29   **Other complications of heart transplant**

     T86.290   **Cardiac allograft vasculopathy**

       EXCLUDES 1   atherosclerosis of coronary arteries (I25.75-, I25.76-, I25.81-)

     T86.298   **Other complications of heart transplant**

√5th T86.3   **Complications of** heart-lung **transplant**

   T86.30   **Unspecified complication of heart-lung transplant**   ▽

   T86.31   **Heart-lung transplant** rejection

   T86.32   **Heart-lung transplant** failure

   T86.33   **Heart-lung transplant** infection

     Use additional code to specify infection

   T86.39   **Other complications of heart-lung transplant**

√5th T86.4   **Complications of** liver **transplant**

   T86.40   **Unspecified complication of liver transplant**   ▽

   T86.41   **Liver transplant** rejection

   T86.42   **Liver transplant** failure

   T86.43   **Liver transplant** infection

     Use additional code to identify infection, such as: cytomegalovirus (CMV) infection (B25.-)

   T86.49   **Other complications of liver transplant**

T86.5   **Complications of** stem cell **transplant**

     Complications from stem cells from peripheral blood
     Complications from stem cells from umbilical cord

√5th T86.8   **Complications of other transplanted organs and tissues**

   √6th T86.81   **Complications of** lung **transplant**

     EXCLUDES 1   complication of heart-lung transplant (T86.3-)

     T86.810   **Lung transplant** rejection

     T86.811   **Lung transplant** failure

     T86.812   **Lung transplant** infection

       Use additional code to specify infection

     T86.818   **Other complications of lung transplant**

     T86.819   **Unspecified complication of lung transplant**   ▽

   √6th T86.82   **Complications of** skin graft (allograft) (autograft)

     EXCLUDES 2   complication of artificial skin graft (T85.693)

     T86.820   **Skin graft (allograft)** rejection

     T86.821   **Skin graft (allograft) (autograft)** failure

     T86.822   **Skin graft (allograft) (autograft)** infection

       Use additional code to specify infection

     T86.828   **Other complications of skin graft (allograft) (autograft)**

     T86.829   **Unspecified complication of skin graft (allograft) (autograft)**   ▽

   √6th T86.83   **Complications of** bone graft

     EXCLUDES 2   mechanical complications of bone graft (T84.3-)

     T86.830   **Bone graft** rejection

     T86.831   **Bone graft** failure

     T86.832   **Bone graft** infection

       Use additional code to specify infection

     T86.838   **Other complications of bone graft**

     T86.839   **Unspecified complication of bone graft**   ▽

   √6th T86.84   **Complications of** corneal **transplant**

     EXCLUDES 2   mechanical complications of corneal graft (T85.3-)

     T86.840   **Corneal transplant** rejection

     T86.841   **Corneal transplant** failure

     T86.842   **Corneal transplant** infection

       Use additional code to specify infection

     T86.848   **Other complications of corneal transplant**

     T86.849   **Unspecified complication of corneal transplant**   ▽

   √6th T86.85   **Complication of** intestine **transplant**

     T86.850   **Intestine transplant** rejection

     T86.851   **Intestine transplant** failure

     T86.852   **Intestine transplant** infection

       Use additional code to specify infection

     T86.858   **Other complications of intestine transplant**

     T86.859   **Unspecified complication of intestine transplant**   ▽

   √6th T86.89   **Complications of other transplanted tissue**

     Transplant failure or rejection of pancreas

     T86.890   **Other transplanted tissue** rejection

     T86.891   **Other transplanted tissue** failure

     T86.892   **Other transplanted tissue** infection

       Use additional code to specify infection

     T86.898   **Other complications of other transplanted tissue**

     T86.899   **Unspecified complication of other transplanted tissue**   ▽

√5th T86.9   **Complication of unspecified transplanted organ and tissue**

   T86.90   **Unspecified complication of unspecified transplanted organ and tissue**   ▽

   T86.91   **Unspecified transplanted organ and tissue rejection**   ▽

   T86.92   **Unspecified transplanted organ and tissue failure**   ▽

EXCLUDES 1 Not coded here   **EXCLUDES 2** Not included here   **N** Newborn Age : 0   **P** Pediatric Age : 0-17   **M** Maternity Age : 12-55   **A** Adult Age : 15-124

1076   ICD-10-CM 2017

T86.93 **Unspecified transplanted organ and tissue infection** ▽
     Use additional code to specify infection

T86.99 **Other complications of unspecified transplanted organ and tissue** ▽

☑4ᵗʰ **T87 Complications peculiar to reattachment and amputation**

☑5ᵗʰ **T87.0 Complications of reattached (part of) upper extremity**

☑6ᵗʰ **T87.0X Complications of reattached (part of) upper extremity**

T87.0X1 **Complications of reattached (part of) right upper extremity**

T87.0X2 **Complications of reattached (part of) left upper extremity**

T87.0X9 **Complications of reattached (part of) unspecified upper extremity** ▽

☑5ᵗʰ **T87.1 Complications of reattached (part of) lower extremity**

☑6ᵗʰ **T87.1X Complications of reattached (part of) lower extremity**

T87.1X1 **Complications of reattached (part of) right lower extremity**

T87.1X2 **Complications of reattached (part of) left lower extremity**

T87.1X9 **Complications of reattached (part of) unspecified lower extremity** ▽

T87.2 **Complications of other reattached body part**

☑5ᵗʰ **T87.3 Neuroma of amputation stump**

T87.30 **Neuroma of amputation stump, unspecified extremity** ▽

T87.31 **Neuroma of amputation stump, right upper extremity**

T87.32 **Neuroma of amputation stump, left upper extremity**

T87.33 **Neuroma of amputation stump, right lower extremity**

T87.34 **Neuroma of amputation stump, left lower extremity**

☑5ᵗʰ **T87.4 Infection of amputation stump**

T87.40 **Infection of amputation stump, unspecified extremity** ▽

T87.41 **Infection of amputation stump, right upper extremity**

T87.42 **Infection of amputation stump, left upper extremity**

T87.43 **Infection of amputation stump, right lower extremity**

T87.44 **Infection of amputation stump, left lower extremity**

☑5ᵗʰ **T87.5 Necrosis of amputation stump**

T87.50 **Necrosis of amputation stump, unspecified extremity** ▽

T87.51 **Necrosis of amputation stump, right upper extremity**

T87.52 **Necrosis of amputation stump, left upper extremity**

T87.53 **Necrosis of amputation stump, right lower extremity**

T87.54 **Necrosis of amputation stump, left lower extremity**

☑5ᵗʰ **T87.8 Other complications of amputation stump**

T87.81 **Dehiscence of amputation stump**

T87.89 **Other complications of amputation stump**
     Amputation stump contracture
     Amputation stump contracture of next proximal joint
     Amputation stump flexion
     Amputation stump edema
     Amputation stump hematoma
     EXCLUDES 2 *phantom limb syndrome (G54.6-G54.7)*

T87.9 **Unspecified complications of amputation stump** ▽

☑4ᵗʰ **T88 Other complications of surgical and medical care, not elsewhere classified**
     EXCLUDES 2 *complication following infusion, transfusion and therapeutic injection (T80.-)*
       complication following procedure NEC (T81.-)
       complications of anesthesia in labor and delivery (O74.-)
       complications of anesthesia in pregnancy (O29.-)
       complications of anesthesia in puerperium (O89.-)
       complications of devices, implants and grafts (T82-T85)
       complications of obstetric surgery and procedure (O75.4)
       dermatitis due to drugs and medicaments (L23.3, L24.4, L25.1, L27.0-L27.1)
       poisoning and toxic effects of drugs and chemicals (T36-T65 with fifth or sixth character 1-4 or 6)
       specified complications classified elsewhere

> The appropriate 7th character is to be added to each code from category T88.
> A   initial encounter
> D   subsequent encounter
> S   sequela

√x7ᵗʰ **T88.0 Infection following immunization**
     Sepsis following immunization

√x7ᵗʰ **T88.1 Other complications following immunization, not elsewhere classified**
     Generalized vaccinia
     Rash following immunization
     EXCLUDES 1 *vaccinia not from vaccine (B08.011)*
     EXCLUDES 2 *anaphylactic shock due to serum (T80.5-)*
       other serum reactions (T80.6-)
       postimmunization arthropathy (M02.2)
       postimmunization encephalitis (G04.02)
       postimmunization fever (R50.83)

√x7ᵗʰ **T88.2 Shock due to anesthesia**
     Use additional code for adverse effect, if applicable, to identify drug (T41.- with fifth or sixth character 5)
     EXCLUDES 1 *complications of anesthesia (in):*
       labor and delivery (O74.-)
       postprocedural shock NOS (T81.1-)
       pregnancy (O29.-)
       puerperium (O89.-)

√x7ᵗʰ **T88.3 Malignant hyperthermia due to anesthesia**
     Use additional code for adverse effect, if applicable, to identify drug (T41.- with fifth or sixth character 5)

√x7ᵗʰ **T88.4 Failed or difficult intubation**

☑5ᵗʰ **T88.5 Other complications of anesthesia**
     Use additional code for adverse effect, if applicable, to identify drug (T41.- with fifth or sixth character 5)

√x7ᵗʰ **T88.51 Hypothermia following anesthesia**

√x7ᵗʰ **T88.52 Failed moderate sedation during procedure**
     Failed conscious sedation during procedure
     EXCLUDES 2 *personal history of failed moderate sedation (Z92.83)*

● √x7ᵗʰ **T88.53 Unintended awareness under general anesthesia during procedure**
     EXCLUDES 2 *personal history of unintended awareness under general anesthesia (Z92.84)*

√x7ᵗʰ **T88.59 Other complications of anesthesia**

√x7ᵗʰ **T88.6 Anaphylactic reaction due to adverse effect of correct drug or medicament properly administered**
     Anaphylactic shock due to adverse effect of correct drug or medicament properly administered
     Anaphylactoid reaction NOS
     Use additional code for adverse effect, if applicable, to identify drug (T36-T50 with fifth or sixth character 5)
     EXCLUDES 1 *anaphylactic reaction due to serum (T80.5-)*
       anaphylactic shock or reaction due to adverse food reaction (T78.0-)

√x7ᵗʰ **T88.7 Unspecified adverse effect of drug or medicament** ▽
     Drug hypersensitivity NOS
     Drug reaction NOS
     Use additional code for adverse effect, if applicable, to identify drug (T36-T50 with fifth or sixth character 5)
     EXCLUDES 1 *specified adverse effects of drugs and medicaments (A00-R94 and T80-T88.6, T88.8)*

√x7ᵗʰ **T88.8 Other specified complications of surgical and medical care, not elsewhere classified**

Use additional code to identify the complication

√x7ᵗʰ **T88.9 Complication of surgical and medical care, unspecified** ▽

EXCLUDES 1 Not coded here   EXCLUDES 2 Not included here   N Newborn Age : 0   P Pediatric Age : 0-17   M Maternity Age : 12-55   A Adult Age : 15-124

1078   ICD-10-CM 2017

Chapter 20. External Causes of Morbidity (V00–Y99)

Chapter Specific Guidelines with Coding Examples

The chapter specific guidelines from the ICD-10-CM Official Guidelines for Coding and Reporting have been provided below. Along with these guidelines are coding examples, contained in the shaded boxes, that have been developed to help illustrate the coding and/or sequencing guidance found in these guidelines.

The external causes of morbidity codes should never be sequenced as the first-listed or principal diagnosis.

External cause codes are intended to provide data for injury research and evaluation of injury prevention strategies. These codes capture how the injury or health condition happened (cause), the intent (unintentional or accidental; or intentional, such as suicide or assault), the place where the event occurred the activity of the patient at the time of the event, and the person's status (e.g., civilian, military).

There is no national requirement for mandatory ICD-10-CM external cause code reporting. Unless a provider is subject to a state-based external cause code reporting mandate or these codes are required by a particular payer, reporting of ICD-10-CM codes in Chapter 20, External Causes of Morbidity, is not required. In the absence of a mandatory reporting requirement, providers are encouraged to voluntarily report external cause codes, as they provide valuable data for injury research and evaluation of injury prevention strategies.

a. General external cause coding guidelines

1) Used with any code in the range of A00.0–T88.9, Z00–Z99

An external cause code may be used with any code in the range of A00.0–T88.9, Z00–Z99, classification that is a health condition due to an external cause. Though they are most applicable to injuries, they are also valid for use with such things as infections or diseases due to an external source, and other health conditions, such as a heart attack that occurs during strenuous physical activity.

> Actinic reticuloid due to tanning bed use
>
> | L57.1 | Actinic reticuloid |
> |---|---|
> | W89.1XXA | Exposure to tanning bed, initial encounter |
>
> *Explanation:* An external cause code may be used with any code in the range of A00.0–T88.9, Z00–Z99, classifications that describe health conditions due to an external cause. Code W89.1 Exposure to tanning bed requires a seventh character of A to report this initial encounter, with a placeholder X for the fifth and sixth characters.

2) External cause code used for length of treatment

Assign the external cause code, with the appropriate 7th character (initial encounter, subsequent encounter or sequela) for each encounter for which the injury or condition is being treated.

Most categories in chapter 20 have a 7th character requirement for each applicable code. Most categories in this chapter have three 7th character values: A, initial encounter, D, subsequent encounter and S, sequela. While the patient may be seen by a new or different provider over the course of treatment for an injury or condition, assignment of the 7th character for external cause should match the 7th character of the code assigned for the associated injury or condition for the encounter.

3) Use the full range of external cause codes

Use the full range of external cause codes to completely describe the cause, the intent, the place of occurrence, and if applicable, the activity of the patient at the time of the event, and the patient's status, for all injuries, and other health conditions due to an external cause.

4) Assign as many external cause codes as necessary

Assign as many external cause codes as necessary to fully explain each cause. If only one external code can be recorded, assign the code most related to the principal diagnosis.

5) The selection of the appropriate external cause code

The selection of the appropriate external cause code is guided by the Alphabetic Index of External Causes and by Inclusion and Exclusion notes in the Tabular List.

6) External cause code can never be a principal diagnosis

An external cause code can never be a principal (first-listed) diagnosis.

7) Combination external cause codes

Certain of the external cause codes are combination codes that identify sequential events that result in an injury, such as a fall which results in striking against an object. The injury may be due to either event or both.

The combination external cause code used should correspond to the sequence of events regardless of which caused the most serious injury.

> Toddler tripped and fell while walking and struck his head on an end table, sustaining a scalp contusion
>
> | S00.03XA | Contusion of scalp, initial encounter |
> |---|---|
> | W01.190A | Fall on same level from slipping, tripping and stumbling with subsequent striking against furniture, initial encounter |
>
> *Explanation:* Combination external cause codes identify sequential events that result in an injury, such as a fall resulting in striking against an object. The injury may be due to either or both events.

8) No external cause code needed in certain circumstances

No external cause code from Chapter 20 is needed if the external cause and intent are included in a code from another chapter (e.g. T36.0X1-Poisoning by penicillins, accidental (unintentional)).

b. Place of occurrence guideline

Codes from category Y92, Place of occurrence of the external cause, are secondary codes for use after other external cause codes to identify the location of the patient at the time of injury or other condition.

Generally, a place of occurrence code is assigned only once, at the initial encounter for treatment. However, in the rare instance that a new injury occurs during hospitalization, an additional place of occurrence code may be assigned. No 7th characters are used for Y92.

Do not use place of occurrence code Y92.9 if the place is not stated or is not applicable.

> A farmer was working in his barn and sustained a foot contusion when the horse stepped on his left foot
>
> | S90.32XA | Contusion of left foot, initial encounter |
> |---|---|
> | W55.19XA | Other contact with horse, initial encounter |
> | Y92.71 | Barn as the place of occurrence of the external cause |
>
> *Explanation:* A place-of-occurrence code from category Y92 is assigned at the initial encounter to identify the location of the patient at the time the injury occurred.

c. Activity code

Assign a code from category Y93, Activity code, to describe the activity of the patient at the time the injury or other health condition occurred.

An activity code is used only once, at the initial encounter for treatment. Only one code from Y93 should be recorded on a medical record.

The activity codes are not applicable to poisonings, adverse effects, misadventures or sequela.

Do not assign Y93.9, Unspecified activity, if the activity is not stated.

A code from category Y93 is appropriate for use with external cause and intent codes if identifying the activity provides additional information about the event.

> Ranch hand who was grooming a horse sustained a foot contusion when the horse stepped on his left foot
>
> | S90.32XA | Contusion of left foot, initial encounter |
> |---|---|
> | W55.19XA | Other contact with horse, initial encounter |
> | Y93.K3 | Activity, grooming and shearing an animal |
>
> *Explanation:* One activity code from category Y93 is assigned at the initial encounter only to describe the activity of the patient at the time the injury occurred.

d. Place of occurrence, activity, and status codes used with other external cause code

When applicable, place of occurrence, activity, and external cause status codes are sequenced after the main external cause code(s). Regardless of the number of external cause codes assigned, generally there should be only one place of occurrence code, one activity code, and one external cause status code assigned to an encounter. However, in the rare instance that a new injury occurs during hospitalization, an additional place of occurrence code may be assigned.

e. If the reporting format limits the number of external cause codes

If the reporting format limits the number of external cause codes that can be used in reporting clinical data, report the code for the cause/intent most related to the principal diagnosis. If the format permits capture of additional external cause codes, the cause/intent, including medical misadventures, of the additional events should be reported rather than the codes for place, activity, or external status.

f. Multiple external cause coding guidelines

More than one external cause code is required to fully describe the external cause of an illness or injury. The assignment of external cause codes should be sequenced in the following priority:

If two or more events cause separate injuries, an external cause code should be assigned for each cause. The first-listed external cause code will be selected in the following order:

External codes for child and adult abuse take priority over all other external cause codes.

See Section I.C.19., Child and Adult abuse guidelines.

External cause codes for terrorism events take priority over all other external cause codes except child and adult abuse.

External cause codes for cataclysmic events take priority over all other external cause codes except child and adult abuse and terrorism.

External cause codes for transport accidents take priority over all other external cause codes except cataclysmic events, child and adult abuse and terrorism.

Activity and external cause status codes are assigned following all causal (intent) external cause codes.

The first-listed external cause code should correspond to the cause of the most serious diagnosis due to an assault, accident, or self-harm, following the order of hierarchy listed above..

30-year-old man accidentally discharged his hunting rifle, sustaining an open gunshot wound to the right thigh, which caused him to fall down the stairs, resulting in closed displaced comminuted fracture of his left radial shaft	
S71.101A	Unspecified open wound, right thigh, initial encounter
W33.02XA	Accidental discharge of hunting rifle, initial encounter
S52.352A	Displaced comminuted fracture of shaft of radius, left arm, initial encounter for closed fracture
W10.9XXA	Fall (on) (from) unspecified stairs and steps, initial encounter

Explanation: If two or more events cause separate injuries, an external cause code should be assigned for each cause.

g. Child and adult abuse guideline

Adult and child abuse, neglect and maltreatment are classified as assault. Any of the assault codes may be used to indicate the external cause of any injury resulting from the confirmed abuse.

For confirmed cases of abuse, neglect and maltreatment, when the perpetrator is known, a code from Y07, Perpetrator of maltreatment and neglect, should accompany any other assault codes.

See Section I.C.19. Adult and child abuse, neglect and other maltreatment

h. Unknown or undetermined intent guideline

If the intent (accident, self-harm, assault) of the cause of an injury or other condition is unknown or unspecified, code the intent as accidental intent. All transport accident categories assume accidental intent.

1) Use of undetermined intent

External cause codes for events of undetermined intent are only for use if the documentation in the record specifies that the intent cannot be determined.

i. Sequelae (late effects) of external cause guidelines

1) Sequelae external cause codes

Sequela are reported using the external cause code with the 7th character "S" for sequela. These codes should be used with any report of a late effect or sequela resulting from a previous injury.

See Section I.B.10 Sequela (Late Effects)

2) Sequela external cause code with a related current injury

A sequela external cause code should never be used with a related current nature of injury code.

3) Use of sequela external cause codes for subsequent visits

Use a late effect external cause code for subsequent visits when a late effect of the initial injury is being treated. Do not use a late effect external cause code for subsequent visits for follow-up care (e.g., to assess healing, to receive rehabilitative therapy) of the injury when no late effect of the injury has been documented.

j. Terrorism guidelines

1) Cause of injury identified by the Federal Government (FBI) as terrorism

When the cause of an injury is identified by the Federal Government (FBI) as terrorism, the first-listed external cause code should be a code from category Y38, Terrorism. The definition of terrorism employed by the FBI is found at the inclusion note at the beginning of category Y38. Use additional code for place of occurrence (Y92.-). More than one Y38 code may be assigned if the injury is the result of more than one mechanism of terrorism.

2) Cause of an injury is suspected to be the result of terrorism

When the cause of an injury is suspected to be the result of terrorism a code from category Y38 should not be assigned. Suspected cases should be classified as assault.

3) Code Y38.9, Terrorism, secondary effects

Assign code Y38.9, Terrorism, secondary effects, for conditions occurring subsequent to the terrorist event. This code should not be assigned for conditions that are due to the initial terrorist act.

It is acceptable to assign code Y38.9 with another code from Y38 if there is an injury due to the initial terrorist event and an injury that is a subsequent result of the terrorist event.

k. External cause status

A code from category Y99, External cause status, should be assigned whenever any other external cause code is assigned for an encounter, including an Activity code, except for the events noted below. Assign a code from category Y99, External cause status, to indicate the work status of the person at the time the event occurred. The status code indicates whether the event occurred during military activity, whether a non-military person was at work, whether an individual including a student or volunteer was involved in a non-work activity at the time of the causal event.

A code from Y99, External cause status, should be assigned, when applicable, with other external cause codes, such as transport accidents and falls. The external cause status codes are not applicable to poisonings, adverse effects, misadventures or late effects.

Do not assign a code from category Y99 if no other external cause codes (cause, activity) are applicable for the encounter.

An external cause status code is used only once, at the initial encounter for treatment. Only one code from Y99 should be recorded on a medical record.

Do not assign code Y99.9, Unspecified external cause status, if the status is not stated.

Chapter 20. External Causes of Morbidity (V00-Y99)

NOTE This chapter permits the classification of environmental events and circumstances as the cause of injury, and other adverse effects. Where a code from this section is applicable, it is intended that it shall be used secondary to a code from another chapter of the Classification indicating the nature of the condition. Most often, the condition will be classifiable to Chapter 19, Injury, poisoning and certain other consequences of external causes (S00-T88). Other conditions that may be stated to be due to external causes are classified in Chapters I to XVIII. For these conditions, codes from Chapter 20 should be used to provide additional information as to the cause of the condition.

This chapter contains the following blocks:

V00-X58	Accidents
V00-V99	Transport accidents
V00-V09	Pedestrian injured in transport accident
V10-V19	Pedal cycle rider injured in transport accident
V20-V29	Motorcycle rider injured in transport accident
V30-V39	Occupant of three-wheeled motor vehicle injured in transport accident
V40-V49	Car occupant injured in transport accident
V50-V59	Occupant of pick-up truck or van injured in transport accident
V60-V69	Occupant of heavy transport vehicle injured in transport accident
V70-V79	Bus occupant injured in transport accident
V80-V89	Other land transport accidents
V90-V94	Water transport accidents
V95-V97	Air and space transport accidents
V98-V99	Other and unspecified transport accidents
W00-X58	Other external causes of accidental injury
W00-W19	Slipping, tripping, stumbling and falls
W20-W49	Exposure to inanimate mechanical forces
W50-W64	Exposure to animate mechanical forces
W65-W74	Accidental non-transport drowning and submersion
W85-W99	Exposure to electric current, radiation and extreme ambient air temperature and pressure
X00-X08	Exposure to smoke, fire and flames
X10-X19	Contact with heat and hot substances
X30-X39	Exposure to forces of nature
▶X50	Overexertion and strenuous or repetitive movements◀
X52-X58	Accidental exposure to other specified factors
X71-X83	Intentional self-harm
▶X92-Y09◀	Assault
Y21-Y33	Event of undetermined intent
Y35-Y38	Legal intervention, operations of war, military operations, and terrorism
Y62-Y84	Complications of medical and surgical care
Y62-Y69	Misadventures to patients during surgical and medical care
Y70-Y82	Medical devices associated with adverse incidents in diagnostic and therapeutic use
Y83-Y84	Surgical and other medical procedures as the cause of abnormal reaction of the patient, or of later complication, without mention of misadventure at the time of the procedure
Y90-Y99	Supplementary factors related to causes of morbidity classified elsewhere

Accidents (V00-X58)

Transport accidents (V00-V99)

NOTE This section is structured in 12 groups. Those relating to land transport accidents ▶(V00-V89)◀ reflect the victim's mode of transport and are subdivided to identify the victim's 'counterpart' or the type of event. The vehicle of which the injured person is an occupant is identified in the first two characters since it is seen as the most important factor to identify for prevention purposes. A transport accident is one in which the vehicle involved must be moving or running or in use for transport purposes at the time of the accident.

Use additional code to identify:
  airbag injury (W22.1)
  type of street or road (Y92.4-)
  use of cellular telephone and other electronic equipment at the time of the transport accident (Y93.C-)

EXCLUDES 1 *agricultural vehicles in stationary use or maintenance (W31.-)*
  assault by crashing of motor vehicle (Y03.-)
  automobile or motor cycle in stationary use or maintenance - code to type of accident
  crashing of motor vehicle, undetermined intent (Y32)
  intentional self-harm by crashing of motor vehicle (X82)

EXCLUDES 2 *transport accidents due to cataclysm (X34-X38)*

NOTE ▶Definitions related to transport accidents:◀

(a) ▶A transport accident (V00-V99) is any accident involving a device designed primarily for, or used at the time primarily for, conveying persons or good from one place to another.◀

(b) A public highway [trafficway] or street is the entire width between property lines (or other boundary lines) of land open to the public as a matter of right or custom for purposes of moving persons or property from one place to another. A roadway is that part of the public highway designed, improved and customarily used for vehicular traffic.

(c) A traffic accident is any vehicle accident occurring on the public highway [i.e. originating on, terminating on, or involving a vehicle partially on the highway]. A vehicle accident is assumed to have occurred on the public highway unless another place is specified, except in the case of accidents involving only off-road motor vehicles, which are classified as nontraffic accidents unless the contrary is stated.

(d) A nontraffic accident is any vehicle accident that occurs entirely in any place other than a public highway.

(e) ▶A pedestrian is any person involved in an accident who was not at the time of the accident riding in or on a motor vehicle, railway train, streetcar or animal-drawn or other vehicle, or on a pedal cycle or animal. This includes, a person changing a tire, working on a parked car, or a person on foot. It also includes the user of a pedestrian conveyance such as a babystroller, ice-skates, skis, sled, roller skates, a skateboard, nonmotorized or motorized wheelchair, motorized mobility scooter, or nonmotorized scooter.◀

(f) A driver is an occupant of a transport vehicle who is operating or intending to operate it.

(g) A passenger is any occupant of a transport vehicle other than the driver, except a person traveling on the outside of the vehicle.

(h) ▶A person on the outside of a vehicle is any person being transported by a vehicle but not occupying the space normally reserved for the driver or passengers, or the space intended for the transport of property. This includes a person travelling on the bodywork, bumper, fender, roof, running board or step of a vehicle, as well as, hanging on the outside of the vehicle.◀

(i) A pedal cycle is any land transport vehicle operated solely by nonmotorized pedals including a bicycle or tricycle.

(j) A pedal cyclist is any person riding a pedal cycle or in a sidecar or trailer attached to a pedal cycle.

(k) ▶A motorcycle is a two-wheeled motor vehicle with one or two riding saddles and sometimes with a third wheel for the support of a sidecar. The sidecar is considered part of the motorcycle. This includes a moped, motor scooter, or motorized bicycle.◀

(l) A motorcycle rider is any person riding a motorcycle or in a sidecar or trailer attached to the motorcycle.

(m) A three-wheeled motor vehicle is a motorized tricycle designed primarily for on-road use. This includes a motor-driven tricycle, a motorized rickshaw, or a three-wheeled motor car.

(n) ▶A car [automobile] is a four-wheeled motor vehicle designed primarily for carrying up to 7 persons. A trailer being towed by the car is considered part of the car. It does not include a van or minivan - see definition (o).◀

(o) A pick-up truck or van is a four or six-wheeled motor vehicle designed for carrying passengers as well as property or cargo weighing less than the local limit for classification as a heavy goods vehicle, and not requiring a special driver's license. This includes a minivan and a sport-utility vehicle (SUV).

(p) A heavy transport vehicle is a motor vehicle designed primarily for carrying property, meeting local criteria for classification as a heavy goods vehicle in terms of weight and requiring a special driver's license.

(q) A bus (coach) is a motor vehicle designed or adapted primarily for carrying more than 10 passengers, and requiring a special driver's license.

(r) A railway train or railway vehicle is any device, with or without freight or passenger cars couple to it, designed for traffic on a railway track. This includes subterranean (subways) or elevated trains.

(s) A streetcar, is a device designed and used primarily for transporting passengers within a municipality, running on rails, usually subject to normal traffic control signals, and operated principally on a right-of-way that forms part of the roadway. This includes a tram or trolley that runs on rails. A trailer being towed by a streetcar is considered part of the streetcar.

(t) ▶A special vehicle mainly used on industrial premises is a motor vehicle designed primarily for use within the buildings and premises of industrial or commercial establishments. This includes battery-powered airport passenger vehicles or baggage/mail trucks, forklifts, coal-cars in a coal mine, logging cars and trucks used in mines or quarries.◀

(u) A special vehicle mainly used in agriculture is a motor vehicle designed specifically for use in farming and agriculture (horticulture), to work the land, tend and harvest crops and transport materials on the farm. This includes harvesters, farm machinery and tractor and trailers.

(v) A special construction vehicle is a motor vehicle designed specifically for use on construction and demolition sites. This

---

☑ Additional Character Required ᵛˣ⁷ᵗʰ Placeholder Alert Manifestation Dx ▽ Unspecified Dx ▶◀ Revised Text ● New Code ▲ Revised Code Title

includes bulldozers, diggers, earth levellers, dump trucks. backhoes, front-end loaders, pavers, and mechanical shovels.

(w) ▶A special all-terrain vehicle is a motor vehicle of special design to enable it to negotiate over rough or soft terrain, snow or sand. Examples of special design are high construction, special wheels and tires, tracks, and support on a cushion of air. This includes snow mobiles, All-terrain vehicles (ATV), and dune buggies. It does not include passenger vehicle designated as Sport Utility Vehicles. (SUV)◀

(x) A watercraft is any device designed for transporting passengers or goods on water. This includes motor or sailboats, ships, and hovercraft.

(y) An aircraft is any device for transporting passengers or goods in the air. This includes hot-air balloons, gliders, helicopters and airplanes.

(z) A military vehicle is any motorized vehicle operating on a public roadway owned by the military and being operated by a member of the military.

Pedestrian injured in transport accident (V00-V09)

INCLUDES person changing tire on transport vehicle
person examining engine of vehicle broken down in (on side of) road
EXCLUDES 1 *fall due to non-transport collision with other person (W03)*
pedestrian on foot falling (slipping) on ice and snow (W00.-)
struck or bumped by another person (W51)

The appropriate 7th character is to be added to each code from categories V00-V09.
A   initial encounter
D   subsequent encounter
S   sequela

√4ᵗʰ **V00**   **Pedestrian conveyance accident**

Use additional place of occurrence and activity external cause codes, if known (Y92.-, Y93.-)

EXCLUDES 1 *collision with another person without fall (W51)*
fall due to person on foot colliding with another person on foot (W03)
fall from non-moving wheelchair, nonmotorized scooter and motorized mobility scooter without collision (W05.-)
pedestrian (conveyance) collision with other land transport vehicle (V01-V09)
pedestrian on foot falling (slipping) on ice and snow (W00.-)

√5ᵗʰ **V00.0**   **Pedestrian on foot injured in collision with pedestrian conveyance**

√x7ᵗʰ **V00.01**   **Pedestrian on foot injured in collision with roller-skater**

√x7ᵗʰ **V00.02**   **Pedestrian on foot injured in collision with skateboarder**

√x7ᵗʰ **V00.09**   **Pedestrian on foot injured in collision with other pedestrian conveyance**

√5ᵗʰ **V00.1**   **Rolling-type pedestrian conveyance accident**

EXCLUDES 1 *accident with babystroller (V00.82-)*
accident with motorized mobility scooter (V00.83-)
accident with wheelchair (powered) (V00.81-)

√6ᵗʰ **V00.11**   **In-line roller-skate accident**

√7ᵗʰ **V00.111**   **Fall from in-line roller-skates**

√7ᵗʰ **V00.112**   **In-line roller-skater colliding with stationary object**

√7ᵗʰ **V00.118**   **Other in-line roller-skate accident**

EXCLUDES 1 *roller-skater collision with other land transport vehicle (V01-V09 with 5th character 1)*

√6ᵗʰ **V00.12**   **Non-in-line roller-skate accident**

√7ᵗʰ **V00.121**   **Fall from non-in-line roller-skates**

√7ᵗʰ **V00.122**   **Non-in-line roller-skater colliding with stationary object**

√7ᵗʰ **V00.128**   **Other non-in-line roller-skating accident**

EXCLUDES 1 *roller-skater collision with other land transport vehicle (V01-V09 with 5th character 1)*

√6ᵗʰ **V00.13**   **Skateboard accident**

√7ᵗʰ **V00.131**   **Fall from skateboard**

√7ᵗʰ **V00.132**   **Skateboarder colliding with stationary object**

√7ᵗʰ **V00.138**   **Other skateboard accident**

EXCLUDES 1 *skateboarder collision with other land transport vehicle (V01-V09 with 5th character 2)*

√6ᵗʰ **V00.14**   **Scooter (nonmotorized) accident**

EXCLUDES 1 *motorscooter accident (V20-V29)*

√7ᵗʰ **V00.141**   **Fall from scooter (nonmotorized)**

√7ᵗʰ **V00.142**   **Scooter (nonmotorized) colliding with stationary object**

√7ᵗʰ **V00.148**   **Other scooter (nonmotorized) accident**

EXCLUDES 1 *scooter (nonmotorized) collision with other land transport vehicle (V01-V09 with fifth character 9)*

√6ᵗʰ **V00.15**   **Heelies accident**

Rolling shoe
Wheeled shoe
Wheelies accident

√7ᵗʰ **V00.151**   **Fall from heelies**

√7ᵗʰ **V00.152**   **Heelies colliding with stationary object**

√7ᵗʰ **V00.158**   **Other heelies accident**

√6ᵗʰ **V00.18**   **Accident on other rolling-type pedestrian conveyance**

√7ᵗʰ **V00.181**   **Fall from other rolling-type pedestrian conveyance**

√7ᵗʰ **V00.182**   **Pedestrian on other rolling-type pedestrian conveyance colliding with stationary object**

√7ᵗʰ **V00.188**   **Other accident on other rolling-type pedestrian conveyance**

√5ᵗʰ **V00.2**   **Gliding-type pedestrian conveyance accident**

√6ᵗʰ **V00.21**   **Ice-skates accident**

√7ᵗʰ **V00.211**   **Fall from ice-skates**

√7ᵗʰ **V00.212**   **Ice-skater colliding with stationary object**

√7ᵗʰ **V00.218**   **Other ice-skates accident**

EXCLUDES 1 *ice-skater collision with other land transport vehicle (V01-V09 with 5th digit 9)*

√6ᵗʰ **V00.22**   **Sled accident**

√7ᵗʰ **V00.221**   **Fall from sled**

√7ᵗʰ **V00.222**   **Sledder colliding with stationary object**

√7ᵗʰ **V00.228**   **Other sled accident**

EXCLUDES 1 *sled collision with other land transport vehicle (V01-V09 with 5th digit 9)*

√6ᵗʰ **V00.28**   **Other gliding-type pedestrian conveyance accident**

√7ᵗʰ **V00.281**   **Fall from other gliding-type pedestrian conveyance**

√7ᵗʰ **V00.282**   **Pedestrian on other gliding-type pedestrian conveyance colliding with stationary object**

√7ᵗʰ **V00.288**   **Other accident on other gliding-type pedestrian conveyance**

EXCLUDES 1 *gliding-type pedestrian conveyance collision with other land transport vehicle (V01-V09 with 5th digit 9)*

√5ᵗʰ **V00.3**   **Flat-bottomed pedestrian conveyance accident**

√6ᵗʰ **V00.31**   **Snowboard accident**

√7ᵗʰ **V00.311**   **Fall from snowboard**

√7ᵗʰ **V00.312**   **Snowboarder colliding with stationary object**

√7ᵗʰ **V00.318**   **Other snowboard accident**

EXCLUDES 1 *snowboarder collision with other land transport vehicle (V01-V09 with 5th digit 9)*

√6ᵗʰ **V00.32**   **Snow-ski accident**

√7ᵗʰ **V00.321**   **Fall from snow-skis**

√7ᵗʰ **V00.322**   **Snow-skier colliding with stationary object**

EXCLUDES 1 Not coded here   **EXCLUDES 2** Not included here   **N** Newborn Age : 0   **P** Pediatric Age : 0-17   **M** Maternity Age : 12-55   **A** Adult Age : 15-124

1082   ICD-10-CM 2017

☑7ᵗʰ **V00.328**   **Other snow-ski accident**
     EXCLUDES 1   *snow-skier collision with other land transport vehicle (V01-V09 with 5th digit 9)*

☑6ᵗʰ **V00.38**   **Other flat-bottomed pedestrian conveyance accident**
   ☑7ᵗʰ **V00.381**   **Fall from other flat-bottomed pedestrian conveyance**
   ☑7ᵗʰ **V00.382**   **Pedestrian on other flat-bottomed pedestrian conveyance colliding with stationary object**
   ☑7ᵗʰ **V00.388**   **Other accident on other flat-bottomed pedestrian conveyance**

☑5ᵗʰ **V00.8**   **Accident on other pedestrian conveyance**
  ☑6ᵗʰ **V00.81**   **Accident with wheelchair (powered)**
   ☑7ᵗʰ **V00.811**   **Fall from moving wheelchair (powered)**
     EXCLUDES 1   *fall from non-moving wheelchair (W05.0)*
   ☑7ᵗʰ **V00.812**   **Wheelchair (powered) colliding with stationary object**
   ☑7ᵗʰ **V00.818**   **Other accident with wheelchair (powered)**

  ☑6ᵗʰ **V00.82**   **Accident with babystroller**
   ☑7ᵗʰ **V00.821**   **Fall from babystroller**
   ☑7ᵗʰ **V00.822**   **Babystroller colliding with stationary object**
   ☑7ᵗʰ **V00.828**   **Other accident with babystroller**

  ☑6ᵗʰ **V00.83**   **Accident with motorized mobility scooter**
   ☑7ᵗʰ **V00.831**   **Fall from motorized mobility scooter**
     EXCLUDES 1   *fall from non-moving motorized mobility scooter (W05.2)*
   ☑7ᵗʰ **V00.832**   **Motorized mobility scooter colliding with stationary object**
   ☑7ᵗʰ **V00.838**   **Other accident with motorized mobility scooter**

  ☑6ᵗʰ **V00.89**   **Accident on other pedestrian conveyance**
   ☑7ᵗʰ **V00.891**   **Fall from other pedestrian conveyance**
   ☑7ᵗʰ **V00.892**   **Pedestrian on other pedestrian conveyance colliding with stationary object**
   ☑7ᵗʰ **V00.898**   **Other accident on other pedestrian conveyance**
     EXCLUDES 1   *other pedestrian (conveyance) collision with other land transport vehicle (V01-V09 with 5th digit 9)*

☑4ᵗʰ **V01**   **Pedestrian injured in collision with pedal cycle**

  ☑5ᵗʰ **V01.0**   **Pedestrian injured in collision with pedal cycle in nontraffic accident**
   ☑x7ᵗʰ **V01.00**   **Pedestrian on foot injured in collision with pedal cycle in nontraffic accident**
     Pedestrian NOS injured in collision with pedal cycle in nontraffic accident
   ☑x7ᵗʰ **V01.01**   **Pedestrian on roller-skates injured in collision with pedal cycle in nontraffic accident**
   ☑x7ᵗʰ **V01.02**   **Pedestrian on skateboard injured in collision with pedal cycle in nontraffic accident**
   ☑x7ᵗʰ **V01.09**   **Pedestrian with other conveyance injured in collision with pedal cycle in nontraffic accident**
     Pedestrian with babystroller injured in collision with pedal cycle in nontraffic accident
     Pedestrian on ice-skates injured in collision with pedal cycle in nontraffic accident
     Pedestrian on nonmotorized scooter injured in collision with pedal cycle in nontraffic accident
     Pedestrian on sled injured in collision with pedal cycle in nontraffic accident
     Pedestrian on snowboard injured in collision with pedal cycle in nontraffic accident
     Pedestrian on snow-skis injured in collision with pedal cycle in nontraffic accident
     Pedestrian in wheelchair (powered) injured in collision with pedal cycle in nontraffic accident
     Pedestrian in motorized mobility scooter injured in collision with pedal cycle in nontraffic accident

  ☑5ᵗʰ **V01.1**   **Pedestrian injured in collision with pedal cycle in traffic accident**

☑7ᵗʰ **V01.10**   **Pedestrian on foot injured in collision with pedal cycle in traffic accident**
     Pedestrian NOS injured in collision with pedal cycle in traffic accident
☑x7ᵗʰ **V01.11**   **Pedestrian on roller-skates injured in collision with pedal cycle in traffic accident**
☑x7ᵗʰ **V01.12**   **Pedestrian on skateboard injured in collision with pedal cycle in traffic accident**
☑x7ᵗʰ **V01.19**   **Pedestrian with other conveyance injured in collision with pedal cycle in traffic accident**
     Pedestrian with babystroller injured in collision with pedal cycle in traffic accident
     Pedestrian on ice-skates injured in collision with pedal cycle in traffic accident
     Pedestrian on nonmotorized scooter injured in collision with pedal cycle in traffic accident
     Pedestrian on sled injured in collision with pedal cycle in traffic accident
     Pedestrian on snowboard injured in collision with pedal cycle in traffic accident
     Pedestrian on snow-skis injured in collision with pedal cycle in traffic accident
     Pedestrian in wheelchair (powered) injured in collision with pedal cycle in traffic accident
     Pedestrian in motorized mobility scooter injured in collision with pedal cycle in traffic accident

☑5ᵗʰ **V01.9**   **Pedestrian injured in collision with pedal cycle, unspecified whether traffic or nontraffic accident**
  ☑7ᵗʰ **V01.90**   **Pedestrian on foot injured in collision with pedal cycle, unspecified whether traffic or nontraffic accident**   ▽
     Pedestrian NOS injured in collision with pedal cycle, unspecified whether traffic or nontraffic accident
  ☑x7ᵗʰ **V01.91**   **Pedestrian on roller-skates injured in collision with pedal cycle, unspecified whether traffic or nontraffic accident**   ▽
  ☑x7ᵗʰ **V01.92**   **Pedestrian on skateboard injured in collision with pedal cycle, unspecified whether traffic or nontraffic accident**   ▽
  ☑x7ᵗʰ **V01.99**   **Pedestrian with other conveyance injured in collision with pedal cycle, unspecified whether traffic or nontraffic accident**   ▽
     Pedestrian with babystroller injured in collision with pedal cycle, unspecified whether traffic or nontraffic accident
     Pedestrian on ice-skates injured in collision with pedal cycle unspecified, whether traffic or nontraffic accident
     Pedestrian on nonmotorized scooter injured in collision with pedal cycle, unspecified whether traffic or nontraffic accident
     Pedestrian on sled injured in collision with pedal cycle unspecified, whether traffic or nontraffic accident
     Pedestrian on snowboard injured in collision with pedal cycle, unspecified whether traffic or nontraffic accident
     Pedestrian on snow-skis injured in collision with pedal cycle, unspecified whether traffic or nontraffic accident
     Pedestrian in wheelchair (powered) injured in collision with pedal cycle, unspecified whether traffic or nontraffic accident
     Pedestrian in motorized mobility scooter injured in collision with pedal cycle, unspecified whether traffic or nontraffic accident

☑4ᵗʰ **V02**   **Pedestrian injured in collision with two- or three-wheeled motor vehicle**

  ☑5ᵗʰ **V02.0**   **Pedestrian injured in collision with two- or three-wheeled motor vehicle in nontraffic accident**
   ☑x7ᵗʰ **V02.00**   **Pedestrian on foot injured in collision with two- or three-wheeled motor vehicle in nontraffic accident**
     Pedestrian NOS injured in collision with two- or three-wheeled motor vehicle in nontraffic accident
   ☑x7ᵗʰ **V02.01**   **Pedestrian on roller-skates injured in collision with two- or three-wheeled motor vehicle in nontraffic accident**
   ☑x7ᵗʰ **V02.02**   **Pedestrian on skateboard injured in collision with two- or three-wheeled motor vehicle in nontraffic accident**

☑ Additional Character Required   ☑x7ᵗʰ Placeholder Alert   Manifestation Dx   ▽ Unspecified Dx   ►◄ Revised Text   ● New Code   ▲ Revised Code Title

☑x7ᵗʰ **V02.09** **Pedestrian with other conveyance injured in collision with two- or three-wheeled motor vehicle in nontraffic accident**

Pedestrian with babystroller injured in collision with two- or three-wheeled motor vehicle in nontraffic accident

Pedestrian on ice-skates injured in collision with two- or three-wheeled motor vehicle in nontraffic accident

Pedestrian on nonmotorized scooter injured in collision with two- or three-wheeled motor vehicle in nontraffic accident

Pedestrian on sled injured in collision with two- or three-wheeled motor vehicle in nontraffic accident

Pedestrian on snowboard injured in collision with two- or three-wheeled motor vehicle in nontraffic accident

Pedestrian on snow-skis injured in collision with two- or three-wheeled motor vehicle in nontraffic accident

Pedestrian in wheelchair (powered) injured in collision with two- or three-wheeled motor vehicle in nontraffic accident

Pedestrian in motorized mobility scooter injured in collision with two- or three-wheeled motor vehicle in nontraffic accident

☑5ᵗʰ **V02.1** **Pedestrian injured in collision with two- or three-wheeled motor vehicle in traffic accident**

☑x7ᵗʰ **V02.10** **Pedestrian on foot injured in collision with two- or three-wheeled motor vehicle in traffic accident**

Pedestrian NOS injured in collision with two- or three-wheeled motor vehicle in traffic accident

☑x7ᵗʰ **V02.11** **Pedestrian on roller-skates injured in collision with two- or three-wheeled motor vehicle in traffic accident**

☑x7ᵗʰ **V02.12** **Pedestrian on skateboard injured in collision with two- or three-wheeled motor vehicle in traffic accident**

☑x7ᵗʰ **V02.19** **Pedestrian with other conveyance injured in collision with two- or three-wheeled motor vehicle in traffic accident**

Pedestrian with babystroller injured in collision with two- or three-wheeled motor vehicle in traffic accident

Pedestrian on ice-skates injured in collision with two- or three-wheeled motor vehicle in traffic accident

Pedestrian on nonmotorized scooter injured in collision with two- or three-wheeled motor vehicle in traffic accident

Pedestrian on sled injured in collision with two- or three-wheeled motor vehicle in traffic accident

Pedestrian on snowboard injured in collision with two- or three-wheeled motor vehicle in traffic accident

Pedestrian on snow-skis injured in collision with two- or three-wheeled motor vehicle in traffic accident

Pedestrian in wheelchair (powered) injured in collision with two- or three-wheeled motor vehicle in traffic accident

Pedestrian in motorized mobility scooter injued in collision with two- or three-wheeled motor vehicle in traffic accident

☑5ᵗʰ **V02.9** **Pedestrian injured in collision with two- or three-wheeled motor vehicle, unspecified whether traffic or nontraffic accident**

☑x7ᵗʰ **V02.90** **Pedestrian on foot injured in collision with two- or three-wheeled motor vehicle, unspecified whether traffic or nontraffic accident** ▽

Pedestrian NOS injured in collision with two- or three-wheeled motor vehicle, unspecified whether traffic or nontraffic accident

☑x7ᵗʰ **V02.91** **Pedestrian on roller-skates injured in collision with two- or three-wheeled motor vehicle, unspecified whether traffic or nontraffic accident** ▽

☑x7ᵗʰ **V02.92** **Pedestrian on skateboard injured in collision with two- or three-wheeled motor vehicle, unspecified whether traffic or nontraffic accident** ▽

☑x7ᵗʰ **V02.99** **Pedestrian with other conveyance injured in collision with two- or three-wheeled motor vehicle, unspecified whether traffic or nontraffic accident** ▽

Pedestrian with babystroller injured in collision with two- or three-wheeled motor vehicle, unspecified whether traffic or nontraffic accident

Pedestrian on ice-skates injured in collision with two- or three-wheeled motor vehicle, unspecified whether traffic or nontraffic accident

Pedestrian on nonmotorized scooter injured in collision with two- or three-wheeled motor vehicle, unspecified whether traffic or nontraffic accident

Pedestrian on sled injured in collision with two- or three-wheeled motor vehicle, unspecified whether traffic or nontraffic accident

Pedestrian on snowboard injured in collision with two- or three-wheeled motor vehicle, unspecified whether traffic or nontraffic accident

Pedestrian on snow-skis injured in collision with two- or three-wheeled motor vehicle, unspecified whether traffic or nontraffic accident

Pedestrian in wheelchair (powered) injured in collision with two- or three-wheeled motor vehicle, unspecified whether traffic or nontraffic accident

Pedestrian in motorized mobility scooter injured in collision with two- or three wheeled motor vehicle, unspecified whether traffic or nontraffic accident

☑4ᵗʰ **V03** **Pedestrian injured in collision with car, pick-up truck or van**

☑5ᵗʰ **V03.0** **Pedestrian injured in collision with car, pick-up truck or van in nontraffic accident**

☑x7ᵗʰ **V03.00** **Pedestrian on foot injured in collision with car, pick-up truck or van in nontraffic accident**

Pedestrian NOS injured in collision with car, pick-up truck or van in nontraffic accident

☑x7ᵗʰ **V03.01** **Pedestrian on roller-skates injured in collision with car, pick-up truck or van in nontraffic accident**

☑x7ᵗʰ **V03.02** **Pedestrian on skateboard injured in collision with car, pick-up truck or van in nontraffic accident**

☑x7ᵗʰ **V03.09** **Pedestrian with other conveyance injured in collision with car, pick-up truck or van in nontraffic accident**

Pedestrian with babystroller injured in collision with car, pick-up truck or van in nontraffic accident

Pedestrian on ice-skates injured in collision with car, pick-up truck or van in nontraffic accident

Pedestrian on nonmotorized scooter injured in collision with car, pick-up truck or van in nontraffic accident

Pedestrian on sled injured in collision with car, pick-up truck or van in nontraffic accident

Pedestrian on snowboard injured in collision with car, pick-up truck or van in nontraffic accident

Pedestrian on snow-skis injured in collision with car, pick-up truck or van in nontraffic accident

Pedestrian in wheelchair (powered) injured in collision with car, pick-up truck or van in nontraffic accident

Pedestrian in motorized mobility scooter injured in collision with car, pick-up truck or van in nontraffic accident

☑5ᵗʰ **V03.1** **Pedestrian injured in collision with car, pick-up truck or van in traffic accident**

☑x7ᵗʰ **V03.10** **Pedestrian on foot injured in collision with car, pick-up truck or van in traffic accident**

Pedestrian NOS injured in collision with car, pick-up truck or van in traffic accident

☑x7ᵗʰ **V03.11** **Pedestrian on roller-skates injured in collision with car, pick-up truck or van in traffic accident**

☑x7ᵗʰ **V03.12** **Pedestrian on skateboard injured in collision with car, pick-up truck or van in traffic accident**

EXCLUDES 1   Not coded here   EXCLUDES 2   Not included here   N Newborn Age : 0   P Pediatric Age : 0-17   M Maternity Age : 12-55   A Adult Age : 15-124

1084   ICD-10-CM 2017

☑x7ᵗʰ **V03.19 Pedestrian with other conveyance injured in collision with car, pick-up truck or van in traffic accident**

Pedestrian with babystroller injured in collision with car, pick-up truck or van in traffic accident

Pedestrian on ice-skates injured in collision with car, pick-up truck or van in traffic accident

Pedestrian on nonmotorized scooter injured in collision with car, pick-up truck or van in nontraffic accident

Pedestrian on sled injured in collision with car, pick-up truck or van in traffic accident

Pedestrian on snowboard injured in collision with car, pick-up truck or van in traffic accident

Pedestrian on snow-skis injured in collision with car, pick-up truck or van in traffic accident

Pedestrian in wheelchair (powered) injured in collision with car, pick-up truck or van in traffic accident

Pedestrian in motorized mobility scooter injured in collision with car, pick-up truck or van in nontraffic accident

☑5ᵗʰ **V03.9 Pedestrian injured in collision with car, pick-up truck or van, unspecified whether traffic or nontraffic accident**

☑x7ᵗʰ **V03.90 Pedestrian on foot injured in collision with car, pick-up truck or van, unspecified whether traffic or nontraffic accident** ▽

Pedestrian NOS injured in collision with car, pick-up truck or van, unspecified whether traffic or nontraffic accident

☑x7ᵗʰ **V03.91 Pedestrian on roller-skates injured in collision with car, pick-up truck or van, unspecified whether traffic or nontraffic accident** ▽

☑x7ᵗʰ **V03.92 Pedestrian on skateboard injured in collision with car, pick-up truck or van, unspecified whether traffic or nontraffic accident** ▽

☑x7ᵗʰ **V03.99 Pedestrian with other conveyance injured in collision with car, pick-up truck or van, unspecified whether traffic or nontraffic accident** ▽

Pedestrian with babystroller injured in collision with car, pick-up truck or van, unspecified whether traffic or nontraffic accident

Pedestrian on ice-skates injured in collision with car, pick-up truck or van, unspecified whether traffic or nontraffic accident

Pedestrian on nonmotorized scooter injured in collision with car, pick-up truck or van, unspecified whether traffic or nontraffic accident

Pedestrian on sled injured in collision with car, pick-up truck or van in nontraffic accident

Pedestrian on snowboard injured in collision with car, pick-up truck or van, unspecified whether traffic or nontraffic accident

Pedestrian on snow-skis injured in collision with car, pick-up truck or van, unspecified whether traffic or nontraffic accident

Pedestrian in wheelchair (powered) injured in collision with car, pick-up truck or van, unspecified whether traffic or nontraffic accident

Pedestrian in motorized mobility scooter injured in collision with car, pick-up truck or van, unspecified whether traffic or nontraffic accident

☑4ᵗʰ **V04 Pedestrian injured in collision with heavy transport vehicle or bus**

EXCLUDES 1 *pedestrian injured in collision with military vehicle (V09.01, V09.21)*

☑5ᵗʰ **V04.0 Pedestrian injured in collision with heavy transport vehicle or bus in nontraffic accident**

☑x7ᵗʰ **V04.00 Pedestrian on foot injured in collision with heavy transport vehicle or bus in nontraffic accident**

Pedestrian NOS injured in collision with heavy transport vehicle or bus in nontraffic accident

☑x7ᵗʰ **V04.01 Pedestrian on roller-skates injured in collision with heavy transport vehicle or bus in nontraffic accident**

☑x7ᵗʰ **V04.02 Pedestrian on skateboard injured in collision with heavy transport vehicle or bus in nontraffic accident**

☑x7ᵗʰ **V04.09 Pedestrian with other conveyance injured in collision with heavy transport vehicle or bus in nontraffic accident**

Pedestrian with babystroller injured in collision with heavy transport vehicle or bus in nontraffic accident

Pedestrian on ice-skates injured in collision with heavy transport vehicle or bus in nontraffic accident

Pedestrian on nonmotorized scooter injured in collision with heavy transport vehicle or bus in nontraffic accident

Pedestrian on sled injured in collision with heavy transport vehicle or bus in nontraffic accident

Pedestrian on snowboard injured in collision with heavy transport vehicle or bus in nontraffic accident

Pedestrian on snow-skis injured in collision with heavy transport vehicle or bus in nontraffic accident

Pedestrian in wheelchair (powered) injured in collision with heavy transport vehicle or bus in nontraffic accident

Pedestrian in motorized mobility scooter injured in collision with heavy transport vehicle or bus in nontraffic accident

☑5ᵗʰ **V04.1 Pedestrian injured in collision with heavy transport vehicle or bus in traffic accident**

☑x7ᵗʰ **V04.10 Pedestrian on foot injured in collision with heavy transport vehicle or bus in traffic accident**

Pedestrian NOS injured in collision with heavy transport vehicle or bus in traffic accident

☑x7ᵗʰ **V04.11 Pedestrian on roller-skates injured in collision with heavy transport vehicle or bus in traffic accident**

☑x7ᵗʰ **V04.12 Pedestrian on skateboard injured in collision with heavy transport vehicle or bus in traffic accident**

☑x7ᵗʰ **V04.19 Pedestrian with other conveyance injured in collision with heavy transport vehicle or bus in traffic accident**

Pedestrian with babystroller injured in collision with heavy transport vehicle or bus in traffic accident

Pedestrian on ice-skates injured in collision with heavy transport vehicle or bus in traffic accident

Pedestrian on nonmotorized scooter injured in collision with heavy transport vehicle or bus in traffic accident

Pedestrian on sled injured in collision with heavy transport vehicle or bus in traffic accident

Pedestrian on snowboard injured in collision with heavy transport vehicle or bus in traffic accident

Pedestrian on snow-skis injured in collision with heavy transport vehicle or bus in traffic accident

Pedestrian in wheelchair (powered) injured in collision with heavy transport vehicle or bus in traffic accident

Pedestrian in motorized mobility scooter injured in collision with heavy transport vehicle or bus in traffic accident

☑5ᵗʰ **V04.9 Pedestrian injured in collision with heavy transport vehicle or bus, unspecified whether traffic or nontraffic accident**

☑x7ᵗʰ **V04.90 Pedestrian on foot injured in collision with heavy transport vehicle or bus, unspecified whether traffic or nontraffic accident** ▽

Pedestrian NOS injured in collision with heavy transport vehicle or bus, unspecified whether traffic or nontraffic accident

☑x7ᵗʰ **V04.91 Pedestrian on roller-skates injured in collision with heavy transport vehicle or bus, unspecified whether traffic or nontraffic accident** ▽

☑x7ᵗʰ **V04.92 Pedestrian on skateboard injured in collision with heavy transport vehicle or bus, unspecified whether traffic or nontraffic accident** ▽

☑ Additional Character Required   ☑x7ᵗʰ Placeholder Alert   Manifestation Dx   ▽ Unspecified Dx   ▶◀ Revised Text   ● New Code   ▲ Revised Code Title

Chapter 20. External Causes of Morbidity

V04.99–V06.01

√x7ᵗʰ **V04.99 Pedestrian with other conveyance injured in collision with heavy transport vehicle or bus, unspecified whether traffic or nontraffic accident** ▽

Pedestrian with babystroller injured in collision with heavy transport vehicle or bus, unspecified whether traffic or nontraffic accident

Pedestrian on ice-skates injured in collision with heavy transport vehicle or bus, unspecified whether traffic or nontraffic accident

Pedestrian on nonmotorized scooter injured in collision with heavy transport vehicle or bus, unspecified whether traffic or nontraffic accident

Pedestrian on sled injured in collision with heavy transport vehicle or bus, unspecified whether traffic or nontraffic accident

Pedestrian on snowboard injured in collision with heavy transport vehicle or bus, unspecified whether traffic or nontraffic accident

Pedestrian on snow-skis injured in collision with heavy transport vehicle or bus, unspecified whether traffic or nontraffic accident

Pedestrian in wheelchair (powered) injured in collision with heavy transport vehicle or bus, unspecified whether traffic or nontraffic accident

Pedestrian in motorized mobility scooter injured in collision with heavy transport vehicle or bus, unspecified whether traffic or nontraffic accident

√4ᵗʰ **V05 Pedestrian injured in collision with railway train or railway vehicle**

√5ᵗʰ **V05.0 Pedestrian injured in collision with railway train or railway vehicle in nontraffic accident**

√x7ᵗʰ **V05.00 Pedestrian on foot injured in collision with railway train or railway vehicle in nontraffic accident**

Pedestrian NOS injured in collision with railway train or railway vehicle in nontraffic accident

√x7ᵗʰ **V05.01 Pedestrian on roller-skates injured in collision with railway train or railway vehicle in nontraffic accident**

√x7ᵗʰ **V05.02 Pedestrian on skateboard injured in collision with railway train or railway vehicle in nontraffic accident**

√x7ᵗʰ **V05.09 Pedestrian with other conveyance injured in collision with railway train or railway vehicle in nontraffic accident**

Pedestrian with babystroller injured in collision with railway train or railway vehicle in nontraffic accident

Pedestrian on ice-skates injured in collision with railway train or railway vehicle in nontraffic accident

Pedestrian on nonmotorized scooter injured in collision with railway train or railway vehicle in nontraffic accident

Pedestrian on sled injured in collision with railway train or railway vehicle in nontraffic accident

Pedestrian on snowboard injured in collision with railway train or railway vehicle in nontraffic accident

Pedestrian on snow-skis injured in collision with railway train or railway vehicle in nontraffic accident

Pedestrian in wheelchair (powered) injured in collision with railway train or railway vehicle in nontraffic accident

Pedestrian in motorized mobility scooter injured in collision with railway train or railway vehicle in nontraffic accident

√5ᵗʰ **V05.1 Pedestrian injured in collision with railway train or railway vehicle in traffic accident**

√x7ᵗʰ **V05.10 Pedestrian on foot injured in collision with railway train or railway vehicle in traffic accident**

Pedestrian NOS injured in collision with railway train or railway vehicle in traffic accident

√x7ᵗʰ **V05.11 Pedestrian on roller-skates injured in collision with railway train or railway vehicle in traffic accident**

√x7ᵗʰ **V05.12 Pedestrian on skateboard injured in collision with railway train or railway vehicle in traffic accident**

√x7ᵗʰ **V05.19 Pedestrian with other conveyance injured in collision with railway train or railway vehicle in traffic accident**

Pedestrian with babystroller injured in collision with railway train or railway vehicle in traffic accident

Pedestrian on ice-skates injured in collision with railway train or railway vehicle in traffic accident

Pedestrian on nonmotorized scooter injured in collision with railway train or railway vehicle in traffic accident

Pedestrian on sled injured in collision with railway train or railway vehicle in traffic accident

Pedestrian on snowboard injured in collision with railway train or railway vehicle in traffic accident

Pedestrian on snow-skis injured in collision with railway train or railway vehicle in traffic accident

Pedestrian in wheelchair (powered) injured in collision with railway train or railway vehicle in traffic accident

Pedestrian in motorized mobility scooter injured in collision with railway train or railway vehicle in traffic accident

√5ᵗʰ **V05.9 Pedestrian injured in collision with railway train or railway vehicle, unspecified whether traffic or nontraffic accident**

√x7ᵗʰ **V05.90 Pedestrian on foot injured in collision with railway train or railway vehicle, unspecified whether traffic or nontraffic accident** ▽

Pedestrian NOS injured in collision with railway train or railway vehicle, unspecified whether traffic or nontraffic accident

√x7ᵗʰ **V05.91 Pedestrian on roller-skates injured in collision with railway train or railway vehicle, unspecified whether traffic or nontraffic accident** ▽

√x7ᵗʰ **V05.92 Pedestrian on skateboard injured in collision with railway train or railway vehicle, unspecified whether traffic or nontraffic accident** ▽

√x7ᵗʰ **V05.99 Pedestrian with other conveyance injured in collision with railway train or railway vehicle, unspecified whether traffic or nontraffic accident** ▽

Pedestrian with babystroller injured in collision with railway train or railway vehicle, unspecified whether traffic or nontraffic

Pedestrian on ice-skates injured in collision with railway train or railway vehicle, unspecified whether traffic or nontraffic

Pedestrian on nonmotorized scooter injured in collision with railway train or railway vehicle, unspecified whether traffic or nontraffic

Pedestrian on sled injured in collision with railway train or railway vehicle, unspecified whether traffic or nontraffic

Pedestrian on snowboard injured in collision with railway train or railway vehicle, unspecified whether traffic or nontraffic

Pedestrian on snow-skis injured in collision with railway train or railway vehicle, unspecified whether traffic or nontraffic

Pedestrian in wheelchair (powered) injured in collision with railway train or railway vehicle, unspecified whether traffic or nontraffic

Pedestrian in motorized mobility scooter injured in collision with railway train or railway vehicle, unspecified whether traffic or nontraffic

√4ᵗʰ **V06 Pedestrian injured in collision with other nonmotor vehicle**

INCLUDES collision with animal-drawn vehicle, animal being ridden, nonpowered streetcar

EXCLUDES 1 pedestrian injured in collision with pedestrian conveyance (V00.0-)

√5ᵗʰ **V06.0 Pedestrian injured in collision with other nonmotor vehicle in nontraffic accident**

√x7ᵗʰ **V06.00 Pedestrian on foot injured in collision with other nonmotor vehicle in nontraffic accident**

Pedestrian NOS injured in collision with other nonmotor vehicle in nontraffic accident

√x7ᵗʰ **V06.01 Pedestrian on roller-skates injured in collision with other nonmotor vehicle in nontraffic accident**

EXCLUDES 1 Not coded here   **EXCLUDES 2** Not included here   N Newborn Age : 0   P Pediatric Age : 0-17   M Maternity Age : 12-55   A Adult Age : 15-124

1086   ICD-10-CM 2017

√x7ᵗʰ **V06.02** **Pedestrian** on skateboard **injured in collision with other nonmotor vehicle in nontraffic accident**

√x7ᵗʰ **V06.09** **Pedestrian** with other conveyance **injured in collision with other nonmotor vehicle in nontraffic accident**

Pedestrian with babystroller injured in collision with other nonmotor vehicle in nontraffic accident

Pedestrian on ice-skates injured in collision with other nonmotor vehicle in nontraffic accident

Pedestrian on nonmotorized scooter injured in collision with other nonmotor vehicle in nontraffic accident

Pedestrian on sled injured in collision with other nonmotor vehicle in nontraffic accident

Pedestrian on snowboard injured in collision with other nonmotor vehicle in nontraffic accident

Pedestrian on snow-skis injured in collision with other nonmotor vehicle in nontraffic accident

Pedestrian in wheelchair (powered) injured in collision with other nonmotor vehicle in nontraffic accident

Pedestrian in motorized mobility scooter injured in collision with other nonmotor vehicle in nontraffic accident

√5ᵗʰ **V06.1** **Pedestrian injured in collision with other nonmotor vehicle in traffic accident**

√x7ᵗʰ **V06.10** **Pedestrian** on foot **injured in collision with other nonmotor vehicle in traffic accident**

Pedestrian NOS injured in collision with other nonmotor vehicle in traffic accident

√x7ᵗʰ **V06.11** **Pedestrian** on roller-skates **injured in collision with other nonmotor vehicle in traffic accident**

√x7ᵗʰ **V06.12** **Pedestrian** on skateboard **injured in collision with other nonmotor vehicle in traffic accident**

√x7ᵗʰ **V06.19** **Pedestrian** with other conveyance **injured in collision with other nonmotor vehicle in traffic accident**

Pedestrian with babystroller injured in collision with other nonmotor vehicle in nontraffic accident

Pedestrian on ice-skates injured in collision with other nonmotor vehicle in traffic accident

Pedestrian on nonmotorized scooter injured in collision with other nonmotor vehicle in traffic accident

Pedestrian on sled injured in collision with other nonmotor vehicle in traffic accident

Pedestrian on snowboard injured in collision with other nonmotor vehicle in traffic accident

Pedestrian on snow-skis injured in collision with other nonmotor vehicle in traffic accident

Pedestrian in wheelchair (powered) injured in collision with other nonmotor vehicle in traffic accident

Pedestrian in motorized mobility scooter injured in collision with other nonmotor vehicle in traffic accident

√5ᵗʰ **V06.9** **Pedestrian injured in collision with other nonmotor vehicle, unspecified whether traffic or nontraffic accident**

√x7ᵗʰ **V06.90** **Pedestrian** on foot **injured in collision with other nonmotor vehicle, unspecified whether traffic or nontraffic accident** ▽

Pedestrian NOS injured in collision with other nonmotor vehicle, unspecified whether traffic or nontraffic accident

√x7ᵗʰ **V06.91** **Pedestrian** on roller-skates **injured in collision with other nonmotor vehicle, unspecified whether traffic or nontraffic accident** ▽

√x7ᵗʰ **V06.92** **Pedestrian** on skateboard **injured in collision with other nonmotor vehicle, unspecified whether traffic or nontraffic accident** ▽

√x7ᵗʰ **V06.99** **Pedestrian** with other conveyance **injured in collision with other nonmotor vehicle, unspecified whether traffic or nontraffic accident** ▽

Pedestrian with babystroller injured in collision with other nonmotor vehicle, unspecified whether traffic or nontraffic accident

Pedestrian on ice-skates injured in collision with other nonmotor vehicle, unspecified whether traffic or nontraffic accident

Pedestrian on nonmotorized scooter injured in collision with other nonmotor vehicle, unspecified whether traffic or nontraffic accident

Pedestrian on sled injured in collision with other nonmotor vehicle, unspecified whether traffic or nontraffic accident

Pedestrian on snowboard injured in collision with other nonmotor vehicle, unspecified whether traffic or nontraffic accident

Pedestrian on snow-skis injured in collision with other nonmotor vehicle, unspecified whether traffic or nontraffic accident

Pedestrian in wheelchair (powered) injured in collision with other nonmotor vehicle, unspecified whether traffic or nontraffic accident

Pedestrian in motorized mobility scooter injured in collision with other nonmotorized vehicle, unspecified whether traffic or nontraffic accident

√4ᵗʰ **V09** **Pedestrian injured in other and unspecified transport accidents**

√5ᵗʰ **V09.0** **Pedestrian injured in** nontraffic **accident involving other and unspecified motor vehicles**

√x7ᵗʰ **V09.00** **Pedestrian injured in** nontraffic **accident involving unspecified motor vehicles** ▽

√x7ᵗʰ **V09.01** **Pedestrian injured in** nontraffic **accident involving military vehicle**

√x7ᵗʰ **V09.09** **Pedestrian injured in** nontraffic **accident involving other motor vehicles**

Pedestrian injured in nontraffic accident by special vehicle

√x7ᵗʰ **V09.1** **Pedestrian injured in unspecified** nontraffic **accident** ▽

√5ᵗʰ **V09.2** **Pedestrian injured in** traffic accident **involving other and unspecified motor vehicles**

√x7ᵗʰ **V09.20** **Pedestrian injured in traffic accident involving unspecified motor vehicles** ▽

√x7ᵗʰ **V09.21** **Pedestrian injured in traffic accident involving military vehicle**

√x7ᵗʰ **V09.29** **Pedestrian injured in traffic accident involving other motor vehicles**

√x7ᵗʰ **V09.3** **Pedestrian injured in unspecified** traffic **accident** ▽

√x7ᵗʰ **V09.9** **Pedestrian injured in unspecified** transport **accident** ▽

Pedal cycle rider injured in transport accident (V10-V19)

INCLUDES   any non-motorized vehicle, excluding an animal-drawn vehicle, or a sidecar or trailer attached to the pedal cycle

EXCLUDES 2   *rupture of pedal cycle tire (W37.0)*

The appropriate 7th character is to be added to each code from categories V10-V19.
A   initial encounter
D   subsequent encounter
S   sequela

√4ᵗʰ **V10** **Pedal cycle rider injured in collision with pedestrian or animal**

EXCLUDES 1   *pedal cycle rider collision with animal-drawn vehicle or animal being ridden (V16.-)*

√x7ᵗʰ **V10.0** **Pedal cycle** driver **injured in collision with pedestrian or animal in** nontraffic **accident**

√x7ᵗʰ **V10.1** **Pedal cycle** passenger **injured in collision with pedestrian or animal in** nontraffic **accident**

√x7ᵗʰ **V10.2** **Unspecified pedal cyclist injured in collision with pedestrian or animal in** nontraffic **accident** ▽

√x7ᵗʰ **V10.3** Person boarding or alighting a pedal cycle **injured in collision with pedestrian or animal**

√x7ᵗʰ **V10.4** **Pedal cycle** driver **injured in collision with pedestrian or animal in traffic accident**

√x7ᵗʰ **V10.5** **Pedal cycle** passenger **injured in collision with pedestrian or animal in traffic accident**

√x7ᵗʰ **V10.9** **Unspecified pedal cyclist injured in collision with pedestrian or animal in traffic accident** ▽

☑ Additional Character Required   √x7ᵗʰ Placeholder Alert   Manifestation Dx   ▽ Unspecified Dx   ►◄ Revised Text   ● New Code   ▲ Revised Code Title

Chapter 20. External Causes of Morbidity

V11–V19.3

✓4th **V11** **Pedal cycle rider injured in collision with other pedal cycle**

✓x7th **V11.0** Pedal cycle driver injured in collision with other pedal cycle in nontraffic accident

✓x7th **V11.1** Pedal cycle passenger injured in collision with other pedal cycle in nontraffic accident

✓x7th **V11.2** Unspecified pedal cyclist injured in collision with other pedal cycle in nontraffic accident ▽

✓x7th **V11.3** Person boarding or alighting a pedal cycle injured in collision with other pedal cycle

✓x7th **V11.4** Pedal cycle driver injured in collision with other pedal cycle in traffic accident

✓x7th **V11.5** Pedal cycle passenger injured in collision with other pedal cycle in traffic accident

✓x7th **V11.9** Unspecified pedal cyclist injured in collision with other pedal cycle in traffic accident ▽

✓4th **V12** **Pedal cycle rider injured in collision with two- or three-wheeled motor vehicle**

✓x7th **V12.0** Pedal cycle driver injured in collision with two- or three-wheeled motor vehicle in nontraffic accident

✓x7th **V12.1** Pedal cycle passenger injured in collision with two- or three-wheeled motor vehicle in nontraffic accident

✓x7th **V12.2** Unspecified pedal cyclist injured in collision with two- or three-wheeled motor vehicle in nontraffic accident ▽

✓x7th **V12.3** Person boarding or alighting a pedal cycle injured in collision with two- or three-wheeled motor vehicle

✓x7th **V12.4** Pedal cycle driver injured in collision with two- or three-wheeled motor vehicle in traffic accident

✓x7th **V12.5** Pedal cycle passenger injured in collision with two- or three-wheeled motor vehicle in traffic accident

✓x7th **V12.9** Unspecified pedal cyclist injured in collision with two- or three-wheeled motor vehicle in traffic accident ▽

✓4th **V13** **Pedal cycle rider injured in collision with car, pick-up truck or van**

✓x7th **V13.0** Pedal cycle driver injured in collision with car, pick-up truck or van in nontraffic accident

✓x7th **V13.1** Pedal cycle passenger injured in collision with car, pick-up truck or van in nontraffic accident

✓x7th **V13.2** Unspecified pedal cyclist injured in collision with car, pick-up truck or van in nontraffic accident ▽

✓x7th **V13.3** Person boarding or alighting a pedal cycle injured in collision with car, pick-up truck or van

✓x7th **V13.4** Pedal cycle driver injured in collision with car, pick-up truck or van in traffic accident

✓x7th **V13.5** Pedal cycle passenger injured in collision with car, pick-up truck or van in traffic accident

✓x7th **V13.9** Unspecified pedal cyclist injured in collision with car, pick-up truck or van in traffic accident ▽

✓4th **V14** **Pedal cycle rider injured in collision with heavy transport vehicle or bus**

    EXCLUDES 1 *pedal cycle rider injured in collision with military vehicle (V19.81)*

✓x7th **V14.0** Pedal cycle driver injured in collision with heavy transport vehicle or bus in nontraffic accident

✓x7th **V14.1** Pedal cycle passenger injured in collision with heavy transport vehicle or bus in nontraffic accident

✓x7th **V14.2** Unspecified pedal cyclist injured in collision with heavy transport vehicle or bus in nontraffic accident ▽

✓x7th **V14.3** Person boarding or alighting a pedal cycle injured in collision with heavy transport vehicle or bus

✓x7th **V14.4** Pedal cycle driver injured in collision with heavy transport vehicle or bus in traffic accident

✓x7th **V14.5** Pedal cycle passenger injured in collision with heavy transport vehicle or bus in traffic accident

✓x7th **V14.9** Unspecified pedal cyclist injured in collision with heavy transport vehicle or bus in traffic accident ▽

✓4th **V15** **Pedal cycle rider injured in collision with railway train or railway vehicle**

✓x7th **V15.0** Pedal cycle driver injured in collision with railway train or railway vehicle in nontraffic accident

✓x7th **V15.1** Pedal cycle passenger injured in collision with railway train or railway vehicle in nontraffic accident

✓x7th **V15.2** Unspecified pedal cyclist injured in collision with railway train or railway vehicle in nontraffic accident ▽

✓x7th **V15.3** Person boarding or alighting a pedal cycle injured in collision with railway train or railway vehicle

✓x7th **V15.4** Pedal cycle driver injured in collision with railway train or railway vehicle in traffic accident

✓x7th **V15.5** Pedal cycle passenger injured in collision with railway train or railway vehicle in traffic accident

✓x7th **V15.9** Unspecified pedal cyclist injured in collision with railway train or railway vehicle in traffic accident ▽

✓4th **V16** **Pedal cycle rider injured in collision with other nonmotor vehicle**

    INCLUDES collision with animal-drawn vehicle, animal being ridden, streetcar

✓x7th **V16.0** Pedal cycle driver injured in collision with other nonmotor vehicle in nontraffic accident

✓x7th **V16.1** Pedal cycle passenger injured in collision with other nonmotor vehicle in nontraffic accident

✓x7th **V16.2** Unspecified pedal cyclist injured in collision with other nonmotor vehicle in nontraffic accident ▽

✓x7th **V16.3** Person boarding or alighting a pedal cycle injured in collision with other nonmotor vehicle in nontraffic accident

✓x7th **V16.4** Pedal cycle driver injured in collision with other nonmotor vehicle in traffic accident

✓x7th **V16.5** Pedal cycle passenger injured in collision with other nonmotor vehicle in traffic accident

✓x7th **V16.9** Unspecified pedal cyclist injured in collision with other nonmotor vehicle in traffic accident ▽

✓4th **V17** **Pedal cycle rider injured in collision with fixed or stationary object**

✓x7th **V17.0** Pedal cycle driver injured in collision with fixed or stationary object in nontraffic accident

✓x7th **V17.1** Pedal cycle passenger injured in collision with fixed or stationary object in nontraffic accident

✓x7th **V17.2** Unspecified pedal cyclist injured in collision with fixed or stationary object in nontraffic accident ▽

✓x7th **V17.3** Person boarding or alighting a pedal cycle injured in collision with fixed or stationary object

✓x7th **V17.4** Pedal cycle driver injured in collision with fixed or stationary object in traffic accident

✓x7th **V17.5** Pedal cycle passenger injured in collision with fixed or stationary object in traffic accident

✓x7th **V17.9** Unspecified pedal cyclist injured in collision with fixed or stationary object in traffic accident ▽

✓4th **V18** **Pedal cycle rider injured in noncollision transport accident**

    INCLUDES fall or thrown from pedal cycle (without antecedent collision)
                 overturning pedal cycle NOS
                 overturning pedal cycle without collision

✓x7th **V18.0** Pedal cycle driver injured in noncollision transport accident in nontraffic accident

✓x7th **V18.1** Pedal cycle passenger injured in noncollision transport accident in nontraffic accident

✓x7th **V18.2** Unspecified pedal cyclist injured in noncollision transport accident in nontraffic accident ▽

✓x7th **V18.3** Person boarding or alighting a pedal cycle injured in noncollision transport accident

✓x7th **V18.4** Pedal cycle driver injured in noncollision transport accident in traffic accident

✓x7th **V18.5** Pedal cycle passenger injured in noncollision transport accident in traffic accident

✓x7th **V18.9** Unspecified pedal cyclist injured in noncollision transport accident in traffic accident ▽

✓4th **V19** **Pedal cycle rider injured in other and unspecified transport accidents**

✓5th **V19.0** Pedal cycle driver injured in collision with other and unspecified motor vehicles in nontraffic accident

    ✓x7th **V19.00** Pedal cycle driver injured in collision with unspecified motor vehicles in nontraffic accident ▽

    ✓x7th **V19.09** Pedal cycle driver injured in collision with other motor vehicles in nontraffic accident

✓5th **V19.1** Pedal cycle passenger injured in collision with other and unspecified motor vehicles in nontraffic accident

    ✓x7th **V19.10** Pedal cycle passenger injured in collision with unspecified motor vehicles in nontraffic accident ▽

    ✓x7th **V19.19** Pedal cycle passenger injured in collision with other motor vehicles in nontraffic accident

✓5th **V19.2** Unspecified pedal cyclist injured in collision with other and unspecified motor vehicles in nontraffic accident

    ✓x7th **V19.20** Unspecified pedal cyclist injured in collision with unspecified motor vehicles in nontraffic accident ▽
            Pedal cycle collision NOS, nontraffic

    ✓x7th **V19.29** Unspecified pedal cyclist injured in collision with other motor vehicles in nontraffic accident ▽

✓x7th **V19.3** Pedal cyclist (driver) (passenger) injured in unspecified nontraffic accident ▽
        Pedal cycle accident NOS, nontraffic
        Pedal cyclist injured in nontraffic accident NOS

EXCLUDES 1 Not coded here   **EXCLUDES 2** Not included here   **N** Newborn Age : 0   **P** Pediatric Age : 0-17   **M** Maternity Age : 12-55   **A** Adult Age : 15-124

1088

ICD-10-CM 2017

√5ᵗʰ **V19.4** Pedal cycle **driver** injured in collision with other and unspecified motor vehicles **in traffic accident**

    √x7ᵗʰ **V19.40** Pedal cycle driver injured in collision with unspecified motor vehicles in traffic accident ▽

    √x7ᵗʰ **V19.49** Pedal cycle driver injured in collision with other motor vehicles in traffic accident

√5ᵗʰ **V19.5** Pedal cycle **passenger** injured in collision with other and unspecified motor vehicles **in traffic accident**

    √x7ᵗʰ **V19.50** Pedal cycle passenger injured in collision with unspecified motor vehicles in traffic accident ▽

    √x7ᵗʰ **V19.59** Pedal cycle passenger injured in collision with other motor vehicles in traffic accident

√5ᵗʰ **V19.6** Unspecified pedal cyclist injured in collision with other and unspecified motor vehicles **in traffic accident**

    √x7ᵗʰ **V19.60** Unspecified pedal cyclist injured in collision with unspecified motor vehicles in traffic accident ▽

        Pedal cycle collision NOS (traffic)

    √x7ᵗʰ **V19.69** Unspecified pedal cyclist injured in collision with other motor vehicles in traffic accident ▽

√5ᵗʰ **V19.8** Pedal cyclist (driver) (passenger) injured in other specified transport accidents

    √x7ᵗʰ **V19.81** Pedal cyclist (driver) (passenger) injured in transport accident with **military vehicle**

    √x7ᵗʰ **V19.88** Pedal cyclist (driver) (passenger) injured in other specified transport accidents

√5ᵗʰ **V19.9** Pedal cyclist (driver) (passenger) injured in unspecified traffic accident ▽

        Pedal cycle accident NOS

Motorcycle rider injured in transport accident (V20-V29)

INCLUDES   moped
        motorcycle with sidecar
        motorized bicycle
        motor scooter

EXCLUDES 1 *three-wheeled motor vehicle (V30-V39)*

The appropriate 7th character is to be added to each code from categories V20-V29.
A   initial encounter
D subsequent encounter
S   sequela

√4ᵗʰ **V20** Motorcycle rider injured in collision with pedestrian or animal

    EXCLUDES 1 *motorcycle rider collision with animal-drawn vehicle or animal being ridden (V26.-)*

    √x7ᵗʰ **V20.0** Motorcycle **driver** injured in collision with pedestrian or animal **in nontraffic accident**

    √x7ᵗʰ **V20.1** Motorcycle **passenger** injured in collision with pedestrian or animal **in nontraffic accident**

    √x7ᵗʰ **V20.2** Unspecified motorcycle rider injured in collision with pedestrian or animal **in nontraffic accident** ▽

    √x7ᵗʰ **V20.3** **Person boarding or alighting** a motorcycle injured in collision with pedestrian or animal

    √x7ᵗʰ **V20.4** Motorcycle **driver** injured in collision with pedestrian or animal **in traffic accident**

    √x7ᵗʰ **V20.5** Motorcycle **passenger** injured in collision with pedestrian or animal **in traffic accident**

    √x7ᵗʰ **V20.9** Unspecified motorcycle rider injured in collision with pedestrian or animal **in traffic accident** ▽

√4ᵗʰ **V21** Motorcycle rider injured in collision with pedal cycle

    √x7ᵗʰ **V21.0** Motorcycle **driver** injured in collision with pedal cycle **in nontraffic accident**

    √x7ᵗʰ **V21.1** Motorcycle **passenger** injured in collision with pedal cycle **in nontraffic accident**

    √x7ᵗʰ **V21.2** Unspecified motorcycle rider injured in collision with pedal cycle **in nontraffic accident** ▽

    √x7ᵗʰ **V21.3** **Person boarding or alighting** a motorcycle injured in collision with pedal cycle

    √x7ᵗʰ **V21.4** Motorcycle **driver** injured in collision with pedal cycle **in traffic accident**

    √x7ᵗʰ **V21.5** Motorcycle **passenger** injured in collision with pedal cycle **in traffic accident**

    √x7ᵗʰ **V21.9** Unspecified motorcycle rider injured in collision with pedal cycle **in traffic accident** ▽

√4ᵗʰ **V22** Motorcycle rider injured in collision with two- or three-wheeled motor vehicle

    √x7ᵗʰ **V22.0** Motorcycle **driver** injured in collision with two- or three-wheeled motor vehicle **in nontraffic accident**

    √x7ᵗʰ **V22.1** Motorcycle **passenger** injured in collision with two- or three-wheeled motor vehicle **in nontraffic accident**

    √x7ᵗʰ **V22.2** Unspecified motorcycle rider injured in collision with two- or three-wheeled motor vehicle **in nontraffic accident** ▽

    √x7ᵗʰ **V22.3** **Person boarding or alighting** a motorcycle injured in collision with two- or three-wheeled motor vehicle

    √x7ᵗʰ **V22.4** Motorcycle **driver** injured in collision with two- or three-wheeled motor vehicle **in traffic accident**

    √x7ᵗʰ **V22.5** Motorcycle **passenger** injured in collision with two- or three-wheeled motor vehicle **in traffic accident**

    √x7ᵗʰ **V22.9** Unspecified motorcycle rider injured in collision with two- or three-wheeled motor vehicle **in traffic accident** ▽

√4ᵗʰ **V23** Motorcycle rider injured in collision with car, pick-up truck or van

    √x7ᵗʰ **V23.0** Motorcycle **driver** injured in collision with car, pick-up truck or van **in nontraffic accident**

    √x7ᵗʰ **V23.1** Motorcycle **passenger** injured in collision with car, pick-up truck or van **in nontraffic accident**

    √x7ᵗʰ **V23.2** Unspecified motorcycle rider injured in collision with car, pick-up truck or van **in nontraffic accident** ▽

    √x7ᵗʰ **V23.3** **Person boarding or alighting** a motorcycle injured in collision with car, pick-up truck or van

    √x7ᵗʰ **V23.4** Motorcycle **driver** injured in collision with car, pick-up truck or van **in traffic accident**

    √x7ᵗʰ **V23.5** Motorcycle **passenger** injured in collision with car, pick-up truck or van **in traffic accident**

    √x7ᵗʰ **V23.9** Unspecified motorcycle rider injured in collision with car, pick-up truck or van **in traffic accident** ▽

√4ᵗʰ **V24** Motorcycle rider injured in collision with heavy transport vehicle or bus

    EXCLUDES 1 *motorcycle rider injured in collision with military vehicle (V29.81)*

    √x7ᵗʰ **V24.0** Motorcycle **driver** injured in collision with heavy transport vehicle or bus **in nontraffic accident**

    √x7ᵗʰ **V24.1** Motorcycle **passenger** injured in collision with heavy transport vehicle or bus **in nontraffic accident**

    √x7ᵗʰ **V24.2** Unspecified motorcycle rider injured in collision with heavy transport vehicle or bus **in nontraffic accident** ▽

    √x7ᵗʰ **V24.3** **Person boarding or alighting** a motorcycle injured in collision with heavy transport vehicle or bus

    √x7ᵗʰ **V24.4** Motorcycle **driver** injured in collision with heavy transport vehicle or bus **in traffic accident**

    √x7ᵗʰ **V24.5** Motorcycle **passenger** injured in collision with heavy transport vehicle or bus **in traffic accident**

    √x7ᵗʰ **V24.9** Unspecified motorcycle rider injured in collision with heavy transport vehicle or bus **in traffic accident** ▽

√4ᵗʰ **V25** Motorcycle rider injured in collision with railway train or railway vehicle

    √x7ᵗʰ **V25.0** Motorcycle **driver** injured in collision with railway train or railway vehicle **in nontraffic accident**

    √x7ᵗʰ **V25.1** Motorcycle **passenger** injured in collision with railway train or railway vehicle **in nontraffic accident**

    √x7ᵗʰ **V25.2** Unspecified motorcycle rider injured in collision with railway train or railway vehicle **in nontraffic accident** ▽

    √x7ᵗʰ **V25.3** **Person boarding or alighting** a motorcycle injured in collision with railway train or railway vehicle

    √x7ᵗʰ **V25.4** Motorcycle **driver** injured in collision with railway train or railway vehicle **in traffic accident**

    √x7ᵗʰ **V25.5** Motorcycle **passenger** injured in collision with railway train or railway vehicle **in traffic accident**

    √x7ᵗʰ **V25.9** Unspecified motorcycle rider injured in collision with railway train or railway vehicle **in traffic accident** ▽

√4ᵗʰ **V26** Motorcycle rider injured in collision with other nonmotor vehicle

    INCLUDES collision with animal-drawn vehicle, animal being ridden, streetcar

    √x7ᵗʰ **V26.0** Motorcycle **driver** injured in collision with other nonmotor vehicle **in nontraffic accident**

    √x7ᵗʰ **V26.1** Motorcycle **passenger** injured in collision with other nonmotor vehicle **in nontraffic accident**

    √x7ᵗʰ **V26.2** Unspecified motorcycle rider injured in collision with other nonmotor vehicle **in nontraffic accident** ▽

    √x7ᵗʰ **V26.3** **Person boarding or alighting** a motorcycle injured in collision with other nonmotor vehicle

    √x7ᵗʰ **V26.4** Motorcycle **driver** injured in collision with other nonmotor vehicle **in traffic accident**

    √x7ᵗʰ **V26.5** Motorcycle **passenger** injured in collision with other nonmotor vehicle **in traffic accident**

    √x7ᵗʰ **V26.9** Unspecified motorcycle rider injured in collision with other nonmotor vehicle **in traffic accident** ▽

✔ Additional Character Required   √x7ᵗʰ Placeholder Alert   Manifestation Dx   ▽ Unspecified Dx   ►◄ Revised Text   ● New Code   ▲ Revised Code Title

ICD-10-CM 2017   1089

✓4th **V27** **Motorcycle rider injured in collision with fixed or stationary object**

  ✓x7th **V27.0** Motorcycle driver injured in collision with fixed or stationary object in nontraffic accident

  ✓x7th **V27.1** Motorcycle passenger injured in collision with fixed or stationary object in nontraffic accident

  ✓x7th **V27.2** Unspecified motorcycle rider injured in collision with fixed or stationary object in nontraffic accident ▽

  ✓x7th **V27.3** Person boarding or alighting a motorcycle injured in collision with fixed or stationary object

  ✓x7th **V27.4** Motorcycle driver injured in collision with fixed or stationary object in traffic accident

  ✓x7th **V27.5** Motorcycle passenger injured in collision with fixed or stationary object in traffic accident

  ✓x7th **V27.9** Unspecified motorcycle rider injured in collision with fixed or stationary object in traffic accident ▽

✓4th **V28** **Motorcycle rider injured in noncollision transport accident**

  INCLUDES fall or thrown from motorcycle (without antecedent collision)
      overturning motorcycle NOS
      overturning motorcycle without collision

  ✓x7th **V28.0** Motorcycle driver injured in noncollision transport accident in nontraffic accident

  ✓x7th **V28.1** Motorcycle passenger injured in noncollision transport accident in nontraffic accident

  ✓x7th **V28.2** Unspecified motorcycle rider injured in noncollision transport accident in nontraffic accident ▽

  ✓x7th **V28.3** Person boarding or alighting a motorcycle injured in noncollision transport accident

  ✓x7th **V28.4** Motorcycle driver injured in noncollision transport accident in traffic accident

  ✓x7th **V28.5** Motorcycle passenger injured in noncollision transport accident in traffic accident

  ✓x7th **V28.9** Unspecified motorcycle rider injured in noncollision transport accident in traffic accident ▽

✓4th **V29** **Motorcycle rider injured in other and unspecified transport accidents**

  ✓5th **V29.0** Motorcycle driver injured in collision with other and unspecified motor vehicles in nontraffic accident

    ✓x7th **V29.00** Motorcycle driver injured in collision with unspecified motor vehicles in nontraffic accident ▽

    ✓x7th **V29.09** Motorcycle driver injured in collision with other motor vehicles in nontraffic accident

  ✓5th **V29.1** Motorcycle passenger injured in collision with other and unspecified motor vehicles in nontraffic accident

    ✓x7th **V29.10** Motorcycle passenger injured in collision with unspecified motor vehicles in nontraffic accident ▽

    ✓x7th **V29.19** Motorcycle passenger injured in collision with other motor vehicles in nontraffic accident

  ✓5th **V29.2** Unspecified motorcycle rider injured in collision with other and unspecified motor vehicles in nontraffic accident

    ✓x7th **V29.20** Unspecified motorcycle rider injured in collision with unspecified motor vehicles in nontraffic accident ▽
      Motorcycle collision NOS, nontraffic

    ✓x7th **V29.29** Unspecified motorcycle rider injured in collision with other motor vehicles in nontraffic accident ▽

  ✓x7th **V29.3** Motorcycle rider (driver) (passenger) injured in unspecified nontraffic accident ▽
    Motorcycle accident NOS, nontraffic
    Motorcycle rider injured in nontraffic accident NOS

  ✓5th **V29.4** Motorcycle driver injured in collision with other and unspecified motor vehicles in traffic accident

    ✓x7th **V29.40** Motorcycle driver injured in collision with unspecified motor vehicles in traffic accident ▽

    ✓x7th **V29.49** Motorcycle driver injured in collision with other motor vehicles in traffic accident

  ✓5th **V29.5** Motorcycle passenger injured in collision with other and unspecified motor vehicles in traffic accident

    ✓x7th **V29.50** Motorcycle passenger injured in collision with unspecified motor vehicles in traffic accident ▽

    ✓x7th **V29.59** Motorcycle passenger injured in collision with other motor vehicles in traffic accident

  ✓5th **V29.6** Unspecified motorcycle rider injured in collision with other and unspecified motor vehicles in traffic accident

    ✓x7th **V29.60** Unspecified motorcycle rider injured in collision with unspecified motor vehicles in traffic accident ▽
      Motorcycle collision NOS (traffic)

    ✓x7th **V29.69** Unspecified motorcycle rider injured in collision with other motor vehicles in traffic accident ▽

  ✓5th **V29.8** Motorcycle rider (driver) (passenger) injured in other specified transport accidents

    ✓x7th **V29.81** Motorcycle rider (driver) (passenger) injured in transport accident with military vehicle

    ✓x7th **V29.88** Motorcycle rider (driver) (passenger) injured in other specified transport accidents

  ✓x7th **V29.9** Motorcycle rider (driver) (passenger) injured in unspecified traffic accident ▽
    Motorcycle accident NOS

Occupant of three-wheeled motor vehicle injured in transport accident (V30-V39)

  INCLUDES motorized tricycle
      motorized rickshaw
      three-wheeled motor car

  EXCLUDES 1 all-terrain vehicles (V86.-)
      motorcycle with sidecar (V20-V29)
      vehicle designed primarily for off-road use (V86.-)

The appropriate 7th character is to be added to each code from categories V30-V39.
A   initial encounter
D   subsequent encounter
S   sequela

✓4th **V30** **Occupant of three-wheeled motor vehicle injured in collision with pedestrian or animal**

  EXCLUDES 1 three-wheeled motor vehicle collision with animal-drawn vehicle or animal being ridden (V36.-)

  ✓x7th **V30.0** Driver of three-wheeled motor vehicle injured in collision with pedestrian or animal in nontraffic accident

  ✓x7th **V30.1** Passenger in three-wheeled motor vehicle injured in collision with pedestrian or animal in nontraffic accident

  ✓x7th **V30.2** Person on outside of three-wheeled motor vehicle injured in collision with pedestrian or animal in nontraffic accident

  ✓x7th **V30.3** Unspecified occupant of three-wheeled motor vehicle injured in collision with pedestrian or animal in nontraffic accident ▽

  ✓x7th **V30.4** Person boarding or alighting a three-wheeled motor vehicle injured in collision with pedestrian or animal

  ✓x7th **V30.5** Driver of three-wheeled motor vehicle injured in collision with pedestrian or animal in traffic accident

  ✓x7th **V30.6** Passenger in three-wheeled motor vehicle injured in collision with pedestrian or animal in traffic accident

  ✓x7th **V30.7** Person on outside of three-wheeled motor vehicle injured in collision with pedestrian or animal in traffic accident

  ✓x7th **V30.9** Unspecified occupant of three-wheeled motor vehicle injured in collision with pedestrian or animal in traffic accident ▽

✓4th **V31** **Occupant of three-wheeled motor vehicle injured in collision with pedal cycle**

  ✓x7th **V31.0** Driver of three-wheeled motor vehicle injured in collision with pedal cycle in nontraffic accident

  ✓x7th **V31.1** Passenger in three-wheeled motor vehicle injured in collision with pedal cycle in nontraffic accident

  ✓x7th **V31.2** Person on outside of three-wheeled motor vehicle injured in collision with pedal cycle in nontraffic accident

  ✓x7th **V31.3** Unspecified occupant of three-wheeled motor vehicle injured in collision with pedal cycle in nontraffic accident ▽

  ✓x7th **V31.4** Person boarding or alighting a three-wheeled motor vehicle injured in collision with pedal cycle

  ✓x7th **V31.5** Driver of three-wheeled motor vehicle injured in collision with pedal cycle in traffic accident

  ✓x7th **V31.6** Passenger in three-wheeled motor vehicle injured in collision with pedal cycle in traffic accident

  ✓x7th **V31.7** Person on outside of three-wheeled motor vehicle injured in collision with pedal cycle in traffic accident

  ✓x7th **V31.9** Unspecified occupant of three-wheeled motor vehicle injured in collision with pedal cycle in traffic accident ▽

✓4th **V32** **Occupant of three-wheeled motor vehicle injured in collision with two- or three-wheeled motor vehicle**

  ✓x7th **V32.0** Driver of three-wheeled motor vehicle injured in collision with two- or three-wheeled motor vehicle in nontraffic accident

  ✓x7th **V32.1** Passenger in three-wheeled motor vehicle injured in collision with two- or three-wheeled motor vehicle in nontraffic accident

  ✓x7th **V32.2** Person on outside of three-wheeled motor vehicle injured in collision with two- or three-wheeled motor vehicle in nontraffic accident

---

EXCLUDES 1 Not coded here   **EXCLUDES 2** Not included here   **N** Newborn Age : 0   **P** Pediatric Age : 0-17   **M** Maternity Age : 12-55   **A** Adult Age : 15-124

1090

ICD-10-CM 2017

✓x7ᵗʰ **V32.3** Unspecified occupant of three-wheeled motor vehicle injured in collision with two- or three-wheeled motor vehicle in nontraffic accident ▽

✓x7ᵗʰ **V32.4** Person boarding or alighting a three-wheeled motor vehicle injured in collision with two- or three-wheeled motor vehicle

✓x7ᵗʰ **V32.5** Driver of three-wheeled motor vehicle injured in collision with two- or three-wheeled motor vehicle in traffic accident

✓x7ᵗʰ **V32.6** Passenger in three-wheeled motor vehicle injured in collision with two- or three-wheeled motor vehicle in traffic accident

✓x7ᵗʰ **V32.7** Person on outside of three-wheeled motor vehicle injured in collision with two- or three-wheeled motor vehicle in traffic accident

✓x7ᵗʰ **V32.9** Unspecified occupant of three-wheeled motor vehicle injured in collision with two- or three-wheeled motor vehicle in traffic accident ▽

✓4ᵗʰ **V33** Occupant of three-wheeled motor vehicle injured in collision with car, pick-up truck or van

✓x7ᵗʰ **V33.0** Driver of three-wheeled motor vehicle injured in collision with car, pick-up truck or van in nontraffic accident

✓x7ᵗʰ **V33.1** Passenger in three-wheeled motor vehicle injured in collision with car, pick-up truck or van in nontraffic accident

✓x7ᵗʰ **V33.2** Person on outside of three-wheeled motor vehicle injured in collision with car, pick-up truck or van in nontraffic accident

✓x7ᵗʰ **V33.3** Unspecified occupant of three-wheeled motor vehicle injured in collision with car, pick-up truck or van in nontraffic accident ▽

✓x7ᵗʰ **V33.4** Person boarding or alighting a three-wheeled motor vehicle injured in collision with car, pick-up truck or van

✓x7ᵗʰ **V33.5** Driver of three-wheeled motor vehicle injured in collision with car, pick-up truck or van in traffic accident

✓x7ᵗʰ **V33.6** Passenger in three-wheeled motor vehicle injured in collision with car, pick-up truck or van in traffic accident

✓x7ᵗʰ **V33.7** Person on outside of three-wheeled motor vehicle injured in collision with car, pick-up truck or van in traffic accident

✓x7ᵗʰ **V33.9** Unspecified occupant of three-wheeled motor vehicle injured in collision with car, pick-up truck or van in traffic accident ▽

✓4ᵗʰ **V34** Occupant of three-wheeled motor vehicle injured in collision with heavy transport vehicle or bus

EXCLUDES 1 *occupant of three-wheeled motor vehicle injured in collision with military vehicle (V39.81)*

✓x7ᵗʰ **V34.0** Driver of three-wheeled motor vehicle injured in collision with heavy transport vehicle or bus in nontraffic accident

✓x7ᵗʰ **V34.1** Passenger in three-wheeled motor vehicle injured in collision with heavy transport vehicle or bus in nontraffic accident

✓x7ᵗʰ **V34.2** Person on outside of three-wheeled motor vehicle injured in collision with heavy transport vehicle or bus in nontraffic accident

✓x7ᵗʰ **V34.3** Unspecified occupant of three-wheeled motor vehicle injured in collision with heavy transport vehicle or bus in nontraffic accident ▽

✓x7ᵗʰ **V34.4** Person boarding or alighting a three-wheeled motor vehicle injured in collision with heavy transport vehicle or bus

✓x7ᵗʰ **V34.5** Driver of three-wheeled motor vehicle injured in collision with heavy transport vehicle or bus in traffic accident

✓x7ᵗʰ **V34.6** Passenger in three-wheeled motor vehicle injured in collision with heavy transport vehicle or bus in traffic accident

✓x7ᵗʰ **V34.7** Person on outside of three-wheeled motor vehicle injured in collision with heavy transport vehicle or bus in traffic accident

✓x7ᵗʰ **V34.9** Unspecified occupant of three-wheeled motor vehicle injured in collision with heavy transport vehicle or bus in traffic accident ▽

✓4ᵗʰ **V35** Occupant of three-wheeled motor vehicle injured in collision with railway train or railway vehicle

✓x7ᵗʰ **V35.0** Driver of three-wheeled motor vehicle injured in collision with railway train or railway vehicle in nontraffic accident

✓x7ᵗʰ **V35.1** Passenger in three-wheeled motor vehicle injured in collision with railway train or railway vehicle in nontraffic accident

✓x7ᵗʰ **V35.2** Person on outside of three-wheeled motor vehicle injured in collision with railway train or railway vehicle in nontraffic accident

✓x7ᵗʰ **V35.3** Unspecified occupant of three-wheeled motor vehicle injured in collision with railway train or railway vehicle in nontraffic accident ▽

✓x7ᵗʰ **V35.4** Person boarding or alighting a three-wheeled motor vehicle injured in collision with railway train or railway vehicle

✓x7ᵗʰ **V35.5** Driver of three-wheeled motor vehicle injured in collision with railway train or railway vehicle in traffic accident

✓x7ᵗʰ **V35.6** Passenger in three-wheeled motor vehicle injured in collision with railway train or railway vehicle in traffic accident

✓x7ᵗʰ **V35.7** Person on outside of three-wheeled motor vehicle injured in collision with railway train or railway vehicle in traffic accident

✓x7ᵗʰ **V35.9** Unspecified occupant of three-wheeled motor vehicle injured in collision with railway train or railway vehicle in traffic accident ▽

✓4ᵗʰ **V36** Occupant of three-wheeled motor vehicle injured in collision with other nonmotor vehicle

INCLUDES collision with animal-drawn vehicle, animal being ridden, streetcar

✓x7ᵗʰ **V36.0** Driver of three-wheeled motor vehicle injured in collision with other nonmotor vehicle in nontraffic accident

✓x7ᵗʰ **V36.1** Passenger in three-wheeled motor vehicle injured in collision with other nonmotor vehicle in nontraffic accident

✓x7ᵗʰ **V36.2** Person on outside of three-wheeled motor vehicle injured in collision with other nonmotor vehicle in nontraffic accident

✓x7ᵗʰ **V36.3** Unspecified occupant of three-wheeled motor vehicle injured in collision with other nonmotor vehicle in nontraffic accident ▽

✓x7ᵗʰ **V36.4** Person boarding or alighting a three-wheeled motor vehicle injured in collision with other nonmotor vehicle

✓x7ᵗʰ **V36.5** Driver of three-wheeled motor vehicle injured in collision with other nonmotor vehicle in traffic accident

✓x7ᵗʰ **V36.6** Passenger in three-wheeled motor vehicle injured in collision with other nonmotor vehicle in traffic accident

✓x7ᵗʰ **V36.7** Person on outside of three-wheeled motor vehicle injured in collision with other nonmotor vehicle in traffic accident

✓x7ᵗʰ **V36.9** Unspecified occupant of three-wheeled motor vehicle injured in collision with other nonmotor vehicle in traffic accident ▽

✓4ᵗʰ **V37** Occupant of three-wheeled motor vehicle injured in collision with fixed or stationary object

✓x7ᵗʰ **V37.0** Driver of three-wheeled motor vehicle injured in collision with fixed or stationary object in nontraffic accident

✓x7ᵗʰ **V37.1** Passenger in three-wheeled motor vehicle injured in collision with fixed or stationary object in nontraffic accident

✓x7ᵗʰ **V37.2** Person on outside of three-wheeled motor vehicle injured in collision with fixed or stationary object in nontraffic accident

✓x7ᵗʰ **V37.3** Unspecified occupant of three-wheeled motor vehicle injured in collision with fixed or stationary object in nontraffic accident ▽

✓x7ᵗʰ **V37.4** Person boarding or alighting a three-wheeled motor vehicle injured in collision with fixed or stationary object

✓x7ᵗʰ **V37.5** Driver of three-wheeled motor vehicle injured in collision with fixed or stationary object in traffic accident

✓x7ᵗʰ **V37.6** Passenger in three-wheeled motor vehicle injured in collision with fixed or stationary object in traffic accident

✓x7ᵗʰ **V37.7** Person on outside of three-wheeled motor vehicle injured in collision with fixed or stationary object in traffic accident

✓x7ᵗʰ **V37.9** Unspecified occupant of three-wheeled motor vehicle injured in collision with fixed or stationary object in traffic accident ▽

✓4ᵗʰ **V38** Occupant of three-wheeled motor vehicle injured in noncollision transport accident

INCLUDES fall or thrown from three-wheeled motor vehicle
overturning of three-wheeled motor vehicle NOS
overturning of three-wheeled motor vehicle without collision

✓x7ᵗʰ **V38.0** Driver of three-wheeled motor vehicle injured in noncollision transport accident in nontraffic accident

✓x7ᵗʰ **V38.1** Passenger in three-wheeled motor vehicle injured in noncollision transport accident in nontraffic accident

✓x7ᵗʰ **V38.2** Person on outside of three-wheeled motor vehicle injured in noncollision transport accident in nontraffic accident

✓x7ᵗʰ **V38.3** Unspecified occupant of three-wheeled motor vehicle injured in noncollision transport accident in nontraffic accident ▽

✓x7ᵗʰ **V38.4** Person boarding or alighting a three-wheeled motor vehicle injured in noncollision transport accident

✓x7ᵗʰ **V38.5** Driver of three-wheeled motor vehicle injured in noncollision transport accident in traffic accident

✓x7ᵗʰ **V38.6** Passenger in three-wheeled motor vehicle injured in noncollision transport accident in traffic accident

✓x7ᵗʰ **V38.7** Person on outside of three-wheeled motor vehicle injured in noncollision transport accident in traffic accident

✓x7ᵗʰ **V38.9** Unspecified occupant of three-wheeled motor vehicle injured in noncollision transport accident in traffic accident ▽

☑ Additional Character Required   ✓x7ᵗʰ Placeholder Alert   Manifestation Dx   ▽ Unspecified Dx   ►◄ Revised Text   ● New Code   ▲ Revised Code Title

Chapter 20. External Causes of Morbidity

V39–V42.9

☑4th **V39 Occupant of three-wheeled motor vehicle injured in other and unspecified transport accidents**

  ☑5th **V39.0** Driver of three-wheeled motor vehicle injured in collision with other and unspecified motor vehicles in nontraffic accident

    √x7th **V39.00** Driver of three-wheeled motor vehicle injured in collision with unspecified motor vehicles in nontraffic accident ▽

    √x7th **V39.09** Driver of three-wheeled motor vehicle injured in collision with other motor vehicles in nontraffic accident

  ☑5th **V39.1** Passenger in three-wheeled motor vehicle injured in collision with other and unspecified motor vehicles in nontraffic accident

    √x7th **V39.10** Passenger in three-wheeled motor vehicle injured in collision with unspecified motor vehicles in nontraffic accident ▽

    √x7th **V39.19** Passenger in three-wheeled motor vehicle injured in collision with other motor vehicles in nontraffic accident

  ☑5th **V39.2** Unspecified occupant of three-wheeled motor vehicle injured in collision with other and unspecified motor vehicles in nontraffic accident

    √x7th **V39.20** Unspecified occupant of three-wheeled motor vehicle injured in collision with unspecified motor vehicles in nontraffic accident ▽

        Collision NOS involving three-wheeled motor vehicle, nontraffic

    √x7th **V39.29** Unspecified occupant of three-wheeled motor vehicle injured in collision with other motor vehicles in nontraffic accident ▽

  √x7th **V39.3** Occupant (driver) (passenger) of three-wheeled motor vehicle injured in unspecified nontraffic accident ▽

        Accident NOS involving three-wheeled motor vehicle, nontraffic

        Occupant of three-wheeled motor vehicle injured in nontraffic accident NOS

  ☑5th **V39.4** Driver of three-wheeled motor vehicle injured in collision with other and unspecified motor vehicles in traffic accident

    √x7th **V39.40** Driver of three-wheeled motor vehicle injured in collision with unspecified motor vehicles in traffic accident ▽

    √x7th **V39.49** Driver of three-wheeled motor vehicle injured in collision with other motor vehicles in traffic accident

  ☑5th **V39.5** Passenger in three-wheeled motor vehicle injured in collision with other and unspecified motor vehicles in traffic accident

    √x7th **V39.50** Passenger in three-wheeled motor vehicle injured in collision with unspecified motor vehicles in traffic accident ▽

    √x7th **V39.59** Passenger in three-wheeled motor vehicle injured in collision with other motor vehicles in traffic accident

  ☑5th **V39.6** Unspecified occupant of three-wheeled motor vehicle injured in collision with other and unspecified motor vehicles in traffic accident

    √x7th **V39.60** Unspecified occupant of three-wheeled motor vehicle injured in collision with unspecified motor vehicles in traffic accident ▽

        Collision NOS involving three-wheeled motor vehicle (traffic)

    √x7th **V39.69** Unspecified occupant of three-wheeled motor vehicle injured in collision with other motor vehicles in traffic accident ▽

  ☑5th **V39.8** Occupant (driver) (passenger) of three-wheeled motor vehicle injured in other specified transport accidents

    √x7th **V39.81** Occupant (driver) (passenger) of three-wheeled motor vehicle injured in transport accident with military vehicle

    √x7th **V39.89** Occupant (driver) (passenger) of three-wheeled motor vehicle injured in other specified transport accidents

  √x7th **V39.9** Occupant (driver) (passenger) of three-wheeled motor vehicle injured in unspecified traffic accident ▽

        Accident NOS involving three-wheeled motor vehicle

Car occupant injured in transport accident (V40-V49)

INCLUDES   a four-wheeled motor vehicle designed primarily for carrying passengers
         automobile (pulling a trailer or camper)

EXCLUDES 1   bus (V50-V59)
         minibus (V50-V59)
         minivan (V50-V59)
         motorcoach (V70-V79)
         pick-up truck (V50-V59)
         sport utility vehicle (SUV) (V50-V59)

The appropriate 7th character is to be added to each code from categories V40-V49.
A   initial encounter
D   subsequent encounter
S   sequela

☑4th **V40 Car occupant injured in collision with pedestrian or animal**

    EXCLUDES 1   car collision with animal-drawn vehicle or animal being ridden (V46.-)

  √x7th **V40.0** Car driver injured in collision with pedestrian or animal in nontraffic accident

  √x7th **V40.1** Car passenger injured in collision with pedestrian or animal in nontraffic accident

  √x7th **V40.2** Person on outside of car injured in collision with pedestrian or animal in nontraffic accident

  √x7th **V40.3** Unspecified car occupant injured in collision with pedestrian or animal in nontraffic accident ▽

  √x7th **V40.4** Person boarding or alighting a car injured in collision with pedestrian or animal

  √x7th **V40.5** Car driver injured in collision with pedestrian or animal in traffic accident

  √x7th **V40.6** Car passenger injured in collision with pedestrian or animal in traffic accident

  √x7th **V40.7** Person on outside of car injured in collision with pedestrian or animal in traffic accident

  √x7th **V40.9** Unspecified car occupant injured in collision with pedestrian or animal in traffic accident ▽

☑4th **V41 Car occupant injured in collision with pedal cycle**

  √x7th **V41.0** Car driver injured in collision with pedal cycle in nontraffic accident

  √x7th **V41.1** Car passenger injured in collision with pedal cycle in nontraffic accident

  √x7th **V41.2** Person on outside of car injured in collision with pedal cycle in nontraffic accident

  √x7th **V41.3** Unspecified car occupant injured in collision with pedal cycle in nontraffic accident ▽

  √x7th **V41.4** Person boarding or alighting a car injured in collision with pedal cycle

  √x7th **V41.5** Car driver injured in collision with pedal cycle in traffic accident

  √x7th **V41.6** Car passenger injured in collision with pedal cycle in traffic accident

  √x7th **V41.7** Person on outside of car injured in collision with pedal cycle in traffic accident

  √x7th **V41.9** Unspecified car occupant injured in collision with pedal cycle in traffic accident ▽

☑4th **V42 Car occupant injured in collision with two- or three-wheeled motor vehicle**

  √x7th **V42.0** Car driver injured in collision with two- or three-wheeled motor vehicle in nontraffic accident

  √x7th **V42.1** Car passenger injured in collision with two- or three-wheeled motor vehicle in nontraffic accident

  √x7th **V42.2** Person on outside of car injured in collision with two- or three-wheeled motor vehicle in nontraffic accident

  √x7th **V42.3** Unspecified car occupant injured in collision with two- or three-wheeled motor vehicle in nontraffic accident ▽

  √x7th **V42.4** Person boarding or alighting a car injured in collision with two- or three-wheeled motor vehicle

  √x7th **V42.5** Car driver injured in collision with two- or three-wheeled motor vehicle in traffic accident

  √x7th **V42.6** Car passenger injured in collision with two- or three-wheeled motor vehicle in traffic accident

  √x7th **V42.7** Person on outside of car injured in collision with two- or three-wheeled motor vehicle in traffic accident

  √x7th **V42.9** Unspecified car occupant injured in collision with two- or three-wheeled motor vehicle in traffic accident ▽

EXCLUDES 1 Not coded here   EXCLUDES 2 Not included here   N Newborn Age : 0   P Pediatric Age : 0-17   M Maternity Age : 12-55   A Adult Age : 15-124

☑4ᵗʰ **V43** **Car occupant injured in collision with car, pick-up truck or van**

  ☑5ᵗʰ **V43.0** **Car** driver **injured in collision with car, pick-up truck or van** in nontraffic accident

    √x7ᵗʰ **V43.01** Car driver injured in collision with sport utility vehicle in nontraffic accident

    √x7ᵗʰ **V43.02** Car driver injured in collision with other type car in nontraffic accident

    √x7ᵗʰ **V43.03** Car driver injured in collision with pick-up truck in nontraffic accident

    √x7ᵗʰ **V43.04** Car driver injured in collision with van in nontraffic accident

  ☑5ᵗʰ **V43.1** **Car passenger injured in collision with car, pick-up truck or van** in nontraffic accident

    √x7ᵗʰ **V43.11** Car passenger injured in collision with sport utility vehicle in nontraffic accident

    √x7ᵗʰ **V43.12** Car passenger injured in collision with other type car in nontraffic accident

    √x7ᵗʰ **V43.13** Car passenger injured in collision with pick-up in nontraffic accident

    √x7ᵗʰ **V43.14** Car passenger injured in collision with van in nontraffic accident

  ☑5ᵗʰ **V43.2** **Person on outside of car injured in collision with car, pick-up truck or van** in nontraffic accident

    √x7ᵗʰ **V43.21** Person on outside of car injured in collision with sport utility vehicle in nontraffic accident

    √x7ᵗʰ **V43.22** Person on outside of car injured in collision with other type car in nontraffic accident

    √x7ᵗʰ **V43.23** Person on outside of car injured in collision with pick-up truck in nontraffic accident

    √x7ᵗʰ **V43.24** Person on outside of car injured in collision with van in nontraffic accident

  ☑5ᵗʰ **V43.3** **Unspecified car occupant injured in collision with car, pick-up truck or van** in nontraffic accident

    √x7ᵗʰ **V43.31** Unspecified car occupant injured in collision with sport utility vehicle in nontraffic accident ▽

    √x7ᵗʰ **V43.32** Unspecified car occupant injured in collision with other type car in nontraffic accident ▽

    √x7ᵗʰ **V43.33** Unspecified car occupant injured in collision with pick-up truck in nontraffic accident ▽

    √x7ᵗʰ **V43.34** Unspecified car occupant injured in collision with van in nontraffic accident ▽

  ☑5ᵗʰ **V43.4** **Person boarding or alighting a car injured in collision with car, pick-up truck or van**

    √x7ᵗʰ **V43.41** Person boarding or alighting a car injured in collision with sport utility vehicle

    √x7ᵗʰ **V43.42** Person boarding or alighting a car injured in collision with other type car

    √x7ᵗʰ **V43.43** Person boarding or alighting a car injured in collision with pick-up truck

    √x7ᵗʰ **V43.44** Person boarding or alighting a car injured in collision with van

  ☑5ᵗʰ **V43.5** **Car** driver **injured in collision with car, pick-up truck or van** in traffic accident

    √x7ᵗʰ **V43.51** Car driver injured in collision with sport utility vehicle in traffic accident

    √x7ᵗʰ **V43.52** Car driver injured in collision with other type car in traffic accident

    √x7ᵗʰ **V43.53** Car driver injured in collision with pick-up truck in traffic accident

    √x7ᵗʰ **V43.54** Car driver injured in collision with van in traffic accident

  ☑5ᵗʰ **V43.6** **Car** passenger **injured in collision with car, pick-up truck or van** in traffic accident

    √x7ᵗʰ **V43.61** Car passenger injured in collision with sport utility vehicle in traffic accident

    √x7ᵗʰ **V43.62** Car passenger injured in collision with other type car in traffic accident

    √x7ᵗʰ **V43.63** Car passenger injured in collision with pick-up truck in traffic accident

    √x7ᵗʰ **V43.64** Car passenger injured in collision with van in traffic accident

  ☑5ᵗʰ **V43.7** **Person on outside of car injured in collision with car, pick-up truck or van** in traffic accident

    √x7ᵗʰ **V43.71** Person on outside of car injured in collision with sport utility vehicle in traffic accident

    √x7ᵗʰ **V43.72** Person on outside of car injured in collision with other type car in traffic accident

    √x7ᵗʰ **V43.73** Person on outside of car injured in collision with pick-up truck in traffic accident

    √x7ᵗʰ **V43.74** Person on outside of car injured in collision with van in traffic accident

  ☑5ᵗʰ **V43.9** **Unspecified car occupant injured in collision with car, pick-up truck or van** in traffic accident

    √x7ᵗʰ **V43.91** Unspecified car occupant injured in collision with sport utility vehicle in traffic accident ▽

    √x7ᵗʰ **V43.92** Unspecified car occupant injured in collision with other type car in traffic accident ▽

    √x7ᵗʰ **V43.93** Unspecified car occupant injured in collision with pick-up truck in traffic accident ▽

    √x7ᵗʰ **V43.94** Unspecified car occupant injured in collision with van in traffic accident ▽

☑4ᵗʰ **V44** **Car occupant injured in collision with heavy transport vehicle or bus**

    EXCLUDES 1   car occupant injured in collision with military vehicle (V49.81)

  √x7ᵗʰ **V44.0** **Car** driver **injured in collision with heavy transport vehicle or bus** in nontraffic accident

  √x7ᵗʰ **V44.1** **Car** passenger **injured in collision with heavy transport vehicle or bus** in nontraffic accident

  √x7ᵗʰ **V44.2** **Person on outside of car injured in collision with heavy transport vehicle or bus** in nontraffic accident

  √x7ᵗʰ **V44.3** **Unspecified car occupant injured in collision with heavy transport vehicle or bus** in nontraffic accident ▽

  √x7ᵗʰ **V44.4** **Person boarding or alighting a car injured in collision with heavy transport vehicle or bus**

  √x7ᵗʰ **V44.5** **Car** driver **injured in collision with heavy transport vehicle or bus** in traffic accident

  √x7ᵗʰ **V44.6** **Car** passenger **injured in collision with heavy transport vehicle or bus** in traffic accident

  √x7ᵗʰ **V44.7** **Person on outside of car injured in collision with heavy transport vehicle or bus** in traffic accident

  √x7ᵗʰ **V44.9** **Unspecified car occupant injured in collision with heavy transport vehicle or bus** in traffic accident ▽

☑4ᵗʰ **V45** **Car occupant injured in collision with railway train or railway vehicle**

  √x7ᵗʰ **V45.0** **Car** driver **injured in collision with railway train or railway vehicle** in nontraffic accident

  √x7ᵗʰ **V45.1** **Car** passenger **injured in collision with railway train or railway vehicle** in nontraffic accident

  √x7ᵗʰ **V45.2** **Person on outside of car injured in collision with railway train or railway vehicle** in nontraffic accident

  √x7ᵗʰ **V45.3** **Unspecified car occupant injured in collision with railway train or railway vehicle** in nontraffic accident ▽

  √x7ᵗʰ **V45.4** **Person boarding or alighting a car injured in collision with railway train or railway vehicle**

  √x7ᵗʰ **V45.5** **Car** driver **injured in collision with railway train or railway vehicle** in traffic accident

  √x7ᵗʰ **V45.6** **Car** passenger **injured in collision with railway train or railway vehicle** in traffic accident

  √x7ᵗʰ **V45.7** **Person on outside of car injured in collision with railway train or railway vehicle** in traffic accident

  √x7ᵗʰ **V45.9** **Unspecified car occupant injured in collision with railway train or railway vehicle** in traffic accident ▽

☑4ᵗʰ **V46** **Car occupant injured in collision with other nonmotor vehicle**

    INCLUDES   collision with animal-drawn vehicle, animal being ridden, streetcar

  √x7ᵗʰ **V46.0** **Car** driver **injured in collision with other nonmotor vehicle** in nontraffic accident

  √x7ᵗʰ **V46.1** **Car** passenger **injured in collision with other nonmotor vehicle** in nontraffic accident

  √x7ᵗʰ **V46.2** **Person on outside of car injured in collision with other nonmotor vehicle** in nontraffic accident

  √x7ᵗʰ **V46.3** **Unspecified car occupant injured in collision with other nonmotor vehicle** in nontraffic accident ▽

  √x7ᵗʰ **V46.4** **Person boarding or alighting a car injured in collision with other nonmotor vehicle**

  √x7ᵗʰ **V46.5** **Car** driver **injured in collision with other nonmotor vehicle** in traffic accident

  √x7ᵗʰ **V46.6** **Car** passenger **injured in collision with other nonmotor vehicle** in traffic accident

  √x7ᵗʰ **V46.7** **Person on outside of car injured in collision with other nonmotor vehicle** in traffic accident

  √x7ᵗʰ **V46.9** **Unspecified car occupant injured in collision with other nonmotor vehicle** in traffic accident ▽

☑4ᵗʰ **V47** **Car occupant injured in collision with fixed or stationary object**

  √7ᵗʰ **V47.0** **Car** driver **injured in collision with fixed or stationary object** in nontraffic accident

  √x7ᵗʰ **V47.1** **Car** passenger **injured in collision with fixed or stationary object** in nontraffic accident

  √x7ᵗʰ **V47.2** **Person on outside of car injured in collision with fixed or stationary object** in nontraffic accident

  √x7ᵗʰ **V47.3** **Unspecified car occupant injured in collision with fixed or stationary object** in nontraffic accident

---

☑ Additional Character Required   √x7ᵗʰ Placeholder Alert   Manifestation Dx   ▽ Unspecified Dx   ▶◀ Revised Text   ● New Code   ▲ Revised Code Title

√x7ᵗʰ **V47.4** **Person boarding or alighting a car injured in collision with fixed or stationary object**

√x7ᵗʰ **V47.5** **Car driver injured in collision with fixed or stationary object in traffic accident**

√x7ᵗʰ **V47.6** **Car passenger injured in collision with fixed or stationary object in traffic accident**

√x7ᵗʰ **V47.7** **Person on outside of car injured in collision with fixed or stationary object in traffic accident**

√x7ᵗʰ **V47.9** **Unspecified car occupant injured in collision with fixed or stationary object in traffic accident**

√4ᵗʰ **V48** **Car occupant injured in noncollision transport accident**

INCLUDES overturning car NOS
overturning car without collision

√x7ᵗʰ **V48.0** **Car driver injured in noncollision transport accident in nontraffic accident**

√x7ᵗʰ **V48.1** **Car passenger injured in noncollision transport accident in nontraffic accident**

√x7ᵗʰ **V48.2** **Person on outside of car injured in noncollision transport accident in nontraffic accident**

√x7ᵗʰ **V48.3** **Unspecified car occupant injured in noncollision transport accident in nontraffic accident** ▽

√x7ᵗʰ **V48.4** **Person boarding or alighting a car injured in noncollision transport accident**

√x7ᵗʰ **V48.5** **Car driver injured in noncollision transport accident in traffic accident**

√x7ᵗʰ **V48.6** **Car passenger injured in noncollision transport accident in traffic accident**

√x7ᵗʰ **V48.7** **Person on outside of car injured in noncollision transport accident in traffic accident**

√x7ᵗʰ **V48.9** **Unspecified car occupant injured in noncollision transport accident in traffic accident** ▽

√4ᵗʰ **V49** **Car occupant injured in other and unspecified transport accidents**

√5ᵗʰ **V49.0** **Driver injured in collision with other and unspecified motor vehicles in nontraffic accident**

√x7ᵗʰ **V49.00** **Driver injured in collision with unspecified motor vehicles in nontraffic accident** ▽

√x7ᵗʰ **V49.09** **Driver injured in collision with other motor vehicles in nontraffic accident**

√5ᵗʰ **V49.1** **Passenger injured in collision with other and unspecified motor vehicles in nontraffic accident**

√x7ᵗʰ **V49.10** **Passenger injured in collision with unspecified motor vehicles in nontraffic accident** ▽

√x7ᵗʰ **V49.19** **Passenger injured in collision with other motor vehicles in nontraffic accident**

√5ᵗʰ **V49.2** **Unspecified car occupant injured in collision with other and unspecified motor vehicles in nontraffic accident**

√x7ᵗʰ **V49.20** **Unspecified car occupant injured in collision with unspecified motor vehicles in nontraffic accident** ▽
Car collision NOS, nontraffic

√x7ᵗʰ **V49.29** **Unspecified car occupant injured in collision with other motor vehicles in nontraffic accident** ▽

√x7ᵗʰ **V49.3** **Car occupant (driver) (passenger) injured in unspecified nontraffic accident** ▽
Car accident NOS, nontraffic
Car occupant injured in nontraffic accident NOS

√5ᵗʰ **V49.4** **Driver injured in collision with other and unspecified motor vehicles in traffic accident**

√x7ᵗʰ **V49.40** **Driver injured in collision with unspecified motor vehicles in traffic accident** ▽

√x7ᵗʰ **V49.49** **Driver injured in collision with other motor vehicles in traffic accident**

√5ᵗʰ **V49.5** **Passenger injured in collision with other and unspecified motor vehicles in traffic accident**

√x7ᵗʰ **V49.50** **Passenger injured in collision with unspecified motor vehicles in traffic accident** ▽

√x7ᵗʰ **V49.59** **Passenger injured in collision with other motor vehicles in traffic accident**

√5ᵗʰ **V49.6** **Unspecified car occupant injured in collision with other and unspecified motor vehicles in traffic accident**

√x7ᵗʰ **V49.60** **Unspecified car occupant injured in collision with unspecified motor vehicles in traffic accident** ▽
Car collision NOS (traffic)

√x7ᵗʰ **V49.69** **Unspecified car occupant injured in collision with other motor vehicles in traffic accident** ▽

√5ᵗʰ **V49.8** **Car occupant (driver) (passenger) injured in other specified transport accidents**

√x7ᵗʰ **V49.81** **Car occupant (driver) (passenger) injured in transport accident with military vehicle**

√x7ᵗʰ **V49.88** **Car occupant (driver) (passenger) injured in other specified transport accidents**

√x7ᵗʰ **V49.9** **Car occupant (driver) (passenger) injured in unspecified traffic accident** ▽
Car accident NOS

Occupant of pick-up truck or van injured in transport accident (V50-V59)

INCLUDES a four or six wheel motor vehicle designed primarily for carrying passengers and property but weighing less than the local limit for classification as a heavy goods vehicle
minibus
minivan
sport utility vehicle (SUV)
truck
van

EXCLUDES 1 heavy transport vehicle (V60-V69)

The appropriate 7th character is to be added to each code from categories V50-V59.
A initial encounter
D subsequent encounter
S sequela

√4ᵗʰ **V50** **Occupant of pick-up truck or van injured in collision with pedestrian or animal**

EXCLUDES 1 pick-up truck or van collision with animal-drawn vehicle or animal being ridden (V56.-)

√x7ᵗʰ **V50.0** **Driver of pick-up truck or van injured in collision with pedestrian or animal in nontraffic accident**

√x7ᵗʰ **V50.1** **Passenger in pick-up truck or van injured in collision with pedestrian or animal in nontraffic accident**

√x7ᵗʰ **V50.2** **Person on outside of pick-up truck or van injured in collision with pedestrian or animal in nontraffic accident**

√x7ᵗʰ **V50.3** **Unspecified occupant of pick-up truck or van injured in collision with pedestrian or animal in nontraffic accident** ▽

√x7ᵗʰ **V50.4** **Person boarding or alighting a pick-up truck or van injured in collision with pedestrian or animal**

√x7ᵗʰ **V50.5** **Driver of pick-up truck or van injured in collision with pedestrian or animal in traffic accident**

√x7ᵗʰ **V50.6** **Passenger in pick-up truck or van injured in collision with pedestrian or animal in traffic accident**

√x7ᵗʰ **V50.7** **Person on outside of pick-up truck or van injured in collision with pedestrian or animal in traffic accident**

√x7ᵗʰ **V50.9** **Unspecified occupant of pick-up truck or van injured in collision with pedestrian or animal in traffic accident** ▽

√4ᵗʰ **V51** **Occupant of pick-up truck or van injured in collision with pedal cycle**

√x7ᵗʰ **V51.0** **Driver of pick-up truck or van injured in collision with pedal cycle in nontraffic accident**

√x7ᵗʰ **V51.1** **Passenger in pick-up truck or van injured in collision with pedal cycle in nontraffic accident**

√x7ᵗʰ **V51.2** **Person on outside of pick-up truck or van injured in collision with pedal cycle in nontraffic accident**

√x7ᵗʰ **V51.3** **Unspecified occupant of pick-up truck or van injured in collision with pedal cycle in nontraffic accident** ▽

√x7ᵗʰ **V51.4** **Person boarding or alighting a pick-up truck or van injured in collision with pedal cycle**

√x7ᵗʰ **V51.5** **Driver of pick-up truck or van injured in collision with pedal cycle in traffic accident**

√x7ᵗʰ **V51.6** **Passenger in pick-up truck or van injured in collision with pedal cycle in traffic accident**

√x7ᵗʰ **V51.7** **Person on outside of pick-up truck or van injured in collision with pedal cycle in traffic accident**

√x7ᵗʰ **V51.9** **Unspecified occupant of pick-up truck or van injured in collision with pedal cycle in traffic accident** ▽

√4ᵗʰ **V52** **Occupant of pick-up truck or van injured in collision with two- or three-wheeled motor vehicle**

√x7ᵗʰ **V52.0** **Driver of pick-up truck or van injured in collision with two- or three-wheeled motor vehicle in nontraffic accident**

√x7ᵗʰ **V52.1** **Passenger in pick-up truck or van injured in collision with two- or three-wheeled motor vehicle in nontraffic accident**

√x7ᵗʰ **V52.2** **Person on outside of pick-up truck or van injured in collision with two- or three-wheeled motor vehicle in nontraffic accident**

√x7ᵗʰ **V52.3** **Unspecified occupant of pick-up truck or van injured in collision with two- or three-wheeled motor vehicle in nontraffic accident** ▽

√x7ᵗʰ **V52.4** **Person boarding or alighting a pick-up truck or van injured in collision with two- or three-wheeled motor vehicle**

EXCLUDES 1 Not coded here | EXCLUDES 2 Not included here | N Newborn Age : 0 | P Pediatric Age : 0-17 | M Maternity Age : 12-55 | A Adult Age : 15-124

1094 | ICD-10-CM 2017

√x7ᵗʰ **V52.5** Driver of pick-up truck or van injured in collision with two- or three-wheeled motor vehicle in traffic accident

√x7ᵗʰ **V52.6** Passenger in pick-up truck or van injured in collision with two- or three-wheeled motor vehicle in traffic accident

√x7ᵗʰ **V52.7** Person on outside of pick-up truck or van injured in collision with two- or three-wheeled motor vehicle in traffic accident

√x7ᵗʰ **V52.9** Unspecified occupant of pick-up truck or van injured in collision with two- or three-wheeled motor vehicle in traffic accident ▽

✓4ᵗʰ **V53** Occupant of pick-up truck or van injured in collision with car, pick-up truck or van

√x7ᵗʰ **V53.0** Driver of pick-up truck or van injured in collision with car, pick-up truck or van in nontraffic accident

√x7ᵗʰ **V53.1** Passenger in pick-up truck or van injured in collision with car, pick-up truck or van in nontraffic accident

√x7ᵗʰ **V53.2** Person on outside of pick-up truck or van injured in collision with car, pick-up truck or van in nontraffic accident

√x7ᵗʰ **V53.3** Unspecified occupant of pick-up truck or van injured in collision with car, pick-up truck or van in nontraffic accident ▽

√x7ᵗʰ **V53.4** Person boarding or alighting a pick-up truck or van injured in collision with car, pick-up truck or van

√x7ᵗʰ **V53.5** Driver of pick-up truck or van injured in collision with car, pick-up truck or van in traffic accident

√x7ᵗʰ **V53.6** Passenger in pick-up truck or van injured in collision with car, pick-up truck or van in traffic accident

√x7ᵗʰ **V53.7** Person on outside of pick-up truck or van injured in collision with car, pick-up truck or van in traffic accident

√x7ᵗʰ **V53.9** Unspecified occupant of pick-up truck or van injured in collision with car, pick-up truck or van in traffic accident ▽

✓4ᵗʰ **V54** Occupant of pick-up truck or van injured in collision with heavy transport vehicle or bus

     EXCLUDES 1 occupant of pick-up truck or van injured in collision with military vehicle (V59.81)

√x7ᵗʰ **V54.0** Driver of pick-up truck or van injured in collision with heavy transport vehicle or bus in nontraffic accident

√x7ᵗʰ **V54.1** Passenger in pick-up truck or van injured in collision with heavy transport vehicle or bus in nontraffic accident

√x7ᵗʰ **V54.2** Person on outside of pick-up truck or van injured in collision with heavy transport vehicle or bus in nontraffic accident

√x7ᵗʰ **V54.3** Unspecified occupant of pick-up truck or van injured in collision with heavy transport vehicle or bus in nontraffic accident ▽

√x7ᵗʰ **V54.4** Person boarding or alighting a pick-up truck or van injured in collision with heavy transport vehicle or bus

√x7ᵗʰ **V54.5** Driver of pick-up truck or van injured in collision with heavy transport vehicle or bus in traffic accident

√x7ᵗʰ **V54.6** Passenger in pick-up truck or van injured in collision with heavy transport vehicle or bus in traffic accident

√x7ᵗʰ **V54.7** Person on outside of pick-up truck or van injured in collision with heavy transport vehicle or bus in traffic accident

√x7ᵗʰ **V54.9** Unspecified occupant of pick-up truck or van injured in collision with heavy transport vehicle or bus in traffic accident ▽

✓4ᵗʰ **V55** Occupant of pick-up truck or van injured in collision with railway train or railway vehicle

√x7ᵗʰ **V55.0** Driver of pick-up truck or van injured in collision with railway train or railway vehicle in nontraffic accident

√x7ᵗʰ **V55.1** Passenger in pick-up truck or van injured in collision with railway train or railway vehicle in nontraffic accident

√x7ᵗʰ **V55.2** Person on outside of pick-up truck or van injured in collision with railway train or railway vehicle in nontraffic accident

√x7ᵗʰ **V55.3** Unspecified occupant of pick-up truck or van injured in collision with railway train or railway vehicle in nontraffic accident ▽

√x7ᵗʰ **V55.4** Person boarding or alighting a pick-up truck or van injured in collision with railway train or railway vehicle

√x7ᵗʰ **V55.5** Driver of pick-up truck or van injured in collision with railway train or railway vehicle in traffic accident

√x7ᵗʰ **V55.6** Passenger in pick-up truck or van injured in collision with railway train or railway vehicle in traffic accident

√x7ᵗʰ **V55.7** Person on outside of pick-up truck or van injured in collision with railway train or railway vehicle in traffic accident

√x7ᵗʰ **V55.9** Unspecified occupant of pick-up truck or van injured in collision with railway train or railway vehicle in traffic accident ▽

✓4ᵗʰ **V56** Occupant of pick-up truck or van injured in collision with other nonmotor vehicle

     INCLUDES collision with animal-drawn vehicle, animal being ridden, streetcar

√x7ᵗʰ **V56.0** Driver of pick-up truck or van injured in collision with other nonmotor vehicle in nontraffic accident

√x7ᵗʰ **V56.1** Passenger in pick-up truck or van injured in collision with other nonmotor vehicle in nontraffic accident

√x7ᵗʰ **V56.2** Person on outside of pick-up truck or van injured in collision with other nonmotor vehicle in nontraffic accident

√x7ᵗʰ **V56.3** Unspecified occupant of pick-up truck or van injured in collision with other nonmotor vehicle in nontraffic accident ▽

√x7ᵗʰ **V56.4** Person boarding or alighting a pick-up truck or van injured in collision with other nonmotor vehicle

√x7ᵗʰ **V56.5** Driver of pick-up truck or van injured in collision with other nonmotor vehicle in traffic accident

√x7ᵗʰ **V56.6** Passenger in pick-up truck or van injured in collision with other nonmotor vehicle in traffic accident

√x7ᵗʰ **V56.7** Person on outside of pick-up truck or van injured in collision with other nonmotor vehicle in traffic accident

√x7ᵗʰ **V56.9** Unspecified occupant of pick-up truck or van injured in collision with other nonmotor vehicle in traffic accident ▽

✓4ᵗʰ **V57** Occupant of pick-up truck or van injured in collision with fixed or stationary object

√x7ᵗʰ **V57.0** Driver of pick-up truck or van injured in collision with fixed or stationary object in nontraffic accident

√x7ᵗʰ **V57.1** Passenger in pick-up truck or van injured in collision with fixed or stationary object in nontraffic accident

√x7ᵗʰ **V57.2** Person on outside of pick-up truck or van injured in collision with fixed or stationary object in nontraffic accident

√x7ᵗʰ **V57.3** Unspecified occupant of pick-up truck or van injured in collision with fixed or stationary object in nontraffic accident ▽

√x7ᵗʰ **V57.4** Person boarding or alighting a pick-up truck or van injured in collision with fixed or stationary object

√x7ᵗʰ **V57.5** Driver of pick-up truck or van injured in collision with fixed or stationary object in traffic accident

√x7ᵗʰ **V57.6** Passenger in pick-up truck or van injured in collision with fixed or stationary object in traffic accident

√x7ᵗʰ **V57.7** Person on outside of pick-up truck or van injured in collision with fixed or stationary object in traffic accident

√x7ᵗʰ **V57.9** Unspecified occupant of pick-up truck or van injured in collision with fixed or stationary object in traffic accident ▽

✓4ᵗʰ **V58** Occupant of pick-up truck or van injured in noncollision transport accident

     INCLUDES overturning pick-up truck or van NOS
            overturning pick-up truck or van without collision

√x7ᵗʰ **V58.0** Driver of pick-up truck or van injured in noncollision transport accident in nontraffic accident

√x7ᵗʰ **V58.1** Passenger in pick-up truck or van injured in noncollision transport accident in nontraffic accident

√x7ᵗʰ **V58.2** Person on outside of pick-up truck or van injured in noncollision transport accident in nontraffic accident

√x7ᵗʰ **V58.3** Unspecified occupant of pick-up truck or van injured in noncollision transport accident in nontraffic accident ▽

√x7ᵗʰ **V58.4** Person boarding or alighting a pick-up truck or van injured in noncollision transport accident

√x7ᵗʰ **V58.5** Driver of pick-up truck or van injured in noncollision transport accident in traffic accident

√x7ᵗʰ **V58.6** Passenger in pick-up truck or van injured in noncollision transport accident in traffic accident

√x7ᵗʰ **V58.7** Person on outside of pick-up truck or van injured in noncollision transport accident in traffic accident

√x7ᵗʰ **V58.9** Unspecified occupant of pick-up truck or van injured in noncollision transport accident in traffic accident ▽

✓4ᵗʰ **V59** Occupant of pick-up truck or van injured in other and unspecified transport accidents

✓5ᵗʰ **V59.0** Driver of pick-up truck or van injured in collision with other and unspecified motor vehicles in nontraffic accident

√x7ᵗʰ **V59.00** Driver of pick-up truck or van injured in collision with unspecified motor vehicles in nontraffic accident ▽

√x7ᵗʰ **V59.09** Driver of pick-up truck or van injured in collision with other motor vehicles in nontraffic accident

---

✓ Additional Character Required   √x7ᵗʰ Placeholder Alert   Manifestation Dx   ▽ Unspecified Dx   ▶◀ Revised Text   ● New Code   ▲ Revised Code Title

☑5ᵗʰ V59.1 Passenger in pick-up truck or van injured in collision with other and unspecified motor vehicles in nontraffic accident

☑x7ᵗʰ V59.10 Passenger in pick-up truck or van injured in collision with unspecified motor vehicles in nontraffic accident ▽

☑x7ᵗʰ V59.19 Passenger in pick-up truck or van injured in collision with other motor vehicles in nontraffic accident

☑5ᵗʰ V59.2 Unspecified occupant of pick-up truck or van injured in collision with other and unspecified motor vehicles in nontraffic accident

☑x7ᵗʰ V59.20 Unspecified occupant of pick-up truck or van injured in collision with unspecified motor vehicles in nontraffic accident ▽

Collision NOS involving pick-up truck or van, nontraffic

☑x7ᵗʰ V59.29 Unspecified occupant of pick-up truck or van injured in collision with other motor vehicles in nontraffic accident ▽

☑x7ᵗʰ V59.3 Occupant (driver) (passenger) of pick-up truck or van injured in unspecified nontraffic accident ▽

Accident NOS involving pick-up truck or van, nontraffic
Occupant of pick-up truck or van injured in nontraffic accident NOS

☑5ᵗʰ V59.4 Driver of pick-up truck or van injured in collision with other and unspecified motor vehicles in traffic accident

☑x7ᵗʰ V59.40 Driver of pick-up truck or van injured in collision with unspecified motor vehicles in traffic accident ▽

☑x7ᵗʰ V59.49 Driver of pick-up truck or van injured in collision with other motor vehicles in traffic accident

☑5ᵗʰ V59.5 Passenger in pick-up truck or van injured in collision with other and unspecified motor vehicles in traffic accident

☑x7ᵗʰ V59.50 Passenger in pick-up truck or van injured in collision with unspecified motor vehicles in traffic accident ▽

☑x7ᵗʰ V59.59 Passenger in pick-up truck or van injured in collision with other motor vehicles in traffic accident

☑5ᵗʰ V59.6 Unspecified occupant of pick-up truck or van injured in collision with other and unspecified motor vehicles in traffic accident

☑x7ᵗʰ V59.60 Unspecified occupant of pick-up truck or van injured in collision with unspecified motor vehicles in traffic accident ▽

Collision NOS involving pick-up truck or van (traffic)

☑x7ᵗʰ V59.69 Unspecified occupant of pick-up truck or van injured in collision with other motor vehicles in traffic accident ▽

☑5ᵗʰ V59.8 Occupant (driver) (passenger) of pick-up truck or van injured in other specified transport accidents

☑x7ᵗʰ V59.81 Occupant (driver) (passenger) of pick-up truck or van injured in transport accident with military vehicle

☑x7ᵗʰ V59.88 Occupant (driver) (passenger) of pick-up truck or van injured in other specified transport accidents

☑x7ᵗʰ V59.9 Occupant (driver) (passenger) of pick-up truck or van injured in unspecified traffic accident ▽

Accident NOS involving pick-up truck or van

Occupant of heavy transport vehicle injured in transport accident (V60-V69)

INCLUDES 18 wheeler
armored car
panel truck
EXCLUDES 1 bus
motorcoach

The appropriate 7th character is to be added to each code from categories V60-V69.
A initial encounter
D subsequent encounter
S sequela

☑4ᵗʰ V60 Occupant of heavy transport vehicle injured in collision with pedestrian or animal

EXCLUDES 1 heavy transport vehicle collision with animal-drawn vehicle or animal being ridden (V66.-)

☑x7ᵗʰ V60.0 Driver of heavy transport vehicle injured in collision with pedestrian or animal in nontraffic accident

☑x7ᵗʰ V60.1 Passenger in heavy transport vehicle injured in collision with pedestrian or animal in nontraffic accident

☑x7ᵗʰ V60.2 Person on outside of heavy transport vehicle injured in collision with pedestrian or animal in nontraffic accident

☑x7ᵗʰ V60.3 Unspecified occupant of heavy transport vehicle injured in collision with pedestrian or animal in nontraffic accident ▽

☑x7ᵗʰ V60.4 Person boarding or alighting a heavy transport vehicle injured in collision with pedestrian or animal

☑x7ᵗʰ V60.5 Driver of heavy transport vehicle injured in collision with pedestrian or animal in traffic accident

☑x7ᵗʰ V60.6 Passenger in heavy transport vehicle injured in collision with pedestrian or animal in traffic accident

☑x7ᵗʰ V60.7 Person on outside of heavy transport vehicle injured in collision with pedestrian or animal in traffic accident

☑x7ᵗʰ V60.9 Unspecified occupant of heavy transport vehicle injured in collision with pedestrian or animal in traffic accident ▽

☑4ᵗʰ V61 Occupant of heavy transport vehicle injured in collision with pedal cycle

☑x7ᵗʰ V61.0 Driver of heavy transport vehicle injured in collision with pedal cycle in nontraffic accident

☑x7ᵗʰ V61.1 Passenger in heavy transport vehicle injured in collision with pedal cycle in nontraffic accident

☑x7ᵗʰ V61.2 Person on outside of heavy transport vehicle injured in collision with pedal cycle in nontraffic accident

☑x7ᵗʰ V61.3 Unspecified occupant of heavy transport vehicle injured in collision with pedal cycle in nontraffic accident ▽

☑x7ᵗʰ V61.4 Person boarding or alighting a heavy transport vehicle injured in collision with pedal cycle while boarding or alighting

☑x7ᵗʰ V61.5 Driver of heavy transport vehicle injured in collision with pedal cycle in traffic accident

☑x7ᵗʰ V61.6 Passenger in heavy transport vehicle injured in collision with pedal cycle in traffic accident

☑x7ᵗʰ V61.7 Person on outside of heavy transport vehicle injured in collision with pedal cycle in traffic accident

☑x7ᵗʰ V61.9 Unspecified occupant of heavy transport vehicle injured in collision with pedal cycle in traffic accident ▽

☑4ᵗʰ V62 Occupant of heavy transport vehicle injured in collision with two- or three-wheeled motor vehicle

☑x7ᵗʰ V62.0 Driver of heavy transport vehicle injured in collision with two- or three-wheeled motor vehicle in nontraffic accident

☑x7ᵗʰ V62.1 Passenger in heavy transport vehicle injured in collision with two- or three-wheeled motor vehicle in nontraffic accident

☑x7ᵗʰ V62.2 Person on outside of heavy transport vehicle injured in collision with two- or three-wheeled motor vehicle in nontraffic accident

☑x7ᵗʰ V62.3 Unspecified occupant of heavy transport vehicle injured in collision with two- or three-wheeled motor vehicle in nontraffic accident ▽

☑x7ᵗʰ V62.4 Person boarding or alighting a heavy transport vehicle injured in collision with two- or three-wheeled motor vehicle

☑x7ᵗʰ V62.5 Driver of heavy transport vehicle injured in collision with two- or three-wheeled motor vehicle in traffic accident

☑x7ᵗʰ V62.6 Passenger in heavy transport vehicle injured in collision with two- or three-wheeled motor vehicle in traffic accident

☑x7ᵗʰ V62.7 Person on outside of heavy transport vehicle injured in collision with two- or three-wheeled motor vehicle in traffic accident

☑x7ᵗʰ V62.9 Unspecified occupant of heavy transport vehicle injured in collision with two- or three-wheeled motor vehicle in traffic accident ▽

☑4ᵗʰ V63 Occupant of heavy transport vehicle injured in collision with car, pick-up truck or van

☑x7ᵗʰ V63.0 Driver of heavy transport vehicle injured in collision with car, pick-up truck or van in nontraffic accident

☑x7ᵗʰ V63.1 Passenger in heavy transport vehicle injured in collision with car, pick-up truck or van in nontraffic accident

☑x7ᵗʰ V63.2 Person on outside of heavy transport vehicle injured in collision with car, pick-up truck or van in nontraffic accident

☑x7ᵗʰ V63.3 Unspecified occupant of heavy transport vehicle injured in collision with car, pick-up truck or van in nontraffic accident ▽

☑x7ᵗʰ V63.4 Person boarding or alighting a heavy transport vehicle injured in collision with car, pick-up truck or van

☑x7ᵗʰ V63.5 Driver of heavy transport vehicle injured in collision with car, pick-up truck or van in traffic accident

☑x7ᵗʰ V63.6 Passenger in heavy transport vehicle injured in collision with car, pick-up truck or van in traffic accident

☑x7ᵗʰ V63.7 Person on outside of heavy transport vehicle injured in collision with car, pick-up truck or van in traffic accident

☑x7ᵗʰ V63.9 Unspecified occupant of heavy transport vehicle injured in collision with car, pick-up truck or van in traffic accident ▽

EXCLUDES 1 Not coded here EXCLUDES 2 Not included here N Newborn Age : 0 P Pediatric Age : 0-17 M Maternity Age : 12-55 A Adult Age : 15-124

1096

ICD-10-CM 2017

√4ᵗʰ **V64** **Occupant of heavy transport vehicle injured in collision with heavy transport vehicle or bus**
> **EXCLUDES 1** *occupant of heavy transport vehicle injured in collision with military vehicle (V69.81)*

√x7ᵗʰ **V64.0** Driver of heavy transport vehicle injured in collision with heavy transport vehicle or bus in nontraffic accident

√x7ᵗʰ **V64.1** Passenger in heavy transport vehicle injured in collision with heavy transport vehicle or bus in nontraffic accident

√x7ᵗʰ **V64.2** Person on outside of heavy transport vehicle injured in collision with heavy transport vehicle or bus in nontraffic accident

√x7ᵗʰ **V64.3** Unspecified occupant of heavy transport vehicle injured in collision with heavy transport vehicle or bus in nontraffic accident ▽

√x7ᵗʰ **V64.4** Person boarding or alighting a heavy transport vehicle injured in collision with heavy transport vehicle or bus while boarding or alighting

√x7ᵗʰ **V64.5** Driver of heavy transport vehicle injured in collision with heavy transport vehicle or bus in traffic accident

√x7ᵗʰ **V64.6** Passenger in heavy transport vehicle injured in collision with heavy transport vehicle or bus in traffic accident

√x7ᵗʰ **V64.7** Person on outside of heavy transport vehicle injured in collision with heavy transport vehicle or bus in traffic accident

√x7ᵗʰ **V64.9** Unspecified occupant of heavy transport vehicle injured in collision with heavy transport vehicle or bus in traffic accident ▽

√4ᵗʰ **V65** **Occupant of heavy transport vehicle injured in collision with railway train or railway vehicle**

√x7ᵗʰ **V65.0** Driver of heavy transport vehicle injured in collision with railway train or railway vehicle in nontraffic accident

√x7ᵗʰ **V65.1** Passenger in heavy transport vehicle injured in collision with railway train or railway vehicle in nontraffic accident

√x7ᵗʰ **V65.2** Person on outside of heavy transport vehicle injured in collision with railway train or railway vehicle in nontraffic accident

√x7ᵗʰ **V65.3** Unspecified occupant of heavy transport vehicle injured in collision with railway train or railway vehicle in nontraffic accident ▽

√x7ᵗʰ **V65.4** Person boarding or alighting a heavy transport vehicle injured in collision with railway train or railway vehicle

√x7ᵗʰ **V65.5** Driver of heavy transport vehicle injured in collision with railway train or railway vehicle in traffic accident

√x7ᵗʰ **V65.6** Passenger in heavy transport vehicle injured in collision with railway train or railway vehicle in traffic accident

√x7ᵗʰ **V65.7** Person on outside of heavy transport vehicle injured in collision with railway train or railway vehicle in traffic accident

√x7ᵗʰ **V65.9** Unspecified occupant of heavy transport vehicle injured in collision with railway train or railway vehicle in traffic accident ▽

√4ᵗʰ **V66** **Occupant of heavy transport vehicle injured in collision with other nonmotor vehicle**
> **INCLUDES** collision with animal-drawn vehicle, animal being ridden, streetcar

√x7ᵗʰ **V66.0** Driver of heavy transport vehicle injured in collision with other nonmotor vehicle in nontraffic accident

√x7ᵗʰ **V66.1** Passenger in heavy transport vehicle injured in collision with other nonmotor vehicle in nontraffic accident

√x7ᵗʰ **V66.2** Person on outside of heavy transport vehicle injured in collision with other nonmotor vehicle in nontraffic accident

√x7ᵗʰ **V66.3** Unspecified occupant of heavy transport vehicle injured in collision with other nonmotor vehicle in nontraffic accident ▽

√x7ᵗʰ **V66.4** Person boarding or alighting a heavy transport vehicle injured in collision with other nonmotor vehicle

√x7ᵗʰ **V66.5** Driver of heavy transport vehicle injured in collision with other nonmotor vehicle in traffic accident

√x7ᵗʰ **V66.6** Passenger in heavy transport vehicle injured in collision with other nonmotor vehicle in traffic accident

√x7ᵗʰ **V66.7** Person on outside of heavy transport vehicle injured in collision with other nonmotor vehicle in traffic accident

√x7ᵗʰ **V66.9** Unspecified occupant of heavy transport vehicle injured in collision with other nonmotor vehicle in traffic accident ▽

√4ᵗʰ **V67** **Occupant of heavy transport vehicle injured in collision with fixed or stationary object**

√x7ᵗʰ **V67.0** Driver of heavy transport vehicle injured in collision with fixed or stationary object in nontraffic accident

√x7ᵗʰ **V67.1** Passenger in heavy transport vehicle injured in collision with fixed or stationary object in nontraffic accident

√x7ᵗʰ **V67.2** Person on outside of heavy transport vehicle injured in collision with fixed or stationary object in nontraffic accident

√x7ᵗʰ **V67.3** Unspecified occupant of heavy transport vehicle injured in collision with fixed or stationary object in nontraffic accident ▽

√x7ᵗʰ **V67.4** Person boarding or alighting a heavy transport vehicle injured in collision with fixed or stationary object

√x7ᵗʰ **V67.5** Driver of heavy transport vehicle injured in collision with fixed or stationary object in traffic accident

√x7ᵗʰ **V67.6** Passenger in heavy transport vehicle injured in collision with fixed or stationary object in traffic accident

√x7ᵗʰ **V67.7** Person on outside of heavy transport vehicle injured in collision with fixed or stationary object in traffic accident

√x7ᵗʰ **V67.9** Unspecified occupant of heavy transport vehicle injured in collision with fixed or stationary object in traffic accident ▽

√4ᵗʰ **V68** **Occupant of heavy transport vehicle injured in noncollision transport accident**
> **INCLUDES** overturning heavy transport vehicle NOS
> overturning heavy transport vehicle without collision

√x7ᵗʰ **V68.0** Driver of heavy transport vehicle injured in noncollision transport accident in nontraffic accident

√x7ᵗʰ **V68.1** Passenger in heavy transport vehicle injured in noncollision transport accident in nontraffic accident

√x7ᵗʰ **V68.2** Person on outside of heavy transport vehicle injured in noncollision transport accident in nontraffic accident

√x7ᵗʰ **V68.3** Unspecified occupant of heavy transport vehicle injured in noncollision transport accident in nontraffic accident ▽

√x7ᵗʰ **V68.4** Person boarding or alighting a heavy transport vehicle injured in noncollision transport accident

√x7ᵗʰ **V68.5** Driver of heavy transport vehicle injured in noncollision transport accident in traffic accident

√x7ᵗʰ **V68.6** Passenger in heavy transport vehicle injured in noncollision transport accident in traffic accident

√x7ᵗʰ **V68.7** Person on outside of heavy transport vehicle injured in noncollision transport accident in traffic accident

√x7ᵗʰ **V68.9** Unspecified occupant of heavy transport vehicle injured in noncollision transport accident in traffic accident ▽

√4ᵗʰ **V69** **Occupant of heavy transport vehicle injured in other and unspecified transport accidents**

√5ᵗʰ **V69.0** Driver of heavy transport vehicle injured in collision with other and unspecified motor vehicles in nontraffic accident

√x7ᵗʰ **V69.00** Driver of heavy transport vehicle injured in collision with unspecified motor vehicles in nontraffic accident ▽

√x7ᵗʰ **V69.09** Driver of heavy transport vehicle injured in collision with other motor vehicles in nontraffic accident

√5ᵗʰ **V69.1** Passenger in heavy transport vehicle injured in collision with other and unspecified motor vehicles in nontraffic accident

√x7ᵗʰ **V69.10** Passenger in heavy transport vehicle injured in collision with unspecified motor vehicles in nontraffic accident ▽

√x7ᵗʰ **V69.19** Passenger in heavy transport vehicle injured in collision with other motor vehicles in nontraffic accident

√5ᵗʰ **V69.2** Unspecified occupant of heavy transport vehicle injured in collision with other and unspecified motor vehicles in nontraffic accident

√x7ᵗʰ **V69.20** Unspecified occupant of heavy transport vehicle injured in collision with unspecified motor vehicles in nontraffic accident ▽
> Collision NOS involving heavy transport vehicle, nontraffic

√x7ᵗʰ **V69.29** Unspecified occupant of heavy transport vehicle injured in collision with other motor vehicles in nontraffic accident ▽

√x7ᵗʰ **V69.3** Occupant (driver) (passenger) of heavy transport vehicle injured in unspecified nontraffic accident ▽
> Accident NOS involving heavy transport vehicle, nontraffic
> Occupant of heavy transport vehicle injured in nontraffic accident NOS

√5ᵗʰ **V69.4** Driver of heavy transport vehicle injured in collision with other and unspecified motor vehicles in traffic accident

√x7ᵗʰ **V69.40** Driver of heavy transport vehicle injured in collision with unspecified motor vehicles in traffic accident ▽

√x7ᵗʰ **V69.49** Driver of heavy transport vehicle injured in collision with other motor vehicles in traffic accident

---

✓ Additional Character Required   √x7ᵗʰ Placeholder Alert   Manifestation Dx   ▽ Unspecified Dx   ►◄ Revised Text   ● New Code   ▲ Revised Code Title

☑5ᵗʰ **V69.5** **Passenger in heavy transport vehicle injured in collision with other and unspecified motor vehicles in traffic accident**

    ✓x7ᵗʰ **V69.50** **Passenger in heavy transport vehicle injured in collision with unspecified motor vehicles in traffic accident** ▽

    ✓x7ᵗʰ **V69.59** **Passenger in heavy transport vehicle injured in collision with other motor vehicles in traffic accident**

☑5ᵗʰ **V69.6** **Unspecified occupant of heavy transport vehicle injured in collision with other and unspecified motor vehicles in traffic accident**

    ✓x7ᵗʰ **V69.60** **Unspecified occupant of heavy transport vehicle injured in collision with unspecified motor vehicles in traffic accident** ▽

        Collision NOS involving heavy transport vehicle (traffic)

    ✓x7ᵗʰ **V69.69** **Unspecified occupant of heavy transport vehicle injured in collision with other motor vehicles in traffic accident** ▽

☑5ᵗʰ **V69.8** **Occupant (driver) (passenger) of heavy transport vehicle injured in other specified transport accidents**

    ✓x7ᵗʰ **V69.81** **Occupant (driver) (passenger) of heavy transport vehicle injured in transport accidents with military vehicle**

    ✓x7ᵗʰ **V69.88** **Occupant (driver) (passenger) of heavy transport vehicle injured in other specified transport accidents**

✓x7ᵗʰ **V69.9** **Occupant (driver) (passenger) of heavy transport vehicle injured in unspecified traffic accident** ▽

        Accident NOS involving heavy transport vehicle

Bus occupant injured in transport accident (V70-V79)

INCLUDES motorcoach
EXCLUDES 1 minibus (V50-V59)

The appropriate 7th character is to be added to each code from categories V70-V79.
A   initial encounter
D   subsequent encounter
S   sequela

☑4ᵗʰ **V70** **Bus occupant injured in collision with pedestrian or animal**

    EXCLUDES 1 bus collision with animal-drawn vehicle or animal being ridden (V76.-)

    ✓x7ᵗʰ **V70.0** **Driver of bus injured in collision with pedestrian or animal in nontraffic accident**

    ✓x7ᵗʰ **V70.1** **Passenger on bus injured in collision with pedestrian or animal in nontraffic accident**

    ✓x7ᵗʰ **V70.2** **Person on outside of bus injured in collision with pedestrian or animal in nontraffic accident**

    ✓x7ᵗʰ **V70.3** **Unspecified occupant of bus injured in collision with pedestrian or animal in nontraffic accident** ▽

    ✓x7ᵗʰ **V70.4** **Person boarding or alighting from bus injured in collision with pedestrian or animal**

    ✓x7ᵗʰ **V70.5** **Driver of bus injured in collision with pedestrian or animal in traffic accident**

    ✓x7ᵗʰ **V70.6** **Passenger on bus injured in collision with pedestrian or animal in traffic accident**

    ✓x7ᵗʰ **V70.7** **Person on outside of bus injured in collision with pedestrian or animal in traffic accident**

    ✓x7ᵗʰ **V70.9** **Unspecified occupant of bus injured in collision with pedestrian or animal in traffic accident** ▽

☑4ᵗʰ **V71** **Bus occupant injured in collision with pedal cycle**

    ✓x7ᵗʰ **V71.0** **Driver of bus injured in collision with pedal cycle in nontraffic accident**

    ✓x7ᵗʰ **V71.1** **Passenger on bus injured in collision with pedal cycle in nontraffic accident**

    ✓x7ᵗʰ **V71.2** **Person on outside of bus injured in collision with pedal cycle in nontraffic accident**

    ✓x7ᵗʰ **V71.3** **Unspecified occupant of bus injured in collision with pedal cycle in nontraffic accident** ▽

    ✓x7ᵗʰ **V71.4** **Person boarding or alighting from bus injured in collision with pedal cycle**

    ✓x7ᵗʰ **V71.5** **Driver of bus injured in collision with pedal cycle in traffic accident**

    ✓x7ᵗʰ **V71.6** **Passenger on bus injured in collision with pedal cycle in traffic accident**

    ✓x7ᵗʰ **V71.7** **Person on outside of bus injured in collision with pedal cycle in traffic accident**

    ✓x7ᵗʰ **V71.9** **Unspecified occupant of bus injured in collision with pedal cycle in traffic accident** ▽

☑4ᵗʰ **V72** **Bus occupant injured in collision with two- or three-wheeled motor vehicle**

    ✓x7ᵗʰ **V72.0** **Driver of bus injured in collision with two- or three-wheeled motor vehicle in nontraffic accident**

    ✓x7ᵗʰ **V72.1** **Passenger on bus injured in collision with two- or three-wheeled motor vehicle in nontraffic accident**

    ✓x7ᵗʰ **V72.2** **Person on outside of bus injured in collision with two- or three-wheeled motor vehicle in nontraffic accident**

    ✓x7ᵗʰ **V72.3** **Unspecified occupant of bus injured in collision with two- or three-wheeled motor vehicle in nontraffic accident** ▽

    ✓x7ᵗʰ **V72.4** **Person boarding or alighting from bus injured in collision with two- or three-wheeled motor vehicle**

    ✓x7ᵗʰ **V72.5** **Driver of bus injured in collision with two- or three-wheeled motor vehicle in traffic accident**

    ✓x7ᵗʰ **V72.6** **Passenger on bus injured in collision with two- or three-wheeled motor vehicle in traffic accident**

    ✓x7ᵗʰ **V72.7** **Person on outside of bus injured in collision with two- or three-wheeled motor vehicle in traffic accident**

    ✓x7ᵗʰ **V72.9** **Unspecified occupant of bus injured in collision with two- or three-wheeled motor vehicle in traffic accident** ▽

☑4ᵗʰ **V73** **Bus occupant injured in collision with car, pick-up truck or van**

    ✓x7ᵗʰ **V73.0** **Driver of bus injured in collision with car, pick-up truck or van in nontraffic accident**

    ✓x7ᵗʰ **V73.1** **Passenger on bus injured in collision with car, pick-up truck or van in nontraffic accident**

    ✓x7ᵗʰ **V73.2** **Person on outside of bus injured in collision with car, pick-up truck or van in nontraffic accident**

    ✓x7ᵗʰ **V73.3** **Unspecified occupant of bus injured in collision with car, pick-up truck or van in nontraffic accident** ▽

    ✓x7ᵗʰ **V73.4** **Person boarding or alighting from bus injured in collision with car, pick-up truck or van**

    ✓x7ᵗʰ **V73.5** **Driver of bus injured in collision with car, pick-up truck or van in traffic accident**

    ✓x7ᵗʰ **V73.6** **Passenger on bus injured in collision with car, pick-up truck or van in traffic accident**

    ✓x7ᵗʰ **V73.7** **Person on outside of bus injured in collision with car, pick-up truck or van in traffic accident**

    ✓x7ᵗʰ **V73.9** **Unspecified occupant of bus injured in collision with car, pick-up truck or van in traffic accident** ▽

☑4ᵗʰ **V74** **Bus occupant injured in collision with heavy transport vehicle or bus**

    EXCLUDES 1 bus occupant injured in collision with military vehicle (V79.81)

    ✓x7ᵗʰ **V74.0** **Driver of bus injured in collision with heavy transport vehicle or bus in nontraffic accident**

    ✓x7ᵗʰ **V74.1** **Passenger on bus injured in collision with heavy transport vehicle or bus in nontraffic accident**

    ✓x7ᵗʰ **V74.2** **Person on outside of bus injured in collision with heavy transport vehicle or bus in nontraffic accident**

    ✓x7ᵗʰ **V74.3** **Unspecified occupant of bus injured in collision with heavy transport vehicle or bus in nontraffic accident** ▽

    ✓x7ᵗʰ **V74.4** **Person boarding or alighting from bus injured in collision with heavy transport vehicle or bus**

    ✓x7ᵗʰ **V74.5** **Driver of bus injured in collision with heavy transport vehicle or bus in traffic accident**

    ✓x7ᵗʰ **V74.6** **Passenger on bus injured in collision with heavy transport vehicle or bus in traffic accident**

    ✓x7ᵗʰ **V74.7** **Person on outside of bus injured in collision with heavy transport vehicle or bus in traffic accident**

    ✓x7ᵗʰ **V74.9** **Unspecified occupant of bus injured in collision with heavy transport vehicle or bus in traffic accident** ▽

☑4ᵗʰ **V75** **Bus occupant injured in collision with railway train or railway vehicle**

    ✓x7ᵗʰ **V75.0** **Driver of bus injured in collision with railway train or railway vehicle in nontraffic accident**

    ✓x7ᵗʰ **V75.1** **Passenger on bus injured in collision with railway train or railway vehicle in nontraffic accident**

    ✓x7ᵗʰ **V75.2** **Person on outside of bus injured in collision with railway train or railway vehicle in nontraffic accident**

    ✓x7ᵗʰ **V75.3** **Unspecified occupant of bus injured in collision with railway train or railway vehicle in nontraffic accident** ▽

    ✓x7ᵗʰ **V75.4** **Person boarding or alighting from bus injured in collision with railway train or railway vehicle**

    ✓x7ᵗʰ **V75.5** **Driver of bus injured in collision with railway train or railway vehicle in traffic accident**

    ✓x7ᵗʰ **V75.6** **Passenger on bus injured in collision with railway train or railway vehicle in traffic accident**

    ✓x7ᵗʰ **V75.7** **Person on outside of bus injured in collision with railway train or railway vehicle in traffic accident**

    ✓x7ᵗʰ **V75.9** **Unspecified occupant of bus injured in collision with railway train or railway vehicle in traffic accident** ▽

EXCLUDES 1 Not coded here   **EXCLUDES 2** Not included here   Ⓝ Newborn Age : 0   Ⓟ Pediatric Age : 0-17   Ⓜ Maternity Age : 12-55   Ⓐ Adult Age : 15-124

√4th **V76** **Bus occupant injured in collision with other nonmotor vehicle**

     INCLUDES collision with animal-drawn vehicle, animal being ridden, streetcar

√x7th **V76.0** Driver of bus injured in collision with other nonmotor vehicle in nontraffic accident

√x7th **V76.1** Passenger on bus injured in collision with other nonmotor vehicle in nontraffic accident

√x7th **V76.2** Person on outside of bus injured in collision with other nonmotor vehicle in nontraffic accident

√x7th **V76.3** Unspecified occupant of bus injured in collision with other nonmotor vehicle in nontraffic accident ▽

√x7th **V76.4** Person boarding or alighting from bus injured in collision with other nonmotor vehicle

√x7th **V76.5** Driver of bus injured in collision with other nonmotor vehicle in traffic accident

√x7th **V76.6** Passenger on bus injured in collision with other nonmotor vehicle in traffic accident

√x7th **V76.7** Person on outside of bus injured in collision with other nonmotor vehicle in traffic accident

√x7th **V76.9** Unspecified occupant of bus injured in collision with other nonmotor vehicle in traffic accident ▽

√4th **V77** **Bus occupant injured in collision with fixed or stationary object**

√x7th **V77.0** Driver of bus injured in collision with fixed or stationary object in nontraffic accident

√x7th **V77.1** Passenger on bus injured in collision with fixed or stationary object in nontraffic accident

√x7th **V77.2** Person on outside of bus injured in collision with fixed or stationary object in nontraffic accident

√x7th **V77.3** Unspecified occupant of bus injured in collision with fixed or stationary object in nontraffic accident ▽

√x7th **V77.4** Person boarding or alighting from bus injured in collision with fixed or stationary object

√x7th **V77.5** Driver of bus injured in collision with fixed or stationary object in traffic accident

√x7th **V77.6** Passenger on bus injured in collision with fixed or stationary object in traffic accident

√x7th **V77.7** Person on outside of bus injured in collision with fixed or stationary object in traffic accident

√x7th **V77.9** Unspecified occupant of bus injured in collision with fixed or stationary object in traffic accident ▽

√4th **V78** **Bus occupant injured in noncollision transport accident**

     INCLUDES overturning bus NOS
         overturning bus without collision

√x7th **V78.0** Driver of bus injured in noncollision transport accident in nontraffic accident

√x7th **V78.1** Passenger on bus injured in noncollision transport accident in nontraffic accident

√x7th **V78.2** Person on outside of bus injured in noncollision transport accident in nontraffic accident

√x7th **V78.3** Unspecified occupant of bus injured in noncollision transport accident in nontraffic accident ▽

√x7th **V78.4** Person boarding or alighting from bus injured in noncollision transport accident

√x7th **V78.5** Driver of bus injured in noncollision transport accident in traffic accident

√x7th **V78.6** Passenger on bus injured in noncollision transport accident in traffic accident

√x7th **V78.7** Person on outside of bus injured in noncollision transport accident in traffic accident

√x7th **V78.9** Unspecified occupant of bus injured in noncollision transport accident in traffic accident ▽

√4th **V79** **Bus occupant injured in other and unspecified transport accidents**

√5th **V79.0** Driver of bus injured in collision with other and unspecified motor vehicles in nontraffic accident

     √x7th **V79.00** Driver of bus injured in collision with unspecified motor vehicles in nontraffic accident ▽

     √x7th **V79.09** Driver of bus injured in collision with other motor vehicles in nontraffic accident

√5th **V79.1** Passenger on bus injured in collision with other and unspecified motor vehicles in nontraffic accident

     √x7th **V79.10** Passenger on bus injured in collision with unspecified motor vehicles in nontraffic accident ▽

     √x7th **V79.19** Passenger on bus injured in collision with other motor vehicles in nontraffic accident

√5th **V79.2** Unspecified bus occupant injured in collision with other and unspecified motor vehicles in nontraffic accident

√x7th **V79.20** Unspecified bus occupant injured in collision with unspecified motor vehicles in nontraffic accident ▽

     Bus collision NOS, nontraffic

√x7th **V79.29** Unspecified bus occupant injured in collision with other motor vehicles in nontraffic accident ▽

√x7th **V79.3** Bus occupant (driver) (passenger) injured in unspecified nontraffic accident

     Bus accident NOS, nontraffic
     Bus occupant injured in nontraffic accident NOS

√5th **V79.4** Driver of bus injured in collision with other and unspecified motor vehicles in traffic accident

     √x7th **V79.40** Driver of bus injured in collision with unspecified motor vehicles in traffic accident ▽

     √x7th **V79.49** Driver of bus injured in collision with other motor vehicles in traffic accident

√5th **V79.5** Passenger on bus injured in collision with other and unspecified motor vehicles in traffic accident

     √x7th **V79.50** Passenger on bus injured in collision with unspecified motor vehicles in traffic accident ▽

     √x7th **V79.59** Passenger on bus injured in collision with other motor vehicles in traffic accident

√5th **V79.6** Unspecified bus occupant injured in collision with other and unspecified motor vehicles in traffic accident

     √x7th **V79.60** Unspecified bus occupant injured in collision with unspecified motor vehicles in traffic accident ▽

         Bus collision NOS (traffic)

     √x7th **V79.69** Unspecified bus occupant injured in collision with other motor vehicles in traffic accident ▽

√5th **V79.8** Bus occupant (driver) (passenger) injured in other specified transport accidents

     √x7th **V79.81** Bus occupant (driver) (passenger) injured in transport accidents with military vehicle

     √x7th **V79.88** Bus occupant (driver) (passenger) injured in other specified transport accidents

√x7th **V79.9** Bus occupant (driver) (passenger) injured in unspecified traffic accident ▽

     Bus accident NOS

Other land transport accidents (V80-V89)

The appropriate 7th character is to be added to each code from categories V80-V89.
A   initial encounter
D   subsequent encounter
S   sequela

√4th **V80** **Animal-rider or occupant of animal-drawn vehicle injured in transport accident**

√5th **V80.0** Animal-rider or occupant of animal drawn vehicle injured by fall from or being thrown from animal or animal-drawn vehicle in noncollision accident

     √6th **V80.01** Animal-rider injured by fall from or being thrown from animal in noncollision accident

         √7th **V80.010** Animal-rider injured by fall from or being thrown from horse in noncollision accident

         √7th **V80.018** Animal-rider injured by fall from or being thrown from other animal in noncollision accident

     √x7th **V80.02** Occupant of animal-drawn vehicle injured by fall from or being thrown from animal-drawn vehicle in noncollision accident

         Overturning animal-drawn vehicle NOS
         Overturning animal-drawn vehicle without collision

√5th **V80.1** Animal-rider or occupant of animal-drawn vehicle injured in collision with pedestrian or animal

     EXCLUDES 1 animal-rider or animal-drawn vehicle collision with animal-drawn vehicle or animal being ridden (V80.7)

     √x7th **V80.11** Animal-rider injured in collision with pedestrian or animal

     √x7th **V80.12** Occupant of animal-drawn vehicle injured in collision with pedestrian or animal

√5th **V80.2** Animal-rider or occupant of animal-drawn vehicle injured in collision with pedal cycle

     √x7th **V80.21** Animal-rider injured in collision with pedal cycle

     √x7th **V80.22** Occupant of animal-drawn vehicle injured in collision with pedal cycle

✔ Additional Character Required   √x7th Placeholder Alert   Manifestation Dx   ▽ Unspecified Dx   ▶◀ Revised Text   ● New Code   ▲ Revised Code Title

ICD-10-CM 2017   1099

√5ᵗʰ **V80.3** Animal-rider or occupant of animal-drawn vehicle injured in collision with two- or three-wheeled motor vehicle

√x7ᵗʰ   **V80.31** Animal-rider injured in collision with two- or three-wheeled motor vehicle

√x7ᵗʰ   **V80.32** Occupant of animal-drawn vehicle injured in collision with two- or three-wheeled motor vehicle

√5ᵗʰ **V80.4** Animal-rider or occupant of animal-drawn vehicle injured in collision with car, pick-up truck, van, heavy transport vehicle or bus

EXCLUDES 1   *animal-rider injured in collision with military vehicle (V80.910)*

occupant of animal-drawn vehicle injured in collision with military vehicle (V80.920)

√x7ᵗʰ   **V80.41** Animal-rider injured in collision with car, pick-up truck, van, heavy transport vehicle or bus

√x7ᵗʰ   **V80.42** Occupant of animal-drawn vehicle injured in collision with car, pick-up truck, van, heavy transport vehicle or bus

√5ᵗʰ **V80.5** Animal-rider or occupant of animal-drawn vehicle injured in collision with other specified motor vehicle

√x7ᵗʰ   **V80.51** Animal-rider injured in collision with other specified motor vehicle

√x7ᵗʰ   **V80.52** Occupant of animal-drawn vehicle injured in collision with other specified motor vehicle

√5ᵗʰ **V80.6** Animal-rider or occupant of animal-drawn vehicle injured in collision with railway train or railway vehicle

√x7ᵗʰ   **V80.61** Animal-rider injured in collision with railway train or railway vehicle

√x7ᵗʰ   **V80.62** Occupant of animal-drawn vehicle injured in collision with railway train or railway vehicle

√5ᵗʰ **V80.7** Animal-rider or occupant of animal-drawn vehicle injured in collision with other nonmotor vehicles

√6ᵗʰ   **V80.71** Animal-rider or occupant of animal-drawn vehicle injured in collision with animal being ridden

√7ᵗʰ   **V80.710** Animal-rider injured in collision with other animal being ridden

√7ᵗʰ   **V80.711** Occupant of animal-drawn vehicle injured in collision with animal being ridden

√6ᵗʰ   **V80.72** Animal-rider or occupant of animal-drawn vehicle injured in collision with other animal-drawn vehicle

√7ᵗʰ   **V80.720** Animal-rider injured in collision with animal-drawn vehicle

√7ᵗʰ   **V80.721** Occupant of animal-drawn vehicle injured in collision with other animal-drawn vehicle

√6ᵗʰ   **V80.73** Animal-rider or occupant of animal-drawn vehicle injured in collision with streetcar

√7ᵗʰ   **V80.730** Animal-rider injured in collision with streetcar

√7ᵗʰ   **V80.731** Occupant of animal-drawn vehicle injured in collision with streetcar

√6ᵗʰ   **V80.79** Animal-rider or occupant of animal-drawn vehicle injured in collision with other nonmotor vehicles

√7ᵗʰ   **V80.790** Animal-rider injured in collision with other nonmotor vehicles

√7ᵗʰ   **V80.791** Occupant of animal-drawn vehicle injured in collision with other nonmotor vehicles

√5ᵗʰ **V80.8** Animal-rider or occupant of animal-drawn vehicle injured in collision with fixed or stationary object

√x7ᵗʰ   **V80.81** Animal-rider injured in collision with fixed or stationary object

√x7ᵗʰ   **V80.82** Occupant of animal-drawn vehicle injured in collision with fixed or stationary object

√5ᵗʰ **V80.9** Animal-rider or occupant of animal-drawn vehicle injured in other and unspecified transport accidents

√6ᵗʰ   **V80.91** Animal-rider injured in other and unspecified transport accidents

√7ᵗʰ   **V80.910** Animal-rider injured in transport accident with military vehicle

√7ᵗʰ   **V80.918** Animal-rider injured in other transport accident

√7ᵗʰ   **V80.919** Animal-rider injured in unspecified transport accident   ▽

Animal rider accident NOS

√6ᵗʰ   **V80.92** Occupant of animal-drawn vehicle injured in other and unspecified transport accidents

√7ᵗʰ   **V80.920** Occupant of animal-drawn vehicle injured in transport accident with military vehicle

√7ᵗʰ   **V80.928** Occupant of animal-drawn vehicle injured in other transport accident

√7ᵗʰ   **V80.929** Occupant of animal-drawn vehicle injured in unspecified transport accident   ▽

Animal-drawn vehicle accident NOS

√4ᵗʰ **V81** Occupant of railway train or railway vehicle injured in transport accident

INCLUDES   derailment of railway train or railway vehicle

person on outside of train

EXCLUDES 1   *streetcar (V82.-)*

√x7ᵗʰ **V81.0** Occupant of railway train or railway vehicle injured in collision with motor vehicle in nontraffic accident

EXCLUDES 1   *occupant of railway train or railway vehicle injured due to collision with military vehicle (V81.83)*

√x7ᵗʰ **V81.1** Occupant of railway train or railway vehicle injured in collision with motor vehicle in traffic accident

EXCLUDES 1   *occupant of railway train or railway vehicle injured due to collision with military vehicle (V81.83)*

√x7ᵗʰ **V81.2** Occupant of railway train or railway vehicle injured in collision with or hit by rolling stock

√x7ᵗʰ **V81.3** Occupant of railway train or railway vehicle injured in collision with other object

Railway collision NOS

√x7ᵗʰ **V81.4** Person injured while boarding or alighting from railway train or railway vehicle

√x7ᵗʰ **V81.5** Occupant of railway train or railway vehicle injured by fall in railway train or railway vehicle

√x7ᵗʰ **V81.6** Occupant of railway train or railway vehicle injured by fall from railway train or railway vehicle

√x7ᵗʰ **V81.7** Occupant of railway train or railway vehicle injured in derailment without antecedent collision

√5ᵗʰ **V81.8** Occupant of railway train or railway vehicle injured in other specified railway accidents

√x7ᵗʰ   **V81.81** Occupant of railway train or railway vehicle injured due to explosion or fire on train

√x7ᵗʰ   **V81.82** Occupant of railway train or railway vehicle injured due to object falling onto train

Occupant of railway train or railway vehicle injured due to falling earth onto train

Occupant of railway train or railway vehicle injured due to falling rocks onto train

Occupant of railway train or railway vehicle injured due to falling snow onto train

Occupant of railway train or railway vehicle injured due to falling trees onto train

√x7ᵗʰ   **V81.83** Occupant of railway train or railway vehicle injured due to collision with military vehicle

√x7ᵗʰ   **V81.89** Occupant of railway train or railway vehicle injured due to other specified railway accident

√x7ᵗʰ **V81.9** Occupant of railway train or railway vehicle injured in unspecified railway accident   ▽

Railway accident NOS

√4ᵗʰ **V82** Occupant of powered streetcar injured in transport accident

INCLUDES   interurban electric car

person on outside of streetcar

tram (car)

trolley (car)

EXCLUDES 1   *bus (V70-V79)*

motorcoach (V70-V79)

nonpowered streetcar (V76.-)

train (V81.-)

√x7ᵗʰ **V82.0** Occupant of streetcar injured in collision with motor vehicle in nontraffic accident

√x7ᵗʰ **V82.1** Occupant of streetcar injured in collision with motor vehicle in traffic accident

√x7ᵗʰ **V82.2** Occupant of streetcar injured in collision with or hit by rolling stock

√x7ᵗʰ **V82.3** Occupant of streetcar injured in collision with other object

EXCLUDES 1   *collision with animal-drawn vehicle or animal being ridden (V82.8)*

√x7ᵗʰ **V82.4** Person injured while boarding or alighting from streetcar

√x7ᵗʰ **V82.5** Occupant of streetcar injured by fall in streetcar

EXCLUDES 1   *fall in streetcar:*

while boarding or alighting (V82.4)

with antecedent collision (V82.0-V82.3)

√x7ᵗʰ **V82.6** Occupant of streetcar injured by fall from streetcar

EXCLUDES 1   *fall from streetcar:*

while boarding or alighting (V82.4)

with antecedent collision (V82.0-V82.3)

√x7ᵗʰ **V82.7** Occupant of streetcar injured in derailment without antecedent collision

EXCLUDES 1   *occupant of streetcar injured in derailment with antecedent collision (V82.0-V82.3)*

EXCLUDES 1   Not coded here   EXCLUDES 2   Not included here   N Newborn Age : 0   P Pediatric Age : 0-17   M Maternity Age : 12-55   A Adult Age : 15-124

√x7ᵗʰ **V82.8 Occupant of streetcar injured in other specified transport accidents**
Streetcar collision with military vehicle
Streetcar collision with train or nonmotor vehicles

√x7ᵗʰ **V82.9 Occupant of streetcar injured in unspecified traffic accident** ▽
Streetcar accident NOS

✓4ᵗʰ **V83 Occupant of special vehicle mainly used on industrial premises injured in transport accident**
INCLUDES battery-powered airport passenger vehicle
battery-powered truck (baggage) (mail)
coal-car in mine
forklift (truck)
logging car
self-propelled industrial truck
station baggage truck (powered)
tram, truck, or tub (powered) in mine or quarry
EXCLUDES 1 *special construction vehicles (V85.-)*
special industrial vehicle in stationary use or maintenance (W31.-)

√x7ᵗʰ **V83.0 Driver of special industrial vehicle injured in traffic accident**

√x7ᵗʰ **V83.1 Passenger of special industrial vehicle injured in traffic accident**

√x7ᵗʰ **V83.2 Person on outside of special industrial vehicle injured in traffic accident**

√x7ᵗʰ **V83.3 Unspecified occupant of special industrial vehicle injured in traffic accident** ▽

√x7ᵗʰ **V83.4 Person injured while boarding or alighting from special industrial vehicle**

√x7ᵗʰ **V83.5 Driver of special industrial vehicle injured in nontraffic accident**

√x7ᵗʰ **V83.6 Passenger of special industrial vehicle injured in nontraffic accident**

√x7ᵗʰ **V83.7 Person on outside of special industrial vehicle injured in nontraffic accident**

√x7ᵗʰ **V83.9 Unspecified occupant of special industrial vehicle injured in nontraffic accident** ▽
Special-industrial-vehicle accident NOS

✓4ᵗʰ **V84 Occupant of special vehicle mainly used in agriculture injured in transport accident**
INCLUDES self-propelled farm machinery
tractor (and trailer)
EXCLUDES 1 *animal-powered farm machinery accident (W30.8-)*
contact with combine harvester (W30.0)
special agricultural vehicle in stationary use or maintenance (W30.-)

√x7ᵗʰ **V84.0 Driver of special agricultural vehicle injured in traffic accident**

√x7ᵗʰ **V84.1 Passenger of special agricultural vehicle injured in traffic accident**

√x7ᵗʰ **V84.2 Person on outside of special agricultural vehicle injured in traffic accident**

√x7ᵗʰ **V84.3 Unspecified occupant of special agricultural vehicle injured in traffic accident** ▽

√x7ᵗʰ **V84.4 Person injured while boarding or alighting from special agricultural vehicle**

√x7ᵗʰ **V84.5 Driver of special agricultural vehicle injured in nontraffic accident**

√x7ᵗʰ **V84.6 Passenger of special agricultural vehicle injured in nontraffic accident**

√x7ᵗʰ **V84.7 Person on outside of special agricultural vehicle injured in nontraffic accident**

√x7ᵗʰ **V84.9 Unspecified occupant of special agricultural vehicle injured in nontraffic accident** ▽
Special-agricultural vehicle accident NOS

✓4ᵗʰ **V85 Occupant of special construction vehicle injured in transport accident**
INCLUDES bulldozer
digger
dump truck
earth-leveller
mechanical shovel
road-roller
EXCLUDES 1 *special industrial vehicle (V83.)*
special construction vehicle in stationary use or maintenance (W31.-)

√x7ᵗʰ **V85.0 Driver of special construction vehicle injured in traffic accident**

√x7ᵗʰ **V85.1 Passenger of special construction vehicle injured in traffic accident**

√x7ᵗʰ **V85.2 Person on outside of special construction vehicle injured in traffic accident**

√x7ᵗʰ **V85.3 Unspecified occupant of special construction vehicle injured in traffic accident** ▽

√x7ᵗʰ **V85.4 Person injured while boarding or alighting from special construction vehicle**

√x7ᵗʰ **V85.5 Driver of special construction vehicle injured in nontraffic accident**

√x7ᵗʰ **V85.6 Passenger of special construction vehicle injured in nontraffic accident**

√x7ᵗʰ **V85.7 Person on outside of special construction vehicle injured in nontraffic accident**

√x7ᵗʰ **V85.9 Unspecified occupant of special construction vehicle injured in nontraffic accident** ▽
Special-construction-vehicle accident NOS

✓4ᵗʰ **V86 Occupant of special all-terrain or other off-road motor vehicle, injured in transport accident**
EXCLUDES 1 *special all-terrain vehicle in stationary use or maintenance (W31.-)*
sport-utility vehicle (V50-V59)
three-wheeled motor vehicle designed for on-road use (V30-V39)

√5ᵗʰ **V86.0 Driver of special all-terrain or other off-road motor vehicle injured in traffic accident**

√x7ᵗʰ **V86.01 Driver of ambulance or fire engine injured in traffic accident**

√x7ᵗʰ **V86.02 Driver of snowmobile injured in traffic accident**

√x7ᵗʰ **V86.03 Driver of dune buggy injured in traffic accident**

√x7ᵗʰ **V86.04 Driver of military vehicle injured in traffic accident**

√x7ᵗʰ **V86.09 Driver of other special all-terrain or other off-road motor vehicle injured in traffic accident**
Driver of dirt bike injured in traffic accident
Driver of go cart injured in traffic accident
Driver of golf cart injured in traffic accident

√5ᵗʰ **V86.1 Passenger of special all-terrain or other off-road motor vehicle injured in traffic accident**

√x7ᵗʰ **V86.11 Passenger of ambulance or fire engine injured in traffic accident**

√x7ᵗʰ **V86.12 Passenger of snowmobile injured in traffic accident**

√x7ᵗʰ **V86.13 Passenger of dune buggy injured in traffic accident**

√x7ᵗʰ **V86.14 Passenger of military vehicle injured in traffic accident**

√x7ᵗʰ **V86.19 Passenger of other special all-terrain or other off-road motor vehicle injured in traffic accident**
Passenger of dirt bike injured in traffic accident
Passenger of go cart injured in traffic accident
Passenger of golf cart injured in traffic accident

√5ᵗʰ **V86.2 Person on outside of special all-terrain or other off-road motor vehicle injured in traffic accident**

√x7ᵗʰ **V86.21 Person on outside of ambulance or fire engine injured in traffic accident**

√x7ᵗʰ **V86.22 Person on outside of snowmobile injured in traffic accident**

√x7ᵗʰ **V86.23 Person on outside of dune buggy injured in traffic accident**

√x7ᵗʰ **V86.24 Person on outside of military vehicle injured in traffic accident**

√x7ᵗʰ **V86.29 Person on outside of other special all-terrain or other off-road motor vehicle injured in traffic accident**
Person on outside of dirt bike injured in traffic accident
Person on outside of go cart in traffic accident
Person on outside of golf cart injured in traffic accident

√5ᵗʰ **V86.3 Unspecified occupant of special all-terrain or other off-road motor vehicle injured in traffic accident**

√x7ᵗʰ **V86.31 Unspecified occupant of ambulance or fire engine injured in traffic accident** ▽

√x7ᵗʰ **V86.32 Unspecified occupant of snowmobile injured in traffic accident** ▽

√x7ᵗʰ **V86.33 Unspecified occupant of dune buggy injured in traffic accident** ▽

√x7ᵗʰ **V86.34 Unspecified occupant of military vehicle injured in traffic accident** ▽

☑ Additional Character Required   √x7ᵗʰ Placeholder Alert   Manifestation Dx   ▽ Unspecified Dx   ►◄ Revised Text   ● New Code   ▲ Revised Code Title

√x7th V86.39 **Unspecified occupant of other special all-terrain or other off-road motor vehicle injured in traffic accident** ▽
Unspecified occupant of dirt bike injured in traffic accident
Unspecified occupant of go cart injured in traffic accident
Unspecified occupant of golf cart injured in traffic accident

√5th V86.4 **Person injured while boarding or alighting from special all-terrain or other off-road motor vehicle**

√x7th V86.41 **Person injured while boarding or alighting from ambulance or fire engine**

√x7th V86.42 **Person injured while boarding or alighting from snowmobile**

√x7th V86.43 **Person injured while boarding or alighting from dune buggy**

√x7th V86.44 **Person injured while boarding or alighting from military vehicle**

√x7th V86.49 **Person injured while boarding or alighting from other special all-terrain or other off-road motor vehicle**
Person injured while boarding or alighting from dirt bike
Person injured while boarding or alighting from go cart
Person injured while boarding or alighting from golf cart

√5th V86.5 **Driver of special all-terrain or other off-road motor vehicle injured in nontraffic accident**

√x7th V86.51 **Driver of ambulance or fire engine injured in nontraffic accident**

√x7th V86.52 **Driver of snowmobile injured in nontraffic accident**

√x7th V86.53 **Driver of dune buggy injured in nontraffic accident**

√x7th V86.54 **Driver of military vehicle injured in nontraffic accident**

√x7th V86.59 **Driver of other special all-terrain or other off-road motor vehicle injured in nontraffic accident**
Driver of dirt bike injured in nontraffic accident
Driver of go cart injured in nontraffic accident
Driver of golf cart injured in nontraffic accident

√5th V86.6 **Passenger of special all-terrain or other off-road motor vehicle injured in nontraffic accident**

√x7th V86.61 **Passenger of ambulance or fire engine injured in nontraffic accident**

√x7th V86.62 **Passenger of snowmobile injured in nontraffic accident**

√x7th V86.63 **Passenger of dune buggy injured in nontraffic accident**

√x7th V86.64 **Passenger of military vehicle injured in nontraffic accident**

√x7th V86.69 **Passenger of other special all-terrain or other off-road motor vehicle injured in nontraffic accident**
Passenger of dirt bike injured in nontraffic accident
Passenger of go cart injured in nontraffic accident
Passenger of golf cart injured in nontraffic accident

√5th V86.7 **Person on outside of special all-terrain or other off-road motor vehicle injured in nontraffic accident**

√x7th V86.71 **Person on outside of ambulance or fire engine injured in nontraffic accident**

√x7th V86.72 **Person on outside of snowmobile injured in nontraffic accident**

√x7th V86.73 **Person on outside of dune buggy injured in nontraffic accident**

√x7th V86.74 **Person on outside of military vehicle injured in nontraffic accident**

√x7th V86.79 **Person on outside of other special all-terrain or other off-road motor vehicles injured in nontraffic accident**
Person on outside of dirt bike injured in nontraffic accident
Person on outside of go cart injured in nontraffic accident
Person on outside of golf cart injured in nontraffic accident

√5th V86.9 **Unspecified occupant of special all-terrain or other off-road motor vehicle injured in nontraffic accident**

√x7th V86.91 **Unspecified occupant of ambulance or fire engine injured in nontraffic accident** ▽

√x7th V86.92 **Unspecified occupant of snowmobile injured in nontraffic accident** ▽

√x7th V86.93 **Unspecified occupant of dune buggy injured in nontraffic accident** ▽

√x7th V86.94 **Unspecified occupant of military vehicle injured in nontraffic accident** ▽

√x7th V86.99 **Unspecified occupant of other special all-terrain or other off-road motor vehicle injured in nontraffic accident** ▽
All-terrain motor-vehicle accident NOS
Off-road motor-vehicle accident NOS
Other motor-vehicle accident NOS
Unspecified occupant of dirt bike injured in nontraffic accident
Unspecified occupant of go cart injured in nontraffic accident
Unspecified occupant of golf cart injured in nontraffic accident

√4th V87 **Traffic accident of specified type but victim's mode of transport unknown**
EXCLUDES 1 collision involving:
pedal cycle (V10-V19)
pedestrian (V01-V09)

√x7th V87.0 **Person injured in collision between car and two- or three-wheeled powered vehicle (traffic)**

√x7th V87.1 **Person injured in collision between other motor vehicle and two- or three-wheeled motor vehicle (traffic)**

√x7th V87.2 **Person injured in collision between car and pick-up truck or van (traffic)**

√x7th V87.3 **Person injured in collision between car and bus (traffic)**

√x7th V87.4 **Person injured in collision between car and heavy transport vehicle (traffic)**

√x7th V87.5 **Person injured in collision between heavy transport vehicle and bus (traffic)**

√x7th V87.6 **Person injured in collision between railway train or railway vehicle and car (traffic)**

√x7th V87.7 **Person injured in collision between other specified motor vehicles (traffic)**

√x7th V87.8 **Person injured in other specified noncollision transport accidents involving motor vehicle (traffic)**

√x7th V87.9 **Person injured in other specified (collision)(noncollision) transport accidents involving nonmotor vehicle (traffic)**

√4th V88 **Nontraffic accident of specified type but victim's mode of transport unknown**
EXCLUDES 1 collision involving:
pedal cycle (V10-V19)
pedestrian (V01-V09)

√x7th V88.0 **Person injured in collision between car and two- or three-wheeled motor vehicle, nontraffic**

√x7th V88.1 **Person injured in collision between other motor vehicle and two- or three-wheeled motor vehicle, nontraffic**

√x7th V88.2 **Person injured in collision between car and pick-up truck or van, nontraffic**

√x7th V88.3 **Person injured in collision between car and bus, nontraffic**

√x7th V88.4 **Person injured in collision between car and heavy transport vehicle, nontraffic**

√x7th V88.5 **Person injured in collision between heavy transport vehicle and bus, nontraffic**

√x7th V88.6 **Person injured in collision between railway train or railway vehicle and car, nontraffic**

√x7th V88.7 **Person injured in collision between other specified motor vehicle, nontraffic**

√x7th V88.8 **Person injured in other specified noncollision transport accidents involving motor vehicle, nontraffic**

√x7th V88.9 **Person injured in other specified (collision)(noncollision) transport accidents involving nonmotor vehicle, nontraffic**

√4th V89 **Motor- or nonmotor-vehicle accident, type of vehicle unspecified**

√x7th V89.0 **Person injured in unspecified motor-vehicle accident, nontraffic** ▽
Motor-vehicle accident NOS, nontraffic

√x7th V89.1 **Person injured in unspecified nonmotor-vehicle accident, nontraffic** ▽
Nonmotor-vehicle accident NOS (nontraffic)

√x7th V89.2 **Person injured in unspecified motor-vehicle accident, traffic** ▽
Motor-vehicle accident [MVA] NOS
Road (traffic) accident [RTA] NOS

√x7th V89.3 **Person injured in unspecified nonmotor-vehicle accident, traffic** ▽
Nonmotor-vehicle traffic accident NOS

☑x7ᵗʰ **V89.9 Person injured in unspecified vehicle accident** ▽
       Collision NOS

Water transport accidents (V90-V94)

The appropriate 7th character is to be added to each code from categories V90-V94.
A   initial encounter
D   subsequent encounter
S   sequela

☑4ᵗʰ **V90 Drowning and submersion due to accident to watercraft**

     EXCLUDES 1   *civilian water transport accident involving military watercraft (V94.81-)*
               fall into water not from watercraft (W16.-)
               military watercraft accident in military or war operations (Y36.0-, Y37.0-)
               water-transport-related drowning or submersion without accident to watercraft (V92.-)

☑5ᵗʰ **V90.0 Drowning and submersion due to watercraft overturning**

   ☑x7ᵗʰ **V90.00 Drowning and submersion due to merchant ship overturning**

   ☑x7ᵗʰ **V90.01 Drowning and submersion due to passenger ship overturning**
       Drowning and submersion due to Ferry-boat overturning
       Drowning and submersion due to Liner overturning

   ☑x7ᵗʰ **V90.02 Drowning and submersion due to fishing boat overturning**

   ☑x7ᵗʰ **V90.03 Drowning and submersion due to other powered watercraft overturning**
       Drowning and submersion due to Hovercraft (on open water) overturning
       Drowning and submersion due to Jet ski overturning

   ☑x7ᵗʰ **V90.04 Drowning and submersion due to sailboat overturning**

   ☑x7ᵗʰ **V90.05 Drowning and submersion due to canoe or kayak overturning**

   ☑x7ᵗʰ **V90.06 Drowning and submersion due to (nonpowered) inflatable craft overturning**

   ☑x7ᵗʰ **V90.08 Drowning and submersion due to other unpowered watercraft overturning**
       Drowning and submersion due to wIndsurfer overturning

   ☑x7ᵗʰ **V90.09 Drowning and submersion due to unspecified watercraft overturning** ▽
       Drowning and submersion due to boat NOS overturning
       Drowning and submersion due to ship NOS overturning
       Drowning and submersion due to watercraft NOS overturning

☑5ᵗʰ **V90.1 Drowning and submersion due to watercraft sinking**

   ☑x7ᵗʰ **V90.10 Drowning and submersion due to merchant ship sinking**

   ☑x7ᵗʰ **V90.11 Drowning and submersion due to passenger ship sinking**
       Drowning and submersion due to Ferry-boat sinking
       Drowning and submersion due to Liner sinking

   ☑x7ᵗʰ **V90.12 Drowning and submersion due to fishing boat sinking**

   ☑x7ᵗʰ **V90.13 Drowning and submersion due to other powered watercraft sinking**
       Drowning and submersion due to Hovercraft (on open water) sinking
       Drowning and submersion due to Jet ski sinking

   ☑x7ᵗʰ **V90.14 Drowning and submersion due to sailboat sinking**

   ☑x7ᵗʰ **V90.15 Drowning and submersion due to canoe or kayak sinking**

   ☑x7ᵗʰ **V90.16 Drowning and submersion due to (nonpowered) inflatable craft sinking**

   ☑x7ᵗʰ **V90.18 Drowning and submersion due to other unpowered watercraft sinking**

   ☑x7ᵗʰ **V90.19 Drowning and submersion due to unspecified watercraft sinking** ▽
       Drowning and submersion due to boat NOS sinking
       Drowning and submersion due to ship NOS sinking
       Drowning and submersion due to watercraft NOS sinking

☑5ᵗʰ **V90.2 Drowning and submersion due to falling or jumping from burning watercraft**

   ☑x7ᵗʰ **V90.20 Drowning and submersion due to falling or jumping from burning merchant ship**

   ☑x7ᵗʰ **V90.21 Drowning and submersion due to falling or jumping from burning passenger ship**
       Drowning and submersion due to falling or jumping from burning Ferry-boat
       Drowning and submersion due to falling or jumping from burning Liner

   ☑x7ᵗʰ **V90.22 Drowning and submersion due to falling or jumping from burning fishing boat**

   ☑x7ᵗʰ **V90.23 Drowning and submersion due to falling or jumping from other burning powered watercraft**
       Drowning and submersion due to falling and jumping from burning Hovercraft (on open water)
       Drowning and submersion due to falling and jumping from burning Jet ski

   ☑x7ᵗʰ **V90.24 Drowning and submersion due to falling or jumping from burning sailboat**

   ☑x7ᵗʰ **V90.25 Drowning and submersion due to falling or jumping from burning canoe or kayak**

   ☑x7ᵗʰ **V90.26 Drowning and submersion due to falling or jumping from burning (nonpowered) inflatable craft**

   ☑x7ᵗʰ **V90.27 Drowning and submersion due to falling or jumping from burning water-skis**

   ☑x7ᵗʰ **V90.28 Drowning and submersion due to falling or jumping from other burning unpowered watercraft**
       Drowning and submersion due to falling and jumping from burning surf-board
       Drowning and submersion due to falling and jumping from burning windsurfer

   ☑x7ᵗʰ **V90.29 Drowning and submersion due to falling or jumping from unspecified burning watercraft** ▽
       Drowning and submersion due to falling or jumping from burning boat NOS
       Drowning and submersion due to falling or jumping from burning ship NOS
       Drowning and submersion due to falling or jumping from burning watercraft NOS

☑5ᵗʰ **V90.3 Drowning and submersion due to falling or jumping from crushed watercraft**

   ☑x7ᵗʰ **V90.30 Drowning and submersion due to falling or jumping from crushed merchant ship**

   ☑x7ᵗʰ **V90.31 Drowning and submersion due to falling or jumping from crushed passenger ship**
       Drowning and submersion due to falling and jumping from crushed Ferry boat
       Drowning and submersion due to falling and jumping from crushed Liner

   ☑x7ᵗʰ **V90.32 Drowning and submersion due to falling or jumping from crushed fishing boat**

   ☑x7ᵗʰ **V90.33 Drowning and submersion due to falling or jumping from other crushed powered watercraft**
       Drowning and submersion due to falling and jumping from crushed Hovercraft
       Drowning and submersion due to falling and jumping from crushed Jet ski

   ☑x7ᵗʰ **V90.34 Drowning and submersion due to falling or jumping from crushed sailboat**

   ☑x7ᵗʰ **V90.35 Drowning and submersion due to falling or jumping from crushed canoe or kayak**

   ☑x7ᵗʰ **V90.36 Drowning and submersion due to falling or jumping from crushed (nonpowered) inflatable craft**

   ☑x7ᵗʰ **V90.37 Drowning and submersion due to falling or jumping from crushed water-skis**

   ☑x7ᵗʰ **V90.38 Drowning and submersion due to falling or jumping from other crushed unpowered watercraft**
       Drowning and submersion due to falling and jumping from crushed surf-board
       Drowning and submersion due to falling and jumping from crushed windsurfer

   ☑x7ᵗʰ **V90.39 Drowning and submersion due to falling or jumping from crushed unspecified watercraft** ▽
       Drowning and submersion due to falling and jumping from crushed boat NOS
       Drowning and submersion due to falling and jumping from crushed ship NOS
       Drowning and submersion due to falling and jumping from crushed watercraft NOS

☑ Additional Character Required   ☑7ᵗʰ Placeholder Alert   Manifestation Dx   ▽ Unspecified Dx   ▶◀ Revised Text   ● New Code   ▲ Revised Code Title

√5ᵗʰ V90.8 Drowning and submersion due to other accident to watercraft

√x7ᵗʰ **V90.80 Drowning and submersion due to other accident to merchant ship**

√x7ᵗʰ **V90.81 Drowning and submersion due to other accident to passenger ship**

Drowning and submersion due to other accident to Ferry-boat

Drowning and submersion due to other accident to Liner

√x7ᵗʰ **V90.82 Drowning and submersion due to other accident to fishing boat**

√x7ᵗʰ **V90.83 Drowning and submersion due to other accident to other powered watercraft**

Drowning and submersion due to other accident to Hovercraft (on open water)

Drowning and submersion due to other accident to Jet ski

√x7ᵗʰ **V90.84 Drowning and submersion due to other accident to sailboat**

√x7ᵗʰ **V90.85 Drowning and submersion due to other accident to canoe or kayak**

√x7ᵗʰ **V90.86 Drowning and submersion due to other accident to (nonpowered) inflatable craft**

√x7ᵗʰ **V90.87 Drowning and submersion due to other accident to water-skis**

√x7ᵗʰ **V90.88 Drowning and submersion due to other accident to other unpowered watercraft**

Drowning and submersion due to other accident to surf-board

Drowning and submersion due to other accident to windsurfer

√x7ᵗʰ **V90.89 Drowning and submersion due to other accident to unspecified watercraft** ▽

Drowning and submersion due to other accident to boat NOS

Drowning and submersion due to other accident to ship NOS

Drowning and submersion due to other accident to watercraft NOS

√4ᵗʰ V91 Other injury due to accident to watercraft

> INCLUDES   any injury except drowning and submersion as a result of an accident to watercraft
>
> EXCLUDES 1 *civilian water transport accident involving military watercraft (V94.81-)*
> *military watercraft accident in military or war operations (Y36, Y37.-)*
>
> EXCLUDES 2 *drowning and submersion due to accident to watercraft (V90.-)*

√5ᵗʰ V91.0 Burn due to watercraft on fire

> EXCLUDES 1 *burn from localized fire or explosion on board ship without accident to watercraft (V93.-)*

√x7ᵗʰ **V91.00 Burn due to merchant ship on fire**

√x7ᵗʰ **V91.01 Burn due to passenger ship on fire**

Burn due to Ferry-boat on fire
Burn due to Liner on fire

√x7ᵗʰ **V91.02 Burn due to fishing boat on fire**

√x7ᵗʰ **V91.03 Burn due to other powered watercraft on fire**

Burn due to Hovercraft (on open water) on fire
Burn due to Jet ski on fire

√x7ᵗʰ **V91.04 Burn due to sailboat on fire**

√x7ᵗʰ **V91.05 Burn due to canoe or kayak on fire**

√x7ᵗʰ **V91.06 Burn due to (nonpowered) inflatable craft on fire**

√x7ᵗʰ **V91.07 Burn due to water-skis on fire**

√x7ᵗʰ **V91.08 Burn due to other unpowered watercraft on fire**

√x7ᵗʰ **V91.09 Burn due to unspecified watercraft on fire** ▽

Burn due to boat NOS on fire
Burn due to ship NOS on fire
Burn due to watercraft NOS on fire

√5ᵗʰ V91.1 Crushed between watercraft and other watercraft or other object due to collision

Crushed by lifeboat after abandoning ship in a collision

> NOTE   Select the specified type of watercraft that the victim was on at the time of the collision

√x7ᵗʰ **V91.10 Crushed between merchant ship and other watercraft or other object due to collision**

√x7ᵗʰ **V91.11 Crushed between passenger ship and other watercraft or other object due to collision**

Crushed between Ferry-boat and other watercraft or other object due to collision

Crushed between Liner and other watercraft or other object due to collision

√x7ᵗʰ **V91.12 Crushed between fishing boat and other watercraft or other object due to collision**

√x7ᵗʰ **V91.13 Crushed between other powered watercraft and other watercraft or other object due to collision**

Crushed between Hovercraft (on open water) and other watercraft or other object due to collision

Crushed between Jet ski and other watercraft or other object due to collision

√x7ᵗʰ **V91.14 Crushed between sailboat and other watercraft or other object due to collision**

√x7ᵗʰ **V91.15 Crushed between canoe or kayak and other watercraft or other object due to collision**

√x7ᵗʰ **V91.16 Crushed between (nonpowered) inflatable craft and other watercraft or other object due to collision**

√x7ᵗʰ **V91.18 Crushed between other unpowered watercraft and other watercraft or other object due to collision**

Crushed between surfboard and other watercraft or other object due to collision

Crushed between windsurfer and other watercraft or other object due to collision

√x7ᵗʰ **V91.19 Crushed between unspecified watercraft and other watercraft or other object due to collision** ▽

Crushed between boat NOS and other watercraft or other object due to collision

Crushed between ship NOS and other watercraft or other object due to collision

Crushed between watercraft NOS and other watercraft or other object due to collision

√5ᵗʰ V91.2 Fall due to collision between watercraft and other watercraft or other object

Fall while remaining on watercraft after collision

> NOTE   Select the specified type of watercraft that the victim was on at the time of the collision

> EXCLUDES 1 *crushed between watercraft and other watercraft and other object due to collision (V91.1-)*
> *drowning and submersion due to falling from crushed watercraft (V90.3-)*

√x7ᵗʰ **V91.20 Fall due to collision between merchant ship and other watercraft or other object**

√x7ᵗʰ **V91.21 Fall due to collision between passenger ship and other watercraft or other object**

Fall due to collision between Ferry-boat and other watercraft or other object

Fall due to collision between Liner and other watercraft or other object

√x7ᵗʰ **V91.22 Fall due to collision between fishing boat and other watercraft or other object**

√x7ᵗʰ **V91.23 Fall due to collision between other powered watercraft and other watercraft or other object**

Fall due to collision between Hovercraft (on open water) and other watercraft or other object

Fall due to collision between Jet ski and other watercraft or other object

√x7ᵗʰ **V91.24 Fall due to collision between sailboat and other watercraft or other object**

√x7ᵗʰ **V91.25 Fall due to collision between canoe or kayak and other watercraft or other object**

√x7ᵗʰ **V91.26 Fall due to collision between (nonpowered) inflatable craft and other watercraft or other object**

√x7ᵗʰ **V91.29 Fall due to collision between unspecified watercraft and other watercraft or other object** ▽

Fall due to collision between boat NOS and other watercraft or other object

Fall due to collision between ship NOS and other watercraft or other object

Fall due to collision between watercraft NOS and other watercraft or other object

EXCLUDES 1 Not coded here   EXCLUDES 2 Not included here   N Newborn Age : 0   P Pediatric Age : 0-17   M Maternity Age : 12-55   A Adult Age : 15-124

1104   ICD-10-CM 2017

Chapter 20. External Causes of Morbidity

V91.3   **Hit or struck by falling object due to accident to watercraft**

Hit or struck by falling object (part of damaged watercraft or other object) after falling or jumping from damaged watercraft

EXCLUDES 2   *drowning or submersion due to fall or jumping from damaged watercraft (V90.2-, V90.3-)*

V91.30   **Hit or struck by falling object due to accident to merchant ship**

V91.31   **Hit or struck by falling object due to accident to passenger ship**

Hit or struck by falling object due to accident to Ferry-boat

Hit or struck by falling object due to accident to Liner

V91.32   **Hit or struck by falling object due to accident to fishing boat**

V91.33   **Hit or struck by falling object due to accident to other powered watercraft**

Hit or struck by falling object due to accident to Hovercraft (on open water)

Hit or struck by falling object due to accident to Jet ski

V91.34   **Hit or struck by falling object due to accident to sailboat**

V91.35   **Hit or struck by falling object due to accident to canoe or kayak**

V91.36   **Hit or struck by falling object due to accident to (nonpowered) inflatable craft**

V91.37   **Hit or struck by falling object due to accident to water-skis**

Hit by water-skis after jumping off of waterskis

V91.38   **Hit or struck by falling object due to accident to other unpowered watercraft**

Hit or struck by surf-board after falling off damaged surf-board

Hit or struck by object after falling off damaged windsurfer

V91.39   **Hit or struck by falling object due to accident to unspecified watercraft** ▽

Hit or struck by falling object due to accident to boat NOS

Hit or struck by falling object due to accident to ship NOS

Hit or struck by falling object due to accident to watercraft NOS

V91.8   **Other injury due to other accident to watercraft**

V91.80   **Other injury due to other accident to merchant ship**

V91.81   **Other injury due to other accident to passenger ship**

Other injury due to other accident to Ferry-boat

Other injury due to other accident to Liner

V91.82   **Other injury due to other accident to fishing boat**

V91.83   **Other injury due to other accident to other powered watercraft**

Other injury due to other accident to Hovercraft (on open water)

Other injury due to other accident to Jet ski

V91.84   **Other injury due to other accident to sailboat**

V91.85   **Other injury due to other accident to canoe or kayak**

V91.86   **Other injury due to other accident to (nonpowered) inflatable craft**

V91.87   **Other injury due to other accident to water-skis**

V91.88   **Other injury due to other accident to other unpowered watercraft**

Other injury due to other accident to surf-board

Other injury due to other accident to windsurfer

V91.89   **Other injury due to other accident to unspecified watercraft** ▽

Other injury due to other accident to boat NOS

Other injury due to other accident to ship NOS

Other injury due to other accident to watercraft NOS

V92   **Drowning and submersion due to accident on board watercraft, without accident to watercraft**

EXCLUDES 1   *civilian water transport accident involving military watercraft (V94.81-)*

drowning or submersion due to accident to watercraft (V90-V91)

drowning or submersion of diver who voluntarily jumps from boat not involved in an accident (W16.711, W16.721)

fall into water without watercraft (W16.-)

military watercraft accident in military or war operations (Y36, Y37)

V92.0   **Drowning and submersion due to fall off watercraft**

Drowning and submersion due to fall from gangplank of watercraft

Drowning and submersion due to fall overboard watercraft

EXCLUDES 2   *hitting head on object or bottom of body of water due to fall from watercraft (V94.0-)*

V92.00   **Drowning and submersion due to fall off merchant ship**

V92.01   **Drowning and submersion due to fall off passenger ship**

Drowning and submersion due to fall off Ferry-boat

Drowning and submersion due to fall off Liner

V92.02   **Drowning and submersion due to fall off fishing boat**

V92.03   **Drowning and submersion due to fall off other powered watercraft**

Drowning and submersion due to fall off Hovercraft (on open water)

Drowning and submersion due to fall off Jet ski

V92.04   **Drowning and submersion due to fall off sailboat**

V92.05   **Drowning and submersion due to fall off canoe or kayak**

V92.06   **Drowning and submersion due to fall off (nonpowered) inflatable craft**

V92.07   **Drowning and submersion due to fall off water-skis**

EXCLUDES 1   *drowning and submersion due to falling off burning water-skis (V90.27)*

drowning and submersion due to falling off crushed water-skis (V90.37)

hit by boat while water-skiing NOS (V91.X)

V92.08   **Drowning and submersion due to fall off other unpowered watercraft**

Drowning and submersion due to fall off surf-board

Drowning and submersion due to fall off windsurfer

EXCLUDES 1   *drowning and submersion due to fall off burning unpowered watercraft (V90.28)*

drowning and submersion due to fall off crushed unpowered watercraft (V90.38)

drowning and submersion due to fall off damaged unpowered watercraft (V90.88)

drowning and submersion due to rider of nonpowered watercraft being hit by other watercraft (V94.-)

other injury due to rider of nonpowered watercraft being hit by other watercraft (V94.-)

V92.09   **Drowning and submersion due to fall off unspecified watercraft** ▽

Drowning and submersion due to fall off boat NOS

Drowning and submersion due to fall off ship

Drowning and submersion due to fall off watercraft NOS

V92.1   **Drowning and submersion due to being thrown overboard by motion of watercraft**

EXCLUDES 1   *drowning and submersion due to fall off surf-board (V92.08)*

drowning and submersion due to fall off water-skis (V92.07)

drowning and submersion due to fall off windsurfer (V92.08)

V92.10   **Drowning and submersion due to being thrown overboard by motion of merchant ship**

☑ Additional Character Required   ✓x7ʰ Placeholder Alert   Manifestation Dx   ▽ Unspecified Dx   ▶◀ Revised Text   ● New Code   ▲ Revised Code Title

ICD-10-CM 2017   1105

√x7ᵗʰ **V92.11** **Drowning and submersion due to being thrown overboard by motion of** passenger ship
     Drowning and submersion due to being thrown overboard by motion of Ferry-boat
     Drowning and submersion due to being thrown overboard by motion of Liner

√x7ᵗʰ **V92.12** **Drowning and submersion due to being thrown overboard by motion of** fishing boat

√x7ᵗʰ **V92.13** **Drowning and submersion due to being thrown overboard by motion of other** powered **watercraft**
     Drowning and submersion due to being thrown overboard by motion of Hovercraft

√x7ᵗʰ **V92.14** **Drowning and submersion due to being thrown overboard by motion of** sailboat

√x7ᵗʰ **V92.15** **Drowning and submersion due to being thrown overboard by motion of** canoe or kayak

√x7ᵗʰ **V92.16** **Drowning and submersion due to being thrown overboard by motion of (nonpowered)** inflatable craft

√x7ᵗʰ **V92.19** **Drowning and submersion due to being thrown overboard by motion of unspecified watercraft** ▽
     Drowning and submersion due to being thrown overboard by motion of boat NOS
     Drowning and submersion due to being thrown overboard by motion of ship NOS
     Drowning and submersion due to being thrown overboard by motion of watercraft NOS

√5ᵗʰ **V92.2** **Drowning and submersion due to being** washed overboard **from watercraft**
     Code first any associated cataclysm (X37.0-)

√x7ᵗʰ **V92.20** **Drowning and submersion due to being washed overboard from** merchant ship

√x7ᵗʰ **V92.21** **Drowning and submersion due to being washed overboard from** passenger ship
     Drowning and submersion due to being washed overboard from Ferry-boat
     Drowning and submersion due to being washed overboard from Liner

√x7ᵗʰ **V92.22** **Drowning and submersion due to being washed overboard from** fishing boat

√x7ᵗʰ **V92.23** **Drowning and submersion due to being washed overboard from other** powered **watercraft**
     Drowning and submersion due to being washed overboard from Hovercraft (on open water)
     Drowning and submersion due to being washed overboard from Jet ski

√x7ᵗʰ **V92.24** **Drowning and submersion due to being washed overboard from** sailboat

√x7ᵗʰ **V92.25** **Drowning and submersion due to being washed overboard from** canoe or kayak

√x7ᵗʰ **V92.26** **Drowning and submersion due to being washed overboard from (nonpowered)** inflatable craft

√x7ᵗʰ **V92.27** **Drowning and submersion due to being washed overboard from** water-skis
     EXCLUDES 1 *drowning and submersion due to fall off water-skis (V92.07)*

√x7ᵗʰ **V92.28** **Drowning and submersion due to being washed overboard from other** unpowered **watercraft**
     Drowning and submersion due to being washed overboard from surf-board
     Drowning and submersion due to being washed overboard from windsurfer

√x7ᵗʰ **V92.29** **Drowning and submersion due to being washed overboard from unspecified watercraft** ▽
     Drowning and submersion due to being washed overboard from boat NOS
     Drowning and submersion due to being washed overboard from ship NOS
     Drowning and submersion due to being washed overboard from watercraft NOS

√4ᵗʰ **V93** **Other injury due to accident on board watercraft, without accident to watercraft**
     EXCLUDES 1 *civilian water transport accident involving military watercraft (V94.81-)*
     other injury due to accident to watercraft (V91.-)
     military watercraft accident in military or war operations (Y36, Y37.-)
     EXCLUDES 2 *drowning and submersion due to accident on board watercraft, without accident to watercraft (V92.-)*

√5ᵗʰ **V93.0** **Burn due to localized fire on board watercraft**
     EXCLUDES 1 *burn due to watercraft on fire (V91.0-)*

√x7ᵗʰ **V93.00** **Burn due to localized fire on board** merchant vessel

√x7ᵗʰ **V93.01** **Burn due to localized fire on board** passenger vessel
     Burn due to localized fire on board Ferry-boat
     Burn due to localized fire on board Liner

√x7ᵗʰ **V93.02** **Burn due to localized fire on board** fishing boat

√x7ᵗʰ **V93.03** **Burn due to localized fire on board other** powered **watercraft**
     Burn due to localized fire on board Hovercraft
     Burn due to localized fire on board Jet ski

√x7ᵗʰ **V93.04** **Burn due to localized fire on board** sailboat

√x7ᵗʰ **V93.09** **Burn due to localized fire on board unspecified watercraft** ▽
     Burn due to localized fire on board boat NOS
     Burn due to localized fire on board ship NOS
     Burn due to localized fire on board watercraft NOS

√5ᵗʰ **V93.1** **Other burn on board watercraft**
     Burn due to source other than fire on board watercraft
     EXCLUDES 1 *burn due to watercraft on fire (V91.0-)*

√x7ᵗʰ **V93.10** **Other burn on board** merchant vessel

√x7ᵗʰ **V93.11** **Other burn on board** passenger vessel
     Other burn on board Ferry-boat
     Other burn on board Liner

√x7ᵗʰ **V93.12** **Other burn on board** fishing boat

√x7ᵗʰ **V93.13** **Other burn on board other** powered **watercraft**
     Other burn on board Hovercraft
     Other burn on board Jet ski

√x7ᵗʰ **V93.14** **Other burn on board** sailboat

√x7ᵗʰ **V93.19** **Other burn on board unspecified watercraft** ▽
     Other burn on board boat NOS
     Other burn on board ship NOS
     Other burn on board watercraft NOS

√5ᵗʰ **V93.2** **Heat exposure on board watercraft**
     EXCLUDES 1 *exposure to man-made heat not aboard watercraft (W92)*
     exposure to natural heat while on board watercraft (X30)
     exposure to sunlight while on board watercraft (X32)
     EXCLUDES 2 *burn due to fire on board watercraft (V93.0-)*

√x7ᵗʰ **V93.20** **Heat exposure on board** merchant ship

√x7ᵗʰ **V93.21** **Heat exposure on board** passenger ship
     Heat exposure on board Ferry-boat
     Heat exposure on board Liner

√x7ᵗʰ **V93.22** **Heat exposure on board** fishing boat

√x7ᵗʰ **V93.23** **Heat exposure on board other** powered **watercraft**
     Heat exposure on board hovercraft

√x7ᵗʰ **V93.24** **Heat exposure on board** sailboat

√x7ᵗʰ **V93.29** **Heat exposure on board unspecified watercraft** ▽
     Heat exposure on board boat NOS
     Heat exposure on board ship NOS
     Heat exposure on board watercraft NOS

√5ᵗʰ **V93.3** **Fall on board watercraft**
     EXCLUDES 1 *fall due to collision of watercraft (V91.2-)*

√x7ᵗʰ **V93.30** **Fall on board** merchant ship

√x7ᵗʰ **V93.31** **Fall on board** passenger ship
     Fall on board Ferry-boat
     Fall on board Liner

√x7ᵗʰ **V93.32** **Fall on board** fishing boat

√x7ᵗʰ **V93.33** **Fall on board other** powered **watercraft**
     Fall on board Hovercraft (on open water)
     Fall on board Jet ski

√x7ᵗʰ **V93.34** **Fall on board** sailboat

√x7ᵗʰ **V93.35** **Fall on board** canoe or kayak

EXCLUDES 1   Not coded here   EXCLUDES 2   Not included here   N   Newborn Age : 0   P   Pediatric Age: 0-17   M   Maternity Age: 12-55   A   Adult Age : 15-124

√x7ᵗʰ **V93.36 Fall on board (nonpowered)** inflatable craft

√x7ᵗʰ **V93.38 Fall on board other** unpowered **watercraft**

√x7ᵗʰ **V93.39 Fall on board unspecified watercraft** ▽

Fall on board boat NOS
Fall on board ship NOS
Fall on board watercraft NOS

✓5ᵗʰ **V93.4 Struck by falling object on board watercraft**

Hit by falling object on board watercraft

EXCLUDES 1 *struck by falling object due to accident to watercraft (V91.3)*

√x7ᵗʰ **V93.40 Struck by falling object on** merchant ship

√x7ᵗʰ **V93.41 Struck by falling object on** passenger ship

Struck by falling object on Ferry-boat
Struck by falling object on Liner

√x7ᵗʰ **V93.42 Struck by falling object on** fishing boat

√x7ᵗʰ **V93.43 Struck by falling object on other** powered **watercraft**

Struck by falling object on Hovercraft

√x7ᵗʰ **V93.44 Struck by falling object on** sailboat

√x7ᵗʰ **V93.48 Struck by falling object on other** unpowered **watercraft**

√x7ᵗʰ **V93.49 Struck by falling object on unspecified** **watercraft** ▽

✓5ᵗʰ **V93.5 Explosion on board watercraft**

Boiler explosion on steamship

EXCLUDES 2 *fire on board watercraft (V93.0-)*

√x7ᵗʰ **V93.50 Explosion on board** merchant ship

√x7ᵗʰ **V93.51 Explosion on board** passenger ship

Explosion on board Ferry-boat
Explosion on board Liner

√x7ᵗʰ **V93.52 Explosion on board** fishing boat

√x7ᵗʰ **V93.53 Explosion on board other** powered **watercraft**

Explosion on board Hovercraft
Explosion on board Jet ski

√x7ᵗʰ **V93.54 Explosion on board** sailboat

√x7ᵗʰ **V93.59 Explosion on board unspecified watercraft** ▽

Explosion on board boat NOS
Explosion on board ship NOS
Explosion on board watercraft NOS

✓5ᵗʰ **V93.6 Machinery accident on board watercraft**

EXCLUDES 1 *machinery explosion on board watercraft (V93.4-)*
machinery fire on board watercraft (V93.0-)

√x7ᵗʰ **V93.60 Machinery accident on board** merchant ship

√x7ᵗʰ **V93.61 Machinery accident on board** passenger ship

Machinery accident on board Ferry-boat
Machinery accident on board Liner

√x7ᵗʰ **V93.62 Machinery accident on board** fishing boat

√x7ᵗʰ **V93.63 Machinery accident on board other** powered **watercraft**

Machinery accident on board Hovercraft

√x7ᵗʰ **V93.64 Machinery accident on board** sailboat

√x7ᵗʰ **V93.69 Machinery accident on board unspecified** **watercraft** ▽

Machinery accident on board boat NOS
Machinery accident on board ship NOS
Machinery accident on board watercraft NOS

✓5ᵗʰ **V93.8 Other injury due to other accident on board watercraft**

Accidental poisoning by gases or fumes on watercraft

√x7ᵗʰ **V93.80 Other injury due to other accident on board** merchant ship

√x7ᵗʰ **V93.81 Other injury due to other accident on board** passenger ship

Other injury due to other accident on board Ferry-boat
Other injury due to other accident on board Liner

√x7ᵗʰ **V93.82 Other injury due to other accident on board** fishing boat

√x7ᵗʰ **V93.83 Other injury due to other accident on board other** powered **watercraft**

Other injury due to other accident on board Hovercraft
Other injury due to other accident on board Jet ski

√x7ᵗʰ **V93.84 Other injury due to other accident on board** sailboat

√x7ᵗʰ **V93.85 Other injury due to other accident on board** canoe or kayak

√x7ᵗʰ **V93.86 Other injury due to other accident on board (nonpowered)** inflatable craft

√x7ᵗʰ **V93.87 Other injury due to other accident on board** water-skis

Hit or struck by object while waterskiing

√x7ᵗʰ **V93.88 Other injury due to other accident on board other** unpowered **watercraft**

Hit or struck by object while surfing
Hit or struck by object while on board windsurfer

√x7ᵗʰ **V93.89 Other injury due to other accident on board unspecified watercraft** ▽

Other injury due to other accident on board boat NOS
Other injury due to other accident on board ship NOS
Other injury due to other accident on board watercraft NOS

✓4ᵗʰ **V94 Other and unspecified water transport accidents**

EXCLUDES 1 *military watercraft accidents in military or war operations (Y36, Y37)*

√x7ᵗʰ **V94.0 Hitting object or bottom of body of water due to fall from watercraft**

EXCLUDES 2 *drowning and submersion due to fall from watercraft (V92.0-)*

✓5ᵗʰ **V94.1 Bather struck by watercraft**

Swimmer hit by watercraft

√x7ᵗʰ **V94.11 Bather struck by** powered **watercraft**

√x7ᵗʰ **V94.12 Bather struck by** nonpowered **watercraft**

✓5ᵗʰ **V94.2 Rider of nonpowered watercraft struck by other watercraft**

√x7ᵗʰ **V94.21 Rider of nonpowered watercraft struck by other** nonpowered **watercraft**

Canoer hit by other nonpowered watercraft
Surfer hit by other nonpowered watercraft
Windsurfer hit by other nonpowered watercraft

√x7ᵗʰ **V94.22 Rider of nonpowered watercraft struck by** powered **watercraft**

Canoer hit by motorboat
Surfer hit by motorboat
Windsurfer hit by motorboat

✓5ᵗʰ **V94.3 Injury to rider of (inflatable) watercraft being pulled behind other watercraft**

√x7ᵗʰ **V94.31 Injury to rider of (inflatable)** recreational watercraft **being pulled behind other watercraft**

Injury to rider of inner-tube pulled behind motor boat

√x7ᵗʰ **V94.32 Injury to rider of** non-recreational **watercraft being pulled behind other watercraft**

Injury to occupant of dingy being pulled behind boat or ship
Injury to occupant of life-raft being pulled behind boat or ship

√x7ᵗʰ **V94.4 Injury to barefoot water-skier**

Injury to person being pulled behind boat or ship

✓5ᵗʰ **V94.8 Other water transport accident**

√6ᵗʰ **V94.81 Water transport accident involving military watercraft**

√7ᵗʰ **V94.810 Civilian watercraft involved in water transport accident with military watercraft**

Passenger on civilian watercraft injured due to accident with military watercraft

√7ᵗʰ **V94.811 Civilian in water injured by military watercraft**

√7ᵗʰ **V94.818 Other water transport accident involving military watercraft**

√x7ᵗʰ **V94.89 Other water transport accident**

√x7ᵗʰ **V94.9 Unspecified water transport accident** ▽

Water transport accident NOS

Air and space transport accidents (V95-V97)

EXCLUDES 1 *military aircraft accidents in military or war operations (Y36, Y37)*

The appropriate 7th character is to be added to each code from categories V95-V97.
A   initial encounter
D   subsequent encounter
S   sequela

✓4ᵗʰ **V95 Accident to powered aircraft causing injury to occupant**

✓5ᵗʰ **V95.0 Helicopter accident injuring occupant**

√x7ᵗʰ **V95.00 Unspecified helicopter accident injuring occupant** ▽

✓ Additional Character Required   √x7ᵗʰ Placeholder Alert   Manifestation Dx   ▽ Unspecified Dx   ►◄ Revised Text   ● New Code   ▲ Revised Code Title

ICD-10-CM 2017   1107

Chapter 20. External Causes of Morbidity

V95.01–V97.810

√x7ᵗʰ **V95.01** **Helicopter crash injuring occupant**

√x7ᵗʰ **V95.02** **Forced landing of helicopter injuring occupant**

√x7ᵗʰ **V95.03** **Helicopter collision injuring occupant**
Helicopter collision with any object, fixed, movable or moving

√x7ᵗʰ **V95.04** **Helicopter fire injuring occupant**

√x7ᵗʰ **V95.05** **Helicopter explosion injuring occupant**

√x7ᵗʰ **V95.09** **Other helicopter accident injuring occupant**

√5ᵗʰ **V95.1** **Ultralight, microlight or powered-glider accident injuring occupant**

√x7ᵗʰ **V95.10** **Unspecified ultralight, microlight or powered-glider accident injuring occupant** ▽

√x7ᵗʰ **V95.11** **Ultralight, microlight or powered-glider crash injuring occupant**

√x7ᵗʰ **V95.12** **Forced landing of ultralight, microlight or powered-glider injuring occupant**

√x7ᵗʰ **V95.13** **Ultralight, microlight or powered-glider collision injuring occupant**
Ultralight, microlight or powered-glider collision with any object, fixed, movable or moving

√x7ᵗʰ **V95.14** **Ultralight, microlight or powered-glider fire injuring occupant**

√x7ᵗʰ **V95.15** **Ultralight, microlight or powered-glider explosion injuring occupant**

√x7ᵗʰ **V95.19** **Other ultralight, microlight or powered-glider accident injuring occupant**

√5ᵗʰ **V95.2** **Other private fixed-wing aircraft accident injuring occupant**

√x7ᵗʰ **V95.20** **Unspecified accident to other private fixed-wing aircraft, injuring occupant** ▽

√x7ᵗʰ **V95.21** **Other private fixed-wing aircraft crash injuring occupant**

√x7ᵗʰ **V95.22** **Forced landing of other private fixed-wing aircraft injuring occupant**

√x7ᵗʰ **V95.23** **Other private fixed-wing aircraft collision injuring occupant**
Other private fixed-wing aircraft collision with any object, fixed, movable or moving

√x7ᵗʰ **V95.24** **Other private fixed-wing aircraft fire injuring occupant**

√x7ᵗʰ **V95.25** **Other private fixed-wing aircraft explosion injuring occupant**

√x7ᵗʰ **V95.29** **Other accident to other private fixed-wing aircraft injuring occupant**

√5ᵗʰ **V95.3** **Commercial fixed-wing aircraft accident injuring occupant**

√x7ᵗʰ **V95.30** **Unspecified accident to commercial fixed-wing aircraft injuring occupant** ▽

√x7ᵗʰ **V95.31** **Commercial fixed-wing aircraft crash injuring occupant**

√x7ᵗʰ **V95.32** **Forced landing of commercial fixed-wing aircraft injuring occupant**

√x7ᵗʰ **V95.33** **Commercial fixed-wing aircraft collision injuring occupant**
Commercial fixed-wing aircraft collision with any object, fixed, movable or moving

√x7ᵗʰ **V95.34** **Commercial fixed-wing aircraft fire injuring occupant**

√x7ᵗʰ **V95.35** **Commercial fixed-wing aircraft explosion injuring occupant**

√x7ᵗʰ **V95.39** **Other accident to commercial fixed-wing aircraft injuring occupant**

√5ᵗʰ **V95.4** **Spacecraft accident injuring occupant**

√x7ᵗʰ **V95.40** **Unspecified spacecraft accident injuring occupant** ▽

√x7ᵗʰ **V95.41** **Spacecraft crash injuring occupant**

√x7ᵗʰ **V95.42** **Forced landing of spacecraft injuring occupant**

√x7ᵗʰ **V95.43** **Spacecraft collision injuring occupant**
Spacecraft collision with any object, fixed, moveable or moving

√x7ᵗʰ **V95.44** **Spacecraft fire injuring occupant**

√x7ᵗʰ **V95.45** **Spacecraft explosion injuring occupant**

√x7ᵗʰ **V95.49** **Other spacecraft accident injuring occupant**

√x7ᵗʰ **V95.8** **Other powered aircraft accidents injuring occupant**

√x7ᵗʰ **V95.9** **Unspecified aircraft accident injuring occupant** ▽
Aircraft accident NOS
Air transport accident NOS

√4ᵗʰ **V96** **Accident to nonpowered aircraft causing injury to occupant**

√5ᵗʰ **V96.0** **Balloon accident injuring occupant**

√x7ᵗʰ **V96.00** **Unspecified balloon accident injuring occupant** ▽

√x7ᵗʰ **V96.01** **Balloon crash injuring occupant**

√x7ᵗʰ **V96.02** **Forced landing of balloon injuring occupant**

√x7ᵗʰ **V96.03** **Balloon collision injuring occupant**
Balloon collision with any object, fixed, moveable or moving

√x7ᵗʰ **V96.04** **Balloon fire injuring occupant**

√x7ᵗʰ **V96.05** **Balloon explosion injuring occupant**

√x7ᵗʰ **V96.09** **Other balloon accident injuring occupant**

√5ᵗʰ **V96.1** **Hang-glider accident injuring occupant**

√x7ᵗʰ **V96.10** **Unspecified hang-glider accident injuring occupant** ▽

√x7ᵗʰ **V96.11** **Hang-glider crash injuring occupant**

√x7ᵗʰ **V96.12** **Forced landing of hang-glider injuring occupant**

√x7ᵗʰ **V96.13** **Hang-glider collision injuring occupant**
Hang-glider collision with any object, fixed, moveable or moving

√x7ᵗʰ **V96.14** **Hang-glider fire injuring occupant**

√x7ᵗʰ **V96.15** **Hang-glider explosion injuring occupant**

√x7ᵗʰ **V96.19** **Other hang-glider accident injuring occupant**

√5ᵗʰ **V96.2** **Glider (nonpowered) accident injuring occupant**

√x7ᵗʰ **V96.20** **Unspecified glider (nonpowered) accident injuring occupant** ▽

√x7ᵗʰ **V96.21** **Glider (nonpowered) crash injuring occupant**

√x7ᵗʰ **V96.22** **Forced landing of glider (nonpowered) injuring occupant**

√x7ᵗʰ **V96.23** **Glider (nonpowered) collision injuring occupant**
Glider (nonpowered) collision with any object, fixed, moveable or moving

√x7ᵗʰ **V96.24** **Glider (nonpowered) fire injuring occupant**

√x7ᵗʰ **V96.25** **Glider (nonpowered) explosion injuring occupant**

√x7ᵗʰ **V96.29** **Other glider (nonpowered) accident injuring occupant**

√x7ᵗʰ **V96.8** **Other nonpowered-aircraft accidents injuring occupant**
Kite carrying a person accident injuring occupant

√x7ᵗʰ **V96.9** **Unspecified nonpowered-aircraft accident injuring occupant** ▽
Nonpowered-aircraft accident NOS

√4ᵗʰ **V97** **Other specified air transport accidents**

√x7ᵗʰ **V97.0** **Occupant of aircraft injured in other specified air transport accidents**
Fall in, on or from aircraft in air transport accident
EXCLUDES 1 accident while boarding or alighting aircraft (V97.1)

√x7ᵗʰ **V97.1** **Person injured while boarding or alighting from aircraft**

√5ᵗʰ **V97.2** **Parachutist accident**

√x7ᵗʰ **V97.21** **Parachutist entangled in object**
Parachutist landing in tree

√x7ᵗʰ **V97.22** **Parachutist injured on landing**

√x7ᵗʰ **V97.29** **Other parachutist accident**

√5ᵗʰ **V97.3** **Person on ground injured in air transport accident**

√x7ᵗʰ **V97.31** **Hit by object falling from aircraft**
Hit by crashing aircraft
Injured by aircraft hitting house
Injured by aircraft hitting car

√x7ᵗʰ **V97.32** **Injured by rotating propeller**

√x7ᵗʰ **V97.33** **Sucked into jet engine**

√x7ᵗʰ **V97.39** **Other injury to person on ground due to air transport accident**

√5ᵗʰ **V97.8** **Other air transport accidents, not elsewhere classified**
EXCLUDES 1 aircraft accident NOS (V95.9)
exposure to changes in air pressure during ascent or descent (W94.-)

√6ᵗʰ **V97.81** **Air transport accident involving military aircraft**

√7ᵗʰ **V97.810** **Civilian aircraft involved in air transport accident with military aircraft**
Passenger in civilian aircraft injured due to accident with military aircraft

EXCLUDES 1 Not coded here   *EXCLUDES 2* Not included here   N Newborn Age : 0   P Pediatric Age : 0-17   M Maternity Age : 12-55   A Adult Age : 15-124

1108   ICD-10-CM 2017

✓7ᵗʰ **V97.811 Civilian injured by military aircraft**

✓7ᵗʰ **V97.818 Other air transport accident involving military aircraft**

✓x7ᵗʰ **V97.89 Other air transport accidents, not elsewhere classified**
Injury from machinery on aircraft

Other and unspecified transport accidents (V98-V99)

EXCLUDES 1   *vehicle accident, type of vehicle unspecified (V89.-)*

The appropriate 7th character is to be added to each code from categories V98-V99.
A   initial encounter
D   subsequent encounter
S   sequela

✓4ᵗʰ **V98 Other specified transport accidents**

✓x7ᵗʰ **V98.0 Accident to, on or involving cable-car, not on rails**
Caught or dragged by cable-car, not on rails
Fall or jump from cable-car, not on rails
Object thrown from or in cable-car, not on rails

✓x7ᵗʰ **V98.1 Accident to, on or involving land-yacht**

✓x7ᵗʰ **V98.2 Accident to, on or involving ice yacht**

✓x7ᵗʰ **V98.3 Accident to, on or involving ski lift**
Accident to, on or involving ski chair-lift
Accident to, on or involving ski-lift with gondola

✓x7ᵗʰ **V98.8 Other specified transport accidents**

✓x7ᵗʰ **V99 Unspecified transport accident**   ▽

Other external causes of accidental injury (W00-X58)

Slipping, tripping, stumbling and falls (W00-W19)

EXCLUDES 1   *assault involving a fall (Y01-Y02)*
fall from animal (V80.-)
fall (in) (from) machinery (in operation) (W28-W31)
fall (in) (from) transport vehicle (V01-V99)
intentional self-harm involving a fall (X80-X81)
EXCLUDES 2   *at risk for fall (history of fall) Z91.81*
fall (in) (from) burning building (X00.-)
fall into fire (X00-X04, X08-X09)

The appropriate 7th character is to be added to each code from categories W00-W19.
A   initial encounter
D   subsequent encounter
S   sequela

✓4ᵗʰ **W00 Fall due to ice and snow**
INCLUDES   pedestrian on foot falling (slipping) on ice and snow
EXCLUDES 1   *fall on (from) ice and snow involving pedestrian conveyance (V00.-)*
fall from stairs and steps not due to ice and snow (W10.-)
AHA: 2016,2Q,4

✓x7ᵗʰ **W00.0 Fall on same level due to ice and snow**

✓x7ᵗʰ **W00.1 Fall from stairs and steps due to ice and snow**

✓x7ᵗʰ **W00.2 Other fall from one level to another due to ice and snow**

✓x7ᵗʰ **W00.9 Unspecified fall due to ice and snow**   ▽

✓4ᵗʰ **W01 Fall on same level from slipping, tripping and stumbling**
INCLUDES   fall on moving sidewalk
EXCLUDES 1   *fall due to bumping (striking) against object (W18.0-)*
fall in shower or bathtub (W18.2-)
fall on same level NOS (W18.30)
fall on same level from slipping, tripping and stumbling due to ice or snow (W00.0)
fall off or from toilet (W18.1-)
slipping, tripping and stumbling NOS (W18.40)
slipping, tripping and stumbling without falling (W18.4-)

✓x7ᵗʰ **W01.0 Fall on same level from slipping, tripping and stumbling without subsequent striking against object**
Falling over animal

✓5ᵗʰ **W01.1 Fall on same level from slipping, tripping and stumbling with subsequent striking against object**

✓x7ᵗʰ **W01.10 Fall on same level from slipping, tripping and stumbling with subsequent striking against unspecified object**   ▽

✓6ᵗʰ **W01.11 Fall on same level from slipping, tripping and stumbling with subsequent striking against sharp object**

✓7ᵗʰ **W01.110 Fall on same level from slipping, tripping and stumbling with subsequent striking against sharp glass**

✓7ᵗʰ **W01.111 Fall on same level from slipping, tripping and stumbling with subsequent striking against power tool or machine**

✓7ᵗʰ **W01.118 Fall on same level from slipping, tripping and stumbling with subsequent striking against other sharp object**

✓7ᵗʰ **W01.119 Fall on same level from slipping, tripping and stumbling with subsequent striking against unspecified sharp object**   ▽

✓6ᵗʰ **W01.19 Fall on same level from slipping, tripping and stumbling with subsequent striking against other object**

✓7ᵗʰ **W01.190 Fall on same level from slipping, tripping and stumbling with subsequent striking against furniture**

✓7ᵗʰ **W01.198 Fall on same level from slipping, tripping and stumbling with subsequent striking against other object**

✓x7ᵗʰ **W03 Other fall on same level due to collision with another person**
Fall due to non-transport collision with other person
EXCLUDES 1   *collision with another person without fall (W51)*
crushed or pushed by a crowd or human stampede (W52)
fall involving pedestrian conveyance (V00-V09)
fall due to ice or snow (W00)
fall on same level NOS (W18.30)
AHA: 2012,4Q,108

✓x7ᵗʰ **W04 Fall while being carried or supported by other persons**
Accidentally dropped while being carried

✓4ᵗʰ **W05 Fall from non-moving wheelchair, nonmotorized scooter and motorized mobility scooter**
EXCLUDES 1   *fall from moving wheelchair (powered) (V00.811)*
fall from moving motorized mobility scooter (V00.831)
fall from nonmotorized scooter (V00.141)

✓x7ᵗʰ **W05.0 Fall from non-moving wheelchair**

✓x7ᵗʰ **W05.1 Fall from non-moving nonmotorized scooter**

✓x7ᵗʰ **W05.2 Fall from non-moving motorized mobility scooter**

✓x7ᵗʰ **W06 Fall from bed**

✓x7ᵗʰ **W07 Fall from chair**

✓x7ᵗʰ **W08 Fall from other furniture**

✓4ᵗʰ **W09 Fall on and from playground equipment**
EXCLUDES 1   *fall involving recreational machinery (W31)*

✓x7ᵗʰ **W09.0 Fall on or from playground slide**

✓x7ᵗʰ **W09.1 Fall from playground swing**

✓x7ᵗʰ **W09.2 Fall on or from jungle gym**

✓x7ᵗʰ **W09.8 Fall on or from other playground equipment**

✓4ᵗʰ **W10 Fall on and from stairs and steps**
EXCLUDES 1   *Fall from stairs and steps due to ice and snow (W00.1)*

✓x7ᵗʰ **W10.0 Fall (on)(from) escalator**

✓x7ᵗʰ **W10.1 Fall (on)(from) sidewalk curb**

✓x7ᵗʰ **W10.2 Fall (on)(from) incline**
Fall (on) (from) ramp

✓x7ᵗʰ **W10.8 Fall (on) (from) other stairs and steps**

✓x7ᵗʰ **W10.9 Fall (on) (from) unspecified stairs and steps**   ▽

✓x7ᵗʰ **W11 Fall on and from ladder**

✓x7ᵗʰ **W12 Fall on and from scaffolding**

✓4ᵗʰ **W13 Fall from, out of or through building or structure**

✓x7ᵗʰ **W13.0 Fall from, out of or through balcony**
Fall from, out of or through railing

✓x7ᵗʰ **W13.1 Fall from, out of or through bridge**

✓x7ᵗʰ **W13.2 Fall from, out of or through roof**

✓x7ᵗʰ **W13.3 Fall through floor**

✓ Additional Character Required	✓x7ᵗʰ Placeholder Alert	Manifestation Dx	▽ Unspecified Dx	▶◀ Revised Text	● New Code	▲ Revised Code Title

✓x7ᵗʰ **W13.4 Fall from, out of or through window**
> EXCLUDES 2   *fall with subsequent striking against sharp glass (W01.110)*

✓x7ᵗʰ **W13.8 Fall from, out of or through other building or structure**
> Fall from, out of or through viaduct
> Fall from, out of or through wall
> Fall from, out of or through flag-pole

✓x7ᵗʰ **W13.9 Fall from, out of or through building, not otherwise specified** ▽
> EXCLUDES 1   *collapse of a building or structure (W20.-)*
> *fall or jump from burning building or structure (X00.-)*

✓x7ᵗʰ **W14 Fall from tree**

✓x7ᵗʰ **W15 Fall from cliff**

✓4ᵗʰ **W16 Fall, jump or diving into water**
> EXCLUDES 1   *accidental non-watercraft drowning and submersion not involving fall (W65-W74)*
> *effects of air pressure from diving (W94.-)*
> *fall into water from watercraft (V90-V94)*
> *hitting an object or against bottom when falling from watercraft (V94.0)*
> EXCLUDES 2   *striking or hitting diving board (W21.4)*

✓5ᵗʰ **W16.0 Fall into swimming pool**
> Fall into swimming pool NOS
> EXCLUDES 1   *fall into empty swimming pool (W17.3)*

    ✓6ᵗʰ **W16.01 Fall into swimming pool striking water surface**

        ✓7ᵗʰ **W16.011 Fall into swimming pool striking water surface causing drowning and submersion**
> EXCLUDES 1   *drowning and submersion while in swimming pool without fall (W67)*

        ✓7ᵗʰ **W16.012 Fall into swimming pool striking water surface causing other injury**

    ✓6ᵗʰ **W16.02 Fall into swimming pool striking bottom**

        ✓7ᵗʰ **W16.021 Fall into swimming pool striking bottom causing drowning and submersion**
> EXCLUDES 1   *drowning and submersion while in swimming pool without fall (W67)*

        ✓7ᵗʰ **W16.022 Fall into swimming pool striking bottom causing other injury**

    ✓6ᵗʰ **W16.03 Fall into swimming pool striking wall**

        ✓7ᵗʰ **W16.031 Fall into swimming pool striking wall causing drowning and submersion**
> EXCLUDES 1   *drowning and submersion while in swimming pool without fall (W67)*

        ✓7ᵗʰ **W16.032 Fall into swimming pool striking wall causing other injury**

✓5ᵗʰ **W16.1 Fall into natural body of water**
> Fall into lake
> Fall into open sea
> Fall into river
> Fall into stream

    ✓6ᵗʰ **W16.11 Fall into natural body of water striking water surface**

        ✓7ᵗʰ **W16.111 Fall into natural body of water striking water surface causing drowning and submersion**
> EXCLUDES 1   *drowning and submersion while in natural body of water without fall (W69)*

        ✓7ᵗʰ **W16.112 Fall into natural body of water striking water surface causing other injury**

    ✓6ᵗʰ **W16.12 Fall into natural body of water striking bottom**

        ✓7ᵗʰ **W16.121 Fall into natural body of water striking bottom causing drowning and submersion**
> EXCLUDES 1   *drowning and submersion while in natural body of water without fall (W69)*

        ✓7ᵗʰ **W16.122 Fall into natural body of water striking bottom causing other injury**

    ✓6ᵗʰ **W16.13 Fall into natural body of water striking side**

        ✓7ᵗʰ **W16.131 Fall into natural body of water striking side causing drowning and submersion**
> EXCLUDES 1   *drowning and submersion while in natural body of water without fall (W69)*

        ✓7ᵗʰ **W16.132 Fall into natural body of water striking side causing other injury**

✓5ᵗʰ **W16.2 Fall in (into) filled bathtub or bucket of water**

    ✓6ᵗʰ **W16.21 Fall in (into) filled bathtub**
> EXCLUDES 1   *fall into empty bathtub (W18.2)*

        ✓7ᵗʰ **W16.211 Fall in (into) filled bathtub causing drowning and submersion**
> EXCLUDES 1   *drowning and submersion while in filled bathtub without fall (W65)*

        ✓7ᵗʰ **W16.212 Fall in (into) filled bathtub causing other injury**

    ✓6ᵗʰ **W16.22 Fall in (into) bucket of water**

        ✓7ᵗʰ **W16.221 Fall in (into) bucket of water causing drowning and submersion**

        ✓7ᵗʰ **W16.222 Fall in (into) bucket of water causing other injury**

✓5ᵗʰ **W16.3 Fall into other water**
> Fall into fountain
> Fall into reservoir

    ✓6ᵗʰ **W16.31 Fall into other water striking water surface**

        ✓7ᵗʰ **W16.311 Fall into other water striking water surface causing drowning and submersion**
> EXCLUDES 1   *drowning and submersion while in other water without fall (W73)*

        ✓7ᵗʰ **W16.312 Fall into other water striking water surface causing other injury**

    ✓6ᵗʰ **W16.32 Fall into other water striking bottom**

        ✓7ᵗʰ **W16.321 Fall into other water striking bottom causing drowning and submersion**
> EXCLUDES 1   *drowning and submersion while in other water without fall (W73)*

        ✓7ᵗʰ **W16.322 Fall into other water striking bottom causing other injury**

    ✓6ᵗʰ **W16.33 Fall into other water striking wall**

        ✓7ᵗʰ **W16.331 Fall into other water striking wall causing drowning and submersion**
> EXCLUDES 1   *drowning and submersion while in other water without fall (W73)*

        ✓7ᵗʰ **W16.332 Fall into other water striking wall causing other injury**

✓5ᵗʰ **W16.4 Fall into unspecified water**

    ✓x7ᵗʰ **W16.41 Fall into unspecified water causing drowning and submersion** ▽

    ✓x7ᵗʰ **W16.42 Fall into unspecified water causing other injury** ▽

✓5ᵗʰ **W16.5 Jumping or diving into swimming pool**

    ✓6ᵗʰ **W16.51 Jumping or diving into swimming pool striking water surface**

        ✓7ᵗʰ **W16.511 Jumping or diving into swimming pool striking water surface causing drowning and submersion**
> EXCLUDES 1   *drowning and submersion while in swimming pool without jumping or diving (W67)*

        ✓7ᵗʰ **W16.512 Jumping or diving into swimming pool striking water surface causing other injury**

    ✓6ᵗʰ **W16.52 Jumping or diving into swimming pool striking bottom**

        ✓7ᵗʰ **W16.521 Jumping or diving into swimming pool striking bottom causing drowning and submersion**
> EXCLUDES 1   *drowning and submersion while in swimming pool without jumping or diving (W67)*

        ✓7ᵗʰ **W16.522 Jumping or diving into swimming pool striking bottom causing other injury**

EXCLUDES 1 Not coded here   EXCLUDES 2 Not included here   N Newborn Age : 0   P Pediatric Age : 0-17   M Maternity Age : 12-55   A Adult Age : 15-124

1110   ICD-10-CM 2017

√6ᵗʰ **W16.53** **Jumping or diving into swimming pool** striking wall

√7ᵗʰ **W16.531** **Jumping or diving into swimming pool striking wall causing** drowning and submersion
EXCLUDES 1 *drowning and submersion while in swimming pool without jumping or diving (W67)*

√7ᵗʰ **W16.532** **Jumping or diving into swimming pool striking wall causing other injury**

√5ᵗʰ **W16.6** **Jumping or diving into** natural body of water
Jumping or diving into lake
Jumping or diving into open sea
Jumping or diving into river
Jumping or diving into stream

√6ᵗʰ **W16.61** **Jumping or diving into natural body of water** striking water surface

√7ᵗʰ **W16.611** **Jumping or diving into natural body of water striking water surface causing** drowning and submersion
EXCLUDES 1 *drowning and submersion while in natural body of water without jumping or diving (W69)*

√7ᵗʰ **W16.612** **Jumping or diving into natural body of water striking water surface causing other injury**

√6ᵗʰ **W16.62** **Jumping or diving into natural body of water** striking bottom

√7ᵗʰ **W16.621** **Jumping or diving into natural body of water striking bottom causing** drowning and submersion
EXCLUDES 1 *drowning and submersion while in natural body of water without jumping or diving (W69)*

√7ᵗʰ **W16.622** **Jumping or diving into natural body of water striking bottom causing other injury**

√5ᵗʰ **W16.7** **Jumping or diving** from boat
EXCLUDES 1 *Fall from boat into water - see watercraft accident (V90–V94)*

√6ᵗʰ **W16.71** **Jumping or diving from boat** striking water surface

√7ᵗʰ **W16.711** **Jumping or diving from boat striking water surface causing** drowning and submersion

√7ᵗʰ **W16.712** **Jumping or diving from boat striking water surface causing other injury**

√6ᵗʰ **W16.72** **Jumping or diving from boat** striking bottom

√7ᵗʰ **W16.721** **Jumping or diving from boat striking bottom causing** drowning and submersion

√7ᵗʰ **W16.722** **Jumping or diving from boat striking bottom causing other injury**

√5ᵗʰ **W16.8** **Jumping or diving into other water**
Jumping or diving into fountain
Jumping or diving into reservoir

√6ᵗʰ **W16.81** **Jumping or diving into other water** striking water surface

√7ᵗʰ **W16.811** **Jumping or diving into other water striking water surface causing** drowning and submersion
EXCLUDES 1 *drowning and submersion while in other water without jumping or diving (W73)*

√7ᵗʰ **W16.812** **Jumping or diving into other water striking water surface causing other injury**

√6ᵗʰ **W16.82** **Jumping or diving into other water** striking bottom

√7ᵗʰ **W16.821** **Jumping or diving into other water striking bottom causing** drowning and submersion
EXCLUDES 1 *drowning and submersion while in other water without jumping or diving (W73)*

√7ᵗʰ **W16.822** **Jumping or diving into other water striking bottom causing other injury**

√6ᵗʰ **W16.83** **Jumping or diving into other water** striking wall

√7ᵗʰ **W16.831** **Jumping or diving into other water striking wall causing** drowning and submersion
EXCLUDES 1 *drowning and submersion while in other water without jumping or diving (W73)*

√7ᵗʰ **W16.832** **Jumping or diving into other water striking wall causing other injury**

√5ᵗʰ **W16.9** **Jumping or diving into unspecified water**

√ₓ7ᵗʰ **W16.91** **Jumping or diving into unspecified water causing** drowning and submersion ▽

√ₓ7ᵗʰ **W16.92** **Jumping or diving into unspecified water causing other injury** ▽

√4ᵗʰ **W17** **Other fall from one level to another**

√ₓ7ᵗʰ **W17.0** **Fall into well**

√ₓ7ᵗʰ **W17.1** **Fall into storm drain or manhole**

√ₓ7ᵗʰ **W17.2** **Fall into hole**
Fall into pit

√ₓ7ᵗʰ **W17.3** **Fall into empty swimming pool**
EXCLUDES 1 *fall into filled swimming pool (W16.0-)*

√ₓ7ᵗʰ **W17.4** **Fall from dock**

√5ᵗʰ **W17.8** **Other fall from one level to another**

√ₓ7ᵗʰ **W17.81** **Fall down embankment (hill)**

√ₓ7ᵗʰ **W17.82** **Fall from (out of) grocery cart**
Fall due to grocery cart tipping over

√ₓ7ᵗʰ **W17.89** **Other fall from one level to another**
Fall from cherry picker
Fall from lifting device
Fall from mobile elevated work platform [MEWP]
Fall from sky lift
AHA: 2015,2Q,6

√4ᵗʰ **W18** **Other slipping, tripping and stumbling and falls**

√5ᵗʰ **W18.0** **Fall due to bumping against object**
Striking against object with subsequent fall
EXCLUDES 1 *fall on same level due to slipping, tripping, or stumbling with subsequent striking against object (W01.1-)*

√ₓ7ᵗʰ **W18.00** **Striking against unspecified object with subsequent fall** ▽

√ₓ7ᵗʰ **W18.01** **Striking against** sports equipment **with subsequent fall**

√ₓ7ᵗʰ **W18.02** **Striking against** glass **with subsequent fall**

√ₓ7ᵗʰ **W18.09** **Striking against other object with subsequent fall**

√5ᵗʰ **W18.1** **Fall from or off toilet**

√ₓ7ᵗʰ **W18.11** **Fall from or off toilet** without subsequent striking against object
Fall from (off) toilet NOS

√ₓ7ᵗʰ **W18.12** **Fall from or off toilet** with subsequent striking against object

√ₓ7ᵗʰ **W18.2** **Fall in (into) shower or empty bathtub**
EXCLUDES 1 *fall in full bathtub causing drowning or submersion (W16.21-)*

√5ᵗʰ **W18.3** **Other and unspecified fall on same level**

√ₓ7ᵗʰ **W18.30** **Fall on same level, unspecified** ▽

√ₓ7ᵗʰ **W18.31** **Fall on same level due to stepping on an object**
Fall on same level due to stepping on an animal
EXCLUDES 1 *slipping, tripping and stumbling without fall due to stepping on animal (W18.41)*

√ₓ7ᵗʰ **W18.39** **Other fall on same level**

√5ᵗʰ **W18.4** **Slipping, tripping and stumbling without falling**
EXCLUDES 1 *collision with another person without fall (W51)*

√ₓ7ᵗʰ **W18.40** **Slipping, tripping and stumbling without falling, unspecified** ▽

√ₓ7ᵗʰ **W18.41** **Slipping, tripping and stumbling without falling due to** stepping on object
Slipping, tripping and stumbling without falling due to stepping on animal
EXCLUDES 1 *slipping, tripping and stumbling with fall due to stepping on animal (W18.31)*

√ₓ7ᵗʰ **W18.42** **Slipping, tripping and stumbling without falling due to** stepping into hole or opening

√ₓ7ᵗʰ **W18.43** **Slipping, tripping and stumbling without falling due to** stepping from one level to another

√ₓ7ᵗʰ **W18.49** **Other slipping, tripping and stumbling without falling**

Chapter 20. External Causes of Morbidity *(side margin)*

√x7th W19 Unspecified fall ▽

    Accidental fall NOS

    AHA: 2012,4Q,95

Exposure to inanimate mechanical forces (W20-W49)

    EXCLUDES 1 *assault ▶(X92-Y09)◀*

        contact or collision with animals or persons (W50-W64)

        exposure to inanimate mechanical forces involving military or war
            operations (Y36.-, Y37.-)

        intentional self-harm (X71-X83)

> The appropriate 7th character is to be added to each code from categories W20-W49.
> A   initial encounter
> D   subsequent encounter
> S   sequela

√4th W20 Struck by thrown, projected or falling object

    Code first any associated:
      cataclysm (X34-X39)
      lightning strike (T75.00)

    EXCLUDES 1 *falling object in machinery accident (W24, W28-W31)*

        falling object in transport accident (V01-V99)

        object set in motion by explosion (W35-W40)

        object set in motion by firearm (W32-W34)

        struck by thrown sports equipment (W21.-)

  √x7th W20.0 Struck by falling object in cave-in

      EXCLUDES 2 *asphyxiation due to cave-in (T71.21)*

  √x7th W20.1 Struck by object due to collapse of building

      EXCLUDES 1 *struck by object due to collapse of burning building*
           (X00.2, X02.2)

  √x7th W20.8 Other cause of strike by thrown, projected or falling object

      EXCLUDES 1 *struck by thrown sports equipment (W21.-)*

√4th W21 Striking against or struck by sports equipment

    EXCLUDES 1 *assault with sports equipment (Y08.0-)*

        striking against or struck by sports equipment with subsequent
           fall (W18.01)

  √5th W21.0 Struck by hit or thrown ball

    √x7th W21.00 Struck by hit or thrown ball, unspecified type ▽

    √x7th W21.01 Struck by football

    √x7th W21.02 Struck by soccer ball

    √x7th W21.03 Struck by baseball

    √x7th W21.04 Struck by golf ball

    √x7th W21.05 Struck by basketball

    √x7th W21.06 Struck by volleyball

    √x7th W21.07 Struck by softball

    √x7th W21.09 Struck by other hit or thrown ball

  √5th W21.1 Struck by bat, racquet or club

    √x7th W21.11 Struck by baseball bat

    √x7th W21.12 Struck by tennis racquet

    √x7th W21.13 Struck by golf club

    √x7th W21.19 Struck by other bat, racquet or club

  √5th W21.2 Struck by hockey stick or puck

    √6th W21.21 Struck by hockey stick

      √7th W21.210 Struck by ice hockey stick

      √7th W21.211 Struck by field hockey stick

    √6th W21.22 Struck by hockey puck

      √7th W21.220 Struck by ice hockey puck

      √7th W21.221 Struck by field hockey puck

  √5th W21.3 Struck by sports foot wear

    √x7th W21.31 Struck by shoe cleats

      Stepped on by shoe cleats

    √x7th W21.32 Struck by skate blades

      Skated over by skate blades

    √x7th W21.39 Struck by other sports foot wear

  √x7th W21.4 Striking against diving board

      Use additional code for subsequent falling into water, if
        applicable (W16.-)

  √5th W21.8 Striking against or struck by other sports equipment

    √x7th W21.81 Striking against or struck by football helmet

    √x7th W21.89 Striking against or struck by other sports
             equipment

  √x7th W21.9 Striking against or struck by unspecified sports ▽
             equipment

√4th W22 Striking against or struck by other objects

    EXCLUDES 1 *striking against or struck by object with subsequent fall*
        (W18.09)

  √5th W22.0 Striking against stationary object

    EXCLUDES 1 *striking against stationary sports equipment (W21.8)*

    √x7th W22.01 Walked into wall

    √x7th W22.02 Walked into lamppost

    √x7th W22.03 Walked into furniture

    √6th W22.04 Striking against wall of swimming pool

      √7th W22.041 Striking against wall of swimming pool
             causing drowning and submersion

          EXCLUDES 1 *drowning and submersion while*
               swimming without striking
               against wall (W67)

      √7th W22.042 Striking against wall of swimming pool
             causing other injury

    √x7th W22.09 Striking against other stationary object

  √5th W22.1 Striking against or struck by automobile airbag

    √x7th W22.10 Striking against or struck by unspecified ▽
             automobile airbag

    √x7th W22.11 Striking against or struck by driver side automobile
             airbag

    √x7th W22.12 Striking against or struck by front passenger side
             automobile airbag

    √x7th W22.19 Striking against or struck by other automobile
             airbag

  √x7th W22.8 Striking against or struck by other objects

      Striking against or struck by object NOS

      EXCLUDES 1 *struck by thrown, projected or falling object (W20.-)*

√4th W23 Caught, crushed, jammed or pinched in or between objects

    EXCLUDES 1 *injury caused by cutting or piercing instruments (W25-W27)*

        injury caused by firearms malfunction (W32.1, W33.1-, W34.1-)

        injury caused by lifting and transmission devices (W24.-)

        injury caused by machinery (W28-W31)

        injury caused by nonpowered hand tools (W27.-)

        injury caused by transport vehicle being used as a means of
           transportation (V01-V99)

        injury caused by struck by thrown, projected or falling object
           (W20.-)

  √x7th W23.0 Caught, crushed, jammed, or pinched between moving
        objects

  √x7th W23.1 Caught, crushed, jammed, or pinched between stationary
        objects

√4th W24 Contact with lifting and transmission devices, not elsewhere classified

    EXCLUDES 1 *transport accidents (V01-V99)*

  √x7th W24.0 Contact with lifting devices, not elsewhere classified

      Contact with chain hoist
      Contact with drive belt
      Contact with pulley (block)

  √x7th W24.1 Contact with transmission devices, not elsewhere classified

      Contact with transmission belt or cable

√x7th W25 Contact with sharp glass

    Code first any associated:
      injury due to flying glass from explosion or firearm discharge
        (W32-W40)
      transport accident (V00-V99)

    EXCLUDES 1 *fall on same level due to slipping, tripping and stumbling with*
        subsequent striking against sharp glass (W01.10)

        striking against sharp glass with subsequent fall (W18.02)

    EXCLUDES 2 *▶glass embedded in skin (W45)◀*

▲√4th W26 Contact with other sharp objects

    EXCLUDES 2 *▶sharp object(s) embedded in skin (W45)◀*

  √x7th W26.0 Contact with knife

    EXCLUDES 1 *contact with electric knife (W29.1)*

  √x7th W26.1 Contact with sword or dagger

  ● **√x7th W26.2 Contact with edge of stiff paper**

      Paper cut

  ● **√x7th W26.8 Contact with other sharp object(s), not elsewhere classified**

      Contact with tin can lid

  ● **√x7th W26.9 Contact with unspecified sharp object(s)** ▽

EXCLUDES 1 Not coded here   *EXCLUDES 2* Not included here   **N** Newborn Age : 0   **P** Pediatric Age : 0-17   **M** Maternity Age : 12-55   **A** Adult Age : 15-124

1112   ICD-10-CM 2017

W19–W26.9 *(side margin)*

✓4ᵗʰ W27 Contact with nonpowered hand tool

  ✓x7ᵗʰ W27.0 Contact with workbench tool

    Contact with auger
    Contact with axe
    Contact with chisel
    Contact with handsaw
    Contact with screwdriver

  ✓x7ᵗʰ W27.1 Contact with garden tool

    Contact with hoe
    Contact with nonpowered lawn mower
    Contact with pitchfork
    Contact with rake

  ✓x7ᵗʰ W27.2 Contact with scissors

  ✓x7ᵗʰ W27.3 Contact with needle (sewing)

    EXCLUDES 1 *contact with hypodermic needle (W46.-)*

  ✓x7ᵗʰ W27.4 Contact with kitchen utensil

    Contact with fork
    Contact with ice-pick
    Contact with can-opener NOS

  ✓x7ᵗʰ W27.5 Contact with paper-cutter

  ✓x7ᵗʰ W27.8 Contact with other nonpowered hand tool

    Contact with nonpowered sewing machine
    Contact with shovel

✓x7ᵗʰ W28 Contact with powered lawn mower

    Powered lawn mower (commercial) (residential)
    EXCLUDES 1 *contact with nonpowered lawn mower (W27.1)*
    EXCLUDES 2 *exposure to electric current (W86.-)*

✓4ᵗʰ W29 Contact with other powered hand tools and household machinery

    EXCLUDES 1 *contact with commercial machinery (W31.82)*
    contact with hot household appliance (X15)
    contact with nonpowered hand tool (W27.-)
    exposure to electric current (W86)

  ✓x7ᵗʰ W29.0 Contact with powered kitchen appliance

    Contact with blender
    Contact with can-opener
    Contact with garbage disposal
    Contact with mixer

  ✓x7ᵗʰ W29.1 Contact with electric knife

  ✓x7ᵗʰ W29.2 Contact with other powered household machinery

    Contact with electric fan
    Contact with powered dryer (clothes) (powered) (spin)
    Contact with washing-machine
    Contact with sewing machine

  ✓x7ᵗʰ W29.3 Contact with powered garden and outdoor hand tools and machinery

    Contact with chainsaw
    Contact with edger
    Contact with garden cultivator (tiller)
    Contact with hedge trimmer
    Contact with other powered garden tool
    EXCLUDES 1 *contact with powered lawn mower (W28)*

  ✓x7ᵗʰ W29.4 Contact with nail gun

  ✓x7ᵗʰ W29.8 Contact with other powered hand tools and household machinery

    Contact with do-it-yourself tool NOS

✓4ᵗʰ W30 Contact with agricultural machinery

    INCLUDES animal-powered farm machine
    EXCLUDES 1 *agricultural transport vehicle accident (V01-V99)*
    explosion of grain store (W40.8)
    exposure to electric current (W86.-)

  ✓x7ᵗʰ W30.0 Contact with combine harvester

    Contact with reaper
    Contact with thresher

  ✓x7ᵗʰ W30.1 Contact with power take-off devices (PTO)

  ✓x7ᵗʰ W30.2 Contact with hay derrick

  ✓x7ᵗʰ W30.3 Contact with grain storage elevator

    EXCLUDES 1 *explosion of grain store (W40.8)*

✓5ᵗʰ W30.8 Contact with other specified agricultural machinery

  ✓x7ᵗʰ W30.81 Contact with agricultural transport vehicle in stationary use

    Contact with agricultural transport vehicle under repair, not on public roadway
    EXCLUDES 1 *agricultural transport vehicle accident (V01-V99)*

  ✓x7ᵗʰ W30.89 Contact with other specified agricultural machinery

  ✓x7ᵗʰ W30.9 Contact with unspecified agricultural machinery ▽

    Contact with farm machinery NOS

✓4ᵗʰ W31 Contact with other and unspecified machinery

    EXCLUDES 1 *contact with agricultural machinery (W30.-)*
    contact with machinery in transport under own power or being towed by a vehicle (V01-V99)
    exposure to electric current (W86)

  ✓x7ᵗʰ W31.0 Contact with mining and earth-drilling machinery

    Contact with bore or drill (land) (seabed)
    Contact with shaft hoist
    Contact with shaft lift
    Contact with undercutter

  ✓x7ᵗʰ W31.1 Contact with metalworking machines

    Contact with abrasive wheel
    Contact with forging machine
    Contact with lathe
    Contact with mechanical shears
    Contact with metal drilling machine
    Contact with milling machine
    Contact with power press
    Contact with rolling-mill
    Contact with metal sawing machine

  ✓x7ᵗʰ W31.2 Contact with powered woodworking and forming machines

    Contact with band saw
    Contact with bench saw
    Contact with circular saw
    Contact with molding machine
    Contact with overhead plane
    Contact with powered saw
    Contact with radial saw
    Contact with sander
    EXCLUDES 1 *nonpowered woodworking tools (W27.0)*

  ✓x7ᵗʰ W31.3 Contact with prime movers

    Contact with gas turbine
    Contact with internal combustion engine
    Contact with steam engine
    Contact with water driven turbine

  ✓5ᵗʰ W31.8 Contact with other specified machinery

    ✓x7ᵗʰ W31.81 Contact with recreational machinery

      Contact with roller coaster

    ✓x7ᵗʰ W31.82 Contact with other commercial machinery

      Contact with commercial electric fan
      Contact with commercial kitchen appliances
      Contact with commercial powered dryer (clothes) (powered) (spin)
      Contact with commercial washing-machine
      Contact with commercial sewing machine
      EXCLUDES 1 *contact with household machinery (W29.-)*
      contact with powered lawn mower (W28)

    ✓x7ᵗʰ W31.83 Contact with special construction vehicle in stationary use

      Contact with special construction vehicle under repair, not on public roadway
      EXCLUDES 1 *special construction vehicle accident (V01-V99)*

    ✓x7ᵗʰ W31.89 Contact with other specified machinery

  ✓x7ᵗʰ W31.9 Contact with unspecified machinery ▽

    Contact with machinery NOS

√4ᵗʰ **W32** **Accidental handgun discharge and malfunction**

INCLUDES   accidental discharge and malfunction of gun for single hand use

accidental discharge and malfunction of pistol

accidental discharge and malfunction of revolver

Handgun discharge and malfunction NOS

EXCLUDES 1   *accidental airgun discharge and malfunction (W34.010, W34.110)*

accidental BB gun discharge and malfunction (W34.010, W34.110)

accidental pellet gun discharge and malfunction (W34.010, W34.110)

accidental shotgun discharge and malfunction (W33.01, W33.11)

assault by handgun discharge (X93)

handgun discharge involving legal intervention (Y35.0-)

handgun discharge involving military or war operations (Y36.4-)

intentional self-harm by handgun discharge (X72)

Very pistol discharge and malfunction (W34.09, W34.19)

√7ᵗʰ **W32.0** **Accidental handgun discharge**

√7ᵗʰ **W32.1** **Accidental handgun malfunction**

Injury due to explosion of handgun (parts)

Injury due to malfunction of mechanism or component of handgun

Injury due to recoil of handgun

Powder burn from handgun

√4ᵗʰ **W33** **Accidental rifle, shotgun and larger firearm discharge and malfunction**

INCLUDES   rifle, shotgun and larger firearm discharge and malfunction NOS

EXCLUDES 1   *accidental airgun discharge and malfunction (W34.010, W34.110)*

accidental BB gun discharge and malfunction (W34.010, W34.110)

accidental handgun discharge and malfunction (W32.-)

accidental pellet gun discharge and malfunction (W34.010, W34.110)

assault by rifle, shotgun and larger firearm discharge (X94)

firearm discharge involving legal intervention (Y35.0-)

firearm discharge involving military or war operations (Y36.4-)

intentional self-harm by rifle, shotgun and larger firearm discharge (X73)

√5ᵗʰ **W33.0** **Accidental rifle, shotgun and larger firearm discharge**

√7ᵗʰ **W33.00** **Accidental discharge of unspecified larger firearm** ▽

Discharge of unspecified larger firearm NOS

√7ᵗʰ **W33.01** **Accidental discharge of shotgun**

Discharge of shotgun NOS

√7ᵗʰ **W33.02** **Accidental discharge of hunting rifle**

Discharge of hunting rifle NOS

√7ᵗʰ **W33.03** **Accidental discharge of machine gun**

Discharge of machine gun NOS

√7ᵗʰ **W33.09** **Accidental discharge of other larger firearm**

Discharge of other larger firearm NOS

√5ᵗʰ **W33.1** **Accidental rifle, shotgun and larger firearm malfunction**

Injury due to explosion of rifle, shotgun and larger firearm (parts)

Injury due to malfunction of mechanism or component of rifle, shotgun and larger firearm

Injury due to piercing, cutting, crushing or pinching due to (by) slide trigger mechanism, scope or other gun part

Injury due to recoil of rifle, shotgun and larger firearm

Powder burn from rifle, shotgun and larger firearm

√7ᵗʰ **W33.10** **Accidental malfunction of unspecified larger firearm** ▽

Malfunction of unspecified larger firearm NOS

√7ᵗʰ **W33.11** **Accidental malfunction of shotgun**

Malfunction of shotgun NOS

√7ᵗʰ **W33.12** **Accidental malfunction of hunting rifle**

Malfunction of hunting rifle NOS

√7ᵗʰ **W33.13** **Accidental malfunction of machine gun**

Malfunction of machine gun NOS

√7ᵗʰ **W33.19** **Accidental malfunction of other larger firearm**

Malfunction of other larger firearm NOS

√4ᵗʰ **W34** **Accidental discharge and malfunction from other and unspecified firearms and guns**

√5ᵗʰ **W34.0** **Accidental discharge from other and unspecified firearms and guns**

√7ᵗʰ **W34.00** **Accidental discharge from unspecified firearms or gun** ▽

Discharge from firearm NOS

Gunshot wound NOS

Shot NOS

√6ᵗʰ **W34.01** **Accidental discharge of gas, air or spring-operated guns**

√7ᵗʰ **W34.010** **Accidental discharge of airgun**

Accidental discharge of BB gun

Accidental discharge of pellet gun

√7ᵗʰ **W34.011** **Accidental discharge of paintball gun**

Accidental injury due to paintball discharge

√7ᵗʰ **W34.018** **Accidental discharge of other gas, air or spring-operated gun**

√7ᵗʰ **W34.09** **Accidental discharge from other specified firearms**

Accidental discharge from Very pistol [flare]

√5ᵗʰ **W34.1** **Accidental malfunction from other and unspecified firearms and guns**

√7ᵗʰ **W34.10** **Accidental malfunction from unspecified firearms or gun** ▽

Firearm malfunction NOS

√6ᵗʰ **W34.11** **Accidental malfunction of gas, air or spring-operated guns**

√7ᵗʰ **W34.110** **Accidental malfunction of airgun**

Accidental malfunction of BB gun

Accidental malfunction of pellet gun

√7ᵗʰ **W34.111** **Accidental malfunction of paintball gun**

Accidental injury due to paintball gun malfunction

√7ᵗʰ **W34.118** **Accidental malfunction of other gas, air or spring-operated gun**

√7ᵗʰ **W34.19** **Accidental malfunction from other specified firearms**

Accidental malfunction from Very pistol [flare]

√x7ᵗʰ **W35** **Explosion and rupture of boiler**

EXCLUDES 1   *explosion and rupture of boiler on watercraft (V93.4)*

√4ᵗʰ **W36** **Explosion and rupture of gas cylinder**

√x7ᵗʰ **W36.1** **Explosion and rupture of aerosol can**

√x7ᵗʰ **W36.2** **Explosion and rupture of air tank**

√x7ᵗʰ **W36.3** **Explosion and rupture of pressurized-gas tank**

√x7ᵗʰ **W36.8** **Explosion and rupture of other gas cylinder**

√x7ᵗʰ **W36.9** **Explosion and rupture of unspecified gas cylinder** ▽

√4ᵗʰ **W37** **Explosion and rupture of pressurized tire, pipe or hose**

√x7ᵗʰ **W37.0** **Explosion of bicycle tire**

√x7ᵗʰ **W37.8** **Explosion and rupture of other pressurized tire, pipe or hose**

√x7ᵗʰ **W38** **Explosion and rupture of other specified pressurized devices**

√x7ᵗʰ **W39** **Discharge of firework**

√4ᵗʰ **W40** **Explosion of other materials**

EXCLUDES 1   *assault by explosive material (X96)*

explosion involving legal intervention (Y35.1-)

explosion involving military or war operations (Y36.-, Y36.2-)

intentional self-harm by explosive material (X75)

√x7ᵗʰ **W40.0** **Explosion of blasting material**

Explosion of blasting cap

Explosion of detonator

Explosion of dynamite

Explosion of explosive (any) used in blasting operations

√x7ᵗʰ **W40.1** **Explosion of explosive gases**

Explosion of acetylene

Explosion of butane

Explosion of coal gas

Explosion in mine NOS

Explosion of explosive gas

Explosion of fire damp

Explosion of gasoline fumes

Explosion of methane

Explosion of propane

✓x7th **W40.8 Explosion of other specified explosive materials**
  Explosion in dump NOS
  Explosion in factory NOS
  Explosion in grain store
  Explosion in munitions
  EXCLUDES 1 *explosion involving legal intervention (Y35.1-)*
        explosion involving military or war operations (Y36.0-,
        Y36.2-)

✓x7th **W40.9 Explosion of unspecified explosive materials**   ▽
  Explosion NOS

✓4th **W42 Exposure to noise**

✓x7th **W42.0 Exposure to supersonic waves**

✓x7th **W42.9 Exposure to other noise**
  Exposure to sound waves NOS

✓4th **W45 Foreign body or object entering through skin**
  INCLUDES ► foreign body or object embedded in skin ◄
        ► nail embedded in skin ◄
  EXCLUDES 2 *contact with hand tools (nonpowered) (powered) (W27-W29)*
        ► *contact with other sharp objects (W26.-)* ◄
        contact with sharp glass (W25.-)
        struck by objects (W20-W22)

✓x7th **W45.0 Nail entering through skin**

✓x7th **W45.8 Other foreign body or object entering through skin**
  Splinter in skin NOS

✓4th **W46 Contact with hypodermic needle**

✓x7th **W46.0 Contact with hypodermic needle**
  Hypodermic needle stick NOS

✓x7th **W46.1 Contact with contaminated hypodermic needle**

✓4th **W49 Exposure to other inanimate mechanical forces**
  INCLUDES exposure to abnormal gravitational [G] forces
        exposure to inanimate mechanical forces NEC
  EXCLUDES 1 *exposure to inanimate mechanical forces involving military or*
        war operations (Y36.-, Y37.-)

✓5th **W49.0 Item causing external constriction**

✓x7th **W49.01 Hair causing external constriction**

✓x7th **W49.02 String or thread causing external constriction**

✓x7th **W49.03 Rubber band causing external constriction**

✓x7th **W49.04 Ring or other jewelry causing external constriction**

✓x7th **W49.09 Other specified item causing external constriction**

✓x7th **W49.9 Exposure to other inanimate mechanical forces**

Exposure to animate mechanical forces (W50-W64)

EXCLUDES 1 *toxic effect of contact with venomous animals and plants (T63.-)*

The appropriate 7th character is to be added to each code from categories
W50-W64.
A   initial encounter
D   subsequent encounter
S   sequela

✓4th **W50 Accidental hit, strike, kick, twist, bite or scratch by another person**
  INCLUDES hit, strike, kick, twist, bite, or scratch by another person NOS
  EXCLUDES 1 *assault by bodily force (Y04)*
        struck by objects (W20-W22)

✓x7th **W50.0 Accidental hit or strike by another person**
  Hit or strike by another person NOS

✓x7th **W50.1 Accidental kick by another person**
  Kick by another person NOS

✓x7th **W50.2 Accidental twist by another person**
  Twist by another person NOS

✓x7th **W50.3 Accidental bite by another person**
  Human bite
  Bite by another person NOS

✓x7th **W50.4 Accidental scratch by another person**
  Scratch by another person NOS

✓x7th **W51 Accidental striking against or bumped into by another person**
  EXCLUDES 1 *assault by striking against or bumping into by another person*
        (Y04.2)
        fall due to collision with another person (W03)

✓x7th **W52 Crushed, pushed or stepped on by crowd or human stampede**
  Crushed, pushed or stepped on by crowd or human stampede with or
  without fall

✓4th **W53 Contact with rodent**
  INCLUDES contact with saliva, feces or urine of rodent

✓5th **W53.0 Contact with mouse**

✓x7th **W53.01 Bitten by mouse**

✓x7th **W53.09 Other contact with mouse**

✓5th **W53.1 Contact with rat**

✓x7th **W53.11 Bitten by rat**

✓x7th **W53.19 Other contact with rat**

✓5th **W53.2 Contact with squirrel**

✓x7th **W53.21 Bitten by squirrel**

✓x7th **W53.29 Other contact with squirrel**

✓5th **W53.8 Contact with other rodent**

✓x7th **W53.81 Bitten by other rodent**

✓x7th **W53.89 Other contact with other rodent**

✓4th **W54 Contact with dog**
  INCLUDES contact with saliva, feces or urine of dog

✓x7th **W54.0 Bitten by dog**

✓x7th **W54.1 Struck by dog**
  Knocked over by dog

✓x7th **W54.8 Other contact with dog**

✓4th **W55 Contact with other mammals**
  INCLUDES contact with saliva, feces or urine of mammal
  EXCLUDES 1 *animal being ridden - see transport accidents*
        bitten or struck by dog (W54)
        bitten or struck by rodent (W53.-)
        contact with marine mammals (W56.-)

✓5th **W55.0 Contact with cat**

✓x7th **W55.01 Bitten by cat**

✓x7th **W55.03 Scratched by cat**

✓x7th **W55.09 Other contact with cat**

✓5th **W55.1 Contact with horse**

✓x7th **W55.11 Bitten by horse**

✓x7th **W55.12 Struck by horse**

✓x7th **W55.19 Other contact with horse**

✓5th **W55.2 Contact with cow**
  Contact with bull

✓x7th **W55.21 Bitten by cow**

✓x7th **W55.22 Struck by cow**
  Gored by bull

✓x7th **W55.29 Other contact with cow**

✓5th **W55.3 Contact with other hoof stock**
  Contact with goats
  Contact with sheep

✓x7th **W55.31 Bitten by other hoof stock**

✓x7th **W55.32 Struck by other hoof stock**
  Gored by goat
  Gored by ram

✓x7th **W55.39 Other contact with other hoof stock**

✓5th **W55.4 Contact with pig**

✓x7th **W55.41 Bitten by pig**

✓x7th **W55.42 Struck by pig**

✓x7th **W55.49 Other contact with pig**

✓5th **W55.5 Contact with raccoon**

✓x7th **W55.51 Bitten by raccoon**

✓x7th **W55.52 Struck by raccoon**

✓x7th **W55.59 Other contact with raccoon**

✓5th **W55.8 Contact with other mammals**

✓x7th **W55.81 Bitten by other mammals**

✓x7th **W55.82 Struck by other mammals**

✓x7th **W55.89 Other contact with other mammals**

✓4th **W56 Contact with nonvenomous marine animal**
  EXCLUDES 1 *contact with venomous marine animal (T63.-)*

✓5th **W56.0 Contact with dolphin**

✓x7th **W56.01 Bitten by dolphin**

✓x7th **W56.02 Struck by dolphin**

✓x7th **W56.09 Other contact with dolphin**

✓ Additional Character Required   ✓x7th Placeholder Alert   Manifestation Dx   ▽ Unspecified Dx   ►◄ Revised Text   ● New Code   ▲ Revised Code Title

ICD-10-CM 2017   **1115**

√5ᵗʰ **W56.1 Contact with** sea lion
  √x7ᵗʰ **W56.11 Bitten by** sea lion
  √x7ᵗʰ **W56.12 Struck by** sea lion
  √x7ᵗʰ **W56.19 Other contact with** sea lion

√5ᵗʰ **W56.2 Contact with** orca
  Contact with killer whale
  √x7ᵗʰ **W56.21 Bitten by** orca
  √x7ᵗʰ **W56.22 Struck by** orca
  √x7ᵗʰ **W56.29 Other contact with** orca

√5ᵗʰ **W56.3 Contact with other marine mammals**
  √x7ᵗʰ **W56.31 Bitten by other marine mammals**
  √x7ᵗʰ **W56.32 Struck by other marine mammals**
  √x7ᵗʰ **W56.39 Other contact with other marine mammals**

√5ᵗʰ **W56.4 Contact with** shark
  √x7ᵗʰ **W56.41 Bitten by** shark
  √x7ᵗʰ **W56.42 Struck by** shark
  √x7ᵗʰ **W56.49 Other contact with** shark

√5ᵗʰ **W56.5 Contact with other fish**
  √x7ᵗʰ **W56.51 Bitten by other fish**
  √x7ᵗʰ **W56.52 Struck by other fish**
  √x7ᵗʰ **W56.59 Other contact with other fish**

√5ᵗʰ **W56.8 Contact with other nonvenomous marine animals**
  √x7ᵗʰ **W56.81 Bitten by other nonvenomous marine animals**
  √x7ᵗʰ **W56.82 Struck by other nonvenomous marine animals**
  √x7ᵗʰ **W56.89 Other contact with other nonvenomous marine animals**

√x7ᵗʰ **W57 Bitten or stung by nonvenomous insect and other nonvenomous arthropods**
  EXCLUDES 1 *contact with venomous insects and arthropods (T63.2-, T63.3-, T63.4-)*

√4ᵗʰ **W58 Contact with crocodile or alligator**

√5ᵗʰ **W58.0 Contact with** alligator
  √x7ᵗʰ **W58.01 Bitten by** alligator
  √x7ᵗʰ **W58.02 Struck by** alligator
  √x7ᵗʰ **W58.03 Crushed by** alligator
  √x7ᵗʰ **W58.09 Other contact with** alligator

√5ᵗʰ **W58.1 Contact with** crocodile
  √x7ᵗʰ **W58.11 Bitten by** crocodile
  √x7ᵗʰ **W58.12 Struck by** crocodile
  √x7ᵗʰ **W58.13 Crushed by** crocodile
  √x7ᵗʰ **W58.19 Other contact with** crocodile

√4ᵗʰ **W59 Contact with other nonvenomous reptiles**
  EXCLUDES 1 *contact with venomous reptile (T63.0-, T63.1-)*

√5ᵗʰ **W59.0 Contact with nonvenomous lizards**
  √x7ᵗʰ **W59.01 Bitten by nonvenomous lizards**
  √x7ᵗʰ **W59.02 Struck by nonvenomous lizards**
  √x7ᵗʰ **W59.09 Other contact with nonvenomous lizards**
    Exposure to nonvenomous lizards

√5ᵗʰ **W59.1 Contact with nonvenomous** snakes
  √x7ᵗʰ **W59.11 Bitten by nonvenomous snake**
  √x7ᵗʰ **W59.12 Struck by nonvenomous snake**
  √x7ᵗʰ **W59.13 Crushed by nonvenomous snake**
  √x7ᵗʰ **W59.19 Other contact with nonvenomous snake**

√5ᵗʰ **W59.2 Contact with** turtles
  EXCLUDES 1 *contact with tortoises (W59.8-)*
  √x7ᵗʰ **W59.21 Bitten by turtle**
  √x7ᵗʰ **W59.22 Struck by turtle**
  √x7ᵗʰ **W59.29 Other contact with turtle**
    Exposure to turtles

√5ᵗʰ **W59.8 Contact with other nonvenomous reptiles**
  √x7ᵗʰ **W59.81 Bitten by other nonvenomous reptiles**
  √x7ᵗʰ **W59.82 Struck by other nonvenomous reptiles**
  √x7ᵗʰ **W59.83 Crushed by other nonvenomous reptiles**
  √x7ᵗʰ **W59.89 Other contact with other nonvenomous reptiles**

√x7ᵗʰ **W60 Contact with nonvenomous plant thorns and spines and sharp leaves**
  EXCLUDES 1 *contact with venomous plants (T63.7-)*

√4ᵗʰ **W61 Contact with birds (domestic) (wild)**
  INCLUDES contact with excreta of birds

√5ᵗʰ **W61.0 Contact with** parrot
  √x7ᵗʰ **W61.01 Bitten by** parrot
  √x7ᵗʰ **W61.02 Struck by** parrot
  √x7ᵗʰ **W61.09 Other contact with** parrot
    Exposure to parrots

√5ᵗʰ **W61.1 Contact with** macaw
  √x7ᵗʰ **W61.11 Bitten by** macaw
  √x7ᵗʰ **W61.12 Struck by** macaw
  √x7ᵗʰ **W61.19 Other contact with** macaw
    Exposure to macaws

√5ᵗʰ **W61.2 Contact with other** psittacines
  √x7ᵗʰ **W61.21 Bitten by other psittacines**
  √x7ᵗʰ **W61.22 Struck by other psittacines**
  √x7ᵗʰ **W61.29 Other contact with other psittacines**
    Exposure to other psittacines

√5ᵗʰ **W61.3 Contact with** chicken
  √x7ᵗʰ **W61.32 Struck by chicken**
  √x7ᵗʰ **W61.33 Pecked by chicken**
  √x7ᵗʰ **W61.39 Other contact with chicken**
    Exposure to chickens

√5ᵗʰ **W61.4 Contact with** turkey
  √x7ᵗʰ **W61.42 Struck by turkey**
  √x7ᵗʰ **W61.43 Pecked by turkey**
  √x7ᵗʰ **W61.49 Other contact with turkey**

√5ᵗʰ **W61.5 Contact with** goose
  √x7ᵗʰ **W61.51 Bitten by goose**
  √x7ᵗʰ **W61.52 Struck by goose**
  √x7ᵗʰ **W61.59 Other contact with goose**

√5ᵗʰ **W61.6 Contact with** duck
  √x7ᵗʰ **W61.61 Bitten by duck**
  √x7ᵗʰ **W61.62 Struck by duck**
  √x7ᵗʰ **W61.69 Other contact with duck**

√5ᵗʰ **W61.9 Contact with other birds**
  √x7ᵗʰ **W61.91 Bitten by other birds**
  √x7ᵗʰ **W61.92 Struck by other birds**
  √x7ᵗʰ **W61.99 Other contact with other birds**
    Contact with bird NOS

√4ᵗʰ **W62 Contact with nonvenomous amphibians**
  EXCLUDES 1 *contact with venomous amphibians (T63.81-R63.83)*
  √x7ᵗʰ **W62.0 Contact with nonvenomous** frogs
  √x7ᵗʰ **W62.1 Contact with nonvenomous** toads
  √x7ᵗʰ **W62.9 Contact with other nonvenomous amphibians**

√x7ᵗʰ **W64 Exposure to other animate mechanical forces**
  INCLUDES exposure to nonvenomous animal NOS
  EXCLUDES 1 *contact with venomous animal (T63.-)*

Accidental non-transport drowning and submersion (W65-W74)

EXCLUDES 1 *accidental drowning and submersion due to fall into water (W16.-)*
accidental drowning and submersion due to water transport accident (V90.-, V92.-)
EXCLUDES 2 *accidental drowning and submersion due to cataclysm (X34-X39)*

The appropriate 7th character is to be added to each code from categories W65-W74.
A initial encounter
D subsequent encounter
S sequela

√x7ᵗʰ **W65 Accidental drowning and submersion while in** bath-tub
  EXCLUDES 1 *accidental drowning and submersion due to fall in (into) bathtub (W16.211)*

☑7ᵗʰ **W67** **Accidental drowning and submersion while in** swimming-pool
     EXCLUDES 1   *accidental drowning and submersion due to fall into swimming pool (W16.011, W16.021, W16.031)*
            accidental drowning and submersion due to striking into wall of swimming pool (W22.041)

☑7ᵗʰ **W69** **Accidental drowning and submersion while in** natural water
     Accidental drowning and submersion while in lake
     Accidental drowning and submersion while in open sea
     Accidental drowning and submersion while in river
     Accidental drowning and submersion while in stream
     EXCLUDES 1   *accidental drowning and submersion due to fall into natural body of water (W16.111, W16.121, W16.131)*

☑7ᵗʰ **W73** **Other specified cause of accidental non-transport drowning and submersion**
     Accidental drowning and submersion while in quenching tank
     Accidental drowning and submersion while in reservoir
     EXCLUDES 1   *accidental drowning and submersion due to fall into other water (W16.311, W16.321, W16.331)*

☑7ᵗʰ **W74** **Unspecified cause of accidental drowning and submersion** ▽
     Drowning NOS

Exposure to electric current, radiation and extreme ambient air temperature and pressure (W85-W99)

EXCLUDES 1   *exposure to:*
     failure in dosage of radiation or temperature during surgical and medical care (Y63.2-Y63.5)
     lightning (T75.0-)
     natural cold (X31)
     natural heat (X30)
     natural radiation NOS (X39)
     radiological procedure and radiotherapy (Y84.2)
     sunlight (X32)

The appropriate 7th character is to be added to each code from categories W85-W99.
A   initial encounter
D   subsequent encounter
S   sequela

☑7ᵗʰ **W85** **Exposure to electric transmission lines**
     Broken power line

☑4ᵗʰ **W86** **Exposure to other specified electric current**
     ☑7ᵗʰ **W86.0** **Exposure to domestic wiring and appliances**
     ☑7ᵗʰ **W86.1** **Exposure to industrial wiring, appliances and electrical machinery**
         Exposure to conductors
         Exposure to control apparatus
         Exposure to electrical equipment and machinery
         Exposure to transformers
     ☑7ᵗʰ **W86.8** **Exposure to other electric current**
         Exposure to wiring and appliances in or on farm (not farmhouse)
         Exposure to wiring and appliances outdoors
         Exposure to wiring and appliances in or on public building
         Exposure to wiring and appliances in or on residential institutions
         Exposure to wiring and appliances in or on schools

☑4ᵗʰ **W88** **Exposure to ionizing radiation**
     EXCLUDES 1   *exposure to sunlight (X32)*
     ☑7ᵗʰ **W88.0** **Exposure to** X-rays
     ☑7ᵗʰ **W88.1** **Exposure to** radioactive isotopes
     ☑7ᵗʰ **W88.8** **Exposure to other ionizing radiation**

☑4ᵗʰ **W89** **Exposure to man-made visible and ultraviolet light**
     INCLUDES   exposure to welding light (arc)
     EXCLUDES 1   ▶*exposure to sunlight (X32)*◀
     ☑7ᵗʰ **W89.0** **Exposure to** welding light (arc)
     ☑7ᵗʰ **W89.1** **Exposure to** tanning bed
     ☑7ᵗʰ **W89.8** **Exposure to other man-made visible and ultraviolet light**
     ☑7ᵗʰ **W89.9** **Exposure to unspecified man-made visible and ultraviolet light** ▽

☑4ᵗʰ **W90** **Exposure to other nonionizing radiation**
     EXCLUDES 1   *exposure to sunlight (X32)*
     ☑7ᵗʰ **W90.0** **Exposure to** radiofrequency
     ☑7ᵗʰ **W90.1** **Exposure to** infrared radiation
     ☑7ᵗʰ **W90.2** **Exposure to** laser radiation
     ☑7ᵗʰ **W90.8** **Exposure to other nonionizing radiation**

☑7ᵗʰ **W92** **Exposure to excessive heat of man-made origin**

☑4ᵗʰ **W93** **Exposure to excessive cold of man-made origin**
     ☑5ᵗʰ **W93.0** **Contact with or inhalation of** dry ice
         ☑7ᵗʰ **W93.01** **Contact with dry ice**
         ☑7ᵗʰ **W93.02** **Inhalation of dry ice**
     ☑5ᵗʰ **W93.1** **Contact with or inhalation of** liquid air
         ☑7ᵗʰ **W93.11** **Contact with liquid air**
            Contact with liquid hydrogen
            Contact with liquid nitrogen
         ☑7ᵗʰ **W93.12** **Inhalation of liquid air**
            Inhalation of liquid hydrogen
            Inhalation of liquid nitrogen
     ☑7ᵗʰ **W93.2** **Prolonged exposure in deep freeze unit or refrigerator**
     ☑7ᵗʰ **W93.8** **Exposure to other excessive cold of man-made origin**

☑4ᵗʰ **W94** **Exposure to high and low air pressure and changes in air pressure**
     ☑7ᵗʰ **W94.0** **Exposure to prolonged high air pressure**
     ☑5ᵗʰ **W94.1** **Exposure to prolonged low air pressure**
         ☑7ᵗʰ **W94.11** **Exposure to residence or prolonged visit at high altitude**
         ☑7ᵗʰ **W94.12** **Exposure to other prolonged low air pressure**
     ☑5ᵗʰ **W94.2** **Exposure to rapid changes in air pressure during** ascent
         ☑7ᵗʰ **W94.21** **Exposure to reduction in atmospheric pressure while surfacing from** deep-water diving
         ☑7ᵗʰ **W94.22** **Exposure to reduction in atmospheric pressure while surfacing from** underground
         ☑7ᵗʰ **W94.23** **Exposure to sudden change in air pressure in** aircraft **during ascent**
         ☑7ᵗʰ **W94.29** **Exposure to other rapid changes in air pressure during ascent**
     ☑5ᵗʰ **W94.3** **Exposure to rapid changes in air pressure during** descent
         ☑7ᵗʰ **W94.31** **Exposure to sudden change in air pressure in** aircraft **during descent**
         ☑7ᵗʰ **W94.32** **Exposure to high air pressure from rapid descent in** water
         ☑7ᵗʰ **W94.39** **Exposure to other rapid changes in air pressure during descent**

☑7ᵗʰ **W99** **Exposure to other man-made environmental factors**

Exposure to smoke, fire and flames (X00-X08)

EXCLUDES 1   *arson (X97)*
EXCLUDES 2   *explosions (W35-W40)*
     lightning (T75.0-)
     transport accident (V01-V99)

The appropriate 7th character is to be added to each code from categories X00-X08.
A   initial encounter
D   subsequent encounter
S   sequela

☑4ᵗʰ **X00** **Exposure to** uncontrolled fire **in building or structure**
     INCLUDES   conflagration in building or structure
     Code first any associated cataclysm
     EXCLUDES 2   *exposure to ignition or melting of nightwear (X05)*
         exposure to ignition or melting of other clothing and apparel (X06.-)
         exposure to other specified smoke, fire and flames (X08.-)
     AHA: 2016,2Q,5
     ☑7ᵗʰ **X00.0** **Exposure to** flames **in uncontrolled fire in building or structure**
     ☑7ᵗʰ **X00.1** **Exposure to** smoke **in uncontrolled fire in building or structure**
     ☑7ᵗʰ **X00.2** **Injury due to collapse of burning building or structure in uncontrolled fire**
         EXCLUDES 1   *injury due to collapse of building not on fire (W20.1)*
     ☑7ᵗʰ **X00.3** **Fall from burning building or structure in uncontrolled fire**
     ☑7ᵗʰ **X00.4** **Hit by object from burning building or structure in uncontrolled fire**
     ☑7ᵗʰ **X00.5** **Jump from burning building or structure in uncontrolled fire**
     ☑7ᵗʰ **X00.8** **Other exposure to uncontrolled fire in building or structure**

☑4ᵗʰ **X01** **Exposure to uncontrolled fire, not in building or structure**
     INCLUDES   exposure to forest fire
     ☑7ᵗʰ **X01.0** **Exposure to** flames **in uncontrolled fire, not in building or structure**
     ☑7ᵗʰ **X01.1** **Exposure to** smoke **in uncontrolled fire, not in building or structure**

☑ Additional Character Required   ☑7ᵗʰ Placeholder Alert   Manifestation Dx   ▽ Unspecified Dx   ▶◀ Revised Text   ● New Code   ▲ Revised Code Title

✓x7ᵗʰ **X01.3** Fall due to **uncontrolled fire, not in building or structure**

✓x7ᵗʰ **X01.4** Hit by object due to uncontrolled fire, not in building or structure

✓x7ᵗʰ **X01.8** Other exposure to uncontrolled fire, not in building or structure

✓4ᵗʰ **X02** Exposure to controlled fire in building or structure

    INCLUDES   exposure to fire in fireplace
           exposure to fire in stove

✓x7ᵗʰ **X02.0** Exposure to flames in controlled fire in building or structure

✓x7ᵗʰ **X02.1** Exposure to smoke in controlled fire in building or structure

✓x7ᵗʰ **X02.2** Injury due to collapse of burning building or structure in controlled fire

      EXCLUDES 1   *injury due to collapse of building not on fire (W20.1)*

✓x7ᵗʰ **X02.3** Fall from burning building or structure in controlled fire

✓x7ᵗʰ **X02.4** Hit by object from burning building or structure in controlled fire

✓x7ᵗʰ **X02.5** Jump from burning building or structure in controlled fire

✓x7ᵗʰ **X02.8** Other exposure to controlled fire in building or structure

✓4ᵗʰ **X03** Exposure to controlled fire, not in building or structure

    INCLUDES   exposure to bon fire
           exposure to camp-fire
           exposure to trash fire

✓x7ᵗʰ **X03.0** Exposure to flames in controlled fire, not in building or structure

✓x7ᵗʰ **X03.1** Exposure to smoke in controlled fire, not in building or structure

✓x7ᵗʰ **X03.3** Fall due to controlled fire, not in building or structure

✓x7ᵗʰ **X03.4** Hit by object due to controlled fire, not in building or structure

✓x7ᵗʰ **X03.8** Other exposure to controlled fire, not in building or structure

✓x7ᵗʰ **X04** Exposure to ignition of highly flammable material

    Exposure to ignition of gasoline
    Exposure to ignition of kerosene
    Exposure to ignition of petrol

      EXCLUDES 2   *exposure to ignition or melting of nightwear (X05)*
            exposure to ignition or melting of other clothing and apparel (X06)

    AHA: 2016,2Q,4

✓x7ᵗʰ **X05** Exposure to ignition or melting of nightwear

      EXCLUDES 2   *exposure to uncontrolled fire in building or structure (X00.-)*
            exposure to uncontrolled fire, not in building or structure (X01.-)
            exposure to controlled fire in building or structure (X02.-)
            exposure to controlled fire, not in building or structure (X03.-)
            exposure to ignition of highly flammable materials (X04.-)

✓4ᵗʰ **X06** Exposure to ignition or melting of other clothing and apparel

      EXCLUDES 2   *exposure to uncontrolled fire in building or structure (X00.-)*
            exposure to uncontrolled fire, not in building or structure (X01.-)
            exposure to controlled fire in building or structure (X02.-)
            exposure to controlled fire, not in building or structure (X03.-)
            exposure to ignition of highly flammable materials (X04.-)

✓x7ᵗʰ **X06.0** Exposure to ignition of plastic jewelry

✓x7ᵗʰ **X06.1** Exposure to melting of plastic jewelry

✓x7ᵗʰ **X06.2** Exposure to ignition of other clothing and apparel

✓x7ᵗʰ **X06.3** Exposure to melting of other clothing and apparel

✓4ᵗʰ **X08** Exposure to other specified smoke, fire and flames

    ✓5ᵗʰ **X08.0** Exposure to bed fire

      Exposure to mattress fire

      ✓x7ᵗʰ **X08.00** Exposure to bed fire due to unspecified burning material   ▽

      ✓x7ᵗʰ **X08.01** Exposure to bed fire due to burning cigarette

      ✓x7ᵗʰ **X08.09** Exposure to bed fire due to other burning material

    ✓5ᵗʰ **X08.1** Exposure to sofa fire

      ✓x7ᵗʰ **X08.10** Exposure to sofa fire due to unspecified burning material   ▽

      ✓x7ᵗʰ **X08.11** Exposure to sofa fire due to burning cigarette

      ✓x7ᵗʰ **X08.19** Exposure to sofa fire due to other burning material

    ✓5ᵗʰ **X08.2** Exposure to other furniture fire

      ✓x7ᵗʰ **X08.20** Exposure to other furniture fire due to unspecified burning material   ▽

      ✓x7ᵗʰ **X08.21** Exposure to other furniture fire due to burning cigarette

---

      ✓x7ᵗʰ **X08.29** Exposure to other furniture fire due to other burning material

    ✓x7ᵗʰ **X08.8** Exposure to other specified smoke, fire and flames

Contact with heat and hot substances (X10-X19)

      EXCLUDES 1   *exposure to excessive natural heat (X30)*
            exposure to fire and flames (X00-X09)

The appropriate 7th character is to be added to each code from categories X10-X19.
A   initial encounter
D   subsequent encounter
S   sequela

✓4ᵗʰ **X10** Contact with hot drinks, food, fats and cooking oils

✓x7ᵗʰ **X10.0** Contact with hot drinks

✓x7ᵗʰ **X10.1** Contact with hot food

✓x7ᵗʰ **X10.2** Contact with fats and cooking oils

✓4ᵗʰ **X11** Contact with hot tap-water

    INCLUDES   contact with boiling tap-water
           contact with boiling water NOS

      EXCLUDES 1   *contact with water heated on stove (X12)*

✓x7ᵗʰ **X11.0** Contact with hot water in bath or tub

      EXCLUDES 1   *contact with running hot water in bath or tub (X11.1)*

✓x7ᵗʰ **X11.1** Contact with running hot water

    Contact with hot water running out of hose
    Contact with hot water running out of tap

✓x7ᵗʰ **X11.8** Contact with other hot tap-water

    Contact with hot water in bucket
    Contact with hot tap-water NOS

✓x7ᵗʰ **X12** Contact with other hot fluids

    Contact with water heated on stove
      EXCLUDES 1   *hot (liquid) metals (X18)*

✓4ᵗʰ **X13** Contact with steam and other hot vapors

✓x7ᵗʰ **X13.0** Inhalation of steam and other hot vapors

✓x7ᵗʰ **X13.1** Other contact with steam and other hot vapors

✓4ᵗʰ **X14** Contact with hot air and other hot gases

✓x7ᵗʰ **X14.0** Inhalation of hot air and gases

✓x7ᵗʰ **X14.1** Other contact with hot air and other hot gases

✓4ᵗʰ **X15** Contact with hot household appliances

      EXCLUDES 1   *contact with heating appliances (X16)*
            contact with powered household appliances (W29.-)
            exposure to controlled fire in building or structure due to household appliance (X02.8)
            exposure to household appliances electrical current (W86.0)

✓x7ᵗʰ **X15.0** Contact with hot stove (kitchen)

✓x7ᵗʰ **X15.1** Contact with hot toaster

✓x7ᵗʰ **X15.2** Contact with hotplate

✓x7ᵗʰ **X15.3** Contact with hot saucepan or skillet

✓x7ᵗʰ **X15.8** Contact with other hot household appliances

    Contact with cooker
    Contact with kettle
    Contact with light bulbs

✓x7ᵗʰ **X16** Contact with hot heating appliances, radiators and pipes

      EXCLUDES 1   *contact with powered appliances (W29.-)*
            exposure to controlled fire in building or structure due to appliance (X02.8)
            exposure to industrial appliances electrical current (W86.1)

✓x7ᵗʰ **X17** Contact with hot engines, machinery and tools

      EXCLUDES 1   *contact with hot heating appliances, radiators and pipes (X16)*
            contact with hot household appliances (X15)

✓x7ᵗʰ **X18** Contact with other hot metals

    Contact with liquid metal

✓x7ᵗʰ **X19** Contact with other heat and hot substances

      EXCLUDES 1   *objects that are not normally hot, e.g., an object made hot by a house fire (X00-X09)*

EXCLUDES 1 Not coded here   EXCLUDES 2 Not included here   Ⓝ Newborn Age : 0   Ⓟ Pediatric Age : 0-17   Ⓜ Maternity Age : 12-55   Ⓐ Adult Age : 15-124

1118   ICD-10-CM 2017

Exposure to forces of nature (X30-X39)

The appropriate 7th character is to be added to each code from categories X30-X39.
A   initial encounter
D   subsequent encounter
S   sequela

✓x7th **X30   Exposure to excessive natural heat**
     Exposure to excessive heat as the cause of sunstroke
     Exposure to heat NOS
     EXCLUDES 1   *excessive heat of man-made origin (W92)*
                 exposure to man-made radiation (W89)
                 exposure to sunlight (X32)
                 exposure to tanning bed (W89)

✓x7th **X31   Exposure to excessive natural cold**
     Excessive cold as the cause of chilblains NOS
     Excessive cold as the cause of immersion foot or hand
     Exposure to cold NOS
     Exposure to weather conditions
     EXCLUDES 1   *cold of man-made origin (W93.-)*
                 contact with or inhalation of dry ice (W93.-)
                 contact with or inhalation of liquefied gas (W93.-)

✓x7th **X32   Exposure to sunlight**
     EXCLUDES 1   *man-made radiation (tanning bed) (W89)*

✓x7th **X34   Earthquake**
     EXCLUDES 2   *tidal wave (tsunami) due to earthquake (X37.41)*

✓x7th **X35   Volcanic eruption**
     EXCLUDES 2   *tidal wave (tsunami) due to volcanic eruption (X37.41)*

✓4th **X36   Avalanche, landslide and other earth movements**
     INCLUDES   victim of mudslide of cataclysmic nature
     EXCLUDES 1   *earthquake (X34)*
     EXCLUDES 2   *transport accident involving collision with avalanche or landslide not in motion (V01-V99)*

   ✓x7th **X36.0   Collapse of dam or man-made structure causing earth movement**

   ✓x7th **X36.1   Avalanche, landslide, or mudslide**

✓4th **X37   Cataclysmic storm**

   ✓x7th **X37.0   Hurricane**
       Storm surge
       Typhoon

   ✓x7th **X37.1   Tornado**
       Cyclone
       Twister

   ✓x7th **X37.2   Blizzard (snow)(ice)**

   ✓x7th **X37.3   Dust storm**

   ✓5th **X37.4   Tidalwave**

     ✓x7th **X37.41   Tidal wave due to earthquake or volcanic eruption**
         Tidal wave NOS
         Tsunami

     ✓x7th **X37.42   Tidal wave due to storm**

     ✓x7th **X37.43   Tidal wave due to landslide**

   ✓x7th **X37.8   Other cataclysmic storms**
       Cloudburst
       Torrential rain
       EXCLUDES 2   *flood (X38)*

   ✓x7th **X37.9   Unspecified cataclysmic storm**   ▽
       Storm NOS
       EXCLUDES 1   *collapse of dam or man-made structure causing earth movement (X36.0)*

✓x7th **X38   Flood**
     Flood arising from remote storm
     Flood of cataclysmic nature arising from melting snow
     Flood resulting directly from storm
     EXCLUDES 1   *collapse of dam or man-made structure causing earth movement (X36.0)*
                 tidal wave NOS (X37.41)
                 tidal wave caused by storm (X37.42)

✓4th **X39   Exposure to other forces of nature**

   ✓5th **X39.0   Exposure to natural radiation**
       EXCLUDES 1   *contact with and (suspected) exposure to radon and other naturally occuring radiation* ▶*(Z77.123)*◀
                 exposure to man-made radiation (W88-W90)
                 exposure to sunlight (X32)

     ✓x7th **X39.01   Exposure to radon**

     ✓x7th **X39.08   Exposure to other natural radiation**

   ✓x7th **X39.8   Other exposure to forces of nature**

▶Overexertion and strenuous or repetitive movements (X50)◀

● ✓x7th **X50   Overexertion and strenuous or repetitive movements**

     The appropriate 7th character is to be added to each code from category X50.
     A   initial encounter
     D   subsequent encounter
     S   sequela

●   ✓x7th **X50.0   Overexertion from strenuous movement or load**
       Lifting heavy objects
       Lifting weights

●   ✓x7th **X50.1   Overexertion from prolonged static or awkward postures**
       Prolonged bending
       Prolonged kneeling
       Prolonged reaching
       Prolonged sitting
       Prolonged standing
       Prolonged twisting
       Static bending
       Static kneeling
       Static reaching
       Static sitting
       Static standing
       Static twisting

●   ✓x7th **X50.3   Overexertion from repetitive movements**
       Use of hand as hammer
       EXCLUDES 2   *overuse from prolonged static or awkward postures (X50.1)*

●   ✓x7th **X50.9   Other and unspecified overexertion or strenuous movements or postures**
       Contact pressure
       Contact stress

Accidental exposure to other specified factors (X52-X58)

The appropriate 7th character is to be added to each code from categories X52-X58.
A   initial encounter
D   subsequent encounter
S   sequela

✓x7th **X52   Prolonged stay in weightless environment**
     Weightlessness in spacecraft (simulator)

✓x7th **X58   Exposure to other specified factors**
     Accident NOS
     Exposure NOS

Intentional self-harm (X71-X83)

Purposely self-inflicted injury
Suicide (attempted)

The appropriate 7th character is to be added to each code from categories X71-X83.
A   initial encounter
D   subsequent encounter
S   sequela

✓4th **X71   Intentional self-harm by drowning and submersion**

   ✓x7th **X71.0   Intentional self-harm by drowning and submersion while in bathtub**

   ✓x7th **X71.1   Intentional self-harm by drowning and submersion while in swimming pool**

   ✓x7th **X71.2   Intentional self-harm by drowning and submersion after jump into swimming pool**

   ✓x7th **X71.3   Intentional self-harm by drowning and submersion in natural water**

   ✓x7th **X71.8   Other intentional self-harm by drowning and submersion**

   ✓x7th **X71.9   Intentional self-harm by drowning and submersion, unspecified**   ▽

☑ Additional Character Required   ✓x7th Placeholder Alert   Manifestation Dx   ▽ Unspecified Dx   ▶◀ Revised Text   ● New Code   ▲ Revised Code Title

Chapter 20. External Causes of Morbidity

√x7th **X72 Intentional self-harm by handgun discharge**
Intentional self-harm by gun for single hand use
Intentional self-harm by pistol
Intentional self-harm by revolver
EXCLUDES 1   Very pistol (X74.8)

√4th **X73 Intentional self-harm by rifle, shotgun and larger firearm discharge**
EXCLUDES 1   airgun (X74.01)

√x7th **X73.0** Intentional self-harm by shotgun discharge
√x7th **X73.1** Intentional self-harm by hunting rifle discharge
√x7th **X73.2** Intentional self-harm by machine gun discharge
√x7th **X73.8** Intentional self-harm by other larger firearm discharge
√x7th **X73.9** Intentional self-harm by unspecified larger firearm discharge ▽

√4th **X74 Intentional self-harm by other and unspecified firearm and gun discharge**

√5th **X74.0** Intentional self-harm by gas, air or spring-operated guns
√x7th   **X74.01** Intentional self-harm by airgun
Intentional self-harm by BB gun discharge
Intentional self-harm by pellet gun discharge
√x7th   **X74.02** Intentional self-harm by paintball gun
√x7th   **X74.09** Intentional self-harm by other gas, air or spring-operated gun
√x7th **X74.8** Intentional self-harm by other firearm discharge
Intentional self-harm by Very pistol [flare] discharge
√x7th **X74.9** Intentional self-harm by unspecified firearm discharge ▽

√x7th **X75 Intentional self-harm by explosive material**

√x7th **X76 Intentional self-harm by smoke, fire and flames**

√4th **X77 Intentional self-harm by steam, hot vapors and hot objects**
√x7th **X77.0** Intentional self-harm by steam or hot vapors
√x7th **X77.1** Intentional self-harm by hot tap water
√x7th **X77.2** Intentional self-harm by other hot fluids
√x7th **X77.3** Intentional self-harm by hot household appliances
√x7th **X77.8** Intentional self-harm by other hot objects
√x7th **X77.9** Intentional self-harm by unspecified hot objects ▽

√4th **X78 Intentional self-harm by sharp object**
√x7th **X78.0** Intentional self-harm by sharp glass
√x7th **X78.1** Intentional self-harm by knife
√x7th **X78.2** Intentional self-harm by sword or dagger
√x7th **X78.8** Intentional self-harm by other sharp object
√x7th **X78.9** Intentional self-harm by unspecified sharp object ▽

√x7th **X79 Intentional self-harm by blunt object**

√x7th **X80 Intentional self-harm by jumping from a high place**
Intentional fall from one level to another

√4th **X81 Intentional self-harm by jumping or lying in front of moving object**
√x7th **X81.0** Intentional self-harm by jumping or lying in front of motor vehicle
√x7th **X81.1** Intentional self-harm by jumping or lying in front of (subway) train
√x7th **X81.8** Intentional self-harm by jumping or lying in front of other moving object

√4th **X82 Intentional self-harm by crashing of motor vehicle**
√x7th **X82.0** Intentional collision of motor vehicle with other motor vehicle
√x7th **X82.1** Intentional collision of motor vehicle with train
√x7th **X82.2** Intentional collision of motor vehicle with tree
√x7th **X82.8** Other intentional self-harm by crashing of motor vehicle

√4th **X83 Intentional self-harm by other specified means**
EXCLUDES 1   intentional self-harm by poisoning or contact with toxic substance - See Table of Drugs and Chemicals
√x7th **X83.0** Intentional self-harm by crashing of aircraft
√x7th **X83.1** Intentional self-harm by electrocution
√x7th **X83.2** Intentional self-harm by exposure to extremes of cold
√x7th **X83.8** Intentional self-harm by other specified means

Assault ▶(X92-Y09)◀

INCLUDES   homicide
injuries inflicted by another person with intent to injure or kill, by any means
EXCLUDES 1   injuries due to legal intervention (Y35.-)
injuries due to operations of war (Y36.-)
injuries due to terrorism (Y38.-)

The appropriate 7th character is to be added to each code from categories X92-Y04 and Y08.
A   initial encounter
D   subsequent encounter
S   sequela

√4th **X92 Assault by drowning and submersion**
√x7th **X92.0** Assault by drowning and submersion while in bathtub
√x7th **X92.1** Assault by drowning and submersion while in swimming pool
√x7th **X92.2** Assault by drowning and submersion after push into swimming pool
√x7th **X92.3** Assault by drowning and submersion in natural water
√x7th **X92.8** Other assault by drowning and submersion
√x7th **X92.9** Assault by drowning and submersion, unspecified ▽

√x7th **X93 Assault by handgun discharge**
Assault by discharge of gun for single hand use
Assault by discharge of pistol
Assault by discharge of revolver
EXCLUDES 1   Very pistol (X95.8)

√4th **X94 Assault by rifle, shotgun and larger firearm discharge**
EXCLUDES 1   airgun (X95.01)
√x7th **X94.0** Assault by shotgun
√x7th **X94.1** Assault by hunting rifle
√x7th **X94.2** Assault by machine gun
√x7th **X94.8** Assault by other larger firearm discharge
√x7th **X94.9** Assault by unspecified larger firearm discharge ▽

√4th **X95 Assault by other and unspecified firearm and gun discharge**
√5th **X95.0** Assault by gas, air or spring-operated guns
√x7th   **X95.01** Assault by airgun discharge
Assault by BB gun discharge
Assault by pellet gun discharge
√x7th   **X95.02** Assault by paintball gun discharge
√x7th   **X95.09** Assault by other gas, air or spring-operated gun
√x7th **X95.8** Assault by other firearm discharge
Assault by Very pistol [flare] discharge
√x7th **X95.9** Assault by unspecified firearm discharge ▽

√4th **X96 Assault by explosive material**
EXCLUDES 1   incendiary device (X97)
terrorism involving explosive material (Y38.2-)
√x7th **X96.0** Assault by antipersonnel bomb
EXCLUDES 1   antipersonnel bomb use in military or war (Y36.2-)
√x7th **X96.1** Assault by gasoline bomb
√x7th **X96.2** Assault by letter bomb
√x7th **X96.3** Assault by fertilizer bomb
√x7th **X96.4** Assault by pipe bomb
√x7th **X96.8** Assault by other specified explosive
√x7th **X96.9** Assault by unspecified explosive ▽

√x7th **X97 Assault by smoke, fire and flames**
Assault by arson
Assault by cigarettes
Assault by incendiary device

√4th **X98 Assault by steam, hot vapors and hot objects**
√x7th **X98.0** Assault by steam or hot vapors
√x7th **X98.1** Assault by hot tap water
√x7th **X98.2** Assault by hot fluids
√x7th **X98.3** Assault by hot household appliances
√x7th **X98.8** Assault by other hot objects
√x7th **X98.9** Assault by unspecified hot objects ▽

√4th **X99 Assault by sharp object**
EXCLUDES 1   assault by strike by sports equipment (Y08.0-)
√x7th **X99.0** Assault by sharp glass

EXCLUDES 1   Not coded here   EXCLUDES 2   Not included here   N   Newborn Age : 0   P   Pediatric Age : 0-17   M   Maternity Age : 12-55   A   Adult Age : 15-124

1120   ICD-10-CM 2017

☑x7ᵗʰ   **X99.1   Assault by** knife

☑x7ᵗʰ   **X99.2   Assault by** sword or dagger

☑x7ᵗʰ   **X99.8   Assault by other sharp object**

☑x7ᵗʰ   **X99.9   Assault by unspecified sharp object**   ▽
         Assault by stabbing NOS

☑x7ᵗʰ   **Y00   Assault by blunt object**
         EXCLUDES 1 *assault by strike by sports equipment (Y08.0-)*

☑x7ᵗʰ   **Y01   Assault by pushing from high place**

☑4ᵗʰ   **Y02   Assault by pushing or placing victim in front of moving object**

     ☑x7ᵗʰ   **Y02.0   Assault by pushing or placing victim in front of** motor vehicle

     ☑x7ᵗʰ   **Y02.1   Assault by pushing or placing victim in front of (subway) train**

     ☑x7ᵗʰ   **Y02.8   Assault by pushing or placing victim in front of other moving object**

☑4ᵗʰ   **Y03   Assault by crashing of motor vehicle**

     ☑x7ᵗʰ   **Y03.0   Assault by being hit or run over by motor vehicle**

     ☑x7ᵗʰ   **Y03.8   Other assault by crashing of motor vehicle**

☑4ᵗʰ   **Y04   Assault by bodily force**
         EXCLUDES 1 *assault by:*
                 submersion (X92.-)
                 use of weapon (X93-X95, X99, Y00)

     ☑x7ᵗʰ   **Y04.0   Assault by** unarmed brawl or fight

     ☑x7ᵗʰ   **Y04.1   Assault by** human bite

     ☑x7ᵗʰ   **Y04.2   Assault by** strike **against or bumped into by another person**

     ☑x7ᵗʰ   **Y04.8   Assault by other bodily force**
            Assault by bodily force NOS

☑4ᵗʰ   **Y07   Perpetrator of assault, maltreatment and neglect**

     NOTE   Codes from this category are for use only in cases of confirmed abuse (T74.-)

            Selection of the correct perpetrator code is based on the relationship between the perpetrator and the victim

     INCLUDES   perpetrator of abandonment
                perpetrator of emotional neglect
                perpetrator of mental cruelty
                perpetrator of physical abuse
                perpetrator of physical neglect
                perpetrator of sexual abuse
                perpetrator of torture

     ☑5ᵗʰ   **Y07.0   Spouse or partner, perpetrator of maltreatment and neglect**
            Spouse or partner, perpetrator of maltreatment and neglect against spouse or partner

         Y07.01   Husband, perpetrator of maltreatment and neglect

         Y07.02   Wife, perpetrator of maltreatment and neglect

         Y07.03   Male partner, perpetrator of maltreatment and neglect

         Y07.04   Female partner, perpetrator of maltreatment and neglect

     ☑5ᵗʰ   **Y07.1   Parent (adoptive) (biological), perpetrator of maltreatment and neglect**

         Y07.11   Biological father, perpetrator of maltreatment and neglect

         Y07.12   Biological mother, perpetrator of maltreatment and neglect

         Y07.13   Adoptive father, perpetrator of maltreatment and neglect

         Y07.14   Adoptive mother, perpetrator of maltreatment and neglect

     ☑5ᵗʰ   **Y07.4   Other family member, perpetrator of maltreatment and neglect**

         ☑6ᵗʰ   **Y07.41   Sibling, perpetrator of maltreatment and neglect**
                EXCLUDES 1 *stepsibling, perpetrator of maltreatment and neglect (Y07.435, Y07.436)*

                Y07.410   Brother, perpetrator of maltreatment and neglect

                Y07.411   Sister, perpetrator of maltreatment and neglect

         ☑6ᵗʰ   **Y07.42   Foster parent, perpetrator of maltreatment and neglect**

                Y07.420   Foster father, perpetrator of maltreatment and neglect

                Y07.421   Foster mother, perpetrator of maltreatment and neglect

         ☑6ᵗʰ   **Y07.43   Stepparent or stepsibling, perpetrator of maltreatment and neglect**

                Y07.430   Stepfather, perpetrator of maltreatment and neglect

                Y07.432   Male friend of parent (co-residing in household), perpetrator of maltreatment and neglect

                Y07.433   Stepmother, perpetrator of maltreatment and neglect

                Y07.434   Female friend of parent (co-residing in household), perpetrator of maltreatment and neglect

                Y07.435   Stepbrother, perpetrator or maltreatment and neglect

                Y07.436   Stepsister, perpetrator of maltreatment and neglect

         ☑6ᵗʰ   **Y07.49   Other family member, perpetrator of maltreatment and neglect**

                Y07.490   Male cousin, perpetrator of maltreatment and neglect

                Y07.491   Female cousin, perpetrator of maltreatment and neglect

                Y07.499   Other family member, perpetrator of maltreatment and neglect

     ☑5ᵗʰ   **Y07.5   Non-family member, perpetrator of maltreatment and neglect**

         Y07.50   Unspecified non-family member, perpetrator of maltreatment and neglect   ▽

         ☑6ᵗʰ   **Y07.51   Daycare provider, perpetrator of maltreatment and neglect**

                Y07.510   At-home childcare provider, perpetrator of maltreatment and neglect

                Y07.511   Daycare center childcare provider, perpetrator of maltreatment and neglect

                Y07.512   At-home adultcare provider, perpetrator of maltreatment and neglect

                Y07.513   Adultcare center provider, perpetrator of maltreatment and neglect

                Y07.519   Unspecified daycare provider, perpetrator of maltreatment and neglect   ▽

         ☑6ᵗʰ   **Y07.52   Healthcare provider, perpetrator of maltreatment and neglect**

                Y07.521   Mental health provider, perpetrator of maltreatment and neglect

                Y07.528   Other therapist or healthcare provider, perpetrator of maltreatment and neglect
                   Nurse perpetrator of maltreatment and neglect
                   Occupational therapist perpetrator of maltreatment and neglect
                   Physical therapist perpetrator of maltreatment and neglect
                   Speech therapist perpetrator of maltreatment and neglect

                Y07.529   Unspecified healthcare provider, perpetrator of maltreatment and neglect   ▽

              Y07.53   Teacher or instructor, perpetrator of maltreatment and neglect
                   Coach, perpetrator of maltreatment and neglect

              Y07.59   Other non-family member, perpetrator of maltreatment and neglect

         Y07.9   Unspecified perpetrator of maltreatment and neglect   ▽

☑4ᵗʰ   **Y08   Assault by other specified means**

     ☑5ᵗʰ   **Y08.0   Assault by strike by** sport equipment

         ☑x7ᵗʰ   **Y08.01   Assault by strike by** hockey stick

         ☑x7ᵗʰ   **Y08.02   Assault by strike by** baseball bat

         ☑x7ᵗʰ   **Y08.09   Assault by strike by other specified type of sport equipment**

     ☑5ᵗʰ   **Y08.8   Assault by other specified means**

         ☑x7ᵗʰ   **Y08.81   Assault by crashing of** aircraft

         ☑x7ᵗʰ   **Y08.89   Assault by other specified means**

     Y09   Assault by unspecified means   ▽
         Assassination (attempted) NOS
         Homicide (attempted) NOS
         Manslaughter (attempted) NOS
         Murder (attempted) NOS

☑ Additional Character Required   ☑x7ᵗʰ Placeholder Alert   Manifestation Dx   ▽ Unspecified Dx   ►◄ Revised Text   ● New Code   ▲ Revised Code Title

ICD-10-CM 2017   **1121**

Event of undetermined intent (Y21-Y33)

Undetermined intent is only for use when there is specific documentation in the record that the intent of the injury cannot be determined. If no such documentation is present, code to accidental (unintentional).

The appropriate 7th character is to be added to each code from categories Y21-Y33.
A   initial encounter
D   subsequent encounter
S   sequela

✓4ᵗʰ **Y21 Drowning and submersion, undetermined intent**

√x7ᵗʰ **Y21.0 Drowning and submersion** while in bathtub, **undetermined intent**

√x7ᵗʰ **Y21.1 Drowning and submersion** after fall into bathtub, **undetermined intent**

√x7ᵗʰ **Y21.2 Drowning and submersion** while in swimming pool, **undetermined intent**

√x7ᵗʰ **Y21.3 Drowning and submersion** after fall into swimming pool, **undetermined intent**

√x7ᵗʰ **Y21.4 Drowning and submersion** in natural water, **undetermined intent**

√x7ᵗʰ **Y21.8 Other drowning and submersion, undetermined intent**

√x7ᵗʰ **Y21.9 Unspecified drowning and submersion, undetermined intent** ▽

√x7ᵗʰ **Y22 Handgun discharge, undetermined intent**
Discharge of gun for single hand use, undetermined intent
Discharge of pistol, undetermined intent
Discharge of revolver, undetermined intent
EXCLUDES 2 *Very pistol (Y24.8)*

✓4ᵗʰ **Y23 Rifle, shotgun and larger firearm discharge, undetermined intent**
EXCLUDES 2 *airgun (Y24.0)*

√x7ᵗʰ **Y23.0 Shotgun discharge, undetermined intent**

√x7ᵗʰ **Y23.1 Hunting rifle discharge, undetermined intent**

√x7ᵗʰ **Y23.2 Military firearm discharge, undetermined intent**

√x7ᵗʰ **Y23.3 Machine gun discharge, undetermined intent**

√x7ᵗʰ **Y23.8 Other larger firearm discharge, undetermined intent**

√x7ᵗʰ **Y23.9 Unspecified larger firearm discharge, undetermined intent** ▽

✓4ᵗʰ **Y24 Other and unspecified firearm discharge, undetermined intent**

√x7ᵗʰ **Y24.0 Airgun discharge, undetermined intent**
BB gun discharge, undetermined intent
Pellet gun discharge, undetermined intent

√x7ᵗʰ **Y24.8 Other firearm discharge, undetermined intent**
Paintball gun discharge, undetermined intent
Very pistol [flare] discharge, undetermined intent

√x7ᵗʰ **Y24.9 Unspecified firearm discharge, undetermined intent** ▽

√x7ᵗʰ **Y25 Contact with explosive material, undetermined intent**

√x7ᵗʰ **Y26 Exposure to smoke, fire and flames, undetermined intent**

✓4ᵗʰ **Y27 Contact with steam, hot vapors and hot objects, undetermined intent**

√x7ᵗʰ **Y27.0 Contact with steam and hot vapors, undetermined intent**

√x7ᵗʰ **Y27.1 Contact with hot tap water, undetermined intent**

√x7ᵗʰ **Y27.2 Contact with hot fluids, undetermined intent**

√x7ᵗʰ **Y27.3 Contact with hot household appliance, undetermined intent**

√x7ᵗʰ **Y27.8 Contact with other hot objects, undetermined intent**

√x7ᵗʰ **Y27.9 Contact with unspecified hot objects, undetermined intent** ▽

✓4ᵗʰ **Y28 Contact with sharp object, undetermined intent**

√x7ᵗʰ **Y28.0 Contact with sharp glass, undetermined intent**

√x7ᵗʰ **Y28.1 Contact with knife, undetermined intent**

√x7ᵗʰ **Y28.2 Contact with sword or dagger, undetermined intent**

√x7ᵗʰ **Y28.8 Contact with other sharp object, undetermined intent**

√x7ᵗʰ **Y28.9 Contact with unspecified sharp object, undetermined intent** ▽

√x7ᵗʰ **Y29 Contact with blunt object, undetermined intent**

√x7ᵗʰ **Y30 Falling, jumping or pushed from a high place, undetermined intent**
Victim falling from one level to another, undetermined intent

√x7ᵗʰ **Y31 Falling, lying or running before or into moving object, undetermined intent**

√x7ᵗʰ **Y32 Crashing of motor vehicle, undetermined intent**

√x7ᵗʰ **Y33 Other specified events, undetermined intent**

Legal intervention, operations of war, military operations, and terrorism (Y35-Y38)

The appropriate 7th character is to be added to each code from categories Y35-Y38.
A   initial encounter
D   subsequent encounter
S   sequela

✓4ᵗʰ **Y35 Legal intervention**
INCLUDES any injury sustained as a result of an encounter with any law enforcement official, serving in any capacity at the time of the encounter, whether on-duty or off-duty. Includes injury to law enforcement official, suspect and bystander

√5ᵗʰ **Y35.0 Legal intervention involving firearm discharge**

√6ᵗʰ **Y35.00 Legal intervention involving unspecified firearm discharge**
Legal intervention involving gunshot wound
Legal intervention involving shot NOS

√7ᵗʰ **Y35.001 Legal intervention involving unspecified firearm discharge, law enforcement official injured** ▽

√7ᵗʰ **Y35.002 Legal intervention involving unspecified firearm discharge, bystander injured** ▽

√7ᵗʰ **Y35.003 Legal intervention involving unspecified firearm discharge, suspect injured** ▽

√6ᵗʰ **Y35.01 Legal intervention involving injury by machine gun**

√7ᵗʰ **Y35.011 Legal intervention involving injury by machine gun, law enforcement official injured**

√7ᵗʰ **Y35.012 Legal intervention involving injury by machine gun, bystander injured**

√7ᵗʰ **Y35.013 Legal intervention involving injury by machine gun, suspect injured**

√6ᵗʰ **Y35.02 Legal intervention involving injury by handgun**

√7ᵗʰ **Y35.021 Legal intervention involving injury by handgun, law enforcement official injured**

√7ᵗʰ **Y35.022 Legal intervention involving injury by handgun, bystander injured**

√7ᵗʰ **Y35.023 Legal intervention involving injury by handgun, suspect injured**

√6ᵗʰ **Y35.03 Legal intervention involving injury by rifle pellet**

√7ᵗʰ **Y35.031 Legal intervention involving injury by rifle pellet, law enforcement official injured**

√7ᵗʰ **Y35.032 Legal intervention involving injury by rifle pellet, bystander injured**

√7ᵗʰ **Y35.033 Legal intervention involving injury by rifle pellet, suspect injured**

√6ᵗʰ **Y35.04 Legal intervention involving injury by rubber bullet**

√7ᵗʰ **Y35.041 Legal intervention involving injury by rubber bullet, law enforcement official injured**

√7ᵗʰ **Y35.042 Legal intervention involving injury by rubber bullet, bystander injured**

√7ᵗʰ **Y35.043 Legal intervention involving injury by rubber bullet, suspect injured**

√6ᵗʰ **Y35.09 Legal intervention involving other firearm discharge**

√7ᵗʰ **Y35.091 Legal intervention involving other firearm discharge, law enforcement official injured**

√7ᵗʰ **Y35.092 Legal intervention involving other firearm discharge, bystander injured**

√7ᵗʰ **Y35.093 Legal intervention involving other firearm discharge, suspect injured**

√5ᵗʰ **Y35.1 Legal intervention involving explosives**

√6ᵗʰ **Y35.10 Legal intervention involving unspecified explosives**

√7ᵗʰ **Y35.101 Legal intervention involving unspecified explosives, law enforcement official injured** ▽

√7ᵗʰ **Y35.102 Legal intervention involving unspecified explosives, bystander injured** ▽

EXCLUDES 1 Not coded here   EXCLUDES 2 Not included here   Ⓝ Newborn Age : 0   Ⓟ Pediatric Age : 0-17   Ⓜ Maternity Age : 12-55   Ⓐ Adult Age : 15-124

1122   ICD-10-CM 2017

√7ᵗʰ **Y35.103** Legal intervention involving unspecified explosives, **suspect injured** ▽

√6ᵗʰ **Y35.11** Legal intervention involving injury by **dynamite**

    √7ᵗʰ **Y35.111** Legal intervention involving injury by dynamite, **law enforcement official injured**

    √7ᵗʰ **Y35.112** Legal intervention involving injury by dynamite, **bystander injured**

    √7ᵗʰ **Y35.113** Legal intervention involving injury by dynamite, **suspect injured**

√6ᵗʰ **Y35.12** Legal intervention involving injury by **explosive shell**

    √7ᵗʰ **Y35.121** Legal intervention involving injury by explosive shell, **law enforcement official injured**

    √7ᵗʰ **Y35.122** Legal intervention involving injury by explosive shell, **bystander injured**

    √7ᵗʰ **Y35.123** Legal intervention involving injury by explosive shell, **suspect injured**

√6ᵗʰ **Y35.19** Legal intervention involving other explosives

    Legal intervention involving injury by grenade

    Legal intervention involving injury by mortar bomb

    √7ᵗʰ **Y35.191** Legal intervention involving other explosives, **law enforcement official injured**

    √7ᵗʰ **Y35.192** Legal intervention involving other explosives, **bystander injured**

    √7ᵗʰ **Y35.193** Legal intervention involving other explosives, **suspect injured**

√5ᵗʰ **Y35.2** Legal intervention involving **gas**

    Legal intervention involving asphyxiation by gas

    Legal Intervention involving poisoning by gas

√6ᵗʰ **Y35.20** Legal intervention involving unspecified gas

    √7ᵗʰ **Y35.201** Legal intervention involving unspecified gas, **law enforcement official injured** ▽

    √7ᵗʰ **Y35.202** Legal intervention involving unspecified gas, **bystander injured** ▽

    √7ᵗʰ **Y35.203** Legal intervention involving unspecified gas, **suspect injured** ▽

√6ᵗʰ **Y35.21** Legal intervention involving injury by **tear gas**

    √7ᵗʰ **Y35.211** Legal Intervention Involving injury by tear gas, **law enforcement official Injured**

    √7ᵗʰ **Y35.212** Legal intervention involving injury by tear gas, **bystander injured**

    √7ᵗʰ **Y35.213** Legal intervention involving injury by tear gas, **suspect injured**

√6ᵗʰ **Y35.29** Legal intervention involving other gas

    √7ᵗʰ **Y35.291** Legal intervention involving other gas, **law enforcement official injured**

    √7ᵗʰ **Y35.292** Legal intervention involving other gas, **bystander injured**

    √7ᵗʰ **Y35.293** Legal intervention involving other gas, **suspect injured**

√5ᵗʰ **Y35.3** Legal intervention involving **blunt objects**

    Legal intervention involving being hit or struck by blunt object

√6ᵗʰ **Y35.30** Legal intervention involving unspecified blunt objects

    √7ᵗʰ **Y35.301** Legal intervention involving unspecified blunt objects, **law enforcement official injured** ▽

    √7ᵗʰ **Y35.302** Legal intervention involving unspecified blunt objects, **bystander injured** ▽

    √7ᵗʰ **Y35.303** Legal intervention involving unspecified blunt objects, **suspect injured** ▽

√6ᵗʰ **Y35.31** Legal intervention involving **baton**

    √7ᵗʰ **Y35.311** Legal intervention involving baton, **law enforcement official injured**

    √7ᵗʰ **Y35.312** Legal intervention involving baton, **bystander injured**

    √7ᵗʰ **Y35.313** Legal intervention involving baton, **suspect injured**

√6ᵗʰ **Y35.39** Legal intervention involving other blunt objects

    √7ᵗʰ **Y35.391** Legal intervention involving other blunt objects, **law enforcement official injured**

    √7ᵗʰ **Y35.392** Legal intervention involving other blunt objects, **bystander injured**

√7ᵗʰ **Y35.393** Legal intervention involving other blunt objects, **suspect injured**

√5ᵗʰ **Y35.4** Legal intervention involving **sharp objects**

    Legal intervention involving being cut by sharp objects

    Legal intervention involving being stabbed by sharp objects

√6ᵗʰ **Y35.40** Legal intervention involving unspecified sharp objects

    √7ᵗʰ **Y35.401** Legal intervention involving unspecified sharp objects, **law enforcement official injured** ▽

    √7ᵗʰ **Y35.402** Legal intervention involving unspecified sharp objects, **bystander injured** ▽

    √7ᵗʰ **Y35.403** Legal intervention involving unspecified sharp objects, **suspect injured** ▽

√6ᵗʰ **Y35.41** Legal intervention involving **bayonet**

    √7ᵗʰ **Y35.411** Legal intervention involving bayonet, **law enforcement official injured**

    √7ᵗʰ **Y35.412** Legal intervention involving bayonet, **bystander injured**

    √7ᵗʰ **Y35.413** Legal intervention involving bayonet, **suspect injured**

√6ᵗʰ **Y35.49** Legal intervention involving other sharp objects

    √7ᵗʰ **Y35.491** Legal intervention involving other sharp objects, **law enforcement official injured**

    √7ᵗʰ **Y35.492** Legal intervention involving other sharp objects, **bystander injured**

    √7ᵗʰ **Y35.493** Legal intervention involving other sharp objects, **suspect injured**

√5ᵗʰ **Y35.8** Legal intervention involving other specified means

√6ᵗʰ **Y35.81** Legal intervention involving **manhandling**

    √7ᵗʰ **Y35.811** Legal intervention involving manhandling, **law enforcement official injured**

    √7ᵗʰ **Y35.812** Legal intervention involving manhandling, **bystander injured**

    √7ᵗʰ **Y35.813** Legal intervention involving manhandling, **suspect injured**

√6ᵗʰ **Y35.89** Legal intervention involving other specified means

    √7ᵗʰ **Y35.891** Legal intervention involving other specified means, **law enforcement official Injured**

    √7ᵗʰ **Y35.892** Legal intervention involving other specified means, **bystander injured**

    √7ᵗʰ **Y35.893** Legal intervention involving other specified means, **suspect injured**

√5ᵗʰ **Y35.9** Legal intervention, means unspecified

    √x7ᵗʰ **Y35.91** Legal intervention, means unspecified, **law enforcement official injured** ▽

    √x7ᵗʰ **Y35.92** Legal intervention, means unspecified, **bystander injured** ▽

    √x7ᵗʰ **Y35.93** Legal intervention, means unspecified, **suspect injured** ▽

√4ᵗʰ **Y36 Operations of war**

    INCLUDES   injuries to military personnel and civilians caused by war, civil insurrection, and peacekeeping missions

    EXCLUDES 1   *injury to military personnel occurring during peacetime military operations (Y37.-)*

    military vehicles involved in transport accidents with non-military vehicle during peacetime (V09.01, V09.21, V19.81, V29.81, V39.81, V49.81, V59.81, V69.81, V79.81)

    AHA: 2014,3Q,4

√5ᵗʰ **Y36.0** War operations involving **explosion of marine weapons**

√6ᵗʰ **Y36.00** War operations involving explosion of unspecified marine weapon

    War operations involving underwater blast NOS

    √7ᵗʰ **Y36.000** War operations involving explosion of unspecified marine weapon, **military personnel** ▽

    √7ᵗʰ **Y36.001** War operations involving explosion of unspecified marine weapon, **civilian** ▽

√6ᵗʰ **Y36.01** War operations involving explosion of **depth-charge**

    √7ᵗʰ **Y36.010** War operations involving explosion of depth-charge, **military personnel**

    √7ᵗʰ **Y36.011** War operations involving explosion of depth-charge, **civilian**

☑ Additional Character Required   √x7ᵗʰ Placeholder Alert   Manifestation Dx   ▽ Unspecified Dx   ►◄ Revised Text   ● New Code   ▲ Revised Code Title

ICD-10-CM 2017   **1123**

√6th **Y36.02 War operations involving explosion of** marine mine

War operations involving explosion of marine mine, at sea or in harbor

√7th **Y36.020 War operations involving explosion of marine mine, military personnel**

√7th **Y36.021 War operations involving explosion of marine mine, civilian**

√6th **Y36.03 War operations involving explosion of** sea-based artillery shell

√7th **Y36.030 War operations involving explosion of sea-based artillery shell, military personnel**

√7th **Y36.031 War operations involving explosion of sea-based artillery shell, civilian**

√6th **Y36.04 War operations involving explosion of** torpedo

√7th **Y36.040 War operations involving explosion of torpedo, military personnel**

√7th **Y36.041 War operations involving explosion of torpedo, civilian**

√6th **Y36.05 War operations involving** accidental detonation of onboard marine weapons

√7th **Y36.050 War operations involving accidental detonation of onboard marine weapons, military personnel**

√7th **Y36.051 War operations involving accidental detonation of onboard marine weapons, civilian**

√6th **Y36.09 War operations involving explosion of other marine weapons**

√7th **Y36.090 War operations involving explosion of other marine weapons, military personnel**

√7th **Y36.091 War operations involving explosion of other marine weapons, civilian**

√5th **Y36.1 War operations involving** destruction of aircraft

√6th **Y36.10 War operations involving unspecified destruction of aircraft**

√7th **Y36.100 War operations involving unspecified destruction of aircraft, military personnel** ▽

√7th **Y36.101 War operations involving unspecified destruction of aircraft, civilian** ▽

√6th **Y36.11 War operations involving destruction of aircraft due to** enemy fire or explosives

War operations involving destruction of aircraft due to air to air missile

War operations involving destruction of aircraft due to explosive placed on aircraft

War operations involving destruction of aircraft due to rocket propelled grenade [RPG]

War operations involving destruction of aircraft due to small arms fire

War operations involving destruction of aircraft due to surface to air missile

√7th **Y36.110 War operations involving destruction of aircraft due to enemy fire or explosives, military personnel**

√7th **Y36.111 War operations involving destruction of aircraft due to enemy fire or explosives, civilian**

√6th **Y36.12 War operations involving destruction of aircraft due to** collision with other aircraft

√7th **Y36.120 War operations involving destruction of aircraft due to collision with other aircraft, military personnel**

√7th **Y36.121 War operations involving destruction of aircraft due to collision with other aircraft, civilian**

√6th **Y36.13 War operations involving destruction of aircraft due to** onboard fire

√7th **Y36.130 War operations involving destruction of aircraft due to onboard fire, military personnel**

√7th **Y36.131 War operations involving destruction of aircraft due to onboard fire, civilian**

√6th **Y36.14 War operations involving destruction of aircraft due to** accidental detonation of onboard munitions and explosives

√7th **Y36.140 War operations involving destruction of aircraft due to accidental detonation of onboard munitions and explosives, military personnel**

√7th **Y36.141 War operations involving destruction of aircraft due to accidental detonation of onboard munitions and explosives, civilian**

√6th **Y36.19 War operations involving other destruction of aircraft**

√7th **Y36.190 War operations involving other destruction of aircraft, military personnel**

√7th **Y36.191 War operations involving other destruction of aircraft, civilian**

√5th **Y36.2 War operations involving other explosions and fragments**

EXCLUDES 1 war operations involving explosion of aircraft (Y36.1-)

war operations involving explosion of marine weapons (Y36.0-)

war operations involving explosion of nuclear weapons (Y36.5-)

war operations involving explosion occurring after cessation of hostilities (Y36.8-)

√6th **Y36.20 War operations involving unspecified explosion and fragments**

War operations involving air blast NOS

War operations involving blast NOS

War operations involving blast fragments NOS

War operations involving blast wave NOS

War operations involving blast wind NOS

War operations involving explosion NOS

War operations involving explosion of bomb NOS

√7th **Y36.200 War operations involving unspecified explosion and fragments, military personnel** ▽

√7th **Y36.201 War operations involving unspecified explosion and fragments, civilian** ▽

√6th **Y36.21 War operations involving explosion of** aerial bomb

√7th **Y36.210 War operations involving explosion of aerial bomb, military personnel**

√7th **Y36.211 War operations involving explosion of aerial bomb, civilian**

√6th **Y36.22 War operations involving explosion of** guided missile

√7th **Y36.220 War operations involving explosion of guided missile, military personnel**

√7th **Y36.221 War operations involving explosion of guided missile, civilian**

√6th **Y36.23 War operations involving explosion of** improvised explosive device [IED]

War operations involving explosion of person-borne improvised explosive device [IED]

War operations involving explosion of vehicle-borne improvised explosive device [IED]

War operations involving explosion of roadside improvised explosive device [IED]

√7th **Y36.230 War operations involving explosion of improvised explosive device [IED], military personnel**

√7th **Y36.231 War operations involving explosion of improvised explosive device [IED], civilian**

√6th **Y36.24 War operations involving explosion due to** accidental detonation and discharge of own munitions or munitions launch device

√7th **Y36.240 War operations involving explosion due to accidental detonation and discharge of own munitions or munitions launch device, military personnel**

√7th **Y36.241 War operations involving explosion due to accidental detonation and discharge of own munitions or munitions launch device, civilian**

√6th **Y36.25 War operations involving** fragments from munitions

√7th **Y36.250 War operations involving fragments from munitions, military personnel**

√7th **Y36.251 War operations involving fragments from munitions, civilian**

EXCLUDES 1 Not coded here   EXCLUDES 2 Not included here   N Newborn Age : 0   P Pediatric Age : 0-17   M Maternity Age : 12-55   A Adult Age : 15-124

1124   ICD-10-CM 2017

✓6ᵗʰ **Y36.26** War operations involving fragments of improvised explosive device [IED]
> War operations involving fragments of person-borne improvised explosive device [IED]
> War operations involving fragments of vehicle-borne improvised explosive device [IED]
> War operations involving fragments of roadside improvised explosive device [IED]

     ✓7ᵗʰ **Y36.260** War operations involving fragments of improvised explosive device [IED], military personnel

     ✓7ᵗʰ **Y36.261** War operations involving fragments of improvised explosive device [IED], civilian

✓6ᵗʰ **Y36.27** War operations involving fragments from weapons

     ✓7ᵗʰ **Y36.270** War operations involving fragments from weapons, military personnel

     ✓7ᵗʰ **Y36.271** War operations involving fragments from weapons, civilian

✓6ᵗʰ **Y36.29** War operations involving other explosions and fragments
> War operations involving explosion of grenade
> War operations involving explosions of land mine
> War operations involving shrapnel NOS

     ✓7ᵗʰ **Y36.290** War operations involving other explosions and fragments, military personnel

     ✓7ᵗʰ **Y36.291** War operations involving other explosions and fragments, civilian

✓5ᵗʰ **Y36.3** War operations involving fires, conflagrations and hot substances
> War operations involving smoke, fumes, and heat from fires, conflagrations and hot substances
> **EXCLUDES 1** war operations involving fires and conflagrations aboard military aircraft (Y36.1-)
> war operations involving fires and conflagrations aboard military watercraft (Y36.0-)
> war operations involving fires and conflagrations caused indirectly by conventional weapons (Y36.2-)
> war operations involving fires and thermal effects of nuclear weapons (Y36.53-)

   ✓6ᵗʰ **Y36.30** War operations involving unspecified fire, conflagration and hot substance

     ✓7ᵗʰ **Y36.300** War operations involving unspecified fire, conflagration and hot substance, military personnel ▽

     ✓7ᵗʰ **Y36.301** War operations involving unspecified fire, conflagration and hot substance, civilian ▽

   ✓6ᵗʰ **Y36.31** War operations involving gasoline bomb
> War operations involving incendiary bomb
> War operations involving petrol bomb

     ✓7ᵗʰ **Y36.310** War operations involving gasoline bomb, military personnel

     ✓7ᵗʰ **Y36.311** War operations involving gasoline bomb, civilian

   ✓6ᵗʰ **Y36.32** War operations involving incendiary bullet

     ✓7ᵗʰ **Y36.320** War operations involving incendiary bullet, military personnel

     ✓7ᵗʰ **Y36.321** War operations involving incendiary bullet, civilian

   ✓6ᵗʰ **Y36.33** War operations involving flamethrower

     ✓7ᵗʰ **Y36.330** War operations involving flamethrower, military personnel

     ✓7ᵗʰ **Y36.331** War operations involving flamethrower, civilian

   ✓6ᵗʰ **Y36.39** War operations involving other fires, conflagrations and hot substances

     ✓7ᵗʰ **Y36.390** War operations involving other fires, conflagrations and hot substances, military personnel

     ✓7ᵗʰ **Y36.391** War operations involving other fires, conflagrations and hot substances, civilian

✓5ᵗʰ **Y36.4** War operations involving firearm discharge and other forms of conventional warfare

   ✓6ᵗʰ **Y36.41** War operations involving rubber bullets

     ✓7ᵗʰ **Y36.410** War operations involving rubber bullets, military personnel

     ✓7ᵗʰ **Y36.411** War operations involving rubber bullets, civilian

✓6ᵗʰ **Y36.42** War operations involving firearms pellets

     ✓7ᵗʰ **Y36.420** War operations involving firearms pellets, military personnel

     ✓7ᵗʰ **Y36.421** War operations involving firearms pellets, civilian

✓6ᵗʰ **Y36.43** War operations involving other firearms discharge
> War operations involving bullets NOS
> **EXCLUDES 1** war operations involving munitions fragments (Y36.25-)
> war operations involving incendiary bullets (Y36.32-)

     ✓7ᵗʰ **Y36.430** War operations involving other firearms discharge, military personnel

     ✓7ᵗʰ **Y36.431** War operations involving other firearms discharge, civilian

✓6ᵗʰ **Y36.44** War operations involving unarmed hand to hand combat
> **EXCLUDES 1** war operations involving combat using blunt or piercing object (Y36.45-)
> war operations involving intentional restriction of air and airway (Y36.46-)
> war operations involving unintentional restriction of air and airway (Y36.47-)

     ✓7ᵗʰ **Y36.440** War operations involving unarmed hand to hand combat, military personnel

     ✓7ᵗʰ **Y36.441** War operations involving unarmed hand to hand combat, civilian

✓6ᵗʰ **Y36.45** War operations involving combat using blunt or piercing object

     ✓7ᵗʰ **Y36.450** War operations involving combat using blunt or piercing object, military personnel

     ✓7ᵗʰ **Y36.451** War operations involving combat using blunt or piercing object, civilian

✓6ᵗʰ **Y36.46** War operations involving intentional restriction of air and airway

     ✓7ᵗʰ **Y36.460** War operations involving intentional restriction of air and airway, military personnel

     ✓7ᵗʰ **Y36.461** War operations involving intentional restriction of air and airway, civilian

✓6ᵗʰ **Y36.47** War operations involving unintentional restriction of air and airway

     ✓7ᵗʰ **Y36.470** War operations involving unintentional restriction of air and airway, military personnel

     ✓7ᵗʰ **Y36.471** War operations involving unintentional restriction of air and airway, civilian

✓6ᵗʰ **Y36.49** War operations involving other forms of conventional warfare

     ✓7ᵗʰ **Y36.490** War operations involving other forms of conventional warfare, military personnel

     ✓7ᵗʰ **Y36.491** War operations involving other forms of conventional warfare, civilian

✓5ᵗʰ **Y36.5** War operations involving nuclear weapons
> War operations involving dirty bomb NOS

   ✓6ᵗʰ **Y36.50** War operations involving unspecified effect of nuclear weapon

     ✓7ᵗʰ **Y36.500** War operations involving unspecified effect of nuclear weapon, military personnel ▽

     ✓7ᵗʰ **Y36.501** War operations involving unspecified effect of nuclear weapon, civilian ▽

   ✓6ᵗʰ **Y36.51** War operations involving direct blast effect of nuclear weapon
> War operations involving blast pressure of nuclear weapon

     ✓7ᵗʰ **Y36.510** War operations involving direct blast effect of nuclear weapon, military personnel

     ✓7ᵗʰ **Y36.511** War operations involving direct blast effect of nuclear weapon, civilian

   ✓6ᵗʰ **Y36.52** War operations involving indirect blast effect of nuclear weapon
> War operations involving being thrown by blast of nuclear weapon
> War operations involving being struck or crushed by blast debris of nuclear weapon

     ✓7ᵗʰ **Y36.520** War operations involving indirect blast effect of nuclear weapon, military personnel

---

☑ Additional Character Required   ✓x7ᵗʰ Placeholder Alert   Manifestation Dx   ▽ Unspecified Dx   ▶◀ Revised Text   ● New Code   ▲ Revised Code Title

✓7ᵗʰ Y36.521 **War operations involving indirect blast effect of nuclear weapon**, civilian

✓6ᵗʰ Y36.53 **War operations involving** thermal radiation **effect of nuclear weapon**

War operations involving direct heat from nuclear weapon

War operation involving fireball effects from nuclear weapon

✓7ᵗʰ Y36.530 **War operations involving thermal radiation effect of nuclear weapon, military personnel**

✓7ᵗʰ Y36.531 **War operations involving thermal radiation effect of nuclear weapon, civilian**

✓6ᵗʰ Y36.54 **War operation involving** nuclear radiation **effects of nuclear weapon**

War operation involving acute radiation exposure from nuclear weapon

War operation involving exposure to immediate ionizing radiation from nuclear weapon

War operation involving fallout exposure from nuclear weapon

War operation involving secondary effects of nuclear weapons

✓7ᵗʰ Y36.540 **War operation involving nuclear radiation effects of nuclear weapon, military personnel**

✓7ᵗʰ Y36.541 **War operation involving nuclear radiation effects of nuclear weapon, civilian**

✓6ᵗʰ Y36.59 **War operation involving other effects of nuclear weapons**

✓7ᵗʰ Y36.590 **War operation involving other effects of nuclear weapons, military personnel**

✓7ᵗʰ Y36.591 **War operation involving other effects of nuclear weapons, civilian**

✓5ᵗʰ Y36.6 **War operations involving biological weapons**

✓6ᵗʰ Y36.6X **War operations involving** biological weapons

✓7ᵗʰ Y36.6X0 **War operations involving biological weapons, military personnel**

✓7ᵗʰ Y36.6X1 **War operations involving biological weapons, civilian**

✓5ᵗʰ Y36.7 **War operations involving chemical weapons and other forms of unconventional warfare**

EXCLUDES 1 *war operations involving incendiary devices (Y36.3-, Y36.5-)*

✓6ᵗʰ Y36.7X **War operations involving** chemical weapons and **other forms of unconventional warfare**

✓7ᵗʰ Y36.7X0 **War operations involving chemical weapons and other forms of unconventional warfare, military personnel**

✓7ᵗʰ Y36.7X1 **War operations involving chemical weapons and other forms of unconventional warfare, civilian**

✓5ᵗʰ Y36.8 **War operations occurring** after cessation of hostilities

War operations classifiable to categories Y36.0-Y36.8 but occurring after cessation of hostilities

✓6ᵗʰ Y36.81 **Explosion of** mine **placed during war operations but exploding after cessation of hostilities**

✓7ᵗʰ Y36.810 **Explosion of mine placed during war operations but exploding after cessation of hostilities, military personnel**

✓7ᵗʰ Y36.811 **Explosion of mine placed during war operations but exploding after cessation of hostilities, civilian**

✓6ᵗʰ Y36.82 **Explosion of** bomb **placed during war operations but exploding after cessation of hostilities**

✓7ᵗʰ Y36.820 **Explosion of bomb placed during war operations but exploding after cessation of hostilities, military personnel**

✓7ᵗʰ Y36.821 **Explosion of bomb placed during war operations but exploding after cessation of hostilities, civilian**

✓6ᵗʰ Y36.88 **Other war operations occurring after cessation of hostilities**

✓7ᵗʰ Y36.880 **Other war operations occurring after cessation of hostilities,** military personnel

✓7ᵗʰ Y36.881 **Other war operations occurring after cessation of hostilities,** civilian

✓6ᵗʰ Y36.89 **Unspecified war operations occurring after cessation of hostilities**

✓7ᵗʰ Y36.890 **Unspecified war operations occurring after cessation of hostilities,** military personnel ▽

✓7ᵗʰ Y36.891 **Unspecified war operations occurring after cessation of hostilities,** civilian ▽

✓5ᵗʰ Y36.9 **Other and unspecified war operations**

✓x7ᵗʰ Y36.90 **War operations, unspecified** ▽

✓x7ᵗʰ Y36.91 **War operations involving unspecified** weapon of mass destruction **[WMD]** ▽

✓x7ᵗʰ Y36.92 **War operations involving** friendly fire

✓4ᵗʰ **Y37 Military operations**

INCLUDES injuries to military personnel and civilians occurring during peacetime on military property and during routine military exercises and operations

EXCLUDES 1 *military aircraft involved in aircraft accident with civilian aircraft (V97.81-)*

military vehicles involved in transport accident with civilian vehicle (V09.01, V09.21, V19.81, V29.81, V39.81, V49.81, V59.81, V69.81, V79.81)

military watercraft involved in water transport accident with civilian watercraft (V94.81-)

war operations (Y36.-)

✓5ᵗʰ Y37.0 **Military operations involving** explosion of marine weapons

✓6ᵗʰ Y37.00 **Military operations involving explosion of unspecified marine weapon**

Military operations involving underwater blast NOS

✓7ᵗʰ Y37.000 **Military operations involving explosion of unspecified marine weapon, military personnel** ▽

✓7ᵗʰ Y37.001 **Military operations involving explosion of unspecified marine weapon, civilian** ▽

✓6ᵗʰ Y37.01 **Military operations involving explosion of** depth-charge

✓7ᵗʰ Y37.010 **Military operations involving explosion of depth-charge, military personnel**

✓7ᵗʰ Y37.011 **Military operations involving explosion of depth-charge, civilian**

✓6ᵗʰ Y37.02 **Military operations involving explosion of** marine mine

Military operations involving explosion of marine mine, at sea or in harbor

✓7ᵗʰ Y37.020 **Military operations involving explosion of marine mine, military personnel**

✓7ᵗʰ Y37.021 **Military operations involving explosion of marine mine, civilian**

✓6ᵗʰ Y37.03 **Military operations involving explosion of** sea-based artillery shell

✓7ᵗʰ Y37.030 **Military operations involving explosion of sea-based artillery shell, military personnel**

✓7ᵗʰ Y37.031 **Military operations involving explosion of sea-based artillery shell, civilian**

✓6ᵗʰ Y37.04 **Military operations involving explosion of** torpedo

✓7ᵗʰ Y37.040 **Military operations involving explosion of torpedo, military personnel**

✓7ᵗʰ Y37.041 **Military operations involving explosion of torpedo, civilian**

✓6ᵗʰ Y37.05 **Military operations involving accidental detonation of** onboard marine weapons

✓7ᵗʰ Y37.050 **Military operations involving accidental detonation of onboard marine weapons, military personnel**

✓7ᵗʰ Y37.051 **Military operations involving accidental detonation of onboard marine weapons, civilian**

✓6ᵗʰ Y37.09 **Military operations involving explosion of other marine weapons**

✓7ᵗʰ Y37.090 **Military operations involving explosion of other marine weapons, military personnel**

✓7ᵗʰ Y37.091 **Military operations involving explosion of other marine weapons, civilian**

✓5ᵗʰ Y37.1 **Military operations involving** destruction of aircraft

✓6ᵗʰ Y37.10 **Military operations involving unspecified destruction of aircraft**

✓7ᵗʰ Y37.100 **Military operations involving unspecified destruction of aircraft, military personnel** ▽

EXCLUDES 1 Not coded here   EXCLUDES 2 Not included here   N Newborn Age : 0   P Pediatric Age : 0-17   M Maternity Age : 12-55   A Adult Age : 15-124

1126   ICD-10-CM 2017

✓7ᵗʰ **Y37.101** Military operations involving
unspecified destruction of aircraft,
civilian   ▽

✓6ᵗʰ **Y37.11** Military operations involving destruction of aircraft
due to enemy fire or explosives
    Military operations involving destruction of aircraft
due to air to air missile
    Military operations involving destruction of aircraft
due to explosive placed on aircraft
    Military operations involving destruction of aircraft
due to rocket propelled grenade [RPG]
    Military operations involving destruction of aircraft
due to small arms fire
    Military operations involving destruction of aircraft
due to surface to air missile

   ✓7ᵗʰ **Y37.110** Military operations involving destruction
of aircraft due to enemy fire or
explosives, military personnel

   ✓7ᵗʰ **Y37.111** Military operations involving destruction
of aircraft due to enemy fire or
explosives, civilian

✓6ᵗʰ **Y37.12** Military operations involving destruction of aircraft
due to collision with other aircraft

   ✓7ᵗʰ **Y37.120** Military operations involving destruction
of aircraft due to collision with other
aircraft, military personnel

   ✓7ᵗʰ **Y37.121** Military operations involving destruction
of aircraft due to collision with other
aircraft, civilian

✓6ᵗʰ **Y37.13** Military operations involving destruction of aircraft
due to onboard fire

   ✓7ᵗʰ **Y37.130** Military operations involving destruction
of aircraft due to onboard fire, military
personnel

   ✓7ᵗʰ **Y37.131** Military operations involving destruction
of aircraft due to onboard fire, civilian

✓6ᵗʰ **Y37.14** Military operations involving destruction of aircraft
due to accidental detonation of onboard munitions
and explosives

   ✓7ᵗʰ **Y37.140** Military operations involving destruction
of aircraft due to accidental detonation
of onboard munitions and explosives,
military personnel

   ✓7ᵗʰ **Y37.141** Military operations involving destruction
of aircraft due to accidental detonation
of onboard munitions and explosives,
civilian

✓6ᵗʰ **Y37.19** Military operations involving other destruction of
aircraft

   ✓7ᵗʰ **Y37.190** Military operations involving other
destruction of aircraft, military personnel

   ✓7ᵗʰ **Y37.191** Military operations involving other
destruction of aircraft, civilian

✓5ᵗʰ **Y37.2** Military operations involving other explosions and fragments

   EXCLUDES 1 *military operations involving explosion of aircraft
(Y37.1-)*
*military operations involving explosion of marine
weapons (Y37.0-)*
*military operations involving explosion of nuclear
weapons (Y37.5-)*

✓6ᵗʰ **Y37.20** Military operations involving unspecified explosion
and fragments
    Military operations involving air blast NOS
    Military operations involving blast NOS
    Military operations involving blast fragments NOS
    Military operations involving blast wave NOS
    Military operations involving blast wind NOS
    Military operations involving explosion NOS
    Military operations involving explosion of bomb NOS

   ✓7ᵗʰ **Y37.200** Military operations involving
unspecified explosion and
fragments, military personnel   ▽

   ✓7ᵗʰ **Y37.201** Military operations involving
unspecified explosion and
fragments, civilian   ▽

✓6ᵗʰ **Y37.21** Military operations involving explosion of aerial
bomb

   ✓7ᵗʰ **Y37.210** Military operations involving explosion
of aerial bomb, military personnel

   ✓7ᵗʰ **Y37.211** Military operations involving explosion
of aerial bomb, civilian

✓6ᵗʰ **Y37.22** Military operations involving explosion of guided
missile

   ✓7ᵗʰ **Y37.220** Military operations involving explosion
of guided missile, military personnel

   ✓7ᵗʰ **Y37.221** Military operations involving explosion
of guided missile, civilian

✓6ᵗʰ **Y37.23** Military operations involving explosion of
improvised explosive device [IED]
    Military operations involving explosion of
person-borne improvised explosive device [IED]
    Military operations involving explosion of
vehicle-borne improvised explosive device [IED]
    Military operations involving explosion of roadside
improvised explosive device [IED]

   ✓7ᵗʰ **Y37.230** Military operations involving explosion
of improvised explosive device [IED],
military personnel

   ✓7ᵗʰ **Y37.231** Military operations involving explosion
of improvised explosive device [IED],
civilian

✓6ᵗʰ **Y37.24** Military operations involving explosion due to
accidental detonation and discharge of own
munitions or munitions launch device

   ✓7ᵗʰ **Y37.240** Military operations involving explosion
due to accidental detonation and
discharge of own munitions or munitions
launch device, military personnel

   ✓7ᵗʰ **Y37.241** Military operations involving explosion
due to accidental detonation and
discharge of own munitions or munitions
launch device, civilian

✓6ᵗʰ **Y37.25** Military operations involving fragments from
munitions

   ✓7ᵗʰ **Y37.250** Military operations involving fragments
from munitions, military personnel

   ✓7ᵗʰ **Y37.251** Military operations involving fragments
from munitions, civilian

✓6ᵗʰ **Y37.26** Military operations involving fragments of
improvised explosive device [IED]
    Military operations involving fragments of
person-borne improvised explosive device [IED]
    Military operations involving fragments of
vehicle-borne improvised explosive device [IED]
    Military operations involving fragments of roadside
improvised explosive device [IED]

   ✓7ᵗʰ **Y37.260** Military operations involving fragments
of improvised explosive device [IED],
military personnel

   ✓7ᵗʰ **Y37.261** Military operations involving fragments
of improvised explosive device [IED],
civilian

✓6ᵗʰ **Y37.27** Military operations involving fragments from
weapons

   ✓7ᵗʰ **Y37.270** Military operations involving fragments
from weapons, military personnel

   ✓7ᵗʰ **Y37.271** Military operations involving fragments
from weapons, civilian

✓6ᵗʰ **Y37.29** Military operations involving other explosions and
fragments
    Military operations involving explosion of grenade
    Military operations involving explosions of land mine
    Military operations involving shrapnel NOS

   ✓7ᵗʰ **Y37.290** Military operations involving other
explosions and fragments, military
personnel

   ✓7ᵗʰ **Y37.291** Military operations involving other
explosions and fragments, civilian

✓5ᵗʰ **Y37.3** Military operations involving fires, conflagrations and hot
substances
    Military operations involving smoke, fumes, and heat from fires,
conflagrations and hot substances

   EXCLUDES 1 *military operations involving fires and conflagrations
aboard military aircraft (Y37.1-)*
*military operations involving fires and conflagrations
aboard military watercraft (Y37.0-)*
*military operations involving fires and conflagrations
caused indirectly by conventional weapons
(Y37.2-)*
*military operations involving fires and thermal effects
of nuclear weapons (Y36.53-)*

✓6ᵗʰ **Y37.30** Military operations involving unspecified fire,
conflagration and hot substance

☑ Additional Character Required   ✓×7ᵗʰ Placeholder Alert   Manifestation Dx   ▽ Unspecified Dx   ▶◀ Revised Text   ● New Code   ▲ Revised Code Title

ICD-10-CM 2017   1127

√7th **Y37.300** **Military operations involving unspecified fire, conflagration and hot substance, military personnel** ▽

√7th **Y37.301** **Military operations involving unspecified fire, conflagration and hot substance, civilian** ▽

√6th **Y37.31** **Military operations involving gasoline bomb**
Military operations involving incendiary bomb
Military operations involving petrol bomb

√7th **Y37.310** **Military operations involving gasoline bomb, military personnel**

√7th **Y37.311** **Military operations involving gasoline bomb, civilian**

√6th **Y37.32** **Military operations involving incendiary bullet**

√7th **Y37.320** **Military operations involving incendiary bullet, military personnel**

√7th **Y37.321** **Military operations involving incendiary bullet, civilian**

√6th **Y37.33** **Military operations involving flamethrower**

√7th **Y37.330** **Military operations involving flamethrower, military personnel**

√7th **Y37.331** **Military operations involving flamethrower, civilian**

√6th **Y37.39** **Military operations involving other fires, conflagrations and hot substances**

√7th **Y37.390** **Military operations involving other fires, conflagrations and hot substances, military personnel**

√7th **Y37.391** **Military operations involving other fires, conflagrations and hot substances, civilian**

√5th **Y37.4** **Military operations involving firearm discharge and other forms of conventional warfare**

√6th **Y37.41** **Military operations involving rubber bullets**

√7th **Y37.410** **Military operations involving rubber bullets, military personnel**

√7th **Y37.411** **Military operations involving rubber bullets, civilian**

√6th **Y37.42** **Military operations involving firearms pellets**

√7th **Y37.420** **Military operations involving firearms pellets, military personnel**

√7th **Y37.421** **Military operations involving firearms pellets, civilian**

√6th **Y37.43** **Military operations involving other firearms discharge**
Military operations involving bullets NOS

EXCLUDES 1 *military operations involving munitions fragments (Y37.25-)*
military operations involving incendiary bullets (Y37.32-)

√7th **Y37.430** **Military operations involving other firearms discharge, military personnel**

√7th **Y37.431** **Military operations involving other firearms discharge, civilian**

√6th **Y37.44** **Military operations involving unarmed hand to hand combat**

EXCLUDES 1 *military operations involving combat using blunt or piercing object (Y37.45-)*
military operations involving intentional restriction of air and airway (Y37.46-)
military operations involving unintentional restriction of air and airway (Y37.47-)

√7th **Y37.440** **Military operations involving unarmed hand to hand combat, military personnel**

√7th **Y37.441** **Military operations involving unarmed hand to hand combat, civilian**

√6th **Y37.45** **Military operations involving combat using blunt or piercing object**

√7th **Y37.450** **Military operations involving combat using blunt or piercing object, military personnel**

√7th **Y37.451** **Military operations involving combat using blunt or piercing object, civilian**

√6th **Y37.46** **Military operations involving intentional restriction of air and airway**

√7th **Y37.460** **Military operations involving intentional restriction of air and airway, military personnel**

√7th **Y37.461** **Military operations involving intentional restriction of air and airway, civilian**

√6th **Y37.47** **Military operations involving unintentional restriction of air and airway**

√7th **Y37.470** **Military operations involving unintentional restriction of air and airway, military personnel**

√7th **Y37.471** **Military operations involving unintentional restriction of air and airway, civilian**

√6th **Y37.49** **Military operations involving other forms of conventional warfare**

√7th **Y37.490** **Military operations involving other forms of conventional warfare, military personnel**

√7th **Y37.491** **Military operations involving other forms of conventional warfare, civilian**

√5th **Y37.5** **Military operations involving nuclear weapons**
Military operation involving dirty bomb NOS

√6th **Y37.50** **Military operations involving unspecified effect of nuclear weapon**

√7th **Y37.500** **Military operations involving unspecified effect of nuclear weapon, military personnel** ▽

√7th **Y37.501** **Military operations involving unspecified effect of nuclear weapon, civilian** ▽

√6th **Y37.51** **Military operations involving direct blast effect of nuclear weapon**
Military operations involving blast pressure of nuclear weapon

√7th **Y37.510** **Military operations involving direct blast effect of nuclear weapon, military personnel**

√7th **Y37.511** **Military operations involving direct blast effect of nuclear weapon, civilian**

√6th **Y37.52** **Military operations involving indirect blast effect of nuclear weapon**
Military operations involving being thrown by blast of nuclear weapon
Military operations involving being struck or crushed by blast debris of nuclear weapon

√7th **Y37.520** **Military operations involving indirect blast effect of nuclear weapon, military personnel**

√7th **Y37.521** **Military operations involving indirect blast effect of nuclear weapon, civilian**

√6th **Y37.53** **Military operations involving thermal radiation effect of nuclear weapon**
Military operations involving direct heat from nuclear weapon
Military operation involving fireball effects from nuclear weapon

√7th **Y37.530** **Military operations involving thermal radiation effect of nuclear weapon, military personnel**

√7th **Y37.531** **Military operations involving thermal radiation effect of nuclear weapon, civilian**

√6th **Y37.54** **Military operation involving nuclear radiation effects of nuclear weapon**
Military operation involving acute radiation exposure from nuclear weapon
Military operation involving exposure to immediate ionizing radiation from nuclear weapon
Military operation involving fallout exposure from nuclear weapon
Military operation involving secondary effects of nuclear weapons

√7th **Y37.540** **Military operation involving nuclear radiation effects of nuclear weapon, military personnel**

√7th **Y37.541** **Military operation involving nuclear radiation effects of nuclear weapon, civilian**

√6th **Y37.59** **Military operation involving other effects of nuclear weapons**

√7th **Y37.590** **Military operation involving other effects of nuclear weapons, military personnel**

√7th **Y37.591** **Military operation involving other effects of nuclear weapons, civilian**

√5th **Y37.6** **Military operations involving biological weapons**

√6th **Y37.6X** **Military operations involving biological weapons**

√7th **Y37.6X0** **Military operations involving biological weapons, military personnel**

✓7ᵗʰ **Y37.6X1　Military operations involving biological weapons, civilian**

✓5ᵗʰ **Y37.7　Military operations involving chemical weapons and other forms of unconventional warfare**
　　　EXCLUDES 1 *military operations involving incendiary devices (Y36.3-, Y36.5-)*

　✓6ᵗʰ **Y37.7X　Military operations involving chemical weapons and other forms of unconventional warfare**
　　　✓7ᵗʰ **Y37.7X0　Military operations involving chemical weapons and other forms of unconventional warfare, military personnel**
　　　✓7ᵗʰ **Y37.7X1　Military operations involving chemical weapons and other forms of unconventional warfare, civilian**

✓5ᵗʰ **Y37.9　Other and unspecified military operations**
　✓×7ᵗʰ **Y37.90　Military operations, unspecified**　　▽
　✓×7ᵗʰ **Y37.91　Military operations involving unspecified weapon of mass destruction [WMD]**　▽
　✓×7ᵗʰ **Y37.92　Military operations involving friendly fire**

✓4ᵗʰ **Y38　Terrorism**

　NOTE　These codes are for use to identify injuries resulting from the unlawful use of force or violence against persons or property to intimidate or coerce a Government, the civilian population, or any segment thereof, in furtherance of political or social objective

　Use additional code for place of occurrence (Y92.-)

✓5ᵗʰ **Y38.0　Terrorism involving explosion of marine weapons**
　　Terrorism involving depth-charge
　　Terrorism involving marine mine
　　Terrorism involving mine NOS, at sea or in harbor
　　Terrorism involving sea-based artillery shell
　　Terrorism involving torpedo
　　Terrorism involving underwater blast
　✓6ᵗʰ **Y38.0X　Terrorism involving explosion of marine weapons**
　　　✓7ᵗʰ **Y38.0X1　Terrorism involving explosion of marine weapons, public safety official injured**
　　　✓7ᵗʰ **Y38.0X2　Terrorism involving explosion of marine weapons, civilian injured**
　　　✓7ᵗʰ **Y38.0X3　Terrorism involving explosion of marine weapons, terrorist injured**

✓5ᵗʰ **Y38.1　Terrorism involving destruction of aircraft**
　　Terrorism involving aircraft burned
　　Terrorism involving aircraft exploded
　　Terrorism involving aircraft being shot down
　　Terrorism involving aircraft used as a weapon
　✓6ᵗʰ **Y38.1X　Terrorism involving destruction of aircraft**
　　　✓7ᵗʰ **Y38.1X1　Terrorism involving destruction of aircraft, public safety official injured**
　　　✓7ᵗʰ **Y38.1X2　Terrorism involving destruction of aircraft, civilian injured**
　　　✓7ᵗʰ **Y38.1X3　Terrorism involving destruction of aircraft, terrorist injured**

✓5ᵗʰ **Y38.2　Terrorism involving other explosions and fragments**
　　Terrorism involving antipersonnel (fragments) bomb
　　Terrorism involving blast NOS
　　Terrorism involving explosion NOS
　　Terrorism involving explosion of breech block
　　Terrorism involving explosion of cannon block
　　Terrorism involving explosion (fragments) of artillery shell
　　Terrorism involving explosion (fragments) of bomb
　　Terrorism involving explosion (fragments) of grenade
　　Terrorism involving explosion (fragments) of guided missile
　　Terrorism involving explosion (fragments) of land mine
　　Terrorism involving explosion of mortar bomb
　　Terrorism involving explosion of munitions
　　Terrorism involving explosion (fragments) of rocket
　　Terrorism involving explosion (fragments) of shell
　　Terrorism involving shrapnel
　　Terrorism involving mine NOS, on land
　　EXCLUDES 1 *terrorism involving explosion of nuclear weapon (Y38.5)*
　　　　　terrorism involving suicide bomber (Y38.81)
　✓6ᵗʰ **Y38.2X　Terrorism involving other explosions and fragments**
　　　✓7ᵗʰ **Y38.2X1　Terrorism involving other explosions and fragments, public safety official injured**
　　　✓7ᵗʰ **Y38.2X2　Terrorism involving other explosions and fragments, civilian injured**

　　　✓7ᵗʰ **Y38.2X3　Terrorism involving other explosions and fragments, terrorist injured**

✓5ᵗʰ **Y38.3　Terrorism involving fires, conflagration and hot substances**
　　Terrorism involving conflagration NOS
　　Terrorism involving fire NOS
　　Terrorism involving petrol bomb
　　EXCLUDES 1 *terrorism involving fire or heat of nuclear weapon (Y38.5)*
　✓6ᵗʰ **Y38.3X　Terrorism involving fires, conflagration and hot substances**
　　　✓7ᵗʰ **Y38.3X1　Terrorism involving fires, conflagration and hot substances, public safety official injured**
　　　✓7ᵗʰ **Y38.3X2　Terrorism involving fires, conflagration and hot substances, civilian injured**
　　　✓7ᵗʰ **Y38.3X3　Terrorism involving fires, conflagration and hot substances, terrorist injured**

✓5ᵗʰ **Y38.4　Terrorism involving firearms**
　　Terrorism involving carbine bullet
　　Terrorism involving machine gun bullet
　　Terrorism involving pellets (shotgun)
　　Terrorism involving pistol bullet
　　Terrorism involving rifle bullet
　　Terrorism involving rubber (rifle) bullet
　✓6ᵗʰ **Y38.4X　Terrorism involving firearms**
　　　✓7ᵗʰ **Y38.4X1　Terrorism involving firearms, public safety official injured**
　　　✓7ᵗʰ **Y38.4X2　Terrorism involving firearms, civilian injured**
　　　✓7ᵗʰ **Y38.4X3　Terrorism involving firearms, terrorist injured**

✓5ᵗʰ **Y38.5　Terrorism involving nuclear weapons**
　　Terrorism involving blast effects of nuclear weapon
　　Terrorism involving exposure to ionizing radiation from nuclear weapon
　　Terrorism involving fireball effect of nuclear weapon
　　Terrorism involving heat from nuclear weapon
　✓6ᵗʰ **Y38.5X　Terrorism involving nuclear weapons**
　　　✓7ᵗʰ **Y38.5X1　Terrorism involving nuclear weapons, public safety official injured**
　　　✓7ᵗʰ **Y38.5X2　Terrorism involving nuclear weapons, civilian injured**
　　　✓7ᵗʰ **Y38.5X3　Terrorism involving nuclear weapons, terrorist injured**

✓5ᵗʰ **Y38.6　Terrorism involving biological weapons**
　　Terrorism involving anthrax
　　Terrorism involving cholera
　　Terrorism involving smallpox
　✓6ᵗʰ **Y38.6X　Terrorism involving biological weapons**
　　　✓7ᵗʰ **Y38.6X1　Terrorism involving biological weapons, public safety official injured**
　　　✓7ᵗʰ **Y38.6X2　Terrorism involving biological weapons, civilian injured**
　　　✓7ᵗʰ **Y38.6X3　Terrorism involving biological weapons, terrorist injured**

✓5ᵗʰ **Y38.7　Terrorism involving chemical weapons**
　　Terrorism involving gases, fumes, chemicals
　　Terrorism involving hydrogen cyanide
　　Terrorism involving phosgene
　　Terrorism involving sarin
　✓6ᵗʰ **Y38.7X　Terrorism involving chemical weapons**
　　　✓7ᵗʰ **Y38.7X1　Terrorism involving chemical weapons, public safety official injured**
　　　✓7ᵗʰ **Y38.7X2　Terrorism involving chemical weapons, civilian injured**
　　　✓7ᵗʰ **Y38.7X3　Terrorism involving chemical weapons, terrorist injured**

✓5ᵗʰ **Y38.8　Terrorism involving other and unspecified means**
　✓×7ᵗʰ **Y38.80　Terrorism involving unspecified means**　▽
　　　Terrorism NOS
　✓6ᵗʰ **Y38.81　Terrorism involving suicide bomber**
　　　✓7ᵗʰ **Y38.811　Terrorism involving suicide bomber, public safety official injured**
　　　✓7ᵗʰ **Y38.812　Terrorism involving suicide bomber, civilian injured**

☑ Additional Character Required　　✓×7ᵗʰ Placeholder Alert　　Manifestation Dx　　▽ Unspecified Dx　　▶◀ Revised Text　　● New Code　　▲ Revised Code Title

Chapter 20. External Causes of Morbidity

✓6ᵗʰ **Y38.89 Terrorism involving other means**

Terrorism involving drowning and submersion

Terrorism involving lasers

Terrorism involving piercing or stabbing instruments

✓7ᵗʰ **Y38.891 Terrorism involving other means, public safety official injured**

✓7ᵗʰ **Y38.892 Terrorism involving other means, civilian injured**

✓7ᵗʰ **Y38.893 Terrorism involving other means, terrorist injured**

✓5ᵗʰ **Y38.9 Terrorism, secondary effects**

NOTE This code is for use to identify conditions occurring subsequent to a terrorist attack not those that are due to the initial terrorist attack

✓6ᵗʰ **Y38.9X Terrorism, secondary effects**

✓7ᵗʰ **Y38.9X1 Terrorism, secondary effects, public safety official injured**

✓7ᵗʰ **Y38.9X2 Terrorism, secondary effects, civilian injured**

Complications of medical and surgical care (Y62-Y84)

INCLUDES complications of medical devices

surgical and medical procedures as the cause of abnormal reaction of the patient, or of later complication, without mention of misadventure at the time of the procedure

Misadventures to patients during surgical and medical care (Y62-Y69)

EXCLUDES 1 ▶surgical and medical procedures as the cause of abnormal reaction of the patient, without mention of misadventure at the time of the procedure (Y83-Y84)◀

EXCLUDES 2 breakdown or malfunctioning of medical device (during procedure) (after implantation) (ongoing use) (Y70-Y82)

✓4ᵗʰ **Y62 Failure of sterile precautions during surgical and medical care**

Y62.0 Failure of sterile precautions during surgical operation

Y62.1 Failure of sterile precautions during infusion or transfusion

Y62.2 Failure of sterile precautions during kidney dialysis and other perfusion

Y62.3 Failure of sterile precautions during injection or immunization

Y62.4 Failure of sterile precautions during endoscopic examination

Y62.5 Failure of sterile precautions during heart catheterization

Y62.6 Failure of sterile precautions during aspiration, puncture and other catheterization

Y62.8 Failure of sterile precautions during other surgical and medical care

Y62.9 Failure of sterile precautions during unspecified surgical and medical care ▽

✓4ᵗʰ **Y63 Failure in dosage during surgical and medical care**

EXCLUDES 2 accidental overdose of drug or wrong drug given in error (T36-T50)

Y63.0 Excessive amount of blood or other fluid given during transfusion or infusion

Y63.1 Incorrect dilution of fluid used during infusion

Y63.2 Overdose of radiation given during therapy

Y63.3 Inadvertent exposure of patient to radiation during medical care

Y63.4 Failure in dosage in electroshock or insulin-shock therapy

Y63.5 Inappropriate temperature in local application and packing

Y63.6 Underdosing and nonadministration of necessary drug, medicament or biological substance

Y63.8 Failure in dosage during other surgical and medical care

Y63.9 Failure in dosage during unspecified surgical and medical care ▽

✓4ᵗʰ **Y64 Contaminated medical or biological substances**

Y64.0 Contaminated medical or biological substance, transfused or infused

Y64.1 Contaminated medical or biological substance, injected or used for immunization

Y64.8 Contaminated medical or biological substance administered by other means

Y64.9 Contaminated medical or biological substance administered by unspecified means ▽

Administered contaminated medical or biological substance NOS

✓4ᵗʰ **Y65 Other misadventures during surgical and medical care**

Y65.0 Mismatched blood in transfusion

Y65.1 Wrong fluid used in infusion

Y65.2 Failure in suture or ligature during surgical operation

Y65.3 Endotracheal tube wrongly placed during anesthetic procedure

Y65.4 Failure to introduce or to remove other tube or instrument

✓5ᵗʰ **Y65.5 Performance of wrong procedure (operation)**

Y65.51 Performance of wrong procedure (operation) on correct patient

Wrong device implanted into correct surgical site

EXCLUDES 1 performance of correct procedure (operation) on wrong side or body part (Y65.53)

Y65.52 Performance of procedure (operation) on patient not scheduled for surgery

Performance of procedure (operation) intended for another patient

Performance of procedure (operation) on wrong patient

Y65.53 Performance of correct procedure (operation) on wrong side or body part

Performance of correct procedure (operation) on wrong side

Performance of correct procedure (operation) on wrong site

Y65.8 Other specified misadventures during surgical and medical care

Y66 Nonadministration of surgical and medical care

Premature cessation of surgical and medical care

EXCLUDES 1 DNR status (Z66)

palliative care (Z51.5)

Y69 Unspecified misadventure during surgical and medical care ▽

Medical devices associated with adverse incidents in diagnostic and therapeutic use (Y70-Y82)

INCLUDES breakdown or malfunction of medical devices (during use) (after implantation) (ongoing use)

EXCLUDES 2 ▶breakdown or malfunctioning of medical device (after implantation) (during procedure) (ongoing use) (Y70-Y82)◀

▶later complications following use of medical devices without breakdown or malfunctioning of device (Y83-Y84)◀

▶misadventure to patients during surgical and medical care, classifiable to (Y62-Y69)◀

▶surgical and other medical procedures as the cause of abnormal reaction of the patient, or of later complication, without mention of misadventure at the time of the procedure (Y83-Y84)◀

✓4ᵗʰ **Y70 Anesthesiology devices associated with adverse incidents**

Y70.0 Diagnostic and monitoring anesthesiology devices associated with adverse incidents

Y70.1 Therapeutic (nonsurgical) and rehabilitative anesthesiology devices associated with adverse incidents

Y70.2 Prosthetic and other implants, materials and accessory anesthesiology devices associated with adverse incidents

Y70.3 Surgical instruments, materials and anesthesiology devices (including sutures) associated with adverse incidents

Y70.8 Miscellaneous anesthesiology devices associated with adverse incidents, not elsewhere classified

✓4ᵗʰ **Y71 Cardiovascular devices associated with adverse incidents**

Y71.0 Diagnostic and monitoring cardiovascular devices associated with adverse incidents

Y71.1 Therapeutic (nonsurgical) and rehabilitative cardiovascular devices associated with adverse incidents

Y71.2 Prosthetic and other implants, materials and accessory cardiovascular devices associated with adverse incidents

Y71.3 Surgical instruments, materials and cardiovascular devices (including sutures) associated with adverse incidents

Y71.8 Miscellaneous cardiovascular devices associated with adverse incidents, not elsewhere classified

✓4ᵗʰ **Y72 Otorhinolaryngological devices associated with adverse incidents**

Y72.0 Diagnostic and monitoring otorhinolaryngological devices associated with adverse incidents

Y72.1 Therapeutic (nonsurgical) and rehabilitative otorhinolaryngological devices associated with adverse incidents

Y72.2 Prosthetic and other implants, materials and accessory otorhinolaryngological devices associated with adverse incidents

Y72.3 Surgical instruments, materials and otorhinolaryngological devices (including sutures) associated with adverse incidents

Y72.8 Miscellaneous otorhinolaryngological devices associated with adverse incidents, not elsewhere classified

EXCLUDES 1 Not coded here   **EXCLUDES 2** Not included here   **N** Newborn Age : 0   **P** Pediatric Age : 0-17   **M** Maternity Age : 12-55   **A** Adult Age : 15-124

1130   ICD-10-CM 2017

✓4ᵗʰ **Y73** **Gastroenterology and urology** devices associated with adverse incidents

    Y73.Ø Diagnostic and monitoring gastroenterology and urology devices associated with adverse incidents

    Y73.1 Therapeutic (nonsurgical) and rehabilitative gastroenterology and urology devices associated with adverse incidents

    Y73.2 Prosthetic and other implants, materials and accessory gastroenterology and urology devices associated with adverse incidents

    Y73.3 Surgical instruments, materials and gastroenterology and urology devices (including sutures) associated with adverse incidents

    Y73.8 Miscellaneous gastroenterology and urology devices associated with adverse incidents, not elsewhere classified

✓4ᵗʰ **Y74** **General hospital and personal-use** devices associated with adverse incidents

    Y74.Ø Diagnostic and monitoring general hospital and personal-use devices associated with adverse incidents

    Y74.1 Therapeutic (nonsurgical) and rehabilitative general hospital and personal-use devices associated with adverse incidents

    Y74.2 Prosthetic and other implants, materials and accessory general hospital and personal-use devices associated with adverse incidents

    Y74.3 Surgical instruments, materials and general hospital and personal-use devices (including sutures) associated with adverse incidents

    Y74.8 Miscellaneous general hospital and personal-use devices associated with adverse incidents, not elsewhere classified

✓4ᵗʰ **Y75** **Neurological** devices associated with adverse incidents

    Y75.Ø Diagnostic and monitoring neurological devices associated with adverse incidents

    Y75.1 Therapeutic (nonsurgical) and rehabilitative neurological devices associated with adverse incidents

    Y75.2 Prosthetic and other implants, materials and neurological devices associated with adverse incidents

    Y75.3 Surgical instruments, materials and neurological devices (including sutures) associated with adverse incidents

    Y75.8 Miscellaneous neurological devices associated with adverse incidents, not elsewhere classified

✓4ᵗʰ **Y76** **Obstetric and gynecological** devices associated with adverse incidents

    Y76.Ø Diagnostic and monitoring obstetric and gynecological devices associated with adverse incidents   ♀

    Y76.1 Therapeutic (nonsurgical) and rehabilitative obstetric and gynecological devices associated with adverse incidents   ♀

    Y76.2 Prosthetic and other implants, materials and accessory obstetric and gynecological devices associated with adverse incidents   ♀

    Y76.3 Surgical instruments, materials and obstetric and gynecological devices (including sutures) associated with adverse incidents   ♀

    Y76.8 Miscellaneous obstetric and gynecological devices associated with adverse incidents, not elsewhere classified   ♀

✓4ᵗʰ **Y77** **Ophthalmic** devices associated with adverse incidents

    Y77.Ø Diagnostic and monitoring ophthalmic devices associated with adverse incidents

    Y77.1 Therapeutic (nonsurgical) and rehabilitative ophthalmic devices associated with adverse incidents

    Y77.2 Prosthetic and other implants, materials and accessory ophthalmic devices associated with adverse incidents

    Y77.3 Surgical instruments, materials and ophthalmic devices (including sutures) associated with adverse incidents

    Y77.8 Miscellaneous ophthalmic devices associated with adverse incidents, not elsewhere classified

✓4ᵗʰ **Y78** **Radiological** devices associated with adverse incidents

    Y78.Ø Diagnostic and monitoring radiological devices associated with adverse incidents

    Y78.1 Therapeutic (nonsurgical) and rehabilitative radiological devices associated with adverse incidents

    Y78.2 Prosthetic and other implants, materials and accessory radiological devices associated with adverse incidents

    Y78.3 Surgical instruments, materials and radiological devices (including sutures) associated with adverse incidents

    Y78.8 Miscellaneous radiological devices associated with adverse incidents, not elsewhere classified

✓4ᵗʰ **Y79** **Orthopedic** devices associated with adverse incidents

    Y79.Ø Diagnostic and monitoring orthopedic devices associated with adverse incidents

    Y79.1 Therapeutic (nonsurgical) and rehabilitative orthopedic devices associated with adverse incidents

    Y79.2 Prosthetic and other implants, materials and accessory orthopedic devices associated with adverse incidents

    Y79.3 Surgical instruments, materials and orthopedic devices (including sutures) associated with adverse incidents

    Y79.8 Miscellaneous orthopedic devices associated with adverse incidents, not elsewhere classified

✓4ᵗʰ **Y80** **Physical medicine** devices associated with adverse incidents

    Y80.Ø Diagnostic and monitoring physical medicine devices associated with adverse incidents

    Y80.1 Therapeutic (nonsurgical) and rehabilitative physical medicine devices associated with adverse incidents

    Y80.2 Prosthetic and other implants, materials and accessory physical medicine devices associated with adverse incidents

    Y80.3 Surgical instruments, materials and physical medicine devices (including sutures) associated with adverse incidents

    Y80.8 Miscellaneous physical medicine devices associated with adverse incidents, not elsewhere classified

✓4ᵗʰ **Y81** **General- and plastic-surgery** devices associated with adverse incidents

    Y81.Ø Diagnostic and monitoring general- and plastic-surgery devices associated with adverse incidents

    Y81.1 Therapeutic (nonsurgical) and rehabilitative general- and plastic-surgery devices associated with adverse incidents

    Y81.2 Prosthetic and other implants, materials and accessory general- and plastic-surgery devices associated with adverse incidents

    Y81.3 Surgical instruments, materials and general- and plastic-surgery devices (including sutures) associated with adverse incidents

    Y81.8 Miscellaneous general- and plastic-surgery devices associated with adverse incidents, not elsewhere classified

✓4ᵗʰ **Y82** **Other and unspecified medical devices associated with adverse incidents**

    Y82.8 Other medical devices associated with adverse incidents

    Y82.9 Unspecified medical devices associated with adverse incidents   ▽

Surgical and other medical procedures as the cause of abnormal reaction of the patient, or of later complication, without mention of misadventure at the time of the procedure (Y83-Y84)

EXCLUDES 1 misadventures to patients during surgical and medical care, classifiable to (Y62-Y69)

EXCLUDES 2 ▶breakdown or malfunctioning of medical device (during procedure) (after implantation) (ongoing use) (Y70-Y82)◀

✓4ᵗʰ **Y83** **Surgical operation and other surgical procedures as the cause of abnormal reaction of the patient, or of later complication, without mention of misadventure at the time of the procedure**

    Y83.Ø Surgical operation with transplant of whole organ as the cause of abnormal reaction of the patient, or of later complication, without mention of misadventure at the time of the procedure

    Y83.1 Surgical operation with implant of artificial internal device as the cause of abnormal reaction of the patient, or of later complication, without mention of misadventure at the time of the procedure

    Y83.2 Surgical operation with anastomosis, bypass or graft as the cause of abnormal reaction of the patient, or of later complication, without mention of misadventure at the time of the procedure

    Y83.3 Surgical operation with formation of external stoma as the cause of abnormal reaction of the patient, or of later complication, without mention of misadventure at the time of the procedure

    Y83.4 Other reconstructive surgery as the cause of abnormal reaction of the patient, or of later complication, without mention of misadventure at the time of the procedure

    Y83.5 Amputation of limb(s) as the cause of abnormal reaction of the patient, or of later complication, without mention of misadventure at the time of the procedure

    Y83.6 Removal of other organ (partial) (total) as the cause of abnormal reaction of the patient, or of later complication, without mention of misadventure at the time of the procedure

    Y83.8 Other surgical procedures as the cause of abnormal reaction of the patient, or of later complication, without mention of misadventure at the time of the procedure

---

☑ Additional Character Required   ✔×7ᵗʰ Placeholder Alert   Manifestation Dx   ▽ Unspecified Dx   ▶◀ Revised Text   ● New Code   ▲ Revised Code Title

Y83.9   Surgical procedure, unspecified as the cause of abnormal reaction of the patient, or of later complication, without mention of misadventure at the time of the procedure ▽

✓4ᵗʰ **Y84**   Other medical procedures as the cause of abnormal reaction of the patient, or of later complication, without mention of misadventure at the time of the procedure

Y84.0   Cardiac catheterization as the cause of abnormal reaction of the patient, or of later complication, without mention of misadventure at the time of the procedure

Y84.1   Kidney dialysis as the cause of abnormal reaction of the patient, or of later complication, without mention of misadventure at the time of the procedure

Y84.2   Radiological procedure and radiotherapy as the cause of abnormal reaction of the patient, or of later complication, without mention of misadventure at the time of the procedure

Y84.3   Shock therapy as the cause of abnormal reaction of the patient, or of later complication, without mention of misadventure at the time of the procedure

Y84.4   Aspiration of fluid as the cause of abnormal reaction of the patient, or of later complication, without mention of misadventure at the time of the procedure

Y84.5   Insertion of gastric or duodenal sound as the cause of abnormal reaction of the patient, or of later complication, without mention of misadventure at the time of the procedure

Y84.6   Urinary catheterization as the cause of abnormal reaction of the patient, or of later complication, without mention of misadventure at the time of the procedure

Y84.7   Blood-sampling as the cause of abnormal reaction of the patient, or of later complication, without mention of misadventure at the time of the procedure

Y84.8   Other medical procedures as the cause of abnormal reaction of the patient, or of later complication, without mention of misadventure at the time of the procedure
    AHA: 2014,4Q,24

Y84.9   Medical procedure, unspecified as the cause of abnormal reaction of the patient, or of later complication, without mention of misadventure at the time of the procedure ▽

Supplementary factors related to causes of morbidity classified elsewhere (Y90-Y99)

NOTE   These categories may be used to provide supplementary information concerning causes of morbidity. They are not to be used for single-condition coding.

✓4ᵗʰ **Y90**   Evidence of alcohol involvement determined by blood alcohol level
    Code first any associated alcohol related disorders (F10)

Y90.0   Blood alcohol level of less than 20 mg/100 ml
Y90.1   Blood alcohol level of 20-39 mg/100 ml
Y90.2   Blood alcohol level of 40-59 mg/100 ml
Y90.3   Blood alcohol level of 60-79 mg/100 ml
Y90.4   Blood alcohol level of 80-99 mg/100 ml
Y90.5   Blood alcohol level of 100-119 mg/100 ml
Y90.6   Blood alcohol level of 120-199 mg/100 ml
Y90.7   Blood alcohol level of 200-239 mg/100 ml
Y90.8   Blood alcohol level of 240 mg/100 ml or more
Y90.9   Presence of alcohol in blood, level not specified ▽

✓4ᵗʰ **Y92**   Place of occurrence of the external cause
    The following category is for use, when relevant, to identify the place of occurrence of the external cause. Use in conjunction with an activity code.
    Place of occurrence should be recorded only at the initial encounter for treatment

✓5ᵗʰ **Y92.0**   Non-institutional (private) residence as the place of occurrence of the external cause
    EXCLUDES 1   abandoned or derelict house (Y92.89)
      home under construction but not yet occupied (Y92.6-)
      institutional place of residence (Y92.1-)

✓6ᵗʰ **Y92.00**   Unspecified non-institutional (private) residence as the place of occurrence of the external cause

    Y92.000   Kitchen of unspecified non-institutional (private) residence as the place of occurrence of the external cause ▽

    Y92.001   Dining room of unspecified non-institutional (private) residence as the place of occurrence of the external cause ▽

    Y92.002   Bathroom of unspecified non-institutional (private) residence single-family (private) house as the place of occurrence of the external cause ▽

    Y92.003   Bedroom of unspecified non-institutional (private) residence as the place of occurrence of the external cause ▽

    Y92.007   Garden or yard of unspecified non-institutional (private) residence as the place of occurrence of the external cause ▽

    Y92.008   Other place in unspecified non-institutional (private) residence as the place of occurrence of the external cause ▽

    Y92.009   Unspecified place in unspecified non-institutional (private) residence as the place of occurrence of the external cause ▽
      Home (NOS) as the place of occurrence of the external cause

✓6ᵗʰ **Y92.01**   Single-family non-institutional (private) house as the place of occurrence of the external cause
    Farmhouse as the place of occurrence of the external cause
    EXCLUDES 1   barn (Y92.71)
      chicken coop or hen house (Y92.72)
      farm field (Y92.73)
      orchard (Y92.74)
      single family mobile home or trailer (Y92.02-)
      slaughter house (Y92.86)

    Y92.010   Kitchen of single-family (private) house as the place of occurrence of the external cause

    Y92.011   Dining room of single-family (private) house as the place of occurrence of the external cause

    Y92.012   Bathroom of single-family (private) house as the place of occurrence of the external cause

    Y92.013   Bedroom of single-family (private) house as the place of occurrence of the external cause

    Y92.014   Private driveway to single-family (private) house as the place of occurrence of the external cause

    Y92.015   Private garage of single-family (private) house as the place of occurrence of the external cause

    Y92.016   Swimming-pool in single-family (private) house or garden as the place of occurrence of the external cause

    Y92.017   Garden or yard in single-family (private) house as the place of occurrence of the external cause

    Y92.018   Other place in single-family (private) house as the place of occurrence of the external cause

    Y92.019   Unspecified place in single-family (private) house as the place of occurrence of the external cause ▽

✓6ᵗʰ **Y92.02**   Mobile home as the place of occurrence of the external cause

    Y92.020   Kitchen in mobile home as the place of occurrence of the external cause

    Y92.021   Dining room in mobile home as the place of occurrence of the external cause

    Y92.022   Bathroom in mobile home as the place of occurrence of the external cause

    Y92.023   Bedroom in mobile home as the place of occurrence of the external cause

    Y92.024   Driveway of mobile home as the place of occurrence of the external cause

    Y92.025   Garage of mobile home as the place of occurrence of the external cause

    Y92.026   Swimming-pool of mobile home as the place of occurrence of the external cause

EXCLUDES 1 Not coded here   **EXCLUDES 2** Not included here   N Newborn Age : 0   P Pediatric Age : 0-17   M Maternity Age : 12-55   A Adult Age : 15-124

1132   ICD-10-CM 2017

Y92.027 Garden or yard of mobile home as the place of occurrence of the external cause

Y92.028 Other place in mobile home as the place of occurrence of the external cause

Y92.029 Unspecified place in mobile home as the place of occurrence of the external cause ▽

✓6ᵗʰ **Y92.03** Apartment as the place of occurrence of the external cause

     Condominium as the place of occurrence of the external cause

     Co-op apartment as the place of occurrence of the external cause

Y92.030 Kitchen in apartment as the place of occurrence of the external cause

Y92.031 Bathroom in apartment as the place of occurrence of the external cause

Y92.032 Bedroom in apartment as the place of occurrence of the external cause

Y92.038 Other place in apartment as the place of occurrence of the external cause

Y92.039 Unspecified place in apartment as the place of occurrence of the external cause ▽

✓6ᵗʰ **Y92.04** Boarding-house as the place of occurrence of the external cause

Y92.040 Kitchen in boarding-house as the place of occurrence of the external cause

Y92.041 Bathroom in boarding-house as the place of occurrence of the external cause

Y92.042 Bedroom in boarding-house as the place of occurrence of the external cause

Y92.043 Driveway of boarding-house as the place of occurrence of the external cause

Y92.044 Garage of boarding-house as the place of occurrence of the external cause

Y92.045 Swimming-pool of boarding-house as the place of occurrence of the external cause

Y92.046 Garden or yard of boarding-house as the place of occurrence of the external cause

Y92.048 Other place in boarding-house as the place of occurrence of the external cause

Y92.049 Unspecified place in boarding-house as the place of occurrence of the external cause ▽

✓6ᵗʰ **Y92.09** Other non-institutional residence as the place of occurrence of the external cause

Y92.090 Kitchen in other non-institutional residence as the place of occurrence of the external cause

Y92.091 Bathroom in other non-institutional residence as the place of occurrence of the external cause

Y92.092 Bedroom in other non-institutional residence as the place of occurrence of the external cause

Y92.093 Driveway of other non-institutional residence as the place of occurrence of the external cause

Y92.094 Garage of other non-institutional residence as the place of occurrence of the external cause

Y92.095 Swimming-pool of other non-institutional residence as the place of occurrence of the external cause

Y92.096 Garden or yard of other non-institutional residence as the place of occurrence of the external cause

Y92.098 Other place in other non-institutional residence as the place of occurrence of the external cause

Y92.099 Unspecified place in other non-institutional residence as the place of occurrence of the external cause ▽

✓6ᵗʰ **Y92.1** Institutional (nonprivate) residence as the place of occurrence of the external cause

Y92.10 Unspecified residential institution as the place of occurrence of the external cause ▽

✓6ᵗʰ **Y92.11** Children's home and orphanage as the place of occurrence of the external cause

Y92.110 Kitchen in children's home and orphanage as the place of occurrence of the external cause

Y92.111 Bathroom in children's home and orphanage as the place of occurrence of the external cause

Y92.112 Bedroom in children's home and orphanage as the place of occurrence of the external cause

Y92.113 Driveway of children's home and orphanage as the place of occurrence of the external cause

Y92.114 Garage of children's home and orphanage as the place of occurrence of the external cause

Y92.115 Swimming-pool of children's home and orphanage as the place of occurrence of the external cause

Y92.116 Garden or yard of children's home and orphanage as the place of occurrence of the external cause

Y92.118 Other place in children's home and orphanage as the place of occurrence of the external cause

Y92.119 Unspecified place in children's home and orphanage as the place of occurrence of the external cause ▽

✓6ᵗʰ **Y92.12** Nursing home as the place of occurrence of the external cause

     Home for the sick as the place of occurrence of the external cause

     Hospice as the place of occurrence of the external cause

Y92.120 Kitchen in nursing home as the place of occurrence of the external cause

Y92.121 Bathroom in nursing home as the place of occurrence of the external cause

Y92.122 Bedroom in nursing home as the place of occurrence of the external cause

Y92.123 Driveway of nursing home as the place of occurrence of the external cause

Y92.124 Garage of nursing home as the place of occurrence of the external cause

Y92.125 Swimming-pool of nursing home as the place of occurrence of the external cause

Y92.126 Garden or yard of nursing home as the place of occurrence of the external cause

Y92.128 Other place in nursing home as the place of occurrence of the external cause

Y92.129 Unspecified place in nursing home as the place of occurrence of the external cause ▽

✓6ᵗʰ **Y92.13** Military base as the place of occurrence of the external cause

     EXCLUDES 1 *military training grounds (Y92.84)*

Y92.130 Kitchen on military base as the place of occurrence of the external cause

Y92.131 Mess hall on military base as the place of occurrence of the external cause

Y92.133 Barracks on military base as the place of occurrence of the external cause

Y92.135 Garage on military base as the place of occurrence of the external cause

Y92.136 Swimming-pool on military base as the place of occurrence of the external cause

Y92.137 Garden or yard on military base as the place of occurrence of the external cause

Y92.138 Other place on military base as the place of occurrence of the external cause

Y92.139 Unspecified place military base as the place of occurrence of the external cause ▽

✓6ᵗʰ **Y92.14** Prison as the place of occurrence of the external cause

Y92.140 Kitchen in prison as the place of occurrence of the external cause

Y92.141 Dining room in prison as the place of occurrence of the external cause

Y92.142 Bathroom in prison as the place of occurrence of the external cause

Y92.143 Cell of prison as the place of occurrence of the external cause

Y92.146 Swimming-pool of prison as the place of occurrence of the external cause

Y92.147 Courtyard of prison as the place of occurrence of the external cause

☑ Additional Character Required   ✓x7ᵗʰ Placeholder Alert   Manifestation Dx   ▽ Unspecified Dx   ▶◀ Revised Text   ● New Code   ▲ Revised Code Title

ICD-10-CM 2017   1133

Y92.148   **Other place in prison** as the place of occurrence of the external cause

Y92.149   **Unspecified place in prison** as the place of occurrence of the external cause   ▽

☑6ᵗʰ   **Y92.15**   **Reform school** as the place of occurrence of the external cause

Y92.150   **Kitchen** in reform school as the place of occurrence of the external cause

Y92.151   **Dining room** in reform school as the place of occurrence of the external cause

Y92.152   **Bathroom** in reform school as the place of occurrence of the external cause

Y92.153   **Bedroom** in reform school as the place of occurrence of the external cause

Y92.154   **Driveway** of reform school as the place of occurrence of the external cause

Y92.155   **Garage** of reform school as the place of occurrence of the external cause

Y92.156   **Swimming-pool** of reform school as the place of occurrence of the external cause

Y92.157   **Garden or yard** of reform school as the place of occurrence of the external cause

Y92.158   **Other place** in reform school as the place of occurrence of the external cause

Y92.159   **Unspecified place** in reform school as the place of occurrence of the external cause   ▽

☑6ᵗʰ   **Y92.16**   **School dormitory** as the place of occurrence of the external cause

> **EXCLUDES 1** *reform school as the place of occurrence of the external cause (Y92.15-)*
> *school buildings and grounds as the place of occurrence of the external cause (Y92.2-)*
> *school sports and athletic areas as the place of occurrence of the external cause (Y92.3-)*

Y92.160   **Kitchen** in school dormitory as the place of occurrence of the external cause

Y92.161   **Dining room** in school dormitory as the place of occurrence of the external cause

Y92.162   **Bathroom** in school dormitory as the place of occurrence of the external cause

Y92.163   **Bedroom** in school dormitory as the place of occurrence of the external cause

Y92.168   **Other place** in school dormitory as the place of occurrence of the external cause

Y92.169   **Unspecified place** in school dormitory as the place of occurrence of the external cause   ▽

☑6ᵗʰ   **Y92.19**   **Other specified residential institution** as the place of occurrence of the external cause

Y92.190   **Kitchen** in other specified residential institution as the place of occurrence of the external cause

Y92.191   **Dining room** in other specified residential institution as the place of occurrence of the external cause

Y92.192   **Bathroom** in other specified residential institution as the place of occurrence of the external cause

Y92.193   **Bedroom** in other specified residential institution as the place of occurrence of the external cause

Y92.194   **Driveway** of other specified residential institution as the place of occurrence of the external cause

Y92.195   **Garage** of other specified residential institution as the place of occurrence of the external cause

Y92.196   **Pool** of other specified residential institution as the place of occurrence of the external cause

Y92.197   **Garden or yard** of other specified residential institution as the place of occurrence of the external cause

Y92.198   **Other place** in other specified residential institution as the place of occurrence of the external cause

Y92.199   **Unspecified place** in other specified residential institution as the place of occurrence of the external cause   ▽

☑5ᵗʰ   **Y92.2**   **School, other institution and public administrative area** as the place of occurrence of the external cause

Building and adjacent grounds used by the general public or by a particular group of the public

> **EXCLUDES 1** *building under construction as the place of occurrence of the external cause (Y92.6)*
> *residential institution as the place of occurrence of the external cause (Y92.1)*
> *school dormitory as the place of occurrence of the external cause (Y92.16-)*
> *sports and athletics area of schools as the place of occurrence of the external cause (Y92.3-)*

☑6ᵗʰ   **Y92.21**   **School** (private) (public) (state) as the place of occurrence of the external cause

Y92.210   **Daycare center** as the place of occurrence of the external cause

Y92.211   **Elementary school** as the place of occurrence of the external cause

Kindergarten as the place of occurrence of the external cause

Y92.212   **Middle school** as the place of occurrence of the external cause

Y92.213   **High school** as the place of occurrence of the external cause

AHA: 2012,4Q,108

Y92.214   **College** as the place of occurrence of the external cause

University as the place of occurrence of the external cause

Y92.215   **Trade school** as the place of occurrence of the external cause

Y92.218   **Other school** as the place of occurrence of the external cause

Y92.219   **Unspecified school** as the place of occurrence of the external cause   ▽

Y92.22   **Religious institution** as the place of occurrence of the external cause

Church as the place of occurrence of the external cause

Mosque as the place of occurrence of the external cause

Synagogue as the place of occurrence of the external cause

☑6ᵗʰ   **Y92.23**   **Hospital** as the place of occurrence of the external cause

> **EXCLUDES 1** *ambulatory (outpatient) health services establishments (Y92.53-)*
> *home for the sick as the place of occurrence of the external cause (Y92.12-)*
> *hospice as the place of occurrence of the external cause (Y92.12-)*
> *nursing home as the place of occurrence of the external cause (Y92.12-)*

Y92.230   **Patient room** in hospital as the place of occurrence of the external cause

Y92.231   **Patient bathroom** in hospital as the place of occurrence of the external cause

Y92.232   **Corridor** of hospital as the place of occurrence of the external cause

Y92.233   **Cafeteria** of hospital as the place of occurrence of the external cause

Y92.234   **Operating room** of hospital as the place of occurrence of the external cause

Y92.238   **Other place** in hospital as the place of occurrence of the external cause

Y92.239   **Unspecified place** in hospital as the place of occurrence of the external cause   ▽

☑6ᵗʰ   **Y92.24**   **Public administrative building** as the place of occurrence of the external cause

Y92.240   **Courthouse** as the place of occurrence of the external cause

Y92.241   **Library** as the place of occurrence of the external cause

Y92.242   **Post office** as the place of occurrence of the external cause

Y92.243   **City hall** as the place of occurrence of the external cause

Y92.248   **Other public administrative building** as the place of occurrence of the external cause

EXCLUDES 1 Not coded here   **EXCLUDES 2** Not included here   🅽 Newborn Age : 0   🅿 Pediatric Age : 0-17   🅼 Maternity Age : 12-55   🅰 Adult Age : 15-124

1134   ICD-10-CM 2017

✓6ᵗʰ **Y92.25** **Cultural building** as the place of occurrence of the external cause

     Y92.250 **Art Gallery** as the place of occurrence of the external cause

     Y92.251 **Museum** as the place of occurrence of the external cause

     Y92.252 **Music hall** as the place of occurrence of the external cause

     Y92.253 **Opera house** as the place of occurrence of the external cause

     Y92.254 **Theater (live)** as the place of occurrence of the external cause

     Y92.258 **Other cultural public building** as the place of occurrence of the external cause

Y92.26 **Movie house or cinema** as the place of occurrence of the external cause

Y92.29 **Other specified public building** as the place of occurrence of the external cause

     Assembly hall as the place of occurrence of the external cause

     Clubhouse as the place of occurrence of the external cause

✓5ᵗʰ **Y92.3** **Sports and athletics area** as the place of occurrence of the external cause

✓6ᵗʰ **Y92.31** **Athletic court** as the place of occurrence of the external cause

     EXCLUDES 1 *tennis court in private home or garden (Y92.09)*

     Y92.310 **Basketball court** as the place of occurrence of the external cause

     Y92.311 **Squash court** as the place of occurrence of the external cause

     Y92.312 **Tennis court** as the place of occurrence of the external cause

     Y92.318 **Other athletic court** as the place of occurrence of the external cause

✓6ᵗʰ **Y92.32** **Athletic field** as the place of occurrence of the external cause

     Y92.320 **Baseball field** as the place of occurrence of the external cause

     Y92.321 **Football field** as the place of occurrence of the external cause

     Y92.322 **Soccer field** as the place of occurrence of the external cause

     Y92.328 **Other athletic field** as the place of occurrence of the external cause

         Cricket field as the place of occurrence of the external cause

         Hockey field as the place of occurrence of the external cause

✓6ᵗʰ **Y92.33** **Skating rink** as the place of occurrence of the external cause

     Y92.330 **Ice skating rink (indoor) (outdoor)** as the place of occurrence of the external cause

     Y92.331 **Roller skating rink** as the place of occurrence of the external cause

Y92.34 **Swimming pool (public)** as the place of occurrence of the external cause

     EXCLUDES 1 *swimming pool in private home or garden (Y92.016)*

Y92.39 **Other specified sports and athletic area** as the place of occurrence of the external cause

     Golf-course as the place of occurrence of the external cause

     Gymnasium as the place of occurrence of the external cause

     Riding-school as the place of occurrence of the external cause

     Stadium as the place of occurrence of the external cause

▲ ✓5ᵗʰ **Y92.4** **Street, highway and other paved roadways** as the place of occurrence of the external cause

     EXCLUDES 1 *private driveway of residence (Y92.014, Y92.024, Y92.043, Y92.093, Y92.113, Y92.123, Y92.154, Y92.194)*

✓6ᵗʰ **Y92.41** **Street and highway** as the place of occurrence of the external cause

Y92.410 **Unspecified street and highway** as the place of occurrence of the external cause ▽

     Road NOS as the place of occurrence of the external cause

Y92.411 **Interstate highway** as the place of occurrence of the external cause

     Freeway as the place of occurrence of the external cause

     Motorway as the place of occurrence of the external cause

Y92.412 **Parkway** as the place of occurrence of the external cause

Y92.413 **State road** as the place of occurrence of the external cause

Y92.414 **Local residential or business street** as the place of occurrence of the external cause

Y92.415 **Exit ramp or entrance ramp** of street or highway as the place of occurrence of the external cause

✓6ᵗʰ **Y92.48** **Other paved roadways** as the place of occurrence of the external cause

     Y92.480 **Sidewalk** as the place of occurrence of the external cause

     Y92.481 **Parking lot** as the place of occurrence of the external cause

     Y92.482 **Bike path** as the place of occurrence of the external cause

     Y92.488 **Other paved roadways** as the place of occurrence of the external cause

✓5ᵗʰ **Y92.5** **Trade and service area** as the place of occurrence of the external cause

     EXCLUDES 1 *garage in private home (Y92.015)*
         schools and other public administration buildings (Y92.2-)

✓6ᵗʰ **Y92.51** **Private commercial establishments** as the place of occurrence of the external cause

     Y92.510 **Bank** as the place of occurrence of the external cause

     Y92.511 **Restaurant or café** as the place of occurrence of the external cause

     Y92.512 **Supermarket, store or market** as the place of occurrence of the external cause

     Y92.513 **Shop (commercial)** as the place of occurrence of the external cause

✓6ᵗʰ **Y92.52** **Service areas** as the place of occurrence of the external cause

     Y92.520 **Airport** as the place of occurrence of the external cause

     Y92.521 **Bus station** as the place of occurrence of the external cause

     Y92.522 **Railway station** as the place of occurrence of the external cause

     Y92.523 **Highway rest stop** as the place of occurrence of the external cause

     Y92.524 **Gas station** as the place of occurrence of the external cause

         Petroleum station as the place of occurrence of the external cause

         Service station as the place of occurrence of the external cause

✓6ᵗʰ **Y92.53** **Ambulatory health services establishments** as the place of occurrence of the external cause

     Y92.530 **Ambulatory surgery center** as the place of occurrence of the external cause

         Outpatient surgery center, including that connected with a hospital as the place of occurrence of the external cause

         Same day surgery center, including that connected with a hospital as the place of occurrence of the external cause

     Y92.531 **Health care provider office** as the place of occurrence of the external cause

         Physician office as the place of occurrence of the external cause

     Y92.532 **Urgent care center** as the place of occurrence of the external cause

     Y92.538 **Other ambulatory health services establishments** as the place of occurrence of the external cause

☑ Additional Character Required   ✓x7ᵗʰ Placeholder Alert   Manifestation Dx   ▽ Unspecified Dx   ▶◀ Revised Text   ● New Code   ▲ Revised Code Title

ICD-10-CM 2017   **1135**

Y92.59   **Other trade areas as the place of occurrence of the external cause**

Office building as the place of occurrence of the external cause

Casino as the place of occurrence of the external cause

Garage (commercial) as the place of occurrence of the external cause

Hotel as the place of occurrence of the external cause

Radio or television station as the place of occurrence of the external cause

Shopping mall as the place of occurrence of the external cause

Warehouse as the place of occurrence of the external cause

√5ᵗʰ **Y92.6**   **Industrial and construction area as the place of occurrence of the external cause**

Y92.61   **Building [any] under construction as the place of occurrence of the external cause**

Y92.62   **Dock or shipyard as the place of occurrence of the external cause**

Dockyard as the place of occurrence of the external cause

Dry dock as the place of occurrence of the external cause

Shipyard as the place of occurrence of the external cause

Y92.63   **Factory as the place of occurrence of the external cause**

Factory building as the place of occurrence of the external cause

Factory premises as the place of occurrence of the external cause

Industrial yard as the place of occurrence of the external cause

Y92.64   **Mine or pit as the place of occurrence of the external cause**

Mine as the place of occurrence of the external cause

Y92.65   **Oil rig as the place of occurrence of the external cause**

Pit (coal) (gravel) (sand) as the place of occurrence of the external cause

Y92.69   **Other specified industrial and construction area as the place of occurrence of the external cause**

Gasworks as the place of occurrence of the external cause

Power-station (coal) (nuclear) (oil) as the place of occurrence of the external cause

Tunnel under construction as the place of occurrence of the external cause

Workshop as the place of occurrence of the external cause

√5ᵗʰ **Y92.7**   **Farm as the place of occurrence of the external cause**

Ranch as the place of occurrence of the external cause

EXCLUDES 1   *farmhouse and home premises of farm (Y92.01-)*

Y92.71   **Barn as the place of occurrence of the external cause**

Y92.72   **Chicken coop as the place of occurrence of the external cause**

Hen house as the place of occurrence of the external cause

Y92.73   **Farm field as the place of occurrence of the external cause**

Y92.74   **Orchard as the place of occurrence of the external cause**

Y92.79   **Other farm location as the place of occurrence of the external cause**

√5ᵗʰ **Y92.8**   **Other places as the place of occurrence of the external cause**

√6ᵗʰ **Y92.81**   **Transport vehicle as the place of occurrence of the external cause**

EXCLUDES 1   *transport accidents (V00-V99)*

Y92.810   **Car as the place of occurrence of the external cause**

Y92.811   **Bus as the place of occurrence of the external cause**

Y92.812   **Truck as the place of occurrence of the external cause**

Y92.813   **Airplane as the place of occurrence of the external cause**

Y92.814   **Boat as the place of occurrence of the external cause**

Y92.815   **Train as the place of occurrence of the external cause**

Y92.816   **Subway car as the place of occurrence of the external cause**

Y92.818   **Other transport vehicle as the place of occurrence of the external cause**

√6ᵗʰ **Y92.82**   **Wilderness area**

Y92.820   **Desert as the place of occurrence of the external cause**

Y92.821   **Forest as the place of occurrence of the external cause**

Y92.828   **Other wilderness area as the place of occurrence of the external cause**

Swamp as the place of occurrence of the external cause

Mountain as the place of occurrence of the external cause

Marsh as the place of occurrence of the external cause

Prairie as the place of occurrence of the external cause

√6ᵗʰ **Y92.83**   **Recreation area as the place of occurrence of the external cause**

Y92.830   **Public park as the place of occurrence of the external cause**

Y92.831   **Amusement park as the place of occurrence of the external cause**

Y92.832   **Beach as the place of occurrence of the external cause**

Seashore as the place of occurrence of the external cause

Y92.833   **Campsite as the place of occurrence of the external cause**

Y92.834   **Zoological garden (Zoo) as the place of occurrence of the external cause**

Y92.838   **Other recreation area as the place of occurrence of the external cause**

Y92.84   **Military training ground as the place of occurrence of the external cause**

Y92.85   **Railroad track as the place of occurrence of the external cause**

Y92.86   **Slaughter house as the place of occurrence of the external cause**

Y92.89   **Other specified places as the place of occurrence of the external cause**

Derelict house as the place of occurrence of the external cause

Y92.9   **Unspecified place or not applicable**   ▽

EXCLUDES 1 Not coded here   EXCLUDES 2 Not included here   N Newborn Age : 0   P Pediatric Age : 0-17   M Maternity Age : 12-55   A Adult Age : 15-124

1136   ICD-10-CM 2017

✓4ᵗʰ **Y93 Activity codes**

NOTE Category Y93 is provided for use to indicate the activity of the person seeking healthcare for an injury or health condition, such as a heart attack while shoveling snow, which resulted from, or was contributed to, by the activity. These codes are appropriate for use for both acute injuries, such as those from chapter 19, and conditions that are due to the long-term, cumulative effects of an activity, such as those from chapter 13. They are also appropriate for use with external cause codes for cause and intent if identifying the activity provides additional information on the event. These codes should be used in conjunction with codes for external cause status (Y99) and place of occurrence (Y92).

This section contains the following broad activity categories:

Y93.0	Activities involving walking and running
Y93.1	Activities involving water and water craft
Y93.2	Activities involving ice and snow
Y93.3	Activities involving climbing, rappelling, and jumping off
Y93.4	Activities involving dancing and other rhythmic movement
Y93.5	Activities involving other sports and athletics played individually
Y93.6	Activities involving other sports and athletics played as a team or group
Y93.7	Activities involving other specified sports and athletics
Y93.A	Activities involving other cardiorespiratory exercise
Y93.B	Activities involving other muscle strengthening exercises
Y93.C	Activities involving computer technology and electronic devices
Y93.D	Activities involving arts and handcrafts
Y93.E	Activities involving personal hygiene and interior property and clothing maintenance
Y93.F	Activities involving caregiving
Y93.G	Activities involving food preparation, cooking and grilling
Y93.H	Activities involving exterior property and land maintenance, building and construction
Y93.I	Activities involving roller coasters and other types of external motion
Y93.J	Activities involving playing musical instrument
Y93.K	Activities involving animal care
Y93.8	Activities, other specified
Y93.9	Activity, unspecified

✓5ᵗʰ **Y93.0 Activities involving walking and running**
EXCLUDES 1 *activity, walking an animal (Y93.K1)*
activity, walking or running on a treadmill (Y93.A1)

Y93.01 Activity, walking, marching and hiking
Activity, walking, marching and hiking on level or elevated terrain
EXCLUDES 1 *activity, mountain climbing (Y93.31)*

Y93.02 Activity, running

✓5ᵗʰ **Y93.1 Activities involving water and water craft**
EXCLUDES 1 *activities involving ice (Y93.2-)*

Y93.11 Activity, swimming
Y93.12 Activity, springboard and platform diving
Y93.13 Activity, water polo
Y93.14 Activity, water aerobics and water exercise
Y93.15 Activity, underwater diving and snorkeling
Activity, SCUBA diving
Y93.16 Activity, rowing, canoeing, kayaking, rafting and tubing
Activity, canoeing, kayaking, rafting and tubing in calm and turbulent water
Y93.17 Activity, water skiing and wake boarding
Y93.18 Activity, surfing, windsurfing and boogie boarding
Activity, water sliding
Y93.19 Activity, other involving water and watercraft
Activity involving water NOS
Activity, parasailing
Activity, water survival training and testing

✓5ᵗʰ **Y93.2 Activities involving ice and snow**
EXCLUDES 1 *activity, shoveling ice and snow (Y93.H1)*

Y93.21 Activity, ice skating
Activity, figure skating (singles) (pairs)
Activity, ice dancing
EXCLUDES 1 *activity, ice hockey (Y93.22)*

Y93.22 Activity, ice hockey
Y93.23 Activity, snow (alpine) (downhill) skiing, snow boarding, sledding, tobogganing and snow tubing
EXCLUDES 1 *activity, cross country skiing (Y93.24)*
Y93.24 Activity, cross country skiing
Activity, nordic skiing
Y93.29 Activity, other involving ice and snow
Activity involving ice and snow NOS

✓5ᵗʰ **Y93.3 Activities involving climbing, rappelling and jumping off**
EXCLUDES 1 *activity, hiking on level or elevated terrain (Y93.01)*
activity, jumping rope (Y93.56)
activity, trampoline jumping (Y93.44)

Y93.31 Activity, mountain climbing, rock climbing and wall climbing
Y93.32 Activity, rappelling
Y93.33 Activity, BASE jumping
Activity, Building, Antenna, Span, Earth jumping
Y93.34 Activity, bungee jumping
Y93.35 Activity, hang gliding
Y93.39 Activity, other involving climbing, rappelling and jumping off

✓5ᵗʰ **Y93.4 Activities involving dancing and other rhythmic movement**
EXCLUDES 1 *activity, martial arts (Y93.75)*

Y93.41 Activity, dancing
AHA: 2012,4Q,108
Y93.42 Activity, yoga
Y93.43 Activity, gymnastics
Activity, rhythmic gymnastics
EXCLUDES 1 *activity, trampolining (Y93.44)*
Y93.44 Activity, trampolining
Y93.45 Activity, cheerleading
Y93.49 Activity, other involving dancing and other rhythmic movements

✓5ᵗʰ **Y93.5 Activities involving other sports and athletics played individually**
EXCLUDES 1 *activity, dancing (Y93.41)*
activity, gymnastic (Y93.43)
activity, trampolining (Y93.44)
activity, yoga (Y93.42)

Y93.51 Activity, roller skating (inline) and skateboarding
Y93.52 Activity, horseback riding
Y93.53 Activity, golf
Y93.54 Activity, bowling
Y93.55 Activity, bike riding
Y93.56 Activity, jumping rope
Y93.57 Activity, non-running track and field events
EXCLUDES 1 *activity, running (any form) (Y93.02)*
Y93.59 Activity, other involving other sports and athletics played individually
EXCLUDES 1 *activities involving climbing, rappelling, and jumping (Y93.3-)*
activities involving ice and snow (Y93.2-)
activities involving walking and running (Y93.0-)
activities involving water and watercraft (Y93.1-)

✓5ᵗʰ **Y93.6 Activities involving other sports and athletics played as a team or group**
EXCLUDES 1 *activity, ice hockey (Y93.22)*
activity, water polo (Y93.13)

Y93.61 Activity, American tackle football
Activity, football NOS
Y93.62 Activity, American flag or touch football
Y93.63 Activity, rugby
Y93.64 Activity, baseball
Activity, softball
Y93.65 Activity, lacrosse and field hockey
Y93.66 Activity, soccer
Y93.67 Activity, basketball
Y93.68 Activity, volleyball (beach) (court)

☑ Additional Character Required   ✓x7ᵗʰ Placeholder Alert   Manifestation Dx   ▽ Unspecified Dx   ▶◀ Revised Text   ● New Code   ▲ Revised Code Title

ICD-10-CM 2017   **1137**

Y93.6A **Activity,** physical games generally associated with school recess, summer camp and children
  Activity, capture the flag
  Activity, dodge ball
  Activity, four square
  Activity, kickball

Y93.69 **Activity,** other involving other sports and athletics played as a team or group
  Activity, cricket

✓5ᵗʰ **Y93.7** **Activities involving other specified sports and athletics**

Y93.71 **Activity,** boxing

Y93.72 **Activity,** wrestling

Y93.73 **Activity,** racquet and hand **sports**
  Activity, handball
  Activity, racquetball
  Activity, squash
  Activity, tennis

Y93.74 **Activity,** frisbee
  Activity, ultimate frisbee

Y93.75 **Activity,** martial arts
  Activity, combatives

Y93.79 **Activity,** other specified sports and athletics
  EXCLUDES 1 *sports and athletics activities specified in categories Y93.0-Y93.6*

✓5ᵗʰ **Y93.A** **Activities involving other cardiorespiratory exercise**
  Activities involving physical training

Y93.A1 **Activity,** exercise machines primarily for cardiorespiratory conditioning
  Activity, elliptical and stepper machines
  Activity, stationary bike
  Activity, treadmill

Y93.A2 **Activity,** calisthenics
  Activity, jumping jacks
  Activity, warm up and cool down

Y93.A3 **Activity,** aerobic and step exercise

Y93.A4 **Activity,** circuit training

Y93.A5 **Activity,** obstacle course
  Activity, challenge course
  Activity, confidence course

Y93.A6 **Activity,** grass drills
  Activity, guerilla drills

Y93.A9 **Activity,** other involving cardiorespiratory exercise
  EXCLUDES 1 *activities involving cardiorespiratory exercise specified in categories Y93.0-Y93.7*

✓5ᵗʰ **Y93.B** **Activities involving other muscle strengthening exercises**

Y93.B1 **Activity,** exercise machines primarily for muscle strengthening

Y93.B2 **Activity,** push-ups, pull-ups, sit-ups

Y93.B3 **Activity,** free weights
  Activity, barbells
  Activity, dumbbells

Y93.B4 **Activity,** pilates

Y93.B9 **Activity,** other involving muscle strengthening exercises
  EXCLUDES 1 *activities involving muscle strengthening specified in categories Y93.0-Y93.A*

✓5ᵗʰ **Y93.C** **Activities involving computer technology and electronic devices**
  EXCLUDES 1 *activity, electronic musical keyboard or instruments (Y93.J-)*

Y93.C1 **Activity,** computer keyboarding
  Activity, electronic game playing using keyboard or other stationary device

Y93.C2 **Activity,** hand held interactive electronic device
  Activity, cellular telephone and communication device
  Activity, electronic game playing using interactive device
  EXCLUDES 1 *activity, electronic game playing using keyboard or other stationary device (Y93.C1)*

Y93.C9 **Activity,** other involving computer technology and electronic devices

✓5ᵗʰ **Y93.D** **Activities involving arts and handcrafts**
  EXCLUDES 1 *activities involving playing musical instrument (Y93.J-)*

Y93.D1 **Activity,** knitting and crocheting

Y93.D2 **Activity,** sewing

Y93.D3 **Activity,** furniture building and finishing
  Activity, furniture repair

Y93.D9 **Activity,** other involving arts and handcrafts

✓5ᵗʰ **Y93.E** **Activities involving personal hygiene and interior property and clothing maintenance**
  EXCLUDES 1 *activities involving cooking and grilling (Y93.G-)*
    activities involving exterior property and land maintenance, building and construction (Y93.H-)
    activities involving caregiving (Y93.F-)
    activity, dishwashing (Y93.G1)
    activity, food preparation (Y93.G1)
    activity, gardening (Y93.H2)

Y93.E1 **Activity,** personal bathing and showering

Y93.E2 **Activity,** laundry

Y93.E3 **Activity,** vacuuming

Y93.E4 **Activity,** ironing

Y93.E5 **Activity,** floor mopping and cleaning

Y93.E6 **Activity,** residential relocation
  Activity, packing up and unpacking involved in moving to a new residence

Y93.E8 **Activity,** other personal hygiene

Y93.E9 **Activity,** other interior property and clothing maintenance

✓5ᵗʰ **Y93.F** **Activities involving caregiving**
  Activity involving the provider of caregiving

Y93.F1 **Activity,** caregiving, bathing

Y93.F2 **Activity,** caregiving, lifting

Y93.F9 **Activity,** other caregiving

✓5ᵗʰ **Y93.G** **Activities involving food preparation, cooking and grilling**

Y93.G1 **Activity,** food preparation and clean up
  Activity, dishwashing

Y93.G2 **Activity,** grilling and smoking food

Y93.G3 **Activity,** cooking and baking
  Activity, use of stove, oven and microwave oven

Y93.G9 **Activity,** other involving cooking and grilling

✓5ᵗʰ **Y93.H** **Activities involving exterior property and land maintenance, building and construction**

Y93.H1 **Activity,** digging, shoveling and raking
  Activity, dirt digging
  Activity, raking leaves
  Activity, snow shoveling

Y93.H2 **Activity,** gardening and landscaping
  Activity, pruning, trimming shrubs, weeding

Y93.H3 **Activity,** building and construction

Y93.H9 **Activity,** other involving exterior property and land maintenance, building and construction

✓5ᵗʰ **Y93.I** **Activities involving roller coasters and other types of external motion**

Y93.I1 **Activity,** rollercoaster riding

Y93.I9 **Activity,** other involving external motion

✓5ᵗʰ **Y93.J** **Activities involving playing musical instrument**
  Activity involving playing electric musical instrument

Y93.J1 **Activity,** piano playing
  Activity, musical keyboard (electronic) playing

Y93.J2 **Activity,** drum and other percussion instrument playing

Y93.J3 **Activity,** string instrument playing

Y93.J4 **Activity,** winds and brass instrument playing

✓5ᵗʰ **Y93.K** **Activities involving animal care**
  EXCLUDES 1 *activity, horseback riding (Y93.52)*

Y93.K1 **Activity,** walking an animal

Y93.K2 **Activity,** milking an animal

Y93.K3 **Activity,** grooming and shearing an animal

Y93.K9 **Activity,** other involving animal care

✓5ᵗʰ **Y93.8** **Activities, other specified**

Y93.81 **Activity,** refereeing a sports activity

Y93.82 **Activity,** spectator at an event

Y93.83 **Activity,** rough housing and horseplay

Y93.84 **Activity,** sleeping

Y93.85 **Activity,** choking game
  Activity, blackout game
  Activity, fainting game
  Activity, pass out game

Y93.89 **Activity,** other specified

Y93.9 **Activity, unspecified**   ▽

EXCLUDES 1 Not coded here   **EXCLUDES 2** Not included here   🅝 Newborn Age : 0   🅟 Pediatric Age : 0-17   🅜 Maternity Age : 12-55   🅐 Adult Age : 15-124

1138   ICD-10-CM 2017

Y95 Nosocomial condition
    AHA: 2013,4Q,119

☑4ᵗʰ **Y99 External cause status**

> NOTE   A single code from category Y99 should be used in conjunction with the external cause code(s) assigned to a record to indicate the status of the person at the time the event occurred.

Y99.Ø Civilian activity done for income or pay
    Civilian activity done for financial or other compensation
    EXCLUDES 1 *military activity (Y99.1)*
                volunteer activity (Y99.2)

Y99.1 Military activity
    EXCLUDES 1 *activity of off duty military personnel (Y99.8)*

Y99.2 Volunteer activity
    EXCLUDES 1 *activity of child or other family member assisting in compensated work of other family member (Y99.8)*

Y99.8 Other external cause status
    Activity NEC
    Activity of child or other family member assisting in compensated work of other family member
    Hobby not done for income
    Leisure activity
    Off-duty activity of military personnel
    Recreation or sport not for income or while a student
    Student activity
    EXCLUDES 1 *civilian activity done for income or compensation (Y99.Ø)*
                military activity (Y99.1)
    AHA: 2012,4Q,108

Y99.9 Unspecified external cause status   ▽

| ☑ Additional Character Required | ☑x7ᵗʰ Placeholder Alert | Manifestation Dx | ▽ Unspecified Dx | ►◄ Revised Text | ● New Code | ▲ Revised Code Title |

ICD-10-CM 2017   **1139**

Chapter 21. Factors Influencing Health Status and Contact with Health Services (Z00–Z99)

Chapter Specific Guidelines with Coding Examples

The chapter specific guidelines from the ICD-10-CM Official Guidelines for Coding and Reporting have been provided below. Along with these guidelines are coding examples, contained in the shaded boxes, that have been developed to help illustrate the coding and/or sequencing guidance found in these guidelines.

Note: The chapter specific guidelines provide additional information about the use of Z codes for specified encounters.

a. Use of Z codes in any healthcare setting

Z codes are for use in any healthcare setting. Z codes may be used as either a first-listed (principal diagnosis code in the inpatient setting) or secondary code, depending on the circumstances of the encounter. Certain Z codes may only be used as first-listed or principal diagnosis.

> Patient with middle lobe lung cancer admitted for initiation of chemotherapy
>
> **Z51.11**   **Encounter for antineoplastic chemotherapy**
>
> **C34.2**   **Malignant neoplasm of middle lobe, bronchus or lung**
>
> *Explanation:* A Z code can be used as first-listed in this situation based on guidelines in this chapter as well as chapter 2, "Neoplasms."

> Patient has chronic lymphocytic leukemia for which the patient had previous chemotherapy and is now in remission
>
> **C91.11**   **Chronic lymphocytic leukemia of B-cell type in remission**
>
> **Z92.21**   **Personal history of antineoplastic chemotherapy**
>
> *Explanation:*The personal history Z code is used to describe a secondary (supplementary) diagnosis to identify that this patient has had chemotherapy in the past.

b. Z codes indicate a reason for an encounter

Z codes are not procedure codes. A corresponding procedure code must accompany a Z code to describe any procedure performed.

c. Categories of Z codes

1) Contact/exposure

Category Z20 indicates contact with, and suspected exposure to, communicable diseases. These codes are for patients who do not show any sign or symptom of a disease but are suspected to have been exposed to it by close personal contact with an infected individual or are in an area where a disease is epidemic.

Category Z77, Other contact with and (suspected) exposures hazardous to health, indicates contact with and suspected exposures hazardous to health.

Contact/exposure codes may be used as a first-listed code to explain an encounter for testing, or, more commonly, as a secondary code to identify a potential risk.

2) Inoculations and vaccinations

Code Z23 is for encounters for inoculations and vaccinations. It indicates that a patient is being seen to receive a prophylactic inoculation against a disease. Procedure codes are required to identify the actual administration of the injection and the type(s) of immunizations given. Code Z23 may be used as a secondary code if the inoculation is given as a routine part of preventive health care, such as a well-baby visit.

3) Status

Status codes indicate that a patient is either a carrier of a disease or has the sequelae or residual of a past disease or condition. This includes such things as the presence of prosthetic or mechanical devices resulting from past treatment. A status code is informative, because the status may affect the course of treatment and its outcome. A status code is distinct from a history code. The history code indicates that the patient no longer has the condition.

A status code should not be used with a diagnosis code from one of the body system chapters, if the diagnosis code includes the information provided by the status code. For example, code Z94.1, Heart transplant status, should not be used with a code from subcategory T86.2, Complications of heart transplant. The status code does not provide additional information. The complication code indicates that the patient is a heart transplant patient.

For encounters for weaning from a mechanical ventilator, assign a code from subcategory J96.1, Chronic respiratory failure, followed by code Z99.11, Dependence on respirator [ventilator] status.

The status Z codes/categories are:

Z14   Genetic carrier

     Genetic carrier status indicates that a person carries a gene, associated with a particular disease, which may be passed to offspring who may develop that disease. The person does not have the disease and is not at risk of developing the disease.

Z15   Genetic susceptibility to disease

     Genetic susceptibility indicates that a person has a gene that increases the risk of that person developing the disease.

     Codes from category Z15 should not be used as principal or first-listed codes. If the patient has the condition to which he/she is susceptible, and that condition is the reason for the encounter, the code for the current condition should be sequenced first. If the patient is being seen for follow-up after completed treatment for this condition, and the condition no longer exists, a follow-up code should be sequenced first, followed by the appropriate personal history and genetic susceptibility codes. If the purpose of the encounter is genetic counseling associated with procreative management, code Z31.5, Encounter for genetic counseling, should be assigned as the first-listed code, followed by a code from category Z15. Additional codes should be assigned for any applicable family or personal history.

Z16   Resistance to antimicrobial drugs

     This code indicates that a patient has a condition that is resistant to antimicrobial drug treatment. Sequence the infection code first.

Z17   Estrogen receptor status

Z18   Retained foreign body fragments

Z19   **Hormone sensitivity malignancy status**

Z21   Asymptomatic HIV infection status

     This code indicates that a patient has tested positive for HIV but has manifested no signs or symptoms of the disease.

Z22   Carrier of infectious disease

     Carrier status indicates that a person harbors the specific organisms of a disease without manifest symptoms and is capable of transmitting the infection.

Z28.3   Underimmunization status

Z33.1   Pregnant state, incidental

     This code is a secondary code only for use when the pregnancy is in no way complicating the reason for visit. Otherwise, a code from the obstetric chapter is required.

Z66   Do not resuscitate

     This code may be used when it is documented by the provider that a patient is on do not resuscitate status at any time during the stay.

Z67   Blood type

Z68   Body mass index (BMI)

     <u>As with all other secondary diagnosis codes, the BMI codes should only be assigned when they meet the definition of a reportable diagnosis (see Section III, Reporting Additional Diagnoses).</u>

Z74.01   Bed confinement status

Z76.82   Awaiting organ transplant status

Z78   Other specified health status

     Code Z78.1, Physical restraint status, may be used when it is documented by the provider that a patient has been put in restraints during the current encounter. Please note that this code should not be reported when it is documented by the provider that a patient is temporarily restrained during a procedure.

Z79   Long-term (current) drug therapy

     Codes from this category indicate a patient's continuous use of a prescribed drug (including such things as aspirin therapy) for the long-term treatment of a condition or for prophylactic use. It is not for use for patients who have addictions to drugs. This subcategory is not for use of medications for detoxification or maintenance programs to prevent withdrawal symptoms in patients with drug dependence (e.g., methadone maintenance for opiate dependence). Assign the appropriate code for the drug dependence instead.

Assign a code from Z79 if the patient is receiving a medication for an extended period as a prophylactic measure (such as for the prevention of deep vein thrombosis) or as treatment of a chronic condition (such as arthritis) or a disease requiring a lengthy course of treatment (such as cancer). Do not assign a code from category Z79 for medication being administered for a brief period of time to treat an acute illness or injury (such as a course of antibiotics to treat acute bronchitis).

Z88	Allergy status to drugs, medicaments and biological substances

Except: Z88.9, Allergy status to unspecified drugs, medicaments and biological substances status

Z89	Acquired absence of limb
Z90	Acquired absence of organs, not elsewhere classified
Z91.0-	Allergy status, other than to drugs and biological substances
Z92.82	Status post administration of tPA (rtPA) in a different facility within the last 24 hours prior to admission to a current facility

Assign code Z92.82, Status post administration of tPA (rtPA) in a different facility within the last 24 hours prior to admission to current facility, as a secondary diagnosis when a patient is received by transfer into a facility and documentation indicates they were administered tissue plasminogen activator (tPA) within the last 24 hours prior to admission to the current facility.

This guideline applies even if the patient is still receiving the tPA at the time they are received into the current facility.

The appropriate code for the condition for which the tPA was administered (such as cerebrovascular disease or myocardial infarction) should be assigned first.

Code Z92.82 is only applicable to the receiving facility record and not to the transferring facility record.

Z93	Artificial opening status
Z94	Transplanted organ and tissue status
Z95	Presence of cardiac and vascular implants and grafts
Z96	Presence of other functional implants
Z97	Presence of other devices
Z98	Other postprocedural states

Assign code Z98.85, Transplanted organ removal status, to indicate that a transplanted organ has been previously removed. This code should not be assigned for the encounter in which the transplanted organ is removed. The complication necessitating removal of the transplant organ should be assigned for that encounter.

See section I.C19. for information on the coding of organ transplant complications.

Z99	Dependence on enabling machines and devices, not elsewhere classified

Note: Categories Z89-Z90 and Z93-Z99 are for use only if there are no complications or malfunctions of the organ or tissue replaced, the amputation site or the equipment on which the patient is dependent.

4) History (of)

There are two types of history Z codes, personal and family. Personal history codes explain a patient's past medical condition that no longer exists and is not receiving any treatment, but that has the potential for recurrence, and therefore may require continued monitoring.

Family history codes are for use when a patient has a family member(s) who has had a particular disease that causes the patient to be at higher risk of also contracting the disease.

Personal history codes may be used in conjunction with follow-up codes and family history codes may be used in conjunction with screening codes to explain the need for a test or procedure. History codes are also acceptable on any medical record regardless of the reason for visit. A history of an illness, even if no longer present, is important information that may alter the type of treatment ordered.

The history Z code categories are:

Z80	Family history of primary malignant neoplasm
Z81	Family history of mental and behavioral disorders
Z82	Family history of certain disabilities and chronic diseases (leading to disablement)
Z83	Family history of other specific disorders
Z84	Family history of other conditions
Z85	Personal history of malignant neoplasm
Z86	Personal history of certain other diseases
Z87	Personal history of other diseases and conditions
Z91.4-	Personal history of psychological trauma, not elsewhere classified
Z91.5	Personal history of self-harm
Z91.8-	Other specified personal risk factors, not elsewhere classified

Exception: Z91.83, Wandering in diseases classified elsewhere

Z92	Personal history of medical treatment

Except: Z92.0, Personal history of contraception

Except: Z92.82, Status post administration of tPA (rtPA) in a different facility within the last 24 hours prior to admission to a current facility

5) Screening

Screening is the testing for disease or disease precursors in seemingly well individuals so that early detection and treatment can be provided for those who test positive for the disease (e.g., screening mammogram).

The testing of a person to rule out or confirm a suspected diagnosis because the patient has some sign or symptom is a diagnostic examination, not a screening. In these cases, the sign or symptom is used to explain the reason for the test.

A screening code may be a first-listed code if the reason for the visit is specifically the screening exam. It may also be used as an additional code if the screening is done during an office visit for other health problems. A screening code is not necessary if the screening is inherent to a routine examination, such as a pap smear done during a routine pelvic examination.

Should a condition be discovered during the screening then the code for the condition may be assigned as an additional diagnosis.

Prostate screening of healthy 50-year-old male patient; PSA noted to be elevated but normal digital rectal exam

Z12.5	**Encounter for screening for malignant neoplasm of prostate**
R97.20	**Elevated prostate specific antigen [PSA]**

Explanation: The patient had no signs or symptoms of any prostate-related illness prior to coming in for the screening. The screening code is appropriately used as the first-listed code to signify that this was for routine screening. The elevated PSA is reported as a secondary diagnosis to reflect that an abnormal lab value was found as a result of the screening procedure(s).

The Z code indicates that a screening exam is planned. A procedure code is required to confirm that the screening was performed.

The screening Z codes/categories:

Z11	Encounter for screening for infectious and parasitic diseases
Z12	Encounter for screening for malignant neoplasms
Z13	Encounter for screening for other diseases and disorders

Except: Z13.9, Encounter for screening, unspecified

Z36	Encounter for antenatal screening for mother

6) Observation

There are **three** observation Z code categories. They are for use in very limited circumstances when a person is being observed for a suspected condition that is ruled out. The observation codes are not for use if an injury or illness or any signs or symptoms related to the suspected condition are present. In such cases the diagnosis/symptom code is used with the corresponding external cause code.

The observation codes are to be used as principal diagnosis only. **The only exception to this is when the principal diagnosis is required to be a code from category Z38, Liveborn infants according to place of birth and type of delivery. Then a code from category Z05, Encounter for observation and evaluation of newborn for suspected diseases and conditions ruled out, is sequenced after the Z38 code.** Additional codes may be used in addition to the observation code but only if they are unrelated to the suspected condition being observed.

Codes from subcategory Z03.7, Encounter for suspected maternal and fetal conditions ruled out, may either be used as a first-listed or as an additional code assignment depending on the case. They are for use in very limited circumstances on a maternal record when an encounter is for a suspected maternal or fetal condition that is ruled out during that encounter (for example, a maternal or fetal condition may be suspected due to an abnormal test result). These codes should not be used when the condition is confirmed. In those cases, the confirmed condition should be coded. In addition, these codes are not for use if an illness or any signs or symptoms related to the suspected condition or problem are present. In such cases the diagnosis/symptom code is used.

Additional codes may be used in addition to the code from subcategory Z03.7, but only if they are unrelated to the suspected condition being evaluated.

Codes from subcategory Z03.7 may not be used for encounters for antenatal screening of mother. *See Section I.C.21. Screening.*

For encounters for suspected fetal condition that are inconclusive following testing and evaluation, assign the appropriate code from category O35, O36, O40 or O41.

The observation Z code categories:

Z03   Encounter for medical observation for suspected diseases and conditions ruled out

Z04   Encounter for examination and observation for other reasons

       Except: Z04.9, Encounter for examination and observation for unspecified reason

Z05   Encounter for observation and evaluation of newborn for suspected diseases and conditions ruled out

7) Aftercare

Aftercare visit codes cover situations when the initial treatment of a disease has been performed and the patient requires continued care during the healing or recovery phase, or for the long-term consequences of the disease. The aftercare Z code should not be used if treatment is directed at a current, acute disease. The diagnosis code is to be used in these cases. Exceptions to this rule are codes Z51.0, Encounter for antineoplastic radiation therapy, and codes from subcategory Z51.1, Encounter for antineoplastic chemotherapy and immunotherapy. These codes are to be first-listed, followed by the diagnosis code when a patient's encounter is solely to receive radiation therapy, chemotherapy, or immunotherapy for the treatment of a neoplasm. If the reason for the encounter is more than one type of antineoplastic therapy, code Z51.0 and a code from subcategory Z51.1 may be assigned together, in which case one of these codes would be reported as a secondary diagnosis.

The aftercare Z codes should also not be used for aftercare for injuries. For aftercare of an injury, assign the acute injury code with the appropriate 7th character (for subsequent encounter).

The aftercare codes are generally first-listed to explain the specific reason for the encounter. An aftercare code may be used as an additional code when some type of aftercare is provided in addition to the reason for admission and no diagnosis code is applicable. An example of this would be the closure of a colostomy during an encounter for treatment of another condition.

Aftercare codes should be used in conjunction with other aftercare codes or diagnosis codes to provide better detail on the specifics of an aftercare encounter visit, unless otherwise directed by the classification. Should a patient receive multiple types of antineoplastic therapy during the same encounter, code Z51.0, Encounter for antineoplastic radiation therapy, and codes from subcategory Z51.1, Encounter for antineoplastic chemotherapy and immunotherapy, may be used together on a record. The sequencing of multiple aftercare codes depends on the circumstances of the encounter.

Certain aftercare Z code categories need a secondary diagnosis code to describe the resolving condition or sequelae. For others, the condition is included in the code title.

Additional Z code aftercare category terms include fitting and adjustment, and attention to artificial openings.

Status Z codes may be used with aftercare Z codes to indicate the nature of the aftercare. For example code Z95.1, Presence of aortocoronary bypass graft, may be used with code Z48.812, Encounter for surgical aftercare following surgery on the circulatory system, to indicate the surgery for which the aftercare is being performed. A status code should not be used when the aftercare code indicates the type of status, such as using Z43.0, Encounter for attention to tracheostomy, with Z93.0, Tracheostomy status.

The aftercare Z category/codes:

Z42   Encounter for plastic and reconstructive surgery following medical procedure or healed injury

Z43   Encounter for attention to artificial openings

Z44   Encounter for fitting and adjustment of external prosthetic device

Z45   Encounter for adjustment and management of implanted device

Z46   Encounter for fitting and adjustment of other devices

Z47   Orthopedic aftercare

Z48   Encounter for other postprocedural aftercare

Z49   Encounter for care involving renal dialysis

Z51   Encounter for other aftercare **and medical care**

8) Follow-up

The follow-up codes are used to explain continuing surveillance following completed treatment of a disease, condition, or injury. They imply that the condition has been fully treated and no longer exists. They should not be confused with aftercare codes, or injury codes with a 7th character for subsequent encounter, that explain ongoing care of a healing condition or its sequelae. Follow-up codes may be used in conjunction with history codes to provide the full picture of the healed condition and its treatment. The follow-up code is sequenced first, followed by the history code.

A follow-up code may be used to explain multiple visits. Should a condition be found to have recurred on the follow-up visit, then the diagnosis code for the condition should be assigned in place of the follow-up code.

The follow-up Z code categories:

Z08   Encounter for follow-up examination after completed treatment for malignant neoplasm

Z09   Encounter for follow-up examination after completed treatment for conditions other than malignant neoplasm

Z39   Encounter for maternal postpartum care and examination

Follow-up for patient several months after completing a regime of IV antibiotics for recurrent pneumonia; lungs are clear and pneumonia is resolved

Z09   Encounter for follow-up examination after completed treatment for conditions other than malignant neoplasm

Z87.01   Personal history of pneumonia (recurrent)

Explanation: Code Z09 identifies the follow-up visit as being unrelated to a malignant neoplasm, and code Z87 describes the condition that has now resolved.

Follow-up for patient several months after completing a regime of IV antibiotics for recurrent pneumonia; pneumonia has recurred, and a new antibiotic regimen has been prescribed

J18.9   Pneumonia, unspecified organism

Explanation: Since the follow-up exam for pneumonia determined that the pneumonia was not resolved or recurred, code Z09 Encounter for follow-up examination after completed treatment for conditions other than malignant neoplasm, no longer applies. Instead the first-listed code describes the pneumonia.

---

9) Donor

Codes in category Z52, Donors of organs and tissues, are used for living individuals who are donating blood or other body tissue. These codes are only for individuals donating for others, not for self-donations. They are not used to identify cadaveric donations.

10) Counseling

Counseling Z codes are used when a patient or family member receives assistance in the aftermath of an illness or injury, or when support is required in coping with family or social problems. They are not used in conjunction with a diagnosis code when the counseling component of care is considered integral to standard treatment.

The counseling Z codes/categories:

Z30.0-   Encounter for general counseling and advice on contraception

Z31.5   Encounter for genetic counseling

Z31.6-   Encounter for general counseling and advice on procreation

Z32.2   Encounter for childbirth instruction

Z32.3   Encounter for childcare instruction

Z69   Encounter for mental health services for victim and perpetrator of abuse

Z70   Counseling related to sexual attitude, behavior and orientation

Z71   Persons encountering health services for other counseling and medical advice, not elsewhere classified

Z76.81   Expectant mother prebirth pediatrician visit

11) Encounters for obstetrical and reproductive services

See Section I.C.15. Pregnancy, Childbirth, and the Puerperium, for further instruction on the use of these codes.

Z codes for pregnancy are for use in those circumstances when none of the problems or complications included in the codes from the Obstetrics chapter exist (a routine prenatal visit or postpartum care). Codes in category Z34, Encounter for supervision of normal pregnancy, are always first-listed and are not to be used with any other code from the OB chapter.

Codes in category Z3A, Weeks of gestation, may be assigned to provide additional information about the pregnancy. **Category Z3A codes should not be assigned for pregnancies with abortive outcomes (categories O00-O08), elective termination of pregnancy (code Z33.32), nor for postpartum conditions, as category Z3A is not applicable to these conditions.** The date of the admission should be used to determine weeks of gestation for inpatient admissions that encompass more than one gestational week.

The outcome of delivery, category Z37, should be included on all maternal delivery records. It is always a secondary code. Codes in category Z37 should not be used on the newborn record.

Z codes for family planning (contraceptive) or procreative management and counseling should be included on an obstetric record either during the pregnancy or the postpartum stage, if applicable.

Z codes/categories for obstetrical and reproductive services:

Z30	Encounter for contraceptive management
Z31	Encounter for procreative management
Z32.2	Encounter for childbirth instruction
Z32.3	Encounter for childcare instruction
Z33	Pregnant state
Z34	Encounter for supervision of normal pregnancy
Z36	Encounter for antenatal screening of mother
Z3A	Weeks of gestation
Z37	Outcome of delivery
Z39	Encounter for maternal postpartum care and examination
Z76.81	Expectant mother prebirth pediatrician visit

12) Newborns and infants

See Section I.C.16. Newborn (Perinatal) Guidelines, for further instruction on the use of these codes.

Newborn Z codes/categories:

Z76.1	Encounter for health supervision and care of foundling
Z00.1-	Encounter for routine child health examination
Z38	Liveborn infants according to place of birth and type of delivery

13) Routine and administrative examinations

The Z codes allow for the description of encounters for routine examinations, such as, a general check-up, or, examinations for administrative purposes, such as, a pre-employment physical. The codes are not to be used if the examination is for diagnosis of a suspected condition or for treatment purposes. In such cases the diagnosis code is used. During a routine exam, should a diagnosis or condition be discovered, it should be coded as an additional code. Pre-existing and chronic conditions and history codes may also be included as additional codes as long as the examination is for administrative purposes and not focused on any particular condition.

Some of the codes for routine health examinations distinguish between "with" and "without" abnormal findings. Code assignment depends on the information that is known at the time the encounter is being coded. For example, if no abnormal findings were found during the examination, but the encounter is being coded before test results are back, it is acceptable to assign the code for "without abnormal findings." When assigning a code for "with abnormal findings," additional code(s) should be assigned to identify the specific abnormal finding(s).

> 12-month-old boy admitted for well-child visit; pediatrician notices some eczema on the child's scalp and back of the knees
>
> **Z00.121**   **Encounter for routine child health examination with abnormal findings**
>
> **L30.9**   **Dermatitis, unspecified**
>
> *Explanation:* The Z code identifying that this is a routine well-child visit is reported first. Because an abnormal finding (eczema) was documented, a code for this condition may also be appended.

Pre-operative examination and pre-procedural laboratory examination Z codes are for use only in those situations when a patient is being cleared for a procedure or surgery and no treatment is given.

The Z codes/categories for routine and administrative examinations:

Z00	Encounter for general examination without complaint, suspected or reported diagnosis
Z01	Encounter for other special examination without complaint, suspected or reported diagnosis
Z02	Encounter for administrative examination
	Except: Z02.9, Encounter for administrative examinations, unspecified
Z32.0-	Encounter for pregnancy test

14) Miscellaneous Z codes

The miscellaneous Z codes capture a number of other health care encounters that do not fall into one of the other categories. Certain of these codes identify the reason for the encounter; others are for use as additional codes that provide useful information on circumstances that may affect a patient's care and treatment.

Prophylactic organ removal

For encounters specifically for prophylactic removal of an organ (such as prophylactic removal of breasts due to a genetic susceptibility to cancer or a family history of cancer), the principal or first-listed code should be a code from category Z40, Encounter for prophylactic surgery, followed by the appropriate codes to identify the associated risk factor (such as genetic susceptibility or family history).

If the patient has a malignancy of one site and is having prophylactic removal at another site to prevent either a new primary malignancy or metastatic disease, a code for the malignancy should also be assigned in addition to a code from subcategory Z40.0, Encounter for prophylactic surgery for risk factors related to malignant neoplasms. A Z40.0 code should not be assigned if the patient is having organ removal for treatment of a malignancy, such as the removal of the testes for the treatment of prostate cancer.

Miscellaneous Z codes/categories:

Z28	Immunization not carried out
	Except: Z28.3, Underimmunization status
Z29	**Encounter for other prophylactic measures**
Z40	Encounter for prophylactic surgery
Z41	Encounter for procedures for purposes other than remedying health state
	Except: Z41.9, Encounter for procedure for purposes other than remedying health state, unspecified
Z53	Persons encountering health services for specific procedures and treatment, not carried out
Z55	Problems related to education and literacy
Z56	Problems related to employment and unemployment
Z57	Occupational exposure to risk factors
Z58	Problems related to physical environment
Z59	Problems related to housing and economic circumstances
Z60	Problems related to social environment
Z62	Problems related to upbringing
Z63	Other problems related to primary support group, including family circumstances
Z64	Problems related to certain psychosocial circumstances
Z65	Problems related to other psychosocial circumstances
Z72	Problems related to lifestyle
	Note: These codes should be assigned only when the documentation specifies that the patient has an associated problem
Z73	Problems related to life management difficulty
Z74	Problems related to care provider dependency
	Except: Z74.01, Bed confinement status
Z75	Problems related to medical facilities and other health care
Z76.0	Encounter for issue of repeat prescription
Z76.3	Healthy person accompanying sick person
Z76.4	Other boarder to healthcare facility
Z76.5	Malingerer [conscious simulation]
Z91.1-	Patient's noncompliance with medical treatment and regimen
Z91.83	Wandering in diseases classified elsewhere
Z91.89	Other specified personal risk factors, not elsewhere classified

Chapter 21. Factors Influencing Health Status and Contact with Health Services

15) Nonspecific Z codes

Certain Z codes are so non-specific, or potentially redundant with other codes in the classification, that there can be little justification for their use in the inpatient setting. Their use in the outpatient setting should be limited to those instances when there is no further documentation to permit more precise coding. Otherwise, any sign or symptom or any other reason for visit that is captured in another code should be used.

Nonspecific Z codes/categories:

Z02.9	Encounter for administrative examinations, unspecified
Z04.9	Encounter for examination and observation for unspecified reason
Z13.9	Encounter for screening, unspecified
Z41.9	Encounter for procedure for purposes other than remedying health state, unspecified
Z52.9	Donor of unspecified organ or tissue
Z86.59	Personal history of other mental and behavioral disorders
Z88.9	Allergy status to unspecified drugs, medicaments and biological substances status
Z92.0	Personal history of contraception

16) Z codes that may only be principal/first-listed diagnosis

The following Z codes/categories may only be reported as the principal/first-listed diagnosis, except when there are multiple encounters on the same day and the medical records for the encounters are combined:

Z00	Encounter for general examination without complaint, suspected or reported diagnosis
	Except: Z00.6
Z01	Encounter for other special examination without complaint, suspected or reported diagnosis
Z02	Encounter for administrative examination
Z03	Encounter for medical observation for suspected diseases and conditions ruled out
Z04	Encounter for examination and observation for other reasons
Z33.2	Encounter for elective termination of pregnancy
Z31.81	Encounter for male factor infertility in female patient
Z31.83	Encounter for assisted reproductive fertility procedure cycle
Z31.84	Encounter for fertility preservation procedure
Z34	Encounter for supervision of normal pregnancy
Z39	Encounter for maternal postpartum care and examination
Z38	Liveborn infants according to place of birth and type of delivery
Z42	Encounter for plastic and reconstructive surgery following medical procedure or healed injury
Z51.0	Encounter for antineoplastic radiation therapy
Z51.1-	Encounter for antineoplastic chemotherapy and immunotherapy
Z52	Donors of organs and tissues
	Except: Z52.9, Donor of unspecified organ or tissue
Z76.1	Encounter for health supervision and care of foundling
Z76.2	Encounter for health supervision and care of other healthy infant and child
Z99.12	Encounter for respirator [ventilator] dependence during power failure

---

Female patient seen at 32 weeks' gestation to check the progress of her first pregnancy

Z34.03   **Encounter for supervision of normal first pregnancy, third trimester**

Z3A.32   **32 weeks gestation of pregnancy**

Explanation: Category Z34 is appropriate as a first-listed diagnosis. Category Z3A helps to clarify at which point in the pregnancy the patient was provided supervision.

Chapter 21. Factors Influencing Health Status and Contact With Health Services (Z00-Z99)

NOTE   Z codes represent reasons for encounters. A corresponding procedure code must accompany a Z code if a procedure is performed. Categories Z00-Z99 are provided for occasions when circumstances other than a disease, injury or external cause classifiable to categories A00-Y89 are recorded as "diagnoses" or "problems." This can arise in two main ways:

(a) When a person who may or may not be sick encounters the health services for some specific purpose, such as to receive limited care or service for a current condition, to donate an organ or tissue, to receive prophylactic vaccination (immunization), or to discuss a problem which is in itself not a disease or injury.

(b) When some circumstance or problem is present which influences the person's health status but is not in itself a current illness or injury.

This chapter contains the following blocks:

Z00-Z13	Persons encountering health services for examinations
Z14-Z15	Genetic carrier and genetic susceptibility to disease
Z16	Resistance to antimicrobial drugs
Z17	Estrogen receptor status
Z18	Retained foreign body fragments
►Z19	Hormone sensitivity malignancy status◄
►Z20-Z29◄	Persons with potential health hazards related to communicable diseases
Z30-Z39	Persons encountering health services in circumstances related to reproduction
Z40-Z53	Encounters for other specific health care
Z55-Z65	Persons with potential health hazards related to socioeconomic and psychosocial circumstances
Z66	Do not resuscitate status
Z67	Blood type
Z68	Body mass index (BMI)
Z69-Z76	Persons encountering health services in other circumstances
Z77-Z99	Persons with potential health hazards related to family and personal history and certain conditions influencing health status

Persons encountering health services for examinations (Z00-Z13)

NOTE   Nonspecific abnormal findings disclosed at the time of these examinations are classified to categories R70-R94.

EXCLUDES 1   *examinations related to pregnancy and reproduction (Z30-Z36, Z39.-)*

√4ᵗʰ   **Z00**   **Encounter for general examination without complaint, suspected or reported diagnosis**

     EXCLUDES 1   *encounter for examination for administrative purposes (Z02.-)*
     EXCLUDES 2   *encounter for pre-procedural examinations (Z01.81-)*
                    special screening examinations (Z11-Z13)

   √5ᵗʰ   **Z00.0**   **Encounter for general adult medical examination**

       Encounter for adult periodic examination (annual) (physical) and any associated laboratory and radiologic examinations

       EXCLUDES 1   *encounter for examination of sign or symptom - code to sign or symptom*
                      general health check-up of infant or child (Z00.12.-)

       Z00.00   **Encounter for general adult medical examination without abnormal findings**   **PDx** **A**
                   Encounter for adult health check-up NOS
                   AHA: 2016,1Q,36

       Z00.01   **Encounter for general adult medical examination with abnormal findings**   **PDx** **A**
                   Use additional code to identify abnormal findings
                   AHA: 2016,1Q,35-36

   √5ᵗʰ   **Z00.1**   **Encounter for newborn, infant and child health examinations**

     √6ᵗʰ   **Z00.11**   **Newborn health examination**

       Health check for child under 29 days old
       Use additional code to identify any abnormal findings
       EXCLUDES 1   *health check for child over 28 days old (Z00.12-)*

       Z00.110   **Health examination for newborn under 8 days old**   **PDx** **N**
                   Health check for newborn under 8 days old

       Z00.111   **Health examination for newborn 8 to 28 days old**   **PDx** **N**
                   Health check for newborn 8 to 28 days old
                   Newborn weight check

     √6ᵗʰ   **Z00.12**   **Encounter for routine child health examination**

       Encounter for development testing of infant or child
       Health check (routine) for child over 28 days old
       EXCLUDES 1   *health check for child under 29 days old (Z00.11-)*
                     health supervision of foundling or other healthy infant or child (Z76.1-Z76.2)
                     newborn health examination (Z00.11-)

       Z00.121   **Encounter for routine child health examination with abnormal findings**   **PDx** **P**
                   Use additional code to identify abnormal findings
                   AHA: 2016,1Q,34-35

       Z00.129   **Encounter for routine child health examination without abnormal findings**   **PDx** **P**
                   Encounter for routine child health examination NOS
                   AHA: 2016,1Q,34

   Z00.2   **Encounter for examination for period of rapid growth in childhood**   **PDx** **P**

   Z00.3   **Encounter for examination for adolescent development state**   **PDx** **P**
       Encounter for puberty development state

   Z00.5   **Encounter for examination of potential donor of organ and tissue**   **PDx**

   Z00.6   **Encounter for examination for normal comparison and control in clinical research program**
       Examination of participant or control in clinical research program

   √5ᵗʰ   **Z00.7**   **Encounter for examination for period of delayed growth in childhood**

     Z00.70   **Encounter for examination for period of delayed growth in childhood without abnormal findings**   **PDx** **P**

     Z00.71   **Encounter for examination for period of delayed growth in childhood with abnormal findings**   **PDx** **P**
       Use additional code to identify abnormal findings

   Z00.8   **Encounter for other general examination**   **PDx**
       Encounter for health examination in population surveys

√4ᵗʰ   **Z01**   **Encounter for other special examination without complaint, suspected or reported diagnosis**

   INCLUDES   routine examination of specific system

   NOTE   Codes from category Z01 represent the reason for the encounter. A separate procedure code is required to identify any examinations or procedures performed

   EXCLUDES 1   *encounter for examination for administrative purposes (Z02.-)*
                  encounter for examination for suspected conditions, proven not to exist (Z03.-)
                  encounter for laboratory and radiologic examinations as a component of general medical examinations (Z00.0-)
                  encounter for laboratory, radiologic and imaging examinations for sign(s) and symptom(s) - code to the sign(s) or symptom(s)

   EXCLUDES 2   *screening examinations (Z11-Z13)*

   √5ᵗʰ   **Z01.0**   **Encounter for examination of eyes and vision**
       EXCLUDES 1   *examination for driving license (Z02.4)*

     Z01.00   **Encounter for examination of eyes and vision without abnormal findings**   **PDx**
       Encounter for examination of eyes and vision NOS

     Z01.01   **Encounter for examination of eyes and vision with abnormal findings**   **PDx**
       Use additional code to identify abnormal findings

   √5ᵗʰ   **Z01.1**   **Encounter for examination of ears and hearing**

     Z01.10   **Encounter for examination of ears and hearing without abnormal findings**   **PDx**
       Encounter for examination of ears and hearing NOS

     √6ᵗʰ   **Z01.11**   **Encounter for examination of ears and hearing with abnormal findings**

       Z01.110   **Encounter for hearing examination following failed hearing screening**   **PDx**

✅ Additional Character Required   ✗7ᵗʰ Placeholder Alert   Manifestation Dx   ▽ Unspecified Dx   ►◄ Revised Text   ● New Code   ▲ Revised Code Title

ICD-10-CM 2017   **1145**

Z01.118 **Encounter for examination of** `PDx`
ears and hearing with other
abnormal findings
Use additional code to identify abnormal
findings

Z01.12 **Encounter for hearing conservation and** `PDx`
treatment

✓5ᵗʰ **Z01.2** **Encounter for dental examination and cleaning**

Z01.20 **Encounter for dental examination and** `PDx`
cleaning without abnormal findings
Encounter for dental examination and cleaning NOS

Z01.21 **Encounter for dental examination and** `PDx`
cleaning with abnormal findings
Use additional code to identify abnormal findings

✓5ᵗʰ **Z01.3** **Encounter for examination of blood pressure**

Z01.30 **Encounter for examination of blood** `PDx`
pressure without abnormal findings
Encounter for examination of blood pressure NOS

Z01.31 **Encounter for examination of blood** `PDx`
pressure with abnormal findings
Use additional code to identify abnormal findings

✓5ᵗʰ **Z01.4** **Encounter for gynecological examination**

EXCLUDES 2 pregnancy examination or test (Z32.0-)
routine examination for contraceptive maintenance (Z30.4-)

✓6ᵗʰ **Z01.41** **Encounter for routine gynecological examination**
Encounter for general gynecological examination
with or without cervical smear
Encounter for gynecological examination (general)
(routine) NOS
Encounter for pelvic examination (annual) (periodic)
Use additional code:
for screening for human papillomavirus, if
applicable, (Z11.51)
for screening vaginal pap smear, if applicable
(Z12.72)
to identify acquired absence of uterus, if applicable
(Z90.71-)
EXCLUDES 1 gynecologic examination status-post
hysterectomy for malignant condition
(Z08)
screening cervical pap smear not a part of
a routine gynecological examination
(Z12.4)

Z01.411 **Encounter for gynecological** `PDx` ♀
examination (general) (routine)
with abnormal findings
▶Use additional code to identify abnormal
findings◀

Z01.419 **Encounter for gynecological** `PDx` ♀
examination (general) (routine)
without abnormal findings

Z01.42 **Encounter for cervical smear to confirm** `PDx` ♀
findings of recent normal smear following
initial abnormal smear

✓5ᵗʰ **Z01.8** **Encounter for other specified special examinations**

✓6ᵗʰ **Z01.81** **Encounter for preprocedural examinations**
Encounter for preoperative examinations
Encounter for radiological and imaging examinations
as part of preprocedural examination

Z01.810 **Encounter for preprocedural** `PDx`
cardiovascular examination

Z01.811 **Encounter for preprocedural** `PDx`
respiratory examination

Z01.812 **Encounter for preprocedural** `PDx`
laboratory examination
Blood and urine tests prior to treatment or
procedure

Z01.818 **Encounter for other** `PDx`
preprocedural examination
Encounter for preprocedural examination
NOS
Encounter for examinations prior to
antineoplastic chemotherapy

Z01.82 **Encounter for allergy testing** `PDx`
EXCLUDES 1 encounter for antibody response
examination (Z01.84)

Z01.83 **Encounter for blood typing** `PDx`
Encounter for Rh typing

Z01.84 **Encounter for antibody response** `PDx`
examination
Encounter for immunity status testing
EXCLUDES 1 encounter for allergy testing (Z01.82)

Z01.89 **Encounter for other specified special** `PDx`
examinations

✓4ᵗʰ **Z02** **Encounter for administrative examination**

Z02.0 **Encounter for examination for admission to** `PDx`
educational institution
Encounter for examination for admission to preschool
(education)
Encounter for examination for re-admission to school following
illness or medical treatment

Z02.1 **Encounter for pre-employment examination** `PDx`

Z02.2 **Encounter for examination for admission to** `PDx`
residential institution
EXCLUDES 1 examination for admission to prison (Z02.89)

Z02.3 **Encounter for examination for recruitment to** `PDx`
armed forces

Z02.4 **Encounter for examination for driving license** `PDx`

Z02.5 **Encounter for examination for participation in sport** `PDx`
EXCLUDES 1 blood-alcohol and blood-drug test (Z02.83)

Z02.6 **Encounter for examination for insurance purposes** `PDx`

✓5ᵗʰ **Z02.7** **Encounter for issue of medical certificate**
EXCLUDES 1 encounter for general medical examination (Z00-Z01,
Z02.0-Z02.6, Z02.8-Z02.9,)

Z02.71 **Encounter for disability determination** `PDx`
Encounter for issue of medical certificate of incapacity
Encounter for issue of medical certificate of invalidity

Z02.79 **Encounter for issue of other medical** `PDx`
certificate

✓5ᵗʰ **Z02.8** **Encounter for other administrative examinations**

Z02.81 **Encounter for paternity testing** `PDx`

Z02.82 **Encounter for adoption services** `PDx`

Z02.83 **Encounter for blood-alcohol and** `PDx`
blood-drug test
Use additional code for findings of alcohol or drugs
in blood (R78.-)

Z02.89 **Encounter for other administrative** `PDx`
examinations
Encounter for examination for admission to prison
Encounter for examination for admission to summer
camp
Encounter for immigration examination
Encounter for naturalization examination
Encounter for premarital examination
EXCLUDES 1 health supervision of foundling or other
healthy infant or child (Z76.1-Z76.2)

Z02.9 **Encounter for administrative examinations,** `PDx` ▽
unspecified

✓4ᵗʰ **Z03** **Encounter for medical observation for suspected diseases and**
conditions ruled out

NOTE This category is to be used when a person without a
diagnosis is suspected of having an abnormal condition,
without signs or symptoms, which requires study, but after
examination and observation, is ruled out. This category is
also for use for administrative and legal observation status.

EXCLUDES 1 contact with and (suspected) exposures hazardous to health
(Z77.-)
newborn observation for suspected condition, ruled out
(P00-P04)
person with feared complaint in whom no diagnosis is made
(Z71.1)
signs or symptoms under study - code to signs or symptoms

Z03.6 **Encounter for observation for suspected toxic effect** `PDx`
from ingested substance ruled out
Encounter for observation for suspected adverse effect from
drug
Encounter for observation for suspected poisoning

EXCLUDES 1 Not coded here *EXCLUDES 2* Not included here `PDx` Primary Dx Only Ⓝ Newborn Age : 0 Ⓟ Pediatric Age : 0-17 Ⓜ Maternity Age : 12-55 Ⓐ Adult Age : 15-124

1146   ICD-10-CM 2017

✓5ᵗʰ **Z03.7** **Encounter for suspected** maternal and fetal conditions **ruled out**

Encounter for suspected maternal and fetal conditions not found

EXCLUDES 1 *known or suspected fetal anomalies affecting management of mother, not ruled out (O26.-, O35.-, O36.-, O40.-, O41.-)*

    Z03.71 **Encounter for suspected problem with** PDx M ♀ **amniotic cavity and membrane ruled out**

        Encounter for suspected oligohydramnios ruled out

        Encounter for suspected polyhydramnios ruled out

    Z03.72 **Encounter for suspected** placental PDx M ♀ **problem ruled out**

    Z03.73 **Encounter for suspected** fetal anomaly PDx ♀ **ruled out**

    Z03.74 **Encounter for suspected problem with** PDx M ♀ **fetal growth ruled out**

    Z03.75 **Encounter for suspected** cervical PDx M ♀ **shortening ruled out**

    Z03.79 **Encounter for other suspected maternal** PDx M ♀ **and fetal conditions ruled out**

✓5ᵗʰ **Z03.8** **Encounter for** observation for other suspected diseases and conditions ruled out

   ✓6ᵗʰ **Z03.81** **Encounter for observation for suspected** exposure to biological agents **ruled out**

      Z03.810 **Encounter for observation for** PDx **suspected exposure to** anthrax **ruled out**

      Z03.818 **Encounter for observation for** PDx **suspected exposure to other biological agents ruled out**

    Z03.89 **Encounter for observation for other** PDx **suspected diseases and conditions ruled out**

✓4ᵗʰ **Z04** **Encounter for examination and observation for other reasons**

INCLUDES encounter for examination for medicolegal reasons

NOTE This category is to be used when a person without a diagnosis is suspected of having an abnormal condition, without signs or symptoms, which requires study, but after examination and observation, is ruled-out. This category is also for use for administrative and legal observation status.

  Z04.1 **Encounter for examination and observation** PDx **following** transport accident

EXCLUDES 1 *encounter for examination and observation following work accident (Z04.2)*

  Z04.2 **Encounter for examination and observation** PDx **following** work accident

  Z04.3 **Encounter for examination and observation** PDx **following other accident**

✓5ᵗʰ **Z04.4** **Encounter for examination and observation following** alleged rape

Encounter for examination and observation of victim following alleged rape

Encounter for examination and observation of victim following alleged sexual abuse

    Z04.41 **Encounter for examination and** PDx A **observation following alleged** adult **rape**

        Suspected adult rape, ruled out

        Suspected adult sexual abuse, ruled out

    Z04.42 **Encounter for examination and** PDx P **observation following alleged** child **rape**

        Suspected child rape, ruled out

        Suspected child sexual abuse, ruled out

  Z04.6 **Encounter for** general psychiatric examination, PDx **requested by authority**

✓5ᵗʰ **Z04.7** **Encounter for examination and observation following** alleged physical abuse

    Z04.71 **Encounter for examination and** PDx A **observation following alleged** adult **physical abuse**

        Suspected adult physical abuse, ruled out

      EXCLUDES 1 *confirmed case of adult physical abuse (T74.-)*

        encounter for examination and observation following alleged adult sexual abuse (Z04.41)

        suspected case of adult physical abuse, not ruled out (T76.-)

    Z04.72 **Encounter for examination and** PDx P **observation following alleged** child **physical abuse**

        Suspected child physical abuse, ruled out

      EXCLUDES 1 *confirmed case of child physical abuse (T74.-)*

        encounter for examination and observation following alleged child sexual abuse (Z04.42)

        suspected case of child physical abuse, not ruled out (T76.-)

  Z04.8 **Encounter for examination and observation for** PDx **other specified reasons**

    Encounter for examination and observation for request for expert evidence

  Z04.9 **Encounter for examination and observation for** PDx ▽ **unspecified reason**

    Encounter for observation NOS

● ✓4ᵗʰ **Z05** **Encounter for observation and evaluation of newborn for suspected diseases and conditions ruled out**

This category is to be used for newborns, within the neonatal period (the first 28 days of life), who are suspected of having an abnormal condition unrelated to exposure from the mother or the birth process, but without signs or symptoms, and which, after examination and observation, is ruled out.

EXCLUDES 2 *newborn observation for suspected condition, related to exposure from the mother or birth process (P00-P04)*

●   **Z05.0** **Observation and evaluation of newborn for suspected** cardiac **condition ruled out**

●   **Z05.1** **Observation and evaluation of newborn for suspected** infectious **condition ruled out**

●   **Z05.2** **Observation and evaluation of newborn for suspected** neurological **condition ruled out**

●   **Z05.3** **Observation and evaluation of newborn for suspected** respiratory **condition ruled out**

● ✓5ᵗʰ **Z05.4** **Observation and evaluation of newborn for suspected** genetic, metabolic or immunologic **condition ruled out**

●   **Z05.41** **Observation and evaluation of newborn for suspected** genetic **condition ruled out**

●   **Z05.42** **Observation and evaluation of newborn for suspected** metabolic **condition ruled out**

●   **Z05.43** **Observation and evaluation of newborn for suspected** immunologic **condition ruled out**

●   **Z05.5** **Observation and evaluation of newborn for suspected** gastrointestinal **condition ruled out**

●   **Z05.6** **Observation and evaluation of newborn for suspected** genitourinary **condition ruled out**

● ✓5ᵗʰ **Z05.7** **Observation and evaluation of newborn for suspected** skin, subcutaneous, musculoskeletal and connective tissue **condition ruled out**

●   **Z05.71** **Observation and evaluation of newborn for suspected** skin and subcutaneous tissue **condition ruled out**

    Z05.72 **Observation and evaluation of newborn for suspected** musculoskeletal **condition ruled out**

    Z05.73 **Observation and evaluation of newborn for suspected** connective tissue **condition ruled out**

●   **Z05.8** **Observation and evaluation of newborn for other specified suspected condition ruled out**

●   **Z05.9** **Observation and evaluation of newborn for** ▽ **unspecified suspected condition ruled out**

  Z08 **Encounter for** follow-up examination after completed treatment for malignant neoplasm

Medical surveillance following completed treatment

Use additional code to identify any acquired absence of organs (Z90.-)

Use additional code to identify the personal history of malignant neoplasm (Z85.-)

EXCLUDES 1 *aftercare following medical care (Z43-Z49, Z51)*

  Z09 **Encounter for** follow-up examination after completed treatment for conditions other than malignant neoplasm

Medical surveillance following completed treatment

Use additional code to identify any applicable history of disease code (Z86.-, Z87.-)

EXCLUDES 1 *aftercare following medical care (Z43-Z49, Z51)*

    surveillance of contraception (Z30.4-)

    surveillance of prosthetic and other medical devices (Z44-Z46)

AHA: 2015,1Q,8

✓ Additional Character Required   ✓x7ᵗʰ Placeholder Alert   Manifestation Dx   ▽ Unspecified Dx   ▶◀ Revised Text   ● New Code   ▲ Revised Code Title

ICD-10-CM 2017   **1147**

✓4ᵗʰ **Z11** **Encounter for** screening for infectious and parasitic diseases

> **NOTE** Screening is the testing for disease or disease precursors in asymptomatic individuals so that early detection and treatment can be provided for those who test positive for the disease.
>
> *EXCLUDES 1* *encounter for diagnostic examination - code to sign or symptom*

Z11.0 **Encounter for screening for** intestinal infectious diseases

Z11.1 **Encounter for screening for** respiratory tuberculosis

Z11.2 **Encounter for screening for other** bacterial diseases

Z11.3 **Encounter for screening for infections with a** predominantly sexual mode of transmission
> *EXCLUDES 2* *encounter for screening for human immunodeficiency virus [HIV] (Z11.4)*
> *encounter for screening for human papillomavirus (Z11.51)*

Z11.4 **Encounter for screening for** human immunodeficiency virus [HIV]

✓5ᵗʰ **Z11.5** **Encounter for screening for other viral diseases**
> *EXCLUDES 2* *encounter for screening for viral intestinal disease (Z11.0)*

Z11.51 **Encounter for screening for** human papillomavirus (HPV)

Z11.59 **Encounter for screening for other viral diseases**

Z11.6 **Encounter for screening for other** protozoal diseases and helminthiases
> *EXCLUDES 2* *encounter for screening for protozoal intestinal disease (Z11.0)*

Z11.8 **Encounter for screening for other infectious and parasitic diseases**
> Encounter for screening for chlamydia
> Encounter for screening for rickettsial
> Encounter for screening for spirochetal
> Encounter for screening for mycoses

Z11.9 **Encounter for screening for infectious and parasitic diseases, unspecified** ▽

✓4ᵗʰ **Z12** **Encounter for** screening for malignant neoplasms

> **NOTE** Screening is the testing for disease or disease precursors in asymptomatic individuals so that early detection and treatment can be provided for those who test positive for the disease.
>
> Use additional code to identify any family history of malignant neoplasm (Z80.-)
>
> *EXCLUDES 1* *encounter for diagnostic examination - code to sign or symptom*

Z12.0 **Encounter for screening for malignant neoplasm of** stomach

✓5ᵗʰ **Z12.1** **Encounter for screening for malignant neoplasm of** intestinal tract

Z12.10 **Encounter for screening for malignant neoplasm of intestinal tract, unspecified** ▽

Z12.11 **Encounter for screening for malignant neoplasm of colon**
> Encounter for screening colonoscopy NOS

Z12.12 **Encounter for screening for malignant neoplasm of rectum**

Z12.13 **Encounter for screening for malignant neoplasm of small intestine**

Z12.2 **Encounter for screening for malignant neoplasm of respiratory organs**

✓5ᵗʰ **Z12.3** **Encounter for screening for malignant neoplasm of** breast

Z12.31 **Encounter for screening** mammogram **for malignant neoplasm of breast**
> *EXCLUDES 1* *inconclusive mammogram (R92.2)*
> **AHA:** 2015,1Q,24

Z12.39 **Encounter for other screening for malignant neoplasm of breast**

Z12.4 **Encounter for screening for malignant neoplasm of cervix** ♀
> Encounter for screening pap smear for malignant neoplasm of cervix
> *EXCLUDES 1* *when screening is part of general gynecological examination (Z01.4-)*
> *EXCLUDES 2* ▶*encounter for screening for human papillomavirus (Z11.51)*◀

Z12.5 **Encounter for screening for malignant neoplasm of prostate** ♂

Z12.6 **Encounter for screening for malignant neoplasm of** bladder

✓5ᵗʰ **Z12.7** **Encounter for screening for malignant neoplasm of** other genitourinary organs

Z12.71 **Encounter for screening for malignant neoplasm of** testis ♂

Z12.72 **Encounter for screening for malignant neoplasm of** vagina ♀
> Vaginal pap smear status-post hysterectomy for non-malignant condition
> Use additional code to identify acquired absence of uterus (Z90.71-)
> *EXCLUDES 1* *vaginal pap smear status-post hysterectomy for malignant conditions (Z08)*

Z12.73 **Encounter for screening for malignant neoplasm of** ovary ♀

Z12.79 **Encounter for screening for malignant neoplasm of other genitourinary organs**

✓5ᵗʰ **Z12.8** **Encounter for screening for malignant neoplasm of other sites**

Z12.81 **Encounter for screening for malignant neoplasm of** oral cavity

Z12.82 **Encounter for screening for malignant neoplasm of** nervous system

Z12.83 **Encounter for screening for malignant neoplasm of** skin

Z12.89 **Encounter for screening for malignant neoplasm of other sites**

Z12.9 **Encounter for screening for malignant neoplasm, site unspecified** ▽

✓4ᵗʰ **Z13** **Encounter for screening for** other diseases and disorders

> **NOTE** Screening is the testing for disease or disease precursors in asymptomatic individuals so that early detection and treatment can be provided for those who test positive for the disease.
>
> *EXCLUDES 1* *encounter for diagnostic examination - code to sign or symptom*

Z13.0 **Encounter for screening for diseases of the** blood and blood-forming organs **and certain disorders involving the immune mechanism**

Z13.1 **Encounter for screening for** diabetes mellitus

✓5ᵗʰ **Z13.2** **Encounter for screening for nutritional, metabolic and other endocrine disorders**

Z13.21 **Encounter for screening for** nutritional disorder

✓6ᵗʰ **Z13.22** **Encounter for screening for** metabolic disorder

Z13.220 **Encounter for screening for** lipoid disorders
> Encounter for screening for cholesterol level
> Encounter for screening for hypercholesterolemia
> Encounter for screening for hyperlipidemia

Z13.228 **Encounter for screening for other metabolic disorders**

Z13.29 **Encounter for screening for other suspected endocrine disorder**
> *EXCLUDES 1* *encounter for screening for diabetes mellitus (Z13.1)*

Z13.4 **Encounter for screening for certain** developmental disorders in childhood P
> Encounter for screening for developmental handicaps in early childhood
> *EXCLUDES 1* *routine development testing of infant or child (Z00.1-)*

Z13.5 **Encounter for screening for** eye and ear **disorders**
> *EXCLUDES 2* *encounter for general hearing examination (Z01.1-)*
> *encounter for general vision examination (Z01.0-)*

Z13.6 **Encounter for screening for** cardiovascular **disorders**

✓5ᵗʰ **Z13.7** **Encounter for screening for** genetic **and** chromosomal **anomalies**
> *EXCLUDES 1* *genetic testing for procreative management (Z31.4-)*

Z13.71 **Encounter for nonprocreative screening for genetic disease carrier status**

Z13.79 **Encounter for other screening for genetic and chromosomal anomalies**

✓5ᵗʰ **Z13.8** **Encounter for screening for** other **specified diseases and disorders**
> *EXCLUDES 2* *screening for malignant neoplasms (Z12.-)*

✓6ᵗʰ **Z13.81** **Encounter for screening for** digestive system **disorders**

Z13.810 **Encounter for screening for** upper gastrointestinal **disorder**

EXCLUDES 1 Not coded here *EXCLUDES 2* Not included here **PDx** Primary Dx Only **N** Newborn Age : 0 **P** Pediatric Age : 0-17 **M** Maternity Age : 12-55 **A** Adult Age : 15-124

Z13.811 Encounter for screening for lower gastrointestinal disorder

EXCLUDES 1   *encounter for screening for intestinal infectious disease (Z11.0)*

Z13.818 Encounter for screening for other digestive system disorders

✓6th **Z13.82** Encounter for screening for musculoskeletal disorder

Z13.820 Encounter for screening for osteoporosis

Z13.828 Encounter for screening for other musculoskeletal disorder

Z13.83 Encounter for screening for respiratory disorder NEC

EXCLUDES 1   *encounter for screening for respiratory tuberculosis (Z11.1)*

Z13.84 Encounter for screening for dental disorders

✓6th **Z13.85** Encounter for screening for nervous system disorders

Z13.850 Encounter for screening for traumatic brain injury

Z13.858 Encounter for screening for other nervous system disorders

Z13.88 Encounter for screening for disorder due to exposure to contaminants

EXCLUDES 1   *those exposed to contaminants without suspected disorders (Z57.-, Z77.-)*

Z13.89 Encounter for screening for other disorder

Encounter for screening for genitourinary disorders

Z13.9 Encounter for screening, unspecified   ▽

Genetic carrier and genetic susceptibility to disease (Z14-Z15)

✓4th **Z14** Genetic carrier

✓5th **Z14.0** Hemophilia A carrier

Z14.01 Asymptomatic hemophilia A carrier

Z14.02 Symptomatic hemophilia A carrier

Z14.1 Cystic fibrosis carrier

Z14.8 Genetic carrier of other disease

✓4th **Z15** Genetic susceptibility to disease

INCLUDES   confirmed abnormal gene

Use additional code, if applicable, for any associated family history of the disease (Z80-Z84)

EXCLUDES 1   *chromosomal anomalies (Q90-Q99)*

✓5th **Z15.0** Genetic susceptibility to malignant neoplasm

Code first, if applicable, any current malignant neoplasm (C00-C75, C81-C96)

Use additional code, if applicable, for any personal history of malignant neoplasm (Z85.-)

Z15.01 Genetic susceptibility to malignant neoplasm of breast

Z15.02 Genetic susceptibility to malignant neoplasm of ovary   ♀

Z15.03 Genetic susceptibility to malignant neoplasm of prostate   ♂

Z15.04 Genetic susceptibility to malignant neoplasm of endometrium   ♀

Z15.09 Genetic susceptibility to other malignant neoplasm

✓5th **Z15.8** Genetic susceptibility to other disease

Z15.81 Genetic susceptibility to multiple endocrine neoplasia [MEN]

EXCLUDES 1   *multiple endocrine neoplasia [MEN] syndromes (E31.2-)*

Z15.89 Genetic susceptibility to other disease

Resistance to antimicrobial drugs (Z16)

✓4th **Z16** Resistance to antimicrobial drugs

NOTE   The codes in this category are provided for use as additional codes to identify the resistance and non-responsiveness of a condition to antimicrobial drugs.

Code first the infection

EXCLUDES 1   *Methicillin resistant Staphylococcus aureus infection (A49.02)*

Methicillin resistant Staphylococcus aureus infection in diseases classified elsewhere (B95.62)

Methicillin resistant Staphylococcus aureus pneumonia (J15.212)

Sepsis due to Methicillin resistant Staphylococcus aureus (A41.02)

✓5th **Z16.1** Resistance to beta lactam antibiotics

Z16.10 Resistance to unspecified beta lactam antibiotics   ▽

Z16.11 Resistance to penicillins

Resistance to amoxicillin

Resistance to ampicillin

Z16.12 Extended spectrum beta lactamase (ESBL) resistance

Z16.19 Resistance to other specified beta lactam antibiotics

Resistance to cephalosporins

✓5th **Z16.2** Resistance to other antibiotics

Z16.20 Resistance to unspecified antibiotic   ▽

Resistance to antibiotics NOS

Z16.21 Resistance to vancomycin

Z16.22 Resistance to vancomycin related antibiotics

Z16.23 Resistance to quinolones and fluoroquinolones

Z16.24 Resistance to multiple antibiotics

Z16.29 Resistance to other single specified antibiotic

Resistance to aminoglycosides

Resistance to macrolides

Resistance to sulfonamides

Resistance to tetracyclines

✓5th **Z16.3** Resistance to other antimicrobial drugs

EXCLUDES 1   *resistance to antibiotics (Z16.1-, Z16.2-)*

Z16.30 Resistance to unspecified antimicrobial drugs   ▽

Drug resistance NOS

Z16.31 Resistance to antiparasitic drug(s)

Resistance to quinine and related compounds

Z16.32 Resistance to antifungal drug(s)

Z16.33 Resistance to antiviral drug(s)

✓6th **Z16.34** Resistance to antimycobacterial drug(s)

Resistance to tuberculostatics

Z16.341 Resistance to single antimycobacterial drug

Resistance to antimycobacterial drug NOS

Z16.342 Resistance to multiple antimycobacterial drugs

Z16.35 Resistance to multiple antimicrobial drugs

EXCLUDES 1   *Resistance to multiple antibiotics only (Z16.24)*

Z16.39 Resistance to other specified antimicrobial drug

Estrogen receptor status (Z17)

✓4th **Z17** Estrogen receptor status

Code first malignant neoplasm of breast (C50.-)

Z17.0 Estrogen receptor positive status [ER+]

Z17.1 Estrogen receptor negative status [ER-]

☑ Additional Character Required   ✓x7th Placeholder Alert   Manifestation Dx   ▽ Unspecified Dx   ►◄ Revised Text   ● New Code   ▲ Revised Code Title

ICD-10-CM 2017   1149

Retained foreign body fragments (Z18)

✓4ᵗʰ **Z18 Retained foreign body fragments**

INCLUDES embedded fragment (status)
embedded splinter (status)
retained foreign body status

EXCLUDES 1 *artificial joint prosthesis status (Z96.6-)*
foreign body accidentally left during a procedure (T81.5-)
foreign body entering through orifice (T15-T19)
in situ cardiac device (Z95.-)
organ or tissue replaced by means other than transplant (Z96.-, Z97.-)
organ or tissue replaced by transplant (Z94.-)
personal history of retained foreign body fully removed Z87.821
superficial foreign body (non-embedded splinter) - code to superficial foreign body, by site

✓5ᵗʰ **Z18.0 Retained radioactive fragments**

    Z18.01 Retained depleted uranium fragments

    Z18.09 Other retained radioactive fragments
        Other retained depleted isotope fragments
        Retained nontherapeutic radioactive fragments

✓5ᵗʰ **Z18.1 Retained metal fragments**

    EXCLUDES 1 *retained radioactive metal fragments (Z18.01-Z18.09)*

    Z18.10 Retained metal fragments, unspecified ▽
        Retained metal fragment NOS

    Z18.11 Retained magnetic metal fragments

    Z18.12 Retained nonmagnetic metal fragments

Z18.2 Retained plastic fragments
    Acrylics fragments
    Diethylhexylphthalates fragments
    Isocyanate fragments

✓5ᵗʰ **Z18.3 Retained organic fragments**

    Z18.31 Retained animal quills or spines

    Z18.32 Retained tooth

    Z18.33 Retained wood fragments

    Z18.39 Other retained organic fragments

✓5ᵗʰ **Z18.8 Other specified retained foreign body**

    Z18.81 Retained glass fragments

    Z18.83 Retained stone or crystalline fragments
        Retained concrete or cement fragments

    Z18.89 Other specified retained foreign body fragments

Z18.9 Retained foreign body fragments, unspecified material ▽

▶Hormone sensitivity malignancy status (Z19)◀

● ✓4ᵗʰ **Z19 Hormone sensitivity malignancy status**
    Code first malignant neoplasm - see Table of Neoplasms, by site, malignant

●   **Z19.1 Hormone sensitive malignancy status**

●   **Z19.2 Hormone resistant malignancy status**
        Castrate resistant prostate malignancy status

Persons with potential health hazards related to communicable diseases ▶(Z20-Z29)◀

✓4ᵗʰ **Z20 Contact with and (suspected) exposure to communicable diseases**

    EXCLUDES 1 *carrier of infectious disease (Z22.-)*
        diagnosed current infectious or parasitic disease - see Alphabetic Index

    EXCLUDES 2 *personal history of infectious and parasitic diseases (Z86.1-)*

✓5ᵗʰ **Z20.0 Contact with and (suspected) exposure to intestinal infectious diseases**

    Z20.01 Contact with and (suspected) exposure to intestinal infectious diseases due to Escherichia coli (E. coli)

    Z20.09 Contact with and (suspected) exposure to other intestinal infectious diseases

Z20.1 Contact with and (suspected) exposure to tuberculosis

Z20.2 Contact with and (suspected) exposure to infections with a predominantly sexual mode of transmission

Z20.3 Contact with and (suspected) exposure to rabies

Z20.4 Contact with and (suspected) exposure to rubella

Z20.5 Contact with and (suspected) exposure to viral hepatitis

Z20.6 Contact with and (suspected) exposure to human immunodeficiency virus [HIV]
    EXCLUDES 1 *asymptomatic human immunodeficiency virus [HIV] HIV infection status (Z21)*

Z20.7 Contact with and (suspected) exposure to pediculosis, acariasis and other infestations

✓5ᵗʰ **Z20.8 Contact with and (suspected) exposure to other communicable diseases**

    ✓6ᵗʰ **Z20.81 Contact with and (suspected) exposure to other bacterial communicable diseases**

        Z20.810 Contact with and (suspected) exposure to anthrax

        Z20.811 Contact with and (suspected) exposure to meningococcus

        Z20.818 Contact with and (suspected) exposure to other bacterial communicable diseases

    ✓6ᵗʰ **Z20.82 Contact with and (suspected) exposure to other viral communicable diseases**

        Z20.820 Contact with and (suspected) exposure to varicella

        Z20.828 Contact with and (suspected) exposure to other viral communicable diseases

    Z20.89 Contact with and (suspected) exposure to other communicable diseases

Z20.9 Contact with and (suspected) exposure to unspecified communicable disease ▽

Z21 Asymptomatic human immunodeficiency virus [HIV] infection status
    HIV positive NOS
    Code first human immunodeficiency virus [HIV] disease complicating pregnancy, childbirth and the puerperium, if applicable (O98.7-)

    EXCLUDES 1 *acquired immunodeficiency syndrome (B20)*
        contact with human immunodeficiency virus [HIV] (Z20.6)
        exposure to human immunodeficiency virus [HIV] (Z20.6)
        human immunodeficiency virus [HIV] disease (B20)
        inconclusive laboratory evidence of human immunodeficiency virus [HIV] (R75)

✓4ᵗʰ **Z22 Carrier of infectious disease**

    INCLUDES colonization status
        suspected carrier

    EXCLUDES 2 *▶carrier of viral hepatitis (B18.-)◀*

Z22.0 Carrier of typhoid

Z22.1 Carrier of other intestinal infectious diseases

Z22.2 Carrier of diphtheria

✓5ᵗʰ **Z22.3 Carrier of other specified bacterial diseases**

    Z22.31 Carrier of bacterial disease due to meningococci

    ✓6ᵗʰ **Z22.32 Carrier of bacterial disease due to staphylococci**

        Z22.321 Carrier or suspected carrier of Methicillin susceptible Staphylococcus aureus
            MSSA colonization

        Z22.322 Carrier or suspected carrier of Methicillin resistant Staphylococcus aureus
            MRSA colonization

    ✓6ᵗʰ **Z22.33 Carrier of bacterial disease due to streptococci**

        Z22.330 Carrier of Group B streptococcus
            EXCLUDES 1 *▶carrier of streptococcus group B (GBS) complicating pregnancy, childbirth and the puerperium (O99.82-)◀*

        Z22.338 Carrier of other streptococcus

    Z22.39 Carrier of other specified bacterial diseases

Z22.4 Carrier of infections with a predominantly sexual mode of transmission

Z22.6 Carrier of human T-lymphotropic virus type-1 [HTLV-1] infection

Z22.8 Carrier of other infectious diseases

Z22.9 Carrier of infectious disease, unspecified ▽

Z23 Encounter for immunization
    Code first any routine childhood examination

    NOTE Procedure codes are required to identify the types of immunizations given

✓4ᵗʰ **Z28 Immunization not carried out and underimmunization status**

    INCLUDES vaccination not carried out

    ✓5ᵗʰ **Z28.0 Immunization not carried out because of contraindication**

        Z28.01 Immunization not carried out because of acute illness of patient

EXCLUDES 1 Not coded here   EXCLUDES 2 Not included here   PDx Primary Dx Only   N Newborn Age : 0   P Pediatric Age : 0-17   M Maternity Age : 12-55   A Adult Age : 15-124

1150   ICD-10-CM 2017

Z28.02   Immunization not carried out because of chronic illness or condition of patient

Z28.03   Immunization not carried out because of immune compromised state of patient

Z28.04   Immunization not carried out because of patient allergy to vaccine or component

Z28.09   Immunization not carried out because of other contraindication

Z28.1   Immunization not carried out because of patient decision for reasons of belief or group pressure

Immunization not carried out because of religious belief

✓5ᵗʰ **Z28.2**   Immunization not carried out because of patient decision for other and unspecified reason

Z28.20   Immunization not carried out because of patient decision for unspecified reason   ▽

Z28.21   Immunization not carried out because of patient refusal

Z28.29   Immunization not carried out because of patient decision for other reason

Z28.3   Underimmunization status

Delinquent immunization status

Lapsed immunization schedule status

✓5ᵗʰ **Z28.8**   Immunization not carried out for other reason

Z28.81   Immunization not carried out due to patient having had the disease

Z28.82   Immunization not carried out because of caregiver refusal

Immunization not carried out because of guardian refusal

Immunization not carried out because of parent refusal

EXCLUDES 1   *immunization not carried out because of caregiver refusal because of religious belief (Z28.1)*

Z28.89   Immunization not carried out for other reason

Z28.9   Immunization not carried out for unspecified reason   ▽

● ✓4ᵗʰ **Z29**   **Encounter for other prophylactic measures**

EXCLUDES 1   *desensitization to allergens (Z51.6)*
prophylactic surgery (Z40.-)

● ✓5ᵗʰ **Z29.1**   Encounter for prophylactic immunotherapy

Encounter for administration of Immunoglobulin

●   **Z29.11**   Encounter for prophylactic immunotherapy for respiratory syncytial virus (RSV)

●   **Z29.12**   Encounter for prophylactic antivenin

●   **Z29.13**   Encounter for prophylactic Rho(D) immune globulin

●   **Z29.14**   Encounter for prophylactic rabies immune globin

●   **Z29.3**   Encounter for prophylactic fluoride administration

●   **Z29.8**   Encounter for other specified prophylactic measures

●   **Z29.9**   Encounter for prophylactic measures, unspecified   ▽

Persons encountering health services in circumstances related to reproduction (Z30–Z39)

✓4ᵗʰ **Z30**   **Encounter for contraceptive management**

✓5ᵗʰ **Z30.0**   Encounter for general counseling and advice on contraception

✓6ᵗʰ **Z30.01**   Encounter for initial prescription of contraceptives

EXCLUDES 1   *encounter for surveillance of contraceptives (Z30.4-)*

Z30.011   Encounter for initial prescription of contraceptive pills   ♀

Z30.012   Encounter for prescription of emergency contraception

Encounter for postcoital contraception

Z30.013   Encounter for initial prescription of injectable contraceptive   ♀

Z30.014   Encounter for initial prescription of intrauterine contraceptive device   ♀

EXCLUDES 1   *encounter for insertion of intrauterine contraceptive device (Z30.430, Z30.432)*

●   **Z30.015**   Encounter for initial prescription of vaginal ring hormonal contraceptive

●   **Z30.016**   Encounter for initial prescription of transdermal patch hormonal contraceptive device

●   **Z30.017**   Encounter for initial prescription of implantable subdermal contraceptive

Z30.018   Encounter for initial prescription of other contraceptives   ♀

▶Encounter for initial prescription of barrier contraception◀

▶Encounter for initial prescription of diaphragm◀

Z30.019   Encounter for initial prescription of contraceptives, unspecified   ♀ ▽

Z30.02   Counseling and instruction in natural family planning to avoid pregnancy

Z30.09   Encounter for other general counseling and advice on contraception

Encounter for family planning advice NOS

Z30.2   Encounter for sterilization

✓5ᵗʰ **Z30.4**   Encounter for surveillance of contraceptives

Z30.40   Encounter for surveillance of contraceptives, unspecified   ▽

Z30.41   Encounter for surveillance of contraceptive pills   ♀

Encounter for repeat prescription for contraceptive pill

Z30.42   Encounter for surveillance of injectable contraceptive   ♀

✓6ᵗʰ **Z30.43**   Encounter for surveillance of intrauterine contraceptive device

Z30.430   Encounter for insertion of intrauterine contraceptive device   ♀

Z30.431   Encounter for routine checking of intrauterine contraceptive device   ♀

Z30.432   Encounter for removal of intrauterine contraceptive device   ♀

Z30.433   Encounter for removal and reinsertion of intrauterine contraceptive device   ♀

Encounter for replacement of intrauterine contraceptive device

Z30.44   Encounter for surveillance of vaginal ring hormonal contraceptive device

Z30.45   Encounter for surveillance of transdermal patch hormonal contraceptive device

Z30.46   Encounter for surveillance of implantable subdermal contraceptive

Encounter for checking, reinsertion or removal of implantable subdermal contraceptive

Z30.49   Encounter for surveillance of other contraceptives   ♀

▶Encounter for surveillance of barrier contraception◀

▶Encounter for surveillance of diaphragm◀

Z30.8   Encounter for other contraceptive management

Encounter for postvasectomy sperm count

Encounter for routine examination for contraceptive maintenance

EXCLUDES 1   *sperm count following sterilization reversal (Z31.42)*
sperm count for fertility testing (Z31.41)

Z30.9   Encounter for contraceptive management, unspecified   ▽

✓4ᵗʰ **Z31**   **Encounter for procreative management**

EXCLUDES 1   *complications associated with artificial fertilization (N98.-)*
female infertility (N97.-)
male infertility (N46.-)

Z31.0   Encounter for reversal of previous sterilization

✓5ᵗʰ **Z31.4**   Encounter for procreative investigation and testing

EXCLUDES 1   *postvasectomy sperm count (Z30.8)*

Z31.41   Encounter for fertility testing

Encounter for fallopian tube patency testing

Encounter for sperm count for fertility testing

Z31.42   Aftercare following sterilization reversal

Sperm count following sterilization reversal

☑ Additional Character Required   ✓x7ᵗʰ Placeholder Alert   Manifestation Dx   ▽ Unspecified Dx   ▶◀ Revised Text   ● New Code   ▲ Revised Code Title

ICD-10-CM 2017

1151

✓6ᵗʰ **Z31.43** **Encounter for genetic testing of female for procreative management**
Use additional code for recurrent pregnancy loss, if applicable (N96, O26.2-)
EXCLUDES 1 *nonprocreative genetic testing (Z13.7-)*

    Z31.430 **Encounter of female for testing for genetic disease carrier status for procreative management** ♀

    Z31.438 **Encounter for other genetic testing of female for procreative management** ♀

✓6ᵗʰ **Z31.44** **Encounter for genetic testing of male for procreative management**
EXCLUDES 1 *nonprocreative genetic testing (Z13.7-)*

    Z31.440 **Encounter of male for testing for genetic disease carrier status for procreative management** ♂

    Z31.441 **Encounter for testing of male partner of patient with recurrent pregnancy loss** Ⓐ ♂

    Z31.448 **Encounter for other genetic testing of male for procreative management** Ⓐ ♂

    Z31.49 **Encounter for other procreative investigation and testing**

Z31.5 **Encounter for genetic counseling**

✓5ᵗʰ **Z31.6** **Encounter for general counseling and advice on procreation**

    Z31.61 **Procreative counseling and advice using natural family planning**

    Z31.62 **Encounter for fertility preservation counseling**
Encounter for fertility preservation counseling prior to cancer therapy
Encounter for fertility preservation counseling prior to surgical removal of gonads

    Z31.69 **Encounter for other general counseling and advice on procreation**

Z31.7 **Encounter for procreative management and counseling for gestational carrier**
EXCLUDES 1 *pregnant state, gestational carrier (Z33.3)*

✓5ᵗʰ **Z31.8** **Encounter for other procreative management**

    Z31.81 **Encounter for male factor infertility in female patient** PDx ♀

    Z31.82 **Encounter for Rh incompatibility status** PDx ♀
AHA: 2015,3Q,40; 2014,4Q,17

    Z31.83 **Encounter for assisted reproductive fertility procedure cycle** PDx ♀
Patient undergoing in vitro fertilization cycle
Use additional code to identify the type of infertility
EXCLUDES 1 *pre-cycle diagnosis and testing - code to reason for encounter*

    Z31.84 **Encounter for fertility preservation procedure** PDx
Encounter for fertility preservation procedure prior to cancer therapy
Encounter for fertility preservation procedure prior to surgical removal of gonads

    Z31.89 **Encounter for other procreative management**

Z31.9 **Encounter for procreative management, unspecified** ▽

✓4ᵗʰ **Z32** **Encounter for pregnancy test and childbirth and childcare instruction**

✓5ᵗʰ **Z32.0** **Encounter for pregnancy test**

    Z32.00 **Encounter for pregnancy test, result unknown** ♀
Encounter for pregnancy test NOS

    Z32.01 **Encounter for pregnancy test, result positive** Ⓜ ♀

    Z32.02 **Encounter for pregnancy test, result negative** ♀

Z32.2 **Encounter for childbirth instruction**

Z32.3 **Encounter for childcare instruction**
Encounter for prenatal or postpartum childcare instruction

✓4ᵗʰ **Z33** **Pregnant state**

Z33.1 **Pregnant state, incidental** Ⓜ ♀
Pregnant state NOS
EXCLUDES 1 *complications of pregnancy (O00-O9A)*
▶*pregnant state, gestational carrier (Z33.3)*◀

Z33.2 **Encounter for elective termination of pregnancy** PDx Ⓜ ♀
EXCLUDES 1 *early fetal death with retention of dead fetus (O02.1)*
late fetal death (O36.4)
spontaneous abortion (O03)

● **Z33.3** **Pregnant state, gestational carrier**
EXCLUDES 1 *encounter for procreative management and counseling for gestational carrier (Z31.7)*

✓4ᵗʰ **Z34** **Encounter for supervision of normal pregnancy**
EXCLUDES 1 *any complication of pregnancy (O00-O9A)*
encounter for pregnancy test (Z32.0-)
encounter for supervision of high risk pregnancy (O09.-)
AHA: 2014,4Q,17

✓5ᵗʰ **Z34.0** **Encounter for supervision of normal first pregnancy**

    Z34.00 **Encounter for supervision of normal first pregnancy, unspecified trimester** PDx Ⓜ♀▽

    Z34.01 **Encounter for supervision of normal first pregnancy, first trimester** PDx Ⓜ ♀

    Z34.02 **Encounter for supervision of normal first pregnancy, second trimester** PDx Ⓜ ♀

    Z34.03 **Encounter for supervision of normal first pregnancy, third trimester** PDx Ⓜ ♀

✓5ᵗʰ **Z34.8** **Encounter for supervision of other normal pregnancy**

    Z34.80 **Encounter for supervision of other normal pregnancy, unspecified trimester** PDx Ⓜ♀▽

    Z34.81 **Encounter for supervision of other normal pregnancy, first trimester** PDx Ⓜ ♀

    Z34.82 **Encounter for supervision of other normal pregnancy, second trimester** PDx Ⓜ ♀

    Z34.83 **Encounter for supervision of other normal pregnancy, third trimester** PDx Ⓜ ♀

✓5ᵗʰ **Z34.9** **Encounter for supervision of normal pregnancy, unspecified**

    Z34.90 **Encounter for supervision of normal pregnancy, unspecified, unspecified trimester** PDx Ⓜ♀▽

    Z34.91 **Encounter for supervision of normal pregnancy, unspecified, first trimester** PDx Ⓜ♀▽

    Z34.92 **Encounter for supervision of normal pregnancy, unspecified, second trimester** PDx Ⓜ♀▽

    Z34.93 **Encounter for supervision of normal pregnancy, unspecified, third trimester** PDx Ⓜ♀▽

Z36 **Encounter for antenatal screening of mother** Ⓜ ♀
EXCLUDES 1 *abnormal findings on antenatal screening of mother (O28.-)*
diagnostic examination - code to sign or symptom
encounter for suspected maternal and fetal conditions ruled out (Z03.7-)
suspected fetal condition affecting management of pregnancy - code to condition in Chapter 15
EXCLUDES 2 *genetic counseling and testing (Z31.43-, Z31.5)*
routine prenatal care (Z34)

✓4ᵗʰ **Z3A** **Weeks of gestation**

NOTE ▶Codes from category Z3A are for use, only on the maternal record, to indicate the weeks of gestation of the pregnancy, if known.◀
Code first complications of pregnancy, childbirth and the puerperium (O00-O9A)
AHA: 2016,2Q,34; 2014,3Q,17; 2014,2Q,9; 2013,2Q,33

✓5ᵗʰ **Z3A.0** **Weeks of gestation of pregnancy, unspecified or less than 10 weeks**

    Z3A.00 **Weeks of gestation of pregnancy not specified** Ⓜ ♀

    Z3A.01 **Less than 8 weeks gestation of pregnancy** Ⓜ ♀

    Z3A.08 **8 weeks gestation of pregnancy** Ⓜ ♀

    Z3A.09 **9 weeks gestation of pregnancy** Ⓜ ♀

✓5ᵗʰ **Z3A.1** **Weeks of gestation of pregnancy, weeks 10-19**

    Z3A.10 **10 weeks gestation of pregnancy** Ⓜ ♀

    Z3A.11 **11 weeks gestation of pregnancy** Ⓜ ♀

    Z3A.12 **12 weeks gestation of pregnancy** Ⓜ ♀

    Z3A.13 **13 weeks gestation of pregnancy** Ⓜ ♀

    Z3A.14 **14 weeks gestation of pregnancy** Ⓜ ♀

    Z3A.15 **15 weeks gestation of pregnancy** Ⓜ ♀

    Z3A.16 **16 weeks gestation of pregnancy** Ⓜ ♀

    Z3A.17 **17 weeks gestation of pregnancy** Ⓜ ♀

    Z3A.18 **18 weeks gestation of pregnancy** Ⓜ ♀

Z3A.19   19 weeks **gestation of pregnancy** Ⓜ ♀

✓5ᵗʰ **Z3A.2 Weeks of gestation of pregnancy, weeks 20-29**

Z3A.20   20 weeks **gestation of pregnancy** Ⓜ ♀
Z3A.21   21 weeks **gestation of pregnancy** Ⓜ ♀
Z3A.22   22 weeks **gestation of pregnancy** Ⓜ ♀
Z3A.23   23 weeks **gestation of pregnancy** Ⓜ ♀
Z3A.24   24 weeks **gestation of pregnancy** Ⓜ ♀
Z3A.25   25 weeks **gestation of pregnancy** Ⓜ ♀
Z3A.26   26 weeks **gestation of pregnancy** Ⓜ ♀
Z3A.27   27 weeks **gestation of pregnancy** Ⓜ ♀
Z3A.28   28 weeks **gestation of pregnancy** Ⓜ ♀
Z3A.29   29 weeks **gestation of pregnancy** Ⓜ ♀

✓5ᵗʰ **Z3A.3 Weeks of gestation of pregnancy, weeks 30-39**

Z3A.30   30 weeks **gestation of pregnancy** Ⓜ ♀
Z3A.31   31 weeks **gestation of pregnancy** Ⓜ ♀
Z3A.32   32 weeks **gestation of pregnancy** Ⓜ ♀
Z3A.33   33 weeks **gestation of pregnancy** Ⓜ ♀
Z3A.34   34 weeks **gestation of pregnancy** Ⓜ ♀
Z3A.35   35 weeks **gestation of pregnancy** Ⓜ ♀
Z3A.36   36 weeks **gestation of pregnancy** Ⓜ ♀
Z3A.37   37 weeks **gestation of pregnancy** Ⓜ ♀
Z3A.38   38 weeks **gestation of pregnancy** Ⓜ ♀
Z3A.39   39 weeks **gestation of pregnancy** Ⓜ ♀

✓5ᵗʰ **Z3A.4 Weeks of gestation of pregnancy, weeks 40 or greater**

AHA: 2014,4Q,23

Z3A.40   40 weeks **gestation of pregnancy** Ⓜ ♀
Z3A.41   41 weeks **gestation of pregnancy** Ⓜ ♀
Z3A.42   42 weeks **gestation of pregnancy** Ⓜ ♀
Z3A.49   Greater than 42 weeks **gestation of pregnancy** Ⓜ ♀

✓4ᵗʰ **Z37 Outcome of delivery**

NOTE This category is intended for use as an additional code to identify the outcome of delivery on the mother's record. It is not for use on the newborn record.

EXCLUDES 1 *stillbirth (P95)*

Z37.0 **Single live birth** Ⓜ ♀
    AHA: 2016,2Q,34; 2014,2Q,9

Z37.1 **Single stillbirth** Ⓜ ♀
Z37.2 **Twins, both liveborn** Ⓜ ♀
Z37.3 **Twins, one liveborn and one stillborn** Ⓜ ♀
Z37.4 **Twins, both stillborn** Ⓜ ♀

✓5ᵗʰ Z37.5 **Other multiple births, all liveborn**

Z37.50   Multiple births, unspecified, all liveborn Ⓜ ♀ ▽
Z37.51   Triplets, all liveborn Ⓜ ♀
Z37.52   Quadruplets, all liveborn Ⓜ ♀
Z37.53   Quintuplets, all liveborn Ⓜ ♀
Z37.54   Sextuplets, all liveborn Ⓜ ♀
Z37.59   Other multiple births, all liveborn Ⓜ ♀

✓5ᵗʰ Z37.6 **Other multiple births, some liveborn**

Z37.60   Multiple births, unspecified, some liveborn Ⓜ ♀ ▽
Z37.61   Triplets, some liveborn Ⓜ ♀
Z37.62   Quadruplets, some liveborn Ⓜ ♀
Z37.63   Quintuplets, some liveborn Ⓜ ♀
Z37.64   Sextuplets, some liveborn Ⓜ ♀
Z37.69   Other multiple births, some liveborn Ⓜ ♀

Z37.7 **Other multiple births, all stillborn** Ⓜ ♀
Z37.9 **Outcome of delivery, unspecified** Ⓜ ♀ ▽
    Multiple birth NOS
    Single birth NOS

✓4ᵗʰ **Z38 Liveborn infants according to place of birth and type of delivery**

NOTE This category is for use as the principal code on the initial record of a newborn baby. It is to be used for the initial birth record only. It is not to be used on the mother's record.

AHA: 2015,2Q,15

✓5ᵗʰ Z38.0 **Single liveborn infant, born in hospital**
    Single liveborn infant, born in birthing center or other health care facility
    Z38.00   **Single liveborn infant, delivered vaginally** ᴾᴰˣ Ⓝ
    Z38.01   **Single liveborn infant, delivered by cesarean** ᴾᴰˣ Ⓝ

Z38.1 **Single liveborn infant, born outside hospital** ᴾᴰˣ Ⓝ
Z38.2 **Single liveborn infant, unspecified as to place of birth** ᴾᴰˣ Ⓝ ▽
    Single liveborn infant NOS

✓5ᵗʰ Z38.3 **Twin liveborn infant, born in hospital**
    Z38.30   **Twin liveborn infant, delivered vaginally** ᴾᴰˣ Ⓝ
    Z38.31   **Twin liveborn infant, delivered by cesarean** ᴾᴰˣ Ⓝ

Z38.4 **Twin liveborn infant, born outside hospital** ᴾᴰˣ Ⓝ
Z38.5 **Twin liveborn infant, unspecified as to place of birth** ᴾᴰˣ Ⓝ ▽

✓5ᵗʰ Z38.6 **Other multiple liveborn infant, born in hospital**
    Z38.61   **Triplet liveborn infant, delivered vaginally** ᴾᴰˣ Ⓝ
    Z38.62   **Triplet liveborn infant, delivered by cesarean** ᴾᴰˣ Ⓝ
    Z38.63   **Quadruplet liveborn infant, delivered vaginally** ᴾᴰˣ Ⓝ
    Z38.64   **Quadruplet liveborn infant, delivered by cesarean** ᴾᴰˣ Ⓝ
    Z38.65   **Quintuplet liveborn infant, delivered vaginally** ᴾᴰˣ Ⓝ
    Z38.66   **Quintuplet liveborn infant, delivered by cesarean** ᴾᴰˣ Ⓝ
    Z38.68   **Other multiple liveborn infant, delivered vaginally** ᴾᴰˣ Ⓝ
    Z38.69   **Other multiple liveborn infant, delivered by cesarean** ᴾᴰˣ Ⓝ

Z38.7 **Other multiple liveborn infant, born outside hospital** ᴾᴰˣ Ⓝ
Z38.8 **Other multiple liveborn infant, unspecified as to place of birth** ᴾᴰˣ Ⓝ ▽

✓4ᵗʰ **Z39 Encounter for maternal postpartum care and examination**

Z39.0 **Encounter for care and examination of mother immediately after delivery** ᴾᴰˣ Ⓜ ♀
    Care and observation in uncomplicated cases when the delivery occurs outside a healthcare facility
    EXCLUDES 1 *care for postpartum complication - see Alphabetic index*

Z39.1 **Encounter for care and examination of lactating mother** ᴾᴰˣ Ⓜ ♀
    Encounter for supervision of lactation
    EXCLUDES 1 *disorders of lactation (O92.-)*

Z39.2 **Encounter for routine postpartum follow-up** ᴾᴰˣ Ⓜ ♀

Encounters for other specific health care (Z40-Z53)

NOTE Categories Z40-Z53 are intended for use to indicate a reason for care. They may be used for patients who have already been treated for a disease or injury, but who are receiving aftercare or prophylactic care, or care to consolidate the treatment, or to deal with a residual state

EXCLUDES 2 *follow-up examination for medical surveillance after treatment (Z08-Z09)*

✓4ᵗʰ **Z40 Encounter for prophylactic surgery**

EXCLUDES 1 *organ donations (Z52.-)*
    therapeutic organ removal - code to condition

✓5ᵗʰ Z40.0 **Encounter for prophylactic surgery for risk factors related to malignant neoplasms**
    Admission for prophylactic organ removal
    Use additional code to identify risk factor
    Z40.00   **Encounter for prophylactic removal of unspecified organ** ▽
    Z40.01   **Encounter for prophylactic removal of breast**
    Z40.02   **Encounter for prophylactic removal of ovary** ♀
    Z40.09   **Encounter for prophylactic removal of other organ**

Z40.8 **Encounter for other prophylactic surgery**
Z40.9 **Encounter for prophylactic surgery, unspecified** ▽

☑ Additional Character Required   ✓7ᵗʰ Placeholder Alert   Manifestation Dx   ▽ Unspecified Dx   ►◄ Revised Text   ● New Code   ▲ Revised Code Title

✓4ᵗʰ Z41 Encounter for procedures for purposes other than remedying health state

    Z41.1 Encounter for cosmetic surgery
        Encounter for cosmetic breast implant
        Encounter for cosmetic procedure
        EXCLUDES 1 encounter for plastic and reconstructive surgery following medical procedure or healed injury (Z42.-)
            encounter for post-mastectomy breast implantation (Z42.1)

    Z41.2 Encounter for routine and ritual male circumcision ♂

    Z41.3 Encounter for ear piercing

    Z41.8 Encounter for other procedures for purposes other than remedying health state

    Z41.9 Encounter for procedure for purposes other than remedying health state, unspecified ▽

✓4ᵗʰ Z42 Encounter for plastic and reconstructive surgery following medical procedure or healed injury

    EXCLUDES 1 encounter for cosmetic plastic surgery (Z41.1)
        encounter for plastic surgery for treatment of current injury - code to relevent injury

    Z42.1 Encounter for breast reconstruction following mastectomy PDx A
        EXCLUDES 1 deformity and disproportion of reconstructed breast (N65.1-)

    Z42.8 Encounter for other plastic and reconstructive surgery following medical procedure or healed injury PDx

✓4ᵗʰ Z43 Encounter for attention to artificial openings

    INCLUDES closure of artificial openings
        passage of sounds or bougies through artificial openings
        reforming artificial openings
        removal of catheter from artificial openings
        toilet or cleansing of artificial openings
    EXCLUDES 1 artificial opening status only, without need for care (Z93.-)
        complications of external stoma (J95.0-, K94.-, N99.5-)
    EXCLUDES 2 fitting and adjustment of prosthetic and other devices (Z44-Z46)

    Z43.0 Encounter for attention to tracheostomy

    Z43.1 Encounter for attention to gastrostomy

    Z43.2 Encounter for attention to ileostomy

    Z43.3 Encounter for attention to colostomy

    Z43.4 Encounter for attention to other artificial openings of digestive tract

    Z43.5 Encounter for attention to cystostomy

    Z43.6 Encounter for attention to other artificial openings of urinary tract
        Encounter for attention to nephrostomy
        Encounter for attention to ureterostomy
        Encounter for attention to urethrostomy

    Z43.7 Encounter for attention to artificial vagina

    Z43.8 Encounter for attention to other artificial openings

    Z43.9 Encounter for attention to unspecified artificial opening ▽

✓4ᵗʰ Z44 Encounter for fitting and adjustment of external prosthetic device

    INCLUDES removal or replacement of external prosthetic device
    EXCLUDES 1 malfunction or other complications of device - see Alphabetical Index
        presence of prosthetic device (Z97.-)

    ✓5ᵗʰ Z44.0 Encounter for fitting and adjustment of artificial arm

        ✓6ᵗʰ Z44.00 Encounter for fitting and adjustment of unspecified artificial arm

            Z44.001 Encounter for fitting and adjustment of unspecified right artificial arm ▽

            Z44.002 Encounter for fitting and adjustment of unspecified left artificial arm ▽

            Z44.009 Encounter for fitting and adjustment of unspecified artificial arm, unspecified arm ▽

        ✓6ᵗʰ Z44.01 Encounter for fitting and adjustment of complete artificial arm

            Z44.011 Encounter for fitting and adjustment of complete right artificial arm

            Z44.012 Encounter for fitting and adjustment of complete left artificial arm

            Z44.019 Encounter for fitting and adjustment of complete artificial arm, unspecified arm ▽

        ✓6ᵗʰ Z44.02 Encounter for fitting and adjustment of partial artificial arm

            Z44.021 Encounter for fitting and adjustment of partial artificial right arm

            Z44.022 Encounter for fitting and adjustment of partial artificial left arm

            Z44.029 Encounter for fitting and adjustment of partial artificial arm, unspecified arm ▽

    ✓5ᵗʰ Z44.1 Encounter for fitting and adjustment of artificial leg

        ✓6ᵗʰ Z44.10 Encounter for fitting and adjustment of unspecified artificial leg

            Z44.101 Encounter for fitting and adjustment of unspecified right artificial leg ▽

            Z44.102 Encounter for fitting and adjustment of unspecified left artificial leg ▽

            Z44.109 Encounter for fitting and adjustment of unspecified artificial leg, unspecified leg ▽

        ✓6ᵗʰ Z44.11 Encounter for fitting and adjustment of complete artificial leg

            Z44.111 Encounter for fitting and adjustment of complete right artificial leg

            Z44.112 Encounter for fitting and adjustment of complete left artificial leg

            Z44.119 Encounter for fitting and adjustment of complete artificial leg, unspecified leg ▽

        ✓6ᵗʰ Z44.12 Encounter for fitting and adjustment of partial artificial leg

            Z44.121 Encounter for fitting and adjustment of partial artificial right leg

            Z44.122 Encounter for fitting and adjustment of partial artificial left leg

            Z44.129 Encounter for fitting and adjustment of partial artificial leg, unspecified leg ▽

    ✓5ᵗʰ Z44.2 Encounter for fitting and adjustment of artificial eye

        EXCLUDES 1 mechanical complication of ocular prosthesis (T85.3)

        Z44.20 Encounter for fitting and adjustment of artificial eye, unspecified ▽

        Z44.21 Encounter for fitting and adjustment of artificial right eye

        Z44.22 Encounter for fitting and adjustment of artificial left eye

    ✓5ᵗʰ Z44.3 Encounter for fitting and adjustment of external breast prosthesis

        EXCLUDES 1 complications of breast implant (T85.4-)
            encounter for adjustment or removal of breast implant (Z45.81-)
            encounter for initial breast implant insertion for cosmetic breast augmentation (Z41.1)
            encounter for breast reconstruction following mastectomy (Z42.1)

        Z44.30 Encounter for fitting and adjustment of external breast prosthesis, unspecified breast ▽

        Z44.31 Encounter for fitting and adjustment of external right breast prosthesis

        Z44.32 Encounter for fitting and adjustment of external left breast prosthesis

    Z44.8 Encounter for fitting and adjustment of other external prosthetic devices

    Z44.9 Encounter for fitting and adjustment of unspecified external prosthetic device ▽

✓4ᵗʰ Z45 Encounter for adjustment and management of implanted device

    INCLUDES removal or replacement of implanted device
    EXCLUDES 1 malfunction or other complications of device - see Alphabetical Index
        presence of prosthetic and other devices (Z95-Z97)
    EXCLUDES 2 encounter for fitting and adjustment of non-implanted device (Z46.-)

    ✓5ᵗʰ Z45.0 Encounter for adjustment and management of cardiac device

EXCLUDES 1 Not coded here   *EXCLUDES 2* Not included here   PDx Primary Dx Only   N Newborn Age : 0   P Pediatric Age : 0-17   M Maternity Age : 12-55   A Adult Age : 15-124

1154   ICD-10-CM 2017

✓6ᵗʰ **Z45.01** **Encounter for adjustment and management of cardiac** pacemaker
►Encounter for adjustment and management of cardiac resynchronization therapy pacemaker (CRT-P)◄
EXCLUDES 1 *encounter for adjustment and management of automatic implantable cardiac defibrillator with synchronous cardiac pacemaker (Z45.02)*

     Z45.010 **Encounter for checking and testing of cardiac pacemaker** pulse generator **[battery]**
Encounter for replacing cardiac pacemaker pulse generator [battery]

     Z45.018 **Encounter for adjustment and management of other part of cardiac pacemaker**

Z45.02 **Encounter for adjustment and management of** automatic implantable cardiac defibrillator
Encounter for adjustment and management of automatic implantable cardiac defibrillator with synchronous cardiac pacemaker
►Encounter for adjustment and management of cardiac resynchronization therapy defibrillator (CRT-D)◄

Z45.09 **Encounter for adjustment and management of other cardiac device**

Z45.1 **Encounter for adjustment and management of** infusion pump

Z45.2 **Encounter for adjustment and management of** vascular access device
Encounter for adjustment and management of vascular catheters
EXCLUDES 1 *encounter for adjustment and management of renal dialysis catheter (Z49.01)*

✓5ᵗʰ **Z45.3** **Encounter for adjustment and management of implanted devices of the special senses**

     Z45.31 **Encounter for adjustment and management of implanted visual substitution device**

✓6ᵗʰ   **Z45.32** **Encounter for adjustment and management of implanted hearing device**
EXCLUDES 1 *Encounter for fitting and adjustment of hearing aide (Z46.1)*

     Z45.320 **Encounter for adjustment and management of bone conduction device**

     Z45.321 **Encounter for adjustment and management of cochlear device**

     Z45.328 **Encounter for adjustment and management of other implanted hearing device**

✓5ᵗʰ **Z45.4** **Encounter for adjustment and management of implanted nervous system device**

     Z45.41 **Encounter for adjustment and management of cerebrospinal fluid drainage device**
Encounter for adjustment and management of cerebral ventricular (communicating) shunt

     Z45.42 **Encounter for adjustment and management of neuropacemaker (brain) (peripheral nerve) (spinal cord)**

     Z45.49 **Encounter for adjustment and management of other implanted nervous system device**
AHA: 2014,3Q,19

✓5ᵗʰ **Z45.8** **Encounter for adjustment and management of other implanted devices**

✓6ᵗʰ   **Z45.81** **Encounter for adjustment or** removal of breast implant
Encounter for elective implant exchange (different material) (different size)
Encounter removal of tissue expander without synchronous insertion of permanent implant
EXCLUDES 1 *complications of breast implant (T85.4-)*
encounter for initial breast implant insertion for cosmetic breast augmentation (Z41.1)
encounter for breast reconstruction following mastectomy (Z42.1)

     Z45.811 **Encounter for adjustment or removal of right breast implant**

     Z45.812 **Encounter for adjustment or removal of left breast implant**

     Z45.819 **Encounter for adjustment or removal of unspecified breast implant** ▽

     Z45.82 **Encounter for adjustment or** removal of myringotomy device (stent) (tube)

     Z45.89 **Encounter for adjustment and management of other implanted devices**
AHA: 2014,4Q,26-28

Z45.9 **Encounter for adjustment and management of unspecified implanted device** ▽

✓4ᵗʰ **Z46** **Encounter for fitting and adjustment of other devices**
INCLUDES removal or replacement of other device
EXCLUDES 1 *malfunction or other complications of device - see Alphabetical Index*
EXCLUDES 2 *encounter for fitting and management of implanted devices (Z45.-)*
issue of repeat prescription only (Z76.0)
presence of prosthetic and other devices (Z95-Z97)

Z46.0 **Encounter for fitting and adjustment of spectacles and contact lenses**

Z46.1 **Encounter for fitting and adjustment of hearing aid**
EXCLUDES 1 *encounter for adjustment and management of implanted hearing device (Z45.32-)*

Z46.2 **Encounter for fitting and adjustment of other devices related to nervous system and special senses**
EXCLUDES 2 *encounter for adjustment and management of implanted nervous system device (Z45.4-)*
encounter for adjustment and management of implanted visual substitution device (Z45.31)

Z46.3 **Encounter for fitting and adjustment of dental prosthetic device**
Encounter for fitting and adjustment of dentures

Z46.4 **Encounter for fitting and adjustment of orthodontic device**

✓5ᵗʰ **Z46.5** **Encounter for fitting and adjustment of other gastrointestinal appliance and device**
EXCLUDES 1 *encounter for attention to artificial openings of digestive tract (Z43.1-Z43.4)*

     Z46.51 **Encounter for fitting and adjustment of gastric lap band**

     Z46.59 **Encounter for fitting and adjustment of other gastrointestinal appliance and device**

Z46.6 **Encounter for fitting and adjustment of urinary device**
EXCLUDES 2 *attention to artificial openings of urinary tract (Z43.5, Z43.6)*

✓5ᵗʰ **Z46.8** **Encounter for fitting and adjustment of other specified devices**

     Z46.81 **Encounter for fitting and adjustment of insulin pump**
Encounter for insulin pump instruction and training
Encounter for insulin pump titration

     Z46.82 **Encounter for fitting and adjustment of non-vascular catheter**

     Z46.89 **Encounter for fitting and adjustment of other specified devices**
Encounter for fitting and adjustment of wheelchair

Z46.9 **Encounter for fitting and adjustment of unspecified device** ▽

✓4ᵗʰ **Z47** **Orthopedic aftercare**
EXCLUDES 1 *aftercare for healing fracture - code to fracture with 7th character D*

Z47.1 **Aftercare following joint replacement surgery**
Use additional code to identify the joint (Z96.6-)

Z47.2 **Encounter for removal of internal fixation device**
EXCLUDES 1 *encounter for adjustment of internal fixation device for fracture treatment - code to fracture with appropriate 7th character*
encounter for removal of external fixation device - code to fracture with 7th character D
infection or inflammatory reaction to internal fixation device (T84.6-)
mechanical complication of internal fixation device (T84.1-)

✓5ᵗʰ **Z47.3** **Aftercare following explantation of joint prosthesis**
Aftercare following explantation of joint prosthesis, staged procedure
Encounter for joint prosthesis insertion following prior explantation of joint prosthesis
AHA: 2015,1Q,16

Z47.31 **Aftercare following explantation of** shoulder **joint prosthesis**
> EXCLUDES 1 *acquired absence of shoulder joint following prior explantation of shoulder joint prosthesis (Z89.23-)*
> *shoulder joint prosthesis explantation status (Z89.23-)*

Z47.32 **Aftercare following explantation of** hip **joint prosthesis**
> EXCLUDES 1 *acquired absence of hip joint following prior explantation of hip joint prosthesis (Z89.62-)*
> *hip joint prosthesis explantation status (Z89.62-)*

Z47.33 **Aftercare following explantation of** knee **joint prosthesis**
> EXCLUDES 1 *acquired absence of knee joint following prior explantation of knee prosthesis (Z89.52-)*
> *knee joint prosthesis explantation status (Z89.52-)*

√5ᵗʰ **Z47.8** **Encounter for other orthopedic aftercare**

Z47.81 **Encounter for orthopedic aftercare** following **surgical amputation**
> Use additional code to identify the limb amputated (Z89.-)

Z47.82 **Encounter for orthopedic aftercare** following **scoliosis surgery**

Z47.89 **Encounter for other orthopedic aftercare**
> AHA: 2015,1Q,8

√4ᵗʰ **Z48** **Encounter for other postprocedural aftercare**
> EXCLUDES 1 *encounter for follow-up examination after completed treatment (Z08-Z09)*
> EXCLUDES 2 *encounter for attention to artificial openings (Z43.-)*
> *encounter for fitting and adjustment of prosthetic and other devices (Z44-Z46)*
> AHA: 2015,4Q,38; 2015,1Q,6-7

√5ᵗʰ **Z48.0** **Encounter for** attention to dressings, sutures and drains
> EXCLUDES 1 *encounter for planned postprocedural wound closure (Z48.1)*

Z48.00 **Encounter for change or removal of** nonsurgical **wound dressing**
> Encounter for change or removal of wound dressing NOS

Z48.01 **Encounter for change or removal of** surgical **wound dressing**

Z48.02 **Encounter for removal of** sutures
> Encounter for removal of staples

Z48.03 **Encounter for change or removal of** drains

Z48.1 **Encounter for planned** postprocedural **wound closure**
> EXCLUDES 1 *encounter for attention to dressings and sutures (Z48.0-)*

√5ᵗʰ **Z48.2** **Encounter for aftercare following** organ transplant

Z48.21 **Encounter for aftercare following** heart **transplant**

Z48.22 **Encounter for aftercare following** kidney **transplant**

Z48.23 **Encounter for aftercare following** liver **transplant**

Z48.24 **Encounter for aftercare following** lung **transplant**

√6ᵗʰ **Z48.28** **Encounter for aftercare following** multiple **organ transplant**

Z48.280 **Encounter for aftercare following heart-lung transplant**

Z48.288 **Encounter for aftercare following** multiple **organ transplant**

√6ᵗʰ **Z48.29** **Encounter for aftercare following other organ transplant**

Z48.290 **Encounter for aftercare following** bone **marrow transplant**

Z48.298 **Encounter for aftercare following other organ transplant**

Z48.3 **Aftercare following** surgery for neoplasm
> Use additional code to identify the neoplasm

√5ᵗʰ **Z48.8** **Encounter for other specified postprocedural aftercare**

√6ᵗʰ **Z48.81** **Encounter for surgical aftercare following** surgery **on specified body systems**
> **NOTE** These codes identify the body system requiring aftercare. They are for use in conjunction with other aftercare codes to fully explain the aftercare encounter. The condition treated should also be coded if still present.
> EXCLUDES 1 *aftercare for injury- code the injury with 7th character D*
> *aftercare following surgery for neoplasm (Z48.3)*
> EXCLUDES 2 *aftercare following organ transplant (Z48.2-)*
> *orthopedic aftercare (Z47.-)*
> AHA: 2015,4Q,38

Z48.810 **Encounter for surgical aftercare following surgery on the** sense organs

Z48.811 **Encounter for surgical aftercare following surgery on the** nervous system
> EXCLUDES 2 *encounter for surgical aftercare following surgery on the sense organs (Z48.810)*

Z48.812 **Encounter for surgical aftercare following surgery on the** circulatory system
> AHA: 2012,4Q,96

Z48.813 **Encounter for surgical aftercare following surgery on the** respiratory system

Z48.814 **Encounter for surgical aftercare following surgery on the** teeth or oral cavity

Z48.815 **Encounter for surgical aftercare following surgery on the** digestive system

Z48.816 **Encounter for surgical aftercare following surgery on the** genitourinary system
> EXCLUDES 1 *encounter for aftercare following sterilization reversal (Z31.42)*

Z48.817 **Encounter for surgical aftercare following surgery on the** skin and subcutaneous tissue

Z48.89 **Encounter for other specified surgical aftercare**

√4ᵗʰ **Z49** **Encounter for care involving renal dialysis**
> Code also associated end stage renal disease (N18.6)

√5ᵗʰ **Z49.0** **Preparatory care for renal dialysis**
> Encounter for dialysis instruction and training

Z49.01 **Encounter for fitting and adjustment of extracorporeal dialysis catheter**
> Removal or replacement of renal dialysis catheter
> Toilet or cleansing of renal dialysis catheter

Z49.02 **Encounter for fitting and adjustment of** peritoneal **dialysis catheter**

√5ᵗʰ **Z49.3** **Encounter for** adequacy testing for dialysis

Z49.31 **Encounter for adequacy testing for** hemodialysis

Z49.32 **Encounter for adequacy testing for** peritoneal **dialysis**
> Encounter for peritoneal equilibration test

▲√4ᵗʰ **Z51** **Encounter for other aftercare and medical care**
> Code also condition requiring care
> EXCLUDES 1 *follow-up examination after treatment (Z08-Z09)*

Z51.0 **Encounter for antineoplastic** radiation therapy   PDx

√5ᵗʰ **Z51.1** **Encounter for antineoplastic chemotherapy and immunotherapy**
> EXCLUDES 2 *encounter for chemotherapy and immunotherapy for nonneoplastic condition - code to condition*

Z51.11 **Encounter for antineoplastic chemotherapy**   PDx
> AHA: 2015,3Q,19

Z51.12 **Encounter for antineoplastic immunotherapy**   PDx

Z51.5 **Encounter for** palliative care

Z51.6 **Encounter for** desensitization to allergens

√5ᵗʰ **Z51.8** **Encounter for other specified aftercare**
> EXCLUDES 1 *holiday relief care (Z75.5)*

Z51.81   **Encounter for** therapeutic drug level **monitoring**
Code also any long-term (current) drug therapy (Z79.-)
   EXCLUDES 1   *encounter for blood-drug test for administrative or medicolegal reasons (Z02.83)*
   DEF: Drug monitoring: Measurement of the level of a specific drug in the body or measurement of a specific function to assess effectiveness of a drug.

Z51.89   **Encounter for other specified aftercare**
AHA: 2012,4Q,95-97

✓4ᵗʰ Z52   Donors of organs and tissues
   INCLUDES   autologous and other living donors
   EXCLUDES 1   *cadaveric donor - omit code*
     examination of potential donor (Z00.5)
   AHA: 2012,4Q,99

   ✓5ᵗʰ Z52.0   Blood donor
     ✓6ᵗʰ Z52.00   Unspecified blood donor
       Z52.000   Unspecified donor, whole blood   PDx ▽
       Z52.001   Unspecified donor, stem cells   PDx ▽
       Z52.008   Unspecified donor, other blood   PDx ▽
     ✓6ᵗʰ Z52.01   Autologous blood donor
       Z52.010   Autologous donor, whole blood   PDx
       Z52.011   Autologous donor, stem cells   PDx
       Z52.018   Autologous donor, other blood   PDx
     ✓6ᵗʰ Z52.09   Other blood donor
       Volunteer donor
       Z52.090   Other blood donor, whole blood   PDx
       Z52.091   Other blood donor, stem cells   PDx
       Z52.098   Other blood donor, other blood   PDx

   ✓5ᵗʰ Z52.1   Skin donor
     Z52.10   Skin donor, unspecified   PDx ▽
     Z52.11   Skin donor, autologous   PDx
     Z52.19   Skin donor, other   PDx

   ✓5ᵗʰ Z52.2   Bone donor
     Z52.20   Bone donor, unspecified   PDx ▽
     Z52.21   Bone donor, autologous   PDx
     Z52.29   Bone donor, other   PDx

   Z52.3   Bone marrow donor   PDx
   Z52.4   Kidney donor   PDx
   Z52.5   Cornea donor   PDx
   Z52.6   Liver donor   PDx

   ✓5ᵗʰ Z52.8   Donor of other specified organs or tissues
     ✓6ᵗʰ Z52.81   Egg (Oocyte) donor
       Z52.810   Egg (Oocyte) donor under age 35, anonymous **recipient**   PDx ♀
         Egg donor under age 35 NOS
       Z52.811   Egg (Oocyte) donor under age 35, designated **recipient**   PDx ♀
       Z52.812   Egg (Oocyte) donor age 35 and over, anonymous **recipient**   PDx ♀
         Egg donor age 35 and over NOS
       Z52.813   Egg (Oocyte) donor age 35 and over, designated **recipient**   PDx ♀
       Z52.819   Egg (Oocyte) donor, unspecified   PDx ♀ ▽
     Z52.89   Donor of other specified organs or tissues   PDx

   Z52.9   Donor of unspecified organ or tissue   ▽
     Donor NOS

✓4ᵗʰ Z53   Persons encountering health services for specific procedures and treatment, not carried out
   ✓5ᵗʰ Z53.0   Procedure and treatment not carried out because of contraindication
     Z53.01   Procedure and treatment not carried out due to patient smoking
     Z53.09   Procedure and treatment not carried out because of other contraindication
   Z53.1   Procedure and treatment not carried out because of patient's decision for reasons of belief and group pressure
   ✓5ᵗʰ Z53.2   Procedure and treatment not carried out because of patient's decision for other and unspecified reasons
     Z53.20   Procedure and treatment not carried out because of patient's decision for unspecified reasons   ▽

     Z53.21   Procedure and treatment not carried out due to patient leaving prior to being seen by health care provider
     Z53.29   Procedure and treatment not carried out because of patient's decision for other reasons
●   **Z53.3   Procedure converted to open procedure**
●   **Z53.31   Laparoscopic surgical procedure converted to open procedure**
●   **Z53.32   Thoracoscopic surgical procedure converted to open procedure**
●   **Z53.33   Arthroscopic surgical procedure converted to open procedure**
●   **Z53.39   Other specified procedure converted to open procedure**
   Z53.8   Procedure and treatment not carried out for other reasons
   Z53.9   Procedure and treatment not carried out, unspecified reason   ▽

Persons with potential health hazards related to socioeconomic and psychosocial circumstances (Z55-Z65)

✓4ᵗʰ Z55   Problems related to education and literacy
   EXCLUDES 1   *disorders of psychological development (F80-F89)*
   Z55.0   Illiteracy and low-level literacy
   Z55.1   Schooling unavailable and unattainable
   Z55.2   Failed school examinations
   Z55.3   Underachievement in school
   Z55.4   Educational maladjustment and discord with teachers and classmates
   Z55.8   Other problems related to education and literacy
     Problems related to inadequate teaching
   Z55.9   Problems related to education and literacy, unspecified   ▽
     Academic problems NOS

✓4ᵗʰ Z56   Problems related to employment and unemployment
   EXCLUDES 2   *occupational exposure to risk factors (Z57.-)*
     problems related to housing and economic circumstances (Z59.-)
   Z56.0   Unemployment, unspecified   ▽
   Z56.1   Change of job   A
   Z56.2   Threat of job loss
   Z56.3   Stressful work schedule
   Z56.4   Discord with boss and workmates
   Z56.5   Uncongenial work environment
     Difficult conditions at work
   Z56.6   Other physical and mental strain related to work
   ✓5ᵗʰ Z56.8   Other problems related to employment
     Z56.81   Sexual harassment on the job
     Z56.82   Military deployment status
       Individual (civilian or military) currently deployed in theater or in support of military war, peacekeeping and humanitarian operations
     Z56.89   Other problems related to employment
   Z56.9   Unspecified problems related to employment   ▽
     Occupational problems NOS

✓4ᵗʰ Z57   Occupational exposure to risk factors
   Z57.0   Occupational exposure to noise
   Z57.1   Occupational exposure to radiation
   Z57.2   Occupational exposure to dust
   ✓5ᵗʰ Z57.3   Occupational exposure to other air contaminants
     Z57.31   Occupational exposure to environmental tobacco smoke
       EXCLUDES 2   *exposure to environmental tobacco smoke (Z77.22)*
     Z57.39   Occupational exposure to other air contaminants
   Z57.4   Occupational exposure to toxic agents in agriculture
     Occupational exposure to solids, liquids, gases or vapors in agriculture
   Z57.5   Occupational exposure to toxic agents in other industries
     Occupational exposure to solids, liquids, gases or vapors in other industries
   Z57.6   Occupational exposure to extreme temperature
   Z57.7   Occupational exposure to vibration
   Z57.8   Occupational exposure to other risk factors
   Z57.9   Occupational exposure to unspecified risk factor   ▽

✔ Additional Character Required   ✓x7ᵗʰ Placeholder Alert   **Manifestation Dx**   ▽ Unspecified Dx   ▶◀ Revised Text   ● New Code   ▲ Revised Code Title

Chapter 21. Factors Influencing Health Status and Contact With Health Services

Z59–Z64.0

✓4ᵗʰ **Z59 Problems related to housing and economic circumstances**
    EXCLUDES 2 *problems related to upbringing (Z62.-)*

Z59.0 Homelessness

Z59.1 Inadequate housing
    Lack of heating
    Restriction of space
    Technical defects in home preventing adequate care
    Unsatisfactory surroundings
    EXCLUDES 1 *problems related to the natural and physical environment (Z77.1-)*

Z59.2 Discord with neighbors, lodgers and landlord

Z59.3 Problems related to living in residential institution
    Boarding-school resident
    EXCLUDES 1 *institutional upbringing (Z62.2)*

Z59.4 Lack of adequate food and safe drinking water
    Inadequate drinking water supply
    EXCLUDES 1 *effects of hunger (T73.0)*
        inappropriate diet or eating habits (Z72.4)
        malnutrition (E40-E46)

Z59.5 Extreme poverty

Z59.6 Low income

Z59.7 Insufficient social insurance and welfare support

Z59.8 Other problems related to housing and economic circumstances
    Foreclosure on loan
    Isolated dwelling
    Problems with creditors

Z59.9 Problem related to housing and economic circumstances, unspecified ▽

✓4ᵗʰ **Z60 Problems related to social environment**

Z60.0 Problems of adjustment to life-cycle transitions
    Empty nest syndrome
    Phase of life problem
    Problem with adjustment to retirement [pension]

Z60.2 Problems related to living alone

Z60.3 Acculturation difficulty
    Problem with migration
    Problem with social transplantation

Z60.4 Social exclusion and rejection
    Exclusion and rejection on the basis of personal characteristics, such as unusual physical appearance, illness or behavior.
    EXCLUDES 1 *target of adverse discrimination such as for racial or religious reasons (Z60.5)*

Z60.5 Target of (perceived) adverse discrimination and persecution
    EXCLUDES 1 *social exclusion and rejection (Z60.4)*

Z60.8 Other problems related to social environment

Z60.9 Problem related to social environment, unspecified ▽

✓4ᵗʰ **Z62 Problems related to upbringing**
    INCLUDES current and past negative life events in childhood
        current and past problems of a child related to upbringing
    EXCLUDES 2 *maltreatment syndrome (T74.-)*
        problems related to housing and economic circumstances (Z59.-)

Z62.0 Inadequate parental supervision and control

Z62.1 Parental overprotection

✓5ᵗʰ **Z62.2 Upbringing away from parents**
    EXCLUDES 1 *problems with boarding school (Z59.3)*

    Z62.21 Child in welfare custody Ⓟ
        Child in care of non-parental family member
        Child in foster care
        EXCLUDES 2 *problem for parent due to child in welfare custody (Z63.5)*

    Z62.22 Institutional upbringing
        Child living in orphanage or group home

    Z62.29 Other upbringing away from parents

Z62.3 Hostility towards and scapegoating of child Ⓟ

Z62.6 Inappropriate (excessive) parental pressure

✓5ᵗʰ **Z62.8 Other specified problems related to upbringing**

    ✓6ᵗʰ **Z62.81 Personal history of abuse in childhood**

        Z62.810 Personal history of physical and sexual abuse in childhood
            EXCLUDES 1 *current child physical abuse (T74.12, T76.12)*
                current child sexual abuse (T74.22, T76.22)

        Z62.811 Personal history of psychological abuse in childhood
            EXCLUDES 1 *current child psychological abuse (T74.32, T76.32)*

        Z62.812 Personal history of neglect in childhood
            EXCLUDES 1 *current child neglect (T74.02, T76.02)*

        Z62.819 Personal history of unspecified abuse in childhood ▽
            EXCLUDES 1 *current child abuse NOS (T74.92, T76.92)*

    ✓6ᵗʰ **Z62.82 Parent-child conflict**

        Z62.820 Parent-biological child conflict
            Parent-child problem NOS

        Z62.821 Parent-adopted child conflict

        Z62.822 Parent-foster child conflict

    ✓6ᵗʰ **Z62.89 Other specified problems related to upbringing**

        Z62.890 Parent-child estrangement NEC

        Z62.891 Sibling rivalry

        Z62.898 Other specified problems related to upbringing

Z62.9 Problem related to upbringing, unspecified ▽

✓4ᵗʰ **Z63 Other problems related to primary support group, including family circumstances**
    EXCLUDES 2 *maltreatment syndrome (T74.-, T76)*
        parent-child problems (Z62.-)
        problems related to negative life events in childhood (Z62.-)
        problems related to upbringing (Z62.-)

Z63.0 Problems in relationship with spouse or partner
    EXCLUDES 1 *counseling for spousal or partner abuse problems (Z69.1)*
        counseling related to sexual attitude, behavior, and orientation (Z70.-)

Z63.1 Problems in relationship with in-laws

✓5ᵗʰ **Z63.3 Absence of family member**
    EXCLUDES 1 *absence of family member due to disappearance and death (Z63.4)*
        absence of family member due to separation and divorce (Z63.5)

    Z63.31 Absence of family member due to military deployment
        Individual or family affected by other family member being on military deployment
        EXCLUDES 1 *family disruption due to return of family member from military deployment (Z63.71)*

    Z63.32 Other absence of family member

Z63.4 Disappearance and death of family member
    Assumed death of family member
    Bereavement
    AHA: 2014,1Q,25

Z63.5 Disruption of family by separation and divorce
    Marital estrangement

Z63.6 Dependent relative needing care at home

✓5ᵗʰ **Z63.7 Other stressful life events affecting family and household**

    Z63.71 Stress on family due to return of family member from military deployment
        Individual or family affected by family member having returned from military deployment (current or past conflict)

    Z63.72 Alcoholism and drug addiction in family

    Z63.79 Other stressful life events affecting family and household
        Anxiety (normal) about sick person in family
        Health problems within family
        Ill or disturbed family member
        Isolated family

Z63.8 Other specified problems related to primary support group
    Family discord NOS
    Family estrangement NOS
    High expressed emotional level within family
    Inadequate family support NOS
    Inadequate or distorted communication within family

Z63.9 Problem related to primary support group, unspecified ▽
    Relationship disorder NOS

✓4ᵗʰ **Z64 Problems related to certain psychosocial circumstances**

Z64.0 Problems related to unwanted pregnancy

Z64.1 Problems related to multiparity

Z64.4 Discord with counselors
Discord with probation officer
Discord with social worker

☑4ᵗʰ **Z65 Problems related to other psychosocial circumstances**

Z65.0 Conviction in civil and criminal proceedings without imprisonment

Z65.1 Imprisonment and other incarceration

Z65.2 Problems related to release from prison

Z65.3 Problems related to other legal circumstances
Arrest
Child custody or support proceedings
Litigation
Prosecution

Z65.4 Victim of crime and terrorism
Victim of torture

Z65.5 Exposure to disaster, war and other hostilities
EXCLUDES 1 target of perceived discrimination or persecution (Z60.5)

Z65.8 Other specified problems related to psychosocial circumstances

Z65.9 Problem related to unspecified psychosocial circumstances   ▽

Do not resuscitate status (Z66)

Z66 Do not resuscitate
DNR status

Blood type (Z67)

☑4ᵗʰ **Z67 Blood type**
AHA: 2015,3Q,40

☑5ᵗʰ **Z67.1 Type A blood**
Z67.10   Type A blood, Rh positive
Z67.11   Type A blood, Rh negative

☑5ᵗʰ **Z67.2 Type B blood**
Z67.20   Type B blood, Rh positive
Z67.21   Type B blood, Rh negative

☑5ᵗʰ **Z67.3 Type AB blood**
Z67.30   Type AB blood, Rh positive
Z67.31   Type AB blood, Rh negative

☑5ᵗʰ **Z67.4 Type O blood**
Z67.40   Type O blood, Rh positive
Z67.41   Type O blood, Rh negative

☑5ᵗʰ **Z67.9 Unspecified blood type**
Z67.90   Unspecified blood type, Rh positive   ▽
Z67.91   Unspecified blood type, Rh negative   ▽

Blood Types

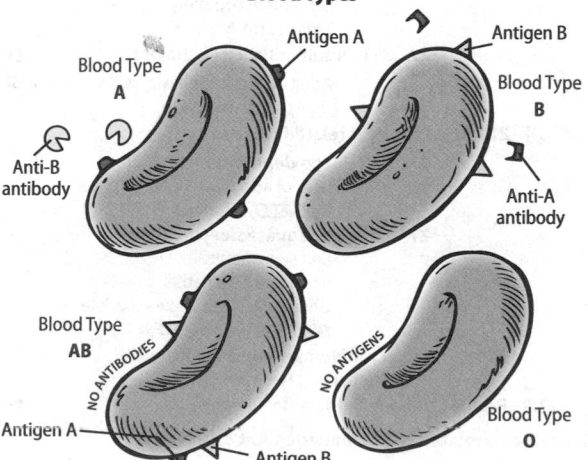

Blood Type A — Antigen A — Anti-B antibody
Blood Type B — Antigen B — Anti-A antibody
Blood Type AB — NO ANTIBODIES — Antigen A — Antigen B
Blood Type O — NO ANTIGENS

Body mass index [BMI] (Z68)

☑4ᵗʰ **Z68 Body mass index [BMI]**
Kilograms per meters squared

NOTE   BMI adult codes are for use for persons 21 years of age or older

BMI pediatric codes are for use for persons 2-20 years of age. These percentiles are based on the growth charts published by the Centers for Disease Control and Prevention (CDC)

Z68.1 Body mass index [BMI] 19 or less, adult   Ⓐ

☑5ᵗʰ **Z68.2 Body mass index [BMI] 20-29, adult**
Z68.20   Body mass index [BMI] 20.0-20.9, adult   Ⓐ
Z68.21   Body mass index [BMI] 21.0-21.9, adult   Ⓐ
Z68.22   Body mass index [BMI] 22.0-22.9, adult   Ⓐ
Z68.23   Body mass index [BMI] 23.0-23.9, adult   Ⓐ
Z68.24   Body mass index [BMI] 24.0-24.9, adult   Ⓐ
Z68.25   Body mass index [BMI] 25.0-25.9, adult   Ⓐ
Z68.26   Body mass index [BMI] 26.0-26.9, adult   Ⓐ
Z68.27   Body mass index [BMI] 27.0-27.9, adult   Ⓐ
Z68.28   Body mass index [BMI] 28.0-28.9, adult   Ⓐ
Z68.29   Body mass index [BMI] 29.0-29.9, adult   Ⓐ

☑5ᵗʰ **Z68.3 Body mass index [BMI] 30-39, adult**
Z68.30   Body mass index [BMI] 30.0-30.9, adult   Ⓐ
Z68.31   Body mass index [BMI] 31.0-31.9, adult   Ⓐ
Z68.32   Body mass index [BMI] 32.0-32.9, adult   Ⓐ
Z68.33   Body mass index [BMI] 33.0-33.9, adult   Ⓐ
Z68.34   Body mass index [BMI] 34.0-34.9, adult   Ⓐ
Z68.35   Body mass index [BMI] 35.0-35.9, adult   Ⓐ
Z68.36   Body mass index [BMI] 36.0-36.9, adult   Ⓐ
Z68.37   Body mass index [BMI] 37.0-37.9, adult   Ⓐ
Z68.38   Body mass index [BMI] 38.0-38.9, adult   Ⓐ
Z68.39   Body mass index [BMI] 39.0-39.9, adult   Ⓐ

☑5ᵗʰ **Z68.4 Body mass index [BMI] 40 or greater, adult**
Z68.41   Body mass index [BMI] 40.0-44.9, adult   Ⓐ
Z68.42   Body mass index [BMI] 45.0-49.9, adult   Ⓐ
Z68.43   Body mass index [BMI] 50-59.9, adult   Ⓐ
Z68.44   Body mass index [BMI] 60.0-69.9, adult   Ⓐ
Z68.45   Body mass index [BMI] 70 or greater, adult   Ⓐ

☑5ᵗʰ **Z68.5 Body mass index [BMI] pediatric**
Z68.51   Body mass index [BMI] pediatric, less than 5th percentile for age
Z68.52   Body mass index [BMI] pediatric, 5th percentile to less than 85th percentile for age
Z68.53   Body mass index [BMI] pediatric, 85th percentile to less than 95th percentile for age
Z68.54   Body mass index [BMI] pediatric, greater than or equal to 95th percentile for age

Persons encountering health services in other circumstances (Z69-Z76)

☑4ᵗʰ **Z69 Encounter for mental health services for victim and perpetrator of abuse**
INCLUDES counseling for victims and perpetrators of abuse

☑5ᵗʰ **Z69.0 Encounter for mental health services for child abuse problems**

☑6ᵗʰ **Z69.01   Encounter for mental health services for parental child abuse**
Z69.010   Encounter for mental health services for victim of parental child abuse   Ⓟ
Z69.011   Encounter for mental health services for perpetrator of parental child abuse
EXCLUDES 1 encounter for mental health services for non-parental child abuse (Z69.02-)

☑6ᵗʰ **Z69.02   Encounter for mental health services for non-parental child abuse**
Z69.020   Encounter for mental health services for victim of non-parental child abuse   Ⓟ

         Z69.021   **Encounter for mental health services for perpetrator of non-parental child abuse**

✓5ᵗʰ **Z69.1**   **Encounter for mental health services for spousal or partner abuse problems**

         Z69.11   **Encounter for mental health services for victim of spousal or partner abuse**

         Z69.12   **Encounter for mental health services for perpetrator of spousal or partner abuse**

✓5ᵗʰ **Z69.8**   **Encounter for mental health services for victim or perpetrator of other abuse**

         Z69.81   **Encounter for mental health services for victim of other abuse**
                Encounter for rape victim counseling

         Z69.82   **Encounter for mental health services for perpetrator of other abuse**

✓4ᵗʰ **Z70**   **Counseling related to sexual attitude, behavior and orientation**

     INCLUDES   encounter for mental health services for sexual attitude, behavior and orientation

     EXCLUDES 2   *contraceptive or procreative counseling (Z30-Z31)*

     Z70.0   **Counseling related to sexual attitude**

     Z70.1   **Counseling related to patient's sexual behavior and orientation**
         Patient concerned regarding impotence
         Patient concerned regarding non-responsiveness
         Patient concerned regarding promiscuity
         Patient concerned regarding sexual orientation

     Z70.2   **Counseling related to sexual behavior and orientation of third party**
         Advice sought regarding sexual behavior and orientation of child
         Advice sought regarding sexual behavior and orientation of partner
         Advice sought regarding sexual behavior and orientation of spouse

     Z70.3   **Counseling related to combined concerns regarding sexual attitude, behavior and orientation**

     Z70.8   **Other sex counseling**
         Encounter for sex education

     Z70.9   **Sex counseling, unspecified**   ▽

✓4ᵗʰ **Z71**   **Persons encountering health services for other counseling and medical advice, not elsewhere classified**

     EXCLUDES 2   *contraceptive or procreation counseling (Z30-Z31)*
               sex counseling (Z70.-)

     Z71.0   **Person encountering health services to consult on behalf of another person**
         Person encountering health services to seek advice or treatment for non-attending third party
         EXCLUDES 2   *anxiety (normal) about sick person in family (Z63.7)*
                expectant (adoptive) parent(s) pre-birth pediatrician visit (Z76.81)

     Z71.1   **Person with feared health complaint in whom no diagnosis is made**
         Person encountering health services with feared condition which was not demonstrated
         Person encountering health services in which problem was normal state
         "Worried well"
         EXCLUDES 1   *medical observation for suspected diseases and conditions proven not to exist (Z03.-)*

     Z71.2   **Person consulting for explanation of examination or test findings**

     Z71.3   **Dietary counseling and surveillance**
         Use additional code for any associated underlying medical condition
         Use additional code to identify body mass index (BMI), if known (Z68.-)

✓5ᵗʰ **Z71.4**   **Alcohol abuse counseling and surveillance**
         Use additional code for alcohol abuse or dependence (F10.-)

         Z71.41   **Alcohol abuse counseling and surveillance of alcoholic**

         Z71.42   **Counseling for family member of alcoholic**
                Counseling for significant other, partner, or friend of alcoholic

✓5ᵗʰ **Z71.5**   **Drug abuse counseling and surveillance**
         Use additional code for drug abuse or dependence (F11-F16, F18-F19)

         Z71.51   **Drug abuse counseling and surveillance of drug abuser**

         Z71.52   **Counseling for family member of drug abuser**
                Counseling for significant other, partner, or friend of drug abuser

     Z71.6   **Tobacco abuse counseling**
         Use additional code for nicotine dependence (F17.-)

     Z71.7   **Human immunodeficiency virus [HIV] counseling**

✓5ᵗʰ **Z71.8**   **Other specified counseling**
         EXCLUDES 2   *counseling for contraception (Z30.0-)*
                counseling for genetics (Z31.5)
                counseling for procreative management (Z31.6-)

         Z71.81   **Spiritual or religious counseling**

         Z71.89   **Other specified counseling**

     Z71.9   **Counseling, unspecified**   ▽
         Encounter for medical advice NOS

✓4ᵗʰ **Z72**   **Problems related to lifestyle**

     EXCLUDES 2   *problems related to life-management difficulty (Z73.-)*
               problems related to socioeconomic and psychosocial circumstances (Z55-Z65)

     Z72.0   **Tobacco use**
         Tobacco use NOS
         EXCLUDES 1   *history of tobacco dependence (Z87.891)*
                nicotine dependence (F17.2-)
                tobacco dependence (F17.2-)
                tobacco use during pregnancy (O99.33-)

     Z72.3   **Lack of physical exercise**

     Z72.4   **Inappropriate diet and eating habits**
         EXCLUDES 1   *behavioral eating disorders of infancy or childhood (F98.2-F98.3)*
                eating disorders (F50.-)
                lack of adequate food (Z59.4)
                malnutrition and other nutritional deficiencies (E40-E64)

✓5ᵗʰ **Z72.5**   **High risk sexual behavior**
         Promiscuity
         EXCLUDES 1   *paraphilias (F65)*

         Z72.51   **High risk heterosexual behavior**
         Z72.52   **High risk homosexual behavior**
         Z72.53   **High risk bisexual behavior**

     Z72.6   **Gambling and betting**
         EXCLUDES 1   *compulsive or pathological gambling (F63.0)*

✓5ᵗʰ **Z72.8**   **Other problems related to lifestyle**

     ✓6ᵗʰ **Z72.81**   **Antisocial behavior**
         EXCLUDES 1   *conduct disorders (F91.-)*

         Z72.810   **Child and adolescent antisocial behavior**   P
                Antisocial behavior (child) (adolescent) without manifest psychiatric disorder
                Delinquency NOS
                Group delinquency
                Offenses in the context of gang membership
                Stealing in company with others
                Truancy from school

         Z72.811   **Adult antisocial behavior**   A
                Adult antisocial behavior without manifest psychiatric disorder

     ✓6ᵗʰ **Z72.82**   **Problems related to sleep**

         Z72.820   **Sleep deprivation**
                Lack of adequate sleep
                EXCLUDES 1   *insomnia (G47.0-)*

         Z72.821   **Inadequate sleep hygiene**
                Bad sleep habits
                Irregular sleep habits
                Unhealthy sleep wake schedule
                EXCLUDES 1   *insomnia (F51.0-, G47.0-)*

         Z72.89   **Other problems related to lifestyle**
                Self-damaging behavior

     Z72.9   **Problem related to lifestyle, unspecified**   ▽

✓4ᵗʰ **Z73**   **Problems related to life management difficulty**

     EXCLUDES 2   *problems related to socioeconomic and psychosocial circumstances (Z55-Z65)*

     Z73.0   **Burn-out**

     Z73.1   **Type A behavior pattern**

     Z73.2   **Lack of relaxation and leisure**

EXCLUDES 1 Not coded here   EXCLUDES 2 Not included here   PDx Primary Dx Only   N Newborn Age : 0   P Pediatric Age : 0-17   M Maternity Age : 12-55   A Adult Age : 15-124

1160   ICD-10-CM 2017

Z73.3   **Stress, not elsewhere classified**
Physical and mental strain NOS
EXCLUDES 1   *stress related to employment or unemployment (Z56.-)*

Z73.4   **Inadequate social skills, not elsewhere classified**

Z73.5   **Social role conflict, not elsewhere classified**

Z73.6   **Limitation of activities due to disability**
EXCLUDES 1   *care-provider dependency (Z74.-)*

✓5ᵗʰ **Z73.8**   **Other problems related to life management difficulty**

    ✓6ᵗʰ **Z73.81**   **Behavioral insomnia of childhood**
      DEF: Behaviors on the part of the child or caregivers that cause negative compliance with a child's sleep schedule; results in lack of adequate sleep.

      Z73.810   **Behavioral insomnia of childhood, sleep-onset association type**   P

      Z73.811   **Behavioral insomnia of childhood, limit setting type**   P

      Z73.812   **Behavioral insomnia of childhood, combined type**   P

      Z73.819   **Behavioral insomnia of childhood, unspecified type**   P ▽

    Z73.82   **Dual sensory impairment**

    Z73.89   **Other problems related to life management difficulty**

Z73.9   **Problem related to life management difficulty, unspecified**   ▽

✓4ᵗʰ **Z74**   **Problems related to care provider dependency**
EXCLUDES 2   *dependence on enabling machines or devices NEC (Z99.-)*

   ✓5ᵗʰ **Z74.0**   **Reduced mobility**

    Z74.01   **Bed confinement status**
      Bedridden

    Z74.09   **Other reduced mobility**
      Chair ridden
      Reduced mobility NOS
      EXCLUDES 2   *wheelchair dependence (Z99.3)*

Z74.1   **Need for assistance with personal care**

Z74.2   **Need for assistance at home and no other household member able to render care**

Z74.3   **Need for continuous supervision**

Z74.8   **Other problems related to care provider dependency**

Z74.9   **Problem related to care provider dependency, unspecified**   ▽

✓4ᵗʰ **Z75**   **Problems related to medical facilities and other health care**

Z75.0   **Medical services not available in home**
EXCLUDES 1   *no other household member able to render care (Z74.2)*

Z75.1   **Person awaiting admission to adequate facility elsewhere**

Z75.2   **Other waiting period for investigation and treatment**

Z75.3   **Unavailability and inaccessibility of health-care facilities**
EXCLUDES 1   *bed unavailable (Z75.1)*

Z75.4   **Unavailability and inaccessibility of other helping agencies**

Z75.5   **Holiday relief care**

Z75.8   **Other problems related to medical facilities and other health care**

Z75.9   **Unspecified problem related to medical facilities and other health care**   ▽

✓4ᵗʰ **Z76**   **Persons encountering health services in other circumstances**

Z76.0   **Encounter for issue of repeat prescription**
Encounter for issue of repeat prescription for appliance
Encounter for issue of repeat prescription for medicaments
Encounter for issue of repeat prescription for spectacles
EXCLUDES 2   *issue of medical certificate (Z02.7)*
      repeat prescription for contraceptive (Z30.4-)

Z76.1   **Encounter for health supervision and care of foundling**   PDx

Z76.2   **Encounter for health supervision and care of other healthy infant and child**   PDx P
Encounter for medical or nursing care or supervision of healthy infant under circumstances such as adverse socioeconomic conditions at home
Encounter for medical or nursing care or supervision of healthy infant under circumstances such as awaiting foster or adoptive placement
Encounter for medical or nursing care or supervision of healthy infant under circumstances such as maternal illness
Encounter for medical or nursing care or supervision of healthy infant under circumstances such as number of children at home preventing or interfering with normal care

Z76.3   **Healthy person accompanying sick person**

Z76.4   **Other boarder to healthcare facility**
EXCLUDES 1   *homelessness (Z59.0)*

Z76.5   **Malingerer [conscious simulation]**
Person feigning illness (with obvious motivation)
EXCLUDES 1   *factitious disorder (F68.1-)*
      peregrinating patient (F68.1-)

✓5ᵗʰ **Z76.8**   **Persons encountering health services in other specified circumstances**

    Z76.81   **Expectant parent(s) prebirth pediatrician visit**
      Pre-adoption pediatrician visit for adoptive parent(s)

    Z76.82   **Awaiting organ transplant status**
      Patient waiting for organ availability

    Z76.89   **Persons encountering health services in other specified circumstances**
      Persons encountering health services NOS
      AHA: 2014,2Q,10

Persons with potential health hazards related to family and personal history and certain conditions influencing health status (Z77-Z99)

Code also any follow-up examination (Z08-Z09)

✓4ᵗʰ **Z77**   **Other contact with and (suspected) exposures hazardous to health**
INCLUDES   contact with and (suspected) exposures to potential hazards to health
EXCLUDES 2   *contact with and (suspected) exposure to communicable diseases (Z20.-)*
      exposure to (parental) (environmental) tobacco smoke in the perinatal period (P96.81)
      ▶*newborn affected by noxious substances transmitted via placenta or breast milk (P04.-)*◀
      occupational exposure to risk factors (Z57.-)
      retained foreign body (Z18.-)
      retained foreign body fully removed (Z87.821)
      toxic effects of substances chiefly nonmedicinal as to source (T51-T65)

✓5ᵗʰ **Z77.0**   **Contact with and (suspected) exposure to hazardous, chiefly nonmedicinal, chemicals**

   ✓6ᵗʰ **Z77.01**   **Contact with and (suspected) exposure to hazardous metals**

      Z77.010   **Contact with and (suspected) exposure to arsenic**

      Z77.011   **Contact with and (suspected) exposure to lead**

      Z77.012   **Contact with and (suspected) exposure to uranium**
        EXCLUDES 1   *retained depleted uranium fragments (Z18.01)*

      Z77.018   **Contact with and (suspected) exposure to other hazardous metals**
        Contact with and (suspected) exposure to chromium compounds
        Contact with and (suspected) exposure to nickel dust

   ✓6ᵗʰ **Z77.02**   **Contact with and (suspected) exposure to hazardous aromatic compounds**

      Z77.020   **Contact with and (suspected) exposure to aromatic amines**

      Z77.021   **Contact with and (suspected) exposure to benzene**

      Z77.028   **Contact with and (suspected) exposure to other hazardous aromatic compounds**
        Aromatic dyes NOS
        Polycyclic aromatic hydrocarbons

Chapter 21. Factors Influencing Health Status and Contact With Health Services

Z77.09–Z79.84

√6th **Z77.09** **Contact with and (suspected) exposure to other hazardous, chiefly nonmedicinal, chemicals**

Z77.090 **Contact with and (suspected) exposure to asbestos**

Z77.098 **Contact with and (suspected) exposure to other hazardous, chiefly nonmedicinal, chemicals**
Dyes NOS

√5th **Z77.1** **Contact with and (suspected) exposure to environmental pollution and hazards in the physical environment**

√6th **Z77.11** **Contact with and (suspected) exposure to environmental pollution**

Z77.110 **Contact with and (suspected) exposure to air pollution**

Z77.111 **Contact with and (suspected) exposure to water pollution**

Z77.112 **Contact with and (suspected) exposure to soil pollution**

Z77.118 **Contact with and (suspected) exposure to other environmental pollution**

√6th **Z77.12** **Contact with and (suspected) exposure to hazards in the physical environment**

Z77.120 **Contact with and (suspected) exposure to mold (toxic)**

Z77.121 **Contact with and (suspected) exposure to harmful algae and algae toxins**
Contact with and (suspected) exposure to (harmful) algae bloom NOS
Contact with and (suspected) exposure to blue-green algae bloom
Contact with and (suspected) exposure to brown tide
Contact with and (suspected) exposure to cyanobacteria bloom
Contact with and (suspected) exposure to Florida red tide
Contact with and (suspected) exposure to pfiesteria piscicida
Contact with and (suspected) exposure to red tide

Z77.122 **Contact with and (suspected) exposure to noise**

Z77.123 **Contact with and (suspected) exposure to radon and other naturally occuring radiation**
EXCLUDES 2 *radiation exposure as the cause of a confirmed condition (W88-W90, X39.0-)*
radiation sickness NOS (T66)

Z77.128 **Contact with and (suspected) exposure to other hazards in the physical environment**

√5th **Z77.2** **Contact with and (suspected) exposure to other hazardous substances**

Z77.21 **Contact with and (suspected) exposure to potentially hazardous body fluids**

Z77.22 **Contact with and (suspected) exposure to environmental tobacco smoke (acute) (chronic)**
Exposure to second hand tobacco smoke (acute) (chronic)
Passive smoking (acute) (chronic)
EXCLUDES 1 *nicotine dependence (F17.-)*
tobacco use (Z72.0)
EXCLUDES 2 *occupational exposure to environmental tobacco smoke (Z57.31)*

Z77.29 **Contact with and (suspected) exposure to other hazardous substances**
AHA: 2016,2Q,33

Z77.9 **Other contact with and (suspected) exposures hazardous to health**

√4th **Z78** **Other specified health status**
EXCLUDES 2 *asymptomatic human immunodeficiency virus [HIV] infection status (Z21)*
postprocedural status (Z93-Z99)
sex reassignment status (Z87.890)

Z78.0 **Asymptomatic menopausal state** A ♀
Menopausal state NOS
Postmenopausal status NOS
EXCLUDES 2 *symptomatic menopausal state (N95.1)*

Z78.1 **Physical restraint status**
EXCLUDES 1 *physical restraint due to a procedure - omit code*

Z78.9 **Other specified health status**

√4th **Z79** **Long term (current) drug therapy**
INCLUDES long term (current) drug use for prophylactic purposes
Code also any therapeutic drug level monitoring (Z51.81)
EXCLUDES 2 *drug abuse and dependence (F11-F19)*
drug use complicating pregnancy, childbirth, and the puerperium (O99.32-)
►*long term (current) use of oral antidiabetic drugs (Z79.84)*◄
►*long term (current) use of oral hypoglycemic drugs (Z79.84)*◄

√5th **Z79.0** **Long term (current) use of anticoagulants and antithrombotics/antiplatelets**
EXCLUDES 2 *long term (current) use of aspirin (Z79.82)*

Z79.01 **Long term (current) use of anticoagulants**

Z79.02 **Long term (current) use of antithrombotics/antiplatelets**

Z79.1 **Long term (current) use of non-steroidal anti-inflammatories (NSAID)**
EXCLUDES 2 *long term (current) use of aspirin (Z79.82)*

Z79.2 **Long term (current) use of antibiotics**

Z79.3 **Long term (current) use of hormonal contraceptives**
Long term (current) use of birth control pill or patch

Z79.4 **Long term (current) use of insulin**

√5th **Z79.5** **Long term (current) use of steroids**

Z79.51 **Long term (current) use of inhaled steroids**

Z79.52 **Long term (current) use of systemic steroids**

√5th **Z79.8** **Other long term (current) drug therapy**

√6th **Z79.81** **Long term (current) use of agents affecting estrogen receptors and estrogen levels**
Code first, if applicable:
malignant neoplasm of breast (C50.-)
malignant neoplasm of prostate (C61)
Use additional code, if applicable, to identify:
estrogen receptor positive status (Z17.0)
family history of breast cancer (Z80.3)
genetic susceptibility to malignant neoplasm (cancer) (Z15.0-)
personal history of breast cancer (Z85.3)
personal history of prostate cancer (Z85.46)
postmenopausal status (Z78.0)
EXCLUDES 1 *hormone replacement therapy (postmenopausal) (Z79.890)*

Z79.810 **Long term (current) use of selective estrogen receptor modulators (SERMs)**
Long term (current) use of raloxifene (Evista)
Long term (current) use of tamoxifen (Nolvadex)
Long term (current) use of toremifene (Fareston)

Z79.811 **Long term (current) use of aromatase inhibitors**
Long term (current) use of anastrozole (Arimidex)
Long term (current) use of exemestane (Aromasin)
Long term (current) use of letrozole (Femara)

Z79.818 **Long term (current) use of other agents affecting estrogen receptors and estrogen levels**
Long term (current) use of estrogen receptor downregulators
Long term (current) use of fulvestrant (Faslodex)
Long term (current) use of gonadotropin-releasing hormone (GnRH) agonist
Long term (current) use of goserelin acetate (Zoladex)
Long term (current) use of leuprolide acetate (leuprorelin) (Lupron)
Long term (current) use of megestrol acetate (Megace)

Z79.82 **Long term (current) use of aspirin**

Z79.83 **Long term (current) use of bisphosphonates**

Z79.84 **Long term (current) use of oral hypoglycemic drugs**
Long term (current) use of oral antidiabetic drugs
EXCLUDES 2 *long term (current) use of insulin (Z79.4)*

EXCLUDES 1 Not coded here   EXCLUDES 2 Not included here   PDx Primary Dx Only   N Newborn Age : 0   P Pediatric Age : 0-17   M Maternity Age : 12-55   A Adult Age : 15-124

1162

ICD-10-CM 2017

✓6ᵗʰ **Z79.89** **Other long term (current) drug therapy**

Z79.890 **Hormone replacement therapy (postmenopausal)**

Z79.891 **Long term (current) use of** opiate analgesic

Long term (current) use of methadone for pain management

EXCLUDES 1 methadone use NOS ▶(F11.9-)◀
use of methadone for treatment of heroin addiction (F11.2-)

Z79.899 **Other long term (current) drug therapy**
AHA: 2015,4Q,34; 2015,3Q,21

✓4ᵗʰ **Z80** **Family history of primary malignant neoplasm**

Z80.0 **Family history of malignant neoplasm of** digestive organs
Conditions classifiable to C15-C26

Z80.1 **Family history of malignant neoplasm of** trachea, bronchus and lung
Conditions classifiable to C33-C34

Z80.2 **Family history of malignant neoplasm of other** respiratory and intrathoracic organs
Conditions classifiable to C30-C32, C37-C39

Z80.3 **Family history of malignant neoplasm of** breast
Conditions classifiable to C50.-

✓5ᵗʰ **Z80.4** **Family history of malignant neoplasm of genital organs**
Conditions classifiable to C51-C63

Z80.41 **Family history of malignant neoplasm of** ovary
Z80.42 **Family history of malignant neoplasm of** prostate
Z80.43 **Family history of malignant neoplasm of** testis
Z80.49 **Family history of malignant neoplasm of other** genital organs

✓5ᵗʰ **Z80.5** **Family history of malignant neoplasm of urinary tract**
Conditions classifiable to C64-C68

Z80.51 **Family history of malignant neoplasm of** kidney
Z80.52 **Family history of malignant neoplasm of** bladder
Z80.59 **Family history of malignant neoplasm of other** urinary tract organ

Z80.6 **Family history of** leukemia
Conditions classifiable to C91-C95

Z80.7 **Family history of other malignant neoplasms of** lymphoid, hematopoietic and related tissues
Conditions classifiable to C81-C90, C96.-

Z80.8 **Family history of malignant neoplasm of other** organs or systems
Conditions classifiable to C00-C14, C40-C49, C69-C79

Z80.9 **Family history of malignant neoplasm, unspecified** ▽
Conditions classifiable to C80.1

✓4ᵗʰ **Z81** **Family history of mental and behavioral disorders**

Z81.0 **Family history of** intellectual disabilities
Conditions classifiable to F70-F79

Z81.1 **Family history of** alcohol abuse and dependence
Conditions classifiable to F10.-

Z81.2 **Family history of** tobacco abuse and dependence
Conditions classifiable to F17.-

Z81.3 **Family history of other** psychoactive substance abuse and dependence
Conditions classifiable to F11-F16, F18-F19

Z81.4 **Family history of other** substance abuse and dependence
Conditions classifiable to F55

Z81.8 **Family history of other** mental and behavioral disorders
Conditions classifiable elsewhere in F01-F99

✓4ᵗʰ **Z82** **Family history of certain disabilities and chronic diseases (leading to disablement)**

Z82.0 **Family history of** epilepsy and other diseases of the nervous system
Conditions classifiable to G00-G99

Z82.1 **Family history of** blindness and visual loss
Conditions classifiable to H54.-

Z82.2 **Family history of** deafness and hearing loss
Conditions classifiable to H90-H91

Z82.3 **Family history of** stroke
Conditions classifiable to I60-I64

✓5ᵗʰ **Z82.4** **Family history of ischemic heart disease and other diseases of the circulatory system**
Conditions classifiable to I00-I52, I65-I99

Z82.41 **Family history of** sudden cardiac death
Z82.49 **Family history of** ischemic heart disease and other diseases of the circulatory system

Z82.5 **Family history of** asthma and other chronic lower respiratory diseases
Conditions classifiable to J40-J47
EXCLUDES 2 family history of other diseases of the respiratory system (Z83.6)

✓5ᵗʰ **Z82.6** **Family history of arthritis and other diseases of the musculoskeletal system and connective tissue**
Conditions classifiable to M00-M99

Z82.61 **Family history of** arthritis
Z82.62 **Family history of** osteoporosis
Z82.69 **Family history of other diseases of the** musculoskeletal system and connective tissue

✓5ᵗʰ **Z82.7** **Family history of congenital malformations, deformations and chromosomal abnormalities**
Conditions classifiable to Q00-Q99

Z82.71 **Family history of** polycystic kidney
Z82.79 **Family history of other congenital malformations, deformations and chromosomal abnormalities**

Z82.8 **Family history of other disabilities and chronic diseases leading to disablement, not elsewhere classified**

✓4ᵗʰ **Z83** **Family history of other specific disorders**
EXCLUDES 2 contact with and (suspected) exposure to communicable disease in the family (Z20.-)

Z83.0 **Family history of** human immunodeficiency virus [HIV] disease
Conditions classifiable to B20

Z83.1 **Family history of other** infectious and parasitic diseases
Conditions classifiable to A00-B19, B25-B94, B99

Z83.2 **Family history of diseases of the** blood and blood-forming organs and certain disorders involving the immune mechanism
Conditions classifiable to D50-D89

Z83.3 **Family history of** diabetes mellitus
Conditions classifiable to E08-E13

✓5ᵗʰ **Z83.4** **Family history of other endocrine, nutritional and metabolic diseases**
Conditions classifiable to E00-E07, E15-E88

Z83.41 **Family history of** multiple endocrine neoplasia [MEN] syndrome
Z83.42 **Family history of** familial hypercholesterolemia
Z83.49 **Family history of other** endocrine, nutritional and metabolic diseases

✓5ᵗʰ **Z83.5** **Family history of eye and ear disorders**

✓6ᵗʰ **Z83.51** **Family history of** eye disorders
Conditions classifiable to H00-H53, H55-H59
EXCLUDES 2 family history of blindness and visual loss (Z82.1)
Z83.511 **Family history of** glaucoma
Z83.518 **Family history of other specified eye** disorder

Z83.52 **Family history of** ear disorders
Conditions classifiable to H60-H83, H92-H95
EXCLUDES 2 family history of deafness and hearing loss (Z82.2)

Z83.6 **Family history of other diseases of the** respiratory system
Conditions classifiable to J00-J39, J60-J99
EXCLUDES 2 family history of asthma and other chronic lower respiratory diseases (Z82.5)

✓5ᵗʰ **Z83.7** **Family history of diseases of the digestive system**
Conditions classifiable to K00-K93

Z83.71 **Family history of** colonic polyps
EXCLUDES 1 family history of malignant neoplasm of digestive organs (Z80.0)
Z83.79 **Family history of other diseases of the digestive system**

✓4ᵗʰ **Z84** **Family history of other conditions**

Z84.0 **Family history of diseases of the** skin and subcutaneous tissue
Conditions classifiable to L00-L99

Z84.1 **Family history of disorders of** kidney and ureter
Conditions classifiable to N00-N29

Z84.2 **Family history of other diseases of the** genitourinary system
Conditions classifiable to N30-N99

Z84.3 **Family history of** consanguinity

✓5ᵗʰ **Z84.8** **Family history of other specified conditions**

Z84.81 **Family history of carrier of** genetic disease

✓ Additional Character Required   ✓x7ᵗʰ Placeholder Alert   Manifestation Dx   ▽ Unspecified Dx   ▶◀ Revised Text   ● New Code   ▲ Revised Code Title

ICD-10-CM 2017   **1163**

Z84.82 Family history of **sudden infant death syndrome**
　　Family history of SIDS

Z84.89 Family history of other specified conditions

✓4th **Z85** **Personal history of malignant neoplasm**
　Code first any follow-up examination after treatment of malignant neoplasm (Z08)
　Use additional code to identify:
　　alcohol use and dependence (F10.-)
　　exposure to environmental tobacco smoke (Z77.22)
　　▶history of tobacco dependence (Z87.891)◀
　　occupational exposure to environmental tobacco smoke (Z57.31)
　　tobacco dependence (F17.-)
　　tobacco use (Z72.0)
　　EXCLUDES 2 personal history of benign neoplasm (Z86.01-)
　　　　　personal history of carcinoma-in-situ (Z86.00-)

✓5th **Z85.0** **Personal history of malignant neoplasm of digestive organs**

　Z85.00 **Personal history of malignant neoplasm of unspecified digestive organ** ▽

　Z85.01 **Personal history of malignant neoplasm of esophagus**
　　　Conditions classifiable to C15

✓6th **Z85.02** **Personal history of malignant neoplasm of stomach**
　　Z85.020 **Personal history of malignant carcinoid tumor of stomach**
　　　　Conditions classifiable to C7A.092
　　Z85.028 **Personal history of other malignant neoplasm of stomach**
　　　　Conditions classifiable to C16

✓6th **Z85.03** **Personal history of malignant neoplasm of large intestine**
　　Z85.030 **Personal history of malignant carcinoid tumor of large intestine**
　　　　Conditions classifiable to C7A.022-C7A.025, C7A.029
　　Z85.038 **Personal history of other malignant neoplasm of large intestine**
　　　　Conditions classifiable to C18

✓6th **Z85.04** **Personal history of malignant neoplasm of rectum, rectosigmoid junction, and anus**
　　Z85.040 **Personal history of malignant carcinoid tumor of rectum**
　　　　Conditions classifiable to C7A.026
　　Z85.048 **Personal history of other malignant neoplasm of rectum, rectosigmoid junction, and anus**
　　　　Conditions classifiable to C19-C21

　Z85.05 **Personal history of malignant neoplasm of liver**
　　　Conditions classifiable to C22

✓6th **Z85.06** **Personal history of malignant neoplasm of small intestine**
　　Z85.060 **Personal history of malignant carcinoid tumor of small intestine**
　　　　Conditions classifiable to C7A.01-
　　Z85.068 **Personal history of other malignant neoplasm of small intestine**
　　　　Conditions classifiable to C17

　Z85.07 **Personal history of malignant neoplasm of pancreas**
　　　Conditions classifiable to C25

　Z85.09 **Personal history of malignant neoplasm of other digestive organs**

✓5th **Z85.1** **Personal history of malignant neoplasm of trachea, bronchus and lung**

✓6th **Z85.11** **Personal history of malignant neoplasm of bronchus and lung**
　　Z85.110 **Personal history of malignant carcinoid tumor of bronchus and lung**
　　　　Conditions classifiable to C7A.090
　　Z85.118 **Personal history of other malignant neoplasm of bronchus and lung**
　　　　Conditions classifiable to C34

　Z85.12 **Personal history of malignant neoplasm of trachea**
　　　Conditions classifiable to C33

✓5th **Z85.2** **Personal history of malignant neoplasm of other respiratory and intrathoracic organs**

　Z85.20 **Personal history of malignant neoplasm of unspecified respiratory organ** ▽

　Z85.21 **Personal history of malignant neoplasm of larynx**
　　　Conditions classifiable to C32

Z85.22 **Personal history of malignant neoplasm of nasal cavities, middle ear, and accessory sinuses**
　　Conditions classifiable to C30-C31

✓6th **Z85.23** **Personal history of malignant neoplasm of thymus**
　　Z85.230 **Personal history of malignant carcinoid tumor of thymus**
　　　　Conditions classifiable to C7A.091
　　Z85.238 **Personal history of other malignant neoplasm of thymus**
　　　　Conditions classifiable to C37

Z85.29 **Personal history of malignant neoplasm of other respiratory and intrathoracic organs**

Z85.3 **Personal history of malignant neoplasm of breast**
　Conditions classifiable to C50.-

✓5th **Z85.4** **Personal history of malignant neoplasm of genital organs**
　Conditions classifiable to C51-C63

　Z85.40 **Personal history of malignant neoplasm of unspecified female genital organ** ♀ ▽

　Z85.41 **Personal history of malignant neoplasm of cervix uteri** ♀

　Z85.42 **Personal history of malignant neoplasm of other parts of uterus** ♀

　Z85.43 **Personal history of malignant neoplasm of ovary** ♀

　Z85.44 **Personal history of malignant neoplasm of other female genital organs** ♀

　Z85.45 **Personal history of malignant neoplasm of unspecified male genital organ** ♂ ▽

　Z85.46 **Personal history of malignant neoplasm of prostate** ♂

　Z85.47 **Personal history of malignant neoplasm of testis** ♂

　Z85.48 **Personal history of malignant neoplasm of epididymis** ♂

　Z85.49 **Personal history of malignant neoplasm of other male genital organs** ♂

✓5th **Z85.5** **Personal history of malignant neoplasm of urinary tract**
　Conditions classifiable to C64-C68

　Z85.50 **Personal history of malignant neoplasm of unspecified urinary tract organ** ▽

　Z85.51 **Personal history of malignant neoplasm of bladder**

✓6th **Z85.52** **Personal history of malignant neoplasm of kidney**
　　EXCLUDES 1 personal history of malignant neoplasm of renal pelvis (Z85.53)
　　Z85.520 **Personal history of malignant carcinoid tumor of kidney**
　　　　Conditions classifiable to C7A.093
　　Z85.528 **Personal history of other malignant neoplasm of kidney**
　　　　Conditions classifiable to C64

　Z85.53 **Personal history of malignant neoplasm of renal pelvis**

　Z85.54 **Personal history of malignant neoplasm of ureter**

　Z85.59 **Personal history of malignant neoplasm of other urinary tract organ**

Z85.6 **Personal history of leukemia**
　Conditions classifiable to C91-C95
　　EXCLUDES 1 leukemia in remission C91.0-C95.9 with 5th character 1

✓5th **Z85.7** **Personal history of other malignant neoplasms of lymphoid, hematopoietic and related tissues**

　Z85.71 **Personal history of Hodgkin lymphoma**
　　　Conditions classifiable to C81

　Z85.72 **Personal history of non-Hodgkin lymphomas**
　　　Conditions classifiable to C82-C85

　Z85.79 **Personal history of other malignant neoplasms of lymphoid, hematopoietic and related tissues**
　　　Conditions classifiable to C88-C90, C96
　　　EXCLUDES 1 multiple myeloma in remission (C90.01)
　　　　　plasma cell leukemia in remission (C90.11)
　　　　　plasmacytoma in remission (C90.21)

✓5th **Z85.8** **Personal history of malignant neoplasms of other organs and systems**
　Conditions classifiable to C00-C14, C40-C49, ▶C69-C75, C7A.098, C76-C79◀

✓6th **Z85.81** **Personal history of malignant neoplasm of lip, oral cavity, and pharynx**
　　Z85.810 **Personal history of malignant neoplasm of tongue**

EXCLUDES 1 Not coded here　*EXCLUDES 2* Not included here　　**PDx** Primary Dx Only　　**N** Newborn Age : 0　　**P** Pediatric Age : 0-17　　**M** Maternity Age : 12-55　　**A** Adult Age : 15-124

Z85.818 **Personal history of malignant neoplasm of other sites of lip, oral cavity, and pharynx**

Z85.819 **Personal history of malignant neoplasm of unspecified site of lip, oral cavity, and pharynx** ▽

✓6ᵗʰ **Z85.82** **Personal history of malignant neoplasm of** skin

Z85.820 **Personal history of malignant** melanoma **of skin**
Conditions classifiable to C43

Z85.821 **Personal history of** Merkel cell carcinoma
Conditions classifiable to C4A

Z85.828 **Personal history of other malignant neoplasm of skin**
Conditions classifiable to C44

✓6ᵗʰ **Z85.83** **Personal history of malignant neoplasm of** bone and soft tissue

Z85.830 **Personal history of malignant neoplasm of** bone

Z85.831 **Personal history of malignant neoplasm of** soft tissue
EXCLUDES 2 *personal history of malignant neoplasm of skin (Z85.82-)*

✓6ᵗʰ **Z85.84** **Personal history of malignant neoplasm of** eye and nervous tissue

Z85.840 **Personal history of malignant neoplasm of** eye

Z85.841 **Personal history of malignant neoplasm of** brain

Z85.848 **Personal history of malignant neoplasm of other parts of nervous tissue**

✓6ᵗʰ **Z85.85** **Personal history of malignant neoplasm of** endocrine glands

Z85.850 **Personal history of malignant neoplasm of** thyroid

Z85.858 **Personal history of malignant neoplasm of other endocrine glands**

Z85.89 **Personal history of malignant neoplasm of other organs and systems**

Z85.9 **Personal history of malignant neoplasm, unspecified** ▽
Conditions classifiable to C7A.00, C80.1

✓4ᵗʰ **Z86** **Personal history of certain other diseases**
Code first any follow-up examination after treatment (Z09)

✓5ᵗʰ **Z86.0** **Personal history of in-situ and benign neoplasms and neoplasms of uncertain behavior**
EXCLUDES 2 *personal history of malignant neoplasms (Z85.-)*

✓6ᵗʰ **Z86.00** **Personal history of** in-situ neoplasm
►Conditions classifiable to D00-D09◄

Z86.000 **Personal history of in-situ neoplasm of breast**

Z86.001 **Personal history of in-situ neoplasm of** cervix uteri ♀
►Personal history of cervical intraepithelial neoplasia III [CIN III]◄

Z86.008 **Personal history of in-situ neoplasm of other site**
►Personal history of vaginal intraepithelial neoplasia III [VAIN III]◄
►Personal history of vulvar intraepithelial neoplasia III [VIN III]◄

✓6ᵗʰ **Z86.01** **Personal history of** benign neoplasm

Z86.010 **Personal history of** colonic polyps

Z86.011 **Personal history of benign neoplasm of the** brain

Z86.012 **Personal history of benign** carcinoid tumor

Z86.018 **Personal history of other benign neoplasm**

Z86.03 **Personal history of** neoplasm of uncertain behavior

✓5ᵗʰ **Z86.1** **Personal history of** infectious and parasitic diseases
Conditions classifiable to A00-B89, B99
EXCLUDES 1 *personal history of infectious diseases specific to a body system*
sequelae of infectious and parasitic diseases (B90-B94)

Z86.11 **Personal history of** tuberculosis

Z86.12 **Personal history of** poliomyelitis

Z86.13 **Personal history of** malaria

Z86.14 **Personal history of** Methicillin resistant Staphylococcus aureus **infection**
Personal history of MRSA infection

Z86.19 **Personal history of other infectious and parasitic diseases**

Z86.2 **Personal history of diseases of the** blood and blood-forming **organs and certain disorders involving the** immune **mechanism**
Conditions classifiable to D50-D89

✓5ᵗʰ **Z86.3** **Personal history of** endocrine, nutritional and metabolic **diseases**
Conditions classifiable to E00-E88

Z86.31 **Personal history of diabetic foot ulcer**
EXCLUDES 2 *current diabetic foot ulcer (E08.621, E09.621, E10.621, E11.621, E13.621)*

Z86.32 **Personal history of gestational diabetes** ♀
Personal history of conditions classifiable to O24.4-
EXCLUDES 1 *gestational diabetes mellitus in current pregnancy (O24.4-)*

Z86.39 **Personal history of other endocrine, nutritional and metabolic disease**

✓5ᵗʰ **Z86.5** **Personal history of mental and behavioral disorders**
Conditions classifiable to F40-F59

Z86.51 **Personal history of** combat and operational stress reaction ▲

Z86.59 **Personal history of other mental and behavioral disorders**

✓5ᵗʰ **Z86.6** **Personal history of diseases of the** nervous system and sense **organs**
Conditions classifiable to G00-G99, H00-H95

Z86.61 **Personal history of** infections of the central nervous system
Personal history of encephalitis
Personal history of meningitis

Z86.69 **Personal history of other diseases of the nervous system and sense organs**

✓5ᵗʰ **Z86.7** **Personal history of diseases of the** circulatory system
Conditions classifiable to I00-I99
EXCLUDES 2 *old myocardial infarction (I25.2)*
personal history of anaphylactic shock (Z87.892)
postmyocardial infarction syndrome (I24.1)

✓6ᵗʰ **Z86.71** **Personal history of** venous thrombosis and embolism

Z86.711 **Personal history of** pulmonary embolism

Z86.718 **Personal history of other venous thrombosis and embolism**

Z86.72 **Personal history of** thrombophlebitis

Z86.73 **Personal history of** transient ischemic attack (TIA), and cerebral infarction without residual deficits
Personal history of prolonged reversible ischemic neurological deficit (PRIND)
Personal history of stroke NOS without residual deficits
EXCLUDES 1 *personal history of traumatic brain injury (Z87.820)*
sequelae of cerebrovascular disease (I69.-)
AHA: 2012,4Q,92

Z86.74 **Personal history of sudden cardiac arrest**
Personal history of sudden cardiac death successfully resuscitated

Z86.79 **Personal history of other diseases of the circulatory system**

✓4ᵗʰ **Z87** **Personal history of other diseases and conditions**
Code first any follow-up examination after treatment (Z09)

✓5ᵗʰ **Z87.0** **Personal history of diseases of the** respiratory system
Conditions classifiable to J00-J99

Z87.01 **Personal history of** pneumonia (recurrent)

Z87.09 **Personal history of other diseases of the respiratory system**

✓5ᵗʰ **Z87.1** **Personal history of diseases of the** digestive system
Conditions classifiable to K00-K93

Z87.11 **Personal history of** peptic ulcer disease

Z87.19 **Personal history of other diseases of the digestive system**

Z87.2 **Personal history of diseases of the** skin and subcutaneous tissue
Conditions classifiable to L00-L99
EXCLUDES 2 *personal history of diabetic foot ulcer (Z86.31)*

☑ Additional Character Required   ✓x7ᵗʰ Placeholder Alert   Manifestation Dx   ▽ Unspecified Dx   ►◄ Revised Text   ● New Code   ▲ Revised Code Title

Chapter 21. Factors Influencing Health Status and Contact With Health Services *(left margin)*

✓5ᵗʰ **Z87.3** **Personal history of diseases of the musculoskeletal system and connective tissue**
Conditions classifiable to M00-M99
EXCLUDES 2   *personal history of (healed) traumatic fracture (Z87.81)*

  ✓6ᵗʰ **Z87.31** **Personal history of (healed) nontraumatic fracture**

    Z87.310 **Personal history of (healed) osteoporosis fracture**
Personal history of (healed) fragility fracture
Personal history of (healed) collapsed vertebra due to osteoporosis

    Z87.311 **Personal history of (healed) other pathological fracture**
Personal history of (healed) collapsed vertebra NOS
EXCLUDES 2   *personal history of osteoporosis fracture (Z87.310)*

    Z87.312 **Personal history of (healed) stress fracture**
Personal history of (healed) fatigue fracture

  Z87.39 **Personal history of other diseases of the musculoskeletal system and connective tissue**

✓5ᵗʰ **Z87.4** **Personal history of diseases of the genitourinary system**
Conditions classifiable to N00-N99

  ✓6ᵗʰ **Z87.41** **Personal history of dysplasia of the female genital tract**
EXCLUDES 1   ▶*personal history of intraepithelial neoplasia III of female genital tract (Z87.001, Z87.008)*◀
personal history of malignant neoplasm of female genital tract (Z85.40-Z85.44)

    Z87.410 **Personal history of cervical dysplasia** ♀

    Z87.411 **Personal history of vaginal dysplasia** ♀

    Z87.412 **Personal history of vulvar dysplasia** ♀

  Z87.42 **Personal history of other diseases of the female genital tract** ♀

  ✓6ᵗʰ **Z87.43** **Personal history of diseases of the male genital organs**

    Z87.430 **Personal history of prostatic dysplasia** ♂
EXCLUDES 1   *personal history of malignant neoplasm of prostate (Z85.46)*

    Z87.438 **Personal history of other diseases of male genital organs** ♂

  ✓6ᵗʰ **Z87.44** **Personal history of diseases of the urinary system**
EXCLUDES 1   *personal history of malignant neoplasm of cervix uteri (Z85.41)*

    Z87.440 **Personal history of urinary (tract) infections**

    Z87.441 **Personal history of nephrotic syndrome**

    Z87.442 **Personal history of urinary calculi**
Personal history of kidney stones

    Z87.448 **Personal history of other diseases of urinary system**

✓5ᵗʰ **Z87.5** **Personal history of complications of pregnancy, childbirth and the puerperium**
Conditions classifiable to O00-O9A
EXCLUDES 2   *recurrent pregnancy loss (N96)*

  Z87.51 **Personal history of pre-term labor** ♀
EXCLUDES 1   *current pregnancy with history of pre-term labor (O09.21-)*

  Z87.59 **Personal history of other complications of pregnancy, childbirth and the puerperium** ♀
Personal history of trophoblastic disease

✓5ᵗʰ **Z87.7** **Personal history of (corrected) congenital malformations**
Conditions classifiable to Q00-Q89 that have been repaired or corrected
EXCLUDES 1   *congenital malformations that have been partially corrected or repair but which still require medical treatment - code to condition*
EXCLUDES 2   *other postprocedural states (Z98.-)*
personal history of medical treatment (Z92.-)
presence of cardiac and vascular implants and grafts (Z95.-)
presence of other devices (Z97.-)
presence of other functional implants (Z96.-)
transplanted organ and tissue status (Z94.-)

  ✓6ᵗʰ **Z87.71** **Personal history of (corrected) congenital malformations of genitourinary system**

    Z87.710 **Personal history of (corrected) hypospadias** ♂

    Z87.718 **Personal history of other specified (corrected) congenital malformations of genitourinary system**

  ✓6ᵗʰ **Z87.72** **Personal history of (corrected) congenital malformations of nervous system and sense organs**

    Z87.720 **Personal history of (corrected) congenital malformations of eye**

    Z87.721 **Personal history of (corrected) congenital malformations of ear**

    Z87.728 **Personal history of other specified (corrected) congenital malformations of nervous system and sense organs**

  ✓6ᵗʰ **Z87.73** **Personal history of (corrected) congenital malformations of digestive system**

    Z87.730 **Personal history of (corrected) cleft lip and palate**

    Z87.738 **Personal history of other specified (corrected) congenital malformations of digestive system**

  Z87.74 **Personal history of (corrected) congenital malformations of heart and circulatory system**

  Z87.75 **Personal history of (corrected) congenital malformations of respiratory system**

  Z87.76 **Personal history of (corrected) congenital malformations of integument, limbs and musculoskeletal system**

  ✓6ᵗʰ **Z87.79** **Personal history of other (corrected) congenital malformations**

    Z87.790 **Personal history of (corrected) congenital malformations of face and neck**

    Z87.798 **Personal history of other (corrected) congenital malformations**

✓5ᵗʰ **Z87.8** **Personal history of other specified conditions**
EXCLUDES 2   *personal history of self harm (Z91.5)*

  Z87.81 **Personal history of (healed) traumatic fracture**
EXCLUDES 2   *personal history of (healed) nontraumatic fracture (Z87.31-)*

  ✓6ᵗʰ **Z87.82** **Personal history of other (healed) physical injury and trauma**
Conditions classifiable to S00-T88, except traumatic fractures

    Z87.820 **Personal history of traumatic brain injury**
EXCLUDES 1   *personal history of transient ischemic attack (TIA), and cerebral infarction without residual deficits (Z86.73)*

    Z87.821 **Personal history of retained foreign body fully removed**

    Z87.828 **Personal history of other (healed) physical injury and trauma**

  ✓6ᵗʰ **Z87.89** **Personal history of other specified conditions**

    Z87.890 **Personal history of sex reassignment**

    Z87.891 **Personal history of nicotine dependence**
EXCLUDES 1   *current nicotine dependence (F17.2-)*

    Z87.892 **Personal history of anaphylaxis**
Code also allergy status such as:
allergy status to drugs, medicaments and biological substances (Z88.-)
allergy status, other than to drugs and biological substances (Z91.0-)

EXCLUDES 1 Not coded here   *EXCLUDES 2* Not included here   **PDx** Primary Dx Only   **N** Newborn Age : 0   **P** Pediatric Age : 0-17   **M** Maternity Age : 12-55   **A** Adult Age : 15-124

Z87.898 **Personal history of other specified conditions**
  AHA: 2013,1Q,21

√4ᵗʰ **Z88 Allergy status to drugs, medicaments and biological substances**
  EXCLUDES 2 *allergy status, other than to drugs and biological substances (Z91.0-)*
  AHA: 2015,3Q,23

Z88.0 **Allergy status to penicillin**
Z88.1 **Allergy status to other antibiotic agents status**
Z88.2 **Allergy status to sulfonamides status**
Z88.3 **Allergy status to other anti-infective agents status**
Z88.4 **Allergy status to anesthetic agent status**
Z88.5 **Allergy status to narcotic agent status**
Z88.6 **Allergy status to analgesic agent status**
Z88.7 **Allergy status to serum and vaccine status**
Z88.8 **Allergy status to other drugs, medicaments and biological substances status**
Z88.9 **Allergy status to unspecified drugs, medicaments and biological substances status** ▽

√4ᵗʰ **Z89 Acquired absence of limb**
  INCLUDES amputation status
    postprocedural loss of limb
    post-traumatic loss of limb
  EXCLUDES 1 *acquired deformities of limbs (M20-M21)*
    congenital absence of limbs (Q71-Q73)

√5ᵗʰ Z89.0 **Acquired absence of thumb and other finger(s)**
  √6ᵗʰ Z89.01 **Acquired absence of thumb**
    Z89.011 **Acquired absence of right thumb**
    Z89.012 **Acquired absence of left thumb**
    Z89.019 **Acquired absence of unspecified thumb** ▽
  √6ᵗʰ Z89.02 **Acquired absence of other finger(s)**
    EXCLUDES 2 *acquired absence of thumb (Z89.01-)*
    Z89.021 **Acquired absence of right finger(s)**
    Z89.022 **Acquired absence of left finger(s)**
    Z89.029 **Acquired absence of unspecified finger(s)** ▽

√5ᵗʰ Z89.1 **Acquired absence of hand and wrist**
  √6ᵗʰ Z89.11 **Acquired absence of hand**
    Z89.111 **Acquired absence of right hand**
    Z89.112 **Acquired absence of left hand**
    Z89.119 **Acquired absence of unspecified hand** ▽
  √6ᵗʰ Z89.12 **Acquired absence of wrist**
    Disarticulation at wrist
    Z89.121 **Acquired absence of right wrist**
    Z89.122 **Acquired absence of left wrist**
    Z89.129 **Acquired absence of unspecified wrist** ▽

√5ᵗʰ Z89.2 **Acquired absence of upper limb above wrist**
  √6ᵗʰ Z89.20 **Acquired absence of upper limb, unspecified level**
    Z89.201 **Acquired absence of right upper limb, unspecified level** ▽
    Z89.202 **Acquired absence of left upper limb, unspecified level** ▽
    Z89.209 **Acquired absence of unspecified upper limb, unspecified level**
      Acquired absence of arm NOS
  √6ᵗʰ Z89.21 **Acquired absence of upper limb below elbow**
    Z89.211 **Acquired absence of right upper limb below elbow**
    Z89.212 **Acquired absence of left upper limb below elbow**
    Z89.219 **Acquired absence of unspecified upper limb below elbow** ▽
  √6ᵗʰ Z89.22 **Acquired absence of upper limb above elbow**
    Disarticulation at elbow
    Z89.221 **Acquired absence of right upper limb above elbow**
    Z89.222 **Acquired absence of left upper limb above elbow**
    Z89.229 **Acquired absence of unspecified upper limb above elbow** ▽

√6ᵗʰ Z89.23 **Acquired absence of shoulder**
  Acquired absence of shoulder joint following explantation of shoulder joint prosthesis, with or without presence of antibiotic-impregnated cement spacer
  Z89.231 **Acquired absence of right shoulder**
  Z89.232 **Acquired absence of left shoulder**
  Z89.239 **Acquired absence of unspecified shoulder** ▽

√5ᵗʰ Z89.4 **Acquired absence of toe(s), foot, and ankle**
  √6ᵗʰ Z89.41 **Acquired absence of great toe**
    Z89.411 **Acquired absence of right great toe**
    Z89.412 **Acquired absence of left great toe**
    Z89.419 **Acquired absence of unspecified great toe** ▽
  √6ᵗʰ Z89.42 **Acquired absence of other toe(s)**
    EXCLUDES 2 *acquired absence of great toe (Z89.41-)*
    Z89.421 **Acquired absence of other right toe(s)**
    Z89.422 **Acquired absence of other left toe(s)**
    Z89.429 **Acquired absence of other toe(s), unspecified side** ▽
  √6ᵗʰ Z89.43 **Acquired absence of foot**
    Z89.431 **Acquired absence of right foot**
    Z89.432 **Acquired absence of left foot**
    Z89.439 **Acquired absence of unspecified foot** ▽
  √6ᵗʰ Z89.44 **Acquired absence of ankle**
    Disarticulation of ankle
    Z89.441 **Acquired absence of right ankle**
    Z89.442 **Acquired absence of left ankle**
    Z89.449 **Acquired absence of unspecified ankle** ▽

√5ᵗʰ Z89.5 **Acquired absence of leg below knee**
  √6ᵗʰ Z89.51 **Acquired absence of leg below knee**
    Z89.511 **Acquired absence of right leg below knee**
    Z89.512 **Acquired absence of left leg below knee**
    Z89.519 **Acquired absence of unspecified leg below knee** ▽
  √6ᵗʰ Z89.52 **Acquired absence of knee**
    Acquired absence of knee joint following explantation of knee joint prosthesis, with or without presence of antibiotic-impregnated cement spacer
    Z89.521 **Acquired absence of right knee**
    Z89.522 **Acquired absence of left knee**
    Z89.529 **Acquired absence of unspecified knee** ▽

√5ᵗʰ Z89.6 **Acquired absence of leg above knee**
  √6ᵗʰ Z89.61 **Acquired absence of leg above knee**
    Acquired absence of leg NOS
    Disarticulation at knee
    Z89.611 **Acquired absence of right leg above knee**
    Z89.612 **Acquired absence of left leg above knee**
    Z89.619 **Acquired absence of unspecified leg above knee** ▽
  √6ᵗʰ Z89.62 **Acquired absence of hip**
    Acquired absence of hip joint following explantation of hip joint prosthesis, with or without presence of antibiotic-impregnated cement spacer
    Disarticulation at hip
    Z89.621 **Acquired absence of right hip joint**
    Z89.622 **Acquired absence of left hip joint**
    Z89.629 **Acquired absence of unspecified hip joint** ▽

Z89.9 **Acquired absence of limb, unspecified** ▽

√4ᵗʰ **Z90 Acquired absence of organs, not elsewhere classified**
  INCLUDES postprocedural or post-traumatic loss of body part NEC
  EXCLUDES 1 *congenital absence - see Alphabetical Index*
  EXCLUDES 2 *postprocedural absence of endocrine glands (E89.-)*
  √5ᵗʰ Z90.0 **Acquired absence of part of head and neck**
    Z90.01 **Acquired absence of eye**
    Z90.02 **Acquired absence of larynx**
    Z90.09 **Acquired absence of other part of head and neck**
      Acquired absence of nose
      EXCLUDES 2 *teeth (K08.1)*

☑5ᵗʰ Z90.1 Acquired absence of breast and nipple

    Z90.10 Acquired absence of unspecified breast and nipple ▽

    Z90.11 Acquired absence of right breast and nipple

    Z90.12 Acquired absence of left breast and nipple

    Z90.13 Acquired absence of bilateral breasts and nipples

Z90.2 Acquired absence of lung [part of]

Z90.3 Acquired absence of stomach [part of]

☑5ᵗʰ Z90.4 Acquired absence of other specified parts of digestive tract

    ☑6ᵗʰ Z90.41 Acquired absence of pancreas

        ▶Code also exocrine pancreatic insufficiency (K86.81)◀

        Use additional code to identify any associated:
        insulin use (Z79.4)
        diabetes mellitus, postpancreatectomy (E13.-)

        Z90.410 Acquired total absence of pancreas
            Acquired absence of pancreas NOS

        Z90.411 Acquired partial absence of pancreas

    Z90.49 Acquired absence of other specified parts of digestive tract

Z90.5 Acquired absence of kidney

Z90.6 Acquired absence of other parts of urinary tract
    Acquired absence of bladder

☑5ᵗʰ Z90.7 Acquired absence of genital organ(s)

    EXCLUDES 1   personal history of sex reassignment (Z87.890)
    EXCLUDES 2   female genital mutilation status (N90.81-)

    ☑6ᵗʰ Z90.71 Acquired absence of cervix and uterus

        Z90.710 Acquired absence of both cervix and uterus ♀
            Acquired absence of uterus NOS
            Status post total hysterectomy

        Z90.711 Acquired absence of uterus with remaining cervical stump ♀
            Status post partial hysterectomy with remaining cervical stump

        Z90.712 Acquired absence of cervix with remaining uterus ♀

    ☑6ᵗʰ Z90.72 Acquired absence of ovaries

        Z90.721 Acquired absence of ovaries, unilateral ♀

        Z90.722 Acquired absence of ovaries, bilateral ♀

    Z90.79 Acquired absence of other genital organ(s)

☑5ᵗʰ Z90.8 Acquired absence of other organs

    Z90.81 Acquired absence of spleen

    Z90.89 Acquired absence of other organs

☑4ᵗʰ Z91 Personal risk factors, not elsewhere classified

    EXCLUDES 2   contact with and (suspected) exposures hazardous to health (Z77.-)
        exposure to pollution and other problems related to physical environment (Z77.1-)
        personal history of physical injury and trauma (Z87.81, Z87.82-)
        occupational exposure to risk factors (Z57.-)

    ☑5ᵗʰ Z91.0 Allergy status, other than to drugs and biological substances

        EXCLUDES 2   Allergy status to drugs, medicaments, and biological substances (Z88.-)

        ☑6ᵗʰ Z91.01 Food allergy status

            EXCLUDES 2   food additives allergy status (Z91.02)

            Z91.010 Allergy to peanuts

            Z91.011 Allergy to milk products
                EXCLUDES 1   lactose intolerance (E73.-)

            Z91.012 Allergy to eggs

            Z91.013 Allergy to seafood
                Allergy to shellfish
                Allergy to octopus or squid ink

            Z91.018 Allergy to other foods
                Allergy to nuts other than peanuts

        Z91.02 Food additives allergy status

        ☑6ᵗʰ Z91.03 Insect allergy status

            Z91.030 Bee allergy status

            Z91.038 Other insect allergy status

        ☑6ᵗʰ Z91.04 Nonmedicinal substance allergy status

            Z91.040 Latex allergy status
                Latex sensitivity status

            Z91.041 Radiographic dye allergy status
                Allergy status to contrast media used for diagnostic X-ray procedure

            Z91.048 Other nonmedicinal substance allergy status

        Z91.09 Other allergy status, other than to drugs and biological substances

    ☑5ᵗʰ Z91.1 Patient's noncompliance with medical treatment and regimen

        Z91.11 Patient's noncompliance with dietary regimen

        ☑6ᵗʰ Z91.12 Patient's intentional underdosing of medication regimen

            Code first underdosing of medication (T36-T50) with fifth or sixth character 6

            EXCLUDES 1   adverse effect of prescribed drug taken as directed - code to adverse effect poisoning (overdose) - code to poisoning

            Z91.120 Patient's intentional underdosing of medication regimen due to financial hardship

            Z91.128 Patient's intentional underdosing of medication regimen for other reason

        ☑6ᵗʰ Z91.13 Patient's unintentional underdosing of medication regimen

            Code first underdosing of medication (T36-T50) with fifth or sixth character 6

            EXCLUDES 1   adverse effect of prescribed drug taken as directed - code to adverse effect poisoning (overdose) - code to poisoning

            Z91.130 Patient's unintentional underdosing of medication regimen due to age-related debility

            Z91.138 Patient's unintentional underdosing of medication regimen for other reason

        Z91.14 Patient's other noncompliance with medication regimen
            Patient's underdosing of medication NOS

        Z91.15 Patient's noncompliance with renal dialysis

        Z91.19 Patient's noncompliance with other medical treatment and regimen

    ☑5ᵗʰ Z91.4 Personal history of psychological trauma, not elsewhere classified

        ☑6ᵗʰ Z91.41 Personal history of adult abuse

            EXCLUDES 2   personal history of abuse in childhood (Z62.81-)

            Z91.410 Personal history of adult physical and sexual abuse Ⓐ
                EXCLUDES 1   current adult physical abuse (T74.11, T76.11)
                  current adult sexual abuse (T74.21, T76.11)

            Z91.411 Personal history of adult psychological abuse Ⓐ

            Z91.412 Personal history of adult neglect Ⓐ
                EXCLUDES 1   current adult neglect (T74.01, T76.01)

            Z91.419 Personal history of unspecified adult abuse Ⓐ ▽

        Z91.49 Other personal history of psychological trauma, not elsewhere classified

    Z91.5 Personal history of self-harm
        Personal history of parasuicide
        Personal history of self-poisoning
        Personal history of suicide attempt

    ☑5ᵗʰ Z91.8 Other specified personal risk factors, not elsewhere classified

        Z91.81 History of falling
            At risk for falling

        Z91.82 Personal history of military deployment Ⓐ
            Individual (civilian or military) with past history of military war, peacekeeping and humanitarian deployment (current or past conflict)
            Returned from military deployment

        Z91.83 *Wandering in diseases classified elsewhere*
            Code first underlying disorder such as:
              Alzheimer's disease (G30.-)
              autism or pervasive developmental disorder (F84.-)
              intellectual disabilities (F70-F79)
              unspecified dementia with behavioral disturbance (F03.9-)

EXCLUDES 1 Not coded here   *EXCLUDES 2* Not included here   **PDx** Primary Dx Only   **N** Newborn Age : 0   **P** Pediatric Age : 0-17   **M** Maternity Age : 12-55   **A** Adult Age : 15-124

1168   ICD-10-CM 2017

   Z91.89   **Other specified personal risk factors, not elsewhere classified**

✓4ᵗʰ **Z92**   **Personal history of medical treatment**
> EXCLUDES 2 *postprocedural states (Z98.-)*

Z92.0   **Personal history of contraception**
> EXCLUDES 1 *counseling or management of current contraceptive practices (Z30.-)*
> *long term (current) use of contraception (Z79.3)*
> *presence of (intrauterine) contraceptive device (Z97.5)*

✓5ᵗʰ **Z92.2**   **Personal history of drug therapy**
> EXCLUDES 2 *long term (current) drug therapy (Z79.-)*

Z92.21   **Personal history of antineoplastic chemotherapy**
Z92.22   **Personal history of monoclonal drug therapy**
Z92.23   **Personal history of estrogen therapy**
✓6ᵗʰ **Z92.24**   **Personal history of steroid therapy**

    Z92.240   **Personal history of inhaled steroid therapy**
    Z92.241   **Personal history of systemic steroid therapy**
       Personal history of steroid therapy NOS

Z92.25   **Personal history of immunosupression therapy**
> EXCLUDES 2 *personal history of steroid therapy (Z92.24)*

Z92.29   **Personal history of other drug therapy**

Z92.3   **Personal history of irradiation**
    Personal history of exposure to therapeutic radiation
> EXCLUDES 1 *exposure to radiation in the physical environment (Z77.12)*
> *occupational exposure to radiation (Z57.1)*

✓5ᵗʰ **Z92.8**   **Personal history of other medical treatment**

Z92.81   **Personal history of extracorporeal membrane oxygenation (ECMO)**
Z92.82   **Status post administration of tPA (rtPA) in a different facility within the last 24 hours prior to admission to current facility**
    Code first condition requiring tPA administration, such as:
      acute cerebral infarction (I63.-)
      acute myocardial infarction (I21.-, I22.-)
      AHA: 2013,4Q,124

Z92.83   **Personal history of failed moderate sedation**
    Personal history of failed conscious sedation
> EXCLUDES 2 *failed moderate sedation during procedure (T88.52)*

Z92.84   **Personal history of unintended awareness under general anesthesia**
> EXCLUDES 2 *unintended awareness under general anesthesia during procedure (T88.53)*

Z92.89   **Personal history of other medical treatment**

✓4ᵗʰ **Z93**   **Artificial opening status**
> EXCLUDES 1 *artificial openings requiring attention or management (Z43.-)*
> *complications of external stoma (J95.0-, K94.-, N99.5-)*

Z93.0   **Tracheostomy status**
    AHA: 2013,4Q,129

Z93.1   **Gastrostomy status**
Z93.2   **Ileostomy status**
Z93.3   **Colostomy status**
Z93.4   **Other artificial openings of gastrointestinal tract status**
✓5ᵗʰ **Z93.5**   **Cystostomy status**

    Z93.50   **Unspecified cystostomy status** ▽
    Z93.51   **Cutaneous-vesicostomy status**
    Z93.52   **Appendico-vesicostomy status**
    Z93.59   **Other cystostomy status**

Z93.6   **Other artificial openings of urinary tract status**
    Nephrostomy status
    Ureterostomy status
    Urethrostomy status

Z93.8   **Other artificial opening status**
Z93.9   **Artificial opening status, unspecified** ▽

✓4ᵗʰ **Z94**   **Transplanted organ and tissue status**
> INCLUDES *organ or tissue replaced by heterogenous or homogenous transplant*
> EXCLUDES 1 *complications of transplanted organ or tissue - see Alphabetical Index*
> EXCLUDES 2 *presence of vascular grafts (Z95.-)*

Z94.0   **Kidney transplant status**

Z94.1   **Heart transplant status**
> EXCLUDES 1 *artificial heart status (Z95.812)*
> *heart-valve replacement status (Z95.2-Z95.4)*

Z94.2   **Lung transplant status**
Z94.3   **Heart and lungs transplant status**
Z94.4   **Liver transplant status**
Z94.5   **Skin transplant status**
    Autogenous skin transplant status
Z94.6   **Bone transplant status**
Z94.7   **Corneal transplant status**
✓5ᵗʰ **Z94.8**   **Other transplanted organ and tissue status**

    Z94.81   **Bone marrow transplant status**
    Z94.82   **Intestine transplant status**
    Z94.83   **Pancreas transplant status**
    Z94.84   **Stem cells transplant status**
    Z94.89   **Other transplanted organ and tissue status**

Z94.9   **Transplanted organ and tissue status, unspecified** ▽

✓4ᵗʰ **Z95**   **Presence of cardiac and vascular implants and grafts**
> EXCLUDES 1 *complications of cardiac and vascular devices, implants and grafts (T82.-)*

Z95.0   **Presence of cardiac pacemaker**
    ▶Presence of cardiac resynchronization therapy (CRT-P) pacemaker◀
> EXCLUDES 1 *adjustment or management of cardiac device ▶(Z45.0-)◀*
> *adjustment or management of cardiac pacemaker (Z45.0)*
> *presence of automatic (implantable) cardiac defibrillator with synchronous cardiac pacemaker (Z95.810)*

Z95.1   **Presence of aortocoronary bypass graft**
    ▶Presence of coronary artery bypass graft◀

Z95.2   **Presence of prosthetic heart valve**
    Presence of heart valve NOS

Z95.3   **Presence of xenogenic heart valve**
Z95.4   **Presence of other heart-valve replacement**
Z95.5   **Presence of coronary angioplasty implant and graft**
> EXCLUDES 1 *coronary angioplasty status without implant and graft (Z98.61)*

✓6ᵗʰ **Z95.8**   **Presence of other cardiac and vascular implants and grafts**

   ✓6ᵗʰ **Z95.81**   **Presence of other cardiac implants and grafts**

     Z95.810   **Presence of automatic (implantable) cardiac defibrillator**
       Presence of automatic (implantable) cardiac defibrillator with synchronous cardiac pacemaker
       ▶Presence of cardiac resynchronization therapy defibrillator (CRT-D)◀
       ▶Presence of cardioverter-defribillator (ICD)◀
     Z95.811   **Presence of heart assist device**
     Z95.812   **Presence of fully implantable artificial heart**
     Z95.818   **Presence of other cardiac implants and grafts**

   ✓6ᵗʰ **Z95.82**   **Presence of other vascular implants and grafts**

     Z95.820   **Peripheral vascular angioplasty status with implants and grafts**
> EXCLUDES 1 *peripheral vascular angioplasty without implant and graft (Z98.62)*
     Z95.828   **Presence of other vascular implants and grafts**
       Presence of intravascular prosthesis NEC

Z95.9   **Presence of cardiac and vascular implant and graft, unspecified** ▽

✓4ᵗʰ **Z96**   **Presence of other functional implants**
> EXCLUDES 2 *complications of internal prosthetic devices, implants and grafts (T82-T85)*
> *fitting and adjustment of prosthetic and other devices (Z44-Z46)*

Z96.0   **Presence of urogenital implants**
Z96.1   **Presence of intraocular lens**
    Presence of pseudophakia
✓5ᵗʰ **Z96.2**   **Presence of otological and audiological implants**

    Z96.20   **Presence of otological and audiological implant, unspecified** ▽
    Z96.21   **Cochlear implant status**

✓ Additional Character Required   ✓x7ᵗʰ Placeholder Alert   Manifestation Dx   ▽ Unspecified Dx   ▶◀ Revised Text   ● New Code   ▲ Revised Code Title

ICD-10-CM 2017   **1169**

Z96.22   Myringotomy tube(s) status

Z96.29   Presence of other otological and audiological implants
- Presence of bone-conduction hearing device
- Presence of eustachian tube stent
- Stapes replacement

Z96.3   Presence of artificial larynx

✓5ᵗʰ **Z96.4**   Presence of endocrine implants

Z96.41   Presence of insulin pump (external) (internal)

Z96.49   Presence of other endocrine implants

Z96.5   Presence of tooth-root and mandibular implants

✓5ᵗʰ **Z96.6**   Presence of orthopedic joint implants

Z96.60   Presence of unspecified orthopedic joint implant ▽

✓6ᵗʰ **Z96.61**   Presence of artificial shoulder joint

Z96.611   Presence of right artificial shoulder joint

Z96.612   Presence of left artificial shoulder joint

Z96.619   Presence of unspecified artificial shoulder joint ▽

✓6ᵗʰ **Z96.62**   Presence of artificial elbow joint

Z96.621   Presence of right artificial elbow joint

Z96.622   Presence of left artificial elbow joint

Z96.629   Presence of unspecified artificial elbow joint ▽

✓6ᵗʰ **Z96.63**   Presence of artificial wrist joint

Z96.631   Presence of right artificial wrist joint

Z96.632   Presence of left artificial wrist joint

Z96.639   Presence of unspecified artificial wrist joint ▽

✓6ᵗʰ **Z96.64**   Presence of artificial hip joint
- Hip-joint replacement (partial) (total)

Z96.641   Presence of right artificial hip joint

Z96.642   Presence of left artificial hip joint

Z96.643   Presence of artificial hip joint, bilateral

Z96.649   Presence of unspecified artificial hip joint ▽

✓6ᵗʰ **Z96.65**   Presence of artificial knee joint

Z96.651   Presence of right artificial knee joint

Z96.652   Presence of left artificial knee joint

Z96.653   Presence of artificial knee joint, bilateral

Z96.659   Presence of unspecified artificial knee joint ▽

✓6ᵗʰ **Z96.66**   Presence of artificial ankle joint

Z96.661   Presence of right artificial ankle joint

Z96.662   Presence of left artificial ankle joint

Z96.669   Presence of unspecified artificial ankle joint ▽

✓6ᵗʰ **Z96.69**   Presence of other orthopedic joint implants

Z96.691   Finger-joint replacement of right hand

Z96.692   Finger-joint replacement of left hand

Z96.693   Finger-joint replacement, bilateral

Z96.698   Presence of other orthopedic joint implants

Z96.7   Presence of other bone and tendon implants
- Presence of skull plate

✓5ᵗʰ **Z96.8**   Presence of other specified functional implants

Z96.81   Presence of artificial skin

Z96.89   Presence of other specified functional implants

Z96.9   Presence of functional implant, unspecified ▽

✓4ᵗʰ **Z97**   **Presence of other devices**

> EXCLUDES 1   complications of internal prosthetic devices, implants and grafts (T82-T85)
> fitting and adjustment of prosthetic and other devices (Z44-Z46)
> EXCLUDES 2   presence of cerebrospinal fluid drainage device (Z98.2)

Z97.0   Presence of artificial eye

✓5ᵗʰ **Z97.1**   Presence of artificial limb (complete) (partial)

Z97.10   Presence of artificial limb (complete) (partial), unspecified ▽

Z97.11   Presence of artificial right arm (complete) (partial)

Z97.12   Presence of artificial left arm (complete) (partial)

Z97.13   Presence of artificial right leg (complete) (partial)

Z97.14   Presence of artificial left leg (complete) (partial)

Z97.15   Presence of artificial arms, bilateral (complete) (partial)

Z97.16   Presence of artificial legs, bilateral (complete) (partial)

Z97.2   Presence of dental prosthetic device (complete) (partial)
- Presence of dentures (complete) (partial)

Z97.3   Presence of spectacles and contact lenses

Z97.4   Presence of external hearing-aid

Z97.5   Presence of (intrauterine) contraceptive device ♀

> EXCLUDES 1   ▶checking, reinsertion or removal of implantable subdermal contraceptive (Z30.46)◀
> ▶checking, reinsertion or removal of intrauterine contraceptive device (Z30.43-)◀

Z97.8   Presence of other specified devices

✓4ᵗʰ **Z98**   **Other postprocedural states**

> EXCLUDES 2   aftercare (Z43-Z49, Z51)
> follow-up medical care (Z08-Z09)
> postprocedural complication - see Alphabetical Index

Z98.0   Intestinal bypass and anastomosis status

> EXCLUDES 2   bariatric surgery status (Z98.84)
> gastric bypass status (Z98.84)
> obesity surgery status (Z98.84)

Z98.1   Arthrodesis status

Z98.2   Presence of cerebrospinal fluid drainage device
- Presence of CSF shunt

Z98.3   Post therapeutic collapse of lung status
- Code first underlying disease

✓5ᵗʰ **Z98.4**   Cataract extraction status
- Use additional code to identify intraocular lens implant status (Z96.1)

> EXCLUDES 1   aphakia (H27.0)

Z98.41   Cataract extraction status, right eye

Z98.42   Cataract extraction status, left eye

Z98.49   Cataract extraction status, unspecified eye ▽

✓5ᵗʰ **Z98.5**   Sterilization status

> EXCLUDES 1   female infertility (N97.-)
> male infertility (N46.-)

Z98.51   Tubal ligation status ♀

Z98.52   Vasectomy status Ⓐ ♂

✓5ᵗʰ **Z98.6**   Angioplasty status

Z98.61   Coronary angioplasty status

> EXCLUDES 1   coronary angioplasty status with implant and graft (Z95.5)

Z98.62   Peripheral vascular angioplasty status

> EXCLUDES 1   peripheral vascular angioplasty status with implant and graft (Z95.820)

✓5ᵗʰ **Z98.8**   Other specified postprocedural states

✓6ᵗʰ **Z98.81**   Dental procedure status

Z98.810   Dental sealant status

Z98.811   Dental restoration status
- Dental crown status
- Dental fillings status

Z98.818   Other dental procedure status

Z98.82   Breast implant status

> EXCLUDES 1   breast implant removal status (Z98.86)

Z98.83   Filtering (vitreous) bleb after glaucoma surgery status

> EXCLUDES 1   inflammation (infection) of postprocedural bleb (H59.4-)

Z98.84   Bariatric surgery status
- Gastric banding status
- Gastric bypass status for obesity
- Obesity surgery status

> EXCLUDES 1   bariatric surgery status complicating pregnancy, childbirth, or the puerperium (O99.84)
> EXCLUDES 2   intestinal bypass and anastomosis status (Z98.0)

Z98.85   Transplanted organ removal status
- Transplanted organ previously removed due to complication, failure, rejection or infection

> EXCLUDES 1   encounter for removal of transplanted organ - code to complication of transplanted organ (T86.-)

Z98.86   Personal history of breast implant removal

EXCLUDES 1   Not coded here   EXCLUDES 2   Not included here   PDx   Primary Dx Only   Ⓝ Newborn Age : 0   Ⓟ Pediatric Age : 0-17   Ⓜ Maternity Age : 12-55   Ⓐ Adult Age : 15-124

☑6ᵗʰ **Z98.87**   **Personal history of** in utero procedure

    Z98.870   **Personal history of in utero**   ♀
       procedure during pregnancy

        EXCLUDES 2 *complications from in utero*
              procedure for current
              pregnancy (O35.7)
              supervision of current pregnancy
              with history of in utero
              procedure during previous
              pregnancy (O09.82-)

    Z98.871   **Personal history of in utero procedure**
       while a fetus

☑6ᵗʰ **Z98.89**   **Other specified postprocedural states**

●   **Z98.890**   **Other specified postprocedural states**

       Personal history of surgery, not elsewhere
       classified

●   **Z98.891**   **History of uterine scar from previous**
       surgery

        EXCLUDES 1 *maternal care due to uterine scar*
              from previous surgery
              (O34.2-)

☑4ᵗʰ **Z99**   **Dependence on enabling machines and devices, not elsewhere classified**

    EXCLUDES 1 *cardiac pacemaker status (Z95.0)*

Z99.0   **Dependence on** aspirator

☑5ᵗʰ **Z99.1**   **Dependence on** respirator

    Dependence on ventilator

    Z99.11   **Dependence on respirator [ventilator] status**

       AHA: 2015,1Q,21

    Z99.12   **Encounter for respirator [ventilator]**   PDx
       dependence during power failure

        EXCLUDES 1 *mechanical complication of respirator*
              [ventilator] (J95.850)

Z99.2   **Dependence on** renal dialysis

    Hemodialysis status
    Peritoneal dialysis status
    Presence of arteriovenous shunt for dialysis
    Renal dialysis status NOS

    EXCLUDES 1 *encounter for fitting and adjustment of dialysis*
          catheter (Z49.0-)

    EXCLUDES 2 ▶*noncompliance with renal dialysis (Z91.15)*◀

    AHA: 2016,1Q,12; 2013,4Q,125

Z99.3   **Dependence on** wheelchair

    Wheelchair confinement status
    Code first cause of dependence, such as:
      muscular dystrophy (G71.0)
      obesity (E66.-)

☑5ᵗʰ **Z99.8**   **Dependence on other enabling machines and devices**

    Z99.81   **Dependence on** supplemental oxygen

       Dependence on long-term oxygen

       AHA: 2013,4Q,129

    Z99.89   **Dependence on other enabling machines and devices**

       Dependence on machine or device NOS

☑ Additional Character Required   ☑x7ᵗʰ Placeholder Alert   Manifestation Dx   ▽ Unspecified Dx   ▶◀ Revised Text   ● New Code   ▲ Revised Code Title

ICD-10-CM 2017   **1171**

Appendixes

Appendix A: 10 Steps to Correct Coding

Follow the 10 steps below to correctly code encounters for health care services.

Step 1: Identify the reason for the visit or encounter (i.e., a sign, symptom, diagnosis and/or condition).

The medical record documentation should accurately reflect the patient's condition, using terminology that includes specific diagnoses and symptoms or clearly states the reasons for the encounter.

Choosing the main term that best describes the reason chiefly responsible for the service provided is the most important step in coding. If symptoms are present and documented but a definitive diagnosis has not yet been determined, code the symptoms. **For outpatient cases, do not code conditions that are referred to as "rule out," "suspected," "probable," or "questionable."** Diagnoses often are not established at the time of the initial encounter/visit and may require two or more visits to be established. Code only what is documented in the available records and only to the highest degree of certainty known at the time of the patient's visit, unless it is an inpatient medical record, in which case uncertain diagnoses may be reported if documented at the time of discharge.

Step 2: After selecting the reason for the encounter, always consult the alphabetic index before verifying code selection in the tabular section.

The most critical rule is to begin code selection in the *alphabetic index*. Never turn first to the tabular list. The index provides cross-references, essential and nonessential modifiers, and inclusion terms not found in the tabular list. To prevent coding errors, always use both the alphabetic index (to identify a code) and the tabular list (to verify a code), as the index does not include the important instructional notes found in the tabular list. An added benefit of using the tabular list, which groups like things together, is that while looking at one code in the list, a coder might see a more specific one that would have been missed had the coder relied solely on the alphabetic index. Additionally, many of the codes require a fourth, fifth, sixth, or seventh, character to be valid, and many of these characters can be found only in the tabular list.

Step 3: Locate the main term entry.

The alphabetic index is a listing of conditions, which may be expressed as nouns or eponyms, with critical use of adjectives. Some conditions known by several names have multiple main entries. Reasons for encounters may be located under general terms such as admission, encounter, and examination. Other general terms such as history of, status post, or presence (of) are used to locate factors influencing health.

Step 4: Read cross-references listed with the main term or the subterm.

Cross-references such as *"see"* and *"see also"* are identified by italicized type and should always be checked to ensure that all alternative terms are researched.

Step 5: Review entries for modifiers.

Nonessential modifiers are the terms in parentheses following the main term entry. These parenthetical terms are supplementary words or explanatory information that may or may not appear in the diagnostic statement and do not affect code selection. The subterms listed under the main term are essential modifiers that do affect coding assignment. Each line of indent represents a more specific code entry. The nonessential modifiers apply to the subterms following a main term except when they are mutually exclusive, in which case the subterm takes precedence. For example, if "acute" is listed as a nonessential modifier but there is a subentry for "chronic," then the nonessential modifier of "acute" does not apply.

Step 6: Interpret abbreviations, cross-references, default codes, additional characters, and brackets.

The abbreviation NEC (not elsewhere classified) that follows some main terms or subterms indicates that there is no specific code for the condition even though the medical documentation may be very specific. The code next to the main term is called the default code. It represents the condition most commonly associated with the main term or the unspecified code for the main term. Additional characters may be required to construct the code; the tabular list must be referenced to determine what those specific characters should be. The alphabetic index uses brackets [] to enclose manifestation codes that can be

used only as secondary codes to the underlying condition code immediately preceding it. Both codes must be reported in this multiple-coding situation.

Step 7: Choose a potential code and locate it in the tabular list.

The coder must follow any Includes, Excludes 1 and Excludes 2 notes, and other instructional notes, such as "Code first" and "Use additional code," listed in the tabular list for the chapter, category, subcategory, and subclassification level of code selection that direct the coder to use a different or additional code. Any codes in the tabular range, A00.0- through T88.9-, may be used to identify the diagnostic reason for the encounter. The tabular list encompasses many codes describing disease and injury classifications (e.g., infectious and parasitic diseases, neoplasms, symptoms, nervous and circulatory system etc.).

Codes that describe symptoms and signs, as opposed to definitive diagnoses, should be used for reporting purposes when an established diagnosis has not been made (confirmed) by the physician. Chapter 18 of the ICD-10-CM code book, "Symptoms, Signs, and Abnormal Clinical and Laboratory Findings, Not Elsewhere Classified" (codes R00.--R99), contains many, but not all, codes for symptoms.

ICD-10-CM classifies encounters with health care providers for circumstances other than a disease or injury using codes in chapter 21, "Factors Influencing Health Status and Contact with Health Services" (codes Z00–Z99). Circumstances other than a disease or injury often are recorded as chiefly responsible for the encounter.

Step 8: Determine whether the code is at the highest level of specificity.

A code is invalid if it has not been coded to the full number of characters (greatest level of specificity) required. Codes in ICD-10-CM can contain from three up to seven alphanumeric characters. A three-character code is to be used only if the category is not further subdivided into four-, five-, or six-character codes. Placeholder character X is used both to allow for future expansion and as a placeholder for empty characters in a code that requires a seventh character but has no fourth, fifth, or sixth character. Certain categories require seventh characters that apply to all codes in that category. Always check the category level for applicable seventh characters for that category.

Step 9: Assign the code.

Having reviewed all relevant information concerning the possible code choices, assign the code that most completely describes the condition.

Repeat steps one through nine for all additional documented conditions that meet the following criteria:

- Conditions that currently exist at the time of the visit
- Conditions that require or affect patient care, treatment, or management

Step 10: Sequence codes correctly.

Sequencing is the order in which the codes are listed on the claim. List first the ICD-10-CM code for the diagnosis, condition, problem, or other reason for the encounter/visit, which is shown in the medical record to be chiefly responsible for the services provided. List additional codes that describe any coexisting conditions. Follow the official coding guidelines (see section II, "Selection of Principal Diagnosis"; section III, "Reporting Additional Diagnoses"; and section IV, "Diagnostic Coding and Reporting Guidelines for Outpatient Services") on proper sequencing of codes.

Coding Examples

Diagnosis: Anorexia

Step 1: The reason for the encounter was the condition, anorexia.

Step 2: Consult the alphabetic index.

Step 3: Locate the main term "Anorexia."

Step 4: There are no cross-references to check.

Step 5: Note that there are two possible subterms (essential modifiers), "hysterical" and "nervosa," neither of which is documented in this instance and therefore cannot be used in code selection. The code listed next to the main term is called the default code selection.

Step 6: There are no abbreviations, cross-references, additional character icons, or brackets.

Step 7: Turn to code R63.Ø in the tabular list and read the instructional notes. In this case the Excludes 1 note indicates that anorexia nervosa and loss of appetite determined to be of nonorganic origin should be coded to a code from chapter 5. The diagnostic statement does not indicate nonorganic origin.

Step 8: There is no further division of the category past the fourth character subcategory. Therefore, the subcategory code level is the highest level of specificity.

Step 9: The default code, R63.Ø Anorexia, is the correct code selection

Step 10: Since anorexia is listed as the chief reason for the health care encounter, the first-listed, or principal, diagnosis is R63.Ø. Note that this is a chapter 18 symptom code but can be assigned since the provider did not establish a more definitive diagnosis.

Diagnosis: Acute bronchitis

Step 1: The reason for the encounter was the condition, acute bronchitis.

Step 2: Consult the alphabetic index.

Step 3: Locate the main term "Bronchitis."

Step 4: There are cross-references to interpret.

Step 5: Review entries for modifiers. Since "acute" is not listed as a nonessential modifier, read past the "with" modifier until you find the subterm "acute or subacute" with a nonessential modifier of "with bronchospasm or obstruction," code J2Ø.9.

Step 6: There are no abbreviations, cross-references, additional character icons, or brackets.

Step 7: Since there are no more appropriate subterms, turn to code J2Ø.9 in the tabular list. The Includes note under category J2Ø does refer to other alternative terms for acute bronchitis. Note that the inclusion term list is not exhaustive but is only a representative selection of diagnoses that are included in the subcategory. The Excludes 1 note refers bronchitis and tracheobronchitis NOS to category J4Ø. There are several Excludes 2 notes that, if applicable, can be coded in addition to this code.

Step 8: Note that the subcategories included in J2Ø represent acute bronchitis due to various infectious organisms that would be selected if identified in the documentation. In this case, the organism was not identified and there is no further division of the category past the fourth character subcategory. Therefore, the subcategory code level is the highest level of specificity.

Step 9: Assign code J2Ø.9 Acute bronchitis, unspecified.

Step 10: Repeat steps 1-9 for any additional code assignments.

Diagnosis: Infectious diarrhea

Step 1: The reason for the encounter was the condition, infectious diarrhea.

Step 2: Consult the alphabetic index.

Step 3: Locate the main term "Diarrhea" in the alphabetic index.

Step 4: There are no cross-references to check.

Step 5: Review entries for modifiers. Note that the nonessential modifiers (in parentheses) after the main term do not include the term "infectious," which means that the coder should search the subterms for the term "infectious." The subterm "infectious" refers to code AØ9.

Step 6: There are no abbreviations, cross-references, additional character icons, or brackets.

Step 7: Locate code AØ9 in the tabular list, and read all instructional notes under the main category and subcategories. The Includes notes does not list the term "infectious diarrhea" under code AØ9; however, as instructed by the alphabetic index, you should code the condition to AØ9. The ICD-1Ø-CM code book implies that infectious diarrhea is the same as infectious gastroenteritis, enteritis, and colitis.

Step 8: There is no further division of the category past the third-character category level. Therefore, the category code level is the highest level of specificity. The final code assignment would be AØ9.

Step 9: Assign code AØ9 Infectious gastroenteritis and colitis, unspecified.

Step 10: Since infectious diarrhea is listed as the chief reason for the health care encounter, the first-listed, or principal, diagnosis is AØ9.

Diagnosis: Decubitus ulcer of right elbow with skin loss and necrosis of subcutaneous tissue

Step 1: The reason for the encounter was the condition, decubitus ulcer.

Step 2: Consult the alphabetic index.

Step 3: Locate the main term "Ulcer" in the alphabetic index.

Step 4: There are no cross-references to check.

Step 5: This entry does not have any important nonessential modifiers; however, there are other terms such as ulcerated, ulcerating, etc., that are included as main terms. Locate the subterm "decubitus" and note that there is an italicized cross-reference to "*see* Ulcer, pressure, by site." Go to the subterm "pressure" and locate "elbow," which refers to code L89.Ø-.

Step 6: Note that the code L89.Ø is followed by a dash and an additional character icon, which indicate that more characters are required. From here, the tabular list can be consulted at code L89.Ø-.

Step 7: Locate code L89.Ø in the tabular list, and check the category level L89 for any instructional, Includes, and Excludes 1 and 2 notes. Note that "decubitus" is an Includes note under L89 Pressure ulcer. Excludes 2 notes indicate that if this were documented as a diabetic pressure ulcer, it would be necessary to use a code from chapter 4.

Step 8: Read through the subcategory codes under L89.Ø and note that the fifth character describes laterality. Locate the right elbow at subcategory L89.Ø1. See that an additional sixth character is now needed to complete the code. The sixth character specifies the stage of the ulcer, which can be determined either by the specific documentation of the stage (e.g., stage 1, stage 2) or in this case, a description that matches one of the Includes notes that follow each stage code. For example, the description in this case of "skin loss and necrosis of the subcutaneous tissue" matches the Includes notes under L89.Ø13 Pressure ulcer of right elbow, stage 3.

Step 9: Assign code L89.Ø13 Pressure ulcer of right elbow, stage 3

Step 10: Since the decubitus ulcer is listed as the chief reason for the health care encounter, the first-listed, or principal, diagnosis is L89.Ø13. However, according to the Code first instructional note at the L89 category level, gangrene would be sequenced before the pressure ulcer if it were documented.

Diagnosis: First visit for bimalleolar fracture of the right ankle due to trauma

Step 1: The reason for the encounter was the condition, bimalleolar fracture of the right ankle.

Step 2: Consult the alphabetic index.

Step 3: Locate the main term "Fracture" in the alphabetic index.

Step 4: Note that the first main term for Fracture is pathological with cross-reference to "*see also* Fracture, traumatic." Locate the main term "Fracture, traumatic."

Step 5: Review entries for nonessential modifiers. Locate the subterms "ankle," "bimalleolar." Note that "displaced" is a nonessential modifier following "bimalleolar," indicating that S82.84- is the default code unless the fracture is specified as nondisplaced.

Step 6: Note that code S82.84- is followed by a dash and an additional character icon, both of which indicate that more characters are required. From here, the tabular list can be consulted at code S82.84.

Step 7: Locate code S82.84 Bimalleolar fracture of lower leg, in the tabular list and check the category level S82 for any instructional, Includes, and Excludes 1 and 2 notes. See the instructional notes indicating that fractures not specified as displaced or nondisplaced default to displaced, and fractures not designated as open or closed default to closed. See also the list of appropriate seventh characters to be added to all codes from category S82.

Step 8: Read through the subcategory codes under S82.84, and note that the sixth character specifies displaced or nondisplaced and laterality. Locate the displaced bimalleolar fracture of the right lower leg at code S82.841. See that an additional seventh character is still needed to complete the code. The seventh character specifies the type of encounter and whether the fracture is open or closed. Use character A listed in the box at the category level to describe initial encounter, closed fracture.

Step 9: Assign code S82.841A Displaced bimalleolar fracture of right lower leg, initial encounter for closed fracture.

Step 10: Since this is an injury code, code additionally any external cause, place of occurrence, and activity codes, with the injury (fracture) sequenced first.

Appendix B: Valid 3-character ICD-10-CM Codes

A09	Infectious gastroenteritis and colitis, unspecified
A33	Tetanus neonatorum
A34	Obstetrical tetanus
A35	Other tetanus
A46	Erysipelas
A55	Chlamydial lymphogranuloma (venereum)
A57	Chancroid
A58	Granuloma inguinale
A64	Unspecified sexually transmitted disease
A65	Nonvenereal syphilis
A70	Chlamydia psittaci infections
A78	Q fever
A86	Unspecified viral encephalitis
A89	Unspecified viral infection of central nervous system
A90	Dengue fever [classical dengue]
A91	Dengue hemorrhagic fever
A94	Unspecified arthropod-borne viral fever
A99	Unspecified viral hemorrhagic fever
B03	Smallpox
B04	Monkeypox
B09	Unspecified viral infection characterized by skin and mucous membrane lesions
B20	Human immunodeficiency virus [HIV] disease
B49	Unspecified mycosis
B54	Unspecified malaria
B59	Pneumocystosis
B64	Unspecified protozoal disease
B72	Dracunculiasis
B75	Trichinellosis
B79	Trichuriasis
B80	Enterobiasis
B86	Scabies
B89	Unspecified parasitic disease
B91	Sequelae of poliomyelitis
B92	Sequelae of leprosy
C01	Malignant neoplasm of base of tongue
C07	Malignant neoplasm of parotid gland
C12	Malignant neoplasm of pyriform sinus
C19	Malignant neoplasm of rectosigmoid junction
C20	Malignant neoplasm of rectum
C23	Malignant neoplasm of gallbladder
C33	Malignant neoplasm of trachea
C37	Malignant neoplasm of thymus
C52	Malignant neoplasm of vagina
C55	Malignant neoplasm of uterus, part unspecified
C58	Malignant neoplasm of placenta
C61	Malignant neoplasm of prostate
C73	Malignant neoplasm of thyroid gland
D34	Benign neoplasm of thyroid gland
D45	Polycythemia vera
D62	Acute posthemorrhagic anemia
D65	Disseminated intravascular coagulation [defibrination syndrome]
D66	Hereditary factor VIII deficiency
D67	Hereditary factor IX deficiency
D71	Functional disorders of polymorphonuclear neutrophils
D77	Other disorders of blood and blood-forming organs in diseases classified elsewhere
E02	Subclinical iodine-deficiency hypothyroidism
E15	Nondiabetic hypoglycemic coma
E35	Disorders of endocrine glands in diseases classified elsewhere
E40	Kwashiorkor
E41	Nutritional marasmus
E42	Marasmic kwashiorkor

E43	Unspecified severe protein-calorie malnutrition
E45	Retarded development following protein-calorie malnutrition
E46	Unspecified protein-calorie malnutrition
E52	Niacin deficiency [pellagra]
E54	Ascorbic acid deficiency
E58	Dietary calcium deficiency
E59	Dietary selenium deficiency
E60	Dietary zinc deficiency
E65	Localized adiposity
E68	Sequelae of hyperalimentation
F04	Amnestic disorder due to known physiological condition
F05	Delirium due to known physiological condition
F09	Unspecified mental disorder due to known physiological condition
F21	Schizotypal disorder
F22	Delusional disorders
F23	Brief psychotic disorder
F24	Shared psychotic disorder
F28	Other psychotic disorder not due to a substance or known physiological condition
F29	Unspecified psychosis not due to a substance or known physiological condition
F39	Unspecified mood [affective] disorder
F53	Puerperal psychosis
F54	Psychological and behavioral factors associated with disorders or diseases classified elsewhere
F59	Unspecified behavioral syndromes associated with physiological disturbances and physical factors
F66	Other sexual disorders
F69	Unspecified disorder of adult personality and behavior
F70	Mild intellectual disabilities
F71	Moderate intellectual disabilities
F72	Severe intellectual disabilities
F73	Profound intellectual disabilities
F78	Other intellectual disabilities
F79	Unspecified intellectual disabilities
F82	Specific developmental disorder of motor function
F88	Other disorders of psychological development
F89	Unspecified disorder of psychological development
F99	Mental disorder, not otherwise specified
G01	Meningitis in bacterial diseases classified elsewhere
G02	Meningitis in other infectious and parasitic diseases classified elsewhere
G07	Intracranial and intraspinal abscess and granuloma in diseases classified elsewhere
G08	Intracranial and intraspinal phlebitis and thrombophlebitis
G09	Sequelae of inflammatory diseases of central nervous system
G10	Huntington's disease
G14	Postpolio syndrome
G20	Parkinson's disease
G26	Extrapyramidal and movement disorders in diseases classified elsewhere
G35	Multiple sclerosis
G53	Cranial nerve disorders in diseases classified elsewhere
G55	Nerve root and plexus compressions in diseases classified elsewhere
G59	Mononeuropathy in diseases classified elsewhere
G63	Polyneuropathy in diseases classified elsewhere
G64	Other disorders of peripheral nervous system
G92	Toxic encephalopathy
G94	Other disorders of brain in diseases classified elsewhere
H22	Disorders of iris and ciliary body in diseases classified elsewhere
H28	Cataract in diseases classified elsewhere
H32	Chorioretinal disorders in diseases classified elsewhere
H36	Retinal disorders in diseases classified elsewhere
H42	Glaucoma in diseases classified elsewhere

I00	Rheumatic fever without heart involvement
I10	Essential (primary) hypertension
I32	Pericarditis in diseases classified elsewhere
I38	Endocarditis, valve unspecified
I39	Endocarditis and heart valve disorders in diseases classified elsewhere
I41	Myocarditis in diseases classified elsewhere
I43	Cardiomyopathy in diseases classified elsewhere
I52	Other heart disorders in diseases classified elsewhere
I76	Septic arterial embolism
I81	Portal vein thrombosis
I96	Gangrene, not elsewhere classified
J00	Acute nasopharyngitis (common cold)
J13	Pneumonia due to Streptococcus pneumoniae
J14	Pneumonia due to Hemophilus influenzae
J17	Pneumonia in diseases classified elsewhere
J22	Unspecified acute lower respiratory infection
J36	Peritonsillar abscess
J40	Bronchitis, not specified as acute or chronic
J42	Unspecified chronic bronchitis
J60	Coalworker's pneumoconiosis
J61	Pneumoconiosis due to asbestos and other mineral fibers
J64	Unspecified pneumoconiosis
J65	Pneumoconiosis associated with tuberculosis
J80	Acute respiratory distress syndrome
J82	Pulmonary eosinophilia, not elsewhere classified
J90	Pleural effusion, not elsewhere classified
J99	Respiratory disorders in diseases classified elsewhere
K23	Disorders of esophagus in diseases classified elsewhere
K30	Functional dyspepsia
K36	Other appendicitis
K37	Unspecified appendicitis
K67	Disorders of peritoneum in infectious diseases classified elsewhere
K77	Liver disorders in diseases classified elsewhere
K87	Disorders of gallbladder, biliary tract and pancreas in diseases classified elsewhere
L00	Staphylococcal scalded skin syndrome
L14	Bullous disorders in diseases classified elsewhere
L22	Diaper dermatitis
L26	Exfoliative dermatitis
L42	Pityriasis rosea
L45	Papulosquamous disorders in diseases classified elsewhere
L52	Erythema nodosum
L54	Erythema in diseases classified elsewhere
L62	Nail disorders in diseases classified elsewhere
L80	Vitiligo
L83	Acanthosis nigricans
L84	Corns and callosities
L86	Keratoderma in diseases classified elsewhere
L88	Pyoderma gangrenosum
L99	Other disorders of skin and subcutaneous tissue in diseases classified elsewhere
N08	Glomerular disorders in diseases classified elsewhere
N10	Acute tubulo-interstitial nephritis
N12	Tubulo-interstitial nephritis, not specified as acute or chronic
N16	Renal tubulo-interstitial disorders in diseases classified elsewhere
N19	Unspecified kidney failure
N22	Calculus of urinary tract in diseases classified elsewhere
N23	Unspecified renal colic
N29	Other disorders of kidney and ureter in diseases classified elsewhere
N33	Bladder disorders in diseases classified elsewhere
N37	Urethral disorders in diseases classified elsewhere
N51	Disorders of male genital organs in diseases classified elsewhere
N62	Hypertrophy of breast
N63	Unspecified lump in breast
N72	Inflammatory disease of cervix uteri
N74	Female pelvic inflammatory disorders in diseases classified

	elsewhere
N86	Erosion and ectropion of cervix uteri
N96	Recurrent pregnancy loss
O68	Labor and delivery complicated by abnormality of fetal acid-base balance
O76	Abnormality in fetal heart rate and rhythm complicating labor and delivery
O80	Encounter for full-term uncomplicated delivery
O82	Encounter for cesarean delivery without indication
O85	Puerperal sepsis
O94	Sequelae of complication of pregnancy, childbirth, and the puerperium
P09	Abnormal findings on neonatal screening
P53	Hemorrhagic disease of newborn
P60	Disseminated intravascular coagulation of newborn
P84	Other problems with newborn
P90	Convulsions of newborn
P95	Stillbirth
Q02	Microcephaly
R05	Cough
R12	Heartburn
R17	Unspecified jaundice
R21	Rash and other nonspecific skin eruption
R32	Unspecified urinary incontinence
R34	Anuria and oliguria
R37	Sexual dysfunction, unspecified
R42	Dizziness and giddiness
R51	Headache
R52	Pain, unspecified
R54	Age-related physical debility
R55	Syncope and collapse
R58	Hemorrhage, not elsewhere classified
R61	Generalized hyperhidrosis
R64	Cachexia
R69	Illness, unspecified
R75	Inconclusive laboratory evidence of human immunodeficiency virus [HIV]
R81	Glycosuria
R99	Ill-defined and unknown cause of mortality
T07	Unspecified multiple injuries
Y09	Assault by unspecified means
Y66	Nonadministration of surgical and medical care
Y69	Unspecified misadventure during surgical and medical care
Y95	Nosocomial condition
Z08	Encounter for follow-up examination after completed treatment for malignant neoplasm
Z09	Encounter for follow-up examination after completed treatment for conditions other than malignant neoplasm
Z21	Asymptomatic human immunodeficiency virus [HIV] infection status
Z23	Encounter for immunization
Z36	Encounter for antenatal screening of mother
Z66	Do not resuscitate

Appendix C: Pharmacology List 2017

This section enables the coder to quickly review drugs, drug actions, and indications that are often associated with overlooked or undocumented diagnoses. The coder should review the patient's medication record and know what condition the physician is treating with the prescribed medication based on documentation in the medical record. When documentation is lacking, the coder can reference this section to locate the drug, determine the drug action, confirm drug indications, and when necessary query the physician.

Drug	Drug Action	Indications
Accupril [quinapril]	ACE inhibitor; antihypertensive	Congestive heart failure; essential hypertension
Acetaminophen and codeine [acetominophen/codeine phosphate]	Analgesic	Pain, moderate to severe
Actemra [tocilizumab]	Antirheumatic	Rheumatoid arthritis
Actonel [risedronate]	Electrolytic and renal agent; bone resorption inhibitor	Decrease bone loss in multiple myeloma patients; Paget's disease; hyperparathyroidism; osteoporosis
Adalat CC [nifedipine]	Calcium channel blocker	Vasospastic angina; chronic stable angina; essential hypertension
Aldactone [spironolactone]	Cardiovascular agent; antihypertensive agent; diuretic; electrolytic and renal agent	Treatment of severe heart failure; ascites associated with cirrhosis; hypokalemia
Allegra [fexofenadine/ hydrochloride pseudoephedrine]	Antihistamine	Seasonal allergic rhinitis
Allopurinol [allopurinol]	Antigout	Gouty arthritis, renal calculus, hyperuricemia, hyperuricemia secondary to leukemia, hyperuricemia secondary to lymphoma
Alphagan P [brimonidine]	Antiglaucoma agent (ophthalmic) antihypertensive, ocular	Open angle glaucoma or another condition in which pressure in the eye is too high (ocular hypertension)
Alprazolam [alprazolam]	Antianxiety; sedative/hypnotic	
Altace [ramipril]	ACE inhibitor; antihypertensive	Congestive heart failure, essential hypertension
Amaryl [glimepiride]	Blood glucose regulator	Diabetes mellitus
Ambien [zolpidem]	Sedative/hypnotic	Insomnia
Abilify [aripiprazole]	Antipsychotic	Depression, bipolar disorder, schizophrenia, autism symptoms
Amikacin [amikacin sulfate]	Aminoglycoside antibiotic	Active in treatment of gram-negative bacterial infections such as *Pseudomonas, Escherichia coli (E. coli), Proteus, Klebsiella-Enterobacter-Serratia*
Aminophylline [aminophylline]	Bronchodilator, pulmonary vasodilator, smooth muscle relaxant	Relief and/or prevention of symptoms from asthma and reversible bronchospasms in bronchitis and emphysema
Amitriptyline hydrochloride [amitriptyline hydrochloride]	Anorexiant/CNS stimulant; antidepressant	Depression
Amoxicillin, Amoxil [amoxicillin]	Penicillin	Effective for infections with a broad spectrum of bactericidal activity against many gram-positive and gram-negative micro-organisms; otitis media, gonorrhea, skin, respiratory, gastrointestinal, and genitourinary infections
Amrix [cyclobenzaprine hydrochloride]	Muscle relaxant	Adjunct to rest and physical therapy for muscle spasms
Ancef [cefazoline sodium]	Semisynthetic cephalosporin antibiotic	Respiratory tract infections due to *Streptococcus pneumoniae, Klebsiella species, Haemophilus influenzae (H. influenzae), Staphylococcus aureus*, and group A betahemolytic streptococci; urinary tract infections due to *E. coli*, Proteus mirabilis, Klebsiella species and some strains of Enterobacter and enterococci; skin and skin structure infections, biliary tract infections, bone and joint infections, genital infections, septicemia, and endocarditis
Antabuse [disulfiram]	Alcohol treatment	Alcoholism
Anzemet [dolasetron mesylate]	Antiemetic/ antinauseant	Management of nausea/vomiting following surgery or from effects of chemotherapy or cancer
Aranesp [darbepoetin alfa]	Erythropoiesis-stimulating agent (ESA)	Treat lower than normal blood cells (anemia) from disorders such as CKD and neoplasms
Aricept [donepezil hydrochloride]	Acetylcholine sterase inhibitor	Symptoms of mild to moderate Alzheimer's disease; can improve thinking ability in some patients
Arthrotec [diclofenac/misoprostol]	Analgesic	Treatment of patients with arthritis who may develop stomach ulcers from taking nonsteroidal anti-inflammatory drugs (NSAIDs) alone; used to help relieve some symptoms of arthritis, such as inflammation, swelling, stiffness, and joint pain

Drug	Drug Action	Indications
Atenolol [atenolol]	Antianginal; antihypertensive; beta blocker	Chronic stable angina pectoris; essential hypertension; reduces cardiovascular mortality in those with definite or suspected acute myocardial infarction
Ativan [lorazepam]	Antianxiety; sedative/hypnotic	Anxiety disorder associated with depressive symptoms; controls tension, agitation, irritability, and insomnia
Atrovent [ipratropium bromide]	Antiasthmatic/bronchodilator	Chronic bronchitis, emphysema; bronchial asthma
Augmentin [amoxicillin/clavulanate]	Antibacterial	Middle ear, lower respiratory, sinus, skin and skin structures, and urinary tract infections
Avapro [irbesartan]	Antihypertensive	Hypertension
Axid [nizatidine]	Histamine H2-receptor antagonist	Acid/peptic disorder; gastroesophageal reflux; duodenal, gastric, and peptic ulcers
Bactrim [sulfamethoxazole trimethoprim]	Antibacterial	Treatment of urinary tract infections, acute otitis media, acute exacerbation of chronic bronchitis, shigellosis, and pneumocystis carinii
Bactroban [mupirocin]	Dermatologic; topical anti-infective	Topical treatment of impetigo
Beconase AQ [beclomethasone dipropionate monohydrate]	Corticosteroids; antiasthmatic	Bronchial asthma, prevention of nasal polyps, perennial allergies, seasonal allergies and vasomotor rhinitis
Betoptic [betaxolol hydrochloride]	Cardioselective beta-adrenergic receptor blocking agent	Lowers intraocular pressure; also used for treatment of ocular hypertension and chronic open-angle glaucoma
Biaxin [clarithromycin]	Macrolide	Acid/peptic disorder or ulcer, acute exacerbation chronic bronchitis, human immunodeficiency virus, lower and upper respiratory tract infection, sinus infection, prophylaxis mycobacterium avium complex, pharyngitis, pneumonia, tonsillitis
Buspirone [buspirone hydrochloride]	Antianxiety	Generalized anxiety disorder
Butorphanol Tartrate [butorphanol tartrate]	Narcotic analgesic	Moderate to severe postsurgical pain
Calan [verapamil hydrochloride]	Antianginal; antiarrhythmic, antiarthritic, antihypertensive, calcium channel blocker	Angina pectoris at rest and chronic stable, arrhythmia, atrial fibrillation, atrial flutter, paroxysmal supraventricular tachycardia, ventricular arrhythmia, essential hypertension
Cardizem CD, Tiazac [diltiazem hydrochloride]	Antianginal, antiarrhythmic, antihypertensive, channel blocker, coronary vasodilator	Chronic stable angina, atrial fibrillation, atrial flutter, essential hypertension, paroxysmal supraventricular tachycardia
Cardura [doxazosin mesylate]	Antihypertensive	Benign prostatic hyperplasia, essential hypertension
Catapres, Clonidine [clonidine]	Antihypertensive	Hypertension
Ceftin [cefuroxime axetil]	Antibiotic: second generation cephalosporins	Acute exacerbation and chronic bronchitis, middle ear infection, sexually transmitted gonorrhea infection, upper respiratory tract infection, urinary tract infection, pharyngitis, tonsillitis
Cefprozil [cefprozil]	Antibiotic: second generation cephalosporins	Acute exacerbation and chronic bronchitis, lower respiratory tract infection, upper respiratory tract infection, pharyngitis, tonsillitis
Celebrex [celecoxib]	Antirheumatic, nonsteroidal anti-inflammatory	Relief of some symptoms caused by arthritis, such as inflammation, swelling, stiffness, and joint pain
Celexa [citalopram hydrobromide]	Antidepressant	Depression
Chantix [varenicline]	Smoking cessation aid	Nicotine addiction, smoking
Cipro [ciprofloxacin]	Anti-infective; quinolone	Cystitis, infectious diarrhea, gonorrhea, bone and joint infection, gastrointestinal tract infection, lower and upper respiratory tract infection, sinus infection, urinary tract infection, nosocomial pneumonia, chronic prostatitis
Claritin [loratadine/ pseudoephedrine sulfate]	Antihistamine	Seasonal allergic rhinitis, chronic idiopathic urticaria
Clonazepam, Klonopin [clonazepam]	Anticonvulsant	Absence, akinetic and myoclonic epilepsy, Lennox-Gastaut syndrome
Cogentin [benztropine mesylate]	Antiparkinsonism	Parkinson's disease
Colace [docusate sodium]	Gastrointestinal agent; laxative, stool softener	Constipation
Combivent [ipratropium bromide/albuterol sulfate]	Antiasthmatic/bronchodilator	Chronic bronchitis, emphysema; bronchial asthma
Compro [prochlorperazine] suppository form only	Antiemetic, antipsychotic	Nausea, vomiting, and manic phase of bipolar syndrome or schizophrenia

Drug	Drug Action	Indications
Cortisporin [hydrocortisone acetate/neomycin sulfate]	Topical anti-infective, topical steroid	Dermatosis
Coumadin [warfarin sodium]	Thrombolytic agent/anticoagulant	Prophylaxis and treatment of venous thrombosis, treatment of atrial fibrillation with embolization (pulmonary embolism), arrhythmias, myocardial infarction, and stroke prevention
Cozaar [losartan]	Antihypertensive	Essential hypertension
Crestor [rosuvastatin calcium]	HMG-CoA reductase inhibitor (statin)	Hypercholesterolemia, hyperlipidemia, hyperproteinemia
Crixivan [indinavir sulfate]	HIV inhibitor	HIV, asymptomatic HIV
Cytomel [liothyronine sodium]	Thyroid hormone	Treatment of hypothyroidism or prevention of euthyroid goiters
Daypro [oxaprozin]	Nonsteroidal anti-inflammatory drug (NSAID)	Osteoarthritis and rheumatoid arthritis
Depakote [divalproex]	Anticonvulsant	Bipolar affective disorder; complex absence, complex partial and mixed pattern epilepsy; migraine headache
Desogen [desogestrel/ethinyl estradiol]	Contraceptive; estrogen/progestin	Contraception
Detrol [tolterodine tartrate]	Muscarinic receptor antagonist	Overactive bladders in patients with urinary frequency, urgency, or urge incontinence
Diflucan [fluconazole]	Antifungal agent	Oropharyngeal and esophageal candidiasis and cryptococcal meningitis in AIDS patients
Digoxin [digoxin]	Cardiotonic glycoside	Heart failure, atrial flutter, atrial fibrillation, and supraventricular tachycardia
Dilantin [phenytoin sodium]	Anticonvulsant	Control of grand mal and psychomotor seizures
Diovan [valsartan]	Ace inhibitor	Essential hypertension
Effexor XR [venlafaxine]	Antidepressant	Depression
Epinephrine [epinephrine]	Bronchodilator, cardiotonic	Most commonly used to relieve respiratory distress due to bronchospasm and to restore cardiac rhythm in cardiac arrest
Epivir, Epivir-HBV [lamivudine]	HIV and HBV inhibitor	HIV, hepatitis B (HBV), asymptomatic HIV
ERY-TAB [erythromycin]	Acne product; macrolide; ocular anti-infective; topical anti-infective	Acne vulgaris, intestinal amebiasis, infectious conjunctivitis, diphtheria, endocarditis, prevention, erythrasma treatment of infections: endocervical, gynecologic, lower and upper respiratory tract, ophthalmic, rectal; skin and skin structures, and urethral; Legionnaires' disease, pelvic inflammatory disease, pertussis, pneumonia, rheumatic fever, prophylaxis, syphilis
Estrace [estradiol]	Estrogen therapy	Vaginal cream used to treat vaginal and vulvar atrophy
Estraderm, Climara [estradiol]	Estrogen therapy	Osteoporosis prevention and to treat menopausal symptoms, vaginal and vulvar atrophy, hypoestrogenism, ovarian failure
Evista [raloxifene hydrochloride]	Estrogen receptor modulator, selective osteoporosis prophylactic	Prevention of thinning of the bones (osteoporosis) only in postmenopausal women
Flavoxate hydrochloride [flavoxate hydrochloride]	Urinary tract spasmolytic	Relief of dysuria, urgency, nocturia, suprapubic pain, frequency, and incontinence associated with cystitis, prostatitis, urethritis, and urethrocystitis/urethrotrigonitis
Flomax [tamsulosin hydrochloride]	Benign prostatic hypertrophy therapy agent	Signs and symptoms of benign enlargement of the prostate (benign prostatic hyperplasia or BPH)
Flonase [fluticasone propionate]	Corticosteroid-inhalation/nasal; topical steroid	Corticosteroid-responsive dermatosis; perennial allergic and seasonal allergic rhinitis
Flovent HFA [fluticasone propionate]	Corticosteroid-inhalation/nasal; topical steroid	Corticosteroid-responsive dermatosis, perennial allergic and seasonal allergic rhinitis
Fosamax [alendronate sodium]	Calcium metabolism	Osteoporosis; Paget's disease
Fosinopril sodium [fosinopril sodium]	ACE inhibitor; antihypertensive	Essential hypertension
Glucophage [metformin hydrochloride]	Blood glucose regulator	Diabetes mellitus antihyperglycemic drug used in the management of non-insulin-dependent diabetes mellitus (NIDDM)
Glucotrol [glipizide]	Oral blood-glucose-lowering agent	Adjunct to diet for the control of hyperglycemia in patients with noninsulin dependent diabetes mellitus (NIDDM, type II)
Glyburide (micronized) [glyburide]	Blood glucose regulator	Diabetes mellitus
Heparin sodium [heparin sodium]	Anticoagulant	Prophylaxis and treatment of venous thrombosis, pulmonary embolism; prevention of cerebral thrombosis, and treatment of consumptive coagulopathies

Drug	Drug Action	Indications
Hydrochlorothiazide [hydrochlorothiazide]	Diuretic, antihypertensive	Management of hypertension and in adjunctive therapy for edema associated with congestive heart failure, hepatic cirrhosis, corticosteroid, and estrogen therapy
Hydrocodone bitartrate and acetaminophen [acetaminophen/ hydrocodone bitartrate]	Analgesic, general; analgesic-narcotic; antitussive/expectorant	Pain, moderate to severe
Hyzaar [hydrochlorothiazide/ losartan/potassium]	Antihypertensive	Hypertension
Imitrex [sumatriptan succinate]	Antimigraine	Migraine headache
Inderal [propranolol hydrochloride]	Beta-adrenergic blocking agent	Management of hypertension, long-term management of angina pectoris due to coronary atherosclerosis, cardiac arrhythmias
Isordil [isosorbide dinitrate]	Smooth muscle relaxant	Acute anginal attacks
Isuprel [isoproterenol hydrochloride]	Adrenergic agent	Bronchodilator for asthma, chronic pulmonary emphysema, bronchitis, and other conditions accompanied by bronchospasm; can be used in cardiogenic shock cases
K-Tab, Klor-Con [potassium chloride]	Replaces potassium and maintains potassium level	Hypokalemia
Keflex [cephalexin]	Antibacterial	Bone, middle ear, skin and skin structures, upper respiratory tract and urinary tract infections; acute prostatitis
Klonopin [clonazepam]	Anticonvulsant, anxiolytic - benzodiazepine	Epilepsy, seizures, panic disorder
Lamisil [terbinafine hydrochloride]	Antifungal	*Tinea cruris* (jock itch), *T. pedis* (athlete's foot), *T. corporis* (ringworm)
Lanoxin [digoxin]	Cardiotonic glycoside	Congestive heart failure
Lasix [furosemide]	Antihypertensive; diuretic	Management of edema associated with congestive heart failure, renal disease, including nephrotic syndrome and hypertension
Lescol [fluvastatin]	HMG-CoA reductase inhibitor (statin)	Hypercholesterolemia; hyperlipidemia; hyperlipoproteinemia
Levaquin [levofloxacin]	Fluoroquinolone antibacterial	Acute exacerbation chronic bronchitis; cellulitis; furuncle; impetigo; infections of the lower and upper respiratory tract, sinus, skin and skin structures, and urinary tract; pneumonia, community-acquired; pyoderma
Levoxyl [levothyroxine sodium]	Synthetic thyroid hormone	Euthyroid goiter; hypothyroidism
Lexapro [escitalopram oxalate]	Antidepressant—selective serotonin reuptake inhibitor (SSRI)	Depression, anxiety
Librium [chlordiazepoxide hydrochloride]	Antianxiety agent	Acute withdrawal symptoms, especially from alcohol, or for other anxiety-producing conditions
Lidocaine [lidocaine hydrochloride]	Antiarrhythmic	Management of ventricular arrhythmias or during cardiac manipulation, such as cardiac surgery
Lipitor [atorvastatin calcium]	HMG-CoA reductase inhibitor (statin)	Hypercholesterolemia, hyperlipidemia, hyperproteinemia
Lithium [lithium carbonate]	Antimanic	Control of manic episodes in bipolar disorders
Lomotil [diphenoxylate hydrochloride with atropine]	Antidiarrheal	Treatment of symptoms of chronic and functional diarrhea
Lopid [gemfibrozil]	Lipid regulating agent	Hypercholesterolemia, hyperlipidemia, hyperlipoproteinemia, hypertriglyceridemia
Lopressor [metoprolol tartrate]	Antihypertensive, betablocker antianginal; antihypertensive; betablocker	Essential hypertension therapy, angina pectoris, and myocardial infarction
Lorazepam [lorazepam]	Antianxiety; sedative/hypnotic	Anxiety disorder associated with depressive symptoms; controls tension, agitation, irritability, and insomnia
Lotensin [benazepril]	ACE inhibitor; antihypertensive	Essential hypertension
Lotrel [amlodipine/benazepril]	Antihypertensive	Hypertension
Lotrisone [clotrimazole/ betamethasone]	Antifungal-corticosteroid	Relief of redness, swelling, itching, and other discomfort of fungus infections
Lovastatin [lovastatin]	HMG-CoA reductase inhibitor (statin)	Hypercholesterolemia; hyperlipidemia, hyperlipoproteinemia
Macrodantin [nitrofurantoin]	Antibacterial	Urinary tract infection; prophylaxis
Meclinzine hydrochloride [meclizine hydrochloride]	Antihistamine	Management of nausea and vomiting, and dizziness associated with motion sickness

Drug	Drug Action	Indications
Medrol [methylprednisolone]	Glucocorticoid; anti-inflammatory	Acute/chronic adrenal insufficiency, congenital adrenal hyperplasia, adrenal insufficiency secondary to pituitary insufficiency; nonendocrine disorders include arthritis, rheumatic carditis, bronchial asthma, cerebral edema, and allergic, collagen, intestinal tract, liver, ocular, renal, and skin diseases
Methergine [methylergonovine maleate]	Oxytocic agent	Routine management of postpartum hemorrhage after delivery of placenta
Miacalcin [calcitonin salmon]	Calcitonin; a peptide hormone	Hypercalcemia, osteoporosis, postmenopausal symptoms, Paget's disease
Monoket [isosorbide mononitrate]	Antianginal; coronary vasodilator, nitrate	Angina pectoris
Motrin [ibuprofen]	Analgesic, general; analgesic, non-narcotic; antiarthritic; antigout; antipyretic; NSAID	Osteoarthritis and rheumatoid arthritis, dysmenorrhea, fever; pain, mild to moderate
Multaq [dronedarone]	Cardiac rhythm regulator	Treatment of patients with recent episodes of atrial fibrillation or atrial flutter
Nabumetone [nabumetone]	Non-steroidal anti-inflammatory drug (NSAID)	Osteoarthritis and rheumatoid arthritis
Naprosyn [naproxen]	Anti-inflammatory analgesic, general; analgesic, non-narcotic; antiarthritic; antigout; NSAID	Rheumatoid, gouty arthritis and osteoarthritis; ankylosing spondylitis; bursitis; dysmenorrhea; pain, mild to moderate; tendonitis
Nefazodone hydrochloride [nefazodone hydrochloride]	Antidepressant	Depression
Nembutal sodium [pentobarbital sodium]	Sedative; hypnotic	Adjunct medication in diagnostic procedures or for emergency use with convulsive disorders
Neurontin [gabapentin]	Anticonvulsant	Epilepsy, partial
Nexium [esomeprazole magnesium]	Proton pump inhibitor	Gastroesophageal reflux disease (GERD), erosive esophagitis
Nitropress [sodium nitroprusside]	Vasodilator	Potent, rapid action in reducing blood pressure in hypertensive crisis or for controlling bleeding during anesthesia by producing controlled hypotension
Nitrostat [nitroglycerin]	Muscle relaxant antianginal; antihypertensive; coronary vasodilator	Prophylaxis and treatment of angina pectoris; heart failure associated with myocardial infarction; hypertension, perioperative; surgery, adjunct
Norpace [dlsopyramide]	Antiarrhythmic	Coronary artery disease, for prevention, recurrence and control of unifocal, multifocal, and paired PVCs
Norvasc [amlodipine besylate]	Calcium channel blocker	Hypertension, chronic stable angina, and vasospastic angina
Onglyza [saxagliptin]	Blood glucose regulator	Adjunct to diet and exercise for the control of hyperglycemia in patients with noninsulin-dependent diabetes mellitus (NIDDM, type II)
Orphenadrine citrate [orphenadrine citrate]	Muscle relaxant	Acute spasms, tension, and post-trauma cases
Ortho-Novum [norethindrone/ethinyl estradiol]	Contraceptive; estrogen/progestin	Contraception
Oxazepam [oxazepam]	Antianxiety	Anxiety, tension, and alcohol withdrawal
Pavabid [papaverine hydrochloride]	Vasodilator	Relief of cerebral and peripheral ischemia
Paxil [paroxetine]	Antidepressant	Anxiety with panic disorder and depression; obsessive-compulsive disorder
Penicillin-VK [penicillin V potassium]	Natural penicillin	Chorea, prevention; endocarditis, prevention, secondary to tooth extraction; erysipelas; infections of the skin and skin structures, upper respiratory tract; rheumatic fever, prophylaxis; scarlet fever; Vincent's gingivitis; Vincent's pharyngitis
Pepcid [famotidine]	Histamine H2-receptor inhibitor	Acid/peptic disorder; adenoma, secretory; gastroesophageal reflux; duodenal and gastric ulcer; Zollinger-Ellison syndrome
Percocet, Roxicet [oxycodone and acetaminophen]	Analgesic, general; analgesic-narcotic	Pain, moderate to severe
Persantine [dipyridamole]	Platelet inhibitor	Therapy for chronic angina pectoris, preventing clots post heart valve surgery
Phenobarbital [phenobarbital sodium]	Barbiturate	Grand mal epilepsy
Pitocin [oxytocin]	Synthetic oxytocin	Induction or stimulation of labor at term

Drug	Drug Action	Indications
Plasmanate [plasma, plasma protein fraction]	Blood volume expander	Hypovolemic shock, burn patients, and hemorrhages when whole blood is unavailable
Plavix [clopidogrel bisulfate]	Antithrombotic platelet aggregation inhibitor	Lessening of the chance of heart attack or stroke
Plendil [felodipine]	Antihypertensive; calcium channel blocker	Essential hypertension
Pravachol [pravastatin]	HMG-CoA reductase inhibitor (statin)	Hypercholesterolemia, hyperlipidemia, hyperlipoproteinemia
Prednisone [prednisone]	Adrenocorticoid, corticosteroid	Used for its immunosuppressant effects and for relief of inflammations; used in arthritis, polymyositis and other systemic diseases
Pregnyl [chorionic gonadotropin]	Gonadotropic hormone	Prepubertal cryptorchidism, hypogonadism, corpus luteum insufficiency and infertility
Premarin [conjugated estrogens]	Antineoplastic; estrogen	Vasomotor symptoms associated with menopause; atrophic vaginitis; kraurosis vulvae, female hypogonadism; primary ovarian failure
Prempro [conjugated estrogens/medroxyproges- terone]	Estrogen/progestin	Menopause, osteoporosis, atrophic vaginitis
Prevacid [lansoprazole]	Proton pump inhibitor (PPI)	Acid/peptic disorder, erosive esophagitis, duodenal ulcer, Zollinger-Ellison syndrome
Prinivil [lisinopril]	Synthetic peptide derivative, long-acting angiotensin converting enzyme inhibitor	Congestive heart failure, essential hypertension
Prilosec [omeprazole]	Proton pump inhibitor	Acid/peptic disorder; endocrine adenoma; erosive esophagitis; systemic mastocytosis; gastroesophageal reflux; duodenal, peptic and gastric ulcer; Zollinger-Ellison syndrome
Procardia [nifedipine]	Antianginal agent; calcium channel blocker	Management of vasospastic angina and chronic stable angina, essential hypertension
Promethazine hydrochloride [promethazine hydrochloride]	Anesthesia, adjunct to; antiemetic; antihistamine; antitussive/expectorant; sedative/hypnotic; vertigo/motion sickness/vomiting	Anesthesia; adjunct; angioedema; conjunctivitis; dermographism; hypersensitivity, motion sickness; pain; perennial, seasonal, and allergic rhinitis; sedation, obstetrical; urticaria
Protonix [pantoprazole]	Proton pump inhibitor (PPI)	Short-term treatment and maintenance therapy of erosive esophagitis associated with gastroesophageal reflux disease (GERD)
Proventil-HFA [albuterol sulfate]	Antiasthmatic/bronchodilator	Asthma
Provera/Depo-Provera [medroxyprogesterone acetate]	Antineoplastic; contraceptive; progestin	Amenorrhea; carcinoma, endometrium, adjunct; carcinoma, renal; contraception; hemorrhage
Prozac [fluoxetine hydrochloride]	Serotonin reuptake inhibitor	Bulimia nervosa; depression; obsessive-compulsive disorder
Qnasl [beclomethasone dipropionate]	Corticosteroid	Perennial allergies, seasonal allergies, and vasomotor rhinitis
Quinidine gluconate [quinidine gluconate]	Antiarrhythmic	Management of cardiac arrhythmias
Qvar [beclomethasone dipropionate]	Corticosteroids; antiasthmatic	Prevention and control of symptoms related to asthma
Restoril [temazepam]	Sedative/hypnotic	Insomnia
Retrovir [zidovudine]	Antiretroviral agent	Indicated in symptomatic HIV infection
Risperdal [risperidone]	Antipsychotic/antimanic	Schizophrenia; bipolar I disorder
Ritalin [methylphenidate hydrochloride]	Central nervous system (CNS) stimulant	Treatment of depression and hyperkinetic activity in children
Sabril [vigabatrin]	Anticonvulsant	Refractory complex partial seizures
Septra [sulfamethoxazole trimethoprim]	Antibacterial	Treatment of urinary tract infections, acute otitis media, acute exacerbations of chronic bronchitis, and shigellosis
Serevent [salmeterol xinafoate]	Bronchodilator	Asthma
Sinemet [carbidopa, levodopa]	Antiparkinsonian	Parkinson's disease
Singulair [montelukast]	Antiasthmatic, leukotriene receptor antagonist	Treatment of mild to moderate asthma to decrease the symptoms of asthma and the number of acute asthma attacks
Soltamox [tamoxifen citrate]	Antineoplastic; hormonal/biological response modifier	Breast cancer
Solu-Medrol [methylprednisolone sodium succinate]	Adrenocorticosteroid	Anti-inflammatory and antiallergenic for shock and ulcerative colitis
Synthroid, Levothroid [levothyroxine sodium]	Thyroid hormone	Treatment of hypothyroidism

Drug	Drug Action	Indications

Drug	Drug Action	Indications
Tagamet [cimetidine]	Acid reducer	Treatment of active duodenal ulcer, short-term treatment of active, benign gastric ulcer, and treatment of pathological hypersecretory conditions
Tegretol [carbamazepine]	Anticonvulsant; analgesic	Epilepsy, especially with complex symptomatology; specific analgesic for trigeminal neuralgia
Tenormin [atenolol]	Antianginal; antihypertensive; beta blocker	Treatment of hypertension; lowering blood pressure lowers the risk of fatal and nonfatal cardiovascular events, primarily strokes and myocardial infarctions
Terazosin hydrochloride [terazosin hydrochloride]	Alphablocker; antihypertensive; diuretic	Benign prostatic hypertrophy; essential hypertension
Tobradex [tobramycin and dexamethasone]	Aminoglycoside ocular anti-infective; anti-inflammatory	Infectious conjunctivitis; dermatosis, corticosteroid-responsive with secondary infection; foreign body in eye; corneal inflammation; uveitis
Toprol-XL [metoprolol succinate]	Antianginal antihypertensive beta blocker	Angina pectoris, essential hypertension
Trazodone hydrochloride [trazodone hydrochloride]	Antidepressant	Depression
Triamterene and hydrochlorothiazide [triamterene/ hydrochlorothiazide]	Antihypertensive, diuretic	Edema; essential hypertension
Trimethoprim [trimethoprim]	Antibacterial	Acute exacerbation chronic bronchitis; travelers' diarrhea; infections of the middle, lower respiratory tract, and urinary tract; pneumonia, pneumocystis; shigellosis
Trivora-28 [ethinyl estradiol/ levonorgestrel]	Contraceptive, estrogen/progestin	Contraception
Ultram [tramadol]	Analgesic, non-narcotic	Pain, moderate to moderately severe
Uniphyl [theophylline]	Bronchodilator, pulmonary vasodilator, smooth muscle relaxant	Treatment of bronchial obstruction in asthma and chronic obstructive pulmonary disease
Valium [diazepam]	Antianxiety, muscle relaxant, anticonvulsant	Anxiety, tension, withdrawal from alcohol, muscle spasms and anticonvulsant therapy; epilepsy, generalized tonic-clonic; status epilepticus; stiff-man syndrome; tetanus
Vasotec [enalaprilat]	ACE inhibitor, antihypertensive	Congestive heart failure; essential hypertension
Ventolin HFA [albuterol, albuterol sulfate]	Antiasthmatic/bronchodilator	Asthma
Verapamil HCL, Calan [verapamil hydrochloride]	Antianginal, antiarrhythmic, antiarthritic, antihypertensive, calcium channel blocker	Angina pectoris, chronic stable angina, atrial fibrillation, atrial flutter, paroxysmal supraventricular tachycardia, ventricular arrhythmia, essential hypertension
Viagra [sildenafil citrate]	Phosphodiesterase-5 (PDE5) inhibitor	Erectile dysfunction
Victoza [liraglutide recombinant]	Glucagon-like peptide-1 (GLP-1) receptor agonist	Adjunct to diet and exercise for the control of hyperglycemia in patients with noninsulin-dependent diabetes mellitus (NIDDM, type II)
Vistaril [hydroxyzine pamoate]	Antianxiety agent, antiemetic	Treatment of nausea and vomiting, for reducing narcotic requirement in surgery and as tranquilizer for tension, anxiety, or agitation states
Wellbutrin SR, Welbutrin XL [bupropion hydrochloride]	Antidepressant; CNS	Depression; smoking cessation
Xalatan [latanoprost]	Prostaglandin F2α analogue	Glaucoma, open-angle; ocular hypertension
Xanax, Xanax XR [alprazolam]	Antianxiety; sedative/hypnotic	Anxiety disorders with panic disorder and depression
Xigris [drotrecogin alfa]	Biologic response modifier	Severe sepsis
Zantac [ranitidine hydrochloride]	Histamine H2-receptors inhibitor	Acid/peptic disorder, erosive esophagitis, gastrointestinal hypersecretion, mastocytosis, gastroesophageal reflux, peptic ulcer, Zollinger-Ellison syndrome
Zestoretic [lisinopril and hydrochlorothiazide]	ACE inhibitor; antihypertensive	Congestive heart failure; essential hypertension
Zestril [lisinopril]	ACE inhibitor; antihypertensive	Congestive heart failure; essential hypertension
Ziac [bisoprolol fumarate/ hydrochlorothiazide]	Antihypertensive	Essential hypertension
Zithromax [azithromycin]	Macrolide	Infections of the cervix, lower respiratory tract, skin and skin structures, urethra, nongonococcal; mycobacterium avium complex; pharyngitis, streptococcal pneumonia; tonsillitis

Drug	Drug Action	Indications
Zocor [simvastatin]	HMG-CoA reductase inhibitor (statin)	Hypercholesterolemia, hyperlipidemia, hyperlipoproteinemia, hypertriglyceridemia
Zoloft [sertraline hydrochloride]	Antidepressant	Anxiety with panic disorder and depression; obsessive-compulsive disorder
Zovirax [acyclovir]	Antiviral	Genital herpes and herpes zoster infections
Zyloprim [allopurinol]	Antigout	Gouty arthritis, renal calculus, hyperuricemia, hyperuricemia secondary to leukemia, hyperuricemia secondary to lymphoma
Zyprexa [olanzapine]	Antipsychotic/antimanic	Psychotic disorders; schizophrenia
Zyrtec [cetirizine hydrochloride]	Antihistamine	Perennial allergic and seasonal allergic rhinitis; chronic urticaria

Drug	Drug Action	Indications

Appendix D: Z Codes for Long-Term Drug Use with Associated Drugs

Z79.01 Long term (current) use of anticoagulants
Arixtra
Coumadin
Eliquis
Heparin
Jantoven
Lovenox
Pradaxa
Warfarin
Xarelto

Z79.02 Long term (current) use of antithrombotics/antiplatelets
Aggrenox
Aggrastat
Clopidogrel
Clopidogrel bisulfate
Effient
Persantine
Plavix
Pletal
Pradaxa
Ticlid

Z79.1 Long term (current) use of non-steroidal anti-inflammatories (NSAID)
Advil
Aleve
Anaprox
Celebrex
Clinoril
Daypro
Feldene
Ibuprofen
Indocin
Lodine
Motrin
Nalfon
Naprosyn
Orudis
Ponstel
Relafen
Tolectin
Toradol
Voltaren

Z79.2 Long term (current) use of antibiotics
Amikin
Amoxicillin
Amoxil
Ampicillin
Ancef

Augmentin
Azactam
Azithromycin
Bactrim
Cefaclor
Ceftriaxone
Cephalexin
Cephalosporin
Cipro
Ciprofloxacin
Clarithromycin
Cleocin
Clindamycin
Co-trimoxazole
Daptomycin
Dificid
Doxycycline
Ertapenem
ERYC
Erythromycin
Factive
Flagyl
Flucloxacillin
Gentamicin
Isoniazid
Invanz
Keflex
Levaquin
Macrobid
Merrem
Metronidazole
Minocin
Nitrofurantoin
Omnipen
Ornidazole
Penicillin G
Penicillin V
Polycillin
Primaxin
Rifampicin
Rocephin
Septra
Streptomycin
Tazicef
Tazocin
Tetracycline HCl
Timentin
Trimethoprim
Tobramycin
Unipen
Vancocin
Vancomycin
Vibramycin

Zinacef
Zithromax
Zosyn
Zyvox

Z79.3 Long term (current) use of hormonal contraceptives
Oral
   Combined oral contraceptive
   Progestin-only pills
Patch
   Ortho Evra
Injectable
   DMPA—depo medroxyprogesterone acetate
Vaginal Ring
   NuvaRing
Implantable rods
   Implanon

Z79.4 Long term (current) use of insulin
Apidra
Humalog
Humulin
Lantus
Levemir
Novolin
NovoLog
Velosulin

Z79.51 Long term (current) use of inhaled steroids
Advair
Aerospan
Alvesco
Asmanex Twisthaler
Dulera
Flovent
Pulmicort
Qvar
Symbicort

Z79.52 Long term (current) use of systemic steroids
Cortef
Cortisone acetate
Depo-Medrol
Dexamethasone
Hydrocortisone
Kenalog
Medrol
Methylprednisolone
Prednisolone
Prednisone
Solu-Medrol

Z79.810 Long term (current) use of selective estrogen receptor modulators (SERMs)
Evista
Fareston
Nolvadex
Osphena
Raloxifene
Soltamox
Tamoxifen
Toremifene

Z79.811 Long term (current) use of aromatase inhibitors
Anastrozole
Arimidex
Aromasin
Exemestane
Femara
Letrozole

Z79.818 Long term (current) use of other agents affecting estrogen receptors and estrogen levels
Eligard
Faslodex
Fulvestrant
Lupron
Megace
Supprelin La
Synarel
Trelstar
Vantas
Viadur
Zoladex

Z79.82 Long term (current) use of aspirin
Bayer
Ecotrin
Bufferin

Z79.83 Long term (current) use of bisphosphonates
Actonel
Aredia
Atelvia
Binosto
Boniva

Didronel
Fosamax
Reclast
Zometa

Z79.890 Hormone replacement therapy (postmenopausal)
Activella
Alora
Angeliq
Climara
Enjuvia
Estrace
Estratest
EstroGel
Femring
Femtrace
Menostar
Premarin
Provera
Vivelle

Z79.891 Long term (current) use of opiate analgesic
Astramorph
Avinza
Buprenex
Buprenorphine
Codeine
Demerol
Dilaudid
Duragesic
Duramorph
Fentanyl
Fentora
Fioricet with codeine
Hydrocodone
Hydromorphone
Kadian
Lorcet
Lortab
Methadone HCL
Methadose
Morphine
MS Contin
Norco
Oxycodone

OxyContin
Percocet
Roxicodone
Sublimaze
Tylenol with codeine
Ultram

Z79.899 Other long term (current) drug therapy]
Actimmune
Antineoplastic/chemotherapy
Astagraf XL
Avonex
Cellcept
Cyclosporin
Envarsus XR
Gengraf
Imuran
Interferon
Monoclonal antibodies
Neoral
Orthoclone OKT3
Peginterferon
Prograf
Protopic
Rapamune
Rebif
Sandimmune
Simulect
Sirolimus
Sylatron
Tacrolimus
Torisel
Zenapax

Appendix E: Z Codes Only as Principal/First-Listed Diagnosis

Z00.00	Z01.20	Z02.3	Z03.810	Z34.00	Z38.4	Z51.11	Z52.4
Z00.01	Z01.21	Z02.4	Z03.818	Z34.01	Z38.5	Z51.12	Z52.5
Z00.110	Z01.30	Z02.5	Z03.89	Z34.02	Z38.61	Z52.000	Z52.6
Z00.111	Z01.31	Z02.6	Z04.1	Z34.03	Z38.62	Z52.001	Z52.810
Z00.121	Z01.411	Z02.71	Z04.2	Z34.80	Z38.63	Z52.008	Z52.811
Z00.129	Z01.419	Z02.79	Z04.3	Z34.81	Z38.64	Z52.010	Z52.812
Z00.2	Z01.42	Z02.81	Z04.41	Z34.82	Z38.65	Z52.011	Z52.813
Z00.3	Z01.810	Z02.82	Z04.42	Z34.83	Z38.66	Z52.018	Z52.819
Z00.5	Z01.811	Z02.83	Z04.6	Z34.90	Z38.68	Z52.090	Z52.89
Z00.70	Z01.812	Z02.89	Z04.71	Z34.91	Z38.69	Z52.091	Z76.1
Z00.71	Z01.818	Z02.9	Z04.72	Z34.92	Z38.7	Z52.098	Z76.2
Z00.8	Z01.82	Z03.6	Z04.8	Z34.93	Z38.8	Z52.10	Z99.12
Z01.00	Z01.83	Z03.71	Z04.9	Z38.00	Z39.0	Z52.11	
Z01.01	Z01.84	Z03.72	Z31.81	Z38.01	Z39.1	Z52.19	
Z01.10	Z01.89	Z03.73	Z31.82	Z38.1	Z39.2	Z52.20	
Z01.110	Z02.0	Z03.74	Z31.83	Z38.2	Z42.1	Z52.21	
Z01.118	Z02.1	Z03.75	Z31.84	Z38.30	Z42.8	Z52.29	
Z01.12	Z02.2	Z03.79	Z33.2	Z38.31	Z51.0	Z52.3	

Illustrations

Chapter 3. Diseases of the Blood and Blood-forming Organs and Certain Disorders Involving the Immune Mechanism (D5Ø–D89)

Red Blood Cells

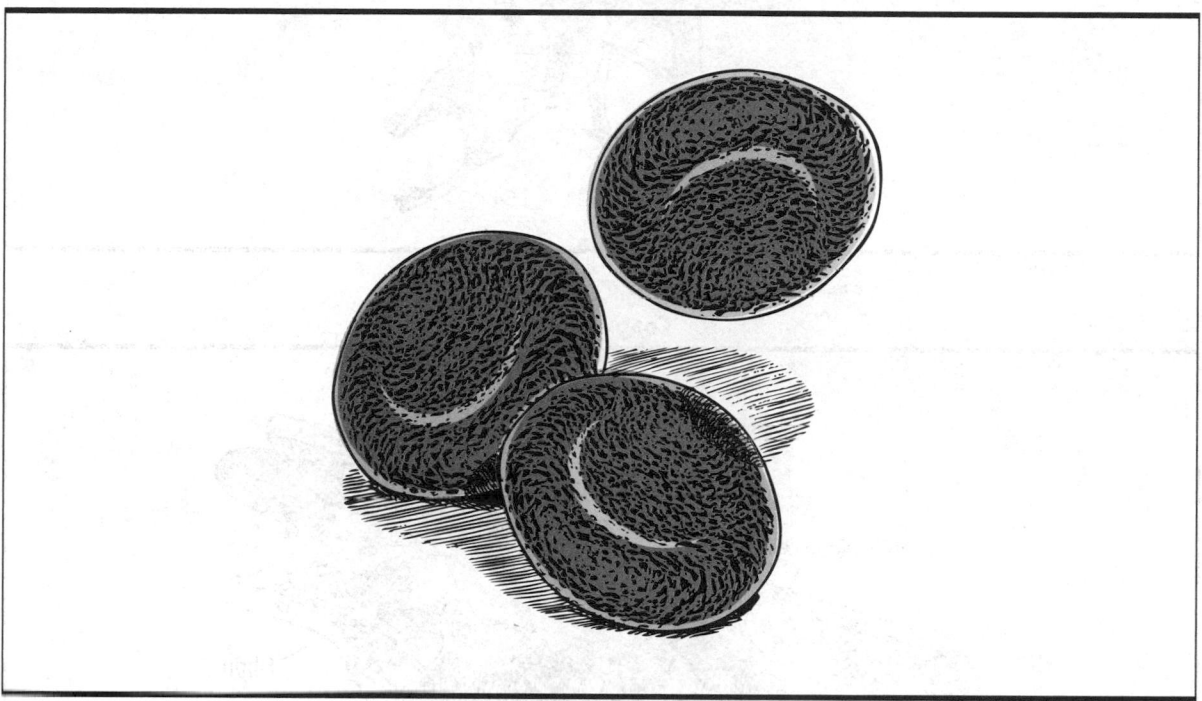

White Blood Cell

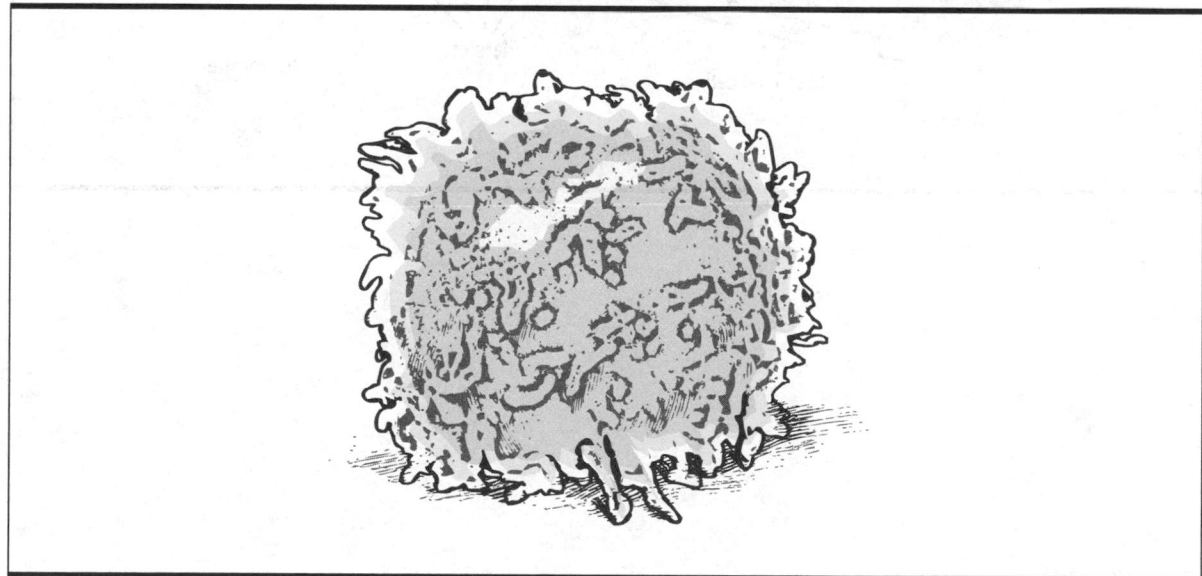

Platelet

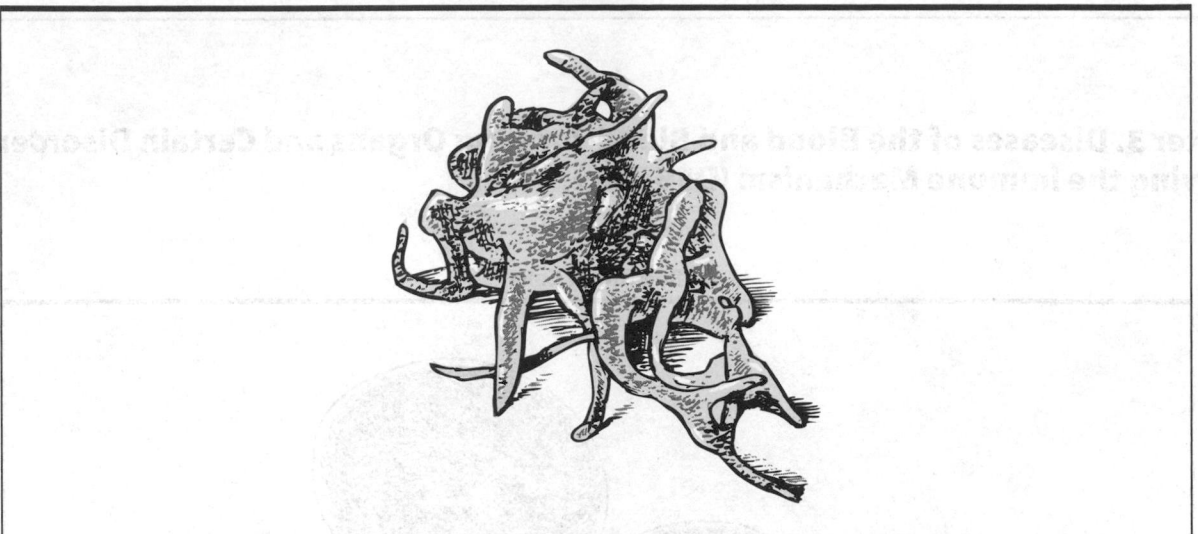

Coagulation

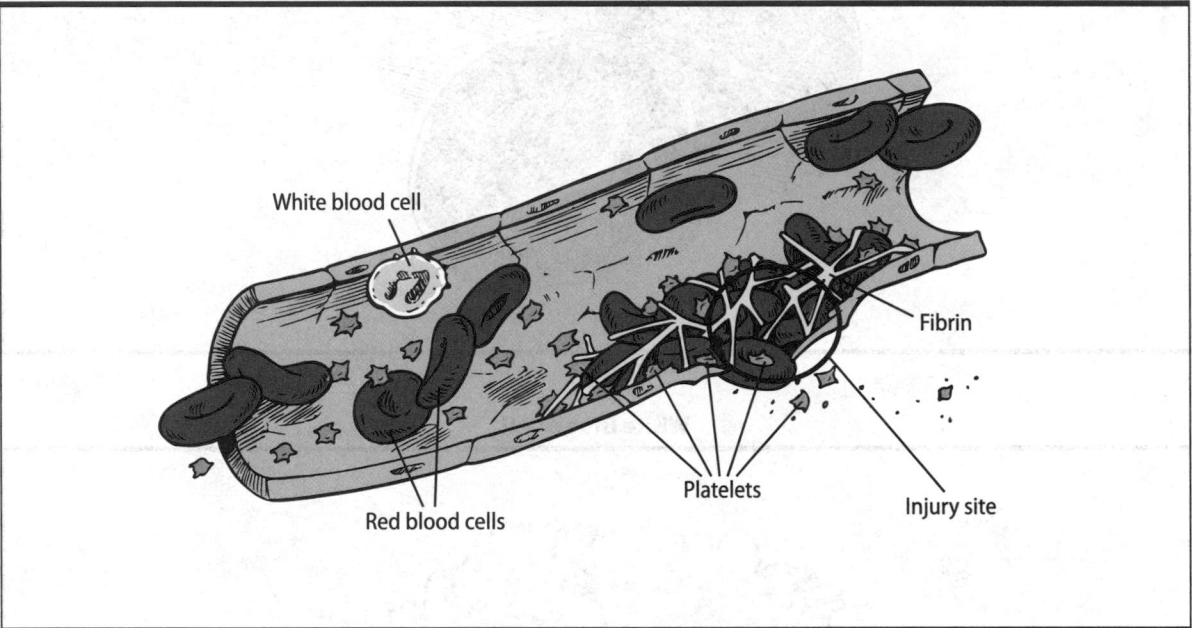

Spleen Anatomical Location and External Structures

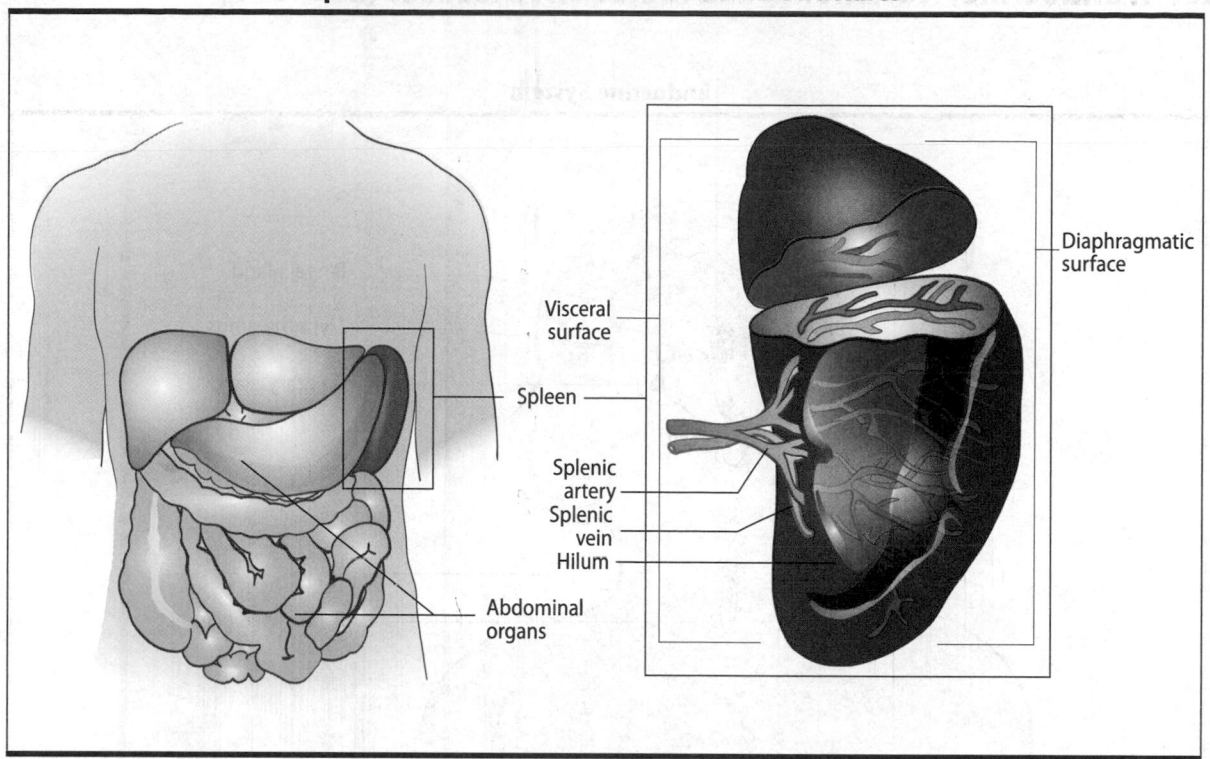

Spleen Interior Structures

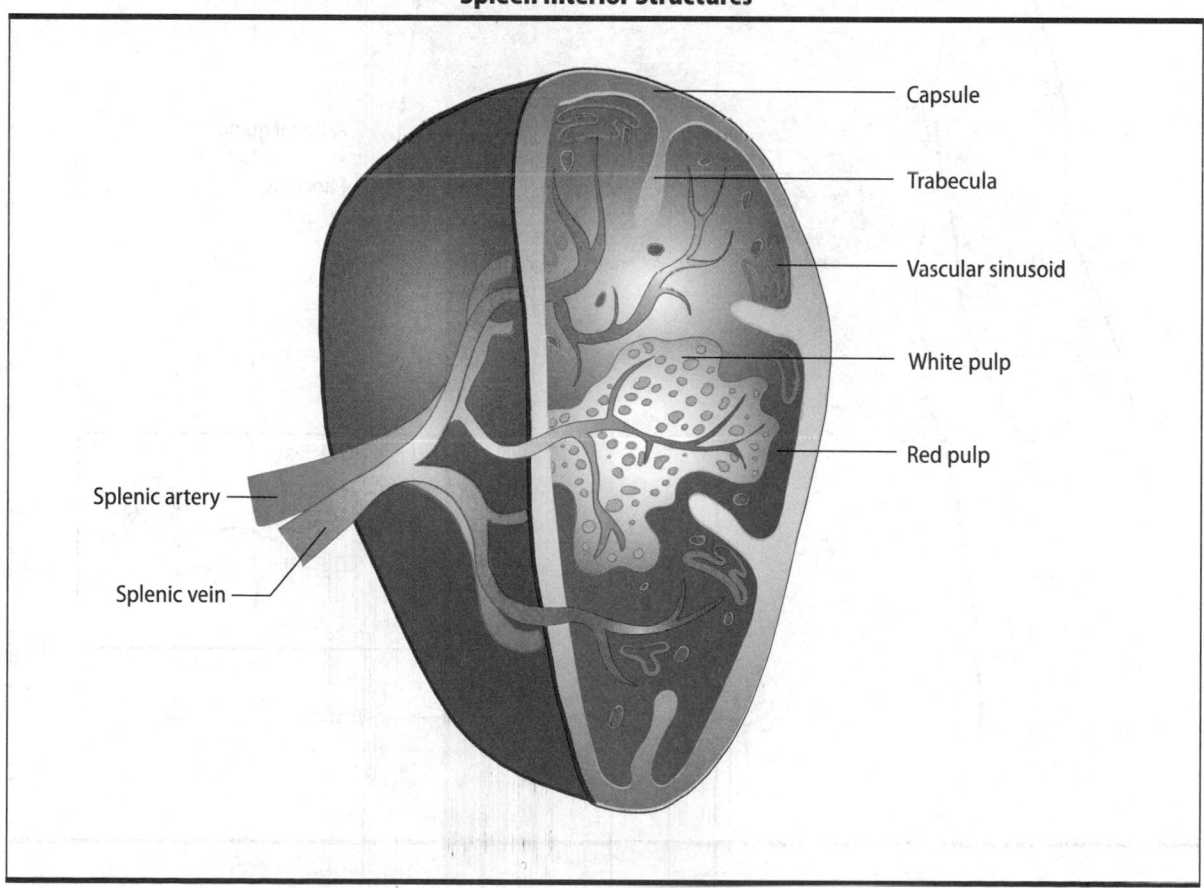

Chapter 4. Endocrine, Nutritional and Metabolic Diseases (EØØ–E89)

Endocrine System

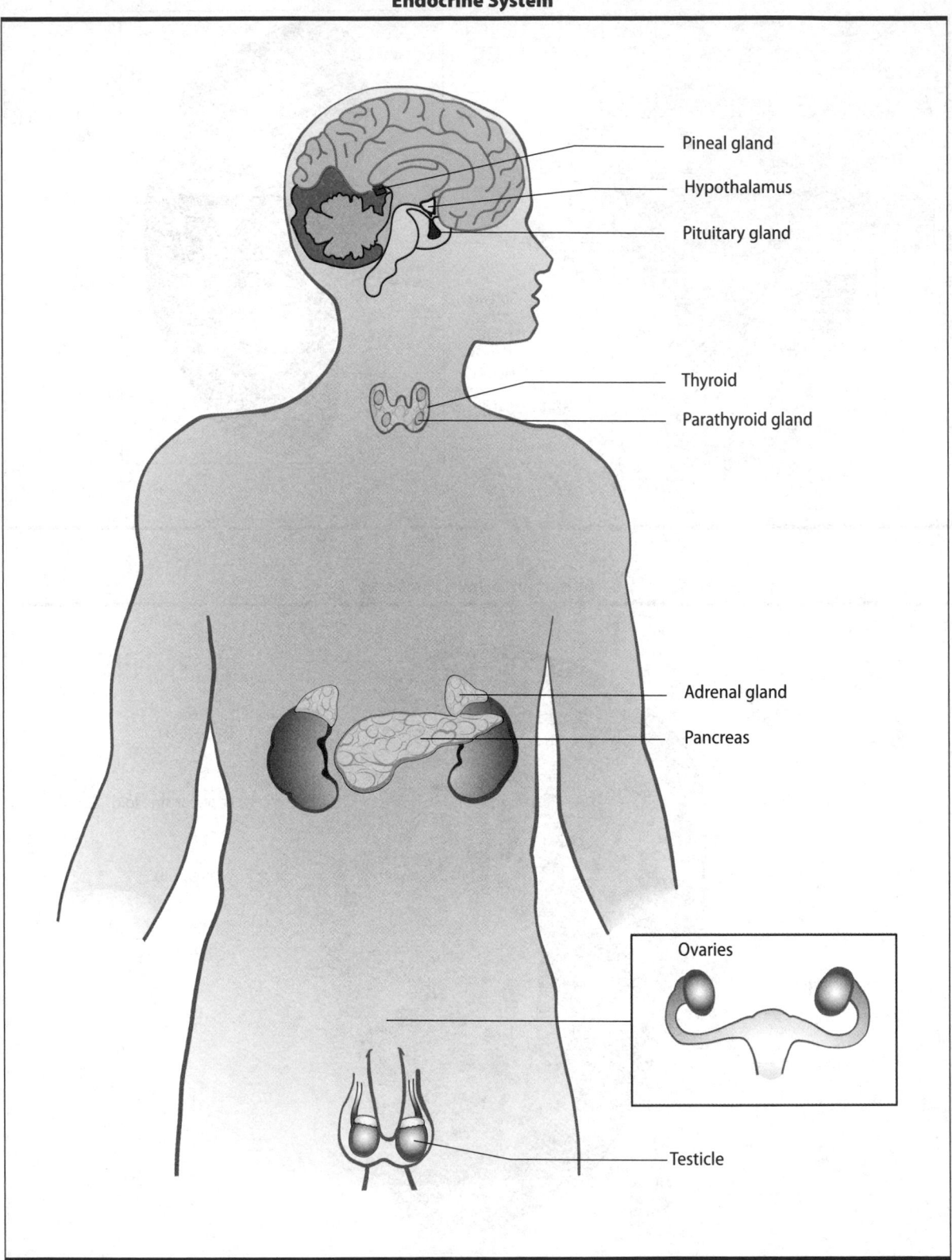

Thyroid

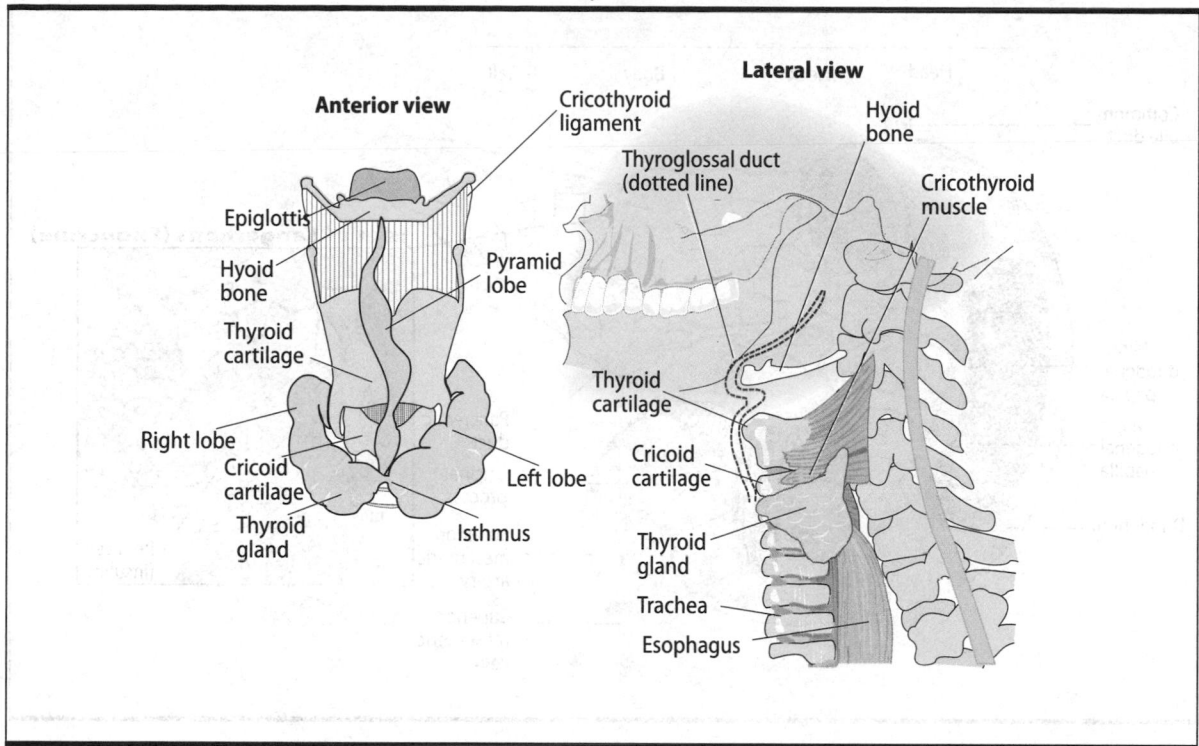

Thyroid and Parathyroid Glands

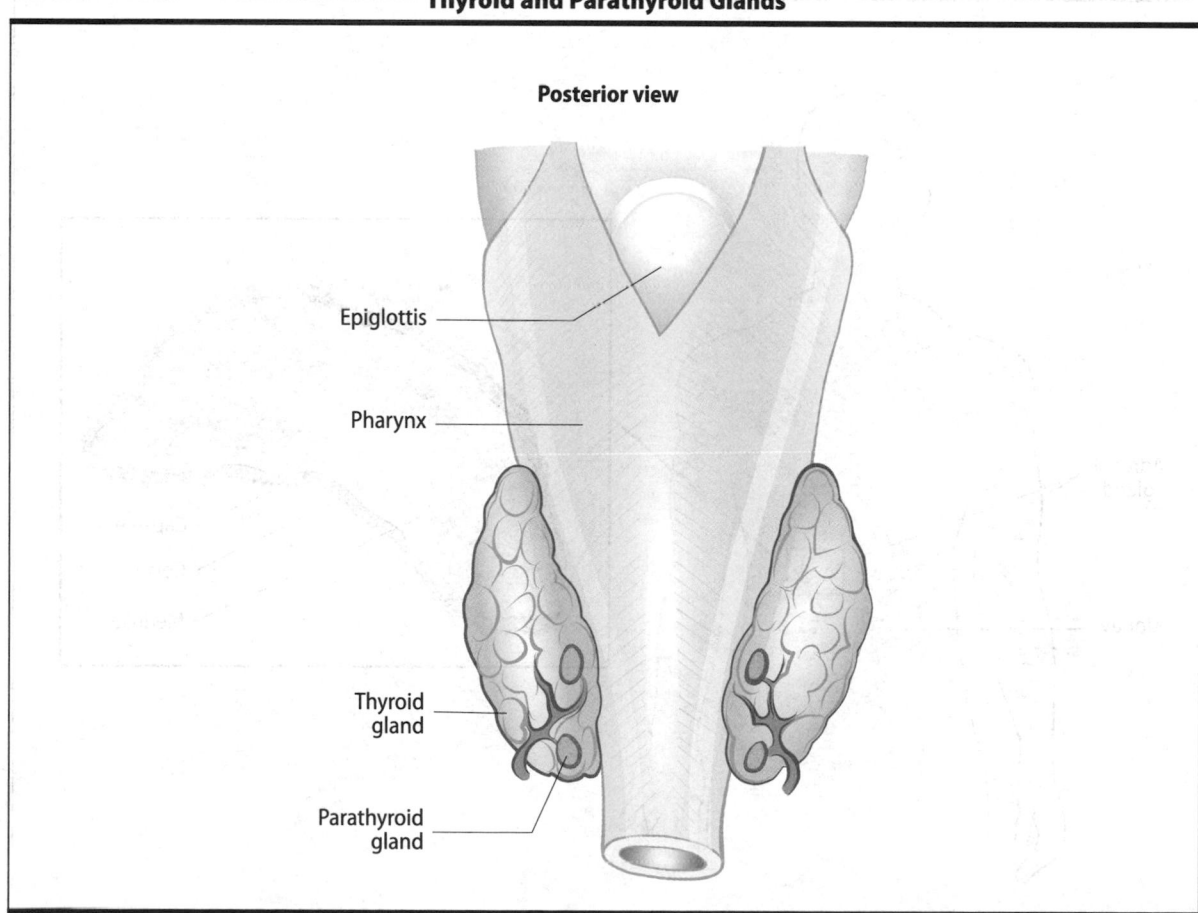

Pancreas

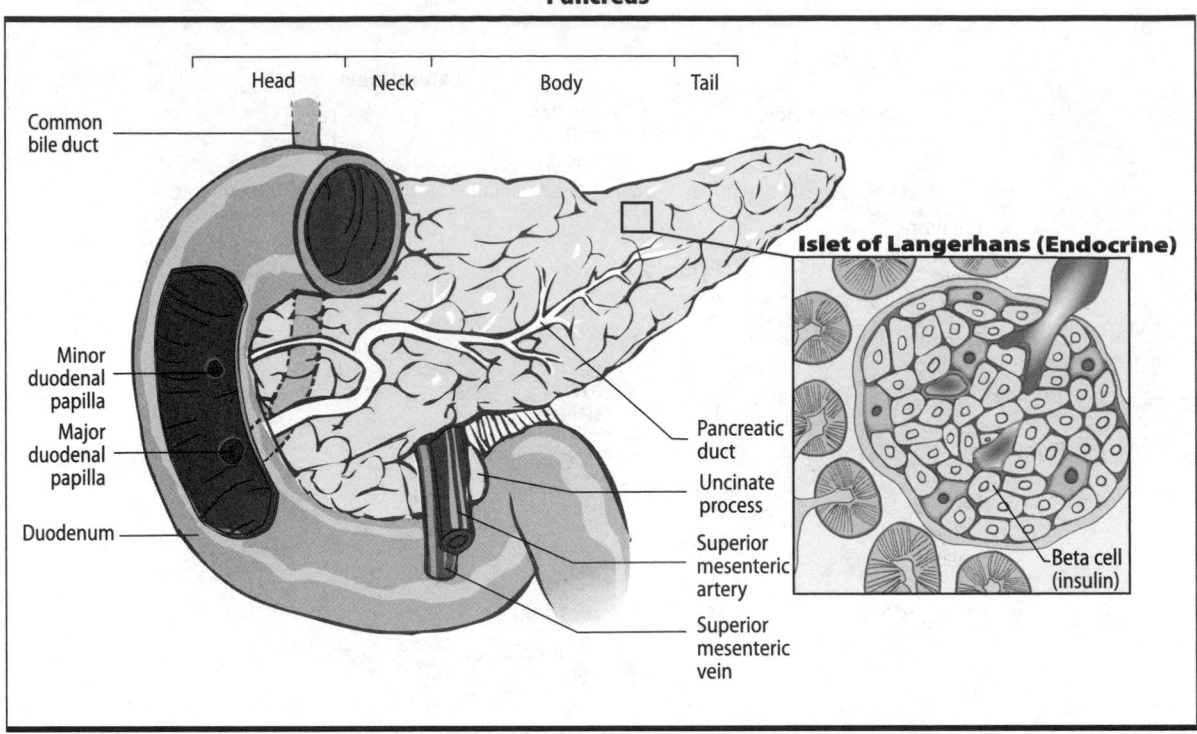

Head Neck Body Tail

Common bile duct

Minor duodenal papilla

Major duodenal papilla

Duodenum

Pancreatic duct

Uncinate process

Superior mesenteric artery

Superior mesenteric vein

Islet of Langerhans (Endocrine)

Beta cell (insulin)

Anatomy of the Adrenal Gland

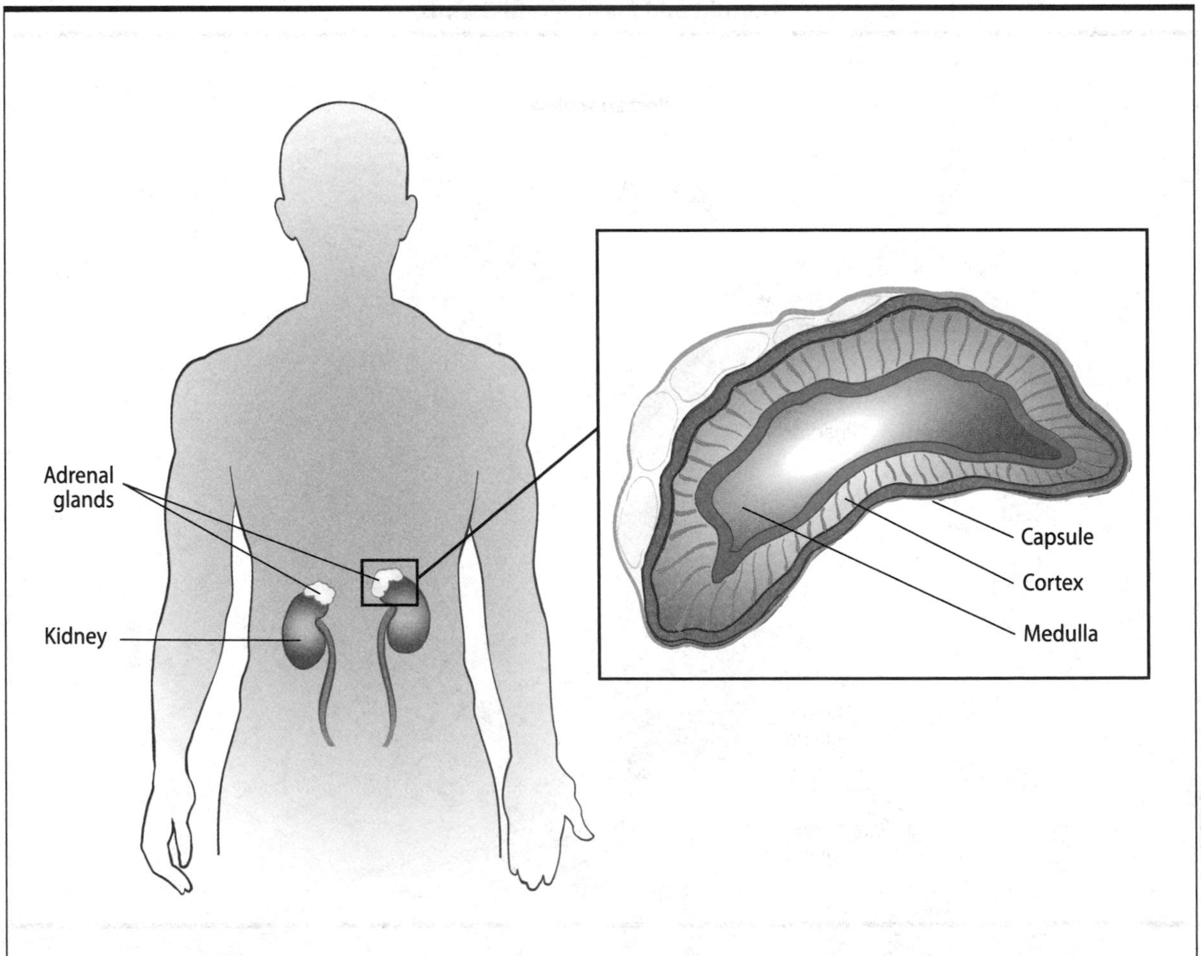

Adrenal glands

Kidney

Capsule

Cortex

Medulla

Structure of an Ovary

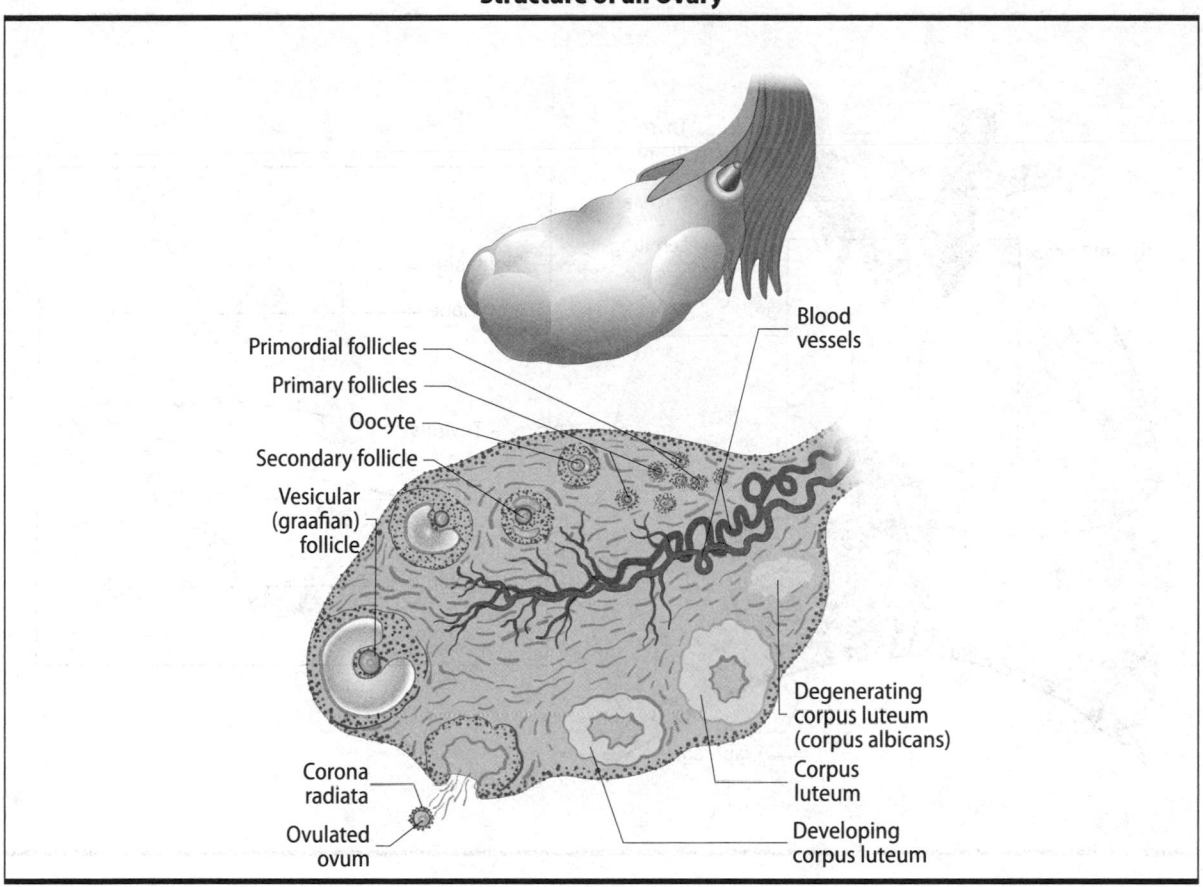

Testis and Associated Structures

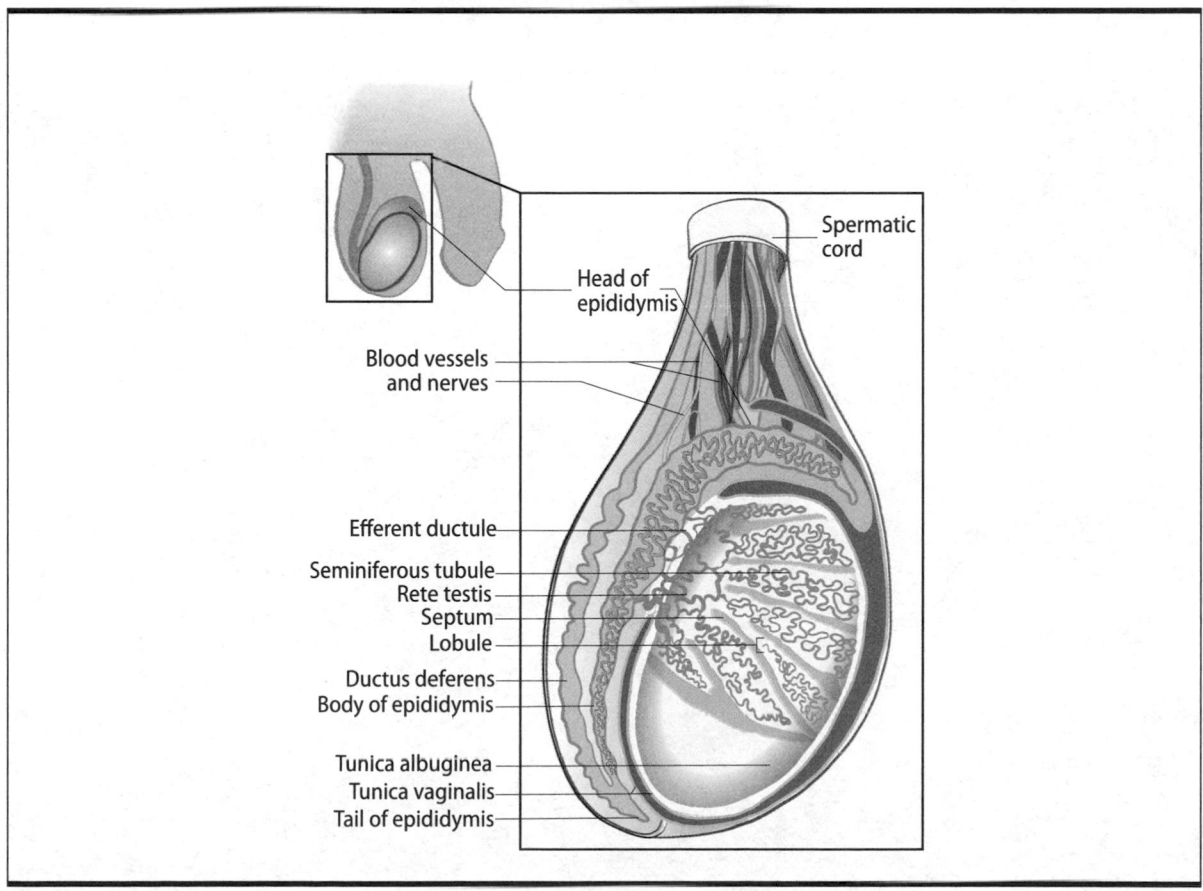

Thymus

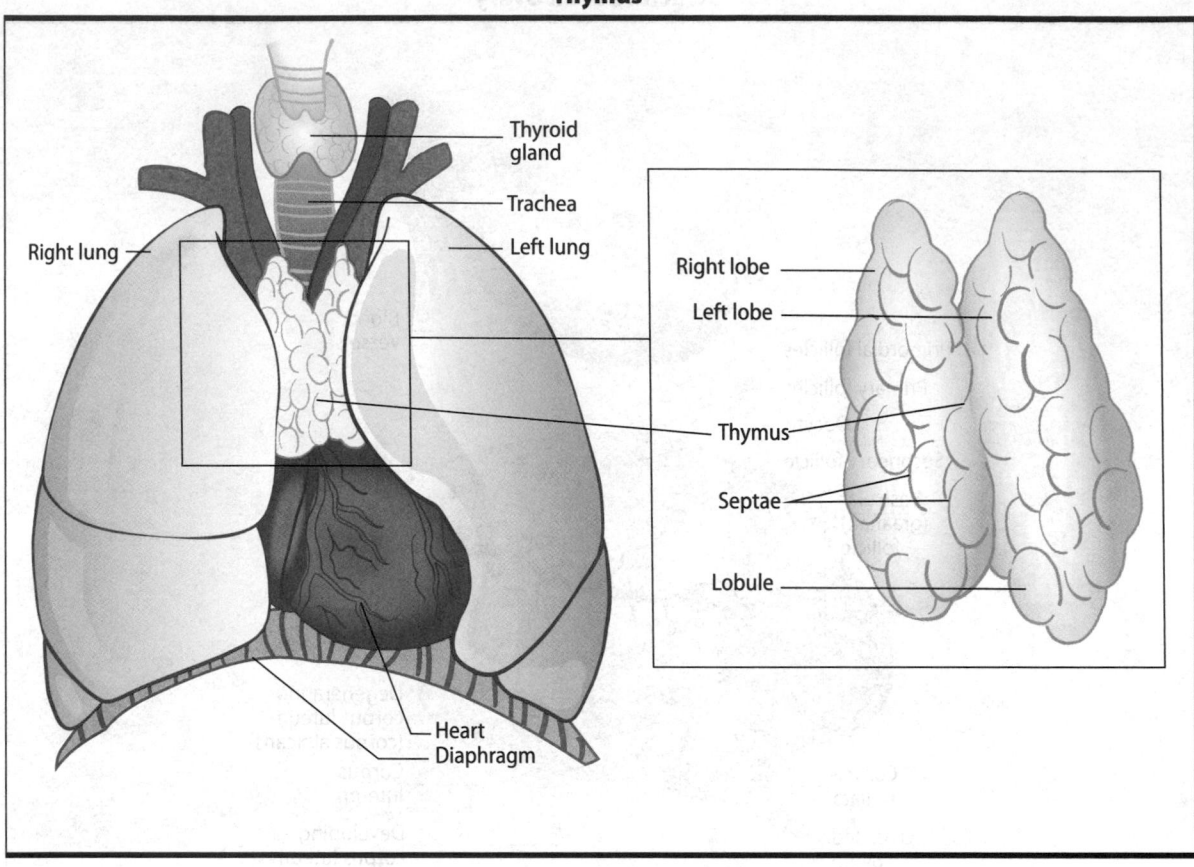

Chapter 6. Diseases of the Nervous System (GØØ–G99)

Brain

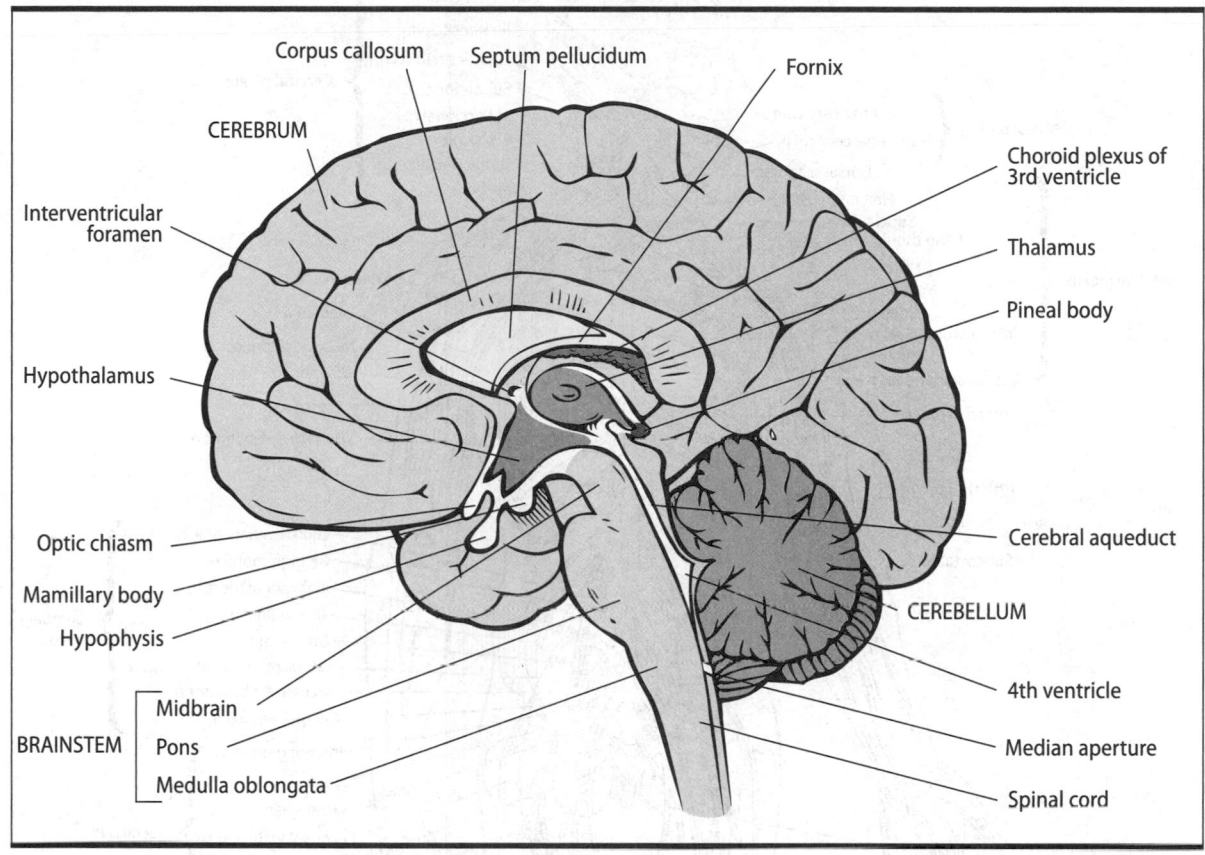

Corpus callosum — Septum pellucidum — Fornix

CEREBRUM

Interventricular foramen

Hypothalamus

Optic chiasm

Mamillary body

Hypophysis

BRAINSTEM — Midbrain — Pons — Medulla oblongata

Choroid plexus of 3rd ventricle

Thalamus

Pineal body

Cerebral aqueduct

CEREBELLUM

4th ventricle

Median aperture

Spinal cord

Cranial Nerves

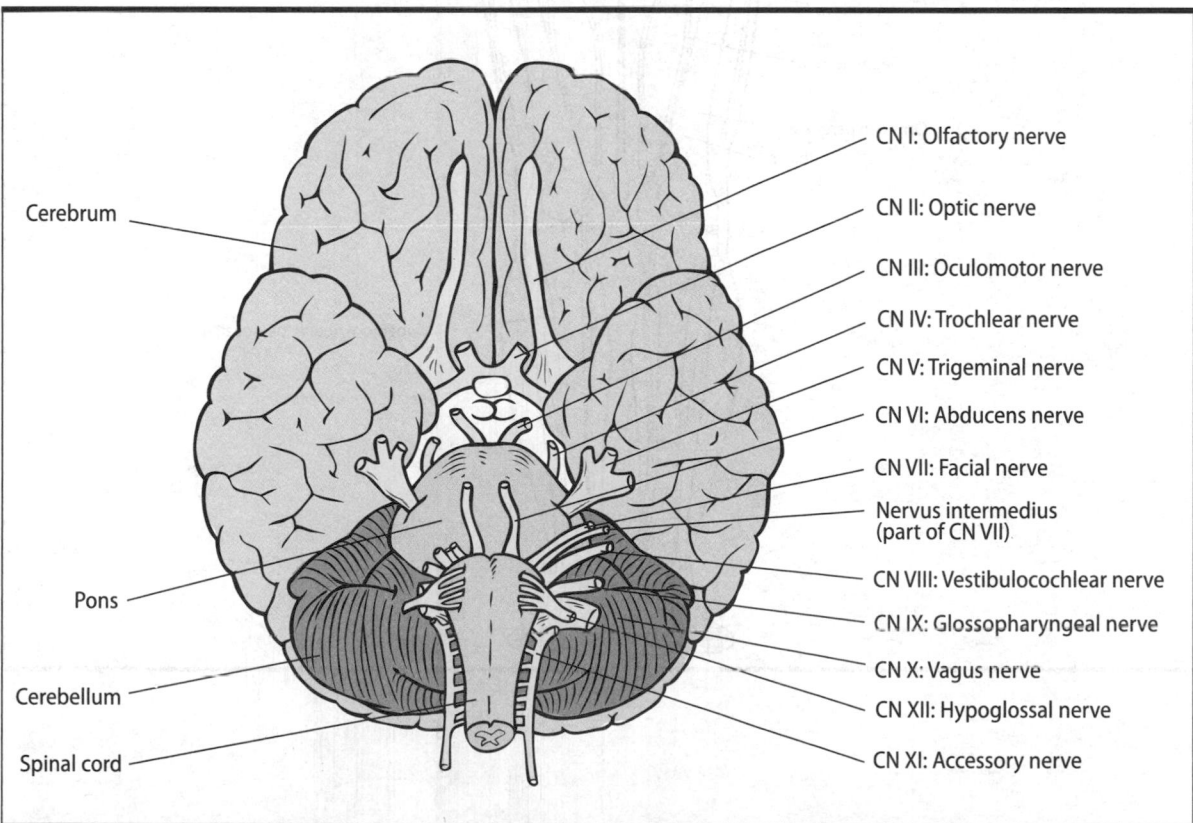

Cerebrum

Pons

Cerebellum

Spinal cord

CN I: Olfactory nerve

CN II: Optic nerve

CN III: Oculomotor nerve

CN IV: Trochlear nerve

CN V: Trigeminal nerve

CN VI: Abducens nerve

CN VII: Facial nerve

Nervus intermedius (part of CN VII)

CN VIII: Vestibulocochlear nerve

CN IX: Glossopharyngeal nerve

CN X: Vagus nerve

CN XII: Hypoglossal nerve

CN XI: Accessory nerve

Peripheral Nervous System

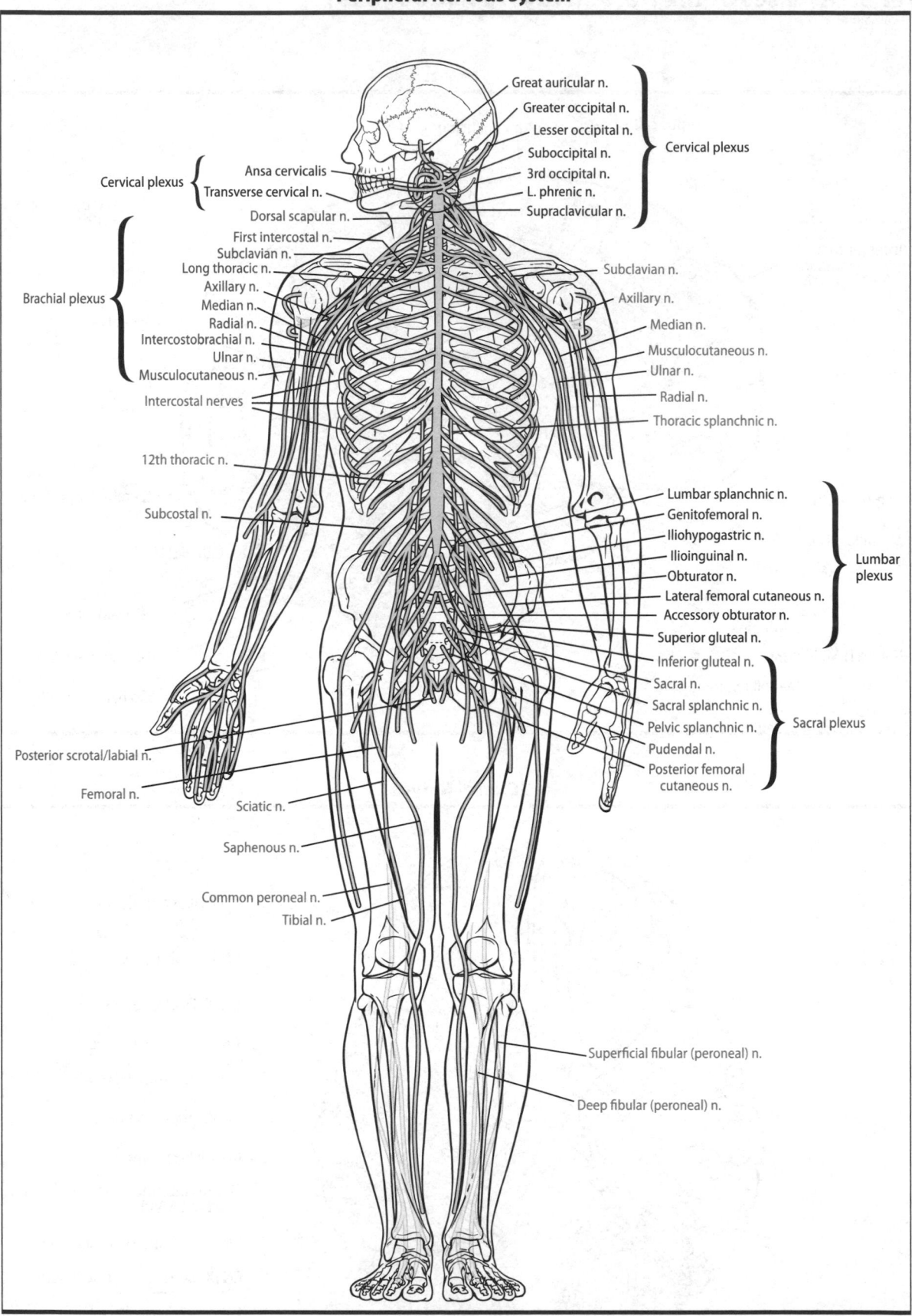

Spinal Cord and Spinal Nerves

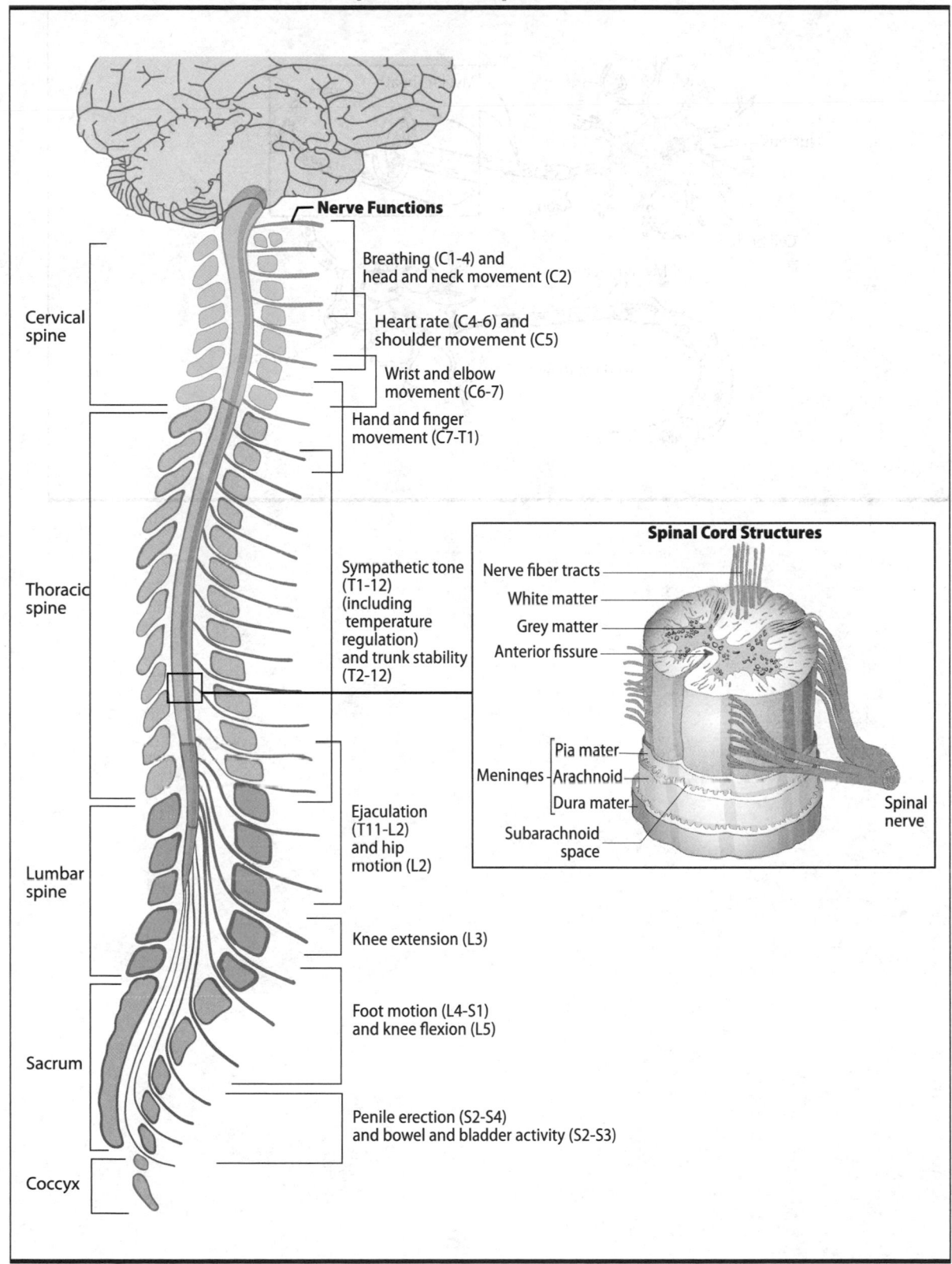

Nerve Functions

Breathing (C1-4) and
head and neck movement (C2)

Heart rate (C4-6) and
shoulder movement (C5)

Wrist and elbow
movement (C6-7)

Hand and finger
movement (C7-T1)

Cervical
spine

Thoracic
spine

Sympathetic tone
(T1-12)
(including
temperature
regulation)
and trunk stability
(T2-12)

Ejaculation
(T11-L2)
and hip
motion (L2)

Lumbar
spine

Knee extension (L3)

Foot motion (L4-S1)
and knee flexion (L5)

Sacrum

Penile erection (S2-S4)
and bowel and bladder activity (S2-S3)

Coccyx

Spinal Cord Structures

Nerve fiber tracts

White matter

Grey matter

Anterior fissure

Meninges — Pia mater
Arachnoid
Dura mater

Subarachnoid
space

Spinal
nerve

Nerve Cell

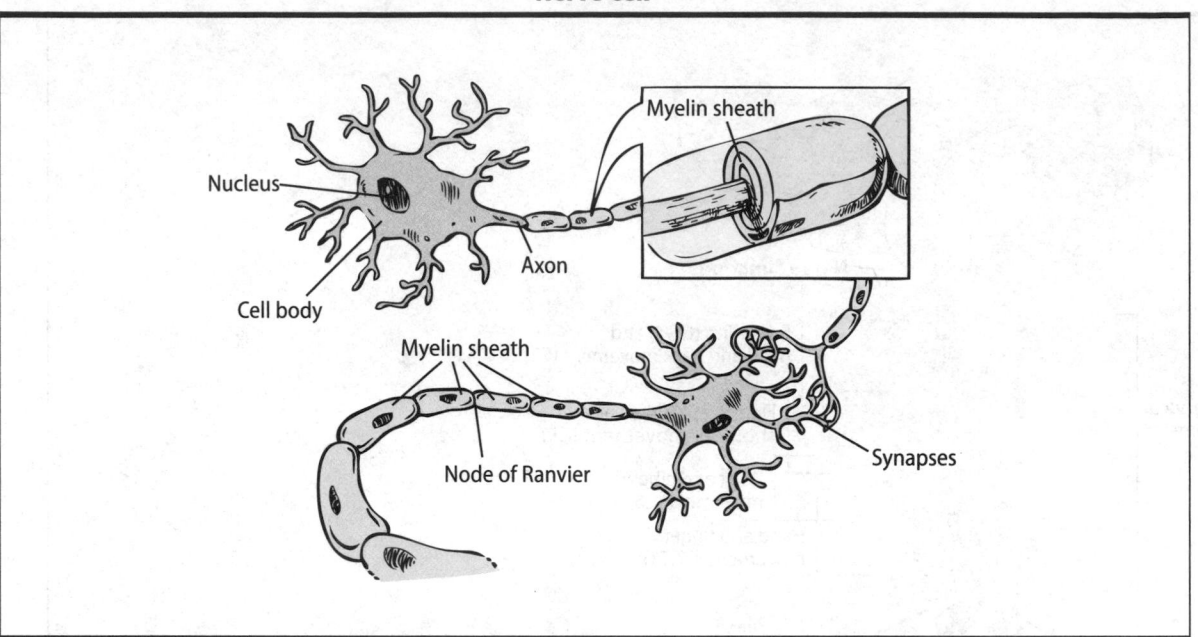

Chapter 7. Diseases of the Eye and Adnexa (H00–H59)

Eye

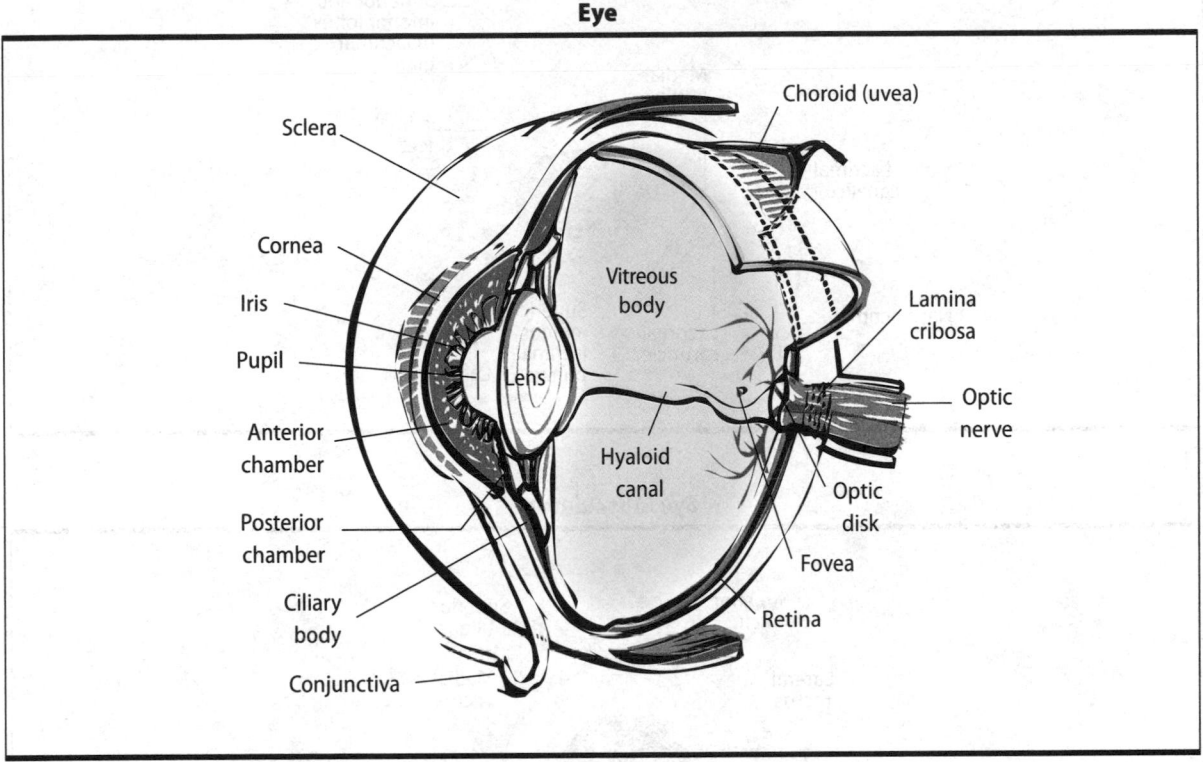

Posterior Pole of Globe/Flow of Aqueous Humor

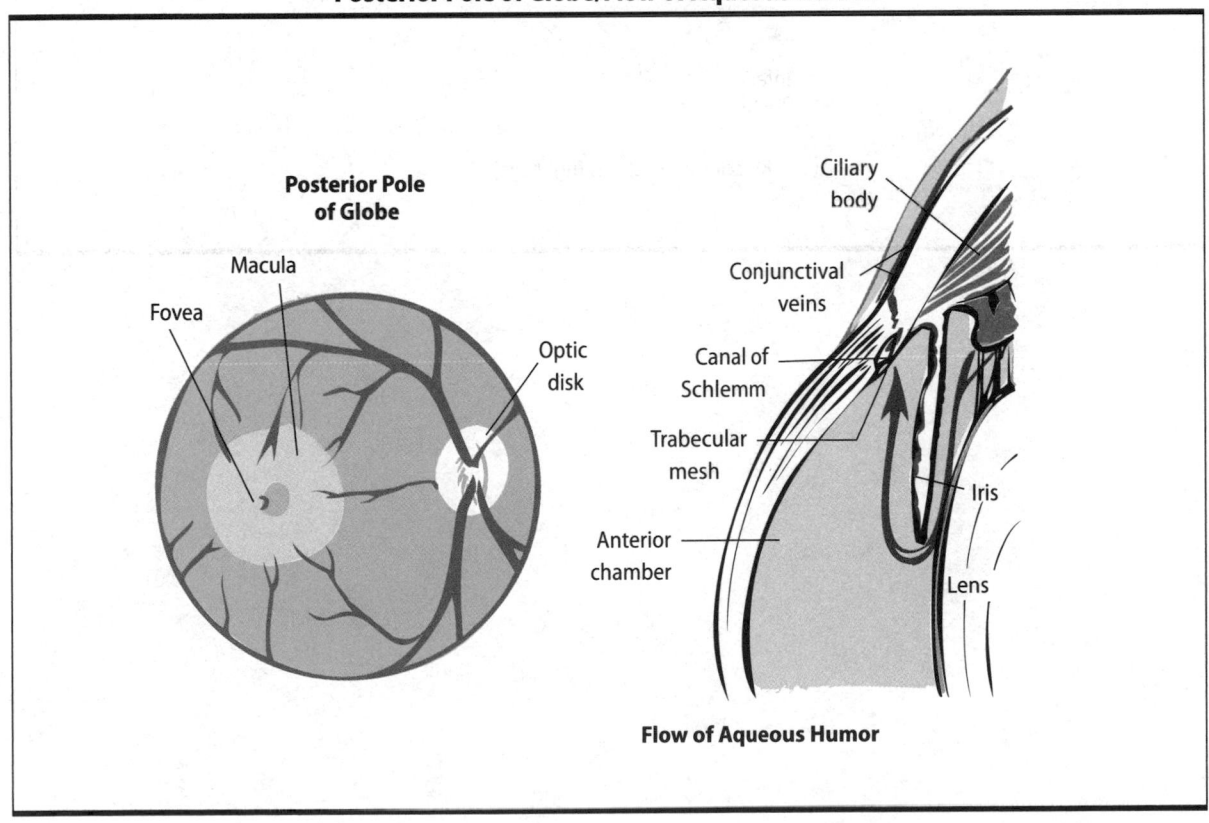

Lacrimal System

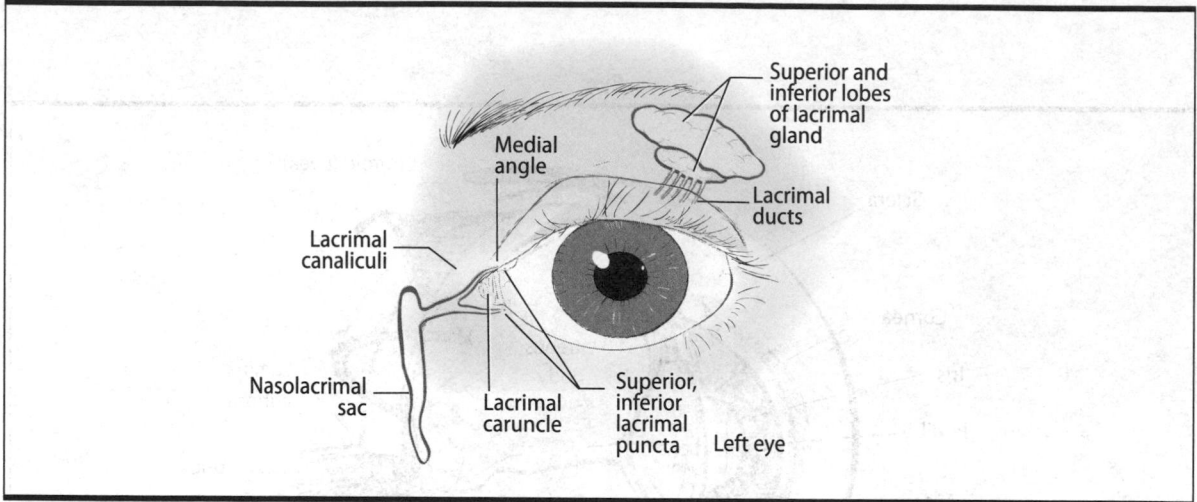

Eye Musculature

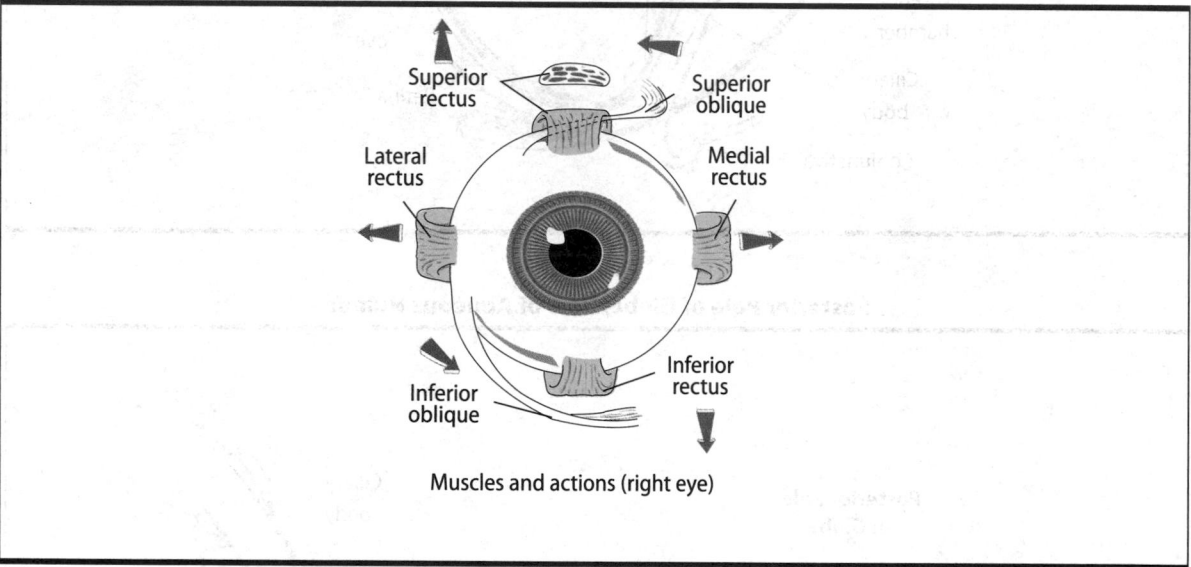

Muscles and actions (right eye)

Eyelid Structures

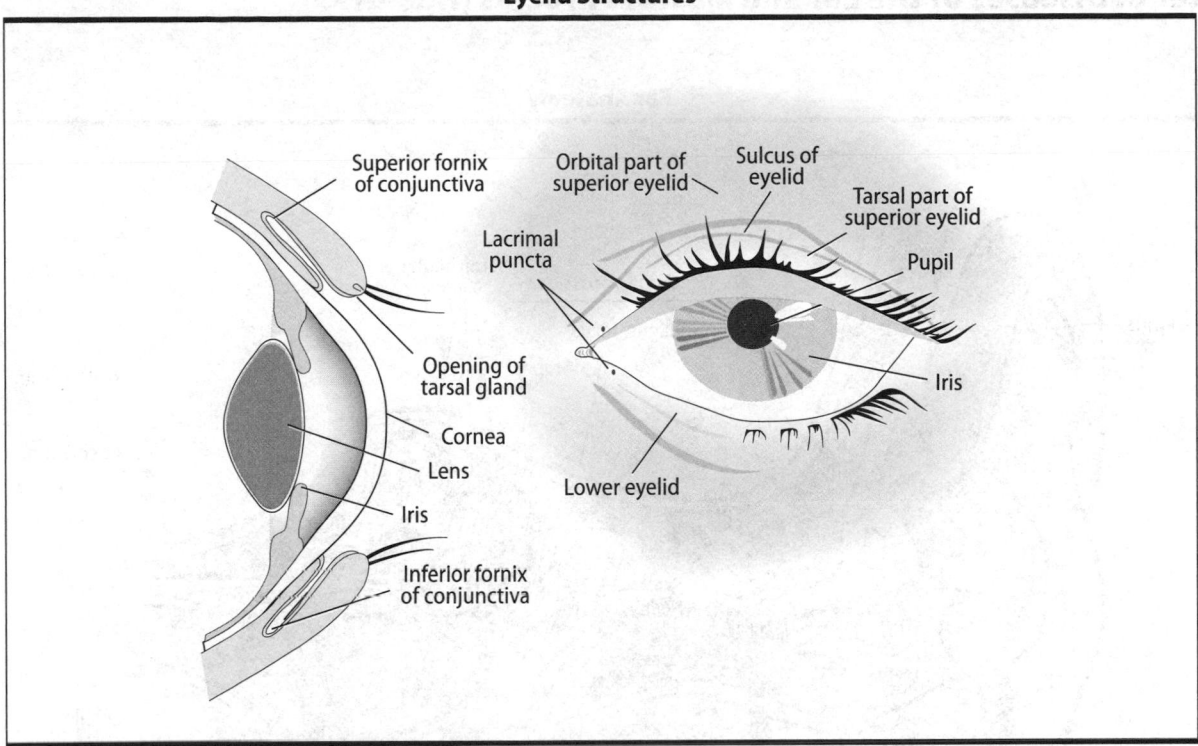

Chapter 8. Diseases of the Ear and Mastoid Process (H60–H95)

Ear Anatomy

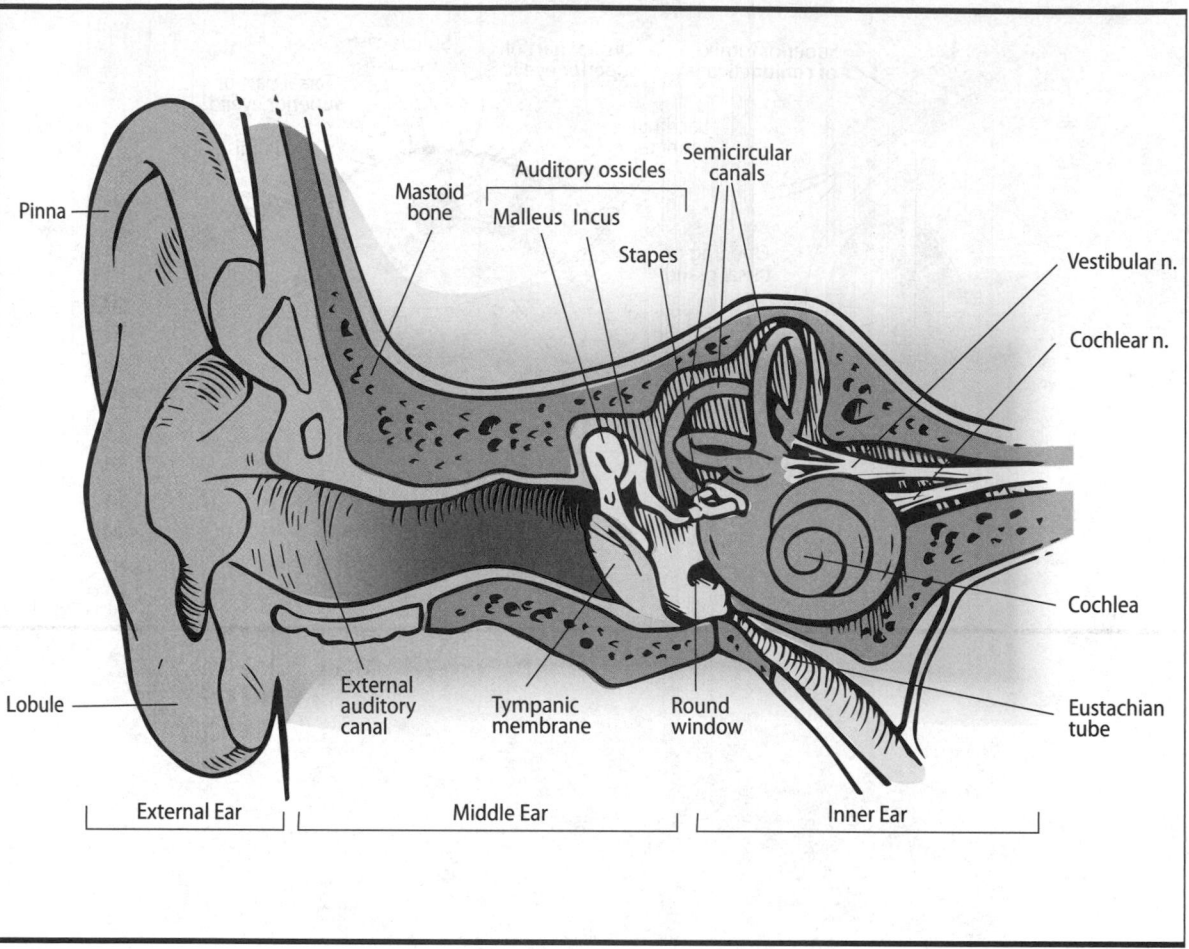

Chapter 9. Diseases of the Circulatory System (I00–I99)

Anatomy of the Heart

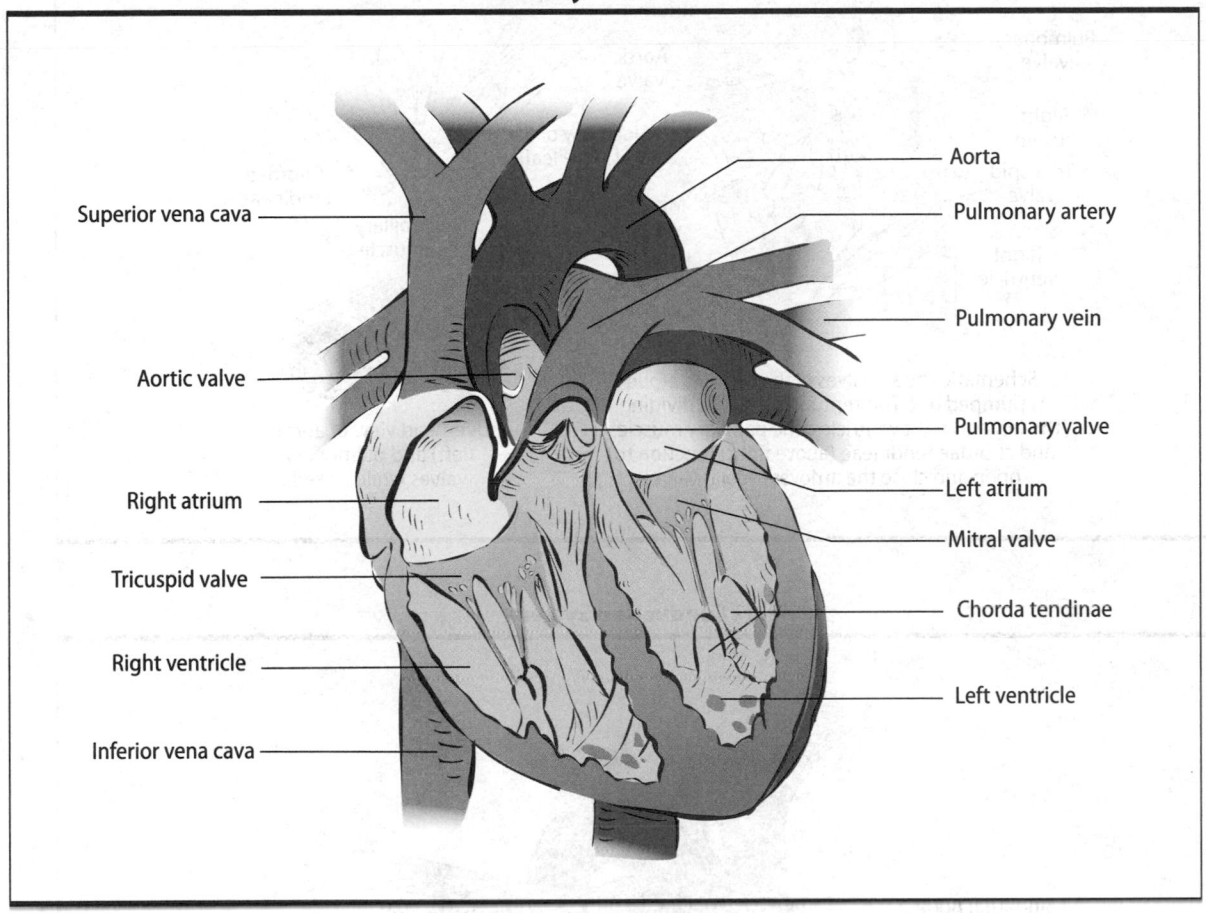

Heart Cross Section

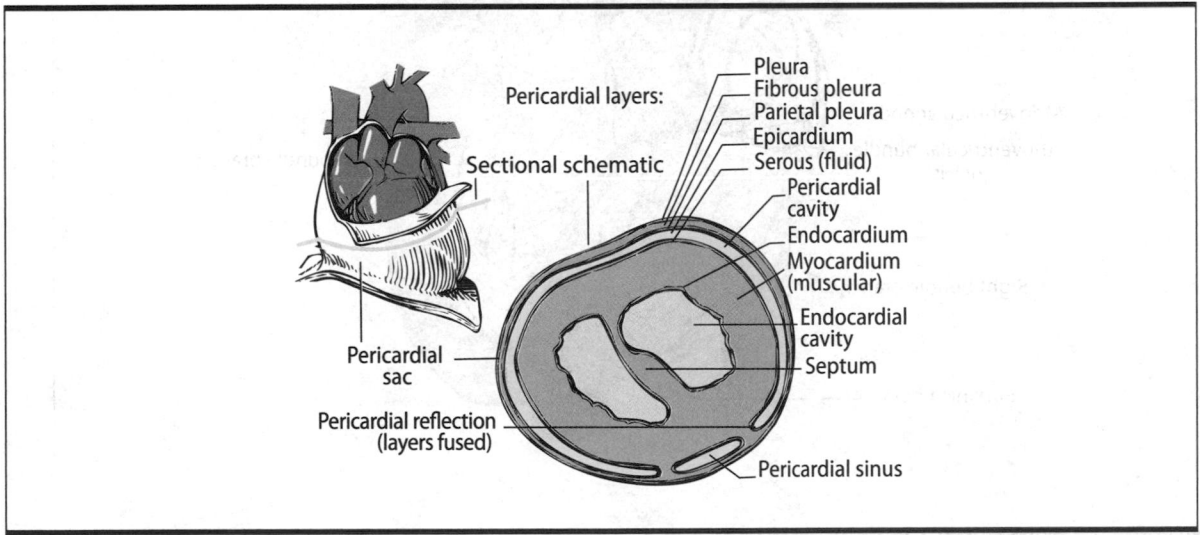

Heart Valves

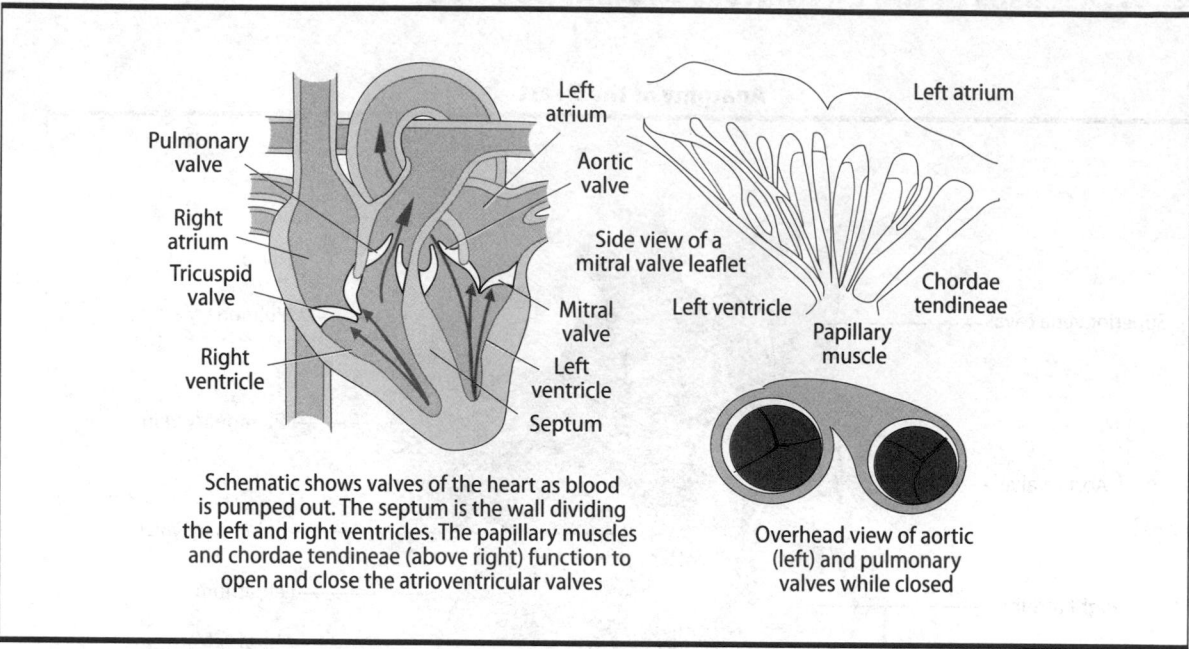

Schematic shows valves of the heart as blood is pumped out. The septum is the wall dividing the left and right ventricles. The papillary muscles and chordae tendineae (above right) function to open and close the atrioventricular valves

Overhead view of aortic (left) and pulmonary valves while closed

Heart Conduction System

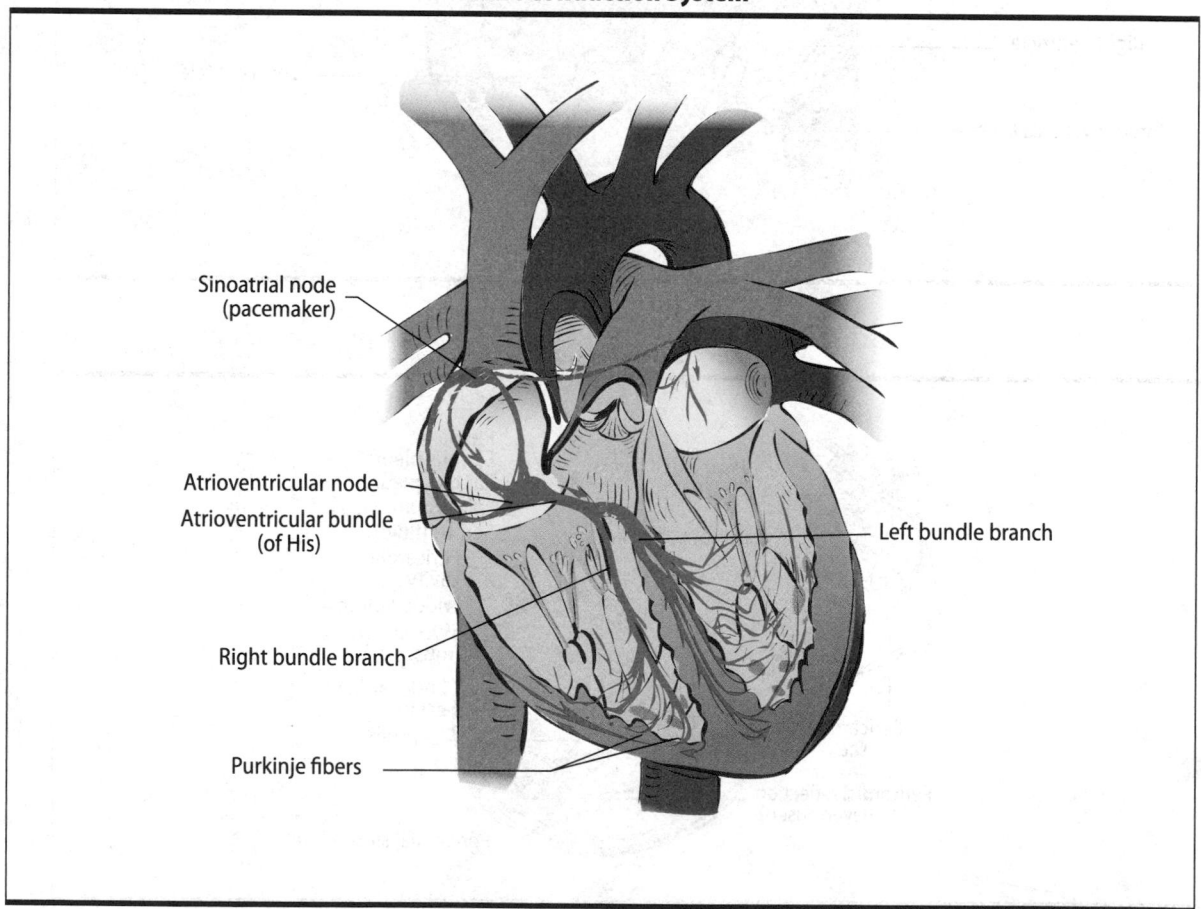

Coronary Arteries

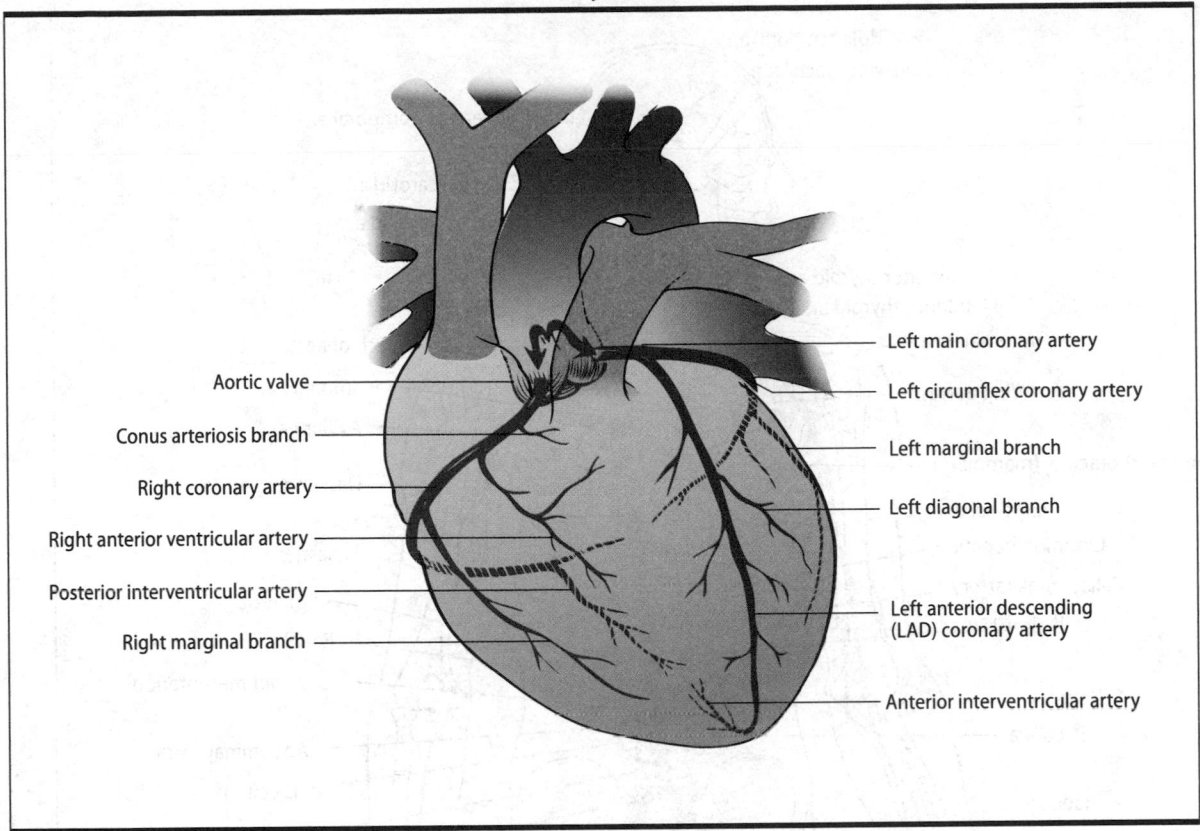

Aortic valve

Conus arteriosis branch

Right coronary artery

Right anterior ventricular artery

Posterior interventricular artery

Right marginal branch

Left main coronary artery

Left circumflex coronary artery

Left marginal branch

Left diagonal branch

Left anterior descending (LAD) coronary artery

Anterior interventricular artery

Arteries

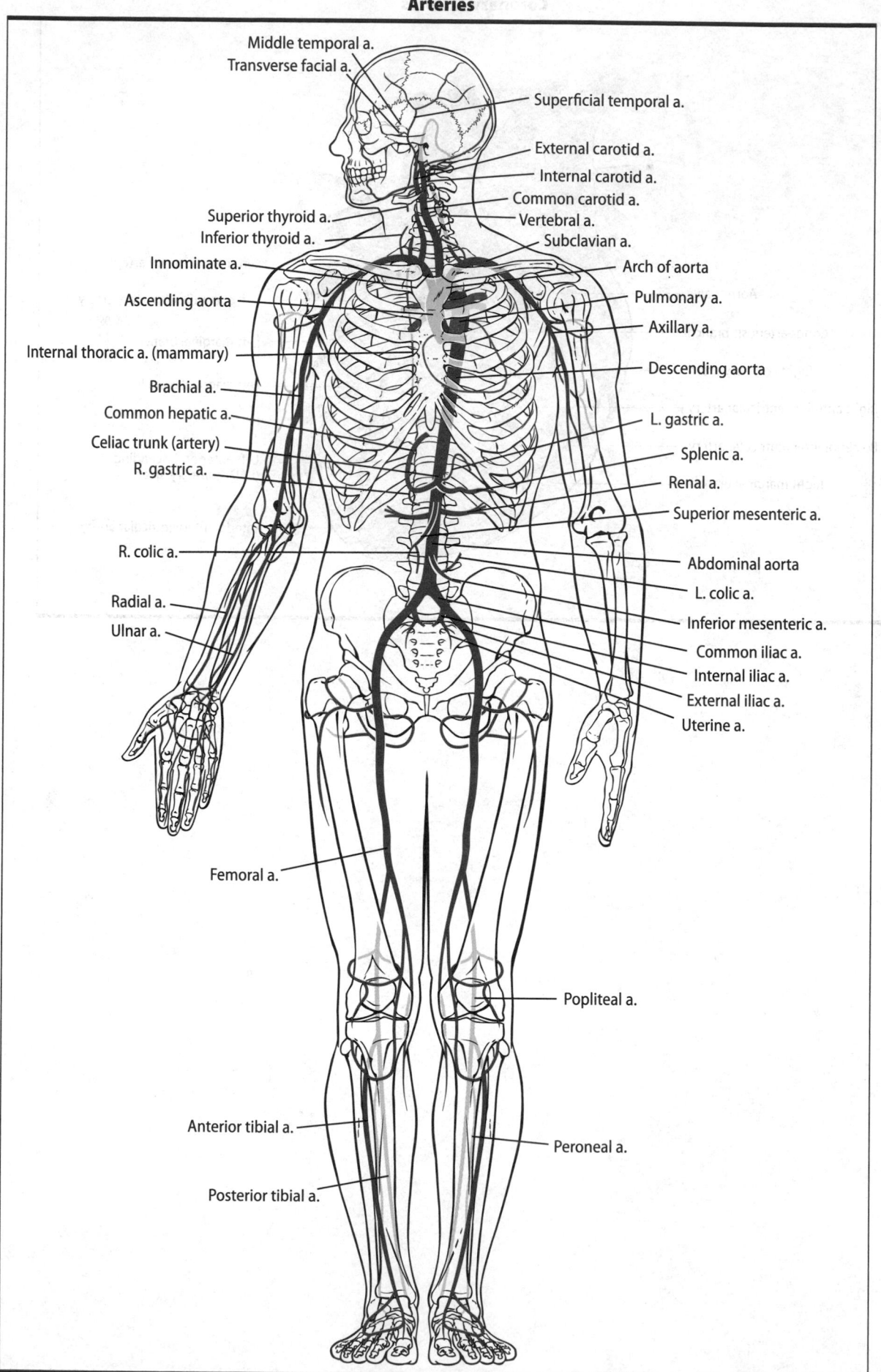

Veins

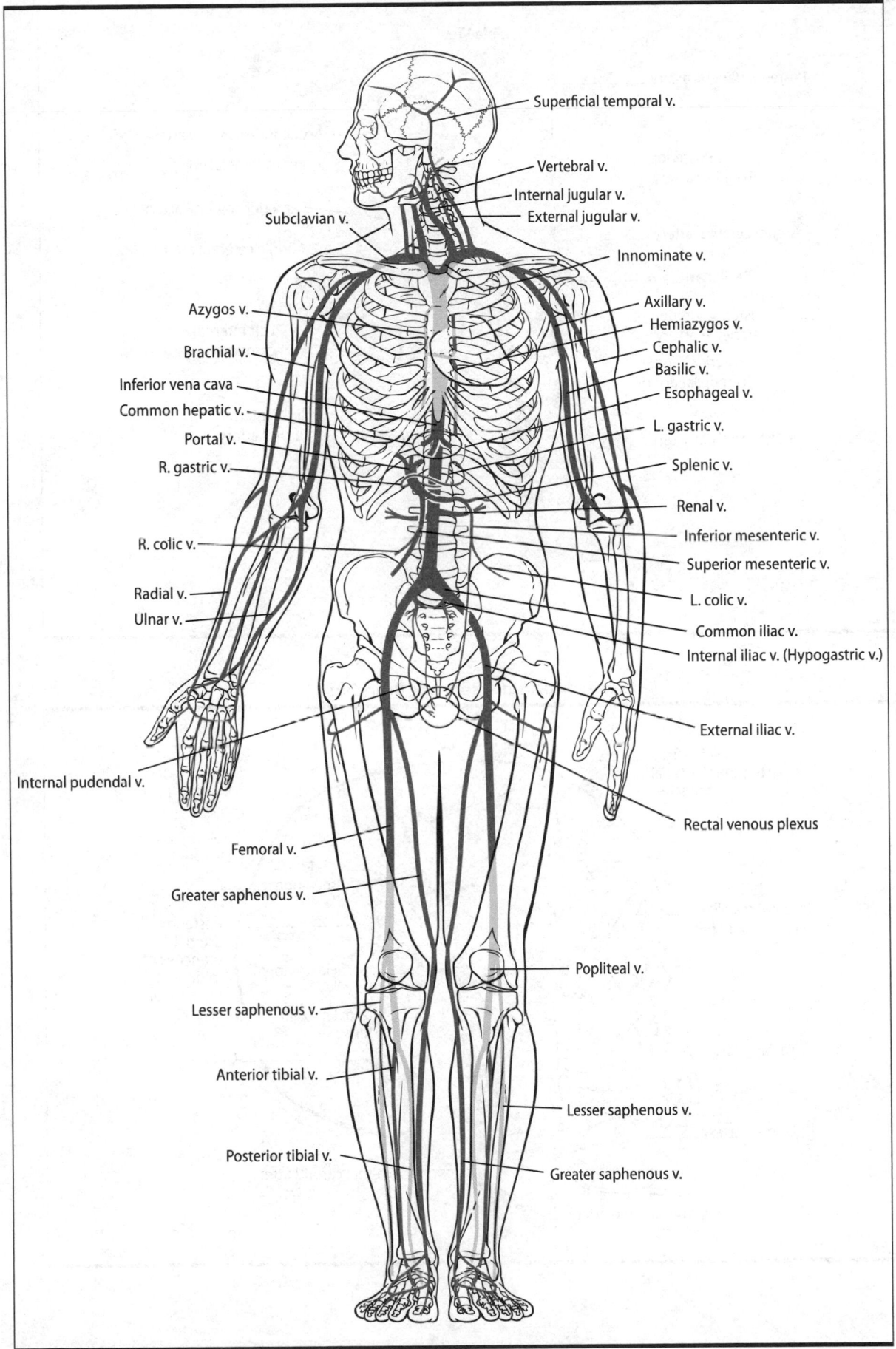

Internal Carotid and Vertebral Arteries and Branches

Side View

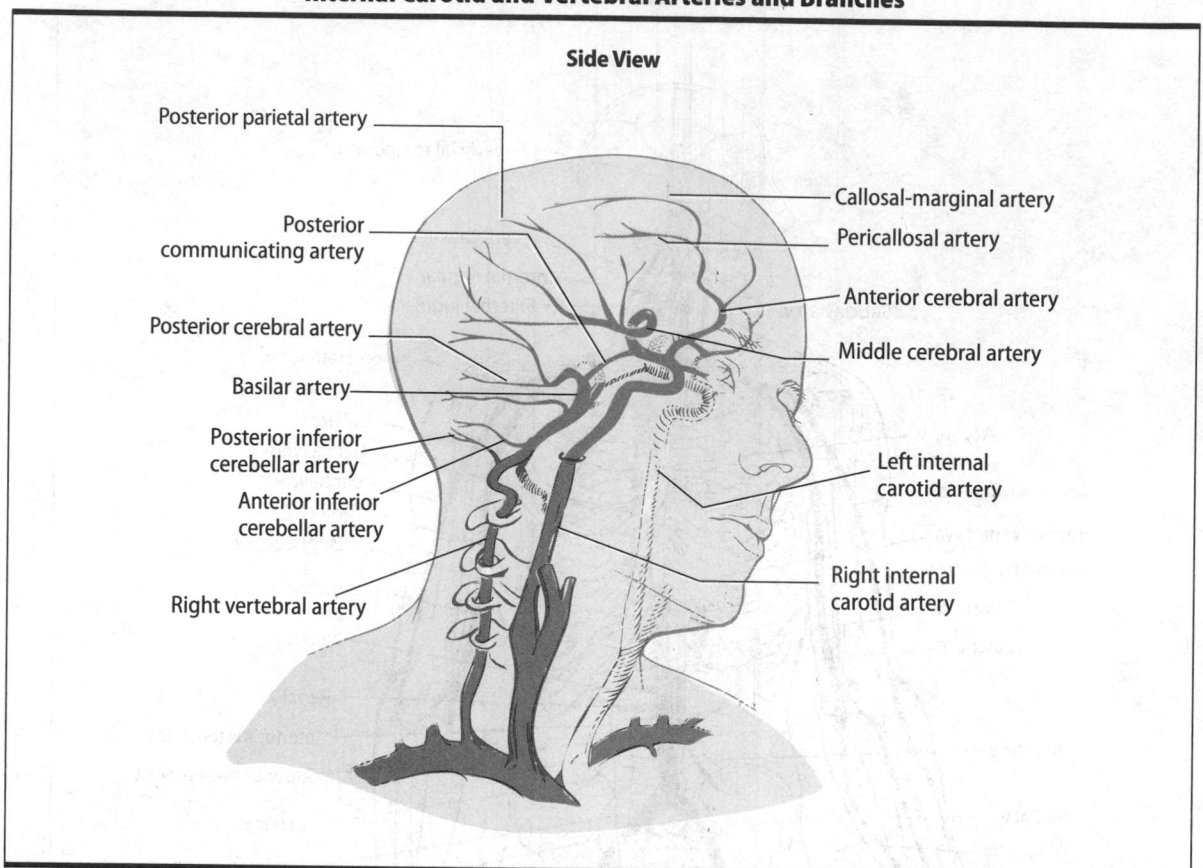

Posterior parietal artery

Posterior communicating artery

Posterior cerebral artery

Basilar artery

Posterior inferior cerebellar artery

Anterior inferior cerebellar artery

Right vertebral artery

Callosal-marginal artery

Pericallosal artery

Anterior cerebral artery

Middle cerebral artery

Left internal carotid artery

Right internal carotid artery

External Carotid Artery and Branches

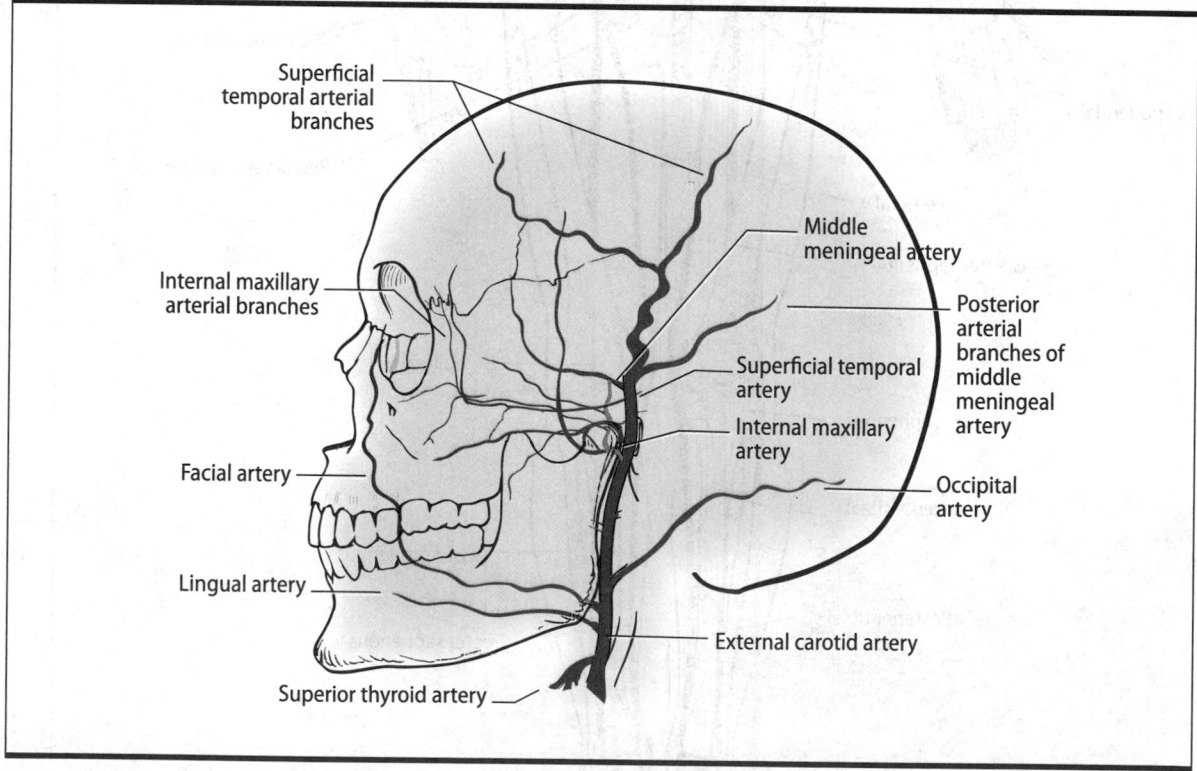

Superficial temporal arterial branches

Internal maxillary arterial branches

Facial artery

Lingual artery

Superior thyroid artery

Middle meningeal artery

Superficial temporal artery

Internal maxillary artery

Posterior arterial branches of middle meningeal artery

Occipital artery

External carotid artery

Branches of Abdominal Aorta

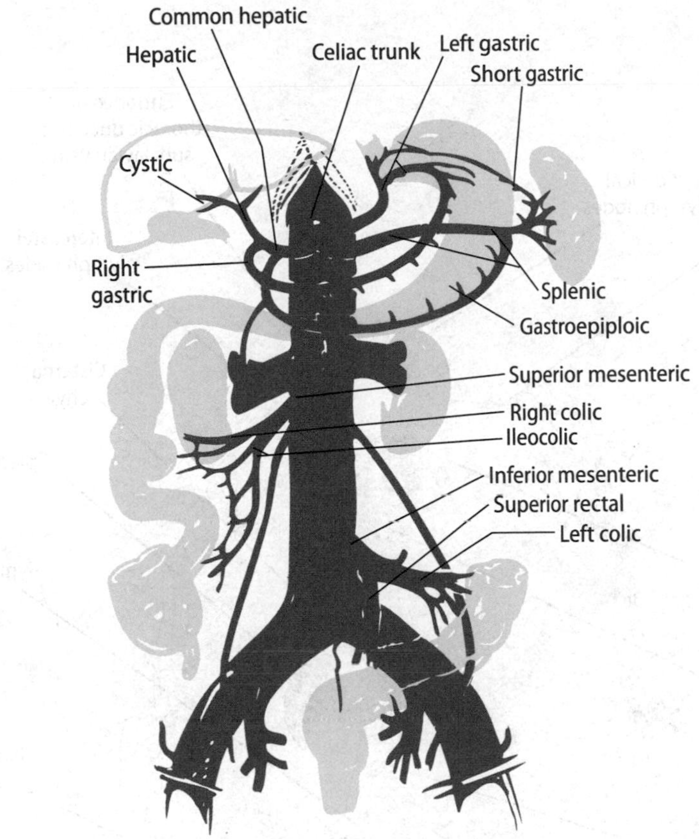

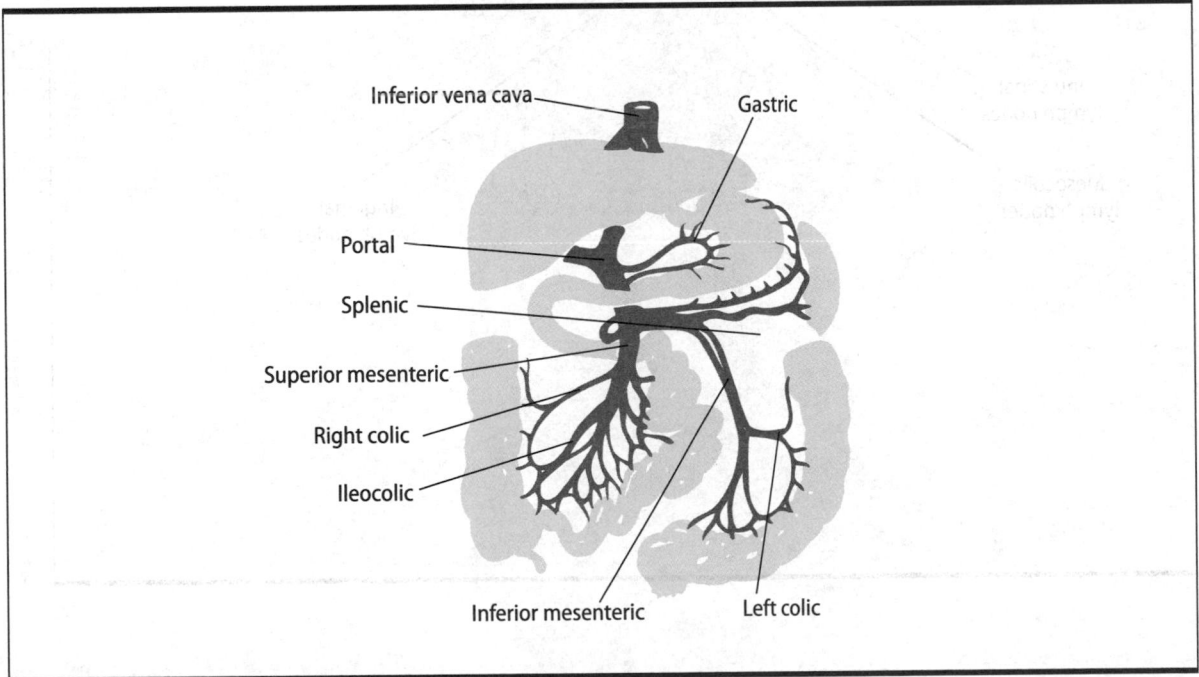

Portal Venous Circulation

Lymphatic System

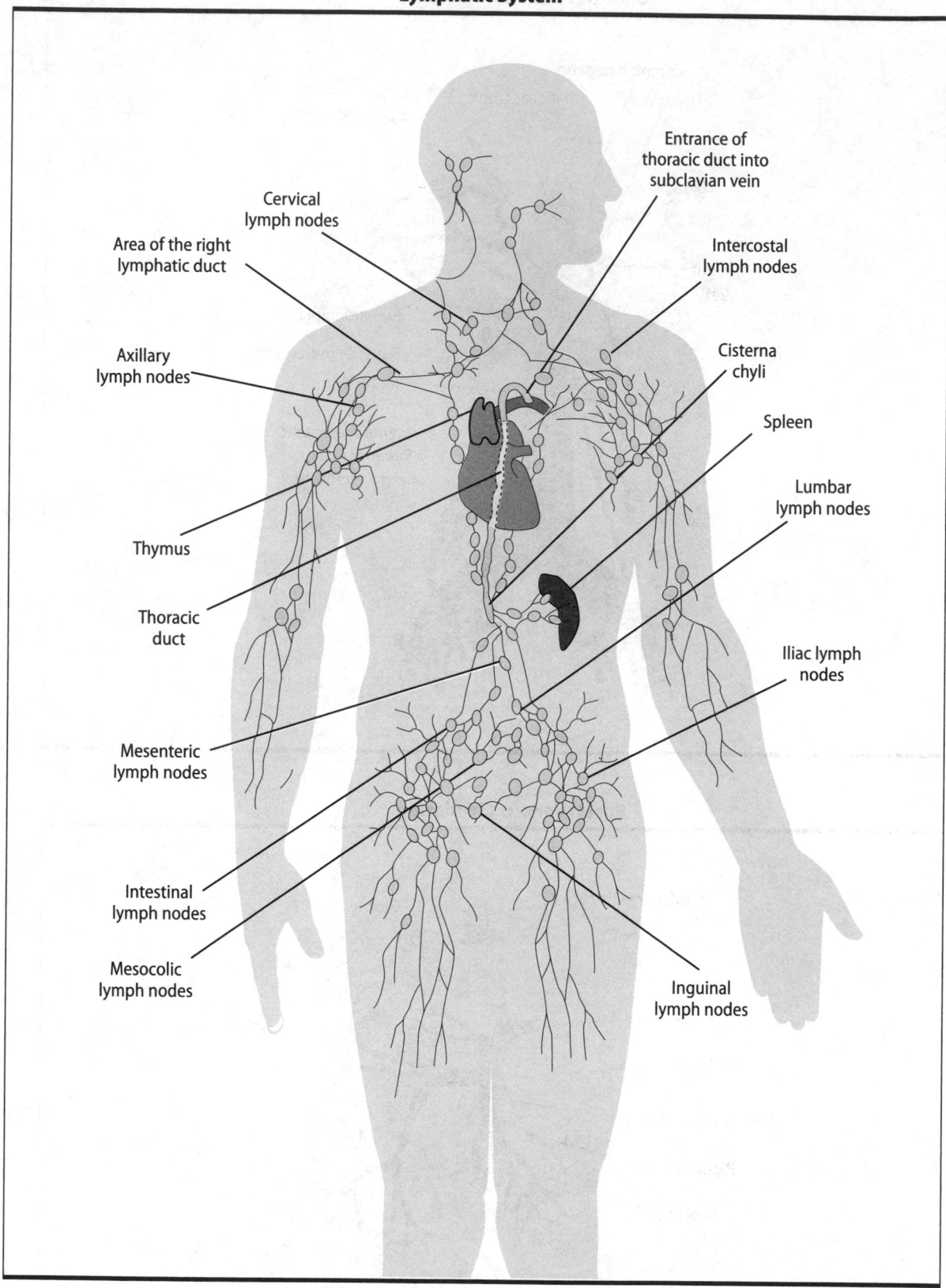

Entrance of
thoracic duct into
subclavian vein

Cervical
lymph nodes

Area of the right
lymphatic duct

Intercostal
lymph nodes

Cisterna
chyli

Axillary
lymph nodes

Spleen

Lumbar
lymph nodes

Thymus

Thoracic
duct

Iliac lymph
nodes

Mesenteric
lymph nodes

Intestinal
lymph nodes

Mesocolic
lymph nodes

Inguinal
lymph nodes

Axillary Lymph Nodes

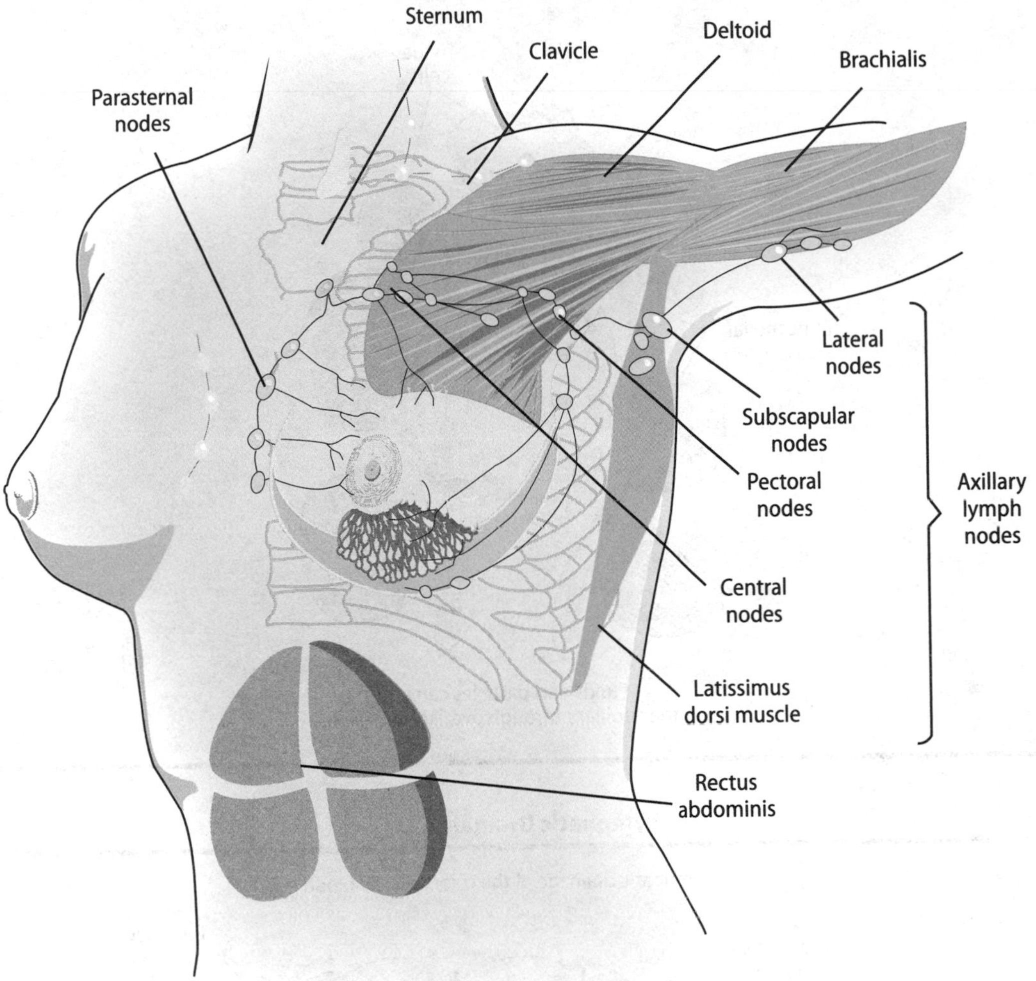

Sternum

Clavicle

Deltoid

Brachialis

Parasternal nodes

Lateral nodes

Subscapular nodes

Pectoral nodes

Axillary lymph nodes

Central nodes

Latissimus dorsi muscle

Rectus abdominis

Lymphatic System of Head and Neck

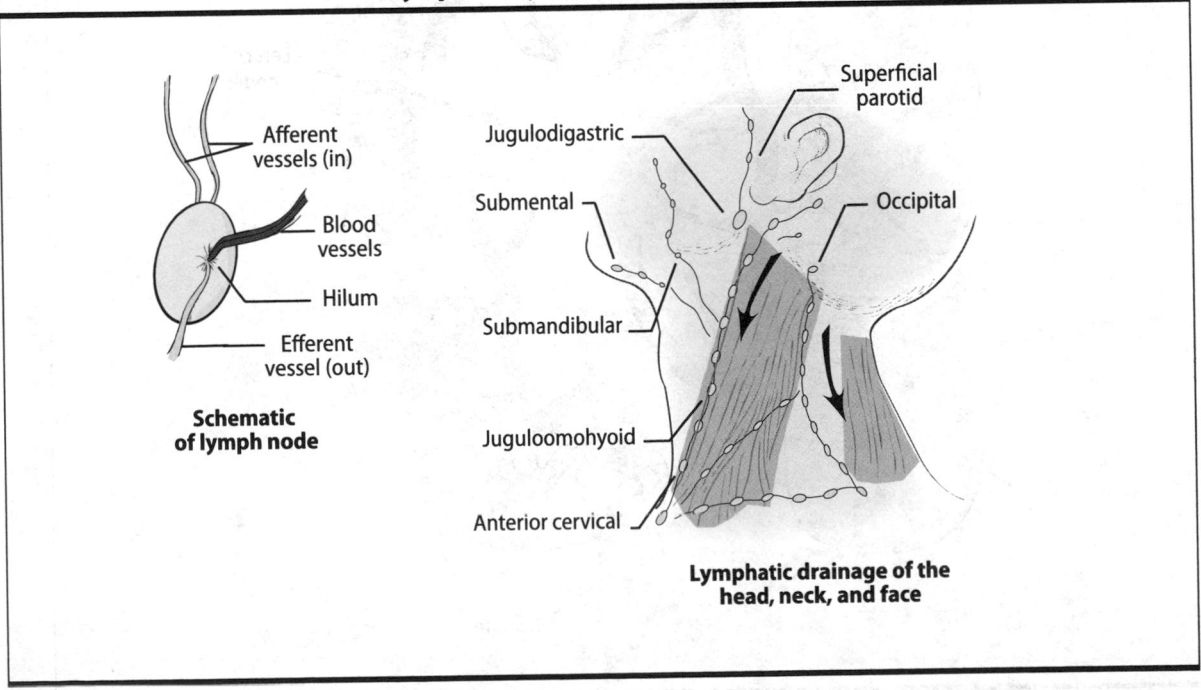

Afferent vessels (in)

Blood vessels

Hilum

Efferent vessel (out)

Schematic of lymph node

Superficial parotid

Jugulodigastric

Submental

Occipital

Submandibular

Juguloomohyoid

Anterior cervical

Lymphatic drainage of the head, neck, and face

Lymphatic Capillaries

Schematic of lymphatic capillaries

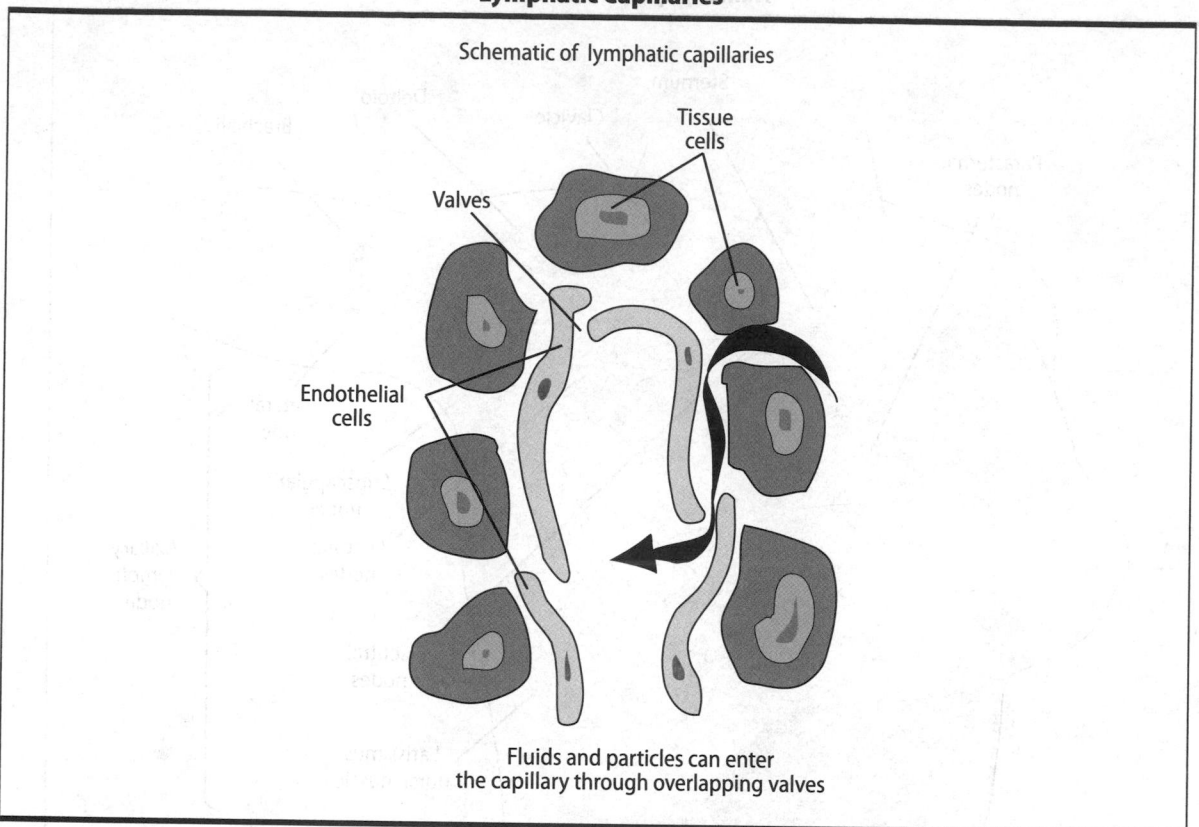

Tissue cells

Valves

Endothelial cells

Fluids and particles can enter the capillary through overlapping valves

Lymphatic Drainage

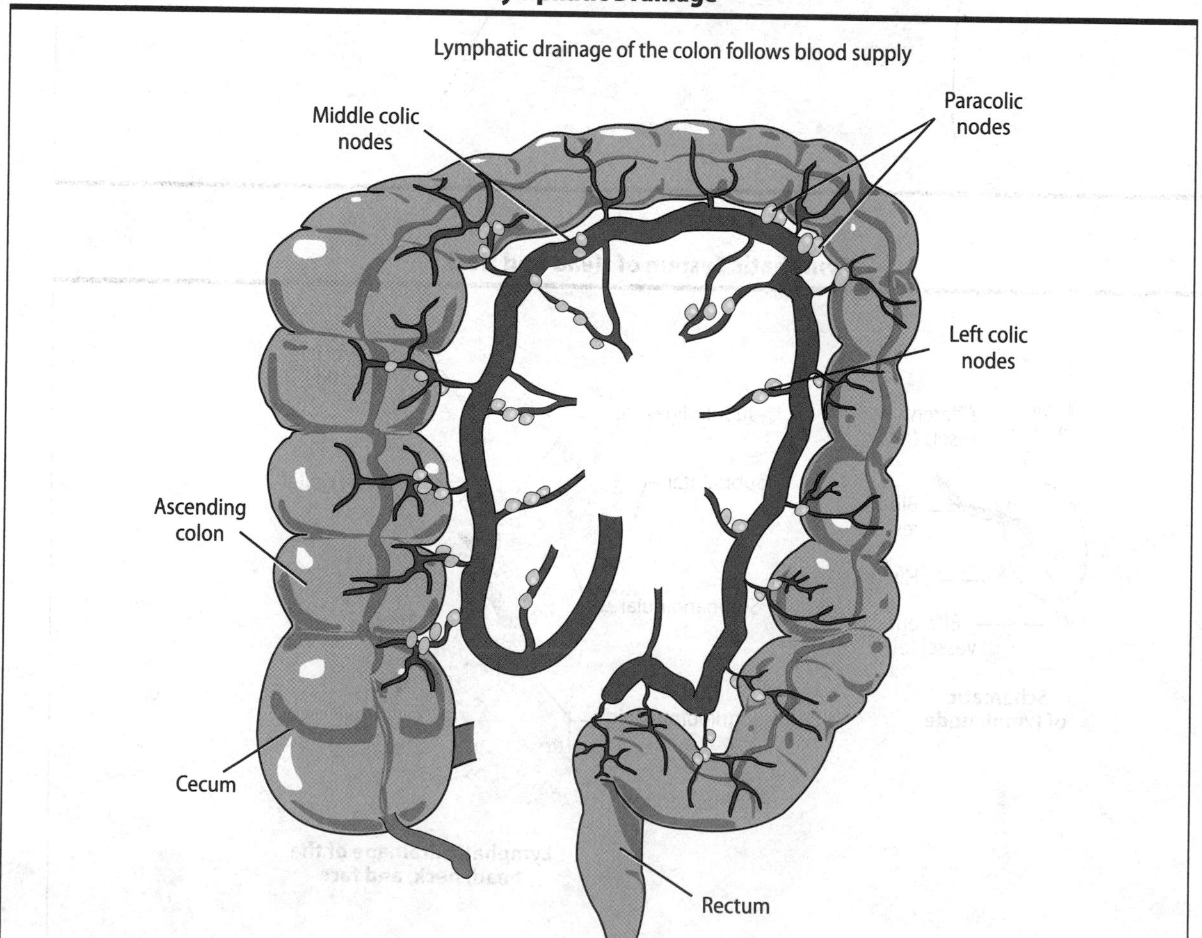

Lymphatic drainage of the colon follows blood supply

Middle colic nodes

Paracolic nodes

Left colic nodes

Ascending colon

Cecum

Rectum

Chapter 10. Diseases of the Respiratory System (JØØ–J99)

Respiratory System

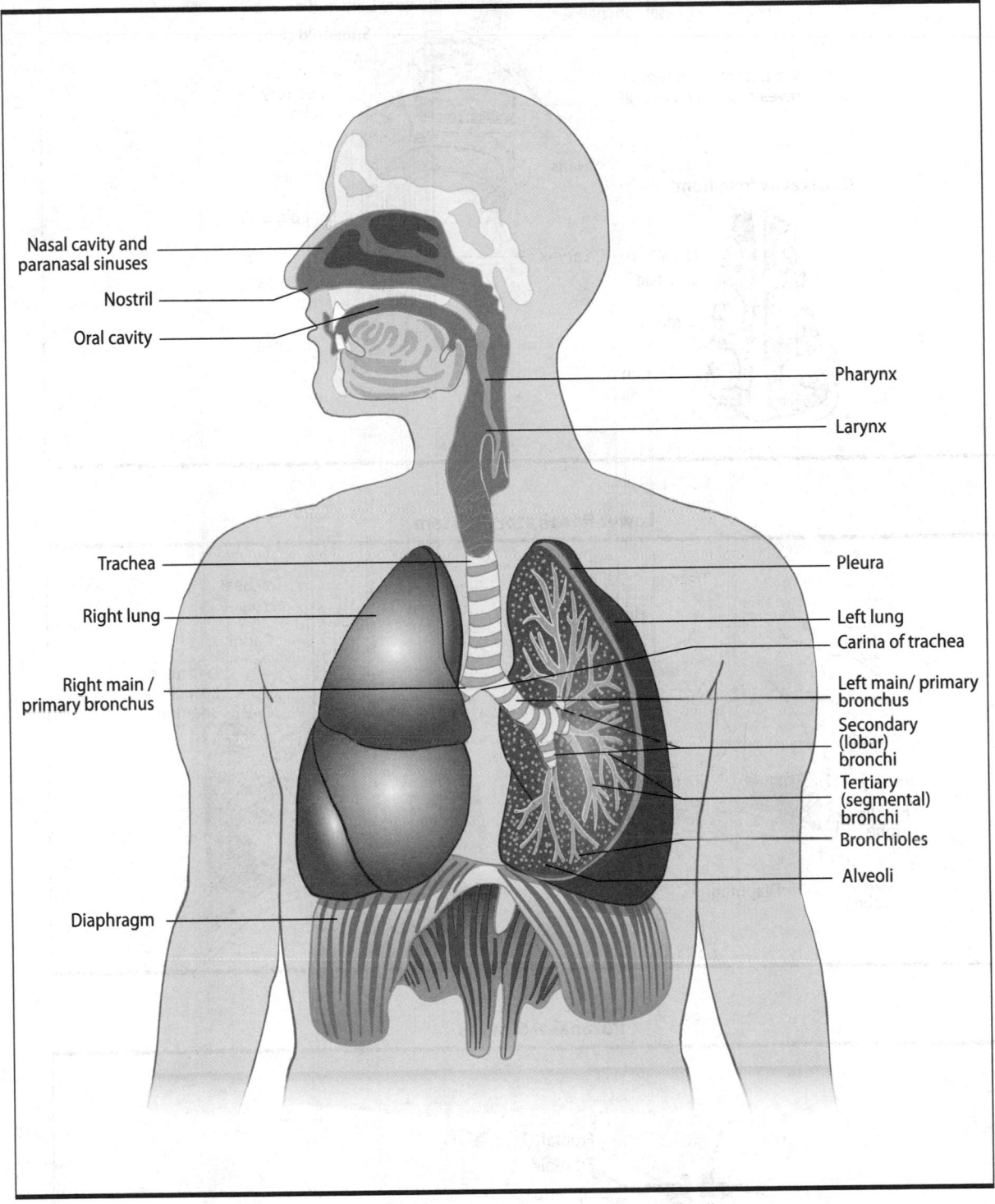

Upper Respiratory System

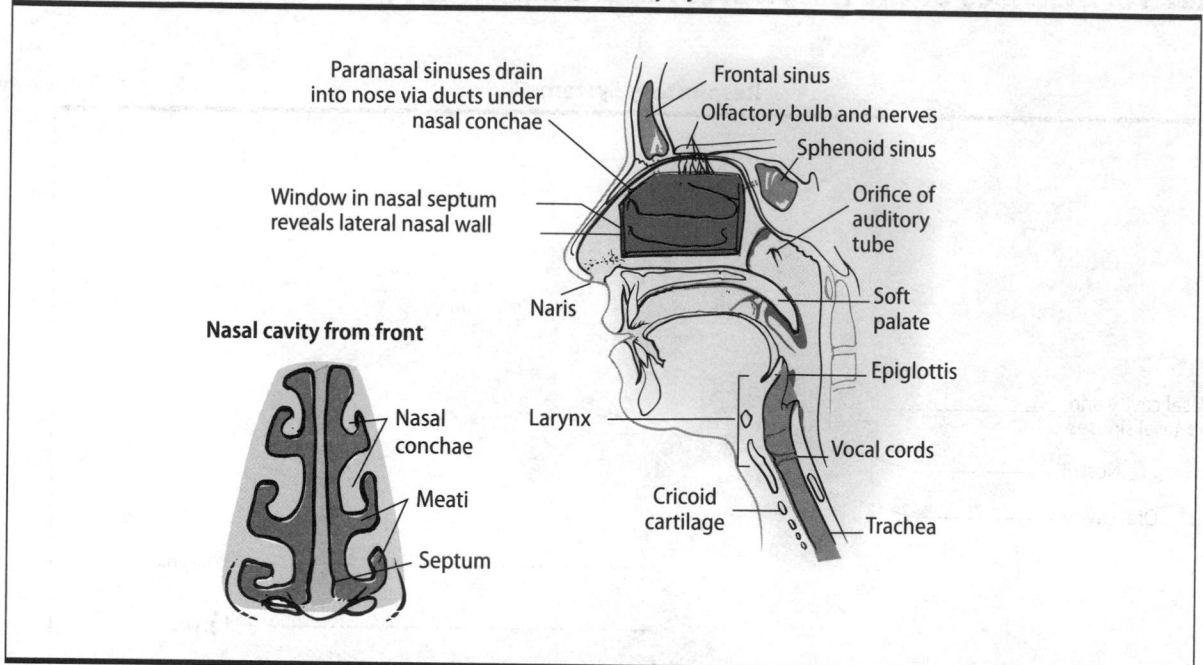

Paranasal sinuses drain into nose via ducts under nasal conchae

Frontal sinus

Olfactory bulb and nerves

Sphenoid sinus

Window in nasal septum reveals lateral nasal wall

Orifice of auditory tube

Naris

Soft palate

Nasal cavity from front

Epiglottis

Larynx

Nasal conchae

Vocal cords

Meati

Cricoid cartilage

Trachea

Septum

Lower Respiratory System

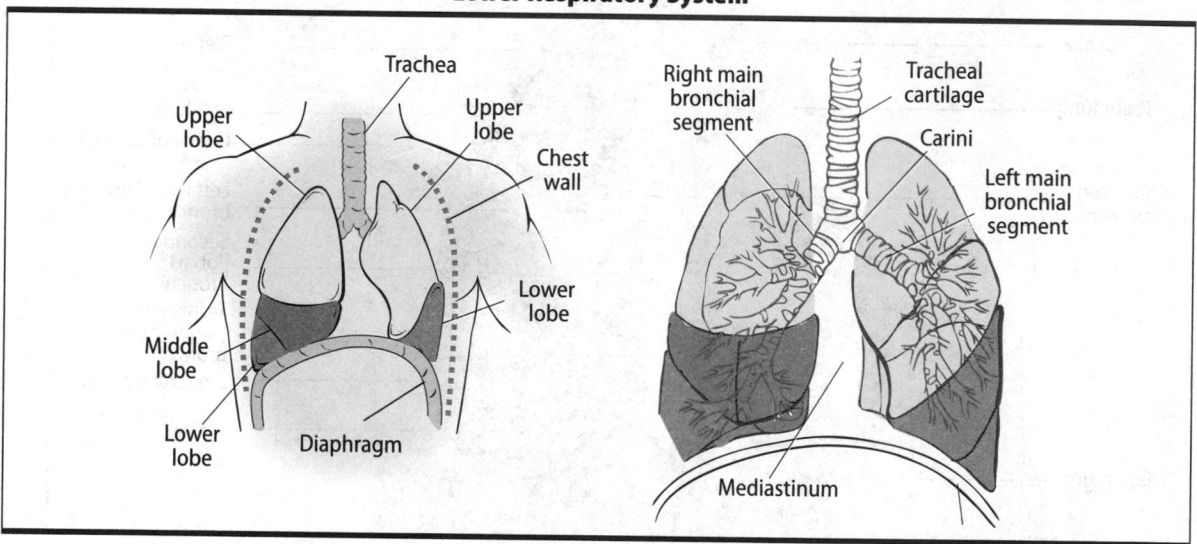

Trachea

Upper lobe

Upper lobe

Chest wall

Right main bronchial segment

Tracheal cartilage

Carini

Left main bronchial segment

Middle lobe

Lower lobe

Lower lobe

Diaphragm

Mediastinum

Paranasal Sinuses

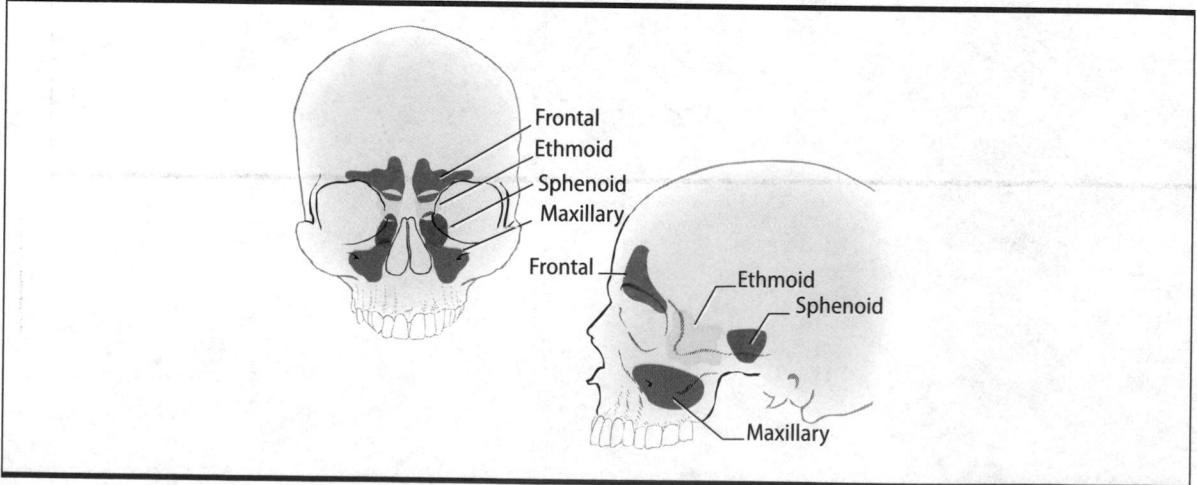

Frontal
Ethmoid
Sphenoid
Maxillary

Frontal

Ethmoid
Sphenoid

Maxillary

Lung Segments

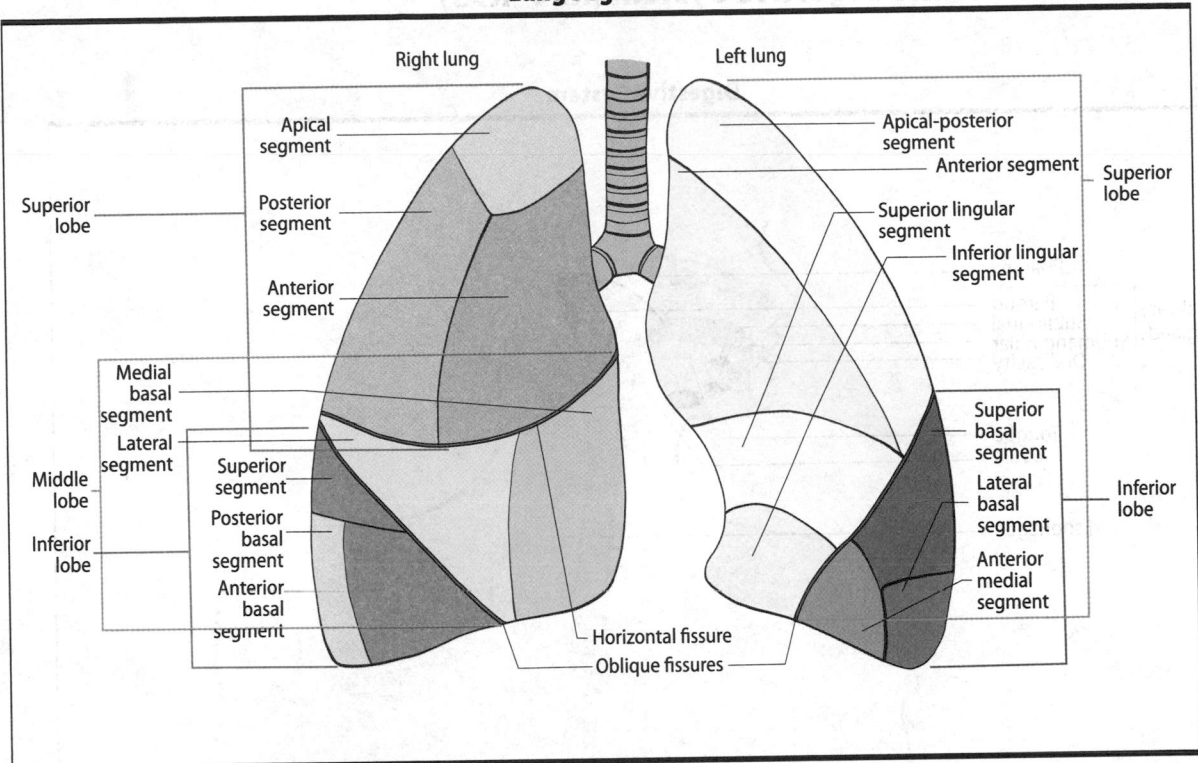

Alveoli

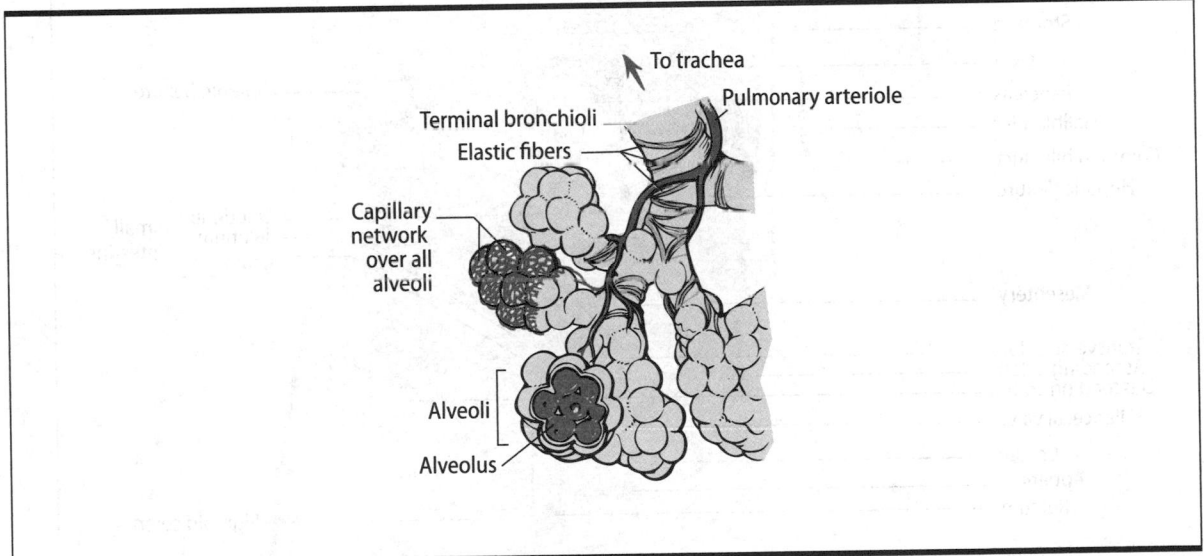

Chapter 11. Diseases of the Digestive System (KØØ–K95)

Digestive System

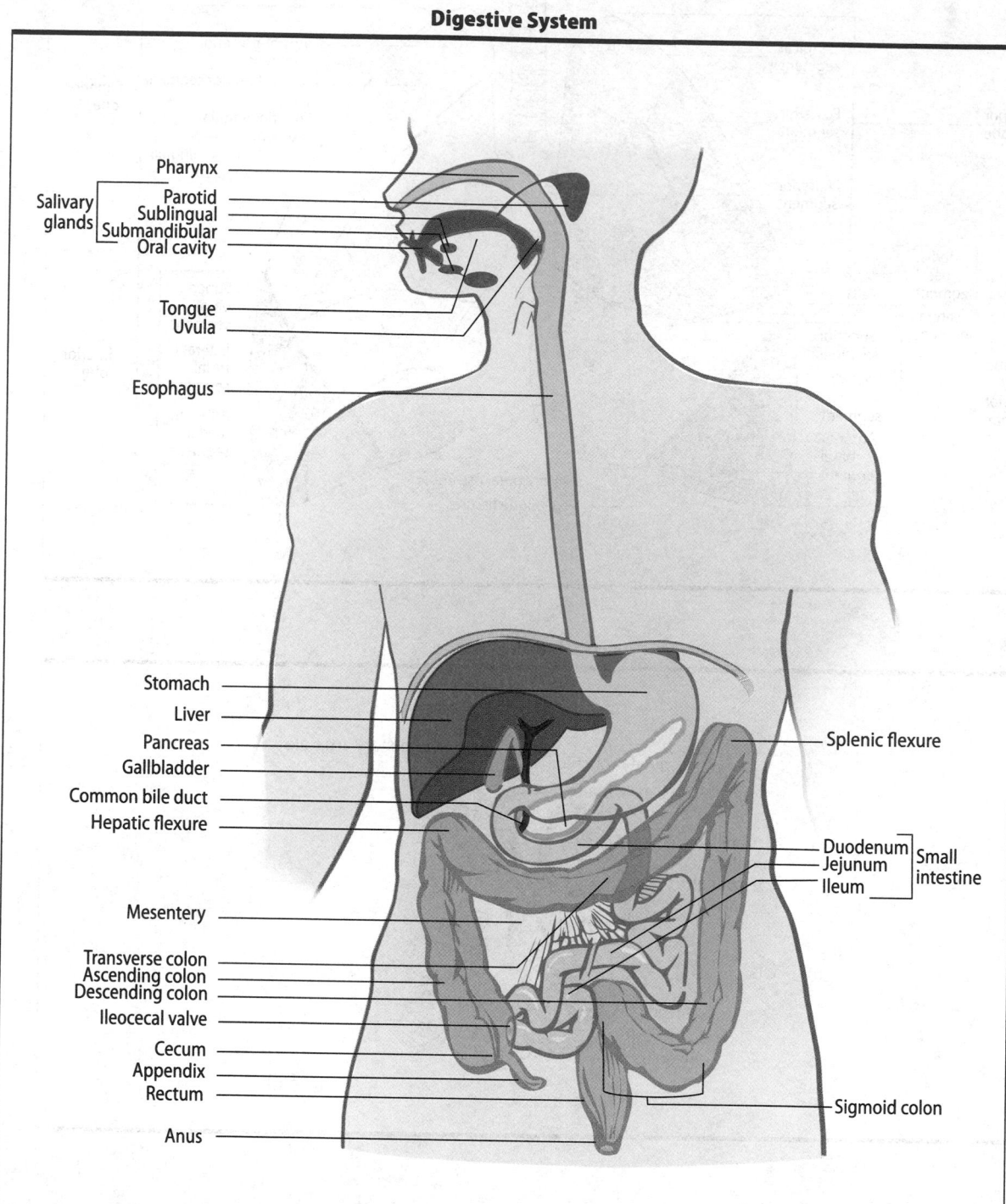

Omentum and Mesentery

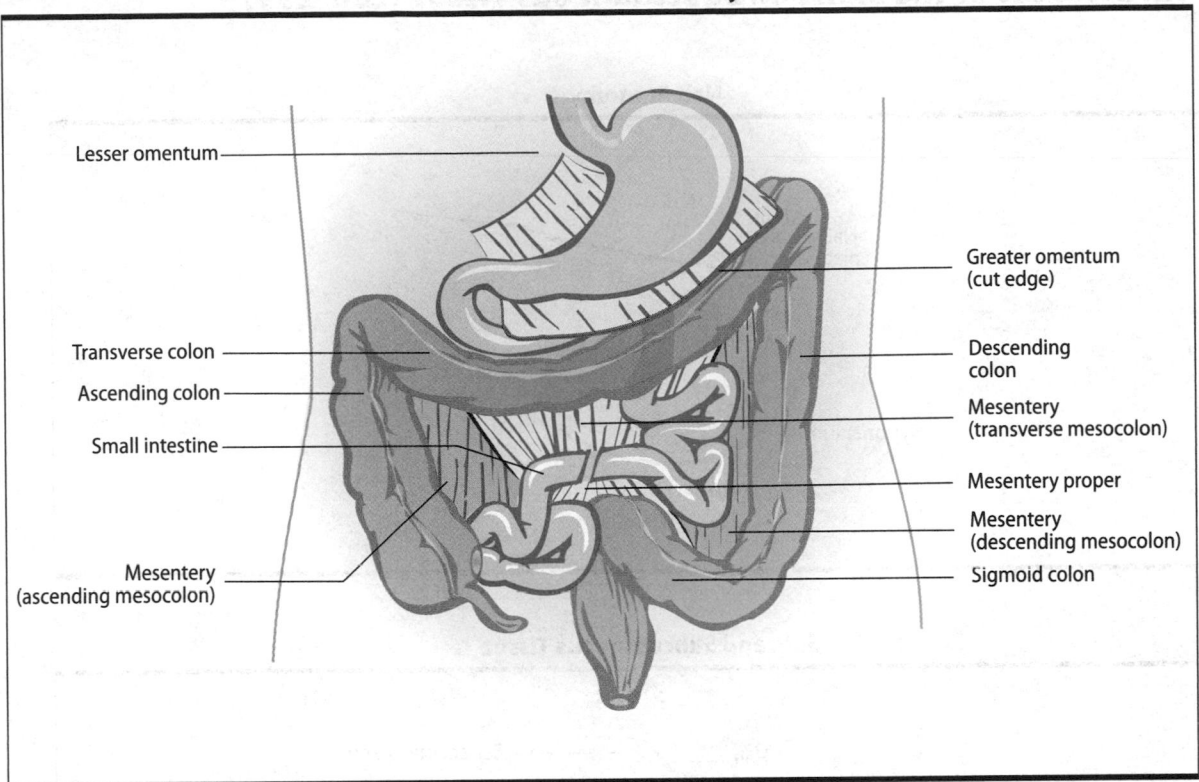

Peritoneum and Retroperitoneum

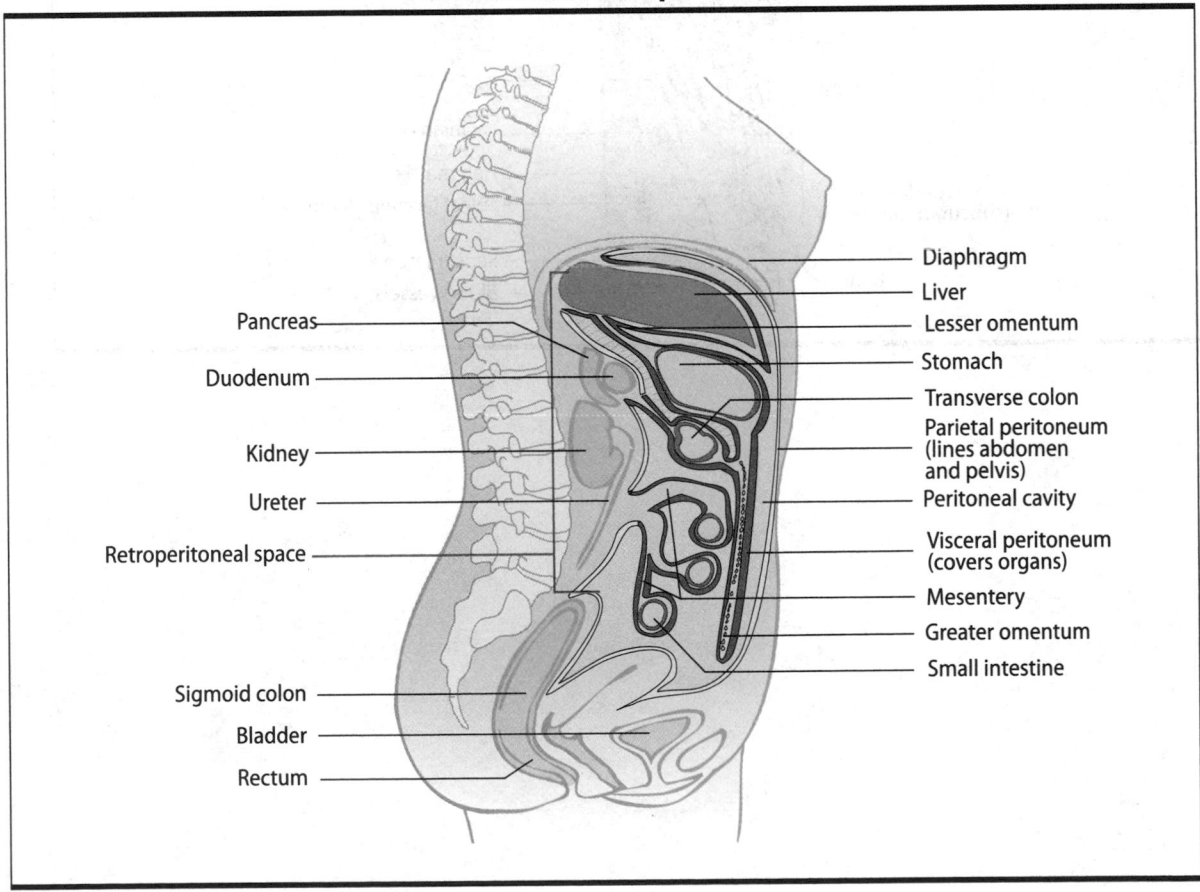

Chapter 12. Diseases of the Skin and Subcutaneous Tissue (L00–L99)

Nail Anatomy

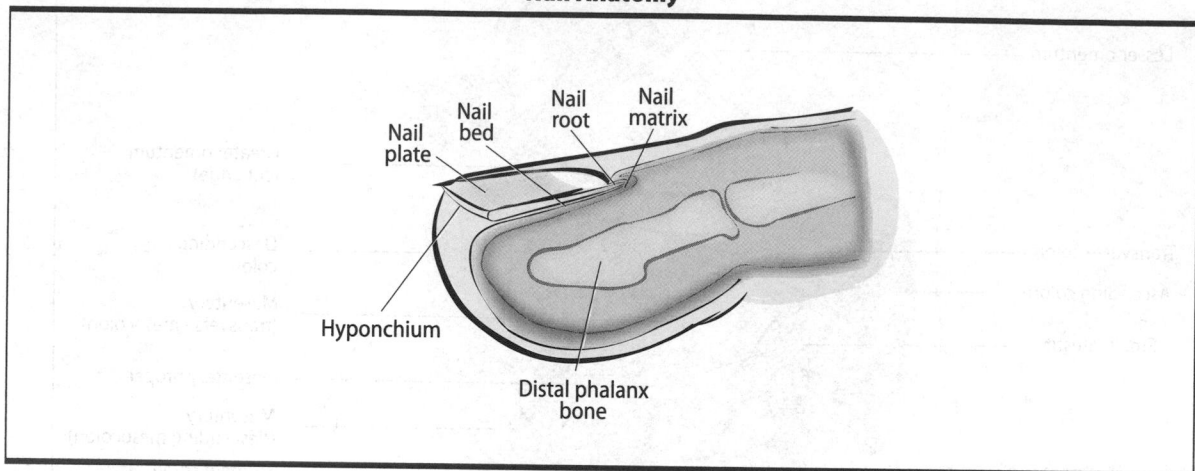

Skin and Subcutaneous Tissue

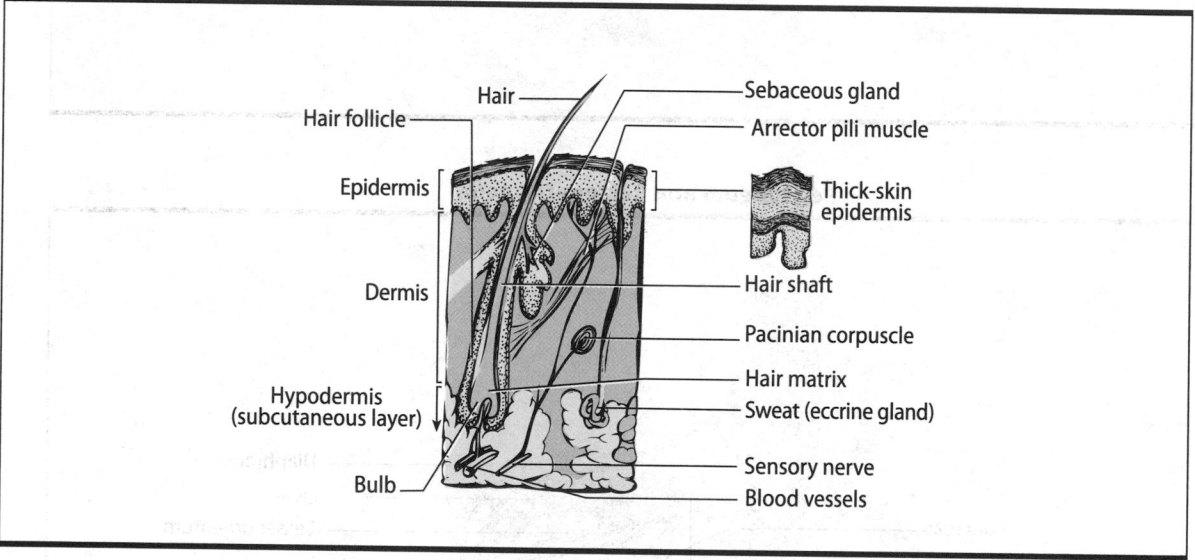

Chapter 13. Diseases of the Musculoskeletal System and Connective Tissue (M00–M99)

Bones and Joints

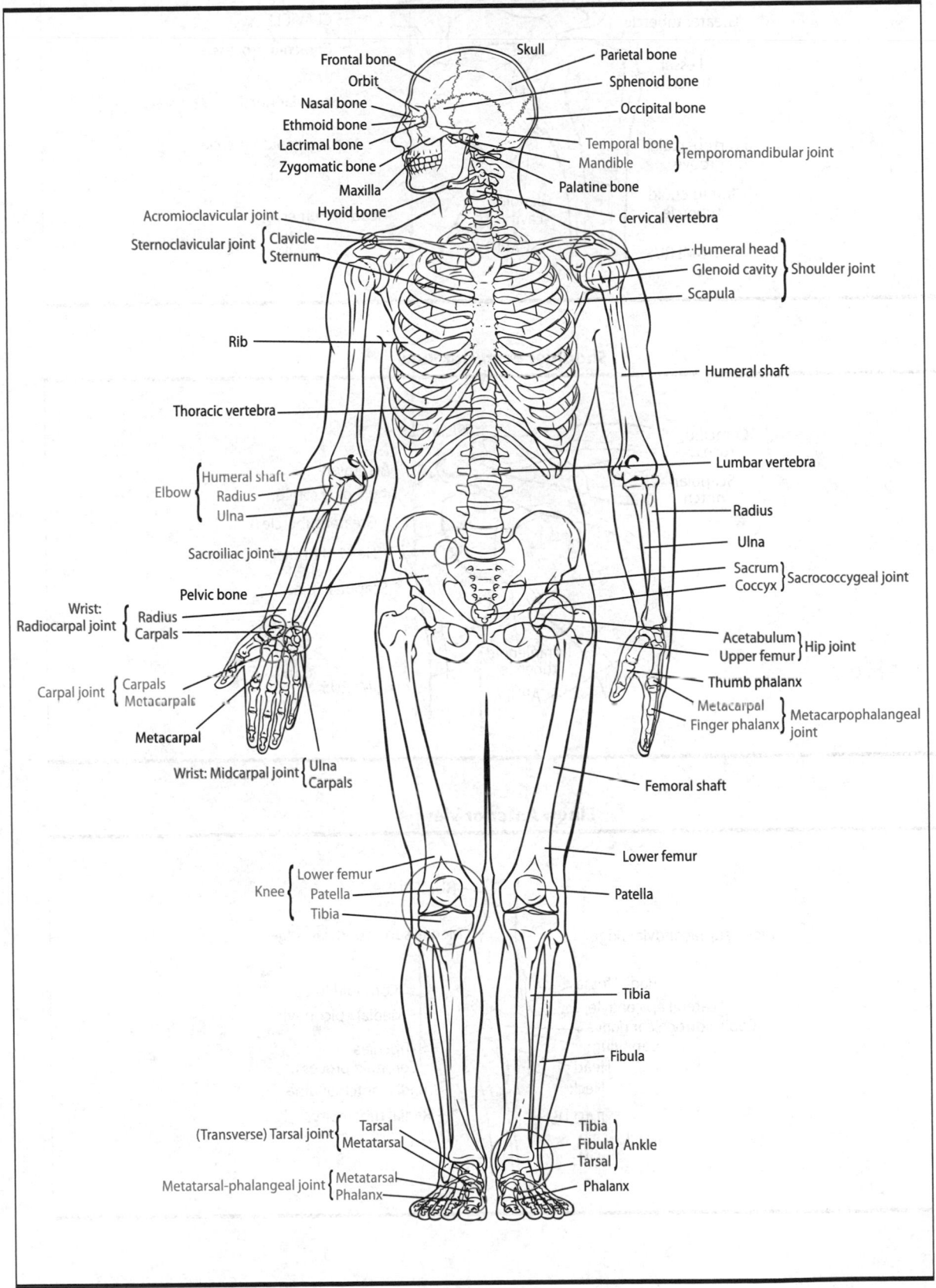

Shoulder Anterior View

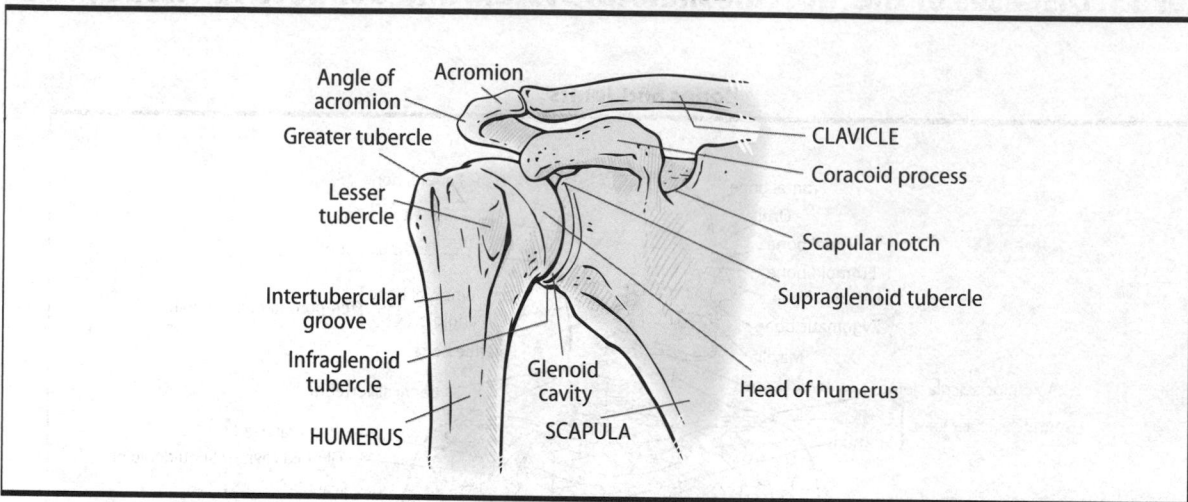

Shoulder Posterior View

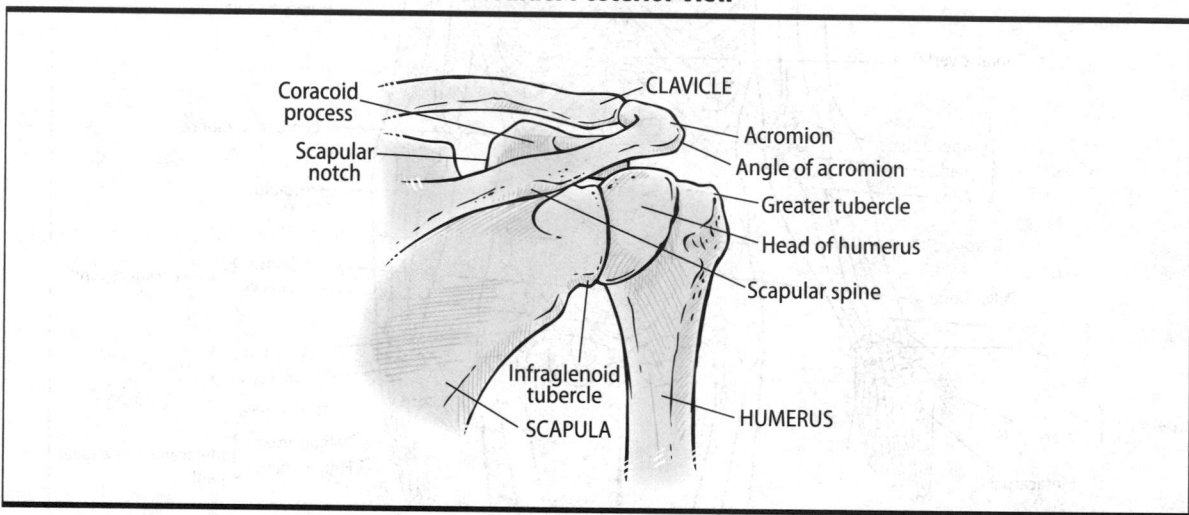

Elbow Anterior View

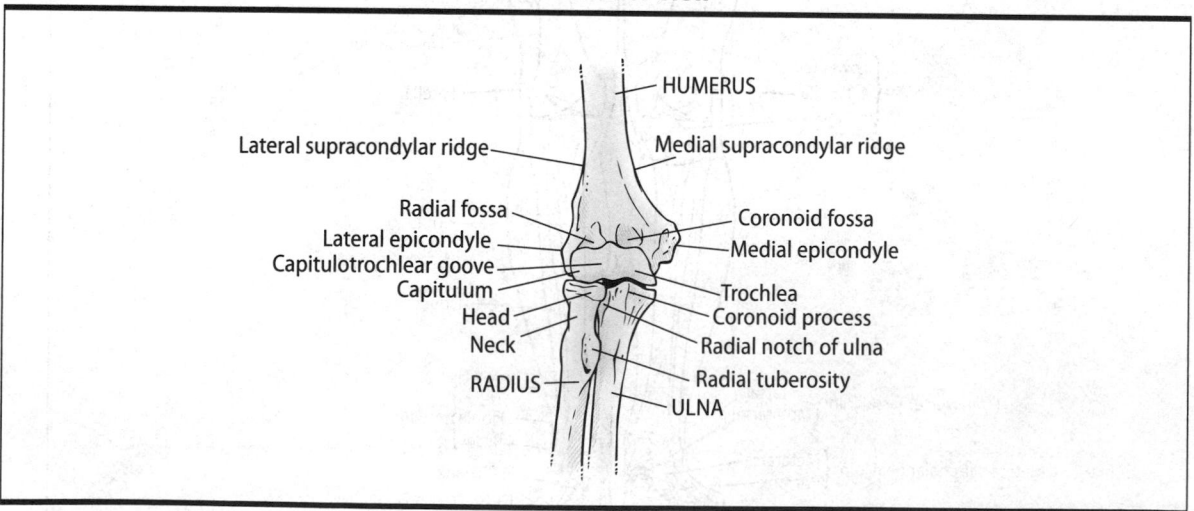

Elbow Posterior View

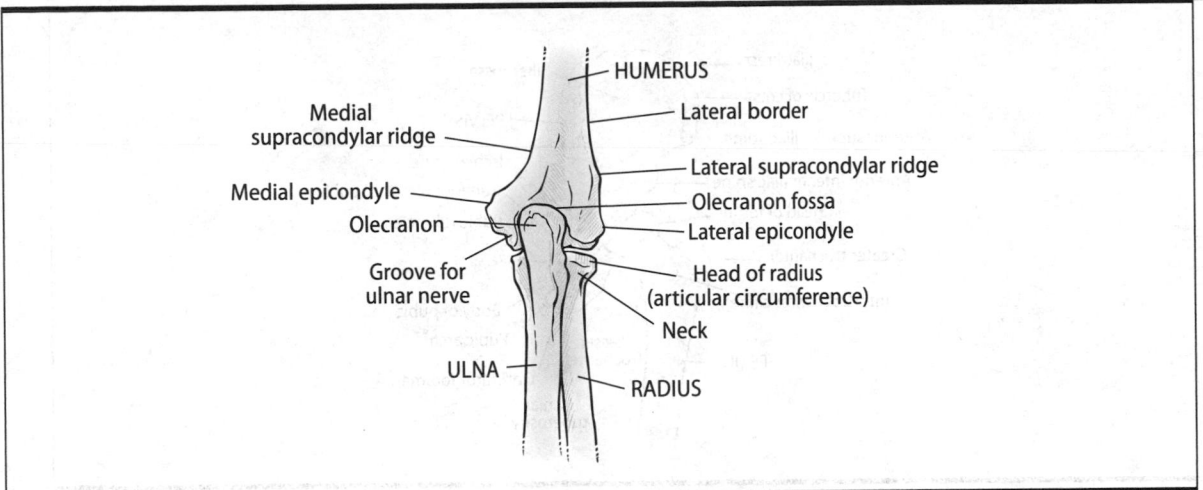

HUMERUS

Medial supracondylar ridge

Lateral border

Lateral supracondylar ridge

Medial epicondyle

Olecranon fossa

Olecranon

Lateral epicondyle

Groove for ulnar nerve

Head of radius (articular circumference)

Neck

ULNA

RADIUS

Hand

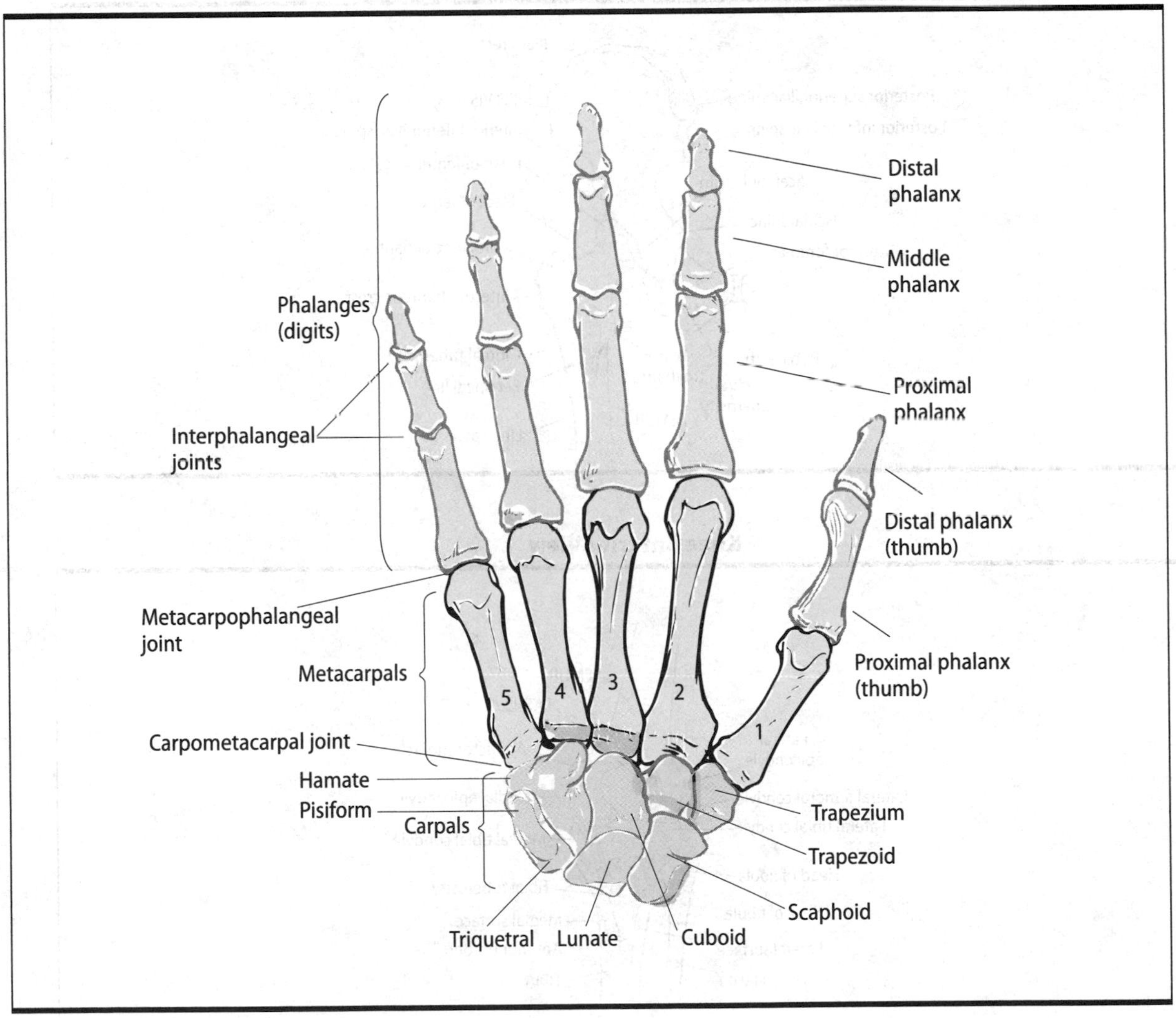

Distal phalanx

Middle phalanx

Phalanges (digits)

Proximal phalanx

Interphalangeal joints

Distal phalanx (thumb)

Metacarpophalangeal joint

Proximal phalanx (thumb)

Metacarpals

5 4 3 2 1

Carpometacarpal joint

Hamate

Pisiform

Carpals

Trapezium

Trapezoid

Scaphoid

Triquetral   Lunate   Cuboid

Hip Anterior View

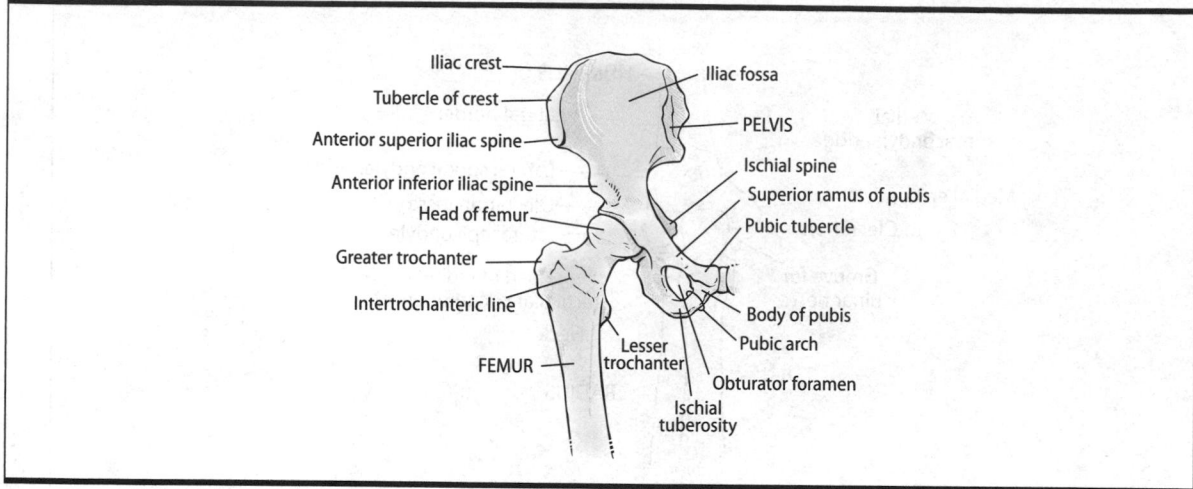

Hip Posterior View

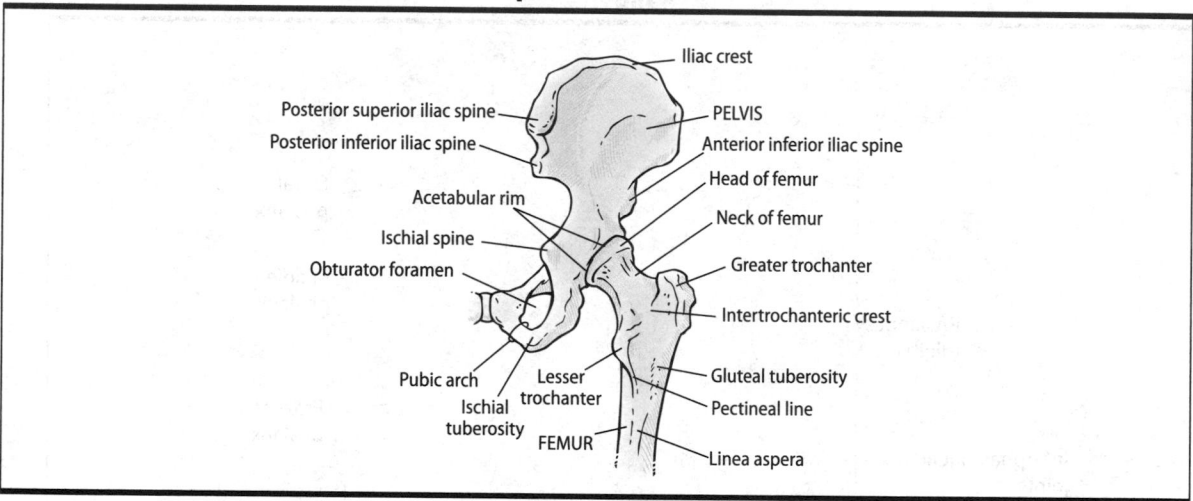

Knee Anterior View

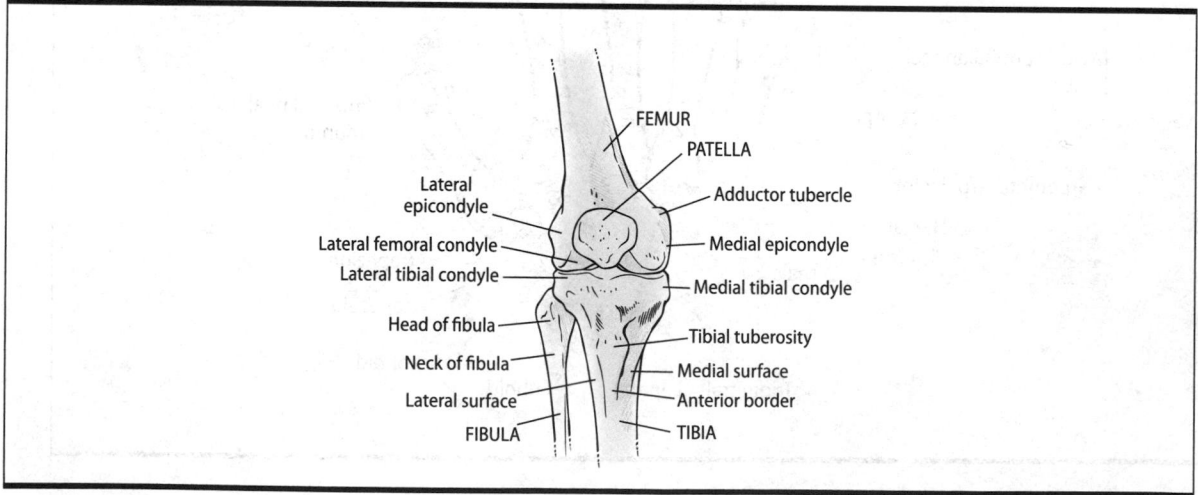

Knee Posterior View

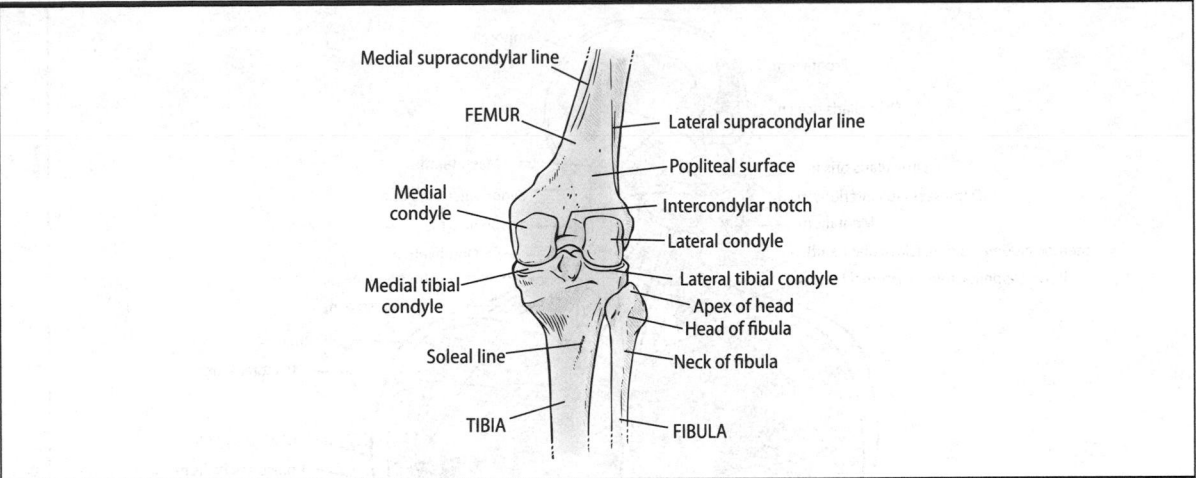

Foot

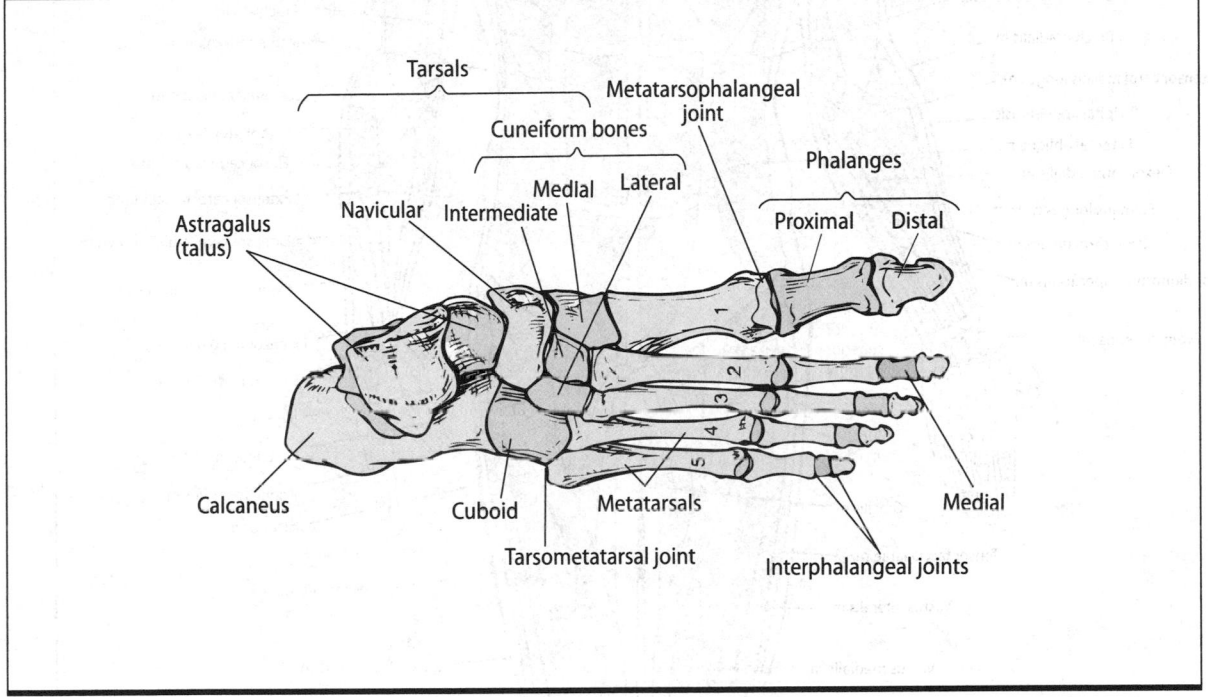

Muscles

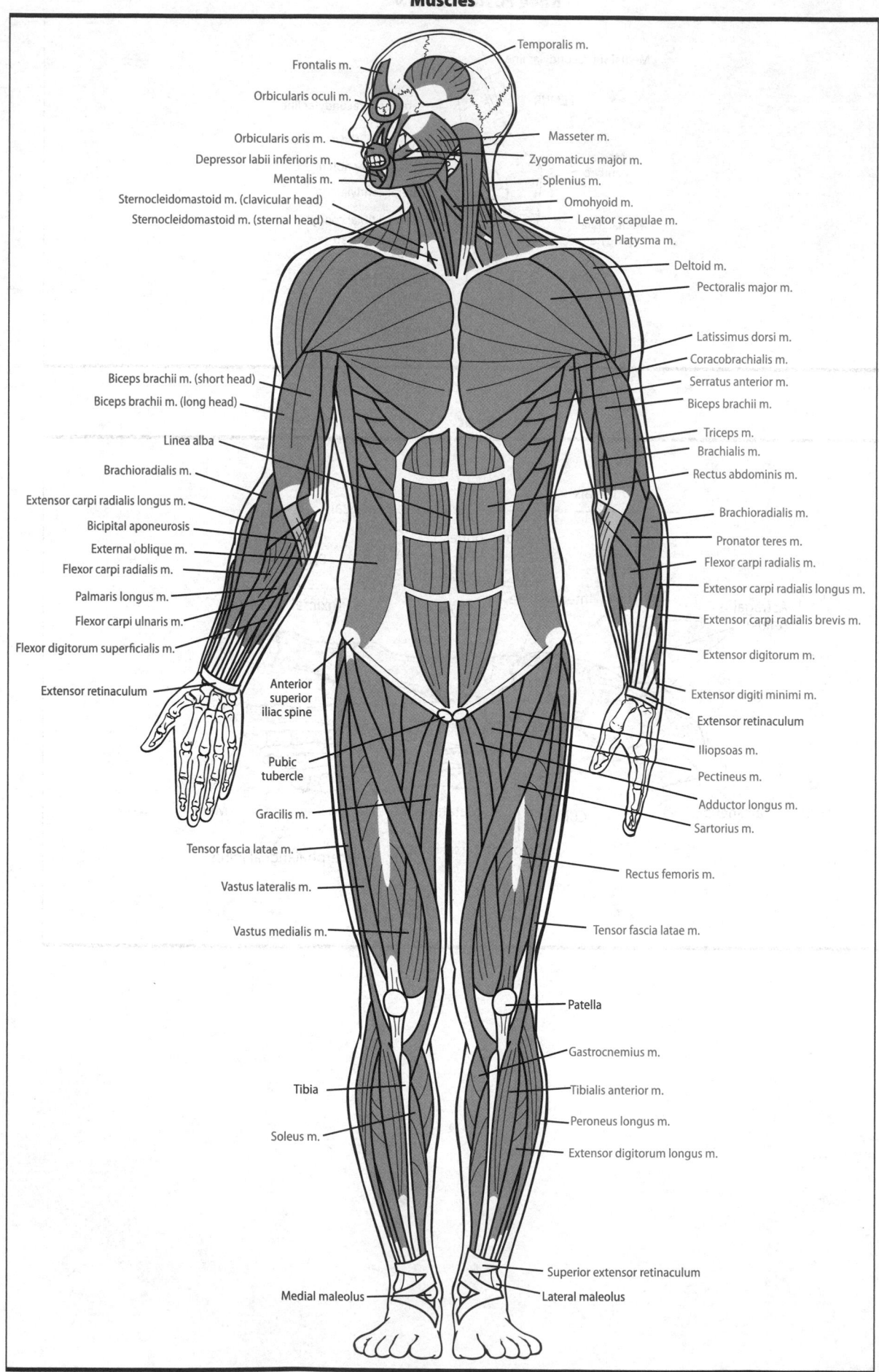

Temporalis m.

Frontalis m.

Orbicularis oculi m.

Orbicularis oris m.

Depressor labii inferioris m.

Mentalis m.

Sternocleidomastoid m. (clavicular head)

Sternocleidomastoid m. (sternal head)

Masseter m.

Zygomaticus major m.

Splenius m.

Omohyoid m.

Levator scapulae m.

Platysma m.

Deltoid m.

Pectoralis major m.

Latissimus dorsi m.

Coracobrachialis m.

Serratus anterior m.

Biceps brachii m.

Triceps m.

Brachialis m.

Rectus abdominis m.

Brachioradialis m.

Pronator teres m.

Flexor carpi radialis m.

Extensor carpi radialis longus m.

Extensor carpi radialis brevis m.

Extensor digitorum m.

Extensor digiti minimi m.

Extensor retinaculum

Iliopsoas m.

Pectineus m.

Adductor longus m.

Sartorius m.

Biceps brachii m. (short head)

Biceps brachii m. (long head)

Linea alba

Brachioradialis m.

Extensor carpi radialis longus m.

Bicipital aponeurosis

External oblique m.

Flexor carpi radialis m.

Palmaris longus m.

Flexor carpi ulnaris m.

Flexor digitorum superficialis m.

Extensor retinaculum

Anterior superior iliac spine

Pubic tubercle

Gracilis m.

Tensor fascia latae m.

Vastus lateralis m.

Vastus medialis m.

Rectus femoris m.

Tensor fascia latae m.

Patella

Gastrocnemius m.

Tibialis anterior m.

Peroneus longus m.

Extensor digitorum longus m.

Tibia

Soleus m.

Superior extensor retinaculum

Medial maleolus

Lateral maleolus

Chapter 14. Diseases of the Genitourinary System (NØØ–N99)

Urinary System

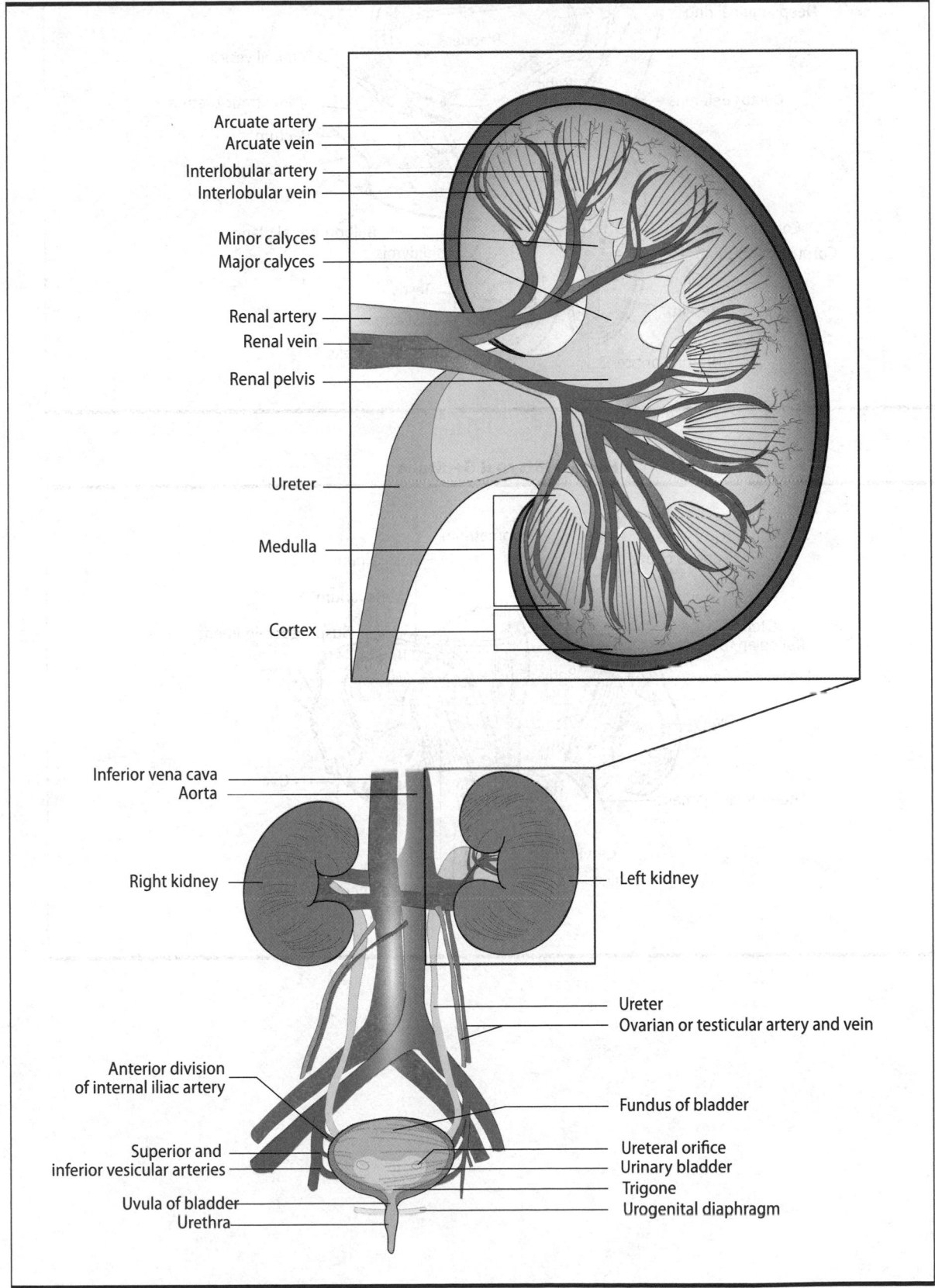

Male Genitourinary System

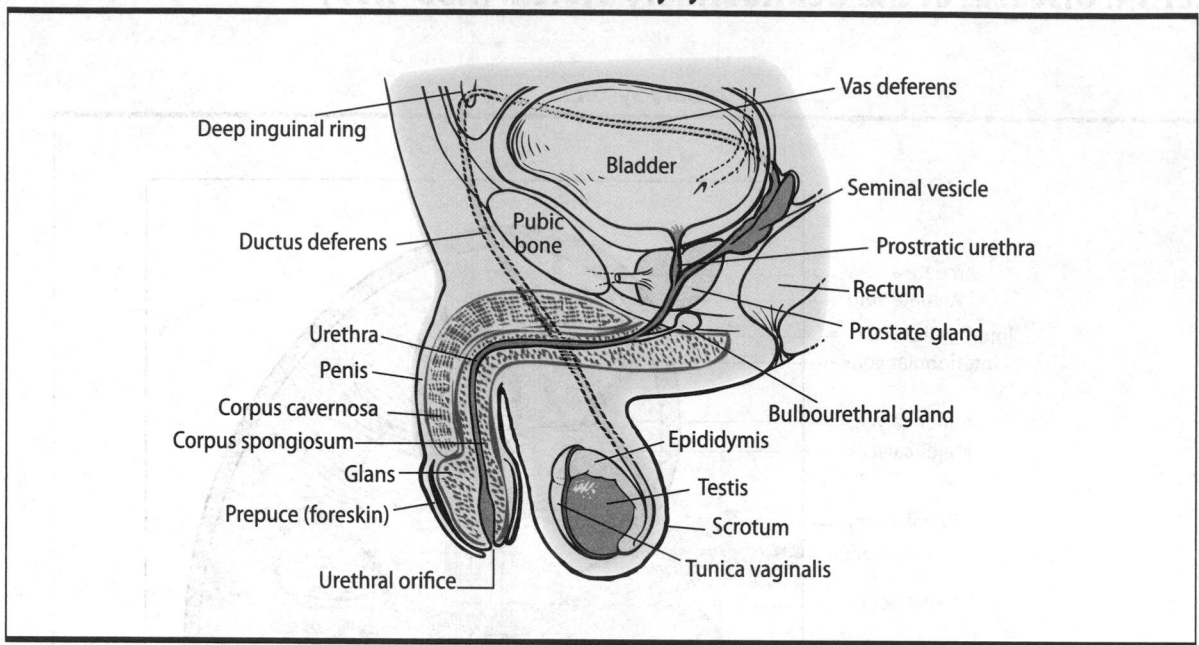

Female Internal Genitalia

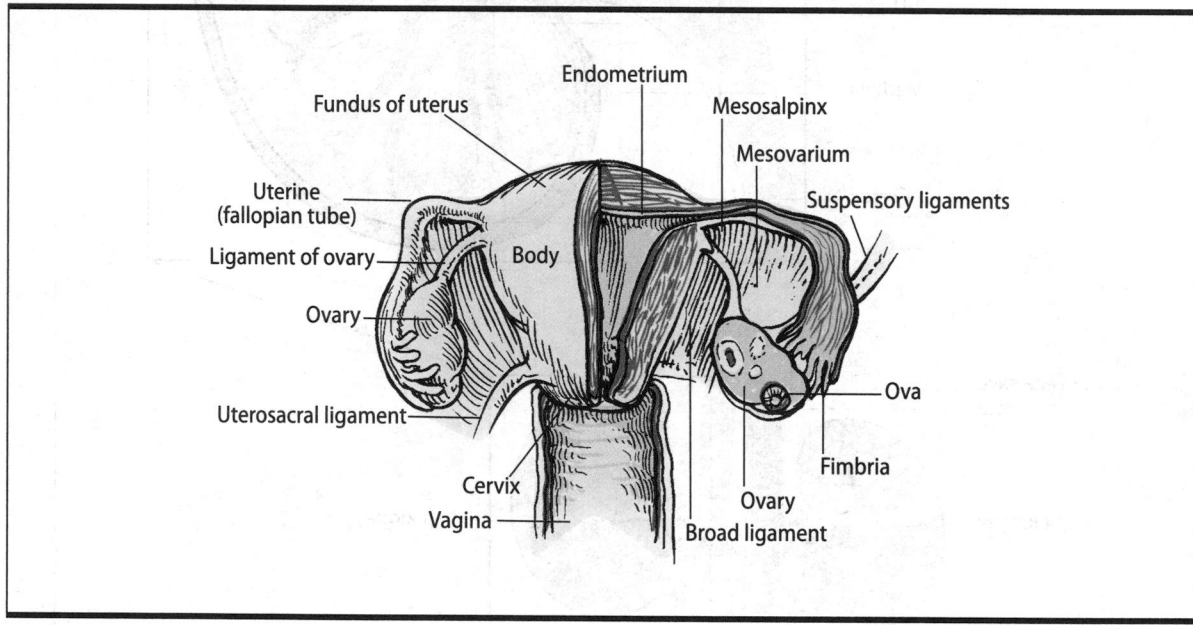

Female Genitourinary Tract Lateral View

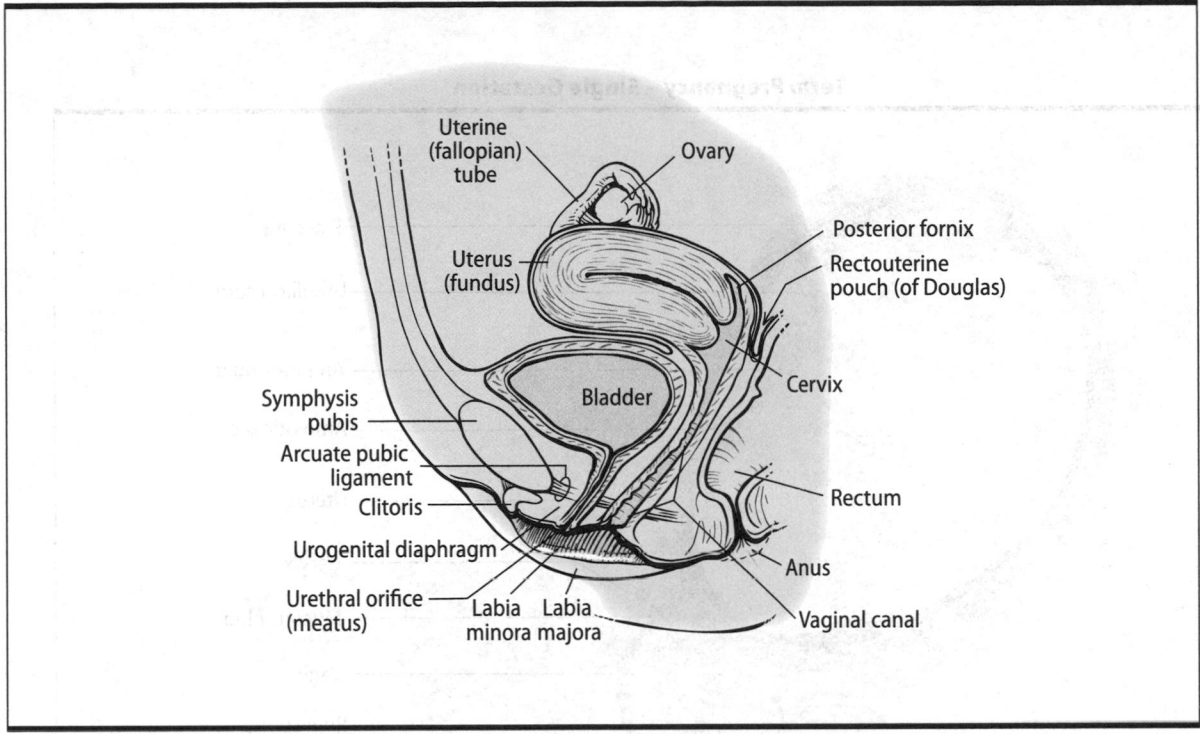

Chapter 15. Pregnancy, Childbirth and the Puerperium (O00–O9A)

Term Pregnancy – Single Gestation

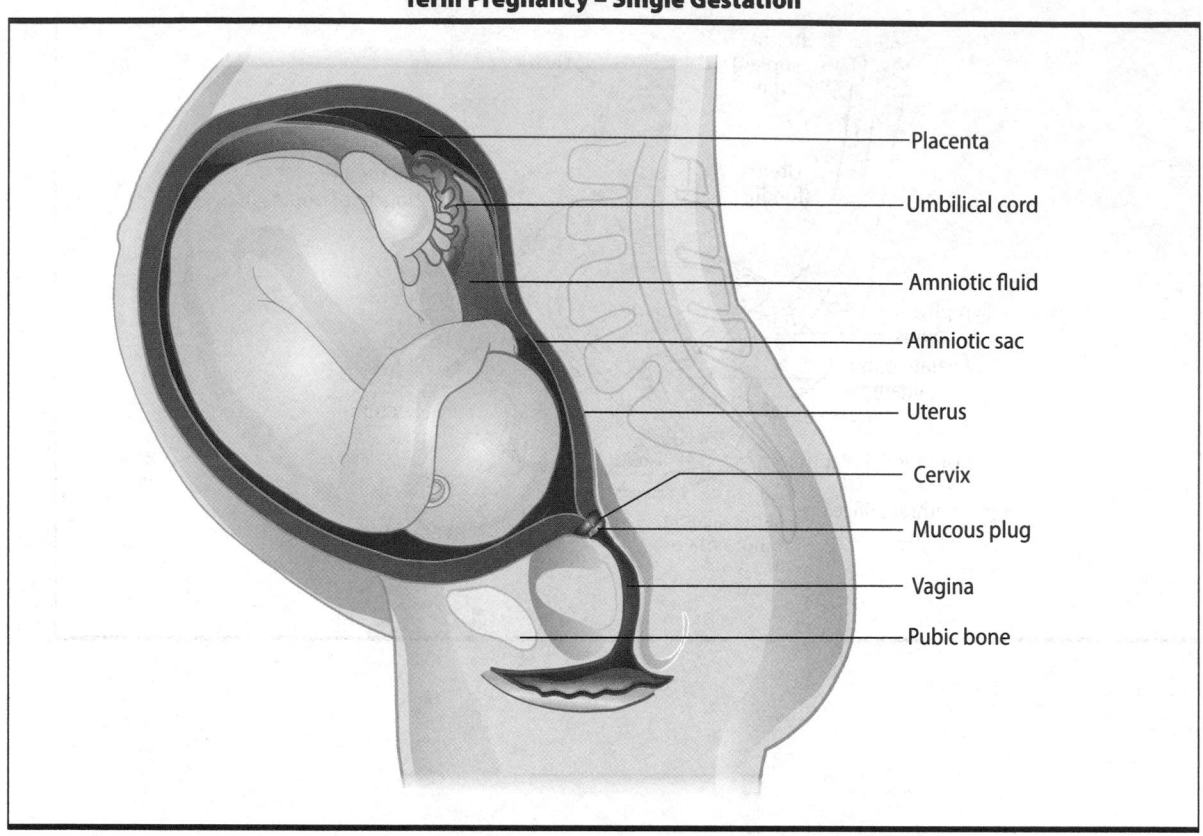

Twin Gestation–Dichorionic–Diamniotic (DI-DI)

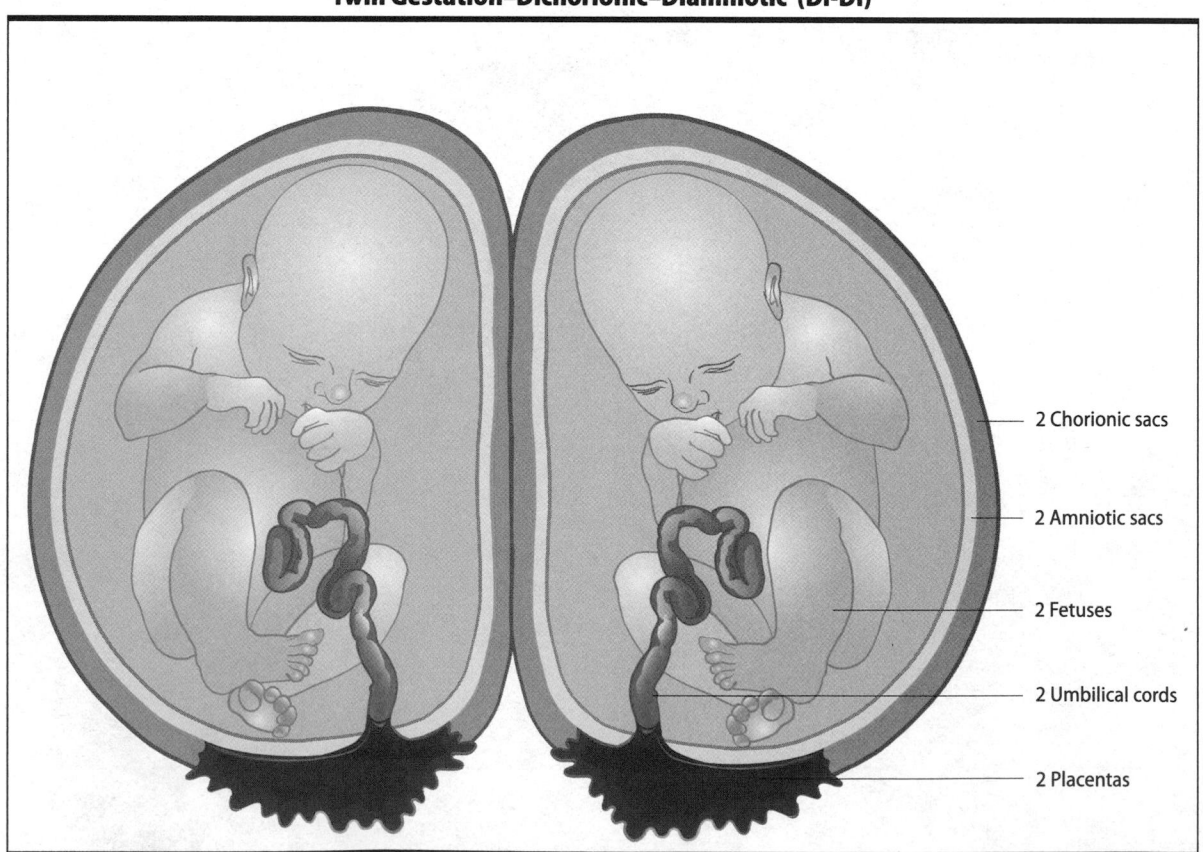

Twin Gestation–Monochorionic–Diamniotic (MO-DI)

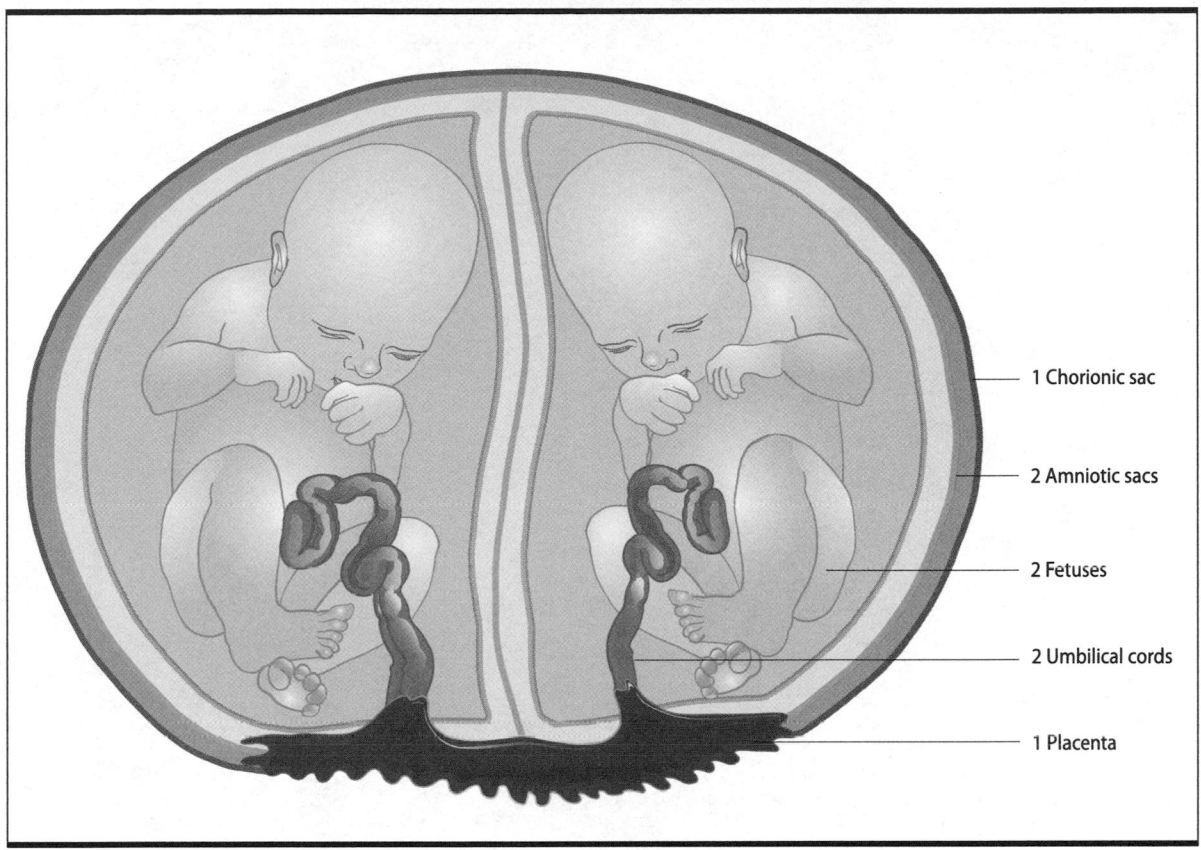

- 1 Chorionic sac
- 2 Amniotic sacs
- 2 Fetuses
- 2 Umbilical cords
- 1 Placenta

Twin Gestation–Monochorionic–Monoamniotic (MO-MO)

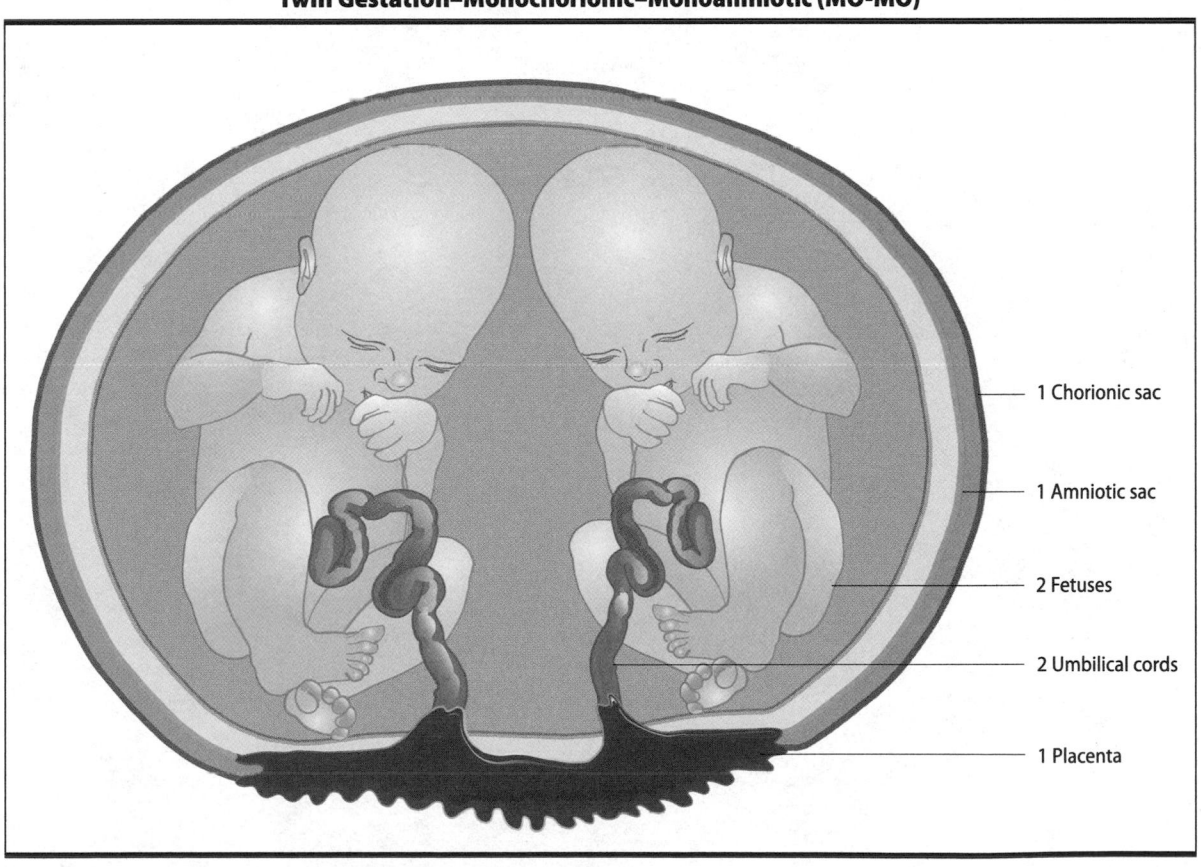

- 1 Chorionic sac
- 1 Amniotic sac
- 2 Fetuses
- 2 Umbilical cords
- 1 Placenta

NOTES

NOTES

NOTES